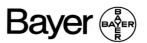

Pharmaceutical Division

Richard K. Goodstein, M.D.
Vice President
Scientific Relations

Dear Doctor:

Bayer Corporation, Pharmaceutical Division, maker of Cipro® (ciprofloxacin HCl) Tablets, Cipro® I.V. (ciprofloxacin), Cipro® HC OTIC (ciprofloxacin HCl and hydrocortisone otic suspension), and Cipro® (ciprofloxacin) 5% and 10% Oral Suspension, is pleased to present you with the 15th edition of *Otorhinolaryngology: Head and Neck Surgery* by John Ballenger and James B. Snow, Jr.

This book is considered a classic in this highly specialized field of medicine. It has been extensively revised and offers comprehensive coverage of diseases of the nose, throat, ear, head, and neck. With many new contributors and nine new chapters added, this outstanding work has been updated with substantial changes reflecting the latest innovations and techniques.

We hope that this addition to your library will become an invaluable ready reference, providing scientific enrichment to you and practical clinical insights for your busy practice.

Sincerely yours,

Richard K. Goodstein, M.D.

Richard K. Goodstein, M.D.
Vice President
Scientific Relations

Bayer Corporation
400 Morgan Lane
West Haven, CT 06516-4175

C07578   BAY-0391   7/98

Otorhinolaryngology:

HEAD AND NECK SURGERY

15th Edition

John Jacob Ballenger

Associate Professor of Otolaryngology—Head and Neck Surgery
Northwestern University School of Medicine
Chief Emeritus, Division of Otolaryngology—Head and Neck Surgery
Evanston Hospital
Evanston, Illinois

James B. Snow, Jr.

Director, National Institute on Deafness and Other Communications Disorders
National Institutes of Health
Bethesda, Maryland

A Lea & Febiger Book

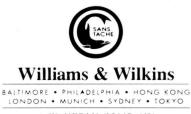

Williams & Wilkins

BALTIMORE • PHILADELPHIA • HONG KONG
LONDON • MUNICH • SYDNEY • TOKYO

A WAVERLY COMPANY

1996

Executive Editor: Darlene Cooke
Senior Managing Editor: Sharon R. Zinner
Production Coordinator: Marette D. Magargle
Project Editor: Susan Rockwell

Copyright © 1996
Williams & Wilkins
Rose Tree Corporate Center
1400 North Providence Road
Building II, Suite 5025
Media, PA 19063-2043 USA

Accurate indications, adverse reactions, and dosage schedules for drugs are provided in this book, but it is possible they may change. The reader is urged to review the package information data of the manufacturers of the medications mentioned.

Printed in the United States of America

First Edition 1908

Library of Congress Cataloging-in-Publication Data

Otorhinolaryngology : head and neck surgery.—15th ed. / [edited by]
    John Jacob Ballenger, James B. Snow.
        p.   cm.
        Rev. ed. of: Diseases of the nose, throat, ear, head, and neck.
    14th. 1991.
        ''A Lea & Febiger book.''
        Includes bibliographical references and index.
        ISBN 0-683-00315-1
        1. Otolaryngology.   I. Ballenger, John Jacob, 1914–   .
    II. Snow, James B. (James Byron), 1932–   .   III. Diseases of the
    nose, throat, ear, head, and neck.
        [DNLM: 1. Otorhinolaryngologic Diseases.   WV 100 0874 1975]
    RF46.D59   1995
    617.5'1—dc20
    DNLM/DLC
    for Library of Congress   95-7241
                                                                  CIP

                                                                          98
                                                            3 4 5 6 7 8 9 10

Reprints of chapters may be purchased from Williams & Wilkins in quantities of 100 or more. Call Isabella Wise, Special Sales Department, (800) 358-3583.

PREFACE

I am pleased, indeed, to have the opportunity again to revise and update this textbook, now renamed *Otorhinolaryngology: Head and Neck Surgery*. It is in the 88th year of continuous use following the first edition in 1908 published by my great uncle, William Lincoln Ballenger. My father, Howard Charles Ballenger, succeeded my great uncle, and I, in 1957, succeeded my father. During the past 14 editions, Lea & Febiger has been the publisher, and now Williams & Wilkins has taken up the task for the 15th edition.

Noting the increasing complexity of otorhinolaryngology and head and neck surgery, in my first edition I elected to invite contributors, each possessing great knowledge in a particular field, to participate in the preparation of the contents of the textbook. This has been a happy decision and has made possible authoritative and current information of the continuously increasing volume of information in the field during these many years. Recent editions of the textbook have been translated into Spanish, Indonesian, Italian, and Portuguese.

For the 15th edition, it has been my good fortune that my invitation to James B. Snow, Jr. to join me in contributing to as well as editing the textbook was accepted. Together with the contributing authors, each an outstanding student of his or her special interest, we have produced an elegant 15th edition that will well serve the students of otorhinolaryngology and head and neck surgery.

The general format has been to present an accurate picture of normal human anatomy and physiology as a basis for the appreciation of altered conditions that underlie disease, its signs, and symptoms. The textbook is directed primarily to resident physicians preparing for the clinical practice of otorhinolaryngology, head and neck surgery, and medicine. Indeed, I believe the textbook will be of great use to all with an abiding interest in this branch of medicine.

I wish enthusiastically to thank James B. Snow, Jr. for joining me and for his many valued suggestions, time-consuming tasks well performed, and his unflagging enthusiasm. Likewise, I consider myself greatly in debt to the many contributors listed elsewhere for the excellent contributions they have made and the integral part they will play in the success of the textbook. Last, I thank Dalia Kleinmuntz and Linda Feinberg of the Webster Library of the Evanston Hospital in Evanston, Illinois, for their cheerful and professional responses to my many requests for help.

John J. Ballenger
Winnetka, Illinois

CONTENTS

III. THE LARYNX
John J. Ballenger

IV. IMAGING OF THE HEAD AND NECK
Galdino E. Valvassori and Mahmood A. Mafee

V. THE EAR
James B. Snow, Jr.

VI. BRONCHOESOPHAGOLOGY
James B. Snow, Jr., and Joyce A. Schild

CONTRIBUTORS

Kedar K. Adour, MD
Senior Consultant and Director of Research,
Dept. of Head and Neck Surgery;
Chairman, Cranial Nerve Research Clinic,
Kaiser Permanente Medical Center
Oakland, California

Peter W. Alberti, MD, MB, PhD, FRCSC, FRCS
Professor of Otolaryngology
University of Toronto
Senior Staff Otolaryngologist
Toronto General Hospital
Toronto, Canada

Simón I. Angeli, MD
Fellow, House Ear Institute
Los Angeles, California

Ellis M. Arjmand, MD
Assistant Professor of Otolaryngology and Pediatrics,
Southern Illinois University School of Medicine,
Springfield, Illinois

Valerie Asher, MD
Department of Otolaryngology
Yale Univesity School of Medicine
New Haven, Connecticut

David F. Austin, MD, FACS
Associate Professor
Otolaryngology, Head, Neck Surgery
Rush Medical School
Chicago, Illinois

John Jacob Ballenger, MD
Associate Profesor of Otolaryngology—Head and Neck
    Surgery
Northwestern University School of Medicine
Chief Emeritus, Division of Otolaryngology—Head and
    Neck Surgery
Evanston Hospital
Evanston, Illinois

Fuad M. Baroody, MD
Assistant Professor
Otolaryngology—Head & Neck Surgery
University of Chicago
Chicago, Illinois

Norman T. Berlinger, MD, PhD
North Memorial Med Center
Abbott Northwestern Hospital
Minneapolis, Minnesota

Joel Bernstein, MD, PhD
Departments of Otolaryngology & Pediatrics,
State University of New York at Buffalo,
Buffalo, New York
Department of Communicative Disorders & Sciences
State University of New York at Buffalo, Buffalo, NY
Division of Infectious Diseases
Children's Hospital of Buffalo
Buffalo, New York

Hugh F. Biller, MD
Chairman and Professor
Department of Otolaryngology
Mount Sinai Medical Center
New York, New York

John L. Boone, MD, Capt MC, USN
Department of Otolaryngology
Naval Medical Center
San Diego, California

William R. Carroll, MD
Assistant Professor
Otolaryngology, Head Neck Surgery
University of Michigan
Ann Arbor, Michigan

Paul F. Castellanos, MD
Assistant Professor of Surgery
Division of Otolaryngology
Director of Voice and Swallowing Disorder Center
University of Maryland
Baltimore, Maryland

Mark Clymer, MD
Department of Otolaryngology
Vanderbilt University School of Medicine
Nashville, Tennessee

Alfred C. Coats, MS, MD
Baylor College of Medicine
Department of Otorhinolaryngology and Commu·
    Sciences
Houston, Texas
Universities Space Research Association,
Division Life Sciences,
Houston, Texas

Jack A. Coleman, Jr., MD, FACS
Assistant Professor
Department of Otolaryngology
Vanderbilt University Medical Center
Nashville, Tennessee

Sharon L. Collins, MS, MD
Associate Professor, Department of
    Otolaryngology—Head & Neck Surgery
Loyola University of Chicago Medical Center
Chief—Section of Otolaryngology, Head & Neck Surgery
Veterans Administration Hospital
Hines, Illinois

Donald N. Cote, MD
Assistant Professor, Department of Otolaryngology
Clinical Assistant Professor, Department of Pediatrics
Tulane University Medical School
New Orleans, Louisiana

Martin Desrosiers, MD, FRCS(C)
Clinical Instructor
Department of Otolaryngology
Universite de Montreal Faculty of Medicine
Attending Surgeon
Hotel-Dieu de Montreal Hospital
Attending Surgeon and Director
Nose and Sinus Care Center
Montreal General Hospital
Montreal, Quebec, Canada

William D. DeWys, MD, FACP
Capital Area Permanente Medical Group
Washington, DC
Fairfax Hospital
Fairfax, Virginia

Paul James Donald, MD, FRCS(C)
Professor, Department of Otolaryngology—Head & Neck
    Surgery
Director, UCDMC Center for Skull Base Surgery
University of California, Davis
Davis, California

Brian P. Driscoll, MD
Assistant Professor of Otolaryngology
University of Texas Branch at Galveston
Department of Otolaryngology
Galveston, Texas

James Patrick Dudley, MD, FACS
Kaiser Permanente
Stockton, California

James A. Duncavage, MD
Vanderbilt University Medical Center
Department of Otolaryngology
Nashville, Tennessee

Carol Gracco, PhD, CCC/SLP
Research Scientist, Haskins Laboratories
Director, Voice and Speech Physiology Laboratory
Yale University School of Medicine
Department of Surgery/Otolaryngology
New Haven, Connecticut

Ray O. Gustafson, MD
Assistant Professor of Otolaryngology
Mayo Medical School
Consultant in Otorhinolaryngology—Head & Neck
    Surgery
Mayo Clinic
Rochester, Minnesota

Troy Hackett, MA
Division of Hearing and Speech Sciences
Vanderbilt University School of Medicine
Nashville, Tennessee

James W. Hall III, PhD
Associate Professor and Director of Audiology
Division of Hearing and Speech Sciences
Department of Otolaryngolgy
Vanderbilt University School of Medicine
Nashville, Tennessee

Jeffrey P. Harris, MD, PhD
University of California
Veteran's Administration Medical Center
San Diego, California

Gerald B. Healy, MD
Childrens Hospital Boston
Otolaryngologist-In-Chief
Surgeon-In-Chief
Professor of Otology & Laryngology
Harvard Medical School
Boston, Massachusetts

Robert A. Hendrix, MD, FACS
Matthews Ear, Nose, and Throat and Communication
    Disorders
Matthews, North Carolina

Douglas M. Hicks, PhD
Head Speech Language Pathology
Department of Otolaryngology &
Communicative Disorders
The Cleveland Clinic Foundation
Cleveland, Ohio

Darrell Hunsaker, MD
Chairman Otolaryngology
Naval Medical Center, San Diego
Associates Professsor, Surgery
Uniformed Services
University of Health Sciences
Assistant Professor, Surgery
University of California, San Diego
San Diego, California

Timothy Kaiser, MD
Fellow, AADHNS
Fellow, American College of Surgeons
Fellow, AAOA
Alton, Illinois

Hidetaka Kanno, MD
Assistant Professor of Otolaryngology
Department of Otolaryngology
Fukushima Medical College
Fukushima, Japan

David W. Kennedy, MD
Professor and Chair
Hospital of the University of Pennsylvania
Philadelphia, Pennsylvania

Kathy Kessler, MS
Speech Language Pathologist and Audiologist
Department of Otolaryngology
Riley Hospital for Children
Indianapolis, Indiana

Janardan D. Khandekar, MD
Head, Division of Hematology/Oncology
Professor of Medicine
Northwestern University Medical School
Kellogg-Scanlon Chair in Oncology
Chicago, Illinois

Charles P. Kimmelman, MD
Clinical Associate Professor
Cornell Medical College
Professor, New York Medical College
Faculty, Manhattan Eye, Ear and Throat Hospital
New York, New York

Howard S. Kotler, MD
Clinical Assistant Professor
Department of Otolaryngology–Head and Neck Surgery
University of Illinois at Chicago
Chicago, Illinois

James A. Koufman, MD, FACS
Director, Center For Voice Disorders
Wake Forest University
Professor of Otolaryngology
Bowman Gray School of Medicine
Winston-Salem, North Carolina

David J. Lim, MD
Chief, Laboratory of Cellular Biology
Division of Intramural Research
National Institute on Deafness and Other Communication
    Disorders, The National Institutes of Health
Professor Emeritus
Department of Otolaryngology
Ohio State University College of Medicine
Columbus, Ohio

Brenda L. Lonsbury-Martin, BA, MS, PhD
Chandler Professor and Director of Research
Department of Otolaryngology
Professor, Departments of Cell Biolgy and Anatomy, and
    Psychology
Professor, Neuroscience Program
University of Miami
Miami, Florida

Christy L. Ludlow, PhD
Voice and Speech Section
National Institute on Deafness and Other Communication
    Disorders
Georgetown University Medical School
University of Maryland, College Park
Bethesda, Maryland

Anne E. Luebke, BS, BA, PhD
Research Assistant Professor
Departments of Physiology & Biophysics and
    Otolaryngology
University of Miami
Miami, Florida

Rodney P. Lusk, MD
St. Louis Children's Hospital
Washington University School of Medicine
St. Louis, Missouri

Mahmood F. Mafee, MD
University of Illinois at Chicago Medical Center
Chicago, Illinois

Glen K. Martin, BS, MS, PhD
Professor and Co-Director of Research
Department of Otolaryngology
Professor, Department of Psychology and Neuroscience
    Program
University of Miami
Miami, Florida

Douglas E. Mattox, MD
Professor and Director
Department of Otolaryngology—Head and Neck Surgery
University of Maryland Medical System
Baltimore, Maryland

Alan G. Micco, MD
Assistant Professor
Otolaryngology, Head & Neck Surgery
Northwestern University Medical School
Chicago, Illinois

Robert H. Miller, MD, FACS
Professor & Chairman
Department of Otolaryngology—Head & Neck Surgery
Tulane University Medical Center
New Orleans, Louisiana

John H. Mills, PhD
Department of Otolaryngology
South Carolina Medical University
Charleston, South Carolina

Fred D. Minifie, PhD
Professor Speech & Hearing Sciences JG-15
Affiliate, Bloedel Hearing Research Center
Seattle, Washington

Richard T. Miyamoto, MD, FACS
Arilla Spence DeVault Professor & Chairman
Department of Otolaryngology—Head and Neck Surgery
Indiana University School of Medicine
Indianapolis, Indiana
Medical Director, Audiology and Speech/Language
    Pathology
Indiana University Hospital
Indianapolis, Indiana

G. Paul Moore, PhD, DS
Distinguished Service Professor Emeritus
Department of Communicative Processes and Disorders
University of Florida
Gainesville, Florida

Juan F. Moscoso, MD
Assistant Professor
Department of Otolaryngology
Mount Sinai School of Medicine
New York, New York

Fabiola Müller, Dr habil rer nat
University of California School of Medicine
Davis, California

Robert M. Naclerio, MD
Professor and Chief
Otolaryngology—Head and Neck Surgery
University of Chicago
Chicago, Illinois

H. Bryan Neel III, MD, PhD, FACS
Professor and Past Chairman
Department of Otorhinolaryngology
Associate Professor, Department of Microbiology
Mayo Medical School, Mayo Medical Center
Rochester, Minnesota

Ronan O'Rahilly, MD, DSc
University of California School of Medicine
Davis, California

Mary Joe Osberger, PhD
Director, Clinical Research
Advanced Bionics Corporation
Sylmar, California

Robert H. Ossoff, DMD, MD
Guy M. Maness Professor and Chairman
Department of Otolaryngology
Vanderbilt University Medical Center
Nashville, Tennessee

Simon C. Parisier, MD
Chairman, Department of Otolaryngology—Head & Neck
    Surgery
Manhattan Eye, Ear and Throat Hospital
Clinical Professor, Otolaryngology
Cornell University Medical Center
New York, New York

Lou Reinisch, PhD
PhD Physics, Surgical Physics Specialty
Director of Laser Research
Vanderbilt University Medical Center
Nashville, Tennessee

Maurice Roth, MD
Assistant Professor of Otolaryngology—Head and Neck
    Surgery
Thomas Jefferson University Medical School
Philadelphia, Pennsylvania

Lee D. Rowe, MD
Associate Clinical Professor of Otolaryngology
Head and Neck Surgery
Jefferson Medical College
Philadelphia, Pennsylvania

Michael J. Ruckenstein, MD MSc, FRCSC
University of California, San Diego
Veteran's Administration Medical Center
Division of Otolaryngology
La Jolla, California

Allen Ryan, PhD
Professor of Surgery and Neurosciences
University of California, San Diego
La Jolla, California

Leonard P. Rybak, MD, PhD
Professor, Department of Surgery
Southern Illinois University School of Medicine
Springfield, Illinois

Stephen J. Salzer, MD
Attending Surgeon, Greenwich Hospital
Greenwich, Connecticut
Instructor in Surgery, Yale–New Haven Hospital
New Haven, Connecticut

Ira Sanders, MD
Director, Grabsheid Voice Center
Associate Professor
Department of Otolaryngology
Mt. Sinai Hospital
New York, New York

Clarence T. Sasaki, MD
Ohse Professor of Surgery
Yale School of Medicine
New Haven, Connecticut

Joyce A. Schild, MD
Professor, Department of Otolaryngology—Head and
    Neck Surgery
University of Illinois at Chicago
Chicago, Illinois

Richard J.H. Smith, MD, FACS, FAAP
Professor, Pediatric Otolaryngology
Director, Molecular Otolaryngology Research Laboratories
Department of Otolaryngology
University of Iowa
Iowa City, Iowa

James B. Snow, Jr, MD
Director, National Institute on Deafness and Other
    Communications Disorders
National Institutes of Health
Bethesda, Maryland

J. Gershon Spector, MD
Washington University School of Medicine
Otolaryngology—Head & Neck Surgery
St. Louis, Missouri

Erich Sturgis, MD
Department of Otolaryngology—Head and Neck Surgery
Tulane University Medical Center
New Orleans, Louisiana

Curtis L. Sutton, MD
Assistant Professor of Radiology and Neurosurgery
Co-Director of Neuroradiology
Tulane University Medical Center
New Orleans, Louisiana

Jonathan M. Sykes, MD
Assistant Professor, Department of Otolaryngology
Head & Neck Surgery
University of California, Davis
Davis, California

M. Eugene Tardy, MD
Professor of Clinical Otolaryngology
Director, Division of Facial, Plastic and Reconstructive
    Surgery
Department of Otolaryngology—Head and Neck Surgery
University of Illinois Medical Center
Chicago, Illinois

Dean M. Toriumi, MD, FACS
Associate Professor
Division of Facial Plastic and Reconstructive Surgery
Department of Otolaryngology—Head and Neck Surgery
University of Illinois at Chicago College of Medicine
Chicago, Illinois

Galdino E. Valvassori, MD
Professor of Radiology & Otolaryngology—Head & Neck
    Surgery
University of Illinois, Chicago
Chicago, Illinois

Richard J. Wiet, MD, FACS
Professor of Clinical Otolaryngology & Neurosurgery
Department of Otolaryngology
Division of Neurosurgery
Northwestern University Medical School
Chicago, Illinois

Gregory T. Wolf, MD
Professor & Chair
Department of Otolaryngology
University of Michigan
Ann Arbor, Michigan

John J. Zappia, MD
The Chicago Otology Group
Assistant Professor, Department of
    Otolaryngology—Head & Neck Surgery
Northwestern University Medical School
Chicago, Illinois

I THE NOSE AND PARANASAL SINUSES

John J. Ballenger

1 Clinical Anatomy and Physiology of the Nose and Paranasal Sinuses

John J. Ballenger

EXTERNAL NOSE

The more or less pointed tip of the nose is known as the apex. Extending posterosuperiorly from the apex is the nasal dorsum. At the junction of the suture between the nasal bones and the frontonasal suture is the nasion (or radix nasi), and between the two superciliary arches is a flattened, slightly elevated area known as the glabella. The rhinion is found at the lower end of the suture between the two nasal bones. The membranous columella extends from the apex posteriorly to the center of the upper lip and is located just distally to the lower or free margin of the nasal septum. The upper lip at this point displays a shallow, rounded, vertically oriented trench, the philtrum. On either side of the columella are the anterior nares or nostrils, bounded by the lower lateral, or alar, cartilages and the floor of the nose.

The upper and lower lateral cartilages form the framework of the distal two thirds of the nose. The lower or caudal margins of the upper lateral cartilages usually overlie the upper or cranial margins of the lower lateral cartilages. On elevation of the tip of the nose (the lower lateral cartilages), the margin or junction can be seen and is spoken of as the limen nasi or nasal valve area. This narrowest part of the nasal airway provides almost half the total airflow resistance. At times, the medial margins of the two lower lateral cartilages may lie close to but separate from the septum and thus provide less support to the nasal dorsum at this point. Between the two alar cartilages laterally are one or more unattached sesamoid cartilages. The lower lateral cartilage has a horseshoe shape. The lateral crus is broad and strong and provides the framework of the nostril. The medial crus is weak and extends within the columella along the medial edge of the nostril (Figs. 1–1 and 1–2).

In the bony skull the pear-shaped nasal opening is the piriform aperture. The superior and lateral margins are formed by the nasal bones and frontal processes of the maxillae and the bases by the alveolar processes of the maxillae. A bony prominence at the midline is called the anterior nasal spine.

There are two sets of alar muscles: the dilators (dilator naris, m. procerus, caput angulare), and the constrictors (m. nasalis and depressor septi). They all receive innervation from cranial nerve (CN) VII.

NASAL SEPTUM

The nasal septum is a midline structure and is formed superiorly by the perpendicular plate of the ethmoid bone, anteriorly by the septal (quadrilateral) cartilage, premaxilla, and the membranous columella, inferiorly by the vomer bone, maxillary, and palatine bones, and by the sphenoidal crest posteriorly (Fig. 1–3). The nasal septum is continuous with the upper lateral cartilages in the cranial third.

NASAL CHAMBERS

The floor of the nose is formed by the palatal processes of the maxilla and the horizontal processes of the palate bones. Moving posteriorly, the roof is composed of the alar cartilages, the nasal bones, the nasal processes of the frontal bones, the body of the ethmoid bones, and the body of the sphenoid bones. The cribriform plate (lamina cribrosa) supplies the major portion of the roof and through it pass the filaments of the olfactory nerve to their distribution on the mucous membrane of the uppermost portion of both the medial and lateral walls of the nose. The lateral wall is formed by the inner

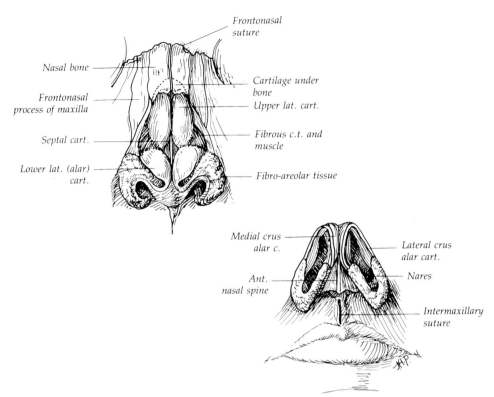

Fig. 1–1. Dorsal and inferior surfaces of the nose.

surfaces of the maxillae, the lacrimal bones, the superior and middle turbinates, the inferior turbinate, and the medial pterygoid plate.

The scroll-like, pitted turbinates divide the nasal fossae into meatus (Fig. 1–4) and increase the nasal mucosal surface to 100 to 200 cm^2. The space between the inferior turbinate and the floor is the inferior meatus, that between the inferior and middle the middle meatus, and that above the superior turbinate the superior meatus. Occasionally, there is a supreme turbinate. The

middle and superior turbinates are extensions of the ethmoid bone, whereas the inferior is a separate bone attached by its superior border to the lateral nasal wall. Both middle and inferior turbinates are covered with pseudostratified ciliated columnar epithelium, except at the anterior ends, where a low cuboidal or squamous type is found. The epithelial stroma of the middle turbinate contains many glands. Sinusoids consist of large, tortuous valveless anastomosing veins, are found mainly in the inferior and middle turbinates,

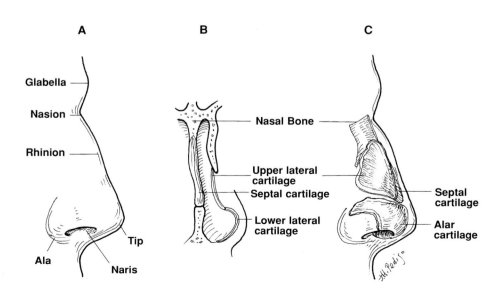

Fig. 1–2. Lateral profile of the nose.

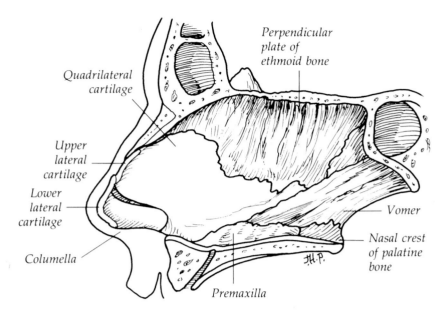

Fig. 1–3. The nasal septum.

and can, by the amount of filling, influence the size of the nasal airway. Physiologically, they are capacitance vessels and respond to neural, mechanical, thermal, psychologic, or chemical stimuli.

Superior Meatus

The superior meatus or ethmoid fissure is a slit-like space between the septum and the ethmoid bone above the middle turbinate. The posterior ethmoid cells drain by one or more orifices into the central portion of the meatus. Above and posterior to the superior turbinate is the sphenoid recess into which the sphenoid sinus drains.

Middle Meatus

This meatus lies between the inferior and middle turbinates. It contains the orifices of the frontal and maxillary sinuses and those of the anterior group of ethmoid cells. Hidden by the anterior half of the overhanging middle turbinate is a deep crescentic groove, the infundibulum. The crescent-shaped opening or fissure leading to the infundibulum is called the hiatus semilunaris (Figs. 1–5 and 1–6). The inferior medial wall of the infundibulum forms a shelf-like ledge known as the uncinate process. Above this is a hemispheric prominence termed the ethmoid bulla and formed by one of the ethmoid cells.

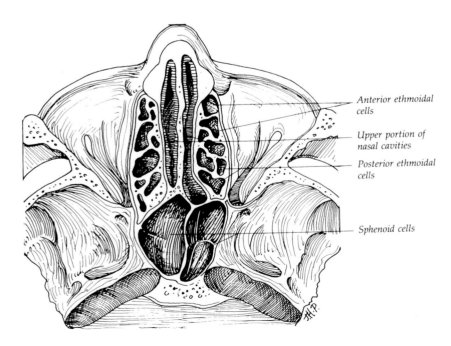

Fig. 1–4. Horizontal section through the nose.

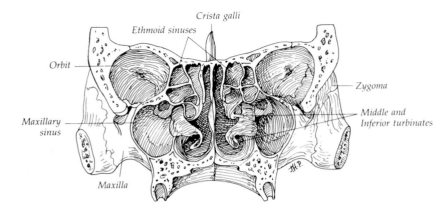

Fig. 1–5. Coronal section through the nose.

The orifices of the frontal, maxillary, and anterior ethmoid cells are usually found in the infundibulum. Certain ethmoid cells may drain above the ethmoid bulla, and the frontonasal duct sometimes has a separate duct.

Inferior Meatus

The inferior meatus, the largest of the three, lies below the inferior turbinates and contains the orifice of the lacrimal duct laterally from 3 to 5 cm posterior to the margin of the nostril.

Nares

The anterior nares or nostrils, defined by the lower lateral cartilages, are about 1.5 by 1 cm transversely, whereas the posterior nares or choanae are 2.5 by 1.5. Each oval-shaped opening of the latter communicates with the nasopharynx and is bordered by the horizontal plate of the palatine bone inferiorly, the vomer medially, the vaginal process of the sphenoid bone superiorly, and the medial pterygoid plate laterally. Just within the nostril is a dilation, the nasal vestibule. It is lined by skin containing coarse hairs (the vibrissae) and sebaceous and sweat glands.

PARANASAL SINUSES

The paranasal sinuses are eight in number, four on the left and four on the right: the frontal, the ethmoid (anterior and posterior), the maxillary, and the sphenoid. Each sinus, under healthful conditions, is filled with air and communicates with the nasal cavity through an ostium. For clinical purposes, the sinuses are divided into two groups, anterior and posterior, depending on their location in reference to the line of attachment of the middle turbinate. The anterior group, consisting of the frontal, maxillary, and anterior ethmoidal cells, drains into or near the infundibulum. The posterior group, made up of the sphenoid and posterior ethmoidal cells, drains above the attachment of the middle turbinate.

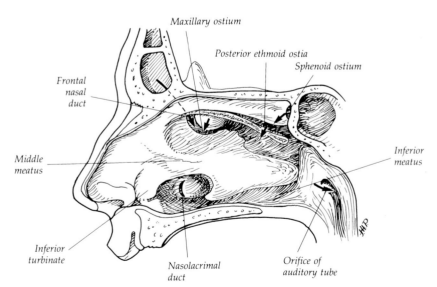

Fig. 1–6. Schematic drawing of the left lateral nasal wall with the entire middle concha and the anterior third of the inferior part of the concha removed.

TABLE 1–1. Maxillary Sinuses

Embryology	First of the paranasal sinuses to develop; begins as a bud along the inferolateral surface of the ethmoid portion of the nasal capsule about gestation day 65
Size	Birth: 7–8 × 4–6 mm Adult: 31–32 × 18–20 mm Volume (adult): 15 ml
Blood supply	Arterial branches of the internal maxillary including the infraorbital, lateral nasal branches of the sphenopalatine, descending palatine, and posterior and anterior superior alveolar arteries; most sinus walls drain into the maxillary vein, which shares communication with the pterygoid plexus
Innervation	Mucosal sensation from the lateroposterior nasal and superior alveolar branches of the infraorbital nerve, all derived from CN V2

TABLE 1–2. Ethmoid Sinuses

Embryology	First appear during the third and fourth fetal month as evaginations of the lateral nasal wall
Size	Adult: 20–24 × 22–24 × 10–12 mm (anterior group) 20–21 × 20–22 × 10–12 mm (posterior group) Number: 10–15 cells each side
Blood supply	Nasal branches of the sphenopalatine artery and anterior and posterior ethmoid arteries, branches of the ophthalmic artery from the internal carotid system; maxillary vein, making connections with the cavernous sinus
Innervation	Posterior nasal branches of the maxillary nerve (CN V2), the anterior and posterior ethmoidal branches of the ophthalmic nerve (CN V1)

Maxillary Sinus (Table 1–1)

Growth of this sinus, the largest of the sinuses, is biphasic. The first period occurs during the first 3 years and the second and final period from 7 to 17 or 18 years. During the second period, much of the growth is related to invasion of the alveolar process following eruption of the permanent dentition.

The maxillary sinus, or antrum of Highmore, occupies the body of the maxilla. It is generally pyramidal, its base formed by the lateral wall of the nasal cavity and its apex directed toward the zygomatic process. The roof separates the sinus from the orbit. The floor is formed by the alveolar process of the maxilla and the hard palate. In children the sinus floor lies at or above the level of the floor of the nasal cavity, whereas in the adult the sinus floor may lie 5 to 10 mm below. The anterior wall corresponds with the canine fossa and separates the sinus from the cheek. The posterior wall separates the sinus from the contents of the infratemporal and pterygomaxillary fossa.

The antrum communicates with the infundibulum by means of an ostium located in the upper and anterior part of the median sinus wall. From 10 to 30% of the time an additional (accessory) ostium is present. The bony orifice is usually larger than the membranous orifice. Most nerves and blood vessels enter the sinus by way of the ostium.

The apices of the second upper bicuspid and first and second molar teeth are located in close relation to the floor of the sinus and may be separated only by mucous membrane and thus permit easy spread from a dental infection. The superior wall or roof of the sinus usually is twice as wide as the floor and is crossed in its central portion by the infraorbital nerve, protected only at times by a thin plate of bone.

Ethmoid Sinus

At birth, usually three or four cells are present and, along with the maxillary sinus, are the only sinus cavities large enough to be of clinical importance. The cells lie on either side of the attachment of the middle turbinate to the lateral wall of the nose, the anterior cells in front of and below it and the posterior above and behind (see Fig. 1–5 and Table 1–2). Generally, the anterior cells are smaller and more numerous than the posterior. They lie on either side of the superior half of the nasal cavity and medial to the orbit. The lateral wall of the ethmoid sinus is the lamina papyracea, which also is the medial wall of the orbit (see Figs. 1–5 and 1–6). The anterior ethmoid cells drain into the infundibulum of the middle meatus and the posterior cells into the superior meatus. The middle turbinate may be the site of an aerated ethmoid cell, a concha bullosa, which can encroach on and interfere with the free sinus drainage. The anterior cells frequently extend into the agar nasi and the uncinate process and may invade the lumen of the frontal sinus (a frontal bulla) or may be found in the body of the sphenoid bone.

Frontal Sinus (Table 1–3)

This sinus can rarely be imaged before the second year of life. At this time, it slowly invades the frontal bone, resulting in much diversity of shape. The sinus usually communicates with the nose by the frontonasal duct

TABLE 1–3. Frontal Sinus

Embryology	Upward extension at about 4 months gestation of the anterior portion of the nasal capsule in the region of the frontal recess
Size	Adult: 3 × 2.5 × 2 cm Volume (adult): 6–7 ml
Blood supply	Supratrochlear and suborbital branches of the ophthalmic artery; venous drainage to the cavernous sinus
Innervation	Mucosal sensation derives from supratrochlear and supraorbital branches of the frontal nerve from CN V1

TABLE 1–4. Sphenoid Sinus

Embryology	Originates during third fetal month as an evagination of mucosa in the sphenoethmoid recess
Size	Adult: 20 × 22 × 16 mm Volume (adult): 7.5 ml
Blood supply	Branches of the sphenopalatine and posterior ethmoid arteries
Innervation	Posterior ethmoidal nerve from CN V1, nasal and sphenopalatine branches of CN V2

near the upper portion of the infundibulum. The anterior plate of the sinus is of diploic bone and separates the skin and periosteum of the forehead from the sinus. The thin posterior compact bony plate separates the content of the cranial fossa from the sinus.

Sphenoidal Sinus (Table 1–4)

Pneumatization of the sphenoid bone occurs during middle childhood, proceeding rapidly after 7 years to its final form at 12 to 15 years. Each sinus communicates with the superior meatus by means of a small aperture of 0.5 to 4 mm that empties into the sphenoethmoidal recess. The meatus is disadvantageously located (for gravity drainage) 10 to 20 mm above the sinus floor or, in other words, 30 mm above the floor of the nasal cavity. The ostium is practically always membranous, its bony circumference larger than its actual orifice.

The optic nerve and the hypophysis lie above the sinus, the pons posteriorly. External and lateral to the sinus are found the cavernous sinus, the superior orbital fissure, and related cranial nerves, as well as the carotid artery, which creates an indentation in the lateral wall of the sinus wall in over 50% of specimens. The nerve of the pterygoid canal (vidian nerve) may encroach on the sinus floor, and so curetting must be done with great care.

Ostiomeatal Unit

The ostiomeatal complex refers to the relationship between the middle meatus and the ostia of the anterior group of paranasal sinuses, particularly the anterior ethmoid cells[1] (Fig. 1–7). If there is an anatomic deformity, e.g., concha bullosa, or a disease process that brings two mucosal layers into direct contact, localized ciliary stasis occurs, free sinus drainage is obstructed, and likely sinus infection is inaugurated.

Function of the Paranasal Sinuses

Prevailing theories of the function of the sinuses, but none generally accepted, include lightening of the skull, vocal resonating box, increased olfaction, humidification of air, and assistance in regulation of intra-

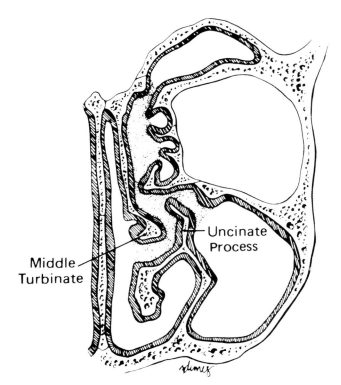

Fig. 1–7. Concept of the ostiomeatal unit (shaded). (Courtesy of David W. Kennedy.)

nasal pressure. Recently, it has been suggested that the sinuses provide a source of environmentally uncontaminated mucus that is delivered to the midportion of the middle and superior meatus and presumably dilutes mucus contaminated by exposure to inspired air.

PTERYGOPALATINE FOSSA

This space, an elongated triangular area with the apex laterally, lies between the rounded posterior border of the maxillary sinus and the pterygoid process. It is bounded medially by the perpendicular plate of the palatal bone and superiorly by the undersurface of the sphenoid bone.

Just medial to the sphenopalatine foramen, an opening in the perpendicular plate opposite the posterior end of the middle turbinate, is the sphenoethmoid recess. Through the foramen, vessels and nerves pass to the nasal cavity. The pterygopalatine ganglion (sphenopalatine ganglion) is located just lateral to the foramen.

Also communicating with the pterygopalatine space are the foramen rotundum and pharyngomaxillary and orbital fissures. A wire passed up the greater or lesser palatine canals enters the fossa from below. Within the fossa also are found the second division of the fifth cranial nerve, the third division of the internal maxillary artery, and the vidian nerve.

NASAL MUCOUS MEMBRANE

The nasal fossa, nasopharynx, and sinuses are lined by a continuous membrane. Within the nasal vestibule it is a tough, keratinized, stratified squamous epithelium containing coarse hairs (vibrissae) and sebaceous and sweat glands. Posteriorly, as the turbinates are approached, the epithelium blends into a cuboidal and then a respiratory type. As the nasopharynx is approached, the respiratory type changes to a moist, non-keratinized, stratified, squamous mucous membrane similar to that of the oral cavity. The nasal mucosa is considered more completely later in this chapter.

The mucosa of the paranasal sinuses contains pseudostratified ciliated columnar to cuboid epithelium but is thinner, contains fewer glands and cilia, and rests on a thin basement membrane. Cilia, somewhat more abundant near the ostia, propel the overlying blanket of mucus to the nasal interior by way of the ostia.

Three types of nasal glands are found in the submucosa and epithelium: serous, located in the vestibule; seromucous; and intraepithelial. Submucosal serous glands are considerably more numerous than mucosal.[2]

NERVE SUPPLY OF THE NOSE

The sensory nerve supply of the nose (in addition to olfactory) consists mainly of the ophthalmic and the maxillary divisions of CN V. The former gives rise to the nasociliary nerve; among its branches are the anterior and posterior ethmoid and the infratrochlear. The anterior ethmoid passes over the anterior part of the cribriform plate (Figs. 1–8 and 1–9) and enters with the anterior ethmoid artery by way of the anterior ethmoid foramen and divides into medial and lateral branches.

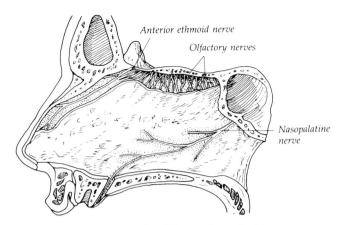

Fig. 1–9. Nerve supply of the medial wall of the nose.

The medial branch passes forward and downward on the nasal septum. The lateral branch supplies a similar part of the lateral nasal wall and also sends a branch, the external nasal nerve, that exists at the distal end of the nasal bone to reach the external surface of the nose. The posterior ethmoid also crosses the cribriform plate to enter the nose along with the artery through the posterior ethmoid foramen to supply the posterior and inferior portions of the septum as well as the olfactory region.

Branches from the maxillary division give rise to the posterior superior nasal nerves that enter the nose by way of sphenopalatine foramen and pass over the anterior face of the sphenoid bone to reach the nasal septum, where the most prominent branch runs forward and downward on the nasal septum as the nasopalatine nerve (n. of Cotunnius) and finally reaches the incisive canal. Laterally a branch, the posterior inferior nasal, passes downward and forward to distribute on the middle and inferior conchae.

The autonomic innervation of the nose consists of parasympathetic and sympathetic fibers. The parasympathetic fibers originate in superior salivary nucleus and travel via the nervus intermedius to the geniculate ganglion, where they join the greater superficial petrosal nerve. As this nerve leaves the temporal bone, it is joined by the deep petrosal nerve to form the nerve of the pterygoid canal, or vidian nerve, to synapse in the sphenopalatine ganglion. The postganglionic fibers distribute over the nasal mucosa via the nasal nerves.

The postganglionic sympathetic fibers follow the internal carotid artery and form the deep petrosal nerve, which joins the aforementioned greater superficial petrosal nerve to form the vidian nerve. Postganglionic sympathetic fibers pass through the sphenopalatine foramen without synapsing to innervate the nasal mucosa via the posterior nasal nerve.

BLOOD SUPPLY OF THE NOSE

The blood supply of the nasal interior comes from the anterior and posterior ethmoid branches of the oph-

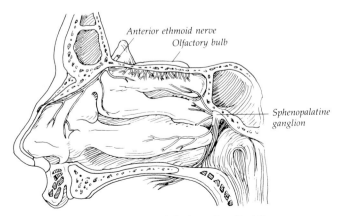

Fig. 1–8. Nerve supply of the lateral wall of the nose.

thalmic arteries and the sphenopalatine artery (the terminal branch of the internal maxillary). The anterior superior portion of the septum and the lateral walls of the nose receive the blood supply from the anterior ethmoid arteries, the smaller posterior ethmoid artery supplying only a small posterior region, including the olfactory region. Both ethmoid branches cross the cribriform plate before entering the nose.

The maxillary artery, usually the penultimate branch of the external carotid, passes lateral to the pterygoid plate to enter the pterygoid fossa and pass, as the sphenopalatine artery, into the nasal cavity through the sphenopalatine foramen at the posterior limit of the middle turbinate. Within the nasal cavity the artery divides into branches that are distributed with branches of the second and third divisions of the trigeminal nerve: the posterior lateral nasal branch, which supplies the turbinates as well as the ethmoid and maxillary sinuses; and the posterior septal branch, which crosses over the nasal roof beneath the sphenoid bone and supplies the entire septum. There is an anastomosis between the lateral nasal arteries and the ethmoid, and thus bleeding can arise from either. Other branches of the sphenopalatine artery descending in the greater palatine canal enter the oral cavity and spread over the undersurface of the palate.

The veins follow a course similar to that of the sphenopalatine artery and drain into the pterygoid plexus. The ethmoidal veins drain into the ophthalmic plexus and part to the cavernous sinus. Furthermore, the nasal veins frequently anastomose with veins of the face and palate. The nasal venous system is without valves and thus predisposes to a retrograde spread of infection to the cavernous sinus.

LYMPHATICS

The nasal vestibule drains toward the external nose, whereas the lymphatics of the nasal fossa drain posteriorly. In the latter situation are two main collecting trunks, one in the olfactory region and one parallel and inferior. They carry the lymph posteriorly to either the lateral retropharyngeal or the subdigastric nodes.

OLFACTION

Above the superior turbinate is the 60- to 70-μm thick olfactory epithelium measuring 200 to 400 mm^2. The sense of smell determines the flavor and palatability of foods and beverages, warns of poisons and spoiled foods, and with the trigeminal system monitors the environment for toxic volatile substances such as leaking gas, smoke, and air pollutants. The influence of olfaction in human social and sexual behavior is less clear than in lower animals. Pheromones are external body secretions that influence behavior and are readily demonstrable in animals and insects but only questionably are present in humans. Aldosterone SO$_4$, human male sweat, and urine have been proposed as sexually attractive pheromones.

In discussing human olfaction, three organs of functional significance in animals must be considered because anatomically they are still represented in part. Moreover, olfaction and taste are perceptively interwoven.

In 1811, Jacobson described a tubular structure on the septum of some animals with afferent nerves projecting to a portion of the olfactory bulb. This became known as Jacobson's or the vomeronasal organ. In humans a remnant of questionable significance is found in the anteroinferior part of the nasal septum. In animals the organ is concerned with pheromonal or sexual detection. The terminal nerve represented in mammals as a plexus of fine branching nerve bundles on the nasal septum is of little or no functional significance in humans. Masera's septal organ, of unknown functional significance, contains bipolar neurons and sends discrete nerve bundles toward the olfactory bulb.

Physiology of Olfaction

The sense of smell is mediated through stimulation of the olfactory receptor cells by airborne volatile chemicals that are lipid soluble. The duration, volume, and velocity of the nasal air currents are important determinants of an odor's stimulating effectiveness. Electrical potentials evoked from the olfactory neuroepithelium with odorants can be measured and are termed the "electro-olfactogram" or EOG.

The molecular receptors are located in the surface membrane of the cilia of the olfactory receptor neurons. The discovery of a huge family of receptor genes that codes for proteins with 7 transmembrane domains has at least explained the ability of the olfactory system to recognize so many different odorants, perhaps 10,000 or more. There may be a gene for each odorant. In this regard the olfactory system is similar to the immune system, with an enormous number of specific genes. When an odorant molecule binds with a receptor protein, a second messenger system is activated and initiates opening of ionic channels that result in depolarization of the receptor. A change in electric potential produced causes an impulse to travel to the olfactory bulb. The shape, duration, and latency are related to the stimulus. The olfactory bulb displays a continuous background of electrical activity and is interrupted by brief or long bursts of activity during stimulation. Olfactory fatigue occurs rapidly with continuous stimulation and recovers promptly at the end of the stimulus. There apparently is no disuse atrophy of CN I.

The stereochemical theory of olfaction presumes that each of the seven primary odors or modalities of the sense of smell possesses a particular electrophilic nature and that the neuro-olfactory epithelium possesses unique sites that are accessible only to certain odorants in a phenomenon of recognition by molecular chemosensitivity.[3] The adsorption of the odorant onto the receptor results in a molecular transformation that results in a change in electrical potential.

The olfactory epithelium is derived from the olfactory placode, first seen at the end of the first month of embryonic life. The lamina propria contains the branched tubuloalveolar glands of Bowman, which produce the thin fluid covering the olfactory surface. This fluid contains odorant-binding proteins, and this clearly separates it from the respiratory mucosa, although otherwise the differences are not known. To be smelled, a substance must be soluble in both water and lipids. The olfactory mucus is not propelled by the underlying cilia in the same sense as is the respiratory mucus but by unknown means, possibly "pulled" by traction of nearby respiratory cilia. The lamina propria contains contains blood vessels, connective tissue, and axons of the ciliated olfactory neurons. The axons of the olfactory neurons coalesce into large bundles and, proceeding centrally, pass through the cribriform plate as cilia olfactoria to synapse with second-order neurons in the glomeruli of the olfactory bulb.

The human olfactory neuroepithelium is located above the superior turbinate in the vault of the nose and occupies about 200 to 400 mm^2 on each side or perhaps 2.5 to 3% of the total nasal mucosa. The olfactory mucosa is constantly being renewed, perhaps in a cycle of 30 to 40 days[4] and is unique in being the only neuroepithelium exposed directly to the external environment. In older adults, there is frequently a replacement of mucosa with respiratory epithelium, likely as a result of aging, environmental insults, infections, or toxic medications.

The epithelium is usually described as consisting of supporting (or sustentacular), basal, and olfactory nerve cells (Fig. 1–10). The nerve cells number about 30,000/mm^2, which is far fewer than the number in animals. In recent years a fourth type, the microvillar cell, has been described.[5]

The supporting (sustentacular) cell is a tall, slender cell with an apically located nucleus. Numerous, branched microvilli extend from the free surface of the cell to form a network entangled with the olfactory cilia and microvilli from adjacent cells. The supporting cells themselves possess no cilia or basal bodies. The supporting cells usually are in intimate contact with the olfactory cells and may facilitate intercellular or metabolic transfer. The supporting cells appear to envelop or "protect" the olfactory axons and dendrites.[6]

Beneath the free surface, the supporting cell contains many organelles, including mitochondria, free ri-

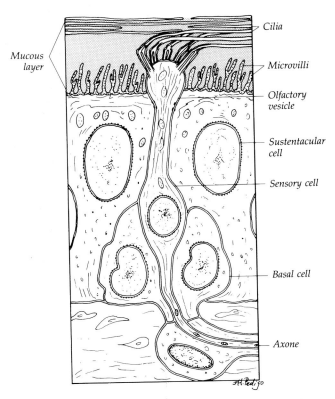

Fig. 1–10. Olfactory mucous membrane (diagrammatic).

bosomes, and membrane-lined vesicular inclusions. The cells produce a secretion into the overlying mucus. The cytoplasm basal to the nucleus is organelle poor.

The ultimate function of the supporting cell is not clear, but these cells probably are not involved in fluid transport as nonciliated cells of the respiratory mucosa may be. It is possible that they participate in the olfactory response by releasing their secretion at least to some odorants.[7] The numerous microvilli greatly increase the surface area, and they may have a phagocytic role in removing the "spent" odorant molecules.

The olfactory neuron is a bipolar cell exposed to the external environment and is continuously renewed in a 30- to 40-day cycle. It uniquely stains with olfactory marker protein. At its apical end is a modified dendrite that extends onto the surface as a thickened, club-shaped form, the olfactory knob or vesicle.

Radiating from the vesicle and bathed by mucus are 10 to 20 olfactory cilia of 50 to 200 μm. On cross-section near the basal end where the diameter is about 250 nm, the "9 plus 2" pattern of tubule pairs characteristic of respiratory cilia usually is present but of unknown significance. The tubules generally do not possess dynein arms, however, probably the reason that olfactory cilia are nonmotile. In the upper part of the cilium, singlets rather than doublets are found. The cilia arise from basal bodies located distally in the cell and are provided with rootlets oriented parallel to the long axis of the cell body. The odorous particles are believed to

Labels on figure: Cilia, Microvilli, Olfactory vesicle, Sustentacular cell, Sensory cell, Basal cell, Axone, Mucous layer be adsorbed onto molecular chemosensitive, intramembranous particles on the free surface of the cell or cilia.[6] Three types of cilia can be identified, 2 of which seem motile and contain adenosine triphosphate as the energy source. The motile cilia are found early in the replacement cycle and before synapse with the olfactory bulb is made. The nonmotile ciliated cell is "mature" and has synapsed with the bulb.

The proximal end of the olfactory neuron tapers into a filament less than 1 μm thick, the axon. As an unmyelinated fiber, it extends below the basal lamina to join axons from adjacent cells to form fascicles that become invested with Schwann cells and penetrate the cribriform plate. The joined fascicles become the grossly visible fila olfactoria, which lead to the olfactory bulbs lying on the upper surface of the cribriform plates and where synapse with the second-order neuron is made. The synapse is with the tufted and mitral cells that are found in tangles of nerve fibers, called olfactory glomeruli (or neuropils).

The olfactory neuroepithelium is also provided with myelinated fibers from the trigeminal nerves. Unmyelinated distal fibers of the fifth nerve, however, arborize between the supporting cells under the epithelial surface. Trigeminal innervation responds to touch, temperature, pain stimuli, and many noxious odorants.

After leaving the olfactory bulb, the second-order neurons form the olfactory tract, which passes along the base of the frontal lobe to enter in a complex pattern in the piriform cortex, the anterior commissure, the caudate nucleus, the olfactory tubercle, and the anterior limbus of the internal capsule with secondary connections.

The flask-shaped microvillar cells are the most numerous cells in the olfactory mucosa. Each cell body tapers upward to a narrow neck at the apex, where it gives rise to 75 to 100 microvilli. Neither cilia nor basal bodies are present. The microvillar cell at its neck is intimately attached to a neighboring supporting cell or a bipolar neuron. At the lower end of the cell, a long, slender cytoplasmic process extends toward the basement membrane and can be said to resemble an axon. Similar cells are found in the vomeronasal organ of animals.

The basal cells are stem cells and are probably the source of the receptor neurons and supporting cells lost during normal cell turnover or after injury. They are located just above the lamina propria, are 4 to 5 μm in diameter, and have a centrally located nucleus.

Olfactory Disorders

Hyposmia implies reduced sensitivity to all or most odorants, and specific anosmia to reduced sensitivity to one or a few odorants. Hyperosmia is an increased sensitivity to all or most odorants, whereas dysosmia

TABLE 1–5. Causes of Smell Impairment

Nasal Trauma
Mucosal Edema
  Allergy
  Polyps
  Vasomotor disorders
  Inflammatory disorders
Mucosal Destruction
  Atrophic rhinitis
  Mucosal aging
  Viral infections
  Ciliary dysfunction
  Toxic chemicals and drugs
Head Trauma
  Fracture of the cribriform plate
  Laceration of the olfactory tract
Intracranial Lesion
  Involvement of the undersurface of the frontal lobe
  Ischemia of the olfactory apparatus
  Infection
  Pressure on the cribriform plate
Endocrine
  Kallmann's syndrome
  Turner's syndrome
Emotional problems and malingering
Alzheimer's and Parkinson's diseases

or parosmia is a distortion of the perceived odor or the presence of an odor that does not exist (Table 1–5).

Accurate clinical evaluation of olfactory function is considerably compromised by the virtual impossibility of clearly separating the perceptual interweaving of cranial nerves V and I and taste and odor. Added to this are the confusions introduced by the aging process, the replacement of olfactory epithelium by a respiratory or squamous type, the loss of olfactory bulb neurons, and the lack of a pure olfactory stimulant.

Tests attempt to measure odor threshold and identification. In the monorhinic method developed by Cain and Gent,[8] the threshold is determined by a forced-choice procedure in which the patient is presented either with a sniff bottle containing a known aqueous concentration of butanol or water alone. Concentrations are increased until the patient correctly identifies the butanol. Cain's odor identification test consists of 10 items presented to each nostril separately. Of the items, 7 are odorants and 3 trigeminal stimulants, and the patient must select from a list containing 10 stimuli and 10 distractor names.

In the University of Pennsylvania Smell Identification Test (UPSIT), each of 40 odors is encapsulated on a pad that, one at a time, the patient "scratches and sniffs."[9] The patient is provided with a list of 4 choices for each pad and from which the correct answer must be chosen or a guess made. The correlation between the 2 tests is good.

Congenital Dysosmia
Berglund and Lindvall suggest a phenomenon of odor blindness loosely akin to color blindness.[10] Kallmann's

syndrome is often associated with hypogonadism and may also involve agenesis of the olfactory bulbs and stalks and faulty development of the hypothalamus. Deafness and other symptoms may be present, but trigeminal response to strong stimulants is retained. Korsakoff's syndrome is often associated with a depression of olfaction, perhaps on the basis of malnutrition, but it is possible that an alcoholic aphasia makes testing unreliable. Decreased olfactory ability is believed to be one of the first signs of Parkinson's disease, although it does not correlate with the severity of the motor affliction.

Kartagener's syndrome involves a congenital disorder of the ultrastructure of the respiratory ciliary axonemal tubules, resulting in the impairment of movement of the cilia and the mucous blanket. Whether this also involves olfactory ciliary malfunction is unknown.

Mechanical Airway Obstruction

An odorous particle may be prevented mechanically from reaching the olfactory mucosa, and thus no stimulus occurs. A modestly deviated nasal septum alone is unlikely to offer enough obstruction to do this. Laryngectomy is frequently accompanied by a seeming loss of smell, but there is no disuse atrophy of the olfaction mucosa. The nasal mucosa may be so inflamed or edematous that obstruction to the airway may occur. Nasal polyps, vasomotor rhinitis, allergic inflammation, and swellings or exudates caused by viral or bacterial disease and tumors are other examples.

Olfactory Mucosal Destruction

Intranasal mucosal destruction may involve the olfactory area and thus may lead to olfactory disturbances. Methotrexate is toxic to rapidly dividing cells and may interfere with taste or smell by reducing turnover. Many antimicrobial and antiproliferative agents can also be harmful by interfering with mitosis or inhibiting protein synthesis. Radiation and hormones are also known to affect turnover of cells.

Atrophic rhinitis is discussed elsewhere. The influenza virus, rhinovirus, herpes simplex virus, and others are associated with destruction of the ciliated respiratory nasal mucous membrane and destruction of the ciliated olfactory receptor cells as well. Insults to the olfactory mucous membrane by environmental pollutants and replacement by respiratory mucous membrane explain to a considerable degree the so-called age-related decline in acuity. The idea of an intrinsic age-related decrease in receptor neurons has not been borne out by animal studies.[11] Topically used chemicals destructive to the nasal mucosa may also be destructive to the olfactory mucosa, including cocaine, HCHO (formaldehyde), tyrothricin, sulfuric acid mist, sulfur dioxide, and chemotherapeutic agents.

Fracture of the cribriform plate or a shearing injury of the olfactory bulb or tract results in obvious damage to olfaction. Intracranial lesions of many sorts involving the undersurface of the frontal lobes and the cribriform plate offer a potential disturbance.

Endocrine Olfactory Problems

In Turner's syndrome, the gonadal activity is at fault. Individuals suffering from Addison's disease, low thyroid function, diabetes mellitus, and other endocrine problems may also complain of dysosmia.

Treatment

Alternatives for treatment of olfactory disturbances are discouragingly few unless there is a specific abnormality, such as abnormal odor conduction pathways or hypothyroidism, to correct. Theoretically, basal cells can replace damaged olfactory neurons, but practically this seems unlikely. Irritants known to damage the olfactory mucosa should be removed.

PHYSIOLOGY OF THE NOSE

The nose serves four essential functions. It is the site of the olfactory epithelium, a rigid airway to the lower respiratory tract, an organ to prepare the inspired air for the pulmonary surfaces, and a self-cleansing structure. The part played by the nose as a resonator is obvious to all who have suffered from the common cold.

Respiratory Mucosa

The pseudostratified respiratory mucosa consists of ciliated, intermediate, basal, and goblet cells. They rest on a well-defined basement membrane supported, in contrast to the olfactory mucosa, by a relatively deep, loose lamina propria containing small blood vessels, venous plexus, ducts of mucous and serous glands, sensory nerves, and blood cells (primarily lymphocytes.) The blood capillaries and venules are thin walled and possess a fenestrated endothelial lining and a porous basement membrane. Basal cells seem to have the capacity to differentiate into goblet or ciliated cells as required.

The tall (15 to 20 μm) columnar ciliated cell is the predominant cell and extends from the basement membrane to the luminal surface, where cilia admixed with microvilli are present. The microvilli are smaller than the cilia (3 μm $\times$ 0.1 μm versus 6 to 7 $\times$ 0.3), and some are branched. The microvilli contain bundles of microfilaments and display hair-like projections characterized as glycalyx. The function of the microvilli is unclear, although they greatly increase cell surface area.

The ciliated cell cytoplasm forms complex interdigitations with adjacent cell membranes, presumably to permit intercellular exchanges. Irregular intercellular spaces exist to accommodate edema fluid and inflammatory cells for implementation of the immune response.

Basal cells lie on the basement membrane and have long been considered the progenitors of the columnar and goblet cells. Recent evidence suggests, however, that the primary progenitor may be a nonciliated columnar cell that can form ciliated cells.

Goblet cells taper upward from the basement membrane to an expanded body at the lumen, where microvilli are found on their exposed surfaces. The nucleus is situated basally, and secretory granules that contain mucin are toward the lumen.

Columnar cells extend from a narrow base at the basement membrane to an expanded surface area covered by microvilli. These cells are related to adjacent cells by tight junctions apically and by interdigitations of the cell membrane. This cell may be the progenitor of the airway epithelium.

Airway

The nose provides a rigid passageway through which incoming and outgoing air passes. Anteriorly the support is provided by the semirigid upper and lower cartilages, posteriorly by the nasal bones.

On entering the nose, the incoming air is directed upward by the anterior nares and the shape of the nasal vault (Fig. 1–11). The airstream turns 80 to 90 degrees posteriorly as it reaches the nasal vault and then traverses a horizontal path until it impacts against the posterior wall of the nasopharynx. At this point, now joined with air from the other side, an 80- to 90-degree downward bend occurs. Each of these two bends are termed impaction points and facilitate the removal of particulate matter. Impaction against the adenoid may enable the adenoid to respond immunologically by "sampling" the particulates. Some of the air, enhanced by sniffing, reaches the olfactory area. The expiratory route is generally the reverse of the inspiratory, and again, some of the expired air also reaches the olfactory area.

Airstream

The anterior nasal valve, or ostium internum, is located at the limen nasi, some 1.5 to 2 cm posterior to the anterior nares. At this point, the cross-section of the airway is 20 to 40 mm^2 on each side and is the narrowest point of the upper respiratory tract and provides about 50% of the total airway resistance. Posterior to this, in the main (horizontal) nasal passage, the cross-section widens while the airstream remains narrow and thus provides a large surface area in intimate contact with the airstream. At the choanae, the cross-section again narrows.

Evidence has accumulated that there is a 2½- to 4-hour cyclic alteration of nasal resistance from one side to the other. Prolonged increase in nasal resistance (e.g., tight nasal packing) can lead to cor pulmonale, cardiomegaly, and pulmonary edema. The most common sequel to increased resistance, however, is mouth breathing with consequent bypassing of the cleansing and air-conditioning function of the nose.

Air Speed

The air speed is greatest at the anterior nasal valve, reaching 3.3 m/sec at an inspiratory flow rate of 200 ml/sec compared to 1 mm/sec in secondary bronchi (Fig. 1–11). Beyond the valve, in the horizontal part of the nasal airway, the air speed slows down. This enables the inspired air to remain in contact longer with a large surface area for warming, humidification, and cleansing.

Particle Removal

The aerodynamic equivalent diameter (AED) is the diameter of a unit density sphere with the same settling speed as the particle in question. Particles of approximately 5 μm AED or greater are 85 to 90% removed by the nose and nasopharynx. Smaller particles penetrate to varying degrees to the lower respiratory tract. Virus-containing droplets coalesce into diameters fre-

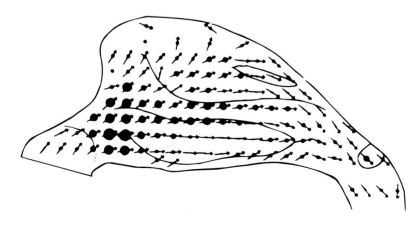

Fig. 1–11. Diagram of the nasal airway and airspeed, the size of the dot indicating the velocity. (From Brau JD, Proctor DF, and Reid LM (eds): Respiratory Defense Mechanisms. Part I. New York, Marcel Dekker, 1977.)

quently exceeding 5 to 6 μm and thus are largely retained in the nose.

Air Conditioning

Tempering and humidification are largely accomplished during the horizontal passage of the inspired air. The air is heated (or cooled) by radiation from the mucosal blood vessels. Humidification occurs by evaporation from the mucous blanket covering the mucosa. That this is an efficient mechanism is attested to by the observation that the inspired air is near normal body temperature and relative humidity near 100% in the nasopharynx. The mucosal blood vessels lie in two layers of more or less parallel rows. The more superficial layer sends capillaries into the epithelium, and the capillaries of the deeper layer below the basement membrane are fenestrated to facilitate fluid movement. The flow of blood is from posterior to anterior, opposite to the flow of inspired air and mucus. The mechanism of a "countercurrent" adds to the efficiency of the system.

The nasal mucous membrane is cooler by varying degrees than the expired air, and thus some condensation on and warming of the membranes occurs—a so-called regenerative exchange. The inferior turbinate, which contains the majority of the blood spaces, acts primarily not as a radiator but as a valve that controls the capacity of the nose.

Respiratory Cilia

In humans, respiratory cilia are found throughout the respiratory tract, except for the extreme anterior part of the nose, the posterior oropharyngeal wall, portions of the larynx, and the terminal ramifications of the bronchial tree. They are located in the eustachian tube, most of the middle ear, and the paranasal sinuses. Cilia in a modified form also occur in the maculae and cristae of the inner ear and in the eye as retinal rods.

Ciliary Ultrastructure

Human cilia extend about 6 μm above the luminal surface of the cell and are about 0.3 μm in width. Perhaps as many as 100 are found on each cell in the nose. Each cilium appears to be anchored to a basal body located just below the cell surface. The structure of the centriole of the a dividing cell is similar to the basal body, the former giving rise to the latter and the basal body to the cilium.[12]

Each cilium is encased by an extension of the cell plasma membrane. Within the cilium is a sheaf of longitudinally arranged microtubules (or fibrils) termed an axoneme. The microtubules are in fact tubule doublets with nine outer pairs arranged in a cartwheel pattern along the periphery of the axoneme. Moreover, two single microtubules are located in the center of the axoneme, creating the characteristic "9 + 2" pattern.

At the distal tip of the cilium is a dense cap or crown from which three to seven "claws" 25 to 35 nm long project. Beneath the cell membrane and the axoneme is a short, cylindrical basal body, and below this the tubules (with a third added to form a triplet) seem to extend into the apical cytoplasm of the cell and are termed "rootlets." They converge into a cone-shaped form and acquire periodic striations. Another structure, the basal foot, pointing in the direction of the effective ciliary beat, projects parallel to the surface from the side of the basal body. The basal foot has a cross-striated appearance resembling that of collagen fibers. In addition, other fine microtubules, which seem to be branched, attach to adjacent basal bodies, to each other, and ultimately to the junctional complex, constituting the terminal web.

The nine outer doublets, looking downward on a cross-section, are each composed of two juxtaposed microtubules: a slightly more centrally located subfiber, A, and a slightly more peripherally located subfiber, B (Fig. 1–12). Two regularly arranged arms composed of adenosine triphosphatase, called dynein arms, extend from a toward b of the adjacent doublet.[13] Also present are links attaching each subfiber a to b of the adjacent doublet and similarly arranged at regular intervals along the length of the subfibers. They are believed to be of an elastic material called nexin. Extending centrally from a to the central pair are radial spokes. At the base of the cilium, the central two microtubules terminate, and each of the peripheral doublets continue downward to enter the basal body as a triplet, with subfiber c added (Fig. 1–12).

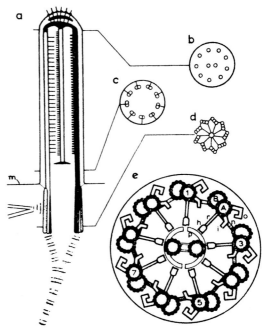

Fig. 1–12. Diagram of the ultra-anatomic arrangement of ciliary tubules at various levels.

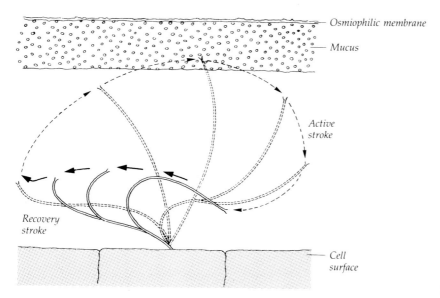

Osmiophilic membrane

Mucus

Active stroke

Recovery stroke

Cell surface

Fig. 1–13. Diagram of the normal ciliary cycle.

The motion of the cilium is caused by the sliding of one tubule past the other, thus creating a shearing force that induces bending. Energy for this work is derived from the breaking down of adenosine triphosphate in the dynein arms. The spokes seem to detach and reattach several times during the bending process. The axis of motion of the cilium is defined by a line perpendicular to a plane connecting the central pair of tubules. Control of ciliary action is poorly understood, but there seems to be a neuroid contact between cells.

Cilary Beat

The to-and-fro movement of the cilium is termed its beat (Fig. 1–13). There is a more forceful forward, effective, stroke in which the cilium is fully extended and the claws at the tip reach the overlying layer of mucus. The recovery stroke is less forceful and slower, and the cilium is curled, somewhat laterally, on itself to be shorter and thus not to reach the overlying flakes of mucus.[14] Beating occurs 1000 or more times per minute and is metachronous. The nature of the nervous coordination is not known.

Mucous Blanket

The mucous blanket is a 12- to 15-μm thick, sticky, tenacious, adhesive sheet consisting of two layers, the mucous and periciliary layers.[15] In health, the pH is slightly acid. Its approximate composition is 2.5 to 3% glycoprotein, 1 to 2% salts, and 95% water. Immunoglobulins comprise about 70% of the protein content. It is found throughout the nose (except the vestibule), sinuses, middle ear, eustachian tube, and bronchial tree (and extending to the alveoli in the form of surfactant). The beating of the underlying cilia propel the blanket of mucus, along with trapped or dissolved ma-

terial, in mostly continuous movement toward the pharyngeal end of the esophagus, where it is swallowed or expectorated. Mucus is produced by the serous and goblet cells.

Mucus from the anterior sinuses is delivered into the middle meatus. The lumina of the sinuses are relatively unexposed to noxious environmental elements and can be said to be uncontaminated. A hitherto unrecognized function of the paranasal sinuses may be the dilution factor this uncontaminated mucus makes to the mucus of the middle meatus.

Enveloping the shafts of the cilia is the thicker, less viscid, and deeper periciliary layer, and above this, interfacing with the luminal surface, is the more viscid and thicker layer of mucus flakes riding on the periciliary fluid below. Insoluble particulate matter caught on the mucus flakes is carried posteriorly to the esophagus. Soluble matter reaches the periciliary fluid and is removed with it. Much more remains to be learned about the rheology and the viscoelastic properties, as well as the thickness, of the mucous blanket (Fig. 1–14).

Mucociliary Transport

The mucociliary transport or clearance system is really two systems working simultaneously. It depends on the actively beating cilia propelling the mucous flakes to the upper end of the esophagus and the deeper periciliary fluid also moving posteriorly by mechanisms poorly understood. Anterior to the inferior turbinates, the mucus may move anteriorly. The speed of the posterior movement varies widely in apparently healthy individuals from 1 to 20 mm/min.[16] Relative mucostasis, however, usually caused by decreased beat frequency, may permit time for noxious elements to inaugurate disease by mucosal penetration.

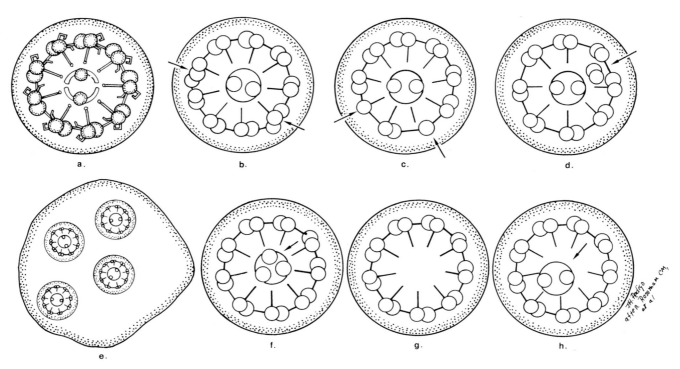

Fig. 1–14. Some observed abnormal alterations of axonemal tubules.

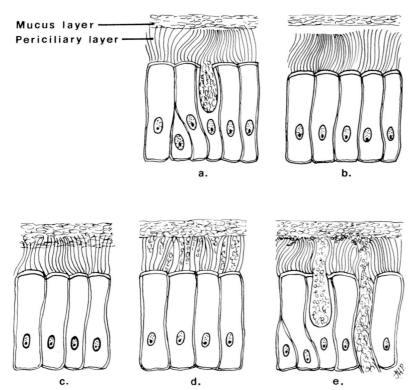

Mucus layer
Periciliary layer

Fig. 1–15. Various possible alterations of the mucous blanket.

Although most bacteria seem to impede ciliary beating little or not at all, Bordetella pertussis, Mycoplasma pneumoniae, and Pseudomonas aeruginosa, among others, do so. Some respiratory viruses and bacteria, notably influenza virus, rhinovirus, adenovirus, herpes simplex virus, and respiratory syncytial viruses, impede mucociliary transport. They can do this by altering either the axonemal ultrastructure or the viscoelastic properties of the blanket of mucus (Figs. 1–14 and 1–15).

Slowing or destruction of the mucociliary transport and the attendant interference with nasal cleansing may prolong nasal and sinus infections.[17] The effect of the environment on the nose, and particularly mucociliary transport, is further considered in Chapters 6 and 7.

SUGGESTED READINGS

1. Messerklinger W: Endoscopy of the Nose. Baltimore, Urban and Schwarzenberg, 1978.
2. Baroody F and Naclerio RM: A Review of Anatomy and Physiology of the Nose. Alexandria, VA, American Academy of Otolaryngology—Head and Neck Surgery, 1990.
3. Pevner J, et al: Molecular cloning of odor-binding protein: member of a ligand carrier family. Science 241:336, 1988.
4. Nakashima CP, Kimmelman CP, and Snow JB: Immunohistopathology of human olfactory epithelium, nerve, and bulb. Laryngoscope 25:391, 1985.
5. Jafek BW: Ultrastructure of human nasal mucosa. Laryngoscope 93:1576, 1983.
6. Moran DT, Powley JC III, Jafek BW, and Lovell MA: The fine structure of the olfactory mucosa in man. J Neurocytol 11:721, 1982.
7. Hornung DE and Mozell MM: Smell: human physiology. In: Clinical Measurement of Taste and Smell. Edited by Meiselman HL and Rivlin RS. New York, Macmillan, 1986.
8. Cain WS and Gent J: Clinical evaluation of olfaction. Am J Otolaryngol 4:2252, 1983.
9. Doty RL, Shaman P, Kimmelman CP, and Dann M: University Pennsylvania smell identification test: a standardized microencapsulized test of olfactory function. Physiol Behav 32:489, 1984.
10. Berglund B and Lindvall TA: Olfaction. In: The Nose. Edited by Proctor DF and Andersen IB. New York, Elsevier Biomedical Press, 1982.
11. Hinds JW and McNally NA: Aging in the rat olfactory system: correlation of the olfactory epithelium and olfactory bulb. J Comp Neurol 203:441, 1981.
12. Carson JL, et al: Morphometric aspects of ciliary distribution and ciliogenesis in human nasal epithelium. Proc Natl Acad Sci USA 78:6996, 1981.
13. Gibbons IR and Rowe AJ: Dynein: a protein with adenosine triphosphate activity from cilia. Science 149:424, 1965.
14. Duchateau G, et al: Correlation between nasal ciliary beat frequency and mucous transport rate in volunteers. Laryngoscope 95:854, 1985.
15. Proctor DF: The mucociliary system. In: The Nose. Edited by Proctor DF and Andersen IB. New York, Elsevier Biomedical Press, 1982.
16. Quinlan MF, et al: Measurement of mucociliary function in man. Am Rev Respir Dis 99:13, 1969.
17. Ballenger JJ: Acquired ultrastructural alterations of respiratory cilia and clinical disease. Ann Otol Rhinol Laryngol 97:252, 1988.

2 Nasal Reconstruction and Rhinoplasty

M. Eugene Tardy and Dean Torilemi

INCISIONS AND EXCISIONS

External nasal and paranasal incision and excision sites should be planned and positioned in areas where scar camouflage is optimum. The varying thickness and mobility of the skin in the upper three fifths of the nose, in contrast to the lower two fifths, dictate different approaches to similar problems of excision. Defects resulting from excision or trauma in the more cephalic nasal regions may be diminished considerably by circumferential dermal undermining and advancement of the thinner mobile skin. The extent of similar defects in the lower nasal regions near the tip is less easily decreased because of thick skin, heavily laden with sebaceous glands and variably dense subcutaneous tissue.

All external nasal incisions should be sited in inconspicuous areas, leading to minimal distortion of nasal features and symmetry. Junctions of facial landmarks hide surgical scars well; therefore, incisions along the nasomaxillary groove, the alar facial junction, and the columellar-labial (or nasolabial) junction heal inconspicuously. Lesion excision in these areas should be preplanned so that the ultimate suture line(s) will symmetrically recreate these natural landmark borders. Strict attention to maintaining or recreating symmetry leads to superior aesthetic results. Local pedicle flaps transposed into these areas should be similarly designed.

Natural folds created by the synergistic interaction of muscle groups at the root of the nose provide ideal sites for incision and excision camouflage. Horizontal, oblique, and vertical wrinkles apparent in this area, blending into the glabellar region, provide wide latitude in scar camouflage in the aging patient (Fig. 2–1). Redundant nasal and glabellar skin allows considerable excisional license without sacrificing normal landmarks. It is usually possible and always preferable to reconstitute these natural folds during the course of repair.

Alternate, but less ideal, incision sites exist. Anterior midcolumellar incisions heal generally with minimal scar evidence, although the lateral columellar incision lends similar surgical access and creates less potential scar. Staggered or W-shaped incisions in the anterior midcolumellar area are acceptable for tumor excision and as an approach to external rhinoplasty procedures.

Congenital nasal tumors (dermoid cysts, lymphangiomas) in children require incisional approaches through the nasal dorsum, with wide exposure required for total excision. A precise midline dorsal incision or semilunar transverse incision creates a visible but symmetric scar that, if meticulously repaired, fades acceptably with time.

Mature nasal scars on exposed nasal epithelium (i.e., not camouflaged in landmark junctions or natural folds) may be rendered less conspicuous with superficial mechanical dermabrasion. Minimal scars resulting from laceration repair or pedicle flap reconstruction of the lower half of the nose respond particularly well to dermabrasion techniques (widened, depressed scars caused by inexact dermal healing require reexcision and meticulous repair; dermabrasion is ineffective in such cases).

A useful technique for diminishing the extent of a large nasal excisional defect is to remove a portion of an existing nasal hump (bone and cartilage), creating a relative excess of skin for repair, proportionally diminishing the defect, and favorably improving the patient's profile and nasal length.

Several areas of nasal anatomy should be considered inviolate because scars there almost always heal with unacceptable results. Incisions or lacerations cutting across the delicate alar rim remain conspicuous (notching is a common sequela), as may incisions cutting across the columella in transverse fashion. Because most incisions bridging a concavity contract and heal as a tight, tethered "bowstring" contracture, transverse incisions crossing the concave upper lateral nasal skin toward the inner canthus must be avoided.

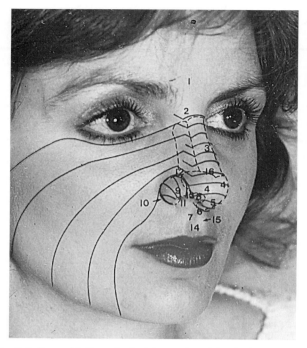

Fig. 2–1. Favorable lines for incision and excision in the nasal and paranasal region.

Finally, the nasal defect created by traumatic laceration or lesion excision provides the surgeon with an unparalleled opportunity to study exposed nasal anatomy and framework, aiding considerably in an understanding of the delicate, precise structural rearrangement necessarily less apparent during septorhinoplasty.

EPITHELIAL RECONSTRUCTION

Epithelial nasal defects commonly result from minor to major excision of nasal lesions, benign or malignant. Occasionally, epithelial reconstitution is necessary for replacement of irradiated nasal skin of poor quality. Traumatic avulsion defects demand immediate repair if aesthetics are to be properly served and unacceptable scarring and contracture avoided. Because it occupies the conspicuous central portion of the face, the nose draws immediate attention to itself, and nasal defects, however minor, accentuate that attention. Therefore, camouflage repair of nasal defects deserves high aesthetic and functional priority, with strict attention to achieving reconstructive symmetry by repair that respects topographic subunit principles (Fig. 2–2).

Until recent decades, the split-thickness or full-thickness skin graft served the surgeon well as an effective tissue for immediate epithelial replacement. Skin is readily available around the head and neck, its rate of successful "take" is high, and one-stage repairs conserve the patient's and the surgeon's time and skills.

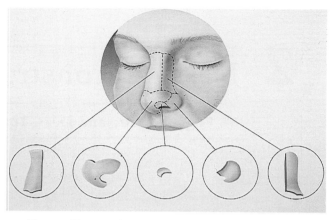

Fig. 2–2. Topographic subunits of the nose (after Burget).

Gradually, however, the multiple advantages of adjacent or regional pedicle flaps become apparent to head and neck surgeons interested and skilled in a higher degree of aesthetic camouflage, effective one-stage (or, on occasion, two-stage) repair and superior defect effacement and color match. Properly designed and executed, flaps should replace missing tissue with like tissue, a fundamental concept in plastic surgery. Furthermore, flaps possess the following distinct advantages over skin grafts:

1. They provide their own blood supply.
2. They contract less than grafts.
3. Cosmetically and chromatically, they are superior to grafts.
4. They provide bulk and lining.
5. They create superior protection for bone and cartilage.
6. They resist infection.
7. They undergo minimal pigment change.
8. They may incorporate cartilage, bone, or skin in composite fashion.

In their simplest form, adjacent flaps may be classified as advancement, rotation, transposition, and interposition flaps, all designed and derived from tissue adjacent to the nasal defect. Regional flaps are best used when more abundant tissue is required for repair or adjacent skin is inadequate or unsatisfactory. They utilize unipedicled flaps of similar texture thickness and color from adjacent regions (glabella, forehead, scalp, cheek, neck). A second stage of repair is required to transect the bridge of the flap, reconstructing both the defect and donor site to render both inconspicuous. Regional flaps are invariably designed and transposed from areas of relative epithelial excess and redundancy in the head and neck.

ADVANCEMENT FLAPS

Advancement flaps are created when tissue is undermined and advanced in a straight line along the same axis as the defect.

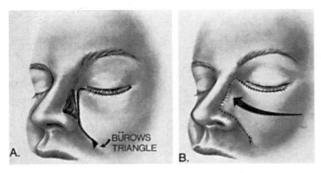

Fig. 2–3. Cheek advancement flap for lateral nasal reconstruction.

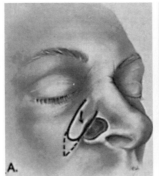
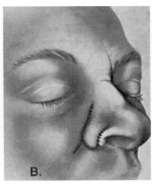

Fig. 2–5. Nasolabial rotation flap for reconstruction of alar nasal defect. Alar-facial junction is reconstituted.

Mobile cheek skin may be undermined and advanced to repair heminasal defects of varying proportions (Fig. 2–3). Design is such that ultimate closure falls in the nasolabial fold and infraciliary area and at the junction of the nose to the face (Fig. 2–4). Where possible, the nasolabial fold should be preserved or reconstituted to achieve bilateral facial symmetry, with incisions falling in the nasolabial crease. The inherent elasticity and redundancy of skin allow a variety of geometric designs in creating advancement flaps with ultimate suture lines lying in favorable areas for camouflage.

Advancement flaps along the dorsum of the nose may be created after transverse fusiform excision of lesions, diminishing the defect when possible by shortening the nose and accomplishing hump removal.

ROTATION FLAPS

A local flap in which the axis is created in a plane different from that of the defect is termed a rotation flap. Rotation flaps are extremely useful in nasal repair, particularly when designed so that the donor site may be closed in an inconspicuous straight line, natural fold, or landmark junction. Typical ideal donor sites are the nasolabial fold (Fig. 2–5) and glabellar regions (Fig. 2–6).

The surgeon should approach any potential nasal defect with several alternative repair techniques in mind, ultimately choosing the flap or technique that possesses the most advantages and fewest risks for defect closure. The extent of almost all excisional defects may be diminished by circumferential undermining. The important concept of reverse planning is used, measuring the final defect size and planning the flap accordingly before creating final incisions. Small local flaps undergo minimal shrinkage during healing (less than 10%); therefore, almost exact flaps may be tailored to reconstitute the nasal defect precisely. Flap thickness should approximate the depth of the defect for full and complete effacement. Suture technique should include key interrupted, buried, absorbable sutures in the dermis and subcutaneous tissue to match the flap precisely to the defect, with nonabsorbable fine sutures used for 3 to 5 days to approximate epithelium. Ten-

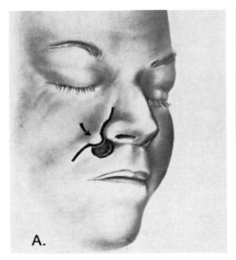
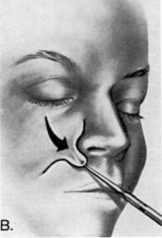
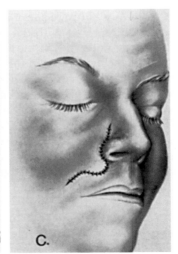

Fig. 2–4. Cheek advancement flap to reconstruct alar-facial junction and tissue void of lateral upper lip.

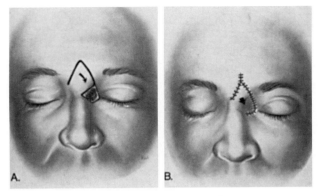

Fig. 2–6. Glabellar rotation flap.

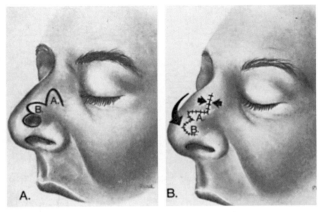

Fig. 2–7. Bilobed transposition flap used for nasal reconstruction.

sion-reducing taping (Steri-strips) or tissue glues (His-toacryl blue) enhance wound approximation and allow earlier removal of sutures. Light compression bandages are used for 24 to 48 hours, then removed and replaced by Neodecadron ophthalmic ointment to keep the suture lines free of debris and clot, maximizing early healing.

Properly designed and executed, rotation flaps of adjacent nasal tissue may be expected to provide superior three-dimensional reconstruction of surgical and traumatic nasal defects within several weeks of repair. Defatting and "touch-up" procedures are rarely necessary. Light dermabrasion of the resulting fine nasal scars, 3 to 4 months later, can favorably enhance the blending effect.

TRANSPOSITION FLAPS

By far the most versatile of adjacent flaps, the transposition flap designs available for nasal repair are varied and reliable. The variety of designs possible with transposed flaps provides the surgeon with many near-equal possibilities for nasal defect repair. Transposition flaps ordinarily allow primary closure of defects larger than those repaired with the simpler advancement and rotation flaps. When the flaps are properly designed, little tension is created on suture lines, and "dog-ears" or "standing cones" are minimized.

In addition to the classic transposition flap design, bilobed transposition flaps, rhomboid transposition flaps, and the standard ubiquitous Z-plasty are superior methods of epithelial nasal reconstruction with adjacent tissue.

The classic transposition flap design is useful in the glabellar area, transposing redundant, lax tissue to upper lateral nasal defects. Proper design allows the ultimate incision lines to fall in or near natural folds, creating effective camouflage. Similar designs can take advantage of redundant nasolabial fold cheek tissue, sliding tissue medially to provide ample cover for lat-

eral nasal tissue deficits; an undesirable side effect of this maneuver is the partial obliteration of the nasolabial groove, which is a highly desirable landmark.

A tissue-abundant and versatile example of transposition flaps is the *bilobed flap* (Fig. 2–7), consisting of two lobes separated by more or less of an angle and based upon a common pedicle. This variety of flap design has several general applications in facial repair and two specific applications in nasal repair. Ideally, the dual flaps used should be similar (although not necessarily exact) in size and designed to rotate no more than 90 degrees for repair. In practice, this angle can vary from 45 to almost 120 degrees, depending on the location of the defect. In the upper half of the nose, in which the primary donor site of the bilobed flap may be easily reduced in size by undermining and advancement of its edges, the required size of the secondary donor flap may be reduced accordingly. The major advantage of the bilobed flap is derived from its use of the laxity (elasticity) and redundancy of tissue along two axes at approximately right angles to each other, compounding these tissues into one flap.

Abundant glabellar skin with vertical wrinkles, common in the aging face, combines favorably with the lax skin of the inner canthus area to supply tissue for the glabellar bilobed flap (Fig. 2–8). The primary lobe of the flap is of ideal thickness and color match for dorsal nasal repair. The glabellar skin, which constitutes the secondary flap, is often thicker than inner canthal skin and must be carefully thinned after undermining to match evenly at the suture line. Heavy, thick eyebrows extending into the glabellar midline may impair the cosmetic effectiveness of this transposition flap.

An extension of this flap design lends itself favorably to the repair of large lesions near the inner canthus and lateral nasal borders (Fig. 2–9). A relaxing incision buried and camouflaged in the nasolabial fold frees an advancement flap of cheek skin to diminish the size of

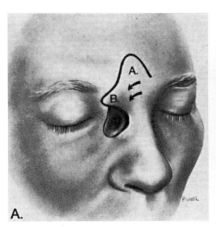
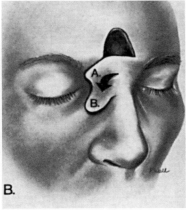
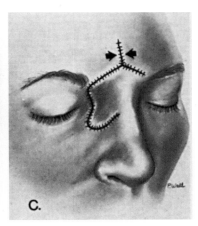

Fig. 2–8. Glabellar bilobed transposition flap.

the primary recipient site, thereby reducing the effective size of the bilobed donor flap.

Similar principles are involved in deriving donor skin for nasal resurfacing from redundant nasolabial fold skin (Fig. 2–10). The secondary donor site is closed primarily in the fold, effectively camouflaging its presence. For large nasal defects especially, the cosmetic appearance of the healed flap is preferable in most situations to free skin or composite grafts. Tissue defects of the nonmobile skin of the nasal tip and infratip lobule are better repaired with full-thickness skin grafts harvested from the nasolabial fold or preauricular skin, however.

The principles involved in bilobed flap design can be used in a variety of reconstructive situations around the head and neck.

REGIONAL FLAPS

Tubed pedicle skin flaps designed and transposed from head and neck regions other than those immediately adjacent to the nose are termed *regional flaps*. They are judiciously used when tissue in more abundance

than that provided by adjacent flaps is required or when flap transport of buried skin, bone, or cartilage is required for framework reconstitution. In the latter incidence, the flap becomes a *composite or compound flap* and always requires delay and staging of 14 to 21 days before total elevation and transposition of the pedicle to the recipient site. Regional flaps are mainly designed around vigorous named vessels in the head and neck to allow nondelayed primary elevation and transposition. As circulatory efficiency in the flaps approaches its optimum level (14 to 21 days), the bridge of the flap is transected, final repair of the recipient site effected, and all or a portion of the unused pedicle either replaced in its previous anatomic bed or discarded if donor site repair is unnecessary. Regional flaps from the midline forehead, scalp, and temple provide excellent tissue of appropriate bulk and near-ideal color match for nasal reconstitution. Furthermore, the ultimate donor sites in these areas are easily and effectively camouflaged, making them the site of choice for regional flap nasal repair. Tissue derived from cervical and more distant unexposed regions (shoulder, arm) lacks this ideal color match potential.

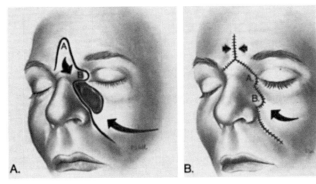

Fig. 2–9. Glabellar bilobed flap combined with advancement cheek flap for repair of large facial defect.

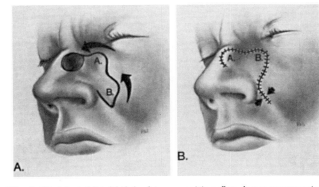

Fig. 2–10. Mesiolabial bilobed transposition flap for reconstruction of lateral nasal defect.

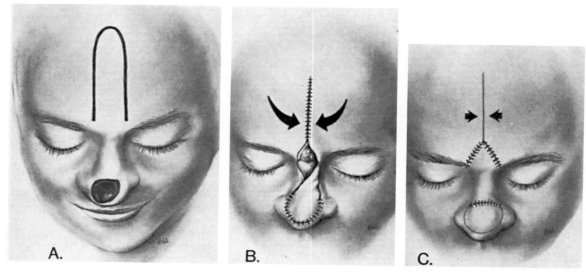

Fig. 2–11. Precise midline forehead flap interposed into large nasal defect.

MIDLINE FOREHEAD FLAP

Of all the subtotal forehead flaps described for nasal reconstitution, the precise midline vertical forehead flap is preferred for immediate transposition (Fig. 2–11). The color match is nearly perfect, the midline donor site defect may be closed immediately by advancing the lateral edges of the defect, and the resultant forehead scar is negligible if closure is meticulous and free of tension. Indeed, a midline vertical wrinkle already exists in many older patients, inviting scar camouflage. A flap width of 2.5 to 4 cm is available, and length is limited only by the extent of the hairline widow's peak. Abundantly nourished by the supratrochlear and dorsal nasal vessels, the midline forehead flap is suitable for primary restoration of defects of lateral nasal epithelium (Fig. 2–12), alar margin, and columella. A dressing of Adaptic gauze and antibiotic ointment substitutes for lining on the undersurface of the flap.

If desirable and appropriate, forehead tissue may be carried as a subcutaneous island pedicle flap beneath the tunnel of skin at the root of the nose; although this design provides one-stage repair, it adds unnecessary vascular hazard to the repair and often unsightly fullness in the tunnel region.

Fourteen to 18 days after primary flap elevation and transfer, the vascular viability of the transposed tissue is challenged by circumferential tourniquet compression; generally, division of the flap bridge is safely accomplished at this time. Most of the flap is discarded, restoring only sufficient tissue to reconstitute the oblique wrinkle lines at the root of the nose (see Fig. 2–11C). Camouflage is excellent.

The aesthetic advantage of the midline flap is apparent to all surgeons who use it regularly. Oblique, transverse, and "off-center" forehead flaps impose a higher penalty in ultimate scar legacy and therefore are poor aesthetic choices. Midline flaps preserve forehead symmetry and expression.

In near-total nasal reconstruction, midline forehead flaps can serve as the internal epithelial lining for the new nose, underlying a scalp flap designed to reconstitute nasal form.

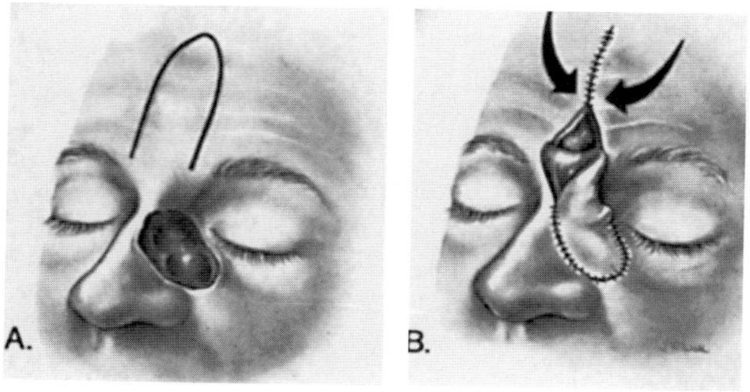

SCALP SICKLE FLAP

Selected facial and nasal reconstructive problems can be solved effectively and aesthetically using a pedicle flap derived from the scalp-forehead junction and designed in sickle or "horseshoe" fashion (Fig. 2–13). A vigorous and tissue-abundant flap based on the superficial temporal vessels with contributions from the postauricular vessels, the sickle flap may be elevated and transposed without delay. The distal tip of the flap is composed of the non-hair-bearing bay of forehead-scalp skin, thereby avoiding major forehead scarring and disfigurement. Ambitious length-to-width ratios

Fig. 2–12. Precise midline forehead flap interposed into large facial-nasal defect.

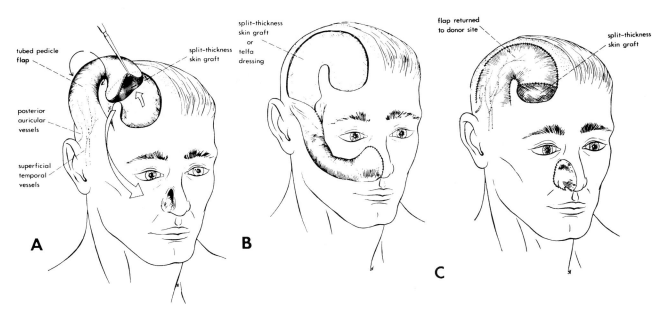

Fig. 2–13. Scalp sickle flap derived from non-hair-bearing bay of forehead skin for major nasal defect reconstruction.

(often 6 or 8 to 1) are commonly feasible. Replacement of the unused bridge of the flap to its previous scalp position effectively camouflages donor site deformity.

The bilateral non-hair-bearing bays of forehead-scalp skin, abundant in normal scalps and more generous in patients with receding hairlines, is a choice site for donor tissue. The requirements of ideal color match and skin texture are admirably fulfilled by the sickle flap tissue. Because the frontal forehead is spared, donor site camouflage is effected by ultimate replacement of the bridge of the flap within the scalp defect, combing adjacent hair over the forehead bay, and, on occasion, lowering the frontal hairline by rotating a small adjacent rhomboid or bilobed hair-bearing flap into the bay defect. Judicious design of the flap thereby creates minimal donor site deformity, all of which may be effectively camouflaged. Normal anatomy is thereby preserved.

Vigorous and reliable nourishment of the flap is derived from the superficial temporal vessels with contributions from postauricular branches, allowing nondelayed flap elevation and transposition to the recipient site. This generous blood supply permits ambitious length-to-width ratios of up to 8 to 1, allowing reconstruction of facial defects at great distances from the scalp. Selected nasal defects of major proportion are ideally suited for sickle flap reconstruction, although the midline forehead flap, if available, may be a preferable choice. Compound sickle flaps, transporting buried skin, bone, or cartilage to a recipient site, routinely require delay to ensure viability. Although based on the same blood supply as the classic forehead flaps, the sickle flap creates less scarring and disfigurement by sparing the central regions of the forehead.

SCALPING FLAPS

Broad exposure of scalp and forehead tissue may be primarily elevated and transposed without fear of vascular embarrassment for near-total nasal reconstitution (Fig. 2–14). In older men with balding tendencies, the donor site portion of the flap is best designed to lie on the scalp, ideally at the vertex of the skull. In younger patients and in women, the laterally placed skin superficial to the frontalis muscle is the donor tissue; a postauricular full-thickness skin graft covers the forehead defect over the intact frontalis muscle. Careful flap design with a reverse planning pattern technique provides ample tissue for alar simulation by enfolding skin edges for both inner and outer nasal lining. Sufficient length must be incorporated into the design for adequate columellar length; failure to provide ample length disallows adequate tip projection. Small local turnover flaps should be developed when possible at the lateral edges of the nasal defect to provide an enhanced vascular bed for side-to-side rather than edge-to-edge suture repair.

SKIN GRAFTS

Although infrequently used, skin grafts of split and full thickness are useful in nasal repair. The alternatives of primary closure or adjacent flap repair are generally preferable because of the inherent advantages previously detailed.

Skin grafts possess several distinct assets when employed for one-stage repair with no sacrifice of surrounding tissue is required: no further incisions are

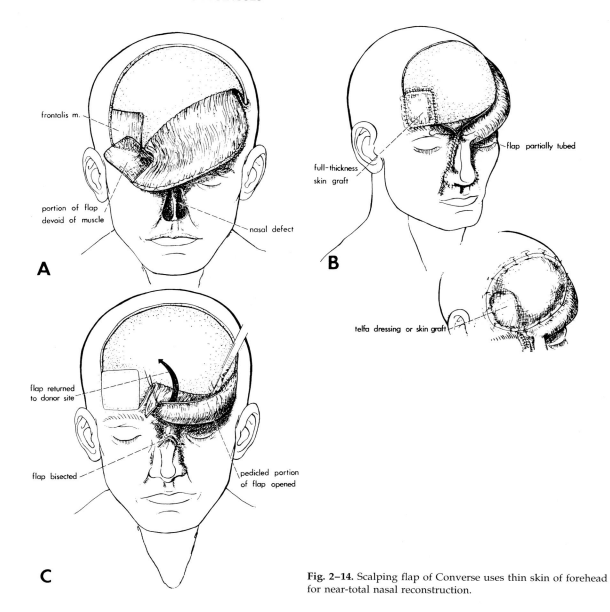

Fig. 2–14. Scalping flap of Converse uses thin skin of forehead for near-total nasal reconstruction.

required adjacent to the defect, and planning is certainly less complex and sophisticated. Normal landmarks are generally undisturbed, and, should the graft fail for any reason, secondary grafting can proceed almost immediately after wound debridement, freshening, and infection control.

Superficial nasal epithelial defects of the lower half of the nose (trauma, burns, surgical excisions) are readily repaired with skin grafts derived from nasolabial, preauricular, or postauricular skin. The postauricular site has been shown by experience to be a less ideal color match than skin derived from the first two sites. An ideal but neglected donor site in older patients is *redundant skin of the nasolabial fold.* Full-thickness skin donated from this site is abundant and of excellent color match and allows camouflage of the donor defect in the nasolabial crease. Full-thickness defects of the

nasal lobule and columella heal beautifully with nasolabial fold full-thickness skin grafts. Similarly, the preauricular and glabellar areas may harbor redundant skin with similar advantages. Seldom does the need arise to graft with skin derived from the more classic distant skin graft sites (inner arm, abdomen, thigh, buttocks).

Deep shave excision repair of the nose afflicted with rhinophyma may dictate the need for near-total skin graft repair of the nose. Shave excision and dermabrasion with preservation of epithelial islands, however, uniformly lead to reepithelialization of remarkable aesthetic appearance, thereby obviating grafting.

Grafts applied to the nose require delicate handling and special attention to detail in the operative and postoperative periods. Human noses are by no means inanimate, and consequently immobilization of skin grafts by means of stents or sutured bolus dressings is necessary for the critical early period of 4 to 5 days. Tie-over bolus dressings compressing the graft dressed with Adaptic or Telfa gauze provide light but reliable immobilization and protection of the graft. In contradistinction, adjacent flaps require no compression dressing and thus provide convenience to the patient and early return to normal activities.

Split-thickness skin grafts seldom satisfy the need for three-dimensional augmentation or effacement of nasal defects, they may become depressed and thinner with time, they seldom provide appropriate covering for implants of bone and cartilage, and they carry with them none of their own blood supply. For these reasons and those previously outlined, adjacent flaps remain the tissue of choice for immediate nasal repair in all areas except the nasal tip and infratip lobule. Specifically, grafts are generally inappropriate in areas of dense scarring and/or irradiation with consequently poor recipient site blood supply.

AESTHETIC SEPTORHINOPLASTY

Patients today seek functional and aesthetic improvements in nasal appearance more than ever before. Rhinoplasty refinements currently allow subtle as well as major modifications with little discomfort, early healing, and predictable results. Perhaps no other surgical procedure blends artistic and technical skills to the degree required in aesthetic rhinoplasty. Although it is one of the more common operations performed, only a few surgeons ever master its subtleties and nuances. An artistic ability to visualize in advance the ultimate result is a critical skill necessary to surgical excellence. Successful rhinoplasty is initially preceded by careful analytic assessment of the nasal configuration, the deformity, and its relationship with the surrounding facial features, that is, deformity diagnosis. A realistic estimate of surgical correction, based on the possibilities and limitations imposed by the characteristics of the nasal tissues, is formulated—the preoperative "game plan." The goal of the surgery is to fashion a natural nose that is in harmony with its surrounding facial features and does not draw attention to itself.

The master surgeon is separated from the novice by the ability to *predict* the favorable and *compensate* for the unfavorable healing factors that influence ultimate nasal appearance evolving over many years. Only with continued experience and study, coupled with a continued impartial analysis of one's own long-term results, can the latter capability be developed and refined.

The truly capable surgeon must have wide knowledge of predictable procedures to be implemented in the unlimited variety of nasal configurations encountered. Strict adherence to basic principles does not nec-

essarily always produce the ideal result. It is essential that an understanding of dynamic nasal structure transcend the components of static bone and cartilage. The relationship of shape and form with muscle tension and skin texture, the relationship of bone and cartilage with surrounding structures, the degree of postoperative thickening and/or relaxation of tissues, and the role of interrelated structures in the production of the deformity must be realized and evaluated.

Variations in rhinoplasty are manifold, ranging from minor corrections to complete reconstruction of the nose. Aesthetic rhinoplasty aims at the creation of a nose that can be considered ideally proportioned; proper physiologic function is essential. In post-traumatic deformities and many developmental and congenital deformities, the correction of respiratory derangements is paramount, and aesthetics, although significant, is secondary. Some congenital deformities, such as the cleft lip or bifid nose, encompass both functional and cosmetic requirements of a special nature.

AESTHETIC RHINOPLASTY

The objective of aesthetic nasal plastic surgery is the creation of a nose that is in harmony with the other features of the face. This simple statement represents a complex problem. The explanation of what is "beautiful" or "ideal" has been an age-old question, and the answer involves a multiplicity of emotional reactions and prejudices. In addition, values and assessments of beauty vary within different age groups and social structures. To evaluate what is beautiful entails a study of physical and cultural anthropology, ethnology, psychology, and aesthetics, the ramifications of which may be endless.

Perhaps Anatole France was right when he declared, "I believe that we shall never know exactly why a thing is beautiful." We may, however, allow ourselves certain elusive generalities by which to gauge the terms "beauty" and "ideal," emphasizing some known facts, one of which was aptly stated by Francis Bacon when he said, "There is no excellent beauty which hath not some strangeness of proportion." It is the slight disproportion that may be entrancing; however, gross disharmony of features is displeasing. The task of plastic surgery is to reduce the disproportionate to "normal" or harmonious proportions, resulting in a patient who is pleased with the outcome.

Multiple factors are involved in studying the face from an artistic viewpoint. As Sir Thomas Browne stated, "It is the common wonder of all men, among so many millions of faces, how there should be none alike." Ability to distinguish people by their facial characteristics is a matter of self-training and the high development of man's innate artistic sense. In all probability, we distinguish faces by variations in facial expression as well as by skeletal differences.

The variations in facial expression are a direct outgrowth of the highly complex development of speech, whereby small muscle fibers are needed superficially to allow multiple variation of facial movement. The muscles involved in facial expression are known as the mimetic muscles and have no real fascial covering such as that of the skeletal muscles of the body. Instead, they are found below and in the panniculus adiposis or superficial fascia, and the fibers are inserted directly into the dermis and cutis of the skin. A thick fascial covering, such as is encountered in the nonmimetic muscle, would leave the face blank and expressionless. Of particular importance in rhinoplasty is the septi depressor muscle, which, if highly developed and strong, results in significant depression of the nasal tip during facial animation.

Anthropometric Factors

The anthropometrist uses basic measurements to divide and subdivide the face; these essentials are shown in Figures 2–15 and 2–16. Designated points in the midline of the face are labeled as follows: the *trichion*, located in the center of the forehead at the hairline; the *nasion*, at the frontonasal suture line; the *subnasale*, a point at the root of the nasal spine; and the *gnathion*, the most anterior point of the symphysis of the mandible. If horizontal lines are drawn through these points, the face is normally divided into three equal parts. If, in profile view, another line is projected from the upper

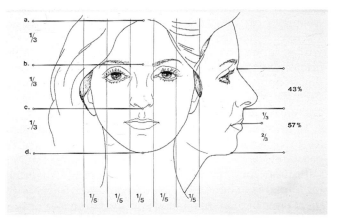

Fig. 2–16. Relatively ideal facial dimensions. (From Tardy ME: Surgical Anatomy of the Nose. New York, Raven Press, 1991.)

rim of the external auditory canal (the auricular point) to the lower rim of the orbit or infraorbital point, a line known as the Frankfort horizontal, or Reid's base line, is formed. This line divides the face into two equal parts from trichion to gnathion (Fig. 2–15).

Many of the basic observations on the divisions of the face were originally described in the fifteenth century by Leonardo da Vinci in the section of his notebooks entitled "Of the Parts of the Face." We use his accepted statement, "The space from the chin to the beginning of the bottom of the nose is the third part of the face, and equal to the nose and to the forehead," and have set up our blocks accordingly. After dividing these three groups into equal spaces, we are immedi-

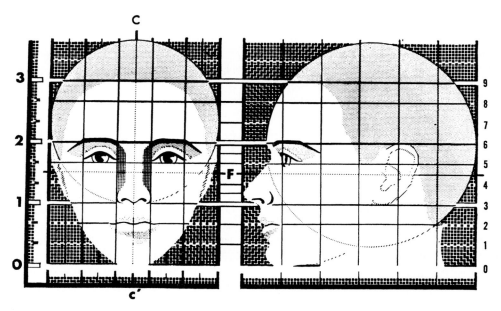

Fig. 2–15. Anthropometric measurements of the "normal" or "ideal" face. Points in the midline of the face (C to c') are the trichion (3), nasion (2), subnasale (1), and gnathion (0), dividing the face into three equal parts. Frankfort horizontal line (F) divides face in half. Further subdivisions of each space into thirds both horizontally and vertically reveal the eye to be a single square, the face to be five squares in width, and the space between the eyes to be one square wide. (From Becker O: Manual of rhinoplasty. Trans Am Acad Ophthalmol Otolaryngol 60:522, 1956.)

ately led to certain observations. Although this spacing is equal, it is not monotonous, for the forms lying next to each other occupy different numbers of spaces. Nevertheless, the proportions are equal, indicating a certain regularity in size, shape, and position of forms. For example, the forehead occupies one entire group, or one third of the height of the face. The eye from the brow to lower lid fills one third of the height of the nose, or, again, one can observe that the upper lip is to the lower lip and the chin as the height of the nostril is to the remainder of the nose. In this manner, one can divide and subdivide and compare indefinitely. It is interesting to notice that the eye tends to group a large area with a small one and to compare this grouping with other similar groupings of large and small areas.

The midline is the most obvious division of the front view. In the midline of the face, the measurement used is the width of one eye, for "the space between the eyes is equal to the size of one eye" (da Vinci). Furthermore, by the size of the eye, the face is divided into five equal vertical sections. These may again be equally divided and mathematical comparisons made, as before, to prove pleasing points of interest. An example is that the alae nasi occupy the space between the two inner canthi, or one eye's breadth.

Aesthetic Values

Can we reduce beauty to a logical or mathematical formula by producing so-called "norm," or is it subject to an intuitive, imaginative, or conceptual image? My opinion is that it involves both a conceptual and a perceptual approach. Certain standards are considered ideal, and this aspect can be considered the logical or intellectual approach; however, this is modified by an overlay of subjective, intuitive, and conditioned thinking. Much is pure projection and association by the viewer, and this projection is largely determined by ethnic and cultural environment. The classical beauty of ancient Greece or Egypt may not fulfill the modern ideal of Western culture, nor is it the standard among Asian or African populations of today.

Our tastes are to a large extent hortatory, fostered by our culture and influenced by multiple factors such as Madison Avenue, the cinema, and television. These factors have a profound influence on our aesthetic judgment and preferences, almost to the point of setting unconscious standards of beauty. They deal in psychologic images and make us feel or sense beauty, rather than understanding how we arrive at these standards or conclusions.

The value of beauty in the fine arts is almost as old as civilization. This includes not only sculpture, painting, architecture, and design, but poetry and music as well. The arts, over the ages, have entailed a monumental effort by man, equal no doubt to the energy expended on war and industry. In modern manufacturing there

is a distinct effort (e.g., motivational research) to make the product appealing to the sense of beauty or to cultivate our senses into believing it is beautiful. As George Santayana stated, "There must be in our nature a very radical and widespread tendency to observe beauty, and to value it. No account of the principles of the mind can be at all adequate that passes over so conspicuous a faculty. That aesthetic theory has received so little attention from the world is not due to the unimportance of the subject of which it treats, but rather to lack of an adequate motive for speculating upon it, and to the small success of the occasional efforts to deal with it."

Psychologic Factors

The importance of beauty and the concept of our own body image, that is, the attitude regarding our physiognomy and body structure, is a potent factor in the emotional and intellectual development of the individual. Paul Schilder, in *The Image and Appearance of the Human Body*, states that we should not underrate the importance of beauty and ugliness in human life. "Beauty can be a promise of complete satisfaction and can lead up to this complete satisfaction. Our own beauty or ugliness will not only figure in the image we get about ourselves, but will also figure in the image others build up about us and which will be taken back again into ourselves. The body-image is the result of social life. Beauty and ugliness are certainly the result of social life. Beauty and ugliness are certainly not phenomena in the single individual, but are social phenomena of the utmost importance. They regulate . . . and thus become the basis for our sexual and social activities."

Beauty is interrelated and identified with the secondary sexual characteristics. Freud, in *Civilization and its Discontents*, states, "The science of esthetics examines the conditions under which we experience beauty. It cannot give an explanation of the nature and genesis of beauty . . . . It is bad that psychoanalysis also can say the least about beauty. Only its origin out of the field of sexual feelings seems assured."

Santayana similarly states, "The attraction of sex could not become efficient unless the senses were first attracted. The eye must be fascinated and the ear charmed by the object which nature intends should be pursued. Both sexes for this reason develop secondary sexual characteristics . . . . "

The nose, being a conspicuous organ, has definite secondary sexual characteristics and is frequently referred to as masculine or feminine. The patient with a poor body image, especially one who has an unconscious sexual or libidinous misidentification, may suffer a severe conflict because of a masculine or feminine appearance or the erroneous belief of such an appearance. Some of the most remarkable psychologic changes in patients are in these individuals, often out of proportion to the surgical result. Regardless of the physical change from a masculine to a feminine nose, if the patient believes that the change has wrought a new identification with his or her sex, the psychic change is spectacular. This psychic change is usually based on unconscious factors, the patient never being aware of the reasons for the dramatic change in attitude.

The psychologic factors basic to an evaluation of one's appearance are instinctive and conditioned; therefore, much of the individual's reaction depends on his or her concept of the *body image*. To a great extent, this is influenced or conditioned in early life, usually by the attitude of the parents. The individual with a distorted and unrealistic self-image is usually an emotionally disturbed person. A *realistic* appraisal of one's own image, within reasonable limits, is usually indicative of a mature individual.

Patients seeking rhinoplastic surgery for a gross deformity usually have a realistic view of themselves and a valid reason for correction of the deformity. The individual with a minor defect may harbor a poor self-image and sometimes exaggerates the deformity. These latter patients are usually, but not always, poor candidates for rhinoplastic surgery. Linn and Goldman have stated: "Psychiatrists are often troubled by the fact that the disruption in the patient's life frequently seems disproportionate to the extent of the actual nasal deformity. It is important to keep in mind that a small but real nasal deformity can immobilize a considerable quantity of psychic energy. The relief which the patient will get from the correction of the defect will be measured not by the size of the deformity but by the quantity of psychic energy bound up by it." Most patients with small or modest nasal deformities are realistic and well adjusted and simply wish improved nasal balance and proportions.

Schulman has contributed to the surgeon's ability to understand the motives and needs of patients seeking aesthetic surgery by summarizing certain exhibited clues and characteristics. Certain diagnostic clues tending to identify the patient with a good prognosis include:

1. Obvious disfigurement.
2. Occupational reason for seeking surgery to improve appearance.
3. Realistic wish to appear younger.
4. A statement that the patient has "wanted to do this for a long time."

A less ideal (or guarded) prognosis might be expected, according to Schulman, in patients who:

1. State an unrealistic motive ("so I can look more masculine").
2. Request surgery on a sudden whim.

3. Expect surgery to be the solution to all their problems (e.g., "to save my marriage").
4. Exhibit a history of hospitalization or treatment of recurrent psychiatric illness.
5. Relentlessly go "surgeon-shopping."
6. Have undergone repeated surgery with consistent dissatisfaction.
7. Are unable or unwilling to follow important instructions provided by surgeon or staff.

In summary, we can state that the motivations for and the psychologic effects of rhinoplastic surgery are a complex subject. A few factors are reviewed, and an evaluation and definition of beauty from a perceptual and conceptual view is attempted.

Beauty of the human face is neither abstract nor absolute; it varies among different ethnic groups and is subject to the projection of the individual. This attitude is based on a multiplicity of factors varying according to the body image and cultural values of individual conditioning, particularly during the formative years, when it often becomes part of the unconscious mind.

In any ethnic group, beauty is the approximation of the so-called norm; for Western civilization we have depicted this norm by mathematical proportions. It is therefore a form of aesthetic ethnocentrism influenced by extraneous factors of culture. A great latitude in the variety and balance of features exists, so there are no absolute rules by which beauty may be determined.

Anatomic Description

The nose on frontal view is in the shape of a pyramid, of which approximately the upper two fifths comprise the bony vault and the lower three fifths the cartilaginous vault (Fig. 2–17). The upper narrow end joins the forehead at the glabella and is called the *radix nasi*, or root of the nose, and its free angle at the lower point is termed the tip or *apex nasi*. The two elliptical orifices, the *nares*, are separated from each other by a skin-carti-

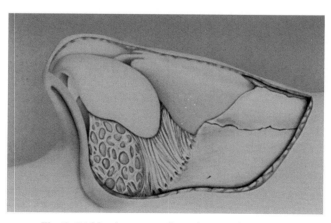

Fig. 2–17. Nasal anatomy (lateral view of the nose).

lage septum known as the *columella*. The lateral surfaces of the nose form the dorsum by their union in the midline. The lateral surface ends below in a rounded eminence, the *ala nasi.*

The bony vault is composed of the two nasal bones, which are set on the nasal process of the frontal bone above, the frontal process of the maxilla laterally, and the perpendicular plate of the ethmoid and the septal cartilage below.

The upper portion of the cartilaginous vault consists of the two *upper lateral cartilages,* which are triangular and fuse with the septum in the midline. The upper margins underride the nasal bones and the frontal process of the maxillae and are attached to them by connective tissue. The lower cartilaginous vault is composed of two *lower lateral* cartilages (alar cartilages), which are of variable shape and more or less frame the nares and help in forming the ala. The two medial crura are attached to each other by fibrous tissue and to the lower end of the septum by skin, making up the columella and the membranous septum. Fairly near the midline, the lateral crura may slightly overlap the upper lateral cartilage and are attached to the lower rim of the upper lateral cartilage and the septum by connective tissue. They are also intimately attached to the overlying skin. The medial crura are loosely attached to the nasal septum and to each other by connective tissue. A few small loose cartilages (minor alar cartilages) are occasionally found laterally or just above the lateral crura (Fig. 2–17).

The septum consists of both cartilage and bone. The septal cartilage is a single quadrilateral plate of cartilage that forms the anterior inferior portion of the septum. It unites with the bony portion of the septum: behind with the perpendicular plate of the ethmoid and rests below on the groove of the vomer, the maxillary crest, and the maxillary spine (Fig. 2–18). A tail-like posterior projection of the cartilage between the perpendicular plate and vomer is known as the sphenoid process. A small strip of cartilage, which is often

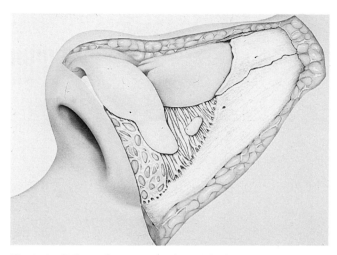

Fig. 2–19. Cadaver dissection displaying thick subcutaneous tissue cushioning nasal skeleton, especially abundant at nasal tip and supratip region.

absent, lies over the nasal spine and maxillary crests and is known as the vomeronasal cartilage of Jacobson.

The skin covering the external nose is thin and contains an areolar type of subcutaneous tissue. It is loosely attached in its upper half, but in its lower portions it is intimately bound to the lower lateral cartilages and may sometimes be thick and fatty and contain many sebaceous glands (Fig. 2–19). The skin continues into the nares to supply lining to the nasal vestibule.

The muscles of the nose lie directly subjacent to the skin, and occasionally muscle bundles are attached to the cutis itself. The muscles comprise the procerus, nasalis, depressor septi, dilator naris posterior, dilator naris anterior, and angular head of the quadratus labii superioris (Fig. 2–20).

The blood supply of the external nose is principally through the angular and lateral nasal branches of the external maxillary artery and the infraorbital branch of the internal maxillary artery. The internal nose is supplied by the sphenopalatine branches of the internal maxillary artery, and the ethmoids from the ophthalmic artery. The veins terminate in the anterior facial and ophthalmic veins.

The motor nerve supply to the nose is by the facial nerve. The sensory supply includes the infratrochlear and nasal branches from the ophthalmic division of the trigeminal nerve and the infraorbital nerves from the maxillary division of the trigeminal nerve. The nasal septum is innervated by the ethmoid and nasopalatine nerves from the first and second divisions of the trigeminal nerve, respectively. The lateral wall of the internal nose receives fibers from the nasal branches of the palatine nerve, the ethmoid nerves, and

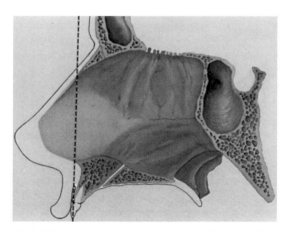

Fig. 2–18. The nasal septum (lateral view of the nose, skeletal).

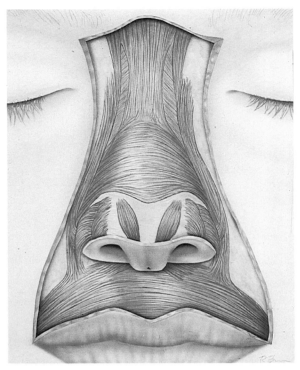

Fig. 2–20. Mimetic musculature of the nose, interconnected in form and function in a superficial muscular aponeurotic system (SMAS).

a small branch from the anterior superior alveolar nerve (Fig. 2–21).

Artistic Anatomy

An artistic anatomic concept must be developed by the rhinoplastic surgeon when approaching the study of nasal anatomy. The surgeon visualizes the nasal structure not only as static bone and cartilage, but also as muscle tension, skin texture, relationship with surrounding structures, and the effect of related and inter-

related structures on the shape of the nose. Furthermore, this concept divides the nose into an upper or immobile portion and a lower or mobile portion.

The immobile or upper portion of the nose is composed of the nasal bones and the upper lateral cartilages. The upper lateral cartilages are firmly attached to the undersurface of the nasal bones and maxillae by dense connective tissue and are fused with the septum in the midline, except for a small area at its lowermost end. The nasal bones are supported by the adjacent maxillae, by the nasal process and spine of the frontal bone, and by the septum below. Covering these structures are periosteum and perichondrium and the procerus and transverse nasalis muscles. The overlying superficial fascia or panniculus adiposus is thin, with scanty fat and fibrous tissue, allowing great mobility of the skin over this area.

The lower or mobile portion of the nose is composed of the two alar (lower lateral) cartilages and occasionally a few sesamoid cartilages superiorly and laterally. These cartilages are curved, thereby shaping the nares (Fig. 2–22). The alar cartilages are more or less free-floating, being suspended and maintained in position by fibrous and muscular attachments to the two upper lateral cartilages, the septum, each other, and the overlying and surrounding skin.

The shape of the nasal tip is basically formed by the alar cartilages. Depending on the thickness of the skin, the amount of subcutaneous fat and areolar tissue, and the activity of the sebaceous glands, however, the configuration of the tip may vary considerably from the basic structure of the alar cartilage. Furthermore, the form of the nasal tip depends on its relative position

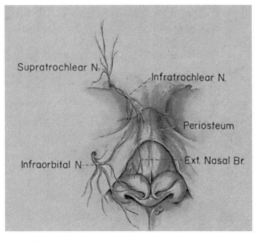

Fig. 2–21. The nerve supply to the nose.

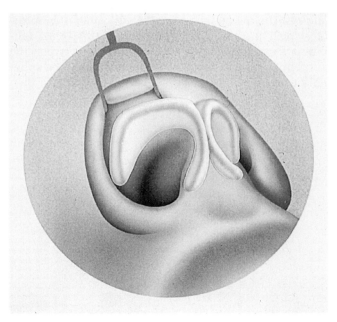

Fig. 2–22. The paired alar (lower lateral) cartilages are more or less free-floating, encased in soft tissues.

to the immobile or fixed structures, which suspend and hold the tip in position by firm fibrous attachments. A long, short, elevated, or depressed septum, long or short upper lateral cartilages, the shape of the nasal bone and maxillary processes, the spine of the maxilla, and the direction and tension of the surrounding muscles and fibrous connective tissue are determining factors in the position and shape of the nasal tip.

We are frequently surprised to note what remarkable changes in shape and position are accomplished by simply dissecting the tip free from the surrounding tissues. A further change is also noted when the last remaining suspensory attachment of the tip is freed by dissection of the alar cartilage from the enveloping skin. The skin at the nasal tip is immobile because of its firm adherence to the cartilage by dense fibrous connective tissue. This firm union aids in suspending and positioning the tip; thus, to mobilize it properly, the alar cartilage is detached from the overlying and surrounding skin. Occasionally, this may be all that is required to change the shape and direction of the tip. This is usually accomplished at the onset of the rhinoplastic operation. With mobilizing of the alar cartilages, the muscle fibers are also detached. The muscles involved are the nasalis (transverse and alar), the dilator nares, the depressor septi, and occasionally a few slips of the caput angularis of the quadratus labii superioris.

The muscles that surround and envelop the nose are part of the mimetic muscles of the face, which have no real fascial covering such as covers the skeletal muscles of the body. Instead, they are found below and in the panniculus adiposus or superficial fascia, and the fibers are inserted directly into the dermis and cutis of the skin. This arrangement of muscle fibers is a direct outgrowth of the highly complex development of speech, whereby small muscle fibers were needed superficially to allow multiple variations of facial movements.

Planning the Correction

In planning the correction of the nasal deformity, the component features of the face and the general body build of the patient must be considered. Frequently, failure to consider the relationship of the nose with the chin, maxilla, and forehead mars an otherwise perfect rhinoplasty and results in a nose that appears unnatural for the particular individual.

Procedures that have been advocated for analysis of deformity include marking angles on photographs, mechanical measuring instruments used directly on the face, and the use of computer imaging. All may be of value. It is, however, difficult to measure so subjective an abstraction as beauty in angles or degrees because of the many variables in physiognomy. Rather, one should strive to attain a harmonious relationship of all the features. A simple but valuable method of

studying the relationship of facial features is by the use of sketches made on the reverse side of the photograph. The photograph is held up to a light or placed on a roentgen film shadow box, and by pencil sketching and shading the ultimate desired result may be depicted.

Whether or not sketches are made on them, pre- and postoperative photographs are an integral part of the surgical routine. In all plastic surgical undertakings, photographs are absolutely essential and should form a part of the patient's record. A series of standardized and uniform photographs is more informative than the most carefully detailed notes, both as a planning and self-instructional device and as a necessary medicolegal record. Series of 5 × 7 black and white prints combined with color 2 × 2 color slides make ideal records in rhinoplasty photography and serve as an ideal immediate reference when projected full-size in the operating room during surgery. Preoperative photographs are followed by postoperative views taken at 1 week, then at 1, 3, 6, 12, 18, and 24 months. This carefully standardized photographic composite provides a clear uniform panorama of the dynamics of healing affecting the ultimate result and is a superior teaching record as well. The Frankfort horizontal line is used in proper positioning of the patient, providing uniformity and standardization from sitting to sitting. The following views are preferred (Fig. 2–23):

1. Frontal.
2. Basal.
3. Right lateral.
4. Left lateral.
5. Right lateral, smiling.

Using single-lens reflex cameras, photographing with properly positioned dual electronic flash units and a pastel background complementary to skin tone (blue or green) is rapid and relatively simple. A fast, sharp lens of approximately 105 mm focal length avoids parallax distortion and provides precise uniformity. Commercial photographers are frequently used, but it is to the surgeon's advantage personally to master the details of precise photography.

Classic Steps of Rhinoplasty

Rhinoplasty remains the most challenging of all aesthetic operations because no two procedures are ever identical. Each patient's nasal configuration and structure require individual and unique operative planning and surgical reconstruction. Therefore, no single technique, even though mastered, will prepare the surgeon for the varied anatomic patterns encountered. It is essential to regard rhinoplasty as one operation planned to *reconstitute and shape* the anatomic features of the nose into a new, more pleasing relationship with one another and the surrounding facial features. Rhinoplasty should be approached as an anatomic dissection

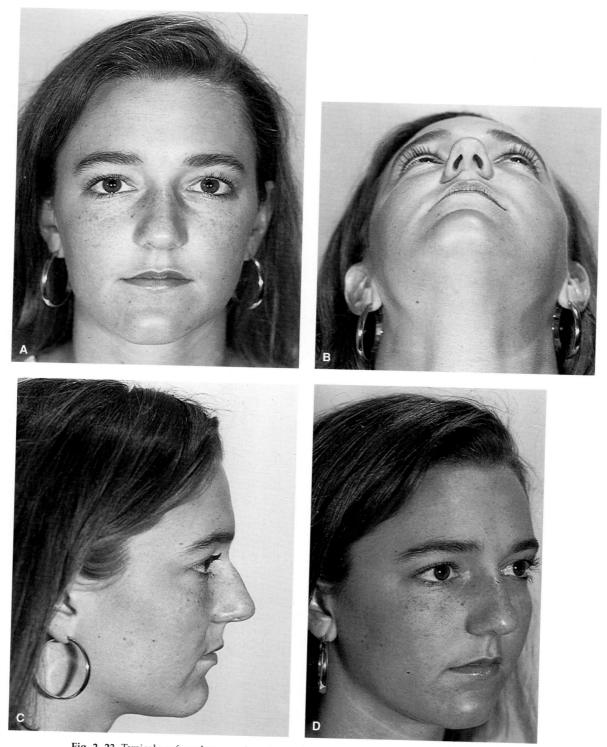

Fig. 2–23. Typical preferred pre- and postoperative rhinoplasty views (smiling view optional).

of the nasal structures requiring alteration, conservatively shaping and repositioning these anatomic elements. Many more problems and complications arise from overcorrection of nasal abnormalities than from conservative correction. Inappropriate technique applied persistently without regard for existing anatomy creates frequent complications. One truism, " . . . it is not what is removed in rhinoplasty that is important, but what is left behind," remains valid. Furthermore, one must comprehend clearly the dynamic aspects of operative rhinoplasty because all surgical steps are interrelated and interdependent, *most maneuvers leading to a temporary deformity to be corrected by the steps that follow.*

Most corrections of the long nose associated with a hump or dorsal prominence follow the basic principles formulated by Jacques Joseph in the first half of the twentieth century. His monumental treatise, *Nasenplastic und Sonstige Gesichtplastik*, published in 1931, has proved its fundamental soundness for over a half century.

The procedure varies in each patient by the amount of tissue excised and/or the relative repositioning of anatomic structures.

Classically, then, rhinoplasty consists of the following interrelated steps (Fig. 2–24):

1. Septoplasty.
2. Tip remodeling, projection, and cephalic rotation.
3. Hump removal (establishing the profile line).
4. Narrowing of the nose with osteotomies.
5. Final correction of subtle deformities.

Preoperative Preparations

Thorough, compulsive preparation by the surgeon before surgery ensures a streamlined operative proce-dure, designed to achieve aesthetic satisfaction and avoid complications. The optimum time for operation in respect to the physiologic and psychologic condition of the patient (and the surgeon) should be chosen. Patients are counseled that the procedure will be a meaningful and exciting event in their lives with long-range implications, rather than a necessarily unpleasant experience.

A complete physical examination is indicated, including routine laboratory tests such as blood count, urinalysis, and chemical and coagulation profiles. Untoward bleeding histories should be comprehensively resolved before proceeding. Recent upper respiratory infections, skin pustules, or allergic exacerbations may be sufficient reasons to postpone surgery. Conditions such as anemia, metabolic disorders, or nutritional deficiency states contraindicate any elective procedure. A patient who is a poor anatomic surgical risk usually heals poorly and unpredictably.

General planning of the operative sequence should be carried out before surgery, with a well-devised "game plan." Intraoperative improvisation may be necessary, but only if complementary to a careful pre-

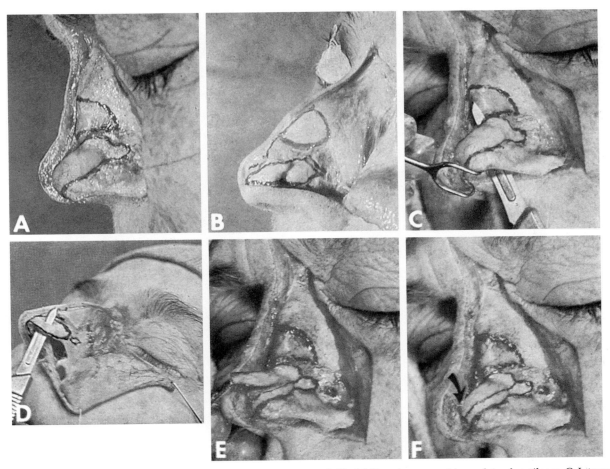

Fig. 2–24. The classic steps of rhinoplasty. A. Surgical anatomy of the nose. B. Variability of upper and lower lateral cartilages. C. Intercartilaginous incision. D. Alternative approach: transcartilaginous incision. E. Volume reduction of lower lateral cartilage. F. Resection of cephalic portion of lower lateral cartilage; intact caudal segment preserved (arrow marks high point of dome).

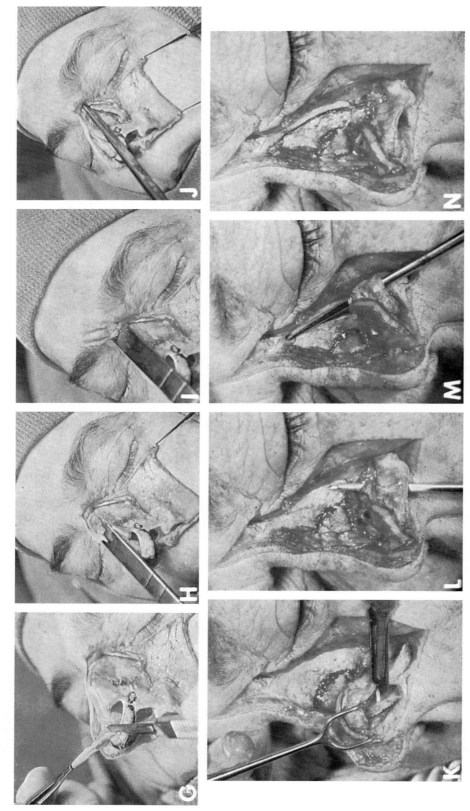

Fig. 2–24. *(continued)* G. Cartilaginous hump removal. H. Bony hump removal initiated. I. Bony hump removal completed. J. Medial oblique osteotomies. K. Caudal septal resection. L. Low curved lateral osteotomy initiated. M. Completion of low curved lateral osteotomy. N. Infracture with nasal narrowing completed.

operative game plan. Photographic evaluation with the patient, clearly defining exact patient expectations and demonstrating realistic expectations as well as anatomic limitations, is mandatory before embarking on surgical repair. The patient must clearly comprehend the details, ramifications, limitations, and potential complications of the procedure. This informed consent discussion is purely a physician-patient encounter; no individual or list of written "helpful hints" supplants this critical part of the preoperative conditioning.

Preoperative Medication

Cardinal rules in preoperative medication of patients are to use as few different categories of drugs as possible and preferably to employ drugs whose actions may be reversed or antagonized. Too often, patients scheduled for rhinoplasty are given a wide array of different drugs, which confuse the pharmacologic picture considerably—certainly a therapeutic error. Reliance on predictable narcotic and phenothiazine drugs only has been found safe and effective, particularly because my colleagues and I perform rhinoplasty with a combination of local infiltration and intravenous analgesia and anesthesia, carefully titrated, controlled, and monitored by a medical anesthesiologist. Individual drug titration in each patient, with the drug slowly infused in minimal intravenous increments, provides a safe and comfortable combination of euphoria, analgesia, and obtundency. Narcotic antagonists (NARCAN) provide a measure of safety, but are rarely required during the operation. The narcotic antagonist is routinely administered at the conclusion of the procedure, however.

One or two small gauze pads (neurosurgical cottonoids) moistened with 5% cocaine solution are placed in each nasal passage. Superb surface anesthesia with intense nasoconstriction and turbinate shrinkage results.

Minimal intranasal subcutaneous infiltration of standard 1% lidocaine (Xylocaine) with 1:100,000 epinephrine is conservatively accomplished. Infiltration occurs only as the No. 27 gauge needle is being withdrawn, to avoid the possibility of direct vessel injection. The intent is to diffuse a thin plane of anesthesia and vasoconstrictive influence *in the plane just above the structured nasal cartilage,* where most dissection will be performed. Small amounts of infiltration anesthesia are added at the alar margins, the pyriform aperture, the columella, and the nasal septum. No attempt is made to create a specific block anesthesia of specific sensory nerves. This method effectively anesthetizes the operative field, creates excellent vasoconstriction, and avoids distortion of the nasal structures (a common error). Seldom is more than 4 to 5 ml of anesthesia solution required. Overaggressive injection leads to tis-

sue ballooning, feature distortion, and consequent impaired surgical judgment.

It is essential that 10 to 15 minutes be allowed to elapse between the completion of injection and the initiation of surgical steps, thereby ensuring *intense vasoconstriction,* minimal bleeding, unrestricted vision, and, consequently, improved surgical technique. The surgeon must use a strong headlight to maximize visualization.

The patient's face and nose are gently cleansed with hexachlorophene the morning of surgery and thoroughly rinsed. Vibrissae are trimmed only if excessively long.

Surgery of the Nasal Tip

Philosophy of Tip Sculpture
Sculpture of the nasal tip is regarded, and properly so, as the most exacting aspect of nasal plastic surgery. The surgeon is challenged by the essentially bilateral, animate, and mobile nasal anatomic components. Because no single surgical technique may be used successfully in correction of the endless anatomic tip variations encountered, the surgeon must analyze each anatomic situation and make a reasoned judgment about which approaches and tip modification techniques will result in a predictably natural appearance. Factored into this judgment decision must be consideration of, among other things, the strength, thickness, and attitude of the alar cartilages, the degree of tip projection, the tip skin and subcutaneous thickness, the columellar length, the length of the nose, the width of the tip, and the tip-lip angulation and relationship.

One fundamental principle of tip surgery is that normal or ideal anatomic features of the tip should be preserved and, if possible, remain undisturbed by surgical dissection, and abnormal features must be analyzed, exposed, reanalyzed, and corrected by reduction, augmentation, or shape modification.

Surgeons have gradually come to understand that radical excision and extensive sacrifice of alar cartilage and other tip-support mechanisms all too frequently result in eventual unnatural or "surgical" tips. What appears pleasant and natural in the early postoperative period may heal poorly because of overaggressive attempts to modify the anatomy more extensively than the tissues allow. Rhinoplasty is, after all, a compromise operation, in which tissue sacrifices are made to achieve a more favorable appearance. It therefore becomes judicious to develop a reasoned, planned approach to the nasal tip based entirely on the anatomy encountered coupled with the final result intended. A philosophy of a *systematic incremental anatomic approach* to tip surgery is highly useful to achieve consistently natural results. Conservative reduction of the volume of the cephalic margin of the lateral crus, preserving a substantially complete, undisturbed strip of residual alar cartilage, is a preferred operation in individuals in whom nasal tip changes are intended to be modest. As the tip deformity or asymmetry encountered becomes more profound, more aggressive techniques are required, from weak and complete strip techniques to significant interruption of the residual complete strip with profound alteration in the alar cartilage size, attitude, and anatomy. Cartilage structural grafts to influence the size, shape, projection, and support of the tip are often invaluable.

Tip sculpture cannot be successfully undertaken, let alone mastered, until the *major and minor tip-support mechanisms* are appreciated, respected, and preserved or, when indicated, reconstructed (Table 2–1). Loss of tip support and projection in the postoperative healing period is one of the most common surgical errors in rhinoplasty. This tip "ptosis" is usually the inevitable result of the sacrifice of nasal tip-support mechanisms.

In the majority of patients the major tip-support mechanisms (Fig. 2–25) consist of (1) the size, shape, and resiliency of the medial and lateral crura, (2) the wrap-around attachment of the medial crural footplates to the caudal end of the quadrangular cartilage, and (3) the soft tissue attachment of the caudal margin of the upper lateral cartilage to the cephalic margin of the alar cartilage. Compensatory reestablishment of major tip support should be considered if, during the operation, any or all of these major tip-support mechanisms are compromised in any fashion.

The minor tip mechanisms (Fig. 2–25) that, in certain anatomic configurations, may assume major support importance include (1) the dorsal cartilaginous septum, (2) the interdomal ligament, (3) the membranous septum, (4) the nasal spine, (5) the surrounding skin and soft tissues, and (6) the alar sidewalls.

Tip projection in every rhinoplasty operation is inevitably enhanced, reduced, or preserved in its original state. Anatomic situations in which each of these outcomes is desirable and intended are regularly en-

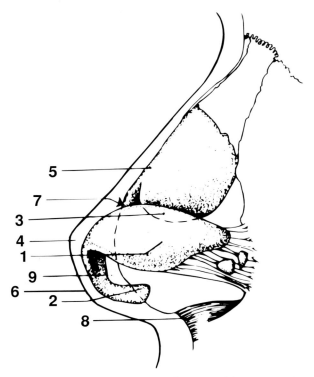

Fig. 2–25. The major tip-support mechanisms of the nose consist of (1) the size, shape, and resiliency of the medial and lateral crura; (2) the wrap-around attachment of the medial-crural footplates to the caudal end of the quadrangular cartilage; and (3) the soft tissue attachment of the caudal margin of the upper lateral cartilage to the cephalic margin of the alar cartilage. The minor tip-support mechanisms, which in certain anatomic configurations may assume major support importance, include (5) the dorsal cartilaginous septum, (4) the interdomal ligament, (9) the membranous septum, (8) the nasal spine, (6) the surrounding skin and soft tissues, and (7) the anterior septal angle.

countered in a diverse rhinoplasty practice. The desirable surgical goal in every operation is preservation of the projection already existent, if, as is true in the majority of rhinoplasty patients, preoperative projection of the tip is satisfactory. Other patients require an increase in the projection of the tip relative to the intended new profile line. A predictable variety of reliable operative methods exist for creating or augmenting tip projection; they are discussed later in this chapter. Finally, in a limited but clearly definable group of patients with overprojecting tips, a calculated intentional reduction of excessive tip projection is desirable to effect intentional retroprojection.

Successfully achieving these diverse surgical results requires an understanding of and a healthy respect for the major and minor tip-support mechanisms, seasoned by the recognition of the intraoperative surgical tip dynamic principles that interact in every tip operation. It clearly follows that the *appropriate tip incisions and approaches should be planned to preserve as many tip supports as possible.* Alar cartilage sculpturing should similarly respect this principle by conserving the vol-

TABLE 2–1. Tip-Support Mechanisms

Major
    Size, shape, and resilience of the medial and lateral crura
    Medial crural footplate attachment to the caudal border of the quadrangular cartilage
    Attachment of the upper lateral cartilages (caudal border) to the alar cartilages (cephalic border)
Minor*
    Ligamentous sling spanning the paired domes of the alar cartilages
    Cartilaginous septal dorsum
    Sesamoid complex extending the support of the lateral crura to the pyriform aperture
    Attachment of the alar cartilages to the overlying skin and musculature
    Nasal spine
    Membranous septum

* On occasion, because of extreme anatomic variability, a "minor" tip support may assume the importance of one of the more major supports.

ume and integrity of the lateral crus and avoiding, in all but the most extreme anatomic situation, radical excision and sacrifice of tip cartilage.

The surgeon should differentiate clearly among *incisions, approaches, and techniques.* Incisions are simply methods of gaining access to the underlying supportive structures of the nose and by themselves have little importance. Approaches to the nasal tip provide important exposure to the skeletal structures and consist of procedures either to deliver the tip cartilages or to avoid complete delivery, or operating on the alar cartilages without removing them from their anatomic beds. Sculpturing techniques are defined as surgical modifications: excision, reconstruction, or orientation of the alar cartilages calculated to cause significant changes in the definition, size, orientation, and projection of the nasal tip. Because of the amazing complexity of anatomic configurations encountered in nasal tip surgery, further modifications are frequently used to ensure stable refinements.

It is important to assess several factors before selecting the appropriate tip procedure. In planning tip remodeling, the surgeon must determine whether or not the tip requires (1) a reduction in the *volume* of the alar cartilages, (2) a change in the *attitude* and *orientation* of the alar cartilages, (3) a change in the *projection* of the tip, and (4) a cephalic *rotation* with a subsequent increase in the columellar inclination (nasolabial angle).

Ideally, conservative reduction of the volume of the cephalic margin of the lateral crus, preserving the majority of the crus while maintaining a complete (uninterrupted) strip of alar cartilage, is preferred. This procedure is satisfactory and appropriately safe when minimal conservational tip refinement and rotation are required. As the tip deformity increases in size and complexity, more aggressive techniques are required. A philosophy of graduated incremental anatomic approach to nasal tip surgery has proved useful. This implies that no routine tip procedure is ever used; instead, the *appropriate incisions, approaches, and tip sculpturing techniques are selected based entirely on an analysis of the varying anatomy encountered.* Whenever possible, a complete strip operation is used, reserving more risky interrupted strip techniques for anatomic situations in which more profound refinement changes and significant rotation are desirable.

Surgical Approaches to the Tip

NONDELIVERY APPROACHES. In anatomic situations in which the nasal tip anatomy is favorable, only conservative refinements are necessary, and nondelivery approaches possess great value. Less dissection and less disturbance of the tip anatomy are necessary, and this reduces the chance for asymmetry, error, and unfavorable healing. Properly executed, nondelivery approaches therefore allow the surgeon to control the healing process more accurately than when more radical approaches and techniques are chosen.

The transcartilaginous approach is preferred because of its simplicity and ease of use (Fig. 2–26). The exact same tip refinements, however, may be accomplished through the retrograde approach. These approaches are chosen in patients whose tip anatomy is fundamentally satisfactory, requiring only volume re-

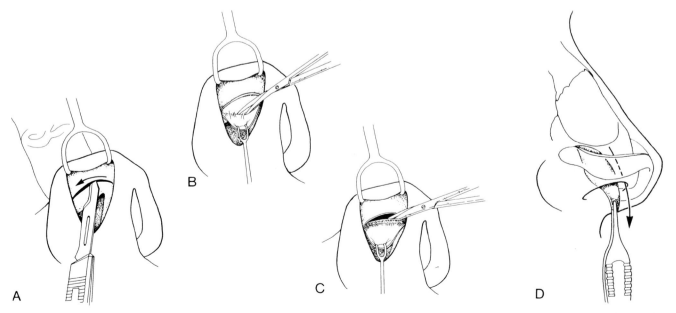

Fig. 2–26. The transcartilaginous approach to the alar cartilages. A. The incision is created through vestibular skin only. B. The cephalic margin of the cartilage is inspected further. C and D. The cephalic margin of the alar cartilage is then excised to the degree required for nasal tip refinement and narrowing.

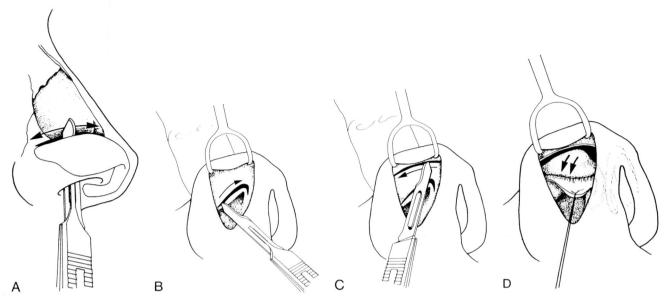

Fig. 2–27. A. The delivery approach to the nasal tip. B and C. Intercartilaginous (B) and marginal (C) incisions are used on either side to free and deliver the alar cartilage for evaluation and refinement. D. Delivery of the lower lateral cartilage.

duction to accomplish a thinning sculpture of the cephalic or medial margin of the lateral crus. When tip projection is to be enhanced by the use of cartilage tip grafts, nondelivery approaches are preferred because precise recipient pockets may be more accurately created in the infratip lobule undisturbed by the minimal dissection inherent in nondelivery approaches. If sutured-in-place tip grafts are required, a delivery or open approach is preferred.

DELIVERY APPROACHES. Delivering the alar cartilages as individual bipedicle chondrocutaneous flaps through intercartilaginous and marginal incisions is the preferred approach when the nasal tip anatomy is more abnormal (broad, asymmetric, etc.) or when more dramatic tip refinements are necessary. Significant modifications in the alar cartilage shape, attitude, and orientation are more predictably attained when the cartilages are delivered (Fig. 2–27). The base photograph is usually helpful in determining which patients may

best be approached in this manner. If the triangularity of the tip from below is satisfactory and only modest volume reduction of the lateral crus appears necessary, the nondelivery approach serves well. If, however, on base and frontal view the alar cartilages flare unpleasantly (Fig. 2–28), tip triangularity is unsatisfactory, or the tip appears too amorphous and bulbous, a delivery approach is chosen to correct these aesthetic deficiencies more thoroughly. Transcartilaginous suture narrowing of broad domes (Fig. 2–29), an effective and preferred technique, is effected by means of the delivery approach. In similar fashion, interrupted strip techniques for more radical tip refinement and cephalic rotation are more efficiently accomplished when the cartilages are delivered. The increased surgical exposure provides the surgeon with an improved binocular view of the tip anatomy and affords the added ease of bimanual surgical modifications.

OPEN (EXTERNAL) APPROACH. The external or open ap-

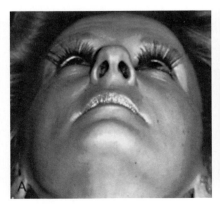
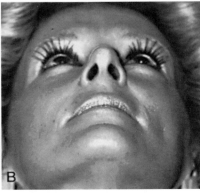

Fig. 2–28. A. Basal view of patient demonstrating a trapezoid amorphous tip, in which the delivery approach is preferred in order to refine the cartilages and achieve additional triangularity. B. Patient after surgery.

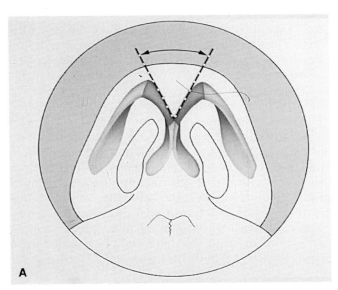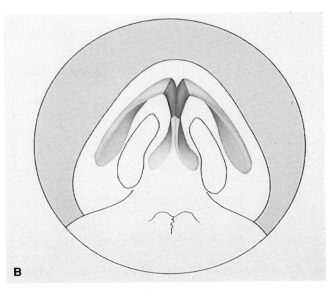

Fig. 2–29. Transdomal suture narrowing of the broad, trapezoid tip configuration.

proach to the nasal tip is in reality a more aggressive form of the delivery approach and is chosen with discretion in specific nasal tip deformities (Fig. 2–30). When the nasal tip is highly asymmetric, markedly overprojected, severely underprojected, or anatomically confusing in its form (as in certain secondary revision cases), the open approach is considered. The transcolumellar scar is of negligible importance in this decision because it routinely heals inconspicuously when meticulously repaired. The anatomic view is unparalleled through this approach, affording the surgeon diagnostic information unavailable through traditional closed approaches. These technical virtues must be balanced with the potential disadvantages of

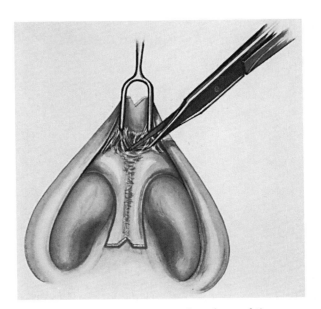

Fig. 2–30. The open approach to the nasal tip.

an enlarged scar bed, slightly delayed healing with some prolongation of tip edema, and an increased operating time. Clearly, when subtle and conservative tip surgery is indicated by the patient's existent anatomy, the open approach is unnecessary.

Alar Cartilage Sculpturing Techniques

The choice of the technique used to modify the alar cartilages and the relationship of the nasal tip with the remaining nasal structures should be based entirely on the anatomy encountered and the predicted result desired, as defined from the known dynamics of long-term healing. The astounding diversity of tip anatomic situations encountered demands a broad diversification of surgical planning and execution by the experienced surgeon.

Three broad categories of nasal tip sculpturing procedures may be identified. Although additional subtle technical variations exist, the three primary categories are (1) volume reduction with residual complete strip, (2) volume reduction with weakened residual complete strip, and (3) volume reduction with interrupted strip.

Preserving intact the major portion of the residual complete strip of the alar cartilage is always preferred when the anatomy of the alar cartilages and their surrounding soft tissue investments allows. This preservative approach retains the supportive advantage of the intact cartilage strip (thus "mimicking" nature), discourages cephalic rotation when it is undesirable, eliminates many of the potential hazards of more radical techniques, and tends to produce a more natural final result (Figs. 2–31 and 2–32).

Techniques involving a weakened (or reoriented) residual complete strip have all the foregoing positive virtues and in addition allow the surgeon to effect re-

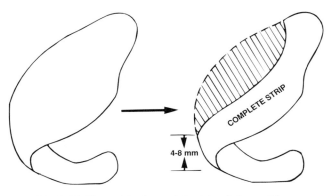

Fig. 2–31. The residual complete strip of alar cartilage.

orientation of the attitude of the wide domal angle, projection modification, and narrowing refinement so desirable in the ideal postoperative appearance (Figs. 2–33 and 2–34). The control of favorable healing is enhanced with these techniques, with the risk of complication diminished considerably.

Despite a laudable desire to preserve the integrity of the residual complete strip whenever possible, ana-

tomic situations are regularly encountered in which the shape, breadth, and orientation of the alar cartilages must be changed more radically by interrupting the complete strip in a vertical fashion somewhere along its extent to refine severe anatomic deficits (Figs. 2–35 and 2–36). When significant cephalic rotation is indicated, interrupted strip techniques are considered. The risks of asymmetric healing are higher when the alar cartilages are divided, however, and initial loss of tip support occurs immediately. The latter problem must be recognized and countermeasures taken during surgery to ensure that sufficient tip support is reconstituted. Shoring struts in the columella, infratip lobule cartilage grafts, and transdomal suturing are the most commonly used tip-support adjuncts. Almost without exception, interrupted strips should be avoided in patients displaying skin with sparse subcutaneous tissue.

Tip Projection and Cartilage Tip Grafts

In addition to the creation of narrowing refinement and symmetry of the nasal tip, most evident in the frontal view, *appropriate projection* must be preserved or newly created to result in the most natural appearance

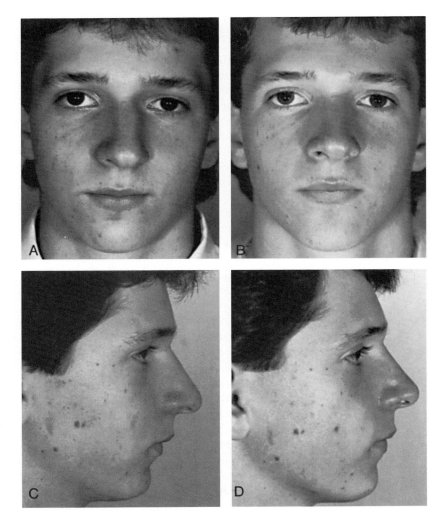

Fig. 2–32. Patient before and 1 year after rhinoplasty using the transcartilaginous approach, preserving a complete strip of alar cartilage. A. Front view before surgery. B. Front view after surgery. C. Profile before surgery. D. Profile after surgery.

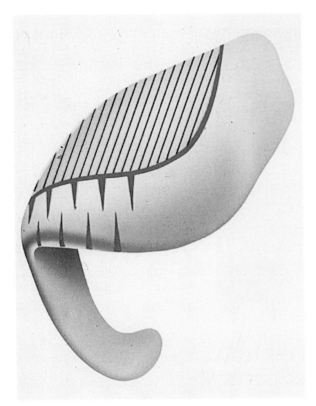

Fig. 2–33. Weakening of residual complete strip by incomplete, non-coalescent incisions through cartilage.

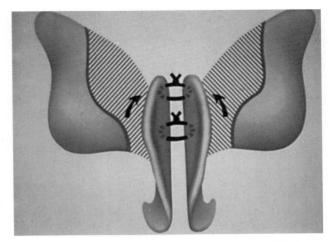

Fig. 2–35. Interruption of the lower lateral cartilage residual complete strip.

possible. Clearly, the most attractive and elegant noses are those in which anterior projection is sufficient to set the tip subtly but distinctly apart from the nasal supratip areas. Ptotic or poorly projected tips produce a snubbed and indistinct appearance.

Ideally on profile view, the nasal tip should be slightly elevated above the cartilaginous dorsum by 1 to 2 mm, blending gently rather than abruptly into the supratip (Fig. 2–37). If the preoperative projection of the tip is normal and adequate, lowering the cartilaginous dorsum into proper alignment will achieve a satisfactory aesthetic appearance, provided no loss of tip support occurs during the operative or postoperative periods. Preserving the major and minor tip-support structures increases this likelihood, whereas their sacrifice without compensatory reestablishment of support inevitably leads to eventual tip ptosis. If preoperative tip projection is inadequate, attempts to overreduce the supratip cartilaginous dorsum to produce pseudoprojection of the tip are inadvisable and lead to apparent flattening or widening of the middle third of the nose.

If tip projection is inadequate, several reliable methods may be used singly or in tandem to establish permanent improvement. All involve reorientation of the alar cartilages or addition of autogenous cartilage grafts to strengthen or sculpture the projection and/or attitude of the tip and infratip lobule.

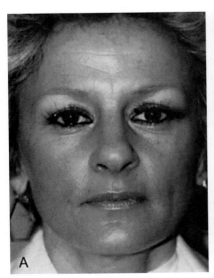
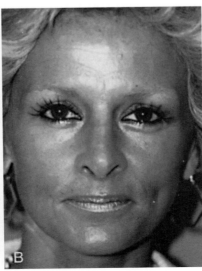

Fig. 2–34. Patient before and 1 year after surgery. Nasal tip has been refined using a weakened complete strip technique with a transdermal suture repair created through a delivery approach. A. Before surgery. B. After surgery.

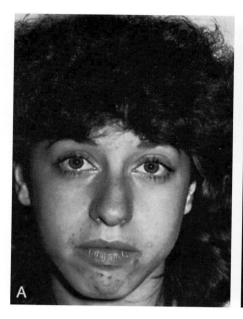

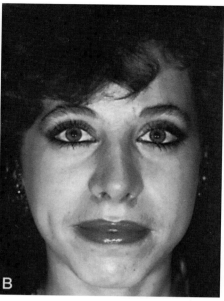

Fig. 2–36. Patient before and 1 year after rhinoplasty using a delivery approach and interrupted strip technique for refinement of the nasal tip. A. Before surgery. B. After surgery.

Because the long-term viability and stability of cartilage tip grafts are well established, they are regularly used with success if the surgical modification of existing alar cartilage configuration is not adequate to produce the desired degree of projection. In revision rhinoplasty in particular, tip cartilage grafts are irreplaceable in skeletal reconstruction beneath scarred skin and asymmetric topography.

Two distinct varieties of tip grafts are preferred: those that directly overlie the dome profile of the alar cartilage, and those that redefine and contour the skeletal anatomy of the infratip lobule. Because these grafts (single or laminated) lie in intimate subcutaneous pockets, exacting sculpture of their size and shape is mandatory. Harvested from septal or auricular cartilage, they are ideally inserted with or without suture fixation into small pockets dissected to accommodate exactly the dimensions of the graft(s) (Fig. 2–38). Bilateral marginal incisions beneath the anatomic dome area facilitate the careful pocket creation and render final positioning and stabilization of the graft easier than if only one unilateral incision is used. Suture fixation to the alar cartilages may be necessary if the tip region has been widely developed in a primary delivery or open approach method, disallowing the creation of a stable, limited defined pocket. Edges of the grafts must be beveled or softened to avoid visible contour irregularities or to offset deformities. Carved in triangular, trapezoid, or shield-like shapes, tip grafts may accentuate favorable tip-defining points and highlights while imparting a more natural appearance to tips with congenital or postsurgical inadequacies (Fig. 2–39).

If additional projection is required, it may be achieved in a variety of ways. Autogenous cartilage struts positioned below and/or between medial crura are effective in establishing permanent tip stability and slight additional projection (Fig. 2–40). Plumping grafts of cartilage fragments, introduced into the base of the columella through a low lateral columellar incision, provide an additional platform for the tip projec-

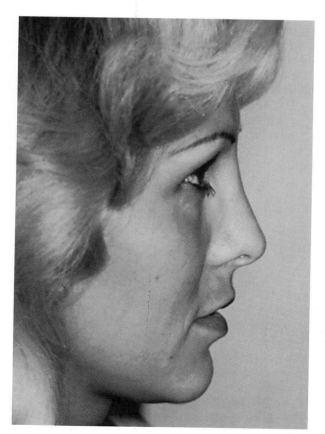

Fig. 2–37. An ideal nasal profile in a woman in which the nasal tip leads the cartilaginous dorsum slightly by 1 to 2 mm.

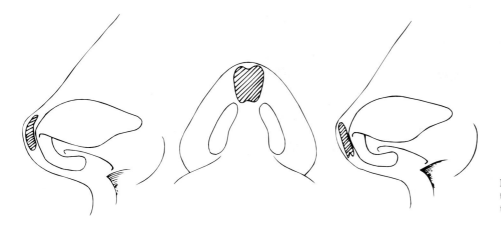

Fig. 2–38. Cartilage grafts positioned in the nasal tip or infratip lobule serve well to contour and create ideal projection.

tion resulting from the strut. Cartilage struts should be shaped with a gentle curve to match the anatomy of the curved columella, at times aiding in the creation of a distinct "double break," but should never extend to the apex of the tip skin lest a visible tent-pole appearance develops. If the medial crural footplates diverge in a widely splayed fashion, further tip projection may be gained by resecting excessive intercrural soft tissue and suturing the medial crura together.

Tip Rotation

In many patients undergoing rhinoplasty, cephalic rotation of the nasal tip complex (alar cartilages, columella, and nasal base) assumes major importance in the surgical event, whereas in other individuals, the *prevention* of upward rotation is vital. Certain well-defined and reliable principles may be invoked by the nasal surgeon essentially to calibrate the degree of tip rotation (or prevention thereof). The dynamics of healing play a critical role in tip rotation principles; the control of these postoperative healing changes distin-

guishes rhinoplasty from less elegant procedures. In the past, overrotation of the nasal tip created an unhealthy stigma for the rhinoplasty procedure. Most individuals recognize and prefer the aesthetic advantages of the stronger nose possessed of sufficient length to impart character and suitable proportions to the face.

The planned degree of tip rotation depends on a variety of factors, which often include:

1. The length of the nose.
2. The length of the face.
3. The length of the upper lip.
4. Facial balance and proportions.
5. The patient's aesthetic desires.
6. The surgeon's aesthetic judgment.

An important distinction must be drawn between *tip rotation* and *tip projection.* Although certain tip rotation techniques may result in desirable increases in tip projection, the converse is not true. Tip rotation and projection, in fact, complement each other, and their proper achievement in individual patients is con-

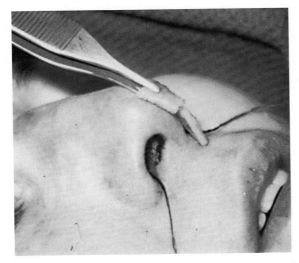

Fig. 2–39. Sculptured tip graft and columellar strut designed for increased tip projection and support.

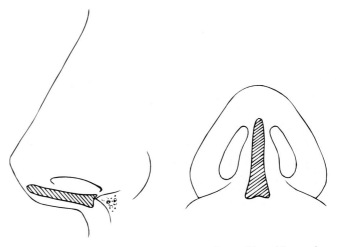

Fig. 2–40. Autogenous cartilage struts may be positioned in precise pockets or sewn into position between the medial crura.

stantly interrelated. A classic example of this interdependent relationship is illustrated by the almost inevitable loss of tip projection when interrupted strip techniques are chosen to enhance cephalic rotation; steps must be planned to restore adequate long-term tip projection by one of the several methods recommended.

Finally, a distinction must be drawn between *true* tip rotation and the *illusion* of tip rotation achieved by contouring cartilage grafts placed in the infratip lobule, columella, and nasolabial angle. Favorable modifications in the tip-lip-complex profile areas with autogenous implants may obviate the need for any actual tip rotation, thus preserving a long, and at times more desirable, nasal appearance. Reduction of the nasal profile, particularly the supratip cartilaginous pyramid, may also impart the illusion of rotation and a shortened nose, although occasionally at the expense of a strong and narrow dorsum.

Nasal tip rotation results fundamentally from planned surgical modifications of the alar cartilages, but increments of rotation may also be realized from additional adjunctive procedures on nasal structures adjacent to the alar cartilages, which exert a favorable influence on calibrated tip rotation methods. Shortening of the caudal septum, excision of overlong caudal upper lateral cartilages, and septal shortening with a high transfixion incision are regularly used to enhance the effects of a planned degree of tip rotation.

Because tip rotation is only one of the many objectives of in rhinoplasty, decisions regarding rotation must be interrelated with planning for tip volume reduction, alar cartilage thinning reduction, and modifications in the attitude and angulation of the alar cartilages.

The techniques and healing dynamics described are not absolute, but are reasonably predictable. Most tip rotation techniques may be incorporated in an organizational scheme that incorporates three procedures preserving a complete, intact strip of alar cartilage (Fig. 2–41) and three additional procedures involving inter-

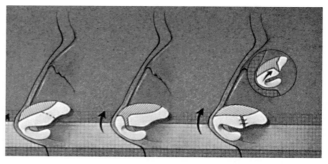

Fig. 2–42. Interrupted strip techniques tend to foster cephalic rotation by weakening the strength of the residual cartilage strip, allowing scar contracture to pull the tip cephalically.

rupted strip techniques (Fig. 2–42). Unique anatomic situations are regularly encountered that require modifications of this scheme to achieve a more refined result, but the fundamental principles elaborated remain constant. In addition, the thickness and strength of the alar cartilages, along with the character of their enveloping soft tissue and skin, dictate, to a degree, which techniques may safely and predictably be used in each anatomic situation.

Complete strip techniques are always preferable tip procedures when the nasal anatomy permits, and the goals of the surgical procedure may be met without resorting to the less predictable interrupted strip procedures. Preserving a complete, uninterrupted segment of alar cartilage remnant contributes to a more stable and better supported nasal tip that tends to *resist* cephalic rotation during healing.

Interrupted strip techniques, combined with volume reduction of excessive alar cartilage, tend to result in a more substantial degree of cephalic rotation of the tip complex. Once the complete strip of residual alar cartilage is divided (interrupted), the result is a relative instability of the nasal tip, on which the forces of upward scar contraction create a variable degree of cephalic rotation, underscoring the principle that during scar contracture tissues are generally moved from areas of instability (in this case, the unstable nasal tip cartilages) toward areas of stability (the bony-cartilaginous nasal pyramid).

Tip Rotation with Complete Strip Techniques

Volume reduction of the alar cartilage causes a tissue deficit of minimal, moderate, or maximal proportions, depending on the degree of cartilage removal indicated or desirable. Essentially no cephalic tip rotation results from minimal volume reduction alone, whereas the greater tissue void resulting from moderate to maximal volume reduction tends to create progressively greater degrees of *minimal* tip rotation (Fig. 2–43). Indeed, preservation of the complete strip is regularly indicated and preferred to resist the forces of upward

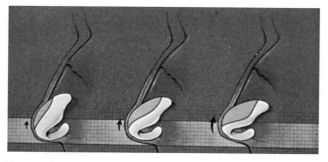

Fig. 2–41. Preserving a complete intact strip of lower lateral cartilage tends to resist upward rotation. The greater the tissue void created, the greater is the tendency of scar tissue contracture to result in slight upward rotation.

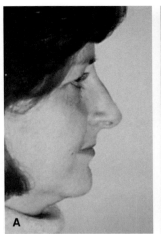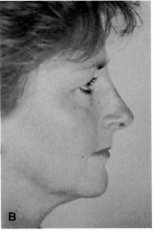

Fig. 2–43. Before and 1 year after rhinoplasty using complete strip technique with tip retroprojection. Cephalic rotation is minimal. A. Before surgery. B. After surgery.

rotation when the preoperative nasal length is to be maintained.

Substantial planned tip rotation when complete strip techniques are used depends therefore on the addition of adjunctive procedures to achieve cephalic elevation of the tip cartilage reduction, on septal shortening with a high septal transfixion, or on designing illusions of tip rotation with a high septal transfixion or the use of cartilage battens, struts, or plumping implants.

Tip Rotation with Interrupted Strip Techniques

When the integrity and spring of the alar cartilage are broken, cephalic rotation is fostered by virtue of upward scar contracture forces acting inexorably on alar cartilage segments, which are now more flail and less supported. These techniques are particularly useful when the attitude of the alar cartilages is one of a profound downward inclination, imparting a depressed or snarl-like appearance to the nose. Caution must be exercised constantly in the use of interrupted strips in patients with thin skin and/or more delicate cartilages because the absence of good tip-supporting structures sets the stage for loss of projection, alar collapse, notching, pinching, and asymmetry.

LATERAL INTERRUPTION TECHNIQUES. In anatomic situations when cephalic rotation is desirable and the anatomy of the bridge between the medial and lateral crus (the "dome") is aesthetically pleasing, lateral interruption of the residual complete strip has merit (see Fig. 2–42). Avoiding interruption of the strip medially fosters symmetric healing and reduces the likelihood that uneven tip-defining points will become evident months after surgery. The lateral interruption allows the reduced alar cartilage to be pulled moderately upward by scar tissue during healing, but because the dividing cut is sited more laterally and therefore more

deeply in the soft tissues of the tip, notching, pinching, and other asymmetries are essentially prevented. If modification of the dome is necessary, transdomal suture techniques to narrow, refine, and even slightly project the tip may be favorably combined with lateral interruption.

MEDIAL INTERRUPTION TECHNIQUES. Many different methods of interruption of the residual complete strip at or near the dome have been described; each predictably leads to some degree of cephalic rotation, and the complete strip is converted to two or more segments of flail cartilage (see Fig. 2–42). Planned rotation with this approach is reserved for patients with thicker skin and supporting structures, to minimize undesirable consequences of asymmetric healing and even overrotation. Elevation of the medial nostril margin, an onerous stigma of nasal surgery, is more common with medial strip interruption.

Medial interruption techniques almost always result in a moderate to major loss of tip projection, and adjunctive procedures are required to restore or augment tip projection to avoid tip ptosis.

LATERAL INTERRUPTION TECHNIQUES WITH SUTURE ROTATION. An ideal method for significant tip rotation would combine lateral strip interruption to preserve the integrity of the strip medially with a calibrated triangular excision of cartilage laterally and stabilization of the cut cartilage edges with suture fixation (Fig. 2–44). The degree of rotation realized here is controlla-

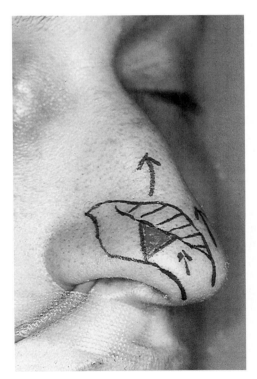

Fig. 2–44. Lateral interruption of the residual lateral crus, with calibrated excision of a base up triangle, allows a *controlled* cephalic rotation dependent on the geometry of the excised triangle.

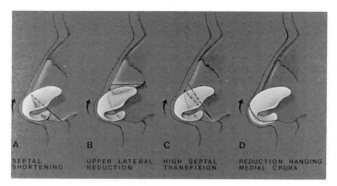

Fig. 2–45. Adjunctive techniques tend to foster cephalic rotation of the nasal tip.

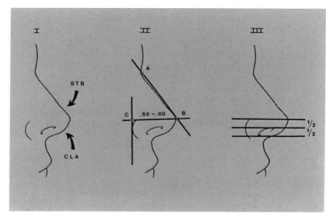

Fig. 2–46. Goode has characterized the guidelines for nasal tip projection. If the tip projects from the alar-facial junction to the nasal tip-defining point more than 0.55 to 0.6 of a line connecting the tip-defining point and nasal frontal angle, the nose may be considered overprojected.

ble by the surgeon, essentially eliminates most of the undesirable sequelae of interrupted strip techniques, and changes in a predictable and permanent way the attitude of the alar cartilages. The suture fixation helps to diminish loss of tip support inherent in most interrupted strip techniques. In individuals with thin or moderately thin skin with more delicate cartilages, this method is highly predictable and desirable.

As with the rotation concepts discussed in connection with complete strip techniques, the same adjunctive techniques for enhancing tip rotation may be useful to combine with interrupted strip techniques. Included among these adjunctive techniques to cephalic rotation are (1) shortening of the caudal septum, (2) shortening of the caudal upper lateral cartilage, (3) high septal incision of wedge excision of septum, and (4) reduction of overly convex medial crura (caudal margin) (Fig. 2–45).

Overrotation, however, must be religiously avoided because the correction of this undesirable postoperative situation is often difficult or impossible.

Correction of the Overprojecting Tip

Profound facial and nasal disharmony may result from the anatomic facial feature variant termed "the overprojecting nose." Because the entire nose, and especially the normal nasal tip, are composed of distinct, interrelated anatomic components, any one or combination of several of these components may be responsible for the tip that projects too far forward of the anterior plane of the face. The guidelines for determining appropriate and inappropriate tip projection are now well accepted (Fig. 2–46). When numerous patients with overprojecting tips are analyzed, it becomes apparent that no single anatomic component of the nose is constantly responsible for overprojection (Table 2–2); therefore, no single surgical technique is uniformly useful in correcting all the problems responsible for the various overprojection deformities.

Accurate anatomic diagnosis allows preoperative development of a logical individualized strategy for correction and tip retropositioning. In almost every in-

stance, *weakening or reducing of normal tip-support mechanisms is required* to achieve normality, supplemented by reduction of the overdeveloped components. The following anatomic variants are commonly responsible individually or collectively for overprojection of the nasal tip.

Overdevelopment of the alar cartilages, commonly associated with thin skin and large nostrils, is frequently encountered in the overprojecting nose. The junction between the medial and lateral crura may form an overlarge dome of significant convexity, or the anatomic dome area may be sharply angulated, twisted, or even buckled, frequently demonstrating significant asymmetry of the entire tip and its tip-defining points. The hypertrophied cartilages must be delivered, their abnormalities visually diagnosed, and overall volume reduction of both the lateral and medial crura accomplished. Portions of the medial crus may require resection to retroposition the nasal tip satisfactorily.

A second common cause of excess nasal tip projection is an overlarge nasal bony spine, which seemingly imparts an upward thrust of the tip components (which may otherwise be of normal dimensions). Compounding this abnormal appearance is often a coexistent blunting of the nasolabial angle, which may appear full, webbed, and excessively obtuse, with no

TABLE 2–2. Causes of Overprojecting Nasal Tip

Alar cartilage overdevelopment
Nasal spine overdevelopment
Caudal septum overdevelopment
Dorsal septum overdevelopment
Elongated columella and medial crura
Combined abnormalities
Iatrogenic overprojection

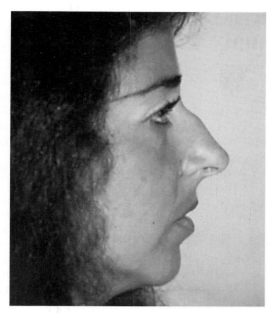

Fig. 2–47. Overprojection of the nose as a result of overdevelopment of the caudal quadrangular cartilage.

obvious demarcation between the tip and columella. The upper lip may appear short, tethered, and tense, often exposing excessive gingiva in facial repose as well as in animation. Rongeur or osteotome reduction of the overlarge spine and associated caudal quadrangular cartilage and soft tissue is a surgical prerequisite to tip retrodisplacement.

A similar deformity of overprojection and obliteration of a definitive nasolabial angle may be the result of overdevelopment of the caudal quadrangular cartilage (Fig. 2–47). The nasal spine may in fact be of normal size, but if it is even slightly overlarge, it compounds the problem of overprojection. In effecting repair, the caudal septal margin abutting the nasal spine should always be inspected and shave reduced to normal proportion before sacrificing any of the nasal spine.

A high anterior septal angle caused by an overdeveloped quadrangular cartilage component may spuriously elevate the tip to an abnormally forward-projecting position (Fig. 2–48), even when associated with otherwise perfectly normal tip anatomy. This condition tends to "tent" the tip away from the face and "tether" the upper lip, producing an indefinite nasolabial angle and, on occasion, creating abnormal exposure of the maxillary gingiva, particularly on smiling. Correction demands a departure from the normal operative sequence of correcting the tip first. The initial surgical steps are planned to lower the cartilaginous profile first, releasing the tip from an abnormal overprojected influence. Further tip-refinement measures can then be carried out as desired and indicated by the alar cartilage anatomy.

Tip overprojection may occur as a result of an overly

long columella associated with excessively long medial crura. In this deformity, the infratip lobule is commonly insufficient, creating the effect of extremely large and disproportionate nostrils. This deformity suggests the use of an external approach to the nasal tip to shorten the columellar length as well as that of the medial crura.

Various combinations of the foregoing hypertrophic anatomic problems may contribute to the overprojecting tip problem. In preoperative analysis, each nasal component must be compulsively identified and analyzed; only then can a definitive plan for natural correction be conceived. Generally, a combination of weakening of the major tip-support mechanisms associated with reduction of the components responsible for the tip overprojection is carried out incrementally and as conservatively as possible to achieve the desired normal final result in a progressive fashion. The various components capable of creating or contributing to overprojection of the nose are shown in Table 2–2.

Iatrogenic overprojection may occur when surgeons intent on profoundly increasing tip projection produce an unnaturally sharp and projected tip configuration (often associated with overrotation of the tip). These misadventures commonly result from overaggressive tip surgery in which portions of the lateral crus are borrowed and rotated medially to increase medial crus

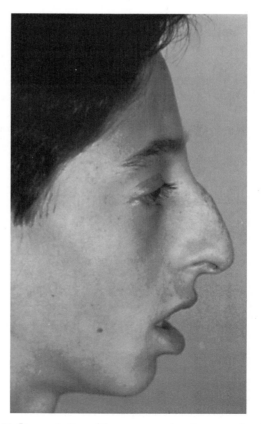

Fig. 2–48. Overprojection of the nose secondary to an overdeveloped dorsal quadrangular cartilage anatomic component.

projection. If this form of interrupted strip technique is carried out in a thin-skinned patient, unpredictable healing may lead to a sharp, narrowed, asymmetric, and overprojected tip with potential collapse of the alar sidewalls early or even late in the postoperative period. Correction requires exploration of the residual nasal tip cartilages through a delivery or open approach to determine the residual anatomy and the precise cause of the deformity. The overprojecting cartilages (usually, the medial crura) are trimmed to a proper position, and when indicated, autogenous cartilage grafts are inserted between the tip skin and the residual alar cartilages to soften and sculpture the tip contours. Sutured-in-place tip grafts may be positioned to camouflage tip irregularities effectively, supplemented by crushed cartilage tip contouring.

Alar Base Reduction

Appropriate reduction of the projecting nose typically requires diminishing the various major and minor tip-support mechanisms to retroposition the tip closer to the face. A concomitant reduction of the alar component length and lateral flare (occasioned by tip repositioning) is usually required to improve nasal balance and harmony. Alar wedge excisions of various geometric designs and dimensions are necessary to balance alar length and position (Fig. 2–49). The exact geometry of these excisions is determined by the present and intended shape of the nostril aperture, the degree and attitude of the lateral alar flare, the width and shape of the nostril aperture, the degree and attitude of the lateral alar flare, the width and shape of the nostril sill, and the thickness of the alae. It is axiomatic that the surgeon creating alar reduction by excision of alar or nostril floor tissue should always err on the side of conservatism and strive for symmetric repair because overaggressive and asymmetric tissue resection leads to an almost irreversible situation of disharmony and even nostril stenosis.

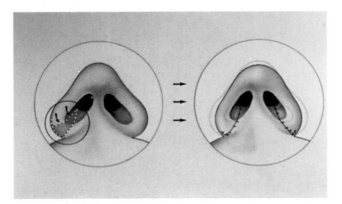

Fig. 2–49. Alar wedge excisions of various geometric designs and dimensions are necessary to improve the alar flaring found in certain patients. The exact design of each tissue removal depends on the dimensions of the alar sidewalls and the nostril itself.

Profile Alignment

Three anatomic nasal components are responsible for the preoperative profile appearance: the nasal bones, the cartilaginous septum, and the alar cartilages. Generally, all three must undergo modification to create a pleasing and natural profile alignment. If the nose is overlarge with a convex profile, reduction of the three segments is required. Less commonly (except in revision rhinoplasty), profile augmentation with autograft materials must be done.

The surgeon visualizes the ultimate intended profile, extending from the nasofrontal angle to the tip-defining point, and then on around the infratip lobule and columella to the nasolabial angle. The extent of reduction of bone, cartilage, and soft tissue always depends on and should be guided by stable tip projection; *therefore, positioning the projection of the tip at the outset of the operative procedure is beneficial.* Because the thickness of the investing soft tissues and skin varies at different areas of the profile and from patient to patient, dissimilar portions of cartilage and bone must be removed to create a straight or slightly concave profile ultimately. Strong, high profiles generally suit the patient best in the long term, contributing to a more elegant nose on profile and oblique views and also a more narrow nasal appearance on frontal view (Fig. 2–50). Overreduced profiles result in a washed-out, indefinite, and widened appearance from the front, separating the eyes inadequately and reflecting light poorly.

In planning profile alignment, the two stable reference points are the existing (or planned) nasofrontal angle and the tip-defining point. Aesthetics are generally best served when profile reduction results in a high, straight-line profile in men and the leading edge of the tip just slightly higher in women. A gentle slope of no more than 2 to 3 mm should exist between the caudal part of the cartilaginous dorsum and the most anteriorly projecting aspect of the nasal tip. Reversal of the usual preoperative tip-supratip relationship is required to achieve this aesthetic ideal.

The degree and angulation of the "hump removal" depends on various factors, the most important of which are the size of the various involved anatomic components and the surgeon's confidence in the stability of postoperative tip projection. These must be balanced with the personal preference for profile appearance combined with the surgeon's value judgment of facial aesthetics.

Surgical access to the nasal dorsum is gained through the transcartilaginous or intercartilaginous incision, depending on which approach was used during tip refinement. The incision is usually extended around the anterior septal angle and into the membranous septum for a distance of 5 to 8 mm to provide full visualization of the nasal skeleton. Complete transfixion incision for exposure is unnecessary and may compromise tip support by sacrificing the attachment of the medial crural footplates to the caudal septum.

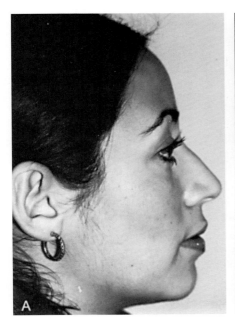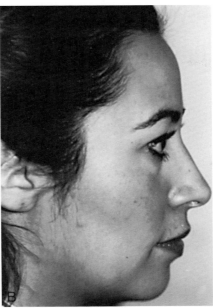

Fig. 2–50. Patient before and 1 year after rhino-plasty. A strong, high profile has been maintained. A. Before surgery. B. After surgery.

The plan of tissue elevation over the nasal dorsum is important for several reasons. A relatively avascular potential plane exists intimate (superficial) to the perichondrium of the cartilaginous vault and just below the periosteum of the bony vault. Elevating the soft tissue flap in this important plane preserves the thickest possible ultimate epithelial-soft tissue covering to cushion the newly formed bony and cartilaginous profile. Generally, only sufficient skin is elevated to gain access to the bony and cartilaginous profile, and therefore wide undermining is unnecessary in the typical rhinoplasty. In older patients with redundant and less elastic skin, or when access is needed for major autograft augmentation, wider undermining is carried out. Even in the latter instance, the periosteal-soft tissue layer over the intended site of the low lateral osteotomies is preserved intact to help stabilize the mobile bony pyramid after in-fracture osteotomy maneuvers.

The soft tissues over the cartilaginous dorsum are elevated by means of scalpel dissection with a No. 15c blade (Fig. 2–51), and the periosteum over the bony

pyramid is lifted from its stable bony attachment with the knife and sharp Joseph elevator (Fig. 2–52). Because the periosteum inserts into the internasal suture line in the midline, the periosteum is lifted on either side of this suture and the space brought into continuity with the sharp scissors. Little or no bleeding should ensue during uncovering of the nasal skeleton in these important planes, allowing direct visual assessment of the anatomy encountered.

Either of two methods of profile alignment is preferred: incremental or en bloc. In the first method, the cartilaginous dorsum is reduced by incrementally

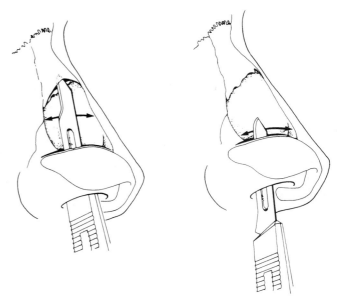

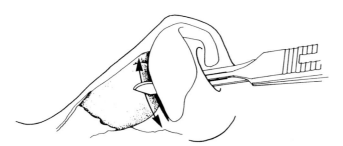

Fig. 2–51. Elevation of the nasal skin and subcutaneous tissue layers by knife dissection, staying intimate to the perichondrium overlying the cartilaginous pyramid.

Fig. 2–52. Elevation of the periosteum overlying the bony pyramid.

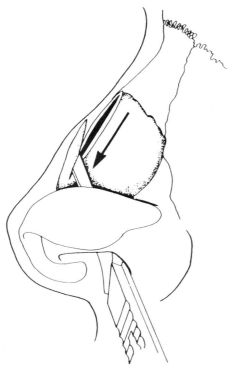

Fig. 2–53. Incremental reduction of the cartilaginous dorsum.

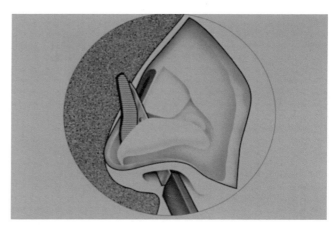

Fig. 2–55. Partial removal of the nasal hump by resection of the cartilaginous dorsum, leaving the osseocartilaginous junction intact. Excision of the nasal hump and alignment of the profile by en bloc resection.

shaving away the cartilaginous dorsum until an ideal tip-supratip relationship is established (Fig. 2–53), followed by sharp osteotome removal of the residual bony hump (Fig. 2–54).

If only minimal hump removal is contemplated, the knife is positioned at the osseocartilaginous junction and plunged through this area, then advanced caudally to and around the anterior septal angle of the caudal septum (Fig. 2–55). In large cartilaginous reductions, a portion of the upper lateral cartilage attach-

ment to the quadrangular cartilage must be removed with the dorsal septum, but leaving these two cartilaginous components attached by the underlying mucoperichondrial bridge.

A Rubin osteotome, honed to razor sharpness for each procedure and seated in the opening made by the knife at the osseocartilaginous junction, is advanced cephalically to remove the desired degree of bony hump in continuity with the cartilaginous hump (Fig. 2–56).

Any remaining irregularities are corrected under direct vision with a knife and sharp tungsten-carbide rasp. Palpating the skin of the dorsum with the examining finger moistened with hydrogen peroxide often provides clues to unseen irregularities, as does intranasal palpation of the profile with the noncutting edge of the No. 15 blade.

Except in large or severely twisted noses, it is unnec-

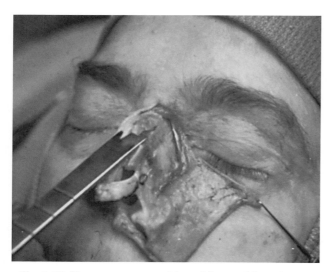

Fig. 2–54. Sharp osteotome excision of the nasal bony hump.

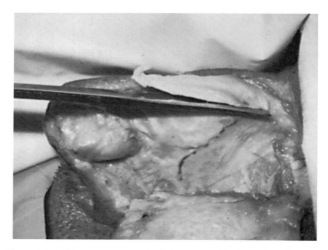

Fig. 2–56. Rubin osteotome seated at osseocartilaginous junction preparatory to en bloc removal of nasal hump.

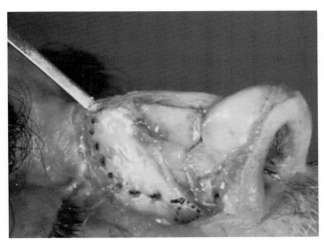

Fig. 2–57. Weakening of the bone at the proposed nasofrontal angle by means of a percutaneous osteotomy using a 2-mm osteotome. The bone is scored and weakened to facilitate ultimate fracture at the intended site of the nasofrontal angle.

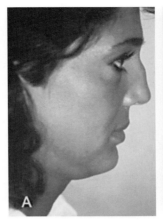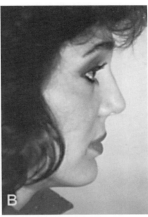

Fig. 2–58. Patient before and 1 year after rhinoplasty, illustrating the benefits of augmentation of the overly deep nasofrontal angle with autogenous cartilage. A. Before surgery. B. After surgery.

essary and potentially harmful to separate the upper lateral cartilages from the septum by cutting through the mucoperichondrial bridge of tissue connecting them at the nasal valve.

Redundant soft tissue around the anterior septal angle may be trimmed away to achieve improved tip-supratip definition. The caudal septum, assessed by stretching the partial transfixion incision posteriorly, lies exposed for geometric shortening or repositioning.

In patients in whom the nasofrontal angle is poorly defined or in need of repositioning, weakening of the bone in the desired area is accomplished before bony hump removal. At the exact site in the midline where the nasofrontal angle is desired, a 2-mm osteotome is plunged transcutaneously into the midline of the nasal bone (Fig. 2–57). By angulating this small osteotome laterally on either side, the exact cephalic extent of bony hump removal may be controlled by scoring the bone in a horizontal line at the nasofrontal angle. During the bony hump removal phase of profile alignment, the nasal bones fracture cephalically where this weakening maneuver has established a bony dehiscence, allowing the surgeon some additional control over the ultimate site of the nasofrontal angle. Creating a more caudally placed angle provides the illusion of a shorter nose without actually shortening, whereas establishing a more cephalically placed angle creates the appearance of a longer nose.

In patients in whom the nasofrontal angle is overly deep, augmentation with residual septal cartilage or remnants of the excised alar cartilages provides a beneficial aesthetic refinement (Fig. 2–58).

Further profile enhancements may be favorably developed with contouring cartilage grafts positioned along the dorsum, supratip area, infratip lobule, columella, and nasolabial angle. In the last site, so-called

"plumping" grafts are commonly used to open an otherwise acute or unsatisfactory nasolabial angle and thereby contribute to improved profile appearance. The illusion of tip rotation and nasal shortening results from this maneuver (Fig. 2–59), reducing the degree of actual shortening required and preserving a longer and often more elegant nose.

Bony Pyramid Narrowing and Alignment

Significant advances have been developed over the past two decades in the reduction of osteotomy trauma in rhinoplasty surgery. Osteotomies, the most traumatic of all nasal surgical maneuvers, are best delayed until the final step in the planned surgical sequence, when vasoconstriction exerts its maximal influence and the nasal splint may be promptly positioned.

Profile alignment in the typical reduction rhinoplasty inevitably results in an excessive plateau-like

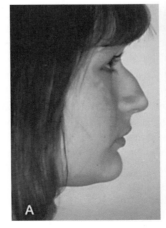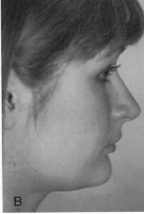

Fig. 2–59. Patient before and 1 year after rhinoplasty whose profile has been improved by cartilaginous grafts positioned at the nasolabial angle and supratip dorsum. A. Before surgery. B. After surgery.

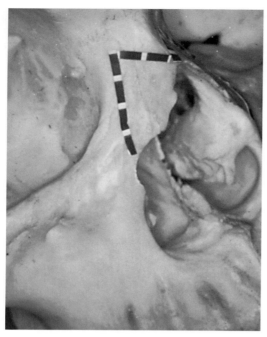

Fig. 2–60. Medial-oblique osteotomies angle laterally, approximately 15 to 20 degrees from the vertical midline.

width of the nasal dorsum, requiring narrowing of the bony and cartilaginous pyramid to restore a natural and more narrow frontal appearance to the nose. The lateral bony sidewalls (consisting of the nasal bones and maxillary ascending processes) must be completely mobilized by nongreenstick fractures and moved medially (exceptions may exist in older patients with more fragile bones in whom greenstick fractures may be acceptable or even preferable). The upper lateral cartilages are also moved medially because of their stable attachment cephalically to the undersurface of the nasal bones.

To facilitate atraumatic low lateral osteotomy execution, medial-oblique osteotomies angled laterally 15 to 20 degrees from the vertical midline are preferred (Fig. 2–60). By creating an osteotomy dehiscence at the intended cephalic apex of the lateral osteotome, the surgeon exerts added control of the exact site of back-fracture in the lateral bony sidewall. A 2- to 3-mm sharp micro-osteotome is positioned intranasally at the cephalic extent of the removal of the bony hump (if no hump removal has been necessary, the site of positioning is at the caudal extent of the nasal bones in the midline). The osteotome is advanced cephalo-obliquely to its intended apex at an angle of 15 to 20 degrees, depending on the shape of the nasal bony sidewall. Little trauma results from medial-oblique osteotomies, which prevent the ever-present possibility of eccentric or asymmetric surgical fractures from developing when lateral osteotomies alone are performed. In addition, bony narrowing to accomplish

desired in-fracture as a consequence of lateral osteotomies combined with medial-oblique osteotomies occurs without strong manual pressure exerted on the nasal bones, a traditional but unnecessary traumatic maneuver.

Trauma may be significantly reduced in lateral osteotomies if 2- or 3-mm micro-osteotomies are used to accomplish a controlled fracture of the bony sidewalls. No need exists for elevation of the periosteum along the pathway of the lateral fractures because the small osteotomies require little space for their cephalic progression. Appropriately, the intact periosteum stabilizes and internally splints the complete fractures, facilitating stable and precise healing. The low curved lateral osteotomy is initiated by pressing the sharp osteotome through the vestibular skin to encounter the margin of the pyriform aperture at or just above the inferior turbinate. This preserves the bony sidewall along the floor of the nose, where narrowing would achieve no favorable aesthetic improvement but might compromise the inferior nasal airway without purpose. The pathway of the osteotome then progresses toward the base of the maxilla, curving next up along the nasal maxillary junction to encounter the previously created small medial-oblique osteotomy (Fig. 2–61). A complete, controlled, and atraumatic fracture of the bony sidewall is thus created, allowing in-fracture without excessive traumatic pressure. Immediate

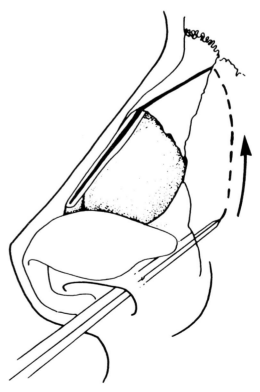

Fig. 2–61. Curved low lateral osteotomies, created with 2- or 3-mm osteotomes, create minimal trauma to the surrounding tissues.

finger pressure is applied bilaterally over the lateral osteotome sites to forestall further extravasation of blood into the soft tissues. *In reality, little or no bleeding occurs during micro-osteotomies because the soft tissues embracing the bony sidewalls remain essentially undamaged.*

In most rhinoplasty procedures, controlled nasal fractures as the result of osteotomy should cause slight but definite mobility of the bony sidewalls stabilized by the internal and external periosteum, which bridges the nasal fragments on either side of the osteotome pathway. Large guarded osteotomies destroy this vital periosteal sling, potentially rendering the bony fragments unstable and susceptible to eccentric or asymmetric healing. In addition, trauma from large osteotomes may produce increased bleeding, edema, and unnecessary ecchymosis.

In deviated noses characterized by essentially convex or concave bony asymmetries, excessively wide or extremely thick bones (including revision rhinoplasty), *double* lateral osteotomies may be considered for improved mobilization and regularization. This decision is best determined preoperatively to allow the higher osteotomy to be accomplished before the low lateral osteotomy. Reversing this order necessitates attempting the higher osteotomy on an already mobilized lateral bony sidewall, a more difficult task.

On completion of satisfactory osteotomies and suitable aesthetic nasal narrowing, the profile line is finally inspected and palpated for irregularities or inadequate alignment. Because the upper lateral cartilages move medially with the bony sidewalls following osteotomies, their dorsal margins should be trimmed to sit flush with or slightly lower than the cartilaginous profile line. Excess soft tissue, if present, is excised and the new nasal dorsum is inspected for and cleaned of any debris. Any profile grafts to be placed to improve the ultimate intended profile line are now scalpel-sculptured to size and placed accordingly. If limited undermining of the overlying dorsal epithelium has occurred, grafts may be placed with no requirement for suture fixation. If a large subcutaneous pocket exists, however, transcutaneous pull-out 5-0 mild chromic catgut sutures are used to fix the grafts into the intended site. The sutures, cut flush with the skin at 5 to 7 days, retract into the subcutaneous space and are absorbed.

Final subtle nasal refinements are now completed and may include caudal septal reduction, resection of excessive vestibular skin and mucous membrane, trimming of the caudal margins of the upper lateral cartilages (only if overlong or projecting into the vestibule), columellar narrowing, and bilateral alar base reduction. These final maneuvers are carried out with the assistant maintaining constant finger pressure over the lateral osteotomy sites to prevent even minimal oozing and intraoperative swelling. All incisions are closed completely with 5-0 chromic catgut suture. No permanent sutures are used.

Nasal dressings are now applied. No intranasal dressing or packing is necessary in routine rhinoplasty. If septoplasty has been an integral part of the operation, a folded strip of Telfa is placed into each nostril along the floor of the nose to absorb drainage. The previously placed transseptal quilting mattress suture acts as a sole internal nasal splint for the septum, completely obliterating the submucoperichondrial dead spaces and fixing the septal elements in place during healing. The external splint consists of a layer of compressed Gelfoam placed along the dorsum and stabilized in place with flesh-colored Micropore tape, extending over and laterally beyond the lateral osteotome sites. A small aluminum and Velcro ("Denver") splint applied firmly over the nasal dorsum completes the operation (Fig. 2-62).

Postsurgical Considerations

The care of the postrhinoplasty patient is directed toward patient comfort, reduction of swelling and edema, patency of the nasal airway, and compression-stabilization of the nose.

Whether the patient is discharged on the afternoon of or the morning after surgery, all intranasal dressings are removed from the nose before the patient leaves. A detailed list of instructions is supplied for the patient or accompanying family member (Fig. 2-63); the important aspects of these "do's" and "don'ts" are emphasized. Prevention of trauma to the nose is clearly the most important consideration. Oral decongestant therapy is helpful, but the value of corticosteroids and antibiotics in routine rhinoplasty is conjectural.

The external splint is removed by the surgeon or surgical nurse 5 to 7 days after surgery. An important consideration should be gentle removal of the tape and splint by bluntly dissecting the nasal skin from the overlying splint with a dull instrument without disturbing or tenting up the healing skin. Failure to follow this policy may lead to disturbance of the newly forming subcutaneous fibroblastic layer over the nasal dorsum, with additional unwanted scarring and even abrupt hematoma.

SEPTUM IN RHINOPLASTY

The role of the septum in rhinoplasty has always been subject to debate. The difficulty arises because of a lack of definition, namely, between the septal operation performed as an entity and its being performed as a combined operation with rhinoplasty. Septal resection without rhinoplasty found many advocates for radical removal of the septum at the turn of the century. In 1937, Peer expressed the opinion that radical removal

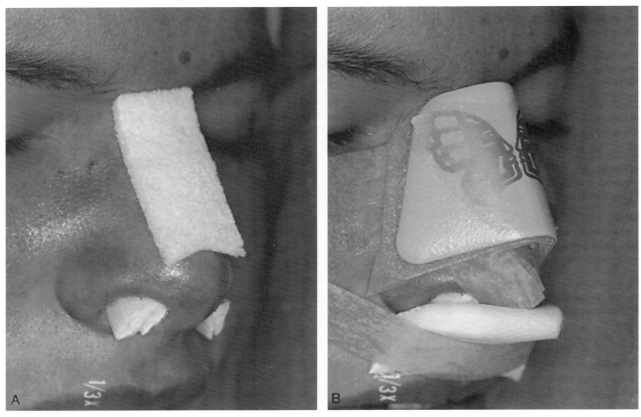

Fig. 2–62. Nasal splint applied to reconstructed nose and maintained for 7 days to support, splint, and protect the nose. A. Gelfoam cushion. B. Velcro-aluminum splint.

might be necessary for certain types of deflection but emphasized the need for a section of cartilage in the anterior position to replace the septum for nasal support. Fomon and associates, in 1946, 1948, and 1951 described a similar method but incorporated the rhinoplastic approach of Joseph. The adherents to this method did not clearly define the limitations of this procedure with regard to rhinoplasty, although this was foreshadowed. These techniques apply primarily to the correction of the deviated-dislocated septum alone and are rarely indicated when combined with rhinoplasty, except in the badly traumatized nose.

A more complex problem arises with combined correction of both an external and a septal deformity. Radical removal of the septum performed with extensive rhinoplasty often results in a depressed nose because of lack of septal support. The exception is the severely traumatized nose. In these cases, the dorsum is depressed, and it is impossible to shift the septum without sacrifice of large sections of cartilage. Radical removal of the septum then may be required, but a dorsal implant of a bone or cartilage graft is necessary to correct the depression.

To correct a deviated-dislocated septum associated with a rhinoplastic correction in the developmental type of deformity safely, techniques advocating the shifting and reconstruction of the septal cartilage with minimal removal of septum are currently considered preferable to radical septal resection.

DEVIATED OR SCOLIOTIC NOSE

Deviation of the entire nose involves both the bony and cartilaginous vaults; deviations of the lower half of the nose are caused mainly by septal derangements accompanied by secondary effects of the cartilaginous vault (Fig. 2–64).

Associated asymmetries and deformities of the upper lateral cartilage commonly accompany severe septal scoliosis. The septal and external deformities are corrected together whenever feasible. Because the procedures are interdependent, a better evaluation of the problem is possible when they are carried out simultaneously, and the patient is saved considerable time and discomfort (Fig. 2–65).

Correction of the cartilaginous component precedes the management of the bony deformity to allow adequate space for readjustment and in-fracturing of the bony vault. Furthermore, seldom can an externally twisted nose be adequately straightened without concomitant septal realignment. The admonition "as goes the septum, so goes the nose" holds much truth.

PATIENT INSTRUCTIONS FOLLOWING NASAL PLASTIC SURGERY

A. INTRODUCTION

Please read and familiarize yourself with these instructions before <u>BEFORE</u> and <u>AFTER</u> surgery. By following them carefully you will assist in obtaining the best possible result from your surgery. If questions arise, do not hesitate to communicate with me and discuss your questions at any time. Take this list to the hospital with you and begin observing these directions on the day of surgery.

B. INSTRUCTIONS

1. Do not blow nose until instructed. Wipe or dab nose gently with kleenex, if necessary.
2. Change dressing under nose (if present) as needed.
3. The nasal cast will remain in place for approximately one week and will be removed in the office. Do NOT disturb it; keep it dry.
4. Avoid foods that require prolonged chewing. Otherwise, your diet has no restrictions.
5. Avoid extreme physical activity. Obtain more rest than you usually get and avoid exertion, including athletic activities and intercourse.
6. Brush teeth gently with a soft toothbrush only. Avoid manipulation of upper lip to keep nose at rest.
7. Avoid excess or prolonged telephone conversations and social activities for at least 10–14 days.
8. You may wash your face—carefully avoid the dressing. Take tub baths until the dressings are removed.
9. Avoid smiling, grinning and excess facial movements for one week.
10. Do not wash hair for one week unless you have someone do it for you. <u>DO NOT GET NASAL DRESSINGS WET.</u>
11. Wear clothing that fastens in front or back for one week. Avoid slipover sweaters, T-shirts and turtlenecks.
12. Absolutely avoid sun or sun lamps for 6 weeks after surgery. Heat may cause the nose to swell.
13. Don't swim for one month, since injuries are common during swimming.
14. Don't be concerned if, following removal of dressing, the nose, eyes and upper lip show some swelling and discoloration—this usually clears in 2–3 weeks. In certain patients it may require 6 months for all swelling to completely subside.
15. Take only medications prescribed by your doctor(s).
16. Do not wear regular glasses or sunglasses which rest on the bridge of the nose for at least 4 weeks. We will instruct you in the method of taping the glasses to your forehead to avoid pressure on the nose.
17. Contact lenses may be worn within 2–3 days after surgery.
18. After the doctor removes your nasal cast, the skin of the nose may be cleansed gently with a mild soap or vaseline intensive care lotion. <u>BE GENTLE.</u> Makeup may be used as soon as bandages are removed. To cover discoloration, you may use "ERACE" by Max Factor, "COVER AWAY" by Adrien Arpel, or "ON YOUR MARK" by Kenneth.
19. <u>DON'T TAKE CHANCES!</u>—If you are concerned about anything you consider significant, call me at 312-472-7559.

Fig. 2–63. Patient instruction sheet.

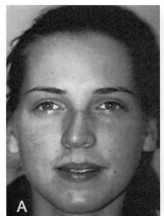
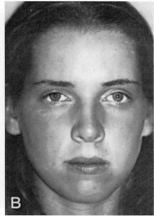

Fig. 2–64. Deviation of the external nose caused by nasal septal deflection. A. Before surgery. B. After surgery.

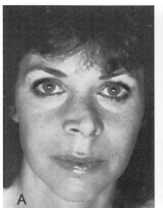
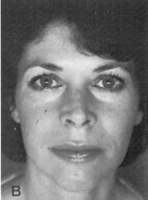

Fig. 2–65. Patient before and 1 year after septal rhinoplasty using preservative reconstruction of the nasal septum. A. Before surgery. B. After surgery.

For a better understanding of the pathologic changes and mechanics involved in correcting this type of nasal deformity, a review of etiologic and anatomic factors is presented.

ETIOLOGIC AND ANATOMIC FACTORS

At birth, the septum is almost completely cartilaginous, with the exception of the vomer and the two premaxillae and their processes. The vomer develops bilaterally on each side of the cartilaginous nasal septum from a pair of ossification centers, which are present at the beginning of the third month of fetal life. The bilateral plates of the vomer unite from behind and grow forward at the expense of the imprisoned cartilage. Their development is completed at age 15. Indication of the bilateral origin of the vomer is evidenced in the infant by a deep groove between the two plates. The groove is somewhat flattened in adults.

The premaxilla parallels the development of the vomer, but after the child is 6 years old, it develops rapidly. The ethmoid bone begins to ossify during the first year of postfetal life and is not completed until the end of the seventeenth year.

At birth, neither the palate bones nor the superior maxillae rise into a crest for the support of the lower edge of the septum, but in the adult these bones have marked crests. The upward growth of the crests, along with the development of the premaxilla and vomer, combined with the downward growth of the septum from the ethmoid ossification centers and the downward expansion of the cranial cavity, may account for many deviations and dislocations of the septum. This disproportion of growth with pressure on the cartilaginous septum has been emphasized as a causative factor in septal deformities.

The vomer and premaxilla are enveloped by a periosteal covering that separates the bony portion of the septum from the cartilaginous septum, which, in turn, is enveloped in perichondrium. Microscopic studies of sections removed from the junction of bone and cartilage in the vomeroseptal maxillary crest region reveal the perichondrial envelopment of the septal cartilage and its fusion with the periosteum of the bone below. The two opposing membranes form a smooth surface between bone and cartilage, especially at the junction of vomer, maxillary crest, and maxillary spine, where the groove of the vomer is usually shallow or flat. This region is therefore a weak point and a frequent site of traumatic dislocations. Furthermore, the bones themselves form a smooth surface. The lower end of the vomer is smooth and rests on the smooth concave surface of the maxillary crest, which, in turn, rests on the smooth concave surface of the nasal spine.

From observations made at the operating table, in the majority of patients a dislocation is usually accompanied by a deviation of the vomer and maxillary crest and spine along with the septal cartilage. These findings are either developmental in origin or traumatic at age 6 or 7. Trauma in early childhood is an important factor because the maxillary crests and vomer are not completely ossified, and a slight shifting of these tissues may cause the crest and vomer, as they develop, to grow to the side. This situation results in a flattening of the vomerian groove and the loss of its lip on the side of deviation. Some of these deviations may have their origin in birth trauma. Cases in which the septal cartilage is displaced from the vomer and maxillary crest are usually traumatic in origin, the injury occurring, in most instances, some time after the child reaches the age of 6 or 7. Complicated septal dislocation, accompanied by buckling, twisting, and reduplication of cartilage and marked internal deformity of depression and deviation, invariably results from trauma.

Some developmental factors in the etiology of the dislocated septum may be gathered from the embryonal description of the nasopalatal relationship and the influence of palatal development on the floor of the septum. Formation of the premaxilla, eruption of the permanent incisor teeth, asymmetric development of the maxillary sinuses, thumb sucking and tongue pressure habits with resultant shifting of the alveolar ridge, mouth breathing, and congenital deformities such as cleft lip and palate are some causative factors that may account for developmental disturbances. The eruption of the permanent incisor teeth and its effect on the septum were well described by Mosher, who believed that deformities of the septum are infrequent and rarely marked in children before the second dentition. The disproportion in growth among the premaxilla, vomer, and ethmoid, with downward encroachment of the cranial cavity, is probably the dominant factor, however.

Nasal Septal Reconstruction

Introduction and Philosophy

The functions of the nasal septum have been described as follows:

1. Support of the external nose.
2. Regulation of air flow.
3. Support of nasal mucosa.

Since the turn of the century, procedures designed to improve the nasal airway while preserving these functions have been developed (and occasionally discarded). The classic "submucous resection (SMR)" with sacrifice of considerable portions of bone and cartilage has fortunately given way to more conservative procedures involving structural preservation and reconstruction. Aside from historical significance, there remains little purpose in retaining the term "SMR" with its more radical implications. The term "RNS" (reconstruction of the nasal septum) or "septoplasty" conveys the meaning of contemporary septal operations more clearly.

Preservative septal surgery is further justified by normal anatomy. Few "normal" septa are perfectly straight, existing without imperfection. Minor septal irregularities after appropriate reconstruction are inconsequential, provided they create no obstruction and contribute to no external nasal deformity. Radical septal resections in pursuit of a "straight" septum are therefore generally without virtue.

Septal reconstruction is usually carried out with (and usually as an integral part of) rhinoplasty. Reduction rhinoplasties invariably diminish breathing space. Reconstructive septoplasty can rescue an airway otherwise potentially compromised by a purely aesthetic procedure. Invariably, the deformed septum contributes to the anatomic deficit inherent in the twisted nose and is best corrected at the outset of septorhinoplasty. It is frequently remarkable at the operating table how initial septoplasty transforms the crooked nose into near-perfect cartilaginous alignment. As in all surgery where perfection is the goal, a secondary procedure of lesser magnitude may be occasionally required (less than 5% of all procedures), and all patients deserve to know that fact before undergoing a reconstructive procedure ("the crooked nose has a memory").

Finally, preservative conservation septal surgery should totally negate the most severe sequelae of more radical septal resections: columellar retraction, saddle nose, airway collapse, loss of tip support, and septal perforation. The latter conditions present complex difficult reconstructive exercises and are better avoided than risked.

Principles of Septal Reconstruction

If the preceding philosophy is accepted, certain precepts emerge as cardinal to all septal surgery. These precepts have as their basis an increasingly detailed, atraumatic dissection and mobilization of the septal components, an assessment of the obstructive problem, and finally, a reconstruction and realignment after minimal tissue sacrifice. These major steps involve the following surgical phases, not always carried out in this sequence:

1. Whenever possible, elevate only one side mucoperichondrial flap.
2. Atraumatically disarticulate the attachment of the quadrangular cartilage to the perpendicular plate of the ethmoid and to the vomer. If a vertical angulation exists just caudal to this articulation, a common site of deviation, the disarticulation can be positioned at this angulation.
3. Mobilize the quadrangular cartilage along the floor of the nose at the maxillary crest. A narrow horizontal strip of cartilage may be removed to

facilitate this mobilization without compromising septal support.
4. Isolate the *bony* septum between its bilaterally elevated mucoperiosteal flaps and medially reposition or resect the portion creating obstruction (bone grafts are commonly taken at this juncture).
5. Realign the cartilaginous septum with the conservative manipulations to be described subsequently.
6. Stabilize all realigned septal segments with quilting mattress transeptal absorbable sutures during the healing phase.

Certain vital fundamental technical concepts are required to accomplish these goals of septal reconstruction:

1. Perform all septal surgery under direct vision. Intense fiberoptic headlighting, long nasal specula, complete septal mobilization, and effective vasoconstriction make this an easily realized surgical prerequisite.
2. Preserve the contralateral mucoperichondrial flap for support, septal cartilage nutrition, and stability. Exceptions to this principle exist but are infrequent.
3. Preserve the caudal septal relationship with the membranous columella and feet of the medial crura. Severe caudal subluxation may negate this principle.
4. Dissect and mobilize the septal components fully before final deformity diagnosis. Only now should the extent of a conservative resection be planned.
5. Resist the temptation to resect more radically in pursuit of a "perfectly straight" septum.
6. In septorhinoplasty of the twisted nose, generally the septal realignment is best created before tip and profile reconstruction. Septoplasty in combined procedures frequently requires more technical ingenuity than rhinoplasty.
7. Religiously avoid removal of septal cartilage contributing important strength to the structure of the external nose.
8. Dissect from the "known to the unknown," to best avoid development of tears and flap perforation. If perforations are created, repair with fine suture technique.
9. Unless it contributes to deformity, preserve the upper lateral cartilage attachment to the septum.
10. Control and stabilize final septal alignment with judiciously placed transeptal sutures, thereby preventing cartilage segment overrides, hematoma, and unfavorable fibrosis. The need for long-term septal splints is thereby lessened or negated.

11. Avoid long-term intranasal packing and tamponade, a more traditional than useful exercise.

12. Constantly reassess and diagnose the obstructive problem during the course of septal surgery with inspection *combined with intranasal palpation.* As in rhinoplasty, the anatomic metamorphosis in septoplasty is dynamic and interdependent, each surgical step often dramatically influencing the next. Remain flexible in ideas and approach, ready to incorporate surgical options as required.

13. Understand that airway improvement, particularly in the twisted nose (or as the sequela of old comminuted fractures) may require nasal osteotomies to achieve optimum breathing space.

Progressive Integrated Technique of Septal Reconstruction

The surgical steps described subsequently have been evaluated over a period of 20 years and found effective in 90% of all septal deformities. They are based on the principles of structural preservation and septal realignment rather than resection, with final suture stabilization of the realigned septal components. Deviation from these principles is not usually required, except in the rarer anatomic circumstances to be described.

ANESTHESIA AND ANALGESIA. With few exceptions, septoplasty and septorhinoplasty are performed under a combination of monitored intravenous analgesia, local infiltration, and topical anesthesia. The patient's comfort is ensured, little bleeding develops, and the patient's condition is constantly monitored by the anesthesiologist. Intravenous sedation is administered in titrated fashion until patient comfort and tranquilization are achieved.

Neurosurgical cottonoids containing 5% cocaine solution (color coded for easy identification) are positioned under direct vision in each nasal cavity. One or two on either side ensures adequate topical anesthesia, vasoconstriction, and nasal tamponade. The mucoperichondrial flap on the intended side of dissection (ordinarily the concave side) is generously infiltrated with a standard solution of 1% lidocaine with epinephrine. Accurately piercing the submucoperichondrial plane with a No. 27 gauge needle provides a "hydraulic dissection," facilitating a rapid and bloodless flap elevation. Additional infiltration anesthesia is used according to the planned extent of septal dissection.

Twelve to 15 minutes of delay should now ensue while vasoconstriction becomes intense. During this period, final inspection and palpation of the cocainized internal nose often reveals irregularities high in the nasal vaults not previously seen. X-ray evaluation at this juncture may aid in surgical planning. The value of *palpation* of the deformed septum and of the structural strength of the nasal tip-supportive elements cannot be overemphasized.

MOBILIZATION OF QUADRANGULAR CARTILAGE. Elevation of the mucoperichondrial septal flap is usually initiated through a vertical incision placed 2 to 3 mm cephalic to the caudal end of the septal cartilage on the concave side of the septum (Fig. 2–66). Actually, it makes little difference on which side this incision is

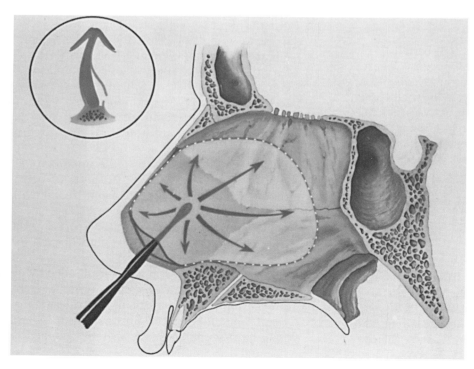

Fig. 2–66. Septal incision is created just cephalic to the mucocutaneous junction.

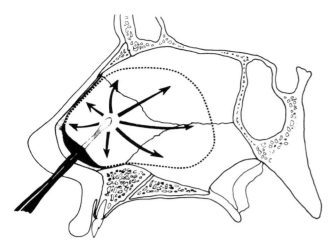

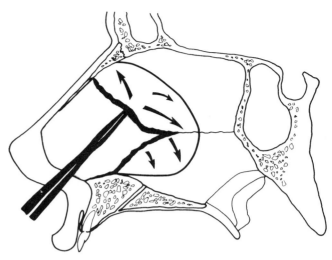

Fig. 2–67. The submucoperichondrial plane up to and in continuity with the subperiosteal plane overlying the perpendicular plate of the ethmoid and vomer is created with semisharp Dunning elevator.

Fig. 2–68. Disarticulation of the bony and cartilaginous septum.

placed. Preserving the normal attachment of the mucoperichondrial flap on the convex side of the septal deformity, however, seems technically easier. If severe caudal septal dislocation exists, a hemitransfixion or complete transfixion incision is generally used.

The submucoperichondrial plane is located and developed with a semisharp Dunning elevator under direct vision (Fig. 2–67). If fracture adhesions, cartilage overlaps, or severe scarring interferes, the dissection is carried out by bypassing these vexing areas and dissecting above or below as required initially to circumvent areas of difficult dissection. Proper hydraulic lidocaine infiltration, as described, facilitates this elevation technique.

This dissection plane is continued onto the ethmoid perpendicular plate and vomer, elevating the continuous ipsilateral mucoperichondrial-mucoperiosteal space. Moderate pressure with the tip of the elevator at the junction (articulation) of the cartilaginous and bony septal components disarticulates these elements and initiates the dissection of the contralateral mucoperiosteal flap (Fig. 2–68). Because this area is a common site of septal fractures and angulation, the disarticulation can also be accomplished in a previous fracture line.

A reassessment of the septal anatomy (and deformity) is now in order. This initial dissection frequently has allowed the quadrangular cartilage to return to the midline without further surgery, being freed from a deviated ethmoid or vomer. The cartilage may be held by a subluxation along the maxillary crest, which is overcome by resecting a horizontal strip of cartilage (and frequently bone) from along the floor of the nose. Any fibrous tissue bands further contributing to a displaced position of the cartilage are divided with sharp knife dissection. These steps will now have completely freed and mobilized the quadrangular cartilage and

usually allow its return to the midline without further surgical manipulation.

CORRECTION OF BONY OBSTRUCTION. Deformities of the bony septum, particularly those high in the nasal vault, are now exposed between the blades of a long nasal speculum; selective resection of obstructing bone is gently carried out with small biting (Takahashi) forceps until the airway is clear (Fig. 2–69). Larger pieces of bone required for graft or implants may be resected

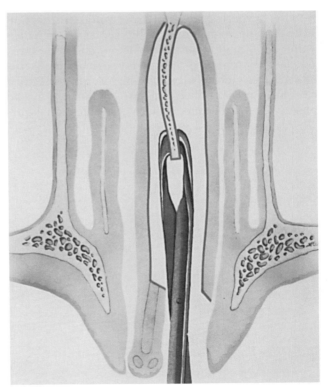

Fig. 2–69. Removal of obstructing portions of the bony septum with a small biting forceps (Takahashi).

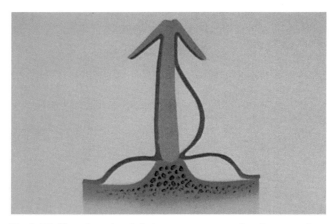

Fig. 2–70. Elevation of an inferior compartment of periosteum along the floor of the nose to gain better access to deviated bony septal components.

with fine osteotomes, heavy scissors, or bone-biting forceps. Great care should be taken in older patients (particularly osteoporotic women) to remove only small portions of the perpendicular plate of the ethmoid. The vomer provides an excellent source of bone-grafting material; flaps should be completely bilaterally elevated to avoid creating flap tears or avulsions during vomerine resection.

These steps in surgical dissection of the septum are relatively routinely carried out in most patients and frequently are all that is required to establish a greatly improved airway. At this point in the septal reconstruction, a *reassessment* is in order before further surgery. Visually and palpably, the septal alignment is evaluated. If alignment is satisfactory and the airway adequate, flap suture-closure is carried out as described later. If the airway remains unsatisfactory, what creates the problem and how is it most easily and conservatively corrected? Once this question is an-

swered, a variety of the following corrections are variously carried out, depending on the existent deformity, its location, and its extent.

ANCILLARY CORRECTIVE PROCEDURES. Significant obstructing deformities along the floor of the nose (cartilaginous or bony spurs and ridges, which often contribute to drying, ulceration, and bleeding) may require an approach created by elevating a second compartment of periosteum along the floor of the nose (Fig. 2–70). The periosteum overlying the premaxilla and maxillary crest is incised and a submucoperiosteal pocket created with the elevator. The two compartments (subperiosteal and subperichondrial) are then connected, exposing the maxillary crest deformity for osteotome and/or rongeur removal.

A vertical angulation of the septum, if contributing to deformity and obstruction (often the site of an old fracture), may be removed with a conservative vertical cartilage strip resection (Fig. 2–71), with realignment carried out by absorbable suture technique.

Similarly, horizontal septal angulations or spurs are resected by means of conservative horizontal strips, again leaving all remaining cartilage segments securely attached to the contralateral undissected mucoperichondrium. *Thinning* the quadrangular cartilage with *shave excision* techniques in a horizontal or vertical plane may contribute to airway improvement without significantly altering the supportive strength of the cartilage (Fig. 2–72).

Significant dislocation of the caudal septum from the midline, whether developmental or traumatic, requires ingenuity in reconstructive techniques to resist the temptation to resect significant caudal segments, thereby risking columellar retraction and loss of tip support.

A vertical incision (or narrow cartilage excision) cephalic to the point of angulation, combined with

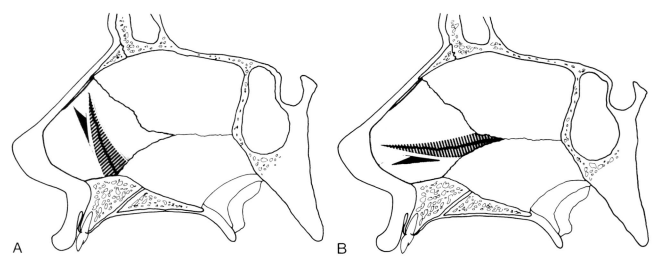

A   B

Fig. 2–71. Vertical (A) or horizontal (B) angulations of the nasal septum may be removed through wedge resection.

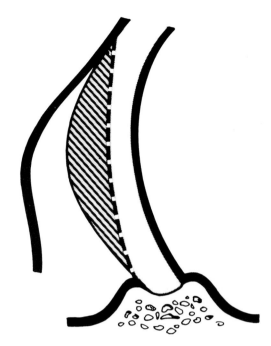

Fig. 2–72. Shave excision techniques in overthick quadrangular cartilages may substantially improve the nasal airway.

freeing the caudal segment from the nasal floor, generally creates a caudal "swinging door" segment that is sutured to the midline columella and occasionally to the midline mucoperiosteum. Further weakening of a deformed caudal segment without total structural sacrifice may be created by generous "cross-hatching," shave excision, and even conservative morselization. Limited contralateral mucoperichondrial flap elevation at the caudal segment facilities its realignment.

An overlong caudal septum, malaligned or not, may require thinning or shortening to facilitate repositioning, particularly during septorhinoplasty procedures.

Occasionally, a previously fractured nasal spine, positioned off the midline, will require refracturing and fixation to the midline to reposition the caudal septum adequately. Unless it deforms the nasolabial angle, the spine is seldom sacrificed, to avoid potential loss of tip support and columellar retraction.

Deformed upper lateral cartilages, the product of maldevelopment or trauma, are occasionally responsible for misalignment of the cartilaginous septum. Inspection and palpation confirm this suspicion. Submucosal dissection and freeing of the upper lateral cartilages from the septum allow further septal mobilization and realignment. This situation, however, is rarely encountered. Preserving the upper lateral septal attachment is preferred.

Final correction of some varieties of badly twisted noses may require realignment of the bony nasal pyramid to mobilize and straighten the septum (and therefore the nose) completely. Such instances are ordinarily the consequence of old trauma (Fig. 2–73).

Persistent airway blockade after careful septal reconstruction is commonly caused by enlargement of the inferior turbinate to partially fill the concavity created by septal deviation. Return of the septum to midline further diminishes the airway. Partial sacrifice of the inferior turbinate (resection, cautery, freezing, crushing, etc.) has never seemed appropriate or physiologic, even when successful. I prefer a submucosal elevation of the turbinate tissue with resection of the bulky bone of the inferior concha (Fig. 2–74). The turbinate is reattached with absorbable sutures and now occupies considerably less space than originally.

Infrequently, in the most severe quadrangular cartilage deformities, extensive cross-hatching, crushing, or morselization of the cartilage is used to "break the spring" totally. These procedures are generally reserved for the more caudal portions of the quadrangular cartilage and are used only in the severest deformities. Bilateral mucoperichondrial flap elevation is usually required, and precise healing is often less predictable than when more conservative measures are employed.

Implantation of autogenous cartilaginous supports in the columella is frequently used, lending support to the tip, correcting retracted columellar deformities, and enhancing the nasolabial angle anatomy. Thin cartilage wafers positioned along the cartilaginous profile line are useful in effacing a slight depression and can be particularly helpful in camouflaging a slightly deviated dorsum without risking breaking the dorsal support with surgical manipulations.

Finally, the complete nasal surgeon should be aware of the occasional reconstructive advantages offered by the technique of *external rhinoplasty.* Advantages include a superb direct vision approach, direct anterior appraisal of the deformed elements, and superior suture realignment of reconstructed septal elements.

PRESERVATION OF REALIGNMENT. With progressive use of the foregoing integrated techniques, most deviated septa may be appropriately reconstructed rather than resected and the septal functions preserved without embarrassing septal support. Controlling the healing process totally is not possible, but it can be favorably influenced by the suture techniques to be described.

All incisions, including any small flap perforations that occasionally occur, are closed with 5–0 absorbable suture.

A series of similar transeptal transperichondrial through and through sutures are now positioned to coapt the septal flap(s), thereby closing all dead space. Hemostasis is promoted and hematoma is avoided. Further fixation sutures to preserve the realignment of cartilage segments are positioned after the manner of Wright to prevent slippage and overriding. The presence of one intact undissected mucoperichondrial flap

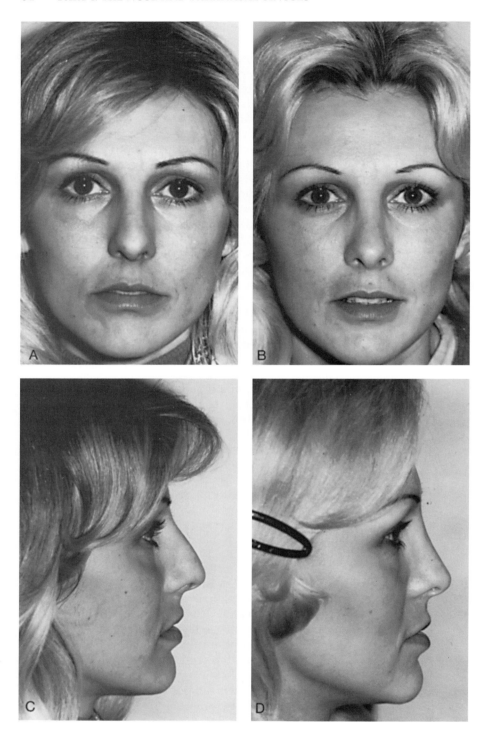

Fig. 2–73. Patient before and 1 year after total septorhinoplasty. A. Front view before surgery. B. Front view after surgery. C. Profile before surgery. D. Profile after surgery.

provides a great advantage in stabilizing the septal reconstruction.

Septal splints are required only rarely when these methods are used. Telfa gauze rolls are placed in each nasal vault to absorb drainage and lightly splint the dissected flaps and are removed in 12 to 24 hours.

If osteotomies have been performed, or after the occasional *external* septorhinoplasty, an external cast is applied for 7 days.

SEPTAL PERFORATIONS: MYOMUCOSAL FLAP REPAIR

Septal perforations present a peculiar challenge to the reconstructive nasal surgeon. They appear as clear tissue voids—at times overt, more often occult—and tantalizingly invite surgical repair. In truth, only selected septal perforations deserve or require repair. All too often, in order to restore septal integrity, the well-in-

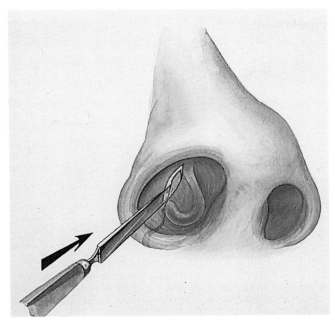

Fig. 2–74. Reduction of enlarged turbinate mass is effected by submucosal resection of enlarged bony concha, preserving the majority of turbinate tissue.

tentioned surgeon attempts repair. Failure of healing is not uncommon (witness the plethora of variable procedures advocated for septal repair), and not infrequently a small perforation assumes larger proportions on failure of the graft (or flap) to survive. Careful selection of patients for septal perforation closure is therefore of critical importance.

Etiology of Septal Perforation

The major causes of septal perforations have changed considerably in past decades (Table 2–3). Septal perforation in conjunction with surgery is uncommon but is still encountered. With the emphasis changing from classic submucous resection surgery to a more progres-

TABLE 2–3. Causes of Septal Perforations

Trauma
  Surgical
  Post-traumatic septal abscess
  Repeated septal cautery
Disease states
  Syphilis
  Tuberculosis
  Wegener's granulomatosis
  Metal poisoning
  Lupus erythematosus
  Chronic relapsing perichondritis
  Atrophic rhinitis
  Cocaine abuse
Nasal neoplasms
Idiopathic causes

sive and conservative septoplasty approach, postoperative septal perforations of any consequence have diminished in frequency. Trauma to the opposing mucoperichondrial flaps, septal hematoma and necrosis, and overzealous tight nasal packing contribute to postoperative perforations. With proper transseptal suture repair after septal reconstruction, nasal packing is unnecessary.

Cocaine abuse represents the current major cause of anterior septal perforations, some astoundingly large.

As nasal trauma increases in all age groups, such as from automobile accidents, muggings, little league baseball, and junior hockey, more unrecognized septal hematomas occur; septal abscess with perforation may result. All patients sustaining nasal trauma deserve immediate intranasal examination by a competent rhinologist, with prompt drainage of significant hematoma.

Repeated septal cautery for epistaxis control not uncommonly is to blame for small to medium-sized anterior septal perforations. Factitious digital trauma (nose picking) predisposes to septal scarring and avascular necrosis.

Various disease states, less commonly, predispose to septal perforations. These include syphilis, tuberculosis, Wegener's granulomatosis, metal poisoning, lupus erythematosus, chronic relapsing perichondritis, and atrophic rhinitis. Patients with coexisting septal perforation and body tattoos should alert the clinician to the possibility of luetic involvement by the contaminated tattooing needle. Nasal neoplasms must be considered and searched for if septal integrity is lost.

Indications for Surgical Repair

In the majority of patients with septal perforations, initial evaluation, elucidation of the cause of the effect, and informed reassurance are indicated. Whistling sounds through small anterior perforations occur but are uncommon and are seldom distressing. Large septal voids are seldom symptomatic and only infrequently create abnormal nasal sounds of any consequence.

The patient with continuous or recurrent severe bleeding and crusting is a candidate for surgical repair. A vicious circle has ordinarily developed in these individuals, with local drying, crusting, bleeding, and scarring. Repair is indicated in such a case, for effective rehabilitation of the patient and control of hemorrhage. Effective symptomatic relief consists of intranasal Neodecadron ophthalmic ointment applied twice daily, but it may not suffice to control symptoms in the long term.

Technique of Repair

During the past 20 years, a pedicle flap of buccal mucosa and muscle from beneath the upper lip has served

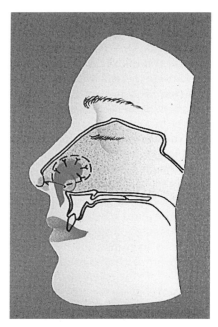

Fig. 2–75. Sublabial myomucosal pedicle flap, tunneled through an oronasal fistula into the nasal cavity, is the technique of choice for repair of significant septal perforations.

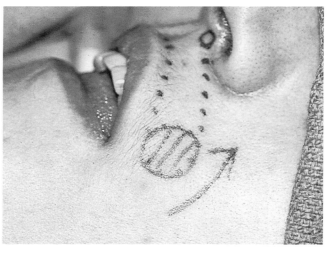

Fig. 2–77. Outline of myomucosal sublabial flap on the upper lip. Circled area indicates region where a disk of cartilage is implanted when a composite flap is planned. The circle at the base of the columella indicates the internal site where the sublabial oronasal fissula is carried out.

admirably in the effective closure of septal perforations of various dimensions. Multiple advantages accrue to the surgeon employing this technique. Because it is based medially near the frenulum of the upper lip, an abundant amount of buccal mucosa is available for transposition to the recipient site. The flap carries its own blood supply, remaining independent of the need for immediate nourishment from an ordinarily poorly vascularized septal host bed. The flap is tunneled through a stab incision in the floor of the adjacent nasal

vestibule, providing immediate access to the perforation.

Formerly, we sutured the contoured flap to the freshened edge of the perforation and applied a buccal mucosa or fascial graft to the opposite side of the septum. More recently, we have avoided the free graft, which has been found to be unnecessary for effective closure of the perforation. The bridge of the flap may be divided in the office under local anesthesia 4 to 6 weeks following primary repair.

For larger perforations (greater than 2.5 cm), a composite flap incorporating ear cartilage into the distal end of the flap is fashioned. A thinned disk of auricular

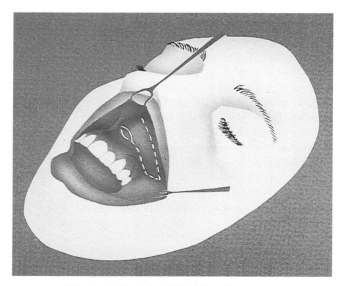

Fig. 2–76. Typical sublabial flap donor site.

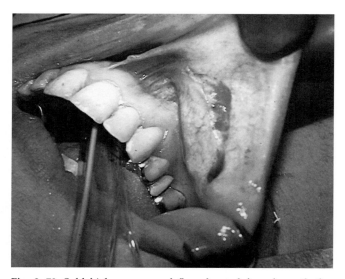

Fig. 2–78. Sublabial myomucosal flap elevated from beneath the upper lip in preparation for tunneling through the oronasal fissula into the nose.

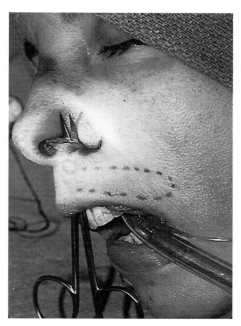

Fig. 2–79. Sublabial oronasal fissula created into the nasal cavity, through which the sublabial flap will be transferred.

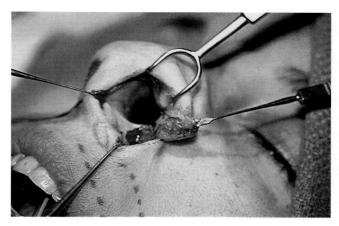

Fig. 2–81. A lateral alotomy of the nose provides useful additional access to the perforation site for appropriate positioning of the flap and careful suture fixation. If the perforation is large and posterior, an open approach to the nose, combined with an alotomy, can be additionally helpful in exposure.

cartilage is harvested and buried in the lateral aspect of the upper lip mucosa. Two weeks later, the flap is elevated and transposed to the perforation site. The security of suture placement is enhanced by the presence of cartilage.

The open rhinoplasty approach, because of the greater exposure provided, may be combined with a

unilateral alotomy to provide unparalleled access to perforations more cephalically located in the septum. Working from above downward as well as below upward through this approach facilitates the ease of bimanual suturing.

Management of the donor site can be individualized. Minimal donor site defects may be closed primarily with mucosal sutures. Larger donor defects, following thorough cautery hemostasis, may be left unrepaired because they heal uneventfully by secondary intention. If required, bilateral sublabial mucosal pedicle flaps may be elevated and transposed primarily to create bilateral reinforcement of a large, scarred perforation.

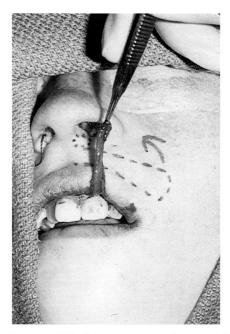

Fig. 2–80. Typical sublabial flap elevated and exposed for demonstration purposes, preparatory to being tunneled through the sublabial oronasal fissula.

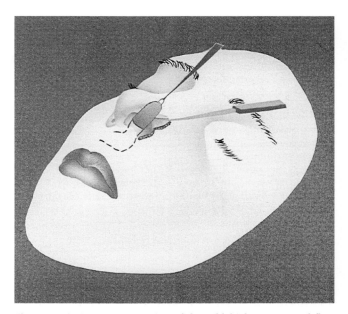

Fig. 2–82. Artist's representation of the sublabial myomucosal flap transposed to the septal perforation.

Experience has led us to prefer this method of pedicle flap repair of perforations of the nasal septum. The technique of repairing septal perforations with the versatile sublabial mucosal flap is shown in Figures 2–75 through 2–82.

SUGGESTED READINGS

Anderson JR: New approach to rhinoplasty. Arch Otolaryngol *93:* 284, 1971.

Becker OJ: Problems of the septum in rhinoplastic surgery. Arch Otolaryngol *53:*622, 1951.

Becker OJ: The routine corrective rhinoplasty operation. Trans Am Acad Ophthalmol Otolaryygol *68:*830, 1964.

Bloom SM: The problem of implants in rhinoplasty, including technique of obtaining iliac crest grafts. Arch Otolaryngol *71:*778, 1960.

Bloom SM: Rhinoplasty in adolescence. Arch Otolaryngol *92:*66, 1970.

Bloom SM: Implants and grafts in nasal reconstruction. In: Plastic and Reconstructive Surgery of the Face and Neck: Proceedings of the First International Symposium, New York. Edited by Conley J and Dickinson J. Stuttgart, Georg Thieme, 1971, p 156.

Book HE: Psychiatric assessment for rhinoplasty. Arch Otolaryngol *94:*851, 1971.

Cinelli JA: Surgical formulae for common nasal tip problems. Eye Ear Nose Throat Monthly *44(May):*99, 1965; *44(June):*96, 1965.

Converse JM: Deviated nose: panel discussion. Trans Am Acad Ophthalmol Otolaryngol *58:*741, 1954.

Converse JM (ed): Reconstructive Plastic Surgery. Vols 1 to 3. Philadelphia, WB Saunders, 1964.

Denecke HJ and Meyer R: Plastic Surgery of the Head and Neck: Corrective and Reconstructive Rhinoplasty. New York, Springer, 1967.

Dingman R and Walter C: Use of composite ear grafts in correction of the short nose. Plast Reconstr Surg *43:*117, 1969.

Farrior RT: The problems of the unilateral cleft-lip nose. Laryngoscope *72:*289, 1962.

Farrior RT: Synthetics in head and neck surgery. Arch Ophthalmol *84:*82, 1966.

Farrior RT: Implant materials restoration of facial contour. Laryngoscope *76:*934, 1966.

Farrior RT: Corrective surgery of the nasal framework. J Fla Med Assoc *45:*276, 1968.

Farrior RT: Septorhinoplasty in children: Otolaryngology Clinics of NH. Pediatr Otolaryngol *3:*345, 1970.

Fomon S, Gilbert JG, Silver AG, and Syracuse VR: Plastic repair of the obstructing nasal septum. Arch Otolaryngol *47:*7, 1948.

Fomon S, Goldman IB, Neivert H, and Schattner A: Management of deformities of the lower cartilaginous vault. Arch Otolaryngol *54:*467, 1951.

Fomon S, Syracuse VR, Bolotow N, and Pullen M: Plastic repair of the defective nasal septum. Arch Otolaryngol *44:*141, 1946.

Freud S: Civilization and Its Discontents. London: Hogart Press, 1930.

Frye H: Interlocked stresses of cartilage. Br J Plast Surg *19:*276, 1966.

Frye H: Cartilage and cartilage grafts: basic properties of tissue and its components responsible for them. Plast Reconstr Surg *40:* 426, 1967.

Frye H: Importance of septal cartilage in nasal trauma. Br J Plast Surg *20:*392, 1967.

Frye H: Nasal skeletal trauma and the interlocked stress of the septal cartilage. Br J Plast Surg *20:*146, 1967.

Gilbert JC and Segal S: Growth of the nose and the septorhinoplastic problems in youth. Arch Otolaryngol *68:*673, 1958.

Goldman IB: Analysis of osseous complications in rhinoplasty. Eye Ear Nose Throat Monthly *42:*78, 1963.

Goldman IB: Nasal plastic surgery: late results. Eye Ear Nose Throat Monthly *42:*88, 1963.

Goldman IB: Nasal tip correction with special reference to the medial crura. Trans Am Acad Ophthalmol Otolaryngol *68:*854, 1964.

Goldman IB: Rhinoplastic sequelae causing nasal obstruction. Arch Otolaryngol *83:*151, 1966.

Hilger J: Internal lateral osteotomy in rhinoplasty. Arch Otolaryngol *88:*211, 1968.

Holmes EM: Restoration of nasal contour lost through deficient septal cartilage. Trans Am Acad Ophthalmol Otolaryngol *68:*874, 1964.

Huffman WC and Lierle D: The deviated nose. Ann Otol Rhinol Laryngol *63:*62, 1954.

Huffman WC and Lierle D: Reduction of the prominent nasofrontal angle. Trans Am Acad Ophthalmol Otolaryngol *68:*838, 1964.

Janeke JB: Studies on the support of the nasal tip. Arch Otolaryngol *93:*458, 1971.

Joseph J: Nasenplastik und sonstige Gesichtplastik: nebst einem Anhang über Mammaplastik und einage weitere Operationen aus dem Gebiete der aussen Korperplastik, Leipzig, Kabitzsch 1931.

Marquit B: Radiated homogenous cartilage in rhinoplasty. Arch Otolaryngol *85:*100, 1967.

Millard DR: Adjuncts in augmentation mentoplasty and corrective rhinoplasty. Plast Reconstr Surg *36:*48, 1965.

Parkes ML and Brennan HG: High septal transfixion to shorten the nose. Plast Reconstr Surg *45:*487, 1970.

Peer LA: An operation to repair lateral displacement of the lower border of the septal cartilage. Arch Otolaryngol *25:*475, 1937.

Rees TD, et al: Secondary rhinoplasty. Plast Reconstr Surg *46:*332, 1970.

Roe J: The deformity termed "plug nose" and its correction by a simple operation. Plast Reconstr Surg *45:*78, 1970.

Rubin FF: Permanent change in shape of cartilage by morselization. Arch Otolaryngol *89:*602, 1969.

Safian J: Deceptive concepts in rhinoplasty. Plast Reconstr Surg *18:* 127, 1956.

Santayana G: The Sense of Beauty. Originality published by Charles Scribner's Sons, 1896. Dover Edition, 1955, unabridged, New York, NY.

Schilder P: The Image and Appearance of the Human Body. New York, NY: Wiley, 1964

Schutz RD: Facial Injuries. Chicago, Year Book, 1971.

Smith HW: Septal bone grafts: correction of saddle nose. Arch Otolaryngol *92:*230, 1970.

Smith TW: The selection of patients for rhinoplasty. Arch Otolaryngol *94:*56, 1971.

Stewart M: Psychological problems of patients requesting rhinoplasty. Trans Am Acad Ophthalmol Otolaryngol *68:*881, 1964.

Tardy ME, et al: Reconstructive Surgery of the Deviated Septum and Nose. Memphis, TN, Richards Manufacturing, 1982.

Tardy ME: Rhinoplasty tip ptosis: etiology and prevention. Laryngoscope *83:*923, 1973.

Tardy ME: Surgical Anatomy of the Nose. New York, Raven Press, 1991.

Unger M: Architectural design of the nasal septum. Laryngoscope *75:*322, 1965.

Walter C: Composite grafts in nasal surgery. Arch Otolaryngol *90:* 622, 1969.

Wright WK: Lateral osteotomy in rhinoplasty. Arch Otolaryngol *78:* 680, 1963.

Wright WK: Study on hump removal in rhinoplasty. Laryngoscope *77:*508, 1967.

Wright WK: General principles of nasal septum reconstruction. Trans Am Acad Ophthalmol Otolaryngol *73:*252, 1969.

3 Etiology of Infectious Diseases of the Upper Respiratory Tract

Darrell H. Hunsaker and John L. Boone

Upper respiratory infection (URI) is one of the most common ailments that patients bring to the primary care physician or otolaryngologist. The importance of understanding the causes of these infections is evident. This chapter is divided into five sections. The first reviews pathogens of URI infections according to anatomic sites. The following sections cover those viral, bacterial, fungal, and protozoan infections that are of special interest or importance.

CAUSES BY ANATOMIC SITE

Pathogens principally responsible for URI are listed by anatomic site in Table 3–1. This listing is not intended to be exhaustive, but is limited to causes that are predominant for each site.

Common Cold

The common cold is an acute, self-limited viral disease characterized by nasal stuffiness, coryza, throat irritation, and no or minimal fever (see Chap. 6). Infection is spread by direct contact with virus-contaminated respiratory secretions. Inoculation occurs at the nasal mucosa and, perhaps, the conjunctiva. Most of the viruses possess surface molecules that bind them to epithelial surfaces. Viral replication follows. Epithelial cell destruction varies according to the virus involved. Among the more constant histopathologic changes are submucosal edema, infiltration by inflammatory cells, and the release of inflammatory mediators such as bradykinin. Infection is opposed by host production of interferon and by the action of cytotoxic cells such as nonspecific natural killer cells and specific T lymphocytes.

More than 200 viruses have been associated with the common cold. The most important of these come from the 5 viral families listed in Table 3–1. Rhinoviruses of the family Picornaviridae account for one third to one half of common colds. More than 100 serotypes have been described. These small, naked viruses contain a single molecule of RNA and are relatively stable in the environment. Rhinovirus infections occur year round, with peaks in the early spring and fall months in the temperate zones, and during the rainy period in the tropics. Coronaviruses are another important cause of colds, accounting for about 10% of infections. These are most prevalent in winter. At least 2 different serotypes cause URIs,[1] and reinfections are common. Parainfluenza viruses and the respiratory syncytial virus are members of the Paramyxoviridae family. They are primarily known as causes of lower respiratory tract infections, but also account for a proportion of common colds. Reinfections occur throughout life.[1] Influenza viruses usually produce a primary influenza-like illness; however, subsequent infections with the same or similar serotype may result in common cold symptoms. Adenoviruses are an important cause of acute upper and lower respiratory tract infections, including the common cold. Specific serotypes are associated with pharyngoconjunctival fever and epidemic keratoconjunctivitis. Adenoviruses are also important causes of pharyngitis and pneumonia, especially in military recruits.

Pharyngitis

In most cases of acute pharyngitis, particularly mild cases, it is not possible to determine a specific microbiologic cause on clinical grounds alone. In a study of pharyngitis in adults, clinical findings such as fever, adenopathy, and exudate correlated imperfectly with microbiologic findings.[2]

TABLE 3–1. Anatomic Sites of Disease

Disease and Site	Causative Agents
Common cold (upper respiratory tract)	Viral Rhinoviruses Coronaviruses Parainfluenza viruses Respiratory syncytial virus Influenza viruses Adenoviruses
Pharyngitis (Pharynx)	Viral Rhinoviruses Coronaviruses Adenoviruses Influenza viruses Parainfluenza viruses Respiratory syncytial virus Coxsackieviruses Bacterial Group A β-hemolytic streptococci (S. pyogenes) Anaerobic bacteria Neisseria gonorrhoeae
Acute supraglottitis (Epiglottis)	Bacterial Haemophilus influenzae type b
Acute laryngotracheobronchitis (Larynx, trachea)	Viral Parainfluenza viruses Influenza viruses
Acute sinusitis (Sinuses)	Bacterial Streptococcus pneumoniae Haemophilus influenzae Moraxella catarrhalis
Chronic sinusitis (Sinuses)	Bacterial (mixed infections common) Streptococcus pneumoniae Haemophilus influenzae Moraxella catarrhalis Anaerobes Staphylococcus aureus α-Hemolytic streptococci
Acute otitis media (Ear)	Bacterial Streptococcus pneumoniae Haemophilus influenzae Moraxella catarrhalis
Chronic otitis media (mixed infections common) (Ear)	Bacterial Streptococcus pneumoniae Haemophilus influenzae Moraxella catarrhalis Anaerobic bacteriae Staphylococcus aureus Pseudomonas aeruginosa

About 70% of acute sore throats are caused by viruses.[3] Most of these occur as part of common cold or influenza syndromes. The most common viral agents are rhinovirus, coronavirus, adenovirus, influenza, and parainfluenza viruses.[4] Other associated viruses include respiratory syncytial virus, herpes simplex virus (types 1 and 2), Coxsackievirus, Epstein-Barr virus, cytomegalovirus, and human immunodeficiency virus (HIV).

Adenoviruses are common agents of acute pharyn-gitis and cause a major share of pharyngitis in military recruits. Sore throat is severe and may be accompanied by cough, hoarseness, and substernal pain. Fever, chills, malaise, myalgias, and headache are generally present. Adenoviruses are also the cause of pharyngo-conjunctival fever, a syndrome characterized by fever, pharyngitis, and follicular conjunctivitis. Community epidemics of this infection most often center around contaminated public swimming pools.

Herpangina is a vesicular and ulcerative condition of the pharynx and is one manifestation of infection by enteroviruses. Coxsackieviruses A and B and, to a lesser extent, echoviruses have been identified as etiologic agents. Infection occurs most frequently in children during summer and fall. Onset is heralded by fever, which is followed by the development of small (1- to 2- mm) mucosal vesicles and ulcers. Over 2 to 3 days these enlarge to 3 to 4 mm and are surrounded by erythematous rings. Lesions are most commonly noted on the anterior tonsillar pillars, as well as the soft palate, tonsils, pharyngeal walls, and posterior buccal mucosa. Uninvolved areas of the pharynx appear normal or are only slightly erythematous. Fever and sore throat are sometimes accompanied by constitutional symptoms, including anorexia and abdominal discomfort. Most cases of herpangina are mild and resolve without complications in 3 to 6 days.

Herpes simplex viruses (types 1 and 2) can cause acute pharyngitis indistinguishable from that caused by other respiratory viruses. More typically, vesicles and shallow ulcers accompany an infection. Herpes simplex virus is to be suspected when palatal or other pharyngeal ulcers are accompanied by gingivostomatitis. Chronic herpetic lesions can occur in immunocompromised patients and are characterized by progressively large, shallow, painful ulcers.

Infectious mononucleosis most often presents with fever, pharyngotonsillitis, fatigue, and cervical adenopathy. The illness is caused predominantly by the Epstein-Barr virus (see Chap. 18). Cytomegalovirus is an occasional cause of infectious mononucleosis-like disease. In such cases, pharyngitis and cervical adenopathy may be mild or absent. These two viruses are addressed in more detail later in this chapter.

Primary infection with HIV may cause an acute febrile pharyngitis.[5] Fever, sore throat, and varying constitutional symptoms precede the onset of adenopathy by about a week.

Group A β-hemolytic streptococcus (GABHS), also known as Streptococcus pyogenes, is the commonest bacterial cause of pharyngitis. Incidence is age-related. In one study of school-aged children, GABHS accounted for 40% of cases of pharyngitis.[6] A prospective study of symptomatic adult patients found 10% with culture-proved GABHS pharyngitis.[7] Although GABHS pharyngitis was previously thought rare in infants, a more recent study found a 25% incidence of

GABHS in children less than 3 years old.[8] As mentioned, attempts to correlate clinical findings with the presence of GABHS in acute pharyngitis have shown imperfect results. Features suggestive of GABHS, however, include pharyngeal exudate, dysphagia, headache, painful cervical adenitis, fever, and the absence of cough, coryza, and hoarseness. Diagnosis may be confirmed by rapid antigen detection tests and/or throat culture. Timely diagnosis is important to prevent suppurative or nonsuppurative complications of GABHS infection. These complications are discussed later in this chapter.

The role of groups B, C, and G streptococci in the pathogenesis of symptomatic pharyngitis is uncertain. These nongroup A streptococci may be responsible for a small portion of pharyngitis cases, but are not associated with the nonsuppurative complications seen in GABHS.

Vincent's angina is an acute oropharyngeal ulcerative condition caused by a combination of anaerobic gram-negative and fusospirochetal microorganisms (see Chap. 17). Fusobacterium necrophorum, Treponema vincentii, peptococcus, bacteroides, and other anaerobic microorganisms have been identified. Poor oral hygiene, fatigue, stress, malnutrition, and endocrine or metabolic disturbances are predisposing factors. Infection typically manifests as unilateral pseudomembranous tonsillar ulceration with pain, fetid breath, and cervical adenopathy. Acute necrotizing ulcerative gingivitis (ANUG), or "trench mouth," is a similar ulcerative process of the gingiva. Penicillin and metronidazole are effective in the treatment of Vincent's angina and ANUG.

Neisseria gonorrhoeae should be considered as a cause of pharyngitis in sexually active patients, especially those with known orogenital contact. In a study of adults with gonorrhea, gonococcal pharyngitis was found in 20% of homosexual men, 10% of women, and 3% of heterosexual men. About 50% of cases were asymptomatic, although odynophagia, low-grade fever, and erythema may occur. Gonococcal pharyngitis may occur without associated urethritis and may serve as a source for disseminated disease.[9]

Corynebacterium diphtheriae is discussed later in this chapter. Other causes of pharyngitis include Arcanobacterium haemolyticum, Yersinia enterocolitica, Mycobacterium tuberculosis, Treponema pallidum (see Chap. 18), and fungal infections.

Acute Supraglottitis (Epiglottitis)

Acute supraglottitis is cellulitis of supraglottic structures including the epiglottis and aryepiglottic folds. Edema progresses rapidly and may result in airway obstruction.

Haemophilus influenzae type b (HIB) is nearly always the cause of acute supraglottitis in children.

Other pathogens, although reported, are distinctly uncommon. In adults, the causes are more varied, although HIB remains the most common agent. Other pathogens include Staphylococcus aureus, Streptococcus pneumoniae, other streptococci, H. influenzae non-type b, and H. parainfluenzae.[10,11] Immunocompromised patients are more likely to have these and other more unusual pathogens. In many adult cases, an agent is not identified. The role of respiratory viruses in acute supraglottitis is unclear.

Acute Laryngotracheobronchitis (Croup)

Acute laryngotracheobronchitis, or croup, produces inflammation of the subglottic areas that results in stridor and respiratory distress. Most patients are children between the ages of 3 months and 3 years.

Parainfluenza virus types 1 and 3 are the most common causes of croup. Influenza A and parainfluenza type 2 virus also cause significant numbers of cases. Influenza A is of special note because it tends to cause more severe disease. Less common pathogens include respiratory syncytial virus, adenoviruses, enteroviruses, rhinoviruses, and Mycoplasma pneumoniae. More recently, bacterial agents such as Streptococcus pneumoniae, Staphylococcus aureus, and Moraxella catarrhalis have been associated with croup. They likely represent superinfection of a preceding viral disease.

Sinusitis

The microbiology of sinusitis varies according to the chronicity of infection, as well as the age and underlying condition of the patient. Accurate culture requires aspiration or irrigation because of the presence of resident microflora in the nasal cavity and nasopharynx (see Chap. 11).

Acute community-acquired sinusitis in adults is most frequently associated with Streptococcus pneumoniae and nontypable Haemophilus influenzae.[12] To these pathogens, in children, may be added Moraxella catarrhalis.[13] Anaerobic bacteria are recovered in about 5 to 10% of cases of acute sinusitis, usually in the presence of dental disease.[12] Anaerobes are rarely recovered from cases of acute sinusitis in children, presumably because of the relative absence of odontogenic infections in the young. Staphylococcus aureus is an uncommon cause of acute sinusitis, found in only about 3% of cases.[12,14] In contrast, S. aureus, α-hemolytic streptococci, and Streptococcus pneumoniae were reported as the predominant pathogens of isolated sphenoid sinusitis. Although this may reflect increased contamination by resident nasal flora, antimicrobial coverage for S. aureus is prudent in patients with acute sphenoid sinusitis. Viral URIs undoubtedly play an important role in predisposing a patient to acute sinusitis;

however, viruses, including rhinoviruses, adenoviruses, influenzae, and parainfluenzae viruses, are isolated in only 15 to 20% of antral aspirates taken from patients with acute sinusitis.[15]

Chronic sinusitis may result from anatomic obstruction that impedes clearance and damages the mucosal lining of the involved sinus.[12] Treatment generally requires surgical drainage in addition to antimicrobial therapy. Infection is often polymicrobial, and anaerobic bacteria play a far greater role in both adults and children than in acute sinusitis.[16] Such anaerobes include bacteroides, peptostreptococci, and fusobacteria. Staphylococcal species, including S. aureus, are also far more frequently encountered in chronic sinusitis, as are α-hemolytic streptococci.[17]

Nosocomial sinusitis, such as that seen following prolonged nasotracheal intubation, is commonly polymicrobial and has a high incidence of Staphylococcus aureus, anaerobes, and gram-negative bacteria such as Pseudomonas aeruginosa, Klebsiella pneumoniae, Proteus mirabilis, and Enterobacter species.[18,19]

In cystic fibrosis patients with acute sinusitis, Pseudomonas aeruginosa and Haemophilus influenzae were the most frequently isolated pathogens[20] (see Chap. 7).

Fungi have been increasingly identified as causes of sinusitis. Acute fungal sinusitis most frequently occurs in the immunocompromised patient, whereas chronic fungal sinusitis generally occurs in an immunocompetent host. Aspergillosis, phaeohyphomycosis, and mucormycosis are the best known examples.

Otitis Media

Otitis media, also discussed in Chapters 47 to 49, is the most common illness diagnosed by pediatricians. Acute otitis media is a suppurative infection of the middle ear with a relatively rapid clinical onset. Recurrent otitis media refers to episodes of repeated acute otitis media separated by a month or more. Chronic otitis media includes the diagnoses of otitis media with effusion, as well as chronic suppurative otitis media with and without cholesteatoma.

The most common bacteria isolated from the middle ear fluid in children with acute otitis media are Streptococcus pneumoniae, Haemophilus influenzae, and Moraxella catarrhalis. In a 10-year review of acute otitis media cases seen at the Pittsburgh Otitis Media Research Center, Bluestone and associates reported isolation of S. pneumoniae in 35%, H. influenzae in 23%, and M. catarrhalis in 14% of cases.[21] An increase in the prevalence of β-lactamase-producing strains of H. influenzae and M. catarrhalis was also noted. Staphylococcus aureus, other streptococci, and Pseudomonas aeruginosa were all found in less than 3% of cases. No bacteria were isolated in 16% of cases. Other studies have documented generally similar results. Bluestone

and colleagues also studied the bacteriology of 34 adults with acute otitis media. S. pneumoniae (21%) and H. influenzae (26%) were again the most frequently isolated micro-organisms. The most common strains of S. pneumoniae associated with acute otitis media are, in descending order, types 19, 23, 6, 14, 3, and 18. This study confirmed the importance of H. influenzae beyond the age of preschool children. Most cases of acute otitis media associated with H. influenzae are due to nontypable strains. Patients with cases associated with H. influenzae type b may have a higher incidence of concomitant bacteremia or meningitis.[22] Recent studies have not assigned a significant role for Mycoplasma pneumoniae in either otitis media or bullous myringitis; however, some patients with lower respiratory tract infection due to M. pneumoniae may have concomitant otitis media. Chlamydia trachomatis may be responsible for some cases of acute otitis media, especially in infants less than 6 months old.

Viruses are found in the middle ear fluid in about one quarter of cases in acute otitis media. Respiratory syncytial virus, influenza virus, enteroviruses, and rhinoviruses are most commonly identified.

Neonatal otitis media is most frequently associated with microorganisms similar to those seen in infants; however, gram-negative enteric organisms and Staphylococcus aureus are more frequently identified than in older patients.[23]

The bacteriology of recurrent otitis media in children with episodes separated by a month or more is essentially that of acute otitis media.

In their 10-year review, Bluestone and associates also studied the bacteriology of otitis media with effusion in children.[21] Haemophilus influenzae (15%), Moraxella catarrhalis (10%), and Streptococcus pneumoniae (7%) were most frequently isolated. Other streptococci, Staphylococcus aureus, and Pseudomonas aeruginosa were isolated in less than 3% of cases. No growth was found in 30%. This and other reports refute previous assumptions that the effusion in otitis media with effusion is sterile.

Chronic suppurative otitis media is defined by the presence of chronic infection in the middle ear and discharge through a central tympanic membrane perforation or patent pressure equalization tube. Mastoiditis is invariably present. Bacteria isolated are seldom those seen in an initial acute otitis media. Polymicrobial infections are common. Pseudomonas aeruginosa is most commonly isolated, and Staphylococcus aureus is seen more frequently than in acute otitis media.[24] Anaerobes, including anaerobic gram-positive cocci, Bacteroides species, and fusobacteria, are present in 50% of cases.[25] In chronic suppurative otitis media with cholesteatoma, Pseudomonas aeruginosa, S. aureus, and anaerobes again predominate.[26]

SPECIFIC VIRUSES

Epstein-Barr Virus

Epstein-Barr virus (EBV), a member of the Herpesvirus family, is a double-stranded DNA virus. Two strains have been identified in humans, the only known natural host. EBV is ubiquitous, infecting more than 90% of the world's population. In less industrialized societies, nearly all inhabitants are infected during childhood, when symptoms of infection are mild. In the United States, western Europe, and other industrialized countries, infection may be delayed until adolescence or young adulthood and may manifest as infectious mononucleosis because of a more mature immune system.

Infection by EBV is largely limited to epithelial cells of the pharynx and to B lymphocytes. The surface receptor for the virus on these cells is the CD21 molecule, which is also the receptor for the CD3 component of complement. Primary infection is initiated in the oropharyngeal epithelium, where replication, cell lysis, and release of virions take place. Adjacent B lymphocytes are infected and disseminate the virus to local and distant lymphoid tissues and to other epithelial cells, including the nasopharynx and salivary glands. Within B lymphocytes, the virus establishes a latent infection. The DNA genome circularizes to form an episome, or extrachromosomal element, in the nucleus of the cell. Transformation of the infected B lymphocytes causes them to become "immortalized," which is to say that they acquire the ability to proliferate indefinitely.[27] The host's immune system responds to infection first with natural killer (NK) cells, then with HLA class I restricted cytotoxic and suppressor T lymphocytes, and by antibody-producing anti-EBV B lymphocytes. The NK and T lymphocytes appear in the peripheral blood as "atypical lymphocytes." Cytokines released from these cells are largely responsible for the clinical manifestations of primary EBV infection. In infants and small children, these immune responses are weak, and symptoms of infection are mild. The immune systems of adolescents and young adults respond more vigorously and cause the syndrome of infectious mononucleosis.

EBV is the predominant cause of infectious mononucleosis, which is characterized by fever, fatigue, pharyngitis, and lymphadenopathy (see Chap. 18). Splenomegaly, mild hepatitis, and cerebritis may also occur. Uncommon manifestations include jaundice, pneumonitis, blood dyscrasias, and central nervous system (CNS) syndromes. The diagnosis is suggested by the clinical features. Abnormal laboratory findings include the presence of atypical lymphocytes in the peripheral blood, elevation of hepatic enzymes, and the presence of positive heterophile antibodies (the "Monospot" or Paul-Bunnell test).

EBV is closely linked to nonkeratinizing nasopharyngeal carcinoma and to Burkitt's lymphoma, a tumor of B lymphocytes limited largely to children in tropical Africa and New Guinea. EBV genomes are also found in about onethird of the non-Hodgkin's B cell lymphomas found in patients with AIDS.

Oral hairy leukoplakia is common in patients with HIV and represents infection by EBV of epithelial cells. It consists of white lesions with a hairy or corrugated appearance located on the lateral surface of the tongue. EBV replication is evident only in the upper layers of the epithelium.

Serologic tests for EBV are outlined in Table 3–2. Specific EBV antibody tests include those to viral capsid antigen (VCA), early antigen (EA), and Epstein-Barr nuclear antigen (EBNA). IgM to VCA indicates current infection, whereas IgG to VCA may indicate active or past infection. Antibodies to EBNA persist for life. IgA to VCA can be used to screen patients at high risk for nasopharyngeal carcinoma because titers may be elevated before clinical symptoms appear (see Chaps. 19, 20, and 35).

TABLE 3–2. Epstein-Barr Virus (EBV) Serology

Laboratory Test	Acute Infectious Mononucleosis (IM)	Carrier State	CMS (reactivation)
IgG: Early antigen diffuse, restricted	1:640	Negative	≥1:640‡
	Positive	Negative†	≥1:640
IgM: Viral capsid antigen (false positive with rheumatoid)	Positive	Negative	?Negative
IgG: Viral capsid antigen	Negative	Positive ≤1:16	^≥1:5120
EBV nuclear antigen	Negative	Positive	33% ≤1:5
Virus in saliva	100% positive	35–50% +	30–50% +
T cells	^T4, n T8	Normal	No change or ^T8
Oligonucleotide synthetase*	+	—	+
Circulating interferon	—	—	—

Oligonucleotide synthetase is an indicator of interferon activity and found to be elevated in chronic active EBV disease. It rises in IM and chronic mononucleosis syndrome (CMS) as an indicator of active viral infection.

† Normal cellular immune response and resolution of acute IM will have normal erythrocyte antibody (EA).

‡ 13% of normal persons 4 years after IM show EA titers >1:40.

Cytomegalovirus

Cytomegalovirus (CMV), the largest member of the Herpesvirus family, consists of a core of double-stranded DNA genome surrounded by a protein coat. The virus is ubiquitous, and serologic evidence suggests that up to 80% of adults have been infected.[28] Most primary infections in immunocompetent persons are asymptomatic. An upsurge in interest in CMV has resulted from an appreciation of its role as an opportunistic pathogen in immunocompromised patients, including those with HIV infection.

The details of pathogenesis in CMV infection are less well understood than for Epstein-Barr virus. Infection may be acquired by contact with the saliva, sputum, urine, or genital fluid of infected persons, through blood transfusion or solid organ transplantation, or by transplacental transfer to a fetus. Ductal epithelial cells of the major salivary glands and proximal renal tubules are especially involved by primary infection. Once acquired, the virus infects nucleated blood cells and spreads systemically. After primary infection, CMV generally remains in an asymptomatic latent state, but immunosuppression may result in reactivation and disease.

CMV is among the most common viral pathogens causing congenital abnormalities. Fetal involvement follows a primary CMV infection of a woman lacking antibody to the virus during pregnancy. Clinical features include mental retardation, hearing loss, jaundice, chorioretinitis, microcephaly, and pneumonitis, among others.

In infants and children, CMV infection generally causes few symptoms. In young adults, however, CMV is responsible for a small proportion of infectious mononucleosis-like disease. Fever, fatigue, and malaise are present, but pharyngitis and lymphadenopathy are less common and severe than in cases caused by EBV. The laboratory features are similar, namely, the presence of atypical lymphocytosis and mild elevations of hepatic enzymes. Patients with infectious mononucleosis caused by CMV, however, have a negative heterophile antibody (Paul-Bunnell) test.

Primary or reactivated CMV infections commonly cause disease in immunosuppressed hosts, such as persons with HIV infection or those who have undergone bone marrow or solid organ transplantation. CMV itself may adversely affect the immune system, causing suppression of NK cell and T lymphocyte function.[29] Clinical features in immunosuppressed patients include encephalitis, chorioretinitis, hepatitis, pneumonitis, colitis, and esophagitis.[30] CMV has also been identified as a cause of oral ulcers in immunosuppressed patients. Diagnosis is based on tissue biopsy, which demonstrates the characteristic histologic findings of intranuclear CMV inclusions surrounded by clear halos ("owl eyes"), as well as clusters of intracytoplasmic inclusions seen with periodic acid-Schiff (PAS) or Gomori's methenamine silver techniques.[31]

Human Immunodeficiency Virus

Human immunodeficiency virus (HIV) is a retrovirus. It is able to convert its own single-stranded RNA to double-stranded DNA for incorporation into a host cell genome. The principal targets are T-helper (CD4) cells, which are central to the function of cell-mediated immunity. Impairment of these cells renders a patient susceptible to a variety of opportunistic infections and unusual malignant diseases (see Chap. 5).

HIV attaches to CD4 receptors and enters T-helper lymphocytes. The single-stranded RNA is converted by the viral enzyme reverse transcriptase into double-stranded DNA. The viral DNA is incorporated into the host cell genome. A latent phase follows that corresponds to clinically quiescent infection. Activation and viral replication lead to cell death and the destruction of large numbers of CD4 cells. It is possible that activation is speeded by presence of DNA viruses such as herpes simplex virus and CMV. The presence or absence of opportunistic infections corresponds with the patient's CD4 counts. A normal level is 700 to 1200 cells/mm^3. Patients with a CD4 count less than 500 cells/mm^3 benefit from antiretroviral therapy. CD4 counts below 200 cells/mm^3 are associated with increased susceptibility to opportunistic infections. Such patients benefit from antibiotic prophylaxis.

Humoral immunity is adversely affected by HIV as well. IgG2 and IgG4 subclass deficiencies predispose patients to recurrent sinopulmonary infections. HIV patients may also develop elevated IgE levels, which may be responsible for an increased incidence of allergic rhinitis.

The reported prevalence of sinusitis in HIV patients varies widely, although clinicians generally agree that the incidence is higher than in immunocompetent patients. Retrospective studies have estimated the prevalence of disease at 10 to 20%. Two small prospective studies placed the incidence at 30 to 68%.[32] Several reports suggest that the incidence of sinus disease increases with progressive immunodeficiency, as measured by declining CD4 counts.[33,34] In addition, IgE levels increase in many HIV-infected patients with disease progression. Sample and associates noted that allergen-specific IgE, as measured by radioallergosorbent test (RAST), and nasal eosinophilia were increased in HIV-infected patients with advanced disease.[35] Such immune dysfunction, with its resultant increase in allergic disease, may predispose HIV-infected patients to recurrent rhinosinusitis. The prevalence of specific pathogens in sinusitis of those HIV-infected patients with a CD4 count greater than 200 cells/mm^3 is similar to that of non-HIV-infected patients. In acute sinusitis, Streptococcus pneumoniae and Haemophilus influenzae are most frequently recovered. In chronic sinusitis, Staphylococcus aureus, anaerobic bacteria, and Pseudomonas aeruginosa are also described.[36] HIV-infected patients with CD4 counts less than 200 cells/mm^3 are more susceptible to unusual pathogens. Infections with P. aeruginosa are more frequent. Other pathogens reported include CMV, Pneumocystis carinii, Acanthamoeba castellanii, and Legionella pneumophila.[36] Fungal pathogens in these patients include Aspergillus species, Pseudallescheria boydii, Candida albicans, and Cryptococcus neoformans.[37] Surprisingly, HIV infection does not appear to be associated with a significantly increased incidence of mucormycosis.

Studies have suggested that children with HIV infection have an increased incidence of otitis media. Moreover, those HIV-infected children with a deteriorating immune system, as indicated by a decline in the CD4 count, are at greater risk for recurrent or chronic disease than those who retain an intact immune system.[38] Causative organisms do not seem to differ from those found in normal hosts. Streptococcus pneumoniae, Haemophilus influenzae, and Moraxella catarrhalis predominate. Unusual pathogens, however, should be suspected when a patient has a severely depressed immune system or responds poorly to standard antibiotic therapy.

Adult HIV-infected patients appear to have an increased incidence of serous otitis media.[39] This may be partly due to poor eustachian tube function. The eustachian tube may be affected by adenoidal hypertrophy, by nasopharyngeal tumors such as Kaposi's sarcoma or non-Hodgkin's lymphoma, or by allergic rhinitis prompted by increased IgE levels. Pneumocystis carinii, recently reclassified as a fungus, is a common cause of pneumonia in AIDS patients. Although extrapulmonary infections are rare, several reports have described otologic involvement.[40] Patients present with aural discharge and the presence of a polyp in the middle ear or external canal. Several patients have had no history of prior P. carinii pneumonia. Diagnosis is made by biopsy of the polyp and demonstration of pneumocystis on Gomori's methenamine silver stain. These otologic infections have responded well to trimethoprim-sulfamethoxazole. Treatment should be directed at possible subclinical pulmonary infection as well as otologic disease. Other unusual pathogens have caused otitis media or mastoiditis, including Aspergillus fumigatus, Candida albicans, and Mycobacterium tuberculosis. Chronic otitis media, cholesteatoma, and intracranial complications of otitis media do not appear to occur more often in the HIV-infected population than in other patients.[39]

Oral candidiasis is a common feature of HIV infection and is often the first finding of the disease. Candidal infections are considered in more detail later in this chapter. As noted earlier, oral hairy leukoplakia is thought to be caused by EBV. The lesion is most frequently located on the lateral surface of the tongue and has a white corrugated or filiform appearance. EBV replication is evident only in the upper layer of the epithelium. Herpes simplex viral infections are more common in HIV-infected patients. Lesions are generally more severe, numerous, and persistent than in immunocompetent patients. Herpes labialis is frequent and may extend onto the face to form a giant herpetic lesion.[41]

Opportunistic infections of the larynx must be considered in HIV-infected patients with stridor or hoarseness. Candidiasis is the most common cause. Laryngeal candidiasis is most often part of a more widespread infection involving the oral cavity or esophagus. Absence of candidiasis in these sites, however, does not exclude laryngeal infection. The vocal folds are most frequently involved. Candidal infection of the epiglottis is much less common, but is capable of causing stridor and airway compromise, especially in children.[42] Laryngeal infections caused by CMV and Cryptococcus neoformans, among others, have been described in HIV-infected patients.[43,44] A series of five HIV-infected patients with supraglottitis was reported by Rothstein and associates.[45] A pale, floppy epiglottis with supraglottic edema, cervical adenopathy, normal to low white blood count without a shift to the left, and rapidly progressive airway obstruction comprised the typical presentation. No unusual pathogens were recovered from epiglottic cultures in these patients. The most common pathogens were Streptococcus pneumoniae and Staphylococcus aureus. Conservative medical management was not successful. Patients required airway intervention with appropriate antibiotic therapy.

SPECIFIC BACTERIA

Group A β-hemolytic Streptococcus (S. pyogenes)

Group A β-hemolytic streptococcus (GABHS), or S. pyogenes, is a chain-forming gram-positive coccus. More than 80 serotypes have been recognized based on a series of distinct surface proteins, the M proteins. The M protein strains of GABHS that cause pharyngitis are generally distinct from those causing impetigo or pyoderma. M proteins inhibit phagocytosis of GABHS by host leukocytes in the absence of type-specific antibodies and therefore play an important role in the virulence of these organisms.[46]

GABHS secretes certain toxins and enzymes that have clinical effects or cause antibodies to be produced that may be used for serologic identification. Streptolysins O and S induce lysis of host cell membranes, including red blood cells. Streptolysin O is antigenic and is the basis of the antistreptolysin O (ASO) antibody assay, the most widely used of the many streptococcal antibody tests. Pyrogenic (also called erythrogenic) exotoxins are produced by some serotypes of GABHS. Three exotoxins have been identified: SPE A, SPE B, and SPE C. These exotoxins are thought to be in part responsible for the clinical manifestations of scarlet fever and the recently described streptococcal toxic shock-like syndrome.

The leading role of GABHS as a cause of pharyngitis is discussed earlier in this chapter. The greater significance of these organisms lies in their capacity to cause complications. These complications may be broadly separated into three categories: suppurative, toxin-mediated, and nonsuppurative.

Suppurative complications of GABHS pharyngitis include peritonsillar abscess, retropharyngeal abscess, suppurative cervical lymphadenitis, sinusitis, otitis media, and mastoiditis. GABHS is a prominent cause of peritonsillar and retropharyngeal abscesses.[47] Similarly, GABHS and Staphylococcus aureus are the most important causes of suppurative cervical lymphadenitis. In contrast, GABHS plays a minor role in the pathogenesis of sinusitis, otitis media, and mastoiditis.

Toxin-mediated complications of GABHS pharyngitis include scarlet fever and streptococcal toxic shock-like syndrome (TSLS). Both are thought to be associated with the release of streptococcal pyrogenic exotoxins by certain M protein serotypes. During the first decades of this century, a decline in the frequency and severity of scarlet fever had been noted. Severe scarlet fever had become uncommon in the United States and western Europe. In the 1980s, however, an increase in the incidence and severity of scarlet fever, as well as the emergence of TSLS, suggested an increase in the numbers of virulent GABHS strains capable of producing pyrogenic exotoxins. Serotypes M-1 and M-3, in particular, were found to be associated with TSLS.[48] Investigators have postulated that manifestations of scarlet fever, including the characteristic rash, are due to host hypersensitivity to these pyrogenic exotoxins.[46]

Initial manifestations of scarlet fever are sore throat, fever, and constitutional symptoms such as vomiting, headache, and malaise. The characteristic rash follows 12 to 48 hours later, beginning on the trunk before quickly becoming generalized. The rash appears diffusely erythematous with fine red papules. It blanches on pressure, may become petechial, and fades in 2 to 5 days, leaving a fine desquamation. Skin folds, such as the groin and axilla, are most intensely involved. The face is flushed, with circumoral pallor. Enlargement and erythema of the papillae of the dorsal tongue produce a characteristic "strawberry tongue."

In the late 1980s, reports emerged of GABHS infections associated with hypotension, progressive multisystem organ failure, and other features suggestive of a toxin-mediated disorder. Because of a partial resemblance to staphylococcal toxic shock syndrome, the new disorder was named "streptococcal toxic shock-like syndrome" (TSLS). The syndrome occurs most often in healthy adults. Most patients have a severe soft tissue focus of infection, such as necrotizing fasciitis and/or myositis; however, 10 to 20% of cases have been associated with pharyngitis.[48] The syndrome most typically consists of hypotension, fever, rash, desquamation, and multisystem organ failure, which is often out of proportion to the extent of local signs and symptoms. Bacteremia is present in about half the cases. In a recently reported series of 50 patients, the mortality rate was 24%.[49] GABHS isolated from patients with TSLS appears to come from a limited group of M protein serotypes. M-1 and M-3 strains, in particular, have been associated with TSLS. These virulent strains more frequently are producers of pyrogenic exotoxins, which are thought to have an important role in the pathogenesis of TSLS.[48] Streptococcal pyrogenic exotoxin A (SPE A) stimulates production of tumor necrosis factor (TNF) by peripheral monocytes in vitro. Cytokine and interleukin 1-β are thought to contribute to the pathophysiology of shock and tissue injury.[50] Treatment of streptococcal TSLS involves support of failing organ systems, appropriate antibiotics, and, if present, aggressive surgical debridement of necrotizing fasciitis or myositis.

Nonsuppurative complications of GABHS pharyngitis include acute poststreptococcal glomerulonephritis and acute rheumatic fever. The pathogenesis of these conditions is unclear, but each is suspected to be immune mediated.

Poststreptococcal acute glomerulonephritis (AGN) is a delayed, nonsuppurative complication resulting in inflammation of the renal glomeruli. AGN may follow either pharyngitis or cutaneous infections caused by GABHS. A limited number of strains are "nephritogenic." M-12 is the M protein serotype most frequently related to pharyngitis-associated nephritis.[51] The pathogenesis of AGN is unclear. Antibodies to antigens of nephritogenic streptococci may cross-react with structurally similar renal antigens, producing injury. Alternatively, inflammation may result from deposition of streptococcal antigen-antibody complexes within the kidney. AGN associated with GABHS pharyngitis occurs most frequently in school-aged children. The latent period following pharyngitis averages 10 days. Clinical features include fever, moderate edema, hypertension, and azotemia. Mild cases may have few symptoms. The urine is smoky or brownish in color with a high specific gravity, proteinuria, and hemoglobinuria. Microscopic examination reveals red blood cells, white blood cells, and hyaline, granular, or red blood cell casts. Other laboratory findings include a mild normocytic normochromic anemia, prolonged erythrocyte sedimentation rate (ESR), decreases in C3 complement, and elevations of the BUN and serum creatinine. Unlike in acute rheumatic fever, recurrences are rare. The long-term prognosis in children is excellent, with few cases leading to residual renal disease. Prognosis in adults is more guarded.[51]

Acute rheumatic fever (ARF) is a nonsuppurative complication of GABHS characterized by inflammatory lesions of the heart, joints, subcutaneous tissues, and CNS. Pyodermic infections are not associated with ARF. The disease has become uncommon in prosperous areas of the world, although local outbreaks thought to be caused by highly rheumatogenic strains of GABHS are periodically reported. In poorer regions, ARF remains prevalent and accounts for a large proportion of cardiac disease in children and young adults.[49] The pathogenesis of ARF is poorly understood. Current evidence supports an immune mechanism. Humoral and cell-mediated immune responses to rheumatogenic antigens of GABHS are thought to cross-react mistakenly with structurally similar antigens in host tissues. Pathologic findings in ARF include inflammatory lesions of connective tissues in the heart, joints, blood vessels, and subcutaneous tissues. A unique feature, seen mainly in the heart, is the Aschoff's nodule—a granuloma that results from injury to collagen. Cardiac findings also include pericarditis, myocarditis, and/or endocarditis. Valvular involvement begins as edema and inflammation of the leaflets and chordae tendineae. With healing, the valves may become thickened and deformed, the chordae shortened, and the valve commissures fused. These changes result in valvular stenosis or insufficiency.[51] The mitral valve is attacked in 75 to 80% of cases, the aortic valve in 30%, and the tricuspid and pulmonary valves in under 5%. ARF occurs most often in children 5 to 15 years of age; it is rare before age 4 or after age 40. Symptoms and signs usually commence 1 to 3 weeks after the streptococcal pharyngitis. No single symptom, sign, or laboratory test is diagnostic of the disease. The Jones criteria, most recently updated in 1992, remain useful in making the diagnosis.[52] If supported by evidence of preceding group A streptococcal infection, the presence of two major manifestations, or of one major and two minor manifestations, a high probability of rheumatic fever is indicated. Supporting evidence includes a positive throat culture, positive rapid streptococcal antigen test, or an elevated or rising streptococcal antibody titer. Major manifestations include carditis, polyarthritis, chorea, erythema marginatum, and subcutaneous nodules. Minor manifestations include clinical findings such as arthralgia or fever, laboratory findings such as an elevated ESR or C-reactive protein, and a prolonged PR interval on an electrocardiogram. Treatment of ARF includes the use of salicylates and corticosteroids to quiet inflammation. Neither agent prevents the development of rheumatic heart disease, the only long-term sequelae of ARF. Rheumatic patients are at extremely high risk of developing recurrent ARF after streptococcal infections and require antibiotic prophylaxis.

Corynebacterium Diphtheriae

The corynebacteria are nonmotile, pleomorphic, unencapsulated, gram-positive bacilli. Diphtheria is caused by toxin-producing strains of Corynebacterium diphtheriae. The infection is now rare in countries with immunization programs, but it remains widespread elsewhere. Arcanobacterium hemolyticum occasionally causes an illness mimicking diphtheria. A. haemolyticum also causes an illness that has been confused with streptococcal scarlet fever.

Diphtheria most frequently manifests in a patient with severe sore throat and erythema of the pharynx, especially the tonsils. The erythema is followed by gray spots that coalesce to form a membrane. Extension beyond the tonsils involves the soft palate, posterior pharynx, and larynx. The membrane is surrounded by a deep red border, and attempts at removal results in bleeding. Cervical lymph nodes are usually enlarged. Severely ill patients may have a bull-necked appearance. Laryngeal or tracheal involvement may occur primarily or may result from pharyngeal extension. Hoarseness and respiratory distress occur. Death may result from airway obstruction, especially in children. Nasal diphtheria initially causes purulent or serosanguinous nasal discharge. Patients with chronic nasal diphtheria may act as transmitters of the disease.

Corynebacterium diphtheriae remains localized to sites of infection. Systemic features of diphtheria result from the effects of a polypeptide toxin absorbed into the blood and lymphatic vessels. After host cell uptake, the toxin inhibits protein synthesis through the inactivation of elongation factor-2 (EF-2). Patients develop fever, pallor, and exhaustion. The organs most affected are the heart, kidneys, and peripheral nerves. Myocarditis usually develops in the first 2 weeks. The toxin's inability to cross the blood-brain barrier explains its preference for involvement of peripheral and cranial nerves. In patients with pharyngeal disease, the most common neurologic finding is palatal paralysis. Swallowing difficulties ensue.

Diphtheria must be suspected in any unimmunized patient with a severe, rapidly spreading pharyngeal exudate. Diagnosis is confirmed by culture on Loeffler's medium and by the demonstration of toxin production by a gel-diffusion precipitin reaction (Elek test). Treatment involves the use of antitoxin and antibiotics (penicillin or erythromycin). Tracheotomy may be required for laryngeal involvement.

Klebsiella Rhinoscleromatis (Scleroma, Rhinoscleroma)

Klebsiella rhinoscleromatis (K. pneumoniae, subspecies rhinoscleromatis) causes a chronic granulomatous disease of the respiratory tract. It is endemic to tropical and subtropical areas of the world. The nose is nearly always involved. Less commonly, the paranasal sinuses, lacrimal sacs, pharynx, larynx, and trachea are involved as well. Nasal lesions often begin at the mucocutaneous junction of the vestibule. The disease usually progresses through three stages. The catarrhal stage is manifested by prolonged purulent rhinorrhea and crusting. In the granulomatous stage, multiple nodules form and coalesce. Severe cases can progress to local destruction and cosmetic deformity. The final fibrotic stage causes cicatrix formation. Nasal or nasopharyngeal stenosis is common. Broadening of the nasal dorsum produces the characteristic Hebra nose. Stenosis of the larynx or trachea can cause airway obstruction. Diagnosis of scleroma is made by clinical findings and biopsy. Histologic findings include granulomatous inflammation and the presence of Mikulicz cells. These findings are most characteristic of the granulomatous stage, in which K. rhinoscleromatis is most easily isolated. Mikulicz cells are "foamy histiocytes" caused by gram-negative bacteria in the cytoplasm of macrophages. They are not pathognomonic for scleroma. Fibrosis is present in advanced disease. Treatment of scleroma is with prolonged antibiotics until repeat cultures are negative. Trimethoprim-sulfamethoxazole is currently favored. Surgery is used to treat stenoses as needed.

Mycobacterium Tuberculosis

Mycobacterium tuberculosis, an acid-fast bacillus, is a cause of infection throughout the upper respiratory tract. Two sites of special interest are the larynx and middle ear.

Tuberculosis is the most common cause of granulomatous disease of the larynx. It is nearly always associated with active pulmonary disease. Spread from lung to larynx is largely ascribed to direct inoculation by bacilli-laden sputum, but hematogenous and lymphatic spread from pulmonary foci is recognized as well. Symptoms of laryngeal tuberculosis may include dysphagia, odynophagia, hoarseness, and referred otalgia. Examination may show edema, submucosal nodules, and shallow ulcerations. Lesions may progress to deeper ulceration, perichondritis, and arytenoid fixation. The true vocal cords and epiglottis are most frequently involved. Laryngeal tuberculosis may mimic carcinoma or chronic laryngitis. Syphilis, mycotic infections, sarcoidosis, and Wegener's disease must also be considered. A chest radiograph is helpful because it is almost always abnormal. A sputum smear may show acid-fast bacilli. The diagnosis may be confirmed by biopsy. Laryngeal tuberculosis responds well to antitubercular chemotherapy. Fibrotic changes from advanced disease may require surgical reconstruction.

Otologic tuberculosis may result either from hematogenous spread from pulmonary foci or from direct inoculation by bacilli-laden sputum refluxed through the eustachian tube. Otorrhea may be scant or profuse. Although the disorder is often painless, many patients experience otalgia. Granulation tissue and occasional polyps are seen in the middle ear. Conductive hearing loss may result from effusion, mucosal thickening, tympanic membrane perforation, or ossicular destruction. Classically, tympanic membrane perforations have been described as initial small multiple perforations that coalesce to a near-total perforation. More recent studies show that simple perforations are more common, however. Denudation and destruction of the ossicular chain are common. Facial nerve paralysis is more common in aural tuberculosis than in otitis media caused by other bacteria. Tuberculosis should always be suspected in children with otitis media complicated by facial paralysis. Otologic tuberculosis can also cause mastoiditis, which, in turn, may progress to subperiosteal abscess and a draining fistula. Other complications may include labyrinthitis, meningitis, and osteomyelitis of the petrous pyramid. The diagnosis of aural tuberculosis is best made by biopsy of granulation tissue or polyps. Histologic presence of caseating granulomata and acid-fast bacilli confirms the diagnosis. Smear and culture of aural discharge are unreliable because the bacilli can be demonstrated in only a minority of patients. A purified protein derivative (PPD) test is almost always positive except in extremely young children and in immunocompromised patients. Chest x-ray abnormalities suggestive of pulmonary disease are present in only 50% of patients with aural tuberculosis.

Treatment of aural tuberculosis consists of longstanding antitubercular chemotherapy. Surgical intervention may be indicated in the presence of facial nerve paralysis, subperiosteal abscess, persistent postauricular fistula, labyrinthitis, or extension of the infection into the CNS. Cortical mastoidectomy may disclose thick granulation tissue and possible bone necrosis. Tympanoplasty or ossicular reconstruction should be delayed until the infection has been controlled.

Mycobacterium Leprae

Mycobacterium leprae is a gram-positive, acid-fast bacillus. It prefers an ambient temperature of less than 37°C and, as a result, has a predilection for skin, peripheral nerves, and the upper aerodigestive tract. Leprosy presents in three general forms. In the lepromatous form, the patient is unable to generate an effective immune response to M. leprae because of a selective unresponsiveness of T lymphocytes. This form of leprosy tends to be the most widespread and destructive. Most upper aerodigestive tract leprosy is of the lepromatous form. In the tuberculoid form, the host has a normal

T-cell response. Tuberculoid form lesions are generally less widespread. They consist of plaques and macules with sharp, raised borders. An intermediate third form of leprosy is the borderline form, which reflects a partial reduction in immune response.

The nose is by far the most frequently involved site in the upper aerodigestive tract. Approximately 95% of patients with lepromatous leprosy have nasal involvement. Lesions begin as a pale, nodular, plaque-like thickening of the nasal mucosa. Untreated lesions can progress to ulceration, septal perforation, and saddle-nose deformity. Symptoms include rhinitis, obstruction, crusting, and bleeding. The anterior end of the inferior turbinate is the site most likely to give a positive biopsy.

The larynx is less commonly involved. Involvement nearly always begins at the tip of the epiglottis. Mucosal thickening is followed by granuloma formation and ulceration. Symptoms may include hoarseness and pain. Laryngeal leprosy can closely mimic carcinoma. Untreated lesions may progress to fibrosis and airway obstruction requiring tracheotomy.

Mycobacterium leprae has never been cultured in vitro. Diagnosis is most reliably made by tissue smear or biopsy, which may show granulomatous changes and the presence of bacilli. Treatment is with dapsone combined with rifampin. Clofazimine is used in dapsone-resistant cases.

SPECIFIC FUNGAL DISEASES

The role of fungi as causes of URI has been increasingly appreciated. Their importance seems destined to increase as the number of immunoincompetent patients continues to increase.

Actinomycosis

Actinomyces israelii is an anaerobic gram-positive bacterium. A filamentous, branching appearance on microscopy caused its initial misidentification as a fungus. A. israelii is an oral saprophyte. It takes advantage of infection, trauma, or surgical injury to penetrate intact mucosa and invade adjacent tissue. Cervicofacial infections commonly follow dental infections or manipulations. Cervicofacial actinomycosis manifests as a phlegmon, "cold" abscess, or draining sinus. The presence of whitish yellow "sulfur granules" is characteristic. Submandibular, submental, and buccal areas are most frequently involved. Infections spread without regard to tissue planes. The mandible is the most common site of bony involvement. Treatment consists of large doses of penicillin over a prolonged period. Surgical treatment involves abscess drainage and the excision of sinus tracts as needed.

Candidiasis

Candida albicans is the most frequent of several species that cause candidiasis. It is a dimorphic fungus with both yeast and hyphal forms. C. albicans is a commensal of the oral cavity and pharynx. Infection usually only follows changes in the local bacterial flora, mucosal integrity, or host immunity. Local factors that may predispose patients to candidiasis include xerostomia and dentures. Systemic factors are numerous and include prolonged antibiotic use, diabetes mellitus, immunocompromised states (e.g., HIV, cytotoxic therapy), pernicious anemia, and hematologic malignant diseases.

Oral candidiasis ("thrush") can vary greatly in appearance. Zegarelli described several variants.[53] The pseudomembranous variant resembles white milk curds overlying an erythematous base. The erythematous variant appears flat, irregular, and dusky red. When candidiasis occurs beneath dentures, it is flat and red, and it extends up to but not beyond the denture border. A hyperplastic variant resembling lichen planus manifests as a true leukoplakia without pseudomembrane or erythematous base. Oral candidiasis is often asymptomatic, but may also cause a "burning" pain. Candidiasis may also be responsible for median rhomboid glossitis, as well as some cases of angular cheilitis.

Candidiasis less commonly infects the larynx and pharynx. When involved, the larynx is covered by a thick, white exudate. Hoarseness is the most common symptom, followed by pharyngeal pain. Severe cases may proceed to airway obstruction and laryngeal scarring. Diagnosis is best made by direct laryngoscopy and biopsy.

Aspergillosis

The Aspergillus species are ubiquitous saprophytic fungi found in soil and decaying organic material. A. fumigatus and A. flavus are the most common of many species to cause disease. Hyphae show regular septa with frequent acute branching. Aspergillus infections are distributed worldwide, although chronic disease is especially prevalent in the Sudan and Saudi Arabia. Infection is acquired by the inhalation of spores. The lungs, nose, and paranasal sinuses are the most commonly affected sites.

Aspergillus is the most common cause of fungal sinusitis. The maxillary and ethmoid sinuses are most frequently involved. Conditions that obstruct sinus drainage such as allergic rhinitis, nasal polyps, and chronic bacterial sinusitis may predispose patients to fungal sinusitis. Infections take one of four forms. Acute fulminant fungal sinusitis occurs primarily in immunocompromised patients. Vascular invasion by hyphae with resultant thrombosis and necrosis may cause a fulminant course resembling craniofacial mucormycosis. Erosion into the orbits, cranium, palate, and skin is common. Chronic invasive fungal sinusitis occurs more frequently in immunocompetent patients. Progression of the infection is generally slow, with mild early signs and symptoms. Extension into the orbit or cranium may produce proptosis, ophthalmoplegia, and headache. The third form of fungal sinusitis is the mycetoma, or "fungus ball." This is a tangle of fungal hyphae within a sinus cavity but without invasion of sinus mucosa. The maxillary sinus is most commonly involved. A fourth form of fungal sinusitis is allergic fungal sinusitis (AFS). Most patients with AFS are immunocompetent and present with features of refractory sinusitis and nasal polyposis. Many also have a history of atopy or asthma. The pathogenesis of AFS is incompletely understood, but evidence supports a Gell and Coombs type I (IgE-mediated) immune response to fungal antigens. Types III and IV immune responses may also be involved. The pathologic hallmark of AFS is "allergic mucin," consisting of eosinophils, Charcot-Leyden crystals, and scattered fungal hyphae. Although AFS is not thought to be invasive, bony erosion is seen on computed tomography (CT) in 20% of reported cases. Laboratory abnormalities include eosinophilia, elevated total serum IgE, and elevated IgE RAST titers to specific fungi.[54] The diagnosis of AFS is confirmed by demonstration of alleric mucin and culture of the fungus.

The presence of aspergillus or other fungi must be suspected in cases of sinusitis that do not respond to the usual medical treatment. CT scans may show a characteristic pattern of alternating high- and low-density signals and may also be of use in determining the extent of disease. Often, the proper diagnosis is suggested only at surgery, with discovery of the mucus-covered, inspissated, cheesy material typical of fungal sinusitis. Diagnosis is confirmed by histology and culture. Treatment of acute fulminant and chronic invasive forms requires surgical drainage, debridement, and the use of systemic antifungal agents. Treatment of a mycetoma requires only surgical removal and aeration of the involved sinus. Systemic antifungal agents are not required. Allergic fungal sinusitis is treated by surgical debridement and aeration of the involved sinus followed by the use of systemic and topical intranasal corticosteroids. Recurrence is common and may be heralded by rising serum total IgE levels.

Phaeohyphomycoses (Dematiaceous Fungi)

Dematiaceous fungi are defined by the presence of melanin in the walls of their hyphae or spores. These fungi are increasingly recognized as causes of fungal sinusitis previously ascribed to Aspergillus species. The list of dematiaceous fungi causing sinusitis is rapidly expanding and currently includes Drechslera, Bi-

polaris, Exserohilum, Curvularia, Alternaria, and Cladosporium species.[55] Signs and symptoms are essentially indistinguishable from those of chronic indolent aspergillus sinusitis. Diagnosis and treatment are similar.

Mucormycosis

Mucormycosis (phycomycosis, zygomycosis) is an infection caused by fungi of the Mucoraceae family, which includes Rhizopus, Mucor, and Absidia species. Nearly all cases occur in patients with diabetes mellitus or who are otherwise immunocompromised. These fungi are found in soil and decaying organic matter. When examined, their hyphae are broad (7 to 15 μm), with few septa and irregular, 90-degree branching.

Craniofacial (rhino-orbital-cerebral) mucormycosis usually originates in the nose or sinuses. Vascular invasion by hyphae leads to thrombosis with resultant ischemic infarction and necrosis. This accounts for the rapid erosion and spread of this infection into the orbit, cranium, palate, or face. Patients may present with purulent or serosanguineous nasal drainage. The lateral nasal wall and turbinates are the most frequent site of initial involvement. Edema and erythema are followed by cyanosis and black necrosis. Orbital extension may cause proptosis and ophthalmoplegia. Cranial involvement may cause cranial neuropathies, focal neurologic deficits, and coma.

Prompt diagnosis requires a high index of suspicion and is confirmed by biopsy. A CT scan delineates the extent of the infection. Treatment requires a prolonged course of amphotericin B, as well as aggressive surgical debridement of all affected tissue. Antifungal azoles are ineffective. The underlying condition must be corrected if possible.

Histoplasmosis

Histoplasma capsulatum is a dimorphic fungus that exists in a mycelial form in the soil and a budding yeast form at body temperature. It is found throughout the world and in the United States is especially prevalent in the Mississippi and Ohio River valleys. The disease is acquired by inhalation of airborne conidia, often during contact with soil contaminated by avian or bat feces. An increased incidence has been seen in patients with AIDS.

Disseminated histoplasmosis occurs most frequently in patients with impaired cell-mediated immunity. In such patients, lesions of the upper aerodigestive tract are most often seen. The larynx is most commonly involved, with preference for the anterior glottis and epiglottis. Symptoms include sore throat, hoarseness, and dysphagia. Other sites of involvement include the tongue, palate, buccal mucosa, and pharynx. Lesions may appear nodular or ulcerative and may mimic carcinoma, syphilis, tuberculosis, or any other granulomatous lesion. Biopsy is a reliable method of diagnosis. It shows a granulomatous response with budding yeast cells.

Blastomycosis

Blastomyces dermatitidis is a dimorphic fungus that grows in a mycelial form at room temperature and as a budding yeast at body temperature. Blastomycosis is most prevalent in the eastern portion of North America and over a wide geographic area of Africa. Infection is thought to be acquired by inhalation of spores. Dissemination occurs by hematogenous seeding from primary pulmonary foci and, when present, is most frequent in skin, bone, and the genitourinary tract. Skin lesions are most commonly located on the face, extremities, scalp, and neck. Appearance of these lesions may vary. Most begin as papules that, over a course of weeks or months, progress to relatively painless ulcerative or verrucous lesions. Long-standing lesions may show central healing with extensive fibrosis. Subcutaneous abscesses and draining sinuses may also be present.

Involvement of the nose, larynx, or mouth may cause well-circumscribed, indurated lesions of the mucosa.[56] As in skin involvement, these lesions are relatively painless, may be ulcerative or verrucous, and may closely mimic squamous cell carcinoma in appearance. Biopsy shows pseudoepitheliomatous hyperplasia of the mucosa with microabscesses, granulomas, and the presence of the fungi. Treatment is with systemic antifungal agents. Amphotericin B is used for severe infections. Oral antifungal azoles may be used for patients with indolent, extracranial blastomycosis.

Cryptococcosis

Cryptococcus neoformans, a yeast with a thick polysaccharide capsule, is saprophytic and distributed worldwide. A common natural source is avian droppings. Many patients with cryptococcosis are immunosuppressed. AIDS is now the most common predisposing factor. Cryptococcosis occurs in about 8% of AIDS patients and is a commonly recognized cause of life-threatening infection. The fungus is acquired by inhalation, with primary pulmonary infection followed by hematogenous spread. The most common site of involvement is the CNS. Other frequently involved sites include the lungs, bones, and skin. The upper respiratory tract is rarely involved. Laryngeal lesions have been described as edematous, exudative, or verrucous.[57,58] Diagnosis is made by biopsy, which shows pseudoepitheliomatous hyperplasia, granulomatous changes, and the presence of encapsulated fungi. The antifungal azoles and amphotericin B are used for treatment.

Coccidioidomycosis

Coccidioides immitis is a dimorphic fungus, growing in mycelial form in the soil and as thick-walled endospore-forming spherules at body temperature. Coccidioidomycosis is endemic to desert and semiarid portions of the southwestern United States and northern Mexico, as well as scattered areas of Central and South America.

Infection is acquired by the inhalation of spores. Most symptomatic patients develop only a mild to moderate flu-like illness that resolves spontaneously. A few patients develop severe pulmonary illness that may include hematogenous dissemination. Immunodeficient hosts are especially at risk. The most frequent sites of spread are to the skin, bones, and meninges. In the upper respiratory tract, the larynx is most frequently involved.[59] Lesions may involve any area of the larynx and may appear nodular or ulcerative. Biopsy shows granulomatous changes. Fungal staining shows the characteristic spherules filled with endospores. Antifungal azoles may be effective in indolent disseminated disease, but amphotericin B is required for severe infections.

Paracoccidioidomycosis

Paracoccidioides brasiliensis is a dimorphic fungus found in mycelial form at cooler temperatures and in yeast form at body temperature. Paracoccidioidomycosis is endemic to those areas of Latin America with hot, humid summers and dry, temperate winters. The greatest number of cases are from Brazil, although the disease has been reported from Mexico to Argentina. The fungus is a saprophyte found in soil and decaying organic matter. Infection is acquired through the respiratory tract. Hematogenous spread may then occur to other areas of the body. The mucous membranes of the oral cavity, nose, pharynx, and larynx are involved in approximately half of all cases. In a smaller number of cases, the fungus may be directly inoculated into the mucosa by chewing or cleaning of the teeth with plant fragments. Pulmonary infection is found in the majority of symptomatic patients. Dyspnea, hemoptysis, and chest pain may occur. Lymphadenitis and hepatosplenomegaly are also common.

Lesions of the mucosa of the oral cavity, nose, pharynx, and larynx are painful and manifest as well-defined areas of hyperemic granulation tissue and ulceration.[55] Hoarseness may result from laryngeal involvement. Destruction of underlying cartilages may lead to nasal collapse. Cutaneous involvement may be present, with the areas of the face around the mouth and nose most frequently involved.

Diagnosis is made by the results of smear, culture, and biopsy. Serologic tests may be helpful. Biopsy demonstrates pseudoepitheliomatous hyperplasia with intraepithelial abscesses, granulomatous changes, and presence of the fungi. Treatment is with antifungal azoles, amphotericin B, and sulfonamides.

Conidiobolomycosis

Conidiobolus coronatus is present in soil and decaying organic matter and is endemic to tropical regions of Africa and America. This chronic granulomatous infection begins in the nasal submucosa before extending to the contiguous facial skin. Nasal symptoms may include obstruction, rhinorrhea, and epistaxis. Infection may then slowly spread bilaterally to the skin of the nose, upper lip, and cheeks or to the paranasal sinuses, orbits, and pharynx. The skin remains intact, but turns shiny and erythematous.[55] Diagnosis is suggested by the clinical picture and the potassium hydroxide (KOH) smear and is confirmed by biopsy and culture. Treatment is with antifungal agents, although long-term results have been disappointing.

Rhinosporidiosis

Rhinosporidium seeberi is thought to be a fungus, although it has yet to be cultured. It is endemic to South Asia and is occasionally seen in tropical Africa and America. It is most frequently contracted by immersion in contaminated water. Rhinosporidiosis is a chronic inflammatory disease that most frequently involves the nasal mucosa. The conjunctiva, oral cavity, and larynx are less commonly involved. In the nose, rhinosporidiosis typically manifests as a friable, painless, polypoid growth. Nasal obstruction and bleeding are the most common symptoms. Histologic findings include chronic inflammatory changes and the presence of sporangia. Surgical excision is the preferred treatment. No effective medical treatment as yet exists.

SPECIFIC PROTOZOA: LEISHMANIA

The leishmaniases are caused by species of the protozoan genus leishmania. These parasites are transmitted from animal hosts to humans by sandflies. The disease is endemic to South and Central America, India, the Middle East, Africa, and the shores of the Mediterranean. Leishmania are obligate intracellular parasites that primarily inhabit macrophages. Expression of the disease can vary and depends on the species of parasite as well as on the immune status of the human host. Three major clinical forms of the disease are recognized: visceral, cutaneous, and mucosal.[60]

Visceral leishmaniasis, also known as kala-azar, reflects parasitic infection of the spleen, liver, bone marrow, and lymph nodes. Fever and weight loss are followed by hepatomegaly and massive splenomegaly. Uncommonly, the mucosa of the upper respiratory tract is involved. Untreated patients with kala-azar may die of hepatic failure.

Cutaneous leishmaniasis progresses from small nodules to ulcers. Healing may be accompanied by considerable scarring. The external nose is frequently involved. Cutaneous lesions of the nose may extend to the skin of the vestibule, but do not ordinarily involve nasal mucosa.

Mucosal (mucocutaneous) leishmaniasis is the least common form of the disease. It occurs as a sequela of the cutaneous form of the disease and appears when the initial skin lesions have healed. The nasal mucosa is most frequently involved. Septal perforation is common, and nasal deformity may result. Advanced lesions may extend onto the external nose, lip, and palate. Mucosal lesions of the oral cavity and larynx have also been described.

The diagnosis of leishmaniasis is confirmed by demonstration of the parasites in biopsy tissue. Serologic tests or a delayed-hypersensitivity skin test (Montenegro test) may help when parasites are not found. Treatment of leishmaniasis relies on pentavalent antimony.

REFERENCES

1. Glezen WP: The common cold. In: Infectious Diseases. Edited by Gorbach SL, Bartlett JG, and Blacklow NR. Philadelphia, WB Saunders, 1992.
2. Huovinen P, et al: Pharyngitis in adults: the presence and coexistence of viruses and bacterial organisms. Ann Intern Med 110: 612, 1989.
3. Mims CA, et al (eds): Medical Microbiology. St. Louis, CV Mosby, 1993.
4. MacMillan JA, et al: Viral and bacterial organisms associated with acute pharyngitis in a school-aged population. J Pediatr 109:747, 1986.
5. Kessler HA, et al: Diagnosis of human immunodeficiency virus infection in seronegative homosexuals presenting with an acute viral syndrome. JAMA 258:1196, 1987.
6. McMillan JA, et al: Viral and bacterial organisms associated with acute pharyngitis. J Pediatr 109:747, 1986.
7. Komaroff AL, et al: The prediction of streptococcal pharyngitis in adults. J Gen Intern Med 1:1, 1986.
8. Schwartz RH, Hayden GH, and Wientzen R: Children less than three years old with pharyngitis. Clin Pediatr 25:185, 1986.
9. Wiesner PJ, et al: Clinical spectrum of pharyngeal gonococcal infection. N Engl J Med 28:181, 1973.
10. Mustoe T and Strome M: Adult epiglottitis. Am J Otolaryngol 4:393, 1983.
11. MayoSmith MF, et al: Acute epiglottitis in adults. N Engl J Med 314:1133, 1986.
12. Gwaltney JM, Scheld WM, Sande MA, and Sydnor A: The microbiological etiology and antimicrobial therapy of adults with acute sinusitis: a fifteen-year experience at the University of Virginia and review of other selected studies. J Allergy Clin Immunol 90:457, 1992.
13. Wald ER, et al: Subacute sinusitis in children. J Pediatr 115:28, 1989.
14. Hamory BH, et al: Etiology and antimicrobial therapy of acute maxillary sinusitis. J Infect Dis 139:197, 1979.
15. Wald ER, et al: Acute maxillary sinusitis in children. N Engl J Med 304:749, 1981.

16. Su WY, Liu C, Hung SY, and Tsai WF: Bacteriological study in chronic maxillary sinusitis. Laryngoscope *93*:931, 1983.

17. Orobello PW, et al: Microbiology of chronic sinusitis in children. Arch Otolaryngol Head Neck Surg *117*:980, 1991.

18. Humphrey MA, Simpson GT, and Gridlinger GA: Clinical characteristics of nosocomial sinusitis. Ann Otol Rhinol Laryngol *96*:687, 1987.

19. Linden BE, Aguilar EA, and Allen SJ: Sinusitis in the nasotracheally intubated patient. Arch Otolaryngol Head Neck Surg *114*:860, 1988.

20. Shapiro ED: Bacteriology of the maxillary sinuses in patients with cystic fibrosis. J Infect Dis *146*:589, 1982.

21. Bluestone CD, Stephenson JS, and Martin LM: Ten-year review of otitis media pathogens. Pediatr Infec Dis J *11*:S7, 1992.

22. Harding AL, et al: Hemophilus influenzae isolated from children with otitis media. In: Hemophilus influenzae. Edited by Sell SH and Karzon DT. Nashville, TN, Vanderbilt University Press, 1973.

23. Berman SA, Balkany TJ, and Simmons MA: Otitis media in infants less than 12 weeks of age: differing bacteriology among in-patients and out-patients. J Pediatr *93*:453, 1978.

24. Kenna MA, Bluestone CD, Reilly JS, and Lusk RP: Medical management of chronic otitis media without cholesteatoma. Laryngoscope *96*:146, 1986.

25. Wald ER: Anaerobes in otitis media and sinusitis. Ann Otol Rhinol Laryngol *154*:14, 1991.

26. Brook I: Aerobic and anaerobic bacteriology of cholesteatoma. Laryngoscope *91*:250, 1981.

27. NIH Conference: Epstein-Barr virus infections: biology, pathogenesis, and management. Ann Intern Med *118*:45, 1993.

28. Berry NJ, et al: Seroepidemiologic studies on the acquisition of antibodies to cytomegalovirus, herpes simplex virus, and human immunodeficiency virus among general hospital patients and those attending a clinic for sexually transmitted diseases. J Med Virol *24*:385, 1988.

29. Rook AH: Interactions of cytomegalovirus with the human immune system. Rev Infect Dis *10*:460, 1988.

30. Drew WL: Cytomegalovirus infection in patients with AIDS. Clin Infect Dis *14*:608, 1992.

31. Jones AC, et al: Cytomegalovirus infections of the oral cavity. Oral Surg Oral Med Oral Pathol *75*:76, 1993.

32. Rubin HS and Honigberg R: Sinusitis in patients with the acquired immunodeficiency syndrome. Ear Nose Throat J *69*:460, 1990.

33. Armstrong M, McArthur JC, and Zinreich JS: Radiographic imaging of sinusitis in HIV infection. Otolaryngol Head Neck Surg *108*:36, 1993.

34. Thompson C, et al: Etiology of acute sinusitis in HIV infection (abstract no. WS-BO8–6). Int Conf AIDS *9*:51, 1993.

35. Sample S, et al: Elevated serum concentrations of IgE antibodies to enviornmental antigens in HIV seropositive male homosexuals. J Allergy Clin Immunol *86*:876, 1990.

36. Tami TA and Wawrose SF: Diseases of the nose and paranasal sinuses in the human immunodeficiency virus-infected population. Otolaryngol Clin North Am *25*:1199, 1992.

37. Meyer RD, et al: Fungal sinusitis in patients with AIDS: report of 4 cases and review of the literature. Medicine *73*:69, 1994.

38. Barnett ED, Klein JO, Pelton SI, and Luginbuhl LM: Otitis media in children born to human immunodeficiency virus-infected mothers. Pediatr Infect Dis J *11*:360, 1992.

39. Lalwani AK and Sooy CD: Otologic and neurotologic manifestations of acquired immunodeficiency syndrome. Otolaryngol Clin North Am *25*:1183, 1992.

40. Sandler ED, et al: Pneumocystis carinii otitis media in AIDS: a case report and review of the literature regarding extrapulmonary pneumocystosis. Otolaryngol Head Neck Surg *103*:817, 1990.

41. Dichtel WJ: Oral manifestations of human immunodeficiency virus infection. Otolaryngol Clin North Am *25*:1211, 1992.

42. Balsam D, Sorrano D, and Barax C: Candida epiglottitis presenting as stridor in a child with HIV infection. Pediatr Radiol *22*:235, 1992.

43. Marelli RA, Biddinger PW, and Gluckman JL: Cytomegalovirus infection of the larynx in the acquired immunodeficiency syndrome. Otolaryngol Head Neck Surg *106*:296, 1992.

44. Browning DG, Schwartz DA, and Jurado RL: Cryptococcosis of the larynx in a patient with AIDS. South Med J *85*:762, 1992.

45. Rothstein SG, Persky MS, Edelman BA, et al: Epiglottitis in AIDS patients. Laryngoscope *99*:389, 1989.

46. Kaplan EL: Group A streptococcal infections. In: Textbook of Pediatric Infectious Diseases. 3rd Ed. Edited by Feigen RD and Cherry JD. Philadelphia, WB Saunders, 1990.

47. Jokipii A, et al: Semiquantitative culture results in peritonsillar abscesses. J Clin Microbiol *26*:957, 1988.

48. Shulman ST: Complications of streptococcal pharyngitis. Pediatr Infect Dis J *13*:S70, 1994.

49. Wood TF, Potter MA, and Jonasson O: Streptococcal toxic shock-like syndrome: the importance of surgical intervention. Ann Surg *217*:109, 1993.

50. Ferrieri P: Microbiological features of current virulent strains of group A streptococci. Pediatr Infect Dis J *10*:S20, 1991.

51. Bisno AL: Nonsuppurative poststreptococcal sequelae: rheumatic fever and glomerulonephritis. In: Principles and Practice of Infectious Disease. 3rd Ed. Edited by Mandell GL, Douglas RG, and Bennett JE. New York, Churchill Livingstone, 1990.

52. Special Writing Group of the American Heart Association: Guidelines for the diagnosis of rheumatic fever: Jones criteria, 1992 update. JAMA *268*:2069, 1992.

53. Zegarelli DJ: Fungal infections of the oral cavity. Otolaryngol Clinic North Am *26*:1069, 1993.

54. Manning SC, et al: Evidence of IgE-mediated hypersensitivity in allergic fungal sinusitis. Laryngoscope *103*:717, 1993.

55. Kwon-Chung KJ and Bennett JE: Medical Mycology. Philadelphia, Lea & Febiger, 1992.

56. Dumich PS and Neel HB: Blastomycosis of the larynx. Laryngoscope *93*:1266, 1983.

57. Smallman LA, et al: Cryptococcus of the larynx. J Laryngol Otol *103*:214, 1989.

58. Browning DG, Schwartz DA, and Jurado RL: Cryptococcosis of the larynx in a patient with AIDS: an unusual cause of fungal laryngitis. South Med J *85*:672, 1992.

59. Boyle JO, Coulthard SW, and Mandel RM: Laryngeal involvement in disseminated cocciodioidomycosis. Arch Otolaryngol Head Neck Surg *117*:433, 1991.

60. Sangueza OP, et al: Mucocutaneous leishmaniasis: a clinicopathologic classification. J Am Acad Dermatol *28*:927, 1993.

4 The Human Immune Response

Joel M. Bernstein

The immune system is charged with the formidable task of protecting the host against infection by potentially pathogenic microorganisms and preventing the development and dissemination of malignant tumors. These objectives are ideally met under conditions in which minimal injury to normal host tissues occurs. Moreover, the immune system must differentiate between "self" and "nonself" and only respond to the latter. Fortunately, immune responses to the majority of bacterial infections are able to eradicate the foreign body with minimal damage to the host; however, prolonged or exuberant immune responses are often associated with significant tissue disease.

Immune responses may be subdivided into two broad divisions, termed *innate* (or natural) *immunity* and *adaptive* (or acquired) *immunity.* These types of immunity differ in certain key properties including specificity and *immunologic memory.* Innate immunity represents an important first line of defense against infectious agents. This type of immunity (1) is present from birth, (2) is not enhanced by prior exposure to an infectious agent, (3) lacks immunologic memory, and (4) does not display antigenic specificity. Innate immune responses entail both cellular and noncellular elements. Physical barriers such as skin and mucous membranes represent a component of innate immunity that infectious agents must breach to gain access to the host. When this initial obstacle has been overcome, the microorganism may then encounter phagocytic cells present in blood and tissues. These include polymorphonuclear leukocytes (PMN), monocyte-macrophages, and a class of lymphocytes termed natural killer (NK) cells. Certain soluble factors also contribute innate immunity. For example, lysozyme, an enzyme found in mucus secretions, can damage the cell walls of many bacteria. Acute-phase proteins found in serum, including C-reactive protein, also contribute to clearance of many bacteria and fungi. The proteins of the complement system (especially the alternative path-

way, as discussed later in this chapter) contribute to innate immunity by generating products that recruit phagocytes into infected tissues, enhance phagocytosis and killing of bacteria, and lysesome microorganisms directly. The α and β interferons play an important role in eradication of virus-infected host cells. These proteins render host cells resistant to infection by viruses and also enhance NK cytotoxicity toward cells already infected by viruses. Interferon-activated NK cells also exhibit increased cytotoxicity toward tumor cells.

Persistence of an infection in spite of innate immune response typically leads to induction of an adaptive immune response. Adaptive immune responses, unlike innate responses, are characterized by (1) exquisite *specificity* for the offending antigen, (2) *memory* (a rapid and heightened response following subsequent encounter with the same or a closely related antigen), (3) *diversity* (the capacity to respond to millions of different antigens present in the environment), and (4) self versus nonself *recognition.* The characteristics of specificity and memory associated with adaptive immunity are often exploited in the development of vaccines designed to provide long-lived protection against pathogenic microorganisms.

CELLULAR ELEMENTS OF THE IMMUNE SYSTEM

The introduction of a foreign molecule or microorganism into an immunocompetent host typically results in the activation of lymphocytes. This adaptive immune response is manifested by an increase in the production of *antibodies* (humoral immunity), *effector lymphocytes* (cellular immunity), or both. In general, humoral immunity plays an important role in host defense against infections due to extracellular pathogens, whereas cellular immunity contributes to eradication of intracellular pathogens, such as virus-infected cells. Humoral and cellular immune responses often function in concert to eliminate infectious agents, however. Thus, cell-mediated reactions help eliminate virus-infected cells, whereas antibodies can block the spread of viruses and prevent reinfection of the host. The key cell types in the acquired immune response include (1) B (bone marrow-derived) lymphocytes, (2) T (thymus-derived) lymphocytes, and (3) antigen-presenting cells.

B Lymphocytes

B lymphocytes are the principal cell type in antibody-mediated, or humoral, immunity. These cells comprise approximately 15 to 30% of the total lymphocyte population in peripheral blood and are readily identified by virtue of their expression of surface immunoglobulins, which serve as a receptor for specific antigen. Following their interactions with antigen, these cells are induced to differentiate into antibody-secreting plasma cells. These antibody molecules exhibit a diverse array of biologic activities that contribute to host immune defense against many species of extracellular bacteria, as well as against certain viruses and tumors. Antibodies are also able to neutralize certain microbial products, particularly toxins, that may be injurious to host tissues.

B lymphocytes are thought to arise from pluripotential stem cells, which subsequently form stem cells committed to differentiation into lymphoid (both T and B cells) or myeloid (granulocytes, erythrocytes, mononuclear phagocytes, and megakaryocytes) cells. The liver is the primary site of B-lymphocyte production during the first trimester of life. Beyond this period, however, the bone marrow is the principal site for production of B lymphocytes.

The development of committed stem cells into mature B lymphocytes and, subsequently, into antibody-secreting plasma cells, involves *antigen-independent* and *antigen-dependent* phases (Fig. 4–1). During antigen-independent maturation, B-lymphocyte precursors undergo a series of changes involving DNA rearrangement of genes encoding for the heavy (H) and light (L) chains that comprise all immunoglobulin molecules. Rearrangements of heavy- and light-chain genes occur independently, with heavy-chain genes rearranging first. Because expression of surface immunoglobulin requires synthesis and assembly of both the heavy and light chains, pre-B cells, which have rearranged and synthesized heavy chains but not light chains, are negative for surface immunoglobulin; however, pre-B cells contain cytoplasmic heavy chains of the IgM class (designated μ chain). Once light-chain gene rearrangements are completed, the immature B cells are able to express surface IgM monomers. More mature B lymphocytes subsequently express both surface IgM and IgD. All these events occur in the absence

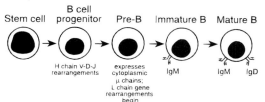

Antigen-independent maturation

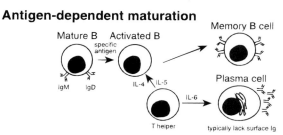

Antigen-dependent maturation

Fig. 4–1. Antigen-independent and antigen-dependent phases of B-lymphocyte development.

of antigen. Virgin B lymphocytes expressing surface immunoglobulin are now poised to bind antigen, which initiates a series of antigen-dependent changes leading to the differentiation of these cells into immunoglobulin-secreting plasma cells. Plasma cells are capable of secreting several thousand immunoglobulin molecules per second for a period of several days. Mature plasma cells are seldom found in the peripheral circulation, being primarily located in lymphoid tissues. These cells express few surface immunoglobulin molecules, consistent with the finding that plasma cells are geared toward immunoglobulin synthesis, rather than antigen-binding activity.

The differentiation of mature B lymphocytes into plasma cells requires multiple signals, the first of which is provided by antigen interaction with surface immunoglobulin (Fig. 4–1). Activated B lymphocytes are able to internalize and process the antigen and subsequently reexpress the antigen on the cell surface in conjunction with glycoproteins encoded in the major histocompatibility complex (MHC). (See the discussions of antigen processing and presentation later in this chapter.) In this manner, the activated B lymphocyte is able to "present" the antigen to T-helper lymphocytes with specificity for the antigen. The T-helper cells, in turn, secrete growth and differentiating factors (particularly interleukin-4 [IL-4] and IL-5) for antigen-stimulated B lymphocytes, which express membrane receptors for these molecules. An additional B-cell differentiation factor, IL-6, is required for terminal differentiation into plasma cells. This factor is produced by a variety of lymphoid and nonlymphoid cells. Thus, although B lymphocytes are the only cells capable of producing antibodies, T lymphocytes play an important role in the process of B-cell activation and differentiation into plasma cells.

Generation of Antibody Diversity

For antibodies to be an effective component of host defense, these molecules must be capable of recognizing a diverse array of antigens. Fortunately, normal individuals produce antibodies capable of combining with more than 10^7 different antigens. This is possible because of the variability and even hypervariability in the primary immunoacid sequences of the antigen-combining sites of immunoglobulin molecules. On the other hand, certain regions of the antibody molecule are structurally conserved. These regions are involved in many of the effector functions of antibodies. The information necessary to produce immunoglobulins of greater than 10^7 different antigenic specificities is encoded in DNA; however, individual genes encoding the heavy and light chains that form each unique antibody do not exist. Rather, B lymphocytes utilize an elaborate scheme involving somatic DNA rearrangements. Through this genetic mechanism, fewer than 10^4 gene segments can be combined in various ways sufficient to generate more than 10^7 antibodies of unique antigenic specificity.

The gene loci encoding sequences for the heavy chain and the two types of light chain (termed kappa [κ] and lambda [λ]) are found in different chromosomes (Fig. 4–2). The heavy- and light-chain loci are divided into multiple gene segments encoding the variable (V) and constant (C) regions of each chain. In the case of the κ and λ light chains, two segments encode the variable region, and one segment encodes the constant region. Heavy-chain synthesis involves three gene segments encoding the variable region and one segment encoding the constant region. The amino-terminal portions of the variable region of heavy and light chains are encoded in one of several variable-region

segments. Each variable-region gene is preceded by a leader sequence involved in the generation of a relatively hydrophobic signal peptide necessary for intracellular transport and secretion of immunoglobulins. Downstream (or in the 3' direction) of the variable-region gene segments are located the constant-region genes. Whereas the κ light-chain locus has a single constant-gene region, the λ light chain has three to six subsegments. Between the variable- and constant-region genes are a variable number of joining (J) region genes and, in the case of heavy chains, a series of diversity (D) segments. Located in the 3' end of the heavy-chain locus is a cluster of constant gene segments encoding the different classes and subclasses of immunoglobulins. As shown in Figure 4–2, there are some differences in the manner in which joining segments are distributed in the κ and λ light-chain loci.

The immunoglobulin gene segments are arranged in a similar germ-line configuration in all cells. Only in B lymphocytes, however, are these genes sequentially rearranged. Light-chain rearrangements begin with the combination of one of several hundred κ variable-region genes or one of approximately 100 λ variable-region genes with a joining segment. The intervening segments between the combined variable and joining segments are deleted. These combined variable-joining segments form the variable region of a light-chain gene. A primary, or nuclear, transcript is generated in which the constant-region genes remain separated from the rearranged variable-joining segments. Through a process termed RNA splicing, the intervening sequences separating the variable-joining and constant genes are eliminated, resulting in the formation of a "mature" messenger RNA. This mRNA can then be translated to yield a single polypeptide containing

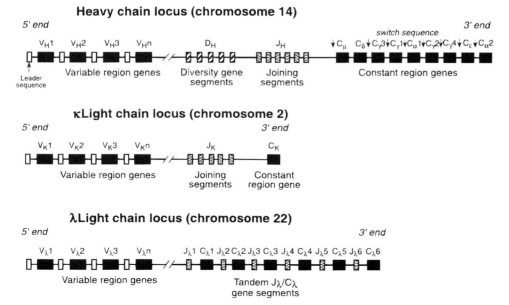

Fig. 4–2. Germline organization of the heavy- and light-chain immunoglobulin genes.

variable and constant-region amino acid sequences. In the case of heavy chains, the process is similar but involves additional gene segments not found in the light-chain loci. The process begins when 1 of approximately 5 to 15 diversity (D) segments recombines with joining segment, during which time any intervening sequences are deleted. This diversity-joining complex then combines with one of nearly 100 variable-region gene segments. Again, intervening sequences between the combined variable and diversity segments are deleted. After a primary RNA transcript is formed, the variable-diversity-joining complex is combined with one of several constant-region genes through RNA splicing. This mature mRNA is then translated into a complete heavy chain.

Rearrangement of variable, diversity, joining, and constant genes is sufficient to generate substantial antibody diversity, although other factors also contribute to this process. For example, *junctional site diversity* can extend the antibody repertoire because slight differences in the point of joining between variable-joining and variable-diversity-joining segments can lead to generation of new codons and, thus, altered amino acid sequences in the variable regions of the heavy and light chains. Second, inasmuch as the heavy and light chains are synthesized independently, the way in which heavy and light chains combine to form a complete immunoglobulin molecule can lead to *combinatorial diversity*. Finally, *somatic mutation* of rearranged genes can extend antibody diversity. This last mechanism is considered to be an important factor in the phenomenon of affinity maturation, as discussed later in this chapter.

Heavy-Chain Isotype Switching

The constant region of the heavy chain defines the class, or isotype, of immunoglobulin. Five such classes have been defined: IgG, IgA, IgM, IgD, and IgE. Studies demonstrated that a single variable region can be associated with different constant regions. Recognition of this fact led to the concept of isotype switching. Recall that mature, resting B lymphocytes display IgM and IgD on their surface. As shown in Figure 4–2, the constant-region genes for IgM (μ) and IgD (δ) heavy chains are in closer proximity to the variable, diversity, and joining segments than are the remaining constant-region genes. In fact, variable-diversity-joining complexes are first transcribed together with the μ constant-region gene. Following initial (primary) exposure to antigen is a lag period in which little or no antibody is present in serum. This is followed by an exponential increase in antibody production, particularly of the IgM isotype. Antibody production reaches a plateau and subsequently declines gradually. On subsequent encounters with the same antigen, the nature of the antibody response is markedly altered. First, the lag period is considerably shortened. Second, the magnitude of antibody production is substantially greater. Both effects are thought to be attributable to the presence of memory B and T lymphocytes. Further, one sees a significant increase (100-fold or greater) in the average affinity of serum antibodies reactive toward the relevant antigen. This has been termed affinity maturation and has been attributed to selection and clonal expansion of B lymphocytes whose surface immunoglobulins exhibit the greatest affinity for the antigen, as well as to somatic mutation of immunoglobulin variable genes.

Apart from the aforementioned quantitative changes that occur during the secondary, or *anamnestic*, response, there is often a quantitative change in which antibody isotypes other than IgM are produced in significant amounts. This latter effect is attributable to isotype switching, a process in which one or more constant heavy-chain genes is irreversibly deleted. The process appears to be mediated by switch sequences (Fig. 4–2) located on the five' side of each constant heavy region gene (except for the δ chain), under the control of cytokines produced by T lymphocytes. Activation of a particular switch sequence results in deletion of all constant region genes located 5' to the expressed heavy-chain gene. That μ and δ heavy-chain genes are not separated by a switch sequence is consistent with the ability of B lymphocytes to coexpress IgM and IgD.

Isotype switching depends on the presence of cytokines elaborated by T lymphocytes. Accordingly, the ability of a given antigen to induce isotype switching depends on the ability of that antigen to activate T lymphocytes. Many carbohydrate antigens, including bacterial lipo-oligosaccharides and pneumococcal polysaccharides, exhibit little or no ability to interact with T lymphocytes via their antigen receptors. Such antigens are termed T-independent antigens. Immunization with T-independent antigens typically results in the production of IgM antibody, with little or no evidence of isotype switching. On the other hand, many protein antigens can be processed and presented to T lymphocytes, resulting in T-lymphocyte activation and elaboration of cytokines involved in B-lymphocyte growth and isotype switching. These types of antigens are termed T-dependent antigens.

T Lymphocytes

A second population of lymphocytes also arises from a pluripotential stem cell in bone marrow. Unlike B lymphocytes, which undergo continued maturation in bone marrow, T lymphocytes differentiate in the thymus. Whereas B lymphocytes recognize antigens via surface immunoglobulins, T lymphocytes are surface-negative for immunoglobulin and do not exhibit DNA rearrangements in immunoglobulin genes. Rather, T lymphocytes express a distinct membrane receptor for antigen that recognizes antigen in conjunction with membrane glycoproteins encoded in the MHC (see later discussion). T lymphocytes play a major role in the initiation and regulation of immune responses and are key elements of cell-mediated immune responses against viruses, intracellular bacteria, and tumors.

T lymphocytes express different membrane antigens at various stages of development and/or cell activation. These surface markers have been useful in the identification of phenotypic and functional diversity among T lymphocytes. These markers were previously identified by means of monoclonal antibodies, which recognize specific antigenic determinants (termed *epitopes*) within a given surface membrane protein. Hence, T-lymphocyte markers were formerly referred to according to their reactivity toward different monoclonal antibodies, for example, OKT4, Leu-15, etc. Because of the structural complexity of membrane proteins, one can generate different monoclonal antibodies that recognize different epitopes within the same molecule. This discovery led to a brief period in which published scientific papers described T lymphocytes on the basis of their reactivity toward a specific monoclonal antibody, rather than on the basis of lymphocyte expression of the entire surface membrane protein. This situation was resolved following a series of International Human Leukocyte Differentiation Antigen Workshops, commencing in 1982. As a consequence of these workshops, a leukocyte surface marker that is reactive toward a group (or cluster) of monoclonal antibodies is now identified according to a *cluster of differentiation* (CD) number (e.g., CD2, CD8).

Certain CD markers are expressed by virtually all peripheral blood T lymphocytes. This is the case with respect to CD2, a 50-kilodalton glycoprotein through which T lymphocytes form rosettes with sheep red blood cells. Other CD markers are useful in segregating T lymphocytes into certain distinct subpopulations. Thus, approximately 60% of peripheral blood T lymphocytes express CD4, a glycoprotein expressed on T cells whose activation depends on recognition of antigen in conjunction with class II MHC molecules (see later). Approximately 30% of peripheral blood T lymphocytes express CD8, a membrane protein expressed by T cells whose activation depends on recognition of antigen in conjunction with class I MHC molecules. The majority of circulating T lymphocytes express either CD4 or CD8, but not both. These two surface markers define subsets of T lymphocytes with significantly different effector functions. Notably, CD4 + T lymphocytes typically function as helper (designated T_H) cells, providing "help" to other T lymphocytes as well as to immunoglobulin-producing B lymphocytes. On the other hand, CD8 + T cells exhibit *cytotoxic/suppressor* (T_C or T_S) activity. These cells elaborate factors that inhibit T_H activity, thereby suppressing immune

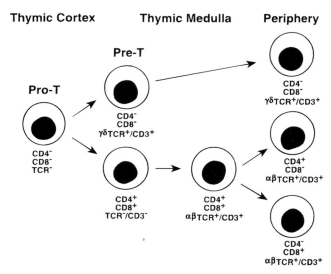

Fig. 4–3. Intrathymic development of T-lymphocyte subpopulations.

responses. CD8 + T lymphocytes also display cytotoxic activity toward numerous virally infected or tumor cells. Whether the suppressor and cytotoxic activities are mediated by the same or distinct subpopulations of CD8 + T cells is unclear.

T-Lymphocyte Ontogeny

T lymphocytes undergo differentiation in the thymus, irrespective of whether they express the CD4 or CD8 phenotype. The process of T-lymphocyte maturation begins with the migration of T-cell precursors from the bone marrow to the cortical regions of the thymus. These cells are thought to be attracted to the thymus by chemical signals provided by thymic epithelial cells. The earliest recognizable thymocyte committed to the T-cell lineage is the *pro-T cell* (Fig. 4–3). These cells bear CD2 (the sheep erythrocyte receptor), but do not express the T-cell antigen receptor. Pro-T cells are also surface-negative for CD4 and CD8. During the next phase of development, maturing cortical thymocytes proceed along one of two alternate pathways. In one instance, the thymocytes begin to rearrange DNA segments encoding for the variable and constant regions of an alternative form of a T-cell antigen receptor (designated γ/δ TCR) and express this receptor in conjunction with a tightly associated complex of five membrane glycoproteins that form the CD3 complex. Most cells expressing the γ/δ TCR fail to express either CD4 or CD8 during further development and release into the peripheral circulation as "double-negative" T lymphocytes. The precise function of these γ/δ TCR expressing cells has not been defined. The majority of pre-T cells follow a different pathway of differentiation. These pre-T cells coexpress both CD4 and CD8, but do not yet express an antigen receptor. Subsequently, these cells undergo DNA rearrangements of genes encoding the constant variable region of the

α/β TCR, which is expressed by the majority of T lymphocytes in the periphery. At this stage, the thymocytes are CD4+ and CD8+ and express the α/β TCR in conjunction with the CD3 complex. During the final stages of development, which occur in the thymic medulla, two important events take place. First, the cells progressively lose either CD4 or CD8. Second, these cells are "educated" by thymic epithelial cells to learn to differentiate between "self" and "nonself" MHC gene products. Those cells that are autoreactive toward self-MHC molecules are eliminated by a process of *clonal deletion,* an important mechanism of self-tolerance. As a consequence of this selection process, only about 10% of the immature T cells that enter the thymus ever reach the peripheral circulation. Mature T cells that survive the selection process leave the thymic medulla through the walls of postcapillary venules. After circulating for a time, these T lymphocytes distribute among various peripheral lymphoid tissues, including the thymus-dependent regions of the inner cortex of lymph nodes, the interfollicular areas of the tonsils and adenoids, the spleen, the mucosa-associated lymphoid tissue, particularly Peyer's patches in the gastrointestinal tract, and the bronchus-associated lymphoid tissue in the lower airway.

Currently, we do not know what signals drive proliferation and differentiation of immature thymocytes. These cells do express receptors for certain cytokines that exhibit growth factor activity, including IL-2 and IL-7 produced by thymocytes and stromal cells, respectively. Alternatively, thymic epithelial cells may induce thymocyte activation via the CD2 molecule, which recognizes a cell-adhesion molecule (LFA-3) expressed on the epithelial cells.

T-Cell Antigen Receptor (TCR) Complex
Unlike B lymphocytes, which recognize soluble antigen through membrane-associated immunoglobulin receptors, T lymphocytes only recognize antigens when displayed on the surface of antigen-presenting cells. The TCR is a heterodimer consisting of a 50-kilodalton acidic α chain and a 42-kilodalton basic β chain, which are linked through an interchain disulfide bond. Genes encoding the α chain are located on chromosome 14, whereas those encoding the β chain reside on chromosome 7. Each chain is composed of a variable region, which interacts with the associated complex of immunogenic peptide plus a histocompatibility molecule, and a constant region. Antigenic diversity among T-lymphocyte antigen receptors is generated through a process of DNA rearrangement similar to those described for the immunoglobulin genes. More than 50 variable-region genes and roughly 100 joining-region genes may encode the α chain. A single constant-region gene for the α chain is located "downstream" of the joining-region segments. The β chain locus consists of 75 to 100 variable-region genes, followed by 2 structur-

ally similar constant-region genes. Upstream of each C_β gene is a cluster of 6 to 7 joining-region gene segments preceded by a diversity-region segment not found in the α chain locus. Through a series of DNA rearrangements, alternative variable-, diversity-, joining-, and constant-region segments are brought into juxtaposition. A primary RNA transcript is formed, which is subsequently processed through RNA splicing to remove intervening gene sequences. The mature messenger RNA thus formed is translated to generate a continuous α or β chain containing variable- and constant-region sequences. Such DNA rearrangements, as well as variable combinations of translated α and β chains, can give rise to a diversity of TCRs capable of recognizing up to 1.7 million antigenic specificities.

The variable regions of the α/β TCR define antigenic specificity. As noted previously, however, T lymphocytes do not recognize antigen alone, but rather "see" processed antigen presented in conjunction with membrane glycoproteins encoded in the MHC. In the case of CD4+ T lymphocytes, antigen is recognized in conjunction with a class II MHC molecule, whereas CD8+ T lymphocytes recognize antigen presented by class I MHC-bearing cells. As shown in Figure 4–4, certain regions of the TCR recognize processed antigen, whereas others recognize variable regions of the class I or class II MHC molecule. In close proximity to the TCR complex is either a CD4 or a CD8 molecule. These molecules do not exhibit structural polymorphism and do not recognize antigen. These cell adhesion molecules recognize conserved regions in either a class I (CD8) or class II (CD4) molecule. The interaction between CD4 or CD8 and the corresponding MHC molecule appears to stabilize TCR interactions with the antigen-MHC complex.

The TCR contains a short cytoplasmic tail (Fig. 4–4). This cytoplasmic domain is thought to be insufficient to participate in signal transduction through the TCR molecule. Tightly associated with the TCR molecule, however, is a group of five molecules that comprise the CD3 complex. Three of the CD3 proteins (γ-δ and ϵ) are members of the immunoglobulin superfamily, each containing a single immunoglobulin-like domain. Two additional proteins, typically consisting of a disulfide-linked homodimer of two ζ chains, comprise the remainder of the CD3 complex. In contrast to the TCR, the proteins of the CD3 complex contain substantial cytoplasmic tails that are thought to play a major role in signal transduction initiated through the TCR.

Functional Properties
T lymphocytes are broadly divided into two subpopulations, T_H and T_C, which exhibit distinct functional characteristics. T_H lymphocytes, which typically display CD4, are essential elements in the development of cell-mediated immunity. Moreover, these cells provide important signals to B lymphocytes producing anti-

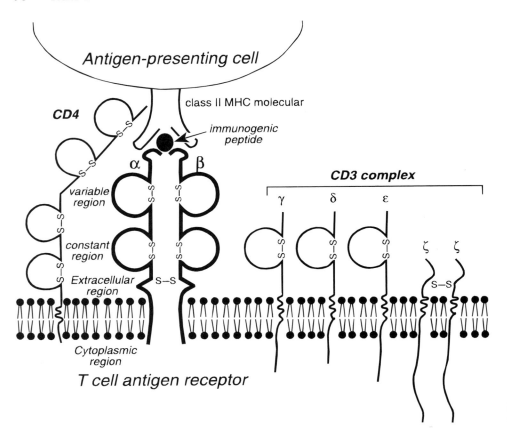

Fig. 4–4. General features of the T-cell antigen receptor/CD3 complex.

bodies. The critical role played by the T_H cell in orchestrating various aspects of the adaptive immune response is demonstrated in patients afflicted with human immunodeficiency virus (HIV), a member of the lentevirus family of animal retroviruses. The envelope of HIV contains a 120-kilodalton serous glycoprotein (gp120) that exhibits high-infinity binding to CD4-bearing cells, including macrophages and T_H lymphocytes. Binding of gp120 to CD4 facilitates insertion of a second viral envelope protein, gp41, into the target cell membrane, thereby initiating viral fusion. This process ultimately leads to the destruction of a substantial number of CD4-bearing lymphocytes, a hallmark of HIV-infected subjects. Depletion of CD4+ lymphocytes leads to the development of the acquired immunodeficiency syndrome (AIDS), in which the patient is markedly susceptible to opportunistic infections, especially pneumonia due to *Pneumocystis carinii*, and neoplastic disease, such as Kaposi's sarcoma. These clinical manifestations result from defects in cytotoxic T-cell, NK-cell and B-lymphocyte functions attributed to the loss of T_H activity.

Activation of T_H lymphocytes requires two distinct signals. The first signal is provided by antigen-presenting cells displaying processed antigen in conjunction with a class II MHC molecule. This signal initiates a series of biochemical changes that lead to the formation of certain second messengers, including inositol tri-

phosphate and diacylglycerol, that cause an increase in cytosolic calcium level and protein kinase activity. These events are necessary but not sufficient to induce T_H activation in the absence of a second signal. The second activation signal is referred to as a *costimulator molecule*, and is provided by the antigen-presenting cell. Some cytokines, including IL-1, tumor necrosis factor (TNF), and IL-6, have been found to exhibit costimulator activity, but which of these provides the critical second signal remains unclear. In any case, T_H lymphocytes respond to these two signals by activating genes encoding for growth factors and growth-factor receptors, particularly IL-2 and IL-2 receptor. IL-2 produced by the activated T_H cell exerts autocrine activity on the same cell that produced it. Expression of IL-2 receptors on the activated T_H cell permits the cell to respond to IL-2 (formally termed T-cell growth factor), resulting in increased cell proliferation. In this way, antigen stimulation of T_H leads to the expansion of the T-cell population capable of responding to the antigen. This clonal expansion is a key factor in the development of heightened immune responses following secondary and subsequent exposure to the same antigen.

Activation of CD4+ T_H lymphocytes also results in the secretion of other cytokines that act on other elements of the immune system. Thus, interferon γ, also called immune interferon, is a potent activator of macrophage microbicidal and tumoricidal activity.

CD4+ lymphocytes also secrete IL-4 and IL-5, which are key growth factors for B lymphocytes. IL-2 also provides the second activation signal for CD8+ T lymphocytes that have been triggered through their TCRs. Under the influence of IL-2 provided by the T_H cell, CD8+ T lymphocytes differentiate into cytotoxic lymphocytes capable of lysing virus-infected and tumor cells.

Recent evidence suggests that CD4+ T_H lymphocytes may be divided into two subsets, based primarily on differences in the patterns of cytokines secreted by human and mouse CD4+ cell lines. CD4+ cells of the T_H1 phenotype secrete IL-2, lymphotoxin, and interferon γ, but not the B-lymphocyte growth factors IL-4 and IL-5. In contrast, CD4+ cells of the T_H2 phenotype secrete IL-4 and IL-5, but not IL-2 lymphotoxin or interferon γ. Cells of the T_H1 phenotype secrete cytokines that appear to be important in delayed hypersensitivity and cytotoxic T-cell reactions, whereas cytokines secreted by the T_H2 phenotype appear to mediate immediate hypersensitivity (allergic reactions) in which B lymphocytes are induced to elaborate IgE. Distinct patterns of cytokines produced in allergic subjects and in patients with certain forms of parasitic infections lend further support to the concept that functional subsets of T_H cells exist. At present, however, no definitive surface markers are available that distinguish CD4+ lymphocytes secreting different patterns of cytokines. Thus, it remains unclear whether the T_H1 and T_H2 phenotypes represent distinct subsets of CD4+ T lymphocytes or merely reflect different stages of activation of a single cell type.

Memory B and T Lymphocytes

The development of a secondary, or anamnestic, humoral immune response depends on the generation of a population of B and T lymphocytes termed *memory* cells. Whether these cells arise during the normal process of antigen-included clonal expansion and activation or are a distinct subset of lymphocytes predestined to become memory cells is unclear. Both memory B and T cells appear to be long-lived, in some instances surviving for as long as three decades. Memory B cells may be distinguished from resting B cells by the isotypes of immunoglobulin displayed on their surface. Notably, whereas resting B cells express surface IgM and IgD, memory B cells express other isotypes including IgG, IgA, and IgE. Differential binding of monoclonal antibodies to two distinct T-cell surface markers, designated CD44 and CD45, has been used to distinguish virgin T lymphocytes from memory T lymphocytes. Memory B and T lymphocytes are responsive to secondary exposure to antigen. In the case of memory B cells, this may be attributable to expression of surface immunoglobulin of high affinity that occurs on resting B cells. Memory T cells, on the other hand, express high-affinity receptors for IL-2.

Cytotoxic Effector Cells

Cell-mediated cytotoxicity (i.e., the capacity of one cell to kill another) is an important process in the elimination of intracellular parasites, as well as virus-infected and malignant host cells. Mononuclear phagocytes activated via the T cell-derived cytokine interferon γ exhibit markedly enhanced microbicidal and tumoricidal killing. Other types of leukocytes are also capable of functioning as cytotoxic effector cells, however. These include (1) *cytotoxic T lymphocytes* (CTL), (2) *NK cells*, and (3) *lymphokine-activated killer* (LAK) cells. Cytotoxic effectors differ in their expression of certain surface markers and in their antigenic specificity toward target cells.

CTL are CD8+ cells and display MHC class I restriction. That is, these cells recognize intracellularly synthesized antigen (produced by virus-infected cells or tumor cells) displayed on the target cell membrane in association with MHC class I molecules. As these cells also display the TCR, they exhibit antigenic specificity toward target cells. NK cells belong to a subset of lymphocytes termed large granular lymphocytes, so named because they possess a round, indented nucleus and abundant cytoplasm containing numerous granules. These cells lack surface markers characteristic of B (surface immunoglobulin) or T (TCR) lymphocytes. They do, however, express CD16, the low-affinity receptor for the Fc region of IgG. NK cells participate in antibody-dependent cell-mediated toxicity (ADCC) toward antibody-coated targets. A third type of cytotoxic effector, the LAK cell, is similar to the NK cell in lacking antigenic specificity. LAK activity is generated following the incubation of freshly isolated lymphoid cells with high concentrations of IL-2. LAK cells display cytolytic activity toward a broader range of target cells than NK cells. Recent evidence indicates that the majority of LAK activity induced by IL-2 derives from NK cells.

CTLs develop from "pre-CTLs," which undergo maturation in the thymus. Pre-CTLs express the TCR/CD3 complex, as well as CD8 but are not competent for cytotoxic activity. On receiving appropriate signals, pre-CTLs undergo differentiation into CTLs. At least two signals are necessary for pre-CTLs to differentiate into CTLs. First, the pre-CTL must bind specific antigen via its membrane TCR. This signal induces expression of IL-2 receptors on the pre-CTL. The pre-CTL is then able to respond to a second signal provided by cytokines by T_H cells. These cytokines include IL-2, IL-4, IL-6, and interferon γ. Certain changes occur as a consequence of differentiation of pre-CTL into the CTL, including the emergence of cytoplasmic granules and the synthesis and secretion of cytokines, particu-

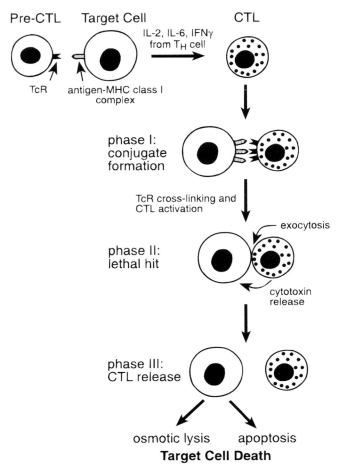

Fig. 4–5. Stages in the activation and function of cytotoxic T lymphocytes.

larly interferon γ and lymphotoxin (TNF β). The cytoplasmic granules contain several proteins that contribute to the cytotoxic properties of CTL, including perforin (a pore-forming protein), serine esterases, and a cytotoxin (either lymphotoxin itself or related protein).

The process of CTL-mediated killing of target cells appears to involve several steps (Fig. 4–5). The first phase entails the firm adhesion (termed *conjugate formation*) of the CTL to an appropriate target. Target specificity is achieved via recognition of the associated complex of antigen and MHC class I macromolecule by the TCR. Cell contact is further reinforced through additional adhesive interactions that lack antigen specificity. In the second (''lethal hit'') phase, cross-linking of TCRs leads to activation of the CTL. One consequence of CTL activation is the exocytosis of cytoplasmic granules in the region of the CTL membrane, which is in direct contact with the target cell. This focused release of cytoplasmic granules probably accounts for the finding that CTL typically do not kill ''innocent bystander'' cells with which they are in contact. Granule exocytosis leads to the release of perforin,

a protein that polymerizes in the target cell membrane to form ion channels. These channels, if sufficient in number, allow the progressive movement of ions and water across the cell membrane, resulting in osmotic lysis. Other cytoplasmic granule constituents also contribute to the ultimate demise of the target cell. During this same period, the activated CTL secretes a cytotoxin, possibly lymphotoxin, which activates certain enzymes in the target cell that uncoil and degrade DNA through a process termed programmed cell death, or *apoptosis*. Under such conditions, cell death occurs without overt lysis of the target cell. Following delivery of the lethal hit, the CTL is released from the target cell, which continues to undergo cytolysis and/or apoptosis. The CTL does not self-annihilate during the process of target cell killing. Rather, these cells recycle and are often capable of attacking additional target cells. Although CTLs appear to participate in acute graft rejection, these cells are thought to play a significant role in the elimination of viral infections.

NK cells, unlike CTLs, do not require prior contact with target cell antigens to develop cytotoxic capability. This is not surprising, because NK cells lack surface immunoglobulins and TCRs necessary for antigen recognition. Moreover, NK cells do not exhibit MHC restriction characteristic of CTLs. NK cells emerge from bone marrow already competent for target cell killing. As in the case of CTLs, however, NK activity can be increased by cytokines such IL-2, TNF, or interferon γ. Moreover, IL-2 induces proliferation of NK cells. Target cell specificity of NK cells is somewhat broader than is true for CTLs, but NK activity is not random; that is, NK cells are capable of killing some tumors but not others. The nature of the target cell structures recognized by NK cells has not been determined. NK activity toward target cells can be enhanced through deposition of specific IgG antibodies to the target surface because NK cells possess receptors for the Fc region of IgG.

The mechanisms utilized by NK cells in target killing appear to be similar to those employed by CTLs. Like CTLs, NK cells contain numerous cytoplasmic granules (hence their morphologic features as large granular lymphocytes) and secrete a cytotoxin. The composition of the granules of CTL and NK cells appears to be similar. Whether the cytotoxin release from NK cells is identical to the protein secreted by CTL is unclear; however, NK cells do not synthesize lymphotoxin. Although the role of NK cells in immunity is poorly understood, these cells may be important in the graft-versus-host reaction seen in patients receiving bone marrow transplants.

Antigen Processing and Presentation

Studies evaluating the specificity of antigen recognition by B and T lymphocytes reveals some fundamen-

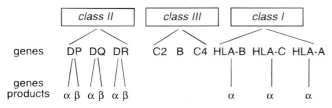

Fig. 4–6. Organization of MHC-encoded molecules in the human leukocyte antigen (HLA) complex.

tal differences in the way these two leukocyte populations recognize various antigens. First, B lymphocytes, via their membrane-bound immunoglobulins, are capable of recognizing carbohydrates, proteins, and nucleic acids, as well as low-molecular-weight chemical (haptens) coupled to carrier proteins. In contrast, T lymphocytes preferentially recognize protein antigens. Second, B lymphocytes often recognize *conformational* determinants in protein antigens, whereas T lymphocytes preferentially recognize *linear* (sequential) determinants. Finally, B lymphocytes (and secreted antibodies) recognize soluble protein antigens, whereas T lymphocytes only respond to protein antigens displayed on the surface of other cells.

We now know that the TCR recognizes peptide fragments of protein antigens, rather than native proteins. Moreover, the T-cell antigen "sees" the peptide fragment in conjunction with membrane glycoproteins encoded in the MHC. The latter conclusion is based on evidence that antigen-specific T lymphocytes only interact with cells expressing the appropriate antigen if the two cells share the same MHC, a phenomenon termed *MHC restriction.* Thus, for a T lymphocyte to recognize a protein antigen, the antigen must be first denatured, partially catabolized into small peptide fragments, become physically associated with a self

MHC-encoded molecule, and be displayed or presented on the surface of a cell as a peptide-MHC complex. This series of events is referred to as *antigen processing.* The MHC molecules that play such a critical role in T-cell antigen recognition are encoded in a multiallelic gene cluster located in the short arm of chromosome 6. The MHC complex in humans is known as the human leukocyte antigen (HLA) complex. The organization of genes associated with the HLA complex is depicted in Figure 4–6. This complex contains loci that encode for three major classes of membrane glycoproteins, termed class I, class II, and class III MHC molecules. The class I and class II gene regions are separated by a region containing genes that encode for certain complement components (C2, C4, and factor B), as well as for certain cytokines (TNF and lymphotoxin). This area is known as the class III gene region. Class I molecules are expressed on the surface of virtually all nucleated cells and include the classic transplantation antigens, which are important in allograft rejection. In contrast, class II molecules are expressed in a restrictive set of leukocytes termed *antigen-presenting cells,* or APCs. The region of the HLA complex encoding class II molecules (HLA-D) controls immunologic responsiveness to certain antigens and is termed the immune response region. Hence, the products of these genes are often referred to as the immune response region-associated antigens.

The general structural features of the MHC class I and II molecules encoded in the HLA complex are depicted in Figure 4–7. Class I MHC molecules have a two-chain structure consisting of a 43-kilodalton α chain encoded in the HLA-A, -B, and -C region and a noncovalently associated 12-kilodalton chain, called β2-microglobulin, which is encoded outside the HLA complex. The α chain is organized into a series of three

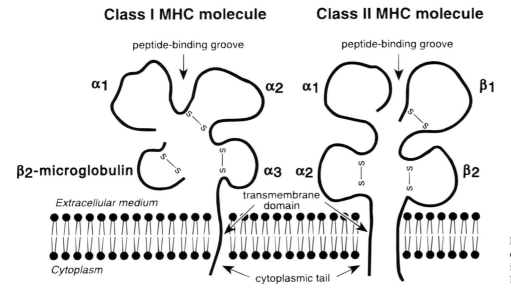

Fig. 4–7. General structural features of MHC class I and class II molecules involved in antigen presentation to T lymphocytes.

extracellular domains (α1, α2, and α3), a single transmembrane domain, and a short cytoplasmic tail. The greatest structural polymorphism among class I molecules is found in the α1 and α2 domains. This region forms the "groove" that serves as the antigen-binding site for processed peptide fragments. β2-Microglobulin, on the other hand, does not exhibit structural polymorphism and does not participate in antigen binding. The association between β2-microglobulin and the α chain appears to be important in maintaining class I molecules in their proper conformation.

Class II MHC molecules also possess a two-chain structure that is organized in a manner analogous to that of class I molecules. These molecules contain a 31- to 35-kilodalton α chain and a 27- to 30-kilodalton β chain, each of which contributes two extracellular domains, a transmembrane domain and a cytoplasmic tail. Both chains are encoded in the HLA-D region. As is the case with class I molecules, the two most extracellular domains (α1 and β1) of class II molecules exhibit the most structural polymorphism and form a groove that appears to participate in peptide binding.

The physical dimensions of the groove present in the extracellular region of MHC class I and class II molecules are consistent with the ability of these molecules to bind small peptides (8 to 10 amino acids) but not large molecules such as globular proteins or complex polysaccharides. Structural polymorphism in the most external regions of MHC class I and class II molecules appears to enable these molecules to bind antigenically distinct peptide fragments. The antigenic specificities of MHC class I and class II are, however, lower than for TCR or immunoglobulins.

Even though MHC class I and class II molecules share certain structural features, these molecules differ in one very significant way. This concerns the nature of the T lymphocytes capable of recognizing class I-peptide and class II-peptide complexes. Specifically, MHC class I molecules present antigens to CD8-bearing T lymphocytes, whereas class II molecules present antigen to CD4-bearing T lymphocytes. There are also differences in the intracellular routes followed by MHC molecules and antigens before their interaction with T lymphocytes, as discussed later.

Pathways of Antigen Processing

The immune system exhibits the capacity to respond to antigens of intracellular as well as extracellular origin. Nature of the immune response in each instance can differ significantly, however. That divergent mechanisms have evolved for the processing and presentation of *intracellular* and *extracellular* antigens is not surprising. The following discussion makes clear that intracellular antigens are presented to CD8+ T lymphocytes by MHC class I molecules, whereas extracellular antigens are presented to CD4+ T lymphocytes by MHC class II molecules.

The processing of intracellular protein antigens, either of host cell origin or encoded by viral nucleic acids, begins in the cytosol (Fig. 4–8). These protein antigens are "shuttled" to the lumen of the endoplasmic reticulum (ER) by transporter proteins. Cleavage of intracellular proteins into smaller peptide fragments is thought to occur during transport through the cytosol, within the lumen of the ER, or both. Peptide fragments of suitable size and composition associate with the peptide-binding groove in the MHC class I molecules located in the lumen of the ER. Class I-peptide complexes are moved to the Golgi apparatus via transport vesicles and subsequently exported to the cell surface. The MHC molecules are anchored to the cell surface by their transmembrane domain. Because virtually all nucleated cells express MHC class I molecules, any cell is capable of processing and presenting intracellular protein antigens in this manner. Intracellular antigens handled via this route are presented to CD8+ T lymphocytes, typically of the cytotoxic-suppressor phenotype, whose antigen receptors have specificity for the antigenic peptide fragment displayed by the MHC molecule. Inasmuch as CD8+ cytotoxic lymphocytes are key effectors against viruses and tumor cells, it makes sense teleologically that intracellular antigens would be presented to CD8+ T cells in this manner.

An alternative pathway is utilized in the processing of extracellular antigens (Fig. 4–9). As currently envisioned, extracellular antigens are first internalized by antigen-presenting cells by means of coated pits and are subsequently shuttled to the endosomal compartment. Within the ER, newly synthesized MHC class II molecules associate with a 30-kilodalton *invariant chain,* which occupies the peptide-binding groove. This interaction prevents class II molecules from binding endogenous peptides. The MHC class II-invariant chain complex is transported to the endosomal compartment, whereupon lysosomal enzymes proteolytically degrade the invariant chain and enable the class II molecule to associate with processed antigen in this same compartment. The peptide-class II complex is transported to the cell surface, where it is available for interaction with CD4+ T lymphocytes bearing TCR of appropriate specificity.

Whereas intracellular antigens are presented to CD8+ T lymphocytes by MHC class I molecules that are found in all nucleated cells, extracellular antigens are presented to CD4+ T lymphocytes by class II molecules found only on a specialized group of antigen-presenting cells (Table 4–1). These cells express class II molecules constitutively. Other cell types, including glial, mesenchymal, and vascular endothelial cells, normally do not express class II molecules unless induced by cytokines such as interferon γ. Once induced

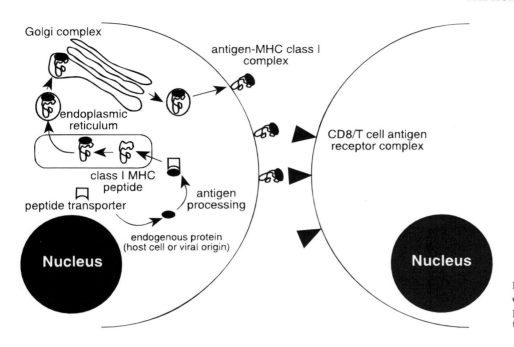

Fig. 4–8. Schematic representation of events involved in processing and presentation of intracellular antigens to CD8 + T lymphocytes.

in this manner, these cells can also function as antigen-presenting cells for CD4 + T lymphocytes.

MHC-restricted antigen presentation is biologically significant for several reasons. First, MHC-encoded molecules, by virtue of the structure of their antigen-binding grooves, determine which antigens will be available for presentation to T lymphocytes. Second, the class of MHC molecule with which the immunogenic peptide fragment is associated determines the

phenotype (CD4 + or CD8 +) of T cell that is ultimately stimulated. Finally, MHC restriction necessitates that intimate contact exist between the antigen-presenting cell and the T lymphocyte. This ensures that signals provided by the antigen-presenting cell are directed to appropriate antigen-specific T cell clones, which preferentially expand. For example, macrophages present antigen to CD4 + T cells in conjunction with class II molecules; however, this is insufficient to cause activa-

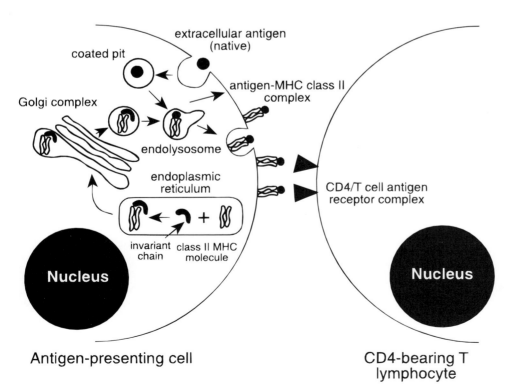

Antigen-presenting cell   CD4-bearing T lymphocyte

Fig. 4–9. Schematic representation of events involved in processing and presentation of extracellular antigens to CD4 + T lymphocytes.

TABLE 4–1. Types of Antigen Presenting Cells Expressing Class II MHC Molecules

Cell Type	Comments
Mononuclear phagocytes	Fixed and wandering mononuclear phagocytes found in most tissues; constitutively express class II MHC molecules, but levels can be markedly increased by mediators such as interferon γ; antigen uptake facilitated by opsonization
Langerhans-dendritic cells (LDC)	Found in high numbers in thymus-dependent regions of peripheral lymphoid organs, as well as skin and epithelia; constitutively express high levels of class II MHC molecules; LDC in skin can process antigen and migrate to lymphoid tissues for subsequent antigen presentation; may be important in processing antigens introduced via skin or epithelia
B lymphocytes	Constitutively express class II MHC molecules; increased class II expression induced by IL-4 but not by interferon γ; antigen uptake may be nonspecific or via membrane immunoglobulin; "resting" B lymphocytes are poor antigen-presenting cells in comparison to B lymphocytes activated by lymphokines or polyclonal B cell activators

tion of the T cell. A second signal is provided in the form of IL-1, a protein secreted by activated macrophages. These two signals induce activation of the CD4 + T cell, which then secretes certain cytokines that promote growth and differentiation of other lymphocytes. Moreover, these cytokines exert an autocrine effect on the T cell, which secreted them, thereby inducing clonal expansion of antigen-specific T cells. In this way, MHC restriction requires that cellular interactions necessary for optimal immune responsiveness take place.

Antigen-presenting cells also play a key role in the development of immature T cells within the thymus. Thymic epithelial cells express both MHC class I and class II molecules on their surface and present these molecules to thymocytes through direct cell-to-cell contact. This interaction appears to be important in "educating" mature thymocytes with respect to differentiation of self versus nonself MHC gene products. Those thymocytes that are capable of recognizing self-MHC molecules are clonally deleted and fail to leave the thymus.

EFFECTOR MECHANISMS OF HOST IMMUNITY

General Features of Immunoglobulins

Investigators have known for many years that a major component of acquired immunity is the production of antibody activity in the fluid phase (plasma) of blood. Antibody activity resides in the heterogenic group of serum proteins that migrate principally as γ-globulins (and, to a lesser degree, as β-globulins) on electrophoresis on agarose gels. For this reason, the term "gamma-globulins" was formerly used to describe the antibody-containing fraction of the serum. This terminology has been abandoned in favor of the term *immunoglobulin*, which is more descriptive of the biologic properties of these molecules.

Immunoglobulins are glycoproteins containing 82 to 96% polypeptide and 4 to 8% carbohydrate and are heterogeneously distributed in various biologic fluids and on the surface of some populations of lymphocytes. These molecules are produced as a consequence of foreign substances reacting with antigen-specific B lymphocytes and are the mediators of humoral immunity. Immunoglobulins are bifunctional molecules that are capable of (1) recognizing specific antigenic determinants and (2) eliciting a diverse array of effector functions that promote neutralization and/or elimination of the antigen. Almost all the biologic activity of immunoglobulins appears to be attributable to the polypeptide component. The role of the carbohydrate moiety in immunoglobulin function is not completely understood. It may, however, be involved in immunoglobulin secretion by plasma cells, as well as in modulation of some of the effector functions of immunoglobulins.

The basic structure of immunoglobulins has been elucidated through several approaches, including the use of proteolytic enzymes (especially pepsin and papain) and chain dissociation techniques (unfolding proteins in 6 M urea and reducing disulfide bonds with mercaptoethanol). The results of these studies have indicated that all immunoglobulins contain a basic monomer structure consisting of two heavy chains and two light chains (Fig. 4–10). The heavy chains contain approximately twice as many amino acid residues as the light chains. Each chain is organized into a series of domains, each consisting of approximately 110 amino acids, generated by intrachain disulfide linkages. The "loop" structure formed through such disulfide bonding is a common characteristic of a broad array of proteins belonging to the immunoglobulin *superfamily*. Immunoglobulins also contain interchain disulfide linkages (heavy-light and heavy-heavy), which can vary in position and number. Comparison of the amino acid sequences of numerous immunoglobulin molecules indicates that the amino termini of each heavy and light chain contain a variable (V) region sequence, whereas the carboxy termini contain more conserved constant (C) region sequences. Hence, the light chain contains a V_L region. The heavy chain also contains a single variable region (V_H), but contains multiple constant (C_H) domains. The latter are numerically ordered from the amino terminus of the heavy chain (e.g., C_H1,

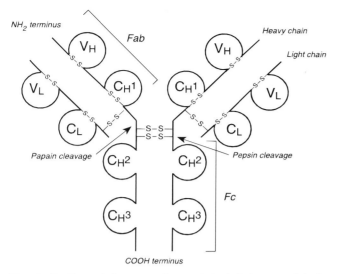

Fig. 4–10. General features of a prototypical immunoglobulin monomer.

C_H2, etc.). The region of the heavy chain between the first (C_H1) and second (C_H2) domains exhibits increased flexibility and susceptibility to proteolytic attack and is termed the *hinge region.*

Within the variable region of each heavy and light chain are certain stretches of amino acids that exhibit marked sequence variation. Such regions are termed *hypervariable regions.* Other segments of the variable region show much less variation and are termed *framework regions.* We now know that the hypervariable regions of the heavy and light chains form the antigen-binding site of the immunoglobulin molecule. Inasmuch as the hypervariable regions possess a structure complementary to that of the antigen that they recognize, these regions are also referred to as *complementarity-determining regions,* or CDRs. Each V_L and V_H segment has three CDRs.

Studies involving limited enzymatic cleavage provide additional insight into the general structure and function of the immunoglobulin molecule. Two enzymes, papain and pepsin, have been particularly useful in this regard. Both enzymes cleave the immunoglobulin molecule in the area between the C_H1 and C_H2 domains, but differ with respect to the precise site of attack relative to the interheavy chain and disulfide linkages (Fig. 4–10). Papain cleaves immunoglobulins on the amino terminal side (i.e., closer to the variable region domain) of the disulfide bonds that link the two heavy chains together. Digestion of the immunoglobulin molecule in this manner yields three fragments. Two of the fragments are of equal molecular mass, each containing all the light chain and the V_H and C_H1 domains. These fragments contain structures capable of binding specific antigen and are termed *Fab* (fragment antigen binding). The remaining fragment, which lacks antigen-binding activity, has a larger mass than the

Fab fragment and tends to crystalize. This fragment has been termed *Fc* (fragment-crystallizable). Pepsin cleaves immunoglobulins on the carboxy-terminal side of the interheavy chain disulfide bonds, producing a single large fragment containing both Fab fragments linked by disulfide bonds and termed F(ab)$_2$. The Fc fragment is extensively degraded by pepsin. The results of these studies indicate that the basic structure of the immunoglobulin monomer is comprised of two antigen-binding Fab fragments and a single Fc fragment, the latter of which is associated with many of the effector functions of immunoglobulins.

Immunoglobulin Heavy Chain Classes (Isotypes)

As noted previously, the constant region of the immunoglobulin heavy chain exhibits considerably less sequence variation than does the variable region; however, subtle structural variations exist in the C_H regions of different immunoglobulin molecules. On the basis of serologic and chemical properties, human immunoglobulins can be differentiated into five distinct classes (or *isotypes*), each containing a different heavy chain. Thus, immunoglobulins are classified as belonging to the IgG, IgA, IgM, IgD, or IgE isotype. The heavy chain associated with each isotype is designated by a Greek letter. Hence, IgG contains a γ heavy chain, IgA an α chain, IgM a μ chain, IgD a δ chain, and IgE an ϵ chain. The immunoglobulin isotype is determined by the structure of the C_H domain, the γ, δ, and α heavy chains each contain a hinge region between the C_H1 and C_H2 domains. The μ and ϵ heavy chains do not have a hinge region, but rather contain an extended C_H2 domain with hinge-like flexibility. Moreover, μ and ϵ heavy chains contain five domains (one variable and four constant), whereas α and γ heavy chains contain four domains (one variable and three constant).

Immunoglobulin Light Chain Types

Structural and antigenic differences in the constant region of light chains are also sufficient to differentiate these molecules into two types (analogous to heavy chain classes), designated kappa (κ) and lambda (λ). A single immunoglobulin molecule always has two identical κ or λ light chains, rather than a mixture of the two types. Both light-chain types are represented in all five immunoglobulin classes, although not equally. Approximately 65% of IgG, IgA, and IgM molecules contain κ light chains, whereas the remaining 35% contain λ light chains (the proportions of these two light-chain types in IgD and IgE are less clear). In general, the $\kappa:\lambda$ ratio among human immunoglobulins is considered 2:1.

Heavy-Chain Subclasses

Based on minor physical, chemical, and serologic differences in the C_H regions of IgG and IgA, the heavy chains of these immunoglobulin isotypes may be further divided into *subclasses.* IgG consists of 4 subclasses (IgG_1, IgG_2, IgG_3, IgG_4), whereas IgA consists of 2 subclasses (IgA_1, IgA_2). The IgG and IgA subclasses differ in their proportional representation in serum. The percentage of each IgG and IgA subclass in serum of normal adults is as follows: IgG_1, 60 to 70%; IgG_2, 19 to 31%; IgG_3, 5 to 8%; and IgG_4, 1 to 4%; IgA_1, 93%; IgA_2, 7%. The IgA and IgG subclasses also differ in number and arrangement of the interchain disulfide linkages (Fig. 4–11). Note, for example, that the light chains of IgA_2 are covalently linked to each other rather than to the heavy chains. Although all 4 IgG subclasses contain covalently linked heavy and light chains, the location of the interchain disulfide linkage varies. The light chain of IgG_1 is linked to the γ heavy chain between C_H1 and C_H2 domains (i.e., closer to the hinge region), whereas the light chains of the remaining 3 IgG subclasses are attached to the heavy chain between the V_H and C_H1 domains. Also note that the number of

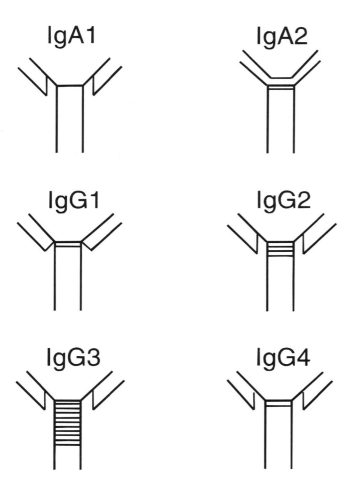

Fig. 4–11. Distribution of interchain disulfide linkages in human IgA and IgG subclasses.

interheavy chain disulfide linkages among the IgG subclasses can vary from 2 IgG_1, IgG_4, to 11 IgG_3. Structural variations can significantly influence the biologic properties of the immunoglobulin classes, as discussed later.

Light-Chain Subtypes

Minor differences in amino acids sequence of the constant region of the light chain have also been identified in humans, permitting classification into subtypes (analogous to heavy chain subclasses). Four subtypes of λ light chains have been identified. κ Light chains, on the other hand, do not exhibit such C_L variation.

Allotypic and Idiotypic Determinants

All normal individuals inherit the set of genes that encode the antigenic determinants in the constant regions of the immunoglobulin molecule that define heavy chain isotype and subclass and light chain type and subtype. Other antigenic determinants are expressed in immunoglobulins in some members of the species but not others. Antigenic variations in the constant regions of some heavy and light chains that differentiate members of the same species are called *allotypic determinants.* Allotypic variations arise because multiple alleles exist for some constant region genes, and these alleles are inherited in a mendelian fashion. Allotypes have been identified on all four human IgG subclasses, for IgA_2 subclass antibodies and for the κ light chain. Allotypic markers on the γ and α heavy chains and the κ light chain are designated as Gm, Am, and Km determinants. Some 20 Gm, 3 Km, and 2 Am allotypes have been identified. Certain allotypic markers are restricted to the constant region of a single IgG subclass, whereas others are shared by 2 or more subclasses, called isoallotypes. IgA_2 molecules bearing the m(1) marker do not contain heavy-light interchain disulfide linkages (Fig. 4–11), whereas those bearing the m(2) marker do.

Allotypic determinants are found on the immunoglobulin molecules of some, but not all, members of a given species. Yet other antigenic determinants distinguish one immunoglobulin molecule from another, even within a single individual. These antigenic markers are termed idiotypic determinants and are found in the variable region of the immunoglobulin molecule. Many of these idiotypic determinants arise as a consequence of the unique amino acid sequences found in the hypervariable regions of the heavy and light chains and are involved in generating the antigen-binding site.

Monomeric versus Polymeric Immunoglobulins

All five classes of immunoglobulins consist of the basic four-chain (two heavy and two light chains) structure.

Nevertheless, the molecular mass of different immunoglobulins can vary considerably, from approximately 150,000 to more than 900,000 daltons, because certain immunoglobulin classes (IgM, IgA) exist as polymers. IgM is a macroglobulin (molecular mass approximately 900,000 daltons) containing five monomer subunits each containing two light chains and two μ chains). IgA can be found in serum in both monomeric (160,000 daltons) and dimeric (415,000 daltons) form, approximately 20% of the total serum IgA being in the dimeric form. All polymeric immunoglobulins are associated with an additional polypeptide approximately 15,000 daltons in size that is termed the J *(joining)* chain. The J chain is synthesized by B lymphocytes producing polymeric immunoglobulins. Although it is not entirely clear how the J chain facilitates assembly of immunoglobulin monomers, this protein appears to forms a disulfide linkage with cysteine residues located in the C-terminal region of the α or μ chain of two adjacent monomer units. Additional monomer subunits (in the case of IgM) are then added, and they polymerize through Fc-Fc interactions. All polymeric immunoglobulins, regardless of the number of monomer subunits, contain the single J-chain molecule.

Secretory Component

IgA comprises only about 20% of the total serum immunoglobulins, but is the principal class of immunoglobulin found in external secretions (saliva, tracheal, bronchial secretions, genital, urinary secretions, sweat, tears, breast milk and colostrum, nasal secretions). IgA present in such secretions possesses a dimeric structure, in which the two IgA monomers are connected via a J chain. However, secretory IgA contains an additional component not found in other immunoglobulins, regardless of whether they are monomeric or polymeric (Fig. 4–12). This protein, termed secretory component, is a 70,000-dalton polypeptide synthesized by epithelial cells, not by B lymphocytes, as is true for the J chain. The secretory component is covalently added

to dimeric IgA during its transport across mucosal epithelial cells and appears to protect secretory IgA from proteolytic cleavage by enzymes present in external secretions. Secretory IgM also occurs in secretions, particularly in the absence of IgA, and also possesses secretory component.

Biologic Properties of Immunoglobulins

The bifunctional nature of immunoglobulins permits these molecules to bind antigen specifically and to initiate certain biologic effector functions. Some of these effector functions are mediated through the antigen-binding region (Fab), whereas others are initiated through the Fc moiety. Moreover, distinct immunoglobulin classes and subclasses are often associated with different biologic activities. Some of the key effector functions performed by immunoglobulins are summarized in Table 4–2. Fab-mediated binding of immunoglobulin to microbial toxins and certain viruses often results in their effective neutralization. For example, if an immunoglobulin molecule binds to a viral surface antigen that is involved in the attachment of the virion to a host cell, the ability of the virus to infect the host is impaired. Similarly, immunoglobulin binding to toxins can inhibit the ability of the toxin to interact with membrane receptors on the host target cell. In both instances, Fab or Fab'$_2$ fragments suffice in mediating these effects.

Other immunoglobulin effector moieties depend on an intact immunoglobulin molecule and are mediated through the Fc moiety. Formation of antigen-antibody complexes involving IgG (but not IgG$_4$) or IgM can lead to activation of the complement system, resulting immunologic and hemodynamic changes associated with the inflammatory response. Complement activation via the classical pathway (see later) results from the interaction between complement component C1 with the C_H2 domain of IgG or the C_H3 domain of IgM. The interaction between immunoglobulins and the iso-

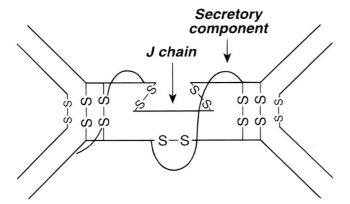

Fig. 4–12. General structure of human secretory IgA.

TABLE 4–2. Biologic Effector Functions of Immunoglobulins

Biologic Property	Antibody Isotype(s)
Toxin neutralization	IgG, IgA, IgM
Virus neutralization	IgG, IgA, IgM
Bacterial agglutination	IgA, IgM
Bacterial opsonization	IgG, IgM
Complement fixation	IgG1, IgG2, IgG3, IgM
Increased vascular permeability	IgE
Antibody-dependent cell-mediated cytotoxicity (ADCC)	
Natural killer (NK) activity toward virus-infected and tumor cells	IgG
Eosinophil-mediated killing of parasites	IgA, IgE
B lymphocyte antigen receptor	IgD, IgM (monomeric)

type-specific Fc receptors on various host cells initiates other biologic effects. For example, deposition of IgG on bacterial surfaces can promote recognition and ingestion of these microorganisms by host phagocytic cells, which bear membrane Fc receptors for IgG. The process through which immunoglobulin binding enhances phagocytic cell function is termed opsonization. Antibody-dependent cell-mediated cytotoxicity (ADCC) plays an important role in the elimination of virus-infected host cells and tumor cells, as well as some types of parasites. In the first instance, IgG binding to virus-infected or neoplastic cells promotes target cell recognition by natural killer cells. In the latter case, IgA and IgE antibodies directed to antigens of helminths such as ascaris and nippostrongylus promote killing of these parasites by eosinophils.

Two remaining effector functions of immunoglobulins involve the association of these molecules with cell membranes before their interaction with specific antigen. Tissue mast cells and basophils in the circulation bear high-affinity surface Fc receptors for IgE. Many of these high-affinity receptors are occupied by IgE in the absence of antigen. Subsequent binding of antigen through surface-found IgE molecules initiates a series of events leading to the release of a broad array of chemical mediators with vasoactive (e.g., histamine) and inflammatory (e.g., prostaglandins, leukotrienes) activity. IgE-mediated degranulation of mast cells and basophils plays a major role in immediate hypersensitivity reactions. Resting B lymphocytes express IgD and monomeric IgM on their surface. These molecules are associated with the lymphocyte membrane through a membrane-spanning domain not found in secreted immunoglobulins. The binding of antigen to membrane IgD or IgM initiates a series of biochemical events that promote the differentiation of B lymphocytes into plasma cells that actively secrete immunoglobulin.

Biologic Properties of the Human IgG Subclasses

Among normal adults, IgG constitutes nearly 75% of the total immunoglobulins present in serum. IgG is also the predominant isotype produced during secondary (anamnestic) immune responses, where it potentially contributes to host defense through diverse mechanisms. Serum IgG consists of four distinct subclasses. Although IgG subclass antibodies have comparable carbohydrate content and do not differ in their electrophoretic mobilities, they exhibit significant structural differences in the hinge region. These differences principally involve the number of amino acid residues and interheavy chain disulfide linkages (see Fig. 4–11) present in the hinge region. Utilization of κ and λ light chains also varies between IgG subclasses. The human IgG subclasses have been found to differ significantly with respect to several biologic properties, as well as in their proportional representation in serum. These differences are summarized in Table 4–3.

As evident in Table 4–3, IgG subclass antibodies differ with respect to two important effector functions, namely, *complement activation* (via the classical pathway) and *Fc receptor binding*. IgG_3 antibodies are most active in fixing complement. Activation of the classical pathway is initiated through binding of the complement component C1 to the C_H2 domain of the immunoglobulin molecule. The greater activity of IgG_3 in fixing complement is thought to be attributable to the finding that the extended hinge region prevents the Fab arms from sterically interfering with C1 access to the C_H2 domain. The extended hinge region of IgG_3 may also be a liability, however, because IgG_3 antibodies exhibit a greater susceptibility to proteolysis and shorter biologic half-life than other IgG subclasses. IgG_1, to a much lesser extent, IgG_2 also activates the classical pathway. In contrast, IgG_4 does not activate the classical pathway, and may actually interfere with the ability of other immunoglobulins to fix complement.

The second important effector function of IgG involves binding to membrane Fc receptors, particularly on mononuclear and polymorphonuclear phagocytes. Phagocyte Fc receptors exhibit preferential binding to IgG_1 and IgG_3. In contrast, IgG_2 antibodies interact only weakly with these receptors.

IgG is the only immunoglobulin isotype capable of crossing the human placenta. It is therefore an impor-

Table 4–3. Biologic and Functional Characteristics of the IgG Subclasses

Characteristic	IgG1	IgG2	IgG3	IgG4
Concentration range in serum (mg/ml)	5–12	2–6	0.5–1	0.2–1
No. of amino acid residues in hinge region	15	12	62	12
No. of H—H disulfide bonds	2	4	11	2
Use of κ and λ L chains ($\kappa:\lambda$ ratio)	2.4	1.1	1.4	8.0
Biologic half-life (days)	21–23	20–23	7–8	21–23
Complement activation (classical pathway)	+ +	+	+ +	none
Fc receptor binding				
Human monocytes	+ +	+	+ +	±
Human neutrophils	+ +	±	+ +	+

Plus signs indicate the presence of the characteristic.

tant source of passive protection of newborn infants during the first weeks of life. Although all four IgG subclasses are subject to placental transport, there appears to be some degree of subclass cell activity. Notably, IgG_2 is transported to a lesser extent than the other three IgG subclasses;. however, the significance of this finding has not been determined.

The IgG subclasses also differ with respect to the nature of the antigens that stimulate their production. This has been demonstrated by evaluating the subclass pattern of IgG antibodies produced against polysaccharides or protein antigens following either a natural infection or vaccination. Bacterial protein antigens preferentially induce IgG_1 antibodies, although detectable amounts of IgG_3 and IgG_4 are produced. Hyperimmunization with protein antigens can, however, result in the production of substantial amounts of IgG_4. Polysaccharide antigens typically induce IgG antibodies that are principally of the IgG_2 subclass, although IgG_1 may also be produced, particularly in children under 2 years of age.

IgA Subclass Antibodies

IgA consists of two distinct subclasses, IgA_1 and IgA_2, which differ in the amino acid composition of the hinge region and in the distribution of interchain disulfide linkages. Structural differences in the hinge region of the two subclasses influence their susceptibility to proteolytic cleavage by microbial enzymes. In particular, certain gram-positive (Streptococcus sanguis) and gram-negative (nontypable Haemophilus influenzae)

mucosal organisms produce an IgA protease that selectively cleaves the hinge region of IgA_1. IgA_2 antibodies are resistant to degradation by this enzyme. Although the nature of the IgA subclass response pattern to protein and polysaccharide antigens is not as well characterized as for IgG subclasses, it appears that protein antigens induce mainly IgA_1, whereas carbohydrate antigens induce IgA_2.

COMPLEMENT SYSTEM

An important mechanism for amplification of immune responses involves a group of more than 20 proteins normally found in plasma, collectively referred to as the *complement system* or complement cascade. Complement activation is linked to certain events associated with inflammatory reactions, including increases in vascular permeability and recruitment of phagocytic cells. In addition, products of complement activation facilitate recognition and ingestion of infectious agents by phagocytic cells, promote direct membranolysis of susceptible gram-negative bacteria, mobilize phagocytes from the bone marrow during acute bacterial infection, and even regulate B- and T-lymphocyte function.

The complement cascade is subdivided into two pathways, termed the *classical* and *alternative* pathways (Fig. 4–13). These two pathways differ in the nature of the substances that trigger their activation and in the proteins involved in the initial steps and activation of each pathway. A recurrent pattern is observed follow-

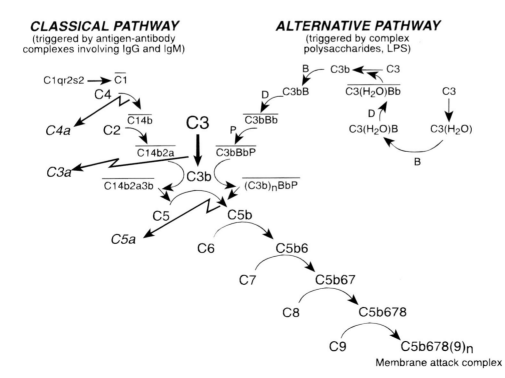

Fig. 4–13. The complement cascade.

ing activation of either pathway, however. Thus, the initial steps in each pathway involve conversion of inactive precursors to their active forms as a consequence of limited proteolysis. The two pathways converge at the C5 cleavage step. Beyond this step, activation of terminal C6 through C9 complement proteins involves *assembly* rather than *proteolysis*.

Classical Pathway

Activation of the classical pathway is typically initiated by soluble antigen-antibody complexes or by deposition of antibody on the surface of particular targets, such as bacteria, viruses. Not all immunoglobulin isotypes are capable of triggering the classical pathway, however. Antigen-antibody complexes containing IgM or certain IgG subclass antibodies (IgG$_1$, IgG$_2$, and IgG$_3$) are effective activators of the classical pathway, whereas complexes containing IgA, IgD, IgE, or IgG$_4$ are not. The initial step in activation of the classical pathway involves binding of macromolecular C1 (consisting of a complex of subunit C1q, C1r, C1s held together by calcium ions) to a single molecule of IgM or to two closely spaced molecules of IgG, termed an IgG *doublet*. C1 binding to the C$_H$2 domain of the antibody molecule occurs via the C1q subunit. C1q bonding results in a conformational change of the associated C1r and C1s subunits, leading to activation of C1s esterase activity. C1 esterase then cleaves C4 into two fragments, C4b and C4a. Cleavage of C4 exposes a binding site on the larger C4b fragment that can form a covalent bond on activating surfaces. Because of the reactivity of this binding site, C4b is typically deposited in close proximity to the C1 complex. C4b facilitates binding of the next component, C2, which is also cleaved by C1 esterase. The larger fragment, C2a, is deposited in the vicinity of C4b, whereas C2b is released into the fluid phase. The C4b2a complex possesses (via the C2a component) enzymatic activity capable of cleaving the next component in the cascade, C3. This complex is referred to as the *classical pathway C3 convertase*, which cleaves C3 into a small fragment (C3a) and a large fragment (C3b). C3b, like C4b, contains a binding site capable of mediating covalent attachment to activating surfaces. Deposition of C3b near the C4b2a complex facilitates binding of the next component, C5, which is also cleaved by this enzyme (now referred to as C3/C5 convertase) into a small fragment (C5a) and a large fragment (C5b). C5b contains an unstable membrane-binding site that can mediate noncovalent association of this fragment with cell surfaces. The membrane-binding site of C5b rapidly decays unless stabilized through binding of the next component, C6. Subsequent binding of C7 results in formation of a more hydrophobic complex (C5b, 6, 7), which inserts into the lipid bilayer of a target cell membrane. Binding of C8 to the C5b, 6, 7 complex results in the formation of a

small pore. The final step in assembly of the membrane attack complex involves polymerization of several molecules of C9 around the C5b, 6, 7, 8 complex, forming a transmembrane pore with a hydrophilic core and a hydrophobic exterior. The effective diameter of the pore increases with the number of C9 molecules polymerizing around the C5b, 6, 7, 8 complex. In the presence of these pores, through which water and small ions can freely move, the target cell is unable to maintain osmotic stability. Continued entry of water and loss of electrolytes eventually lead to osmotic lysis of susceptible cells.

C5b, 6, 7 complexes can form in the fluid phase. Alternatively, these complexes can form on, and be released from, immune complexes or the surfaces of noncellular targets. Once released, the C5b, 6, 7 complexes can bind to nearby cells. Following assembly of C8 and C9, these can be lysed via the membrane attack complex. This phenomenon, known as "innocent bystander lysis," appears to contribute to tissue injury seen in certain immune complex diseases.

Alternative Pathway

A second pathway for activation of complement leads to cleavage of C3 and C5, as well as to assembly of the membrane attack complex, but bypasses the classical pathway component C1, C4, and C2. This pathway, termed the *alternative pathway*, is triggered *in the absence of antibody* by complex polysaccharides, lipopolysaccharides from gram-negative bacteria, and teichoic acids from gram-positive bacteria, as well as by less well characterized components on the surface of fungi and certain viruses. Although antibody is not required for alternative pathway activation, aggregated immunoglobulins, as well as antigen-antibody complexes involving IgA, IgD, and IgE, are capable of activating this pathway. Interestingly, alternative pathway activation by immunoglobulins involves the F(ab)$_2$ region of molecule, rather than the Fc domain involved in C1q binding activation in the classical pathway. The alternative pathway may be particularly important in facilitating host defense during the preimmune phase of infection, when insufficient quantities of specific IgM and IgG are available to activate complement via the classical pathway.

Activation of the alternative pathway begins with the slow, spontaneous hydrolysis of an unstable thioester in the native C3 molecule, resulting in formation of a protein termed C3 (H$_2$O). This conformationally altered form of C3 is capable of interacting with factor B (C3 proactivator), forming C3 (H$_2$O) B complex. Bound factor B is then cleaved by factor D (C3 proactivator convertase), resulting in formation of C3 (H$_2$O) Bb complex, which expresses C3 convertase activity. The spontaneous hydrolysis of C3, with ensuing formation of a C3 convertase, has been termed C3 "tickover" and is thought to provide the initial C3b necessary to prime the alternative pathway. Once formed, C3b binds factor B to form a C3bB complex, which is subsequently cleaved by factor D to form second alternative pathway C3 convertase, C3bBb. Deposition of additional C3b molecules in proximity to the C3bBb complex facilitates binding and subsequent cleavage of C5. The C3bBb complex is unstable and Bb readily dissociates from C3b; however, binding of the serum protein properdin to C3bBb decreases the rate of dissociation of this complex and thereby prolongs convertase activity. As in the classical pathway, cleavage of C5 by C3bBb generates a C5a and C5b fragment, the latter of which contributes to assembly of the terminal complement proteins.

Despite the C3 tickover phenomenon, only a small percentage of the total serum C3 actually exists in the form of C3b. This is due to the presence of two regulatory proteins that coordinately act to limit C3bBb convertase formation and activity. These two proteins consist of factor H and factor I. In the presence of factor I, C3b is rapidly degraded to iC3b, which is unable to associate with the factor B and thus no longer participates in the complement cascade. Factor I is unstable to cleave C3b when the latter is complexed with factor B, however. This problem is overcome through the presence of factor H, a cofactor for factor I. Factor H competitively inhibits binding of both B and Bb to C3b

and enhances the rate of dissociation of C3bB and C3bBb complexes, exposing the unassociated C3b to factor I-mediated cleavage.

Biologic Effects of Complement Activation

Activation of complement produces certain responses that are integral to the inflammatory process (Fig. 4–14). For example, enzymatic cleavage of component C3, C4, and C5 results in the generation of large fragments (C3b, C4b, and C5b) that participate in the next step in the complement cascade and the concurrent release of smaller fragments (C3a, C4a, and C5a), which are released into the fluid phase. These smaller fragments, collectively termed *anaphylatoxins*, are able to trigger release of a variety of inflammatory mediators (including histamine) from mast cells and basophils, leading to smooth muscle contraction and increased capillary leakage. In addition to its activity as an anaphylatoxin, C5a also has effects on phagocytic cells, promoting directed migration (chemotaxis), increased adherence, and respiratory burst activity of neutrophils. The larger C3b fragment generated during the cleavage of C3 was discussed previously with respect to its role in generating convertase activity in both the classical and alternative pathways. Covalent deposition of C3b on the surface can also promote phagocytosis of the target, however, because phago-

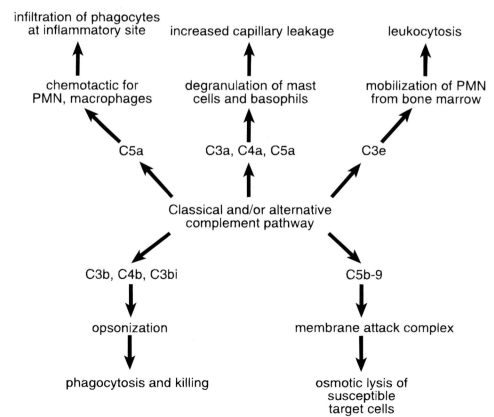

Fig. 4–14. Biologic properties associated with activation of the complement cascade.

cytes express plasma membrane receptors through C3b. This same receptor recognizes C4b fragments bound to the activating surface. The process whereby deposition of complement fragments on a target promotes receptor-mediated phagocytosis is termed *opsonization.* Although cleavage of C3b by factor I inactivates this fragment with respect to further participation in the complement cascade, iC3b retains significant opsonic activity. Recognition of iC3b-coated particles involves a phagocyte membrane receptor distinct from that of the receptor for C3b. Finally, assembly of the terminal complement component C5b, C6, C7, C8, C9 on the surface of numerous species of gram-negative bacteria is sufficient to promote osmotic lysis of these microorganisms through formation of the membrane attack complex. Less well characterized biologic activities of complement include (1) effects of Ba and Bb fragments on B-lymphocyte proliferation and differentiation, (2) effects of C3a and C5a on T-lymphocyte function, and (3) C3e-mediated mobilization of mature PMNs from bone marrow during acute bacterial infection.

Regulation of the Complement Cascade

Given the multiple proinflammatory effects of complement, one should readily appreciate that excessive or prolonged generation of complement fragments can be deleterious to the host. To minimize the proinflammatory properties of complement, several regulatory mechanisms have evolved. These regulatory proteins are broadly subdivided into (1) fluid-phase regulator proteins and (2) membrane-bound regulatory proteins. An additional level of complement regulation entails the spontaneous decay of metastable membrane-binding sites (as on C3b, C4b, and C5b) and the decay-dissociation of enzyme complexes (e.g., C4b 2a, C3bBb). Some regulatory proteins (e.g., C1 inhibitor) exert their effects through stoichiometric inhibition of the proteolytic activity of complement components, whereas other proteins inactivate complement fragments via enzymatic degradation (e.g., factor I-mediated inactivation of C3b and C4b). As noted previously, certain membrane-bound regulatory proteins have also been identified. Two such examples are decay-accelerating factor and C8-binding protein, which appear to interfere with effective assembly of the membrane attack complex on host cell membranes, thereby limiting complement-mediated host cell cytotoxicity.

PHAGOCYTIC CELLS

Phagocytes are nonlymphoid leukocytic cells that are capable of engulfing and subsequently ingesting particulate matter, including foreign microorganisms, dead or injured host cells, and cellular debris. Moreover, these cells secrete numerous cytokines involved in the initiation and regulation of immune and inflammatory responses. Various types of phagocytes are distributed throughout the body, being present in blood, tissues, and serous cavities (e.g., plural and peritoneal cavities), where they play a major role in clearance of microorganisms.

The chief types of phagocytes found in the body include PMNs and mononuclear phagocytes (monocytes and macrophages). As the name suggests, these cells are classified, at least in part, on the basis of cellular morphology. PMNs contain a segmented, multilobed (2 to 5) nucleus (Fig. 4–15), whereas mononuclear phagocytes contain a round or indented nucleus. Both types of phagocytes are produced in the bone marrow during hematopoiesis and are subsequently released into the peripheral blood. Once in the blood, these cells circulate for several hours before migrating into various tissues, either randomly or in response to specific chemical signals.

The principal phagocytic cell found in peripheral circulation is the PMN, comprising 50 to 70% of the total circulating white blood cell pool. PMNs include neutrophils, eosinophils, and basophils, which are collectively also known as granulocytes because of the presence of numerous granules in the cytoplasm; however, circulating neutrophils vastly outnumber both

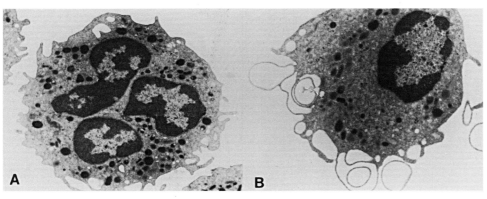

Fig. 4–15. A. Transmission electron micrograph of a resting human neutrophil. ×3000. B. Transmission electron micrograph of a resting human neutrophil treated with cytochalasin B (cytochalasin B destroys outer membrane of neutrophil). ×3000.

eosinophils and basophils, which represent only 1 to 3% and less than 1% of the total white blood cell pool, respectively. For this reason, the terms PMN and neutrophil are often used interchangeably. Given its numerical predominance in the circulation, the neutrophil is considered the first line of defense against infection due to extracellular bacteria.

Cells of the mononuclear phagocyte system include circulating monocytes and tissue macrophages. Although monocytes exhibit phagocytic activity comparable to that of the neutrophil, these cells comprise only 3 to 8% of the circulating white blood cell pool. Hence, the monocyte is considered less important in host resistance to acute bacterial infection than the neutrophil. The greater significance of circulating monocytes lies in that these cells migrate into various tissues, where they undergo further differentiation into macrophages. Macrophages differ from their precursor monocytes in enzymatic, phagocytic, and microbicidal activity, as well as in cell surface membrane characteristics. In addition, macrophages in various tissues exhibit properties that are unique to the environment in which they differentiate, probably as a result of local factors. For this reason, macrophages are named according to their tissue location (Table 4–4), and they may either be "fixed" in certain tissues (e.g., Kupffer cells in liver and microglia in brain) or "wandering" in serous cavities (e.g., alveolar macrophages in lung).

Resting macrophages possess considerably phagocytic and microbicidal activity. This activity can, however, be further enhanced as a consequence of exposure to cytokines (especially interferon γ) produced by T lymphocytes. These activated macrophages are characterized by increased size and metabolic and phagocytic activity, and they exhibit an enhanced ability to kill intracellular pathogens as well as tumor cells. Mononuclear phagocytes, like PMNs, function as phagocytic cells eliminating foreign protein, bacteria, and other debris. We now know, however, that mononuclear phagocytes contribute in other important ways to the

immune response. Notably, these cells participate in *immune induction* by virtue of their ability to internalize, process, and present antigen, in conjunction with MHC class II molecules, to T-helper lymphocytes. In addition, mononuclear phagocytes, especially activated macrophages, elaborate certain proteins that play a key role in the development of an immune response. These factors include the following: (1) IL-1 (formerly referred to as lymphocyte-activating factor), which promotes activation of helper T cells and maturation of B-lymphocyte precursors; (2) TNF, which is capable of killing certain tumor cells; (3) colony-stimulating factors (CSFs), which enhance production of macrophages and neutrophils in bone marrow; and (4) IL-6, which promotes differentiation of mature B lymphocytes into antibody-secreting plasma cells and induces hepatic synthesis of acute-phase proteins (involved in innate immunity).

Circulating neutrophils are rapidly mobilized to the extravascular compartment in response to acute inflammation or infection. In fact, marked neutrophil infiltration is a cardinal feature of the acute inflammatory response. On leaving the circulation, neutrophils must then be capable of recognizing, internalizing, and degrading foreign protein, bacteria, or other noxious agents. Fortunately, neutrophils, as well as mononuclear phagocytes, which are more important in chronic inflammatory states, are well equipped to perform these functions.

Within the peripheral blood of normal individuals, the measured neutrophil count is actually an underestimation of the total number of neutrophils in the circulation. This is because neutrophils are distributed between two more or less distinct "pools," termed circulating and marginating pools. Standard venipuncture techniques typically sample only the circulating pool; however, approximately half to two thirds of peripheral blood neutrophils are found in a marginated pool of cells that is sequestered in postcapillary venules, where they remain in association with the vascular endothelium. The latter pool provides the primary source of neutrophils exiting the circulation during the inflammatory response. In the absence of inflammation, marginated neutrophils remain loosely, reversibly associated with the surface of vascular endothelium. In fact, neutrophils can actually be seen "rolling" on the surface of endothelial cells (Fig. 4–16A). In areas of inflammation, however, biochemical changes in both the neutrophil and endothelial cell result in the firm adhesion between these two cells, followed by the movement of a leukocyte through the endothelial barrier and into the extravascular space (Fig. 4–16B). The latter process has been termed transendothelial migration or *diapedesis*. The adhesive events involved in the interaction between circulating phagocytes and vascular endothelium are complex; however, significant progress has been made in understanding the na-

TABLE 4–4. Cells of the Mononuclear Phagocyte System

Cell Type	Location
Monocytes	Bone marrow, blood
Macrophages, free	
Alveolar macrophages	Lung
Pleural macrophages	Pleural cavity
Peritoneal macrophages	Peritoneal cavity
Histiocytes	Connective tissue
Macrophages, fixed	
Kupffer cells	Liver
Osteoclasts	Bone
Microgial cells	Central nervous system
Other fixed tissue macrophages	Spleen (red pulp macrophages), lymph nodes, bone marrow, thymus, etc.

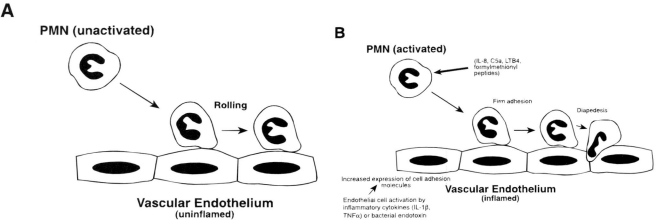

Fig. 4–16. Interaction between circulating neutrophils and vascular endothelium in uninflamed (A) and inflamed (B) sites.

ture of these interactions at a molecular level. At least three major superfamilies of adhesion molecules have been found to participate in the phagocyte-endothelium interactions. These include (1) integrins, (2) members of the immunoglobulin super gene family (particularly intercellular adhesion molecules or ICAMs), and (3) selectins.

Once phagocytes have traversed the endothelial barrier, they must then move toward the target particle to be ingested and eliminated. This objective is met by virtue of the ability of phagocytes to migrate unidirectionally along the chemical concentration gradient generated between inflamed or infected tissues and blood vessels. The chemical substances capable of eliciting such behavior by phagocytes are termed *chemoattractins,* or *chemotaxins,* and a directed migration of phagocyte toward these agents is referred to as *chemotaxis.* Certain substances, both host-derived and bacterially derived, have been found to promote directed migration of phagocytes (Table 4–5).

Phagocytic cells are actively motile even in the ab-

sence of chemotactic substances. Under such conditions, phagocytes exhibit *random migration* (i.e., movement occurring with an equal probability in all directions) (Fig. 4–17A). Following exposure to a chemoattractin, these cells lose their typically round appearance in favor of an oriented configuration with a distinct "head" (lamellipodium) and "tail" (uropod). The process through which phagocytes adopt an orientation in the direction of a chemotactic gradient is termed *polarization.* Once this orientation has been established, the phagocyte is able to move unidirectionally toward the source of the chemical gradient (Fig. 4–17B). Chemotactic agents can increase the speed of migration of phagocytic cells even if a chemical gradient is not established. This effect is termed *chemokinesis* (Fig. 4–17C). Chemotaxis is initiated through the interaction between chemoattractins and specific receptors on the phagocyte plasma membrane. Chemoattractin receptor expression along the cell is not uniform. Rather, chemoattractin receptors are present in comparatively higher density at the anterior of the cell than at the uropod, thus enabling the migrating cell to maintain its orientation. By regulating the distribution of chemoattractin receptors on the cell surface, phagocytes are able to recognize gradients as small as 1% across the length of a cell. Phagocytes "crawl," rather than swim. Phagocyte locomotion is therefore critically dependent on cell-cell or cell-substrate (e.g., connective tissue matrix protein) interactions that promote cell adhesion. Phagocytic cells of patients with congenital or acquired defects in leukocyte adhesion often exhibit impaired chemotactic activity.

A key property of phagocytic cells is their ability to recognize and ingest particulate matter. The process of ingestion involves direct contact between the phagocyte and particle, followed by formation of finger-like projections (pseudopodia) that surround the target. The pseudopods fuse on the distal surface of the particle, which is now enveloped in a membranous sack

TABLE 4–5. Chemoattractants for Phagocytic Cells

Chemotatic Agent	Source(s)
C5a	Complement activation and cleavage of C5
Leukotriene B4 (LTB4)	Product of cellular arachidonate metabolism via the lipoxygenase pathway
Platelet-activating factors (PAF)	Platelets, leukocytes (including PMN, monocyte/macrophages and NK cells)
Interleukin-8 (IL-8)	Mainly mononuclear phagocytes, but also fibroblasts, T lymphocytes, endothelial cells, and keratinocytes
N-formylmethionyl peptides	Products of bacterial protein synthesis

termed a phagocytic vacuole, or *phagosome* (Fig. 4–18). The phagosome moves to the interior of the cell, where fusion with cytoplasmic granules results in the formation of a phagolysosome. Within the phagolysosomal compartment, efficient killing of many microorganisms occurs.

Phagocytic cells are capable of recognizing and ingesting a diverse array of particulate matter. Their phagocytic activity is not indiscriminant, however. While targeting numerous species of bacteria and

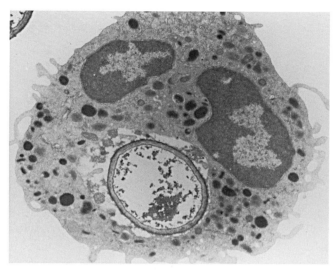

Fig. 4–18. Transmission electron micrograph of a human neutrophil phagocytizing opsonized zymosan (yeast cell wall) particles. Original magnification ×6000.

A

B

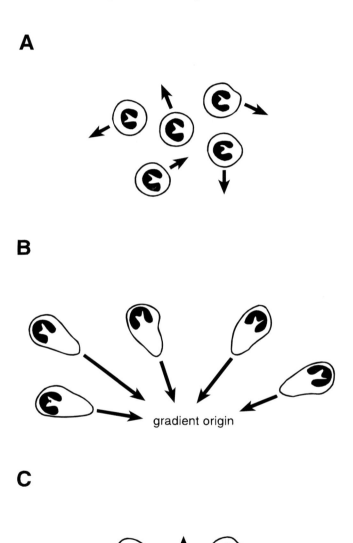

gradient origin

C

Fig. 4–17. General types of phagocyte motility. A. Random migration (absence of chemotactic agent). B. Chemotaxis (chemotactic agent present, gradient established). C. Chemokinesis (chemotactic agent present, but no gradient established).

fungi, as well as damaged or senescent host cells, phagocytes display little interest in viable autologous cells or tissues. Particle-recognition ingestion involves specific interactions between the phagocyte membrane and one or more components of the particle surface. Efficient phagocytosis often requires that the particle be coated with one or more host serum proteins through a process termed opsonization (meaning "to prepare for eating"). The two principal types of serum proteins, referred to as *opsonins*, involved in this process are immunoglobulin G antibodies and cleavage fragments of complement component C3 (iC3b, C3b). Targets opsonized with IgG and/or C3 fragments are recognized through specific receptors located on the phagocyte membrane. The sequential interaction between opsonins and their corresponding receptors results in an engulfment of the particle through a process termed "zippering."

Opsonic requirements can vary for different bacterial species or even different strains of a single species. In general, however, three principal mechanisms of opsonization are known (Fig. 4–19). *Complement-dependent opsonization* results from the covalent attachment of C3b and iC3b on the bacterial surface following complement activation, primarily via the alternative pathway. Phagocyte membranes possess distinct receptors for each of these fragments. Complement receptor type 1 (CR1) mediates binding of C3b-coated targets, whereas complement receptor type 3 (CR3) recognizes iC3b-coated targets. The extent to which covalently bound C3b is susceptible to cleavage by the complement regulatory proteins factor H and factor I determines whether C3b or iC3b is the predominant form presented to the phagocyte. *Antibody-dependent opsonization* results from the binding of specific IgG antibody

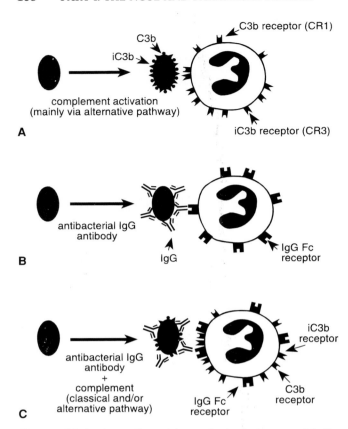

Fig. 4–19. Mechanisms of bacterial opsonization by immunoglobulin and/or complement. A. Complement-dependent opsonization. B. Antibody-dependent opsonization. C. Antibody- and complement-dependent opsonization.

to bacterial surface structures via the antigen-binding domain (Fab), leaving the Fc domain exposed. Phagocytic cells possess membrane receptors capable of binding the Fc region of the IgG molecule. These receptors are distinct from C3 receptors. All four human IgG subclasses can bind to IgG Fc receptors on neutrophils, although these cells exhibit preferential binding of IgG_1 and IgG_3. Only IgG_1 and IgG_3 appear to bind to monocyte Fc receptors. In many instances, antibody and *complement-dependent opsonization* may be required for efficient phagocytosis to occur. IgG antibodies can be particularly effective in such cases, in that they are directly opsonic (being recognized via Fc receptors) and are able to activate complement through the classical pathway (thereby enhancing C3 receptor-mediated phagocytosis). Antibodies of the IgM isotype lack direct opsonic activity because neither PMNs nor mononuclear phagocytes have Fc receptors for IgM.

IgM deposited on a bacterial surface can be particularly effective in triggering the classical pathway of complement, however, thereby enhancing C3 deposition on the target surface. The opsonized target is recognized by the phagocyte solely through the membrane C3 receptors. For this reason, IgM is considered an indirect *opsonin*.

Recent studies indicate that some microorganisms may be ingested through nonopsonic phagocytosis, that is, in the absence of antibody or C3 fragments. For example, certain microorganisms possess fimbria that contain lectins (carbohydrate-binding proteins) capable of recognizing phagocyte membrane glycoproteins. One target for these bacterial lectins appears to be a glycoprotein component of the iC3b (CR3) receptor itself. Macrophages possess surface lectins capable of recognizing specific carbohydrate moieties found on bacterial surfaces. Thus, interactions between lectins on one cell and carbohydrates on the other can lead to phagocytosis in the absence of opsonization.

The process of particle uptake initiates certain events linked to the microbicidal properties of phagocytic cells, including the fusion of cytoplasmic granules with a newly formed phagocytic vacuole and an increase in cellular oxidative metabolism. Cytoplasmic granules contain proteins, both enzymatic and nonenzymatic, which are bactericidal or bacteriostatic for many microorganisms. The two major classes of cytoplasmic granules present in neutrophils are the *primary* (azurophil) and *secondary* (specific) granules. The contents of these two cytoplasmic granule populations vary (Table 4–6). As a group, these antimicrobial proteins display a wide range of activity against gram-positive and gram-negative bacteria and fungi. Degranulation of cytoplasmic granules into the phagocytic vacuole compartment results in the formation of a phagolysosome containing high concentrations of neutral and acid proteases, as well as other microbicidal constituents. This leads to effective intracellular killing with minimal damage to the host. Under conditions in which extracellular degranulation occurs, however, these enzymes are also capable of inflicting injury on host tissues. Extracellular degranulation

TABLE 4–6. Subcellular Distribution of Enzymes and Other Constituents of PMN Cytoplasmic Granules

Class of Constituents	Primary Granules	Secondary Granules
Microbicidal enzymes	Myeloperoxidase Lysozyme	Lysozyme
Neutral proteinases	Elastase Cathepsin G Proteinase 3	Collagenase
Acid hydrolases	N-acetyl-β-glucosaminidase Cathepsin B Cathepsin D β-Glucuronidase β-Glycerophosphatase α-Mannosidase	
Other	Defensins Cationic proteins Bactericidal/permeability increasing factor	Lactoferrin Vitamin B_{12}-binding protein C3bi receptor (CR3) Cytochrome b_{245}

plays a key role in the proinflammatory properties of phagocytic cells. Stimulation of phagocytic cells by particular agents, or certain soluble factors (e.g., complement fragment C5a), leads to an increase in cellular consumption of molecular oxygen (O_2), a process termed the *respiratory burst*. This respiratory burst is associated with the generation of certain oxygen metabolites that are injurious to many species of microorganisms. The majority of O_2 consumed by the phagocyte is converted directly to superoxide ion (O_2-) through the action of a membrane-bound reduced form of nicotinamide-adenine dinucleotide phosphate (NADPH) oxidase, which catalyzes the transfer of an electron from NADPH to O_2. Superoxide radicles (O_2-), in turn, may undergo spontaneous or enzyme-catalyzed (via superoxide dismutase) conversion to hydrogen peroxide (H_2O_2), a two-electron reduction product of molecular oxygen. Alternatively, superoxide anions may react with H_2O_2 in the presence of iron to form hydroxal radicles ($OH-$). These various oxygen species appear to contribute significantly to the microbicidal activity of phagocytic cells. Additional oxidant species (hypochlorous acid toxic aldehydes) are generated as a consequence of the interaction between H_2O_2 and the azurophil enzyme myeloperoxidase (MPO) in the presence of a suitable halide, chloride being most physiologically relevant.

Collectively, phagocyte bactericidal mechanisms are broadly characterized as oxygen-independent or oxygen-dependent. O_2-dependent bactericidal activity is further subdivided into MPO-dependent and MPO-independent. Although these various components often work in concert to promote destruction of ingested bacteria, certain mechanisms may be relatively more important in the intracellular killing of specific microbes. Moreover, availability of O_2 may limit oxidative bactericidal activity, particularly at sites of tissue necrosis in which blood flow may be compromised. Fortunately, phagocytic cells are able to kill many species of bacteria in the complete absence of oxygen.

PMNs and mononuclear phagocytes constitute an important mechanism for elimination of extracellular bacteria, particularly those that engender a strong antibody response. These cells are less effective in the elimination of infections due to intracellular microorganisms (both viral and bacterial) or microorganisms that elicit a poor humoral response, however. Additional host response mechanisms are called into action in such instances. These mechanisms involve stimulation of cellular immunity, in which T cell-derived cytokines induce activation of mononuclear phagocytes with enhanced microbicidal activity as well as cytotoxic T cells.

CYTOKINES

The interaction between various cells of the immune system often involves direct cell-to-cell contact; however, one of the principal ways in which cells communicate with each other is via the production and secretion of protein hormones termed *cytokines*. These hormones play an important role in the effector phases of both innate and acquired immune responses. Certain cytokines that contribute to innate immunity are produced by mononuclear phagocytes and are thus referred to as *monokines*. Other cytokines are produced by antigen- or mitogen-stimulated T lymphocytes and help to orchestrate specific immune responses. These protein hormones are termed *lymphokines*. Some cytokines of this type promote growth and differentiation of immature leukocytes in bone marrow through effects of hemopoietic stem cells and are termed *colony-stimulating factors* (CSFs) Cytokines are not stored preformed in cells, but rather are synthesized de novo following cell activation. In addition, receptors for certain cytokines are also induced during cell stimulation. The latter feature may serve to limit the number of cells responding to specific antigen.

Cytokines exert their biologic effects through binding to specific receptors on the membrane of target cells. In some instances, the cytokine acts as an autocrine hormone, stimulating the same cell from which it was secreted. Cytokines may also stimulate cells in close proximity to the cells that secreted them (paracrine effect). Finally, these protein hormones may enter the circulation, where they can interact with immune cells of some distance from their point of origin (endocrine effect). Many of the cytokines share certain common features. First, cytokines often exhibit *pleiotropic activity*; that is, a single cytokine possesses the ability to stimulate certain different cell types. For example, IL-1 activates T cells, induces maturation of pre-B lymphocytes, promotes osteoclastic-mediated bone resorption, and induces expression of cell adhesion molecules on vascular endothelium. Second, different cytokines often evoke similar biologic responses (*redundancy*), as is the case with respect to the antiviral properties of interferons and TNF. Third, certain cytokines may influence the production of other cytokines; thus, IL-1 promotes IL-2 synthesis and secretion by T lymphocytes. Finally, cytokines may exhibit either *synergy* or *antagonism* toward other cytokines. Thus, IL-4 and IL-5 are B cell growth factors that act sequentially to promote B-cell growth and differentiation, whereas interferon γ antagonizes the ability of IL-4 to induce class switching (from IgM to IgE production) by B lymphocytes.

More than 20 cytokines have been identified to date (Table 4–7). Their biologic properties may be broadly subdivided into four categories. The first includes cytokines that serve as mediators of *innate immunity*. For example, interferons α and β increase resistance of host cells to infection by certain viruses and also stimulate natural killer activity of large granular lymphocytes. TNF also exhibits antiviral activity. In addition, these

TABLE 4–7. Cytokines and Their Biologic Properties

Cytokine	Cell Source(s)	Key Activities
IL-1	Mainly macrophages and keratinocytes; also fibroblasts, endothelial cells, smooth muscle, and others	Stimulates acute phase reactions; general stimulation of immune system; augments hematopoiesis
IL-2	T lymphocytes	Promotes T lymphocyte growth and activity, enhances activity of NK cells, lymphockine-activated killer cells, and macrophages, enhances Ig production by B lymphocytes
IL-3	T lymphocytes	Promotes growth of early myeloid (but not lymphoid) progenitor cells in bone marrow
IL-4	T_H lymphocytes (especially T_H2 phenotype)	B lymphocyte growth factor; induces expression of MHC class II molecules on B cells; promotes class switch to IgE; promotes growth of helper and cytotoxic T lymphocytes
IL-5	T_H lymphocytes	Stimulates growth and differentiation of eosinophils; promotes IgA production by B lymphocytes; promotes growth of activated B lymphocytes
IL-6	Lymphocytes, monocytes, fibroblasts, endothelial cells, others	Promotes final differentiation of B lymphocytes into plasma cells; induces acute-phase protein synthesis in hepatocytes
IL-7	Bone marrow stromal cells	Promotes growth of early lymphoid precursors of T and B lineage
IL-8	Mononuclear phagocytes, endothelial cells, fibroblasts, T cells keratinocytes	Chemotactic for PMN (but not mononuclear phagocytes); pan-activator of PMN
IL-9	T_H lymphocytes	Promotes mast cell growth; induces proliferation of some T_H lymphocytes in the absence of antigen
IL-10	T_H2 subset of T lymphocytes	Inhibits antigen presentation to T_H1 cells and release of T_H1-derived cytokines
IL-11	Bone marrow stomal cells	Potentiates IL-3 induced growth of megakarocytes; promotes T cell-dependent IgG secretion by B cells
IL-12	B lymphocytes	Synergizes with IL-2 in generating cytotoxic T lymphocyte and lymphokine-activated killer activity
TNFα	Mononuclear phagocytes	Key mediator of endotoxic shock; induces wasting (cachexia); activates mononuclear phagocytes and PMN; increases cell adhesion molecules expression on vascular endothelium; promotes tumor necrosis; antiviral activity
TNFβ	T lymphocytes	Shares many properties with TNFα, including toxicity for tumor cells
TGFβ	T and B lymphocytes	Increases IgA production by B lymphocytes; promotes wound healing; antagonizes actions of IL-2, IL-4 and IFN-γ
Granulocyte CSF	Mononuclear phagocytes, endothelial cells, fibroblasts	Promotes generation of PMN from bone marrow progenitors
Macrophage CSF	Mononuclear phagocytes, endothelial cells, fibroblasts	Promotes generation of monocytes from bone marrow progenitors
Granulocyte/ Macrophage CSF	T lymphocytes, mononuclear phagocytes, endothelial cells, fibroblasts	Promotes growth and differentiation of granulocytes and mononuclear phagocytes from bone marrow progenitors
IFNα	Macrophages, epithelial cells, other cell types	Inhibits viral replication in host cells; promotes NK activity; induces expression of MHC class I molecules
IFNβ	Fibroblasts	Activities similar to IFNα
IFNγ	T lymphocytes	Antiviral activity; activator of macrophage function; increases expression of MHC class I and II molecules; increases activity of NK and cytotoxic T cells; antagonizes effects of IL-4

factors promote inflammation by stimulating phagocyte adherence to vascular endothelium and cause hemorrhagic necrosis of tumors. Another cytokine, IL-6, induces synthesis of acute-phase proteins that contribute to innate immunity.

A second group includes cytokines that regulate the *growth and differentiation of lymphocytes.* IL-2 is mainly secreted by T cells, particularly T-helper cells (which have been stimulated by antigen or mitogen). IL-2 induces proliferation of antigen-primed T-helper and T-cytotoxic cells. This cytokine also enhances the activity

of cytotoxic and NK cells. Moreover, IL-2 promotes differentiation of antigen-stimulated B cells into immunoglobulin-secreting cells. Another T cell-derived cytokine, IL-4, promotes the activation, proliferation, and differentiation of B lymphocytes. B lymphocytes stimulated by this cytokine exhibit increased expression of MHC class II molecules, which are important in the interaction between T helper cells and B cells. IL-4 also promotes class switching of B cells from IgM production to IgG_1 and IgE production.

Although not as potent as IL-2 as a growth factor

for T cells, IL-4 does induce T-cell proliferation and T-cytotoxic activity. Another cytokine belonging to this group, transforming growth factor β (TGF β), inhibits activation and proliferation of T lymphocytes by antagonizing the actions of other cytokines including IL-2, IL-4, and interferon γ. The "anti-cytokine" activity of TGF-β may be important in restricting the magnitude and/or duration of immune responses, thereby facilitating the process of wound healing.

Erythrocytes and leukocytes are produced from stem cells and bone marrow at a rate sufficient to replace cells lost through normal attrition or consumption, particularly inflammatory cells such as PMNs. The process through which the various formed elements of blood (leukocytes, erythrocytes, and platelets) are produced in bone marrow from stem cells is termed *hematopoiesis.* Hematopoietic activity in bone marrow is regulated through the action of a third group of cytokines, collectively referred to as CSFs, produced by stromal cells or by antigen-stimulated T lymphocytes. Certain CSFs have been identified including GM-CSF (granulocyte monocyte CSF), G-CSF (granulocyte CSF), M-CSF (monocyte CSF), and multi-CSF (IL-3 and IL-7). Whereas other cytokines, such as IL-2 and IL-4, promote growth and differentiation of mature leukocytes, CSFs stimulate growth and differentiation of immature leukocytes. Multi-CSF appears to act on the most primitive progenitor cells in bone marrow, possibly at the level of the pluripotent stem cell, to induce formation of all nonlymphoid cells. Other cytokines in this group, such as G-CSF and macrophage CSF, act at a later stage, promoting formation of lineage-specific cells. IL-7 acts on B- and T-lymphoid precursors that are at a stage of development comparable to IL-3-sensitive nonlymphoid progenitors.

A final group of cytokines shares the common property of being *activators of inflammatory cell function.* Notable in this group is interferon γ, also known as immune interferon, a T cell-derived cytokine that is a potent activator of mononuclear phagocyte function and has phagocytic, microbicidal, and tumoricidal activity, as well as antigen-presenting activity. Interferon γ also stimulates vascular endothelial cells to increase expression of certain cell adhesion molecules that play a major role in trafficking of inflammatory cells to sites of inflammation. Another member of this group, TNF β, also activates PMN and vascular endothelium to promote the egress of circulating leukocytes.

Cytokines influence host defense capabilities at several levels. First, these peptide mediators stimulate the generation of mature leukocytes from their precursors in bone marrow. Second, they promote the growth and terminal differentiation of mature leukocytes. Further, certain cytokines are responsible for activating leukocytes. Given their influence in orchestrating immune responses, it is not surprising that cytokines can also play an important role in the pathogenesis of disease.

For example, increased production of IL-1 and TNF is observed in gram-negative septic shock, and good evidence suggests that these cytokines are important mediators of the hematologic and hemodynamic changes seen in septic patients. This has promoted efforts to develop effective antagonists of IL-1 and TNF in the treatment and management of sepsis. The anti-inflammatory properties of IL-1 receptor antagonist and soluble IL-1 receptor are also being evaluated in patients with rheumatoid arthritis.

The therapeutic effects of certain recombinant human cytokines are currently under investigation, particularly in the treatment of cancer. Clinical trials involving IL-2, interferon γ, or TNF α have met with mixed success; combination therapies capitalizing on the often synergistic actions of these cytokines may ultimately prove more beneficial. Recombinant human CSFs may also have therapeutic benefit. For example, G-CSF shows promise in boosting circulating granulocyte levels in cancer patients receiving cytotoxic chemotherapy. Elevation of the circulating granulocyte count induced by G-CSF or GM-CSF may also be useful in preventing lethal bacterial sepsis.

ADVERSE IMMUNOLOGIC RESPONSES: HYPERSENSITIVITY REACTIONS

Immune responses are often able to provide protection with minimal injury to host tissues. In some instances, however, immune responses are associated with a significant pathologic process. This may occur as a result of an excessive or inappropriate response to a foreign antigen. Immune reactions that are overtly injurious to the host are termed *hypersensitivity reactions.* The clinical manifestations of hypersensitivity reactions depend on the host's immune response to antigen and not on the nature of the antigen itself. The mechanisms of hypersensitivity can be as diverse as the various elements of the immune system. All hypersensitivity reactions have one important feature in common, however; these individuals had previously mounted an immune response to the offending antigen.

Nearly four decades ago, Gell and Coombs devised a classification scheme for describing hypersensitivity reactions on the basis of the immune reactions elicited, rather than on the clinical symptoms of the disease. Based on differences in the mechanisms of initiation and chemical-cellular mediators, hypersensitivity reactions were divided into four types (Table 4–8). As our understanding of the organization and function of the immune system has expanded, it has become evident that many immunopathologic reactions involve both cellular and humoral responses and several effector mechanisms. Nevertheless, the Gell and Coombs classification scheme remains a useful tool for description of hypersensitivity reactions.

TABLE 4–8. Classification of Pathologic Processes

Reaction Type/Description	Immune Component(s)	Inflammatory Response	Disease Manifestations
Type I: immediate hypersensitivity reactions	IgE	Release of phamacologic mediators from mast cells	Anaphylaxis/atopy
Type II: cytolytic reactions	IgM, IgM	Binding of immunoglobulin to target cells with destruction mediated by complement or other antibody effectors	ABO incompatibility; myasthenia gravis; autoimmune hemolytic anemia
Type III: immune complex reactions	IgG, IgM	Formation of antigen-antibody complexes deposited in various tissues; leads to complement activation and recruitment of phagocytes	Rheumatoid arthritis; Arthus reaction; immune complex glomerulonephritis
Type IV: delayed hypersensitivity reactions	T lymphocytes (CD4$^+$)	T lymphocytes activation leads to release of cytokines, which activate macrophages and stimulates other T lymphocytes	Contract dermatitis; tuberculin-type reactions

The first three types of hypersensitivity phenomena are antibody-mediated, although the immunoglobulin isotype responsible varies. Type IV hypersensitivity reactions, on the other hand, involve cell-mediated immune responses. Hypersensitivity reactions also vary with respect to the time frame in which clinical manifestations of the reaction become apparent. In type I (immediate) reactions, maximum response can occur within 5 to 15 minutes after antigen exposure, and the response fades within 1 to 2 hours thereafter. Type II reactions develop during a period of 5 to 8 hours after antigen exposure, whereas type III reactions develop within 2 to 8 hours. In contrast, type IV reactions require 24 to 72 hours to develop, prompting their description as *delayed hypersensitivity reactions.*

Type I (Immediate Hypersensitivity) Reactions

Type I reactions are considered to be mediated by IgE antibodies. The discovery of IgE as the principal mediator of immediate hypersensitivity in allergy was made in 1966 by Kimishige and Teruko Ishizaka. Two years later, IgE was formally recognized as a distinct class of immunoglobulin. IgE, produced on clinical contact with antigen, binds to the surface of human mast cells and basophils, which possess high-affinity

receptors for the Fc region of the ϵ heavy chain. IgE binding to these cells does not require the presence of specific antigen. Once bound to mast cells and basophils (which are then referred to as being "sensitized"), IgE serves as an antigen receptor. Subsequent exposure of sensitized mast cells and basophils to specific antigen results in the "cross-linking" of adjacent membrane-bound IgE molecules and their associated Fc ϵ receptors. Receptor cross-linking activates a G (guanosine triphosphate-binding) protein, which, in turn, stimulates the production of secondary messengers involved in mast cell and basophil activation. The consequence of the signal transduction process is mast cell and basophil degranulation and the de novo synthesis and release of other inflammatory mediators. The release of these pharmacologically activate mediators produces the clinical manifestations of immediate hypersensitivity. A partial list of the chemical mediators released by mast cells is provided in Table 4–9. These mediators are broadly divided into two categories: *preformed* (granule-associated) and *newly synthesized* (particularly lipid-derived) mediators.

All normal (nonatopic) individuals produce limited amounts of IgE in response to various antigens. These antibodies bind to high-affinity IgE receptors and mast cells and basophils as previously described. Neverthe-

TABLE 4–9. Mast Cell-derived Mediators of Immediate Hypersensitivity

Class of Mediator	Pharmacologic Properties
Preformed	
Histamine	Capillary dilatation; increased vascular permeability; constriction of bronchial smooth muscle
Eosinophil chemotactic factor of anaphylaxis (ECF-A)	Chemoattraction of eosinophils
Neutrophil chemotactic factor of anaphylaxis (NCF-A)	Chemoattraction of neutrophils
Newly Synthesized	
Platelet-activating factor (PAF)	Constriction of bronchial smooth muscle; aggregation and degranulation of platelets
Prostaglandins (especially PGD$_2$)	Constriction of central and peripheral airways; vasodilatation
Leukotrienes (LTC$_4$, LTD$_4$, and LTE$_4$)	Contraction of bronchial smooth muscle; increased vascular permeability

less, nonatopic subjects are not prone to immediate hypersensitivity reactions. This is attributable to the finding that, on a given mast cell or basophil, receptor-bound IgE molecules are directed to distinct antigens. Therefore, a single antigen has a low probability of bridging two adjacent IgE molecules with specificity for that antigen. Patients with atopic disease *(atopy)* are individuals who exhibit abnormal hypersensitivity to antigens that do not affect the general population, and in contrast, produce significant amounts of antigen-specific IgE. In such individuals, the likelihood that mast cells and basophils may be sensitized with IgE antibodies and a common antigenic specificity is significantly increased (and thus, the opportunity for antigen-induced IgE cross-linking).

Clinically significant atopic disease occurs in approximately 10 to 20% of the United States population and shows a strong familial clustering of cases. The most common form of atopic disease is *allergic rhinitis*, or hayfever, in which the hypersensitivity reactions are localized to the nasal mucosa and conjunctiva. Clinical symptoms include rhinorrhea, sneezing, and nasal obstruction. Afflicted subjects often complain of itching of the eyes, nose, and throat. The disease may be seasonal, coinciding with the appearance of pollens in the environment, or perennial, such as when caused by house dust or mites (see Chap. 8).

Other localized type I reactions include atopic dermatitis and asthma. Atopic dermatitis, also known as allergic eczema, is a cutaneous form of type I hypersensitivity that often accompanies allergic rhinitis and asthma. Although the cause is unknown, nearly 75% of patients with this disease have a familial history of atopic disease. Serum IgE concentrations can be markedly elevated in these patients. The essential features of atopic dermatitis include dry, itchy skin, which results in frequent scratching and rubbing. This rubbing produces typical features of eczema and may lead to secondary infection. It is not within the scope of this chapter to discuss bronchial asthma except to say that most bronchial asthma probably is not related to IgE-mediated hypersensitivity. Finally, the relationship between IgE-mediated hypersensitivity and otitis media has long been a controversial area in our field. The general consensus of opinion of those who have objectively studied this disease is that IgE-mediated hypersensitivity is indeed related to the pathogenesis of otitis media, but most likely by the production of allergic rhinitis, blockage of the eustachian tube, and the development of gas absorption in the middle ear secondary to eustachian tube obstruction.

Immediate hypersensitivity reactions typically involve IgE-mediated release of chemical mediators from sensitized mast cells and basophils. Clinical symptoms typically become apparent within minutes of allergen exposure and usually fade within 1 to 2 hours. In approximately 50% of atopic patients, however, this immediate reaction is followed by a so-called *late-phase reaction*, which develops some 3 to 4 hours after allergen challenge, peaks at 6 to 12 hours, and resolves within 24 to 72 hours. Late-phase reaction is an inflammatory reaction that involves accumulation of several cell types including neutrophils, eosinophils, and basophils. Variable evidence indicates that the late-phase reaction is caused by IgE-mediated degranulation of sensitized basophils rather than mast cells, which contain substances that are chemotactic for neutrophils and eosinophils.

Type II (Cytolytic) Reactions

Type I hypersensitivity reactions involving binding of antibody to target cells, which are then destroyed through the action of membrane attack complex of complement or through cellular effectors of antibody-dependent cell-mediated cytoxicity. Clinical manifestations of these cytolytic reactions depend on which cell types are damaged. Type II reactions generally involve IgG or IgM antibodies, inasmuch as these are the isotypes capable of activating the classical pathway of complement.

Hemolysis caused by the production of antierythrocyte antibody, as occurs in *erythroblastosis fetalis,* is an example of type II hypersensitivity reaction. This hemolytic disorder results from an Rh incompatibility between an Rh-negative mother and an Rh-positive fetus. An Rh-negative mother can become ''sensitized'' to the Rh antigen during the carriage of an Rh-positive fetus. This sensitization occurs particularly during delivery, at which time the Rh-positive fetal erythrocytes are able to enter the mother's circulation. On subsequent pregnancies involving carriage of an Rh-positive fetus, maternal IgG antibodies cross the placenta, causing substantial lysis of fetal erythrocytes. Intravascular hemolysis can result in severe anemia and central nervous system damage caused by accumulation of bilirubin. Hemolytic reactions resulting from transfusion of ABO-incompatible erythrocytes are a similar example of type II hypersensitivity.

In other instances, inadvertent lysis of host cells occurs as a consequence of adsorption of certain drugs to these cells, especially antibiotics such as penicillin and cephalosporins. Production of antibody against the drug-host cell complex results in antibody deposition on the target cell, which is subsequently lysed by complement. Examples of this type of hypersensitivity include drug-induced hemolytic anemia and drug-induced thrombocytopenia.

The production of autoantibodies directed against cellular components can also result in damage characteristic of type II hypersensitivity. For example, in Goodpasture's syndrome, autoantibodies are produced against the basement membrane of the lung and renal glomerulus. Deposition of autoantibodies in these organs leads to tissue injury resulting from complement activation and infiltration by inflammatory cells, especially neutrophils. In the field of otology, autoimmune sensorineural hearing loss may be related to the development of autoantibody developed against type II collagen, which may be present in the otic capsule (otosclerosis) and possibly in the stria vascularis or other parts of the inner ear and may be related to progressive autoimmune sensorineural hearing loss.

Type III (Immune Complex) Reactions

Type III hypersensitivity reactions are initiated by the formation of antigen-antibody complexes that precipitate in various tissues. These immune complexes activate complement, thereby generating chemotactic factors (e.g., C5a) that promote infiltration by phagocytic cells, particularly neutrophils. The tissue damage that ensues is principally due to the production of toxic oxygen metabolites and the release of histolytic enzymes by neutrophils during their unsuccessful attempt to ingest the deposited immune complexes. The type of tissue damage observed depends on the anatomic location in which the immune complexes are deposited.

Antibodies in immune complex-mediated tissue injury belong to the IgG (IgG$_1$, IgG$_2$, and IgG$_3$ only) or IgM class, inasmuch as these are the isotypes capable of activating complement via the classical pathway. The size of the immune complex is an important variable influencing the potential for tissue injury. Immune complexes of intermediate size (formed by one or two molecules of antigen and one or two molecules of antibody) pose the greatest threat. This is because small complexes are relatively ineffective in activating complement, whereas large complexes are readily cleared by mononuclear phagocytes in the liver and spleen.

Immune complex-mediated injury may either be localized or generalized, depending on the manner in which antigen and antibody react. A classic example of localized type III hypersensitivity is the *Arthus* reaction, an acute immune complex-mediated vasculitis. In this reaction, antigen is injected into the skin of an immune ("sensitized") individual who has circulating antibodies against the antigen. Immune complexes form along blood vessel walls. These complexes activate complement, liberating anaphylatoxins (C3a, C5a), which induce degranulation of mast cells and thereby enhance vascular permeability. This facilitates penetration of the immune complexes, which eventually become lodged in the basement membrane of affected blood vessels. Complement-derived chemotactic factors (C5a) promote subsequent infiltration by circulating neutrophils, which migrate toward the immune complexes. The phagocytic cells are unable to ingest the entrapped immune complexes but are able to bind the complexes via their membrane receptors for IgG and opsonic C3 fragments. Through a process termed "frustrated phagocytosis," the neutrophils adhere tightly to the noningestible surface and release the contents of their cytoplasmic granules into the underlying extracellular space. Lysosomal enzymes, as well as oxygen metabolites produced during the attendant respiratory burst, cause local tissue damage. This leads to hemorrhagic necrosis and eventual vessel occlusion.

The combination of antigen and antibody within the vascular compartment can result in a more generalized form of immune complex disease, an example of which is serum sickness. Sites of deposition of these circulating immune complexes are subject to the influence of several factors, including hydrostatic pressure and turbulence. Capillaries in the renal glomeruli and synovia represent regions of increased hydrostatic pressure and turbulence, and in these tissues circulating immune complexes tend to be localized. Accordingly, glomerulonephritis and arthritis are common manifestations of generalized immune complex-mediated hypersensitivity reactions. Investigators are also recognizing that other areas of hydrodynamic tissue are the stria vascularis of the inner ear, the choroid plexus of the brain, and the iris of the eyes. Therefore, it is conceivable that circulating immune complexes may nonspecifically deposit in the stria vascularis and cause a type of autoimmune sensorineural hearing loss.

Type IV (Delayed Hypersensitivity) Reactions

In contrast to the first three types of hypersensitivity, which are antibody mediated, type IV hypersensitivity reactions are mediated by T lymphocytes. Delayed-type hypersensitivity reactions are due to antigen-induced stimulation of CD4 + T helper cells, particularly those of the T$_H$1 phenotype. T-helper cells of this phenotype elaborate certain cytokines, including IL-2 and interferon γ, which promote infiltration and activation of machrophages at the affected site. The tissue damage that ensues is a consequence of a release of lysosomal enzymes and toxic oxygen metabolites by the activated macrophages.

A common example of delayed-type hypersensitivity is contact dermatitis seen in subjects who are sensitive to cosmetics, poison ivy, poison oak, or metals such as nickel. Such substances are able to form complexes with various proteins in the skin. These complexes are subsequently internalized by antigen-presenting cells present in skin, including Langerhans cells and epidermal keratinocytes. The internalized complexes are processed and reexpressed on the surface of the antigen-presenting cell in conjunction with MHC class II macromolecules. Antigen-specific CD4 + lymphocytes present in the sensitized individual are activated by the antigen-presenting cells, resulting in the secretion of inflammatory cytokines.

The delayed-type hypersensitivity reaction likely plays a significant role in the elimination of parasites and intracellular bacteria, with the activated macrophage representing a key effector cell. Persistence of the offending antigen can, however, lead to the development of a chronic form of delayed-type hypersensitivity that is injurious to the host. One example of such a chronic reaction is the granulomatous skin lesion observed in patients infected with Mycobacterium leprae. Because of the host's inability to eliminate this microorganism, infiltrating macrophages and fibroblasts proliferate and produce collagen in an effort to "wall off" the mycobacteria. In addition, macrophages often fuse to form giant cells. The granuloma that forms is a consequence of the prolonged recruitment of macrophages and can result in significant tissue destruction.

AUTOIMMUNITY

Hypersensitivity reactions produce tissue injury as a consequence of an immune response to *exogenous* antigens. The immune system does not typically respond to *autologous* (self) antigens because of the induction of tolerance, either through clonal deletion (elimination of autoreactive T and B lymphocytes) or clonal anergy (in which autoreactive lymphocytes persist but are rendered unresponsive). Nevertheless, in some instances unresponsiveness to self-antigens is altered, resulting in the state termed autoimmunity. The existence of an autoimmune response is not necessarily deleterious to the host. In certain instances autoimmune reactions are clearly beneficial in immune function and regulation. Two key examples of physiologic autoimmunity are the recognition of MHC-encoded macromolecules by T lymphocytes and the production of anti-idiotypic antibodies.

Thus, CD4+ T lymphocytes recognize exogenous antigens displayed on the surface of antigen-presenting cells in association with MHC class II macromolecules. Were it not for the ability of the T lymphocyte to recognize self-MHC encoded molecules the immune system would be unable to differentiate between self and nonself extracellular antigens. Anti-idiotype antibodies appear to participate in a regulatory network that can enhance or suppress immune responsiveness. Anti-idiotype antibodies are produced in response to unique variable-region determinants present in immunoglobulins, including determinants involved in formation of complementarity-determining regions. These anti-idiotypic antibodies can enhance the immune response by either stimulating idiotype-bearing T-helper lymphocytes or by eliminating specific T-suppressor lymphocytes. Alternatively, such antibodies may stimulate T-suppressor activity and thereby negatively influence production of the first (idiotypic) antibody.

A breakdown in the mechanisms that control the proliferation and activity of autoreactive lymphocytes can result in abnormal autoimmune reactions. The clinical manifestations of autoimmune disease may be organ-specific or systemic, depending on the distribution of the antigen responsible for stimulating the immune response. Moreover, the reaction may involve production of autoantibody, autoreactive T lymphocytes, or both. Three principal mechanisms appear to account for the majority of autoimmune diseases in humans. In the first instance, autoantibodies are produced that are reactive toward modified or unmodified cell surface antigen. This may lead to cellular destruction through complement-mediated lysis or antibody-dependent cell-mediated cytotoxicity, or to noncytotoxic alteration of cellular function. For example, in Graves' disease, a form of organ-specific autoimmunity, autoantibodies directed against the receptor for thyroid-stimulating hormone (TSH) are produced. These antibodies mimic TSH-mediated stimulation of the thyroid, resulting in overproduction of thyroid hormones.

A second pathogenetic mechanism entails the formation of autoantigen-autoantibody complexes. The antigen-antibody complexes may form in the circulation, ultimately being deposited in tissue such as the renal glomerulus or in the intercellular spaces. Tissue damage associated with this reaction, which is analogous to type III hypersensitivity as mentioned previously, is mediated by complement activation and/or infiltration by phagocytic cells. A notable example of this type of systemic autoimmunity is *rheumatoid arthritis*, a disease characterized by the presence of antibodies (termed *rheumatoid factors*) that react with the Fc region of the patient's IgG molecules. Rheumatoid factors are usually of the IgM isotype, although IgG autoantibodies are not uncommon. Rheumatoid factors have been found in middle ear effusions. Complexes formed between the rheumatoid factor and the patient's own IgG circulate for a time before being deposited in tissue such as synovial membranes. Complement activation in phagocytic infiltration produces damage associated with chronic joint inflammation. Similarly, there appears to be increasing evidence that this type of mechanism may be a cause of progressive sensorineural hearing loss, particularly in the potential of autoantibodies directed against type II collagen in the inner ear.

A final mechanism of tissue injury caused by autoimmune reactions involves the generation of autoreactive T lymphocytes. On activation by autoantigen, these T lymphocytes secrete various cytokines that promote the infiltration and activation of mononuclear phagocytes, the products of which mediate damage to host tissues. An example of this form of autoimmunity is multiple sclerosis, a disease associated with sensory and motor abnormalities. The pathogenesis of this disease is associated with demyelination of nerve cells in the central nervous system. The areas of demyelination are associated with accumulations of lymphocytes and mononuclear phagocytes. It is conceivable that autoreactive T lymphocytes may also be a mechanism for the development of autoimmunity in the inner ear.

The basis for development of autoimmune disease is incompletely understood, but it appears to be multifactorial. Factors that appear to contribute to the development of autoimmune diseases include: (1) release of antigens normally sequestered from immunocompetent cells (and that, therefore, do not induce tolerance); (2) molecular mimickery, such as occurs when antibodies form in response to microbial infection cross-react with host components; (3) alterations in MHC class II molecules (possibly by drugs or infectious agents), which are recognized in a manner analogous to that of other allogeneic MHC molecules; and (4) polyclonal B lymphocyte activation, such as may be induced by microbial constituents (including lipopolysaccharides), certain viruses (Epstein-Barr virus) or parasites (Plasmodium malariae). In general, autoantibodies induced by polyclonal B-lymphocyte activators are of the IgM isotype, inasmuch as these agents bypass T-helper lymphocytes that provide signals for isotype switching. Nonimmune factors also appear to have propensity for the development of autoimmune diseases. These include genetic (HLA alleles) and hormonal (sex hormone) factors.

Evidence for a hormonal association derives from the observation that the incidence of systemic lupus erythematosus in postpubertal women is nearly ninefold greater than in men. On the other hand, the incidence of ankylosing spondylitis is higher among men than women.

SUGGESTED READINGS

Abbas AK, Lichtman AH, and Pober JS: Cellular and molecular immunology. Philadelphia, WB Saunders Company, 1991.

Gallin JI, Goldstein IM, and Snyderman R: Inflammation: Basic Principles and Clinical Correlates. New York, Raven Press, 1988.

Golub ES and Green DR: Immunology: A Synthesis. 2nd Ed. Sunderland, MA, Sinauer Associates, 1991.

Klebanoff SJ and Clark RA: The Neutrophil: Function and Clinical Disorders. Amsterdam. Elsevier/North-Holland Publishing, 1978.

Kuby J: Immunology. New York, WH Freeman, 1992.

Monaco JJ: A molecular model of MHC class I-restricted antigen processing. Immunol Today 13:173, 1992.

Neefjes JJ and Ploegh HL: Intracellular transport of MHC class II molecules. Immunol Today 13:179, 1992.

Paul WE: Fundamental Immunology. 2nd Ed. New York, Raven Press, 1989.

Shakib F: The Human IgG Subclasses: Molecular Analysis of Structure, Function and Regulation. Oxford, Pergamon Press, 1990.

Stites DP and Terr AI: Basic and Clinical Immunology. 7th Ed. Norwalk, CT, Appleton and Lange, 1991.

von Boehmer H and Kisielow P: How the immune system learns about self. Sci Am 265:74, 1991.

5 Current Concepts of the Acquired Immunodeficiency Syndrome (AIDS)

Norman Berlinger

The acquired immunodeficiency syndrome (AIDS) has emerged as one of the most extraordinary diseases in human history. We have seen the unfolding of a medical mystery in which an apparently new disease has appeared,[1] first recognized in the United States and now in existence worldwide. The common denominator of the disease is a profound quantitative and qualitative deficiency of a specific set of thymus-derived (T) lymphocytes, designated by the phenotypic marker CD4. These cells are responsible for the helper-inducer function of the immune system. The immune defect is apparently remarkably selective for the CD4 subpopulation of lymphocytes, although other cells, such as monocytes and central nervous system cells, have some CD4 receptors on their surface that are also involved in this defect. Because of the central and critical role that the CD4 population of lymphocytes plays in the orchestration of the human immune response, however, its gradual but inevitable destruction is associated with a profound immune deficiency. Although this deficiency is most readily appreciated in the cell-mediated limb of the immune system, the defects that are noted are both broad and heterogeneous, reflecting the major influence of the CD4 subset on the entire scope of the immune response.

The immune defect in AIDS leads to a constellation of secondary complications manifested predominantly by opportunistic infections and the development of unusual neoplasms such as Kaposi's sarcoma. The syndrome, for the most part, has remained confined to well-defined risk groups in accordance with the modes of transmission, which are predominantly sexual contact and exposure to contaminated blood or blood products.

The impact of AIDS on the afflicted population has been devastating because there are no recognized cases of spontaneous or therapeutically induced recovery of immune function. Although the overall mortality of the disease is reported to be about 50 to 60%, the eventual mortality in patients with the full-blown disease is likely to be 100%.

EPIDEMIOLOGY

AIDS is still a rapidly growing problem in the United States and other developed countries, and its prevalence in the developing world is even more problematic. The World Health Organization estimates that 13 million persons are now infected worldwide, and approximately 38 to 100 million will be infected by the year 2000.

The AIDS problem may truly be called a pandemic, and it is probably best viewed as a series of separate epidemics that overlap in both time and place.[2] Three kinds of epidemiologic patterns are recognized. One kind is that seen in the United States, Canada, western Europe, and northern Africa in which the human immunodeficiency virus (HIV) is spread predominantly by homosexual or bisexual men and by intravenous drug abusers. There is a male preponderance, and spread of HIV among heterosexual contacts is uncommon. A second epidemiologic pattern is seen in the rest of Africa and most of South America, where the majority of people have been infected heterosexually, with no apparent sex predilection. Rates of infection are devastating in these regions, with about 8 million infected persons living in sub-Saharan Africa. A third pattern is beginning to develop in Asia and the Middle East in which three groups of individuals have successively been infected: (1) intravenous drug abusers; (2) female commercial sex workers (CSWs); and (3) young heterosexual men. Thailand is probably the best studied and most alarming example of this third wave

117

in the AIDS pandemic. HIV seropositivity among brothel-based CSWs can be as high as 40%, and studies of male army conscripts reveal that up to 75% have had sex with female CSWs. Condom usage in this latter group may be only about 60%, and so young Thai men are clearly at high risk for becoming infected with HIV. Sadly, a majority of Thai people surveyed believe themselves to be at low risk for HIV infection because the epidemic in Thailand is relatively new and few people have developed the visibility of full-blown AIDS. Therefore, it will be difficult to convince apparently healthy young men and women to practice safe sex.

As the African experience suggests, the Asian epidemic will bring about large numbers of orphaned children. The workforce will gradually fall ill, and food production will diminish. The educational system will break down, and the medical system will be strapped with increased costs. Two thirds of the world's cases of tuberculosis (TB) are in Asia, and thousands of cases of latent TB infections will be activated as the immunodeficiency spreads.

In the United States through 1992, over one million people have become seropositive, and 300,000 have progressed to full-blown AIDS. The type 1 epidemiologic pattern seen in this country in the past decade is now changing in the 1990s. The annual incidence rates among homosexual or bisexual men and among intravenous drug abusers seems to have leveled off. Other risk groups are experiencing increases in HIV seropositivity and AIDS incidence, most notably heterosexual females and infants infected perinatally.

Now 12 years into the epidemic in the United States, women are the fastest growing group of AIDS patients. The Centers for Disease Control and Prevention (CDC) now report 40,000 cases of AIDS among women, still far fewer than the 340,000 cases among men. From 1991 to 1992, however, the number of cases in women increased 9.1%, compared with a rise of 2.5% in men, and in 1992, for the first time, the number of women infected through heterosexual contact exceeded the number infected through intravenous drug abuse. AIDS is now the fourth leading cause of death among women aged 25 to 44 in the United States.

To date, almost 5000 cases of AIDS in children have been reported to the CDC, and the number of children infected with HIV who have not yet demonstrated full-blown clinical AIDS must be much higher. The principal risk factor, present in most cases of childhood AIDS, is HIV infection in the mother. Given the increasing incidence of heterosexual transmission of HIV and the rapidly rising rate of infection among women of childbearing age, many more cases of pediatric AIDS seem inevitable.

Some infants infected with HIV become rapidly and severely ill and die within the first year of life.[3] Although not yet proved, these are probably the children who were infected early in utero. Children who acquire their infection closer to delivery have higher birthweights, later onset of symptoms, and higher CD8 counts. Many children go on to become long-term survivors, and severe intercurrent illnesses, low CD4 counts, and p24 antigenemia do not preclude long-term survival. In fact, 10% are completely aysmptomatic, and another 30% display only minimal clinical features. Lymphadenopathy and parotitis are more frequent among the long-term survivors. These signs seem to be positive predictors of survival in children and are part of the diffuse infiltrative lymphocytosis syndrome (DILS), which is associated with a milder form of disease in adults and is possibly due to a genetically determined response to HIV.[4]

TRANSMISSION

The known routes of transfer of the AIDS virus are blood, blood products, intimate sexual activity, and transmission from mother to child perinatally. Careful tissue culture studies have documented the amounts of free HIV and HIV-infected cells in a variety of body fluids including blood, genital secretions, cerebrospinal fluid (CSF), amniotic fluid, bronchial lavage fluids, urine, milk, tears, and saliva. Essentially, aside from blood, genital fluids, and CSF, other body fluids contain little free infectious virus. HIV can be found in genital fluid from vasectomized men and in preejaculatory fluid indicating virus secretions from other glands besides the testes. Virus-infected cells may be the most important source of HIV transmission because they are more numerous in body fluids than free virus. Other venereal diseases causing the accumulation of numerous inflammatory cells in the vagina or seminal ejaculate could influence HIV transmission by transferring more virus-infected cells to the receptive host. This parameter of venereal infection could be a major cause of the high frequency of heterosexual spread of HIV in Africa. Considering the relatively large size of a cell, an intact condom would seem to provide reasonably effective protection against viral transmission.

Currently, the blood supply in developed countries is well protected by both donor deferral and screening for antibodies to HIV. In the United States, the present risk of acquiring an HIV infection from screened blood has been estimated at 1/225,000 units. The rare infection is caused by blood from individuals who have recently been infected but have not yet seroconverted.

HIV can survive the treatments needed to produce cryoprecipitates or lyophilized factor VIII or IX preparations, with the virus remaining stable in the lyophilized powder for several years. Previously, patients with hemophilia became infected as a result of the transfusion of these contaminated blood products.

Now hemophiliacs are virtually protected from infection because of the heat treatment that is required of all factor VIII and factor IX preparations.

Several studies have clearly shown that the receptive partner in homosexual anal-genital contact is the more susceptible individual for HIV infection. Abrasions in the anal canal are not necessary for virus entry, because bowel mucosa contains columnar and goblet cells that can be directly infected by HIV. Tissue culture studies show that HIV-infected monocytes and lymphocytes can pass virus directly to epithelial cells by cell-to-cell contact.

In addition to anal-genital contact in heterosexual relationships, vaginal intercourse carries a substantial risk for transmission of HIV. Infection in women usually occurs by virus-infected cells entering the cervical os and then interacting with macrophages, lymphocytes, or the epithelial cells lining the uterine cavity. The vaginal squamous epithelial cells constitute a relatively strong barrier for virus infection unless affected with abrasions or excoriations from venereal diseases or trauma. Infection may take place at the cervix, especially if it is irritated with spermicidal compounds such as nonoxynol 9. The male partner in vaginal intercourse could become infected by having female infected cells enter the penile urethra and come into contact with macrophages or epithelial cells of the urethral canal. If the female partner has a concurrent veneral disease, HIV infection would be even more likely because she would transfer more infected inflammatory cells. Similarly, venereal disease in the male, especially with ulceration of the penis, would increase the likelihood of viral transmission.

There seem to be three ways of transmitting the HIV infection from mother to child: (1) prenatally in utero during any trimester; (2) during delivery; and (3) postnatally through breast milk.[5] Even though the fetus and infant seem at great risk, most infants are spared, with infection rates of only about 20 to 30%.[6] These children with HIV infection (and the remaining 70 to 80% who escape infection) have mothers who will more than likely die of their own HIV infection before their children do. Investigators estimate that about 80,000 children in the United States will lose their mothers to AIDS by the year 2000.[7]

VIRUS

The AIDS virus is a retrovirus, meaning that the virus possesses a single strand of RNA as its genetic material, which it can then convert to a double strand of DNA for incorporation into the genome of the cell that it infects. This synthesis of DNA from an RNA template is accomplished by the enzyme reverse transcriptase (RNA-dependent DNA polymerase). HIV-2 is also a retrovirus that causes a milder form of AIDS. It is found almost exclusively in Africa, with only a few cases reported in the United States.

The spherical virus attaches to the CD4 receptor on T-helper cells with high affinity. Other cells have a few CD4 receptors and can serve as targets for infection. These include circulating and fixed macrophages, gut epithelial cells, and perhaps glial cells.

The outer envelope of the virion is a typical lipid bilayer with a glycoprotein moiety, gp120, protruding from its surface. The gp120 functions as the actual binding site to the CD4 receptor of the host cell to bring about infection (Fig. 5–1). As a consequence, trials are underway to determine whether gp120 can be used as a vaccine or can be administered to patients already infected to bring about an antibody response to gp120.

The inner envelope, or capsid, encircles the viral RNA and reverse transcriptase and is composed of

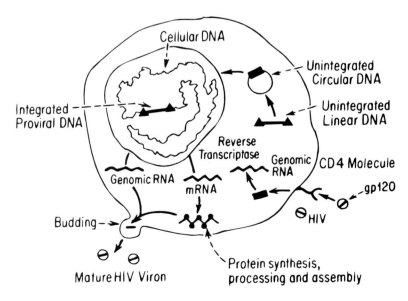

Fig. 5–1. Representation of the life cycle of the HIV-1 virus. On the right side of the diagram, the glycoprotein 120 epitope of the virus has an atropism for the CD_4 molecule, and the virus is uncoded at the periphery of the CD_4 cell. Genomic RNA is then transcribed to DNA by reverse transcriptase and becomes integrated into the cellular DNA as a provirus. It can then remain dormant for years or, when it is activated by another viral infection or mitogen as described in the text, becomes activated and starts to transcribe for messenger and genomic RNA of the virus. The virus is then assembled at the periphery and buds off as a mature HIV variant. (Adapted from Fauci AS: The human immunodeficiency virus: infectivity and mechanisms of pathogenesis. Science 239:617, 1988.)

four distinct nucleocapsid proteins. These proteins are synthesized as a single progenitor, which is ultimately cleaved by a viral protease into the four distinct subunits: p7, p9, p17, and p24. The protease cleavage is vital to the life cycle of the virus, and attempts are being made to synthesize clinically useful inhibitors of the protease. The p17 protein must undergo myrisylation with a fatty acid to be incorporated into the capsid. Inhibitors of myrisylation impair virion assembly and infectivity and may find clinical utility.

The enzyme reverse transcriptase has no close analogue in the human host cell. Nucleoside analogues such as zidovudine have already been used as reasonably successful, albeit palliative, therapies for AIDS infections. The nucleoside analogues compete with the usual nucleoside substrates of reverse transcriptase to bring about termination of the elongating DNA strand. Inhibitors of reverse transcriptase that are not nucleosides are also undergoing clinical trials for possible therapeutic effectiveness.

HIV may kill its host cell by budding from the cell surface and incorporating portions of the host cell membrane into the glycoprotein envelope of the virion. This seems to destroy the integrity of the host cell membrane and brings about cell death. Single-cell killing may also result from the accumulation of unincorporated viral DNA or from the inhibition of host cell protein synthesis after HIV infection. Some evidence indicates that another type of cytopathic effect results from infected CD4 cells forming syncytia, which are ultimately short lived.

IMMUNOPATHOLOGY AND CLINICAL COURSE

The clinical course of HIV infection is similar for most patients. Up to 70% of patients with primary acute HIV infection develop an infectious mononucleosis-like syndrome several weeks after the infectious event, and high titers of virus are found in the blood. During the period of marked viremia, the virus widely disseminates and in particular seeds the lymphoid organs (lymph nodes, tonsils, and adenoids). In several more weeks, easily detectable humoral and cellular immune responses to the virus occur. Plasma viremia soon becomes difficult to detect, and HIV mRNA is virtually absent in peripheral blood lymphocytes. Although the viremia is then markedly curtailed, the immune responses are usually inadequate to suppress viral replication completely, and HIV expression persists in lymphoid organs.

Most patients then enter a long period of clinical latency (median, 10 years) during which symptoms are usually absent. This concept is misleading, because during this time immune functions, particularly those mediated by CD4 T-helper cells, are deteriorating. Al-

though not much virus is detectable in plasma, virus replication is occurring in lymphoid tissue and is probably the major cause of the gradual depletion of CD4 lymphocytes.

After this period of clinical latency, constitutional signs and symptoms appear first, and then clinically apparent disease (AIDS). Death usually occurs within 2 years even with treatment. The profound immunosuppression that occurs during this period is the end result of the immunopathologic events that began at the time of primary infection and continued through the clinically latent but virologically active subsequent years.

The resulting immune deficiency with HIV infection is due to both qualitative and quantitative defects of CD4 T-helper cells. As mentioned before, single-cell killing and syncytia formation are two mechanisms to explain the deletion of these crucial immune cells.

Paradoxically, the very immune mechanisms directed against the virus may actually accelerate the development of the immune deficit, because these immune attacks against the virus can destroy the CD4 cells harboring it. Some anti-HIV antibodies directed against envelope glycoprotein moieties elicit an antibody-dependent cellular cytotoxicity reaction, after binding to natural killer cells, that will destroy the CD4 cell expressing viral envelope proteins on its surface. In this manner, CD4 lymphocytes, follicular dendritic cells of lymph nodes, and macrophages may be progressively eliminated.[8]

Some lines of experimentation seem to indicate that antibodies directed against the gp120 envelope glycoprotein of the virion will cross-react with class II molecules of the major histocompatibility complex (MHC) on immunocompetent cells. Antigen-presenting cells with MHC class II molecules on their surface may then not be able to interact appropriately with CD4 cells. The antigen-specific functions of CD4 cells may thus be inhibited, leading to a functional deficit in the helper role of these cells. The CD4 cells can even become anergic when complexes of gp120 antigen and antibody bind to CD4 molecules, thus making them refractory to further stimulation.[9]

Considerable experimental evidence seems to indicate that superantigens encoded by the retrovirus perturb many T-cell subgroups. These superantigens, unlike conventional antigenic peptides, bind to nearly all T cells that have a specific variable region of the ß-chain of the T-cell antigen receptor, rather than in the groove of the MHC class II molecules. As such, the superantigens bind almost indiscriminately to many more T cells. These superantigens can therefore induce massive stimulation and expansion of T cells, which are unfortunately followed by cell deletion and anergy. Moreoever, while stimulated, T cells are much more susceptible to infection with the virus.

Apoptosis, or programmed cell death, is a mechanism whereby the body eliminates clones of T cells that are autoreactive. Investigators now speculate that cross-linking of the CD4 receptor by HIV gp120 or by gp120-anti-gp120 immune complexes prematurely prepares the cell for apoptosis as soon as a MHC class II molecule in complex with an antigen binds to the T-cell antigen receptor. In this manner, an HIV virion can cause the death of a CD4 cell even without infecting it.

The lymphoid organs appear to be the major anatomic site for the establishment as well as the propagation of HIV infection. Throughout the period of so-called clinical latency, the amount of virus in the lymphoid organs is much greater than in the peripheral blood, and therefore, blood studies may generate an incorrect impression of a quiescent infection that is actually rapidly establishing itself within solid lymphoid tissue. Virions accumulate within lymph nodes, where they are trapped by follicular dendritic cells in the germinal centers. These latter cells trap antigens during the normal immune response and present them to immuncompetent cells within the germinal centers. As the infection progresses, the network of follicular dendritic cells progressively degenerates. Consequently, the lymphoid organs lose their ability to trap HIV particles, and virus titers in the peripheral blood increase. These events help explain the dichotomy of absence of HIV in the blood but presence in the lymphoid organs during the many years of latency.

ANTIRETROVIRAL THERAPY

The Food and Drug Administration has approved three antiretroviral drugs for use in HIV infections.

Zidovudine (formerly known as azidothymidine, or AZT) was originally developed as an anticancer drug in 1964. Virion reverse transcriptase incorporates the zidovudine into the elongating nucleic acid chain, competitively inhibiting the incorporation of thymidine. Early trials of zidovudine clearly indicated prolonged survival, fewer opportunistic infections, more normal body weight, greater functional capacities, more normal scores on tests of cognition, and transient inprovement in peripheral blood CD4 counts.[10] Zidovudine is used at a dose of 500 to 600 mg daily in adults and 180 mg/m^2 every 6 hours in children over 3 months of age.

Although no definitive statements can be made about the optimal time to begin zidovudine, good evidence indicates that it should be started in asymptomatic individuals whose CD4 counts have dropped below 500/mm^3.[11] This strategy delays the progression of the disease, as manifested by the delayed onset of opportunistic infections, neurologic problems, and tumors.

The ability of zidovudine to reduce maternal-fetal transmission of the virus during pregnancy is being evaluated. What is most encouraging is how well tolerated zidovudine is during pregnancy without causing fetal distress, malformations, or premature birth. The use of zidovudine prophylaxis is being called into question because several infections have occurred among occupationally exposed health care workers despite the drug's administration soon after exposure to the virus.

The efficacy of zidovudine decreases over time, perhaps because HIV-1 develops resistance to the drug as a result of amino acid substitutions in its reverse transcriptase. A majority of patients have zidovudine-resistant HIV-1 strains after 12 months of treatment.

These zidovudine-resistant strains usually remain susceptible to the nucleosides didanosine and zalcitabine or to non-nucleoside reverse transcriptase inhibitors. Didanosine is usually given as later management to symptomatic patients whose CD4 counts are below 300/mm^3. HIV-1 isolates resistant to didanosine also occur after prolonged therapy.

Zalcitabine tends to be used in combination with zidovudine for patients whose CD4 counts are less than 300/mm^3 and who are deteriorating immunologically or clinically. Its use results in weight gain, decreased levels of p24 antigenemia, and increased CD4 counts.

Foscarnet is the non-nucleoside, noncompetitive inhibitor of HIV reverse transcriptase that has so far gained the most clinical exprience. Foscarnet serves to prolong life in AIDS patients, but it is associated with considerable toxicity such as electrolyte abnormalities, seizures, and renal failure.

OPPORTUNISTIC INFECTIONS

Pneumocystis carinii pneumonia (PCP) occurs in 75% of patients with AIDS and used to be the most common serious opportunistic infection. Owing to widespread chemoprophylaxis of PCP in patients with full-blown AIDS and in patients with CD4 counts less than 200/mm^3, the incidence of PCP significantly decreased after 1988. Trimethoprim-sulfamethoxazole (TMP-SMZ) for 21 days is the therapeutic regimen of choice for clinically manifest disease. If the PCP is more severe, with PaO$_2$ less than 70 mm Hg, a 21-day tapering course of prednisone is added. Alternative drugs include atovaquone or pentamidine. Although not approved by the United States Food and Drug Administration for treatment of PCP, trimethoprim with dapsone, aerosolized pentamidine, primaquine with clindamycin, and trimetrexate with leucovorin are showing efficacy in clinical trials. Any patient with a prior episode of PCP or with a CD4 count less than 200/mm^3 should receive chemoprophylaxis with TMP-SMZ indefinitely.

By delaying death from PCP without actually stopping the deterioration of immune function, chemoprophylaxis of PCP has shifted the clinical manifestations of HIV infection to illnesses that occur when immune function is even more suppressed. PCP prophylaxis also seems to have delayed the first AIDS-related illness by 6 to 12 months. Commonly seen now are infections due to microorganisms that are common in humans or in the environment: cytomegalovirus (CMV), candida, and Mycobacterium avium complex (MAC).[12]

Only when CMV causes significant disease such as retinitis, esophagitis, or colitis is treatment warranted.[13] The drug of choice is ganciclovir, which does not eradicate the virus but can often suppress the clinical manifestations. An alternative is foscarnet, which is equally effective but more toxic.

In AIDS patients, candidiasis is usually limited to mucosal surfaces and rarely disseminates to deep organs. Oral and vaginal infections usually respond well to topical nystatin or clotrimazole, but esophageal candidiasis requires systemic drugs, with fluconazole being highly effective. No established recommendations exist for prophylaxis of candida infections.

Disseminated MAC is now the most common systemic bacterial infection seen among patients with advanced HIV disease in the United States. Up to 40% of patients ultimately develop it, and the patients at greatest risk are those with CD4 counts less than 100/ mm³. MAC causes fever, night sweats, abdominal pain, weight loss, diarrhea, lymphadenopathy, hepatosplenomegaly, and anemia with significant mortality. Rifabutin has been approved for the prophylaxis of MAC bacteremia. Once MAC becomes disseminated, a multidrug regimen is required. A combination of clarithromycin, ciprofloxacin, ethambutol, clofazimine, and amikacin for 2 to 8 weeks has been suggested.

Toxoplasmosis is treated with pyrimethamine plus sulfadiazine. Herpes simplex and varicella-zoster virus infections respond to acyclovir, with foscarnet being a good alternative. No one drug seems particularly effective against cryptosporidiosis, but azithromycin, paromomycin, and octreotide acetate have some benefit.

OTOLARYNGOLOGIC MANIFESTATIONS

More than 50% of patients with AIDS will present with a symptom or physical finding in the head and neck.[14]

Otitis media is relatively frequent and is usually due to the pathogens common in patients who are immunologically normal. Kaposi's sarcoma, molluscum contagiousum, and seborrheic dermatitis are the common dermatologic processes affecting the pinna. Sensorineural hearing loss can occur in up to 69% of AIDS patients; CMV is often implicated because CMV inclusion-bearing cells can sometimes be found in cranial nerve VIII in the internal auditory canal, in the cochlea, or in vestibular endolymphatic epithelium. Facial pa-

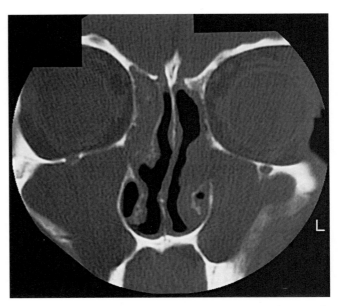

Fig. 5–2. Coronal CT section of a 26-year-old homosexual man with AIDS and a long history of therapeutically resistant sinusitis. Sinusitis was due to a mixed infection with pseudomonas and cytomegalovirus.

ralysis is common and is probably a reflection of the higher incidence of viral infections.

Nasal obstruction is common and is often due to enlarged adenoids because the virus replicates in this lymphoid organ. Sinusitis is frequent and can be due to routine pathogens, anaerobes, opportunistic microorganisms, or even a combination of bacteria and viruses (Fig. 5–2).

Oral candidiasis can take either the usual form, with white patches easily detachable from a hyperemic base, or a purely erythematous form, with the mucosa appearing uniformly smooth and inflamed. This latter form is sometimes referred to as "candidosis." Angular cheilitis, giant herpetic ulcers, and gingivitis are also common. The Epstein-Barr virus seems to cause an oral finding unique to AIDS that has been called "hairy leukoplakia." This consists of white patches along the lateral borders of the tongue and occurs early in the course of HIV infections, sometimes being the first hint that the patient may indeed be seropositive. Kaposi's sarcoma is overwhelmingly the most frequent oral tumor and can occur anywhere in the oral cavity, whereas B-cell lymphomas are common and tend to be restricted to the gingivae.[15]

Candidal esophagitis, as previously mentioned, is becoming increasingly common and can cause significant dysphagia, odynophagia, and dehydration. Kaposi's sarcoma can involve the esophagus extensively and can cause identical symptoms.

Neck masses are frequent in AIDS patients. Most commonly, this finding represents cervical lymphadenopathy, but parotid gland cysts (Fig. 5–3) and infectious processes (Fig. 5–4) are also common.

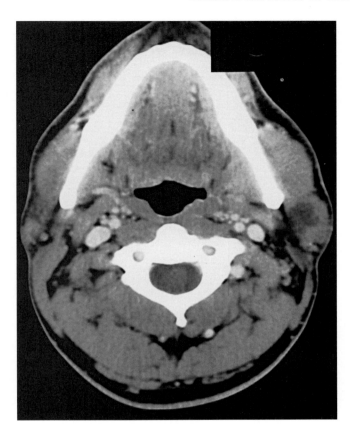

Fig. 5–3. Axial CT section of a 32-year-old homosexual man with a 2-month history of a progressively enlarging, nontender, soft mass in the left cheek. It has the typical radiographic appearance of a lympho-epithelial cyst. Aspiration cytology revealed fluid-containing epithelial cysts and benign lymphocytes. These do not need to be excised if the radiographic and cytologic characteristics are as described. Excision seems necessary only in the face of diagnostic uncertainty because the course of these cysts does not appreciably change the patient's clinical condition.

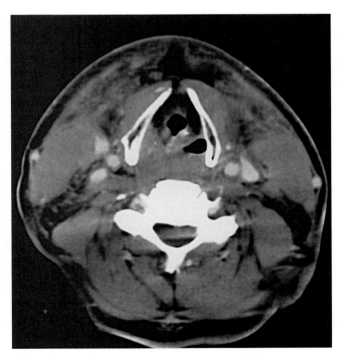

Fig. 5–4. Axial CT section of a 32-year-old homosexual man with diffuse cellulitis of the anterior neck. No organism was ever cultured, and he slowly responded to broad-spectrum antibiotics.

SUGGESTED READINGS

1. Allen JR and Curran JW: Epidemiology of the acquired immunodeficiency syndrome. In: Advances in Host Defense Mechanisms. Edited by Gallin JI and Fauci AS. New York, Raven Press, 1985, p 1.
2. Editorial. AIDS: The third wave. Lancet *343*:186, 1994.
3. Flynn PM: Pediatric HIV infection and the primary care physician. Postgrad Med *95*:59, 1994.
4. Itescu S, et al: HLA-B35 is associated with accelerated progression to AIDS. J AIDS *5*:37, 1991.
5. Falloon J, et al: Human immunodeficiency virus in children. J Pediatr *114*:1, 1989.
6. Gabiano C, et al: Mother-to-child transmission of human immunodeficiency virus type 1: risk of infection and correlates of transmission. Pediatrics *90*:369, 1992.
7. Michaels D and Levine C: Estimates of the number of motherless youth orphaned by AIDS in the United States. JAMA *268:* 3456, 1992.
8. Pantaleo G, Graziosi C, and Fauci AS: The immunopathogenesis of human immunodeficiency virus infection. N Engl J Med *328*:327, 1993.
9. Golding H, et al: Common epitope in human immunodeficiency virus (HIV) 1-gp41 and HLA class II elicits immunosuppressive autoantibodies capable of contributing to immune dysfunction in HIV 1-infected individuals. J Clin Invest *83*:1430, 1989.
10. Hirsch MS and D'Aquila R: Therapy for human immunodeficiency virus infection. N Engl J Med *328*:1686, 1993.

11. Lancaster DJ and Lancaster LL: Antiretroviral therapy in HIV-infected adults. Postgrad Med *95*:47, 1994.

12. Hoover DR, et al: Clinical manifestations of AIDS in the era of pneumocytis carinii prophylaxis. N Engl J Med *329*:1922, 1993.

13. Hughes WT: Opportunistic infections in AIDS patients. Postgrad Med *95*:81, 1994.

14. Marcusen DL and Sooy CD: Otolaryngologic and head and neck manifestations of the acquired immunodeficiency syndrome (AIDS). Laryngoscope *95*:401, 1985.

15. Dichtel WJ: Oral manifestations of human immunodeficiency virus infection. Otolaryngol Clin North Am *25*:1211, 1992.

6 Acute Infections of the Nose and Face

John J. Ballenger

THE COMMON COLD

The common cold (acute coryza) is an acute, common, relatively mild infection of the upper respiratory tract with symptoms centered in and around the nose. It is a frequent reason for a visit to the physician. Causative agents are most often a rhinovirus or coronavirus (see Chap. 3), although a bacterial rhinitis is occasionally found in young children.

Most colds occur in the winter months, perhaps because transmission from person to person is facilitated by more crowded winter, indoor conditions. Chilling, either local or general, does not increase the frequency of experimentally induced colds. Evidence indicates that the presence of psychologic stress increases the susceptibility to the common cold.[1] Transmission is more likely from contaminated fomites deposited by the infected individual on a table, spoon, door handle, etc. A finger, contaminated by touching the fomite, then transmits the infection by touching the mucosa of the eye, nose, or mouth of an until-then uncontaminated person. The fomite is spread less frequently by inhaled infected droplets coughed or sneezed into the air by an infected individual.[2]

The onset of a cold may be heralded by a sense of dryness, tickling, or burning in the nose, throat, or nasopharynx. Brief chills are followed by malaise, sneezing, and a watery nasal discharge, with a full-blown cold developing in 24 to 48 hours. Variably, as the symptoms develop, the patient may have a husky voice, suffusion of the eyes, a profuse watery nasal discharge, nasal blockage, slight vertigo, and temporary loss of smell and hearing. The mucosae of the paranasal sinuses and nose participate in the inflammatory reaction and may lead to a sense of fullness about the eyes and forehead. The osteomeatal complex is obstructed in the more severe infections.[3]

Most colds last 7 to 10 days, but the course is prolonged if a secondary bacterial infection exists, particularly if this infection interferes with the efficiency of the mucociliary cleansing system. When the cold is complicated by secondary bacterial invaders, the nasal discharge becomes creamy and yellow green.

Physical examination during the first few days of a cold reveals a hyperemic, dry, and even glazed nasal mucosa that becomes progressively "wet" with a clear, watery discharge. Later, the mucosa is pale and boggy, resembling the allergic state. Frequent "blowing" of the nose may excoriate the skin of the nares.

Histologic studies of the nasal and nasopharyngeal mucosae exhibit edema and hypersecretion with little cellular infiltration. Desquamation of the ciliated epithelium occurs, particularly in influenza. Viral shedding is common. The slowing of the nasal mucociliary transport during a cold has been frequently noted.[4] Certain bacteria, viruses, and environmental pollutants are more damaging to the mucociliary transport system than others and may prolong the time before efficient mucociliary cleansing is regained for as long as 6 or 7 weeks.[5,6] The earliest sign of measles (Koplik's spots), rubella, chickenpox, and smallpox may closely mimic the common cold—a so-called exanthematous rhinitis.

The treatment of the common cold is largely symptomatic, with bed rest in the more serious infections and fluids. In the absence of bacterial complications, antibiotics and sulfonamides are not indicated, and the use of antihistamines gains nothing therapeutically but, symptomatically, promotes nasal dryness. Headache, fever, and myalgia can be controlled by short-term use of aspirin or other mild analgesic in patients without sensitivity to the medication. Studies of some patients with experimental rhinovirus infections have suggested that aspirin and acetaminophen may increase nasal symptoms, can suppress the formation of neutralizing antibodies, and may also increase viral shedding.[7] Prophylaxis of the common cold has been discouraging, and the development of a vaccine for prophylaxis is unlikely because of the myriad viruses capable of causing the malady.

Extreme nasal congestion, a most distressing symptom, can be relieved somewhat by the judicious use of vasoconstricting nose drops and sprays four to five times a day for 3 to 4 days (see Chap. 7). The pH of the "drops" should be 7 or slightly acid because an alkaline pH may inactivate nasal lysozyme. Nasal congestion may be relieved by oral administration of a vasoconstricting medication such as ephedrine, 30 mg every 4 hours, without danger of invoking the "rebound" phenomenon.

A promising approach to control of colds is through the development of interferon or the use of virucidal preparations for use on the hands.[8] Keeping the hands of both the patient and the uninfected individual clean breaks the transmission cycle of infected fomite to a receptive mucous membrane.

ORBITAL CELLULITIS

This acute infection of the orbital contents surrounding the globe is most commonly caused by a bacterium, although, in immunodeficient or debilitated patients, it may follow infection with fungi. Most infections spread to the orbit from contiguous structures including the paranasal sinuses and injuries to the lamina papyracea.

Fever, eyelid edema, and rhinorrhea are early signs and are followed by orbital pain, tenderness of the eyelids, and headache. As the infection progresses, the eyelids become discolored to a dark red. Conjunctival hyperemia, chemosis, and proptosis follow. The patient may have limitation of ocular motion with increased resistance to retropulsion, although vision is normal in the early stages. In posterior cellulitis, the situation is more serious and is not discussed here. The differentiation from an orbital abscess is made with the use of computed tomography (CT). With use of antibiotics, the prognosis is good. If an abscess forms, it must be drained, usually through an incision posterior to the inner canthus.

INFLUENZAL RHINITIS

Influenza, usually during an epidemic, is occasionally encountered as a subclinical influenzal rhinitis and is detected by serologic testing. Myxoviruses A, B, and C are the responsible agents and are discussed in Chapter 3. Symptoms in the nose early are much like those of the common cold or coryza. With influenza, however, desquamation of the ciliated epithelium is marked, secondary bacterial infection is common, and recovery prolonged. Protective vaccines are available and should be used for patients at risk.

NASAL DIPHTHERIA AND OTHER BACTERIAL RHINITIDES

The onset of nasal diphtheria, although rare nowadays, is much like that of the common cold. A serous nasal discharge occurs early, and later a white-yellow membranous exudate covers the mucous membrane of the respiratory tract and may obstruct the airway. Other specific bacterial infections (e.g., tuberculosis, rhinoscleroma, syphilis, and leprosy) involving the nose and face are discussed in Chapters 3 and 7. In apparently healthy individuals, recovery of staphylococci, Haemophilus influenzae, and Branhamella catarrhalis may be "normal" nasal or nasopharyngeal inhabitants and difficult to interpret.[9]

PYODERMA

Streptococci (group A) can produce localized purulent skin infections or pustules known as pyoderma, streptococcal impetigo, or impetigo contagiosa. Ecthyma is a more severe form of pyoderma. Definitive diagnosis requires cultures.

A good therapeutic response is frequently gained simply by local cleansing with soap and water after removal of the crusts. Topical use of antibiotics has been disappointing. If response is poor, parenteral use of antibiotic medication is advisable.

ERYSIPELAS

Erysipelas, also known as St. Anthony's fire, is an acute β-hemolytic streptococcus infection of the skin of the face and head, although infection can occur elsewhere. A portal of entry, created by an abrasion or surgical procedure, is common.

The onset is usually abrupt, with fever, redness, tenderness, and induration of the involved skin. Characteristically, one sees an elevated, well-demarcated ("rolled"), advancing border from which the streptococci can best be cultured. To the rear of the advancing border, the skin may regain its normal appearance. In the face, the infection frequently displays a "butterfly" pattern of inflammation covering the nose, adjacent cheeks, and upper lip.

Erysipelas responds well to penicillin or erythromycin. The disease must be differentiated from cellulitis, which is a more generalized, deeper infection of the skin and subcutaneous tissue but also caused by a staphylococcus or streptococcus.

Cellulitis is a spreading, bacterial infection of the skin and subcutaneous tissues that may or may not be preceded by injury. It is evidenced by local pain, tenderness, edema, and erythema. The border between the infected and uninvolved skin is indistinct, however, with the erythema gradually fading into normal-appearing skin. Cellulitis may be accompanied by systemic manifestations such as fever, chills, malaise, and toxicity. Lymphangitis is an inflammation of lymphatic channels in the subcutaneous tissues and first manifests as visible red streaks. Cellulitis and lymphangitis can be treated by antibiotics.

NASAL VESTIBULITIS

Common among adults is the occurrence of nasal vestibulitis. A portal of entry through the nasal vestibular skin is required and results in a diffuse, usually mild, recurrent inflammation caused by a staphylcoccus that is almost always already resident in the area awaiting the portal of entry. Surprisingly painful fissures or pustules, although disarmingly simple in appearance, can be found in the skin of the rim of the nostril. The area should not be squeezed or manipulated. Heat and topical antibiotics usually help.

FURUNCLES

Again, if a portal of entry through the vestibular skin is present, the resident bacteria, almost always Staphylococcus aureus, gain entrance, usually in the hair-bearing area, to the subepithelial tissue, and a small abscess is created. The abscess or furuncle is surrounded by localized cellulitis. The lesion is sometimes excruciatingly tender because the vestibular skin is tightly bound to the subjacent lower lateral cartilage and thus provides no room for edema. Furuncles of the nasal vestibule, the upper lip, and the nasal apex, are potentially dangerous because of the possibility of rupture into the valveless venous channels leading to the cavernous sinus.

Improvement of nasal hygiene and avoidance of digital manipulation of the nasal vestibule is important in prophylaxis. Main reliance in active treatment should be placed on heat to the area and antibiotic therapy. If the abscess is localized to a clearly defined, fluctuant "head," consideration can be given to gentle and careful incision of the fluctuant area only.

TOXIC SHOCK SYNDROME AND SEPTAL ABSCESS

Toxic shock symptoms have been reported following occlusive postoperative nasal packing[10] and also after occlusive nasal packing to control epistaxis. A toxin-producing staphylococcus is present, the toxin is absorbed, and shock symptoms appear: headache, myal-

gia, lethargy, nausea, vomiting associated with fever, tachycardia, hypotension, redness of the skin, and delayed desquamation of the skin of the hands. The onset is usually within a few days but may be delayed a week or more after the surgery. Rarely, nasal surgery without packing is followed by toxic shock.

At the first sign of the syndrome, the packing must be removed and cultures taken for Staphylococcus aureus. A β-lactamase-resistant antistaphylcoccal antibiotic must be administered. Prophylaxis clearly requires that a preoperative patient be free of infection.

A septal abscess may follow septal surgery or may be associated with trauma. If infected, the hematoma enlarges and nasal obstruction occurs, and if untreated, it may erode the septal cartilage so that significant loss of septal cartilaginous support to the nasal dorsum and saddle deformity occur. Incision and drainage of an abscess is required, as well as use of an appropriate antibiotic.

CAVERNOUS SINUS THROMBOSIS

The cavernous sinus is a venous sinus situated on either side of the body of the sphenoid bone with communication across the midline to the adjacent sinus. It is irregular in shape and broken up by trabeculae into many venous cavernous spaces. Within its walls are found the third, fourth, and first two divisions of the fifth cranial nerves, as well as the sixth cranial nerve and internal carotid artery. An extensive, valveless, venous drainage connects the nose and adjacent face, nasopharynx, pharynx, orbit, and paranasal sinuses to the cavernous sinus such that a spread of an infection from these areas occurs readily, most frequently from the oculonasal area. The symptoms of an infection of the sinus and thrombosis are an acutely ill patient with orbital edema, chemosis, and variable evidence of palsy of the foregoing nerves. Papillary edema may occur, and the globe may be proptosed. The cerebrospinal fluid is frequently normal unless the patient has an associated meningitis. The differentiation of this entity from a periorbital cellulitis is accomplished by CT. Vigorous antibiotic treatment should be instituted at once. The use of anticoagulant therapy should be considered, but the value has not been clearly proved.

SUGGESTED READINGS

1. Cohen S, Tyrrell DAJ, and Smith VAP: Psychological stress and susceptibility to the common cold. N Engl J Med 325:606, 1991.
2. Gweltney JB and Hendley JO: Transmission of experimental rhinovirus infection by contaminated surfaces. Am J Epidemiol 116:825, 1982.
3. Gwaltney JM, et al: Computed tomographic study of the common cold. N Engl J Med 330:15, 1994.

4. Sakakura Y: Changes of mucociliary functions during colds. Eur J Respir Dis *64:*348, 1983.

5. Carson JL, Collier AM, and Clyde WA Jr: Ciliary membrane alterations occurring in experimental mycoplasma pneumonia infection. Science *206:*3494, 1979.

6. Ballenger JJ: Acquired ultrastructural alterations of respiratory cilia and clinical disease: a review. Ann Otolaryngol *206:*253, 1988.

7. Graham NMHJ, et al: Adverse effects of aspirin, acetaminophen, and ibuprofen or immune function, viral shedding, and clinical status in rhinovirus-infected volunteers. J Infect Dis *162:* 1277, 1990.

8. Hendley JO and Gweltney J Jr: Mechanism of transmission of rhinovirus infections. Epidemol Rev *10:*242, 1988.

9. Wald ER, Cheponis D, and Ledesma-madina J: Comparative effectiveness of amoxicillin and amoxicillin-clavulamate potassium in acute sinus infections in children; a double-blind, placebo-controlled trial. Pediatrics *77:*795, 1986.

10. Thomas SW, Baird IM, and Frazier RD: Toxic shock following submucous resection and rhinoplasty JAMA *247:*2402, 1982.

7 Chronic Rhinitis and Nasal Obstruction

John J. Ballenger

Increases in nasal resistance resulting from mucosal congestion or airway deformity are the main factors in producing the complaint of nasal obstruction. Rhinomanometry attempts to measure this resistance by simultaneously recording on an x-y graph the transnasal pressure and flow of air. When the airflow is laminar, the relationship is linear and equals the pressure divided by the airflow. The nasal valve, the narrowest part of the nasal airway, causes the airflow to become turbulent, and the relationship then becomes more difficult to assess accurately.

In anterior rhinomanometry, the method commonly used today, the pressure-measuring device is sealed in one nostril while the patient actively breathes through the opposite side. In posterior rhinomanometry, the tip of a catheter measuring pressure is placed posteriorly in the patient's mouth (held there by the teeth) while the patient breathes through both sides of the nose and refrains from raising the palate against the posterior wall of the pharynx. Rather than have the patient actively breathe, air may passively be forced through the nasal airway by external means. Pressure transducers are appropriately connected.

PHYSIOLOGIC CONSIDERATIONS

Direct measurement of the airflow at the nasal outlet can also be accomplished by a snugly fitting face mask fitted with a pneumotachograph. Plethysmography is another way to assess airflow. In acoustic rhinometry, a shock wave is presented to the nasal airway, and the reflected sound measured.

Because the veins of the nose have few valves, the blood seeks its own level and physiologically congests the lower side when a person is in the recumbent position. About 80% of people also have a physiologic 2½-to 4-hour cycle of congestion-decongestion of one side of the nasal airway and then the other, although the total airway resistance does not change. Individuals who have undergone a laryngectomy wrongly sense a congested nose, although the nasal cycle does seem to continue. Horner's syndrome, by interrupting the sympathetic innervation, leaves the vasodilating parasympathetic nerves unopposed, and nasal congestion may occur. A discomfort referred to the face from contraction of the scalp muscles, from the temporomandibular joint, or from emotional problems may be interpreted by the patient as a chronic "rhinitis."

ANATOMIC OR STRUCTURAL FACTORS

An open nasal airway depends, in part, on a physiologic stiffness of the upper and lower lateral cartilages. If this stiffness is lost, the nasal airway suffers by an in-drawing of the cartilages on inspiration. This is particularly apparent when the nasal valve area is compromised. If the airway is improved by pulling the skin upward and laterally opposite the lower third of the nose (Cottle's sign), the obstruction likely is located in the valve area. If the nasal septum deviates significantly from the midline, the nasal airway suffers. Perforation of the nasal septum and the accompanying crusts may compromise the airway. Nasal obstructions produced by an endonasal scar (synechia), an anatomically narrow nose, and stenosis of the nasopharynx are usually postoperative or traumatic in origin. Obstructing, enlarged adenoids or tonsils are described elsewhere (see Chap. 1).

Foreign bodies in the nose, found most frequently in children, can obstruct the airway. Myiasis is an infestation of the nose by larvae of nonbloodsucking flies. The most common animate foreign bodies found are maggots. The symptoms of a long-lasting foreign body usually consist of an odorous, bloody, unilateral nasal discharge. Mucosal and bone destruction may be marked.

Rhinoliths are composed of concretions of calcium, magnesium, phosphates, and carbonates adhering to a nucleus of bacteria, blood, pus cells, or foreign material. Usually unilateral, they begin in childhood and become evident after years of development. For inanimate foreign bodies located posteriorly, the tip of a probe tip bent into an L-shape is passed under direct vision beyond the object and the foreign body teased forward until it can be easily grasped.

CHOANAL ATRESIA

Choanal atresia is the persistence after birth of a membranous or bony closure of one or both posterior choanae. Because the neonate is a near-obligate nasal breather, the bilateral condition requires emergency provision of an oral airway. The diagnosis can readily be made by noting the failure to pass a nasal catheter into the mouth. A membranous occlusion may require no more than perforation with a probe. The condition is considered in Chapter 19.

IMMOTILE CILIA SYNDROME

Ultrastructural ciliary abnormalities, either congenital or acquired, may result in a chronic rhinitis because of inefficient ciliary cleansing of the nasal mucosal and other respiratory surfaces. An important example is Kartagener's syndrome.[1] The defect is usually in the dynein arms, although abnormalities of the ciliary spokes and of the number and placement of the axonemal tubules also have been reported. The syndrome is characterized by situs inversus (50%), bronchiectasis, and chronic rhinitis (sinusitis) and, frequently, immotile spermatozoa. The cilia of the oviducts and fimbrae, the eustachian tube, and middle ear may also be affected.

NASAL POLYPS

The most common benign tumor in the nose is a polyp. Overall, the ratio in men to women is 2:1, but if asthma is present the ratio is 1:1. Polyps are rare in children.

Etiology

The cause is obscure. Cystic fibrosis and allergy have been associated with polyps, as well as with the use of aspirin and other nonsteroidal anti-inflammatory medication, and with chronic paranasal sinusitis. The relationship of cystic fibrosis is probably only incidental. Patients undergoing nasal polypectomy, however, seem to have no greater incidence of allergy than the general public. Polyps occur in about half of aspirin-intolerant patients, and about one third of patients with polyps have asthma. Patients with aspirin intolerance, asthma, and sinusitis ("the aspirin triad") seem to be at greater risk. Asthma may follow nasal polypectomy; however, withholding aspirin does not reduce the incidence of polyps. A relationship may exist between nasal mastocytosis and nasal polyps. Many patients complaining of nasal polyps have a history of perennial rhinitis or nasal congestion following exposure to nonspecific noxious stimuli such sudden temperature changes, dust, and air pollutants.

Polyp tissue contains all the cellular and chemical elements found in normal respiratory mucosa. The inflammatory exudate in the nose often contains many eosinophils, and this finding suggests an allergic background, but the attempt to use skin tests to elicit an allergen usually have failed. Tos and Mogensen believe that edema within the mucosa due to inflammation ruptures the epithelium, and the lamina propria then prolapses into the lumen.[2] Polyps contain more histamine than does normal nasal mucosa.

Clinical Features

The most common symptoms are nasal obstruction, frequently with an associated anosmia, and clear, watery secretions unless superimposed infection has occurred. Nasal examination reveals one or more rounded, smooth, grayish pear-shaped masses within the nose. They are stalked, mobile, do not bleed, and are not sensitive to manipulation. They may occur at the posterior choanae (antrochoanal polyp) or may project slightly out of the anterior nares. Imaging techniques frequently reveal the origin to be in the paranasal sinuses. Differentiation must be made from inverting papillomas, encephaloceles, carcinoma, sarcomas, and angiofibromas.

If an allergic background is found, appropriate treatment should be instituted. A salicylate- and tartrazine-free regimen should be followed. Corticosteroids, either topical or systemic, may be tried. The goal of surgical treatment is to remove the polyps completely, and this may require opening the maxillary or ethmoid sinuses. For a single, readily accessible polyp, removal with a snare is feasible. In a patient with aspirin sensitivity, precautions to avoid bronchospasm must be made. Recurrences are common, but beclomethasone and flunisolide, used topically, may be useful in treatment and prevention of recurrence.

PAPILLOMAS

Simple papillomas are benign, wart-like tumors that occur on both the septum and the lateral wall of the nose and may obstruct the airway and bleed spontaneously. Inverting papillomas arise on the lateral wall of the nose, have a pronounced tendency to recur after removal, and bleed readily. They are associated with malignancy 5 to 15% of the time, but usually are benign, locally destructive lesions.

GLIOMAS AND ENCEPHALOCELES

Both these lesions are rare. Gliomas are deposits of glial tissue in extradural sites, usually with no attachment to the central nervous system, and can be readily removed. If intranasal, they are firm, pink-red masses obstructing the airway. Extranasal gliomas usually occur along the nasomaxillary suture line. Encephaloceles maintain a connection to the central nervous system, but otherwise are similar to gliomas.

VASOMOTOR RHINITIS

Vasomotor rhinitis (perennial nonallergic rhinitis) represents a perennial imbalance of the sympathetic and parasympathetic nerve control of the blood supply of the nasal mucosa and is characterized by perennial rather than seasonal symptoms, lack of eosinophilia in the nasal smear, and absence of positive allergy skin tests. The symptoms are not reagin or IgE mediated. Nonspecific stimuli are thought to act on the autonomic nervous system. Aspirin sensitivity and environmental irritants may play an unrecognized part. Endocrine abnormalities and nonallergic rhinitis must be ruled out. The nasal mucosa is found to be "wet," the turbinates are congested, and, in long-standing cases, the nasal mucosa may be irreversibly hypertrophied.

Treatment is symptomatic. All irritants must be eliminated, nasal polyps managed, and hormonal or glandular problems corrected. Aspirin should be avoided. Vidian neurectomy occasionally provides short-term relief. Oral decongestants can be tried, and reduction in the size of an obstructing turbinate, perhaps by cryosurgery, may be required.

EOSINOPHILIC NONALLERGIC RHINITIS

This perennial watery rhinitis mimics allergic rhinitis and is characterized by sneezing and a prominent eosinophilia but negative skin tests, normal serum IgE levels, and negative aspirin and methacholine challenges.[3] It seems to be caused by undefined irritants, and treatment is symptomatic.

NASAL MASTOCYTOSIS

Found mostly in adults, this is a rare type of rhinitis with an idiopathic increase in the nasal mucosal mast cells but with few eosinophils. Skin tests and IgE levels are normal.

RHINITIS MEDICAMENTOSA

A drug-induced rhinitis, this represents perhaps 5% of cases in patients complaining of nasal obstruction. Frequent and prolonged use of topical nasal vasoconstrictor medication results in a vascular atony in the nasal vessels, with persistent "rebound" vasodilation and nasal obstruction. Topical use of cocaine, in addition to a vasoconstrictive effect, causes crusting and ulceration and may even lead to septal perforation. The patient must discontinue topical medication and resort to oral decongestants. Beclomethasone and flunisolide also may be used carefully.

The treatment of hypertension with derivatives of rauwolfia is occasionally associated with turbinate congestion, as is the use of methyldopa, guanethidine, hydralazine, and prazosin. Some β blockers and antidepressants also have this side effect. Oral contraceptives, nonsteroidal anti-inflammatory agents, antithyroid drugs, and alcohol may be associated with this problem.

WEGENER'S GRANULOMATOSIS

This uncommon, necrotizing, granulomatous vasculitis of both the upper and lower respiratory and the urinary tract is most commonly found in middle-aged patients. Pansinusitis with destruction of bone, septal perforation, saddle nose, nasal obstruction, and a bloody rhinorrhea are frequently present. Otic, laryngeal, and ocular involvement may occur. The skin may show nodules and frank ulceration. The cause is unknown, but the disorder may be related to an abnormal host immune response.

Histopathologically, the lesions in extrarenal locations are characterized by necrotizing granulomatous inflammation and vasculitis, typically most common in the respiratory tract. The most common renal lesion is a focal, segmental, necrotizing glomerulonephritis. In as many as 80% of patients, antineutrophil cytoplasmic antibodies (ANCA, originally called ACPA) are found. Biopsy is the best way to make the diagnosis.

The most effective drug in treatment is a cytotoxic agent, especially cyclophosphamide, with or without corticosteroids.[4] Trimethoprim-sulfamethoxazole may be sufficient in less-advanced situations.

POLYMORPHIC RETICULOSIS

An uncommon disease once known as "lethal midline granuloma," polymorphic reticulosis is manifested by a relentless, locally destructive process predominantly in the paranasal sinus, nasal, and palatal areas. The cause is unknown, although the tissue reaction suggests localized hypersensitivity or an immunologically mediated process.

Pathologically, one sees a noncaseating, nonspecific necrosis. Histologically, a dense infiltrate of mature lymphocytes, simulated lymphocytes, plasma cells, histiocytes, and immunoblasts is found and suggests a lymphoma. The cells seem to orient around blood vessels, although a primary vasculitis is rare. Distinguishing the lesion from Wegener's granulomatosis is difficult.

Corticosteroid treatment is largely ineffective. Radiation therapy brings about the greatest improvement.

ENVIRONMENTAL FACTORS

Human beings, in northern climes at least, spend perhaps 95% of the day in the home, office, or work place or traveling in vehicles (20 to 22 hours per day), and thus indoor environmental factors are significant: sulfur dioxide (SO_2), cigarette smoke (including passive smoking), and formaldehyde.

SO_2 increases the nasal resistance and depresses the nasal mucociliary transport time (MCT) beginning at about 5 parts per million (ppm). This suggests that inefficient cleansing of the mucosal surfaces will occur, increasing the resident time in the nose of inhaled irritants and leading to an irritative "environmental" watery rhinitis. SO_2 may react with other pollutants in the outside atmosphere and form such irritants as SO_3, sulfurous acid (H_2SO_3), and sulfuric acid (H_2SO_4). Some natural (outdoor) sources also emit SO_2 and hydrogen sulfide. The allergic environment is considered in Chapter 8.

Togias and associates found that when a cold-sensitive individual was challenged by cold, dry air at -3 to $-10°C$, there was a release of inflammatory mediators in the nose, probably from the mast cells or the basophils.[5] The pharmacologic action of this release causes symptoms of rhinitis as well as constriction of the bronchioles. Warm, moist air failed to reproduce these symptoms.

Room smoke consists of the mainstream smoke that is exhaled from the smoker's respiratory tract and the sidestream smoke released directly into the room from the burning tip of the cigarette itself. Both types are inhaled nasally ("passive smoking") by nonsmoking occupants of the room.[6] Increased nasal irritation be-

gins at about 0.1 ppm. Slower respiratory MCTs are recorded in long-time smokers than in nonsmokers.[7,8] Other investigators suggest that the problem is due to a loss of nasal cilia and possibly an increase in depth or a change in viscoelastic properties of the nasal mucous blanket. "Smokeless" tobacco is harmful as well.

Environmental formaldehyde is a nasal carcinogen in rats and mice. At 2 ppm (a realistic level in human affairs), rhinitis has been observed in humans. In monkeys, rhinitis can be found at 0.1 ppm.[9] The effect of low-level human exposure to formaldehyde of years' duration is unknown.

Industrial factors such as chromium, arsenic, copper, zinc, nitric acid mist, and other substances are capable of depressing ciliary function. Little evidence indicates that positive air ions have a deleterious effect on the nose. The development of an increased risk of nasal disease (including cancer) after years of exposure to wood dust is well documented.

ASPIRIN TRIAD

In the aspirin-sensitive asthmatic patient, aspirin can provoke severe asthma. Occasionally, a similar thing can happen with other nonsteroidal anti-inflammatory agents. Most of these asthmatic patients have nasal polyps and lack IgE-mediated allergies. A few aspirin-sensitive patients react similarly to tartrazine added to foods or drugs.

ENDOCRINE PROBLEMS

The nasal congestion of pregnancy is estrogen induced and is likely to occur in the second and third trimesters. Similar congestion may occur in the premenstrual or menstrual periods and also may be associated with the use of oral contraceptives. Changes in the viscoelastic properties of the nasal mucous blanket in hypothyroid states may simulate a rhinitis by interfering with the cleansing ability of the nasal cilia.

CYSTIC FIBROSIS

In this hereditary disease of exocrine dysfunction, the primary target organs are the lungs, pancreas, and gastrointestinal tract. The respiratory ciliary activity becomes impaired by excess viscid mucus, and the sweat contains high sodium concentrations.

SARCOIDOSIS

Sarcoidosis is a noncaseating, granulomatous multisystem disorder of unknown cause commonly affecting young adults and manifesting with pulmonary infiltrates, skin lesions, and occasionally, enlargement of the parotid gland. If the lesion is examined with great care, acid-fast bacilli may be found. Immunologically, the disease displays normal or enhanced B-lymphocyte activity and at the same time depressed T-lymphocyte function. The Kveim reaction is usually positive. By an unknown mechanism, the angiotension-converting enzyme is usually elevated. The disease may disappear spontaneously.

Most patients with sarcoidosis come to medical attention because of intrathoracic involvement. Granulomatous skin lesions occur in 10 to 30% of patients and are especially common in blacks. The common lesion in the skin is the plaque-like lupus pernio—a persistent, violaceous, painless plaque seen in skin of the nose, cheek, and ears. The larynx may be involved. Epistaxis, nasal pain and obstruction,[10] and anosmia may be found. Peripheral neuropathies of cranial nerves V, VII, and VIII may occur. The disease seems to be associated in some way with uveoparotid fever (Heerfordt's disease). Corticosteroids are helpful in controlling the disease.

AMYLOIDOSIS

Amyloidosis consists of an extracellular deposit of the fibrous protein amyloid in various sites in the body. The etiology is unknown. Secondary amyloidosis is suspected when the condition of a patient with a chronic inflammatory disease progressively deteriorates and proteinuria develops. Lesions of the skin are characteristic and consist of slightly raised, waxy papules that may be found in the face and neck and on mucosal areas of the tongue, lips, nose, sinuses, larynx, and trachea. Hepatomegaly and splenomegaly are common. Diagnosis by labial salivary gland biopsy has a high degree of sensitivity.[11] Colchicine may be useful in treatment.

ATROPHIC RHINITIS (OZENA)

Atrophic rhinitis is recognized by a sclerotic change of the respiratory mucous membrane to a cuboidal or squamous type, obstruction of the nasal airway by crusts, and an offensive odor. Frequently, the condition is associated with a gram-negative organism, Klebsiella pneumoniae subspecies ozaenae. Treatment requires gentle removal of the crusts by nasal irrigations. Careful use of intravenous or topical aminoglycosides has been recommended.

TUBERCULOSIS

Mycobacterium tuberculosis is rarely found first on the nasal floor or septum as a granulation. Septal perfora-

tions and spread up the eustachian tube to involve the ear may occur. In the past, involvement of the larynx was common. Lupus vulgaris may be an attenuated form of tuberculosis. In the nose, it usually begins in the anterior portion of the cartilaginous septum and produces small, discrete nodules that slowly spread, coalesce, and ulcerate (see Chap. 3).

SYPHILIS

Syphilis, acquired almost invariably by sexual contact, is a general infection of the blood and lymph caused by Treponema pallidum. The primary lesion, or chancre, occurs at the point of initial inoculation, and occasionally, this may be just within the nostril or mouth. After several weeks, if the chancre is in the nose, it becomes a 1- to 2-cm erosive, scabbed, impetiginous lesion obstructing the airway.

The clinical signs of congenital syphilis include saddle nose, a high palatal arch, Hutchinson's incisors, and mulberry molars. In tertiary syphilis, destructive gummatous lesions occur in the nose (saddling), and perforation of the palate or nasal septum may occur.

YAWS

Yaws (frambesia) is a chronic, tropical, infectious disease of childhood that may disfigure the face and nose by deep gummatous nodules. Its cause, Treponema pertenue, is indistinguishable from T. pallidum and is effectively treated by penicillin.

LEPROSY

Leprosy (or Hansen's disease) is acquired by prolonged, intimate contact with the disease by a susceptible person. It is caused by Mycobacterium leprae. Extensive skin lesions may occur and may create facial distortion, the so-called "leonine faces." Nasal obstruction, epistaxis, and hoarseness are common. Destruction of the nasal septum may occur (see Chap. 3).

RHINOSPORIDOSIS

Presumably caused by the yeast-like Rhinosporidium seeberi, the characteristic lesion is a painless, bleeding polyp in the nose, nasopharynx, or rarely, the larynx. Surgical polypectomy is effective. Dapsone and electrodesiccation of the polyp are useful.

MUCORMYCOSIS

The fungus mucor, order Mucorales, causes invasive sinusitis in diabetics and immunocompromised hosts (see Chaps. 3 and 11).

BLASTOMYCOSIS

This entity, also known as Gilchrist's disease, is caused by the fungus Blastomyces dermatitidis. Uncommonly, one sees verrucous, granulating ulcers in the oropharynx, nose, larynx, or skin resembling a well-differentiated carcinoma (see Chap. 3).

TABLE 7–1. Causes of Rhinitis

Specific rhinitus
   Viral, bacterial infections
   Nasal septal deformities
   Nasal valve obstruction
   Hypertrophied turbinates
   Obstructing tonsils, adenoids
   Choanal atresia, nasopharyngeal stenosis
   Collapsed alar cartilages
   Tumors, benign and malignant
   Nasal polyps
   Foreign bodies
   Tuberculosis and lupus vulgaris
   Syphilis, yaws
   Leprosy
   Rhinosporidosis
   Mucormycosis
   Blastomycosis
   Rhinoscleroma
   Wegener's granulomatosis
   Polymorphic reticulosis
   Nasal diphtheria
   Aspergillosis
   Leishmaniasis
Nonspecific rhinitis
   Recumbent position
   Allergic rhinitis
   Referred head pain
   Nasal cycle
   Vasomotor rhinitis
   Environmental Factors
   ASA triad
   Cold, dry air
   Endocrine factors
   Cystic fibrosis
   Sarcoidosis
   Atrophic Rhinitis (ozena)
   Amyloidosis

RHINOSCLEROMA

Rhinoscleroma is a chronic, slowly progressive, granulomatous, nodular disease caused by the gram-negative bacterium Klebsiella pneumoniae subspecies rhinoscleromatis (von Frisch's bacillus) (see Chap. 3). Usually, the disease begins as an indolent, chronic, purulent rhinitis, and later, the skin and mucous membrane become smooth, nodular, brownish red, and of cartilaginous consistency. Eventually, nasal obstruction occurs. Gamea found that topical rifampicin helpful.[12] Oral ciprofloxacin and trimethoprim-sulfamethoxazole have been of benefit.

Table 7–1 is a list of causes of specific and nonspecific rhinitis. Other diseases occasionally obstructing the nasal airway are aspergillosis, brucellosis, glanders (melioidosis), actinomycosis, malaria, and leishmaniasis and are further discussed in Chapter 3.

SUGGESTED READINGS

1. Imbrie DJ: Kartagener's syndrome. Am J Otolaryngol 2:215, 1981.
2. Tos M and Mogensen C: Mucus glands in nasal polyps. Arch Otolaryngol 103:407, 1977.
3. Mullarkey MF: Eosinophilc non-allergic rhinitis. J Allergy Clin Immunol 82:941, 1988.
4. Kornblutt AD, Wolff S, DeFries HO, and Fauci AS: Wegener's granulomatosis. Laryngoscope 90:1453, 1980.
5. Togias AG, et al: Nasal challenge with cold, dry air results in release of mediators: possible mast cell involvement. J Clin Invest 76:1375, 1985.
6. Respiratory Health Effects of Passive Smoking: Lung Cancer and Other Disorders. Washington, D.C., United States Department of Health and Human Services. NIH Publication No. 93–3605, 1993, p 223.
7. Stanley P, et al: Effect of cigarette smoking on nasal mucociliary clearance and ciliary beat frequency. Thorax 41:519, 1986.
8. Stanley J, et al: Effect of cigarette smoke on nasal mucociliary clearance in apparently healthy subjects. Eur J Respir Dis 64 (suppl 26):482, 1983.
9. Rusch GM, et al: A 25-week inhalation toxicity study with formaldehyde in the monkey, rat, and hamster. Toxicol Appl Pharmacol 68:329, 1983.
10. McCaffrey TV and McDonald TH: Sarcoidosis of the nose and paranasal sinuses. Laryngoscope 93:1281, 1983.
11. Delgado WA and Mosqueda A: A highly sensitive method for diagnosis of secondary amyloidosis by labial salivary gland biopsy. J Oral Pathol 18:310, 1989.
12. Gamea AM: Local rifampicinin treatment of rhinoscleroma. J Laryngol Otol 102:319, 1988.

8 Allergic Rhinitis

Martin Desrosiers, Fuad M. Baroody, and Robert M. Naclerio

Allergic rhinitis, a benign but chronic disease of the upper airway, is increasingly recognized as an important public health problem. It is the sixth most prevalent chronic condition in the United States, and its prevalence exceeds that of heart disease.[1] The overall prevalence of allergic rhinitis is about 15%, and therefore, about 40 million people are affected by this disease in the United States.[2] In 1975, a United States national health survey estimated that Americans suffered 28 million restricted days and lost 2 million school days because of allergic rhinitis alone. Even if the cost of decreased productivity is not considered, Americans still spend in excess of 500 million dollars a year on physician fees and medications to alleviate the symptoms of allergic rhinitis. In an otolaryngologist's practice, the prevalence of allergic rhinitis in patients coming to the office exceeds that of the general population.

Evidence supporting an increase in the incidence of allergic rhinitis comes from studies of Swedish military conscripts, using skin testing to document the existence of atopy.[3] The prevalence of allergic rhinitis was 4.4% in this 18-year-old Swedish population in 1971 and increased to 8.1% by 1981. Similar trends have been observed in a recent statistical survey performed in Canada. The cause of the increasing prevalence of allergic rhinitis is not clear. Pollution may play a role by increasing nasal responsiveness to environmental allergens. Common outdoor pollutants include sulfur dioxide (SO_2), nitrogen dioxide (NO_2), and ozone, whereas indoor pollutants include sidestream cigarette smoke. Exposure to high levels of SO_2, NO_2, and ozone leads to bronchial hyperresponsiveness and potentiates the pulmonary response to allergen, perhaps converting asymptomatic to symptomatic asthmatic patients.[4,5] Similarly, skin test-positive subjects who lack clinical symptoms of allergic rhinitis may be converted into symptomatic patients by exposure to environmental pollutants. Another purported role for pollution is as an adjuvant in the development of IgE antibodies, which are central to the allergic reaction.[6] Evidence against the role of outdoor pollutants comes from a German study comparing the prevalence of rhinitis and asthma in genetically similar populations in a West and East German city.[7] Despite higher levels of SO_2 and particulate matter in the air in the East German city, the incidence of rhinitis and asthma were considerably lower than in the comparable city in West Germany.

Another potential explanation for the apparent increased prevalence of allergic rhinitis involves the role of indoor allergens. Evaluation of specific IgE antibodies suggests that increased rates of sensitization occur more frequently to common indoor allergens such as dust mites and household pets, but not to outdoor allergens, such as grass pollens. This study suggests that "Western" style housing with better weatherproofing and decreased ventilation may be increasing the indoor allergen burden, leading to an increased rate of sensitization.[8] In support of this notion is a study of allergen avoidance in children of atopic parents.[9] Compared with a control group, reduction of allergen load in the first 2 years of life led to a lower-than-expected incidence of allergic rhinitis at age 2 years.

Symptoms of allergic rhinitis can begin at any age but are most frequently first reported in adolescence or young adulthood.[2] Rates of prevalence are similar for males and females, and no racial or ethnic variations are reported.[10] The incidence of developing an allergic diathesis is higher in children whose parents suffer from allergic rhinitis. If one parent has allergies, the chances of the child's having rhinitis are 29% and increase to 47% when both parents have the disease.[11] The rate of loss of allergic rhinitis symptoms has been estimated to be about 10% and occurs in patients with the mildest form of the disease.[12]

Part of the clinical importance of allergic rhinitis lies in its association with complications related to chronic nasal obstruction. Total nasal obstruction regardless of etiology can cause sleep disturbances. Whether interference with sleep or the effects of systemically released mediators contribute to the fatigue associated with the disease is unknown. Nasal obstruction resulting from allergic rhinitis causes the hyposmia reported by some allergic patients.[13] Sinusitis often occurs in conjunction with allergic rhinitis. For example, the prevalence of abnormal sinus x-ray studies is greater in patients with perennial allergic rhinitis, compared with those with seasonal disease and approaches 50%.[14] Whether nasal polyps result from allergic rhinitis remains an open question. Settipane and Chafee, in an allergy practice setting, found that 2.1% of patients with allergic rhinitis had nasal polyps.[15] Although this is higher than the 0.3% incidence of nasal polyposis reported for the general population in the 1980 American Health Survey, it is less than the 12.5% incidence noted by Settipane and Chafee in nonallergic asthmatic patients.[15] The contribution of allergic rhinitis to middle ear disease is debated. Studies by Friedman and colleagues suggest that an induced allergic reaction can cause eustachian tube dysfunction.[16] Other data provide less support for a significant role of allergic rhinitis in the pathophysiology of otitis media.[17]

PATHOPHYSIOLOGY

The distinguishing characteristic of allergic rhinitis is the involvement of IgE immunoglobulins. In an individual with a susceptibility for developing allergic disease, an initial contact with allergen leads to the production of specific IgE molecules, a process termed sensitization. This begins when macrophages and other antigen-presenting cells process the allergen before presenting it to T-helper cells, which then interact with B lymphocytes, leading to their differentiation into IgE-producing plasma cells, a process involving interleukin-4 (IL-4). These newly formed IgE molecules bind to high-affinity receptors principally located on mast cells and basophils and to low-affinity receptors located on eosinophils, monocytes, and platelets. The high-affinity IgE receptors on mast cells mediate the initial allergic response. In the nasal mucosa of allergic subjects, mast cells are usually found within the mucosal connective tissue stroma, in the vicinity of blood vessels and glandular structures.[18] Seasonal exposure increases the number of mast cells located close to the surface and in the nasal epithelium without affecting their overall number, suggesting that these cells migrate from the deeper to the more superficial layers of the nasal mucosa during the pollen season.[18]

In a sensitized individual, another encounter with the same allergen provokes an immediate (early) allergic reaction. Within seconds of entering the nasal cavity, antigens interact with specific IgE molecules on the surface of mast cells. Cross-linking of two adjacent IgE

molecules by antigen initiates a sequence of intracellular events resulting in mast cell degranulation and the subsequent release of preformed and newly generated mediators into the nasal milieu. The preformed mediators are stored within granules in the cytoplasm and include histamine, tryptase, heparin, and chondroitin sulfate. The newly generated mediators are synthesized from the phospholipids of the cell membrane subsequent to mast cell activation. These include platelet-activating factor (PAF), prostaglandins, and leukotrienes. Evidence suggests that mast cells may also produce interleukins by IgE-mediated mechanisms, and these, unlike the lipid and granule mediators, require hours to be synthesized and released.[19,20] Released mediators can also initiate extracellular events that generate additional mediators; for example, the generation of kinins depends, in part, on the transudation of precursor proteins, kininogens, from the plasma that increase as a result of the action of histamine on vascular H_1 receptors. Other nonmast cell mediators are also associated with this early response to antigen. To ascertain the importance of any mediator in the pathophysiology of allergic rhinitis, it should satisfy three criteria: (1) the mediator should be present during the allergic reaction; (2) instilling the mediator in the nasal cavity should mimic part of the pathophysiology and symptoms of the disease; and (3) a mediator antagonist must partially or totally attenuate disease expression. To establish the importance of different mediators in allergic rhinitis, several investigators have attempted to satisfy one or more of these criteria.

Multiple mediators have been recovered in increased levels in nasal secretions following allergen challenge, and these include histamine,[21] kinins,[22] plasma and glandular kallikrein,[23,24] mast cell tryptase,[25] prostaglandin D_2 (PgD_2),[22] leukotriene C_4 (LTC_4),[26] leukotriene B_4 (LTB_4),[27] and MBP[28] (Fig. 8–1). Furthermore, several of these mediators have been used to challenge the nasal mucosa and observe resultant responses. Histamine provocation, for example, produces rhinorrhea, congestion, pruritus, and sneezing by stimulating receptors on sensory nerves and blood vessels.[29] Instillation of serotonin produces sneezing,[30] whereas PgD_2,[31] LTD_4,[32] and kinins[33] all produce nasal congestion.[34] The other approach to establishing the importance of a mediator involves the use of antagonists, and the best example is H_1 antihistamines: the clinical utility of H_1 receptor antagonists serves to demonstrate the importance of this inflammatory mediator.

Whereas mast cell degranulation and the released inflammatory mediators mimic most of the symptoms of allergic disease, the short duration of these events, as opposed to the prolonged symptoms of clinical disease, suggests that additional inflammatory processes are probably important in clinical disease. Furthermore, increased responsiveness and mucosal cellular

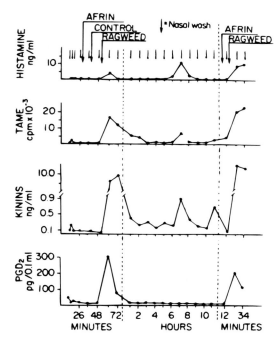

Fig. 8–1. The nasal response to allergen provocation in allergic subjects challenged with ragweed extract. The abscissa depicts the time after allergen provocation = minutes: time points of the early response, hours = time points of the late response and minutes (to the right) = time points of the rechallenge response. Short arrows at the top of the graph represent nasal lavages, and long arrows represent times of administration of different substances into the nasal cavities. There was a rise in all measured mediators during the early reaction. After a quiescent phase, there was a recurrence in elevations in the levels of histamine, tosyl-L-arginine methyl ester (TAME)-esterase, kinins but not PgD$_2$ in nasal lavages. During rechallenge, there was an exaggeration of the nasal response to challenge with a dose identical to that used during the early reaction for histamine, TAME-esterase and kinins. This is an illustration of the priming response, whereby subjects respond more vigorously to a dose of allergen after previous stimulation. (From Naclerio RM, et al: Inflammatory mediators in late antigen-induced rhinitis. N Engl J Med 313:65, 1985.)

changes that accompany chronic allergen exposure cannot be explained by this mechanism alone. Many of these phenomena are thought to be related to the cellular infiltration that is a hallmark of the inflammatory response.[35]

Various techniques of experimental nasal allergen provocation, in addition to being useful to an understanding of the events of the early response, assist investigators in understanding subsequent inflammatory events. Following challenge is an increase in symptoms and mediator levels characteristic of the early allergic reaction, which soon return to baseline. If one continues to monitor the response for several hours, symptoms recur, associated with an elevation of levels of inflammatory mediators in approximately 50% of the patients, the late-phase response[36,37] (Fig. 8–1). During the late-phase response, subjects have a recurrence of sneezing, rhinorrhea, and congestion,

with congestion predominating.[38] The late reaction is also accompanied by increases in some, but not all, of the inflammatory mediators associated with the early reaction.[36]

As in clinical disease, a striking characteristic of the late-phase response is cellular inflammation. One sees an increase in basophils, eosinophils, neutrophils, and mononuclear inflammatory cells in nasal secretions, as recovered by nasal lavage.[39] Nasal mucosal biopsies, performed 24 hours after topical allergen provocation, also show increases in the number of inflammatory cells, but in contrast to the nasal secretions, in which eosinophils and neutrophils account for the majority of recovered cells, mononuclear cells predominate.[40] These are mostly of the T-helper category, as evidenced by positive staining with antibodies against CD4, and a portion of them are activated as documented by IL-2 receptor expression (CD25 +).[41] The cellular changes observed after allergen provocation are similar to observations of nasal cytology during seasonal disease. In separately conducted studies, Bryan and Bryan and Okuda and Otsuka observed basophilic cells in nasal secretions during seasonal pollen exposure of allergic individuals.[42–46] In contrast to nasal secretions, which represent the most superficial compartment of the nasal mucosa, examination of nasal mucosal scrapings[46,47] or biopsies[18,46,47] which sample deeper layers, showed that the majority of metachromatic cells in these compartments were mast cells. Enerbäck and colleagues, using biopsies and cytologic imprints to examine the cellular content of the nasal mucosa during the birch pollen season in Sweden, showed a seasonal increase in mast cell number on the surface of the nasal epithelium after 4 or 5 days of pollen exposure.[18] The consensus of most studies is that basophils predominate in nasal secretions, whereas mast cells are more abundant in the epithelium and lamina propria of allergic subjects exposed to antigen either experimentally or naturally. Bentley and colleagues also reported significant seasonal increases in total MBP$^+$ and activated (EG2$^+$) eosinophils in the submucosa of allergic patients when compared with preseasonal biopsies or biopsies from nonallergic control subjects.[48]

Recent studies have also demonstrated increases in endothelial adhesion molecules, namely, vascular cell adhesion molecule-1 (VCAM-1) in nasal biopsies obtained from allergic subjects 24 hours after nasal allergen challenge.[49] This molecule is expressed on the surface of vascular endothelial cells and interacts with a counterligand, very late antigen-4 (VLA-4), which is present on the surface of several leukocytes including lymphocytes, monocytes, eosinophils, and basophils, but not neutrophils.[50,51] The VLA-4/VCAM-1 adhesion pathway has been suggested as a mechanism for specific eosinophil, as opposed to neutrophil, migration from the circulation into allergic inflammatory sites.[50,52,53] Other adhesion molecules thought to be important in the recruitment of inflammatory cells from the intravascular compartment into tissue sites of allergic inflammation are intercellular adhesion molecule-1 (ICAM-1), which is constitutively expressed in the nasal mucosa, and E-selectin, which is modestly upregulated 24 hours after allergen provocation.[49] ICAM-1, a ligand for the β_2 integrin molecules LFA-1 and Mac-1, which are present on the surface of leukocytes, mediates the attachment of all classes of leukocytes to endothelial cells,[51] and E-selectin binds to sialyl Lewis X expressed on the surface of leukocytes.[54]

The expression of adhesion molecules has also been studied by Montefort and colleagues, who compared the expression of endothelial cell adhesion molecules in nasal biopsies from subjects with perennial allergic rhinitis and normal control subjects. These investigators found enhanced expression of ICAM-1 and VCAM-1, but not E-selectin, in the mucosa of allergic subjects.[55]

In addition to the role of inflammatory mediators in allergic disease, cytokines are increasingly recognized as important mediators of allergic inflammation and have been shown to have proinflammatory effects in vitro. Such effects include increasing the production of cells in the bone marrow, aiding in the survival of cells in the nasal mucosa, synergizing with other cellular activators, and acting as chemoattractants. Although initially thought to originate exclusively from lymphocytes, other inflammatory cells such as mast cells, basophils, and eosinophils can also produce them.[56,57] Inflammatory cell recruitment enhances the interactions among cells and leads to additional cytokine production, thereby amplifying the reaction and causing further cellular recruitment and increasing survival of already recruited inflammatory cells.[58] Some of these inflammatory cells elaborate substances that can cause local damage and mucosal modifications characteristic of chronic rhinitis. The presence of cytokines in nasal secretions and tissues after allergen provocation and natural allergen exposure is beginning to be recognized. Durham and colleagues have demonstrated an increase in the number of cells bearing mRNA for IL-3, IL-4, IL-5, and granulocyte macrophage-colony stimulating factor (GM-CSF) in nasal mucosal biopsies after allergen challenge.[59] Furthermore, increased levels of IL-1β and GM-CSF have been measured in nasal secretions during the late-phase reaction, and these elevations peaked at the fifth hour after allergen provocation.[60]

Besides the development of recurrent symptoms hours after a nasal challenge, the inflammatory cellular influx is accompanied by increased nasal reactivity. This has been demonstrated as increased responsiveness to specific stimuli, such as the antigen that initiated the reaction, and to nonspecific stimuli, such as the secretagogues histamine and methacholine. In the 1960s, John Connel coined the term "priming" to refer to increased specific responsiveness. Priming may explain why patients become more symptomatic to the same amounts of pollen in the environment later during the allergy season. Nonspecific reactivity implies increased responsiveness to nonantigenic substances and has been studied by provoking individuals with methacholine, with histamine, and more recently, with cold, dry air and bradykinin. Like priming, nonspecific reactivity is not obligatorily linked to the appearance of a late reaction. Walden and colleagues found increased sensitivity to histamine 24 hours after antigen challenge.[61] The response to histamine challenge returned to baseline 10 days later, suggesting that increased responsiveness to histamine was reversible. Other studies noted a positive correlation between the number of eosinophils 24 hours after antigen challenge and the magnitude of responsiveness to histamine, and this hyperresponsiveness was inhibited by pretreatment with topical corticosteroids.[62,63] Majchel and colleagues examined the effect of seasonal exposure on nasal responsiveness to histamine by challenging allergic subjects with histamine before, at the peak of, near the end of, and 2 weeks after the ragweed pollen season.[64] These investigators observed a significant increase in symptoms at the peak of the pollen season that returned to baseline with the disappearance of pollen. The increase above baseline at the peak of the season was not significant for any of the parameters measured, however, suggesting that increased reactivity to histamine with seasonal exposure appears to represent a change in baseline rather than an increased sensitivity to histamine itself. This change in baseline reactivity was inhibited in subjects who were receiving immunotherapy.

Similar studies demonstrate nasal hyperresponsiveness to the cholinomimetic agonist methacholine.[65] Klementsson and colleagues measured the volume of nasal secretions after intranasal administration of 6 mg of methacholine before and after antigen challenge of allergic subjects out of allergy season and observed significant increases in methacholine-induced secretions at 2, 4, 6, 8, 10, and 24 hours after antigen challenge, compared to baseline.[66] Although eosinophils in nasal secretions increased significantly after antigen challenge, no correlation was seen between their numbers and the increase in nonspecific hyperresponsiveness to methacholine. These workers also showed that premedication with two different H$_1$ antihistamines (terfenadine and cetirizine) resulted in inhibition of both the acute allergic reaction and the allergen-induced increase in responsiveness to methacholine without affecting eosinophil influx after antigen.[67] In contrast, corticosteroids, given topically or orally, have dramatic inhibitory effects on cellular infiltration and both specific and nonspecific hyperresponsiveness.[62,63,68] An important consequence of nonspecific hyperactivity is the increased symptoms on exposure

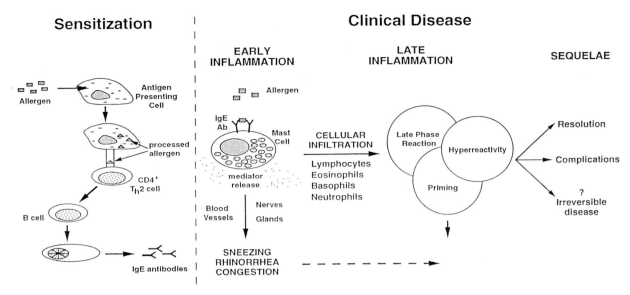

Fig. 8–2. Pathophysiology of allergic rhinitis. On the left side of the schematic, sensitization to allergen is depicted and involves the production of specific IgE antibodies to a certain allergen. Upon subsequent exposure to the allergen, depicted on the right, there is cross-linking of specific IgE receptors with resultant degranulation of mast cells and the release of inflammatory mediators. Subsequent to the early reaction, inflammatory cells infiltrate the nasal mucosa and the late-phase response develops. This is accompanied by a state of increased reactivity that renders the nasal mucosa more responsive to subsequent exposure to allergen (priming) or other stimuli (hyperreactivity). Finally, natural allergic disease might resolve or lead to complications such as sinus infections or otitis media. (From Naclerio RM: Allergic rhinitis. N Engl J Med 325:860, 1991.)

to irritants, such as gasoline odors, reported by patients during their allergy season.

One can summarize the pathophysiology of allergic rhinitis as follows: After sensitization of the nasal mucosa to a certain allergen, subsequent exposure leads to cross-linking of specific IgE receptors on mast cells and their resultant degranulation, with the release of a host of inflammatory mediators that are responsible for allergic nasal symptoms (Fig. 8–2). Proinflammatory substances produced by other inflammatory cells are also generated after antigen exposure. Cytokines are thought to be generated, in part, by lymphocytes, which are found in abundance in both resting and stimulated nasal mucosa. Cytokines can upregulate adhesion molecules on the vascular endothelium and possibly on marginating leukocytes, leading to the migration of these cells into tissues. Other cytokines also promote chemotaxis and survival of recruited inflammatory cells. All these changes lower the threshold of mucosal responsiveness and amplify it to a variety of specific and nonspecific stimuli, making allergic individuals more responsive to stimuli to which they are exposed in daily life (Fig. 8–2).

ALLERGENS

Allergens are foreign substances capable of provoking an IgE-mediated response. Most allergens are between 5 and 20 μm in diameter, a size that permits their com-

plete removal by the nose. They are proteins with molecular weights between 10 and 40 kilodaltons. No distinguishing surface characteristics appear to differentiate allergens from nonantigenic substances.

We often categorize allergens into indoor and outdoor. In general, outdoor allergens are responsible for seasonal allergic rhinitis, whereas indoor allergens usually cause perennial rhinitis. Pollens causing allergy in temperate climates are released into the air from plants, trees, weeds, and grasses and are carried great distances. Thus, cutting down trees around a suburban home in an effort to reduce the amount of pollen has little effect. About 75% of patients with seasonal allergens have symptoms due to ragweed, 40% have them to grasses, and 5% to trees alone. Approximately 25% have allergies to both grass and ragweed, and 5% have allergies to all three pollens.[2] Trees clearly have geographic variations; for example, Western red cedar is limited to the Northwest. Grasses are diverse and include timothy grass, often used for feeding horses, Kentucky bluegrass, widely used in lawn grass mixtures, orchard grass, rye grass, and English plantain. Common short ragweed is found throughout North America, with the exception of Newfoundland, and is conspicuously absent from the European continent.

Pollination, and hence the allergy season, occurs in a predictable annual pattern for different regions of the country.[69] The pattern, however, varies throughout the country. In the Northeast, trees pollinate in mid-March to late April, grasses follow in May and June, and ragweed flowers from mid-August until the first frost. In the South, tree blooming begins in early February. In contrast to the sharply demarcated grass season that occurs to the north, in the south grasses may pollinate from March through September, and in some parts, pollination may be a year-round process. The pattern in the central United States resembles the patterns seen on the eastern coast. In the California lowlands, grass pollen is present from early March through November, and trees and short ragweed are present as in other regions. In the Northwest coastal region, trees and grass pollen are present, but the region is ragweed-free. In the traditionally arid Southwest, previously a haven for allergy sufferers, increased urbanization and irrigation have contributed to increasing the pollen load.

The most frequent perennial allergens are animal danders, dust mites, cockroach, and molds. Dust mites are microscopic, eight-legged organisms of the genus Dermatophagoides, including Dermatophagoides pteronyssinus, Dermatophagoides farinae, and Euroglyphus maynei. They are the major allergens in "house-dust." Dust mites are found throughout the world, with the exception of extremely dry climates such as northern Sweden, central Canada, and areas at elevations over 10,000 feet. These mites feed on human epithelial scales and thrive in warm, humid environments (60 to 70% relative humidity, temperatures 65° to 80°F). Bedding provides an ideal environment for proliferation of dust mites. Other sites for mite accumulation are upholstered furniture, carpets, and stuffed toys. Dust mite feces, the source of the allergen, are relatively large particles that remain airborne for short periods, unlike outdoor pollens. When an individual sits on a bed, the particles become airborne and are inhaled. Because these particles are large, they settle from the air rapidly, and air filtration systems cannot effectively remove them.

Animal danders are an important source of indoor allergens. Cat and dog danders are the most frequent, but mice, guinea pigs and horses can all be responsible for allergic symptoms. Laboratory workers can become allergic to animals at work. In most cases, the allergen is found in secretions. In cats, *Fel d I* is the principal allergen secreted in cat saliva. It dries on fur and is spread to furniture, bedding, and carpets. When these reservoirs are disturbed, allergen becomes airborne and can provoke symptoms.

Cockroach is an important source of allergen in inner city populations. Both American (Periplaneta americana) and German cockroach (Blatella germanica) have been identified as important allergens in asthma. Allergenicity occurs to body parts and to feces. Molds, although less well studied, are sources of allergens, particularly in warm, humid environments. They tend to be found inside older homes in areas of decreased ventilation or increased dampness. Although

a phenomenal variety of molds exists, alternaria and cladosporium are principally responsible for symptoms to outdoor exposure, and aspergillus and penicillium are most prevalent indoors.

The patient's work environment may also be a source of allergens. Symptoms occurring only at work and subsiding on weekends may reflect an occupational disorder. At risk are flour handlers, workers in paint and plastic industries, woodworkers, fish and shellfish processors, and animal handlers. Unfortunately, few specific tests exist for the diagnosis of these disorders.

CLINICAL PRESENTATION

History

Antigen exposure causes itching within seconds that is soon followed by sneezing. Rhinorrhea follows, and within about 15 minutes nasal congestion peaks. Besides nasal symptoms, patients often complain about ocular pruritus, tearing, pharyngeal itching, throat clearing, cough, and ear popping. Itching is the symptom most suggestive of allergic disease. The relative importance of each symptom may vary among individuals, but each symptom is usually present at least to some degree. When obtaining the history, the physician should attempt to link exposure to allergens temporally with the occurrence of symptoms. Symptoms immediately following exposure to a potential source of allergen, such as a cat, strongly suggest an allergy to that allergen. Patients with seasonal allergies complain only of recurrent symptoms at specific times of each year that coincide with pollination periods. In contrast, a history of year-round symptoms may indicate sensitivity to a perennial allergen or multiple seasonal allergens. The presence of domestic pets (including birds) and whether these sleep in the patient's room must be determined. Exposure to perennial allergens tends to be accentuated in winter in colder climates, where ventilation is reduced. Symptoms occurring only at work or during the work week and subsiding on weekends may reflect an occupationally related disorder. Additional considerations in history taking include the response to prior therapy and evidence of complications. Nasal obstruction may lead to mouth breathing. In children, this may be manifested as adenoid facies, with a high palatal arch and abnormal dental development. In adults, nasal obstruction may contribute to snoring and sleep apnea. Obstruction of sinus ostia may predispose to sinusitis. Eustachian tube dysfunction may occur,[70] but this has not been shown to lead to an increased incidence of otitis media or otitis media with effusion.[71,72]

A general medical history remains important. Past medical history may document systemic disorders that affect the nose, such as hypothyroidism. Pregnancy can produce nasal congestion and may require modification of treatment strategies. The presence of pulmonary disease such as asthma should be sought. Between 5 and 10% of asthmatic subjects may have an intolerance to aspirin and nonsteroidal anti-inflammatory drugs. A family history of allergic rhinitis increases the chances of the patient's having an allergic disorder. Nasal symptoms might also be due to intake of medications such as β blockers, which may contribute to nasal congestion through interference with adrenergic mechanisms. Tricyclic antidepressants may produce dryness of the nasal mucosa by virtue of their anticholinergic effects. Angiotensin-converting enzyme inhibitors can produce a chronic cough. Birth control pills can cause nasal congestion, and topical eye drops can also induce nasal symptoms.

Examination

The classic description of allergic facies includes mouth breathing, allergic "shiners" (resulting from periorbital venous stasis from chronic nasal obstruction), and a transverse supratip nasal crease from long-term rubbing of the nose upward to relieve itching. These classic presentations occur more often in children, but absence of these signs does not exclude the disease. Allergic rhinitis shares features of other nasal disease entities. Attentive history taking and physical examination, combined with appropriate diagnostic tests, are required to establish the correct diagnosis.

Physical examination must be complete. Ocular examination may demonstrate injection of the conjunctiva or swelling of the eyelids. Examination of the nose begins with observing the external appearance for gross deformities such as a deviation suggesting previous trauma or expansion of the nasal bridge suggestive of nasal polyps. A nasal speculum permits evaluation of the anterior third of the internal nasal architecture and character of the nasal mucosa. Structural anomalies providing an anatomic basis for obstruction or recurrent infections such as septal deviations or spurs should be sought. Character and consistency of nasal secretions should be noted. These can vary from thin and clear to thick and whitish. The nasal mucosa may be swollen and pale bluish, although these signs are not pathognomonic of the disease, as previously thought. The examination of allergic individuals often appears normal, and the primary importance of the physical examination is to rule out other causes of or contributors to the symptoms.

Decongestion of swollen nasal mucosa with a topical decongestant improves visualization and allows the differentiation of reversible from irreversible changes. Combining the vasoconstrictor with a topical anesthetic allows complete examination with an endoscope. The choanae and the nasopharynx can be visualized in this manner. The region of the middle meatus should also be examined carefully because secretions there might be suggestive of acute or chronic sinusitis. Nasal polyps that were not visualized by anterior rhinoscopy may be seen during a careful endoscopic examination. Nasal polyps are infrequent in allergic rhinitis (< 2%), but are found in up to 20% of patients with cystic fibrosis.[15] The presence of nasal polyps in children suggests the diagnosis of cystic fibrosis, because polyps are rarely found in this age group.

DIAGNOSIS

The identification of allergen(s) responsible for the patient's symptoms is important both for establishing the diagnosis and for the institution of avoidance measures. Symptoms occurring in temporal relation to allergen exposure suggest sensitization but are not diagnostic. Sensitization implies the presence of elevated levels of IgE directed against a specific allergen and can be demonstrated by a wheal and flare response to skin testing with allergen extracts or by measuring the level of antigen-specific IgE antibodies in the serum. Moreover, individuals can show evidence of sensitization by a positive skin test or elevated specific antibody levels in the serum without having evidence of clinical disease. This emphasizes the importance of a good history in the evaluation of patients with suspected allergic disorders.

Skin Testing

Skin testing furnishes an excellent in vivo method to demonstrate sensitivity to a given allergen. This test evaluates the presence of specific IgE antibodies on skin mast cells, the reactivity of these cells, and the reaction of the end organ to released mediators. Its advantages include greater sensitivity, the rapidity with which results can be obtained, and low cost. Like all diagnostic tests, skin testing also has disadvantages, which include the inability to perform the test in patients with dermatologic problems such as dermatographism and extensive eczema, poor tolerance of many children for multiple needle pricks, the inhibitory effect of certain ingested drugs such as antihistamines on skin test reactivity,[73,74] the need to maintain the potency of the allergen extracts, and the possibility of systemic reactions.

Skin testing often begins with puncture testing, which provides low-dose allergen exposure. A small drop of concentrated allergen is placed on the skin (usually the volar surface of the forearm or the back), and a minute quantity is introduced into the dermis with a sharp object. Positive responses occur within 10 to 15 minutes and produce a characteristic raised central area of induration (wheal), with a surrounding zone of erythema (flare). The response is graded in comparison with a positive histamine response, and a negative control with the diluent for the allergen extracts is also included to control for nonspecific reactivity to the vehicle. The positive control ensures that the patient can mount a cutaneous reaction to histamine, and the absence of a reaction can unmask interference by medications, decreased skin reactivity, or technical problems with the procedure. Skin testing is valid in infants and young children, but the criteria for a positive reaction need to be adjusted because the reactions are smaller.[75] Measurement of serum-specific IgE levels is also valid in this younger age group.[76]

Negative puncture tests are usually confirmed by intradermal tests, which are more sensitive. In an intradermal test, a small (0.01 to 0.05 ml) quantity of dilute allergen is injected into the superficial dermis, and the same wheal and flare responses are observed and graded in comparison with a positive histamine control. Because antihistamines can interfere with the results of skin testing, most H_1 receptor antagonists are withheld for 2 days before skin testing, but in the case of astemizole, the test can be affected for up to 6 weeks, as a result of the long half-life of this agent. Tricyclic antidepressants can suppress responses for several weeks, as can tranquilizers and antiemetics of the phenothiazine class through intrinsic anti-H_1 activity. Short-term oral corticosteroid treatment has no effect on skin test reactivity, but it may have an inhibitory effect if the agent is taken for long periods.

In Vitro IgE Measurements

Drawing blood for the measurement of specific IgE can circumvent some of the disadvantages of skin testing. False-positive results may occur if patients have elevated IgE levels in their sera because of nonspecific binding. Therefore, although IgE levels alone are of limited usefulness in the diagnosis of allergic rhinitis, and because elevated levels can also exist in patients with nonallergic conditions, these levels must be obtained in conjunction with a determination of specific IgE levels. False-negative results may also occur from inhibition by IgG antibodies with similar affinities as in patients receiving immunotherapy. Data from clinical studies comparing results of skin testing and one of the in vitro tests for specific IgE determination (the radioallergosorbent assay) in allergic subjects suggest a good correlation between the two,[77] with a higher sensitivity for skin testing.[78] Therefore, both determinations of specific IgE levels and skin testing are useful in the diagnosis of allergic disorders, but their results should always be interpreted in the context of clinical symptoms.

Other Diagnostic Tests

Peripheral eosinophilia, although nonspecific, may indicate the presence of other atopic diseases. Nasal cytologic examination allows the identification of eosinophils and other inflammatory cells in nasal secretions and may be helpful in differentiating an infectious from an allergic cause during a clinical exacerbation of symptoms. In normal individuals, smears show the presence of epithelial cells, including some ciliated and goblet cells, with few eosinophils, neutrophils, basophils, or bacteria. In subjects with an infection, neutrophils increase in nasal secretions, and in symptomatic allergic subjects, the percentage of eosinophils increases. A value greater than 10% is suggestive of allergic disease.[79–83] Eosinophils may also be present in the absence of IgE-mediated disease, however. Approximately 25% of patients with chronic rhinitis and negative skin tests demonstrate eosinophilia on nasal cytologic study, and this entity is known as the nonallergic rhinitis with eosinophilia syndrome (NARES). Regardless of the cause, the presence of eosinophilia usually implies a favorable clinical response to corticosteroid therapy.[84]

Soft tissue radiography of the neck can evaluate adenoid size, a major consideration in the differential diagnosis of rhinitis in children, especially when the predominant symptom is nasal obstruction. Sinus disease often complicates perennial allergic rhinitis and may be a consideration in the differential diagnosis. Although plain sinus films can help evaluate the maxillary and frontal sinuses for evidence of opacification, their role has greatly decreased since the development of computed tomography (CT), which is now standard for the evaluation of the presence and extent of sinus abnormalities. The common association of upper and lower airway disease makes the use of tests of pulmonary functions useful adjuvants. This statement applies to such diverse disorders as cystic fibrosis, asthma, and bronchopulmonary aspergillosis.

THERAPY

Environmental Modifications

The most potent treatments cannot eliminate symptoms in the face of overwhelming allergen load. Furthermore, evidence is accumulating that increasing allergen load may be responsible for the rising prevalence of allergic rhinitis in the general population and may contribute to the development of allergic rhinitis in the children of allergic patients.

Complete avoidance of the allergen(s) to which the patient is sensitive eliminates symptoms of the disease. Thus, measures aimed at reducing allergen load from the patient's environment are effective in reducing symptoms. In seasonal allergic rhinitis, patients can reduce exposure by keeping windows closed on days when pollen counts are high and limiting physical activity outdoors in the early morning and evening, when pollen counts peak. Air conditioning can help, and the addition of special filters can prevent pollen grains and mold spores from entering the home. Pollen counts are often given during daily weather reports, and the previous day's pollen counts are the best predictor of the next day's. Rain, however, profoundly reduces the levels of outdoor pollens.

Measures to reduce exposure to dust mites concentrate on the bedding.[85] These include replacing feather pillows and bedspreads with synthetic ones that can be washed in hot water (hotter than 130°F) and covering mattresses with commercially available plastic covers. Removing carpets and frequent vacuuming also help. Where carpets cannot be removed, acaricidal products can directly kill mites.

In subjects with allergies to animal dander, removal of a domestic pet is a first step. Reduction in the allergen load after pet removal may take up to 6 months, however, and thus symptoms may persist. Furthermore, complete removal of a pet may be difficult, but eliminating the animal from the bedroom, where we spend an average 8 hours per day, is a helpful alternative. In the case of cats, regular washing of the animal may help decrease allergen load.[86]

Humidifiers must be cleaned regularly to avoid becoming a source of mold allergens, which thrive in moist environments. The humidity should not exceed 40 to 45% because higher levels encourage the growth of dust mites and molds. The use of high-efficiency particulate air (HEPA) filters and of electrostatic filters effectively removes particulates larger than 1 μm in diameter. Particles, however, must be airborne for removal, such as pollens, whereas heavy particles that settle from the air rapidly, such as dust mites, are not eliminated by these measures.[87]

Pharmacologic Therapy

Antihistamines

Three receptors exist for histamine. H_1 receptors are found on blood vessels, on sensory nerves, on smooth muscles of the respiratory and digestive tracts, and in the central nervous system. Stimulation leads to vasodilatation, increased vascular permeability, sneezing, pruritus, glandular secretion, and increased intestinal motility. H_2 receptors have a distribution similar to that of H_1 receptors, but are principally involved in the regulation of gastric acid secretion. H_3 receptors are principally located in the brain and seem to be involved in the regulation of histamine synthesis and release. The contribution of histamine to the early allergic response, largely mediated by the H_1 receptor, has long been recognized and is the rationale for the large number of H_1 antagonists in clinical use.

H_1 antihistamines have recently been classified into first-generation, or sedating, and second-generation, or nonsedating, antihistamines. The first generation of antihistamines are effective, but they have some undesirable side effects because of their lack of selectivity and subsequent nonspecific stimulation of other receptors. Among these side effects are sedation, anticholinergic effects, and gastrointestinal distress. When applied topically, some act as local anesthetics. The most important of the side effects is sedation, which is reported in approximately 20% of patients.[88] Recent objective studies of performance have documented the problem. The correlation with the subjective reporting of sedation was weak, however, and the problem appeared more significant than previously believed; that is, a larger number of subjects developed impaired performance compared with the number reporting sedation. Furthermore, impaired performance can persist after the subjective feeling of somnolence dissipates, hence the importance of warning patients who are taking these medications not to perform some tasks such as operating heavy machinery or driving. Although some side effects may be useful, such as the use of diphenhydramine for treating insomnia, they are usually a nuisance and limit compliance.

Second-generation antihistamines are less lipophilic than first-generation H_1 antihistamines and do not penetrate the blood-brain barrier. Therefore, they produce no more somnolence than placebo. Their greater receptor selectivity also reduces the incidence of anticholinergic side effects. In addition to antagonizing histamine at the H_1 receptor, some antihistamines, such as azatadine, of the piperidine class, and terfenadine, a nonsedating antihistamine, inhibit histamine release after intranasal antigen challenge.[89,90] Treatment with some antihistamines also reduces the production of leukotrienes and kinins, mediators with proinflammatory effects,[90,91] as well as the allergen-induced increased responsiveness to methacholine.[67]

Oral antihistamines are readily absorbed. Their onset of action is rapid, usually within 60 minutes, and maximum benefit occurs within hours, with the exception of astemizole.[92] Metabolism of most antihistamines primarily occurs through the hepatic cytochrome P-450 system. Drugs interfering with this system, such as antifungal agents, can lead to the accumulation of antihistamines in toxic levels. Cetirizine, an H_1 receptor antagonist currently being reviewed by the United States Food and Drug Administration (FDA) for approval, is primarily excreted in the urine and does not depend on the cytochrome P-450 system. Clinical effectiveness of antihistamines exceeds the duration of measurable serum levels. This phenomenon may be due to the presence of active metabolites; for example, astemizole is degraded to desmethylastemizole, which has a half-life of 9.5 days. Another explanation for prolonged efficacy of H_1 receptor antagonists beyond their measurable serum levels relates to extended tissue levels.

Rarely, cardiac arrhythmias have been reported

with terfenadine and astemizole and seem to be associated with increased serum levels. Toxic levels can occur with overdoses or when either of these two antihistamines is taken concomitantly with macrolide antibiotics or the imidazole family of systemic antifungal agents that interfere with the cytochrome P-450 system. Toxicity occurs through prolongation of the QT interval, leading to the development of torsades de pointes. The frequency of cardiac arrests from terfenadine and astemizole is probably about one in a million and therefore occurs less frequently than being struck by lightning. Before prescribing these two antihistamines, however, physicians need to make sure that their patients do not have hepatic dysfunction or a previous history of cardiac arrhythmias and are not receiving macrolide antibiotics or systemic antifungal agents of the imidazole family, notably ketoconazole or itraconazole. This prolongation of the QT interval has not been reported with loratadine, cetirizine, or acrivastine. Cardiac arrhythmias were reported in the past with first-generation antihistamines, but these compounds have been less extensively studied.

Levocabastine is a topical antihistamine available in Canada and in Europe. It is currently available in the United States as an ophthalmic preparation. Intranasal levocobastine's effectiveness is comparable to that of oral antihistamines and, like these agents, it does not affect nasal congestion.[93] Its principal advantage is a rapid onset of action.

All antihistamines are effective in the treatment of allergic rhinitis and differ principally in their side effects, duration of action, and cost. In equipotent doses, they are equally effective in suppressing histamine-induced skin wheals.[94] H_1 receptor antagonists are most effective in treating sneezing, nasal and ocular pruritus, and rhinorrhea associated with allergic rhinitis, but have little or no effect on nasal congestion. They are thus often combined with an oral decongestant. Generic first-generation H_1 blockers are considerably less expensive than their nonsedating counterparts: a month's supply of generic chlorpheniramine costs approximately $2.46, compared with a similar supply of terfenadine ($51.00) or loratadine ($51.00). Some clinicians have tried to circumvent the sedation caused by first-generation antihistamines by directing that they be taken before bedtime, when somnolence is not a problem. The next day, prolonged tissue levels provide continued efficacy without the undesirable side effect of drowsiness.[95]

Decongestants

Decongestants exert their effect through stimulation of α_1 or α_2 adrenergic receptors. These receptors are present on resistance vessels, where they control blood flow, and on capacitance vessels, where they control blood volume. In capacitance vessels, α_2 outnumber α_1 receptors.[96] In resting conditions, sympathetic nervous activity regulates nasal patency by maintaining the sinusoids contracted to approximately half maximal capacity. The resting state is affected by the nasal cycle, a periodic, reciprocal alteration of nasal cavity congestion and decongestion that affects about 80% of normal individuals. Increased sympathetic stimulation, such as occurs during exercise, reduces nasal congestion.

Oral decongestants exert their effects directly and by stimulating norepinephrine release. The two major decongestants are pseudoephedrine and phenylpropanolamine, which can be prescribed separately or in combination with antihistamines. These decongestants stimulate α_1 and α_2 receptors, leading to decreased nasal blood flow. Because oral decongestants also stimulate adrenergic receptors other than those in the nasal vasculature, overdosage has been associated with hypertensive crisis. When given in prescribed doses, however, they do not induce hypertension in normotensive patients, nor do they alter the pharmacologic control of stable hypertensive patients. Current recommendations suggest that decongestants should not be used in patients with uncontrolled hypertension, in those with severe coronary artery disease, or in patients receiving monoamine oxidase inhibitors. Decongestants should be prescribed with caution in patients with diabetes, hyperthyroidism, closed-angle glaucoma, coronary artery disease, cardiac insufficiency, prostatic hypertrophy, or urinary retention.[97] Their major side effect is insomnia, which occurs in approximately 25% of patients.

Topical decongestants are effective in reducing nasal congestion, regardless of the cause, and these include catecholamines (such as phenylephrine) and imidazoline derivatives (such as xylometazoline or oxymetazoline). Prolonged use can bring about rhinitis medicamentosa, which is characterized by reduced duration of action and rebound nasal congestion after cessation of therapy. Because this phenomenon can appear even after a short period, use of these agents should be limited to a few days. These agents are best reserved for cases where nasal congestion is so severe that it precludes the use of other topical preparations such as intranasal corticosteroids or to allow more restful sleep during acute exacerbations of disease.

Disodium Cromoglycate and Nedocromil Sodium

Disodium cromoglycate exerts a protective effect on the allergic response when given four to six times daily beginning before the development of symptoms.[98] Although it was initially thought to prevent mast cell degranulation, the exact mechanism of action of this agent is unknown. Its effectiveness approximates that of antihistamines,[99] but the need for frequent dosing limits compliance. Like antihistamines, cromolyn is more helpful for sneezing, rhinorrhea, and nasal itching than it is for nasal congestion.[100]

Nedocromil sodium, the disodium salt of a pyranoquinoline dicarboxylic acid, has been approved for the treatment of asthma in the United States. Corrado and colleagues demonstrated that pretreatment of allergic subjects with nedocromil sodium resulted in significant reductions in allergen-induced sneezing and elevations in nasal airway resistance and secretion weights, compared with placebo.[101] In clinical studies, 1% nedocromil sodium solution, given four times daily, was found to relieve symptoms of allergic rhinitis within 2 hours of administration[102] and was significantly more effective than placebo in controlling allergic symptoms during pollen exposure.[103] In a clinical trial during the ragweed pollen season, nedocromil was found to be at least as effective as cromolyn in improving rhinitis symptoms, and both treatments were more effective than placebo.[104] Studies of patients with perennial allergic rhinitis also suggest that nedocromil is effective in the treatment of this condition.[105] Nedocromil sodium is not yet available as a nasal or an ophthalmic preparation in the United States.

Anticholinergic Agents

Ipratropium bromide and atropine for topical intranasal use are both available in Canada and Europe. Anticholinergic agents inhibit parasympathetic stimulation of glandular secretion by competing for muscarinic receptors on glands. They are highly effective in reducing rhinorrhea, but they have no effect on the other symptoms of allergic rhinitis.[106,107] The clinical benefit of anticholinergic agents is primarily limited to the treatment of patients with rhinitis in whom rhinorrhea is the predominant complaint. This could occur in a variety of nasal conditions such as allergic and nonallergic rhinitis, as well as the rhinorrhea precipitated by exposure to cold, windy environments, often referred to as "skiers' nose."[108] Dosage should be titrated to avoid excessive drying of the nasal mucosa and epistaxis, which are the most frequent side effects.

Topical Intranasal Corticosteroids

Topical intranasal glucocorticosteroids are potent medications for the treatment of allergic rhinitis. These agents profoundly reduce multiple aspects of the inflammatory response to allergen. Corticosteroids penetrate the interior of the cell, where they are bound by a glucocorticoid receptor in the cytoplasm. The glucocorticoid-receptor complex then penetrates the nucleus, where it inhibits the synthesis of the proinflammatory cytokines IL-1, 2, 3, 5, 6, interferon γ, tumor necrosis factor α, and GM-CSF[109] and induces the synthesis of other anti-inflammatory substances such as vasocortin and lipocortin. These agents reduce eosinophil survival and function induced by IL-1, 3, and 5.[109,110] Corticosteroid-induced cellular modifications require several hours to appear, and this might explain why their onset of action is gauged in days.

Topical corticosteroids effectively suppress the response to allergen provocation. In contrast to systemic corticosteroids, pretreatment with topical corticosteroids reduces the acute nasal response to allergen challenge, as shown by a reduction in symptoms and levels of recovered inflammatory mediators in nasal secretions[111] (Fig. 8–3). Treatment with topical corticosteroids also reduces symptoms, the levels of mediators and cellular infiltration during the late-phase reaction to allergen challenge, and the priming response to antigen[39,111] (Fig. 8–3). These agents also inhibit priming

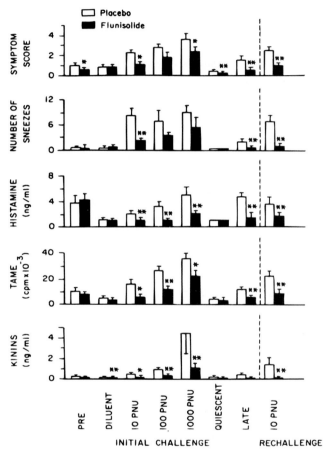

Fig. 8–3. The effect of intranasal corticosteroids (flunisolide) on the nasal response to allergen. The protocol of challenge is seen on the abscissa: Pre = prewash at the initiation of the allergen challenge protocol, Diluent = challenge with the diluent for the allergen extract to control for nonspecific reactivity, 10, 100, and 1000 protein nitrogen units (PNU) = increasing doses of allergen used for challenge, Quiescent = the initial hours after allergen provocation, Late = the late phase response, 10 PNU = rechallenge with the lowest dose of allergen 10 hours after the initial challenge. As can be seen from the response with the subjects on placebo (open bars), there was a significant increase over diluent in all the parameters measured both during the early and late responses. There was also an increase in responsiveness to the lowest dose of allergen (10 PNU) as assessed by levels of histamine, TAME-esterase and kinins in nasal lavages, indicative of the priming response. Pretreatment with flunisolide (closed bars) resulted in inhibition of the early, late and rechallenge responses to allergen. (Adapted from Pipkorn U, et al: Inhibition of mediator release in allergic rhinitis by pretreatment with topical glucocorticosteroids. N Engl J Med *316*:1506, 1987.)

and hyperresponsiveness to nonantigenic stimuli such as histamine.[62] Topical corticosteroids also prevent the increase in mast cells and inflammatory cells seen during seasonal exposure to allergen.[80] Furthermore, they also resulted in suppression of the seasonal increase in specific IgE antibodies during the ragweed season.[112] A direct vasoconstrictor effect of topical glucocorticosteroids, found in the skin, does not occur in the nasal mucosa.[113]

Currently, topical forms of corticosteroids include dexamethasone, flunisolide, beclomethasone dipropionate, triamcinolone, budesonide, and fluticasone, although not all are available in the United States. Although differences in strength among these molecules can be demonstrated in vitro assays and certain in vivo models, none of these variations have been shown to translate into major clinical differences. They are principally distinguished by the form of administration (pressurized aerosol, meter-dose inhaler, powder), by the frequency of administration (either once or twice daily), and by the potential to cause systemic toxicity. Their onset of action has been reported to be as short as 1 day, with most preparations having a noticeable clinical effect by 3 days and a peak effect by 2 weeks. These medications work best with continued usage, as opposed to intermittent, as needed, use.[114]

Side effects are relatively rare.[115] The most frequent is nasal irritation, which occurs in approximately 10% of patients. This is manifested as a nasal burning sensation or sneezing. Two percent of patients have blood-tinged secretions either because of the medication or because of the delivery system.[116] Although septal perforations have been reported, they are extremely rare.[117] Nasal biopsies after prolonged use of these agents have not shown thinning of the nasal epithelium or abnormalities in the nasal mucosa.[118-120] Mucosal superinfection with Candida albicans, occasionally found with the use of topical, orally inhaled, corticosteroids in the treatment of asthma, has not been a problem in the nose.[121]

Systemic side effects have long been a concern. Dexamethasone, the first available topical corticosteroid in the United States, had measurable systemic absorption, leading to adrenal suppression after prolonged use.[122] The newer preparations now available on the market have lower systemic absorption, and at the standard doses used for the treatment of allergic rhinitis, no detectable effects on the hypothalamic-pituitary-adrenal axis have been found. One report of the development of retrocapsular cataract during beclomethasone therapy appeared, but some of these patients had also received systemic corticosteroids.[123] A reduction in bone growth in children has been a concern of pediatricians.[124] This potential problem has been studied best in asthmatic children, and the majority of studies suggest no effect and are confounded by the effect of asthma itself on growth in these patients. Therefore,

for long-term use, a topical corticosteroid with a low bioavailability, administered in the lowest dose necessary to provide relief of symptoms, seems advisable and safe.[115]

In comparative trials, topical corticosteroids are more potent in relieving nasal symptoms than cromolyn[105] or antihistamines.[125,126] The addition of antihistamines to intranasal corticosteroids benefits ocular symptoms and adds more rapid onset of effectiveness at the initiation of treatment. In the only study comparing intranasal corticosteroids with immunotherapy, budesonide was found to be superior to Pollinex-R (Bencard Allergy Service, Weston, Ontario, Canada). Pollinex-R is not a standard, accepted form of immunotherapy, however, and further investigation is warranted in that regard.[127]

Systemic Corticosteroids

Clinical practice confirms the impression that oral corticosteroids reduce symptoms during seasonal allergies, but this has not been documented in placebo-controlled trials.[128] These agents are usually administered to patients during severe exacerbations of allergic symptoms, when total nasal obstruction prevents the introduction of a topical intranasal corticosteroid. Furthermore, these agents are used successfully in combination with antibiotics to treat sinus infections complicating allergic exacerbations. Depot injections of corticosteroids have efficacy comparable with short-term oral prednisone therapy and enjoy some popularity in Europe, including Scandinavia.[129] Corticosteroid injections into the turbinates are also perceived as clinically effective but have rarely been practiced in North America since the advent of intranasal corticosteroids and because of a small associated risk of blindness.[130] Although this complication can be minimized by using a corticosteroid with small particle size, the need to take this infrequent risk in lieu of alternative successful therapies has led to a decline in the popularity of this form of treatment.

Immunotherapy

The exact mode by which immunotherapy achieves efficacy remains to be elucidated.[131] Immunotherapy produces several immune modifications in peripheral blood and the nasal mucosa that probably contribute to its efficacy.[132,133] Treatment causes a rise in serum-specific IgG antibodies, a suppression in the usual seasonal rise in specific IgE antibodies with a decline over years and an increase in IgA and IgG antibodies in nasal secretions.[134,135] It reduces in vitro lymphocyte responsiveness to antigen[136] and decreases IL-2 release by inflammatory cells.[137] In experimental models of nasal provocation, immunotherapy reduces both early and late responses to ragweed antigen challenge, cellular influx into nasal secretions, and priming.[138] During the allergy season, immunotherapy leads to an inhibition of eosinophil migration into nasal secretions[139] and a reduction in nonspecific hyperreactivity to histamine.[140]

Indications for immunotherapy have not been established by experimental studies, but rather have evolved over years of clinical experience.[141] The primary indication is symptoms not adequately controlled by avoidance measures and pharmacotherapy. Patients with perennial symptoms may prefer immunotherapy over year-long daily medication. In making their selection, patients must be advised that immunotherapy offers control of symptoms but is slow in onset and, unlike pharmacotherapy, is effective only for the allergens to which the patient is treated. Whether years of successful therapy cure the disease after discontinuation of immunotherapy is an important but unanswered question.

Immunotherapy begins with low-dose injections of allergen extracts and builds to a maintenance dose. Injections usually begin at weekly intervals and are then reduced in frequency when maintenance doses are reached. The choice of allergens for treatment must be made after a careful diagnostic workup to increase the probability that treatment is started with extracts from all the allergens responsible for symptoms. Treatment should not be given if evidence of an IgE-mediated mechanism cannot be confirmed by skin or serum testing. Whereas excellent relief can be expected with pollen allergens, dust mites, and some animal danders, treatment with molds is less reliable. Immunotherapy with too many allergens is impractical, and usually treatment with no more than 6 to 10 allergens is attempted. Enzymes from some allergens can destroy other extracts, reducing the expected potency of the treatment.[141] Furthermore, combining allergens of different clinical sensitivities may interfere with reaching adequate maintenance doses for all allergens. Patients who are taking β blockers should not receive immunotherapy because, if anaphylaxis occurs, patients cannot be resuscitated. Immunotherapy in symptomatic asthmatic patients should be administered with extreme caution because these patients have the greatest frequency of morbidity.

Improvement of symptoms may begin as soon as 12 weeks, but optimal effect usually takes 1 year to attain.[141] Effectiveness of immunotherapy requires administration of sufficient amounts of allergen. For ragweed, this has been shown to be between 6 and 12 μg of *Amb a 1* (the major antigen in ragweed) per injection. The effect is antigen specific; thus, selection of relevant antigens for treatment is paramount. Patients who do not achieve symptomatic improvement after 2 years of immunotherapy should have it discontinued. No information is available on the length of time effective immunotherapy should be pursued, but most physicians treat from 2 to 5 years.

Allergen injections should be administered under the supervision of a qualified medical practitioner, and patients should be observed for at least 30 minutes after every injection. Local reactions at the site of injection are frequent with effective dosages and require no therapy. Repeated strong reactions (greater than 4 cm in diameter) persisting for 24 hours should lead to consideration of dose reduction. Proper resuscitative equipment should be present because anaphylactic reactions can occur at any time during treatment, even in patients receiving maintenance dosages. Factors that seem to contribute to increased complications, including fatalities, seem to be labile, corticosteroid-dependent asthma that has required prior hospitalizations, high sensitivity to allergen (as demonstrated by serum-specific IgE tests or skin test), and a history of prior systemic reactions.[142] Therefore, although death from immunotherapy is uncommon (risk estimated at one fatality for every two million injections), special precaution needs to be taken in patients with asthma, and a waiting period of at least 20 minutes after administration of the injection is recommended for all patients, with longer intervals (30 minutes) appropriate for high-risk patients.[142] Concern over mortality in the United Kingdom has led to decreased usage.[143]

TOWARD A RATIONAL CHOICE OF THERAPY

Prevention remains the mainstay of treatment of allergic rhinitis (Fig. 8–4). If allergen exposure can be reduced, this should be part of long-term management. Short-term avoidance does not result in an instant resolution of symptoms and is rarely completely achievable.

Pharmacotherapy provides the quickest relief. Antihistamines begin to take effect within 1 hour and traditionally constitute the first line of intervention. They are excellent for the treatment of sneezing and watery rhinorrhea. When cost is not an issue, nonsedating antihistamines should always be prescribed. To minimize cost, one can administer a long-acting, sedating antihistamine around bedtime and allow its efficacy to persist into the next day without its sedative side effect. Decongestants can be added to antihistamines in fixed combinations or as separate agents to relieve nasal congestion. Cromolyn sodium is an alternative to antihistamines as an initial treatment, but the need for frequent dosing, with the resultant reduction in compliance, should be kept in mind.

When antihistamines and/or decongestants are insufficient in relieving symptoms, or when the patient requires daily medication, topical corticosteroids should be recommended. They are highly effective in reducing all the nasal symptoms of allergic rhinitis, including congestion. They are nonsedating, have few

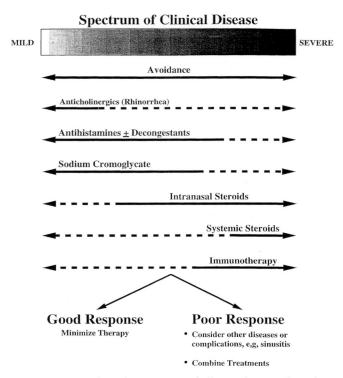

Fig. 8–4. Approach to the treatment of allergic rhinitis. This schematic depicts the different treatments available for allergic rhinitis and establishes some guidelines for the use of these therapies in different stages of severity of the disease. Avoidance should be used in all stages. Anticholinergics have limited use for the control of rhinorrhea. Antihistamines and/or decongestants as well as sodium cromoglycate are usually used for allergic rhinitis of mild to moderate severity. Severe disease usually warrants more aggressive treatment such as intranasal corticosteroids or immunotherapy. Systemic corticosteroids are reserved for severe allergic rhinitis leading to complete nasal obstruction. Clearly, these guidelines need to be varied in the context of different clinical settings as some patients with mild disease might benefit from intranasal corticosteroids while some other patients with more severe disease might respond well to antihistamine/decongestant combinations.

side effects, and are well tolerated by patients. The daily cost of treatment with nasal corticosteroids is less than that of the daily use of nonsedating antihistamines. Topical corticosteroids are initially given at the dose recommended in the PDR. Patients should be seen 2 weeks after initiating therapy to monitor for the development of local side effects. Superficial septal erosions can occur secondary to trauma from the nozzle, and the application technique should be carefully reviewed with these patients. The dosage is adjusted depending on the response: if a patient is better but continues to have breakthrough symptoms, the frequency of administration is increased; if excellent control is achieved, the frequency or the dose should be reduced.

Furthermore, periods of exacerbations can be predicted, based on a patient's pattern of allergies, and therefore, medication dosage can be varied accord-

ingly. Ocular symptoms are minimally controlled by intranasal corticosteroids, and thus adding an ophthalmic preparation or an oral antihistamine may be necessary.

In children, the long-term use of topical corticosteroids is approved in patients above the age of 6 years. For most topical corticosteroids, it is recommended to reduce the dose by half in young children. Because of the small possibility that intranasal corticosteroids can interfere with growth, these medications should always be given in the lowest effective dose.[115] Treatment with topical corticosteroids requires patient education. Their slow onset of action compared with that of antihistamines must be appreciated. An explanation of the mechanism of action may help the patient to understand the importance of using the product on a regular rather than an as-needed basis. The physician often must reassure patients as to the safety of intranasal corticosteroids, compared with oral preparations.

Initiation of immunotherapy depends on patient preference and the response to pharmacotherapy. Immunotherapy has not been shown to be more effective than intranasal corticosteroids.

Treatment of rhinitis during pregnancy poses special problems. Rhinitis and nasal congestion frequently occur during pregnancy (30%) and relate to hormonal change.[144,145] Patients with allergic rhinitis may also manifest symptoms during pregnancy. The management of rhinitis in pregnancy remains controversial. Ideally, no medication should be used, particularly during the first trimester. Avoidance measures should be implemented first. If symptoms of rhinitis interfere with maternal well-being, pharmacologic management is considered.[146] The patient must be advised that no drug can be considered absolutely safe because most drugs cross the placenta and can be measured in fetal blood.

The Group Health Cooperative Safety Study on medication use in pregnancy makes the following recommendations.[147] Tripelennamine, a first-generation H_1 blocker, has not been associated with teratogenic effects in humans or animals. Clorpheniramine, diphenhydramine, and hydroxyzine have been available for years and have not been associated with an increased incidence of fetal malformations. Pseudoephedrine is the preferred oral decongestant in pregnancy, although overdosage may be associated with reduced uterine blood flow. Oxymetazoline can also be used safely at recommended doses. Sodium cromoglycate is a safe drug during pregnancy and should be considered in the treatment of allergic rhinitis before corticosteroids. No teratogenicity of nasal topical corticosteroids has been reported in animal studies; however, no data exist on the teratogenicity of these products in humans.[97] Given their effectiveness in allergic disease and the lack of systemic effects of topical corticosteroids, therapy with these agents may be considered. Newer forms with lower bioavailability may be a more prudent choice.

Maintenance immunotherapy may be safely continued during pregnancy in patients who are not prone to systemic reactions. Because of the increased risk of systemic reactions, immunotherapy should not be initiated during pregnancy.

Surgical management of nasal obstruction is covered in Chapters 2 and 9. Major septal deviations should be corrected because they may interfere with the delivery of intranasal medications. Less severe obstructions should be corrected only if symptoms persist after adequate control of allergic symptoms. Similarly, turbinate reduction by means of submucous resection, vaporization with the laser, cryotherapy, or electrocautery may be adjuvant procedures in patients with allergic rhinitis, but more often find use in the management of nonallergic rhinitis. Functional endoscopic sinus surgery, covered in Chapter 12, can be used for the treatment of chronic rhinosinusitis, which frequently complicates perennial rhinitis.[148] Vidian neurectomy interrupts the parasympathetic and sympathetic neural supply to the nasal mucosa.[149] It causes a reduction in rhinorrhea, an effect that appears transitory. The availability of anticholinergic agents and the adverse effects on lacrimation will probably further decrease the use of this procedure in allergic rhinitis.

SUGGESTED READINGS

1. Collins J, ed: Prevalence of Selected Chronic Conditions, United States, 1983–1985. Hyattsville, MD, United States Public Health Service, Advance Data from Vital and Health Statistics, No. 155; Vol DHHS Pub No (PHS) 88–1250.
2. Evans RI: Epidemiology and natural history of asthma, allergic rhinitis, and atopic dermatitis. In: Allergy: Principles and Practice. 4th Ed. Edited by Middleton EJ Jr, et al. St Louis, Mosby-Year Book, 1993.
3. Åberg N: Asthma and allergic rhinitis in Swedish conscripts. Clin Exp Allergy 19:59, 1989.
4. Bascom RB, et al: Effect of ozone inhalation on the response to nasal challenge with antigen of allergic subjects. Am Rev Respir Dis 142:594, 1990.
5. Molfino NA, Slutsky AS, and Zamel N: The effects of air pollution on airway hyperresponsiveness. Clin Exp Allergy 22:667, 1992.
6. Matsumura Y: The effects of ozone, nitrogen dioxide, and sulfur dioxide on the experimentally induced allergic respiratory disorders in guinea pigs. 1. The effect on sensitization with albumin through the airway. Am Rev Respir Dis 102:430, 1970.
7. von Mutius E, et al: Prevalence of asthma and atopy in two areas of West and East Germany. Am J Respir Crit Care Med 149:358, 1994.
8. Magnussen H, Jörres R, and Nowak D: German reunification and the prevalence of asthma and allergy. Thorax 48:879, 1993.
9. Hide DW, et al: Effect of allergen avoidance in infancy on allergic manifestations at age two years. J Allergy Clin Immunol 93:842, 1994.
10. Malmberg H: Symptoms of chronic and allergic rhinitis and occurrence of nasal secretion granulocytes in university students, school children and infants. Allergy 36:209, 1981.
11. Zeiger RS: Development and prevention of allergic disease in childhood. In: Allergy: Principles and Practice. 4th Ed. Edited by Middleton EJ Jr, et al. St. Louis, Mosby-Year Book, 1993.
12. Åberg N and Engstrom I: Natural history of allergic diseases in children. Acta Paediatr Scand 79:206, 1990.
13. Church JA, et al: Hyposmia associated with atopy. Ann Allergy 40:105, 1978.
14. Binder E, Holopainen E, Malmberg K, and Salo OP: Clinical findings in patients with allergic rhinitis. Rhinology 22:255, 1984.
15. Settipane GA and Chafee FH: Nasal polyps in asthma and rhinitis: a review of 6,037 patients. J Allergy Clin Immunol 59:17, 1977.
16. Friedman RA, et al: Immunologic-mediated eustachian tube obstruction: a double-blind crossover study. J Allergy Clin Immunol 71:442, 1983.
17. Bernstein JM, et al: Role of IgE mediated hypersensitivity in recurrent otitis media with effusion. Am J Otol 5:66, 1983.
18. Enerbäck L, Pipkorn U, and Olofsson A: Intraepithelial migration of mucosal mast cells in hay fever: ultrastructural observations. Int Arch Allergy Appl Immunol 81:289, 1986.
19. Plaut M, et al: Mast cell lines produce lymphokines in response to cross-linkage of FcεRI or to calcium ionophores. Nature 339:64, 1989.
20. Bradding P, et al: Interleukin 4 is localized to and released by human mast cells. J Exp Med 716:1381, 1992.
21. Naclerio RM, et al: Mediator release after airway challenge with antigen. Am Rev Respir Dis 128:597, 1983.
22. Baumgarten CR, et al: Influx of kininogens into nasal secretions following antigen challenge of allergic individuals. J Clin Invest 76:191, 1985.
23. Baumgarten CR, et al: Plasma kallikrein during experimentally induced allergic rhinitis: role in kinin formation and contribution of TAME-esterase activity. J Immunol 137:977, 1986.
24. Baumgarten CR, Nichols RC, Naclerio RM, and Proud D: Concentration of glandular kallikrein in human nasal secretions increases during experimentally induced allergic rhinitis. J Immunol 137:1323, 1986.
25. Castells M and Schwartz LB: Tryptase levels in nasal lavage fluid as an indicator of the early allergic reaction. J Allergy Clin Immunol 82:348, 1988.
26. Creticos PS, et al: Peptide leukotriene release after antigen challenge in patients sensitive to ragweed. N Engl J Med 310:1626, 1984.
27. Freeland H, et al: The role of leukotriene B4 (LTB4) in human allergic late phase reactions (abstract). J Allergy Clin Immunol 77:244, 1986.
28. Bascom R, et al: Major basic protein and eosinophil-derived neurotoxin concentrations in nasal lavage fluid after antigen challenge: Effect of systemic corticosteroids and relationship to eosinophil influx. J Allergy Clin Immunol 84:338, 1989.
29. Togias AG, et al: Studies on the relationships between sensitivity to cold dry air, hyperosmolar solutions and histamine in the adult nose. Am Rev Respir Dis 141:1428, 1990.
30. Tønnesen P and Mygind N: Nasal challenge with serotonin and histamine in normal persons. Allergy 40:350, 1985.
31. Karim SMM, Adaikian PG, and Kunaratnam N: Effect of topical prostaglandins on nasal patency in man. Prostaglandins 15:457, 1978.
32. Bisgaard H, Olsson P, and Bende M: Effect of leukotriene D4 on nasal mucosal blood flow, nasal airway resistance and nasal secretions in humans. Clin Allergy 16:289, 1986.
33. Proud D, et al: Nasal provocation with bradykinin induces symptoms of rhinitis and a sore throat. Am Rev Respir Dis 137:613, 1988.
34. Doyle WJ, Boehm S, and Skoner DP: Physiologic responses to intranasal dose-response challenges with histamine, metacholine, bradykinin, and prostaglandin in adult volunteers with

and without nasal allergy. J Allergy Clin Immunol *86:*924, 1990.

35. Gleich G: The late phase of the immunoglobulin E-mediated reaction: a link between anaphylaxis and common allergic disease? J Allergy Clin Immunol *70:*160, 1982.

36. Naclerio RM, et al: Inflammatory mediators in late antigen-induced rhinitis. N Engl J Med *313:*65, 1985.

37. Iliopoulos O, et al: Relationship between the early, late, and rechallenge reaction to nasal challenge with antigen: observations on the role of inflammatory mediators and cells. J Allergy Clin Immunol *86:*851, 1990.

38. Taylor G and Shivalkar PR: "Arthus-type" reactivity in the nasal airways and skin in pollen sensitive subjects. Clin Allergy *1:*407, 1971.

39. Bascom R, et al: Basophil influx occurs after nasal antigen challenge: Effects of topical corticosteroid pretreatment. J Allergy Clin Immunol *81:*580, 1988.

40. Lim-Mombay M, Baroody FM, Taylor R, and Naclerio RM: Mucosal cellular changes after nasal antigen challenge (abstract). J Allergy Clin Immunol *89:*205, 1993.

41. Varney VA, et al: Immunohistology of the nasal mucosa following allergen-induced rhinitis. Am Rev Respir Dis *146:*170, 1992.

42. Bryan WTK and Bryan MP: Significance of mast cells in nasal secretions. Trans Am Acad Ophthalmol Otolaryngol *63:*613, 1959.

43. Okuda M and Otsuka M: Basophilic cells in allergic nasal secretions. Arch Otorhinolaryngol *214:*283, 1977.

44. Okuda M, Kawabori S, and Otsaka H: Electron microscope study of basophilic cells in allergic nasal secretions. Arch Otorhinolaryngol *221:*215, 1978.

45. Hastie R, Heroy JH, and Levy DA: Basophil leukocytes and mast cells in human nasal secretions and scrapings studied by light microscopy. Lab Invest *40:*554, 1979.

46. Okuda M, Otsuka H, and Kawabori S: Basophil leukocytes and mast cells in the nose. Eur J Respir Dis *64(suppl 128):*7, 1983.

47. Otsuka H, et al: Heterogeneity of metachromatic cells in the human nose: significance of mucosal mast cells. J Allergy Clin Immunol *76:*695, 1985.

48. Bentley AM, et al: Immunohistology of the nasal mucosa in seasonal allergic rhinitis: increases in activated eosinophils and epithelial mast cells. J Allergy Clin Immunol *89:*877, 1992.

49. Lee BJ, et al: Nasal challenge with allergen upregulates the local expression of vascular endothelial adhesion molecules. J Allergy Clin Immunol (in press).

50. Walsh GM, et al: Human eosinophil, but not neutrophil, adherence to IL-1 stimulated human umbilical vascular endothelial cells is a 4β1 (very late antigen-4) dependent. J Immunol *146:*3419, 1991.

51. Lobb RR: Integrin-immunoglobulin superfamily interactions in endothelial-leukocyte adhesion. In: Adhesion: Its Role in Inflammatory Disease. Edited by Harlan JM and Liu DY. New York, WH Freeman, 1992.

52. Schleimer RP, et al: Interleukin-4 induces adherence of human eosinophils and basophils but not neutrophils to endothelium: association with expression of VCAM-1. J Immunol *148:*1086, 1992.

53. Bochner BS, et al: Adhesion of human basophils, eosinophils, and neutrophils to IL-1-activated human vascular endothelial cells: contributions of endothelial cell adhesion molecules. J Exp Med *173:*1553, 1991.

54. Phillips ML, et al: ELAM-1 mediates cell adhesion by recognition of a carbohydrate ligand, sialyl-Le^x. Science *250:*1130, 1990.

55. Montefort S, et al: The expression of leukocyte-endothelial adhesion molecules is increased in perennial allergic rhinitis. Am J Respir Cell Mol Biol *7:*393, 1992.

56. Robinson DS: Interleukin-5, eosinophils and bronchial hyperreactivity. Clin Exp Allergy *23:*1, 1993.

57. Altman L, Ayars G, Baker C, and Luchtel D: Cytokines and

58. Holgate S: Mediator and cytokine mechanisms in asthma. Thorax *48:*103, 1993.

59. Durham SR, et al: Cytokine messenger RNA expression for IL-3, IL-4, IL-5, and granulocyte/macrophage-colony-stimulating factor in the nasal mucosa after local allergen provocation: relationship to tissue eosinophilia. J Immunol *148:*2390, 1992.

60. Alam R, et al: Development of a new technique for recovery of cytokines from inflammatory sites in situ. J Immunol Methods *155:*25, 1992.

61. Walden SM, et al: Antigen-provoked increase in histamine reactivity: observations on mechanisms. Am Rev Respir Dis *144:*642, 1991.

62. Andersson M, Andersson P, and Pipkorn U: Allergen-induced specific and non-specific nasal reactions: reciprocal relationship and inhibition by topical glucocorticosteroids. Acta Otolaryngol (Stockh) *107:*270, 1989.

63. Baroody FM, et al: Intranasal beclomethasone inhibits antigen-induced nasal hyperresponsiveness to histamine. J Allergy Clin Immunol *90:*373, 1992.

64. Majchel AM, et al: The nasal response to histamine challenge: effect of the pollen season and immunotherapy. J Allergy Clin Immunol *90:*85, 1992.

65. Druce HM, et al: Cholinergic nasal hyperreactivity in atopic subjects. J Allergy Clin Immunol *76:*445, 1985.

66. Klementsson H, et al: Changes in non-specific nasal reactivity and eosinophil influx and activation after allergen challenge. Clin Exp Allergy *20:*539, 1990.

67. Klementsson H, Andersson M, and Pipkorn U: Allergen-induced increase in nonspecific nasal reactivity is blocked by antihistamines without a clear-cut relationship to eosinophil influx. J Allergy Clin Immunol *86:*466, 1990.

68. Klementsson H, et al: Eosinophils, secretory responsiveness and glucocorticoid-induced effects on the nasal mucosa during a weak pollen season. Clin Exp Allergy *21:*705, 1991.

69. Solomon WR: Aerobiology and inhalant allergens: pollens and fungi. In: Allergy: Principles and Practice. 4th Ed. Edited by Middleton EJ Jr, et al. St Louis, Mosby-Year Book, 1993.

70. Skoner DP, Doyle WJ, Boehm S, and Fireman P: Priming of the nose and eustachian tube during natural pollen season. Am J Rhinol *3:*53, 1989.

71. Reisman PE and Bernstein JM: Allergy and secretory otitis media. Pediatr Clin North Am *22:*251, 1975.

72. Van Cauwenberge P: Secretory otitis media. Een Epidemiologische, Klinische en Experimentale Stuie. Ghent, 1988.

73. Long W, et al: Skin test suppression by antihistamines and the development of subsensitivity. J Allergy Clin Immunol *76:*113, 1985.

74. Bousquet J and Michel FB: In vivo methods for the study of allergy: skin tests. In: Allergy: Principles and Practice. 4th Ed. Edited by Middleton EJ Jr, et al. St Louis, Mosby-Year Book, 1993.

75. Menardo JL, et al: Skin test reactivity in infancy. J Allergy Clin Immunol *75:*646, 1985.

76. Ownby DR: Allergy testing: in vivo versus in vitro. Pediatr Clin North Am *35:*995, 1988.

77. Norman P: Correlations of RAST with in vivo and in vitro assays. In: Advances in Diagnosis of Allergy, RAST. Edited by Evans R. Miami, Symposia Specialists, 1975.

78. Berg TLO and Johansson SGO: Allergy diagnosis with the radioallergosorbent test: a comparison with the results of skin and provocation tests in an unselected group of children with asthma and hay fever. J Allergy Clin Immunol *54:*209, 1974.

79. Bickmore J: Nasal cytology in allergy and infection. ORL Allergy *40:*39, 1978.

80. Meltzer E, Orgel H, and Bronsky E: A dose ranging study of

fluticasone propionate aqueous nasal spray for seasonal allergic rhinitis assessed by symptoms, rhinomanometry and nasal cytology. J Allergy Clin Immunol 86:221, 1990.

81. Lans D, et al: Nasal eosinophilia in allergic and non-allergic rhinitis: usefulness of the nasal smear in the diagnosis of allergic rhinitis. Allergy Proc 10:275, 1989.

82. Miller R, et al: The nasal smear for eosinophils. Am J Dis Child 136:1009, 1982.

83. Meltzer EO, Orgel HA, and Jalowayski A: Cytology. In: Allergic and Non-allergic Rhinitis: Clinical Aspects. Edited by Naclerio RM and Mygind NM. Copenhagen, Munksgaard, 1993.

84. Mullan Key MF, Hill JS, and Webb DR: Allergic and nonallergic rhinitis: their characterization with attention to the meaning of nasal eosinophilia. J Allergy Clin Immunol 65:122, 1980.

85. Kniest FM, et al: Clinical evaluation of a double-blind dust-mite avoidance trial with mite-allergic rhinitic patients. Clin Exp Allergy 21:39, 1991.

86. De Blay F, Chapman MD, and Platts Mills TAE: Airborne cat allergen (Fel d I): Environmental control with cat in situ. Am Rev Respir Dis 143:1334, 1991.

87. Reisman RE, et al: A double blind study of the effectiveness of a high-efficiency particulate air filter in the treatment of patients with perennial allergic rhinitis and asthma. J Allergy Clin Immunol 85:1050, 1990.

88. Drovin MA: H1 antihistamines: perspective on the use of conventional and new agents. Ann Allergy 55:797, 1985.

89. Togias AG, et al: Demonstration of inhibition of mediator release from human mast cells by azatadine base: In vivo and in vitro evaluation. JAMA 255:225, 1986.

90. Naclerio RM, et al: Terfenadine, an H1 antihistamine, inhibits histamine release in vivo in man. Am Rev Respir Dis 142:167, 1990.

91. Naclerio RM, et al: The effect of cetirizine on early allergic response. Laryngoscope 99:596, 1989.

92. Simons FER and Simons KJ: Antihistamines. In: Allergy: Principles and Practice. Edited by Middleton EJ Jr, et al. St Louis, Mosby-Year Book, 1993.

93. Sohoel P, et al: Topical levocabastine compared with orally administered terfenadine for the prophylaxis and treatment of seasonal rhinoconjunctivitis. J Allergy Clin Immunol 92:73, 1993.

94. Simons F, McMillan J, and Simons K: A double-blind, single dose, cross over comparison of cetirizine, terfenadine, loratadine, astemizole, and chlorpheniramine versus placebo: suppressive effects on histamine-induced wheal and flares during 24 hours in normal subjects. J Allergy Clin Immunol 86:540, 1990.

95. Majchel AM, et al: Evaluation of a bedtime dose of a combination antihistamine/analgesic/decongestant product on antigen challenge the next morning. Laryngoscope 102:330, 1992.

96. Lacroix J: Adrenergic and non-adrenergic mechanisms in the sympathetic vascular control of the nasal mucosa. Acta Physiol Scand 136:1, 1989.

97. Compendium of Pharmaceuticals and Specialties. 29th Ed. Toronto, CK Productions, 1994.

98. Orie N, Booij-Nord H, and Pelikan Z: Protective effect of disodium cromoglycate on nasal and bronchial reactions after allergen challenge. In: Disodium Cromoglycate in Airways Disease. Edited by Pepys J and Frankland A. London, Butterworth, 1970.

99. Lindsay-Miller A and Chambers A: Group comparative trial of cromolyn sodium and terfenadine in the treatment of seasonal allergic rhinitis. Ann Allergy 58:23, 1987.

100. Coffman DA: A controlled trial of disodium cromoglycate in seasonal allergic rhinitis. Br J Clin Pract 25:403, 1971.

101. Corrado OJ, et al: The effect of nedocromil sodium on nasal provocation with allergen. J Allergy Clin Immunol 80:218, 1987.

102. Donnelly MA and Casale TB: Nedocromil sodium is rapidly effective in the therapy of seasonal allergic rhinitis. J Allergy Clin Immunol 91:997, 1993.

103. Bellioni P, Salvinelli F, Patalano F, and Ruggieri F: A double-blind group comparative study of nedocromil sodium in the treatment of seasonal allergic rhinitis. Rhinology 26:281, 1988.

104. Schuller DE, et al: A multicenter trial of nedocromil sodium, 1% nasal solution, compared with cromolyn sodium and placebo in ragweed seasonal allergic rhinitis. J Allergy Clin Immunol 86:554, 1990.

105. Ruhno J, Denburg J, and Dolovich J: Intranasal nedocromil sodium in the treatment of ragweed allergic rhinitis. J Allergy Clin Immunol 81:570, 1988.

106. Borum P, Larsen FS, and Mygind N: Nasal methacholine provocation and ipratropium therapy of perennial rhinitis. Acta Otolaryngol Suppl 360:35, 1979.

107. Mygind N and Borum P: Anticholinergic treatment of watery rhinorrhea. Am J Rhinol 4:1, 1990.

108. Østberg B, Winther B, and Mygind N: Cold air-induced rhinorrhea and high-dose ipratropium. Arch Otolaryngol 113:160, 1987.

109. Schleimer R: Glucocorticosteroids: their mechanisms of activation and use in allergic diseases. In: Allergy: Principles and Practice. Edited by Middleton EJ Jr, et al. St Louis, Mosby-Year Book, 1993.

110. Cox G, et al: Promotion of eosinophil survival by human bronchial epithelial cells and its modulation by steroids. Am J Respir Cell Mol Biol 4:525, 1991.

111. Pipkorn U, et al: Inhibition of mediator release in allergic rhinitis by pretreatment with topical glucocorticosteroids. N Engl J Med 316:1506, 1987.

112. Naclerio RM, et al: Intranasal steroids inhibit seasonal increases in ragweed-specific Immunoglobulin E antibodies. J Allergy Clin Immunol 92:717, 1993.

113. Bende M, Lindqvist N, and Pipkorn U: Effect of a topical glucocorticoid, budesonide, on nasal mucosal blood flow as measured with ^{133}Xe wash-out technique. Allergy 38:461, 1983.

114. Juniper EF, Guyatt GH, O'Byrne PM, and Vivieros M: Aqueous beclomethasone dipropionate nasal spray: regular versus "as required" use in the treatment of seasonal allergic rhinitis. J Allergy Clin Immunol 86:380, 1990.

115. Bryson H and Faulds D: Intranasal fluticasone propionate: a review of its pharmacodynamic and pharmacokinetic properties, and therapeutic potential in allergic rhinitis. Drugs 43:760, 1992.

116. Naclerio RM and Mygind N: Intranasal steroids. In: Allergic and Non-allergic Rhinitis: Clinical Aspects. Edited by Mygind NM and Naclerio RM. Copenhagen, Munksgaard, 1993.

117. Soderberg-Warner M: Nasal septal perforation associated with topical corticosteroid therapy. J Pediatr 105:840, 1984.

118. Sahay JN, et al: Long-term study of flunisolide treatment in perennial rhinitis with special reference to nasal mucosal histology and morphology. Clin Allergy 10:451, 1980.

119. Orgel H, Meltzer E, and Bierman W: Intranasal fluorocortin butyl in patients with perennial rhinitis: a 12 month efficacy and safety study including nasal biopsy. J Allergy Clin Immunol 88:257, 1991.

120. Klemi PJ, Virolainen E, and Puhakka H: The effect of intranasal beclomethasone dipropionate on the nasal mucosa. Rhinology 18:19, 1980.

121. Sorenson H, Mygind N, Pedersen C, and Prytz S: Long term treatment of nasal polyps with beclomethasone dipropionate aerosol. III. Morphological studies and conclusions. Acta Otolaryngol (Stockh) 182:260, 1976.

122. Norman PS, Winkerwerder WL, Agbayon BF, and Migeon CJ: Adrenal function during the use of dexamethasone aerosols in the treatment of ragweed hay fever. J Allergy Clin Immunol 40:57, 1967.

123. Frauenfelder F and Myer S: Posterior subcapsular cataracts associated with nasal or inhalational steroids. Am J Ophthalmol 109:489, 1990.

124. Wolthers O and Pedersen S: Growth of asthmatic children during treatment with budesonide: a double blind trial. Br Med J 303:163, 1991.

125. Beswick K, Kenyon G, and Cherry J: A comparative study of beclomethasone dipropionate aqueous nasal spray with terfenadine tablets in seasonal allergic rhinitis. Curr Med Res Opin 9:560, 1985.

126. Juniper E, et al: Comparison of beclomethasone dipropionate aqueous nasal spray, astemizole, and the combination in the prophylactic treatment of allergen-induced rhinoconjunctivitis. J Allergy Clin Immunol 83:627, 1989.

127. Juniper E, Kline P, Ramsdale E, and Hargreave FE: Comparison of efficacy and side effects of aqueous steroid nasal spray (budesonide) and allergen injection therapy (Pollinex-R) in the treatment of seasonal allergic rhinoconjunctivitis. J Allergy Clin Immunol 85:606, 1990.

128. Mygind N: Glucocorticosteroids and rhinitis. Allergy 48:476, 1993.

129. Borum P, Grøndberg H, and Mygind N: Seasonal allergic rhinitis and depot injection of a corticosteroid. Allergy 42:26, 1987.

130. Mabry R: Intranasal corticosteroid injection: indications, technique and complications. Otolaryngol Head Neck Surg 87:207, 1979.

131. Creticos PS, et al: Responses to ragweed-pollen nasal challenge before and after immunotherapy. J Allergy Clin Immunol 84:197, 1989.

132. Bousquet J, et al: Differences in clinical and immunologic reactivity of patients allergic to grass pollens and to multiple pollen species. J Allergy Clin Immunol 88:43, 1991.

133. Brunet C, et al: Allergic rhinitis to ragweed pollen. II. Modulation of histamine-releasing factor production by specific immunotherapy. J Allergy Clin Immunol 89:87, 1992.

134. Platt-Mills T, et al: IgA and IgG anti-ragweed antibodies in nasal secretions. J Clin Invest 57:1041, 1976.

135. Creticos PS, Van Metre TE, and Mardiney MR: Dose response of IgE and IgG antibodies during ragweed immunotherapy. J Allergy Clin Immunol 73:94, 1984.

136. Rocklin RE, Sheffer AL, Greineder DK, and Melmon DK: Generation of antigen-specific suppressor cells during allergy desensitization. N Engl J Med 302:1213, 1980.

137. Hsieh K-H: Altered interleukin-2 (IL-2) production and responsiveness after hyposensitization to house dust. J Allergy Clin Immunol 76:188, 1985.

138. Iliopoulus O, et al: Effects of immunotherapy on the early, late and rechallenge nasal reaction to provocation with allergen: changes in inflammatory mediators and cells. J Allergy Clin Immunol 87:855, 1991.

139. Furin MJ, et al: Immunotherapy decreases antigen-induced eosinophil cell migration into the nasal cavity. J Allergy Clin Immunol 88:27, 1991.

140. Majchel AM, et al: The nasal response to histamine challenge—effect of the pollen season and immunotherapy. J Allergy Clin Immunol 90:85, 1992.

141. Van Metre T and Adkinson FN: Immunotherapy for aeroallergen disease. In: Allergy: Principles and Practice. Edited by Middleton EJ Jr, et al. St Louis, Mosby-Year Book, 1993.

142. Reid MJ, Lockey RF, Turkeltaub PC, and Platts-Mills TAE: Survey of fatalities from skin testing and immunotherapy 1985–1989. J Allergy Clin Immunol 92:6, 1993.

143. Kay A: Allergen injection immunotherapy (hyposensitization) on trial. Clin Exp Allergy 19:591, 1989.

144. Mabry R: Rhinitis of pregnancy. South Med J 79:965, 1986.

145. Toppozada H, Michaels L, and El-Ghazzourri I: The human respiratory nasal mucosa in pregnancy. J Laryngol Otol 96:613, 1982.

146. Schatz M, et al: The course and management of asthma and allergic diseases in pregnancy. In: Allergy: Principles and Practice. 4th Ed. Edited by Middleton EJ Jr, et al. St Louis, Mosby-Year Book, 1993.

147. Aselton P, et al: First trimester drug use and congenital disorders. Obstet Gynecol 65:451, 1985.

148. Stammberger H: Endoscopic endonasal surgery-concepts in treatment of recurring rhinosinusitis. Part I. Anatomic and pathophysiologic considerations. Otolaryngol Head Neck Surg 94:143, 1986.

149. Konno A and Togawa K: Role of the vidian nerve in nasal allergy. Ann Otol Rhinol Laryngol 88:258, 1979.

9 Epistaxis, Septal Perforation, and Skin of the Face

John J. Ballenger

EPISTAXIS

Most patients developing epistaxis cope with the problem without recourse to a physician. Whereas anterior bleeding is more common in children and young adults, posterior bleeding is more common in older individuals. Wintertime living in heated homes where the air is dry seems to predispose to epistaxis. Some acute infectious diseases are characterized by nasal bleeding and are described in chapters that discuss the particular disease. Epistaxis is more common in vascular purpura, thrombocytopenic purpura, and diseases complicated by various coagulation defects. Anticoagulants, used in the treatment of some diseases, promote a tendency to bleed, and aspirin, in sensitive individuals, induces ease of bleeding. Epistaxis may follow sudden mechanical decompression (caisson's disease), extreme high altitude, and violent exercise.

The blood supply of the nose is discussed in Chapter 1. The nasal septal vessels (from which most bleeding occurs) lack a muscular coat, have no thick protecting mucosal cover, and, lying closely adjacent to the cartilage and bone, have only scant submucosa into which to retract and "self-seal." In caring for an epistaxis, the physician and assistants should immediately don a gown, face mask, eye protection, and rubber gloves to protect against blood-borne diseases. The next step is to gain rapport with the patient to assess the degree of blood loss more accurately and to ascertain the site of the bleeding. If the patient has undergone trauma, the airway must be considered. With the patient in a semisitting position, the patient can be more cooperative because blood does not run down the throat as frequently.

Anterior bleeding frequently arises in the anteroinferior part of the septum where branches of the anterior ethmoid, sphenopalatine, and superior labial arteries anastomose—known as Kiesselbach's plexus or Little's area. Posterior bleeding often arises behind the middle turbinate where the sphenopalatine artery enters the nose and courses down the septum. Severe posterior epistaxis in the elderly with cardiovascular problems is likely to arise from a branch of the sphenopalatine artery far posteriorly in the inferior meatus.

Most important in treatment of epistaxis is the use of rigid-tube spot suction and bright, shadow-free illumination to facilitate accurate location of the bleeding point. If it is from a readily accessible, relatively dry, small area, as is usual in anterior bleeding, it can be controlled by application of chemical cautery (e.g., 10% silver nitrate) to the bleeding point and surrounding area. Electrocautery is also an effective way, and, in this case, topical anesthesia may be desirable. The cautery tip is heated to cherry redness and the bleeding vessel lightly singed until the outlines have disappeared. Deep cautery may result in septal perforation. Electrodesiccation is preferable but requires a combination suction-desiccation unit to provide a dry field.

If the bleeding is vigorous and the location uncertain, general packing of the nose, preceded by topical anesthesia, with half-inch petrolatum gauze is necessary. The gauze is first inserted well above the posterior end of the middle turbinate and, working forward and downward, the entire nasal space is filled, yet leaving space on the opposite side for breathing. For comfort the gauze should not be allowed to enter the nasopharynx. The pack may be left in place for 3 to 4 days, and antibiotic coverage is prudent.

A posterior pack frequently is used to control posterior epistaxis or, in some cases, to enhance an ineffective anterior pack. This can be accomplished by a No. 16 or 18 Foley catheter, passed through the nose, and, after inflation, pulled anteriorly so it rests against the vomer and sphenoid rostrum. Forward traction must be maintained by a clamp or tape. Gottschalk has devised a more effective balloon.[1]

Another way of packing the nasopharynx is to fashion a gauze roll approximately 3 × 5 cm. A long suture is tied around the pack, leaving two long, dangling ends. A small rubber catheter is passed through the bleeding side of the nose, brought out through the mouth, and attached to one of the suture ends. The catheter is then withdrawn, along with the suture, and the pack is positioned in the nasopharynx. The suture is secured to the patient's cheek to maintain the position of the pack. The second suture, allowed to dangle in the pharynx, is useful when the pack is removed.

Tight occlusive packing of the nose carries the danger, particularly if used in patients with marginal cardiovascular and pulmonary disease, of a decreased arterial oxygen tension with little change in the carbon dioxide.[2] In addition, the total airway resistance may be increased. The toxic shock syndrome has been reported with occusive nasal packing.

Ligation of the vascular supply, near the bleeding point, may be required if other methods fail. The approach to the sphenopalatine artery is most readily done via the maxillary sinus. After gaining entry to the sinus by a Caldwell-Luc procedure, the posterior, mediosuperior wall is removed to expose the pterygopalatine fat where the artery is found, usually coursing horizontally, at the level of the posterior end of the middle turbinate. It is doubly clipped as near the sphenopalatine foramen as convenient. Intraoral ligation of the maxillary artery has been proposed by Stepnick and associates.[3]

The anterior ethmoid artery is approached through an incision medial to the inner canthus of the eye on the bleeding side. The periosteum is elevated, beginning posterior to the lacrimal bone, until the vessel is found at a depth of 3 to 4 cm. It is doubly ligated with a clip or suture. Further posterior is the posterior ethmoid, but its ligation adds little.

OSLER-WEBER-RENDU DISEASE

This is a hereditary, autosomnal dominant, hemorrhagic telangiectasia that occurs throughout the aerogastrointestinal tract but is particularly obvious in the mucosa of the nose, the inner surface of the lips, gingiva, buccal mucosa, palate, tongue, conjunctivae, and skin of the face. The sexes are affected equally. The arterioles, venules, and capillaries form into small, nonpulsating, 1- to 3-mm angiomas where even slight trauma leads to bleeding. The pathologic feature is loss of subendothelial structures, notably the muscle coat, of the blood vessels. Abnormal tests of platelet and bleeding times and factor VIII deficiencies are rarely encountered.

Treatment of the nasal bleeding in this disease, if primarily affecting the nose, is by replacing the mucosa with dermis. The use of laser photocoagulation has also shown promising results.[4]

PERFORATION OF THE NASAL SEPTUM

Most septal perforations, particularly in the adult, arise out of an operative procedure on the nasal septum, including primarily submucous septal resection or cautery of some sort. The septal cartilage depends on the covering mucosa for its blood supply, and thus, if the cartilage is bare the potential for perforation is present. In children, repeated digital trauma (nose picking) may be the cause. Syphilis, tuberculosis, Wegener's granuloma, typhoid, diphtheria, lupus erythematosus, tumors, sarcoidosis, and recreational sniffing of cocaine all may be accompanied by septal perforation. Prolonged exposure to industrial pollutants, particularly sulfuric acid fumes but also arsenicals, mercury, phosphorus, copper, and steroid sprays, may play a part.

Crusting of the margins of the perforation is commonplace and may give rise to a sensation of foreign body. If the crusts are forcefully removed, streaking of blood is common. As the air passes the perforation, it may give rise to a bothersome "whistling."

Prophylaxis requires that no septal cartilage be left uncovered by mucosa following a surgical procedure. Nonsurgical closure can be obtained with a "winged" Silastic button or grommet tailored to fit the perforation exactly and then inserted in such a fashion that it is held in place semipermanently by the wings on either side of the septum. Surgical closure is covered in Chapter 2.

LUPUS ERYTHEMATOSUS AND OTHER DISEASES AFFECTING THE FACE

Systemic lupus erythematosus (SLE) is a disease of probable immunologic origin. Affecting women more than men in a ratio of 9:1, it frequently is associated with arthritis and arthralgia. In 40 to 50%, a butterfly eruption over the nose and malar area occurs, consisting of erythema and edema in the acute stages and atrophy and telangiectasis in the chronic stage. Ulcers may be encountered in the nasal and oral mucosa. Laryngeal lupus may occur. Positive tests to antinuclear antibodies are essential for the diagnosis. Corticosteroids are useful in the treatment.

Lupus vulgaris is likely an attenuated form of tuberculosis and frequently appears as firm, discrete nodules that coalesce and ulcerate in and around the nasal orifice. The disease readily attacks cartilage but not bone.

Leprosy, or Hansen's disease, caused by Mycobacterium leprae, can be acquired by prolonged, intimate contact with a leper. Lepromatous leprosy is characterized by extensive skin lesions in the form of macules, papules, and nodules of the cheeks, nose, eyebrows, ears, and forehead. Eventually, the skin becomes thickened and corrugated to produce the so-called lionine facies. The lesions may be intranasal and may cause considerable obstruction. Dapsone, rifampin, and clofazimine are useful in treatment.

Glanders and actinomycosis occasionally cause facial lesions, the former as purulent nodules appearing in either the skin or the mucosa of the nose, depending on the site of infection. The cervicofacial area is the site in 50% of the cases of actinomycosis. The lesion is a nontender, reddish-purple, indurated area. Draining tracts may be present.

BENIGN SKIN LESIONS OF THE FACE

Warts, benign lesions that are caused by the human papilloma virus, can occur anywhere on the skin of the face and neck. They may be refractory to treatment, but the body usually recognizes them as "foreign" and develops an antibody.

The lesion of seborrheic keratosis is irregularly rounded, readily movable, brownish to black, slightly elevated but occasionally pedunculated, smooth to touch, sharply demarcated, painless, and often first appears in middle life. If removal is desirable for cosmetic considerations, it can be done by shave excision or local application of nitrogen freezing.

Solar Radiation

The ultraviolet (UV) radiation is arbitrarily divided into three catagories: C, B, and A. UV-C includes wavelengths shorter than 290 nm that do not reach the earth because of absorption by the stratosphere ozone. UV-B consists of wavelengths between 290 and 320 nm and is the likely cause of "sunburn and tanning" and "aging" of the skin following repeated acute exposures to the sun. Following long-term exposure, UV-B is considered to be involved in the initiation, promotion, and conversion of benign precursors in the skin into malignant lesions, a process likely requiring additional genetic alterations in already transformed cells. Likely UV-2 immunologically compromises the capability of the skin to reject cancer cells. UV-A (wavelengths between 400 and 700 nm) is much less efficient in inducing skin damage.

Sunscreens (para-aminobenzoic acid), applied to the skin, have the potential to protect against UV-B and, to a less extent, UV-A (acute sunburn reactions), but protection against carcinogenic effects and alterations of DNA is not clear. The presumed efficiency is given by the SPF (sun protective factor) number.

Actinic Keratosis

Clinically, actinic keratosis (senile or solar keratosis) is a flat, reddened, slightly rough area that fades into the adjacent skin, rather than possessing a sharply defined border. Some studies indicate that 5 to 20% of persistently invoked actinic keratoses develop basal or squamous cell carcinoma. Signs of developing malignancy are elevation of the lesion, ulceration, recent enlargement, or other sudden change.

Keratoacanthoma is a rapidly growing benign tumor derived from hair follicles. It occurs most commonly in the elderly on sun-exposed areas. Microscopy reveals a keratin-filled crater, surrounded by strands of epidermis, that grows rapidly for 6 to 8 weeks to a size of 1 to 2.5 cm, and it generally involutes in about 6 months. Malignant transformation is unlikely. Treatment usually is surgical.

Bowen's disease, occurring in sun-exposed or covered skin, is an irregular, scaly, dull red patch that spreads by peripheral extension. Histology reveals an intraepidermal squamous cell carcinoma with an intact basal layer.

Nevi

Congenital nevi are present at birth, whereas the more common "acquired" nevi are typically first noted at puberty. The risk of malignant change in the former is about 4%. A nevus may be junctional, intradermal, or a combination of the two. The first named is a benign, nonpalpable, tan to brownish macule with uniform color of 1 cm or more in size. By definition, the nevus cells in dermal nevi are all within the dermis (the common mole) and, in addition, may contain coarse hair. The mole may be flat or raised and warty, pigmented or skin color, sessile or pedunculated. Treatment, if desired, is by shave excision if pedunculated and hairless and by deep excision in other suspicious lesions.

Lentigo senilis, also known as a liver spot, is found on the skin of the face and dorsum of the hands, particularly in elderly persons. These lesions do not derive from nevocytes or melanocytes. They are smooth, noninfiltrating, uniformly dark brown, irregular in outline, and from a few millimeters to 1 to 2 cm in outline. They do not undergo malignant degeneration. Treatment of these lesions with topical 0.1% tretinoin has been encouraging.

ROSACEA AND RHINOPHYMA

Rosacea, a chronic hyperemic disease of the "flush" areas of the skin of the face, is characterized by telangiectasis and persistent erythema. It tends to occur in women between the ages of 30 and 50 and is largely limited to the middle third of the face, but the more severe manifestations, rhinophyma, are found only in men. Patients with rosacea often have acute episodes of edema, papules, and pustules. The skin may be oily.

Rhinophyma is usually limited to the lower half of the face but spares the configuration of the margin of the lower lateral cartilage. It may involve distortion of the cheeks (buccalphyma) or ears (otophyma). Although the presence of the mite, Demodex folliculorum, in the depths of the skin creases is commonplace, it is not considered to be the cause.

Histologically, rhinophyma is a benign hypertrophy and hyperplasia of the sebaceous glands and ducts, telangiectasis, and inflammatory cell infiltration into the skin.

No definite, effective medical treatment for rosacea exists, but it is well to avoid factors that contribute to facial flushing and vasodilation. The acneiform elements respond to topical applications of antibiotics and to tetracycline systemically.

Disfiguring rhinophyma is usually best treated by surgical removal of excess tissue by sharp dissection, electrosurgery, or the laser. The pathologic tissue is removed down to but not exposing the cartilage or bone, (called decortication) and then regrowth of epithelium recurs from the numerous remaining skin follicles. If the nasal cartilages are injured, skin grafts should be used to cover them. Dermabrasion may be useful in the final contouring of the nose. A rim of untouched skin should be left around the free margin of the anterior nares, if possible, to avoid a cicatricial contracture.

MALIGNANT TUMORS OF THE FACE

Malignant melanomas arise from melanocytes. If recognized early and well treated, the outlook is good. They commonly arise from existing nevi but may arise de novo; they appear more frequently in men (1.5:1) and in individuals with a fair complexion. The incidence of melanoma is higher in areas of intense sunlight, and solar radiation is considered to a cocarcinogen. Other causative agents include ionizing radiation, genetic susceptibility, arsenic, and other environmental hazards. The incidence increased 80% between 1973 and 1980.

The borders of a melanoma, as compared with a nevus, are irregular, scalloped, poorly demarcated, roughened, and nodular. The color displays shades of red, white, and blue. In general, if a stable mole or nevus changes in color, size, border, or surface characteristics, biopsy is indicated. The depth of invasion of the melanoma is the most important predictive feature.

Malignant melanomas can be divided into three types. Hutchinson's freckle is a premalignant, spreading, macular, pigmentation with grossly irregular borders that occurs most commonly on the skin of the temple or malar regions in elderly patients. The development of a noticeable, thickened, elevated nodule

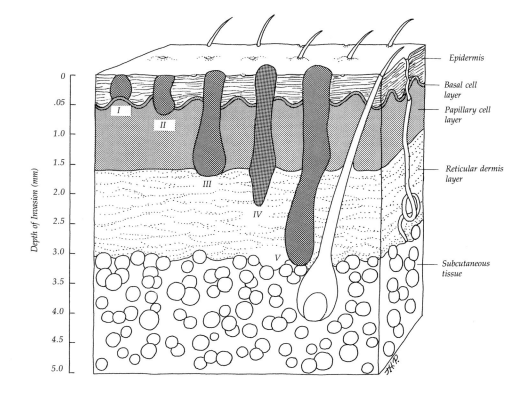

Fig. 9–1. Schematic representation of depths of invasion of cutaneous melanoma, described by Clark (Roman numerals) and depth in millimeters (Breslow).

within the freckle may indicate degeneration into lentigo maligna melanoma (Fig. 9–1).

Superficial spreading melanoma, the second type, comprises about 75% of the total. The major features are a spreading pigmentation containing a variety of colors ranging from tan-black and blue-gray to pink. Eventually, ulceration and bleeding herald dermal invasion.

Nodular melanomas are the most invasive and constitute 7 to 8% of the total. They present as blue-black nodules that bleed easily and grow rapidly. Melanomas metastasize via the lymphatic system.

The depth of invasion of the melanoma is the most important parameter in treatment.[5] For localized lesions of less than 0.75 mm in thickness (Clark I and II) (Fig. 9–1), the 5-year survival after adequate excision should exceed 90%, with a rapid decline of this figure as the lesion penetrates more deeply. Lesions penetrating more than 1.5 mm require an elective neck dissection. In the future, stimulation of the immune system may be an important adjunct to treatment.

Squamous cell carcinoma is less common than melanoma, but both seem to respond to many of the same etiologic factors. Bowen's disease, a variant of a usually noninvasive squamous cell carcinoma, is found more frequently in association with ingestion of arsenic. Total cumulative lifetime exposure to the sun seems to bear a direct relation to the development of squamous cell carcinoma. Actinically induced squamous cell carcinomas are associated with a low (less than 1%) incidence of metastasis, whereas the figure for nonsolar lesions is 2 to 3%.

A squamous cell carcinoma is frequently found in the sun-exposed areas of skin as a slow growing, hyperkeratotic, scaly, elevated patch. The lesion may be ulcerated, with a rolled border, or vegetative and nodular, and at times pigmented so as to make it difficult to distinguish from a basal cell tumor. Any change in size, nodularity, or color should arouse suspicion of a malignant process.

Treatment of both squamous and basal cell carcinomas of the face and neck can be done by several methods and, when well done, should provide 5-year disease-free states of more than 90%. These methods include electrodesiccation (fulgeration), excision, cryosurgery, radiation therapy, and Mohs' surgery.[6]

Basal cell carcinoma or "rodent ulcer" is a common malignant tumor in humans and one of the most successfully treated if done early when still localized. Many studies indicate that excessive exposure to sunlight is a primary factor in its origin, but genetic predisposition and carcinogens such as tars, arsenic, and ionizing radiation play a part. Suspicion of a "rodent ulcer" should be aroused by a painless, enlarging, pruritic, non-healing, scaly nodule on the face or neck that forms a plaque and seems to be developing a centrally located ulcer. The tumor may slowly extend after being stationary for years. Those that grow downward, rather than vertically upward or horizontally, are difficult to treat and metastasize more frequently.

Histopathologic examination reveals collections of cells with dark-staining nuclei and scant cytoplasm. Some of the cell masses seem to resemble basal layers of the epidermis.

Treatment is by complete surgical excision, destruction by electrodesiccation, radiation therapy, or Mohs' technique, all with an adequate margin of normal tissue monitored by histopathologic examination. Recurrent basal cell carcinomas are more difficult to treat.

SUGGESTED READINGS

1. Gottschalk GH: Epistaxis and the nasostat. J Am Coll Emerg Physicians 5:793, 1976.
2. Cassisi NJ: Changes in arterial oxygen tension and pulmonary mechanics with use of posterior packing in epistaxis. Laryngoscope 81:1261, 1971.
3. Stepnick DW, et al: Intraoral-extramaxillary approach for ligation of the maxillary artery. Laryngoscope 100:1166, 1990.
4. Parkin JL and Dixon JA: Laser photocoagulation in hereditary hemorrhagic telangiectasis. Otolaryngol Head Neck Surg 89:204, 1981.
5. Wolf GT and Sullivan MJ: Management of head and neck melanoma. In: Otolaryngology: Head and Neck Surgery. Edited by Cummings CW, et al. St. Louis, CV Mosby, 1993.
6. Swanson NA and Johnson TM: Management of basal and squamous cell carcinoma. In: Otolaryngology: Head and Neck Surgery. Edited by Cummings CW, et al. St. Louis, CV Mosby, 1993.

10 Headache and Neuralgia of the Face

John J. Ballenger

Headache ranks ninth among complaints that lead patients to a physician's office. Most are either migraine or so-called tension headaches. Table 10–1 is a simplified classification of this disorder.

ORIGIN OF HEAD PAIN

With the exception of the slightly pain-sensitive periosteum of the skull, all extracranial structures covering the head are pain-sensitive. Of particular importance are the scalp, fascia, and muscles of the head and neck, the orbital contents, the external and middle ear, and the mucosa of the upper respiratory tract and of the paranasal sinuses, particularly near the ostia. Pain originating in the conchae or paranasal sinuses is frequently referred by the first and second divisions of the fifth cranial nerve (CN V).

Structures sensitive to painful stimuli include the skin of the scalp and its appendages and the caliber of the blood vessels, the cerebral and other intracranial arteries, the great venous sinuses and their tributaries, parts of the dura at the base of the brain, the dural arteries, the CN V, CN VI, and CN VII, and the upper three cervical nerves. Insensitive to pain are the brain parenchyma, most of the pia and dura mater, the ependymal lining of the ventricles, the choroid plexus, and the cranium.

Generally, head pain located anterior to a vertical plane through the external auditory meatus, if from an intracranial source, is transmitted by one or more branches of CN V, has its origin above the tentorium cerebelli, and is appreciated by the patient in the frontal, temporal, and parietal regions of the head. Head pain originating posterior to this plane is carried chiefly by the CN X, but also by the ninth, eleventh, and upper three cervical nerves; it has its origin below the tentorium and is referred to the occipital regions of the head. When the headache is clearly localized

behind one ear, homolateral acoustic neuromas and cerebellopontine angle tumors must be considered.

PATHOPHYSIOLOGY OF HEADACHE

Extracranial mechanisms in the generation of a headache include distension of cranial arteries, sustained muscle contraction about the face, scalp, and upper neck muscles (particularly near the occiput), various disease processes of the eyes, ears, teeth, nose, and paranasal sinuses, the cranial neuralgias, nonspecific inflammations of the cranial arteries, and pain incident to injury and tumors. The majority of extracranial headaches are thought to arise from either distension of arteries ("vascular headache") or sustained scalp or neck muscle contraction ("tension headache"). Vasoconstriction of an intracranial vessel may occur preceding an attack, but its reference to an aura is uncertain. If the vascular headache is remittent, it is termed a migraine headache; if nonrecurrent, it frequently is associated with fever and systemic infection (toxic headache). Also associated with nonrecurrent vasodilating head pain are hypoxic states, carbon monoxide poisoning, vasodilating chemical agents, caffeine withdrawal, postconcussion and postconvulsive states, "hangover" reactions, hypoglycemia, hypercapnia, acute pressor reactions, oral contraceptives, and foods containing sodium nitrate, monosodium glutamate, or tyramine. This list could be extended.

Harold Wolff considered migraine to be a vascular problem in which a reduction of regional cerebral blood flow (rCBF) occurred during the aura of migraine headaches, followed by a hyperemic phase in which extracranial vasodilation caused the pulsating headache.[1] Other studies have suggested that the explanation is more complicated.[2] Sequential flow measurements performed before, during, and after a classic migraine attack demonstrated only a mild reduction

TABLE 10–1. Classification of Headache and Facial Neuralgia

Migraine-type
    Classic
    Common
    Complicated
    Toxic vascular
    Hypertensive
Cluster
Tension-type
Traction
Post-traumatic
Temporal neuritis
Neuralgia of Face and Head
    Trigeminal neuraligia
    Glossopharyngeal neuralgia
    Paratrigeminal neuralgia
    Pterygopalatine neuralgia
Temporomandibular joint syndrome

in cerebral flow (oligemia) beginning in the parietal-occipital region and gradually spreading anteriorly to involve the entire hemisphere and lasting throughout the aura and headache phases.[3] This suggests correlation of the spreading metabolic (neuronal) depression during migraine of Leao in animals,[4] and it implies an instability of the cortical blood supply. Other studies suggest that a cerebral hyperemia follows the oligemia.[5] Olsen and associates question whether the variations in the vasospasm cause the differing symptoms.[6,7]

Cephalic blood vessels contain afferent fibers emanating from the trigeminal ganglion that transmits nociceptive impulses, and a hypothesis based on this information has been proposed. Serotonin (5-hydroxytryptamine, 5-HT) is believed to play a role: drugs that deplete brain 5-HT provoke migraine, and 5-HT agonists relieve migraine. Sumatriptan, a 5-HT agonist, also is being studied.

Migraine is likely a disease of cerebral hemodynamics involving many vessels and affecting neurogenic, chemical, metabolic, and myogenic factors. The final explanation is yet to be developed.

Vascular headaches of the migraine types are characterized by recurrent episodes of throbbing head pain, at least at the outset.[8] Occipital neuralgia is likely caused by dilation of the postauricular and occipital arteries. Distension of the extracranial portion of the middle meningeal and internal maxillary may lead to Sluder's "lower half headache." Also included in the vasodilating group are cluster headaches.

In addition to the instability of the cerebral circulation, the principal intracranial mechanisms that may lead to a head pain include inflammation or irritation of the pain-sensitive structures of the head or portions of the dura and pia at the base of the skull, direct pressure on a pain-sensitive nerve or structure, traction or displacement of the pain-sensitive arteries, including the middle meningeal, and traction on or displacement of the veins that are tributary to the venous sinuses from the surface of the brain. Studies of the endogenous opiates suggest a possible lessened ability of the migraineur to mobilize the body's pain control mechanism.[9]

"Complicated" migraine headaches are associated with prolonged focal neurologic symptoms such as numbness of the face or hand, difficulty in speech or writing, hemiplegia, and ophthalmoplegia.

Hypertensive headaches are not common, and when they do occur they usually are associated with encephalopathy.

Pseudotumor cerebri (benign intracranial hypertension) is a disorder in which increased intracranial pressure is present but intracranial masses, infection, and hypertensive encephalopathy are excluded. The cerebrospinal fluid is unremarkable except for the elevated pressure, and cerebral function is good. The patient usually presents with a generalized headache made worse by coughing, with blurred vision and papilledema. It is associated with endocrine and metabolic disorders.

Recurrent headaches are not a symptom of unruptured aneurysms. The headache produced by leaks of blood from an aneurysm or the occurrence of a subarachnoid hemorrhage may be abrupt and severe. Brief headaches may be associated with temporary ischemic attacks (TIAs). Traumatic headaches are discussed later in this chapter.

MIGRAINE HEADACHE

A migraine headache is probably hereditary, neurogenic, vasomotor, pulsatile, unilateral or bilateral, recurrent cephalgia of some hours' duration, with virtually complete freedom from headache between attacks.

Classic migraine usually begins in childhood, adolescence, or early adult life and recurs with decreasing frequency in later years. Women are more frequently afflicted and seem to be genetic carriers. It may be introduced by an aura consisting of scotomata, hemianopsia, speech defects, paresthesia, or other neurologic defects that subside in 30 or more minutes (and may overlap the headache) and is followed abruptly by the headache, which may last for 6 to 8 or more hours. The headache is typically pounding and located unilaterally in the temple, forehead, or aural areas but may become generalized. It may be found on the side opposite to the visual defect. Nausea and vomiting may occur. After the headache has disappeared, the head pain can be replaced by other body disturbances known as "migraine equivalents."

Common migraine is considerably more common than classic. The aura is absent but the headache is more frequent and prolonged, often lasting days at a time, frequently present on awakening and intensifying as the day passes. A darkened, quiet room often relieves the pain. The headaches commonly appear first in the teens and increase in frequency over the years. A majority of women with migraine experience relief to some degree during pregnancy. Many women develop migraine for the first time after beginning the use of oral contraceptives.

Disturbance of water metabolism is frequently a concomitant symptom. Before and during an attack the face and eyelids become edematous, and a watery nasal discharge and lacrimation may occur. Weight loss occurs after the attack. Attacks may be precipitated by missed sleep, stress, or foods rich in tyramine, sodium nitrite, or phenylethylamine. Excess intake of alcohol may play a part.

Basilar migraine consists of vertigo and tinnitus, bilateral visual blurring, diplopia, dysarthria, unsteadiness, paresthesias, and occasionally loss of consciousness. The presumed cause is functional disturbances of the posterior cerebral circulation.

Ophthalmoplegic and hemiplegic migraine are uncommon. Onset of the former is usually in childhood after the history of periodic headaches is well established. The oculomotor nerve is almost always involved, giving rise to ptosis, muscle weakness, and pupillary changes. Symptoms may last for days.

Treatment

A discussion of the nature of migraine should be had with the patient and reassurance provided. Nonspecific factors such as fatigue, alcohol use, dietary indiscretion, depression, and stress should be removed from the patient's life. Potential allergies should be investigated and allergens removed if possible.

The most widely used drug for the treatment of disabling migraine is ergotamine tartrate, with or without caffeine, belladonna, or barbituates, taken orally, rectally, or intramuscularly. Ergonovine maleate, an amine derivative of ergot, is useful for prophylaxis. All ergot preparations should be withdrawn occasionally to prevent ergotism. Sumatriptan has been used successfully for the treatment of migraine headache, but it must be used cautiously if cardiac function is compromised significantly.[10]

CLUSTER HEADACHE

A variety of vasodilating pain, cluster headache (Horton's cephalgia or histamine cephalgia), is less common than migraine, but the pain is more severe and there is no aura. The disorder begins in the third or fourth decade but does not become well established until middle age. The attacks come in clusters of one to several each day or night for a period of a week or more, and then symptom-free intervals of weeks or months follow. Men are afflicted more commonly than women.

Typically, an attack is in and about the eye or temple and occurs at the same time each night, waking the patient from the REM stage of sleep. It reaches a maximum intensity in 2 to 15 minutes and lasts 1 to 2 hours. Nasal congestion, coryza, lacrimation, flushing of the face, ptosis, and miosis may occur. Occasionally, the patient has an ipsilateral Horner's sign. Nausea and vomiting are absent. Cluster vertigo is known to occur. An attack may be precipitated by oral ingestion of alcohol or injection of histamine base. Mathew has proposed prophylaxis with oral use of ergotamine or intravenous administration of dihydroergotamine.[11] Some patients are improved by inhaling 100% oxygen. Lithium may be helpful. Sumatriptan injected subcutaneously during an attack is reported by some investigators to be helpful.[12]

TENSION HEADACHE

Considerable doubt exists that "tension" headache is caused by prolonged contraction of the scalp and posterior neck muscles. Heightened electromyographic activity of these muscles is found in approximate equal percentages of both control and patient groups. The headache is often, however, associated with conditions of emotional duress and worry. Perhaps vascular and tension headaches represent different degrees of severity of the same pathologic process.

The onset of tension headache is usually gradual. The headache is bilateral and may last weeks or months at a time. Its onset is usually in the middle years. The headache is frequently localized to the occipital-nuchal area, and usually it is constant, rather than throbbing.

Treatment of tension headache is nonspecific. The best modalities are explanation and reassurance, heat, massage, and the use of nonsteroidal anti-inflammatory medication. Biofeedback mechanisms to promote relaxation may yield benefit. Narcotic medication is rarely necessary.

TRACTION AND INFLAMMATORY HEADACHES

Traction headache results from traction, either direct or indirect, on pain-sensitive intracranial structures by tumors or masses. Headache that follows lumbar puncture is a traction headache. The loss of spinal fluid leads to intracranial hypotension, caudal displacement of the brain, and traction on the various pain-sensitive structures that anchor it to the cranium. Such postpuncture headaches are relieved by elevation of the pressure to normal and assumption of the horizontal position.

PARANASAL SINUS PAIN AND HEADACHE

If pain arises from the ear, nose, throat, and paranasal sinuses, other signs of infection are usually present. Probably not more than 10% of all headaches are caused by verifiable sinus disease. Head pain emanating from the frontal or maxillary sinuses is located over the sinus itself and that of an ethmoid or sphenoid sinus posterior to and between the eyes, with a tendency to refer to the vertex.[13] Sinus pain, if moderately severe, tends to be pulsatile and is made worse by conditions that increase the engorgement of the nasal and sinus mucosa. Sinal barotrauma or "vacuum sinusitis" is related to a history of flying or water diving.

The gravamen for pain in glaucoma is more the rate of increase of the intraocular pressure than the pressure itself and may range from self-limited ocular discomfort and blurred vision to excruciating pain with a rock-hard globe.

Uveitis is an inflammatory condition of the iris and ciliary body, usually associated with a deep-seated eye pain made worse by exposure to light. Examination reveals a perilimbal inflammation with a small pupil. In retrobulbar neuritis, the pain is mild to severe, worsened by eye movements and pressure on the globe, and usually precedes the advent of blurred vision. Orbital cellulitis, pseudotumor of the eye, and metastatic cancer in the orbit are all painful eye diseases.

Eye strain (asthenopia) or visual discomfort may occur with uncorrected astigmatism or presbyopia. Rarely, eye muscle imbalance leads to asthenopia.

TEMPOROMANDIBULAR JOINT SYNDROME (TMJS)

TMJS and myofascial pain dysfunction syndrome (MPDS) are closely related and incorrectly are called neuralgias. In the former, the patient usually has some malocclusion or improper positioning of the mandibular condyle within the glenoid fossa, but not infrequently there is pain in and around the joint with no demonstrable disorder. Innervation occurs from the auriculotemporal and masseteric nerves. The discomfort of MPDS arises from prolonged and painful contraction of the masticatory muscles, probably the source of the pain, and may be part of a tension headache. Bruxism plays a part.

Treatment is by correcting organic disease, if present, moist heat, joint rest, massage, muscle relaxant exercises, and biofeedback.

POST-TRAUMATIC HEADACHES

Headache frequently occurs in immediate post-trauma periods, but usually is gone in a week or so. Occasionally, however, an ill-defined dizziness and difficulty in concentration persists, perhaps explained by secondary scar formation. Evaluation should seek to uncover neurologic defects, and appropriate treatment should be offered.

TEMPORAL ARTERITIS

Temporal neuritis (giant cell neuritis) is marked by an intense cephalgia in the region supplied by the superficial temporal artery, although other vessels may also be involved. The walls of the vessel are edematous and palpable. Anorexia, fever, and intermittent jaw claudication may be present. The most dreaded complication is an irreversible blindness.

On histologic examination of the superficial temporal artery, necrosis of the vessel's media and fragmentation of the elastic lamina are found, along with macrophage infiltration and giant cell formation. Typically, the erythrocyte sedimentation rate (ESR) is elevated. Prednisone should begun at once, to avoid eye complications until the ESR has fallen and other signs have improved greatly. Resection of the diseased vessel may aid in the diagnosis as well as provide therapeutic benefit.

RAMSAY HUNT NEURALGIA

In this rarely encountered syndrome (also known as the geniculate ganglion syndrome or herpes zoster oticus), the herpes virus invades variously the geniculate ganglion or CN VII or CN VIII.

The most obvious symptom is an intense, boring ear pain that persists after disappearance of the associated vesicular eruption along the sensory cutaneous nerves of the external auditory canal and the concha. At times, perhaps by way of the sensory root of the nervus intermedius (Wrisberg), lesions are seen on the tonsils and in the nasopharynx. Herpes viral involvement of the geniculate ganglion can produce hyperacusis, facial paralysis, decrease in taste, and impairment of secretory functions.

POSTHERPETIC NEURALGIA

Herpes zoster virus is responsible for several neuralgias of the head and face. The same organism causes varicella and the intercostal neuralgia known as shingles. In herpetic neuralgia, the patient has an erythematous, maculopapular eruption in the distribution of the affected cranial nerves. Painful vesicles develop and become pustular. Long after the skin lesions disappear the pain persists (postherpetic neuralgia). The most commonly involved cranial nerve is the first division of the trigeminal. Such infections occur at age 45 to 50 years over half the time, and in 10 to 15% the lesions are on the face. The prognosis for complete recovery of a paralyzed fifth or seventh nerve in herpetic neuralgia is poor. Acyclovir has been shown to prevent the local spread of the virus but is less effective in lessening the postherpetic neuralgia. For otalgia, symptomatic treatment should be followed, although hydantoin and carbamazepine may help.

TRIGEMINAL NEURALGIA

Also known as "tic douloureux," this is a disorder of mainly the second and third divisions of CN V and the most common of the cranial neuralgias. The average age of onset is about 50 years. The cause is unknown. The incidence of multiple sclerosis among patients with trigeminal neuralgia is about 3%.

The pain is a severe, darting, lancinating pain of 10 to 30 seconds' duration along the course of one or more branches of CN V, but almost never crossing the midline. The frequency of attacks varies from a few times daily to a few times a month. The patient has no objective loss of motor or sensory function. Touching a so-called "trigger zone" incites the pain. These areas are usually located around the ala, upper lips, gums, and hard palate.

Treatment is usually symptomatic. Hydantoin, phenytoin, and carbamazepine may be of use.

GLOSSOPHARYNGEAL NEURALGIA

Except for location, the symptoms of this uncommon entity are similar to those of tic douloureux. Men are more affected than women, and the onset is most frequently in the fourth or fifth decades. The burning, stabbing pain occurs in paroxysms in the region of the tonsils, posterior pharynx, back of the tongue, and middle ear. It may occur spontaneously, but more often seems to be precipitated by swallowing, talking, or touching the tonsils or posterior pharynx. The attacks last for only a few seconds, and the frequency varies from many times daily to long remissions. Carbamazepine alone or in combination with phenytoin is effective.

PARATRIGEMINAL NEURALGIA (RAEDER'S SYNDROME)

The paratrigeminal space is a small area containing components of CN V, including the gasserian ganglion, CN III, CN IV, and the carotid artery. This uncommon neuralgia is characterized by retro-orbital pain, although sensation is intact. The pupil is dilated. On surgical exploration, an encroachment on the paratrigeminal area by blood vessels has occasionally been found.

PTERYGOPALATINE NEURALGIA

The pterygopalatine ganglion is parasympathetic in function and seems to be suspended from the maxillary nerve by two or three branches. The cause of this disorder is unknown. It occurs more frequently in women, usually between 20 and 50 years of age.

The clinical picture consists of nonpulsating pain around the eye, lower jaw, and teeth, extending to the zygoma and temple. It has been termed the "lower half" headache of Sluder. The patient seems to respond to local anesthesia of the ganglion, perhaps because of its effect on CN V.

SUGGESTED READINGS

1. Dalessio DJ (ed): Wolff's Headache and Other Head Pain. 6th Ed. New York, Oxford University Press, 1993.
2. Raskin NH: Headache. New York, Churchill Livingstone, 1988.
3. Olesen J, Larsen B, and Lauritzen M: Focal hyperemia followed by spreading oligemia and impaired activation of rCBF in classic migraine. Ann Neurol 9:344, 1981.
4. Leao AP: Spreading depression in activity in the cerebral cortex. J Neurophysiol 7:359, 1944.
5. Andersen AR, Friberg L, Olsen ST, and Olsen J: Delayed hyperemia following hypoperfusion in classic migraine. Arch Neurol 45:154, 1988.
6. Olsen ST, Friberg L, and Lassen NA: Ischemia may be the primary cause of the neurological deficits in classical migraine. Arch Neurol 44:156, 1987.
7. Olsen ST: Migraine with and without aura: the same disease due to cerebral vasospasm of different intensity. Headache 30: 269, 1990.
8. Dalessio DJ (ed): Wolff's Headache and Other Head Pain. 6th Ed. New York, Oxford University Press, 1993.
9. Ansemi B, Baldi E, Cassaci F, and Salman S: Endogenous opinoids in cerebrospinal fluids and blood in idiopathic headache sufferers. Headache 20:294, 1988.
10. Subcutaneous Sumatriptan International Study Group: Treatment of migraine attacks with sumatriptan. N Engl J Med 325: 316, 1991.
11. Mathew NT: Cluster headache. Neurology 42(suppl):22,1992.
12. Sumatriptan Cluster Study Group: Treatment of acute cluster headache with sumatriptan; Sumatriptan Cluster Study Group. N Engl J Med 325:322, 1991.
13. Levine H: Otorhinolaryngologic causes of head and facial pain. In: The Practicing Physician's Approach to Headache. Edited by Diamond S and Dalessio DL. Baltimore, Williams & Wilkins, 1992.

11 Paranasal Sinus Infections

James Dudley

Sinusitis can sometimes be a difficult entity to pin down; it can mean something different to otolaryngologists, primary care physicians, and the general public. Lay persons, for instance, often use the term "sinus" to describe any change from normal sensation in the sinus and nose area. They use this term to cover such symptoms as nasal stuffiness, fullness in the nose and sinus areas, and pain or discomfort in these same areas. Sometimes "sinus" is synonymous for them with what physicians term sinusitis. Physicians, presented with the same set of symptoms, may or may not make a similar presumptive diagnosis.

If physicians want to confirm their suspicions, they will order a paranasal sinus roentgenogram or computed tomography (CT). Physicians have always had a certain attachment to this kind of diagnostic study they believe that a positive finding on a roentgenogram or CT will provide the necessary proof of infection to confirm their clinical impression. This fail-safe method of determining the presence or absence of sinusitis has been delivered a blow by a recent study. This study, using CT, demonstrated paranasal sinus mucosal edema in the osteomeatal complex occurring soon after onset of a cold. In fact, this change was noted in two thirds of subjects with virally induced common colds during the first 24 to 48 hours after symptoms of a cold developed.[1] This information would seem to imply that mucosal edema happens simultaneously in the maxillary sinus and nasal cavity. This finding is not as startling as it would appear because the sinuses and the nasal cavity are a continuum. More than imaging is needed to understand what sinusitis is and what it is not.

PATHOGENESIS

The mechanisms of infection in the paranasal sinuses are better understood because of research done on other mucous membrane surfaces. Because all mucous membranes have a resident population of microorganisms that colonize them, the dynamics of host infection by these same microorganisms and others is gradually unfolding. Most upper respiratory bacteria live in harmony with the host until something happens to change the equilibrium. That change in equilibrium results in the appearance of bacterial virulence, which can be defined as the capacity to overcome available defenses.[2] That change in equilibrium can, on a ciliated epithelial surface, be induced by something that alters the effectiveness of the cilia and its overlying mucus layer. Viral infection can be a facilitator in this process.[3] This study found that nasal mucociliary function during a common cold was diminished in subjects whose mucociliary function was normal before and after the cold. This temporary alteration in mucociliary function may be a significant factor in the pathogenesis of sinusitis (see Chap. 1). A recent study, previously cited, lends further weight to this line of thought.[1] This study followed subjects who developed symptoms compatible with the common cold. Viral cultures from the nose were obtained, whereas the progress of the symptom complex was followed by obtaining paranasal sinus CT.

Positive viral cultures were found in 41% of all subjects in the study, and in 77% of these virus-positive patients the osteomeatal complex was occluded. The osteomeatal complex is the area on the lateral wall of the nasal cavity where the the maxillary, ethmoid, and frontal sinuses drain. This finding indicates that a routine virally induced common cold, by decreasing mucociliary transport, can result in the occlusion of the orifices of the sinuses and can provide a mechanism for the possible development of sinusitis.

What may be unique about respiratory membranes is this dual protection afforded by mucus enveloping most of the cilia shafts. The cilia shaft, or axoneme, is an organelle of the respiratory cell and is an extension

163

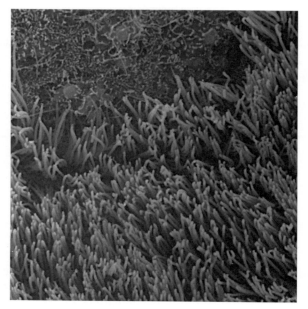

Fig. 11–1. The 6 μm above the cell surface plus the suprajacent mucus layer can provide a formidable barrier to a potential pathogen.

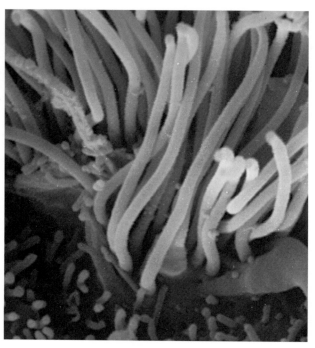

Fig. 11–2. Damaged ciliated cells after exposure to a toxic microorganism.

of the cell membrane. The 6 μm (Fig. 11–1) above the cell surface plus the suprajacent mucus layer can provide a formidable barrier to a potential pathogen. For pathogenic bacteria to cause damage to the cell and thus start the process of infection, they must first penetrate the mucociliary layer. The act of breaking through this barrier is made easier if an antecedent viral infection causes damage to this vital blanket of protection.[4] An example of this can be seen in damaged ciliated cells after exposure to a toxic microorganism (Fig. 11–2). Once microorganisms can breach this barrier, they can become adherent to cell surfaces and multiply (Fig. 11–3). This newly created environment permits bacteria to overwhelm other natural defense mechanisms of the respiratory membrane surface and enter a growth stage that expands the destructive process. Experiments in the middle ear show this effect. Adenovirus and Haemophilus influenzae were placed in the nose of an animal model, the chinchilla. When adenovirus was placed 1 week before the bacteria, H. influenzae persisted much longer in the nasopharynx and middle ear and the middle-ear infection was more severe when compared with the animal given H. influenzae alone.[5] Although similar studies have not been performed for maxillary sinusitis, the mechanics of initiation of infection in the maxillary sinus and the middle ear would not appear to be too dissimilar. Each of these cavities is connected through an ostium to the nasal cavity (the maxillary sinus) and through the eustachian tube to the nasopharynx (the middle ear). The development of the maxillary sinus and the middle ear in the fetus is similar, with both areas arising from an ingrowth of epithelium.

A second step in the development of sinusitis or any infection on the surface of a membrane is the process of microbial adherence.[6] Attachment to the cell surface is crucial if bacterial growth is to occur in sufficient numbers to overwhelm any defense mounted by the host. Bacterial cell surface proteins known as adhesins

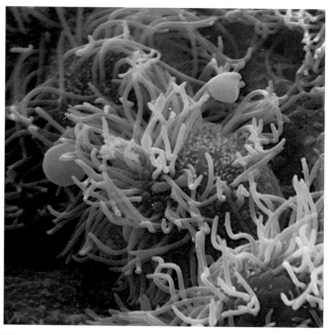

Fig. 11–3. Once microorganisms breach this barrier, they can adhere to cell surfaces and multiply.

mediate the attachment to the host's cells. This adherence mechanism gives bacteria a kind of "permanance" that prevents them from being swept away. Because most bacteria that can be pathogenic for respiratory membrane are not invasive,[7] with the exception of Neisseria meningitidis, Streptococcus pyogenes, and some pneumococci,[8] the host has to begin the process of controlling infection by mounting a neutrophil-mediated defense directed toward the cell surface. These phagocytes may be effective in preventing infection from gaining a foothold on respiratory cell surfaces and thus may prevent the development of acute sinusitis. Neutrophils may, in certain instances, be of special importance. The same proteolytic enzymes and oxygen metabolites used to kill bacteria can also damage respiratory membrane.[9] If the damage is severe, respiratory membrane at the site of infection could be permanently damaged. This may, in fact, be a mechanism that allows an infection to persist after an acute infection.

Another possible mechanism by which chronic infection may be induced is the toxic effect of killed bacteria such as pneumococci. Experiments with Streptococcus pneumoniae have shown that cell wall elements in the middle ear produce an inflammatory response.[10] Thus, it appears that even when S. pneumoniae, the most common bacterial pathogen causing sinusitis, has been inactivated, cell wall elements of this bacteria can continue to produce inflammatory changes on respiratory membranes in the upper respiratory tract even leading to the development of maxillary sinus polyps. This outcome, the development of polyps, has been demonstrated in rabbit maxillary sinuses when they were infected with S. pneumoniae.[11]

ETIOLOGY

The bacteria responsible for acute maxillary sinusitis are for the most part the same bacteria responsible for acute otitis media (see Chap. 3). They are Streptococcus pneumoniae, Haemophilus influenzae, Moraxella catarrhalis, Streptococcus pyogenes, and α-hemolytic streptococci. Up to 40% of episodes of acute maxillary sinusitis fail to reveal evidence of any bacteria,[12] but this same study showed a recovery rate for viruses of approximately 8%. The recovered viruses were found in mixed bacterial and viral combinations and in pure culture. The isolated viruses were rhinovirus, influenza A, and parainfluenzae viruses. Adenoviruses have also been isolated in other carefully performed studies. Although the presence of a virus and a bacterium in acute otitis media has been associated with a poor treatment outcome, no information leads to the same conclusion in maxillary sinusitis. Anaerobic bacteria are occasionally isolated in acute maxillary sinusitis, but they are frequently isolated in chronic sinusitis. In fact, they may be the only isolates in many cases of chronic sinusitis.[13]

In chronic sinusitis the bacterial flora is usually polymicrobial, with streptococcal species and Staphylococcus aureus as the chief aerobic and facultative bacteria. Many patients, however, have chronic sinusitis from which no bacteria can be recovered. One study, in which careful aerobic and anaerobic techniques were utilized, demonstrated sterile maxillary sinuses in 50% of the samples obtained.[14]

Fungi can also be an etiologic factor in sinusitis. Because all invasive fungi, except candida, use the respiratory tract for their portal of entry,[15] it is remarkable that fungi are not a frequent cause of sinusitis. Aspergillus, the most common fungus associated with sinusitis, can produce disease in healthy hosts. In the United States, Aspergillus fumigatus is the most frequent fungus associated with sinus disease. This fungus can be be noninvasive, that is, relatively benign, or it can be invasive. Aspergillus has been identified as a contaminant of marijuana, and its isolation from infected maxillary sinuses of marijuana smokers has provided information about a possible source for the fungus. Bipolaris species, Scedosporium (Monosporium) apiospermum, and curvularia are among other fungi capable of causing sinusitis in healthy as well as immunocompromised hosts. Even the fungi Blastomycocis dermatitidis and Cryptococcus neoformans have been isolated from infected maxillary sinuses. Fungi belonging to the order Mucorales are the cause fungal disease commonly known as mucormycosis. This type of fungal sinusitis, first noted in diabetics, is also found in patients who are or have been rendered immunocompromised. Other fungi that can produce a syndrome of allergic bronchopulmonary aspergillosis with sinusitis are alternaria, aspergillus, bipolaris, chrysoporium, dreschlera, and exserohilum.[16] Allergic aspergillus sinusitis can be associated nasal polyps and asthma.

In addition to fungi, other unusual microorganisms have been found to cause sinusitis. One report described the isolation of Corynebacterium botulinum from the maxillary sinus of a patient with a severe case of clinical botulism.[17]

DIAGNOSIS

Few clinical guidelines are universally accepted in helping to make the diagnosis of sinusitis except an imaging study. Too often, the symptoms of sinusitis are little different from those of an acute upper respiratory tract infection. In fact, changes in the sinuses begin shortly after the onset of the common cold.[1] Information obtained from sinus CT during the first 24 hours of a cold implicates the sinuses as an area of the upper respiratory tract contributing to the symptoms of the cold. If sinus discomfort can be present during the early stages of a common cold, then a sign such as the presence of purulent secretions might be suggested as a marker for acute sinusitis. Apparently, however, the presence or absence of purulence should not be relied on. Analysis of antral punctures performed in patients with symptoms of acute sinusitis and roentgenographic suspicion of the same found bacteria in 81% of purulent secretions, but also found bacteria in 77% of nonpurulent secretions.[18]

If symptoms appear to be present beyond 7 to 10 days that are usually associated with an uncomplicated cold, a diagnosis of sinusitis can be entertained.

Just as the diagnosis of acute sinusitis is made by prolongation of the symptoms associated with the common cold, the diagnosis of chronic sinusitis is made in the same way. In an effort to bring some uniformity to the diagnosis of chronic sinusitis, a special committee of the American Academy of Otolaryngology—Head and Neck Surgery (AAO-HNS) is making an attempt to develop guidelines for the diagnosis of acute and chronic sinusitis.[19] This AAO-HNS committee has classified symptoms as major and minor. In the major symptom category are facial pain, nasal obstruction, purulent discharge, and impaired sense of smell. In the minor symptom category are fever, halitosis, dental pain, fatigue, and cough. The AAO-HNS committee believes that a strong clinical history of chronic sinusitis is dominated by symptoms in the major category. Those patients whose symptoms go beyond 2 months would be categorized as having chronic sinusitis. Although these preliminary suggestions are not meant to be absolute guidelines for making a clinical diagnosis of chronic sinusitis, they do provide a first step in helping clinicians in this process.

Physical examination is the next step in the evaluation of the patient. Some physicians believe that anterior rhinoscopy is "insufficiently sensitive" to identify sinus disease;[20] however, it is a necessary but often unrevealing examination. Do midfacial or frontal palpation and percussion add anything to the physical diagnosis of sinusitis? These maneuvers are suggested in many otolaryngologic textbooks and in most textbooks written for practitioners of internal medicine and family medicine. No one has ever investigated whether this diagnostic tool is of any real value, however. It seems logical to assume that pressure over an infected sinus would produce pain, as when pressure is applied over an abscess elsewhere in the body. Unfortunately, pressure applied over the maxillary sinus and frontal sinus also places pressure on the infraorbital nerve and the supraorbital nerve. For the patient to differentiate discomfort or pain caused by compression of a nerve from pain produced by digital pressure over an infected sinus may be difficult.

Infection within the ethmoid sinuses may be no easier to detect clinically than infection within the maxillary sinuses. Occasionally in pediatric patients and less frequently in adults, infection within the ethmoid sinus

may break through the lateral bony wall of the ethmoid sinus complex. The result may be abscess formation under the periosteum.

Infections of the sphenoid sinus may occur when other sinuses are infected, but isolated infections are extremely rare. The patient may experience headaches in the midline at the junction of the frontal and parietal bones. If an isolated infection is present, physical examination may be unrevealing.

Frontal sinus infection may go hand in hand with maxillary and ethmoid sinusitis. It may cause frontal headache or, as is more likely, it may be asymptomatic. If infection within the sinus takes on a life of its own, periosteal swelling over the frontal bone may occur. When infection in the sinus overwhelms local defense mechanisms, a subperiosteal abscess may form. The swelling produced by this collection of pus is called Pott's puffy tumor. Edema of the periosteum or subperiosteal abscess is an indication of severe and potentially fatal disease requiring surgical intervention. It is not seen as commonly as in the past, but frontal sinus infection of this magnitude, once diagnosed, must be treated surgically.

Although minimal frontal and sphenoid sinus involvement often occurs in tandem with infections in the maxillary and ethmoid sinuses, symptomatic frontal and sphenoidal sinusitis is probably uncommon. On the other hand, headache in the frontal and parietal areas is exceedingly common and is usually associated with muscle tension and anxiety. The differentiation between these so-called tension headaches, which are part of the human experience, and infection in either of these two sinus complexes, the frontal and the sphenoidal, may at times be difficult.

For otolaryngolgists, the endoscopic examination of the nose is an important part of the diagnostic workup of a patient with suspected sinusitis. This examination, whether done with a flexible or a rigid endoscope, can provide valuable information about the presence or absence of mucopus in the middle meatus or in area around the sphenoid ostium. Polyps and small septal spurs, which may also be found, can be a contributing factor in the development of sinusitis.

Sinus imaging, the next step in diagnosis, includes roentgenograms, CT, magnetic resonance (MR) imaging, and ultrasound. Plain sinus films, although providing some information, often do not provide enough detail. If a maxillary or frontal sinus is opacified, information will be sufficient to make a diagnosis. Some investigators have suggested that measuring the thickness of maxillary sinus mucosa at the inferior lateral border of the sinus film (Waters' view) may provide valuable information. A 5- to 6-mm thickness usually correlates with the presence of bacteria at a titer of 10^4.[21] Accurate measurement of mucosal thickening in this location may prove difficult. The value of plain sinus films is diminished by poor technique. If technique or patient positioning is poor, the ability to measure mucosal thickness or indeed to interpret the film as a whole may be placed in jeopardy. A major problem associated with the use of plain sinus films may be the high rate of false-negative results, that is, the presence of infection despite a negative reading. These false-negative results have been reported to be as high as 55% for the sphenoid and ethmoid sinuses when surgical results were compared with preoperative films.[22] MR imaging tends to "magnify" changes in mucosal thickness. An example of this is the demonstration in a recent study that mucosal thickening persists for as long as 8 weeks after the onset of acute sinusitis. In all these cases, symptoms had resolved weeks before.[23] The greatest drawback of MR imaging as a diagnostic tool is its cost.

Sinus CT, on which otolaryngologists have come to depend, is expensive. The advantage of CT scans is the clarity with which they depict the relationship of nasal and sinus mucosa with the underlying bone of the sinuses themselves. These scans can also provide useful information in chronic sinusitis. The detail of the ethmoid and maxillary sinuses provided by CT has been used by a variety of staging systems that have been formulated to provide a tool for following chronic sinusitis as well as providing a coherent way of measuring various therapeutic modalities.[24]

Ultrasonography is a less expensive tool to help to make the diagnosis and to follow the course of disease. Although it has been used extensively in parts of Europe for the diagnosis of sinusitis, it has been generally ignored in the United States. This may be because ultrasonography does not provide the detail many of us are used to, and most otolaryngologists in the United States have not been trained to read sinus ultrasound studies. Considering that sinus utrasonography is a familiar tool in parts of Europe and is even taught to medical students,[25] its use in the United States needs to be explored further. One study in this country has begun this process.[26] The authors compared sinus CT with sinuses evaluated with B-mode ultrasonography. They found a 100% correlation between the two techniques.

TREATMENT

Discussion of nonsurgical treatment of sinusitis has to begin with a disclaimer that the value of treatment modalities has never been thoroughly explored. Evidence in animal experiments, for instance, indicates that pneumococcal sinusitis can be a brief, self-limiting infection.[27] Studies have compared the use of one antibiotic with another, but no study has been undertaken to compare no antibotic treatment with an antibiotic or antibiotic combinations. Because of this lack of hard information, one investigator has made the statement that antibiotics are used in the treatment of acute sinusitis "to prevent complications of sinusitis such as osteomyelitis and meningitis,"[28] and this statement reflects mild skepticism about the role of antibiotics in the treatment of acute sinusitis.

Currently, once a diagnosis of sinusitis is made, antibiotics are prescribed. The mechanism by which antibiotics are able to diminish sinus mucosal infection is apparently their ability to reach the mucosal cells' surface. This is the only way they can make contact with microorganisms because most sinus microbial pathogens are not invaders of this respiratory epithelium. This characteristic seems a shame, because the concentration of many antibotics in sinus mucosal cells exceeds the minimum inhibitory concentration (MIC) of most bacteria associated with sinusitis.[29] The ability of antibiotics to reach the surface of respiratory cell surface is a function of the level of the antibiotic in the serum and edema of the sinus mucosa[30] and other factors that are not as easily controlled. In the case of some antibiotics, such as cefotaxime, increasing the antibiotic serum concentration does not increase the concentration in respiratory secretions.[31]

In the case of doxycycline and other lipid soluble antibiotics, higher levels of the drug can be found in respiratory secretions than are present in the serum.[30] Thus, a variability exists in antibiotic concentration reaching the cell surface. Penicillin levels have been measured in the maxillary sinus after oral administration. These concentrations range from 0.2 to 1.2 μg/ml, but in this same study 40% of sinuses had no detectable level.[32] From a theoretic standpoint, a way around this problem would be to place the antibiotic directly on the surface of the mucosa. Instilling antibiotic directly into a maxillary sinus cavity during an episode of acute sinusitis represents an intriguing method of handling some maxillary sinus infections. This is akin to putting antibiotic ointment directly on a noninvasive skin infection. Despite the observation that an "increased rate of healing" has been noted in patients with acute maxillary sinusitis when this treatment regimen was used,[33] it seems unlikely that this approach, irrespective of its theoretic appeal, will be adopted by many otolaryngologists. It has been descibed for use in chronic infection, as discussed later in this chapter.

Antibiotics appear to be effective in sinusitis despite antibiotic levels in the sinus below many microorganisms' MIC, however, for several reasons. Antibiotics are frequently used in episodes of sinusitis that might resolve without treatment. Although no information permits an estimate of how often spontaneous resolution occurs, most busy clinicians have been witness to this phenomenon. The previously cited experiments demonstrating spontaneous resolution of pneumococcal sinusitis in an animal model can be offered as experimental evidence that a sinus may possibly return to normal without antibiotics.[27]

Another mechanism may well be the effect of subinhibitory concentrations. Subinhibitory concentrations are antibiotic levels below the MIC of that antibiotic for a particular bacterium. Because most bacteria need to adhere to a mucosal surface to cause damage to that surface and ultimately to the host, inhibition of this attachment would be beneficial to the host. Although poorly understood, this is what some antibiotics are capable of doing.[34] By preventing adherence, they diminish access of bacteria to mucosal cells and in so doing prevent bacteria from overwhelming the natural defense mechanisms of the sinus mucosa.

The most frequently associated bacteria isolated in acute sinusitis are Streptococcus pneumoniae, Haemophilus influenzae, and Moraxella catarrhalis. S. pyogenes is a less common cause of acute sinusitis (see Chap. 3).

How does a clinician know which of these bacteria is responsible for an episode of acute sinusitis? The usual way might be to obtain a culture, but from where? Obtaining a culture of nasal secretions would seem to be a first and easy step; however, this method, although relatively simple, may not provide an accurate answer. Despite some evidence from early investigators of fair to good correlation between nasal cultures and cultures taken from inside the sinus itself, present information appears to dispute this finding.[21] A sample of secretions obtained directly from the sinus would be the ideal, although that is not something a nonotolaryngologic physician would want to or should do. Middle-meatus culture, a culture taken from area of the natural ostium of the maxillary sinus, does provide an 80% correlation with those bacteria present in the sinus.[35] This technique can be done by otolaryngologists, but it does not lend itself to easy use by nonotolaryngologists. The question is this: If it is so difficult to obtain a meaningful culture, is it necessary to obtain a culture in an uncomplicated case of acute sinusitis before instituting therapy? The answer is no. Because the first three microorganisms listed previously are the ones most frequently isolated, the use of an antibiotic that might be effective against all three bacteria would be the way to proceed. The gradual acquisition of plasmid-mediated β-lactamase production by Haemophilus influenzae and Moraxella catarrhalis has made 20% of the former and up to 80% or more of the latter resistant to the semisynthetic penicillins. In the last 20 years, increasing penicillin resistance of pneumococcus has become more of a problem in the United States.[36] This resistance, unrelated to β-lactamase production, has not reached the levels associated with H. influenzae and M. catarrhalis, but increasing pneumococcal resistance is a problem with no end in sight at present. Because of this resistance problem, the choice of an antibiotic is more difficult than in the past. Because of the relatively benign course of most cases of acute sinusitis, however, the use of amoxicillin can be advocated as a starting antibiotic because of its low cost and because it is well tolerated. It is effective against sensitive pneumococci, the most frequently isolated bacteria from acute sinusitis, and it is effective against 80% of H. influenzae, the second most frequently isolated.

Although the duration of therapy has not been determined by a controlled study, custom has placed the length of therapy from 10 to 14 days. If some improvement is noted but more is thought to be necessary, continuing the drug for another 10 to 14 days is recommended. If no improvement occurs or if the improvement is not thought to be significant, another drug should be used. Trimethoprim-sulfamethoxazole may be considered as an alternative. Although it may not be as effective against some pneumococci, it is effective against H. influenzae and M. catarrhalis. The duration of therapy should be 14 to 21 days. The fluoroquinolones offer another alternative. Some newer fluoroquinolones awaiting introduction have even greater effectiveness against gram-positive bacteria than ciprofloxacin,[37] but in the meantime, ciprofloxacin appears to offer another alternative for penicillin-allergic patients, albeit an expensive one.

The addition of antihistamines has no proven efficacy in sinusitis, but patients often take them on their own. These drugs as a class have a drying effect on respiratory secretions. By their interference with histamine, however, they may decrease mucociliary activity in the maxillary sinus.[38] Oral decongestant agents are used by patients because they may help to decrease a sense of nasal congestion. As is the case with antihistamines, however, no information exists about whether they help speed recovery. Caution should be exercised in suggesting the use of antihistamines by men over 50 years of age, because antihistamines may diminish urinary bladder muscle function.

The benchmark of therapeutic efficacy in most cases of sinusitis should be the disappearance of symptoms. Although symptomatic relief and absence of disease in the sinuses are not always the same thing, the correlation is reasonable. This benchmark is more practical than obtaining sinus imaging. With 25 to 50 million or more patients with suspected acute sinusitis in the United States each year, obtaining sinus roentgenograms on completion of therapy in all patients treated for sinusitis would be impractical. For those patients whose symptoms do not fully resolve after 4 weeks of antibiotic therapy, referral to an otolaryngologist should be the next step.

Treatment of chronic sinusitis, that is, sinusitis that has been present 2 months or longer despite treatment, can present a more difficult therapeutic problem, and surgical intervention is an option. Imaging the sinuses may become necessary during this stage of disease. Sinus roentgenograms may fill this need most of the time, but coronal CT may be needed.

If disease is seen on these films, the physician will need to consider the same antibiotics that would be used for the treatment of acute sinusitis. The bacteria are basically the same as those that cause acute sinusitis, with two additions: Staphylococcus aureus and anaerobes. Two factors may make antibiotic treatment of these infections more difficult. One is the presence of β-lactamase secreting anaerobes.

The other factor may be that bacteria in many chronic infections are categorized as "slow growing." Slow-growing bacteria have a slower metabolism that may make them less susceptible to antibiotics, most of which are aimed at interrupting the metabolism of bacteria that are experiencing log-phase growth.[39] Another peculiarity of slow-growing bacteria is the protective shield that develops around them. This shield is to a large extent formed by the host's own neutrophils. These cells, which are called on to destroy these invaders, often end up walling them off and thus make it difficult for antibiotics to reach these dormant bacteria. Therefore, surgical intervention may need to be considered.

Maxillary sinus irrigation was used to treat chronic sinusitis earlier in this century. It has recently been resurrected.[40] The placement of a specially designed in-dwelling polyethylene catheter in the maxillary sinus permits irrigation to be done by any physician. This study found that two thirds of patients suffering from chronic sinusitis who were treated in this fashion avoided surgery.

Experimental evidence has indicated that the combined use of corticosteroids and antibiotics in the treatment of middle ear infections in an animal model lessens the chances for the development of chronic ear infections.[41] Perhaps at some future date treatment similar to this might provide the same protection for the sinuses.

When the diagnosis of acute frontal sinusitis is made because of an unsually severe frontal headache accompanied by roentgenologic evidence of frontal sinus opacification, antibiotic treatment is required. Because of the possible intracranial complications of untreated or undertreated frontal sinusitis, it is imperative to begin treatment immediately and continue it until total resolution of symptoms occurs, as evidenced by absence of headache accompanied by normal frontal sinuses on roentgenogram or CT. The choice of antibiotics is the same as for maxillary sinusitis. In severe cases, intravenous antibiotics may be needed. Patients with frontal sinusitis who do not appear to be responding to nonsurgical therapy should be considered for surgical drainage.

PEDIATRIC SINUSITIS

The concept of pediatric sinusitis took a giant leap forward with the introduction of CT. This tool provided a look at the sinus cavities of children, which plain sinus films were never able to do. For the first time, the small sinus cavities were visualized in a manner that allowed clinicians to see the degree of sinus mucosal disease. Plain sinus films have remained the primary tool for the diagnosis of pediatric sinusitis, however.

Unfortunately for the clinician, interpreting plain sinus films is often extraordinarily difficult. Not only does small sinus size make it difficult to judge what is seen on the film, but also technique and patient cooperation play roles in what ends up on the film. As children grow older, the value of these films may increase because of increased cooperation of the patient and the gradually increasing size of the sinuses. In fact, some physicians believe that, in patients over the age of 1 year, the presence of normal sinuses on plain sinus films indicates that no sinusitis is present.[42] The quality of these films varies, and hence their interpretation is often difficult. The use of CT to solve this dilemma is not at present a viable alternative. Expense alone makes CT a tool that will be infrequently employed.

In attempting to bring some order into the discussion of pediatric sinusitis, reports of some studies have appeared. The publication of an article in 1981 in the *New England Journal of Medicine* helped to develop a place for acute pediatric sinusitis as an entity separate from acute upper respiratory tract infection.[43] This study found that the major symptoms were cough and nasal discharge and that these were present in 75% of patients. Although the authors found that headache and facial pain were present one third of the time, most clinicians might not agree with these data, especially when applied to young children. In this benchmark study, the age range of the children was 1½ to 16 years. One of the problems of dealing with information on pediatric sinusitis is that statistics of all pediatric age groups may be lumped together. This is not always a good thing, for preteens and teenagers have sinuses that have more in common with sinuses of an adult than they do with the sinuses of a younger child. In addition to this often overlooked fact is that young children have adenoids, which preteens and teens do not have. The adenoids are probably a major reason that so many young children have prolonged rhinosinusitis, because these lymphoid elements in the nasopharynx, by their very size, can prevent the efficient drainage of secretions from the nasal cavity. This bottleneck to drainage can produce a "backup" and then spillover into the maxillary and ethmoid sinuses. A CT study of children with the diagnosis of sinusitis indicated that this might be the mechanism, at least for ethmoid sinus infection. A decreasing involvement of the ethmoid sinus was noted with increasing age.[44] Because adenoids usually diminish in size as children grow older, the effect of impeding the flow of nasal secretions also lessens with increasing age. Another study that may give some credence to this theory demonstrated the isolation of Streptococcus pneumoniae (titer 10^4) from two thirds of children with opacified maxillary sinuses and adenoid hyperplasia.[45]

The physical examination of children in whom sinusitis is suspected is even less rewarding than it is in adults. One may have little to see other than mucopus in the nose. In older children, as in adults, no mucopus may be found.

Thus, the history from a parent of cough, nasal congestion, and rhinorrhea lasting longer than 10 days is the key to making the diagnosis of acute sinusitis (up to 28 days of symptoms) or chronic sinusitis (over 28 days of symptoms). Because plain sinus films are costly, they will probably not be part of the workup of an average patient. A-mode ultrasound has been found to be valuable in helping to make the diagnosis of sinusitis in some children. B-mode ultrasound has been found to be unreliable.

Because the microorganisms found in pediatric sinusitis are identical to those found in adult sinusitis, that is, Streptococcus pneumoniae, Haemophilus influenzae, and S. pyogenes, as well as Moraxella catarrhalis, the recommended antibiotics are the same. Although no studies provide guidelines to duration of therapy in either acute or chronic sinusitis, it seems reasonable to treat for a minimum of 2 weeks in acute sinusitis and 3 to 4 weeks or longer in chronic sinusitis. In a study of chronic sinusitis, 60% of S. pneumoniae isolates were found to be relatively resistant to penicillin.[46] Thus, even in chronic pediatric sinusitis, the presence of resistant S. pneumoniae has to be kept in mind.

In some children, the symptoms continue unabated despite antibiotic treatment. In these patients, adenoidectomy should be considered, and plain sinus films and even CT may need to be considered. Although the value of sinus surgery in children has yet to be proven, perhaps consideration of this modality might be necessary for recalcitrant disease. Evidence even indicates spontaneous resolution of chronic nasal and sinus infection in children. One retrospective study found that 24 of 26 children who were described as having "therapy-resistant" chronic maxillary sinusitis were found to have a spontaneous cure by the age of 7.[47] Apparently, no prospective studies have dealt with the problem of recalcitrant infection and with whether any serious complications are associated with failure to treat stubborn sinus infections.

COMPLICATIONS

Intracranial infections have been a major concern because of the proximity of the paranasal sinuses to the cranial cavity. Similarly, the orbital contents can become infected, because the eye shares a common wall with the ethmoid sinuses. The resulting infection can cause a loss of vision or intracranial sequelae such as severe neurologic deficits or death. Apparently, the incidence of these complications may be decreasing, but when intracranial complications occur, the mortality rate may be as high as 20%.[48] The incidence of intraorbital infections also seem to be decreasing. As an example, a recent report covering a 10-year period found only 19 children with perioribital abscess.[49]

The most frequent complication of sinusitis is what is called, by some clinicians, orbital cellulitis. Preseptal cellulitis is an infection involving the soft tisues of the orbit that lie anterior to the orbital septum. This structure, the orbital septum, separates the soft tissues of the eyelids from the orbital contents themselves and is firmly bound to the bony orbital rim. Because preseptal infection is anterior to the tough tissue of the orbital septum, it does not involve the orbital contents themselves. Although these infections are 100 times more frequent than postseptal infections,[50] they may present a diagnostic dilemma on the basis of physical examination alone. Both preseptal cellulitis and orbital abscess/cellulitis, in their early stages, may look the same. In both conditions the eyelids may be swollen. In preseptal cellulitis the movement of the extraocular muscles is intact, but the movement of the same muscles may also be normal in the early stages orbital subperiosteal abscess. If one has any question about the differentiation of preseptal abscess from infection of the orbital contents, CT should be done. It is more useful if the study is done in the axial plane. Bulging of the medial orbital wall or edema of the medial orbital contents will signal that the infection is in the orbit itself.

Treatment of these intraorbital infections is by a combination of intravenous antibiotics and surgery. Sometimes, in the right clinical setting, antibiotics alone can be used. Because intraorbital infections are usually caused by Haemophilus influenzae, intravenous antibiotics should be those effective against this bacterium, remembering that 20% or more of these microorganisms produce β-lactamase.

Thoughtful clinical judgment needs to be brought to bear on the treatment options for these infections. The clinician should not be lulled into a sense of security by the absence of intraorbital findings on CT. This is demonstrated by a recent retrospective study reporting blindness in four patients with "orbital infection," normal visual acuity, and CT showing no intraorbital mass. All these patients had subperiosteal abscesses at surgery, and in all of them the blindness was permanent.[51]

No cookbook mentality is appropriate when approaching this problem. Clinical judgment is of paramount importance in dealing with these patients. If the slightest question exists in the physician's mind, surgery should be considered.

Complications of frontal sinusitis are sometimes more difficult to prevent. Because the frontal sinus is "buried" beneath the dense bone of the frontal plate, one may see no external manifestations of disease within the sinus. Although infection in the frontal sinus begins with an infection of the maxillary and ethmoid sinuses, those infections may no longer be present.

The patient may develop a swelling over the frontal sinus caused by periosteal edema or a soft swelling in the same area caused by the erosion of anterior wall of the sinus and the formation of a collection of pus subcutaneously (Pott's puffy tumor). In patients with either of these two presentations or the presence of a prolonged frontal headache with evidence of frontal sinus opacification on an imaging study, frontal sinus surgery is indicated. Severe frontal sinus disease leading to intracranial complications is not common today, but its infrequent occurrence should not lull clinicians into thinking it has disappeared. The question arises why frontal sinusitis requiring surgical treatment is not seen more fequently. This is especially baffling considering that bacteria at a titer of 10^4 can be present in the frontal sinus without producing any symptoms.

One additional complication that bears mentioning is the sinusitis that follows an oroantral fistula resulting from tooth extaction. If the tooth root is close to the floor of the maxillary sinus, a communication is made into the sinus cavity. This allows bacteria, mainly anaerobes, from the oral cavity to enter the the maxillary sinus. Chronic maxillary sinusitis associated with an oroantral fistula is usually symptomatic and can cause serious complications such as blindness (unpublished observation) and brain abscess.

SUGGESTED READINGS

1. Gwaltney JM, et al: Computed tomographic study of the common cold. N Engl J Med *330:*25, 1994.
2. Sparling PF: Bacterial virulence and pathogenesis: an overview. Rev Infect Dis *5(suppl 4):*S637, 1983.
3. Sakakura Y, et al: Nasal mucociliary function in man. J Otolaryngol Jpn *83:*1592, 1980.
4. Henderson FW, Collier AM, and Sanyai MA: A longitudinal study of respiratory viruses and bacteria in the etiology of acute otitis media with effusion. N Engl J Med *306:*1377, 1982.
5. Suzuki K and Bakaletz LO: Synergistic effect of adenovirus type 1 and nontypeable Hemophilus influenzae in a chinchilla model of experimental otitis media. Infect Immun *65:*1710, 1994.
6. Dudley JP: Adherence of microorganisms in infections of the respiratory tract. Laryngoscope *92:*68, 1982.
7. Lundberg C and Engquist S: Pathogenesis of maxillary sinusitis. Scand J Infect Dis *39(suppl):*53, 1983.
8. McGee ZA, et al: Mechanisms of mucosal invasion by pathogenic Neisseria. Rev Infect Dis *5(suppl):*S708, 1983.
9. Weiss SJ: Tissue destruction by neutrophils. N Engl J Med *320:*365, 1989.
10. Ripley-Pezoldt ML, et al: The contributions of pneumococcal cell wall to the pathogenesis of experimental otitis media. J Infect Dis *157:*245, 1988.
11. Norlander T, et al: Formation of mucosal polyps in the nasal and maxillary sinus cavities. Otolaryngol Head Neck Surg *109:*522, 1993.
12. Hamory BH, et al: Etiology and antimicrobial therapy of acute maxillary sinusitis. J Infect Dis *139:*197, 1979.
13. Brook I: Bacteriology of chronic maxillary sinusitis in adults. Ann Otol Rhinol Laryngol *98:*426, 1989.
14. Goldenhersh MJ, et al: The microbiology of chronic sinus disease in children with respiratory allergy. J Allergy Clin Immunol *85:*1030, 1990.
15. Levitz SM: Overview of host defenses in fungal infections. Clin Infect Dis *14(suppl 1):*S37, 1992.
16. Goldstein MF and Dunsley EH. Allergic fungal sinusitis. Am J Rhinol *8:*13, 1994.
17. Public Health Letter. Los Angeles, Los Angeles County Department of Health Services, 1979.
18. Savolainen S, Ylikski J, and Jousimies-Somer H: Differential diagnosis of purulent and non-purulent acute maxillary sinusitis in young adults. Rhinology *27:*53, 1989.
19. Am Acad Otolaryngol Head Neck Surg Bull *Oct:*12, 1994.
20. Loury MC and Kennedy DW: Chronic sinusitis and nasal polyposis. In: Smell and Taste in Health and Disease. Edited by Getchell TV et al. New York, Raven Press, 1991, p 517.
21. Evans FO, et al: Sinusitis of the maxillary antrum. N Engl J Med *293:*735, 1975.
22. Skinner DW and Richards SH: A comparison between sinus radiographic findings and the macroscopic appearances of para-nasal sinus mucosa. Ear Nose Throat J *70:*169, 1991.
23. Leopold DA, et al: Clinical course of acute maxillary sinusitis documented by sequential MRI scanning. Am J Rhinol *8:*19, 1994.
24. Friedman WH, Katsantonis GP, Sivore M, and Kay S: Computed tomography staging of the paranasal sinuses in chronic hyperplastic sinusitis. Laryngoscope *100:*1161, 1990.
25. Revonta M and Kuuliala I: The diagnosis and follow-up of pediatric sinusitis: Water's view radiography versus ultrasonography. Laryngoscope *99:*321, 1989.
26. Gianoli GJ, Mann WJ, and Miller RH: B-mode ultrasonography of the paranasal sinuses compared with CT findings. Otolaryngol Head Neck Surg *107:*713, 1992.
27. Westrin KM, Stierna P, Carlsoo B, and Nord CE: Mucosubstance histochemistry of the maxillary sinus mucosa in experimental sinusitis: a model study on rabbits. ORL J Otorhinolaryngol Relat Spec *53:*299, 1991.
28. Lundberg C, Gullers K, and Malmberg AS: Antibiotics in sinus secretions. Lancet *2:*107, 1968.
29. Ekedahl C, Holm SE, and Bergholm AM: Penetration of antibiotics into normal and diseased maxillary sinus mucosa. Scand J Infect Dis *14:*279, 1978.
30. Eneroth CM, Lundberg C, and Wretlind B: Antibiotic concentrations in maxillary sinus secretions and in the sinus mucosa. Chemotherapy *21(suppl 1):*1, 1975.
31. Bergogne-Berezin E, et al: Penetration of cefotaxime into bronchial secretions. Rev Infect Dis *suppl 4:*392, 1982.
32. Lundberg C, Gullers K, and Malmborg AS: Antibiotics in sinus secretions. Chemotherapy *14:*303, 1969.
33. Bjorkwall T: Local treatment with antibiotics in cases of maxillary sinusitis. Acta Otolaryngol Suppl (Stockh) *224:*338, 1966.
34. Visser MR, et al: Changes in adherence of respiratory pathogens to HEp-2 cells induced by subinhibitory concentrations of sparfloxacin, ciprofloxacin, and trimethoprim. Antimicrob Agents Chemother *37:*885, 1993.
35. Orobello PW Jr, et al: Microbiology of chronic sinusitis in children. Arch Otolaryngol Head Neck Surg *117:*980, 1991.
36. Breiman RF, et al: Emergence of drug-resistant pneumococcal infections in the United States. JAMA *271:*1831, 1994.
37. Piddock LJV: New quinolones and gram-positive bacteria. Antimicrob Agents Chemother *38:*163, 1994.
38. Dolata J, Lindberg S, and Mercke U: Histamine stimulation of mucociliary activity in the rabbit maxillary sinus. Ann Otol Rhinol Laryngol *99:*666, 1990.

39. Eng RH, et al: Bactericidal effects of antibiotics on slowly growing and nongrowing bacteria. Antimicrob Agents Chemother 35:1824, 1991.

40. Bertrand B and Eloy P: Temporary nasosinal drainage and lavage in chronic maxillary sinusitis. Ann Otol Rhinol Laryngol 102:858, 1993.

41. Kawana M, Kawana C, and Giebink GS: Penicillin treatment accelerates middle ear inflammation in experimental pneumococcal otitis media. Infect Immun 60:1908, 1992.

42. Kovatch AL, et al: Maxillary sinus radiographs in children with nonrespiratory complaints. Pediatrics 73:306, 1984.

43. Wald ER, et al: Acute maxillary sinusitis in children. N. Engl J Med 304:749, 1981.

44. van der Veken PJV, et al: CT-scan study of the incidence of sinus involvement and nasal anatomic variations in 196 children. Rhinology 28:177, 1990.

45. Arruda LK, et al: Abnormal maxillary sinus radiographs in children: do they represent bacterial infection? Pediatrics 85:553, 1990.

46. Tinkelman DG and Silk HJ: Clinical and bacteriologic features of chronic sinusitis in children. Am J Dis Child 143:938, 1989.

47. Otten FWA and Grote JJ: Treatment of chronic maxillary sinusitis in children. Int J Pediatr Otolaryngol 15:269, 1988.

48. Maniglia AJ, Goodwin J, Arnold JE, and Ganz E: Intracranial abscesses secondary to nasal, sinus, and orbital infections in adults and children. Arch Otolaryngol Head Neck Surg 115:1424, 1989.

49. Clary RA, Cunningham MJ, and Eavey RD: Orbital complications of acute sinusitis: comparison of computed tomography scan and surgical findings. Ann Otol Rhinol Laryngol 101:598, 1992.

50. Spires JR and Smith RJH: Bacterial infections of the orbital and periorbital soft-tissues in children. Laryngoscope 96:763, 1986.

51. Patt BS and Manning SC: Blindness resulting from orbital complications of sinusitis. Otolaryngol Head Neck Surg 104:789, 1991.

12 Functional Endoscopic Sinus Surgery

David W. Kennedy and Maurice Roth

Almost 100 years have passed since the first nasal endoscopy was performed by Hirschmann, utilizing a modified cystoscope. Since then, major advances in optics, biomechanics, and radiographic imaging have allowed otorhinolaryngologists to evaluate and treat paranasal sinus disorders with greater precision.

Naumann recognized the relationship between the middle meatal-anterior ethmoid complex, termed the osteomeatal unit (Fig. 12–1), and the pathogenesis of maxillary and frontal sinus disease.[1] After decades of painstaking work, Messerklinger demonstrated that relieving the osteomeatal unit of obstruction and inflammation could reverse mucosal disease within the frontal and maxillary sinuses, thus rejecting the "irreversibility" theory.[2] Functional endoscopic sinus surgery is the natural extension of his labors. Through the work of Kennedy and associates,[3,4] Stammberger,[5] and others, advanced endoscopic techniques are now used to treat an extended list of medical problems in addition to inflammatory processes of the paranasal sinuses (Table 12–1).

Even though visualization and instrumentation have improved, endoscopic sinus surgery carries the same risks as traditional sinus surgery. The use of endoscopes has not decreased the complication rate. Surgeons performing endoscopic sinus surgery must understand the anatomy, physiology, technique, and complications related to this surgical procedure.

ANATOMY

Four, roughly parallel, bony laminae are attached to the lateral nasal wall. Each lamella represents an important landmark usually encountered during endoscopic sphenoethmoidectomy (Fig. 12–2). The uncinate is the bony process of the lateral nasal wall that covers the ethmoidal infundibulum. The uncinate arises anterior and superior from the agger nasi and extends pos-

terior and inferior along the superior border of the inferior turbinate. Variability in the size, shape, and attachments of the uncinate is considerable. Bolger and associates found a direct correlation between uncinate development and maxillary hypoplasia.[6] Also important is the degree of uncinate rotation in relation to the lateral nasal wall. Lateral rotation brings the uncinate against the medial orbital wall and thereby places the orbit at risk during surgery.

Two dehiscences in the lateral nasal wall, termed fontanelles, are described in relation to the free margin of the uncinate. The anterior fontanelle is found anterior and inferior, and the posterior is found posterior and superior.

The bulla ethmoidalis is the most constant of the ethmoidal cells. Suspended laterally from the medial orbital wall, it can usually be seen following removal of the uncinate. The crescent-shaped space formed between the bulla and the uncinate is the hiatus semilunaris inferioris. Posterior to the bulla lies the sinus lateralis. When present, it forms the hiatus semilunaris superioris and represents the most posterior of the anterior group of ethmoidal cells.

The basal lamella of the middle turbinate separates the anterior ethmoidal cells from the posterior ethmoidal cells. Beginning from an almost vertical position attached laterally to the medial orbital wall, it slopes inferior and posterior to lie in a more horizontal plain. The sphenopalatine neurovascular bundle emerges from the sphenopalatine foramen and projects into the horizontal portion of the middle turbinate at its posterolateral end. Injection at this site provides excellent anesthesia and hemostasis.

The posterior ethmoid cells are larger and fewer in number than the anterior group. Pneumatization of the sphenoid bone from the posterior ethmoid is known as an Onodi cell. The incidence of Onodi cells ranges from 12 to 42%, and they are more prevalent in Asians.[7] Kainz and Stammberger found the average thickness

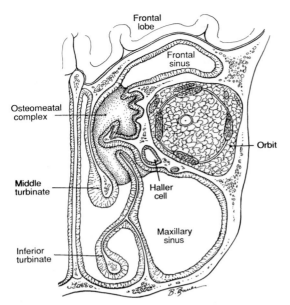

Fig. 12–1. The osteomeatal unit (shaded). Obstruction of this area leads to disease within the maxillary and frontal sinuses.

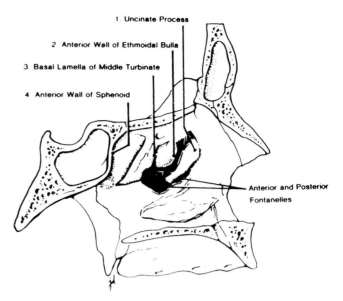

Fig. 12–2. Bony anatomy of the lateral nasal wall demonstrating four bony laminae encountered during endoscopic ethmoidectomy. The numbers indicate the surgical order of bony landmarks during approach in the unoperated patient.

of the bony wall covering the optic nerve in Onodi cells to be 0.28 mm, with dehiscence noted in 12% of specimens.[8] Knowledge of these cells is important for preventing visual complications.

The sphenoid sinus begins to pneumatize by age 3 years. Hamberger and associates described three different degrees of sphenoid pneumatization and classified them as sellar 86%, presellar 11%, and conchal 3%.[9] In a well-pneumatized sphenoid sinus, the optic nerve and internal carotid artery canals can be seen as convexities of the walls of the sinus (Fig. 12–3) and are therefore at risk during sphenoid sinus surgery. Kennedy and colleagues found a clinical dehiscence of the internal carotid canal in 22% of specimens examined.[10]

TABLE 12–1. Possible Indications for Functional Endoscopic Sinus Surgery

Recurrent acute sinusitis
Chronic sinusitis
Nasal polyposis
Fungal sinusitis
Barosinusitis
Advanced techniques
  Tumor removal
  Antral choanal polyp removal
  Dacryocystorhinostomy
  Encephalocele repair
  CSF leak repair
  Pituitary surgery
  Mucocele removal
  Orbital abscess/cellulitis management
  Orbital decompression
  Septal reconstruction
  Choanal atresia repair
  Epistaxis control

The frontal sinus begins to pneumatize from within the frontal recess during the first few years of life, but the sinus does not appear on plain radiographs until age 7 years. Seventeen percent of people have aplastic frontal sinuses. Unilateral aplasia occurs in 3% of the population. According to Lang, the frontal sinus may drain into the frontal recess from either a duct (77%)

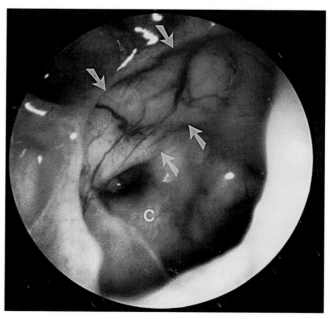

Fig. 12–3. Endoscopic view of a postoperative sphenoid sinus. Arrows, optic nerve; C, internal carotid artery. (From Kennedy D: Prognostic factors, outcomes, and staging in ethmoid sinus surgery. Laryngoscope 102(suppl 57):5, 1992.)

or an ostium (23%).[11] Montgomery stated, however, that only 15% of people have a nasofrontal duct.[12] The discrepancy may be related to one's definition of a true duct. The diameter of the frontal os ranges from 2 to 11 mm. Patients with smaller frontal sinuses usually have smaller ostia and therefore may be at increased risk of stenosis.

The natural ostium of the maxillary sinus is found in the semilunar hiatus in relation to the anteroinferior aspect of the bulla ethmoidalis. The anterior edge of the ostium is in close proximity to the lacrimal duct. Occasionally, only mucosa separates the duct from the ostium. The ostium leading to the maxillary sinus may be narrowed by a large air cell in the roof of the sinus—a so-called Haller cell.

PHYSIOLOGY

Functional endoscopic sinus surgery is supported from observations regarding mucociliary clearance. Mucociliary clearance is the process by which the ciliated

TABLE 12–2. Anatomic Obstruction

Concha bullosa
Septal deviation
Haller cell
Rotated uncinate
Paradoxic middle turbinate
Scar tissue

epithelium of the paranasal sinuses clears mucus and debris. Hilding,[13] and later Messerklinger,[14] demonstrated that the mucus blanket covering the epithelium was propelled in an organized pattern from within the sinuses through natural ostia and then into the nose and nasopharynx (Fig. 12–4). Osteomeatal obstruction precipitated by mucosal contact points or bony abnormalities inhibits mucociliary clearance and produces chronic mucosal changes (Table 12–2). In most cases, these changes can be reversed after the obstruction has been removed. Failure to address osteomeatal obstruction prevents the restoration of mucociliary clearance and ultimately leads to treatment failure (Fig. 12–5) see also Chap. 1).

In addition to obstruction, mucociliary clearance can be inhibited if the respiratory epithelium is injured or dysfunctional (Table 12–3). Patients with injured or dysfunctional epithelium are not cured with surgery alone and require specific treatment aimed at restoring healthy epithelium.

The etiology of sinusitis is multifactorial (Fig. 12–6); however, most factors result in paranasal sinus obstruction with subsequent postobstructive mucosal disease. Therefore, even if the underlying cause is resolved, the patient's sinusitis can still persist if the osteomeatal obstruction is not removed.

PREOPERATIVE ASSESSMENT

History

A complete history is essential. We use a detailed questionnaire that, in addition to containing specific ques-

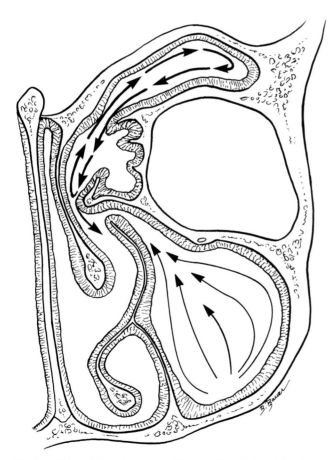

Fig. 12–4. Mucociliary clearance patterns within the frontal and maxillary sinuses. (Modified from Kennedy D: Endoscopic sinus surgery. In: Otolaryngology Update I. Edited by Cummings CW. St. Louis, CV Mosby, 1989.)

TABLE 12–3. Causes of Epithelial Injury

Primary ciliary dyskinesia
Environmental injury (pollution, extreme weather)
Allergy
Toxins (cocaine, phenylephrine, flunisolide)
Infection
Trauma
Radiation
Dehydration
Foreign body
Hypoxia
Genetic predisposition

(Modified from Knops JL, et al: Physiology, clinical applications. Otolaryngol Clin North Am 26:529, 1993.)

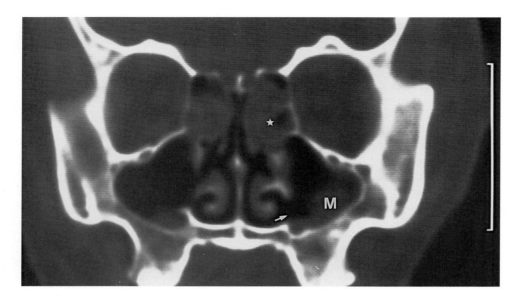

Fig. 12–5. Coronal CT demonstrating anterior ethmoid disease (*), patent nasal antral window (arrow), and persistent maxillary sinus disease (M).

tions relating to sinus infections, identifies allergic symptoms, smell and taste dysfunction, and pressure-related discomfort. The questionnaire serves as an objective assessment of the patient's clinical complaints and as a data base for future reference. Patients are considered for surgery after extensive medical management has failed.

During the interview, the patient's commitment to participate in his or her own care is ascertained. The perioperative period requires frequent clinic visits and, in some cases, life-style changes. Patients who are not motivated to quit smoking or to adhere to other medical recommendations are poor candidates for sinus surgery. In addition, patients with unreasonable expectations from surgery are less likely to benefit.

Examination

The examination of the nose begins with inspection of the vestibular skin and nasal valve area. Anterior

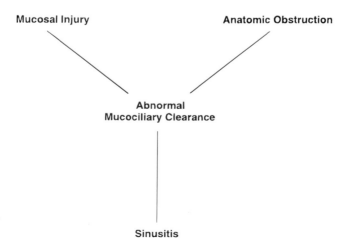

Fig. 12–6. Multiple factors result in abnormal mucociliary clearance, which leads to chronic sinusitis.

rhinoscopy is performed before the application of decongestants. This gives the surgeon an unaltered overview of the nasal mucosa and gives the patient confidence that the examiner has observed the nose before changes occur with decongestion.

Nasal endoscopy has markedly improved our ability to visualize and evaluate nasal disease. Directed cultures can be obtained to help in antibiotic selection. In addition, medical and surgical treatments can now be judged not only by patient history and radiographic findings, but also by direct inspection of the nose and paranasal sinuses.

Adult nasal endoscopy is performed with a 30-degree 4-mm telescope. Occasionally, a 2.7-mm telescope is required for the patient with a septal deviation or a narrow nasal passage. The nasal cavity is decongested with aerosolized phenylephrine or ephedrine and anesthetized with a topical anesthetic. If necessary, 4% cocaine on cotton-tip applicators is inserted endoscopically to sensitive areas. Three passes are made. The first pass is along the floor of the nose and brings the inferior turbinate, inferior meatus, and eustachian tube orifice into view. The second pass is made between the inferior turbinate and the middle turbinate and allows inspection of the middle meatus, sphenoethmoidal recess, and sphenoid sinus ostium. The third pass is performed on withdrawal of the telescope. Remember that the telescopic view is directed 30 degrees and that certain structures will not be seen if the telescope is not rotated during the examination. That is why, during the third pass, the telescope is gently rolled superiorly and laterally. The middle meatus can now be examined in more detail, noting the bulla ethmoidalis, hiatus semilunaris, and any accessory ostia.

Radiography

The technologic advances in radiology, including computed tomography (CT), have greatly enhanced our

TABLE 12–4. Radiography Review

Presence of bony abnormalites producing osteomeatal obstruction
Slope and integrity of the skull base along with the depth of the olfactory fossa
Uncinate and maxillary sinus development
The vertical height of the posterior ethmoid in relation to the postero-medial roof of the maxillary sinus
The presence of Onodi cells
The attachment of the sphenoid sinus septa to the skull base in relation to the optic canal and internal carotid artery

ability to evaluate disease of the paranasal sinuses.[15] CT is excellent for evaluating bone anatomy. Coronal CT scans of the paranasal sinuses are obtained in 3-mm intervals beginning at the anterior edge of the frontal sinus and extending through the sphenoid sinus (Table 12–4 and Fig. 12–7). Windowing is adjusted for maximal viewing of the uncinate, bulla, and ethmoid complex. Obstruction of the osteomeatal unit, frontal sinus disease, and pneumatization of the maxillary sinus are noted. Additional anatomic detail of the frontal recess and sphenoid sinus can be obtained through axial or direct sagittal images.

Magnetic resonance (MR) imaging has been shown to be useful in certain situations. MR provides better visualization of soft tissue than CT. With T2-weighted MR, inflammatory mucosal lesions within the frontal, maxillary, and sphenoid sinuses display high signal intensity, whereas neoplasms display medium signal intensity. Fungal and desiccated sinus concretions display hypointense signal on T2-weighted images. MR can also be used to evaluate intracranial extension of paranasal sinus disease.

TECHNIQUE

Instrumentation

The instruments necessary for a safe and complete operation are pictured in Figure 12–8. The majority of the dissection is carried out using the 0-degree endoscope because the angulation of the other telescopes can be disorienting. The 30-degree endoscope is usually required for examination and manipulation of the maxillary sinus ostia and frontal recess. The 70-degree endoscope is excellent for viewing the antrum and for identification of an anterior frontal sinus. Attaching a commercially available endoscope washer facilitates surgery by defogging and clearing secretions from the tip of the telescope.

Anesthesia

The operation can be performed under local or general anesthesia. Local anesthesia with intravenous sedation is preferable because sensory information remains intact along the periorbita and skull base. Allowing the patient to listen to favorite music during surgery reduces the amount of anxyiolytics necessary during the procedure.

Before the patient enters the operating suite, oxymetazoline hydrochloride nasal spray is used for initial mucosal shrinking. The nasal mucosa is then decongested and anesthetized, one side at a time, with 150 mg of topical cocaine followed by injections of 1% lidocaine with 1:100,000 epinephrine (Fig. 12–9). Septal

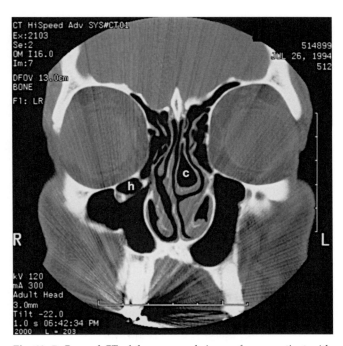

Fig. 12–7. Coronal CT of the paranasal sinuses from a patient with recurrent acute sinusitis and septal deviation. The CT is obtained 4 to 6 weeks after initiating medical therapy. Table 12–4 lists anatomic highlights to review before surgery. h, Haller cell; c, concha bullosa.

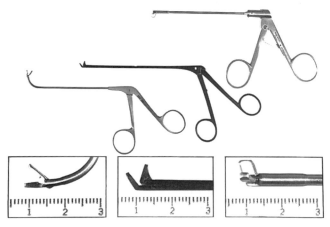

Fig. 12–8. Micro-through cutting instruments with varying angles allow mucosal sparing dissection throughout all regions of the paranasal sinuses. The Stammberger down-biting punch is excellent for enlarging the maxillary ostium.

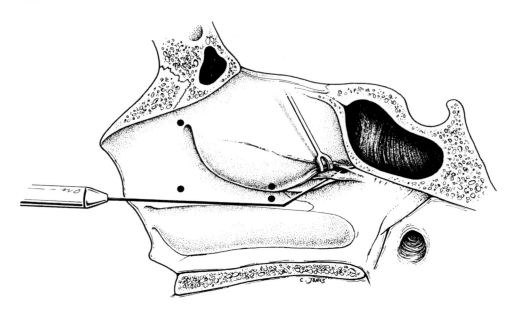

Fig. 12–9. Recommended injection sites for endoscopic sinus surgery. Angled tonsil needle is used for intranasal injection of the sphenopalatine neurovascular bundle.

abrasions should be avoided; otherwise, visualization becomes difficult from repeated soiling of the telescope. In addition, the sphenopalatine ganglion is anesthetized through the nose or through the greater palatine foramen. Allowing at least 10 minutes for maximal vasoconstriction decreases bleeding. The second side of the nose is anesthetized when surgery on the first side is near completion.

Procedure

The surgeon should be comfortable and relaxed during the dissection. The preoperative CT should be readily available in the operating room for repeated viewing. The surgeon must perform a meticulous dissection with adequate visualization if complications are to be avoided.

To begin, an infundibulotomy is made using a sickle knife along the anterior and inferior edge of the uncinate process. The uncinate is grasped with Blakesley forceps and removed, taking care not to strip mucosa from the lateral nasal wall. Gentle medial displacement of the uncinate during the infundibulotomy helps define the line of the incision. If possible, the location of the maxillary sinus ostium is noted along with any accessory ostia. Extent of surgery is based on the preoperative assessment; however, for purposes of instruction, a description of a sphenoethmoidectomy with frontal sinusotomy and antrostomy follows.

The bulla ethmoidalis is entered and removed. The medial orbital wall should be identified as early as possible during the dissection. Every attempt at preserving the mucosa along the medial orbital wall is made to improve and hasten postoperative healing. The posterior ethmoid is entered through the inferior and medial area of the basal lamella. The skull base is most

easily identified within the posterior ethmoidectomy and serves as the superior boundary for the dissection. We have found that the safest way to remove bony partitions within the ethmoid is to feel behind the partitions with Blakesley forceps prior to removal (Fig. 12–10). This technique assists in avoiding orbital or intracranial penetration.

The sphenoid ostium is located and, if necessary, widened beginning inferior and medially. The ostium is usually a few millimeters from the posteroinferior edge of the superior turbinate. The free edge of the superior turbinate may be difficult to appreciate when

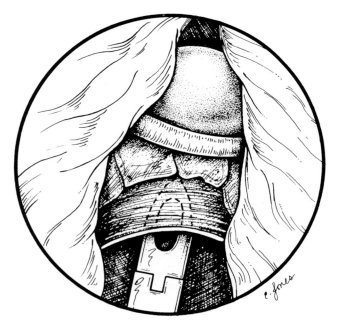

Fig. 12–10. Blakesley forceps are used to palpate behind bony partitions before removal.

working in the ethmoid sinus. Placing the endoscope medial to the middle turbinate usually brings the free edge of the superior turbinate in view. The sphenoid sinus can also be entered by amputating the inferior aspect of the superior turbinate. Care must be taken not to remove this turbinate completely because olfactory fila could be injured. Absolutely no blind tissue removal is performed within the sphenoid because this may lead to optic nerve or carotid artery injury.

At this point, the dissection is continued anterior along the skull base, with care not to injure the anterior and posterior ethmoid arteries. The mucosa along the skull base is also preserved. The frontal recess is dissected only if required because manipulation of this region can lead to stenosis of the frontal ostium. In addition, frontal recess surgery increases the requirement for postoperative care.

Operating within the frontal recess is the most challenging segment of the operation. Changing to the 30-degree endoscope is helpful for dissecting this area. The dome of the ethmoid should be identified and followed anteriorly as the skull base ascends. The skull base represents the posterior limit of dissection in this area. All motions should be made away from the skull base in an anterior direction. Anteromedial ethmoid cells as well as agger cells can be removed with a frontal recess curette. Eicken curved suction is helpful in this area. The size of the frontal ostium should be recorded for postoperative reference.

Finally, attention is turned toward the maxillary sinus ostium. The 30-degree telescope is usually required to identify the natural ostium of the maxillary sinus. If necessary, the ostium is enlarged posteriorly and inferiorly. Beginning from within the ostium, the mucosa of the posterior fontanelle is split and then removed with the aid of a back-biting instrument. The remaining uncinate is removed at this time to prevent postoperative scarring in this area.

At the conclusion of the operation, an expandable sponge covered with a water-soluble antibacterial ointment is placed lateral to the middle turbinate. Additional packing is rarely required. Most patients are released the day of surgery and return to the clinic on the first postoperative day for removal of the sponge.

POSTOPERATIVE CARE

The overall success of functional endoscopic sinus surgery is in large part due to appropriate postoperative care. The goal during this period is to promote mucosal generation within the sinus cavities. To facilitate this generation, sinus cavities are examined and cleaned of blood, fibrin clots, and crusts at regular intervals following surgery. Endoscopes should be used, as opposed to blind manipulation, to prevent injury to

healthy mucosa and for directed debridement. This is especially true for the frontal recess.

Patients are instructed to irrigate the nose with saline solution twice daily. For many patients with chronic sinusitis, surgery alone is not enough. Long-term, culture-directed, systemic antibiotics are usually required. Occasionally, antibiotics are added to the nasal irrigation solution for patients with recalcitrant chronic sinusitis.

COMPLICATIONS

Although the potential complications from functional endoscopic sinus surgery are severe, the overall complication rate for experienced surgeons is low.[16] The most common problem following endoscopic sinus surgery is postoperative scarring. Scarring within the ethmoid cavity can lead to continued sinus obstruction, decreased mucociliary clearance, and nasal obstruction. Scarring can be minimized with meticulous cleanings during the postoperative period.

Visual loss following endoscopic sinus surgery can result from direct trauma to the optic nerve or from orbital hematoma.[17] Direct trauma is most likely to occur in the posterior ethmoid or sphenoid sinus and is generally irreversible. Orbital hematoma is usually caused by injury to the lamina papyracea or periorbita. The bony orbit has a fixed volume, so as blood enters,

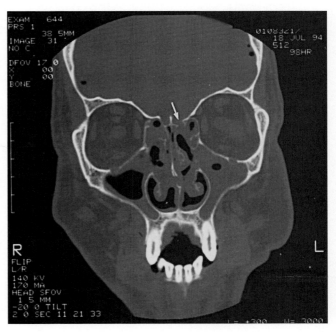

Fig. 12–11. Coronal CT of the paranasal sinuses from a patient referred for postoperative evaluation of a cerebrospinal fluid leak and pneumocephalus. The arrow demonstrates a common area of intracranial penetration where the anterior ethmoidal artery penetrates the lateral lamella of the cribriform plate.

orbital pressure rises. Lid edema, ecchymosis, chemosis, proptosis, and, eventually, visual loss develop. Immediate action is necessary to prevent blindness. The nasal packing should be removed. If gentle massage, ice, and diuretics do not reverse the ocular injury, a lateral canthotomy and cantholysis should be performed.

Cerebrospinal fluid leak most commonly occurs where the anterior ethmoidal artery penetrates the lateral lamella of the cribriform plate (Fig. 12–11). If the leak is identified during surgery, it should be repaired. A free mucosal graft from the septum or a middle turbinate flap works well.[18]

Bolger and associates reported a 15% incidence of lacrimal drainage system injury using intraoperative fluorescein in 24 patients undergoing functional endoscopic sinus surgery with middle meatal antrostomy.[19] None of the patients in this series developed epiphora, however, a finding suggesting that the lacrimal system recannulized into the middle meatus. The overall rate of postoperative epiphora is less than 2% for experienced surgeons. Epiphora may be prevented by enlargement of the maxillary ostium into the posterior fontanelle, as opposed to removing the anterior wall.

LONG-TERM CARE

Following surgery, intensive medical management is continued until the inflammation within the sinus cavities has resolved and all surfaces have remucosalized. One of the great advantages of using endoscopes in the practice of rhinology is that an objective assessment of the patient's paranasal sinuses can be obtained and medical therapy adjusted accordingly. Patients are reevaluated on a regular schedule based on the severity of their disease. Asymptomatic recurrent mucosal disease can then be detected and treated before clinical sinusitis develops. In addition, small areas of persistent inflammation or adhesions can be removed more readily before recurrent obstruction and further symptoms occur.

SUGGESTED READINGS

1. Naumann H: Pathologische Anatomie der chronischen Rhinitis and Sinusitis. In: Proceedings of the VIIIth International Congress of Otorhinolaryngology. Amsterdam, Excerpta Medica, 1965, p 80.
2. Messerklinger W: Endoscopy of the Nose. Baltimore, Urban & Schwarzenberg, 1978.
3. Kennedy D, Goodstein M, Miller N, and Zinreich J: Endoscopic transnasal orbital decompression. Arch Otolaryngol Head Neck Surg 116:275, 1990.
4. Kennedy D, et al: Endoscopic sinus surgery for mucoceles: a viable alternative. Laryngoscope 99:885, 1989.
5. Stammberger H: Functional Endoscopic Sinus Surgery. Philadelphia, BC Decker, 1991.
6. Bolger W, Woodruff W, Morehead J, and Parsons D: Maxillary sinus hypoplasia: classification and description of associated uncinate process hypoplasia. Otolaryngol Head Neck Surg 103: 759, 1990.
7. Yeoh K and Tan K: The optic nerve in the posterior ethmoid in Asians. Acta Otolaryngol 114:329, 1994.
8. Kainz J and Stammberger H: Danger areas of the posterior rhinobasis. Acta Otolaryngol 112:852, 1992.
9. Hamberger C, et al: Transantrosphenoidal hypophysectomy. Arch Otolaryngol 74:2, 1961.
10. Kennedy D, Zinreich J, and Hassab M: The internal carotid artery as it relates to endonasal sphenoethmoidectomy. Am J Rhinol 4:7, 1990.
11. Lang J: Clinical Anatomy of the Nose, Nasal Cavity, and Paranasal Sinuses. New York, Thieme, 1989.
12. Montgomery W: Frontal sinus anatomy. In: Surgery of the Upper Respiratory System. Edited by Montgomery W. Philadelphia, Lea & Febiger, 1979, p 117.
13. Hilding A: The physiology of drainage of nasal mucus: IV. Drainage of the accessory sinuses of man. Ann Otol Rhinol Laryngol 53:35, 1932.
14. Messerklinger W: On the drainage of the normal frontal sinus of man. Acta Otolaryngol (Stockh) 63:176, 1967.
15. Zinreich J: Imaging of inflammatory sinus disease. Otolaryngol Clin North Am 26:535, 1993.
16. May M, Levine H, Schaitkin B, and Mester S: Complications of Endoscopic Sinus Surgery. In: Endoscopic Sinus Surgery. Edited by Levine H and May M. New York, Thieme, 1993, p 193.
17. Stankiewicz J: Blindness and intranasal endoscopic ethmoidectomy: prevention and management. Otolaryngol Head Neck Surg 101:320, 1989.
18. Maddox D and Kennedy D: Endoscopic management of cerebrospinal fluid leaks and cephaloceles. Laryngoscope 100:857, 1990.
19. Bolger W, Parsons D, Mair E, and Kuhn F: Lacrimal drainage system injury in functional endoscopic sinus surgery. Arch Otolaryngol Head Neck Surg 118:1179, 1992.

13 Open Operations for Paranasal Sinusitis

Robert H. Miller and Donald N. Cote

The evolution of the treatment of sinus disease, from the origins of sinus trephination, as practiced by prehistoric man in Peru,[1] to modern developments including endoscopic techniques, has advanced the treatment of sinus infections, tumors of the sinuses, and access of deeper spaces of the head and face via the paranasal sinuses (pterygomaxillary space, hypophysis). Functional endoscopic sinus surgery, as discussed in detail in Chapter 12, is the most recent advance in the progression of treatment of inflammatory sinus diseases. Whereas endoscopic sinus surgery has assumed a leading role in the care of chronic sinusitis, open sinus procedures have stood the test of time, and our experience with these techniques mandates that the sinus surgeon consider them in selected situations. In addition, open sinus procedures are often required when acute sinusitis is complicated by orbital and/or intracranial involvement. Although endoscopic surgery has for the most part become the first line of surgical therapy, external and intranasal procedures are still important. This chapter focuses on these nonendoscopic surgical methods of treating inflammatory diseases of the sinuses.

GENERAL PRINCIPLES

Surgery for sinus infections is indicated in patients who have not responded to appropriate medical therapy. If antibiotics and decongestants in acute infections or antibiotics, decongestants, and adequate allergic management in chronic sinusitis have failed to relieve the infection and obstruction of the paranasal sinuses, then surgical intervention is indicated.

The sinus surgeon's priorities are to prevent progression or development of a complication of sinusitis and to prevent the persistence or recurrence of chronic sinusitis. This is accomplished by: (1) precise and complete excision of disease tissue, sparing healthy tissue;

(2) providing free gravitational drainage from the sinuses or promoting drainage from normal physiologic pathways into the nose and inviting ingrowth of healthy nasal mucosa while preserving normal intranasal physiology; (3) obliteration, if creating adequate drainage from the frontal sinus is impossible or doubtful; and (4) considering the cosmetic end result of the surgical procedure.

The surgeon should perform simple intranasal procedures to establish better drainage if physical examination, radiographic analysis, and the medical therapeutic course indicate a simple solution. More radical surgery is required if simple drainage procedures fail or if the disease is extensive, however. Nonetheless, the sinus surgeon must tailor the operation to the type and extent of the disease, as well as to the desires of the well-informed patient. The patient may prefer repeated maxillary sinus lavage, allergy management, and pharmacologic therapy for chronic sinusitis over a surgical procedure. The open procedures for inflammatory diseases of each sinus (Table 13–1) are addressed separately, recognizing that the interrelationship among the sinuses cannot be ignored.

MAXILLARY SINUS

An adequate trial of conservative therapy is the treatment of choice for acute and chronic maxillary sinusitis, as discussed in Chapter 11. Appropriate antibiotics and local and/or systemic decongestants are administered for a minimum of 10 days and up to 6 weeks. If physical examination, radiographs, and symptoms fail to improve, surgical intervention is considered. This can range from simple maxillary sinus lavage to the more aggressive Caldwell-Luc procedure. Once medical therapy has been determined to be unsuccessful, then attempts to facilitate drainage of the maxillary sinus or removal of diseased tissue must be performed.

TABLE 13–1. Open Sinus Procedures

Maxillary
    Antral lavage
    Nasal antrostomy
    Caldwell-Luc procedure
    Oroantral fistula repair
Ethmoid
    Intranasal ethmoidectomy
    Transantral ethmoidectomy
    External ethmoidectomy
Frontal
    Trephination
    Frontal sinus septectomy
    Frontoethmoidectomy
    Osteoplastic frontal sinus obliteration
Sphenoid
    Intranasal sphenoidotomy
    Sphenoethmoidectomy
    Transseptal sphenoidectomy

Antral Lavage

Failure of the maxillary sinus infection to clear with adequate medical therapy implies damage to the mucociliary blanket or obstruction of the natural ostium. This creates retention of mucopus and infectious products within the antrum. In these cases, irrigation of the maxillary sinus removes the retained products of the infection such as necrotic tissue, the infecting microorganism and their toxins, and the cellular debris, but it does not reverse the anatomic or physiologic obstruction. Moreover, specimens for culture and, if indicated, cytologic study can be obtained. Patients with defects of the orbital floor should not undergo lavage because of the introduction of irrigation and bacteria into the orbit. The first antral irrigation was performed by Hartmann in 1885 via the membranous portion of the middle meatus.[2] Subsequent to this, the maxillary sinus has also been lavaged through the natural ostium, puncture through the inferior meatus, and puncture through the anterior wall of the maxillary sinus in the canine fossa. Most otolaryngologist prefer to irrigate via the inferior meatus.

Technique

Anesthesia and decongestion are obtained by the application of topical 4% cocaine solution on cotton pledget introduced intranasally into the middle or inferior meatus, depending on the approach selected. Local infiltration of the mucosa with lidocaine with epinephrine will aid in hemostasis and in achieving anesthesia of the lateral nasal wall.

To cannulate the natural ostium, a curved cannula (sharp or blunt) is inserted superiorly and posteriorly to the midportion of the middle meatus. The tip of the cannula is rotated laterally and then pulled anteriorly to slide into the natural ostium. Once in the ostium, the cannula is pointed inferiorly, anteriorly, and laterally.

According to Van Alyea,[2] 80% of patients should be cannulated with minimal trauma. Prolonged probing should be avoided because this trauma may cause stenosis of the ostia, thereby offsetting the benefits of cannulation. The advantages of the cannulation of the natural ostium technique are absence of injury to structures of the medial wall of the antrum and decreased tendency to spread infection. The major disadvantage is the technical difficulty in performing the procedure without the use of an endoscope.

The direct puncture technique is performed using a curved trocar, positioned in the inferior meatus approximately 1.5 to 2 cm behind the attachment of the inferior turbinate (Fig. 13–1). The trocar is directed superiolaterally toward a point midway between the ear and lateral canthus of the eye. The trocar is then gently advanced with mild pressure. If resistance is met, the cannula is repositioned. Care must be taken not to traverse the antrum and puncture the superior or lateral walls. Once in position, the trocar is aspirated. If the trocar is positioned too far anteriorly, blood may be aspirated from the soft tissue of the cheek, and repositioning of the cannula will be necessary.

After the cannula is in the proper position, the antrum is irrigated. The patient is asked to lean forward and breathe through the mouth, and a bowl is placed beneath the chin. Warm saline is injected slowly, and the return is collected in the bowl until clear of grossly infected material. The irrigation is then terminated, and the trocar is removed. Air should never be injected because fatalities secondary to air embolism have been reported.[3]

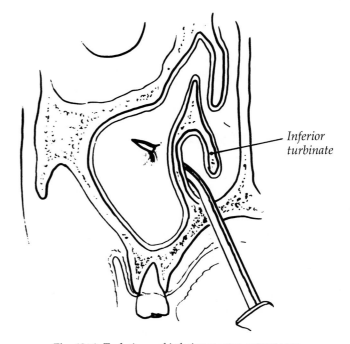

Inferior turbinate

Fig. 13–1. Technique of inferior meatus antrostomy.

An alternative method of antral lavage is via the anterior wall of the maxillary sinus above the canine fossa. The anterior wall is locally anesthetized, and the trocar is placed above the premolar teeth and below the infraorbital nerve foramen. The trocar is then rotated into the antrum with slight pressure. Aspiration and irrigation are performed as previously described. This variation can be performed with the patient in the recumbent position, and it can be used in children.[4]

Complications

As previously mentioned, fatal air embolus has been reported. In addition, infiltration with irrigant and/ or emphysema of the cheek can occur. Blindness or proptosis can result from injection into the orbit; this complication is more likely to occur in patients with a dehiscent orbital floor. Bacteremia and sepsis have also been reported. Hemorrhage with epistaxis can result after puncture, especially in patients with a coagulopathy. Injury to the nasolacrimal duct can also occur if the puncture is done in the most anterior portion of the inferior meatus.

Intranasal Antrostomy

When irrigation fails, surgical drainage of the maxillary sinus is required. An inferior meatal nasoantral window may be indicated in patients with recurrent or chronic infection with stenosis or occlusion of the natural ostium. The creation of a large antrostomy has the benefits of providing gravitational drainage of the antrum, thereby reducing infection and allowing visual inspection of the sinus and access for antral lavage and removal of necrotic debris (patients receiving radiotherapy for tumors) or a foreign body. It is also used concomitantly with repair of an oroantral fistula. The nasoantral window functions through dependent drainage as mucociliary flow continues toward the natural ostia.

Technique

The nasoantral window can be performed with the patient under general or local anesthesia. The inferior meatus is anesthetized with 4% cocaine solution on cotton pledgets. This also provides decongestion for better visualization. The inferior turbinate is pushed medially (in-fractured) and can be packed in this position for exposure. An inferior-based mucosal flap on the lateral wall is created, and the flap is laid onto the floor of the nose to be used later. An opening is made in the midportion of the lateral wall of the inferior meatus with a punch or curved hemostat. This opening is then enlarged to at least 2 cm with biting forceps, mainly posteriorly to avoid injury to the nasolacrimal duct, which lies in the anterior portion of the inferior meatus. The antral wall must be removed down to the level of the nasal floor. The mucosal flap is rotated into the

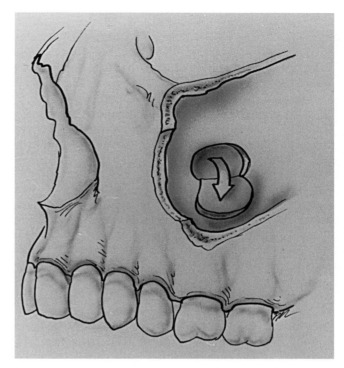

Fig. 13–2. Nasal mucosal flap rotated into nasoantral window.

defect to help prevent stenosis of the antrostomy, which occurs within 2 years in 30 to 45% of patients (Fig. 13–2).[5] Packing is not necessary unless troublesome bleeding occurs.

The antrostomy can be performed through the middle meatus and the natural ostium of the maxillary sinus. With the area under local anesthesia, the natural ostium is identified behind the uncinate process in the hiatus semilunaris of the middle meatus. The ostium is enlarged with biting forceps. If the middle turbinate was in-fractured, it is returned to its normal position after the antrostomy.

Complications

Complications of nasal antrostomy include bleeding, closure of the window, synechia formation, and injury to the nasolacrimal duct.

Caldwell-Luc Procedure

In 1893, Caldwell described a procedure of making an opening into the maxillary sinus through the canine fossa. He did this in combination with an intranasal antrostomy. In 1897, Luc reported a similar operation, and eventually the procedure became known as the Caldwell-Luc operation.[6]

Indications for the external approach include failure of the nasoantral antrostomy to resolve the infection, hypertrophic rhinosinusitis (polyps) filling the antrum, neoplasm of the maxillary sinus, presence of an oroantral fistula, osteonecroses of the maxilla, and complicated fractures of the maxilla and/or orbital floor. The Caldwell-Luc procedure also provides access to the ethmoid and sphenoid sinuses through the superiomedial wall, to the orbit for orbital decompression, and to the pterygomaxillary space through the posterior wall for internal maxillary artery ligation, vidian neurectomy, sphenopalatine ganglionectomy, and sectioning of the second division of the trigeminal nerve.

Technique

The Caldwell-Luc operation may be performed with the patient under either general or local anesthesia. Local anesthesia has the advantage of less operative bleeding and the absence of a general anesthetic risk. Regional anesthesia can be accomplished by an infraorbital nerve block, sphenopalatine nerve block by way of the greater palatine foramen, posterosuperior alveolar nerve block, and local infiltration of the gingiva. A 4% cocaine solution on a cotton pledget is placed intranasally to block the anterior ethmoid nerve and the medial wall of the maxillary sinus topically. The head of the patient is elevated approximately 30 degrees to decrease bleeding and swelling.

A horizontal incision is made several millimeters above the junction of the gingiva in the gingivobuccal sulcus (Fig. 13–3) and extends from the canine tooth area posterolaterally to the second molar area. It is made through the mucosa and periosteum down to the bone. Using a periosteal elevator or a Kitner dissector, the mucoperiosteal flap is elevated to the level of the infraorbital foramen, identifying and avoiding injury to the neurovascular bundle. Lateral retraction of an L-shaped flap described by Yarington helps to avoid

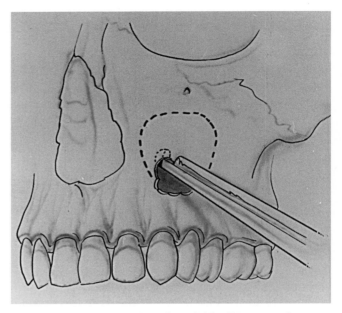

Fig. 13–4. Removal of bone for a Caldwell-Luc procedure.

this complication.[7] Elevating the periosteum to the edge of the pyriform aperture increases the surgical exposure.

The anterior wall of the sinus is fenestrated with a gouge, osteotome, or a cutting bur. The opening is enlarged with a Kerrison rongeur until adequate exposure of the interior of the sinus has been obtained (Fig. 13–4). The surgeon must be careful to avoid damaging the roots of the teeth or the developing tooth buds in children. If a free bone graft is needed, a small drill or gouge is used to outline the donor area needed, and the dots are connected to remove the intact anterior lateral wall of the maxillary sinus. The diseased mucosa, mucopus, and other cysts or polyps are removed with elevators, curettes, and/or tissue forceps. Care is taken in the roof of the sinus to avoid injury to the infraorbital nerve.

A nasoantral window is created below the inferior turbinate and the nasal mucosal flap rotated into the sinus as previously described. The gingivobuccal incision is closed with absorbable suture. Bleeding is controlled by packing with antibiotic impregnated gauze or a balloon catheter in the sinus by way of the intranasal antrostomy. If packing is used, it is removed on the first or second postoperative day.

Complications

The most common complication of radical antral procedures is paresthesia or anesthesia of the cheek, teeth, and gingiva secondary to stretch injury of the infraorbital nerve. Fortunately, this is usually temporary and resolves in 3 to 6 months. Hemorrhage with hematoma and massive facial swelling can occur. Injury to the superior alveolar nerve may devitalize the upper teeth.

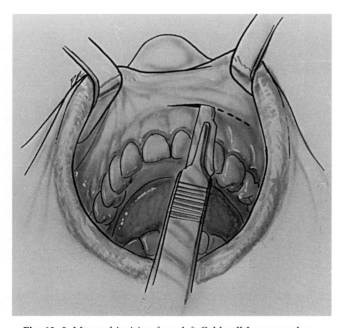

Fig. 13–3. Mucosal incision for a left Caldwell-Luc procedure.

This procedure should not be performed in children whose upper teeth have not erupted because of the risk of injury to unerupted permanent teeth. The lacrimal apparatus can be injured during resection of the medial wall. Blindness from direct injury to the optic nerve or an intraorbital hematoma have been reported. Chronic pain or neuroma can occur from damage to neural structures, and an oroantral fistula can occur in the suture line. Postoperative ethmoiditis has been reported as well as pulmonary atelectasis.[7] Revision surgery increases the likelihood of all complications, especially injury to the infraorbital nerve.

Oroantral Fistula

The maxillary sinus cavity is separated from the upper molar teeth by a thin layer of bone that is particularly thin and occasionally absent in the region of the first molar tooth, in which case the root may extend into the sinus. An oroantral fistula most commonly occurs following the extraction of a tooth that is intimately involved with the floor of the maxillary sinus. The risk of fistula formation is increased if the patient has an apical abscess or cyst.

Escape of liquids into the nose during swallowing is the most common symptom. Other symptoms include pain over the maxillary sinus, purulence at the fistula site, foul taste, and malodorous nasal discharge. Conservative treatment, consisting of antibiotics and irrigation, is worthwhile if the oroantral fistula is discovered early. If this is unsuccessful after 2 to 4 weeks, surgery should be considered.

Technique

With the patient under local or general anesthesia, the fistula is completely excised. If an adjacent tooth root is involved, the tooth must be extracted. A buccal mucoperiosteal flap, as described in Berger,[8] is elevated, including the alveolus exposing the canine fossa. The flap is advanced over the exposed fistula site and sutured in place. A palatal rotational flap based on the greater palatine artery is another popular method to close the fistula.[9] This flap has the advantage of not obliterating the gingivobuccal sulcus, which is important in denture wearers but lacks the pliability of the buccal flap. The raw donor site on the palate is left to heal by secondary intention. Both palatal and buccal flaps may be necessary to close large fistulas. A nasoantral window should be performed at the time of repair to prevent an episode of maxillary sinusitis from causing breakdown of the flap. Postoperative care includes a soft diet. The patient is advised not to blow the nose and to sneeze with the mouth open.

Complications

Breakdown of the flap and recurrence of the fistula are the most common complications. If this occurs, then the health of the antrum must be suspected.

ETHMOID SINUS

The ethmoid sinus is the keystone of the paranasal sinuses because of its central location and its vital role in nasal and sinus infection. All the sinuses, the orbits, the nasal cavity, and the cranium share common borders with the ethmoid sinus. Because of the proximity of the anterior ethmoid sinus to the ostia of the frontal, maxillary, and sphenoid sinuses, disease in the ethmoid sinus can cause obstruction of these ostia and subsequent sinusitis.

Surgery of the ethmoid sinus dates back to Hippocrates.[10] In 1884, Jansen probably performed the first transantral ethmoidectomy.[11] Mosher described the anatomy of the ethmoid sinus and intranasal ethmoidectomy in 1912.[12] Smith is credited with the first external ethmoidectomy.[12]

The most common indication for open surgery of the ethmoid sinus is nasal polyposis, frequently arising in the middle-meatal region. Also known as hyperplastic rhinosinusitis, the diseased mucosa can range from thickened mucosa to isolated polyps. Nasal polypectomy alone has limited usefulness in controlling nasal polyps; therefore, more radical surgery is recommended with complete exenteration of the ethmoid labyrinth. Ethmoidectomy with removal of the lamina papyracea may also be used for decompression of the orbit in cases of exophthalmos secondary to Graves' disease.

The specific ethmoidectomy approach depends on the surgeon's familiarity with the procedure, the degree of visualization needed, and the presentation of the disease. Intranasal, transantral, and external ethmoidectomies each have specific advantages and disadvantages. The anterior cranial fossa approach to the ethmoid sinus is used for neoplasms and is discussed elsewhere. Intranasal ethmoidectomy allows bilateral access and direct entry to the ethmoid cells, but the visualization is not as good as with other techniques. The transantral approach gives access to both the maxillary and ethmoid sinuses. Its disadvantages are unilateral access and limited visualization of the anterior air cells. External ethmoidectomy allows direct visualization of the orbital contents. Its disadvantages are unilateral access, poor inferior nasal visualization, and an external scar. These approaches can be done alone or, if necessary, in combination.

Intranasal Ethmoidectomy (Sphenoethomoidectomy)

The procedure can be performed with the patient under either local or general anesthesia. The nasal mucosa is anesthetized with 4% cocaine solution on cotton pledgets and mucosal injection of lidocaine with epinephrine. If necessary for exposure, a submucous re-

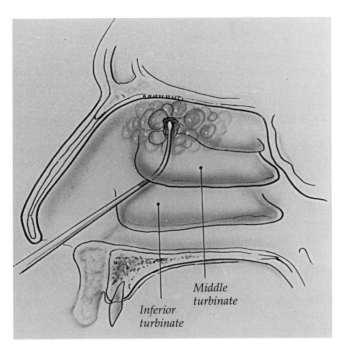

Fig. 13–5. Removal of ethmoid disease during intranasal ethmoidectomy.

Inferior turbinate

Middle turbinate

section of the septum or nasal septoplasty is performed initially. A sharp curette is used to enter the anterior ethmoid cells in the area of the agger nasi and the infundibulum. Angulated sharp loop curettes are used to remove the anterior cells (Fig. 13–5). If bleeding becomes bothersome, the area is packed and attention is turned to the other side of the nose because this procedure is usually performed bilaterally.

Minimal resection of the middle turbinate is important because the attachment of the middle turbinate is a landmark for the cribriform plate, which is just medial to it.

A curette or forceps is inserted into the posterior cells, which are opened carefully. The posterior limit of the ethmoid labyrinth is the anterior wall of the sphenoid sinus, which is slightly inferior to the posterior ethmoid cells. If indicated, the sphenoid sinus is entered and a portion of the anterior wall is removed. Full visualization of the roof and lateral wall of the sphenoid enables the surgeon to remove the posterior and anterior ethmoid cells in a three-dimensional block, always working posterior to anterior. The medial boundary is the plane of the middle turbinate, the lateral boundary is the plane of the lateral sphenoid wall and lamina papyracea, and the superior boundary is the plane of the sphenoid sinus roof and cribriform plate. The lateral wall of the sphenoid is not always visible; however, the optic nerve, carotid canal, cribriform plate, lamina papyracea, fovea ethmoidalis, and cavernous sinus should not be at risk as long as the forceps are never used outside the extension of the planes of the roof and lateral sphenoid wall.

Attempts are made to exteriorize each ethmoid cell individually. Packing with antibiotic-impregnated gauze or lining the surgical defect with antibiotic ointment is performed. Postoperative care consists of saline irrigations. The crusts that form are not removed until they can be removed gently with suctioning or forceps approximately 1 week later. Care is taken to prevent formation of synechiae. If they form, they are lysed and Telfa splints can be placed intranasally for a few days to prevent recurrence.

Transantral Ethmoidectomy

Transantral ethmoidectomy may also be performed with the patient under either local or general anesthesia. When the procedure is performed for orbital decompression, general anesthesia is usually used. A Caldwell-Luc procedure is performed as previously described. When the interior of the maxillary sinus is visualized, the upper medial wall of the maxillary sinus is approached halfway down the border between the medial and superior walls of the antrum. At this point, the ethmoid labyrinth may be noted to bulge into the maxillary sinus (bulla ethmoidalis). This area is entered with bone-cutting forceps, and the anterior ethmoid cells are opened, although the anterior most cells are often difficult to remove with this approach. Exenteration of cells is carried posteriorly. Care is taken not to damage the orbital rim. The middle turbinate serves as the medial margin of the dissection, and the lamina papyracea is the lateral margin. The roof of the ethmoids (fovea ethmoidalis) must be maintained under direct vision. After removal of the ethmoid cells, a nasoantral window is not necessary because the middle meatal wall has been removed. Packing is not necessarily required.

External Ethmoidectomy

External ethmoidectomy is the traditional approach for acute ethmoiditis complicated by orbital abscess. It is also indicated for frontoethmoid disease requiring simultaneous access to the ethmoid and frontal sinuses. Mucocele, pyocele, and tumors of the ethmoid are also approached by the external method.

Technique

External ethmoidectomy is best done under general anesthesia because the orbital contents, which are very sensitive, must be retracted. A 2- to 3-cm curvilinear incision is made halfway between the inner canthus and the anterior aspect of the nasal bones (Fig. 13–6). This incision can be extended laterally beneath the eyebrow for frontal sinus exposure. Troublesome bleeding from the angular vessel lying superficial to the periosteum is controlled with ligation or cauterization. The

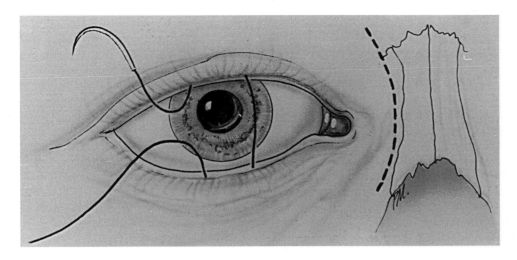

Fig. 13–6. Incision for external ethmoidectomy.

periosteum over the frontal process of the maxilla is incised and elevated laterally until the lacrimal crest is identified. The orbital contents are retracted, taking care not to injure the lacrimal sac in the medioinferior portion of the operative field. If the medial canthal ligament is incised, it must be reattached to avoid blunting or telecanthus. The lamina papyracea, which is the lateral wall of both anterior and posterior ethmoid labyrinths, is exposed. Approximately 2 cm posterior to the posterior lacrimal crest in the frontoethmoid suture line is the anterior ethmoid artery. The posterior ethmoid artery is approximately another 1 cm posterior to this, and the optic nerve is approximately 0.5 cm posterior to the posterior ethmoid artery.[13] The anterior ethmoid artery is usually clipped, ligated, or cauterized. Cautery should be used with caution as there

are reports of blindness from transfer of the current to the optic nerve. The posterior ethmoid artery is identified but not necessarily ligated, to help prevent injury to the optic nerve.

When the operative field is fully visualized, the lamina papyracea is entered and the ethmoid cells taken down with rongeur (Fig. 13–7). The ethmoid cells can be removed while keeping the limits of the procedure anterior to the posterior ethmoid artery. The vessels correspond with the level of the cribriform plate. The middle turbinate is identified and preserved, although some surgeons remove the inferior half of the middle turbinate. The posterior limit of the ethmoid is the anterior wall of the sphenoid sinus. If diseased, the sphenoid is opened and the anterior wall is removed. Diseased mucosa and polyps are removed if present.

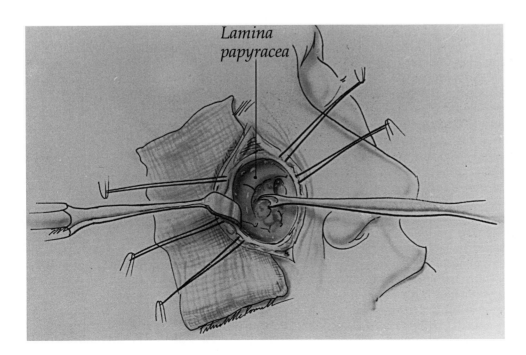

Lamina papyracea

Fig. 13–7. Removal of ethmoid disease during external ethmoidectomy.

Complications

If the surgeon visualizes the important landmarks and observes the appropriate planes of dissection, then complications should be minimal.

In external ethmoidectomy, a poorly placed incision can result in medial canthal webbing or hypertrophic scar. Making a Z-plasty at the time of the original incision can prevent this complication. Injury to the lacrimal apparatus and blunting of the medical canthus can occur. Deep dissection in the orbit can result in damage to the second, third, fourth, fifth, and sixth cranial nerves. Visual loss secondary to retrobulbar hematoma or direct injury to the optic nerve can occur. Cerebrospinal fluid leakage secondary to damage to the cribriform plate and fovea ethmoidalis can occur.

Transantral ethmoidectomy may result in numbness of the gingivobuccal sulcus, alveolar ridge, and distribution of the infraorbital nerve. Damage to the cribriform plate and roof of the ethmoid with cerebrospinal fluid leakage have been reported. Damage to tooth roots and the creation of an oroantral fistula are possible complications.

Intranasal ethmoidectomy has the same complications as the external and transantral procedures. Other complications include orbital cellulitis, sinusitis, and prolonged crusting (atrophic rhinitis).

FRONTAL SINUS

Surgery of the frontal sinus is performed to treat acute and chronic frontal sinusitis and its complications including orbital and intracranial extension, pyocele, mucocele, and osteomyelitis. The first frontal sinus procedure was trephination, followed by techniques using internal and external approaches. The lack of universal success indicates that no single operation is adequate for the broad spectrum of frontal sinus disease. The factors that can lead to surgical failure are inadequate opening or stenosis of the frontal ostium, frontal sinus septa that obstructs drainage, narrow extension of the frontal sinus superiorly and posteriorly forming isolated pockets of infection, inadequate removal of mucosa from the sinus walls, supraorbital ethmoid cells obstructing the frontal ostium, reinfection from adjacent infected sinuses, persistence of resistant microorganisms, and foci of osteomyelitis. The operations performed for frontal sinusitis can be separated into intranasal and external procedures. Intranasal procedures strive to create drainage from the frontal sinus by eliminating obstruction of the nasofrontal ostium within the nasal cavity and removal of disease in the adjacent paranasal sinuses. Endoscopes have proved valuable in assisting with the visualization of the nasofrontal duct during intranasal procedures (see Chap. 12). External procedures can be classified as follows: (1) drainage procedures via a

trephination; (2) removal of the anterior and/or orbital wall for access to the sinus and nasofrontal ostium; (3) creation of an osteoplastic flap for access to the sinus and frontal ostium; (4) obliteration of the sinus cavity; and (5) various combinations of these procedures.

Intranasal Procedures

The intranasal procedures of submucous resection of the septum or septoplasty, removal of intranasal polyps, excision of the anterior portion of the middle turbinate, and intranasal ethmoidectomy are used to promote drainage of the frontal sinus. Nonendoscopic intranasal trephination of the frontal sinus is extremely dangerous. Cannulation of the nasofrontal ostium is difficult because of its inconsistent location and tortuosity. Injury of the nasofrontal ostium may result in scarring and stenosis. Therefore, most intranasal attempts to improve the function of the nasofrontal ostium directly are not recommended unless performed under direct vision with an endoscope.

External Procedures

Trephination

Trephination is usually indicated for acute frontal sinusitis unresponsive to antibiotics. Other indications include an empyema or the presence of an intracranial or orbital complication of acute sinusitis.

Trephination can be carried out with the patient under either local or general anesthesia. A 1- to 2-cm curvilinear incision is made beneath the medial aspect of the patient's unshaven eyebrow. This is carried through the skin, subcutaneous tissue, and the periosteum over the floor of the frontal sinus. The periosteum is elevated, and the floor of the frontal sinus is penetrated because the floor is the thinnest and has no marrow spaces. Care must be taken to avoid the diploic bone of the anterior wall because the marrow spaces here can serve as a route for spread of infection leading to osteomyelitis. A curette or, preferably, a rotating cutting bur is used to make a 6- to 8-mm opening in the floor of the frontal sinus (Fig. 13–8). Specimens are taken for culture and, if indicated, for histologic study. Catheters to be used for irrigating the sinus are inserted and sutured in place. The nasofrontal ostium is noted to be functioning when the irrigant comes out the nose, at which time the drains can be removed.

Frontal Sinus Septectomy

A frontal sinus septectomy is considered in patients who have unilateral disease. By establishing drainage from the diseased side to the normal side, a more extensive procedure can be avoided, although the results with this procedure are inconsistent. This procedure, however, can make a unilateral problem bilateral.

The approach is identical to trephination, but the

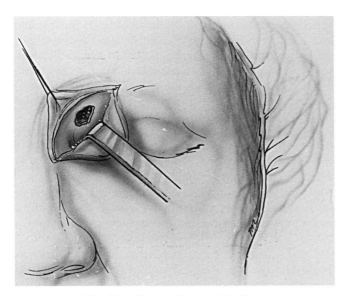

Fig. 13–8. Frontal sinus trephination.

opening in the floor is enlarged to 1 to 1.5 cm with the drill or rongeurs until the intrasinus septum is visualized. The septum is taken down with the bur or rongeurs. Care is taken not to injure the contralateral nasofrontal ostium. A catheter is sutured in place, and the sinus is irrigated until one sees evidence of nasal drainage. After drainage via the nose is established, the catheter is removed.

Frontoethmoidectomy Procedures

Of the numerous external frontal sinus procedures, the most commonly used are those described by Riedel, Killian, Lothrop, and Lynch. The anatomic changes created by each are shown in Fig. 13–9, with a comparison with the osteoplastic approach. Initial attempts to control frontal sinus disease were made by obliterating the cavity by collapsing the overlying skin onto the posterior wall. In 1898, Riedel described an operation that consisted of removing the anterior wall and floor of the frontal sinus that offered wide exposure of the sinus, but was successful only in small frontal sinuses.[14] The Riedel procedure, however, is disfiguring and offers no better success rate than the Lynch procedure discussed later. In 1903, Mosher modified Riedel's procedure by removing the posterior wall of the frontal sinus as well.[15] In 1903, Killian described another modification of the Riedel procedure in an attempt to avoid postoperative disfigurement.[16] His procedure removed the anterior and inferior wall but left the supraorbital rim intact. An anterior ethmoidectomy and middle turbinectomy were also performed. Although cosmetically acceptable, the preservation of the supraorbital rim did not obliterate the sinus. Again, the results of this procedure offered no advantage over the Lynch procedure.

Lothrop, in 1912, proposed a unique procedure that

consisted of unilateral or bilateral ethmoidectomy and middle turbinectomy.[17] The intersinus septum of the frontal sinus was removed, resulting in a large opening from the frontal sinus into the nasal cavity by connecting the two nasofrontal ostia.

The Lynch procedure, described in 1920, consists of an external ethmoidectomy, resection of the middle turbinate, and removal of the floor of the frontal sinus.[18] The sinus mucosa is removed by curettage.

The advantages of the Lynch procedure include a small and cosmetically acceptable incision and access to the frontal, ethmoid, and sphenoid sinuses, and because only the floor of the frontal sinus is removed, it is not deforming. The disadvantage of this technique is stenosis or closure of the reconstructed nasofrontal ostium, leading to recurrent infection or formation of a mucocele. Furthermore, exposure of the frontal sinus is limited.

The major cause of failure of the external frontal ethmoidectomy is stenosis of the nasofrontal ostium. Recurrent infection rates of up to 31% and mucocele development of 22% have been reported.[19] Reepithelization of the ostium with free grafts and rotational flaps has been attempted to prevent stenosis, but these attempts have been generally unsuccessful.

TECHNIQUE. The procedure is usually performed with the patient under general anesthesia. A tarsorrhaphy is performed to protect the cornea. A 4- to 6-cm

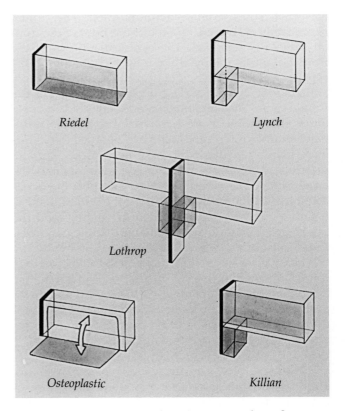

Fig. 13–9. Result of various frontal sinus procedures. See text.

curvilinear incision similar to that for an external ethmoidectomy is extended under the floor of the frontal sinus. The periosteum is incised and elevated from the floor of the frontal sinus. This elevation is most easily begun at the junction of the superior and medial orbital walls. The elevation is extended inferiorly, and the lacrimal crest and fossa are identified. The medial canthal ligament is identified, and the lacrimal sac is retracted laterally, exposing the cribriform lacrimal bone and, more posteriorly, the lamina papyracea of the ethmoid bone. Periosteal elevation upward identifies the frontoethmoid suture line. The anterior and posterior ethmoid vessels run through this and serve as a key landmark for the level of the cribriform plate. The anterior ethmoid artery lies 2 to 2.5 cm posterior to the lacrimal crest, whereas the posterior ethmoid artery is another 1 to 1.5 cm posterior to the anterior ethmoid artery. The optic nerve is approximately 0.5 cm behind the posterior ethmoid artery.[13] After the anterior ethmoid artery is identified, it is clipped or cauterized and divided. Next, the posterior ethmoid artery is identified but usually not divided.

The ethmoid sinus is entered by removing the thin bone in the posterior aspect of the lacrimal fossa with a sharp curette or straight punch. The underlying mucous membrane is preserved. The opening is enlarged posteriorly and superiorly with a Kerrison rongeur. The anterior ethmoid cells are encountered as the bony opening is enlarged. A mucous membrane flap is created to be turned up later for epithelization of the reconstructed nasofrontal communication. The frontal sinus cavity is entered, and the entire floor of the frontal sinuses is removed. The diseased mucosa of the frontal sinus is removed completely by curette, forceps, elevator, or burs. This can be difficult if there are superior, lateral, and posterior projections of the frontal sinus. The remaining anterior ethmoid and posterior ethmoid cells are removed. The middle turbinate, another important landmark because the cribriform plate is medial to it, may need to be partially resected to establish an adequate opening into the nasal cavity. The anterior wall of the sphenoid is encountered at the posterior limit of the ethmoid sinus. If indicated, the sphenoid cavity is entered, and the opening is enlarged with rongeurs. Polyps and diseased mucosa are removed.

The mucous membrane flap created earlier is then turned upward to line the medial wall of the newly formed nasofrontal opening. This is kept in place with a Silastic tube, 1 cm in diameter, and is sutured in place intranasally. The tube is maintained for 6 to 8 weeks. The periosteum is reapproximated, and the skin is closed.

COMPLICATIONS. The most likely cause of failure after a frontoethmoidectomy is subsequent stenosis of the reconstructed nasofrontal ostium resulting in obstruction of the frontal sinus with recurrent infection or mucocele. Other complications include (1) incomplete control of the ethmoid vessels or damage to the ciliary veins resulting in periorbital hematoma and visual loss, (2) injury to the lacrimal sac leading to epiphora or dacryocystitis, and (3) injury to the dura with cerebrospinal fluid leakage and possible meningitis. Visual loss may also occur from direct injury to the optic nerve if dissection or cautery is performed too far posteriorly in the orbit.

Osteoplastic Frontal Sinus Procedure

More recently, frontal sinus surgery has returned to efforts to obliterate the sinus because of the difficulty of maintaining a patent nasofrontal ostium postoperatively. Unlike the earlier obliterative procedures of Riedel and Mosher, today's procedure spares the patient postoperative deformity. This operation is best performed by means of the direct approach to the frontal sinus using a hinged osteoperiosteal flap of the anterior wall of the frontal sinus, as was first reported by Schonburn in Europe in 1894.[20] In the United States, Goodale and Montgomery popularized the procedure in 1958.[21]

Advantages of the osteoplastic flap procedure are direct visualization of both frontal sinuses, direct access to the supraorbital ethmoid sinus, elimination of the need to reconstruct the nasofrontal ostium for drainage, easy obliteration of the sinus cavity if required, and minimal cosmetic deformity. The disadvantages of the operation include a more extensive procedure with a potential for greater blood loss, potential supraorbital nerve injury with hypesthesia of the forehead, possible abnormal healing of the bone flap (frontal bossing), and a larger scar.

The procedure can be performed through an incision directly above the eyebrows (gullwing incision if bilateral) or through a coronal approach (placing the incision behind the hairline [Fig. 13–10]). Obliteration of the sinus has also become an integral part of this procedure and is usually accomplished with implanted autogenous fat based on studies by Montgomery.[22] MacBeth[23] and Bosley,[24] however, rely on natural obliteration resulting from osteoneogenesis. Other materials that have been used to obliterate the sinus include muscle, bone dust, plaster, and hydroxyapatite. Cranialization, removal of the posterior wall of the frontal sinus, is another suggested method of obliteration, most commonly utilized when the posterior wall of the sinus is fractured or dehiscent.[25]

The osteoplastic flap provides the best visualization of the frontal sinus, but it does not provide exposure of the other sinuses. Patients with pansinusitis require additional intranasal or external approaches to remove inflamed or diseased tissue from the other sinuses. The osteoplastic approach can be used to remove osteomas without obliteration of the sinus unless the nasofrontal ostium is injured during the resection. The osteoplastic

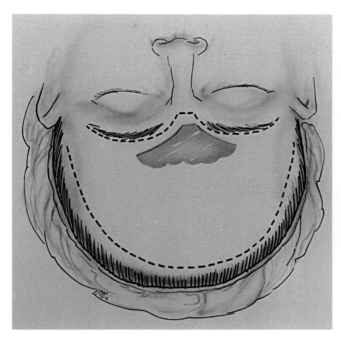

Fig. 13–10. Incision used for osteoplastic approach to the frontal sinus.

flap is used frequently for revision of frontal sinus surgery.

TECHNIQUE. A 6-foot Caldwell radiograph of the paranasal sinuses is obtained preoperatively, and a template of the frontal sinus is fashioned and sterilized. If the sinus is to be obliterated, the periumbilical abdomen is prepared and draped. The patient's face and hair are prepared and draped for a coronal incision, whereas only the face is prepared for the eyebrow incision.

In the unilateral procedure, the incision extends along the entire length of the upper border of the unshaven eyebrow. If the procedure is bilateral, the incision is arched downward to cross the root of the nose horizontally onto the contralateral side in a gullwing fashion. The subcutaneous tissue and frontalis muscle are divided. The flap is elevated superiorly superficial to the periosteum in the areolar tissue between the frontalis muscle and periosteum. The incision is elevated inferiorly to expose the supraorbital ridges. The flaps are elevated sufficiently to permit placement of the x-ray template and insertion of the oscillating saw.

If the coronal incision is chosen (usually for bilateral procedure and for all trauma cases), the surgeon is positioned at the head of the patient, and the incision is placed approximately 2 cm behind the hairline. The incision is curved laterally toward the ears bilaterally. Hemostasis is obtained by fine-point cautery and Raney clips. Cautery should be avoided in the scalp because it may result in alopecia. The flap is elevated in a plane just superficial to the periosteum to the supraciliary ridges and the root of the nose. Care must

be taken to prevent injury to the supraorbital neurovascular bundle.

The sterilized template is carefully positioned over the nasal root and supraorbital ridges. Transillumination of the frontal sinus with an endoscope through a trephination has also been used to delineate the margins of the frontal sinus. The periosteal incision is made with electrocautery around the template to the supraorbital ridges and is elevated only 1 to 2 mm (Fig. 13–11). The periosteum along the supraorbital rims is not disturbed, to preserve an adequate blood supply for the osteoplastic flap. The bone cuts are made along the outline created by the periosteal incision using an oscillating saw held at an angle of approximately 45 degrees and directed toward the frontal sinus cavity. Beveling the bone cut is used to ensure entering the frontal sinus cavity and aid in repositioning the osteoplastic flap. Extreme care must be observed at this stage because of the possibility of a shallow frontal sinus. The intersinus septum needs to be cut to elevate the flap in a bilateral approach. The bone flap is carefully elevated with an osteotome. The bone flap, which is hinged inferiorly by periosteum, is rotated inferiorly, exposing the sinus cavity. The interior of the frontal sinus is inspected and cultures are taken. The diseased mucosa is stripped from the sinus and all of its recess. The bone of the sinus walls is denuded using a bur with visualization with the operating microscope to ensure complete removal of the sinus mucosa. This facilitates the establishment of the blood supply to nourish the adipose autograph. Extensions of the frontal sinus and any supraorbital ethmoid cells are opened. Strips of pericranium or temporalis muscle are used to obliterate the nasofrontal ostium. An abdominal fat graft harvested through a periumbilical incision is used to fill the sinus cavity, the bone flap is repositioned, and the periosteum is reapproximated with sutures. If the flap is unstable, it may need to be wired or plated in place. Drains are placed, and the flap is closed in layers.

COMPLICATIONS. Operative and postoperative complications occur in approximately 18% of cases.[26] These include hematoma, infection or abscess of the abdominal or frontal wound, bony cuts outside the sinus resulting in dural tears, skin necrosis, anosmia, ptosis of the eyelids, loss of frontalis muscle function, frontal pain secondary to neuroma of the supraorbital nerve or sectioning of the supraorbital nerve, hypesthesia of the forehead (temporary or permanent), unacceptable scar with the gullwing incision, depression or elevation of the flap (especially in unilateral procedure), fistula, fat necrosis of the implant with infection, pyocele, chronic pain, chronic sinusitis, osteomyelitis, recurrent infection, mucocele, depilation of the eyebrow on the gullwing incision or alopecia around the coronal incision, frontal nerve injury, and embossment (hyperostosis) of the bone flap.

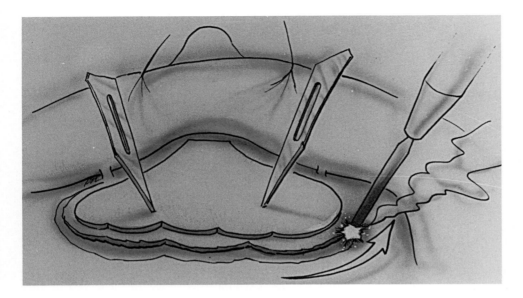

Fig. 13–11. Periosteal incision being made around margins of template. The arrow indicates the direction of the periosteal incision made by the cautery handpiece.

SPHENOID SINUS

In 1949, Van Alyea described the sphenoid sinus as the "most neglected by disease at its deep location within the skull, and neglected by the physician because of its subtle presentation."[2] Thirteen important structures are adjacent to the sphenoid. These are the dura, pituitary gland, optic nerve, cavernous sinus, internal carotid artery, abducens nerve, oculomotor nerve, trochlear nerve, ophthalmic nerve, maxillary nerve, sphenopalatine ganglion, sphenopalatine artery, and the nerve of the pterygoid canal.

When the sphenoid sinus is involved with a disease process, history and physical examination offer little to establish a correct diagnosis. Once a disease process has been identified, it is difficult to determine a primary from a secondary process or benign from malignant lesions. The most frequent symptoms in sphenoid sinus disease are retro-orbital headache, followed by headache in the frontal, vertex, and temporal areas. Diplopia and altered vision are the next most common complaints.

The most common disease of the sphenoid sinus is sinusitis. The complications of sphenoid sinusitis, although uncommon, include cavernous sinus thrombosis, retrobulbar neuritis, meningitis, blindness, orbital apex syndrome, and carotid artery occlusion. Early diagnosis and treatment of sphenoid sinusitis are the most important factors in reducing morbidity and mortality. The CT scan has improved the accuracy of diagnosing sphenoid sinus disease and should be obtained when the physician suspects this diagnosis.

Many of the surgical approaches to the sphenoid were developed for transsphenoidal surgery of sellar lesions. The sphenoid can be approached by several routes, including intranasal through the natural ostia, transethmoid during an external, transantral, or intra-

nasal ethmoidectomy, and transseptal. The transnasal route was first used by Schloffer in 1907.[27] In 1910, Cushing, using the best features of several techniques, performed a submucosal nasal septal resection via the sublabial incision.[28] Hirsch introduced an intranasal route to the sphenoid sinus.[29]

Technique

The patient is placed under general anesthesia regardless of which technique is used because of the extent of dissection. The intranasal route involves opening and enlarging the natural ostia, which is located just medial to the superior turbinate. The anterior wall of the sphenoid sinus is between 6.5 to 8 cm from the anterior nasal spine and is at a 20 to 30 degree angle from the nasal floor. The endoscope has proved to be invaluable in finding the ostia. The ostia can be enlarged using a rongeur, thereby improving drainage. Biopsies and cultures can also be obtained.

For the transseptal approach that is used in transsphenoidal surgery, the patient's head is slightly elevated and turned to the side of the operating surgeon. A C-arm is recommended for localization and is positioned before the patient is prepared and draped. The nasal septum and nose are treated with topical vasoconstrictors, and lidocaine with epinephrine is injected into the septal mucosa. A sublabial incision is made in the gingiva well above the gingival margin down through the periosteum of the maxilla. An elevator elevates the periosteum superiorly, exposing the anterior nasal spine, nasal floor, and piriform aperture. The mucoperiosteal flap is elevated from the floor of the nose up to the nasal septum. Following this, a unilateral mucoperichondrial flap is elevated back to the bony septum. An incision in the cartilaginous/bony septum is made, and the anterior septum is displaced laterally but not resected. The nasal spine and maxillary crest attachments need to be separated, and occasionally the nasal spine needs to be removed. The mucoperiosteal flap is elevated along the bony septum bilaterally until the rostrum of the sphenoid sinus is encountered. The bony septum is removed to the keel of the sphenoid sinus. A radiograph with the C-arm confirms the correct anatomic location for the sphenoidotomy. The anterior wall of the sphenoid sinus is opened, and the intrasinus septum is taken down. This gives wide exposure of the sinus, facilitating procedures on the sphenoid sinus itself or to the sella, just behind the posterior sphenoid wall. An operating microscope improves visualization. The indentation of the internal carotid artery and optic nerve can often be seen in the superolateral wall of the sphenoid. At the completion of the procedure, the nasal flaps and cartilaginous septum are returned to the midline. The sublabial incision is closed with absorbable suture, and the nose is packed. The packing is removed in 24 to 48 hours. The transethmoid approach to the sphenoid sinus is simply an extension of an ethmoidectomy, as previously described.

Complications

Complications include nasal septal perforation, bleeding, cerebrospinal fluid leakage, meningitis, and recurrent sinusitis. Cosmetic complications such as saddlenose deformity, deviated septum, and nasal-tip deformities have been reported. The most serious complications are related to damage to surrounding neurovascular structures. Injury to the second, third, fourth, fifth, and sixth cranial nerves can occur. The internal carotid artery and cavernous sinus can be damaged. An air embolus can occur, as well as venous hemorrhage from injury to the cavernous sinus.

SUGGESTED READINGS

1. Canalis RF, Cabieses F, Hemenway WG, and Aragon R: Prehistoric trephination of the frontal sinus. Ann Otol Rhinol Laryngol 90:186, 1981.
2. Van Alyea OF: Nasal Sinuses: An Anatomic and Clinical Consideration. Baltimore, Williams & Wilkins, 1951.
3. Bacher JA: Fatal air embolism after puncture of the maxillary antrum-Autopsy. Calif State Med J 21:433, 1923.
4. Peterson RJ: Canine fossa puncture. Laryngoscope 83:369, 1973.
5. Lund VJ: Fundamental considerations of the design and function of intranasal antrostomies. Rhinology 23:231, 1985.
6. Goodman WS: The Caldwell-Luc procedure. Otolaryngol Clin North Am 9:187, 1976.
7. Yarington CT: The Caldwell-Luc operation revisited. Ann Otol Rhinol Laryngol 93:380, 1984.
8. Berger A: Oroantral openings and their surgical correction. Arch Otolaryngol Head Neck Surg 30:400, 1939.
9. Girgis IH and Mourice M: Mobilization of the greater palatine artery in closure of oro-antral fistulae. J Laryngol Otol 95:707, 1981.
10. Harrison DFN: Surgery in allergic sinusitis. Otolaryngol Clin North Am 4:83, 1971.
11. Jansen A: Fur Eriffang der Nebenhohlen der Nase bei Chronischer Eiterung. Arch Laryngol Rhinol 1:135, 1894.
12. Mosher HP: The surgical anatomy of the ethmoidal labyrinth. Ann Otol Rhinol Laryngol 38:869, 1929.
13. Kirchner JA, Yanagisawa E, and Crelin ES: Surgical anatomy of the ethmoid arteries. Arch Otolaryngol 74:382, 1961.
14. Riedel: In: Schenke: Inang Dissertation, Jena, 1898.
15. Mosher HP and Judd DK: An analysis of seven cases of osteomyelitis of the frontal bone complicating frontal sinusitis. Laryngoscope 43:153, 1933.
16. Killian G: Die Killianische Radicoloperation Chronischer Stirnhohlenes Terungen: II. Weiteres Kasuistisches Material und Zusammenfassung. Arch Laryngol Rhinol 13:59, 1903.
17. Lothrop HA: Frontal sinus suppuration. Ann Surg 59:937, 1912.
18. Lynch RC: The technique of a radical frontal sinus operation which has given me the best results. Laryngoscope 31:1, 1921.
19. Goodale RL: Some cause for failure in frontal sinus surgery. Ann Otol Rhinol Laryngol 51:648, 1942.
20. Schonborn, cited by Wilkop A: Ein Beitrag Zur Casuistik der Erkrankungen des Sinus Frontalis. Wurzberg, F. Frome, 1894.
21. Goodale RL and Montgomery WW: Experience with the osteoplastic anterior wall approach to the frontal sinus. Arch Otolaryngol 68:271, 1958.
22. Montgomery WW and Pierce DL: Anterior osteoplastic fat obliteration for frontal sinus: clinical experience and animal studies. Trans Am Acad Ophthalmol Otolaryngol 67:46, 1963.
23. MacBeth RG: The osteoplastic operation for chronic infection of the frontal sinus. J Laryngol Otol 68:465, 1954.
24. Bosley WA: Osteoplastic obliteration of the frontal sinus: a review of 100 patients. Laryngoscope 82:1463, 1972.
25. Malecki J: New trends in frontal sinus surgery. Acta Otolaryngol 50:137, 1959.
26. Donald PJ and Bernstein L: Compound frontal sinus injuries with intracranial penetration. Laryngoscope 88:225, 1978.
27. Schloffer H: Erfolgreiche Operatione Eines Hypophysentumors auf Nasalem Wege. Wein Klin Wochenschr 20:G21, 1907.
28. Levine E: The sphenoid sinus: the neglected nasal sinus. Arch Otolaryngol 104:585, 1978.
29. Hirsch O: Eine Neuen Methode der Endonasalem Operation von Lypophysentumoren. Wien Med Wochenschr 59:636, 1902.

14 Neoplasms of the Nose and Paranasal Sinuses

Robert H. Miller, Erich M. Sturgis, and Curtis L. Sutton

Neoplasms of the nose and paranasal sinuses are rare if contrasted to inflammatory disease of these structures. Because the signs and symptoms of the two may be similar, the former may not be recognized until far advanced, and thus the differential diagnosis of sinonasal complaints must include neoplasms, particularly if the response to treatment is poor.

EPIDEMIOLOGY AND ETIOLOGY

Neoplasms of the sinonasal tract represent less than 1% of all malignant tumors and approximately 3% of malignant tumors of the upper areodigestive tract. Although only 100 cases of malignant disease of the sinuses occur in the United States each year, rates are higher in Japan and parts of Africa. There is a 2:1 male to female distribution. Most (80%) of these malignant tumors are squamous cell carcinomas.[1] The site of origin is usually the maxillary sinus (50 to 70%), followed by the nasal cavity (15 to 30%) and the ethmoid sinuses (10 to 20%), with the frontal or sphenoid sinuses accounting for less than 5%.

Various industrial exposures have been linked to malignant tumors of the sinonasal tract, including nickel, wood dust, leather, formaldehyde, mineral oils, chromium, isopropyl oils, lacquer paint, soldering/welding, and radium paint. Although most of these exposures have been linked to epithelial malignancies, especially squamous cell carcinoma, hardwood dust has a particular association with adenocarcinoma of the ethmoid sinuses.[1,2] There also seems to be a long latent period of two to four decades.

Although the link of sinonasal malignant disease to tobacco exposure was weak in the past, a recent case-control study demonstrated a doubling of risk in long-term or heavy smokers. Also noted were associations between certain dietary factors and cancer of the sinonasal tract, with alcohol and salted/smoked foods linked to increased risk and fruits and vegetables linked to decreased risk.[2] Although some authors believe that chronic sinusitis is associated with the development of cancer, the link appears weak or may represent prior misdiagnosis.[3]

EVALUATION

History

The symptoms of malignant tumors of the sinuses are not necessarily different from those of inflammatory disease and frequently do not develop until the tumor is quite advanced. Facial swelling is the most common presenting symptom of patients with maxillary sinus cancer. Nasal obstruction, the next most common symptom of antral neoplasms, is the most common complaint of patients with ethmoid malignant disease. Pain and epistaxis are relatively common symptoms and should increase the clinician's index of suspicion for malignancy. Abnormalities of the eye, numbness of the cheek, and trismus are ominous symptoms.

Examination

Although the most common finding is a nasal mass, less advanced tumors may not be visible. Certainly, endoscopy provides advantages over anterior rhinoscopy. Second, the surrounding anatomic areas should be evaluated because up to 75% have extended beyond the nose and paranasal sinuses. Proptosis or epiphora occurs in up to 45% of patients with ethmoid neoplasms. The overlying skin and palate should be checked for swelling. Cranial neuropathies have been reported in approximately one third of patients with sinonasal malignant disease.[4] Neck and distant metastasis rates are generally reported as approximately 15% and 5%, respectively.[5] Second primary malignancy rates are less than 5%, with the contralateral antrum being the most common site.[6]

Radiology

Following a detailed physical examination and an accurate history, an imaging evaluation of the paranasal sinuses is performed. Imaging techniques include plain films, computed tomography (CT), and magnetic resonance imaging (MR).

In patients with neoplastic involvement of the sinuses, the most common finding on plain radiographs is opacification (> 90%) of the involved sinus, which may be difficult to distinguish from inflammatory disease.[7] If bone destruction is observed, however, "run of the mill" inflammatory disease is less likely, and neoplasm should be suspected. Bone destruction is the second most common plain film finding in patients with sinus neoplasms, occurring in approximately 69% of cases.[7] Other aggressive, nonmalignant processes, such as sinonasal polyposis and Wegener's granulomatosis, can cause bone erosion and destruction.

Because plain films are reported as normal in 7% and interpreted as inflammatory disease in 17% of patients with malignant sinus disease, high-resolution, thin-section CT and MR have largely replaced plain radiographs in the initial evaluation if neoplastic disease is suspected. CT, because of the excellent depiction of soft tissue and bony structures, provides a detailed picture of tumor extent and degree of bone destruction (Fig. 14–1). A standard CT currently includes thin-section (3- to 5-mm thickness) axial and direct coronal (patient in prone position if possible) scans.

Critical bony structures and surrounding areas assessed by CT include orbital walls, cribiform plate, fovea ethmoidalis, bony confines of the sphenoid sinus, posterior walls of the frontal and maxillary sinuses, pterygopalatine fossa, pterygomaxillary fissure, and infratemporal fossa. Accuracy rates of 78 to 85% have been reported for CT prediction of the extent of the neoplasm when compared with the ultimate surgical findings.[8] One important limitation of CT, however, is distinction among neoplasm, soft tissue edema, and retained secretions resulting from sinus obstruction by the neoplasm. In such cases, overestimation of the extent of the neoplasm may occur.

MR can provide a distinction among inspissated mucus or retained secretions, soft tissue edema, and neoplasm, thereby providing a more accurate delineation of the true extent of the neoplasm (Fig. 14–2). Edema and secretions generally exhibit low signal intensity on T1-weighted images and high signal intensity on T2-weighted sequences, basically because of high water content. When the fluid secretions become more proteinaceous with reduced water content, the signal intensity can be variable, with high signal intensity seen on T1-weighted imaging. When complete desiccation occurs, signal intensity can be low on both T1- and T2-weighted images. Carcinomas involving the sinuses tend to have intermediate to low signal intensity on both T1- and T2-weighted images, owing to their highly cellular content with little free water. Intravenous gadolinium-DTPA (diethylenetriamine pentaacetic acid) can be used as a contrast agent to assist in evaluating margins of the neoplasm and in detecting intracranial or intraorbital extension.

MR's major limitation is poor assessment of bony erosion or destruction. A second limitation is the diagnostic confusion that arises when evaluating osteogenic and chondrogenic neoplasms, as well as the nonneoplastic conditions, such as fibrous dysplasia, that can involve the paranasal sinuses. In such cases, CT evaluation is essential to refine the differential diagnosis. The critical structures best assessed by MR are the soft tissues and include the pterygoid muscles, ocular muscles, optic nerve, brain and meninges, cavernous sinus, and prevertebral fascia. In comparison with surgical findings, accuracy rates of 94% for MR and 98% for MR with gadolinium have been reported.[9] When CT and MR were compared in evaluating the extent of neoplasm, false-positive and false-negative results occurred simultaneously, suggesting that CT and MR did not differ significantly in staging neoplasms of the nasal cavity and paranasal sinuses.[10] As expected, MR was better in evaluating soft tissue structures and large bony structures, whereas CT was superior in evaluating fine bony detail.[10] CT and MR are often comple-

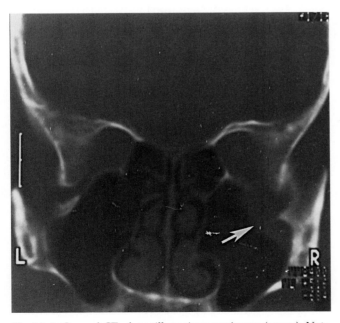

Fig. 14–1. Coronal CT of maxillary sinus carcinoma (arrow). Note erosion of orbital floor.

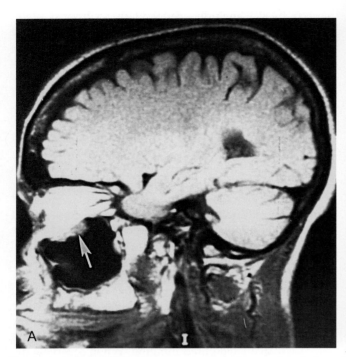

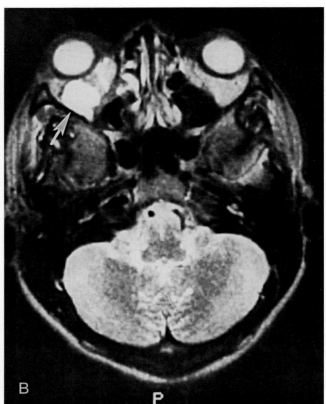

Fig. 14–2. A. Sagittal MR of squamous cell carcinoma of roof of maxillary sinus (arrow). B. Axial MR of squamous cell carcinoma of sinus extending into orbit (arrow). The carcinoma appears bright on T2-weighted imaging.

mentary in evaluating neoplasms of the paranasal sinuses and nasal cavity and may often together offer an extremely detailed picture of the amount and extent of the neoplasm. MR is often reserved for cases in which the margin of the neoplasm is unclear on CT, however.[8]

Biopsy

If the patient has an intranasal mass and the clinician is confident that the tumor is neither vascular nor a congenital lesion with intracranial extension, the mass can be biopsied in the office. Imaging usually should be performed before biopsy, however, because it provides information about vascularity and origin, and the trauma of biopsy may complicate the radiologic interpretation of margins. If the mass is small, the accuracy of the biopsy can be improved using optical biopsy forceps available with sinus endoscopic instruments. If no intranasal mass is present, tissue from the antrum or ethmoid sinuses must be obtained.

To obtain material from the maxillary sinus, the surgeon was traditionally required to perform a nasoantral window or even a Caldwell-Luc procedure. With the advent of endoscopic sinus instruments, it is possible to perform a puncture of the anterior wall of the maxillary antrum with a trocar and to examine the sinus endoscopically. This allows an accurate biopsy, which can be performed in the office or operating room. Ethmoid tumors can also be biopsied endoscopically after a partial ethmoidectomy is performed for exposure.

STAGING

The American Joint Committee on Cancer has established a classification system for neoplasms of the maxillary antrum (Table 14–1).[11] The traditional basis of staging has been Ohngren's line, which runs from the medial canthus of the eye to the angle of the mandible.[12] In general, tumors below this line (infrastructure) have a better prognosis than those located above it (suprastructure).

Lymph node metastases from squamous carcinomas are uncommon at the time of presentation. The most common site of metastasis is the lung. The primary echelon nodes for maxillary sinus cancers include the retropharyngeal, submandibular, and jugular nodes. If the neoplasm invades the oral cavity, however, it behaves more like an oropharyngeal carcinoma, and the frequency of nodal metastases is dou-

TABLE 14–1. Maxillary Sinus Tumor Classification

TX	Primary tumor cannot be assessed
T0	No evidence of primary tumor
Tis	Carcinoma in situ
T1	Tumor limited to the antral mucosa
T2	Tumor with erosion of the bone of the infrastructure (palate, medial or anterior wall of antrum)
T3	Tumor invading the skin or bone of the suprastructure (posterior wall of antrum, floor or medial wall of orbit, anterior ethmoid)
T4	Tumor invading orbital contents, cribriform plate, posterior ethmoid, sphenoid, nasopharynx, soft palate, pterygomaxillary fossa, temporal fossa, base of skull

(From Beahrs OH, Henson DE, Hutter RVP, and Kennedy BJ (eds): Manual for Staging of Cancer: American Joint Committee on Cancer. 4th Ed. Philadelphia, JB Lippincott, 1992.)

TABLE 14–2. Regional Lymph Node Classification

NX	Regional lymph nodes cannot be assessed
N0	No regional lymph node metastasis
N1	Metastasis in a single ipsilateral lymph node, 3 cm or less in greatest dimension
N2a	Metastasis in a single ipsilateral lymph node more than 3 cm, but not more than 6 cm in greatest dimension
N2b	Metastasis in muliple ipsilateral lymph nodes, none more than 6 cm in greatest dimension
N2c	Metastasis in bilateral or contralateral lymph nodes, none more than 6 cm in greatest dimension
N3	Metastasis in a lymph node more than 6 cm in greatest dimension

(From Beahrs OH, Henson DE, Hutter RVP, and Kennedy BJ (eds): Manual for Staging of Cancer: American Joint Committee on Cancer. 4th Ed. Philadelphia, JB Lippincott, 1992.)

TABLE 14–3. Stage Grouping

	T1	T2	T3	T4
N0	Stage I	Stage II		
N1			Stage III	
N2				
N3				Stage IV

(From Beahrs OH, Henson DE, Hutter RVP, and Kennedy BJ (eds): Manual for Staging of Cancer: American Joint Committee on Cancer. 4th Ed. Philadelphia, JB Lippincott, 1992.)

bled. Only 10 to 15% have palpable lymphadenopathy at the time of diagnosis, whereas after treatment this incidence has been reported to increase to 20 to 30%.[5] Ten percent of patients ultimately develop distant metastases.[5] The classification of nodal metastases is outlined in Table 14–2, and the stage groups are listed in Table 14–3.[11]

TREATMENT

Surgery has been the cornerstone of therapy for neoplasms of the paranasal sinuses. The extent of the dis-

section varies with the histopathologic features and extension and includes the surgical continuum from simple endoscopic excision to radical maxillectomy with orbital exenteration. The standard incision used for the open approaches is the Weber-Fergusson incision (Fig. 14–3), and this may be combined with the Dieffenbach extension for orbital exenteration or the Lynch extension for better access to the upper nasal cavity, the ethmoid sinus, or the floor of the frontal sinus. The lip split or infraorbital extensions may not be necessary for small anterior lesions.

Endoscopic excision may be possible for certain benign lesions, but complete removal may be sacrificed. Similarly, the Caldwell-Luc approach may be adequate for certain types of neoplasms, but en bloc removal is essential for malignant lesions. Medial maxillectomy is the classic procedure for inverted papilloma and involves en bloc removal of the lateral nasal wall from the roof of the ethmoid to the floor of the maxillary sinus (Fig. 14–4). The ethmoid labyrinth can be exenterated completely, and with it a portion of the floor of the orbit. Although frequently performed by way of Weber-Fergusson incision, a facial degloving approach through the superior gingivobuccal sulcus provides excellent exposure of all but the most superior limits of the resection. A Caldwell-Luc antrotomy is used in

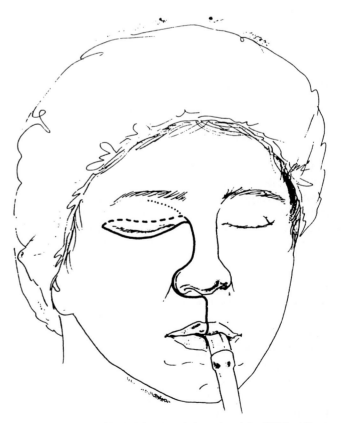

Fig. 14–3. Various skin incisions used: (– – –) standard Weber-Fergusson, (-----) Dieffenbach extension, and (.....) Lynch extension.

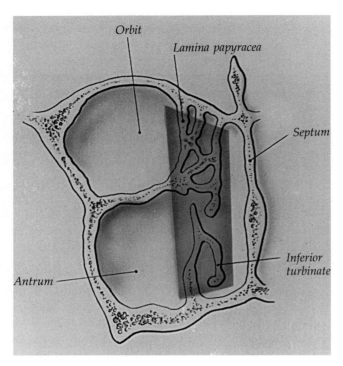

Fig. 14–4. Structures removed by a medial maxillectomy (shaded area).

section is in the area posterior to the sinus and is usually associated with considerable blood loss. Some surgeons prefer to use hypotensive anesthesia for this part of the procedure. If the neoplasm has not traversed the posterior wall of the sinus, a curved chisel can be passed between the pterygoid plates and the posterior wall of the sinus. The pterygoid plates can, however, be removed if necessary. Following the posterior cuts, Mayo scissors are used to free any remaining soft tissue attachments. Rather than trying to ligate or cauterize bleeding vessels at this time, the surgeon should pack the pterygomaxillary space and wait for several minutes. The packing can then be carefully removed and hemostasis obtained in a controlled fashion. Frequently, suture ligatures are required for the diffuse bleeding of the pterygoid venous plexus. The internal surface of the skin flap is lined with a split-thickness skin graft, and a palatal splint, fabricated preoperatively, is placed. This allows the patient to resume eating in the immediate postoperative period. In a partial maxillectomy, an attempt is generally made to preserve the orbital floor, whereas in a radical maxillectomy, the body of the zygoma is removed with the maxilla. Elective neck dissection is not performed be-

transecting the medial maxilla inferiorly and anteriorly. The medial orbital wall is freed after retracting orbital contents laterally, and finally the medial maxilla is freed posteriorly and removed. Reapproximation of the medial canthus is important in preventing postoperative telecanthus. Experience has demonstrated that the nasolacrimal duct can be transected as it exits the lacrimal fossa, allowing the anteriormost portion of the lateral nasal wall to be removed with minimal problems of epiphora.

Maxillectomy is the standard surgical procedure for maxillary sinus cancer. Partial maxillectomy is possible for early lesions, but they are rare. Therefore, most patients undergo total maxillectomy, and if orbital involvement is present, radical maxillectomy with orbital exenteration (Fig. 14–5). The maxillary sinus is approached through a Weber-Fergusson incision. The skin is elevated from the anterior wall of the maxillary sinus in a plane determined by the level of invasion of the neoplasm. Although several bone cuts are required, the bone is usually thin and easy to transect. An incisor tooth is removed, and a right-angle clamp is passed from the nose behind the posterior margin of the hard palate through the oral mucosa into the mouth. A Gigli saw is grasped and pulled through the nose, and the hard palate is divided. Similarly, the Gigli saw is passed through the lateral edge of the inferior orbital fissure, and the lateral buttress of the maxilla is cut. The lamina papyracea is cut with a chisel back to the medial edge of the inferior orbital fissure. The last dis-

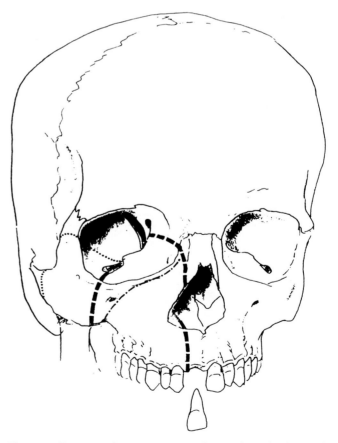

Fig. 14–5. Bone cuts for various surgical procedures (-·-·-) partial maxillectomy, (-----) total maxillectomy, and (.....) radical maxillectomy.

TABLE 14–4. Five-Year Survival for Radiation Therapy Only

Author	Patients	% T3/T4	Local Control (%)	5-Year Survival (%)
Amendola et al[14]	20	90	50	35
Lee & Ogura[15]	35	91	14	0
Frich[16]	22	86	55	39
Bush & Bagshaw[17]	22	100	23	22
Shibuya et al[18]	78	NR	NR	30
Issacs et al[19]	22	92	28 (2 yr)	10
Average (range)			32 (14–55)	23 (0–39)

NR (not reported)

cause of the low incidence of occult nodal metastasis and an inability to clear the retropharyngeal space adequately.

Neoplasms of the ethmoid and frontal sinuses and upper nasal cavity can also be approached through a Weber-Fergusson incision and a lateral rhinotomy, but these lesions often require craniofacial resection. If access to the intracranial cavity is required for complete removal, a small midline craniotomy through the forehead or a bitemporal craniotomy can be used.

A survival advantage appears to exist with combined therapy using both radiation and surgery, although the sequence has varied (see Chap. 34). One technique is to use 55 to 65 Gy of radiation therapy and then perform exploration of the sinus (frequently through a hard palatectomy) to determine whether any residual disease is present. If not, the sinus can be examined for recurrences on a regular basis through the fenestra. Another approach is to perform a maxillectomy followed by postoperative radiation therapy, usually in the 50- to 60-Gy range. Although some authors have suggested the use of preoperative radiation for globe salvage, the superiority in tumor control has not been defined between preoperative and postoperative radiation. Primary radiation is reserved for the rare early lesion or lymphoreticular lesions, but generally this modality serves an important adjuvant role.

The value of chemotherapy in the primary treatment of maxillary sinus cancer is still undetermined. In lymphoreticular lesions and some sarcomas, chemotherapy is used in an adjuvant or palliative manner. Some Japanese researchers have reported higher control rates with concomitant intra-arterial chemotherapy and radiation therapy with weekly cryotherapy and debridement via antrostomy and maxillectomy for salvage.[13]

Despite the use of surgery, radiation, and chemotherapy, the results of treatment of malignant tumors have been discouraging. Comparison of various treatment modalities has been difficult, however, because series are small and retrospective and because some authors lump all neoplasms together regardless of histologic features. The results of treatment of carcinoma of the paranasal sinuses are not good, particularly in advanced lesions. Overall, in examining series since 1980 with more than 20 patients, the reported 5-year survival rates have been 0 to 39% (average, 23%) for radiation only,[14–19] and 35 to 64% (average, 44%) for combined surgery and radiation therapy[15,18,20–24] (Tables 14–4 and 14–5). The addition of radiation has generally been thought to boost the surgical 5-year survival rates by 10 to 15%.[25]

Recent successes in organ preservation in laryngeal cancer have instigated the adaptation of this philosophy to sinus cancer. In a small pilot study, Swedish investigators administered to 12 patients with advanced sinus cancer, including 5 with orbital involvement and 3 with intracranial involvement, 3 courses of cisplatin and 5-fluorouracil, followed by preoperative 48 Gy of radiation and a surgical procedure taking tumor response into account. Local control was achieved in 11 of 12 patients, and no evidence of disease was found in 10 of 12, with a median follow-up of 22.5 months with no reported functional or cosmetic

TABLE 14–5. Five-Year Survival for Combined* Therapy

Author	Patients	% T3/T4	Local Control (%)	5-Year Survival (%)
Lee & Ogura[15]	61	66	69	38
Shibuya et al[18]	35	NR	NR	40
Korzeniowski et al[20]	57	86	51	35
Tsujii et al[21]	116	97	NR	44
Sisson et al[22]	35	73	49	64
Lavertu et al[23]	31	68	52	51
Zamora et al[24]	39	78	NR	45
Average (range)			57 (49–69)	44 (35–64)

Surgery plus radiation; NR (not reported)

loss.[26] Although this study is small, with a limited follow-up, it does provide an impetus for further studies addressing therapy from the point of view of the patient's quality of life.

TUMOR DIFFERENTIAL DIAGNOSIS

Primary tumors involving the nose and paranasal sinuses are generally divided into benign versus malignant and epithelial versus nonepithelial, with epithelial by far the most common (Table 14–6). Moreover, metastatic lesions, chiefly renal cell, breast, and lung carcinoma, may involve the sinonasal tract.

Benign Epithelial Tumors

Inverted Papilloma
Inverted papillomas or transitional papillomas account for approximately half of schneiderian papillomas. The fungiform papillomas make up most of the remainder, with the cylindric papilloma being a rare form of the schneiderian papilloma. Keratotic papillomas, the nasal equivalent of the simple cutaneous wart, occur in the nasal vestibule, whereas fungiform papillomas are generally found on the septum. Inverted papillomas usually arise from the lateral nasal wall, and the most common presenting symptom is nasal obstruction. Physical examination reveals a unilateral mass that frequently resembles an easily bleeding inflammatory polyp. Inflammatory polyps are usually bilateral, however, so the presence of a unilateral polyp should make the clinician suspicious of an inverted papilloma.

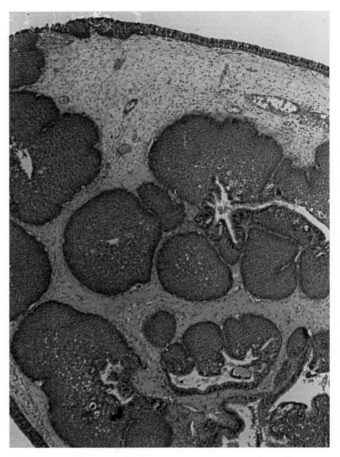

Fig. 14–6. Histopathologic appearance of inverted papilloma.

These tumors are slow growing and gradually erode bone to involve the ethmoid and maxillary sinuses, the orbit, and even the intracranial cavity.

Histopathologically, the tumor is characterized by hyperplastic respiratory epithelium with an exophytic or inverting pattern of growth (Fig. 14–6). The epithelial areas are composed of squamous cell epithelium with or without keratin formation. Micromucinous cysts are frequently present, and inflammatory cells are found in the stroma. Malignant transformation can occur in approximately 5% of patients and is usually squamous cell carcinoma or occasionally adenocarcinoma.[27,28]

The key to the successful treatment of an inverted papilloma is complete excision. Because of its location, this can be technically difficult, and therefore, recurrence rates are reported to be over 40% for intranasal excision and under 30% for extranasal excision.[27,28] Although the surgical procedure must be tailored to each neoplasm, most tumors can be removed completely by medial maxillectomy, with recurrence rates in the 0 to 22% range.[27,28] Although recently some investigators have reported endoscopic excision of inverted papillomas, including some advanced lesions with reasonable recurrence rates, most believe that standard medial

TABLE 14–6. Tumor Differential Diagnosis

Benign Epithelial	Malignant Epithelial
Keratatic papilloma	Squamous cell carcinoma
Fungiform papilloma	Transitional cell carcinoma
Inverted papilloma	Adenocarcinoma
Cylindric papilloma	Adenoid cystic carcinoma
Adenoma	Mucoepidermoid carcinoma
Ameloblastoma	Esthesioneuroblastoma
	Melanoma
	Undifferentiated carcinoma

Benign Nonepithelial	Malignant Nonepithelial
Ossifying fibroma	Rhabdomyosarcoma
Chondroma	Leiomyosarcoma
Osteoma	Fibrosarcoma
Neurilemmoma	Liposarcoma
Neurofibroma	Angiosarcoma
Hemangioma	Myxosarcoma
Giant cell granuloma	Hemangiopericytoma
Giant cell tumor	Chondrosarcoma
Nasopharyngeal angiofibroma	Osteosarcoma
	Lymphoma
	Plasmacytoma

maxillectomy should remain the procedure of choice, with the only possible exception being extremely early lesions.[27,28] No matter what approach or procedure is used, we cannot emphasize too strongly that complete removal of the neoplasm should be achieved at the time of the first operation because, otherwise, the success of all subsequent procedures is diminished significantly.[28] Radiation therapy should not be used because of the potential for malignant degeneration of the neoplasm.

Ameloblastoma

Neoplasms of dental origin occasionally manifest as a mass in the sinus. Although most tumors and cysts of dental origin respond to simple curettage, ameloblastoma, despite its benign histologic features, must be treated more aggressively to achieve a cure. The neoplasm is locally aggressive and, if not completely removed, can involve vital structures and cause death. A few cases of metastases have been reported, but these seem to occur only after multiple surgical procedures or radiation therapy.

Only 20% of ameloblastomas (also sometimes called adamantinomas) occur in the maxilla, usually in the region of the third molar. They may, however, extend into the maxillary sinus, nose, orbit, or even the base of the skull. Radiographically, the neoplasm is a multilocular lucency, although the appearance can vary. Histologically, the neoplasm can have both follicular and plexiform patterns, but the hallmark finding is its tendency to mimic the enamel organ (Fig. 14–7).

Treatment is complete surgical excision with adequate margins of normal tissue, with an associated recurrence rate of less than 5%. Less radical surgery and

radiation therapy are associated with a recurrence rate of 60 and 40%, respectively.

Benign Nonepithelial Tumors

Osteoma

Osteomas occur most frequently in the frontal (80%) and ethmoid (16%) sinuses, with the balance found in the maxillary sinuses. They are more common in men and are frequently discovered as an incidental finding on radiographs. Their radiographic appearance is characterized by a sharply defined bony margin (Fig. 14–8). The base may be broad or narrow. Two types of osteoma exist, although mixtures of the two types have been reported. The eburnated type is a uniformly radiodense structure, whereas the cancellous type, which has a central core of cancellous bone, appears radiographically as a bony rim with a more radiolucent center.

Most osteomas are asymptomatic. Some authors have suggested that osteomas can cause headaches that are not due to secondary sinus disease or involvement of any other structures. In these cases, removal of the osteoma has generally relieved the symptoms. More commonly, when symptoms are present, they are usually caused by the osteoma-induced sinusitis or erosion into other anatomic areas, usually the orbit. The patient complains of diplopia, and with larger lesions, lateral and inferior displacement of the globe occurs. Although the clinical picture mimics that of a frontoethmoid mucocele, radiographs reveal the osteoma. Osteomas may also cause sinus obstruction with subsequent sinusitis and even mucocele formation. Expansion inferiorly may cause nasal obstruction. Growth may also occur superiorly into the intracranial cavity and may cause displacement of the brain. Leakage of cerebrospinal fluid, meningitis, and brain abscess can result.

If a small osteoma is noted on a routine radiograph in an otherwise asymptomatic patient, the osteoma must be evaluated radiographically on a periodic basis to monitor its growth. If symptoms are present, however, removal of the osteoma should be considered. The surgical approach must be tailored to the size and location of the tumor. Osteomas of the frontal sinus are best approached through an osteoplastic flap, which allows excellent visualization of the tumor and permits careful removal. If the patency of the nasofrontal ostium can be maintained, simple removal is sufficient. If the ostium has been obstructed, however, the sinus should be obliterated with fat after careful removal of the mucosa. Ethmoid osteomas are approached through an external ethmoidectomy, and a Caldwell-Luc procedure is used to remove osteomas of the maxillary sinus.

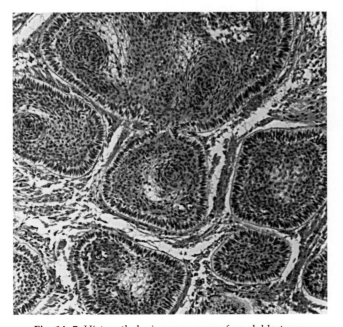

Fig. 14–7. Histopathologic appearance of ameloblastoma.

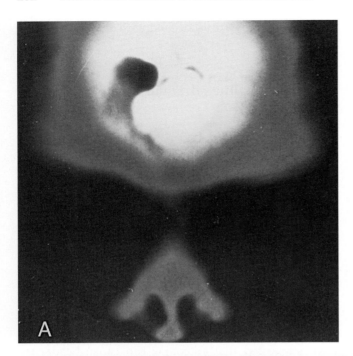

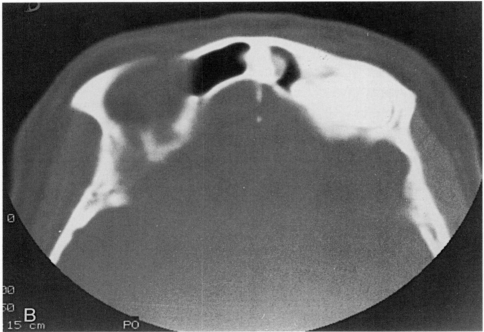

Fig. 14–8. A. Coronal CT view of a frontal sinus osteoma. B. Axial CT view.

Ossifying Fibroma and Fibrous Dysplasia

The correct classification of the fibro-osseus lesions has been a source of debate for years. One of the most controversial areas has been the differentiation between fibrous dysplasia and ossifying fibroma.[29] The latter is a benign neoplasm that is thought to originate from periosteum or periodontal membrane. Its peak incidence is the second through the fourth decades, and it is more common in women than in men. Although it can involve any site in the head and neck, it involves the mandible more commonly than the maxilla. It

rarely involves long bones and is rarely polyostotic. Radiographically, it is well demarcated, with decreased density or an eggshell appearance. It is usually enucleated easily, and microscopic examination reveals woven and lamellar bone with smooth borders and rimming osteoblasts. A characteristic finding is parallel birefringence with polarized light.

Fibrous dysplasia represents a developmental maturation defect or fibro-osseus metaplasia. It usually occurs in the first decade and is more common in girls than in boys. It involves the maxilla more frequently than the mandible and can involve other cranial sites and the long bones, the latter particularly in its polyostotic form. Radiographically, one sees a poorly demarcated density in the facial skeleton. The lesion is difficult to remove, and contouring is usually the only therapy when it causes significant deformity or impinges on vital structures. The histopathologic appearance of fibrous dysplasia is distinct from that of ossifying fibroma; only woven bone is present, with feathery, irregular borders often described as Chinese characters. One sees random birefringence with polarized light.

Juvenile Nasopharyngeal Angiofibroma

Juvenile nasopharyngeal angiofibroma, a benign tumor, develops exclusively in boys, usually around the age of puberty. The presenting symptoms are nasal obstruction and bleeding, which can be massive (also see Chap. 19). Any boy in the appropriate age range who has recurrent nosebleeds should be carefully examined for an angiofibroma. The tumor usually arises from the lateral wall of the nasopharynx and can extend anteriorly into the nose. It frequently extends superiorly into the sphenoid sinus, and in some cases intracranial extension may develop. It can pass laterally through the pterygomaxillary fissure into the pterygomaxillary space and, if untreated, into the face. As the tumor expands in the pterygomaxillary space, it produces a characteristic anterior bowing of the posterior wall of the maxillary sinus (Holman-Miller sign).

The tumor is pale to beefy red. Although it may be tempting to biopsy the mass, profuse bleeding will ensue, so the diagnosis is better made radiographically. CT with contrast demonstrates an enhancing mass. Angiography is not usually necessary for diagnosis, but is used for preoperative embolization.

Giant Cell Lesions

Giant cell granuloma, which has also been termed giant cell reparative granuloma, is a rare tumor of the sinuses. It occurs most frequently in younger patients, with a peak incidence in the second to fourth decades. The most common location is the region of the premolar teeth. The major symptom is usually the presence of a mass or deformity of the maxilla. Radiographically, one sees opacification of the sinus with thinning and expansion of the bone. CT demonstrates calcifications in the soft tissue and therefore may resemble ossifying fibroma. True giant cell tumors resembling those of long bones have also been described in the sinuses, although they are exceedingly rare. Whereas traditionally giant cell granulomas and tumors were thought to represent separate entities, some investigators now believe that they are merely a continuum of aggressiveness from low to high. Clinical features of aggressiveness are pain, rapid growth, cortical bone perforation, tooth root resorption, and paresthesias. All giant cell

lesions should be resected with wider margins considered for those with an aggressive picture.[30]

Malignant Epithelial Tumors

Carcinoma of the Nasal Vestibule and Septum

Malignant tumors of the nasal vestibule and nasal septum are extremely uncommon. They are usually low-grade squamous cell carcinomas and arise most commonly at the anterior portion of the septum. Most patients present with a nonhealing lesion of the anterior septum or vestibule. Although metastases are unusual, the particular danger with these lesions is their propensity to invade the planes of the nose (such as the subperichondrial plane along the nasal septum), which allows undetected spread to areas well away from the primary tumor. If nodal metastasis occurs, it is usually to the prevascular nodes along the facial artery near the border of the mandible.

Radiation therapy and surgery have been used with equal effectiveness, with 5-year survival rates ranging from 38 to 63%. Prophylactic neck dissection is not warranted because the incidence of nodal metastasis is approximately 10%.

Carcinoma of the Paranasal Sinuses

Most malignant tumors of the paranasal sinus are carcinomas; consequently, their epidemiology, etiology, evaluation, and treatment are discussed throughout this chapter. Squamous cell carcinomas make up 50 to 80% in most studies, with salivary type carcinomas accounting for most of the remainder. Adenocarcinomas are the most common salivary type and make up 4 to 8% of sinonasal malignant tumors, whereas adenoid cystic carcinoma is the second most common salivary malignant tumor in the nose and paranasal sinuses. The rare mucoepidermoid carcinoma is a distant third in frequency among malignant salivary tumors in the sinonasal tract.[1]

Melanoma

Melanomas arise from rests of melanocytes normally found throughout the nose and paranasal sinuses and account for 3% of sinonasal malignant tumors. Almost one quarter of all melanomas occur in the head and neck, but fewer than 1% occur in the sinonasal tract (see Chap. 9). As with most malignant tumors of the nose and paranasal sinuses, these are more common in men than in women. Although the presenting symptoms are similar to those of other tumors in this area, with obstruction and epistaxis common, occasionally patients have a history of a black nasal discharge. On physical examination, one may see a pigmented, necrotic, hemorrhagic nasal mass and, rarely, regional or distant metastasis at the time of diagnosis. The lateral nasal wall and septum are the most common sites of

TABLE 14–7. Staging for Esthesioneuroblastoma

A	Tumor confined to the nasal cavity
B	Tumor in nasal cavity extending to paranasal sinus
C	Tumor extending beyond the nasal cavity and paranasal sinuses or having metastasis

(Adapted from Kadish S, Goodman M, and Wang CC: Olfactory neuroblastoma. Cancer 37:1571, 1976.

origin. Combined therapy offers the best chance at cure, although 5-year survival rates are about 25%.[31]

Esthesioneuroblastoma

Esthesioneuroblastoma is a rare tumor that arises from the olfactory neuroepithelium. It can occur in any age group, but is more common under age 40 years. The histologic appearance can mimic that of various small cell tumors, but the characteristic finding consists of an intercellular matrix of neurofibrils with clusters of round to ovoid cells grouped in nests by vascular septa. Symptoms are usually nasal obstruction and epistaxis, but diplopia and other eye findings may occur with more advanced lesions. Kadish and associates developed a clinical grouping system for esthesioneuroblastomas that has been helpful in analyzing treatment results (Table 14–7).[32]

The treatment of choice is combined radiation and surgery, including resection of the cribriform plate. Most surgeons now prefer a craniofacial resection, which provides the best exposure of the anterior cranial fossa. Levine and colleagues have found that preoperative chemotherapy in more advanced lesions produces better survival.[33] The most common site of failure is local, but metastases to the cervical lymph nodes and lungs are not uncommon.

Malignant Nonepithelial Tumors

Rhabdomyosarcoma

Rhabdomyosarcoma is the most common sarcoma of the head and neck and the most common soft tissue sarcoma in the pediatric population. One out of 10 occurs in the sinonasal tract, and most affect children. A recent trial in children demonstrated improved survival with nonradical surgery followed by radiation and intrathecal chemotherapy.[34] This has not been duplicated in adults, in whom combined therapy including wide surgical resection remains the therapy of choice. Prognosis correlates with clinical groupings based on amount of residual disease after resection.[34]

Hemangiopericytoma

Fifteen to 20% of hemangiopericytomas occur in the head and neck, with the origin in the nose and paranasal sinuses reported in 50% of cases. This highly vascular tumor develops from the pericytes of Zimmermann and invades locally, with 10 to 15% metastasizing.

These tumors tend to be radioresistant and consequently are treated surgically. Prognosis is related to size, number of mitoses, and presence of metastases.[35]

Lymphoma

Lymphomas (generally Non-Hodgkin's) represent approximately 8% of sinonasal malignant tumors, with the maxillary sinus being the most common site. Extranodal sites are much more common in children, in whom 16% occur in the oral cavity, nose, and paranasal sinuses. Presenting signs and symptoms are similar to those of other sinonasal malignant tumors. Up to one third of patients present with cervical adenopathy, and 6% demonstrate intracranial involvement. Evaluation should include a CT of the head, paranasal sinuses, chest, and abdomen, bone marrow biopsy, and lumbar puncture for cytologic study. Three staging systems have been used for lymphomas of the nose and paranasal tract (Ann Arbor Classification, Wollner Classification, and TNM-American Joint Committee on Cancer [AJCC] Staging, in which TNM means extent of tumor [T], condition of regional lymph nodes [N], and presence or absence of lymph nodes [M]). Treatment is accomplished with chemotherapy and radiation to the primary site. Prognosis is worse in adults and in patients with lymphadenopathy, larger primary tumors, tumors of T-cell origin, and dissemination during treatment.[36]

Extramedullary Plasmacytoma

Virtually all extramedullary plasmacytomas occur in the head and neck, and almost half occur in the sinonasal tract. They are more common in elderly men, and one third are associated with multiple myeloma. Treatment is 40 to 50 Gy of radiation therapy, and survival is about 50% unless the tumor is associated with multiple myeloma.[37]

EMERGING INTERESTS

From an etiologic point of view, human papilloma virus (HPV) appears to have a role in inverted papilloma and in some sinonasal malignant tumors. Using polymerase chain reaction, HPV types 6 and 11 have been identified in inverted papillomas and types 16 and 18 in squamous cell carcinomas, both de novo and in association with inverted papilloma.[38]

SUGGESTED READINGS

1. Krause DH, et al: Nonsquamous cell malignancies of the paranasal sinuses. Ann Otol Rhinol Laryngol 99:5, 1990.
2. Zheng W, et al: Risk factors for cancers of the nasal cavity and paranasal sinuses among white men in the United States. Am J Epidemiol 138:965, 1993.

3. Lareo AC, et al: History of previous nasal diseases and sinonasal cancer: a case-control study. Laryngoscope 102:439, 1992.

4. Weisberger EC and Dedo HH: Cranial neuropathies in sinus disease. Laryngoscope 87:357, 1977.

5. Robin PE and Powell DJ: Regional node involvement and distant metastases in carcinoma of the nasal cavity and paranasal sinuses. J Laryngol Otol 94:301, 1980.

6. Miyaguchi M, Sakai S, Mori N, and Kitaoku S: Multiple primary malignancies in patients with malignant tumors of the nasal cavities and paranasal sinuses. J Laryngol Otol 104:696, 1990.

7. Lewis JS and Castro EB: Cancer of the nasal cavity and paranasal sinuses. J Laryngol Otol 86:255, 1972.

8. Chow JM, Leonetti JP, and Mafee MF: Epithelial tumors of the paranasal sinuses and nasal cavity. Radiol Clin North Am 31: 61, 1993.

9. Lund VS, et al: Magnetic resonance imaging of paranasal sinus tumor for craniofacial resection. Head Neck 11:279, 1989.

10. Hunink MGM, et al: CT and MR assessment of tumors of the nose and paranasal sinuses, the nasopharynx and the parapharyngeal space using ROC methodology. Neuroradiology 32:220, 1990.

11. Beahrs OH, Henson DE, Hutter RVP, and Kennedy BJ (eds): Manual for Staging of Cancer: American Joint Committee on Cancer. 4th Ed. Philadelphia, JB Lippincott, 1992.

12. Ohngren LG: Malignant tumors of the maxillo-ethmoidal region. Acta Otolaryngol 19(suppl):1, 1993.

13. Sakai S, Hohki A, Fuchihata H, and Tanaka Y: Multidisciplinary treatment of maxillary sinus carcinoma. Cancer 52:1360, 1983.

14. Amendola BE, et al: Carcinoma of maxillary antrum: surgery or radiation therapy? Int J Radiat Oncol Biol Phys 7:743, 1981.

15. Lee F and Ogura JH: Maxillary sinus carcinoma. Laryngoscope 91:133, 1981.

16. Frich JC: Treatment of advanced squamous carcinoma of the maxillary sinus by irradiation. Int J Radiat Oncol Biol Phys 8:1453, 1982.

17. Bush SE and Bagshaw MA: Carcinoma of the paranasal sinuses. Cancer 50: 154, 1982.

18. Shibuya H, et al: Maxillary sinus carcinoma: results of radiation therapy. Int J Radiat Oncol Biol Phys 10:1021, 1984.

19. Isaacs JH, Mooney S, Mendenhall WM, and Parsons JT: Cancer of the maxillary sinus treated with surgery and/or radiation therapy. Am Surg 56:327, 1990.

20. Korzeniowski S, Reinfuss M, and Skokyszewski J: The evaluation of radiotherapy after incomplete surgery in patients with carcinoma of the maxillary sinus. Int J Radiat Oncol Biol Phys 11:505, 1985.

21. Tsujii H, et al: The role of radiotherapy in the management of maxillary sinus carcinoma. Cancer 57:2261, 1986.

22. Sisson GA, Toriumi DM, and Atiyah RA: Paranasal sinus malignancy: a comprehensive update. Laryngoscope 99:143, 1989.

23. Lavertu P, et al: Squamous cell carcinoma of the paranasal sinuses: the Cleveland Clinic experience 1977–1986. Laryngoscope 99:1130, 1989.

24. Zamora RL, et al: Clinical classification and staging for primary malignancies of the maxillary antrum. Laryngoscope 100:1106, 1990.

25. Osguthorpe JD: Sinus neoplasia. Arch Otolaryngol Head Neck Surg 120:19, 1994.

26. Bjork-Eriksson T, Mercke C, Petruson B, and Ekholm S: Potential impact on tumor control and organ preservation with cisplatin and 5-fluorouracil for patients with advanced tumors of the paranasal sinuses and nasal fossa. Cancer 70:2615, 1992.

27. Stankiewicz JA and Girgis SJ: Endoscopic treatment of nasal and paranasal sinus inverted papilloma. Otolaryngol Head Neck Surg 109:988, 1993.

28. Bielamowicz S, Calcaterra TC, and Watson D: Inverting papilloma of the head and neck: the UCLA update. Otolaryngol Head Neck Surg 109:71, 1993.

29. Kridel RWH, Miller RH, and Greenberg SD: Ossifying fibroma: diagnostic clarification. Otolaryngol Head Neck Surg 91:568, 1983.

30. Stolovitzky JP, Waldron CA, and McConnel FMS: Giant cell lesions of the maxilla and paranasal sinuses. Head Neck 16:143, 1994.

31. Lund VJ: Malignant melanoma of the nasal cavity and paranasal sinuses. Ear Nose Throat J 72:285, 1993.

32. Kadish S, Goodman M, and Wang CC: Olfactory neuroblastoma. Cancer 37:1571, 1976.

33. Levine PA, McLean WC, and Cantrell RW: Esthesioneuroblastoma: the University of Virginia experience 1960–1985. Laryngoscope 96:742, 1986.

34. Raney RB, et al: Improved prognosis with intensive treatment of children with cranial soft tissue sarcomas arising in nonorbital parameningeal sites. Cancer 59:147, 1987.

35. Abdel-Fattah HM, Adams GL, and Wick MR: Hemangiopericytoma of the maxillary sinus and skull base. Head Neck 12:77, 1990.

36. Bumpous JM, Martin DS, Curran P, and Stith JA: Non-Hodgkin's lymphoma of the nose and paranasal sinuses in the pediatric population. Ann Otol Rhinol Laryngol 103:294, 1994.

37. Kapadia SB, Desai U, and Cheng VS: Extramedullary plasmacytoma of the head and neck. Medicine 61:317, 1982.

38. Kashima HK, et al: Human papillomavirus in sinonasal papillomas and squamous cell carcinoma. Laryngoscope 102:973, 1992.

II NECK, PHARYNX, OROPHARYNX AND NASOPHARYNX, MAXILLA AND MANDIBLE

John J. Ballenger

15 Congenital Anomalies of the Head and Neck

Lee Rowe

Congenital head and neck anomalies represent a diverse group of clinical disorders. Frequently, these present as upper aerodigestive tract neoplasms and neck masses, with thyroglossal duct abnormalities most common, followed by branchial arch defects, lymphangiomas (cystic hygromas), and subcutaneous vascular anomalies (hemangiomas, arteriovenous malformations). Less common are teratomas, heterotopic neural tissue, and nasopharyngeal neoplasms. Additional disorders encountered include congenital disorders of the oral cavity including cleft lip and palate, Pierre Robin sequence, and other aberrations such as primary ciliary dyskinesia, Kartagener's syndrome, and craniofacial anomalies.

CONGENITAL DISORDERS OF THE NECK

Branchial Cleft Anomalies

Lateral cervical lesions termed branchial cleft cysts are congenital developmental defects that arise from the primitive branchial apparatus (branchial arch, cleft, and pouches). First branchial cleft anomalies are discussed elsewhere in this chapter.

Embryogenesis

The branchial arches consist of five parallel mesodermal bars, each with its own nerve supply and blood vessel (primitive aortic arches that develop during the third and fourth embryonic weeks). The branchial arches are separated externally by branchial clefts consisting of ectoderm and internally by endodermis-lined branchial (pharyngeal) pouches. A branchial plate is located between each arch separating pouch from cleft. The nerves are anterior to their respective arteries, except in the fifth arch, where the nerve is posterior to

the artery. Caudal to all the arches is the twelfth nerve. The sternocleidomastoid muscle is derived from cervical somites posterior and inferior to the foregoing arches. In each arch, a central artery develops connecting the two ventral and two dorsal aortas. The two ventral aortas fuse completely, whereas the two dorsal aortas only fuse caudally. With continued development, the ventral aortas become the external and common carotid arteries, whereas the arteries of the first and second arch degenerate. Segments of the dorsal aorta persist as the internal carotid artery along with the artery of the third arch. The left fourth arch artery becomes the arch of the aorta, and the right fourth arch artery becomes the proximal subclavian artery. The primitive clefts pass between the corresponding arteries.[1] The most widely accepted theory of the genesis of branchial cleft anomalies is that fistulas and cysts result from incomplete closure of the connection between the cleft and the pouch, with rupture of the branchial plate. These anomalies are generally lined with stratified squamous epithelium containing subepithelial lymphoid follicles, keratin, hair follicles, sweat glands, cartilage, and sebaceous glands.

Clinical Presentation

Typically, branchial clefts present as smooth, round, fluctuant, nontender masses along the anterior border of the sternocleidomastoid muscle, anywhere from the external auditory canal to the clavicle. During upper respiratory tract infections, a painful increase in size is common and occasionally may be associated with external drainage through an unrecognized fistula. Small cysts may not be recognized until the second decade in life. Male and female incidences are equal, and nearly all these lesions are recognized by time the patient reaches 30 years of age.

Second Branchial Cleft Anomalies

Second branchial cleft lesions are the most common anomalies and are encountered most frequently in the anterior triangle of the neck along the anterior border of the sternocleidomastoid muscle.[2] The fistula tract, if present, ascends along the carotid sheath, crosses over the hypoglossal and glossopharyngeal nerves, and courses between the internal and external carotid arteries. It ends in the tonsillar fossa, a second branchial pouch derivative.

Third Branchial Cleft Anomalies

Third branchial cleft anomalies are unusual. The external ostium occurs at the same position as the second branchial cleft anomaly, and the cyst may be located anywhere along the fistula. The fistula tract ascends along the carotid sheath behind the internal carotid artery and over the hypoglossal nerve, and it enters the pyriform sinus, piercing the middle constrictor muscle below the glossopharyngeal nerve. Clinically, the anomaly may mimic suppurative thyroiditis or symptoms of an external laryngocele and can cause recurrent infection, discharge, and, rarely, stridor.

Fourth Branchial Cleft Anomalies

Fourth branchial cleft anomalies are extremely rare. Only 31 cases have been reported. The fistula tract descends along the carotid sheath, enters the chest passing under either the aortic arch on the left or the subclavian artery on the right, and ascends in the neck to open at the apex of the pyriform sinus.

Treatment

Complete surgical excision is the treatment of choice for branchial cleft anomalies and is indicated for recurrent infection, cosmetic deformity, and potential for malignant degeneration. Preoperative assessment with computed tomography (CT) scanning or magnetic resonance (MR) imaging is essential and may be combined with a fistulogram or pharyngoesophagram when indicated. A ''stepladder'' surgical approach is used to avoid long, cosmetically deforming incisions, paralleling the sternocleidomastoid muscle.

Branchiogenic Carcinoma

Branchiogenic carcinoma is an extraordinarily rare squamous cell carcinoma arising exclusively from branchial apparatus remnants. The physician must completely rule out an occult primary malignant tumor of the head and neck, chest, or gastrointestinal tract, to prove conclusively that the neoplasm is not metastatic. The treatment of choice is wide excision and radical neck dissection.

LYMPHANGIOMAS, HEMANGIOMAS, AND VASCULAR MALFORMATIONS

Congenital lymphangiomatous malformations of the head and neck represent a wide clinical spectrum.

Lymphangiomas result from abnormal development of the lymphatic system, with obstruction of lymph drainage from the affected area causing multicystic endothelium-lined spaces. The neck is the most common site (25% of all cases). Over half these lesions are present at birth, with 90% manifesting by 2 years of age.

Cystic Hygroma

Cystic hygromas are large lymphangiomas most commonly found in the posterior triangle of the neck and axilla in children. Cervical cystic hygromas commonly appear before 30 weeks' gestation and are usually associated with chromosomal or structural abnormalities. Prognosis is poor for these types of hygromas. By contrast, cystic hygroma developing late in pregnancy has a more favorable outcome and is more likely to be encountered by the head and neck surgeon. Cystic hygromas are soft, painless, and compressible masses that may increase when the patient cries. Two thirds are asymptomatic. After an upper respiratory tract infection, however, sudden enlargement with inflammation, infection, dysphagia, and stridor may develop. This is more commonly seen if the anterior triangle of the neck is involved or in patients with pharyngolaryngeal extension or intraoral involvement.

Vascular Lesions

Other congenital vascular lesions of the head and neck include hemangiomas and arteriovenous malformations or lymphovenous lesions. Diagnostic imaging of these anomalies is based on the need for surgical treatment. Only those lesions that cause functional impairment or developmental disturbance are surgically addressed. Angiography, combined with MR imaging, allows separation into low-flow lesions (hemangiomas, venous, and lymphatic malformations) and high-flow lesions (arteriovenous malformations and invasive, combined lymphovascular malformations).[3] Treatment of small cystic hygromas and true hemangiomas that have not regressed, but have enlarged, is by surgical excision with staged debulking of larger cystic hygromas. Neural structures such as the facial nerve, vagus nerve, and phrenic nerves should not be sacrificed. Recurrence is uncommon when gross neoplasm is removed.

For low-flow lesions, sclerosant therapy is effective, either alone in small lesions or combined with surgical resection or embolization. Preoperative embolization at the time of selective angiography and surgical excision is the treatment of choice in high-flow malformations.[4]

ABERRANT THYROID TISSUE

Ectopic thyroid tissue can occur anywhere from the foramen cecum to the lower neck (Fig. 15–1). Most fre-

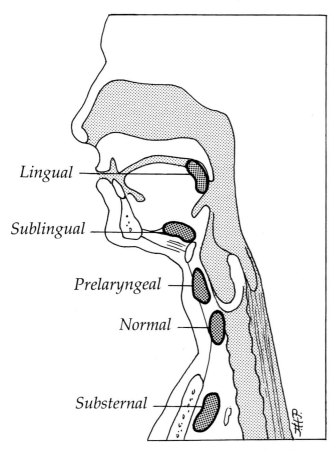

Fig. 15–1. Most common locations of midline aberrant thyroid tissue, schematically illustrated.

quently, it occurs as a thyroglossal duct cyst associated with a normal thyroid gland. Less common is total ectopia, manifesting as a lingual thyroid or occurring laterally in the neck.

Embryology

In the 4-week-old embryo, the primitive thyroid gland begins as a ventral diverticulum of endodermal origin, arising in the floor of the pharynx between the tuberculum impar and the copula. Ultimately, it becomes the foramen cecum, and the copula becomes the posterior third of the tongue. The thyroid descends caudally through or adjacent to the primitive hyoid bone. The developing thyroglossal duct reaches its final position in the midline of the neck and develops into the median lobe of the thyroid. It normally persists as a hollow stalk for 6 weeks and then atrophies. Thyroglossal duct anomalies result from a failure of complete obliteration of the thyroglossal duct and are located anywhere along the descent of the gland.

Lingual Thyroid

Lingual thyroid presents in the midline as a sessile, nontender reddish mass in the base of the tongue, ante-

rior to the vallecula. It is the most frequent benign mass encountered in the oropharynx and, unlike other aberrant thyroid anomalies, has a female preponderance. Symptoms may include dysphagia, cough, dysphonia, dyspnea, and hemorrhage. Lingual thyroid may become apparent during pregnancy because of increased thyroid function.

Lingual thyroid is covered with squamous epithelium and often exhibits an abundant aberrant vascular supply. The mass consists of normal or immature thyroid tissue, which may be either functional or dysfunctional. Indications for surgical removal include uncontrollable hyperthyroidism, hemorrhage, symptomatic enlargement, or question of malignancy.[5] Preoperatively, a thyroid uptake study and scan should be obtained to determine whether functioning thyroid tissue exists in its normal cervical location. MR imaging may also be of value because it allows multiplanar imaging and provides the best soft tissue definition. Excision is performed by the transhyoid or transoral route.

Thyroglossal Duct Anomalies

Signs and Symptoms
A thyroglossal duct cyst is the most common congenital neck mass and the second most common of all childhood cervical neck masses. Cysts, sinuses, and fistulas of the thyroglossal duct manifest as anterior midline neck masses from the foramen cecum to the thyroid gland, typically before 20 years of age (most before 10 years), with an equal male and female incidence. Thyroglossal ducts and fistulas are often asymptomatic. They may also become recurrently infected during upper respiratory tract infections, which can cause cyst enlargement, abscess development, and rupture with external sinus formation. Thyroglossal duct cysts most commonly are found below the hyoid bone and above the thyroid gland, displaying movement with anterior tongue protrusion and swallowing. Usually, the cysts are 1 to 3 cm in diameter and are smooth, round, and fluctuant.

Histopathologic Features
Thyroglossal duct cysts and fistulas are lined with squamous, ciliated columnar, or transitional cell epithelium. They may be surrounded by fibrous tissue with infiltrating inflammatory cells lacking organized lymphoid tissue. Islands of ectopic thyroid tissue and mucus glands are not uncommonly identified. The cyst or sinus tract is filled with mucoid or mucopurulent material.

Differential Diagnosis
The differential diagnosis includes dermoid cyst, pyramidal lobe hyperplasia or cyst, teratomas, hamartoma, lipomas, sebaceous cysts, cavernous hemangiomas,

hyperplastic lymph nodes, and malignant primary or metastatic neoplasms.

Treatment

As with lingual thyroid, a preoperative thyroid scan and uptake study are mandatory, even though concomitant agenesis of the thyroid is extremely rare.[6] Malignant degeneration, recurrent infections, undesirable cosmetic appearance, and, rarely, intermittent upper airway obstruction are indications for surgical excision of thyroglossal duct cysts and fistulas. Incision and drainage may be necessary in the interim if an abscess has developed. Because of the high recurrence rate after excision, the Sistrunk procedure is recommended to prevent recurrence. This involves a transverse incision over the cyst or a fusiform incision over an external fistula opening. All abnormal tissue including the cyst, fistula, body of the hyoid bone (preferably more than 15 mm), and the fibrous cord extending to the foramen cecum should be resected. Recurrence develops up to 20% of cases, a result of failure to remove all abnormal tissue including accessory ducts.[7] Papillary carcinoma arising in a thyroglossal duct cyst has been reported, as well as Hürthle cell adenoma. Most patients with papillary carcinoma are in their forties, although 20% are less than 20 years of age. Typically, the tumor is small and clinically unsuspected, and in rare cases it may be associated with regional or distant metastasis. Rarely, squamous cell carcinoma arising directly from the lining epithelium in a thyroglossal duct remnant has been reported and, as a rule, has a poor prognosis.

Lateral Aberrant Thyroid

Previously, surgical dictum stated that the so-called lateral aberrant thyroid represented metastatic thyroid cancer. Recent evidence points to a nonmalignant histologic picture. Histologic analysis of the aberrant tissue and intraoperative examination of the ipsilateral thyroid lobe are used to guide therapy. If papillary carcinoma is found in an ectopic thyroid nodule, then either ipsilateral thyroid lobectomy with isthmusectomy or total thyroidectomy is performed.

THYMIC CYST

Cystic lesions of the thymus are rare. In a large series of over 200 mediastinal cysts, only 2 cases of thymic cysts were reported. Cervical thymic cysts are so rare that only 31 cases have been documented in the English-language literature. Treatment is surgical excision.

NEUROGENIC NEOPLASMS

Congenital neurogenic lesions involving the head and neck include all neoplasms or anomalies originating in the neural tissue or its covering. Two groups have been recognized: (1) heterotopic brain lesions with developmental defects, which are discussed in the next section; and (2) neoplasms of neurogenic origin including neurinomas, neurofibromas, ganglioneuromas, and meningiomas. Neurinomas originating from the connective tissue sheath of the nerve are termed schwannomas and may appear as multiple neurofibromas arising from cutaneous, visceral, and cranial nerves in neurofibromatosis type I or II.

Typically, neuromas appear as solitary, encapsulated lesions with elongated spindle-shaped cells with an oval or flattened nucleus. Ganglioneuromas, rarely seen in the head or neck, are characterized by ganglion and glial cells. Meningiomas are usually benign and arise from embryonic arachnoid rests. They may appear extracranially at the nasal root or in the sinuses. Whorl-like fibroblastic neuclei with hyaline formations producing a sand-like appearance may be present (psammoma body). Pharyngeal neuromas are rare and appear as a smooth, firm, rounded, and yellow mass. Symptoms depend on the size and location of the tumor. If multiple brown discolorations of the skin or café au lait spots are present, neurofibroma may be suggested. Treatment is surgical excision and must be complete because recurrence is common.

CONGENITAL DISORDERS OF THE NOSE AND PARANASAL SINUSES

Heterotopic Neural Tissue

Heterotopic neural tissue or glioma may manifest as isolated ectopic brain tissue with only a fibrous band connecting it to the endocranium. A glioma may be of the external or endonasal type. The external nasal glioma is typically found in the nasion as a red, relatively firm, mobile mass located subcutaneously that does not increase in size when the patient cries. The endonasal glioma is less common and arises from the middle turbinate or the lateral nasal vault, where it may be mistaken for a polyp. By contrast, a meningocoele is a hernial protrusion of the meninges, and if it contains brain tissue, it is called an encephalocele. An encephalocele is caused by a defect of the fetal skull and contains an ependyma-lined cavity filled with cerebrospinal fluid. Two basic types of hernial protrusions are identified: (1) the sincipital type; and (2) the basal type. The sincipital type is rare and is associated with termination of the meninges near the base of the nose. This type has three different forms: (1) nasofrontal, in which the encephalocele extends between the nasal and frontal bones, resulting in a midline swelling at the base of the nose; (2) nasoethmoidal, in which a defect among the nasal, frontal, and ethmoid bones allows the encephalocele to appear as a mass beneath the skin of the bony-cartilaginous junction; and (3) naso-orbital protrusion of the encephalocele through the suture line among the lacrimal, frontal, and ethmoidal bones appearing as a conjunctival mass. The basal type, in which the hernia extends into the naso-orbital and pharyngeal region, is less common than the sincipital. Three varieties have been identified: (1) sphenoid-pharyngeal, in which the encephalocele extends through the ethmoid or sphenoid bones or their suture lines into the nasal or nasopharyngeal cavity; (2) sphenoid-orbital, in which the encephalocele extends through the spheno-orbital fissure into the posterior aspect of the orbit, resulting in pulsatile exophthalmos; and (3) sphenomaxillary, in which the encephalocele herniates through the spheno-orbital fissure into the orbit, with extension inferiorly through the inferior orbital fissure into the pterygopalatine fissure. This results in a mass bulging into the cheek or into the oropharynx, medial to the ramus of the mandible. In all cases, unlike with gliomas, pulsations and an increase in size of the mass can be observed when the patient coughs or strains. CT and MR imaging are necessary to determine the appropriate combined transfacial and intracranial approach for surgical resection.[8]

Dermoid Cysts

Dermoid cysts occasionally occur in the neck, usually in the midline. Overall, fewer than 10% of all dermoid cysts occur in the head and neck. One fourth are found in the floor of the mouth, with the remainder in the periorbital region. These lesions are seen primarily in children and adolescents during the second decade of life, but they also may occur in infants. Cyst walls consist of squamous cell epithelium containing epidermal appendages. These cysts are thought to originate from displacement of epidermal elements during the intramembranous growth phase of the nasal bones in the embryo. Because of the variability in clinical presentation and contiguous structure involvement, segregation of periorbital lesions into three distinct subgroups is helpful: (1) brow region dermoid cysts; (2) orbital region dermoid cysts; and (3) nasoglabellar dermoid cysts. Midline nasoglabellar cysts may have associated sinus tracts, which, in rare cases, may have intracranial extensions. In those patients with intracranial extension, the sinus tract traverses either the cribriform plate or foramen cecum and is attached to the dura, falx cerebri, or other intracranial structures.[9]

The treatment of choice is surgical excision after CT and MR imaging to evaluate intracranial extension. All tissue must be removed to prevent recurrences. In patients with intracranial extension, a bicoronal flap is employed to facilitate removal and to prevent postoperative meningitis and abscess formation.[10]

Other congenital midface cysts are those associated with the facial clefts, including the nasoethmoidal cleft cyst, nasolabial cyst, subalar cleft cyst, globulomaxillary cyst, cysts connected with cleft lip or palate, premaxillary cyst, nasopalatine cyst, foraminal incisor cyst, and Jacobson's organ cysts.

Choanal Atresia

Bilateral atresia of the posterior choanae is the most frequently encountered congenital nasal anomaly (1 in 8000 live births) and is a common cause of neonatal respiratory distress. Unilateral atresia is twice as common as bilateral disease, and 80% of these anomalies are bony or membrano-osseous, with 20% membranous. A female predisposition is seen in choanal atresia, and recent evidence points to an autosomal recessive mode of inheritance.

Failure of breakdown of the buccopharyngeal membrane on gestational day 45 is considered to be the cause of choanal atresia. Other theories include abnormalities in the migration of the cephalic neural crest following neural tube closure. Several craniofacial abnormalities including skull base defects and systemic malformations have been described in association with choanal atresia, including the CHARGE association (Table 15–1). The CHARGE association refers to a problem of multiple congenital anomalies that occur in nonrandom association with choanal atresia (C, coloboma; H, congenital heart disease; A, atresia choanae; R, retarded growth and development; G genital anomalies in males; E, ear abnormalities and deafness). Almost all patients have malformed pinnae and exhibit hypoplastic incudes and semicircular canals on CT scan, and the majority demonstrate severe conductive or mixed hearing loss. In addition, half exhibit facial nerve palsies. Laryngotracheal anomalies occur in one third of cases.[11]

Symptoms

Respiratory distress at birth is the sine qua non of bilateral choanal atresia. In spite of vigorous attempts at respiration, effective air exchange does not occur until

TABLE 15–1. Congenital Anomalies Associated with Choanal Atresia

Branchial Anomalies
CHARGE Association
Humeroradial synostosis
Mandibulofacial synostosis
Microcephaly
Micrognathia
Nasopharyngeal anomalies
Palatal defects

the neonate begins to cry, bypassing the nasal obstruction. Once the crying ceases, however, the patient's mouth closes, and a pattern of cyclic obstruction gradually develops, resulting in increasing respiratory failure. Because neonates are obligatory nasal breathers, placement of an oral airway or McGovern nipple is lifesaving. By contrast, children with unilateral choanal atresia present later in life with unilateral rhinorrhea without respiratory distress.

Diagnosis

The diagnosis of bilateral choanal atresia is confirmed by the inability to pass a No. 5 or 6 French feeding catheter at least 3 cm through the nose into the nasopharynx. In addition, direct observation with nasofiberoptic endoscopy and CT scan is essential to determine the type of obstruction. Specifically, the CT scan demonstrates the thickness of the atretic plate as well as its medial encroachment of the posterior aspect of the medial maxilla.

Treatment

Multiple methods are available to repair choanal atresia. The appropriate method is determined by the age of the patient and whether the atresia is bilateral or unilateral. In all methods, the challenge is to provide adequate mucosal lining to the new posterior choana and to prevent granulation tissue formation and subsequent stenosis. Treatment requires perforation of the atresia plate followed by stenting for 4 to 12 weeks with preservation of mucosal flaps.

TRANSNASAL APPROACH. The most direct and simplest route for choanal atresia repair is transnasal, using a No. 2 Lempert or similar curette inserted 3 to 3.5 cm beyond the nares along the nasal floor, and exerting firm pressure against the bony atresia plate until it is perforated. The anterior nasal mucous membrane is sacrificed after satisfactory enlargement of the posterior choana, to permit placement of 3.5-mm Silastic endotracheal tube as a stent. Posterior membranous flaps are developed in a stellate fashion to cover the denuded bone (Figs. 15–2 and 15–3). Care must be taken to prevent injury to the roof of the choana and the skull base because reported complications of this approach have included meningitis, cerebrospinal fluid leaks, brain injuries, Gradenigo's syndrome, and cervical vertebral subluxation. Other methods include the use of the carbon dioxide laser, endoscopic endonasal approach, and neodymium:yttrium-aluminum-garnet (Nd:YAG) laser technique.[12] After effective stenting and removal, and the use of topical corticosteroids to diminish granulation tissue formation, stenosis may still occur, and dilatation may be necessary. If this fails, a transpalatal approach will be required. A transseptal approach, which is reserved for older children with unilateral atresia, offers better exposure of the posterior vomer without risk of palatal injury and

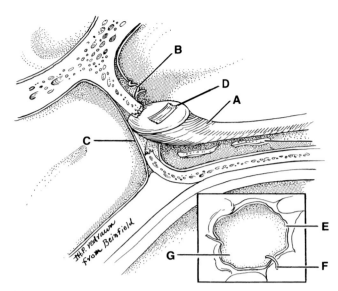

Fig. 15–2. A, Curette; B, shreds of nasal mucous membrane; C, intact nasopharyngeal mucous membrane; D, spicule of bone; E, bony atresia almost completely removed; F, shreds of mucous membrane; and G, intact pharyngeal mucous membrane.

impairment of growth. This approach can be modified either via sublabial extension or by an external rhinoplasty approach to improve visualization.

TRANSPALATAL APPROACH. The transpalatal approach provides superior visualization of membranous or bony atresia and may be useful for both bilateral and unilateral atresia. Although impaired palatal growth

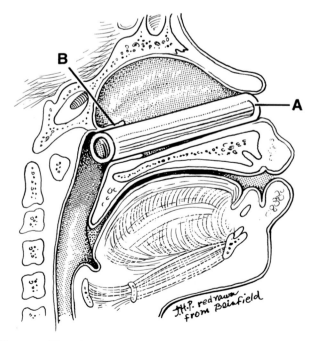

Fig. 15–3. The tube in place. A, The anterior end of the tube lying just within the nares; B, pharyngeal mucous membrane covering the raw bony surface.

is a potential problem in the neonate, the procedure can be safely used in patients older than 8 months of age if one takes great care to avoid injury to the posterior palatine canals.

The procedure is carried out with the patient in the supine position and the head hyperextended. After infiltration of local anesthesia, a horseshoe-type incision is developed several millimeters posterior to the alveolar ridge, and a mucoperiosteal flap is then raised based on the greater palatine vessels. Once the posterior edge of the hard palate is reached, the mucosa is divided, providing access to the atretic plate. An attempt is made to maintain mucosal flaps on both sides of the atretic plate. The atretic plate, posterior vomer, and medial aspect of the posterior maxilla are removed with a diamond bur, otologic curette, or rongeur. After removal of bone, mucosal flaps are transposed to cover the superior and inner surfaces of the choana, with stents placed as previously described. The palatal flap is reapproximated anteriorly with absorbable sutures. If stenosis occurs after surgical repair, patients generally slowly develop progressive respiratory difficulties. Revision surgery and/or dilatation may be necessary.

CONGENITAL DISORDERS OF THE NASOPHARYNX AND OROPHARYNX

Thornwaldt's Cyst and Rathke's Pouch Cyst

If the pharyngeal segments of the primitive notochord remain connected to the entoderm in the nasopharynx, a bursa or embryonic pouch occurs. In approximately 3% of individuals, this invaginated connection persists, and the resulting sac and canal, located in the posterior midline of the nasopharynx, extends posteriorly and cephalad toward the occipital bone. If the bursa is occluded by inflammation, a cyst will develop, and if the cyst becomes infected, an abscess will result. Anterior to the invagination and above the bursa is a small pharyngeal hypophysis developed from Rathke's pouch, which sometimes persists as the craniopharyngeal canal running from the sella turcica through the body of the sphenoid.

Most Thornwaldt's cysts appear clinically in the second and third decades of life, with males and females affected equally. Symptoms include intermittent or persistent postnasal discharge of tenacious mucous or purulent material, associated with odynophagia, halitosis, unpleasant taste, and occasionally, a dull occipital headache exacerbated by head movement with associated stiffness of the posterior cervical muscles. Nasopharyngoscopy reveals a smooth, submucosal, 1- to 2-cm midline cystic mass, superior to the adenoidal pad. Frequently, a central dimple or fistula is identified. CT scan demonstrates a soft tissue mass located high on the posterior nasopharyngeal wall with sharp borders (see Chap. 19). Microscopically, Thornwaldt's cyst is lined by respiratory epithelium with minimal amounts of lymphoid tissue in the wall. Treatment requires either excision to the periosteum or wide marsupialization. Rathke's pouch cysts, on the other hand, are basically cysts lined by columnar or cuboidal, ciliated epithelium that appear intracranially and are most commonly associated with headache followed by galactorrhea, visual field loss, and hypopituitarism. Treatment is transsphenoidal drainage of the cyst with biopsy of the wall. Radiation therapy is not indicated.

Chordomas

Chordomas are rare malignant neoplasms arising from primitive notochordal remnants. Fifty percent occur in the spheno-occipital area. The mean patient age is 40 to 45 years. Chordomas may become clinically apparent in childhood and adolescence. Males and females are approximately equally affected. Presenting signs and symptoms include an expanding nasopharyngeal mass, frontal headaches, cranial nerve palsies (sixth nerve involvement is seen in 60% of patients, followed equally by ninth and tenth nerve involvement), and pituitary abnormalities.

MR imaging with gadolinium is essential to evaluate the extent of the tumor, and it may be helpful in distinguishing classic chordoma from the chondroid variant. CT scanning frequently reveals extensive bone destruction at the skull base and is used to plan surgical resectability. Treatment is surgical resection via a skull base approach combined with postoperative radiation therapy. The overall prognosis in patients with chordomas is unfavorable, with median 5-year survival rates at 50% for patients undergoing resection.[13] Patients undergoing postoperative radiation therapy tend to have longer disease-free survival times. A younger age is the single most important factor associated with longer survival. Unfortunately, chordomas in children are more histologically variable and may pursue a more aggressive clinical course than chordomas in adults.[14] The lung and lymph nodes are the most common distant metastatic sites for chordomas in children.

Craniopharyngioma

Craniopharyngiomas arise from Rathke's pouch and are composed of well-differentiated epithelial elements including bone, cysts, and ameloblasts. Rarely, this lesion is first seen in the nasopharynx, but most commonly it occurs intracranially above the sella turcica. It accounts for approximately 10 to 15% of all childhood and adolescent intracranial neoplasms. Clinical manifestations include visual field defects, sudden blindness, extraocular motor paralysis, and hypopituitarism. The median age at presentation in children is 7.5 years, with an approximately equal female-to-male ratio. MR imaging with gadolinium or gadodiamide injection is mandatory for pretreatment assessment. Management of craniopharyngiomas has been controversial. Currently, surgical resection followed by radiation therapy achieves long-term control with low morbidity for tumors smaller than 5 cm.[15] Ten-year actuarial overall survival rates are 90%.[16]

Teratomas

Teratomas are true neoplasms that contain tissues foreign to the site in which they arise. The haphazard arrangement of tissue with asynchronous maturation is believed to escape the controlling influence of the primitive streak notochord or adjacent structures. Teratomas grow aggressively, and in the head and neck, they most commonly occur in the cervical area, followed by the nasopharynx.[17] Nasophargneal teratomas occur with a female-to-male ratio of 6:1. Overall, teratomas of the head and neck comprise approximately 2 to 9% of all teratomas.

Teratomas of the nasopharynx typically arise on the lateral or superior wall. Four basic types were recognized: (1) dermoid cyst, the most common form, composed of ectoderm and mesoderm arising as an epithelium-lined cavity with variable numbers of skin appendages; (2) teratoid cyst, derived from all three germ layers but poorly differentiated; (3) true teratoma, composed of ectoderm, mesoderm, and endoderm, with specific tissue and organ differentiation; and (4) epignathus, in which well-developed fetal parts are recognizable; this type of teratoma arises from the soft or hard palate and is frequently incompatible with life.

Clinically, dermoids are more common than true teratomas, and in the nasopharynx, the dermoid cyst is the most common developmental anomaly found. Known as "hairy polyps," these lesions appear at birth as a pedunculated mass filling the nasopharynx, often with oropharyngeal extension. Patients with teratomas have nasal obstruction, dysphagia, and copious secretions. CT and MR imaging are critical to define the extent of the neoplasm and to exclude either a nasoencephalomeningocele or intracranial extension of a sphenoid-based teratoma through the craniopharyngeal canal.[18] Most cervical teratomas occur in the neonate and are benign. The tumor can surround or encroach on the airway, thereby causing progressive dysphagia and airway obstruction.

Surgical removal must be carefully planned to ensure a controlled airway throughout the intraoperative and postoperative periods. Tracheotomy is generally not necessary if orotracheal intubation is combined with a transoral removal of pedunculated nasopharyngeal teratomas or with early excision of cervical terato-

mas. Operative and postoperative bleeding in patients with nasopharyngeal teratomas is usually only slight because these tumors are poorly vascularized, and if removal is complete, recurrences are rare. More sessile tumors arising in the nasopharynx require a transpalatal approach. Malignant metastasizing cervical teratoma is extremely rare.

CONGENITAL DISORDERS OF THE ORAL CAVITY AND LIP

Numerous congenital defects of the oral cavity and related structures may occur. Common major anomalies, such as cleft lip and palate, are described in detail, whereas less common deformities are mentioned for completeness.

Congenital lesions of the tongue include aglossia, microglossia, and macroglossia (secondary to lymphangioma, hemangiomas, or as commonly found in Down's syndrome). Ankyloglossia due to varying degrees of underdevelopment of the lingual frenulum is not uncommon. Indications for frenuloplasty with Z-plasty are notching of the protruding tongue tip, inability to contact the maxillary alveolus, and/or restriction of protrusion beyond the mandibular alveolus. Other glossal anomalies include dermoid cysts, hamartomas, lingual thyroid, fissured (scrotal) tongue, median rhomboid "glossitis," and enteric duplication cysts.

Nonodontogenic cysts derived from epithelial remnants trapped in embryonic fusion lines during the developmental stage include midline maxillary cysts (median alveolar, nasal palatal, median palatal) and lateral maxillary cysts (globomaxillary, nasolabial). Treatment varies from simple incision and drainage to removal of the cysts from the palatal side, with or without adjacent teeth. Noncleft lip congenital anomalies encountered include microstomia, congenital pits, and "double lip."

Finally, congenital epulis or gingival granular cell tumor arises exclusively from the alveolus and is a rare lesion of unknown origin found in newborn female infants.

Cleft Lip and Palate

Cleft lip and palate are the most common congenital malformations of the head and neck, occurring approximately once in every 700 births. The risk of additional siblings' having a defect increases when an older sibling is affected. Both cleft lip with or without cleft palate and isolated cleft palate may be further classified into those classes associated with (syndromic) or without (nonsyndromic) a recognized malformation. The cause of syndromic clefting may be single gene transmission, chromosomal aberrations, teratogenicity, or environmental factors. Associated head and neck anomalies such as maxillary or malar hypoplasia, abnormal pinnae or atresia, facial nerve paresis or paralysis, mandibular dysmorphism, or abnormal excursion may be identified. Nonsyndromic clefting is associated with no obvious first or second arch anomalies or systemic organ malformation. Multifactorial inheritance is the cause of these clefts, and calculated risk rates are essential to provide genetic counseling to families.

Anatomy

The lips are a movable muscular sphincter composed primarily of orbicularis oris muscle with motor supply from the seventh cranial nerve. The lips are covered by skin on the outer surface and mucosa on the inner. The vermillion or lip edge forms a junction with the skin (white line) that creates a gentle arching in the upper lip or "Cupid's bow." The cephalic extension from the handle of the Cupid's bow encloses a small depressed area at the base of the columella called the philtrum. These anatomic landmarks plus the protrusion of the vermillion below Cupid's bow or the tubercle are used for orientation in cleft lip repair.

The palate is composed of a hard anterior portion and a soft muscular posterior portion. The anterior primary palate is formed by the alveolar ridge and four incisor teeth plus the triangular premaxilla. The remaining hard palate is formed by the palatine processes of the maxillary and palatine bones, which, with the soft palate, comprise the secondary palate. The soft palate is a muscular curtain formed by the tensor veli palatini muscle innervated by the fifth cranial nerve and the levator veli palatini muscle, musculae uvulae, and glossopalatine and palatopharyngeus muscles innervated by the pharyngeal plexus.

Embryogenesis

Clefts of the lip, alveolus, or palate are midfacial soft tissue and skeletal fusion abnormalities. In the normally developing fetus, the median nasal process fuses with the maxillary processes to form the upper lip, the premaxilla, and the corresponding segments of the alveolar process. Together, the premaxilla and the alveolus form the primary palate. The palatal processes fuse with each other to form the secondary palate, along with the nasal septum and premaxilla in the vicinity of the incisive foramen between gestational weeks 8 and 10. Palatal growth proceeds posteriorly toward the uvula. Failure of ingrowth of mesodermal tissue at this point results in a lack of cohesion of the palatal segments, causing a cleft palate, which may be seen in conjunction with clefts of the lip and/or alveolar process or alone. Interruption in the migration of mesodermal tissue during the first 2 months of embryonic life results in cleft lip deformities. Ultimately, a lack of fusion of the median nasal processes with the maxillary processes causes a cleft of the upper lip, premaxilla,

and alveolus. The incidence of cleft palate increases in the presence of a cleft lip, which occurs in an earlier stage than cleft palate. Moreover, the tongue is positioned higher in the oral cavity in cleft lip, further interfering with palatal fusion and leading to greater palatal clefting.

Management

The head and neck surgeon is part of a cleft palate or craniofacial team that includes pediatrics, ophthalmology, general plastic surgery, neurosurgery, audiology, speech and language pathology, orthodontics, prosthodontics, oral surgery, genetics, dentistry, cytology, psychiatry, social work, and nursing. The goals of this team are to restore normal anatomy and physiology, with an emphasis on muscular reconstruction of the lip and/or palate to allow normal facial development and to minimize growth disturbance.[19]

The initial priority for infants with clefts is to establish adequate feeding and nutrition. Infants with a unilateral or bilateral cleft lip and alveolus feed generally well by either breast or bottle. Infants with bilateral cleft lip, alveolus, and palate have significant feeding problems and require modified nipples, with feeding in the upright position to minimize nasal regurgitation.

Although the timing of surgical repair is controversial, most experts perform cleft lip repair at 3 months of life and cleft palate repair at 12 months, to establish a competent velopharyngeal sphincter. Surgical treatment is dictated by the anatomic defect, and a classification scheme is helpful in planning surgical repair: (1) cleft lip, unilateral or bilateral; (2) cleft palate, either with unilateral or bilateral cleft lip; and (3) isolated cleft palate.

UNILATERAL CLEFT LIP. In the basic complete defect, the floor of the nose communicates with the oral cavity, and the alveolar defect passes through the developing dentition. One sees significant nasal deformity, including columella displacement, nasal dome deformity, and alar flattening and retrodisplacement. The goals of surgical repair are restoration of orbicularis muscle function, alar base, and columellar height and creation of symmetry of philtral columns, tip height, Cupid's bow, and vermillion. This can be accomplished with a Millard rotation advancement procedure in concert with either preoperative orthodontic appliances or lip adhesion.

BILATERAL CLEFT LIP. The floor of the nose is absent bilaterally, and the nasal and oral cavities communicate freely. The central alveolar arch is displaced forward and superiorly, whereas the nasal tip is widened and the columella is short. The goals of bilateral cleft lip repair are the same as for unilateral defects. Bilateral lip adhesion, if indicated is performed when the patient is 2 to 4 weeks old, with definitive lip repair followed at 4 to 6 months of age. If no lip adhesion is necessary to align the underlying maxillary segments before definitive lip repair, bilateral lip repair is performed at 3 months.

CLEFT PALATE. The basic defect, absence of the nasal floor, may be complete or incomplete, with or without associated cleft lip. The goals of cleft palate repair are to close the defect without inhibiting maxillary arch growth, to achieve adequate velopharyngeal function, and to normalize oronasal resonance and speech patterns.[20] Although the exact timing of the repair is controversial, the procedure is performed when the patient is 10 to 18 months old, and it may require preoperative orthopedic devices used as an alternative to move the premaxilla posteriorly and to expand the lateral maxillary segments, facilitating surgical closure of the lip. Of the many techniques described for bilateral cleft palate repair, the two-flap palatoplasty by Bardach is commonly employed: (1) complete two-layer closure (oral and nasal sides); and (2) dissection, redirection, and suturing of the soft palatal musculature.

Secondary problems of cleft lip and palate that require subsequent treatment include correction of nasal airway impairment, cosmetic nasal defects, velopharyngeal insufficiency with associated hypernasality, and recurrent acute and chronic otitis media with effusion.[21]

PIERRE ROBIN SEQUENCE

"Pierre Robin" is one of the most recognized diagnostic eponyms. It is a poorly understood, nonspecific grouping of malformations, however, which as yet have no prognostic significance. The classic Pierre Robin sequence (PRS) of glossoptosis, micrognathia, and cleft palate (50% of cases) may occur as an isolated, nonsyndromic congenital disorder or as part of a larger anomaly that may include facial dysmorphism, cardiac defects, mental retardation, and/or musculoskeletal anomalies.[22] Möbius syndrome or nonprogressive congenital facial diplegia is such an example of PRS, with concomitant brachial and thoracic muscle aplasia along with cranial neuropathies (six and seven). PRS has no sex predilection, and it may be secondary to an intrauterine insult during the fourth month of gestation or due to hereditary causes. Syndromic PRS is often associated with ocular anomalies (detached retina or glaucoma) or aural abnormalities (chronic otitis media and low-set pinna).

Infants with PRS are at increased risk of airway obstruction and resulting hypoxemia, cor pulmonale, failure to thrive, and cerebral anoxia. Obstructive sleep apnea and snoring are common. Aspiration is a primary cause of death. Aerophagia associated with vomiting frequently results in aspiration. When compared with normal infants, infants with PRS exhibit a shorter tongue and mandibular length, with a narrow airway and a posteroinferior position of the hyoid bone resulting in airway compromise. Patients are initially given a trial of prone positional management with high-calorie gavage feeding. When continued respiratory distress and failure to thrive develop, a modified glossopexy, attaching the tongue at the mandibular alveolus and the lower lip, is performed. The genioglossus is also released to lengthen the tongue.[23] Bedside polysomnography may help to identify those infants without clinically severe airway obstruction who may benefit from a modified tongue lip adhesion. Tracheostomy is reserved for those patients following tongue lip adhesion who have continued failure to thrive and respiratory embarrassment.

CONGENITAL DISORDERS OF THE SALIVARY GLANDS

Congenital anomalies of the salivary gland are uncommon. Rarely, the parotid gland may be absent in the first and second branchial arch syndromes. Congenital sialoadenitis with cystic dilatation of the salivary ducts can occur, resulting in single or multiple cystic spaces. Sialography in the infant under sedation may help to demonstrate ductal ectasia. If obstruction and stasis develop, recurrent infections may result, necessitating parotidectomy with seventh nerve preservation. Congenital cysts may also appear in or adjacent to the salivary glands. They may develop from a defect in the growth of the ductal system or in relation to first branchial cleft anomalies.

First Branchial Cleft Anomalies

First branchial cleft anomalies have been classified into two groups: type 1 and type 2. Type 1 anomalies are first cleft ectodermal defects or duplication anomalies of the membranous external auditory canal. Type 1 cysts are found anterior and inferior to the pinnae in association with the parotid gland. The fistulous tract extends superiorly along the facial nerve and parallel to the external auditory canal, where it terminates. Type 2 branchial cysts are primarily first cleft and arch defects (ectodermal and mesoderm) with duplication of the external canal and pinnae. Type 2 cysts are found below the angle of the mandible along the sternoclerdomastoid muscle. The fistulous tract, like in type 1 anomalies, is variable and may run lateral to, medial to, or between the main branches of the facial nerve, ultimately ending in the external auditory canal.

Clinically, first branchial cleft cysts are associated with repeated infection and may require incision and drainage of an apparent neck abscess. Occasionally, purulent otorrhea may occur in the absence of demonstrable middle ear disease. Microscopically, the cyst is lined with hair follicles, apocrine or sweat glands, and sebaceous glands. Treatment is surgical excision of the cyst, sinus tract, and skin surrounding the sinus tract orifice. Because of the intimate relationship between the seventh nerve and the sinus tract, it is critical to expose the seventh nerve as in a parotidectomy, using the bony landmarks (styloid process, mastoid tip, and tympanomastoid suture line) to help identify the nerve, instead of the tragal pointer. A nerve integrity monitoring system may prove exceedingly beneficial in these difficult cases.

Hemangiomas and lymphangiomas are congenital lesions that may involve the salivary glands and are discussed earlier in this chapter.

PRIMARY CILIARY DYSKINESIA (KARTAGENER'S SYNDROME)

Primary ciliary dyskinesia syndrome is an inherited disorder characterized by recurrent upper and lower respiratory tract infections secondary to abnormal ciliary structure and function. Also termed immotile cilia syndrome, its most recognizable form is in Kartagener Syndrome's (bronchiectasis, chronic sinusitis, situs inversus, and sterility). It has also been recognized in Usher's syndrome type I, congenital heart disease, congenital esophageal dysfunction, and cutaneous abnormalities including folliculitis, nummular eczema, and pyoderma gangrenosum (see Chap. 7).

SUGGESTED READINGS

1. Todd NW: Common congenital anomalies of the neck: embryology and surgical anatomy. Surg Clin North Am 73:599, 1993.
2. Ford GR, Balakrishan A, Evans JN, and Bailey CM: Branchial cleft and pouch anomalies. J Laryngol Otol 106:137, 1992.
3. Baker LL, et al: Hemangiomas and vascular malformations of the head and neck: MR characterization. Am J Neuroradiol 14:307, 1993.
4. Jackson IT, Carreno R, Potparic Z, and Hassain K: Hemangiomas, vascular malformations, and lymphovenous malformations: classification and methods of treatment. Plast Reconstr Surg 91:1216, 1993.
5. Kozol RA, Geelhoed GW, Flynn SD, and Kinder B: Management of ectopic thyroid nodules. Surgery 114:1103, 1993.
6. Radkowski D, et al: Thyroglossal duct remnants: pre-operative evaluation and management. Arch Otolaryngol Head Neck Surg 117:1378, 1991.
7. Horisawa M, Niinomi N, and Ito T: What is the optimal depth for core-out toward the foramen cecum in a thyroglossal duct cyst operation? J Pediatr Surg 27:710, 1992.
8. Carpenter LM and Martin DF: Radiographic manifestations of congenital anomalies affecting the airway. Radiol Clin North Am 29:219, 1991.
9. Wardinsky TD, et al: Nasal dermoid sinus cysts: association with intracranial extension and multiple malformations. Cleft Palate Craniofac J 28:87, 1991.
10. Bartlett SP, Lin KY, Grossman R, and Katowitz J: The surgical management of orbitofacial dermoids in the pediatric patient. Plast Reconstr Surg 91:1208, 1993.
11. Morgan D, et al: Ear, nose, throat abnormalities in the CHARGE association. Arch Otolaryngol Head Neck Surg 119:49, 1993.
12. el-Guindy A, el-Sherief S, Hagrass M, and Gamea A: Endoscopic, endonasal surgery of posterior choanal atresia. J Laryngol Otol 106:528, 1992.
13. Forsyth PA, et al: Intracranial chordomas: a clinicopathological and prognostic study of 51 cases. J Neurosurg 78:741, 1993.
14. Mitchell A, et al: Chordoma and chondroid neoplasms of the sphenoocciput: an immunohistochemical study of 41 cases with prognostic and nosologic implications. Cancer 72:2943, 1993.
15. Rajan B, et al: Craniopharyngioma: long term results following limited surgery and radiotherapy. Radiother Oncol 26:1, 1993.
16. Hetelekidis S, et al: 20 year experience in childhood craniopharyngioma. Int J Radiat Oncol Biol Phys 27:189, 1993.
17. Fearon JA, Munro IR, Bruce DA, and Whitaker LA: Massive teratomas involving the cranial base. Treatment and outcome: a two center report. Plast Reconst Surg 91:223, 1993.
18. Barkovich AJ, Vandermarck P, Edwards MS, and Cogen PH: Congenital nasal masses: CT and MR imaging features in 16 cases. Am J Neuroradiol 12:105, 1991.
19. Nguyen PN and Sullivan PK: Issues and controversies in the management of cleft palate. Clin Plast Surg 20:671, 1993.
20. Witt PD and D'Antonio LL: Velopharyngeal insufficiency and secondary palatal management: a new look at an old problem. Clin Plast Surg 20:707, 1993.
21. Sadove AM and Eppley BL: Correction of secondary cleft lip and nasal deformities. Clin Plast Surg 20:793, 1993.
22. Shprintzen RJ: The implications of the diagnosis of Robin sequence. Cleft Palate Craniofac J 29:205, 1992.
23. Argamaso RV: Glossopexy for upper airway obstruction in Robin sequence. Cleft Palate Craniofac J 29:232, 1992.

Anatomy and Physiology of the Oral Cavity and Pharynx

John J. Ballenger

The nasopharynx is located above the palate, the oropharynx between the palate and hyoid bone, and the laryngopharynx from the hyoid to the lower border of the cricoid cartilage. The oral cavity lies immediately anterior to the oropharynx and is subdivided into the anteriorly located vestibule and the oral cavity proper. The vestibule is bounded by the alveolar ridges of the two jaws and externally by the lips and cheeks. The oral cavity proper contains the tongue and is bounded superiorly by both the hard and soft parts of the palate, below by floor of the mouth, and laterally by the cheeks; it communicates posteriorly directly with the oropharynx through the isthmus of the fauces. The bony hard palate is covered by a dense mucosa firmly adherent to the underlying periosteum.

TONGUE

Except for the muscles, the anterior two thirds of the tongue is derived from the first branchial arch, and the posterior third from the third arch. The muscles, deriving from mesodermal tissue, fall into two groups, extrinsic and intrinsic. The former, three in number, originate on the mandible, styloid, and hyoid processes and are able to pull the tongue in different directions. The intrinsic muscles are the superior and inferior longitudinal, transverse, and vertical, and because of the muscle orientation can impart great diversity to the movements of the tongue. Ventrally, the tongue is attached to the floor of the mouth and anteriorly to the centrally located frenulum linguae.

Approximately at the junction of the anterior two thirds and posterior third of the tongue is a V-shaped groove, the terminal sulcus, with the apex directed posteriorly. At the apex of the sulcus is found the foramen cecum, marking the origin of the thyroglossal duct.

Anteriorly, the tongue is covered by a thin mucous membrane closely attached to the underlying muscles. Posteriorly, the mucosa is thick and freely movable. Near the midline posteriorly is found an aggregate of lymph nodules known as the lingual tonsil.

INNERVATION OF THE TONGUE

Except for the palatoglossus muscle (the pharyngeal plexus), the motor nerve to the tongue is the hypoglossal, which turns forward above the greater cornu of the hyoid bone and runs on the outer surface of the hyoglossus muscle accompanied by the lingual vein (Fig. 16–1). The two major sensory nerves of the tongue are the glossopharyngeal for the posterior third and the lingual for the anterior two thirds. The latter, a branch of the mandibular division of the fifth cranial nerve (CN V), also receives the chorda tympani from the CN VII. The lingual nerve runs above the submandibular gland and the hypoglossal nerve. The glossopharyngeal nerve passes around the posterior border and lateral surface of the stylopharyngeal muscle to reach the posterior part of the tongue deep to the hypoglossus muscle (see Chap. 17).

Together, the two lingual nerves supply the mucosa of the anterior two thirds of the tongue. CN V provides general sensation and reaches some of the facial fibers of the taste buds. The glossopharyngeal nerves supply both general sensation and taste from the vallate papillae to the epiglottic valleculae.

The innervation of the tongue can be understood embryologically.[1] The lingual branch of the trigeminal, the nerve of the first branchial arch, supplies the epithelium of the anterior two thirds of the tongue. Taste buds in the anterior tongue are supplied by the chorda tympani branch of the facial nerve, the nerve of the

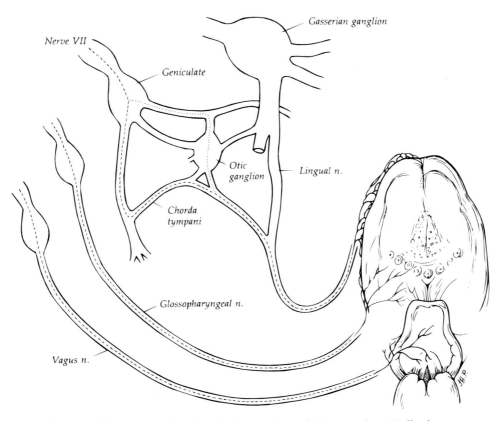

Fig. 16–1. The nerve supply and central connections of taste are schematically shown.

second arch, however. The circumvallate papillae on the posterior border of the anterior tongue are supplied by the glossopharyngeal nerve of the third arch.

TASTE

The sense of taste is subserved by taste buds broadly distributed on the epithelial surfaces of the tongue, soft palate, epiglottis, and three types of gustatory papillae that contain buds. The fungiform papillae are found on the anterior two thirds of the tongue (Fig. 16–2). The 8 to 12 vallate (circumvallate) papillae are found in a V formation in front of the terminal sulcus. They are flattened structures, each surrounded by a moat-like trench and richly supplied with taste buds. Ebner's glands (serous) open into the bottom of some of the trenches surrounding the papillae. Peg-like foliate papillae, studded with taste buds, form ridges on the posterior and lateral parts of the tongue. They, too, lie in a "moat."[2] Filiform papillae are keratinized structures distributed over the entire tongue dorsum and are not gustatory, but rather function in the tactile aspects of feeding.

Taste buds in the anterior walls of the foliate papillae are innervated by the chorda tympani, and buds in the posterior walls are innervated by the lingual

branch of the glossopharyngeal nerve. This latter branch also supplies the taste buds in the circumvallate papillae. Taste buds in the soft palate are innervated by the greater superficial branch of the facial nerve and in the epiglottis by the superior laryngeal branch of

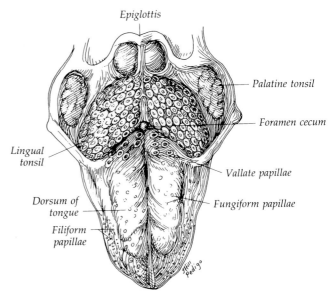

Fig. 16–2. Note the lingual and palatine tonsils, the two principal members of Waldeyer's Ring.

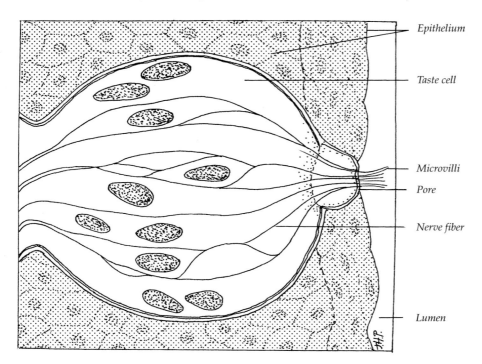

Epithelium

Taste cell

Microvilli

Pore

Nerve fiber

Lumen

Fig. 16–3. A schematic drawing of a taste bud.

the vagus. CN X probably mediates taste from buds on the epiglottis and upper larynx, and the CN IX and X mediate taste from buds in the larynx. Free endings from the trigeminal nerve also are found on the tongue and oral cavity.

TASTE BUDS

Taste buds consist of taste, sustentacular, and basal epithelial cells arranged to form a barrel-shaped organ. The taste cells at the apical ends contain microvilli 2 to 3 μm in length that connect with the luminal surface through a pore-like opening (Fig. 16–3). Several taste buds can be innervated by a single chorda tympani fiber, and one fiber can innervate more than one bud. Adsorption of the tastant onto the surface of the microvillus may be the mechanism initiating the electrophysiologic phenomenon perceived as taste. The epithelial taste buds have a life span of about 10 to 12 days and then are replaced by adjacent cells. This is reminiscent of the bipolar neurosensory olfactory cells, the first-order neuron, which is replaced about every 30 days.[2]

FLOOR OF THE MOUTH

The floor of the mouth contains the submandibular and sublingual glands (see Chap. 22) and the extrinsic musculature of the tongue. Clinically, the paired mylohyoid muscles constitute the muscular floor of the mouth. They arise from the body of the mandible and insert into a median raphe that extends posteriorly to the anterior surface of the hyoid bone. The firmness of this muscle, when inflammation occurs above it, directs edema upward and thus may encroach on the airway.

PALATE

The palate consists of a bony part anteriorly and an attached soft part posteriorly. The palate forms the roof of the mouth and the floor of the nose. It is covered by stratified squamous epithelium on its oral and pseudostratified columnar on the nasal surfaces. The "primary palate" is part of the premaxilla, or the bone that contains the incisor teeth, and its union with the posterior part of the hard palate is marked in the midline by the incisive foramen. Posterior to this, the palatine bone's horizontal lamina extends medially from the upper alveolar ridge to meet its fellow in the midline to form the "secondary palate" (Fig. 16–4).

Posterior to the bony palate is found the fibromuscular soft palate. The interior, fibrous portion of the soft palate is called the palatine aponeurosis. It is continuous with the periosteum of the hard palate, is firmly attached to the posterior margins of the bony palate, and continues laterally to blend with the tendons of the tensor veli palatini muscle. All the muscles of the palate insert into the aponeurosis. Posteriorly in the midline is a tubular extension of the soft palate, the uvula, containing the musculus uvulae.

At the junctions of the soft and hard palate are two

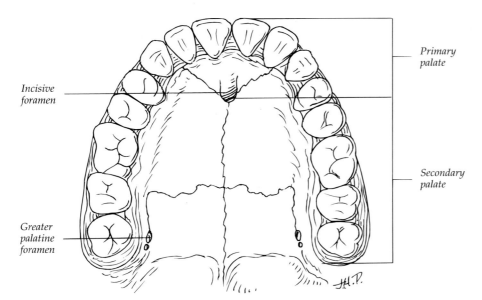

Fig. 16–4. The divisions of the hard palate.

or more foramina laterally representing the lower ends of the pterygopalatine canal. The larger and more anterior is the greater palatine foramen, and posteriorly are one or two lesser palatine foramina, together carrying blood vessels and nerves to the hard and soft palates. The hard palate receives its blood supply from the terminal vessels of the sphenopalatine vessels, the nasopalatine artery and vein issuing from the foramina. The nasopalatine nerve, CN V2, descends through the incisive canal and innervates the primary palatal plate. Most of the lymphatic vessels drain into the upper deep jugular or lateral retropharyngeal nodes.

The retromolar trigone is the gingiva attached to the overlying ascending ramus of the mandible. The distal surface of posterior lower molar tooth forms the base of a triangle, and its apex terminates at the maxillary tuberosity. Malignant tumors arising in the area may easily infiltrate the mandible. The lymphatic drainage of the retromolar trigone is similar to that of the tonsillar fossa.

The function of the soft palate is primarily to occlude the nasopharynx during swallowing and speech production. Contraction of the upper fibers of the superior pharyngeal constrictor muscle forms a muscular pad, known as Passavant's pad, on the posterior wall of the pharynx, and with this pad, the soft palate makes contact to occlude the nasopharynx.

PHARYNX

The pharynx, extending from the base of the skull and the styloid process to the lower border of the cricoid bone, is a muscular, cone-shaped tube that serves as a passageway for both air and food. At its lower end, it is continuous with the esophagus posteriorly and wraps around the larynx anteriorly by forming the piriform sinuses. In the nasopharynx, it receives the opening from the nose, the choanae, and in the oropharynx, the opening from the mouth. The pharynx is approximately 13 cm long, 3.5 cm wide superiorly, and 1.5 cm inferiorly. The mucosa is ciliated columnar in the nasopharynx and stratified columnar in both the oropharynx and laryngopharynx. The muscular layer of the pharynx consists of both circular and longitudinal fibers.

BLOOD SUPPLY OF THE PHARYNX AND TONSIL

The chief blood supply is derived from the ascending pharyngeal and faucial branches of the external carotid artery and from the superior palatine branch of the internal maxillary artery. The tonsillar artery, a branch of the external maxillary artery, is the chief vessel to the tonsil, although the ascending palatine sometimes takes its place. The tonsillar artery (or the ascending pharyngeal) passes upward through the superior constrictor muscle, giving branches to the soft palate and tonsil (Fig. 16–5). The dorsalis lingualis, a branch of the lingual artery, ascends to the base of the tongue and sends branches to the tonsil and to the pillars of the fauces. The descending or posterior palatine artery, a branch of the internal maxillary, supplies the tonsil and soft palate from above, forming an anastomsis with the ascending palatine. The small meningeal artery sends unimportant branches to the tonsil. A venous plexus is found at the base of the tongue, and varicosities may occur. The arterial supply is from the external carotid through the dorsal lingual branch of the lingual artery.

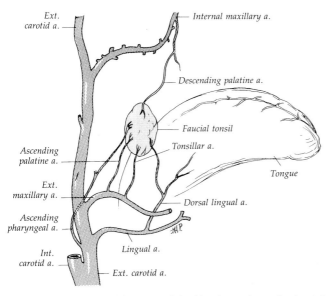

Fig. 16–5. The essential features of the blood supply to the faucial tonsil are depicted.

TONSILS AND ADENOID

The palatine (or faucial) tonsils are almond-shaped masses of lymphoid tissue lying between the anterior pillar (palatoglossus muscle) and the posterior pillar (palatopharyngeus muscle). They are covered on the lateral surface by the pharyngeal fascia and thus are loosely attached to the superior constrictor muscle. The pharyngeal fascia sends trabeculae carrying blood vessels, nerves, and efferent lymphatic vessels into the parenchyma of the tonsil. No afferent lymphatic vessels are present. Contractions of the superior constrictor, palatoglossus, and palatopharyngeus muscles compress the tonsil. The free surface is covered by a closely adherent stratified squamous epithelium that extends into blind pouches or crypts of the tonsil. The epithelium lining the crypts is thin and, in fact, may be a semipermeable membrane that "lends" itself to sampling by the tonsil of ingested material. The crypts, 8 to 10 in number, are usually compound and extend deep into the substance of the tonsil and come into intimate contact with the lymphatic structures, suggesting permeability. The germinating follicles are centers in which mother cells of the leukocytic group undergo karyokinesis and form young lymphoid cells. The interfollicular tissue is made up of lymphoid cells in various stages of development. Above the tonsil and between the 2 pillars a space, the supratonsillar fossa, is found.

The pharyngeal tonsil or adenoid is a lobulated mass of lymphoid tissue found chiefly on the upper and posterior walls of the nasopharynx and is arranged like separate segments of an orange with clefts in between. The adenoid (Luschka's tonsil) has no crypts,

but folds lined by respiratory epithelium. It is composed of lymphoid tissue in a delicate reticulum of fibers and acts as a peripherally placed lymph node from which efferent lymph ducts pass to the cervical chain. The adenoid is covered by pseudostratified epithelium. Groups of the lympoid cells are differentiated in the form of more or less rounded or oval areas with pale centers and darker margins—the follicles or "germ centers" of Goodsir. The incoming air from the nose contacts the adenoid, and speculatively, the adenoid can "sample" the air and respond immunologically. These lymphoid structures are capable of considerable hyperplasia with obstruction of the nasal airway under adverse conditions.

In the midline of the nasopharynx and surrounded by the adenoid is a depressed structure, the bursa pharyngea, that represents the remnants of the notochord. Thornwaldt's disease is an infection of the bursa.

The lingual tonsil, a sessile, midline lymphoid structure covered by squamous epithelium, is situated at the base of the tongue and extends from the foramen cecum to the epiglottis. Separated from the musculature of the tongue by a layer of fibrous tissue, it consists of numerous rounded or crater-like elevations of lymphoid tissue in the center of which a duct of a mucous gland opens.

WALDEYER'S RING

The pharyngeal tonsils and adenoid together comprise the most important members of Waldeyer's ring of lymphoid tissue. The other elements are the lingual tonsil, the lateral pharyngeal bands, scattered lymphoid nodules located in Rosenmueller's fossa, and nodules near the orifice of the eustachian tube (Gerlach's tonsil). Waldeyer's ring is involved in the development of nonthymus-related or B cells, particularly in the first few years of life. Production of all major classes of immunoglobulins and T lymphocytes with intact effector function of cell-mediated or "delayed" immunity can be attributed to elements of the ring.

LYMPHATICS OF THE ORAL CAVITY

The lymphatic drainage of the oral cavity is composed of both superficial and deep vessels that ultimately drain into the submandibular, upper jugular, and, occasionally, spinal accessory nodes. Cancers arising in the buccal mucosa primarily drain into the preglandular nodes of the submandibular triangle and secondarily drain into the upper jugular nodes of the deep jugular chain. Contralateral metastases are infrequent.

The lymphatic network overlying the gingiva of the maxillary and mandibular bones joins the lingual and

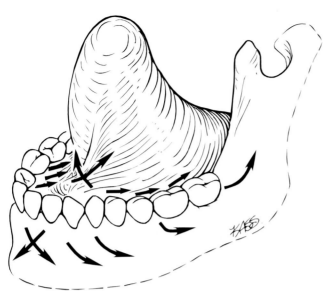

Fig. 16–6. Artist's drawing of the superficial lymphatic vessels of the floor of the mouth. Note that the vessels of the floor of the mouth connect with the gingival vessels.

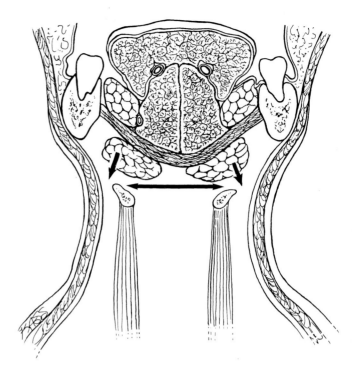

Fig. 16–7. Drawing demonstrating the lymphatic efferent upper jugular communicating pathway when the submandibular group of nodes has been bypassed.

buccal surfaces. The preglandular submandibular nodes represent the primary drainage route for both systems.

The superficial lymphatic vessels of the floor of the mouth connect with the gingival system before draining to the preglandular submandibular nodes (Fig. 16–6). The superficial system located in the anterior floor of the mouth crosses the midline and drains into either the ipsilateral or contralateral preglandular nodes (see Fig. 16–5). The deep collecting system drains into the same preglandular nodes before draining into the subdigastric nodes of the internal jugular chain. A second pathway bypasses the submandibular nodes and drains into the jugular omohyoid nodes. Additionally, an efferent upper jugular pathway crosses the midline and bypasses the submandibular nodes (Fig. 16–7).

The tongue possesses both a superficial and a deep system. No midline separation is present, so crossover into contralateral lymphatics is not uncommon. Lymphatic capillaries in the anterior portion of the tongue tend to drain into the submental and midjugular nodes, the lymphatics from the middle third to the submandibular or digastric nodes, and those from the base of the tongue to the upper jugular nodes (Fig. 16–8). The normal anatomic configuration of the lymphatics can be altered by obstruction from cancerous growths, by previous surgery, or by irradiation.

PHYSIOLOGY OF THE OROPHARYNX AND LARYNGOPHARYNX

These structures serve collectively not only as a rigid passageway for air, but also as a channel for food taken

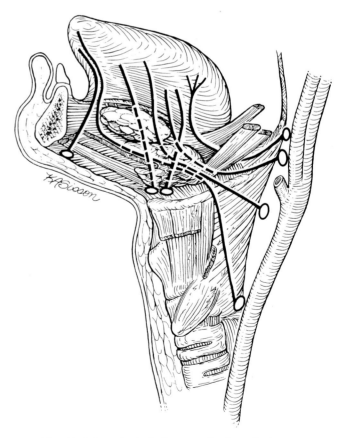

Fig. 16–8. Lymphatic drainage routes from the tongue.

into the mouth. The pharynx is open to air at all times except during swallowing and vomiting. Difficulty in swallowing is called dysphagia.

Swallowing consists essentially of three phases. The first, or voluntary, phase occurs when the bolus of food or drink introduced into the mouth is forced (after mastication in the case of food) through the fauces by the tongue and contraction of the tonsil pillars. As this occurs, the soft palate elevates and makes contact with Passavant's pad to close the nasopharynx. The cranial nerves involved are primarily CN V, VII, IX, X, and XII.

The second, or pharyngeal, stage is involuntary and encompasses the passage of the bolus, under control of the same nerves, from the fauces to the entrance to the esophagus. Peristaltic actions of superior, middle, and inferior constrictor muscles aid in the movement of the bolus. A final stage, also involuntary, occurs when the relaxation of the cricopharyngeus muscle allows the bolus to enter the esophagus. Food passage down the esophagus is assisted by gravity, positive external pressure, peristaltic esophageal waves, and negative intraesophageal pressure. The fibers of the inferior sphincter contribute to the cricopharyngeal sphincter.

PHYSIOLOGY OF TASTE

The simplest catagories of taste are sweet, salt, sour, and acid (bitter), and these combined with tactile and olfactory cues in various combinations account for taste perception. The term "flavor" includes components contributed by gustatory, olfactory, and somatic stimuli.[3]

Taste receptor cells are epithelial cells usually described as capable of stimulus by the foregoing catagories. This occurs likely by adsorption of the tastant onto the microvilli found in the pores of the taste buds and initiates a change in polarity that passes to the first-order neruon.[4] A sour taste is usually related to the hydrogen ion. Substances producing a sweet taste are commonly exemplified by glucose and sucrose. A common salty taste is sodium chloride. Bitter tastes usually involve long chains of organic substances or an alkaloid such as quinine, caffeine, or strychnine. Taste blindness or specific ageusia does occur on a genetic basis. The perception of taste can sometimes be stimulated by the injection of substances into the blood.

PATHOLOGY OF TASTE

Taste disorders fall into two broad classifications: taste distortions and taste losses. The former, dysgeusia, likely is the result of a fully active but malfunctioning taste system, whereas the latter, ageusia, reflects an absence or reduction of taste function. As with olfac-

tion, taste declines with age, but studies suggest that taste buds are not lost in substantial numbers and the loss may relate more to environmental problems.[5] Destruction of the oral or the upper aerodigestive mucosa can interfere with taste by its effect on neural pathways or on the taste buds and cells themselves. Irradiation and antirheumatic, antimicrobic, antiproliferative, and other drugs similarly can reduce acuity. Some drugs such as penicillamine, captopril, levamisole, and the aminoglycosides may have a depressive effect on the cells.[6] Gymnemic acid selectively blocks the capacity to appreciate sweetness.

Various disease states may be related to decreased gustatory function.[7] These include erythema multiforme, Addison's disease, Turner's syndrome, diabetes mellitus, hypothyroidism, Bell's palsy, multiple sclerosis, and herpes simplex infection. Sjögren's syndrome and irradiation-induced xerostomia adversely affect taste, probably because dryness of the tongue prevents a solution of the tastant. Various dental diseases must be evaluated in relation to dryness of the mouth. Inflammation of the tongue and mouth may form an exudate that imparts a "bad" taste. During ear surgery, the chorda tympani nerve may be severed, and depression of taste sensitivity may be produced. Moreover, ageusia may follow skull base surgery, but multiple nerve supply to the gustatory system makes it relatively resistant to traumatic destruction, compared with the olfactory system.[8]

Electrogustometry involves the application of weak electric current to taste fields in the oral cavity. In subjects with normal taste function, anodal (+) and cathodal (−) currents produce sour-metallic and indistinct bitter-sweet sensations, respectively, but in practice, anodal stimuli is used almost exclusively. In comparison with chemical solutions, electrical stimuli can be used more precisely and do not activate olfactory receptors retronasally, but they do not separately activate sweet, salty, sour, and bitter modalities. The problem of separating somatic sensations from taste also remains.

The taste threshold is usually sought in electrogustometry, and the tongue and oral cavity can be mapped. Localized testing with solutions of known concentration on standardized sizes of filter paper can be directed toward areas of known innervation.

CLINICAL MEASUREMENT OF TASTE

Odor identification has been shown to be a clinical useful procedure, but a comparable approach regarding taste is not yet available. The clinical measurement usually takes the form of detection of recognition thresholds, using a staircase method combined with a forced-choice procedure to ensure a bias-free measurement. This provides only a limited assessment of sensory capacity. Measurement of suprathreshold intensities can be done, but differences in individuals rating the strength of the same solution compromise the accuracy.

Perhaps the greatest promise lies in a psychophysical procedure known as magnitude matching. In this procedure, several concentrations of sodium chloride, sucrose, citric acid, or quinine hydrochloride and loudness levels of a 1000-Hz tone are compared. The taste solutions, presented in medicine cups, are sipped and then expectorated, and the tone is presented through headphones. The psychophysical function of taste can then be compared and graded in relation to the loudness of the 1000-Hz tone. The patient's hearing is presumed to be normal, at least for this tone. The procedure involves whole-mouth data and awaits development of normative figures.

The degree of taste function of the tongue and oral cavity can also be assessed by small squares of filter paper saturated with the tastant placed on one of the quarters of the tongue, rather than obtaining whole-mouth data.[9]

SUGGESTED READINGS

1. Getchell TV (ed): Smell and Taste in Health and Disease. New York, Raven Press, 1991.
2. West JB (ed): Best and Taylor: Physiological Basis of Medical Practice. 12th Ed. Baltimore, Williams & Wilkins, 1991.
3. Christensen CM: Role of saliva in human taste perception. In: Clinical Measurement of Taste and Smell. Edited by Meiselman HL and Rivlin RS. New York, MacMillan, 1986.
4. Teeter JH and Johnson P: Peripheral mechanisms of gustation: physiology and biochemistry. In: Neurobiology of Taste and Smell. Edited by Finger TE and Silver WL. New York, John Wiley & Son, 1987.
5. Murphy C: Taste and smell in the elderly. In: Clinical Measurement of Taste and Smell. Edited by Meiselman M and Rivlin RS. New York, MacMillan, 1986.
6. Bartoshuk LM: Chemosensory alteration and cancer therapies. NCI Mongr 9:179, 1990.
7. Schiffman SS: Taste and smell in disease. N Engl J Med 308: 1275 and 1337, 1983.
8. Smith DV: Taste and smell dysfunction. In: Otolaryngology. 3rd Ed. Edited by Paparella MM. Philadelphia, WB Saunders, 1988.
9. Bartoshuk LM, Gent J, Catalanotto FA, and Goodspeed RB: Clinical evaluation of taste. Am J Otolaryngol 4:257, 1983.

17 Diseases of the Oral Cavity

John J. Ballenger

Diseases of the oral cavity and those of the oropharynx (see Chap. 18) should be considered together.

PLUMMER-VINSON SYNDROME

The otolaryngologist may be the first to recognize this syndrome of dysphagia, glossitis, fissures at the corners of the mouth (perleche), cheilitis, and essential hypochromia. The patient should be referred to a gastroenterologist.

BURNING MOUTH SYNDROME

Patients afflicted with burning mouth syndrome complain of "burning" in the mouth, frequently worse at the tip of the tongue (glossodynia) despite a normal-appearing mucosa. In the past, it was frequently ascribed to psychogenic problems, but more recent information suggests a central or peripheral causalgic dysfunction of small afferent nerve fibers in the tongue.

A strawberry tongue is an exudative glossitis with prominent, beefy red papillae poking through. It is found in scarlet fever, Kawasaki's disease, Plummer-Vinson's disease, and toxic shock syndromes.

In Kawasaki's disease, patients, usually children, present with an ulcerative gingivitis, rhinitis, fever, and cervical adenitis. On about the third day, a generalized macular rash, erythema, and edema of the palms of the hand appear. The cause is unknown and the course self-limited.

BLACK HAIRY TONGUE

Excessively long, blackish filiform papillae that grow on the posterior tongue and extend toward the tip are found in this disorder. The cause likely is related to tobacco abuse, poor oral hygiene, or use of systemic antibiotics.

GEOGRAPHIC TONGUE

Typically, one sees a white margin of desquamating epithelium of various size and shape on the dorsum of the tongue surrounding a central red, atrophic area. The lesions are asymptomatic or slightly uncomfortable and may "migrate" across the surface of the tongue. The cause is unknown and no treatment is necessary.

SYPHILIS

Syphilis (lues) is a venereal disease caused by the spirochete Treponema pallidum. The chancre of primary syphilis is usually in the genital region but occasionally is found in oropharyngeal sites, where the lesion appears about 3 weeks after exposure as an ulcerated, painless papule with regional adenopathy. Syphilis can lead to interstitial glossitis, endarteritis, epithelial atrophy, and loss of papillae.

GONORRHEA

Gonorrhea, a common venereal disease, is caused by the gonococcus Neisseria gonorrhoeae and may affect the oral mucosa, lips, tongue, and palate with an ulcerative, pseudomembranous reaction.

AIDS

Acquired immunodeficiency syndrome (AIDS) is discussed in Chapter 5. Thirty-five percent of these patients display the giant oral and pharyngeal ulcers of Kaposi's sarcoma. Opportunistic infections may be found.[1] Differentiation from Hodgkin's and non-Hodgkin's lymphoma must be made.

LEUKEMIA

Leukemia suggests a group of neoplastic diseases of unknown cause arising from a malignant proliferation of hemopoietic cells. Malaise, fever, purpura, and epistaxis are common presenting symptoms. Petechial and ulcerative lesions of the nasal mucosa associated with bleeding, swollen gums are frequently noted. Epistaxis is best managed by avoiding packing and cautery when possible.

CHEMOTHERAPY AND IRRADIATION

Chemotherapy and irradiation used for treatment of various diseases may cause severe oral stomatitis and ulceration, either directly or as a result of depression of the bone marrow. Such ulcers are deep, necrotic, and persistent, and they lack a surrounding zone of inflammation.

PEMPHIGUS

Pemphigus (pemphigus vulgaris and pemphigus vegetans), pemphigoid (bullous pemphigoid), and benign mucous membrane pemphigoid are primarily autoimmune vesiculobulous disorders of the skin.[2] One sees a loss of cohesion among epidermal cells (acantholysis), with a resulting cleft and accumulation of intradermal fluid or blisters. In pemphigus, the cleft is in the suprabasal layer and, in pemphigoid, at the basement membrane zone. In pemphigus Nikolsky's sign can be elicited by sliding the skin sideways adjacent to a lesion, thus creating a cleft and a fluid-filled bulla, but not in pemphigoid. In pemphigus, tattered, shallow, bullous lesions appear on the buccal mucosa, mouth, and lips in about two thirds of patients, so confusion with Stevens-Johnson syndrome is possible. Treatment of pemphigus vulgaris is with glucocorticosteroids and persisting and careful attempts to prevent infection. Bullous pemphigus and pemphigoid are treated with systemic corticosteroids, usually taken orally, and long remissions may occur.

STEVENS-JOHNSON SYNDROME

Stevens-Johnson syndrome is generally recognized as a severe form of erythema multiforme. Erythema multiforme is an immune reaction in the skin and mucous membranes that evolves in response to certain antigenic stimuli (infections, drugs, connective tissue disease) and causes the development of erythematous plaques, blisters, and target (bull's-eye) skin lesions.[3] The mucous membrane of the eye and mouth may be involved. In Stevens-Johnson syndrome the skin is more widely involved, and the patient looks and feels ill with fever, prostration, and odynophagia. In about half the cases, the cause remains obscure, but agents that may trigger the reaction include drugs (penicillin, barbiturates, phenytoin, sulfonamides) and infections (herpes simplex, streptococcus, Mycoplasma pneumoniae). The majority of cases seem to relate to prior infection with herpes simplex virus-1 or 2. For treatment, offending agents should be withdrawn. The value of corticosteroids is controversial. A fluid balance must be maintained.

HERPESVIRUS

Of the more than 50 herpesviruses, humans are particularly susceptible to herpes simplex virus (HSV), varicella-zoster virus (VZV), and Epstein-Barr virus (EBV). Of the 2 types of HSV, HSV-1 causes oral and pharyngeal infections, and HSV-2 causes genital infections. The primary HSV-1 infection is almost always subclinical, in an infant, and resembles a "cold." The physician who inserts an ungloved finger into the mouth of an infected patient runs the risk of acquiring an ulcerous infection on the finger (a whitlow) accompanied by lymphadenitis and regional adenopathy. Recurrent herpes simplex (RHS) is to be distinguished from recurrent aphthous stomatitis (RAS) and occurs in patients who have previously experienced herpes simplex infections. Clinically, RHS is associated with herpes labialis (cold sores, fever blisters, and vesicles of 1 to 2 mm). HSV-1 is sensitive to acyclovir.

In RAS, recurrent ulcers form on the oral mucosa and heal within 1 to 2 weeks. A more severe form (Sutton's disease) require months to heal and does so with scars. In RAS, the lesions are confined to the oral mucosa, consist of 2 to 6 round, 2- to 3-mm shallow ulcers not preceded by vesicles. Treatment is palliative.

Herpangina is a relatively minor disease, sometimes of an epidemic nature. It causes fever, chills, anorexia, and odynophagia. Bilateral, discrete, small ulcerated vesicles involve the posterior pharynx and soft palate. Supportive therapy is indicated.

VZV is the etiologic agent of varicella (chickenpox) and herpes zoster (shingles). Rarely, it attacks the fifth cranial nerve and the geniculate ganglion (see Ramsay-Hunt syndrome, Chap. 10).

BEHÇET'S DISEASE

Behçet's disease is of uncertain origin and is characterized by aphthous ulcers. It may be associated with uveitis, cutaneous vasculitis, synovitis, meningitis, or genital ulcerations. In the mouth the ulcerations are sharply demarcated by a surrounding red halo. Acyclovir and chlorambucil have been described as helpful in treatment.

ROOT OR RADICULAR DISEASE

A root or periosteal cyst arises from death of the tooth pulp, with subsequent development of a granuloma or cyst, and accounts for perhaps 80% of dental cysts. Dentigerous cysts are frequently found in the mandible and probably represent an expanded tooth follicle. The cyst, thin walled and lined with squamous cell epithelium, expands progressively with displacement of adjacent structures. The most effective treatment is extirpation. Cysts encroaching on the anterior portion of the hard palate are rare and presumably result from incomplete closure of the premaxilla and maxilla. Ranula is a degenerative cyst formation of the salivary glands in the sublingual region near the frenum. Treatment consists of complete extirpation.

AMELOBLASTOMAS

Ameloblastomas (adamantinomas) are benign tumors that can be locally aggressive. They arise from paradental epithelial debris and are solid in the early stages, but cystic degeneration and softening occur later. Hard odontomas are composed of one or more elements of dentin, cement, or enamel. Odontomas grow by direct expansion, whereas ameloblastoma do so by infiltration.

WHITE LESIONS OF THE ORAL CAVITY

"Leukoplakia" indicates the presence of a white patch on the mucous membrane and raises the possibility of a precancerous lesion (2 to 6%, long-term risk). The presence or absence of keratosis or adherence to the underlying mucosa is critical. If both are present, the likelihood of malignancy is heightened. Of final importance, always, is the finding on microscopy of the presence or absence of cellular atypia (also called dyskeratosis and dysplasia). Suspicioun of malignancy is heightened if a red, granular, atrophic-base erythroplasia is noted. Hairy leukoplakia, often associated with AIDS, displays a slightly raised, corrugated ("hairy") surface. Isotretinoin and β-carotene show some promise in the treatment of oral leukoplakia.

LICHEN PLANUS

The primary cutaneous lesion of lichen planus is a linear arrangement of polygonal, white, reticulated pap-

ules. The primary oral lesion is a small papule with a painless, glistening white, sky-blue, or gray lesion, frequently with bilateral symmetry. The white, sponge-like, hereditary oral lesion of Cannon appears in infancy.

VINCENT'S ANGINA

This disease, caused by a spirochete and a fusiform bacillus, is most often found in adverse social as well as wartime conditions. The lesion commonly is an acute, pseudomembranous involvement of the pharynx or tonsils or an acute necrotizing disease of the interdental papillae (trench mouth). Collectively, these lesions are known as Vincent's disease or angina. In the pharynx, the disorder is characterized by sore throat, fetor ex ore, and gingival or tonsil bleeding. A pseudomembrane is present and progresses to a gangrenous stomatitis. The disease usually responds readily to penicillin. Dental care is necessary.

LYMPHATICS OF THE ORAL CAVITY

The lymphatic drainage from the oral cavity is to superficial and deep vessels that ultimately reach the submandibular, upper jugular, and occasionally, spinal accessory nodes. Channels from the buccal mucosa primarily reach the preglandular nodes of the submandibular triangle and secondarily the upper jugular nodes of the deep jugular chain. The gingiva overlying the maxillary bones has a network that joins the lingual and buccal surfaces, and a similar relation exists for

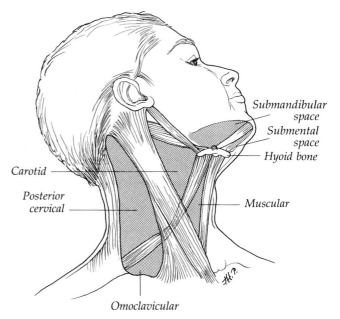

Fig. 17–1. Schematic representation of the triangles of the neck.

the mandibular gingiva as well. The preglandular submandibular nodes represent the primary drainage route for both these systems.

The mucosa and underlying soft tissues of the floor of the mouth have abundant superficial and deep lymphatics. The superficial vessels connect with the gingival system before draining into the preglandular nodes. The superficial system located in the anterior floor of the mouth crosses the midline and drains into either the ipsilateral or contralateral preglandular submandibular nodes. The deep collecting system drains into the same preglandular nodes before draining into the subdigastric nodes of the internal jugular chain. A secondary pathway bypasses the submandibular nodes and drains into the jugulomohyoid nodes. An efferent upper jugular pathway has also been demonstrated.

The tongue possesses both deep and superficial lymphatic vessels with no midline demarcation. In the anterior portion, the vessels tend to drain into the submental and midjugular nodes, those from the middle third to the submandibular and subdigastric nodes, and those from the base to the upper jugular nodes.

FASCIAL PLANES OF THE NECK

For descriptive purposes, the sternocleidomastoid muscle divides the neck into an anterior triangle, lying anterior, and a posterior triangle, lying posterior, to the muscle. These areas are further divided as indicated in Figure 17–1.

The fascia of the neck consists of the superficial or investing layer and the deep cervical fascia. The superficial fascial layer lies just below the skin of the neck and is continuous with that of the face, including in-

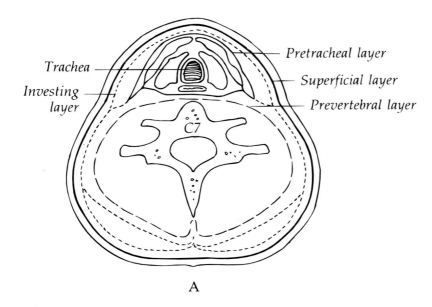

A

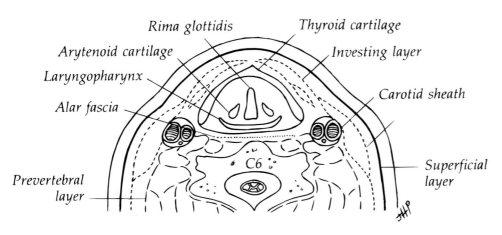

B

Fig. 17–2. Schematic representation of the fascial planes of the neck.

vestment of the submandibular and parotid glands. In the deepest layers of the superficial fascia are found the fibers of the platysma muscle.

The deep cervical fascia has three principal layers: the enveloping (investing) or anterior layer, the pretrachial or middle layer, and the prevertebral or posterior layer. The carotid sheath, containing the carotid artery, internal jugular vein, and vagus nerve, can be considered a separate fascial compartment but also is intimately involved with the second and third layers (Figs. 17–2 and 17–3).

The so-called fascial spaces of the neck are potential spaces or clinical tracts less resistant to the spread of infection. The visceral space lies between the pretracheal and prevertebral fascias and extends downward into the anterior mediastinum, laterally along the subclavian vessels into the axillary space, and upward into the retromandibular space. The prevertebral fascia lies anterior to the cervical vertebral bodies, extends laterally to the tips of the transverse processes, and covers the paraspinous muscles. The prevertebral space and fascia of the superior constrictor muscle become firmly attached with the prevertebral muscles to the occiput at about the level of the prominence of the second cervical vertebra (Fig. 17–4). This tends to confine abscesses to the upper portion. The suprahyoid space, between the investing fascia and the mylohyoid muscle, communicates with the submandibular space as well as the visceral space. The lateral pharyngeal space is found lateral to the pharynx and is also known as the peripharyngeal or pharyngmaxillary space. The ca-

rotid sheath, which pierces the cone-shaped lateral pharyngeal space at its apex, provides a direct conduit for infection to the mediastinum. The parotid gland is encased by the splitting of the superficial layer of the deep cervical fascia. The medial part of the split is thin and abuts the lateral pharyngeal space, and infections within the parotid gland extend more easily medially than laterally where the fascia is thicker.

DEEP NECK INFECTIONS

Deep neck infections commonly are of odontogenic origin but they may result from a penetrating injury or the implantation of organisms by needle injections. Extension of tonsillar and peritonsillar infections is still one of the more common causes.

In the past, about 50% of deep neck infections were in the lateral pharyngeal space. Such a patient complains of fever, trismus, and edema involving the submandibular regions and the parotid gland. Trismus is severe, and neck motion is limited. Intraorally, swelling of lateral pharyngeal wall is marked, and the tonsils are displaced anteriorly and medially. Neurologic deficits involving cranial nerves IX, X, and XII occur. Horner's syndrome may be present (Figs. 17–5 to 17–7).

Treatment of lateral pharyngeal space infections should be aggressive, with antibiotics, fluid replacement, and careful observation. Surgical intervention may be required, particularly if the patient has hemor-

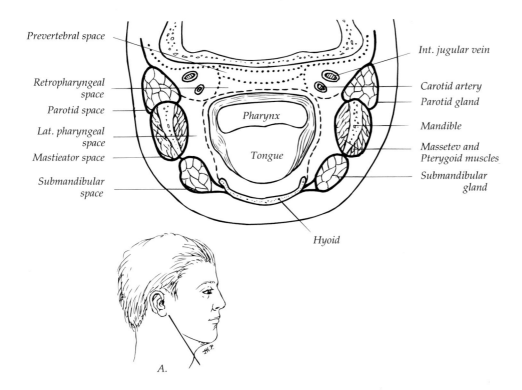

Prevertebral space

Retropharyngeal space

Parotid space

Lat. pharyngeal space

Mastieator space

Submandibular space

Int. jugular vein

Carotid artery
Parotid gland

Mandible

Massetev and Pterygoid muscles

Submandibular gland

Pharynx

Tongue

Hyoid

A.

Fig. 17–3. The neck spaces as indicated in A.

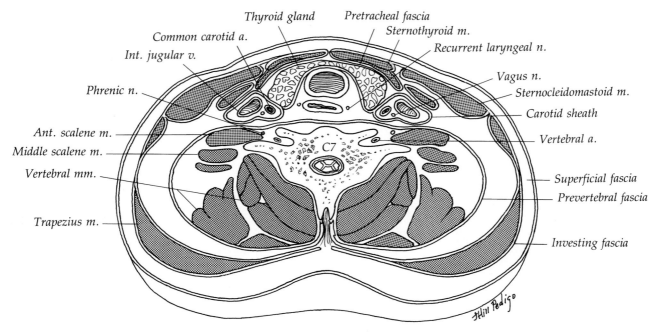

Fig. 17–4. Cross-section of the neck at level C7.

rhage, subcutaneous emphysema, neurologic deficits, dyspnea suggestions of internal jugular vein thrombosis, or pus formation. Cellulitis can be easily distinguished from abscess formation by computed tomography (CT) or magnetic resonance (MR) imaging.

Ludwig's angina, commonly found in young adults, is a rapidly spreading cellulitis of the submandibular space. This space comprises the submaxillary and sublingual spaces, the latter containing the submental space lying between the anterior bellies of the digastric

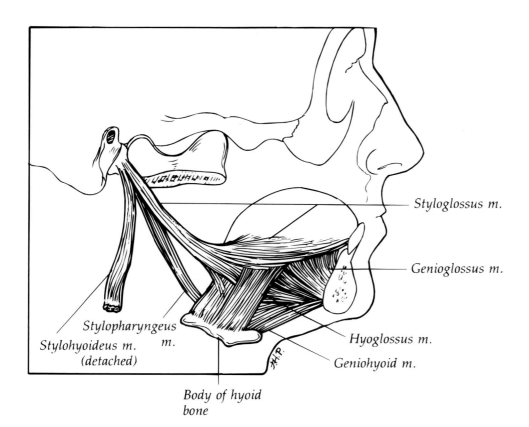

Fig. 17–5. Diagram of muscles related to the tongue.

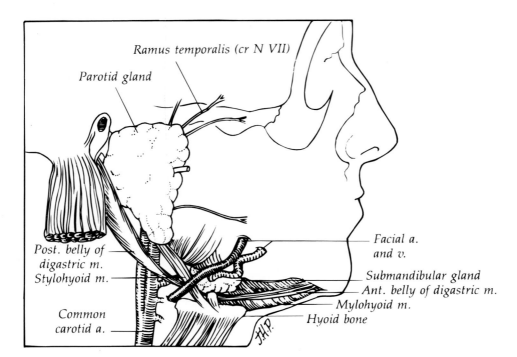

Fig. 17–6. Note the location of the submandibular gland.

muscles. The submaxillary space lies below the myelohyoid muscle, and the sublingual space is above, but below the tongue. Both spaces communicate with each other via the space between the mylohyoid and geniohyoid muscles. Orodental disease, particularly of the second and third lower molars, whose roots extend inferior to the attachment of the myelohyoid muscle to the body of the mandible, frequently inaugurates Ludwig's angina. Bacteria, including anaerobic types, are usually the cause.

Symptoms of Ludwig's angina are related to the site of the infection. If it is above the firm, unyielding mylohyoid muscles, the edema displaces the tongue upward and posteriorly, presenting a threat to the airway. The floor of the mouth is tender and edematous and has a board-like induration. Trismus may be marked. Involvement of the submandibular spaces produces a tense, brawny suprahyoid swelling of the neck and submental areas. The infection, if unchecked, may travel to the lateral pharyngeal and retropharyngeal spaces or downward to the mediastinum.

Treatment of Ludwig's angina must be aggressive, with antibiotics selected to control the infecting organism. Attention to the adequacy of the airway must never be relaxed because airway compromise is the major cause of death. At times an infected tooth must be removed. Abscesses must be drained.

DIFFERENTIAL DIAGNOSIS OF A NECK MASS

The differential diagnosis of a neck mass, particularly if metastatic, can be difficult and occasionally cannot be made with certainty even after an autopsy.[4] All neck masses should be recorded by tenderness, size, location, fixation, compressibility, displacement, consistency, and the presence of bruit, thrills, odor, or anything else that seems pertinent. After a careful history and physical examination, a thorough mirror examination of all mucosal surfaces of the upper aerodigestive tract should again be made, taking particularly into account the source of the lymph channels leading to

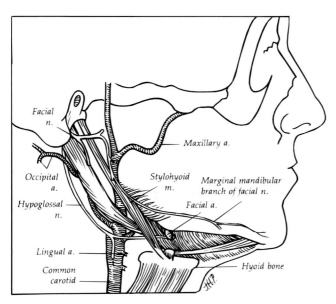

Fig. 17–7. Diagram of the branches of the external carotid artery.

TABLE 17–1. Differential Diagnosis of a Neck Mass*

Age 0–15	16–40	41 +
Congenital/ Developmental	Congenital/ Developmental	Congenital/ Developmental
Thyroglossal duct cyst	Branchial cleft cyst	Lymphangioma
	Thymic cyst	
Dermoid		
Laryngocele	Sialadenopathy	
	Ectopic thyroid	
	Pharyngeal diverticulum	
Inflammatory	Inflammatory	Inflammatory
Adenitis (viral, bacterial)	Adenitis (viral, bacterial)	Adenitis (viral, bacterial)
Granuloma	Granuloma	Granuloma
	Sialadenitis	
Neoplastic*	Neoplastic	Neoplastic
Thyroid	Lymphoma	Lymphoma
Lymphoma	Metastatic cancer	Metastatic cancer

* Does not include neurogenic or vascular masses.

the area of the mass. Flexible fiber endoscopy aids considerably in areas difficult to visualize with a mirror. It usually is helpful to organize the search from the point of view of both the age of the patient and the location of the mass.

In the pediatric population (age 15 and younger), neck masses are almost always viral or bacterial inflammatory lymph nodes, followed in frequency by congenital and developmental problems, and finally, by neoplastic lesions. Cat scratch disease and atypical tuberculosis may on occasion be found.

In adults (16 to 40 years), an inflammatory origin is less frequent, and congenital and developmental origins are more likely, as well as sialadenopathies. In older adults (41 +), the first consideration must always be suspicion of a metastatic lesion, although granulomatous (e.g., actinomycosis and tuberculosis) and congenital or developmental diseases may first be detected at this time. Primary malignant tumors rarely appear in the neck at any age, particularly in children; however, Hodgkin's disease, lymphoma, and leukemia should be kept in mind in all age groups. Table 17–1 is a simplified age-related representation of common neck lesions.

For all age groups, congenital and developmental masses are usually found in the anterior midline or anterior triangle of the neck (see Fig. 17–1), whereas metastatic malignant tumors are distributed along the pathways of the cervical lymphatic channels (see Chap. 16). Knowing what lymph vessels drain a particular region frequently suggests where to look for the primary tumor. The congenital and developmental struc-

tures include sebaceous, dermoid, and thymic cysts and branchial cleft and thyroglossal duct cysts, as well as lymphangiomas, hemangiomas, ectopic thyroid tissue, laryngoceles, and pharyngeal diverticula. These disorders are considered in Chapter 15.

Information so far accumulated provides the examiner with a general idea of the nature of the lesion, so various tests appropriate to the lesion can now be employed to refine the problem. These include examination of the blood, skin tests, radiography, sialography, ultrasonography, CT, MR imaging, and biopsy. Positron emission tomography (PET) with 2-(18F)-fluoro-2-deoxy-D-glucose (FDG) has been shown to measure uptake in lymphatic tissues of Waldeyer's ring, in lymph nodes, and in mucosal surfaces. Because an important characteristic of neoplastic tissue is its increased rate of cell division, this increased uptake of glucose is likely indicative of a primary or metastatic tumor.

An open biopsy is usually undesirable because of the disturbance to the local lymph nodes. Moreover, if an open biopsy is done, provision for immediate neck dissection must be made in the event that frozen sections reveal the presence of a malignant tumor. In the young child, greater latitude is present because so many glands are inflammatory (or congenital) in nature and malignancy is rare.

Alternatively, a 23-gauge needle aspiration biopsy can be safely and accurately done, provided a competent cytopathologist is available. If no primary malignant tumor, or other explanation, can be found to explain a neck mass, it may be necessary to resort to a guided biopsy of suspicious "remote" areas. The location of the node and knowledge of the anatomic area it drains should guide the surgeon to the likely primary sites for biopsy. Statistically for the otolaryngologist, these remote areas include the nasopharynx, the tonsil (tonsillectomy), the base of the tongue, and the pyriform sinus. Panendoscopy may be required.

SUGGESTED READINGS

1. Pindborg JJ, Odont HC: Classification of oral lesions associated with HIV infection. Oral Surg Oral Med Oral Pathol 67:292, 1989.
2. Venning VA, et al: Ocular and oral involvement in bullous and cicatricial phemphigoid: a clinical and immunopathological study. Br J Dermatol 115(suppl 30):19, 1986.
3. Lozada F and Silverman S: Erythema multiforme: clinical characteristics and natural history in 50 patients. Oral Surg 46:628, 1978.
4. McGirt WF: Differential diagnosis of neck masses. In: Otolaryngology: Head and Neck Surgery. Edited by Cummings CW. St. Louis, Mosby-Year Book, 1993.

18 Diseases of the Oropharynx

John J. Ballenger

A simple, acute oropharyngitis may accompany a "common cold" and is discussed in Chapter 6.

ADENOTONSILLITIS

"Sore throat" is a term that suggests a painful condition in the oropharynx but usually, in children, is associated with adenotonsillitis. The etiology is discussed in Chapter 3.

Symptoms

Often the onset of an acute adenotonsillitis is abrupt, particularly in children, and is manifested by chills and low-grade fever, malaise, thirst, odynophagia, dysphagia, nasal speech, and swollen, tender cervical lymph nodes. Examination of the oropharynx reveals the tonsils to be swollen (even to the point, occasionally, of contact across the midline and thus a threat to the airway) and red and frequently to display yellowish white spots or follicles (follicular or lacunar tonsillitis) or, in more severe situations, a membranous or pseudomembranous tonsillitis if the spots coalesce. The tongue may be coated with a grayish covering, and mucus be thick and tenacious. Fetor ex ore may be evident. The adenoid also may be acutely enlarged and add to the threat to the adequacy of the airway. Bacterial cultures should be taken. When viral tonsillitis is suspected, specific agglutination tests can be done, but they usually are not warranted and are not cost effective.

Although acute bacterial tonsillitis is usually self-limited, rarely, it may persist and be complicated by peritonsillar edema with airway obstruction, peritonsillar abscess, deep neck infections, septicemia, rheumatic fever, and possibly glomerulonephritis if neglected. The disease must be differentiated primarily from diphtheria, scarlet fever, Vincent's angina or trench mouth, and various viral afflictions. An abscess of the tonsil itself is rare but could result from acute follicular tonsillitis with obstruction of the crypts or from spontaneous rupture of a peritonsillar abscess into the tonsil.

Treatment

Treatment of acute adenotonsillitis includes bed rest, adequate fluid intake, analgesics, and antipyretic medications. Systemic antibiotics are necessary for the treatment of bacterial adenotonsillitis, particularly if a group A hemolytic streptococcus infection is present. Usually, penicillin taken in adequate doses for 10 days is sufficient in patients with such a streptococcal infection, and frequently treatment is begun before the culture reports are returned. Care must be taken that β-lactamase is not present, and if so, appropriate changes must be made in the antibiotic regimen (see Chap. 3). Erythromycin or tetracycline may be used as a second choice, although tetracycline should not be used in children whose teeth have not yet erupted because of possible dental staining.

CHRONIC PHARYNGITIS

This nonspecific entity must be distinguished from recurrent infection. If the sore throat persists, the irritative effects of the environment on the nasal and oropharyngeal mucosa must be considered, as well as passive and active tobacco smoking. The complaint is frequently a sense of a foreign body in the pharynx, and consideration must be given to concomitant hyperkeratosis, a tonsillar calculus, an elongated styloid process, or a persisting viral infection. Discomfort in the pharynx may represent pain referred from disease elsewhere in the head.

LINGUAL TONSILLITIS

The odynophagia in this situation is usually unilateral, and the discomfort is made worse by depression or protrusion of the tongue. By mirror laryngoscopy, the presence of an acutely inflamed and tender mass, usually with white exudate, at the base of the tongue makes the diagnosis. Treatment by antibiotics is usually sufficient. The disease must be distinguished from a lingual thyroid, a thyroglossal duct cyst, a dermoid cyst, and tumors.

DIFFERENTIAL DIAGNOSIS OF ADENOTONSILLITIS

In addition to the foregoing, adenotonsillitis can be confused with diphtheria, scarlet fever, and Vincent's angina or trench mouth. Although the onset is frequently gradual, with less-pronounced systemic symptoms, in diphtheria, hoarseness, stridor, and a croupy cough do occur and are similar to the signs and symptoms of adenotonsillitis. The diphtheritic membrane is firm, leathery, grayish, and firmly adherent to the tonsils and pharyngeal mucosa. Attempts to remove the membrane produce bleeding. Airway obstruction by the diphtheritic membrane is possible, and the organism can produce an exotoxin that is both neurotoxic and cardiotoxic. The diagnosis is made by demonstrating Klebs-Löffler bacteria on culture or by stain (see Chap. 3).

Scarlet fever also may result in membranous tonsillitis, as well as a marked erythema of the oropharyngeal mucosa. A characteristic "strawberry" tongue with prominent lingual papillae may occur, along with a diffuse erythematous papular skin rash. Diagnosis is made by the demonstration of β-hemolytic streptococci and by immune testing (Dick's test or the Schultz-Charlton blanching phenomenon). Vincent's angina is discussed in Chapter 17.

KERATOSIS OF THE TONSIL

Cornification of the epithelial lining of the tonsil crypts with minute horny projections from the surface occurs in this situation, and sometimes the horny projections arise in other lymphoid masses. A sense of foreign body can be a complaint with no other symptoms. The bacterium Leptotrichia buccalis was at one time thought to have a causal relationship, but it probably does not. The cause may be related to some metabolic disturbance. Local removal of the keratosis is easily done, but recurrence is common.

TONSILLAR HYPERTROPHY

Hypertrophy occurs physiologically, beginning in early childhood and continuing until puberty, after which a slow atrophy, or involution, usually occurs. Enlargement is due to an overall increase in the cells of the parenchyma, and prominent cellular activity is found in the germinal centers. When tonsillar hypertrophy follows inflammatory activity, the size increase occurs primarily in the tonsil's connective tissue stroma. The size of the tonsil is of little clinical significance unless large enough to produce mechanical obstruction of the airway or present difficulties in swallowing. Enlarged tonsils of moderate size alone usually are insufficient reason for removal.

ADENOID HYPERTROPHY

Adenoidal enlargement is common in preadolescent or adolescent children. The enlarged adenoid can obstruct the nasopharyngeal airway, particularly at night when the patient is in the recumbent position. During the day, elevation of the upper lip improves the airway, if an obstructing adenoid is present, and this elevation combined with an open mouth is called the "adenoid facies." An enlarged adenoid and Gerlach's tonsil can obstruct the eustachian tubes, with resulting conductive hearing loss. The presence of fluid in the middle ear suggests an inefficient eustachian tube, either from blockage or for other reasons. If from blockage, the significance of the loss of hearing to the young schoolchild must be assessed.

Alveolar hypotension may follow pronounced and prolonged interference with the oral and nasopharyngeal airway and may lead to hypertension of the pulmonary artery, cor pulmonale, and hypercapnia.[1] Establishment of an adequate airway permits return to a normal condition.

Treatment of modestly enlarged tonsils and adenoid in the absence of frequent and marked infections is one in which the physician tries to "tide" the patient over until involution occurs. The use of x-irradiation, particularly in the young, is fraught with danger and should not be used in most cases. The indications for tonsillectomy and adenoidectomy are given later in this chapter.

TONSILLOLITH

A tonsillolith is a calculus of the tonsil. Quantities of caseous, gritty, and light yellow or yellow-gray material, filling a crypt, may be up to 1 cm in size. Leptothrichia buccalis may be found but is of little significance. More likely, previous tonsillar infections, which effectively seal the mouth of the crypt, allow epithelial debris to collect in the crypt. Sudden, spontaneous extrusion of a tonsillolith may be followed by spotting of blood for short periods. Treatment consists of expressing the material with a flat or rounded, blunt instrument under no or minimal local anesthesia. Recurrences are common.

INFECTIOUS MONONUCLEOSIS

The Epstein-Barr virus (EBV) is a ubiquitous member of the human herpesvirus group, is worldwide in distribution, and causes a largely subclinical disease in early childhood. It is passed from one individual to another by the interchange of oral fluids and causes infectious mononucleosis (IM), usually in young adults. This heterophile antibody-positive disease is also known as "glandular fever." EBV has also been implicated in Burkitt's lymphoma, nasopharyngeal carcinoma, and a variety of B-cell disorders.

After an incubation period of 3 or 4 to 14 days, fever, cervical adenopathy, typically in the posterior two thirds of the chain, sore throat, and frequently profound malaise occur. A striking feature in about one third of cases is a scattered, gray-white membranous pharyngotonsillitis. Tonsillar hyperplasia may be so pronounced as to justify concern about the airway. Fleeting scarlatiniform rashes may develop, usually in association with the use of ampicillin or other antibiotic. Occasionally, fusospirochetal or streptococcal secondary invaders are found. In 50%, one sees splenomegaly and, in 10%, hepatomegaly. Neurologic complications occur rarely, and most recover completely.

The white blood cell count (WBC) is elevated to 10,000 to 15,000, of which 50% or more are lymphocytes containing "atypical" oval, kidney-shaped nuclei with vacuolated cytoplasm. The EBV-specific heterophile-antibody serologic test is positive. The test is based on the removal of sheep antibodies by prior absorption with beef red blood cells but not with guinea pig kidney. B lymphocytes are infected and stimulate the production of suppressor T cells. The antibodies usually persist for years. Thrombocytopenia is common. Monospot tests for IM are directed against heterophile antibodies and are the tests most frequently employed in diagnosis. In most cases, the disease resolves completely in 1 to 3 weeks, but occasionally persists longer.

A confusing relationship exists between IM and an infection with cytomegalovirus (CMV).[2] Symptoms mimic those of IM. Heterophile antibodies are not formed. CMV-induced mononucleosis is usually more insidious in onset and is slower to resolve than EBV-induced mononucleosis. The diagnosis must be made by isolating the CMV virus. Most patients recover without sequelae, although postviral fatigue may be marked and may persist for months.

Treatment of IM is supportive, including bed rest until the fever is gone and then a gradual return to physical activity. If the liver or spleen is involved, patients must be monitored carefully. The administration of corticosteroids may be helpful if airway obstruction is marked, but these drugs are rarely necessary. Specific antiviral agents (e.g., acyclovir and ganciclovir) may be of some value.

SLEEP APNEA

Sleep apnea (SA) is defined as an intermittent cessation of air flow at both the nose and mouth during sleep. A healthy adult may expect apneic periods of 10 seconds or less several times an hour during sleep without significant clinical disturbances. People who do have significant disturbances report perhaps 15 or more events per hour, each lasting 20 to 30 seconds, but they may last as long as 2 to 3 minutes.[3,4]

The respiratory disturbance is marked by repetitive reduction in breathing (hypopnea) or cessation of breathing (apnea). If an obstruction to the upper airway causes the symptoms, the disorder is termed obstructive sleep apnea (OSA), and if the cause is in the brain stem (uncommon), central sleep apnea (CSA). In OSA, airflow ceases, but the patient makes vigorous effort to overcome the obstruction. In CSA, the central neural drive to the respiratory muscles is transiently abolished and little physical effort is made to breathe. Mixed sleep apnea (MSA) is a combination of the two.

Patients with OSA complain infrequently of difficulty in breathing, but the person within earshot of the sleeping patient is acutely aware of noisy breathing, increased sleep movements, and the apnea. The apnea leads to progressive asphyxia until it causes a brief arousal from sleep, whereupon airway patency is restored and airflow resumes. Snoring and daytime somnolence are common in these patients, but personality change, mental deterioration, decrease in efficiency, sexual dysfunction, headache, and other symptoms occur frequently as well. Sleep disruption (arousals) occur 50 or more times an hour.

Pathophysiology

In healthy individuals, patency of the oropharynx and hypopharynx is maintained by tonic activity of the pharyngeal dilatory muscles. Sleep results in a decrease in the behavioral responses that maintain these muscles. The rapid eye movement (REM) stage of sleep is particularly associated with loss of tone of many inspiratory muscles (other than the diaphragm). Relaxation of the muscles thus creates an obstruction by narrowing the airway and is a common component of the problem. Structural abnormalities such as micrognathia or retrognathia, macroglossia, nasal obstruction, or gross enlargement of the pharyngeal tonsils or adenoid are less frequently the cause of the narrowing. Alcohol predisposes patients to SA by exaggerating the relaxation of the upper respiratory muscles. SA must be distinguished from narcolepsy.[5] Obesity, chronic obstructive pulmonary disease, hypothyroidism, androgens, and the postmenopausal state are risk factors. CSA may be associated with myasthenia gravis, muscular dystrophy, various lesions of the brain stem, and central alveolar hypoventilation ("Ondine's curse"). Pure CSA is rare.

The pathophysiology of this disorder is most easily explained in physical terms. The Venturi effect describes the acceleration of air as the current of air enters a narrowed passageway and the Bernoulli principle states that a negative pressure or partial vacuum exists at the outer edge of a current of flowing air; the faster the flow, the greater the negative pressure. Thus, the indrawn air meets an obstructing structure, the airway narrows, and the velocity of the air increases. The resulting decreased pressure at the edge of the airway (the Bernoulli effect) "pulls" the airway wall inward and further decreases the patency. In addition, the increased speed of the airway produces vibration of some of the loose anatomic structures of snoring. The levels at greatest risk for obstruction are the nasopharynx, base of the tongue, and supraglottis.

Symptoms

Patients (males much more often than females) with SA often complain of frequent nocturnal arousal periods and a feeling of asphyxia, excessive daytime somnolence, loss of memory and judgment, and fatigue. Many also have related hypertension. Most of these patients have a long history of snoring antedating the SA and that may be so severe as to endanger family relationships, but all snorers do not develop SA. The hypoxia and carbon dioxide retention associated with SA can eventually lead to polycythemia, pulmonary hypertension, right-sided heart failure, and cardiac dysrhythmias.

The diagnosis of SA is confirmed by overnight respiratory monitoring by polysomnography. The frequency of apneas per hour (apnea index), apneas and hypopneas per hour (apnea-hypopnea index), and arousals per hour (arousal index) are recorded. Moreover, one should also measure the frequency and grade of associated cardiac dysrhythmias, the degree of hypercapnia, and the severity of oxygen desaturation.

Treatment

All identifiable anatomic and significant obstructions to the supraglottic airway tract should be noted. Medical management consists of weight reduction in the obese and control of alcohol ingestion. Medroxyprogesterone or protriptyline orally may be tried. Use of respiratory stimulants has not been of much benefit. Tongue-retaining devices are not well tolerated but, in the short run, are helpful.

Continuous positive airway pressure during the sleeping hours by a well-fitting nasal mask (nCPAP) now is a commonly prescribed treatment that corrects or considerably alleviates the situation in 80% of the patients by providing a pneumatic "stenting" in the open position of the nasopharyngeal airway. The amount of pressure (5 to 20 cm H_2O) required must be determined empirically during all phases of sleep.

Surgical measures to remove airway obstructions include hyoid section, mandibular osteotomy or advancement, adenotonsillectomy to improve the nasal

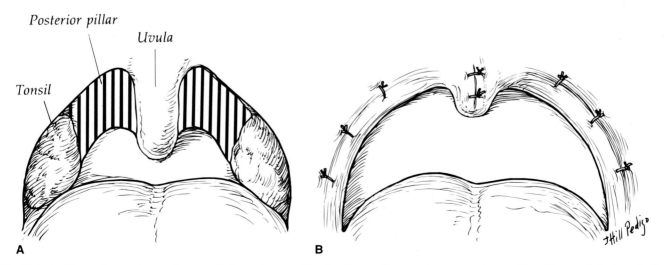

Fig. 18–1. A. Obstruction to the oropharyngeal airway is caused by the abnormally prominent posterior tonsillar pillars and the large bulky uvula. B. An improved airway has been created by reduction in size of these structures.

airway, and removal of redundant tonsilloglossal folds or trimming of a low-hanging palate, for example. In pressing and acute situations, tracheostomy must be considered. Reports indicate that success in surgical procedures is more likely to reduce snoring than clearly improving OSA as measured by polysomnography.

One of the procedures advocated, the uvulopalatopharyngoplasty (UPPP), is illustrated diagrammatically in Figure 18–1. Demonstration that the uvulopalatal narrowing of the nasopharyngeal airway is the predominate cause of the obstruction identifies the group most likely to be helped by UPPP.[6] The carbon dioxide laser has been used as an office procedure to remove redundant and obstructing membranes in the posterior pharynx. The disadvantage is that several procedures are required. Recently, submucosal midline resection of palatoglossus and palatopharayngeus muscles (uvulopalatal myotomy or UPM), with preservation of all mucosa has been suggested. This procedure is thought to be effective by releasing the sphincter effect produced by these muscles.

BEHÇET'S DISEASE

Behçet's disease is a chronic relapsing syndrome of oral ulceration, painful genital ulcers, and uveitis. Pathologically, the disease is marked by a non-necrotizing perivascular infiltrate of lymphocytes and monocytes. The disease can be treated with chlorambucil and acyclovir.

KAWASAKI'S DISEASE

The cardinal features of Kawasaki's disease (mucocutaneous lymph node syndrome) are fever, conjunctival congestion, dry red lips, erythematous palms and soles, cervical lymphadenopathy, desquamation at the fingertips, and various rashes of the trunk. In some respects, the disease must be differentiated from Stevens-Johnson syndrome. γ-Globulin has been used in treatment.

EAGLE'S SYNDROME

Reichert's cartilage gives rise to the styloid process, the ligament, and the upper half of the body of the hyoid bone. In the adult, the styloid is about 12.5 cm in length and lies between the internal and external carotid arteries and lateral to the tonsilar fossa. Because of its location, it may cause discomfort in the pharynx and hypopharynx by impinging on either the artery or the fossa, particularly if the process is elongated. The diagnosis can be made by palpation of the process deep to the

tonsillar fossa or by radiologic imaging. Short-term relief can be obtained by injecting the appropriate area with an anesthetic solution, and long-term relief can be effected by surgical shortening of the styloid process.

WALDEYER'S RING

Encircling the junctions of the nasopharynx, the oropharynx, and hypopharynx is a ring of lymphoid tissue known as Waldeyer's ring (also see Chap. 18). The essential elements are the faucial tonsil, the adenoid, the lingual tonsil, and a collection of lymphoid tissue at the entrance to the eustachian tubal (Gerlach's tonsil). This ring functions in the production of B-cell lymphocytes. Controversy exists regarding decreased competence of the immune system, particularly in the young, by surgical removal of parts (e.g., the faucial tonsils and adenoid) of this structure.

TONSILLECTOMY AND ADENOIDECTOMY

Indications

No absolute set of indications for removal of the tonsils and adenoid can be made. As a generalization, one can say that the amount of obstruction the enlarged tonsils and adenoid offer to normal function of the eustachian tube, the pharynx, the nasopharynx, and the airway is the criterion on which the advisability of removal is made. Obstruction of the nasopharynx is associated with a nasal voice (rhinolalia clausa). Frequent ear infections with middle ear effusions and a conductive loss of hearing may occur and represent likely indications for removal of the adenoid. If the obstruction to the airway is marked, cor pulmonale may occur and is an absolute indication.[7,8]

Evaluation of recurrent infections of the tonsils and adenoid is more difficult. Recurrent pyrexial bacterial pharyngotonsillitis and adenoiditis, despite adequate antimicrobial therapy, are relative indications. In general, a history of four such marked infections with cervical adenopathy in the previous 6 months is considered a probable indication. If the infection is repeatedly associated with β-hemolytic, group A streptococci, the indication is more persuasive. Removal of the tonsils in the very young must be balanced against the contribution the tonsillar B cells make to the immunocompetence of the body. The anatomy and physiology of the tonsil and adenoid are considered in Chapter 16.

Procedure

General anesthesia is given to all children and is preferable in nervous or uncooperative older patients. A local anesthetic (e.g., 1% lidocaine with epinephrine 1:

200,000) is injected in several sites between the capsule and the body of the tonsil. More than 5 to 7 ml is rarely needed. The patient is supine in the Rose position (head low to minimize the chances of aspiration of blood) if a general anesthetic is used and in a semisitting position if a local anesthetic is sufficient.

The "dissection-snare" method is commonly employed today. The "guillotine" technique has largely been abandoned. The tonsil is grasped near the upper pole with vulsellum forceps and is displaced medially (Fig. 18–2A). The incision is begun at the upper pole just posterior to the free anterior pillar margin and carried downward and is then repeated on the other pillar. It is important to preserve the integrity of the pillars, particularly the posterior.[9]

Curved Metzenbaum scissors, or other dissecting instrument, or the finger is then used to separate the capsule of the tonsil from its bed (Fig. 18–2B). The dis-

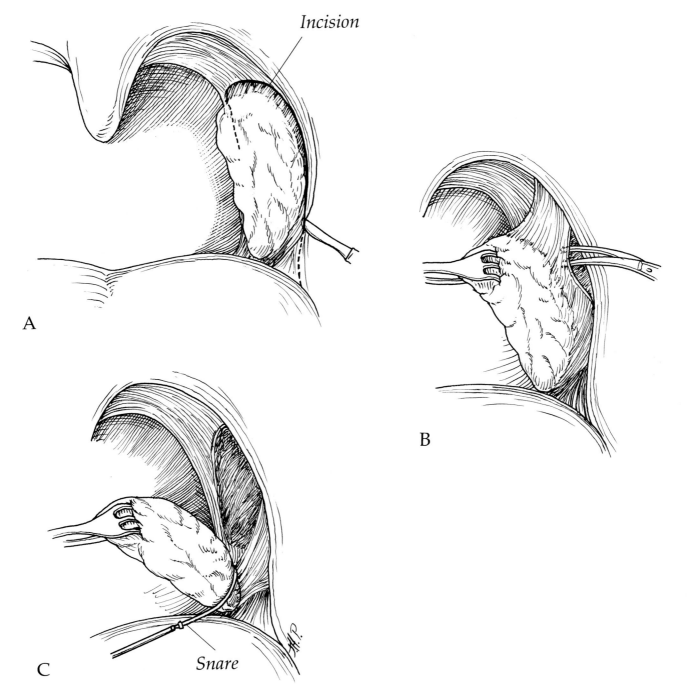

Incision

A

B

C   *Snare*

Fig. 18–2. Dissection-snare method of tonsillectomy. A. The initial incision. B. Freeing the upper pole. C. The snare has encircled the inferior pole of the tonsil.

section is carried progressively (Fig. 18–2B) inferiorly until only the lower pole remains, and at this point a wire snare is conveniently used. The vulsellum forceps are passed through the loop of the snare and the tonsil again is grasped. The snare is then depressed over the instrument to encircle the inferior pole of the tonsil, and the snare is closed to amputate the tonsil flush with the tongue. Bleeding points can be controlled by suture (Fig. 18–2C), ligature, or electrodesiccation.

The adenotome is a box-like instrument with a retractable blade on one side. With the blade retracted, the open box is lowered over the adenoid so when the blade is advanced to close the box, the bulk of the adenoid is removed and retained in the box. Finally, a curette is used to scrape out bits of adenoid tissue that have been missed, including tissue obstructing the eustachian tube.

Laser tonsillectomy and adenoidectomy are effective and involve less postoperative pain, less blood loss, and more rapid healing. The main drawback is the greater expense.[10]

Complications

Nationwide, fatality rates in the United States have been reported as approximately 1 in 16,000.[11,12] The complications are almost always from bleeding during or after surgery, complications of anesthesia, or unidentified complications.[13]

Nasal speech for a few days following tonsillectomy is not unusual because of temporary limitation of motion of the pillars and soft palate because of pain. If, however, the posterior pillar has been too widely removed, more marked changes occur (rhinolalia operta), resulting from an undue patency of the posterior nares and nasopharynx. Surgery should be considered with extreme caution if a palatal submucous cleft or a frank cleft exists. The teeth are at some risk as a result of mounting a mouth gag to facilitate surgery, but the risk is low if care is observed.

Rarely, following inexpert surgery, the pillars and palate may adhere to the posterior pharyngeal wall, creating a stenosis of the nasopharynx and nasal airway. Treatment consists in surgical removal of the cicatrix and covering the raw areas with a split-thickness graft. The use of the carbon dioxide laser may decrease the amount of grafting needed.

PERITONSILLAR ABSCESS (QUINSY)

This situation likely arises out of an infection in the crypts of the upper part of the tonsil. The disease is more common among young adults and is rare in children.

First, cellulitis occurs that develops into an abscess extending beyond the tonsillar capsule into the potential space between the buccopharyngeal fascia and the capsule itself. Abscess of the tonsil itself is rare. The cellulitis causes marked swelling and edema of the soft palate and displaces the tonsil medially, forward, and downward. The pus may burrow downward, leading to edema of the posterior pillar. The patient may have pain on rotating the neck. If the superior constrictor muscle is penetrated, an infection of the parapharyngeal space may result, with potential damage to the great vessels of the neck.

The overwhelming complaint is unilateral, extreme soreness of the throat, with odynophagia so severe it prevents opening the mouth adequately for examination and swallowing so painful that dehydration occurs. Characteristically, viscid saliva dribbles from the mouth and is found in the throat. Elevation of the temperature is modest. The oral airway may be reduced, so concern about the airway is justified.

Digital examination of the tonsil usually finds a more or less fluctuant area superior and 2 to 4 mm external to the free border of the anterior pillar. In the past, the custom was to incise and probe the fluctuant area for drainage and follow with tonsillectomy 6 weeks later. Excellent results, however, have been obtained with needle aspiration of the abscess alone or, instead, with early tonsillectomy on the affected side.[14] In all cases, the patient must be rehydrated and placed on antibiotics.

RETROPHARYNGEAL SPACE INFECTIONS

The retropharyngeal space, lying just anterior to the prevertebral space, extends from the anterior face of the basiocciput into the posterior mediastinum, and laterally, a potential connection exists with the lateral pharyngeal space. The prevertebral space clinically is two spaces. The first, usually the one infected, ends at about the level of the second thoracic vertebra and tends to confine infections to the upper portion. Extension may extend downward, however, into the posterior mediastinum. The retropharyngeal lymph nodes, usually two to five in number, are located behind the posterior pharyngeal mucosa near the outer edge and are in close relation externally to the great vessels of the neck.

Diagnosis

An aneurysm of an artery in the region can be mistaken for a retropharyngeal abscess, but pulsation and bruit present in the former and not the latter differentiate the two conditions. The ability to aspirate blood with a fine needle from the aneurysm further separates the two. Also confusing are the bony hard and prominent or malformed vertebral bodies. The greatest danger, particularly in the young, if the disorder is neglected, is the rupture of the abscess with aspiration. The classic symptom in past years of a retropharyngeal bulge and neck stiffness are now noted in fewer than half the cases.

Treatment

In the past, incision and drainage of an abscess were common, but using strategically selected antibiotics, this method now is infrequent.[15]

LATERAL PHARYNGEAL SPACE INFECTIONS

The lateral pharyngeal, or parapharyngeal, space extends from the base of the skull inferiorly to the level of the hyoid bone. Posterolaterally, the space contains the medial portion of the carotid sheath, posteromedially, there is potential communication with the retropharyngeal space, and anteriorly and inferiorly, the space communicates with the submandibular spaces. The lateral pharyngeal space is further divided by the styloid process into anterior and posterior compartments. The posterior contains the internal carotid artery, the internal jugular vein, cranial nerves IX, X, and XII, and the cervical sympathetic trunk.

ETIOLOGY OF DEEP NECK INFECTIONS

In the past, the frequent cause of deep neck infections was extension of an infection from the pharynx and tonsils, but currently, infections of dental origin are the major source. In some cases, no obvious site of origin can be found. Extensions of infections have occurred from aerodigestive trauma, retropharyngeal lymphadenitis, Pott's disease, sialadenitis, Bezold's apicitis, congenital cysts and fistulas, and intravenous drug injection.

Symptoms

Pain, fever, trismus, neck swelling, and limitation of neck movement are usually found and suggest cervical space involvement. Dyspnea may be a late symptom and should not be neglected. Fluctuance should be looked for, but with antibiotics is not common. A change in the voice may occur in lateral and retropharyngeal infections. Mediastinal extension is heralded by chest pain and severe dyspnea. The use of computed tomography and magnetic resonance imaging helps to locate the site and extent of involvement of the infection.

Treatment

Once the airway is secured, appropriate antibiotic therapy, tailored to the individual patient and the infecting organism, may be sufficient. If medical management fails, and particularly if fluctuance or a threat to the airway develops, surgical drainage is appropriate. Surgical drainage in the case of Ludwig's angina usually is a decompression of the suprahyoid region through the submental region.

Surgical drainage of the retropharyngeal space may be done intraorally in patients who have no dyspnea and whose infection is localized to the posterior wall of the pharynx. This is done by a transoral incision with the patient in the Rose (head down) position to avoid aspiration. If the infection is more complicated, an approach along the anterior border of the sternocleidomastoid muscle can be used.

An intraoral surgical approach to infections of the lateral pharyngeal space usually is confined to treatment of offending teeth or to drainage of a peritonsillar abscess. The external approach below the inferior margin of the mandible provides more adequate entry in more advanced situations to the lateral pharyngeal space. Fortunately, advanced situations have become relatively rare since the advent of penicillin and other antimicrobial drugs.

SUGGESTED READINGS

1. Levy AM, et al: Hypertrophic adenoids causing pulmonary hypertension and severe congestive heart failure. N Engl J Med 277:506, 1967.
2. Holmes GP: A cluster of patients with chronic mononucleosis-like symptoms: is Epstein-Barr the cause? JAMA 257:2297, 1988.
3. Snyderman NL, Reynolds CF, and Johnson JT: Evaluation of the adult with sleep apnea. Ann Otol Rhinol Laryngol 92:518, 1983.
4. Iber C and Ingram TH: Sleep apnea syndrome. Sci Am Med 14:5, 1994.
5. Kales A, Vela-Bueno A, and Kales JD: Sleep disorders and narcolepsy. Ann Intern Med 106:434, 1987.
6. Simmons FB, Guilleminault C, and Miles LF: The palatopharyngoplasty operation for snoring and sleep apnea. Otolaryngol Head Neck Surg 92:375, 1984.
7. Spaur RC: The cardiorespiratory syndrome. Cor pulmonale secondary to chronic upper airway obstruction for hypertrophied tonsils and adenoids: a review. Ear Nose Throat J 62:562, 1982.
8. Brown OE, Manning SC, and Ridenour B: Cor pulmonale secondary to tonsillar and adenoidal hypertrophy: management considerations. Int J Pediatr Otorhinolaryngol 16:131, 1988.
9. Koopman CF: Avoiding the complications of tonsillectomy and adenoidectomy. J Respir Dis 9:84, 1988.
10. Martinez SA and Akin DP: Laser tonsillectomy and adenoidectomy. Otolaryngol Clin North Am 20: 371, 1987.
11. Pratt LW and Gallagher RA: Tonsillectomy and adenoidectomy: incidence and mortality. Otolaryngol Head Neck Surg 87:159, 1979.

12. Colclasure JB and Graham SS: Complications of out-patient tonsillectomy and adenoidectomy: a review of 3340 cases. Ear Nose Throat J *69:*155, 1990.

13. Crysdale WS and Russel D: Complications of tonsillectomy and adenoidectomy in 9409 children observed overnight. Can Med Assoc J *135:*1139, 1986.

14. Kronenberg J, Wolf M, and Leverton G: Peritonsillar abscess recurrence rate and the indication for tonsillectomy. Am J Otolaryngol *8:*82, 1987.

15. Thompson JW, Cohen SR, and Reddix P: Retropharyngeal abscess in children: a retrospective and historical analysis. Laryngoscope *98:*589, 1988.

19 Diseases of the Nasopharynx

John J. Ballenger

ANATOMY OF THE NASOPHARYNX

The nasopharynx extends from the base of the skull to the soft palate. Above, it is formed by the body of the sphenoid and the basilar process of the occipital bones and posteriorly by the cervical vertebrae. Inferiorly, it is continuous with the oropharynx. Situated on the lateral walls of the nasopharynx, posterior to the inferior conchae, are the eustachian tube orifices. These tubes pass laterally through a defect just above the upper edge of the superior constrictor muscle known as the sinus of Morgagni. Just posterior to the tube is a prominent cartilaginous lip, the torus tubarius, and extending downward from this lip is a fold of mucous membrane, the salpingopharyngeal membrane. A less prominent fold, the salpingopalatine membrane, passes downward anterior to the eustachian orifice (Figs. 19–1 and 19–2).

The deep pocket formed at the angle of the nasopharynx between the posterior ridge of the eustachian cartilage and the posterior wall is known as the fossa of Rosenmüller, and above this is found the foramen lacerum. Other foramina leading from the nasopharynx are the foramen ovale, foramen spinosum, the carotid canal, and the jugular canal, and any of these may provide a conduit for extension of disease from the nasopharynx to the skull interior (Figs. 19–1 and 19–2). Lymphoid tissue is frequently found around the orifice of the eustachian tube (Gerlach's tonsil) and where the roof of the nasopharynx joins the posterior wall, the adenoid, or Luschka's tonsil.

PHYSIOLOGY OF THE NASOPHARYNX

This structure functions as a rigid tube for respired air. During swallowing, vomiting, belching, and gagging, the nasopharynx is completely separated from the oropharynx by elevation of the palate against Passavant's pad, a prominence created on the posterior pharyngeal wall by contraction of the upper fibers of the superior constrictor muscle.

The eustachian tube and the nose drain into the nasopharynx. As a resonating chamber, it, along with the nose, contributes to the quality of the voice. Loss of the resonating capacity produces a "nasal" voice or rhinolalia operta. For certain vowels adequate functional closure of the soft palate is necessary to avoid non-nasal speech. When such vowels are uttered the nasopharynx acts as a resonating chamber. When the mouth is closed and the vibrating column of air is blown out through the nose, nasal consonants are formed (see Chap. 26).

The mucous membrane of the nasopharynx is mostly of the ciliated columnar type, changing to stratified columnar below the level of the soft palate. In addition, the mucosa in the nasopharynx contains lymphoid tissue of the B-cell type, epithelial tissue, and minor salivary gland tissue. Because of this variety of cell types, many different lesions may occur. Efferent lymph channels flow to the lateral retropharyngeal nodes of Rouvière (node of Krause), the jugulodigastric nodes, and the spinal accessory chain. There is free communication across the midline. Infections of the upper respiratory tract readily extend by contiguity to the nasopharynx (see Chaps. 3, 6, and 7). The nasopharynx is a relatively "silent" area, and primary diseases limited to the nasopharynx may be surprisingly advanced before symptoms are produced and draw attention to the nasopharynx.

BENIGN LESIONS OF THE NASOPHARYNX

Rathke's pouch, Thornwaldt's bursa, chordomas, teratomas, and other benign lesions are discussed in Chapter 14. Rathke's pouch may develop when remnants of

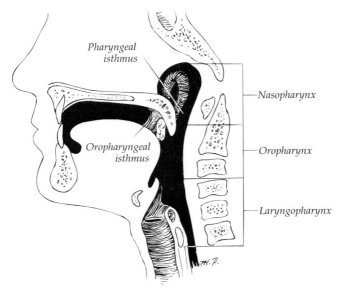

Fig. 19–1. The regions of the nasopharynx are diagrammatically depicted.

the buccal mucosal invagination of early life to form the anterior lobe of the pituitary remain. It is represented clinically by a dimple high in the nasopharynx (see Fig. 19–2). Rarely, a tumor may arise in these cells, a craniopharyngioma. Symptoms take the form of pituitary-hypothalmic derangements.

The nasopharyngeal bursa of Thornwaldt is a midline structure situated more inferiorly than Rathke's pouch, found in the adenoid mass, and representing the end of the notochord. It may be filled with jelly-like notochordal tissue, may perhaps rupture spontaneously, and may drain into the nasopharynx. Recur-

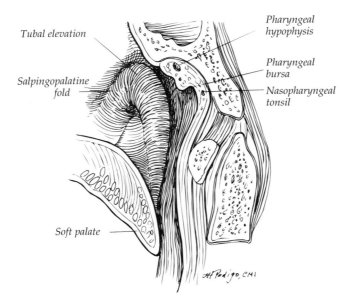

Fig. 19–2. An enlarged view of the nasopharynx is shown.

rent infection of the bursa is known as Thornwaldt's disease.

Chordoma is a rare tumor arising from the remnants of the notochord, and about 45% of these are found in the nasopharynx. The tumor is histologically benign but locally aggressive and often far advanced at the time of discovery and thus difficult to treat successfully. The so-called chondroid chordoma has a better prognosis.

Teratomas, occasionally found in the nasopharynx, are usually present at birth. An intra-adenoid cyst, usually located in the midline, is a retention cyst and may occur elsewhere in the nasopharynx as well. Choristomas and hamartomas are not true tumors, but overgrowth of normal nasopharyngeal tissue. Branchial cleft cysts of the nasopharynx are rare.

Stenosis of the nasopharynx may be acquired from an uncontrolled disease such as syphilis, diphtheria, or occasionally a granuloma. Postoperative stenosis of the nasopharynx is the usual cause and is considered with tonsillectomy and adenoidectomy (see Chap. 18).

ATRESIA OF THE POSTERIOR CHOANAE

Atresia of the posterior choanae is a persistent, usually congenital, partial or complete, membranous or bony closure of one or both choanae, usually located immediately anterior to the posterior border of the hard palate. It occurs in about 1 in 8000 births and reflects a familial tendency. About half the infants with this abnormality display other congenital problems. In adults, unilateral atresia may long be unrecognized because it does not cause nasal obstruction or significant dyspnea. The most striking symptoms and danger of choanal atresia occur in an infant. The newborn is a near-obligate nasal breather, and the absence of a nasal airway is an emergency requiring quick provision of an oral airway.

The diagnosis can by made by failure to pass a nasal catheter into the pharynx and can be confirmed by digital palpation of the nasopharynx or, in an older individual, by mirror nasopharyngoscopy. A membranous occlusion may require no more than perforation with a probe and subsequent dilations to maintain patency.

Atresia of the choanae and its treatment are considered in Chapter 15. The approach can be made transpalatally or transnasally, but in each case the obstructing bone is removed and the raw edges are covered with mucosa to thwart stenosis. A stent frequently is used in the nasopharynx postoperatively for 3 to 4 weeks for this purpose. The carbon dioxide laser may be employed to remove either a bony or membranous occlusion.

FIBROMA

Fibroma in the nasopharynx occurs most frequently in males between the ages of 10 and 25. These lesions are usually single. Softer varieties are called polypoid fibromas or fibromatous polyps. As age advances, the growths tend to undergo spontaneous involution.

ANGIOFIBROMA OF THE NASOPHARYNX

Nasopharyngeal angiofibroma is the most common benign tumor of the nasopharynx and yet represents only 0.05% of head and neck tumors. In the past, the term "juvenile" nasopharyngeal angiofibroma was used, but this term is inappropriate because the neoplasms occur in older patients as well. It is a morphologically benign but clinically aggressive and destructive tumor, most frequently found in boys of 12 to 16 years of age. The cause is unknown. Untreated tumors may grow to a substantial size, penetrate the cranial cavity through the various foramina, and cause considerable structural and functional damage.

The usual presenting complaints are a progressive nasal obstruction and recurrent epistaxis for no apparent reason. Clinically, the lesion appears as a firm, reddish-purple, mucosa-covered, and friable or granular mass in the nasopharynx or nose. As the tumor enlarges, interference with eustachian tube function and attendant conductive hearing loss follow. The tumor arises typically from a point above the superior margin of the sphenopalatine foramen, and from there may extend into the nose, the nasopharynx, the paranasal sinuses, the temporal or infratemporal fossae, or the cranium. Cranial nerves likely to be involved with extended tumors are CN II, III, IV, V, and VI. Although this finding has not been clearly authenticated, some investigators believe that an unoperated angiofibroma undergoes regression when the patient reaches puberty.

On imaging, opacification of one or more paranasal sinuses is generally seen, most commonly the maxillary sinus. The presence of anterior bowing of the posterior wall of the maxillary sinus is considered virtually pathognomic. Other common radiographic signs include erosion of the greater wing of the sphenoid bone, erosion of the medial wall of the antrum or hard palate, and displacement of the nasal septum.

Histologically, the mass consists of connective tissue stroma containing numerous immature fibroblasts, thin-walled blood vessels with little or no muscular layer, and large vascular lacunar spaces filled with blood, resembling a hemangioma (Fig. 19–3).

The diagnosis can usually be made preoperatively on the physical and roentgenologic findings, so biopsy and the accompanying danger of vigorous bleeding are avoided. If biopsy is considered necessary, it preferably should be done with the patient under general anesthesia in the operating room with preparations for immediate tumor removal. Opacification of one or more sinuses, usually the maxillary, is frequently

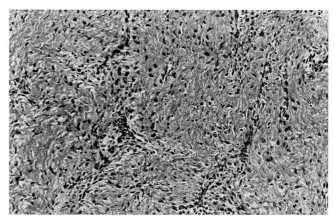

Fig. 19–3. Nasopharyngeal angiofibroma consisting of an admixture of vascular tissue and fibrous stroma. The blood vessels are thin walled, of variable size and shape, and are compressed by the fibrous component which consists of stellate fibroblasts and thick collagen bundles. (Courtesy of the Department of Pathology, Evanston Hospital, Evanston, IL.)

found with forward bowing of the posterior wall. The nasal septum frequently is crowded to the opposite side. Because of the diverse blood supply and because of the danger involved, arteriography is usually not done. The dominant arterial supply is usually the ipsilateral internal maxillary artery, however. The extent of the growth can be assessed by contrast-enhanced computed tomography and magnetic resonance imaging. Preoperative arteriography to determine the source of the blood supply is wise. If it originates in part from the internal carotid artery system, surgery likely will be contraindicated.

Staging

Analagous to the staging of cancer suggested by the American Joint Committee, an attempt has been made by Chandler and associates (Table 19–1).[1]

Treatment

The indication for surgery is hemorrhage, nasopharyngeal obstruction, or orbital encroachment. Although controversy exists, the goal of treatment should be re-

TABLE 19–1. Staging of Angiofibroma

   I: Tumor confined to the nasopharynx
  II: Tumor extending into the nasal cavity and/or the sphenoid sinus
 III: Tumor extending into one or more locations: the antrum, ethmoid sinus, pterygomaxillary and infratemporal fossa, orbit, and cheek
  IV: Tumor extending into the cranial cavity

(From Chandler JR, Moskowitz L, Goulding R, and Quencer RM: Nasopharyngeal angiofibromas: staging and management. Ann Otol Rhinol Laryngol 93:322, 1984.)

lief of symptoms and not total and meticulous removal of all tumor regardless of risk.

The treatment of choice for most patients without intracranial extension is surgical excision. Brisk bleeding must be anticipated, and preparation for adequate amounts of preoperatively donated autologous blood for replacement made.

The approach provided by a lateral rhinotomy is preferred by many surgeons because it allows direct and wide exposure of the bulk of the tumor. This approach and its variations are cosmetically acceptable and allow removal of the tumor from the nose, the nasopharynx, the paranasal sinuses, the pterygomaxillary fossa, the infratemporal and temporal fossae, the orbit, and the middle cranial fossa. Some surgeons rely on intra-arterial embolization to decrease the vascularity, and some favor preoperative treatment with stilbestrol for 5 weeks to reduce the vascularity. Some investigators favor primary treatment with radiation for patients with known intracranial extension.[2] Briant and associates reported success with radiation therapy as a primary mode.[3] Without question, the vascularity of the tumor can be reduced by radiation, but, in the case of the young, the potential exists for later osteoradionecrosis, delayed or abnormal bone growth, or malignant induction and thus represents a contraindication for many to its use in a benign disease.

An angiofibroma extending to the cavernous sinus is generally considered unresectable because of the attendant bleeding. The overall recurrence rate is 15 to 16%, but if the lesion is extracranial, recurrence is considerably less frequent.

Malignant tumors of the nasopharynx are considered in Chapter 20.

SUGGESTED READINGS

1. Chandler, JR, Moskowitz L, Goulding R, and Quencer RM: Nasopharyngeal angiofibromas: staging and management. Ann Otol Rhinol Laryngol 93:322, 1984.
2. Gates GL: Angiofibroma. In: Current Therapy in Otolaryngology: Head and Neck Surgery. Edited by Sessions RB and Humphrey D. Philadelphia, BC Decker, 1984–1985.
3. Briant TD, Fitzpatrick PJ, and Berman J: Nasopharyngeal angiofibroma: a twenty year study. Laryngoscope 88:1247, 1978.

20 Squamous Cell Carcinoma of the Oral Cavity, Oropharynx, Pharyngeal Wall, and Nasopharynx

Sharon L. Collins

Squamous cell carcinoma (SCC) in the various sites discussed in this chapter has many features in common: tumor biology (basic principles of solid tumor oncology), pathophysiology (causes, histopathology, natural history of treated and untreated SCC of the head and neck, mechanisms of cancer spread, cancer patterns in recurrent disease, and prognostic factors), and treatment principles.[1] Relevant particulars of the individual sites (lips, gums, buccal mucosa, palate, floor of mouth (FOM), tongue, oropharynx, pharyngeal wall, and nasopharynx) are discussed with emphasis on surgical techniques applicable to each, including reconstruction of defects in the mouth and throat and complications of treatment.

In the sites under discussion (defined in Table 20–1 with International Classification of Diseases (ICD) codes), the primary tumor (T) is classified on the basis of surface dimension, except for pharyngeal wall neoplasms arising in the hypopharynx. Neck staging is the same regardless of primary tumor site. Certain T and N conditions are grouped to define four stages, presumably representing a progressively graver prognosis. Classification and staging of neoplasms in these sites are shown in Table 20–2.

In earlier years, the staging system was clinical. Tumor status was defined on the basis of what could be seen and felt in the patient. The new system allows inclusion of data obtained from pretreatment radiologic and other studies (e.g., computed tomographic [CT] scan, mandibular radiographs, chest radiographs). This sometimes allows better definition of disease at the primary site, in the neck, and distantly. Findings based on histologic examination of excised specimens (neck lymph nodes, positive or negative)

are also now admissible in initial staging. This eliminates the well-known significant clinical error in staging neck lymph nodes,[2] and elective neck dissection has become important as a biopsy staging procedure. The patient's clinical status may be upgraded or downgraded on the basis of histopathologic findings. Although the histologic grade of the tumor and the status of surgical margins at the primary site do not enter into staging of the tumor, they should be recorded.

TUMOR BIOLOGY

Despite improvement in surgical and radiotherapeutic techniques and the addition of multimodality therapy, SCCs of the mouth and throat continue to have a fatal outcome in about half the patients.

Accepted surgical oncology principles of the late 1800s and early 1900s (which persist today in many places) held that carcinomas spread from the primary site to the regional lymph nodes by direct continuity and permeation of lymphatic vessels. The capacity of carcinoma to spread by way of the circulation was not appreciated, although this route was widely accepted for sarcomas. Clinicians assumed that the regional lymphatics formed a protective blockade (filter mechanism) between the primary site and the systemic circulation. This concept of the method of cancer spread dictated the surgical goals and therefore the types of operations performed, which were pioneered by Halsted in carcinoma of the breast.

In fact, because of the many communications between the lymphatic and venous systems in the body (thoracic duct at subclavian vein, lymphaticovenous

TABLE 20–1. Definition of Sites in the Oral Cavity and Pharynx

The oral cavity extends from the skin-vermilion junction of the lips to the junction of the hard and soft palate above and to the line of circumvallate papillae below, and is divided into the following specific areas:

Lip (ICD-O 140). The lip begins at the junction of the vermilion border with the skin and includes only the vermilion surface or the portion of the lip that comes into contact with the opposing lip. It is well defined into an upper and lower lip joined at the commissures of the mouth.

Buccal Mucosa (ICD-O 145.0). This includes all the membrane lining of the inner surface of the cheeks and lips from the line of contact of the opposing lips to the line of attachment of mucosa of the alveolar ridge (upper and lower) and pterygomandibular raphe.

Lower Alveolar Ridge (ICD-O 143.1). This ridge includes the alveolar process of the mandible and its covering mucosa, which extends from the line of attachment of mucosa in the buccal gutter to the line of free mucosa of the floor of the mouth. Posteriorly, it extends to the ascending ramus of the mandible.

Upper Alveolar Ridge (ICD-O 143.0). The upper ridge is the alveolar process of the maxilla and its covering mucosa, which extends from the line of attachment of mucosa in the upper gingival buccal gutter to the junction of the hard palate. Its posterior margin is the upper end of the pterygopalatine arch.

Retromolar Gingiva (Retromolar Trigone or Pterygomandibular Raphe) (ICD-O 145.6). This is the attached mucosa overlying the ascending ramus of the mandible from the level of the posterior surface of the last molar tooth to the apex superiorly, adjacent to the tuberosity of the maxilla.

Oropharynx. The oropharynx extends from the plane of the hard palate, superiorly, to the plane of the hyoid bone, inferiorly, and is continuous with the oral cavity. The faucial arch includes both the surfaces of the entire soft palate and the uvula, the anterior border and base of the anterior tonsillar pillar, and the line of the circumvallate papillae. The base of the tongue extends from the line of the circumvallate papillae to the junction with the base of the epiglottis (the vallecula) and includes the pharyngoepiglottic and glossoepiglottic folds. The lateral wall of the oropharynx is comprised largely of the tonsil and tonsillar fossae. The posterior tonsillar pillar, the narrow lateral wall, and the posterior wall comprise the pharyngeal wall.

Floor of the Mouth (ICD-O 144). This semilunar space over the mylohyoid and hyoglossus muscles, extend from the inner surface of

the lower alveolar ridge to the undersurface of the tongue. Its posterior boundary is the base of the anterior pillar of the tonsil. It is divided into two sides by the frenulum of the tongue and contains the ostia of the submandibular and sublingual salivary glands.

Hard Palate (ICD-O 145.2). This is the semilunar area between the upper alveolar ridge and the mucous membrane covering the palatine process of the maxillary palatine bones. It extends from the inner surface of the superior alveolar ridge to the posterior edge of the palatine bone.

Anterior Two Thirds of the Tongue (Oral Tongue) (ICD-O 141.1 to 141.4). This freely mobile portion of the tongue extends anteriorly from the line of circumvallate papillae to the undersurface of the tongue at the junction of the floor of the mouth. It is composed of four areas: the tip, the lateral borders, the dorsum, and the undersurface (nonvillous surface of the tongue). The undersurface of the tongue is considered a separate category by the World Health Organization (WHO) (ICD-O 141.3).

Oropharynx (ICD-O 141.0; 145.3; 145.4; 146.1–146.3; 146.4; 146.6–146.7)

Anterior wall (glossoepiglottic area)
  Tongue posterior to the vallate papillae (base of tongue or posterior third) (ICD-O 141.0)
  Vallecula (ICD-O 146.3)
Lateral wall (ICD-O 146.6)
  Tonsil (ICD-O 146.0)
  Tonsillar fossa (ICD-O 146.1) and faucial pillars (ICD-O 146.2)
  Glosso-tonsillar sulci (ICD-O 146.2)
Posterior wall (ICD-O 146.7)
Superior wall
  Inferior surface of soft palate (ICD-O 145.3)
  Uvula (ICD-O 145.4)

(Modified from American Joint Committee on Cancer: Manual for Staging of Cancer. 4th ed. Philadelphia, JB Lippincott, 1992, p. 362.)

communications within lymph nodes, for example), the two vascular systems are basically inseparable, and access of tumor cells to one essentially allows simultaneous access to the other. Contemporary thought as exemplified by the "alternate hypothesis" of the Fishers (contrasted with Halsted's principles of breast carcinoma in Table 20–3) strongly supports the concept that solid carcinomas are *not* simply local-regional diseases (primary tumor site and draining lymphatics), but rather *systemic* diseases, in the case of breast carcinoma, because of the early access to the circulation.[3,4]

Unfortunately, in carcinoma of the breast, the stage at which metastasis occurs is likely to be preclinical, occurring before the primary tumor becomes apparent.[3] Therefore, the extent of surgery in the local-

regional area (in otolaryngology this includes the primary site and the neck), although a *necessary* prerequisite for long-term survival and important with respect to maintenance of local hygiene and function, is not *sufficient* to ensure the survival of the patient because the "horse has already gotten out of the barn" in the form of occult (not clinically evident) distant metastases (DM).

Surgery and radiotherapy (RT) are local-regional treatment modalities, and the person practicing these specialties operates within their limited scope. Because neither therapeutic technique addresses the problem of systemic disease (DM), practitioners of both have limited ability to "cure" the patient. The realization of this limitation is sometimes shocking, especially to

TABLE 20–2. TNM Classification and Staging of Tumors in the Oral Cavity, Lip, Oropharynx, and Pharynx

Oral Cavity	Pharynx

Lips:
  Upper
  Lower
Buccal mucosa
Floor of mouth
Oral tongue
Hard palate
Gingivae:
  Upper
  Lower
  Retromolar trigone
	Nasopharynx
	  Posterosuperior wall
	  Lateral wall
	Oropharynx
	  Faucial arch
	  Tonsillar fossa, tonsil
	  Base of tongue
	  Pharyngeal wall
	Hypopharynx
	  Piriform fossa
	  Postcricoid area
	  Posterior wall
	Primary Tumor (T)

Primary Tumor (T)
  TX Primary tumor cannot be assessed
  T0 No evidence of primary tumor
  Tis Carcinoma in situ
  T1 Tumor 2 cm or less in greatest dimension
  T2 Tumor more than 2 cm but not more than 4 cm in greatest dimension
  T3 Tumor more than 4 cm in greatest dimension
  T4 (lip) Tumor invades adjacent structures, e.g., through cortical bone, tongue, skin of neck
  T4 (oral cavity) Tumor invades adjacent structures, e.g., through cortical bone, into deep (extrinsic) muscle of tongue, maxillary sinus, skin
	Oropharynx
	  T1 Tumor 2 cm or less in greatest dimension
	  T2 Tumor more than 2 cm but not more than 4 cm in greatest dimension
	  T3 Tumor more than 4 cm in greatest dimension
	  T4 Tumor invades adjacent structures e.g., through cortical bone, soft tissues of neck, deep (extrinsic) muscle of tongue
	Hypopharynx
	  T1 Tumor limited to one subsite of hypopharynx
	  T2 Tumor invades more than one subsite of hypopharynx or an adjacent site, without fixation or hemilarynx
	  T3 Tumor invades more than one subsite of hypopharynx or an adjacent site, with fixation of hemilarynx
	  T4 Tumor invades adjacent structures, e.g., cartilage or soft tissues of neck

Lymph Node (N)
  NX Regional lymph nodes cannot be assessed
  N0 No regional lymph node metastasis
  N1 Metastasis in a single ipsilateral lymph node, 3 cm or less in greatest dimension
  N2 Metastasis in a single ipsilateral lymph node, more than 3 cm but not more than 6 cm in greatest dimension, or multiple ipsilateral lymph nodes, none more than 6 cm in greatest dimension, or bilateral or contralateral lymph nodes, none more than 6 cm in greatest dimension
    N2a Metastasis in a single ipsilateral lymph node more than 3 cm but not more than 6 cm in greatest dimension
    N2b Metastasis in multiple ipsilateral lymph nodes, none more than 6 cm in greatest dimension
    N2c Metastasis in bilateral or contralateral lymph nodes, none more than 6 cm in greatest dimension
  N3 Metastasis in a lymph node more than 6 cm in greatest dimension
Distant Metastasis (M)
  Presence of distant metastasis cannot be assessed
  No distant metastasis
  Distal metastasis
	Stage Grouping
	[ ] 0 Tis N0 M0
	[ ] I T1 N0 M0
	[ ] II T2 N0 M0
	[ ] III T3 N0 M0
	         T1 N1 M0
	         T2 N1 M0
	         T3 N1 M0
	[ ] IV T4 N0 M0
	         T4 N1 M0
	         Any T N2 M0
	         Any T N3 M0
	         Any T Any N M1

From American Joint Committee on Cancer: Manual for Staging of Cancer. *4th Ed. Philadelphia, JB Lippincott, 1992.*

surgeons. The appropriate goal for a surgeon or radiotherapist is *control of disease in the treated volume.* Cure of the patient depends on other currently ill-defined aspects of the tumor-host relationship related to control of metastasis in the individual patient.

Although the surgeon or radiotherapist is not in complete control of the patient's curability, it is still vitally important to the patient to attempt to achieve local-regional control of disease. In the head and neck, for example, death from uncontrolled local-regional cancer can be preceded by such manifestations as cosmetic disfigurement, causing separation from society; malodorous and frequently painful tumors growing out of the face and neck and interfering with respira-

TABLE 20–3. Two Divergent Hypotheses of Tumor Biology

Halstedian	Alternative
Tumors spread in an orderly defined manner based on mechanical consideration	No orderly pattern of tumor cell dissemination occurs
Tumor cells traverse lymphatics to lymph nodes by direct extension supporting en bloc dissection	Tumor cells traverse lymphatics by emolization challenging the merit of en bloc dissection
Positive lymph node is an indicator of tumor spread and is the instigator of distant disease	Positive lymph node is an indicator of a host-tumor relationship that permits development of metastases rather than being the instigator of distant disease
Regional lymph nodes are barriers to the passage of tumor cells	Regional lymph nodes are ineffective as barriers to tumor cell spread
Regional lymph nodes are of anatomic importance	Regional lymph nodes are of biologic importance
The circulation is of little significance as a route of tumor dissemination	The circulation is of considerable importance in tumor dissemination
A tumor is autonomous of its host	Complex host-tumor interrelationships affect every facet of the disease
Operable breast cancer is a local-regional disease	Operable breast cancer is a systemic disease
The extent and nuances of operation are the dominant factors influencing patient outcome	Variations in local-regional therapy are unlikely to substantially affect survival

(Modified from Fisher B, et al: The contribution of recent NSABP clinical trials of primary breast cancer therapy to an understanding of tumor biology: an overview of findings. Cancer 46:1009, 1980.)

tion, speech, and deglutition; and bleeding, with the potential for exsanguinating hemorrhage. On the other hand, death from distant metastatic disease is relatively asymptomatic, frequently associated with cachexia but with no dramatic premortem events.

The goal of controlling local-regional disease is most likely to be accomplished with an appropriately aggressive *initial* treatment plan. One general principle of solid tumor oncology is that the first attack on the cancer is the best chance to control the disease. SCC of the head and neck is treacherous and difficult to control, and salvage treatment for recurrent disease is notoriously unsuccessful.

Unfortunately, no reliably effective treatments are yet available for metastatic SCC of the head and neck. It was hoped that chemotherapy would solve this dilemma because of promising early experimental studies in rodent systems, in which the incidence of DM was favorably affected by drugs. Such has not proved to be the case for human solid tumors, however, and the survival of patients with cancers that metastasize is limited for this reason until an effective systemic treatment becomes available.

Another concept, an additional "fly in the ointment" in respect to curing patients with carcinomas, is that of *tumor cell heterogeneity*. It was originally thought that solid tumors arose from a single cell by means of monoclonal expansion resulting in a mass of identical progeny. We now know, based on the pioneering work of Fidler[5] and others, that solid tumors are composed of a heterogeneous population of cells with diverse and currently ill-defined intratumoral interactions.

This concept is important with respect to the utility of various therapeutic modalities. Any treatment method that fails to remove the entire tumor at once (i.e., nonsurgical treatments such as RT and chemotherapy) acts on a heterogeneous tumor cell population as a *selective agent*. Any of three cancer growth patterns can be seen in response to such treatment: the tumor can remain the same, it can decrease in size, or it can grow. Although many cells in the tumor mass are killed over time, some resistant cells remain. When released from the intratumoral controls of the original population, these resistant cells have the potential to act in an uncontrolled manner. Wildly anaplastic behavior of residual cancer is one possible negative outcome. When surgery is the initial treatment, the entire clinically apparent tumor mass is mechanically removed at one time. Therefore, surgery has the theoretic advantage of being the least selective of any of the major treatment modalities currently available.

A particular behavior pattern and outcome can generally be predicted to some extent when tumor site, size, histologic features, and spread are defined. Patients with "identical" tumors (based on these parameters), however, manifest a biologic spectrum with respect to outcome, based on tumor-host factors that are currently unknown and undoubtedly operate at molecular and genetic levels, as well as at the levels of cells and organs. For example, most patients with T1 vocal cord carcinomas can be "cured" with surgery or RT. Occasional patients, however, usually those treated with RT with curative intent, develop persistent or recurrent disease, which progresses inexorably to death despite heroic salvage attempts. Conversely, some patients who present with neck metastases only (who are therefore at high risk to die of DM), without evidence of a primary tumor, may survive. Thus, an apparent element of "biologic predeterminism" influences the outcome of each cancer patient and may not be greatly altered by the type of treatment.

These variabilities are relevant to the treatment manager. The individual patient must be assessed, not merely as a representative of a certain type and location of tumor, but on the basis of the demonstrated positive or negative characteristics of his or her individual tumor. For example, some patients with head and neck cancer apparently live well in symbiosis with multiple primary tumors in the upper aerodigestive tract (UADT) mucosa and are long-term survivors, whereas, in other patients with putatively easily "curable" (low-stage) tumors, the outcome is sometimes rapidly fatal. The treatment planner must decide whether or not the patient is trying to act like a survivor, and the patient who is may benefit from continuing aggressive treatment. This is especially true in patients without neck metastases because control of the local disease is potentially possible owing to the low risk of developing DM (see the following paragraph). Conversely, if salvage surgery for recurrent cancer is quickly followed by recurrence, an unfavorable disease pattern is manifested, and the goal of additional treatment might reasonably be palliation (relief of symptoms), rather than probably futile heroic surgery.

Patients who present with positive neck lymph nodes are likely to develop DM within 2 years, and this can be important in deciding the extent of surgery at the primary site. For example, an operation to preserve important functions such as voice and swallowing (*conservation* surgery) can be appropriate in patients with limited survivability, so their quality of remaining life will be optimal. Clearly, such decisions in treatment planning require considerable experience and are usually "best guesses." Only vision through the "retrospectoscope" is infallible.

Treatment planning is further complicated by the virtual absence of scientifically valid objective data in the field of head and neck cancer. Treatment is typically predicated on tradition and on the treatment planner's individual experience and biases. For this reason, questions that have been debated for the past 80 years remain unanswered, and pendulum swings of opinion persist. Because of the relatively small number of head and neck cancer patients, cancer treatment results are usually presented in the format of retrospective series compiled over many years to accrue sufficient patient numbers. This format incorporates the physicians' biases that influenced the selection of treatment and also variables related to advances in treatment technology. Therefore, many uncontrolled variables affect the conclusions in such reports.

Another major flaw that interferes with data interpretation is the method of reporting end results. Surgeons typically report patient *survival*, whereas radiotherapists (correctly) tend to report *tumor control in the treated volume*. The second reporting method is appropriate when discussing a local-regional treatment modality such as surgery or RT. Survival is a "contaminated" end point affected by many factors other than the treatment used. Survival is variously reported as determinate (death from local, regional, or distant cancer), indeterminate (death from unrelated causes or lost to follow-up), or absolute (determinate plus indeterminate). The last two types of survival obscure cancer-related mortality. Because survival data derived from retrospective studies provide only a vague indication of therapeutic efficacy, numeric data derived from such studies are minimized in favor of emphasizing treatment principles.

Scientifically valid cancer treatment data should ideally be collected by treating through randomized prospectively controlled clinical trials. Treatments are allocated randomly, eliminating treatment selection bias and ensuring that differences in treatment outcomes are attributable to variations in the treatment "arms."

The study should also be designed to test a hypothesis of intrinsic interest with respect to tumor biology, so the outcome will provide information of biologic importance regardless of the result. An excellent prototype for testing through clinical trials is exemplified by the National Surgical Adjuvant Breast and Bowel Project (NSABBP), started in 1952.[3] A similar scientific basis for clinical trials has been delayed for an additional 30 years in the case of head and neck cancer, and the recent trend toward acceptance of this strategy has been introduced, not by surgeons, but by chemotherapists in multimodality treatment protocols for advanced head and neck cancer patients. In this era, surgeons have the responsibility not only to modify their decisions on the basis of new information, but also to participate in scientific acquisition of such information by submitting their patients to clinical trials.

With the exception of studies including chemotherapy trials, the randomized prospective studies dealing with head and neck cancers can be numbered on fewer than the fingers of one hand, and most have originated in Europe. The difficulty and logistic problems associated with performing such trials adequately are not to be underestimated, but the attempt is worthwhile if scientifically valid treatment guidelines are ever to evolve. In their absence, certain treatment methods have been accepted as advanced based on circumstantial data, for example, the efficacy of *combined* surgery and RT over either alone for advanced head and neck cancer.

Because of the unscientific methods used in accumulating head and neck cancer treatment data, almost every statement in this chapter is controversial to a greater or lesser extent. Articles can be found to support both sides of almost all issues. The information and recommendations represent guidelines that, in my opinion, are generally valid.

PATHOPHYSIOLOGY

Under this general heading are discussed the causes, histopathology, "natural history," mechanisms of spread, and prognostic factors of SCC in the mouth and throat. These topics all provide important information for the physician treating head and neck cancer because, without an understanding of underlying mechanisms, no rational basis exists on which to formulate treatment guidelines in the individual case.

Causes

In the United States, approximately 19,500 new cases of oral cancer and 8000 of pharyngeal cancer are expected each year. At the time of diagnosis, most are large, symptomatic, stage III and IV lesions, and at least 50% of patients have metastatic lymphadenopathy. Although better combinations of local-regional treatment modalities have improved the quality of life after diagnosis, the relative 5-year survival of 30 to 50% has not changed much over the years. The estimated new cancer cases broken down by sex for some UADT sites (mouth, and pharynx, esophagus, larynx, lung) and the estimated cancer deaths for 1995 are tabulated in Table 20–4, along with the survival trends for the same sites from 1960 to 1990.

The most significant causative factor associated with SCC of the mouth and throat is use of tobacco products; only rarely does this type of cancer arise in people who have never smoked.[6]

In the United States, head and neck cancer comprises only 5 to 8% of all cancer, whereas in Southeast Asia and the Indian subcontinent, the incidence is 40 to 50%, directly reflecting the higher use of various types of tobacco products. Smoking short-stemmed clay pipes or cigarettes with high concentrations of toxins (known as bidi) and placing a mixture of chewing tobacco combined with slaked lime wrapped in a betel leaf (known as pan) in the gingivobuccal sulcus are predisposing factors for oral cancer. Chewing of betel nuts uncombined with tobacco apparently does not cause oral cancer. Moreover, in the habit of ''reverse'' smoking practiced in South America, India, the Philippines, and Sardinia, which consists of placing the lighted end of the cigarette or cigar inside the mouth (to protect the lit end from wind currents), little smoke is inhaled, but tremendous heat is generated, and carcinogens drop off and accumulate at the base of tongue and in the hypopharynx.

Cancer risk increases dramatically when five cigars or pipebowls of tobacco or more than one pack of cigarettes are used daily. Tobacco smoke condensate is a complete carcinogen experimentally. It contains substances that act as both initiators and promoters of carcinogenesis and also enhance the local absorption of carcinogens.

The risk of developing cancer remains significant if

TABLE 20–4. Cancer Statistics

A. Estimated New Cancer Cases by Sex for All Sites, United States, 1995*

	Total	Male	Female
All Sites	1,252,000	677,000	575,000
Buccal cavity and pharynx (oral)	28,150	18,800	9,350
Lip	2,500	1,900	600
Tongue	5,550	3,600	1,950
Mouth	11,000	6,900	4,100
Pharynx	9,100	6,400	2,700
Digestive organs	223,000	118,800	105,000
Esophagus	12,100	8,800	3,300
Respiratory system	186,300	108,400	77,900
Larynx	11,600	9,000	2,600
Lung	169,900	96,000	73,900
Other and unspecified respiratory	4,800	3,400	1,400

B. Trends in Cancer Survival by Race and Years of Diagnosis, United States, 1960–1990

	Relative Five-Year Survival Rates (%)									
	1960–1963†		1970–1973†		1974–1976‡		1980–1982‡		1983–1990‡	
Site	White	Black	White	Black	White	Black	White	Black	White	Black
All Sites	39	27	43	31	50	39	52	39	56§	40
Oral cavity and pharynx	45	—	43	—	55	36	55	31	55	34
Esophagus	4	1	4	4	5	4	7	5	11§	6§
Larynx	53	—	62	—	66	59	69	58	69§	53
Lung and bronchus	8	5	10	7	12	11	14	12	14§	11

* Excludes basal and squamous cell skin cancers and in situ carcinomas except bladder. The difference in rates between 1974 to 1976 and 1983 to 1990 is statistically significant (P < 0.05). The standard error of the survival rate is between 5 and 10 percentage points. The standard error of the survival rate is greater than 10 percentage points. A dash indicates that a valid survival rate could not be calculated.

† Rates are based on End Results Group data from a series of hospital registries and one population-based registry.

‡ Rates are based on SEER data from Connecticut, New Mexico, Utah, Iowa, Hawaii, Atlanta, Detroit, Seattle-Puget Sound, and San Francisco-Oakland. Rates are based on follow-up of patients through 1991.

the habit has been discontinued for less than 5 years; after that time, the risk decreases. When 15 years of tobacco abstinence have been achieved, the odds ratio for developing cancer is not elevated. Nonsmoking men and women seem to be at no increased risk related to alcohol consumption.[7] Quitting the smoking habit is difficult, and new medical assistance is being investigated.[8] The smoker must really want to quit for personal reasons, and "cold turkey" is the most successful way. Emphasis is placed on cancer prevention,[9] focusing on the head and neck cancer population and on the "chemoprevention" of second primary tumors.[10,11]

Assessing the individual effects of alcohol is difficult because most heavy drinkers are also heavy smokers. The largest case-controlled study conducted to date concluded that smoking and drinking together accounted for about three quarters of the cases of oropharyngeal cancer in the United States.[12]

In cigarette smokers, 75% of oral cancers develop in the dependent drainage areas of the mouth (Figs. 20–1 and 20–2). These oral reservoirs pool and concentrate dissolved carcinogens, promoting prolonged contact with the mucosa. These sites may be more vulnerable to carcinogenic agents because they are devoid of a protective keratin layer. Absorption by sebaceous glands underlying the mucosa may enhance chemical carcinogenesis. Alcohol probably acts synergistically with tobacco as a cocarcinogen (promoter). Alcohol

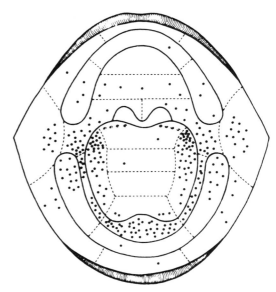

Fig. 20–2. Scattergram showing sites of predilection for development of cancer in the oral cavity and oropharynx. (From Mashberg A and Myers H: Cancer *37*:2149, 1976.)

may act directly on the mucosa or indirectly by promoting malnutrition and cirrhosis. Hepatocellular dysfunction interferes with detoxification of systemically active oral carcinogens.[13]

Whether or not smokeless tobacco products cause

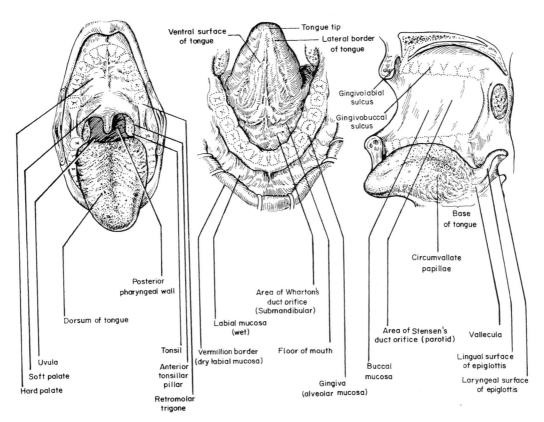

Fig. 20–1. Relevant topographic anatomy of the oral cavity and oropharynx.

oral cancer is attracting much attention because of the alarming increase in the use of smokeless tobacco by young Americans.[14] Young people typically begin to use smokeless tobacco between the ages of 10 to 12 years, and the habit is being promoted as the safest alternative to smoking.[15]

Snuff-dipping involves placing powdered tobacco in the gingivobuccal sulcus and is practiced mainly in Scandinavia, in the southeastern United States, and by sports figures.

The role of snuff-dipping as causative agent of oral cancer has been controversial for many years. A definite association between the use of smokeless tobacco and oral and pharyngeal cancer has apparently been established.[16] A 4-fold excess of oral and pharyngeal cancer was linked to snuff use among nonsmoking white women, and the exceptionally high mortality from this cancer among white women in the South was related primarily to the long-term use of snuff. For cancers in the gingival and buccal mucosa, the risk was nearly 50-fold among long-term users. Most women who dipped snuff did not smoke cigarettes or consume alcohol.

The spectrum of precancerous changes (discussed in this paragraph) can be seen in snuff-related oral lesions. Some individuals never develop oral cancer, even after lifelong use. Others may not develop malignant disease until they have used smokeless tobacco for 20 to 40 years, and even with this length of use, discontinuing the habit can revert extensive mucosal changes to normal in 2 weeks or less. Some individuals, however, develop oral cancer after a relatively short period of snuff use. This demonstrates the biologic spectrum of disease expression discussed in the section of this chapter on tumor biology. A leukoplakic lesion does not necessarily precede a premalignant or malignant area. Erythroplasia may be the first observed change, and this carries an extremely high potential for malignancy unless it is completely excised promptly. Red patches, ulceration, and extensive surface roughness in leukoplakias induced by smokeless tobacco use are suspicious signs. Homogeneous leukoplakias that disappear after discontinuation of the habit should be monitored monthly for 6 months. Pictures of typical snuff-induced oral changes can be found in an article by Wood.[17]

Other than use of tobacco and alcohol, risk factors associated with an increased chance of forming cancer in the mouth and throat include vitamin deficiency (especially vitamin A), malnutrition, and poor oral hygiene. The roles of these factors has not been well defined. Studies have shown that vitamin A and its retinoid analogues (retinol, retinoic acid) can inhibit the development of some epithelial tumors through the mediation of specific intracellular binding proteins. Such agents show promise as prophylactic or therapeutic agents against spontaneous and chemically in-duced tumors, and one hopes that such compounds may be useful in the chemoprevention of carcinogenesis in humans.[10]

Increased vulnerability of textile workers to the development of oral cancer is possibly related to exposure to cotton and wool dust. The role of oral trauma is unclear. The most severely traumatized areas of the oral cavity are infrequent sites of neoplasia. Syphilis was commonly associated with oral leukoplakia and cancer in the preantibiotic era, and this association has decreased dramatically to about 0.3%. Syphilitic infection leads to interstitial glossitis, end-arteritis, atrophy of the overlying epithelium, and loss of papillae. These changes presumably make the area more vulnerable to carcinogenesis.

Patients with compromised immune systems, especially those with compromise of cell-mediated immunity, usually develop cancers of the lymphoreticular system; however, SCC is the second most common type.[18,19] Evidence suggests a connection between herpes simplex virus type 1 and cancer. The virus may act as a promotor or a cofactor.[20]

Histopathology

Oral Mucosa Topography

Embryologically, the ectodermally lined stomodeum gives rise to the mucosa of the lips, buccal mucosa, gingiva, FOM, retromolar trigone, and oral tongue. Endodermally derived structures (originating from the foregut) include the nasopharynx, oropharynx, base of tongue, hypopharynx, larynx, trachea, bronchi, and esophagus.

The oral mucosa (except the hard palate, tongue, gingiva, and tonsil) rests on a loose submucosa, which invests salivary glands, blood vessels, and nerves and is permeated by a rich lymphatic system. The masticatory mucosa is keratinized and firm, whereas the lining mucosa is nonkeratinized and distensible. The color of the mucosa is related to the thickness of its epithelium and the degree of keratinization. The FOM, ventrolateral tongue, and soft palate are lined by a fine layer of squamous cell epithelium devoid of keratin. In contrast, the gingiva, hard palate, and dorsum of the tongue are keratinized structures. Little or no submucosa is present in the tongue. The epithelium of the mucous membranes is mainly stratified, nonkeratinizing squamous cell epithelium containing intercellular bridges. There is no stratum granulosum.

The response to irritation in this area is thickening of the malpighian layer and development of a nonnucleated keratin layer that clinically appears as leukoplakia. Lining mucosa that lacks a protective keratin layer is subject to the action of carcinogenic agents with decreased resistance to injury, early atrophy, and delayed healing. Vitamin deficiencies (particularly A, B, and C deficiencies) are known to lead to subepithelial inflammation resulting in glossitis, glossodynia, stomatitis, and gingivitis. Iron deficiency anemia predisposes to the development of hyperkeratotic lesions in the mouth.

The posterior regions of the oral cavity and oropharynx contain the lingual, palatine, and pharyngeal tonsils. Deep in the tonsillar and adenoidal crypts are nonmaturing, poorly differentiated epithelial cells. The absence of basement membranes or typical epithelial desmosomes permits free migration of lymphocytes.

Melanocytes occur in all areas of the mucous membrane. They are numerous in the gingiva, hard palate, and buccal mucosa. Melanomas have been described in all areas.

"Minor" salivary glands (mucous and serous) line most of the oral cavity, including the tongue and hard palate. Sebaceous glands are present in the buccal and lip submucosa.[21,22]

Oral Precancer

A precancerous lesion is morphologically altered tissue in which cancer is more likely to occur than in its normal counterpart. Friability (easy surface bleeding) or a scraped mucosal area is highly suggestive of malignant change in the UADT. Precancerous lesions include leukoplakia, erythroplasia, and submucous fibrosis.[23] These terms are clinical descriptions of the appearance of the lesion. Biopsy is necessary to define histologic features.

Leukoplakia is a white patch or plaque that will not rub off and cannot be attributed to other definable pathologic processes. It appears white because of hyperkeratosis. Keratinized epithelium seldom exhibits leukoplakia. The incidence and location of leukoplakias depend on the geographic population studied and reflect the positioning of the irritating influence that causes them. In India, most occur on the buccal mucosa. In North America and Europe, FOM and lingual sites are more common (see also Chaps. 16 and 17).

The natural course of leukoplakia is variable. If smoking (or other definable irritation such as snuff-dipping) is discontinued, most leukoplakias will disappear, whereas if the habit is only decreased, few will disappear. Studies show that 10 to 45% of leukoplakias regress without change in oral habits.

The transformation of leukoplakia into carcinoma is a controversial topic. Earlier reports cited the incidence of oral cancer development in 10 to 100% of leukoplakias. Investigators now consider that about 2% (0.13 to 6%) transform into cancer.[24,25]

Erythroplasia appears as a flat or slightly elevated granular, sharply circumscribed, asymptomatic, red plaque.[25] The red color is caused by the absence of the normal surface keratin and engorged capillaries close to the surface. It has also been attributed to a round

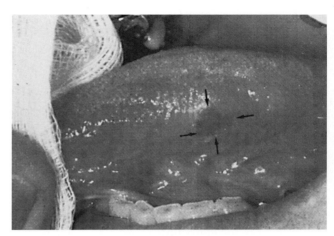

Fig. 20–3. Erythroplasia of lateral tongue (arrows).

cell infiltrate (Fig. 20–3). The most dangerous precancerous lesions are red. Almost every case of erythroplasia is associated at least with dysplasia and frequently with carcinoma in situ or invasive carcinoma. The incidence of malignant transformation is about 17 times higher than with leukoplakia. Size does not predict invasiveness.[26] Characteristics suggestive of invasion include a granular, roughened surface, elevation, induration, erythema of the mucosa adjacent to the lesion, discomfort, and ulceration. The lesions tend to occur in a horseshoe-shaped area including the FOM, ventral and lateral tongue, and soft palate anterior pillar complex[27] (see Fig. 20–2). "Speckled" (nodular) leukoplakia is associated with Candida albicans, which is considered the cause. Most speckled leukoplakias occur at the oral commissures and have both red and white components. Their transforming potential is consistent with the presence of a red component.[23] Various studies have reported an incidence of carcinoma in 14 to 65% of these lesions.

Submucous fibrosis is a precancerous lesion occurring mainly in India and Pakistan, and rarely among North Americans or Europeans. This insidious chronic disease affects the mucosa of the oral cavity, pharynx, and esophagus. An inflammatory reaction and fibroblastic changes in the lamina propria lead to epithelial atrophy; the oral mucosa becomes stiff, and trismus results.

Lichen planus is typically a lacy, white, striated lesion occurring on the buccal mucosa. Erosive and atrophic forms, also recognized, can have the appearance of invasive cancer. Lichen planus is rarely thought to be associated with malignant transformation.[23,28]

White lesions of the palate are either leukoplakia or *nicotinic stomatitis* (leukokeratosis nicotina palati). Palatal changes associated with nicotinic stomatitis include diffuse palatal keratosis, umbilicated excrescences, red or white patches, amelanotic areas, and ulcerated areas. This lesion is considered by many not to be precancerous, although dysplasia and microinvasive carcinomas are occasionally seen in palatal keratoses.[29]

Excellent photographs of these and many other oral conditions can be found in Pindborg's atlas.[30]

Variants of Squamous Cell Carcinoma

SCC (synonymous with epidermoid carcinoma) constitutes 95% of cancers in the oral cavity and oropharynx. There are several ways of classifying SCC. On a gross morphologic basis, one sees exophytic, ulcerative, or verrucous (warty with a papillary surface) types. Infiltration and invasion are associated with a higher histologic grade and early metastasis.

The continuum of SCC progresses from individual cell changes in the epithelium (atypia) to a generalized disturbance of the epithelium (dysplasia) to carcinoma in situ. The frank tumor consists of nests, columns, or strands of malignant epithelial cells infiltrating subepithelially, with the border typically characterized as "pushing" or "infiltrating." The tumor may resemble any or all of the layers of stratified squamous cell epithelium. Intercellular bridges and tonofilaments are present. Desmosomes are visible on electron microscopy and can help distinguish SCC from undifferentiated carcinomas.

Classification by histologic features includes the following varieties:

A. Keratinizing.
B. Nonkeratinizing (transitional cell carcinoma, lymphoepithelioma).
C. Verrucous.
D. Spindle cell (pseudosarcoma, carcinosarcoma).
E. Adenoid squamous carcinoma (adenoacanthoma, pseudoglandular SCC).
F. Basaloid squamous carcinoma.[31]

Nonkeratinizing carcinomas tend to arise from respiratory-type mucosa whose cells are endodermally derived and may be well to poorly differentiated. These cancers are frequently associated with a lymphoid tissue stroma that is not an integral component of the tumor. They occur frequently in the nasopharynx, pharynx, and larynx. Nonkeratinizing tumors show mainly submucosal spread and have "pushing" margins in 50% of cases.[32]

Keratinizing SCC occurs in all areas of the UADT, with the greatest frequency in structures derived from the ectodermally lined stomadeum. In general, these carcinomas are ulcerative or fungating, show infrequent submucosal spread, have sharp infiltrating margins, and are well differentiated in 20% of cases. No differences exist with respect to lymph node metastases or survival based on the feature of keratinization.[32]

SPINDLE CELL CARCINOMA. In this rare variant of SCC, tumors tend to be polypoid or pedunculated masses attached to the larynx, pharynx, tongue, FOM, gingiva, esophagus, and bronchi. Symptoms result from the bulk and anatomic location of the tumors. They are friable, and patients may cough up parts of the tumor or have spotty bleeding.

Histologically, spindle cell carcinoma consists of bizarre, spindle-shaped mesenchymal cells giving the impression of a highly anaplastic sarcoma with an overlying epidermoid carcinoma. The epidermoid component can be missed unless multiple sections are examined. Electron microscopy supports the classification of spindle cell carcinoma as a variant of SCC with no evidence of malignant degeneration of connective tissue.[33] The carcinoma component is usually small and well differentiated.

Tumor metastases are present in 50% of cases, usually in the regional lymph nodes. The metastases may demonstrate the epithelial or spindle pattern or both. The primary tumor tends to remain localized. In a study of 20 patients, the major prognostic factor was considered to be tumor invasiveness, with tumor location and prior radiation also having prognostic significance. Oral cavity tumors fared worse than those in the pharynx, larynx, or nose. After RT with curative intent, 5 of 6 tumors were fatal.[34]

Failure to control local disease occurs 50% of the time, and one third of patients die of local disease. One series of 8 patients had an average survival of 9 years and a 75% overall cure rate.[35] Low-grade tumors can be treated by wide surgical excision, but poorly differentiated and invasive tumors should probably be treated with planned combined operation and RT.

ADENOID SQUAMOUS CELL CARCINOMA. This rare variant of SCC occurs primarily on the vermilion border of the lips and more rarely on the tongue and gingiva. The basic cell is of the keratinizing squamous type. This lesion can be distinguished from salivary gland or metastatic tumor by acid mucopolysaccharide stains. The pathogenesis of this lesion is unknown. Adenoid SCCs of the lip are associated with a good prognosis and no regional metastases or deaths. Within the oral cavity, these tumors behave similarly to SCC and have a greater proclivity toward lymph node metastasis.[36]

VERRUCOUS CARCINOMA. The diagnosis of this interesting variant of well-differentiated SCC requires concurrence between the pathologist and the clinician; that is, the diagnosis is clinicopathologic, and microscopic and clinical features must both be consistent with the diagnosis. In Ackerman's original series, 60% were in the buccal mucosa, 30% on the alveolar ridges and gingivae, and 10% in the FOM.[37] The lesion is soft and circumscribed at first, but becomes indurated as it advances. This exophytic and warty growth occurs in areas of leukoplakia and consists of well-differentiated keratinized epithelium thrown up into long, papillomatous folds (Fig. 20–4).

Histologically, the tumor consists of large, heavily keratinized fronds and downward, sharply projecting,

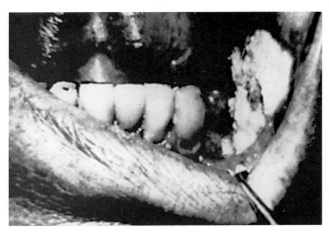

Fig. 20–4. Verrucous carcinoma.

circumscribed, bulbous rete pegs. The border is typically pushing rather than infiltrating. A dense inflammatory reaction occurs in the adjacent stroma. Cytologic features of malignancy (cellular atypism, mitoses) are lacking, and the basement membrane may appear intact.

Biopsies of the surface of the lesion are interpreted repeatedly as benign hyperkeratosis, delaying diagnosis and treatment. The differential diagnosis includes pseudoepitheliomatous hyperplasia, keratoacanthoma, and squamous cell papilloma. Verrucous carcinoma and well-differentiated SCC with a verrucoid appearance are considered separate entities. Deep biopsy at the base of the lesion is required to show the foregoing diagnostic features.

Verrucous "carcinoma" acts in a benign manner. Growth of the primary tumor is indolent, with erosion of underlying structures including bone, but little surface spread. The slow-pushing nature of growth yields few symptoms. This clinical pattern is interesting in view of tissue culture findings, which show that the typical growth pattern is rapid.[38] Indeed, primary tumors can recur rapidly and repeatedly when incompletely excised.[39]

The benign nature of this entity is further documented by the finding that, although regional lymph nodes can be enlarged, this is presumably caused by an inflammatory response to the heavy keratin deposits rather than by metastatic disease, and Batsakis and associates believe that true verrucous carcinoma has no metastatic ability. DMs have never been reported.[40]

High recurrence rates and anaplastic transformation of verrucous carcinoma leading to rapid metastatic dissemination and death of the patient have been reported following RT.[41] This has led to a long treatment controversy, and reevaluation of this topic has resulted in changing treatment recommendations.[39] Anaplastic transformation of verrucous carcinoma after RT has mainly been reported for lesions in the oral cavity, and

only one such occurrence has been reported in the larynx. The risk of anaplastic transformation after RT has received widespread acceptance, so using this treatment modality is almost considered malpractice. One review reported that 30% of cases undergo anaplastic transformation after RT,[42] but this review was a compilation of papers that reported anaplastic transformation. Most papers do not mention this process, and therefore the review reflected a reporting bias. A more accurate incidence is probably 7 to 10%.

Theoretic rationales for this transformation have included development of a highly aggressive neoplasm and the coexistence of a hidden area of less well-differentiated SCC in the tumor. In one series,[43] no evidence of SCC was found in 140 specimens reviewed. Such "hybrid" verrucous SCC was reported, however, by Batsakis and colleagues,[40] in 3 of 7 laryngeal specimens and in 20% of 104 verrucous lesions of the oral cavity.[44]

The existence of hybrid tumors may explain the findings of McDonald and collaborators that only four cases of anaplastic transformation following RT have been properly documented in the literature, and a further six cases of transformation of verrucous carcinoma to a less well-differentiated SCC occurred either spontaneously or after treatment with surgery alone.[42] These findings suggest that RT may not be the instigator of, but only the scapegoat for, a transformation process that can occur without it.

In any event, avoidance of this risk has resulted in the preferred management of verrucous carcinoma with surgery alone. The conclusion of one review was that, although verrucous carcinoma is moderately radiosensitive, the major contraindication to RT with curative intent is the high recurrence rate rather than anaplastic transformation.[42] Another study supports the use of RT for a different reason.[39] A good response to RT with a low recurrence rate is seen for small laryngeal lesions, and RT was advocated in this context without undue concern for changes in biologic behavior. The chance of recurrence when RT is used to treat verrucous carcinoma in the oral cavity as a single modality is high. Another report, however, showed favorable results when 52 patients with oral verrucous carcinoma were treated by RT in India, with no comment regarding anaplastic transformation.[45]

In the series reported by Medina and associates, 82% of oral cavity verrucous carcinomas were controlled with one surgical procedure, and control rates were satisfactory even for T4 lesions.[44] No case of anaplastic transformation after RT was found in this series; however, a definite tendency was noted for recurrences to assume a less differentiated, nonverrucoid SCC pattern regardless of the treatment used. The hybrid verrucous-squamous cell group showed clinical characteristics similar to those of the pure verrucous carcinomas, and all patients were treated by surgery alone. The local recurrence rate was 30% for hybrid tumors and 18% for pure verrucous carcinomas.

Medina and co-workers' series concluded that surgery was a remarkably effective mode of therapy for verrucous carcinomas of the oral cavity, providing tumor control in more than 80% of patients after the initial surgery and in 95% after surgical salvage of recurrences.[44] This finding is at variance with McClure and co-workers' series of 15 cancers, in which a high recurrence rate was noted in tumors of the oral cavity treated with RT or surgery alone.[39] Medina and associates concluded that surgery was more effective than RT for verrucous carcinoma, but the diagnosis of verrucous carcinoma of the oral cavity should not constitute an absolute contraindication to RT in selected patients (presumably medically inoperable). Similarly, McClure and co-workers' conclusion was that extensive lesions might benefit from combined therapy, and RT should be considered in the management of this tumor without undue concern for change in biologic behavior.

The occasional appearance of apparent anaplastic transformation can be explained on the basis of tumor heterogeneity cited earlier in this chapter, and such behavior is undoubtedly not unique to verrucous carcinoma. RT can act as a selective agent on a heterogeneous tumor cell population, and this can unmask especially malignant activity.

BASALOID SQUAMOUS CELL CARCINOMA. Basaloid SCC (BSCC) is an aggressive, histologically distinctive variant of SCC that has a predilection for the UADT (base of tongue, pyriform sinus, supraglottic larynx), although other sites including the anus, esophagus, and uterine cervix have also been reported. Since its first description in 1986, only about 90 patients have been reported in the English literature.

BSCC tends to occur in older populations, with male predominance. Its aggressive biologic behavior is characterized by a high incidence of cervical lymph node metastases (64%), DMs (44%), primarily to the lungs, liver, bones, brain, and skin, and death from disease: 38% mortality at 17 months median follow-up.[31] The tumors are usually hard and centrally ulcerated, with submucosal infiltration.

Histopathologically, BSCC is distinctive. Microscopically, one sees a dual population of cells, and characteristic growth patterns consist of lobules, nests, and cords of basaloid cells, comedonecrosis, nuclear palisading around the periphery of tumor lobules, small cyst-like spaces surrounding material that resembles mucin, hyalinosis, prominent mitotic activity, and a surface component of dysplastic in situ or frankly invasive SCC. Some reports note multifocal origin in overlying mucosa. Perineural invasion does not appear to be a prominent feature of the process.

Keratin positivity is seen in the squamous cell component. Studies of oncogene expression in BSCC suggest that it is a distinct variant of SCC characterized by a poorly differentiated cell population. Assessment of tumor ploidy by flow cytometry provides no additional prognostic information beyond that available by routine histologic evaluation. BSCC may well originate from cells located in the basal area of the mucous membrane or in the proximal ducts of minor salivary glands. Smoking and drinking alcohol appear to be risk factors, and second primary tumors have been reported in association with BSCC, as is typical of other patients with head and neck cancer.

In BSCC, basaloid and squamous cells are intimately admixed, but the cellular composition is heterogeneous, and establishing the correct diagnosis on biopsy may be difficult or impossible. The two tumors that cause the most difficulty in differential diagnosis are adenoid cystic carcinoma (particularly the solid variant) and small cell undifferentiated (neuroendocrine) carcinoma.[31]

Methods of Tissue Diagnosis

Direct biopsy is the standard method of obtaining tissue from lesions in the oral cavity and oropharynx. Panendoscopy is performed to define the extent of large and posteriorly located lesions using vision and palpation (the base of tongue and nasopharynx should always be palpated carefully) and to look for simultaneous primary tumors in the mucosal "nooks and crannies" of the UADT. Multiple biopsies at the apparent limits of the tumor are not used to help define its extent because induced inflammation can interfere with margin interpretation at definitive operation. Rather, one should "go for the money" and obtain the biopsy from the most suspicious, central, non-necrotic portion of the tumor. The tissue biopsy should be obtained with sharp instruments to avoid crush artifacts. Biopsies have the potential to evaluate the invasiveness and depth of tumor, but this is limited by sampling error.

Toluidine blue (tolonium chloride) applied in situ has been used as a diagnostic adjunct in the detection of asymptomatic, multifocal, oral SCC and to define tumor margins. The mechanism of action is unknown, but the dye is thought to be preferentially taken up by areas of carcinoma with increased nuclear DNA content. Alternatively, the dye may preferentially stain cancer because it penetrates the haphazardly arranged cell layers more readily than it does organized epithelium with intact architecture.[46] A positive stain is dark or royal blue. Normal mucosa is colorless or light blue. Asymptomatic erythroplastic lesions stain well, but the stain does not penetrate keratotic areas. Because of the a high percentage of false-positive results with inflammatory lesions, the technique is not good for mass screening, and Mashberg, the pioneer of the technique, recommends that, if a mucosal alteration is identified with toluidine blue rinse, 10 to 14 days should elapse, during which withdrawal of all irritating factors allows inflammatory lesions to subside.[47,48] The area should then be restained. The rinse sequence is as follows:

1. Rinse mouth with 1% acetic acid for 20 seconds.
2. Rinse mouth with water for 20 seconds, twice.
3. Rinse mouth with 5 to 10 ml of 1% toluidine blue solution and then gargle.
4. Rinse with 1% acetic acid for 1 minute. Solutions should not be swallowed.
5. Rinse with water.

Natural History

The term "natural history" is used to indicate the usual course of events in the untreated patient with head and neck SCC. The clinician must be aware of the behavior patterns of the histopathologic entities encountered to be able to tell whether a clinical situation is usual or unexpected. As brought to attention by Bouquot, Weiland, and Kurland,[49] the clinical course and natural history of SCC of the UADT may have been misrepresented in the literature because of the disproportionate referral of more severely affected patients to academic medical centers, from which most of the medical literature emanates. This may result in inadvertent confusion of referral factors with disease presentation and may yield an overstatement of features of disease that are associated with poor prognostic outcomes. Community-based studies are suggested as necessary to reduce or eliminate these biases and to develop figures that are more representative of the general population than are hospital-based statistics. (Treatment biases would probably be present between the two milieus, with relatively more single-modality RT in the private sector.)

The longevity of the patient with head and neck SCC is limited by three cancer-related events that typically occur within 18 to 24 months of treatment of the first cancer ("index primary"):

1. Recurrence of disease at the primary site, in the neck, or both.
2. Development of another primary tumor in the mucosa of the UADT.
3. Development of DM.

Multiple primary tumors of the UADT were first described by Billroth. In the head and neck, multiple primary tumors develop in the "condemned mucosa" of the UADT, which had presumably been uniformly exposed to the carcinogens in tobacco smoke and possibly in alcohol, dissolved in saliva. This phenomenon is also known as "field cancerization."[50] Multiple primary tumors are spoken of as being simultaneous (diagnosed at the same time as the index tumor), synchronous (diagnosed within 6 months of the index tumor), or metachronous (diagnosed more than 6 months after the index cancer).

Therefore, the UADT mucosa is carefully examined with panendoscopy (laryngoscopy, bronchoscopy, and esphagoscopy) at the time of initial tumor mapping under general anesthesia. The chance of finding a second primary tumor in the lung in the presence of a normal chest radiograph is only 1%, and therefore rigid bronchoscopy is not frequently done.[51]

The risk of developing multiple primary cancers seems generally greatest in patients with a history of high consumption of both alcohol and tobacco and has been reviewed.[52,53] One study noted that the risk of developing a second primary cancer was six times greater in patients who continued to smoke after diagnosis of the index tumor than in those who stopped smoking. The decreased risk of second cancers with cessation of smoking has not been found by others. For lung cancer, the risk of developing a tumor does not revert to normal in smokers until 15 years after discontinuing the smoking habit.

Multiple primary cancers of the UADT occur in 10 to 20% of patients with head and neck cancer. At initial panendoscopy, 10% of patients have a second primary tumor.[51] The lung and esophagus are the two most common sites.[52] About 6% of simultaneous primary cancers occur in the esophagus, especially with pharyngeal primary cancers. Patients with pharyngeal wall primary cancers have a higher incidence of multiple primary tumors than do patients with SCC in other head and neck sites, namely, 30 to 50%. Epithelial carcinoma of the UADT rarely sheds identifiable tumor cells into the tracheobronchial tree. When malignant cells are found in bronchial washings, the likely source is a second primary cancer in the lung.[53a]

One study showed a 5-year survival of 9% for head and neck cancer patients with multiple primary tumors,[54] which is intuitively logical because the chance for cure diminishes with each subsequent recurrence. One subset of patients, however, seems to live well in symbiosis with multiple primary tumors over time, and physicians who specialize in the treatment of head and neck cancer have seen patients who survive long enough to develop 8 or 10 primary cancers. These survivors tend to have small superficial mucosal lesions and seem to truly be manifesting the pattern of neoplastic transformation in "condemned mucosa." When this disease pattern is recognized, RT should be held in reserve when possible in favor of managing the patient with repeated surgical excisions.

Some investigators have suggested that multiple primary tumors may be induced by RT; however, the coexistent process of "field cancerization" is a much more likely explanation. In fact, RT to the head and neck is thought neither to promote nor to inhibit formation of additional mucosal primary tumors.[55]

Patients with malignant tumors of the reticuloendothelial system develop head and neck cancers as second primary cancers in 5 to 20% of cases.[56]

SCC of the head and neck is locally aggressive and difficult to control. This fact and the phenomenon of multiple primary tumors provide some interesting dilemmas for treatment management. If the first tumor is not adequately treated, the patient will, of course, not live long enough to develop other tumors. Consideration should, nevertheless, be given to holding something in reserve for treatment of future primary tumors, if treatment of the index tumor is not thereby compromised. For example, if the first tumor is small and in a location associated with a low incidence of cervical metastases, surgery as single-modality therapy might be considered, rather than automatically adding RT "insurance." Elective functional neck dissection is useful in this context, too. If no positive lymph nodes are found in the individual, then "prophylactic" neck irradiation can reasonably be held in reserve for future need. Similar considerations apply when deciding on reconstructive methods. Many options exist for reconstructing small defects rather than immediately resorting to a myocutaneous flap (see subsequent section), which could then be held in reserve for future need.

Sites of Cancer Failure

In recent years, the "natural history" of head and neck SCC has been altered by treatment at first-rate institutions in the United States.[57,58] For decades, the results of ineffective control of local-regional disease were seen: progression of disease above the clavicle killed the patient within a relatively short time. More recently, as technologic advances have allowed better combinations of standard therapy, less local-regional disease recurs. Patients are now dying more frequently of DM or the consequences of multiple primary tumors, but overall survival (about 50%) has not changed.[58] The incidence of second malignant tumors as the cause of death has remained at 14%.[53]

In 1923, Crile reported that only 1% of patients with head and neck SCC had DM at autopsy. More recent series have shown a clinical incidence of DM in 5 to 25% of patients (rarely at presentation, however) and in 17 to 60% (average 32%) of autopsies.[59]

In earlier decades, when local-regional disease was only transiently or never controlled, other contributors to mortality (DM, multiple primary tumors) were rarely seen, either because the patients did not live long enough or because the diagnosis was not made because of the lack of sophisticated diagnostic technology and close follow-up with radiologic examination. Failure of local-regional cancer control is still the major cause of death in patients with head and neck SCC in the United States and certainly worldwide. In India, for example, the incidence of DM in head and neck cancer patients is recorded at only 3 to 5% because the majority of patients still present with advanced disease and quickly die of local-regional disease, and sophisticated diagnostic capability is absent.[60] In most developing countries, lack of medical resources precludes definitive cancer treatment, and patients are usually sent home to die, possibly with a feeding tube and analgesics when available.

Distant Metastases

In patients who die of DM with disease controlled above the clavicle, death seems to occur at about 2 years (but sometimes as at 4 to 6 months) after treatment of the index primary cancer: the same time as previously seen when death occurred from uncontrolled local-regional disease. Thus, it seems that DMs are concomitantly progressing at the subclinical level, consistent with the current view that solid carcinomas are systemic from their inception (see the section of this chapter on tumor biology).

As emphasized elsewhere in this chapter, the development of DM is most strongly predicted by the presence of positive cervical lymphadenopathy. DMs are also frequently seen in association with certain recurrence patterns in the head and neck. When patients develop uncontrolled local-regional disease, DMs often appear almost simultaneously, representing an apparent "systemic derepression" that allows diffuse cancer progression. Development of recurrent disease at the skull base also appears to be a harbinger of DM within 3 to 4 months. A Radiation Therapy Oncology Group (RTOG) cancer control report showed that local-regional cancer control was the most significant variable affecting the development of DMs for all tumor sites, except for primary tumors of the hypopharynx and nasopharynx.[61] By implication, survival could be improved by increasing local-regional control, except for the last two sites, where improved cure awaits effective treatments for DMs.

The most common sites for DM from head and neck SCC are the lung (50 to 70%) and bone (20 to 25%). The older literature stated that about 80% of DM were detected within 2 years of treatment of the index cancer, and 90% of patients died within 2 years, the average survival after diagnosis of DM being 9 months.[61] Younger patients without multisystem disease did not die as soon, however.

Because the lungs are the most frequent sites of DM and second primary tumors, a chest radiograph is recommended every 6 months for follow-up. Suspicious lesions are evaluated by CT and are confirmed, if indicated, by CT-guided fine-needle aspiration and cytologic examination (any resultant pneumothorax can be reexpanded with the small Heimlich tube, rather than placing traditional chest tubes). An isolated central lesion is usually treated as a second primary tumor, and multiple lesions, either unilateral or bilateral, are assumed to represent metastatic disease. Metastatic lesions are typically more peripheral and are not as accessible to cytologic diagnosis by way of bronchoscopy. Metastatic lung disease is generally not treated unless it becomes symptomatic, which occurs rarely. RT is most reliable for palliation. Chemotherapy is not generally useful for palliation of gross metastatic disease. Excision of selected pulmonary metastases resulting from head and neck SCC appears promising in selected patients.[62,63]

Because of the low incidence of metastatic disease at presentation (2%), routine bone and liver scanning is not cost-effective. A liver scan (CT) is indicated when the patient is symptomatic and has an enlarged or nodular liver and abnormal liver function tests. Heat-stable alkaline phosphatase is elevated in 50% of patients with proved liver metastases. Some clinicians believe that no reliable information can be obtained from enzyme elevations because of the high incidence of cirrhosis and malnutrition in patients with head and neck cancer.

Bone pain is a good indication for bone scintigraphy, although osteoblastic lesions may not produce pain. The increased metabolic turnover of bone minerals in areas of tumor invasion is detected earlier by scintigraphy than by radiography. Metastatic lesions detected on bone scan generally predate plain film abnormalities by 3 to 6 months.[63a] An elevated heat-labile alkaline phosphatase is indicative of bone metastases. A normal level occurs in fewer than 5% of patients with bony DM. An elevated calcium level is a relatively late indicator of bone metastases. Bone pain can be palliated with a short course of RT. The clinical picture is generally characteristic enough that the diagnosis does not have to be confirmed with bone biopsy.

Mechanisms of Cancer Spread

Understanding the mechanisms of cancer spread is vitally important to the head and neck surgeon to allow rational planning of excisions, whether radical or conservative. The term "conservation surgery" implies excising the cancer in a manner that spares functionally significant portions of the organ territory while achieving a local control rate equivalent to or better than that accomplished by more radical ablation and is particularly relevant in the complex and compact anatomy of the head and neck. The head and neck surgeon is always trying to reach an appropriate compromise between achieving adequate negative cancer margins and preserving structures to optimize breathing, voice, swallowing, and appearance. Extensive studies in the patterns of spread of laryngeal cancer provided the groundwork that led to formulation of principles of conservation surgery, but similar studies and definitions are largely lacking for cancer of the oral cavity, oropharynx, and pharynx. A few studies have appeared from which useful information can be extrapolated,[64-68] and these are discussed in subsequent sections of this chapter.

Concerning general concepts, spread by *permeation* implies contiguous extension as an unbroken front of cancer cells (spread in continuity), whereas spread by *embolization* denotes discontinuous spread of individual tumor cells or small "packets" of tumor cells, which break off and are separately carried into the interstitium or regional fluid channels. The surgical attack on cancer that spreads by permeation is different from that used for cancer that spreads by embolization.

Microscopic cancer spread can cause subtle changes in the quality of tissue planes, which are recognized by the experienced surgeon in previously untreated patients. (These changes are more difficult to detect in the context of postradiation fibrosis.) Abnormal tissue planes in the neck have sclerotic, "congealed," or hypervascular characteristics (the last representing tumor angiogenesis unless the patient has a coagulopathy). This spread can occur as microscopic permeation from the primary tumor or as extracapsular spread from positive neck lymph nodes, which may be occult. In this situation, not every cancer cell can be removed (or necessarily killed by postoperative RT), and local-regional disease recurrence is likely.

Spread at the Primary Site

Head and neck SCC usually spreads by permeation from the primary focus into the surrounding tissue, where it encounters structures that it follows as paths of least resistance, such as blood vessels, nerves, and bone or cartilage. The direct spread of tumors along tissue planes is generally accepted and was a major determinant of Halsted's principles of surgical oncology. Embolic spread in the interstitial tissues can also occur, however, and attention has been redirected to this almost completely ignored route of spread by Scanlon.[69]

The initial spread of a malignant tumor is through the interstitial fluid with extension into the interstitial space immediately below the basement membrane, where anatomic structures are soon encountered. Flow from the interstitial space into lymphatics and capillaries is facilitated by pressure gradients related to gravity and muscular activity.

With respect to the *mucosal* component of the primary tumor, most SCCs of the mouth and throat arise as surface lesions that tend to spread horizontally rather than vertically. A vertical growth pattern is more typical of tongue cancers, in which spread is not limited by underlying barriers and may be enhanced by muscular contraction of the organ. The phenomenon of mucosal "field cancerization"[50] is discussed earlier in this chapter.

Submucosal spread is a well-recognized pattern, said to be typical of tumors in the pharynx, although histopathologic confirmation is lacking in the literature. If carcinoma appears *submucosally* in the oral cavity or oropharynx, the differential diagnosis will also include lymphoma, a minor salivary gland neoplasm, and DM from an infraclavicular primary tumor.[70] According to a survey of the literature,[49] investigators have estimated that 1% of all human cancers metastasize to the jaws, 1 to 8% of all oral cancers represent metastatic foci, and 0.1% of patients dying of cancer have metastatic disease within the oral soft tissues. The survey of the authors in Rochester, Minnesota demonstrated that 3.6% of all UADT carcinomas were, in fact, metastases to the index site, and the UADT lesion was the first evidence of malignancy in approximately half of all such patients. (Overall, the event occurred approximately 0.6 times annually per 100,000 persons and thereby qualifies as an uncommon occurrence in the general population, although it is not uncommon among UADT cancer patients.)

SCC of the head and neck frequently extends by irregular, finger-like projections from its epicenter, as attested by the important report of Davidson and associates,[68] in which Moh's technique was applied to excision of mucosal SCC of the head and neck. With this technique, the entire excision margin of the tumor is monitored intraoperatively by horizontal sectioning and frozen section analysis, which is theoretically a thousand times more likely to detect tumor extensions than conventional vertical histologic examination, in which only areas suspicious to the surgeon or, typically, four-quadrant mucosal margins are checked. Davidson and colleagues found that 70% of tumors had microscopic tumor at least 1 cm beyond clinically evident margins by vision and palpation.

As Davidson and co-workers point out, assessment of margins using Moh's technique can be done only when surgery is the *primary* treatment modality because this technique cannot detect *discontinuous* tumor spread.[68] Preoperative treatment with RT or chemotherapy leaves nests of discontinuous tumor, a multifocal pattern of diffuse contamination of the entire field occupied by the original tumor.[71–73] In addition, about 25% of patients with head and neck SCC show a pattern of embolic spread at the primary site, as can be documented from literature reporting the histologic criteria of Jakobsson and associates,[74] in which the pattern of invasion at the tumor-host interface is assessed (see the discussion in this chapter on diagnostic factors).

These studies provide explanations for the mechanism of local recurrence with negative margins, which is stated to be 15 to 35% (average 30%) in the literature. One explanation is that the random sampling of margins misses positive foci, and therefore the margins are reported as falsely negative when Moh's technique is not used. Similarly, discontinuous spread of the tumor is also not reliably identified by assessment of the margins. (These explanations are more logical than the attribution of local recurrence to malignant transformation at the margins of excision in an area of field cancerization.)

Both the existence of discontinuous spread at the primary site and subclinical pseudopodial extensions inhibit the surgeon's ability to remove every cancer cell. Attempts to compensate for this deficit (i.e., to achieve negative margins) include Moh's technique intraoperatively, but this is not logistically feasible at most centers. Some surgeons compensate for this limitation by leaving the wound open for several days until total circumferential margin assessment can be made based on permanent sections. If a margin is reported as positive, however, it is unlikely that the surgeon will be able to identify the appropriate spot to remove additional tissue in this delayed manner because the open wound has been undergoing contraction during the interim. Delayed reexcision of a positive margin shows no residual tumor in at least 50% of cases,[75] either because the location of the positive margin was missed (likely) or because residual cancer had been removed in the previous margin (unlikely).

Harrison also noted discontinuous cancer spread up to 1.2 cm from the apparent clinical margin of tongue cancers, based on careful examination of the total glossectomy specimens of 14 patients.[64] His response to this finding is to suggest that an appropriate margin, at least for tongue cancers, is at least 2 cm. Encompassing any tumor of significant size with this suggested margin would result in total glossectomy more frequently than is currently performed (based on the dimensions of the average tongue, 6.5 cm × 11 cm), and some reports in the literature favor this approach.[64,76]

Controversy exists over the appropriate method of managing microscopic residual disease, which is known to exist frequently at the primary site. Surgeons are naturally reluctant to remove an entire organ to encompass the theoretic discontinuous spread of cancer because of the severe functional consequences to the patient in the confined and compact anatomy of the head and neck.

Muscle tissue is said to be relatively resistant to tumor invasion, with spread typically occurring longitudinally along the axis of the overlying fascia, although actual invasion of muscle with extension along the sarcolemma can occur.

Perineural Spread

With respect to "*nerve-related spread*" (terminology suggested by McGregor and MacDonald[67]) some cancers of the head and neck (adenoid cystic carcinomas of salivary gland origin) have a specific predilection for this mode of spread, known as neurotropism. SCC, however, seems to spread along nerve bundles as a path of least resistance[77] (Fig. 20–5). Although spread in relation to nerves is often perineural, endoneural spread can also be seen.

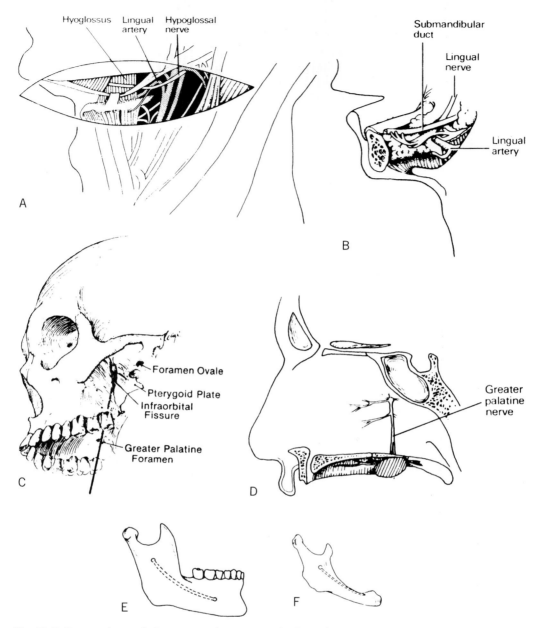

Fig. 20–5. Routes of spread along nerves from cancers in the oral cavity and oropharynx. (A, B, D, E, and F, from Barron JN and Saad MN (eds): Operative Plastic and Reconstructive Surgery. New York, Churchill Livingstone, 1981; C, from Konrad HR, et al: Arch Otolaryngol *104*:209, 1978.)

In the literature, only 30 to 40% of patients with pathologic evidence of perineural invasion are reported to present with related signs or symptoms, and they may represent a subset of patients with a particularly poor prognosis. The first symptom experienced by the patient frequently is a sensation of ants or worms crawling under the skin (formication), progressing to pain, numbness, or motor deficits. The early signs and symptoms of perineural invasion are frequently missed by the physician if leading questions or neurologic testing are omitted from the history and physical examination. Although the tumor usually

tracks in an antegrade direction (toward the central nervous system), tumors following a cranial nerve near the meninges may extend along adjacent cranial nerves and peripherally in a retrograde manner, giving rise to confusing signs and symptoms and bizarre patterns of recurrence.[77–80]

At surgery, nerves may be seen to contain tumor cells and still function and appear normal, or involved nerves may appear enlarged and stiff. Figure 20–5 shows the primary nerves along which a tumor can spread from sites in the oral cavity and oropharynx. Note the varying relationship of the inferior alveolar nerve with the alveolar rim in mandibles with and without teeth. Because of resorption of the alveolar ridge, the nerve is superficial in edentulous mandibles and is more prone to involvement from overlying mucosal tumor (discussed later).

Nerve-related spread usually seems to be continuous,[67,81] but skip lesions have also been described.[82] Which of these is the predominant pattern is unanswerable because of inadequate investigations. Nerve-related spread in the mandible is discussed in more detail in the following paragraph. Lymphatics are associated with neurovascular bundles, but lymphatic channels within the nerve sheath probably do not exist.[82]

Nerve-related spread is considered a poor prognostic sign, although some investigators believe that cures can be effected if the involved tissues can be treated. Surgical excision and inclusion of the course of nerves to the base of skull in radiation ports are treatment options, the efficacy of which has not been compared. Undoubtedly, gross tumor involvement is best managed by surgical excision. The extent of resection necessary to encompass the path of most nerves in the head is, however, potentially mutilating with severe functional consequences, and for microscopic disease, postoperative RT may well be an appropriate option. Suspicion of perineural invasion should be raised when a complaint of burning, stinging or shooting pains, or numbness along the distribution of a nerve (paresthesia or hyperthesia) is elicited on history. Sensory complaints may precede recognition of cancer by many months, and specific tests should be done.

Historically, radiographic evidence of neural involvement was evidenced by enlargement of nerve foramina at the base of the skull (ovale, rotundum, jugular) on plain films or widened mandibular nerve canals on panoramic radiographs (Panorex). These have been superseded by CT and magnetic resonance (MR) imaging; MR imaging can sometimes detect microscopic perineural spread if gadolinium enhancement is used.

Vascular Spread

Varied prognostic significance has been attributed to vascular invasion at the primary site.[83] In one study,[84] it was found to have the greatest impact on survival in uni- and multivariate analysis, as well as correlating statistically with local recurrence, neck recurrence, and DM. Although veins are easily invaded and occluded by tumor ingrowth from adjacent positive cervical lymph nodes (whereas arteries typically are not), the demonstration of tumor emboli in veins is now thought by many to reflect the tumor burden in the individual, representing the presence of enormous numbers of cells in the circulation, rather than being a measure of tumor aggressiveness with vein wall invasion.

Bone and Cartilage Invasion

Bone and cartilage are generally thought to be barriers to tumor spread and are invaded only in advanced lesions. Scientifically acceptable studies have emerged that provide information relating to the patterns of involvement of facial bones by intraoral SCC. This information is of use to the surgeon in resection planning. Useful work has come from Carter's group at the Royal Marsden Hospital in London,[80,85,86] although data are flawed by initial reports of studies on resected mandibles that had been previously irradiated. The bone and soft tissue interface was generally distorted by patchy new bone formation, presumably related to infection and previous RT. The bone surface was irregular, and tumor cells appeared initially to penetrate through natural defects, often following small blood vessels. Once the tumor had breached the cortex, it evoked an intense bone cell response with osteoclasts accumulating in front of the tumor and eroding local bone. Parallel activation of osteoblasts gave a mixed picture of osteolysis and osteogenesis, but bone destruction predominated. Bone absorption by osteoclasts proceded anterior to the advancing tumor, which infiltrated deeply and occasionally laterally inside the intact cortical bone in a manner reminiscent of submucosal spread. The osteoclasts eventually disappeared, and only at this stage carcinoma cells impinged directly on the eroded bone surface, where they appeared to take over the resorptive process unaided. Stimulation by carcinoma cells of local osteoclasts was presumably related to their possession of prostaglandin-like material, commonly found in SCC of the head and neck.[87]

The implication of this work was that, because SCCs tend to infiltrate laterally beneath intact cortical bone, the bony resection line should be examined histologically to exclude lateral tumor infiltration and also spread in perineural spaces. Moreover, prostaglandin inhibitors might eventually have a place in the management of these patients.

McGregor's group studied both reactive changes in the mandible in the presence of SCC[66] and patterns of frank tumor spread within the mandible.[67] Their material consisted of 80 mandibles that had been removed as part of a composite resection for primary intraoral SCC, both irradiated and nonirradiated. Osteoblastic activity producing new bone was much greater than that reported by Carter, presumably because of the lack of radiation in some specimens. McGregor's observations allowed definition of a temporal sequence. The first change is deposition of new bone, especially on the periosteal surface as carcinoma approaches the mandible. As invasion becomes imminent, the hematopoietic marrow is replaced by fibrous tissue, and osteoclasts may appear in relation to the bone. These changes progress as early invasion develops. With further invasion, new bone deposition is seen.

Applications for the surgeon operating on both irradiated and nonirradiated mandibles can be extrapolated from these studies. Marchetta and co-workers showed that when *any* normal soft tissue was present between the tumor and bone, the periosteum was never involved, and therefore, bony resection was not needed in this situation.[88,89] The problem arises when tumor abuts bone, usually along the alveolus or inner table of the mandible. Intraoperatively, dissection between the periosteum and the cortical bone of the mandible (subperiosteal plane) can be carried out to assess whether carcinoma has spread through the periosteum to involve the bone. Such spread provokes a fibrous tissue reaction, and the periosteum adheres to the underlying cortical bone and does not strip away from it cleanly. This can be produced by any stimulus inducing a focal inflammatory reaction in the periosteum, but with SCC close to the mandible, the surgeon must assume that adherence is caused by the presence of tumor.

Dissection of the periosteum from the mandible often reveals small, roughening areas or pitting of the cortical surface of the bone. These areas probably represent areas of periosteal new bone deposition; however, this has not been proved. Periosteal new bone formation generally occurs in advance of tumor spread, but the surgical margins should be in sound bone beyond any areas of reactive periosteal new bone.

McGregor's information that fibrosis in the marrow in nonirradiated mandibles extends no more than 5 mm beyond the invading tumor is also useful. If bone resection margins show fibrous marrow, the tumor should be considered likely to be at least adjacent to the margin. In nonirradiated mandibles, the pathologist may see active new bone formation and osteoclastic resorption at some distance beyond the invading tumor.

In irradiated mandibles, loss of osteoblastic activity was noted (in contrast to the findings in Carter's work) and indicates, among other things, that osteotomy carried through previously irradiated mandibles may heal by fibrous rather than bony union. Any new bone formation seen is probably a response to SCC close to or invading the mandible before the mandible was irradiated. Moreover, in irradiated mandibles, changes in the marrow, bone resorption, and osteoclast distribution are extensive and diffuse, rather than localized in relation to the cancer, and are therefore of no help in assessing the margins of excision.

In the subset of mandibles invaded by SCC, nerve-related spread and intramedullary spread were also studied. SCC was found extending along the inferior alveolar nerve in 10% of partially dentate, nonirradiated specimens; in 42% of edentulous, nonirradiated specimens; and in 25% of irradiated mandibles. No significant difference was noted in the frequency of nerve-related spread in irradiated versus nonirradiated mandibles, but a highly significant difference in this pattern

was seen between edentulous and partially dentate mandibles, presumably caused by reduction of the vertical height of the occlusal ridge above the mandibular canal containing the inferior alveolar nerves. Resorption of the alveolus in edentulous mandibles can be so severe that the inferior alveolar neurovascular bundle lies on the occlusal surface, immediately beneath the mucosa, and is thereby more accessible to direct spread of SCC from the occlusal surface. No skip lesions were seen in nerve-related spread in either irradiated or nonirradiated mandibles. In a few cases, massive tumor was seen around the nerve without evidence of propagation by perineural spread.

With respect to spread within medullary bone, little spread of tumor was seen deep to intact overlying alveolar mucosa or intact cortical bone in either irradiated or nonirradiated mandibles. This was in contradiction to Carter's reported subcortical lateral extension. In the few cases in which lateral spread did occur beneath normal tissue, spread was no more than 4 to 5 mm beyond the overlying tumor mass, suggesting that an adequate surgical excision margin would include 5 to 10 mm of apparently normal bone on either side of the tumor mass.

These histopathologic studies are relevant to developing appropriate guidelines for conservation surgery of the mandible and now must be correlated clinically with the cancer control rates associated with various types of limited mandibular resection. Local recurrences must be assessed with respect to occurrence in the vicinity of retained structures. The prototype of this approach is presented in the literature.[90]

Regional Spread

Once tumor cells encounter a lymphatic or venous channel, access to the other side of the system is virtually simultaneous because *lymphaticovenous anastomoses* occur all over the body. The largest are the junctions of the right lymphatic duct or left-sided thoracic duct with the venous circulation; however, many anastomoses occur among small vessels and within lymph nodes. It may well be, therefore, that the main source of venous dissemination of tumor is through these lymphaticovenous anastomoses, although direct invasion of either lymphatic or venous channels is certainly possible.

Traditionally, the principal mode of spread of SCC of the head and neck has been thought to be by way of lymphatics to the cervical lymph nodes. Lymphatic metastasis relates mechanically to the depth of tumor invasion and the richness of lymphatic drainage at the primary site. Any tumor having access to capillary lymphatics, regardless of histologic type, can spread by way of the lymphatic system. The transit time of metastatic emboli depends on lymphatic channel caliber and associated muscle contraction. The potential for metastasis increases when larger-caliber vessels are breached in areas where lymphatic flow is rapid and muscular contraction aids propulsion (tongue). Embolization is difficult and rare when the tumor involves only the superficial lymphatic network of small-caliber vessels. Occurrence of cervical metastasis is unpredictable, however, because other host and tumor factors interact in the formation of metastases.[1,91]

Whether the lymph nodes serve as an immune depot to trap and kill tumor cells or whether they are a rich source of nutrients for cancer cells is controversial.[1] Initiation of systemic tumor immunity by the regional lymph node may, in fact, depend on the antigenicity of the individual tumor. Evidence indicates that the efficiency of filtering and trapping of tumor cells in regional lymph nodes is decreased by tumor growth in the node, inflammation, and RT-induced fibrosis.

Spread along lymphatic channels that connect the primary tumor with the regional lymph nodes typically occurs by embolization, rather than by permeation, in previously untreated patients. Because lymphatic metastasis is typically discontinuous, the tradition of removing the tumor and metastatic disease en bloc is not as important as previously thought,[92] except in the rare cases of massive cancers at the primary site and in the neck connected by direct tumor extension.

The primary drainage sites (first-echelon nodes) in the neck for primary tumors in different head and neck sites are predictable[93] (Table 20–5). Indeed, the drainage pathway from the tonsil is so characteristic that the subdigastric node is frequently called the "tonsillar node." For many years, spread through the cervical lymphatics was believed to occur in an orderly progression down the jugular chain. In fact, neoplasms of the oral cavity and oropharynx do not metastasize in orderly or predictable patterns, and "skip" metastases are frequently seen.

The nodal groups involved in cancer of the mouth and throat are diagrammed in Figure 20–6. The primary-echelon drainage from most tumor sites in the mouth is through the upper deep jugular chain (subdigastric, jugulocarotid) and submandibular triangle. The jugular chain lymph nodes extend from the base of skull to the root of the neck. It is particularly important to remove node-bearing tissue from the "submuscular recess," which is frequently neglected during neck dissection: the area beneath the upper sternocleidomastoid, the posterior belly of the digastric, and the tail of the parotid. Some surgeons include the tail of the parotid and the posterior belly of the digastric muscle in a neck dissection to encompass this area adequately.

The retropharyngeal lymph nodes (Fig. 20–7) are closest to the oropharynx but are less frequently involved than the high jugular lymph nodes. They lie in the crotch between the styloid process and the internal carotid artery, are difficult to palpate without direct

TABLE 20–5. Incidence of Cervical Lymph Node Metastases by Site and Size of Primary Tumor Based on Clinical Examination of 1155 Patients Presenting with Palpable Nodes. Percent of Nodal Metastasis by T Stage Squamous Cell Carcinoma, 1948 through 1965

		N0	N1	N2 to N3
Oral tongue	T1	86	10	4
	T2	70	19	11
	T3	52.5	16.5	31
	T4	23.5	10	66.5
Floor of mouth	T1	89	8.7	2.3
	T2	71	18.5	10.5
	T3	56.5	20	23.5
	T4	46.5	10.5	43
Retromolar trigone-anterior faucial pillar	T1	88.5	2.5	9
	T2	62.5	18	19.5
	T3	46	21	33
	T4	32.5	17.5	50
Soft palate	T1	92	0	8
	T2	63.5	12	24.5
	T3	35	26	39
	T4	33	11	56
Tonsillar fossa	T1	29.5	41	29.5
	T2	32.5	14	53.5
	T3	30	18	52
	T4	10.5	13	76.5
Base of tongue	T1	30	15	55
	T2	29	14.5	56.5
	T3	25.5	23	51.5
	T4	15.5	8.5	76
Oropharyngeal walls	T1	75	0	25
	T2	70	10	20
	T3	33	22.5	44.5
	T4	24	24	52
Supraglottic larynx	T1	61	10	29
	T2	58.5	16	25.5
	T3	35.5	25	39.5
	T4	41	18	41
Hypopharynx	T1	37	21	42
	T2	30.5	20.5	49
	T3	21	25.5	53.5
	T4	26.5	15	58.5
Nasopharynx	T1	7.5	11	81.5
	T2	15.5	12.5	72
	T3	11.5	9	79.5
	T4	17.5	5.5	77.5

(From Lindberg R: Cancer 37:1901, 1976.)

surgical exposure, and are discontinuous from the jugular chain and not encompassed in a routine neck dissection.

The remainder of the jugular chain is divided into upper, middle, and lower groups. These lie in intimate relation to the internal jugular vein. Neck dissections that preserve this vessel must strip the adventitia of the vein. The lowest jugular nodes removed during routine neck dissection lie about two fingerbreadths above the clavicle (to avoid damaging the large lymphatics at the root of the neck), and this is at the level of the omohyoid muscle tendon. Therefore, the important regions of the jugular chain are removed with supra-

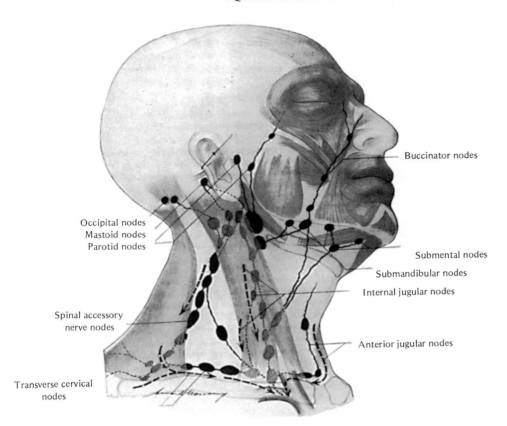

Buccinator nodes

Occipital nodes
Mastoid nodes
Parotid nodes

Submental nodes

Submandibular nodes

Internal jugular nodes

Spinal accessory
nerve nodes

Anterior jugular nodes

Transverse cervical
nodes

Fig. 20–6. Cervical lymph node groups involved from cancers of the head and neck. (From Rouvière H: Anatomie des lymphatiques de l'homme. Paris, Masson, 1932.)

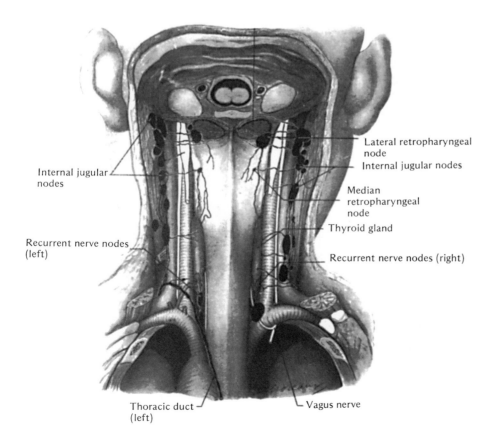

Lateral retropharyngeal
node

Internal jugular nodes

Internal jugular
nodes

Median
retropharyngeal
node

Thyroid gland

Recurrent nerve nodes
(left)

Recurrent nerve nodes (right)

Thoracic duct
(left)

Vagus nerve

Fig. 20–7. Lymphatic drainage of the pharynx. (From Rouvière H: Anatomie des lymphatiques de l'homme. Paris, Masson, 1932.)

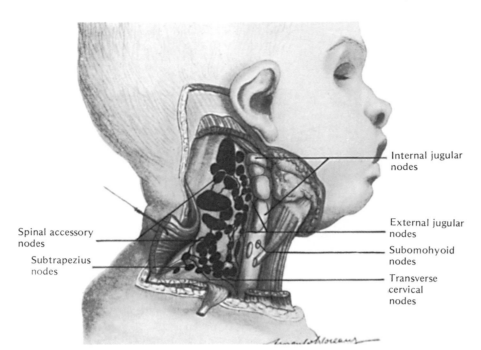

Fig. 20–8. Detail of posterior triangle and supraclavicular lymph nodes. (From Rouvière H: Anatomie des lymphatiques de l'homme. Paris, Masson, 1932.)

omohyoid neck dissection (see subsequent paragraphs).

Lymph nodes of the spinal accessory chain are distributed along the course of the eleventh cranial nerve in the posterior triangle and tend to be superficial (Fig. 20–8). In general, with primary cancers of the oral cavity, posterior triangle nodes are involved only when cancer cells are carried retrograde in lymphatics blocked by massive infestation of the jugular lymph nodes.[94] The posterior triangle nodes can be involved with primary tumors of the tonsil, base of the tongue, and posterior pharyngeal wall (rarely).

Several lymph nodes occur in association with the submandibular gland, the undersurface of the mandible, and the facial vein. These lie outside the substance of the gland and are referred to as pre- and postglandular nodes. They drain the lips, FOM, buccal mucosa, upper and lower gingivae, nasal vestibule, and skin of the anterior face. Excision of the submandibular gland in neck dissection is done primarily to allow clearance of these nodes because the gland itself is rarely involved by cancer.[95]

Submental lymph nodes lie in the midline between the anterior bellies of the digastric muscles external to the mylohyoid muscle. They drain the lip, chin, cheeks, and to a lesser extent the FOM, lower anterior gingivae, and tip of the tongue. Efferent vessels drain to the submandibular and subdigastric lymph nodes. The submental nodes are seldom involved primarily (Fig. 20–9). In nodal staging, midline lymph nodes are considered homolateral to the primary lesion.

Bilateral lymphatic metastases occur where lymphatics are abundant or when lesions invade muscle, and they tend to occur with midline primary sites where lymphatic drainage is bilateral, such as the soft palate, base of the tongue, posterior pharyngeal wall, and FOM.

Cancer spread to the contralateral side of the neck can occur in three ways[96]:

1. By way of crossing efferent lymphatic vessels.
2. By way of efferent lymphatic vessels after regional lymph nodes are involved by cancer and collateral lymphatic flow occurs.
3. In areas without a discrete midline barrier and with a rich lymphatic network: anterior FOM, na-

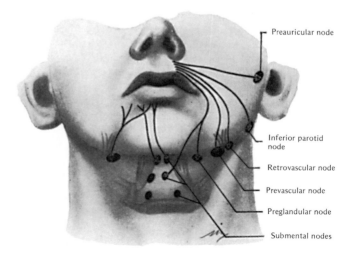

Fig. 20–9. Submental and submandibular lymph nodes. (From Rouvière H: Anatomie des lymphatiques de l'homme. Paris, Masson, 1932.)

sopharynx, soft palate, base of the tongue, base of the epiglottis, thyroid, cervical esophagus, trachea, postcricoid larynx.

Contralateral spread may occur from lateralized lesions in the vicinity of large lymphatics with cross-communications (lip, FOM, base of tongue). Although cervical lymphatics contain valves, retrograde flow may occur after distal lymphatic obstruction, which can occur secondary to tumor infiltration or scarring from RT or surgery. Unusual metastatic patterns in previously untreated patients may represent "skip" metastases or metastasis from a second primary tumor (which should be sought).

Spread to mediastinal nodes is rare from SCC of the head and neck, occurring in about 3% of cases.

Two patterns of cancer spread to cervical lymph nodes deserve special mention: (1) supraclavicular metastases and (2) the situation of the "unknown primary tumor."[70,97] The supraclavicular lymph nodes (transverse cervical chain) lie above the clavicle posterior to the sternocleidomastoid muscle origin and communicate with the spinal accessory chain (see Fig. 20–8). They receive lymphatic flow from the head and neck, ipsilateral upper extremity, breast, thorax, and abdomen. Disease in Virchow's node is palpable in the left supraclavicular area.

The significance of spread to the supraclavicular lymph nodes is that it rarely occurs as the *only* manifestation of the primary SCC of the head and neck, and it usually represents metastatic spread from an *infraclavicular* primary tumor. In this situation, tissue diagnosis can be achieved by fine-needle aspiration cytology and generally reveals either SCC or adenocarcinoma. Workup includes a chest radiograph, blood chemistry, history, and physical examination; findings determine the need for additional studies. CT scan of the chest and abdomen is considered worthwhile by some clinicians, but usually, in the absence of laboratory abnormalities or signs and symptoms that would indicate an organ source, extensive radiologic workup to look for the primary tumor is a case of diminishing returns. The infraclavicular "unknown primary tumor" frequently does not manifest itself before the patient's death, which is typically within 6 months of diagnosis of neck metastases. The standard treatment for the neck metastasis is palliative RT.

The situation of the "unknown primary tumor" refers to a patient presenting with cervical metastases with no apparent primary carcinoma detectable in the mucosa of the UADT. This occurs in about 10% of UADT SCCs. One literature review showed an incidence, compiled from the clinicopathologic literature, of 4% (range, 1 to 9%).[49] As Martin and Morfit pointed out in the 1940s, it was "not generally realized that cervical metastasis frequently occurs as the initial, and, for a time, the only symptom from an otherwise silent primary malignant tumor in the upper respiratory or alimentary tracts,"[97] and this misconception persists to a lesser extent today. Patients are frequently referred by internists to surgeons who are not familiar with the manifestations of head and neck SCC for neck node biopsy. A tissue diagnosis is obtained, but the primary tumor may not be searched for, much to the patient's detriment.

A firm, lateralized neck mass in a smoker can be assumed to represent metastatic SCC from a primary tumor originating in the mucosa of the UADT above the clavicle until proved otherwise. The first step is for a specialist to perform a complete head and neck examination. The primary tumor is identified in 90 to 95% of patients without difficulty. If no tumor is identifiable, panendoscopy is usually performed next, and some surgeons perform random (not "blind") biopsies from the sites shown to be the likely origins of occult primary tumors: nasopharynx, tonsil, base of the tongue, and piriform sinus. Random biopsy can reveal microscopic cancer, but it is generally a low-yield procedure unless mucosal friability is present. A serially sectioned upsilateral tonsillectomy specimen can reveal a microscopic primary tumor. In such a situation, the patient can be spared bilateral wide-field RT with its attendant morbidity of profound xerostomia.

If no tumor is identified by these methods, tissue from the neck mass must be obtained by needle aspiration or open biopsy. A large-bore needle biopsy is not recommended because of the potential for tumor seeding of the needle tract. A fine-needle aspiration biopsy is an acceptable technique that is accurate for certain types of cancer, including SCC, when interpreted by an experienced cytopathologist.[98] Negative aspiration cytology does not rule out cancer in a clinically suspicious lesion, and open biopsy should then be performed.

An open-neck biopsy should be excisional if possible. One should be prepared to do a neck dissection at the time of diagnostic biopsy if metastatic SCC is revealed on frozen section. Alternatively, the incision may be closed and RT administered to both sides of the neck and the likely sites for occult primary tumor. A full course of RT to both sides of the neck and the "unknown primary ports" is associated with much morbidity, which results from drying out of all the salivary glands (specifically *both* parotids), and local control of the tumor is equivalent with neck dissection (or total excisional biopsy) and postoperative RT to the affected side of the neck, with close observation of likely primary sites for eventual tumor development.[99]

Biopsy of metastatic cervical SCC without concomitant care of the entire neck and any associated primary lesion has been associated with increased wound complications, local recurrence, and DM and is therefore detrimental to the patient's survival.[100–102] The attribution of this detrimental outcome to an incisional versus excisional biopsy of the metastatic neck cancer[100] is erroneous, if proper definitive treatment follows within a short period of diagnosis.[103,103a] The detrimental outcome in respect to survival is related more to the metastatic neck cancer than to biopsy, which, as is mentioned elsewhere, is the primary predictor of DM and a fatal outcome.

Various series show that only 30 to 40% of occult ("unknown primary") tumors are identified within a 5-year period after initial treatment of the neck metastasis if the primary sites remain untreated. In such a situation, two thirds of all lesions appear during the first 18 months. The prognosis for these patients is said to be worse than for those for in whom the primary tumor remains undetected. The ultimate poor prognosis, however, is related to the presentation of the tumor in metastatic form. The 3-year survival rate after single-modality RT or surgery to the primary sites and the neck is 35 to 40%.[104]

Neck masses in children are usually inflammatory or congenital. Neoplasms are almost always nonsquamous cell.[105] An open biopsy is more often appropriate because many of the entities are difficult to identify by needle aspiration cytology alone (e.g., lymphoma).

Distant Metastases

DMs, presumably derived from contamination of the circulation (lymphatic and hematogenous) with cancer cells, are discussed in the sections of this chapter on tumor biology and natural history.

Cancer Patterns in Recurrent Disease

Regrowth of cancer at the *primary* tumor site most likely results from residual tumor cells that were not removed or killed by previous treatment (surgery, RT, or chemotherapy). Theoretic sources of regrowth at the primary site include the following:

1. "Field cancerization," which is malignant transformation in an adjacent area of "condemned mucosa."
2. "Seeding" of operative wounds. In the 1960s, studies were performed on the cells obtained from wound washings, and the aggregate conclusions support the finding that this mechanism occurs rarely, if at all.[106] Most experienced head and neck surgeons, however, have seen tumor regrowth patterns in a previously operated field that are almost unequivocally related to this mechanism, such as regrowth in the area undermined during elevation of a local rotation-advancement flap or seeding of an incision without other associated recurrent disease. Methods to decrease intraoperative seeding by cancer cells have been summarized.[107]
3. Inflammatory oncotaxis is another theoretic

method of regrowth of tumor at the primary site in which dormant or circulating tumor cells are attracted to an area of inflammation that can result from surgery or RT.[108]

Regrowth of tumor in the neck can originate from seeding from an uncontrolled or recurrent primary tumor, tumor regrowth in lymph nodes not removed during neck dissection, or regrowth of cancer cells that contaminated the soft tissues of the neck (extracapsular spread).

Recurrent massive disease at the primary site or in the neck often causes retrograde spread through the lymphatics resulting in atypical patterns of disease presentation such as spread to the contralateral neck or skull base. In the context of recurrent disease, direct permeation is found more often than embolization. When cancer recurs after previous treatment, one must assume that the entire field occupied by the original tumor remains contaminated by cancer cells because, after chemotherapy or RT, the tumor does not shrink in a cohesive centripetal manner but rather leaves multifocal cancer nests throughout the extent of the previous tumor. Similarly, after surgery, any scar present must be assumed to be contaminated with cancer cells.

It is frequently difficult to assess the extent of recurrent disease in a previously treated field. A significant submucosal component may exist at the primary site, and recurrent neck disease often seems to originate deeply and sometimes has surrounded critical structures (carotid artery, brachial plexus) by the time it is unequivocally demonstrable at the surface. The examiner generally has a sensation of a "vague fullness" in both situations before the recurrent tumor becomes obvious. Compression of structures can cause problematic symptoms such as syncope[109] and pain.

Histologic confirmation of recurrent tumor may also be difficult to obtain because of the scattered nature of the cells and the histologic changes caused by previous surgery and RT. Repeat biopsies may be necessary, and occasionally reoperation must be performed based on clinical suspicion without a tissue diagnosis (with appropriately detailed informed consent, of course).

Obtaining a baseline post-treatment CT or MR scan can provide a useful reference point to assess changes if clinical suspicion of recurrent cancer arises. This is usually performed about a month after the end of postoperative RT and documents post-treatment anatomy, which can later be used for comparison to diagnose recurrent tumor.

Two disease patterns frequently associated with massive recurrence at the primary site or in the neck deserve special mention: dermal metastases and skull base recurrences. Dermal or skin metastases typically occur in previously treated patients with advanced recurrent SCC (Fig. 20–10) and presumably represent embolic cancer deposits carried by retrograde flow in

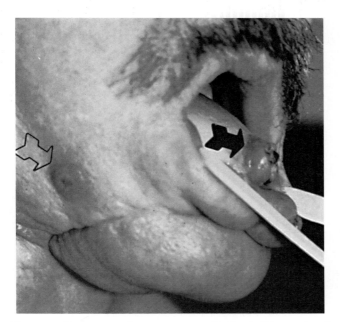

Fig. 20–10. Recurrent oral cancer at pectoralis flap (solid arrow) and dermal metastasis (open arrow).

the capillary lymphatics to the dermis. Once dermal penetration has occurred, spread is diffuse, and the treatment goal is palliation, usually with RT or chemotherapy. Surgery is unwarranted because cancer quickly regrows at the margins of even wide excisions. Unless the skin manifestation is thought to represent isolated disease in a surgical scar arising from tumor implantation at the time of prior excision, reoperation is pointless. Differentiating between these two forms of skin recurrence is obviously difficult.

Disease at the skull base occurs rarely in previously untreated patients or, much more commonly, as a manifestation of recurrent disease either alone or in combination with recurrence at the primary site or in the neck. In previously untreated patients, it presumably represents cancer in retropharyngeal lymph nodes (see Fig. 20–7) and should be searched for on preoperative CT (Fig. 20–11) and by specific questioning during history taking. Lateralized head pain, particularly in the retro-orbital and ipsilateral forehead areas, is suspicious, as is pain on neck flexion or extension.[110]

In the context of recurrent disease, the appearance of skull base disease is frequently a harbinger of DM (within 3 to 4 months). This failure pattern may have the appearance of discrete, circumscribed lymphadenopathy or of a more diffuse tissue involvement with or without bone erosion. The pathogenesis of cancer regrowth at the skull base includes growth of cancer in undissected retropharyngeal lymph nodes, retrograde spread through lymphatics or Batson's venous plexus, or direct cephalad extension from recurrent disease elsewhere in the head and neck. Risk factors for development of disease in retropharyngeal lymph nodes include the following:

1. A primary tumor of any size in the posterior pharyngeal wall.
2. Positive cervical lymphadenopathy.
3. A massive tumor anywhere in the oral cavity or oropharynx that may obstruct local lymphatics and result in retrograde embolization to skull base lymph nodes.

Because patients with recurrent cancer are generally heavily pretreated, additional treatment options are limited, and, in a personal series, chemotherapy was found to be more effective than additional RT in palliating these patients' frequently excruciating pain. Neurosurgical percutaneous cordotomy is an option for nerve compression-related pain (e.g., brachial plexus) uncontrolled by analgesics. Stereotactic radiosurgery ("gamma knife") is a new option under investigation.[111] Principles of managing chronic cancer pain are different from those for acute (e.g., postoperative) pain and are reviewed elsewhere.[112–115]

Prognostic Factors

Prognostic factors are those that presumably help to predict the outcome in an individual cancer patient. An *individual* cancer patient is not a *series* of cancer patients. In an individual patient, a relevant factor is either present or absent—the "all-or-none" phenomenon. For example, neck lymph nodes are either positive or negative in an individual, whereas in a series of 100 patients with similar primary tumors, 20 might manifest metastatic spread to the neck. Any maneuver that helps to define the prognosis in an individual definitively, therefore, has at least theoretic use over the application to the individual of statistics that relate to a series of patients derived from retrospective analysis.

For example, the literature may indicate that patients with T2N0 SCCs of the tongue have a 30% chance of harboring occult metastases in neck lymph nodes. A properly performed and processed elective functional neck dissection specimen, however, objectively answers whether or not a particular patient has cancer in the neck lymph nodes. Knowing this can influence treatment planning. For example, planned postoperative RT, which seemed indicated initially to sterilize a putatively significant likelihood of occult neck cancer, may no longer be indicated if the neck operation has proved that no positive lymph nodes are present.

TNM staging has not proved adequate to predict *individual* prognosis, namely, which patients will have a favorable and which will have an unfavorable outcome.[116] This is because many relevant aspects of the tumor-host interaction are not taken into account by simple TNM staging. Moreover, each stage includes biologically diverse subcategories. For example, a patient with head and neck cancer is placed in stage IV if he or she has a large primary tumor with no evidence

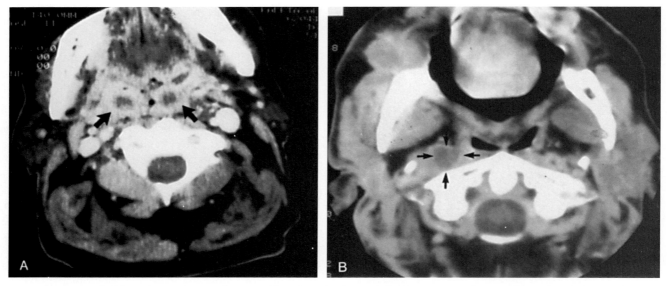

Fig. 20–11. A. Bilateral necrotic retropharyngeal lymph nodes (arrows). B. Necrotic retropharyngeal lymph node (arrows).

of metastases to the neck or distantly, *or* a small primary tumor with large neck metastases, *or* a small primary tumor without neck metastases but with DMs. Each of these three subcategories is associated with progressively less likelihood of survival, although they are all grouped within stage IV. Probably, prognosis will ultimately be defined by molecular and genetic parameters that remain to be defined.[117] Intermediate between the imprecision of TNM staging and the theoretic accuracy of the future lie a variety of useful histopathologic parameters (see subsequent paragraphs).

For patients with head and neck SCC, certain *tumor* (primary and neck) and *patient* variables are cited as having prognostic significance. Attributing survival significance to an *individual* prognostic variable is probably invalid in view of the complexity of the tumor-host interaction and the many factors (tumor, patient, treatment) that inevitably influence the outcome. Studies that assess certain factors in a multivariate regression analysis overcome this objection to some extent, but still suffer from the defects of retrospective analysis.

Tumor Variables
For cancers in the oral cavity, oropharynx, and pharyngeal wall, "significant" prognostic factors with respect to the primary tumor include the tumor's *site, size,* and, to some extent, *histopathology.* Clinicians generally accept (again, with dissenting data available in the literature) that as the *size* of the primary tumor increases, the patient's curability decreases. This undoubtedly relates at least partly to the finding that large tumors are generally deeply infiltrative and therefore presumably have greater access to regional lymphatics and a greater opportunity to metastasize. The proclivity to metastasize is not determined simply by anatomic

proximity to lymphatic or vascular channels because metastasis involves a complex cascade of events.[91]

Traditional dogma holds that as the *site* of the primary tumor progresses from anterior to posterior (oral tongue to base of tongue to oropharynx to pharynx), the prognosis becomes worse. The initial attribution of this phenomenon to the finding that posteriorly located tumors have inherently greater malignant potential has been questioned.[118] Rather than relating to inherent biologic aggressiveness, this may merely indicate that posteriorly located tumors tend to have achieved a large size (which correlates with increased incidence of neck metastases) because they originate in clinically "silent" areas and do not cause symptoms until they become large.

Of all prognostic parameters, *histologic grade* of the primary tumor is considered to be the least informative for head and neck SCC. Poorly differentiated tumors generally tend to have a faster growth rate and a greater tendency to metastasize early and more frequently than well- or moderately well-differentiated tumors.[119]

Clinicians generally accept that endophytic invasive tumors are less favorable than exophytic superficial lesions.[32] Deep tumors presumably gain access to blood and lymph vessels favoring diffuse local and regional and distant spread and are also more resistant to RT because of the anoxic environment.[120–122]

Other histopathologic features also appear to be of significance. The pattern of invasion at the tumor-host interface has been correlated with prognosis (mainly in the European literature, "Jakobsson criteria"[74]). Once again, this is related to the proclivity for metastatic spread. An ill-defined, jagged pattern at the interface with dissociated clumps of cells penetrating the adjacent interstitium has greater likelihood for local recurrence and metastatic spread than a tumor with a well-circumscribed, smooth, pushing border.[123–125]

In the literature, attention is also being directed to the measured depth of the tumor as a significant prognosticator for an SCC of the head and neck, similar to Breslow's[126] melanoma staging.[127–129] At this point, no agreement exists on what constitutes a worrisome thickness (2 to 10 mm), and evaluation of such parameters is subject to sampling error.

The most significant prognosticator for head and neck SCC is the presence or absence of cervical lymph node metastases.[1] A widely accepted adage is that the cure rate for SCC of the head and neck decreases by at least 50% when cervical metastases are present. In previous decades, this reflected relative inability to control cervical disease, and patients often died *because of* the cancer in their neck. Although our ability to control local-regional disease has improved (see subsequent paragraphs), cervical metastases are still a poor prognostic sign, but *not* because they serve as depots that shed cells and are thereby instigators of DM, or because the patient's death is necessarily related to disease of the neck. Rather, the presence of cervical metastases (clinically palpable or occult) indicates that the tumor has the ability to spread in that particular individual, and in most of these individuals, DM will appear if the patients survive long enough. Thus, the presence of positive cervical adenopathy is an indicator of systemic disease in the individual patient and therefore of a likely fatal outcome in the current absence of effective treatment against the systemic cancer component.

Certain features of the primary tumor tend to predict spread to the neck (Tables 20–5 through 20–8); these features are size, histologic differentiation, and site. One large study,[119] which looked at the histologic rather than the clinical status of neck nodes, defined three site clusters as having increasing metastatic potential:

Cluster 1: Lip, buccal mucosa, hard palate, gingiva.
Cluster 2: Oral tongue (anterior two thirds), FOM.
Cluster 3: Oropharynx, base of tongue.

The incidence of neck metastases as related to primary tumor site is shown in Tables 20–5 through 20–8.

Increase in the size of the primary tumor has been correlated with increased frequency of multiple unilateral, bilateral, and "fixed" neck metastases for cancers of the tongue, FOM, retromolar trigone, anterior faucial pillar, soft palate, and oropharyngeal wall.[93] This correlation was not seen for tumors of the tonsillar fossa and base of tongue (see Table 20–5).

The ultimate significance of cervical metastases is related to their importance as predictors of systemic disease, but in the literature on head and neck cancer, certain individual features of neck disease have been imbued with prognostic significance. Because results are usually reported as survival rather than as sites of treatment failure, it is unclear whether the poor prognosis associated with individual neck lymph node variables is related to patients' dying from disease in the neck or from DMs. Poor prognosis has been associated with positive lymph nodes in the inferior jugular chain and posterior triangle, contralateral or bilateral posi-

TABLE 20–6. Incidence of Clinically Palpable Cervical Metastases Present Initially and Later in the Course of Disease, and of Occult Cervical Metastases by Site of Primary Tumor

Site	Percentage of Patients		
	N+ at Presentation	N0 Clinically N+ Pathologically	N0 Clinically → N+ Clinically with N0 Neck Treatment
Floor of mouth	30–59	40–50	20–35
Gingiva	18–52	19	17
Hard palate	13–24		22
Buccal mucosa	9–31		16
Oral tongue	34–65	25–54	38–52
Nasopharynx	86–90		19–50
Anterior tonsillar pillar/retromolar trigone	39–56		
Soft palate/uvula	37–56		16–25
Tonsillar fossa	58–76		22
Base of tongue	50–83	22	
Pharyngeal walls	50–71	66	
Supraglottic larynx	31–54	16–26	33
Hypopharynx	52–72	38	

* T1 N0 patients only.

† Patients received preoperative radiation.

(From Mendenhall WM, et al: Head Neck Surg 3:15, 1980.)

TABLE 20–7. Incidence of Cervical Metastases by Site Based on Histologic Examination of the Primary Lesion in 699 Cases from Memorial-Sloan Kettering Hospital

Primary Site	Patients with Negative Nodes	Patients with Clinically and Histologically Positive Nodes	Patients with Clinically Negative and Histologically Positive Nodes	Total Number of Patients
Tongue	62	113	38	213
Floor of mouth	73	60	23	156
Tonsil	33	62	18	113
Gingiva	59	27	16	102
Palate	31	17	7	55
Buccal mucosa	25	23	5	53
Lip	4	3		7
Totals	287	305	107	699

(From Strong EW and Spiro RH: Arch Surg 107:382, 1972.)

TABLE 20–8. Incidence of Cervical Metastases Related to Several Characteristics of the Primary Tumor Based on Histological Study of 898 Cases

By Site of Primary

Site	Metastases Absent		Metastases Present		Total No.
	No.	Percentage (%)	No.	Percentage (%)	
Lip	32	63	19	37	51
Anterior tongue	74	41	107	59	181
Posterior tongue	20	17	97	83	117
Mouth floor	66	48	77	52	143
Cheek mucosa	32	50	32	50	64
Hard palate	8	47	9	53	17
Gingiva	40	54	34	46	74
Oropharynx	56	22	195	78	251
	328	37	570	63	898

By Size of Primary

Size (cm)	Metastases Absent		Metastases Present		Total No.
	No.	Percentage (%)	No.	Percentage (%)	
<1	12	55	10	45	22
1 to <2	27	49	28	51	55
2 to <3	87	53	78	47	165
3 to <4	93	38	152	62	245
4 or more	109	27	302	73	411
	328	37	570	63	898

By Differentiation of Primary

	Metastases Absent		Metastases Present		Total No.
	No.	Percentage (%)	No.	Percentage (%)	
Well differentiated	33	52	31	48	64
Moderately differentiated	243	43	324	57	567
Poorly differentiated	52	19	215	81	267
	328	37	570	63	898

(Modified from Shear M, et al: Cancer 37:1901, 1976.)

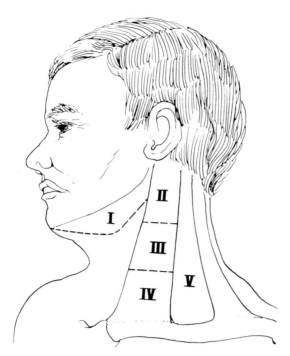

Fig. 20–12. Levels of lymph node involvement that have been designated for prognostic significance. (From Strong EW and Spiro RH: Cancer of the oral cavity. In: Cancer of the Head and Neck. Edited by Suen J and Myers E. New York, Churchill Livingstone, 1981.)

tive lymph nodes, and multiple lymph nodes at multiple levels or in noncontiguous areas. (The neck is frequently divided into levels I through V for purposes of description; Fig. 20–12.)

The literature has particularly directed attention to the significance of extranodal or extracapsular cancer spread.[130] This denotes involvement of or rupture of the lymph node capsule and extension of tumor into the soft tissue of the neck. Disease in the soft tissue of the neck is aggressive, with potential for recurrence leading directly to decreased survival because of major vessel rupture, for example.[131] Although a "node" larger than 3 cm usually represents confluence of multiple lymph nodes or soft tissue extension, studies have shown that lymph node rupture can be present in a significant proportion of N0 necks (where no disease is palpable). In one study, 50% of clinically N0 necks contained tumors and 13% showed capsular rupture.[132] In other series, neck lymph nodes 1 cm or less in size were associated with a 22% incidence of extracapsular spread, whereas lymph nodes greater than 3 cm showed such spread in almost 75% of cases.[2,133]

Patient Variables

Clinicians widely believe that young patients with SCC have a poorer prognosis than elderly patients. Many papers have addressed the topic of SCC of the head and neck in patients 30 to 40 years old.[134,135] Many treatment managers hold the belief that young patients tend to have biologically aggressive tumors and disproportionately poorer survival rates; however, the literature differs on this issue.

Most articles stress the similarities in cancer behavior in young and older age groups. Despite an age of 30 to 40 years, many of these patients have accumulated the requisite 15- to 20-pack-year history of tobacco product use, which is the primary etiologic agent for SCC of the head and neck. No one has suggested that SCC in the young age group is *less* aggressive than in elderly patients, and treatment should certainly be equally aggressive. Reports from tertiary-care referral centers tend to present results that are distorted when compared with the unreferred or "general" cancer population because they are composed of a larger proportion of patients with advanced or previously treated tumors or other unfavorable situations. Whether the prognosis of younger patients with head and neck SCC is worse than that of their older counterparts at a similar disease stage, provided both receive equally aggressive treatment, is a question that remains unanswered.

Patients with significant tobacco and alcohol habits have decreased survival rates because of intercurrent disease, tumor problems, and second primary cancers, and according to one series,[136] this difference between users and nonusers is not explained by difference in tumor stage, patient age, or type of therapy. Decreased immunocompetence in tobacco and alcohol users may be relevant in this regard. These data contradict another belief, held by many, that the relatively rare SCC of the head and neck occurring in nonsmokers is biologically more aggressive. In fact, almost no data have been accumulated on this point.

TREATMENT PRINCIPLES

An infrequently expressed truth is that the prognosis of patients with SCC of the head and neck also depends on the expertise of the people treating them. Surgeons must be able to remove tumors with a margin of normal tissue while, one hopes, preserving function whenever possible, and radiotherapists must be able to treat the wide fields necessary without compromising tumor dose or causing unusual regional morbidity. The patient's treatment plan should never be dictated by limitations of the physician's ability. Because head and neck cancer is relatively rare and difficult to control, many clinicians believe that these patients are best served by being referred to physicians who specialize in head and neck oncology, rather than being treated by general otolaryngologists who are "occasional" cancer surgeons.[137,138] Special expertise on the part of the radiotherapist is also vital.

Overview

Tumor biology principles relevant to deciding treatment for head and neck cancer patients are described earlier in this chapter. The first treatment principle is that the initial therapy of any cancer offers the best chance for cure. Salvage attempts in recurrent cancers are notoriously unsuccessful. One must decide whether the treatment goal in the individual patient is palliation or cure. Treatment with curative intent is generally appropriate in previously untreated patients, especially those without positive neck lymph nodes. On rare occasions, a previously untreated patient presents with massive disease that is considered technically unresectable, and in this case, the patient is unlikely to be cured. The definition of resectability varies with the experience and expertise of the surgeon. The treatment goal in patients with recurrent cancer is more often palliation. Repeated aggressive treatment attempts, however, are occasionally rewarded by long-term survival of the patient. Deciding the appropriate treatment for the individual patient requires considerable experience on the part of the treatment manager. One hopes that in the future a scientific basis for treatment planning will emerge, based on data accumulated from prospective randomized clinical trials.

The overall goal of palliation or cure is decided on the basis of tumor factors and patient factors.[139]

Tumor factors include histologic diagnosis, anatomic site, extent and invasiveness of primary tumor, presence or absence of cervical adenopathy, likelihood of occult metastasis or DMs, and history or presence of multiple primary tumors. *Patient factors* include medical condition, smoking and alcohol habits, reliability in follow-up, intelligence, motivation to cooperate with therapy and rehabilitation, overall attitude (positive, negative), and family support structure.

As explained previously, the role of the surgeon or radiotherapist is to control local-regional disease, and the "curability" of patients is limited by the phenomenon of DM and by intercurrent disease (deaths unrelated to cancer), significant in this patient population, which has typically abused multiple organ systems with the effects of smoking and alcohol habits. Because overall survivability is limited, secondary treatment considerations related to the patient's occupation and hobbies should be taken into consideration because one should preserve optimal function for as long as possible.

In the absence of randomized prospective trials to provide a scientific underpinning for treatment, fluctuations in treatment philosophy persist. Full-course RT appears to be giving way to initial operation for oral cancer because of poor control rates and high postradiation complication rates. More mandible-sparing operations are being undertaken with planned postoperative RT.[140,141]

The patient should be involved in making the treatment decision and should be told which treatment plan is recommended as most likely to achieve local-regional control and that all possible treatments are not equally effective. A description of the unpleasant consequences of failure to control disease in the head and neck helps give the patient perspective and motivation to cooperate with the difficult treatment and post-treatment course.

Although many cancers are technically resectable, not every patient is a suitable candidate for radical "high-tech" operations because of both physical and psychologic considerations. The patient must be intelligent enough to appreciate the possible risks and complications and must be able to cooperate in a motivated way with postoperative rehabilitation. Similar understanding and support from family members is also highly desirable. Patients who lack the educational and socioeconomic background to participate in their own rehabilitation or to understand the reasons for the treatment undertaken or who, for example, are influenced by unscientific personal beliefs (such as that if cancer is "opened to the air" it spreads like wildfire and an unfavorable outcome is inevitable) probably do better in adjusting to treatment that emphasizes nonsurgical modalities.

The surgeon should also be sure that the patient and the family fully understand the nature of the proposed treatment and rehabilitation. In my experience, the trauma of being informed of the diagnosis of cancer interferes with the patient's ability to comprehend the technical details of the treatment plan initially, and I personally attempt to have three lengthy sessions with each patient before performing any surgery. With each subsequent session, additional details "register" in the patient's mind, and preoperatively the patient should be able to outline (without coaching) the treatment plan and goals and the type of operation to be performed, with its potential risks, complications, and possible postoperative sequelae in respect to cosmesis and function. These considerations are seldom addressed in the literature, but head and neck surgical oncology involves many aspects other than learning surgical technique. In each case, the tumor is growing in an individual who has many fears and concerns that must be addressed in addition to simply planning appropriate treatment on the basis of tumor characteristics.

Therapeutic Modalities

Therapeutic modalities in common use for treating SCC of the head and neck include surgery, RT, and chemotherapy. In treatment planning, the pros and cons of each modality must be evaluated.

Generally, stage I and II tumors (T1, T2, N0) can be controlled equally well with surgery *or* RT as single modalities. Determinant survivals for this magnitude of disease are favorable (in the range of 65 to 75%) because of the small size of the primary tumor and the lack of metastatic spread. The decision for surgery or RT is influenced by a variety of tumor and patient factors. For example, RT might be the best choice for a small lesion anatomically related to any neurovascular bundle, which has a pathway to the base of skull (e.g., small palate cancer adjacent to greater palatine neurovascular bundle) because the entire course of the nerve could be encompassed in the RT port. Similarly, all other things being equal, a gainfully employed patient might prefer an operation with a short convalescent period rather than appearing for daily treatments for 7 weeks.

The ability to control local-regional disease or to cure the patient decreases as the primary tumor increases in size (T3 or T4) and with the addition of positive cervical adenopathy. A *planned* combination of surgery and RT is generally considered necessary for the physician to have any chance to control stage III and IV disease. Long-term survival for patients with stage III and IV disease is in the range of 20 to 30% at best because of large primary tumors and the presence of positive lymph nodes. The frequent inadequacy of this combination has led in recent years to the addition of chemotherapy in an attempt to control advanced disease (see subsequent paragraphs). The failure of adjuvant chemotherapy to provide a survival advantage to patients with advanced SCC of the head and neck makes the following statement accurate: planned combined surgery with RT is the treatment of choice for advanced SCC of the head and neck.

For disease extent of which either surgery or RT has an equal likelihood of achieving local control, patients usually choose RT because of the presumed cosmetic and functional consequences of surgery. With modern technology (laser), conservation ablative surgery, and sophisticated reconstructive techniques, this difference is no longer so compelling. Moreover, the morbidity of RT with curative intent to the head and neck (dry mouth, etc.) is not insignificant, and for other theoretic and actual reasons, surgery may, in fact, be preferable (see subsequent paragraphs).

Clinicians generally accept that RT with curative intent or "full-course" RT is most likely to succeed in small, superficial cancers. Many surgeons believe that if a tumor is big enough to see and feel (with the possible exception of superficial mucosal disease at the primary site and N1 disease in the neck), RT cannot reliably control the disease. When RT is used alone for more advanced disease, the goal is often palliation, with cures expected in only 10% of cases. The philosophy held by some of using initial RT with curative intent for *all* lesions and holding surgery in reserve for recurrent or persistent cancer is risky because salvage surgery is usually unsuccessful, and the complications associated with full-course RT to the oral cavity can be significant. The use of "elective" RT for subclinical disease at the primary site and the neck is discussed in the subsequent sections of this chapter on surgery, combined therapy, and management of neck disease.

Surgery should be used for large lesions or those with invasive characteristics in the soft tissue and bone. Surgery is also advantageous for extensive areas of dyskeratoses and diffuse mucosal changes, especially when the laser is used.[142] Surgery is theoretically preferable in young patients, who may survive long enough to develop RT-induced cancers later in life.[143] As a staging procedure, surgery can define the extent of disease in the individual patient. Operation or reoperation is generally chosen for recurrent cancer in the head and neck.

If the decision is for initial surgery, either alone or to be followed by RT, the operation should ideally be performed soon after the diagnosis is made, allowing time for adequate patient preparation. If RT is to be the initial treatment, the patient's dental situation needs to be evaluated, and any teeth that require extraction should be removed at least 10 (and probably 21) days before beginning treatment, based on Marx and Johnson's work.[144]

Radiotherapy With Curative Intent

A basic principle in deciding to choose RT for a patient is that exophytic, well-oxygenated tumors are more radioresponsive than erosive, infiltrative, hypoxic tumors. Small, superficial mucosal lesions are potentially curable by RT, whereas invasive tumors with bone and deep soft tissue involvement are generally not, although this dogma has been challenged in the literature.[145] Single-modality RT is generally considered inadequate for palpable neck disease greater than N1.

Full-course RT for head and neck SCC typically consists of a total dose of 60 to 70 Gy delivered in fractionated doses of 2 Gy per day on weekdays over 6½ to 7 weeks. For principles of RT, see the general references.

X-rays and electrons generated by machines and gamma photons generated by large isotope sources can be used to treat the body at a distance from the source of radiation (teletherapy). These forms of external beam radiation are used to irradiate the majority of cancer patients who receive RT. Other methods of applying radiation are intracavitary insertion and interstitial implantation of isotopes (brachytherapy). The external beam component is directed against the superficial mucosal extent. The application of an interstitial form of radiation is designed to deliver a high dose to the penetrating, presumably hypoxic, tumor core. SCCs of the tongue and FOM are often treated (especially in Europe) by external beam radiation plus interstitial implantation of the tumor with radium needles or more commonly iridium wire in an afterloading form.[141,146] Afterloading refers to implantation of the tumor by plastic catheters (for head and neck SCC, usually under general anesthesia in the operating room), which are later loaded with active sources. This method, unlike direct implantation, prevents undue exposure of operators and personnel to radiation. Sutures loaded with iodine-125 (^{125}I) "seeds" that can be placed in a wound intraoperatively is another method of delivering interstitial radiation[147,148] (see subsequent section on recurrent disease).

Other methods of delivery of external beam RT currently under investigation, and unproved for SCC of the head and neck, include altered fractionation schemes which delivers more or less than 2 Cy per fraction and/or 2 more doses per day. The latter format is sometimes used in emergency RT for rapidly enlarging tumors (lymphomas). Delivery of radiation in multiple daily doses over shorter total periods reduces the possibility that the tumor can divide between fractions and has proved efficacy for tumors with a short doubling time and rapid cellular turnover.[149,150]

One may protect dose-limiting normal tissues by using a shrinking field technique. For example, for head and neck RT, the spinal cord is typically shielded after 40 Gy, and the total tumor dose up to the limit (65 to 70 Gy) is delivered by a "boost" to the smaller field.

Radiation does not cure all tumors, for a multitude of reasons related to the tumor, the host, and the treatment. Tumor factors that explain RT failures include the following:

1. Excessive numbers of clonogenic cells (too large a tumor burden).
2. Hypoxia-induced radioresistance.
3. Protraction of treatment time that allows cancer cell regeneration sometimes required to relieve acute RT morbidity.
4. Intrinsic radioresistance of the tumor cells.[151] (That radiation acts as a selective treatment modality on a heterogeneous cancer cell population is discussed in the section on tumor biology.)

The acute effects of radiation develop during or immediately after RT and tend to subside during the month following the end of RT. Late effects start after about 6 months and progress over time. Acute morbidity results from the effects of radiation on rapidly dividing cell populations and includes moist desquamation of skin and exudative mucositis of mucous membranes.

Late effects, on the other hand, develop in tissues with slowly dividing cell populations. Late radiation injury to vasculoconnective tissue is caused by excessive production of collagen, obliteration of small blood vessels, and luminal narrowing of large blood vessels. Compromise of blood supply to an irradiated area leads to poor wound healing after salvage surgery.

Collagen deposition secondarily entraps and obstructs lymphatic vessels and causes swelling of tissues (post-obstructive lymphedema) because interstitial fluid is normally drained by the obstructed lymphatic vessels. The collagen deposition also tends to stenose the lumen of any hollow viscus in the irradiated field. Damaged blood vessels result in ischemia, atrophy of mucous membranes, and sometimes ulceration of soft tissues and eventual necrosis of the irradiated tissue[144] (see subsequent section on complications of treatment).

After about 7 to 10 days of treatment, a local "tumoritis" develops at the primary site and demarcates the actual limits of the tumor clearly. Because of the potential for acute problems requiring nutritional support and analgesia, patients undergoing full-course RT should be seen by the head and neck surgeon every 2 weeks during their treatment. Patients usually lose about 10 pounds during full-course RT for SCC in the oral cavity, oropharynx, and pharynx. In patients who receive full-course RT, tumor response is evaluated 6 to 8 weeks after completion of RT because the tumor continues to shrink after the total dose is delivered.

When full-course RT is delivered as a combination of external beam and implants, the total dose delivered is frequently between 80 and 90 Gy. An external dose of 40 to 50 Gy is usually delivered first, followed by 20 to 25 Gy interstitially. Centers specializing in these techniques report phenomenal control of local disease. The long-term survival, however, is much poorer because of limiting factors reviewed earlier. For example, Pierequin and associates reported a 95% 4-year local control rate with 50% survival in patients with tongue cancers treated in this way.[146]

Heavy smokers and drinkers do not tolerate full-course RT well because of the already compromised status of their UADT mucosa. Full-course RT is indicated in patients who have prohibitive surgical risks (medically inoperable), a situation that is increasingly rare today when sophisticated medical care is available. In this situation, chemotherapy is sometimes an option as initial treatment (see subsequent section). Preoperative RT may also be needed in the rare patients whose lesions are technically unresectable because of massive primary tumor or "fixed" neck disease: 50 Gy is generally administered and, depending on the response (favorable or unfavorable), additional radiation progressing to full course or definitive surgery is then undertaken, respectively. Implantation techniques can also be considered in the latter context as a more effective way of delivering radiation to gross persistent disease.

With respect to complications of RT, of which the patient should be apprised, a profoundly dry mouth results unless one parotid gland is excluded from the radiation field because atrophy of all the salivary glands occurs when radiation is delivered to the primary site and both sides of the neck. The dry mouth, which persists for the rest of the patient's life, is the major morbidity accompanying full-course RT to the head and neck. The sensation is like that resulting from using a permanent scopolamine patch. This problem seems trivial only to those who do not have it. Because it can be avoided by sparing one parotid gland, the radiotherapist should investigate the actual status of neck disease in the ipsilateral or contralateral neck by means of elective functional neck dissection (see subsequent section) to spare the patient the necessity of having both sides of the neck irradiated postoperatively for prophylaxis against theoretically present occult disease. Sometimes the requirements for adequately irradiating the primary site necessitate that both parotid glands be irradiated; however, experienced head and neck radiotherapists can sometimes develop an innovative oblique beam delivery plan.

Another problem that results from full-course RT to the head and neck is in diagnosing persistent or recurrent disease. The area irradiated tends to be persistently edematous to some extent (most pronounced after larynx irradiation in the area of the arytenoid mucosa), and this can interfere with postoperative follow-up. Recurrences tend to have a major submucosal component, and persistent edema or induration is suspicious. A large biopsy must be taken, including tissue underneath the mucosa. This can expose underlying bone or cartilage, however, and predisposes the patient to the development of radionecrosis (see subsequent section). In addition, the histopathologic diagnosis is not always confirmed by biopsy because of radiation changes and the scattered nature of recurrent or persistent tumor cell foci, causing the clinical dilemma to persist. Woody induration in the neck progresses over time because of postradiation fibrosis and makes early determination of residual disease difficult.

Obstructive lymphedema in the irradiated tissues is also of concern to patients and can have consequences such as airway obstruction, which may require placing a tracheostomy. After RT for head and neck cancer, an almost guaranteed sequel is the development of a radiation "dewlap" in the submental area. The lymphedema is intermittent and fluctuates for no apparent reason for the duration of the patient's life. Patients should be advised that intermittent swelling is generally a consequence of the treatment and does not typically signal regrowth of cancer, although examination of the patient with head and neck cancer who has a change in status is never amiss. The problem can reach massive and troublesome proportions ("pumpkin head") in patients in whom scarring is significant because of previous surgery or RT to both sides of the neck, which creates a constrictive collar obstructing lymphatic outflow from the head to the body. Attempts to relieve this condition (usually by internists unfamiliar with the cause) with corticosteroids and diuretics are not worthwhile because the mechanical source of the problem is not addressed.

Surgery With Curative Intent

The "occasional" head and neck cancer surgeon, a dying breed one hopes,[137,138] should probably err on the side of radicality (i.e., standard rather than conservation operations, or radical rather than functional neck dissection—see subsequent section). Saving anatomy while removing cancer effectively requires the experience of physicians who subspecialize in head and neck surgical oncology to properly select and operate on patients and achieve results comparable to those of standard "radical" operations. Preferably, patients with head and neck cancer are referred to such subspecialists, so the least possible normal anatomy and function are sacrificed.

A theoretic advantage of surgery is that it is a relatively nonselective modality, as discussed previously in the section on tumor biology. In small tumors, surgery frequently provides the same local control rate as RT alone, with little or no disability after a brief hospitalization (or none) and convalescence, and fewer long-term complications, contrary to popular belief among patients and physicians who are not head and neck cancer surgeons. Unreliable patients are better treated with surgery or surgery plus RT than with RT alone. Patients who have demonstrated the phenomenon of "field cancerization" with development of multiple small primary tumors in the UADT mucosa are best approached with repeated wide local excisions, if possible, with RT held in reserve.

When surgery as a single modality is considered adequate initially, it may be wise to perform additional treatment based on the findings of the pathology report on the excised specimen, for example, if positive margins are returned. Additional treatment options in this case could involve more surgery or postoperative RT in the form of implants or external beam. This is not meant to imply that postoperative RT can compensate for grossly inadequate excision.

The question of what constitutes an adequate margin for excision of SCC of the head and neck has never been scientifically addressed. The reported incidence of positive margins in the literature after major head and neck cancer surgery is 3 to 33% and is probably underreported because of the discontinuous nature of disease spread in at least 25% of cases and selective sampling of margins. It is intuitively logical that "positive margins" favor local recurrence.[75,152–154] The incidence of recurrence is higher, 70 to 80%, when surgical margins are positive than when they are negative, although the incidence in the latter situation is not zero but rather 15 to 30%. This reflects the error of focal margin sampling and the discontinuous nature of tumor spread discussed previously.

I find it useful to cut my own margins as soon as

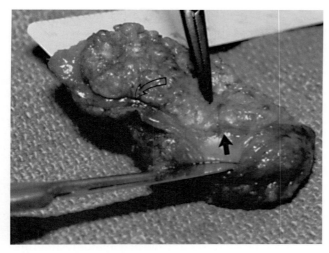

Fig. 20–13. Freshly excised specimen, margins being cut. Solid arrow, Edge of cancer; open arrow, retracting mucosal margin.

the specimen is removed rather than leaving this important activity for surgical pathologists to perform. Pathologists are seldom familiar with the anatomy or operative nuances, and the margins have usually dried out and contracted against the cancer by the time the pathologists receive the specimen (Fig. 20–13).

Davidson and co-workers' attribution of an enhanced local control rate to use of Moh's technique for margin control is untenable because the patients in their series also underwent postoperative RT.[68] The local control rates were exactly the same as in patients (reported from a different institution) who had not had this type of margin control but had undergone combination therapy.[155] Therefore, the result cannot be attributed to the addition of fastidious intraoperative control of margins at the primary site because two variables were uncontrolled.

A reasonable goal in excising head and neck mucosal SCC is to remove all gross (visible and palpable) disease with a 1 cm margin of surrounding normal tissue while simultaneously attempting to conserve the function of the organ territory in question. The surgeon must not leave gross disease in the patient and assume that postoperative RT will cure it. The effect of postoperative RT on positive margins remains to be scientifically validated. One article purporting to elucidate the significance of "cut-through" of SCC of the head and neck (leaving gross or microscopic residual disease) unfortunately does not present adequate data to answer the question.[156] One article indirectly addressed this issue.[141] Sixteen patients who underwent presumably incomplete excisional biopsy of oral tongue cancers were referred for RT. Eight had interstitial implants only, and 8 had implants plus external megavoltage treatments. Local control was achieved in 14 of 15 patients. The disadvantage of RT in cancers of the oral cavity, namely, the development of soft tissue

necrosis or bone exposure in a significant number of patients, was noted.

Patients who underwent only surgical treatment had a local recurrence rate of 73% if the margins were positive and 39% if margins were negative.[153] When surgery and RT were used as a planned combination, the respective incidences of local recurrence were 10.5 and 2%. Other series have not shown this marked difference based on margin status, however, and several series report local recurrence rates of 25 to 40% even with combined therapy.

It is unfortunate to have to add postoperative RT with its attendant complications because the initial surgery was inadequate. For example, performing a partial glossectomy, which risks positive margins, rather than a hemiglossectomy, which would more likely guarantee negative margins, is not warranted if such a result would necessitate adding adjuvant RT because the functional consequences to the patient are similar with both operations (i.e., the surgeon should err on the side of larger resections for tongue cancers).

Survival rate after transoral resection of carcinoma of the oral cavity—"transorectomy"—varies in the literature. Once again, control of local disease is the proper end point to evaluate the efficacy of a surgical procedure. In one series, the subsequent incidence of neck metastases was low, and the incidence of second primary cancers was high (20 to 40%). Therefore, RT and neck dissection were reserved as treatment for the subsequent appearance of neck metastases and additional primary cancers.[157] In another series of 65 patients operated on between 1956 and 1967 (including 3 patients who had discontinuous radical neck dissection), a local control rate of 82% occurred, with a 5-year cure rate of 67% in patients without positive lymph nodes. The cure rate was 23% in patients with clinically positive lymph nodes.[158] Retrospectively attributing a survival result to extent of local-regional treatment is impossible in a situation also influenced by other prognostic factors, and tailoring the extent of surgery to the lesion seems reasonable. Appropriately selected soft tissue tumors in the oral cavity, oropharynx, and pharynx are suitable for transoral resection.

Another basic principle is that, although it is reasonable to tailor the extent of surgery to the size of the primary cancer, adequate removal is facilitated by appropriate access and exposure. This decreases the incidence of local recurrence.

In rare instances, massive disease may be technically unresectable, and a nonsurgical treatment modality is necessary at the beginning. If the tumor responds, one may be tempted to attempt resection. Whether this plan is valid (i.e., can technically unresectable cancer be rendered resectable?) has not been established. The "operating principle," however, is that the operation should be the same as would have been required initially regardless of the tumor response to chemotherapy or RT because tumors do not shrink in a cohesive centripetal manner, but rather leave nests of cancer cells throughout the entire territory of the original tumor. When a nonsurgical treatment modality is used first, the margins of resection should be tattooed with India ink (not at the edge of the cancer, to avoid implanting cancer cells into underlying structures), so they will not be undercut at any subsequent operation.

Special mention should be made of the use of the *laser* in cancer surgery of the mouth and throat. The laser is simply a cutting tool and has no magic cancer-curing properties (contrary to the image sometimes propagated in the lay press). The laser does seal small lymphatics and blood vessels during dissection, and this may theoretically decrease dissemination of cancer cells. Viable tumor cells are unlikely to be dispersed in the products of carbon dioxide laser tumor vaporization.[159] Using the laser in "continuous" mode avoids impact shock and cell scatter. The issue of health hazard from laser smoke and its contained particles is reviewed by Nezhat and colleagues.[160]

In my opinion, any lesion suitable for a transoral excision should be removed with the laser because of the decreased morbidity of this technology in respect to swelling, pain, and scarring. It facilitates examination for recurrent cancer. Early reports suggested that the laser should be used only for small and superficial tumors and when adjunctive RT or neck dissection was

not necessary. Cancer treatment results that have accumulated in the literature show comparability between laser excision and standard "cold steel" excision methods.[161,162] The main factor that determines the suitability of the lesion for laser excision is whether it can be adequately exposed through the open mouth (Fig. 20–14), as determined by both characteristics of the tumor and the individual patient's anatomy. The size and depth of the tumor are not absolute contraindications to use of the laser, and the issues of neck dissection and the need for adjunctive RT can be decided separately on their own merits.

Leaving the wound open to reepithelialize is appropriate for FOM and some oropharynx excisions, but resections involving the papillated surface of the tongue should be closed primarily to decrease scar contracture (Fig. 20–15). Covering such wounds with a skin or dermal graft is not compatible with the unique features of laser wound healing.[163] Healing is generally uncomplicated if the surgical indications and technique were appropriate, and postoperative RT can commence 3 weeks later. Moderate scar contracture is not unusual, and this tendency is best counteracted by mouth-opening or tongue-stretching exercises by the patient.

The laser should be used at an appropriate power density to decrease the contact time of the beam with the tissue, thus minimizing the deposition of carbon-

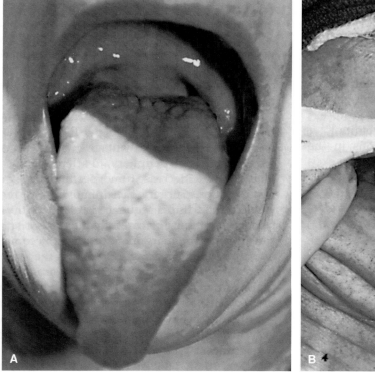 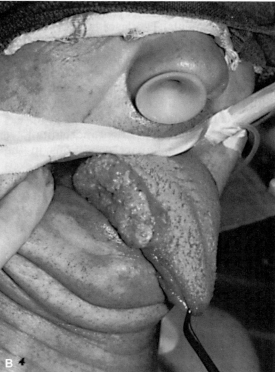

Fig. 20–14. A, Exposure and anatomy favorable for transoral laser excision of lesion in oral cavity or oropharynx. B, Tongue cancer suitable for transoral laser excision.

predict which patients will have a favorable response. Sufficient time has now elapsed to state that, unfortunately, the addition of chemotherapy to surgery and RT conveys no survival advantage to the patient with advanced SCC of the head and neck when one evaluates data from randomized prospective controlled trials,[174–177] which is the only valid format. In fact, when chemotherapy was given in the neoadjuvant setting, some patients' survival was poorer because the planned surgery and RT to follow were not given because patients who had a complete response to chemotherapy often refused additional treatment. Unless consolidated with additional treatment, chemotherapy alone does not cure, and the tumor that regrows is typically resistant to the drugs that caused the initial response. When such tumors recur, many are technically unresectable.

Another problem that arose from anterior chemotherapy was that the drugs were widely given in the community as the initial treatment, and only then were patients referred to a surgeon, who had never seen the initial extent of tumor. Operations were therefore impossible to plan properly and were frequently inadequate. The question whether "up front" chemotherapy can convert technically unresectable disease to resectable disease has not been definitively answered. Because tumors shrink in a discontinuous manner after chemotherapy (or RT), however, the general principle holds that the magnitude of the operation planned before chemotherapy must be the same regardless of the response of the tumor to drugs, to avoid undercutting the margins. Chemotherapy does not seem to lead to increased wound-healing complications when followed by surgery, although surgery following concomitant chemoradiotherapy is associated with a 50% incidence of severe wound healing complications.[178]

Patients who are complete responders to "up front" chemotherapy and who then have RT occasionally achieve long-term disease control. This appears to be the only category of initial response in which surgery as the next step can be eliminated, and this has only been scientifically shown for larynx cancers,[176] a group of tumors with a favorable natural history in comparison with other head and neck cancers in sites. A partial or minimal response to chemotherapy predicts a similar response to subsequent irradiation.

Chemotherapy was hoped to be advantageous as a systemic treatment modality to inhibit the process of DM. In at least one study in which patients received triple therapy, the incidence of DM was *increased* in those who received chemotherapy over those who did not.[179] Therefore, current chemotherapy is apparently not the hoped-for panacea for the systemic component of solid carcinoma spread, although large randomized studies show a "trend" toward significant systemic activity.[176,177]

The aggressive local-regional nature of head and neck squamous cancer is attested to by the recurrence of local-regional disease in some patients who responded completely to "up front" chemotherapy and then underwent the planned resection and showed no tumor in the specimen (and who then underwent RT).[73,180]

The current uses of chemotherapy for SCC of the head and neck include palliation of recurrent disease in which subjective pain relief can sometimes be achieved despite failure of objective tumor shrinkage, and possibly in the rare patient with technically unresectable massive disease or who refuses other treatment. In this latter situation, RT with curative intent is likely to meet with failure (although a criticism of the prospective, randomized trials of chemotherapy is that they have not included an RT-only arm for comparison), and chemotherapy might be tried as the first treatment in the hope that the patient will select himself or herself into the favorable "complete response" category, which can then be followed by additional treatment (surgery or RT) in an attempt to gain an occasional durable remission.

Chemotherapy as an adjunct to surgery plus RT for advanced SCCs of the head and neck is *not* part of standard treatment,[181] except *possibly* for advanced glottic-transglottic carcinoma.[176,182] Because interest in "neoadjuvant" regimens has waned, various combinations of simultaneous chemoradiotherapy are being investigated, but they are difficult to manage in the fragile population of patients with head and neck cancer.[183] Chemotherapy or chemoradiotherapy should be used only as part of protocol studies, so any utility can be properly defined. The future of chemotherapy (for some types of cancers) may include dose intensification with autologous bone marrow support.

Although conservation surgery for laryngeal cancer was the original "organ-preservation" strategy for head and neck cancer, modifications of traditional radical operations for head and neck cancer in other sites are only starting to be proposed as viable alternatives to nonsurgical "cytoreductive" strategies. Theoretic and practical considerations on combining multimodality therapy for head and neck cancer are presented elsewhere.[184,185]

Management of Cancer in the Neck

Management of cancer in any of the UADT mucosa primary site is automatically related to management of cancer in the neck because of the proclivity of SCC in all sites of the UADT mucosa to spread regionally. This massive and controversial topic has been comprehensively presented in a review that summarizes the relevant clinical data and relates it to tumor biology principles.[1]

What is the ability of various treatment modalities to control disease in the neck? The literature is difficult to evaluate because the end result reported is usually apy or RT because tumors do not shrink in a cohesive centripetal manner, but rather leave nests of cancer cells throughout the entire territory of the original tumor. When a nonsurgical treatment modality is used first, the margins of resection should be tattooed with India ink (not at the edge of the cancer, to avoid implanting cancer cells into underlying structures), so they will not be undercut at any subsequent operation.

Special mention should be made of the use of the *laser* in cancer surgery of the mouth and throat. The laser is simply a cutting tool and has no magic cancer-curing properties (contrary to the image sometimes propagated in the lay press). The laser does seal small lymphatics and blood vessels during dissection, and this may theoretically decrease dissemination of cancer cells. Viable tumor cells are unlikely to be dispersed in the products of carbon dioxide laser tumor vaporization.[159] Using the laser in "continuous" mode avoids impact shock and cell scatter. The issue of health hazard from laser smoke and its contained particles is reviewed by Nezhat and colleagues.[160]

In my opinion, any lesion suitable for a transoral excision should be removed with the laser because of the decreased morbidity of this technology in respect to swelling, pain, and scarring. It facilitates examination for recurrent cancer. Early reports suggested that the laser should be used only for small and superficial tumors and when adjunctive RT or neck dissection was

not necessary. Cancer treatment results that have accumulated in the literature show comparability between laser excision and standard "cold steel" excision methods.[161,162] The main factor that determines the suitability of the lesion for laser excision is whether it can be adequately exposed through the open mouth (Fig. 20–14), as determined by both characteristics of the tumor and the individual patient's anatomy. The size and depth of the tumor are not absolute contraindications to use of the laser, and the issues of neck dissection and the need for adjunctive RT can be decided separately on their own merits.

Leaving the wound open to reepithelialize is appropriate for FOM and some oropharynx excisions, but resections involving the papillated surface of the tongue should be closed primarily to decrease scar contracture (Fig. 20–15). Covering such wounds with a skin or dermal graft is not compatible with the unique features of laser wound healing.[163] Healing is generally uncomplicated if the surgical indications and technique were appropriate, and postoperative RT can commence 3 weeks later. Moderate scar contracture is not unusual, and this tendency is best counteracted by mouth-opening or tongue-stretching exercises by the patient.

The laser should be used at an appropriate power density to decrease the contact time of the beam with the tissue, thus minimizing the deposition of carbon-

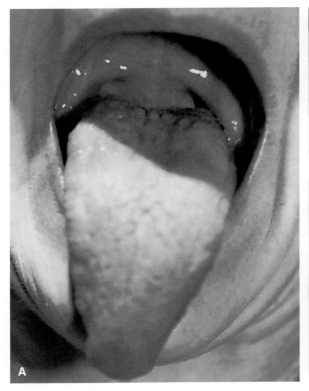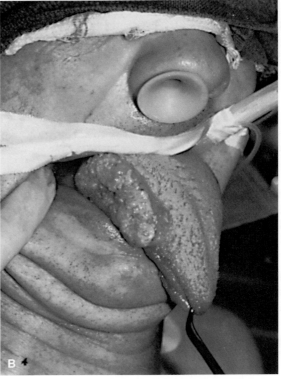

Fig. 20–14. A, Exposure and anatomy favorable for transoral laser excision of lesion in oral cavity or oropharynx. B, Tongue cancer suitable for transoral laser excision.

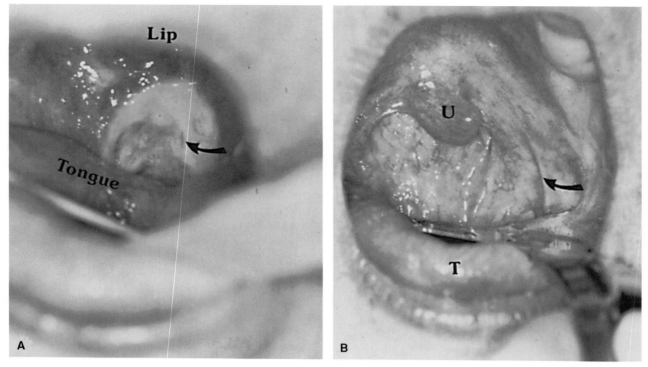

Fig. 20–15. Laser excision site. A. Arrow, Fibrinous exudate covering left tonsil laser excision site. B. Arrow, Same area healed 4 weeks later; U, uvula; T, tongue.

ized particles, which can interfere with the assessment of histologic margins and with wound healing of the resection bed. Using the laser with the handpiece on continuous power at low wattage (10 to 15 watts) subserves these requirements. The laser should be used only to excise soft tissue, and bone of the mandible should *not* be exposed during such procedures. Mandible that has been exposed to the laser beam tends to be devitalized and sequesters to constitute a nonhealing focus. Failure to follow these guidelines can lead to wound-healing complications that can delay postoperative RT and cause significant patient morbidity.[164]

For cancers and premalignant conditions in the mouth and throat, the laser should be used as an excision tool rather than in the vaporization mode. This provides a specimen for pathologic evaluation to confirm the diagnosis and to assess the status of margins. A detailed description of the use of the laser for excising cancers in the mouth and throat is provided.[142]

Combination Therapy

The rationale for combining radical surgery and RT in varying sequences resulted from the inadequacy of either modality alone to control large primary tumors and palpable neck disease. Combining therapy is done in two ways, planned and unplanned. In *planned* combination therapy, the initial treatment modality is followed within a defined period by the second. In *unplanned* combination therapy, one treatment modality is used with curative intent and the second for "salvage" in recurrent disease.

In planned combined therapy, surgery removes all visible and palpable disease including the hypoxic tumor core with a 1- to 2-cm margin of normal tissue, and RT eradicates microscopic residual disease (at least theoretically). Hypoxic cells have been found in the smallest observable animal tumors and are expected to exist in the subclinical tumor that is the target of postoperative RT.

Either surgery or RT can be performed first. In former years, it was common to give RT preoperatively to provide the theoretic advantage of inactivating cancer cells at the tumor periphery, to sclerose and seal lymphatics, and to decrease tumor seeding during surgical manipulation. Surgery then removed any remaining viable tumor. If this sequence is planned, the original tumor extent must be carefully mapped or tattooed in situ because the margins of resection become inaccurate after tumor shrinkage. Observing the fibrinous exudate ("tumoritis") developing from superficial necrosis of tumor cells 5 to 10 days after the initiation of preoperative RT can also help outline tumor extent.

Surgeons believe that RT followed by radical surgery in the head and neck is frequently complicated by significant wound healing problems such as oropharyngocutaneous fistulas, wound sloughs, and vascular ruptures. In the mid-1970s, a gradual shift occurred from administering RT preoperatively to administering it postoperatively, and this sequence is still generally favored. The reason that the literature does not scientifically bear out the increased incidence of wound-healing problems after RT[165] may be that operating soon after RT (when the treatments are given in a planned sequence) is a relatively favorable situation because the blood supply to the area is normal or even enhanced. When salvage surgery follows RT at least 6 months after the radiation is delivered (unplanned combination), the vascularity of the wound is decreased and the fibrosis is increased (and this progresses over time), resulting in the typical wound-healing problems dreaded by surgeons.

When surgery is the initial modality in a planned combination, dogma states that RT should follow within 6 weeks, according to one study,[166] which showed a 5% local recurrence rate when postoperative RT was delivered 6 weeks or less after surgery but a 30% rate if therapy was delayed (a bias here is that delay in RT usually results from wound healing problems typically associated with large tumors and resections). A subsequent report was unable to verify the "magic" 6-week number, however.[167]

With uneventful wound healing, one can generally to begin RT 3 weeks postoperatively. In fact, at least this amount of time should be allowed to elapse after surgical wounding.[144] The usual postoperative dose is 50 to 65 Gy, depending on the number of positive lymph nodes in the neck and the status of margins at the primary site. When surgery is performed first, necessary tooth extractions are performed intraoperatively. Depending on the location of the tumor, it may be wise to remove the tumor and irrigate the site first, to avoid cancer cell seeding of the sockets.[107]

Most head and neck oncologists would agree that the best method of controlling advanced local-regional SCC (stages III and IV) is planned combined surgery and RT. Strictly speaking, this is still in the realm of belief—now deeply ingrained, however, on the basis of heavy circumstantial evidence—rather than based on scientifically valid data from randomized prospective studies. The issue is controversial; some articles indicate that surgical therapy alone achieves survival equivalent to combined therapy, and some even show that survival of patients in combined therapy programs is poorer than that for patients treated with surgery alone, even when treatment groups are compared by stage of lesion.[168–172] Confusion persists to some extent because "survival" is an inappropriate end point to use when evaluating local-regional treatment modalities such as surgery and RT, as discussed previously.

One randomized study showed that, for sites in the oral cavity and oropharynx (small numbers), no statistically significant differences were seen in local-regional control or survival in patients undergoing combined therapy (preoperative or postoperative RT) versus full-course RT (with surgical salvage).[172] Local-regional control was, however, significantly better for patients receiving postoperative than preoperative RT.

Studies supporting the benefit of combination therapy indicate that combination of the two modalities produces local-regional disease control in twice as many patients as single-modality therapy.[57,58,155,173] A concomitant survival advantage is not seen, however, but this is not an indictment of combination therapy because one expects these local-regional treatments only to be able to improve local-regional disease control.

Vikram concluded that local-regional control had been considerably increased by using planned combined therapy,[57] when compared with a historical series from the same institution using surgery only, accumulated between 1960 and 1964. In the surgery-only comparison group, the relapse rate in the head and neck was 50 to 75%. In the series reporting combination therapy, local-regional failure occurred in only 18%. When the surgery-only series was compiled, patients presented with relatively more advanced disease, and treatment techniques were archaic in comparison with current methods. Changes in the patient population and treatment techniques in the intervening years are important variables that may make this comparison group inappropriate. Overall, tumors recurred in 9.5% of patients at the primary site and in 8.5% in the neck. The result in the combined treatment group was duplicated by another series composed of almost the same number of total patients and of patients in each stage.[68]

In general, postoperative RT seems to be indicated when the margins of excision at the primary site are unsatisfactory, based on pathologic examination, or when the patient has multiple pathologically positive lymph nodes. These findings presumably indicate a high-risk group for local-regional recurrence.

Chemotherapy

Traditionally, chemotherapy for SCC of the head and neck has been used to treat recurrent disease. Fibrosis from previous treatment decreases the blood supply to the tumor and impedes delivery of antitumor drugs yielding an overall, generally short-term response rate of 30 to 40%. A basic principle is that rapidly growing tumors are relatively more sensitive to chemotherapy or RT than are slow-growing tumors. Most patients with recurrent head and neck cancer are nutritionally depleted and anorexic, suffer from xerostomia, have dysphagia and odynophagia, and are poor candidates for vigorous chemotherapy.

Agents have been developed with particular activity against head and neck SCC (cisplatin and 5-fluorouracil) that shrink massive tumors (both advanced primary cancers and large masses in the neck) when given before any other treatment ("up front," anterior, or "neoadjuvant" therapy), although it is not possible to predict which patients will have a favorable response. Sufficient time has now elapsed to state that, unfortunately, the addition of chemotherapy to surgery and RT conveys no survival advantage to the patient with advanced SCC of the head and neck when one evaluates data from randomized prospective controlled trials,[174–177] which is the only valid format. In fact, when chemotherapy was given in the neoadjuvant setting, some patients' survival was poorer because the planned surgery and RT to follow were not given because patients who had a complete response to chemotherapy often refused additional treatment. Unless consolidated with additional treatment, chemotherapy alone does not cure, and the tumor that regrows is typically resistant to the drugs that caused the initial response. When such tumors recur, many are technically unresectable.

Another problem that arose from anterior chemotherapy was that the drugs were widely given in the community as the initial treatment, and only then were patients referred to a surgeon, who had never seen the initial extent of tumor. Operations were therefore impossible to plan properly and were frequently inadequate. The question whether "up front" chemotherapy can convert technically unresectable disease to resectable disease has not been definitively answered. Because tumors shrink in a discontinuous manner after chemotherapy (or RT), however, the general principle holds that the magnitude of the operation planned before chemotherapy must be the same regardless of the response of the tumor to drugs, to avoid undercutting the margins. Chemotherapy does not seem to lead to increased wound-healing complications when followed by surgery, although surgery following concomitant chemoradiotherapy is associated with a 50% incidence of severe wound healing complications.[178]

Patients who are complete responders to "up front" chemotherapy and who then have RT occasionally achieve long-term disease control. This appears to be the only category of initial response in which surgery as the next step can be eliminated, and this has only been scientifically shown for larynx cancers,[176] a group of tumors with a favorable natural history in comparison with other head and neck cancers in sites. A partial or minimal response to chemotherapy predicts a similar response to subsequent irradiation.

Chemotherapy was hoped to be advantageous as a systemic treatment modality to inhibit the process of DM. In at least one study in which patients received triple therapy, the incidence of DM was *increased* in those who received chemotherapy over those who did not.[179] Therefore, current chemotherapy is apparently not the hoped-for panacea for the systemic component of solid carcinoma spread, although large randomized studies show a "trend" toward significant systemic activity.[176,177]

The aggressive local-regional nature of head and neck squamous cancer is attested to by the recurrence of local-regional disease in some patients who responded completely to "up front" chemotherapy and then underwent the planned resection and showed no tumor in the specimen (and who then underwent RT).[73,180]

The current uses of chemotherapy for SCC of the head and neck include palliation of recurrent disease in which subjective pain relief can sometimes be achieved despite failure of objective tumor shrinkage, and possibly in the rare patient with technically unresectable massive disease or who refuses other treatment. In this latter situation, RT with curative intent is likely to meet with failure (although a criticism of the prospective, randomized trials of chemotherapy is that they have not included an RT-only arm for comparison), and chemotherapy might be tried as the first treatment in the hope that the patient will select himself or herself into the favorable "complete response" category, which can then be followed by additional treatment (surgery or RT) in an attempt to gain an occasional durable remission.

Chemotherapy as an adjunct to surgery plus RT for advanced SCCs of the head and neck is *not* part of standard treatment,[181] except *possibly* for advanced glottic-transglottic carcinoma.[176,182] Because interest in "neoadjuvant" regimens has waned, various combinations of simultaneous chemoradiotherapy are being investigated, but they are difficult to manage in the fragile population of patients with head and neck cancer.[183] Chemotherapy or chemoradiotherapy should be used only as part of protocol studies, so any utility can be properly defined. The future of chemotherapy (for some types of cancers) may include dose intensification with autologous bone marrow support.

Although conservation surgery for laryngeal cancer was the original "organ-preservation" strategy for head and neck cancer, modifications of traditional radical operations for head and neck cancer in other sites are only starting to be proposed as viable alternatives to nonsurgical "cytoreductive" strategies. Theoretic and practical considerations on combining multimodality therapy for head and neck cancer are presented elsewhere.[184,185]

Management of Cancer in the Neck

Management of cancer in any of the UADT mucosa primary site is automatically related to management of cancer in the neck because of the proclivity of SCC in all sites of the UADT mucosa to spread regionally. This massive and controversial topic has been comprehensively presented in a review that summarizes the relevant clinical data and relates it to tumor biology principles.[1]

What is the ability of various treatment modalities to control disease in the neck? The literature is difficult to evaluate because the end result reported is usually *survival,* rather than *control of disease in the neck.* To assess the ability of a treatment to control neck disease, the primary tumor must remain controlled because neck disease can develop through seeding from a recurrent primary tumor. The end result seen is then related to uncontrolled primary tumor, rather than to the type of neck treatment initially undertaken.

One must also define the context of neck treatment. Two terms are typically used: *elective,* referring to treatment of the N0 neck, and *therapeutic,* referring to treatment directed at clinically palpable (N+) disease in the neck. The term "prophylactic" is frequently used to describe treatment in the elective context, but this implies a therapeutic benefit to the patient that is not proved. The N0 neck was formerly defined as one with no clinically palpable disease, but with the new staging system, the results of scans can now be used to define the neck status. Because of the altered method of definition, new and old retrospective series concerning issues related to neck disease will be even less comparable than heretofore.

Some studies that apparently support treatment in the elective rather than therapeutic context for neck disease are invalid because they report the response of *clinically* palpable neck disease without *histologic* confirmation of cancer in the neck. Because the incidence of false-positive (and false-negative) clinical adenopathy is significant,[2,133] such conclusions are suspect. Patients who had no histologic disease in their necks were included in these reports and skewed the results toward a more favorable conclusion because they would not be expected either to die of recurrent disease in the neck (if the primary tumor remained controlled) or to develop DM. The clinical and histologic incidence of neck metastases related to various features of the primary tumor is presented in Tables 20–5 and 20–6.

The ability of full-course RT (65 to 70 Gy) to control positive neck disease (clinically staged and therefore subject to the errors described) from top-level institutions is 91% for N1, 78% for N2, and 67% for N3.[186] A dose of 50 Gy, which is considered adequate to eradicate 95% of subclinical (occult) neck disease,[187–189] controls only 50% of 2- to 3-cm neck nodes. When RT is planned to be the curative treatment for tumor at the primary site, positive necks can be included in the RT ports, and the response to treatment assessed about 6 to 8 weeks after the completion of RT. For persistent palpable disease, neck dissection should be performed. If disease in the neck has completely disappeared, holding neck dissection in reserve for recurrent disease is an option, although salvage results in this context are poor.

The standard classic operation for metastatic cancer in the neck is radical neck dissection. In the few papers that report neck disease control rates with primary tumor also controlled, recurrence after radical neck dissection ranges from 11% for N1 disease and 19% for

N2 disease to 25 to 30%. One paper reported a series of patients with head and neck cancer who underwent neck dissection; 75% were treated with primary surgery alone.[190] The recurrence rates in dissected necks at 2 years were 7.5%, 20.2%, and 37.4% for N0, N1, and N2 necks, respectively. Most neck recurrences were noted before primary recurrence was found, but this variable was not strictly controlled. These results seemed to confirm the intuitively logical conclusion that the efficacy of radical neck dissection decreases as the amount of disease in the neck increases and as it spreads from containment in lymph nodes into the adjacent soft tissue.[131] Radical neck dissection is by no means an ineffective treatment modality, however. The lack of control attributed to the operation is largely related to lack of control of the primary tumor.

Head and neck cancer surgeons have been using various types of modified neck dissection since the 1920s. These have been given standard definitions by the American Academy of Otolaryngology—Head and Neck Surgery.[191] The standard for comparison is the work of Bocca's group in Italy.[192] Since the 1960s, this group has been using routine elective functional neck dissection, which removes the lymph node-bearing contents of the neck but preserves the normal structures (sternocleidomastoid muscle, internal jugular vein, spinal accessory nerve, submandibular gland). Modified or conservation neck dissections have come continually under fire because they deviate from Halsted's principles, which dictate that radical neck dissection is necessary for the best removal of all cancer in the neck. Disapproval of conservation operations was expressed by Conley, a preeminent authority in the field, in 1975.[193]

Bocca maintains that the radicality of a neck operation should be directed against the cancer rather than against the neck and has presented data confirming that this modified procedure is as oncologically radical as any traditional neck dissection, provided the lymph nodes are still mobile and that some technical details are respected: the dissection consists of removing the aponeurotic sheaths with the areolar tissues that they surround, as beautifully illustrated by Calearo and Teatini.[194] When so performed, functional neck dissection offers oncologic safety comparable to that of radical neck dissection while avoiding unnecessary mutilation.[192,195,196]

No significant difference in neck tumor recurrence has been found after functional or radical neck dissection regardless of the stage of neck disease.[197,198] General guidelines from that institution (in which modified neck dissection is generally supplemented by postoperative RT) indicate that a modified procedure is adequate for N1 to N2a disease in combination with postoperative RT, but it is inadequate for N2b and N3a disease (institutional neck staging system), and radical neck dissection with postoperative RT is indicated for patients with these advanced stages. If an elective neck dissection specimen is histologically positive, 50 Gy are delivered postoperatively. Neck dissection without postoperative RT can be considered for specimens containing a single positive lymph node without extracapsular spread. Other reports generally favor using single-modality surgery in preference to combination treatment and tend to present results that support this philosophy.[190]

Functional neck dissection, *when performed competently*, can serve as a biopsy procedure with virtually no negative functional or cosmetic consequences to the patient and is therefore an acceptable alternative to elective neck irradiation. If no nodes are histologically positive, it may be possible to hold postoperative RT in reserve, and this may be a significant maneuver with respect to treatment of future primary tumors.[52] When excision of the primary tumor requires entering the neck, one should probably perform an elective neck dissection.

The issue of whether treatment to the neck should be performed *electively* (N0) or *therapeutically* (N+) merits further discussion. Currently, no statistically significant evidence in the head and neck cancer literature indicates any detriment to patient survival by delaying neck treatment until lymph nodes become clinically evident in patients who present with N0 necks. Several retrospective series have reached this conclusion.[199,200] These studies have generally evaluated survival as it relates to the method of treatment, rather than to the amount of disease in the neck. One randomized prospective trial in the literature addresses this issue.[132] Between 1966 and 1973, 75 patients were accrued with T1 to T3, N0 SCC of the oral cavity. Half of them underwent elective radical neck dissection within 2 months of treatment of the primary tumor (which was itself treated by interstitial implantation). The other patients, who were treated similarly at the primary site, underwent therapeutic radical neck dissection when and if nodes became clinically palpable later. The percentage of patients in each group with histologically positive or negative nodes was the same; however, patients undergoing therapeutic neck dissection had twice the incidence of extracapsular spread. Patients with histologically positive neck nodes received postoperative RT. On the basis of a careful 5-year follow-up, no difference in survival was noted between the two groups, and this persisted when histologic node parameters, such as extracapsular spread, were assessed. In the delayed-treatment group, the condition of the patient or the tumor precluded operation when lymph nodes became palpable in only 2 patients.

A study from India looked at the issue of elective versus therapeutic neck dissection in a prospective randomized format.[129] Nearly 100 patients with T1 to T2, N0 SCC of the oral tongue were studied. Of the 70 patients who had been followed for at least 12 months

at the time of reporting, 40 underwent hemiglossectomy and 30 had hemiglossectomy and radical neck dissection. In the former group (surgery to primary site only), 58% subsequently developed ipsilateral positive nodes, and 5 of 23 were inoperable at that time. In the latter group (surgery to primary tumor and neck), one third of the N0 patients had *histologically* positive nodes. Note the lack of comparability between the expected (histologically 30%) and actual (60%) incidence of neck metastases, despite a presumably homogeneous group with respect to primary tumor homogeneity. Twenty of the 25 patients who died in this group did so as a result of uncontrolled neck disease. Overall, however, no significant difference was noted in disease-free *survival* between the two groups. Whether the tumor biology of the study population is comparable with that of a similar group in the United States is questionable. About 25 of the 100 patients had never used tobacco products, and 5 developed cancer presumably as a result of submucous fibrosis. A subsequent report of this study with 2- to 3-year follow-up is awaited with interest and, one hopes, will report end points other than survival.

According to the "alternate hypothesis" (see previous section), the only risk when adopting a wait-and-see policy for N0 disease is that patients who have developed contraindications to surgery or in whom disease has become inoperable die as a result of cancer in the neck, whereas this might have been prevented by elective treatment. These findings support the contention that *elective* treatment of the neck is not "prophylactic" because it does not prevent cancer-related deaths or increase survival. Once again, we see that survival is an inappropriate end point for evaluating the efficacy of a *regional* treatment modality. The tendency to attribute survival results to the method of treatment is probably also a major misinterpretation. The survival difference may well be related more significantly to the pathologic condition of the lymph nodes or to intrinsic tumor biology than to the type or timing of the operation performed.

Despite this evidence to the contrary, if the patient has a 20 to 30% likelihood of occult cancer spread to the neck based on the size or site of the primary tumor, many treatment managers consider elective treatment to the neck indicated, and irradiation seems much simpler than operation to many. Clinicians generally accept that 50 Gy eradicates more than 90% of occult (subclinical) neck disease.[187–189] Elective neck irradiation theoretically decreases the need for subsequent radical neck dissection from 1 in 3 to 1 in 50 when the primary cancer is controlled. The data that support the efficacy of elective neck irradiation derive from an apparent decrease in the expected incidence of delayed neck metastases in patients, in comparison with the histologically demonstrated incidence of cervical disease in radical neck dissection specimens related to the size and site of the primary tumor *or* in comparison with the observed conversion rate of N0 to N+ in untreated necks. The flaw in interpreting all the data on elective neck irradiation lies in that no histologic specimen is available from the individual patient to tell whether positive lymph nodes were actually (rather than theoretically) present. An individual patient is not a series, and lymph nodes are either positive *or* negative—an all-or-none phenomenon. Moreover, actual and theoretic reasons exist to avoid using RT frivolously in patients with head and neck cancer,[1] and the study of Fakih and associates showed that, even in a prospectively randomized group of patients who presumably therefore had comparable primary tumors, the *observed* incidence of delayed clinical neck metastases (60%) did not always approximate that *expected* based on the incidence of histologically positive nodes (30%).[129] Most of the studies from which the putative value of elective neck dissection has been extrapolated were uncontrolled and retrospective, therefore comprising a heterogeneous patient population.

Nevertheless, situations for which elective neck dissection has been recommended in the literature include the following:

1. Large primary tumors.
2. Small invasive tumors.
3. Poorly differentiated primary tumors.
4. Primary tumors in the nasopharynx, oropharynx, hypopharynx, or supraglottic larynx and large invasive tumors of the oral cavity.
5. Patients with necks that are difficult to examine (short, fat).
6. Anticipation of poor patient follow-up.

Treatment to the entire neck bilaterally is recommended for all lesions except those that are lateralized and have a low probability of bilateral spread (buccal mucosa, gingiva, hard palate). This means tremendous morbidity to the patient in terms of xerostomia and limits treatment options for future cancers. Clearly, elective neck dissection is almost always recommended, and this trend has been widely accepted on the basis of circumstantial evidence. Alternatives to this philosophy have been mentioned repeatedly in this section. If patients are reliable, that is, if follow-up holding RT in reserve to follow is delayed,[201] therapeutic neck dissection is my preferred method of treatment for tumors with a low likelihood of spread to the neck.

NECK DISSECTION: TECHNICAL CONSIDERATIONS. In previously untreated patients, normal structures whose sacrifice would entail morbidity to the patient can be preserved unless these structures are directly invaded by cancer.

The morbidity of radical neck dissection is related to sacrifice of the spinal accessory nerve (XI), resulting in shoulder drop, musculoskeletal pain, and limitation of neck and limb motion,[202,203] and this disadvantage

favors use of modified neck dissection whenever possible.

Many types of modified neck dissection have been described and illustrated in the literature.[204–206] These preserve various combinations of the structures normally removed in radical neck dissection: the sternocleidomastoid muscle, internal jugular vein, submandibular gland, and spinal accessory nerve. A true *"functional"* neck dissection removes the superficial and deep cervical fascias with the enclosed lymph nodes but leaves the sternocleidomastoid muscle, omohyoid muscles, internal jugular vein, spinal accessory nerve, and submandibular gland.[194] The lymphatic content of the posterior triangle may be removed also (Fig. 20–16). (I now prefer to leave fascial coverings in situ.[107])

Supraomohyoid neck dissection is a type of functional anterior neck dissection in which the parajugular lymphatic compartment enclosed by the superficial and deep cervical fascia at and above the level of the omohyoid muscle tendon is removed. Because the low jugular nodes correspond to the level of the omohyoid tendon and are normally left in situ even in radical neck dissection, this is a valid oncologic procedure.[196,204]

Suprahyoid neck dissection is *not* a valid oncologic procedure because the route of cervical metastatic spread is unpredictable. With its limited extent, suprahyoid dissection is unreliable as therapy for clinically palpable upper neck nodes *or* as a biopsy technique in assessing the status of occult lymph nodes. Suprahyoid dissection merely enhances the adequacy of excision of large primary lesions of the lip and FOM.[207]

It is no longer necessary to perform neck dissection in continuity (en bloc) with excision of the primary tumor. Discontinuous neck dissection is not detrimental,[92] and continuous dissection is necessary only in rare cases in which direct extension of cancer occurs between the primary site and the neck and the intervening tissue is permeated with cancer cells. Discontinuous neck dissection is permissible as a standard procedure in previously untreated patients because the mechanism of spread between the primary site and the neck is embolic.

Bilateral neck disease can present synchronously[208] or metachronously. Surgical options for synchronous bilateral cervical metastases include simultaneous or staged radical or modified neck dissection. The morbidity of simultaneous neck dissection relates to sacrificing the major venous drainage from the head, which can result in dangerous corneal and cerebral edema. A pathophysiologic basis for decreasing these problems has been presented by McQuarrie and colleagues.[209]

Because collateral vessels in the occipital and posterior cervical venous systems gradually open after ve-

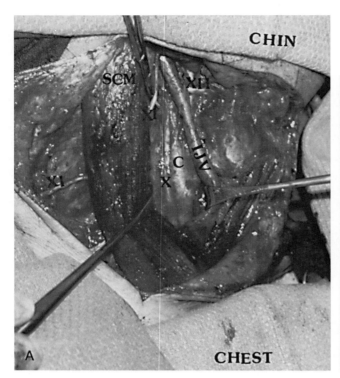
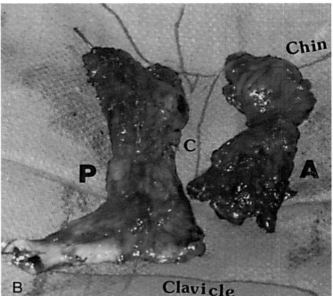

Fig. 20–16. A. Neck structures remaining after right functional neck dissection (FND). C, Carotid; IJV, internal jugular vein; SCM, sternocleidomastoid muscle; X, vagus nerve; XI, spinal accessory nerve; XII, hypoglossal nerve. B. Tissue removed at FND. A, Anterior lymph node-bearing tissue and submandibular gland; P, posterior neck contents; C, relationship to carotid.

nous interruption in the neck, the complications associated with a delayed contralateral neck dissection are generally less, but they vary according to the extent to which these venous channels have formed. A 6-week delay is generally traditionally recommended, and simultaneous bilateral neck dissections are preferred from an oncological viewpoint. Clearly, preserving the internal jugular vein on the second side greatly diminishes circulatory embarrassment.[210]

The time involved in performing bilateral neck dissections can be decreased if surgical teams can operate on both sides simultaneously. If the surgeon anticipates that one internal jugular vein can be preserved, this should be ascertained before the opposite vein is sacrificed. Sometimes the intraoperative situation is the opposite of that anticipated preoperatively, or it may be possible to preserve both internal jugular veins.

To decrease the risk of implanting cancer cells, I prefer to excise the primary tumor performing neck dissection(s),[107] a reversal of the traditional order of procedure intraoperatively.

In clinically N0 necks, when the neck is to be entered in removal of the primary tumor, it is then worthwhile to ''explore'' both sides of the neck to look for lymphadenopathy. This is accomplished by bluntly dissecting the sternocleidomastoid off the internal jugular vein. The internal jugular vein is skeletonized, and the jugular chain is carefully (lightly) palpated from the subdigastric area to the level of the omohyoid tendon. Unless these maneuvers are carried out, occult disease can be easily missed. It is not adequate merely to palpate over the sternocleidomastoid muscle after elevation of the cervical skin flaps if one is serious about exploring the neck. If palpable lymph nodes are found, it is reasonable, depending on the extent of disease found, either to perform a functional neck dissection or, in the case of an isolated lymph node, to excise the node and send it for frozen section (many lymph nodes palpable in this situation are reactively enlarged in response to the contaminated primary tumor). If cancer is found in the lymph node, the extent of optimal treatment has not been defined. Some surgeons have stated that, in this case, they would not hesitate to proceed with a radical neck dissection. Some type of modified neck dissection seems more reasonable, however, in occult disease. Only rarely does occult disease require sacrifice of major structures in the vicinity. In my experience, sacrifice of the internal jugular vein has been necessary on only two occasions for occult neck disease that was not appreciated either by palpation or CT scan.

Decision-Making in Previously Untreated Versus Recurrent Disease

Sometimes patients are declared ''medically inoperable'' without exhaustive and serious evaluation and proceed to RT with curative intent for this reason. Often the cancer is not controlled, and surgery is then reevaluated. In this difficult setting, the initial decision is frequently reversed, and patients suddenly become operable. Because the extent of tumor is then difficult to ascertain (especially if the initial treatment plan was generated in a community setting and the tertiary-care surgeon never saw the original lesion), salvage surgery seldom removes all neoplastic cells, and it is not unusual for cancer to regrow quickly at the excision margins or in the surgical scars.

For these reasons, patients with lesions that are unlikely to be radiocurable should have every effort made initially to make them surgical candidates. In the population of elderly patients with head and neck cancer, this might include performing a cardiac bypass or (rarely) a carotid endarterectomy as a preliminary operation, for example. Hoping that RT alone will cure a lesion of significant extent is "magical thinking." The patient's eventual fate is usually determined by the appropriateness of the initial treatment plan.

Successful conservation surgery can be more frequent in previously untreated than in treated patients because postoperative RT is available to control microscopic residual disease. For previously treated patients, additional RT, at least external beam, is usually no longer an option. The apparent extent of recurrent cancer is frequently only the "tip of the iceberg," and appropriate resection margins are difficult to determine. Therefore, the magnitude of reoperation is generally greater. In previously operated patients, all areas of scarring should be assumed to be contaminated with cancer cells and should be removed even if they are beyond the apparent palpable borders of the recurrent tumor.

The goal of surgery for recurrent neck disease should be to remove all of the gross disease, although this may require "peeling" the cancer from important neck structures. If this is accomplished and the UADT mucosa has not been violated, the literature suggests a benefit to placement of [125]I "seeds" loaded into suture intraoperatively in areas of suspected microscopic residual disease.[147,148] The incidence of complications in the neck after ^{125}I seeding is not reported to be prohibitive, but because an additional 100 Gy is delivered to the implanted area (during the ensuing 12 months), a pectoralis myofascial flap[211] should be used to protect against necrosis of the overlying cervical neck flaps and carotid rupture. Personal experience with ^{125}I seeds has not been favorable because resultant soft tissue fibrosis is painful, and cancer quickly regrows outside the implanted area.[212]

Some forms of RT may still be available to patients with recurrent disease who have had full-course external beam therapy as part of their previous treatment. In the United States, it is still usually possible to use interstitial implants and, in some cases, additional external beam therapy in combination with hyperthermia, especially for disease that is relatively superficial. A second course of external beam radiation is also possible at expert centers if dose-limiting structures such as larynx or hemimandible are removed with the resection of recurrent cancer, to decrease the risk of radionecrosis.[213]

The treatment of recurrent disease involves many philosophic and ethical issues, and the approach varies among surgeons as related to their experience.[214-216] Treatment for recurrent disease is more often palliative than curative; however, control of disease is still a goal in some circumstances, especially in patients who live long enough to develop multiple primary tumors. Repeated resections of local-regional disease are occasionally rewarded by long-term survival.

Historically, palliation of recurrent head and neck SCC has consisted of a tracheostomy tube, a feeding tube[217] (which can be placed percutaneously unless cancer in the UADT mucosa could be implanted at the G-tube site[217a]), and radical radiation. Cryosurgery has occasionally been used with the objectives of decreasing tumor bulk, bleeding, and pain and facilitating deglutition and respiration.[218] The laser is occasionally used in a similar context, although both measures are temporary and not too useful. Optimizing pain control is important.[112-115]

In some cases, radical resection may represent the most effective means of alleviating symptoms of uncontrolled local-regional cancer. Such attempts are warranted as long as the balance favors salvageable life. Current reconstructive technology allows single-stage ablation and reconstruction; patients can be rehabilitated quickly and their lives comfortably prolonged.[219] These advantages allow radical surgery with palliative intent to be considered even in the face of coexistent metastatic disease in selected patients. Young patients without multisystem failure can live for more than 2 years with DMs, and radical surgery for uncontrolled local-regional disease may be particularly warranted in this group. Radical surgery in elderly patients with head and neck cancer is also generally well tolerated, and most patients are willing to undertake such procedures to obtain the best quality of remaining life.[220,221]

Whether it is worthwhile to sacrifice the carotid artery in an attempt to remove recurrent cancer is controversial. Historically, majority opinion has found this to be a case of diminishing returns; however, an occasional dissenter has arisen. A meta-analysis of literature reports has concluded that elective carotid resection allows significant local-regional control of disease and that carotid artery involvement is not an unusually poor prognostic factor in patients with advanced head and neck cancer.[222] Tests to assess the patient's ability to withstand carotid ligation or bypass (not an option if the UADT has been entered or gross disease is left in the neck) without major neurologic sequelae[223] have included examination for neck bruits, the invasive Matas test,[224] ocular plethysmography,[225] and panangiography of carotid and vertebral vessels bilaterally with carotid cross-compression. Intraoperative carotid stump pressures (and EEG recording) are of use. Recent advances in skull base surgery permit a more radical approach to this problem, and this trend has been seen in the literature.[226] Parallel development of reliable diagnostic tests has occurred, including the currently most accurate predictor of CNS outcome after carotid occlusion: preoperative balloon occlusion of the internal carotid artery followed by xenon flow studies with CT.[227,228] Even with normal studies preoperatively, 10% or more of patients undergoing carotid sacrifice sustain significant neurologic sequelae. An alternative to operative occlusion of a bleeding carotid artery is preoperative neuroradiologic balloon occlusion.[229] In most cases, however, the nature of the recurrent disease is still too extensive and diffuse to warrant operative intervention. Death from carotid rupture is quick and painless. The patient should be in an inpatient hospice setting at this point, at a comfortable level of sedation.

MANAGEMENT OF SQUAMOUS CARCINOMA IN INDIVIDUAL SITES IN THE MOUTH AND THROAT

The bibliography includes general references concerning cancer categorized by individual sites not referenced in the text.

Cancer of the Lip

The lips consist of (1) dry mucosa known as the vermilion border (exposed mucosa), (2) wet (labial) mucosa, and (3) the cutaneous surfaces. Strictly speaking, lip cancers include only those arising on the vermilion border, although most series include heterogeneous locations. My "utility" incision for cancers of the mouth and throat requiring a transcervical approach is a transversely oriented "W"; the midpoint is above the thyroid notch and the low points bilaterally are halfway between the lower border of the jaw and the clavicle. This is consistent with the blood supply to the neck skin and affords exposure for tumor excision, neck dissection, and pectoralis flap reconstruction without the need for dropping a vertical limit that avoids trifurcation points.

The literature states that lip cancer is the most common cancer of the head and neck (25 to 30%), although it is infrequently seen by specialists in otolaryngology and head and neck surgery. The majority (95%) occur on the lower lip, 5% on the upper lip, and 2% at the labial commissures. Lip cancer typically occurs in elderly, blond, light-complexioned white men who have occupations associated with sun exposure. The predominance of *lower* lip cancer is because of the lip's protrusion. In the United States, men outnumber women 10 to 20:1 for lower lip cancer, presumably because of the protection afforded women by lipstick. The incidence of lip cancer in dark-skinned people is low because melanin blocks ultraviolet absorption. Populations with the highest incidence of lip cancer have the lowest incidence of intraoral cancer, and the converse is also true. Patients with lip cancer are usually cigarette smokers. The presenting age is in the sixth or seventh decade. The incidence in patients under 40 years old is about 15%.

Lip changes that predispose to cancer include chronic cheilitis, senile elastosis, leukoplakia, and hyperkeratosis. Malignant transformation in an area of leukoplakia occurs in 2 to 15% of patients. Actinic keratosis may transform to SCC in 20% of patients. Another premalignant lesion is keratoacanthoma.[230] This lesion is elevated and umbilicated, has a central core filled with keratin, and can regress spontaneously.

The lip is a site of "field cancerization"—multicentricity of lip lesions is common. Synchronous or metachronous cancers occur in 5 to 15% of patients. Fifty percent are simultaneous at presentation. The average elapsed time between metachronous primary cancers is 10 years.[231] A tendency exists for 13 to 30% of patients to develop second primary cancers, usually in the skin and lung.

Immunosuppressed renal transplant patients have a tendency to develop neoplasms of the lip. Ninety percent of these patients have an active herpesvirus infection that may explain the proclivity for this site.[232] An association between cancer of the lip and syphilis has been noted in 2 to 3% of cases,[231] although this was more common in earlier decades.

About 95% of lip cancers are well-differentiated SCCs. Basal cell carcinomas arise in the adjacent skin and may secondarily involve the lip. They are more common on the upper lip. Most upper lip tumors originate on the skin rather than the mucous membrane. Malignant salivary gland neoplasms can present in the lip submucosally.

The spindle cell variant of SCC occurs more frequently on the lip than in any other head and neck site (60%). It occurs on the lower lip, tends to be polypoid or ulcerative, and is associated with a poor prognosis, especially if preceded by trauma or radiation.

Adenoid SCC occurs predominantly on the vermilion border and is indolent—generally present for about 5 years. These lesions are ulcerated, with a rolled and indurated margin, and tend to recur. The prognosis is good, similar to that for well-differentiated SCC.

The typical SCC of the lower lip is a painless growth

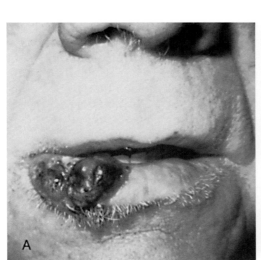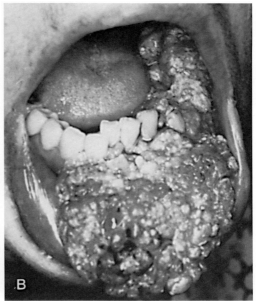

Fig. 20–17. A and B. Lip cancers. (Courtesy of Dr. GJ Spector.)

that is crusted or cracked and fails to heal (Fig. 20–17A). The lesions are usually present for 6 to 24 months before treatment. They grow slowly and metastasize rarely. They tend to spread laterally rather than deeply. Vertical growth is associated with metastases. The overall prognosis is excellent for small tumors.

SCC of the lower lip spreads to cervical lymph nodes in 15% of cases. The primary site of drainage is to the ipsilateral submandibular, submental, and upper jugular areas (see Fig. 20–9). The lymphatics arise on the vermilion margin and coalesce in the collecting trunks over the mandible ("Fu Manchu" pattern, see Fig. 20–9). Lymphatic crossovers in the midline provide a pathway for occasional contralateral spread. The submandibular and submental lymph nodes seldom reach large size before bursting and seeding the loose areolar subplatysmal tissues. Indeed, in one study showing a 13% incidence of cervical metastases, 70% demonstrated extracapsular spread and 63% involved bone.[233]

Cancer of the upper lip has a relatively poor prognosis. It can arise spontaneously, metastasizes early, and spreads more quickly by way of abundant lymphatics. Cervical metastases occur in 20% of primary tumors at the commissures and in 50% of upper lip tumors. Drainage from upper lip primary tumors is to the preauricular, intraparotid, facial, and submandibular lymph nodes.

At presentation, about 10% of patients with lip cancer have clinically positive cervical metastases. The incidence of clinically false-positive cervical lymph nodes is higher with lip cancer than with cancer of other sites in the oral cavity except FOM primary cancers. Late cervical metastases after successful treatment of the primary occur in 5 to 15% of patients. Cervical metastases present initially are cured more frequently than those with delayed onset (60% versus 40%). In one series of patients, 10% presented with cervical metastases. Of these, 25% died of recurrent cancer, whereas 75% of the patients with delayed appearance of positive neck nodes died of recurrent cancer. Forty percent of the delayed metastases were in stage I tumors.[235] Therefore, although lip cancer is generally considered to have an excellent prognosis for small tumors and a low incidence of spread to the neck, biologic variability is demonstrated as with all other sites.

The best prognosis accompanies a small, well-differentiated tumor of the lower lip without deep invasion or cervical metastases. In this category, 5-year survival is greater than 90% with adequate treatment. The majority of lip cancers fall into this category; more than 90% are T1 or T2 and grade I or II at initial presentation. Prognosis decreases in stage III and IV disease to the 10 to 15% 5-year survival typical of SCC in other sites.

Low-grade tumors metastasize rarely (6%), and high-grade tumors metastasize frequently (50%). Verrucous lesions rarely metastasize. Poorly differentiated and spindle cell tumors tend to spread along neural pathways and involve cervical lymph nodes. Regional hyperesthesia or pain indicate perineural spread. Perineural invasion is associated with an 80% metastatic rate.

Tumors less than 2 cm metastasize rarely (2 to 5%), whereas tumors greater than 2 cm metastasize as frequently as those in the anterior two thirds of the tongue and FOM (50 to 70%). Sack and Ford reported cervical metastases in 9 of 27 patients with T1 or T2 lesions.[233]

In the same series, 75% of patients who had T1 lesions with positive margins at initial surgery later developed metastases.

Advanced lip cancers (Fig. 20–17B) may spread along the mylohyoid muscle to the larynx and FOM, along the FOM and medial pterygoid muscles to the pterygoid fossa, along the hypoglossus muscle to the intrinsic muscles of the tongue, in the perineural spaces of the regional nerves (hypoglossal, lingual) to mylohyoid and anterior belly of digastric, along the inferior alveolar nerve and mental nerve to the middle cranial fossa, and along the infraorbital nerve to the foramen rotundum. Advanced tumors can invade the mandible by direct extension from the primary or spread from infested submandibular lymph nodes. The overlying skin and buccal mucosa may also be involved. The worst prognostic factors are fixation to or invasion of the mandible or FOM, spread along the mental nerves, and skin infiltration.[234]

Most local recurrences appear in the first year after treatment. Failure of treatment for cancer of the lip usually results from local persistence rather than metastatic spread. Recurrence rates are higher for the upper than the lower lip (25% versus 14%). Involvement of the labial commissures doubles the recurrence rate (in patients who have had surgery, this may reflect a tendency of the surgeon to "cheat" at this area because it is difficult to reconstruct). Local recurrence also increases as the size of the primary tumor increases.

After surgery, most recurrences develop in the neck. Postirradiation recurrences are more evenly divided between the lip and the neck. One major center was able to salvage 80% of patients with local recurrences: 60% with cervical lymph node recurrence and 25% with local-regional recurrence.[235]

Treatment

Small lip cancers can be treated with similar survival rates using surgery *or* RT as single modalities. Surgery provides a better cosmetic result and more rapid rehabilitation.

RT can produce a dry lip and mucosal atrophy. Recurrences are more difficult to identify, and the mucosa is more susceptible to carcinogenic agents such as sun and smoke. When large lesions are treated with RT, the area may take several months to heal, and a soft tissue defect, atrophic scar, and "whistle" deformity can result. RT for large invasive lesions can result in significant soft tissue and mandibular necrosis. Some authors favor wide-field RT if the mental nerve is involved, to encompass its course to the base of the skull. RT can be used for surgical failures, but salvage of scar recurrences is poor.[234]

RT may be considered preferentially as the initial treatment of lesions at the commissures and for superficial T2 or T3 lesions. RT may be administered as external beam, interstitial implants,[236] or a combination of both. For small lesions, kilovoltage (orthovoltage) radiation may be adequate, although this technique is generally considered outmoded. Electron beam or external megavoltage therapy is used for larger lesions. An appropriate sequence for invasive tumors is 30 Gy of external beam therapy followed by implants of equal amounts. Alternatively, small lesions may be treated with a dose of 45 Gy of external beam therapy.

Planned combined therapy should be used for surgical failures, massive tumors, and cervical metastases. General principles of surgical ablation[237] include a "lip shave" in cases with extensive multicentric dyskeratosis. Total vermilionectomy can be resurfaced with mucosa advanced from the inner moist mucosa as a bipedicled flap. Wedge resection is used for small to medium-sized tumors. For tiny superficial lesions, a normal margin of 4 to 5 mm may suffice. Large lip cancers tend to spread beyond palpable and visible tumor limits, and margins should be at least 1 cm. The margins of resection should be checked with frozen section.

In previously untreated patients, enlarged facial lymph nodes can often be removed incontinuity with mandibular periosteum leaving the underlying bone intact. With mandibular invasion, the involved bone should be removed at the primary resection. If involvement is in the vicinity of upper neck lymph nodes "fixed" to the mandible, it may be possible to perform a marginal (rim) resection of the lower half of the jawbone, preserving the upper alveolus and thereby avoiding segmental resection.

Nerve involvement (mental nerve) should be checked using frozen section. Resection should be extended to encompass gross extension of tumor associated with regional nerves. With respect to the mental nerve, which continues into the inferior alveolar canal, Byers has suggested drilling out the canal by removing the bone lateral to it and peeling the involved nerve out of the canal, leaving the surrounding bone intact. Wide-field postoperative radiation to the base of skull is presumably an acceptable alternative for microscopic perineural involvement.

For large lip cancers, bilateral suprahyoid neck dissection may be indicated to encompass the primary tumor adequately. Formal clearance of the submental and submandibular areas with primary tumors of the lip should include removal of the platysma muscle and anterior belly of the digastric muscles, and all tissue down to the mylohyoid muscle.

Elective neck treatment is not necessary for small lip cancers because of the low likelihood of metastatic spread. If lymph nodes are clinically positive, it has been suggested that an ipsilateral or bilateral suprahyoid neck dissection be performed as a biopsy technique. If the lymph nodes are histologically positive, a full neck dissection is completed at the same time. The inadequacy of this approach because of "skip metastases" has been alluded to previously. Palpable jugular chain disease should be treated with a full neck dissection.

When surgery to both the primary cancer and neck is necessary, Barbosa recommends staged procedures.[238] Excision and reconstruction of the primary lesion is carried out first, with the neck dissection performed at least 2 weeks later. This preserves the facial arteries long enough to supply the regional flaps used in reconstruction of the primary site; however, it is possible to perform a neck dissection, including submandibular gland excision, without transecting the facial arteries if care is taken and if no cancer extends directly into the neck. The arteries are related to the superior aspect of the submandibular glands and do not penetrate the substance of the gland.

Some authors suggest that the indications for elective neck treatment should be liberalized for lip primary cancers.[239] Patients with primary tumors of advanced stage or histologic grade, or those requiring surgical entry into the neck, may well benefit from neck dissection at the time of the primary surgery. Postoperative RT is added, based on the state of disease in the removed specimen. These authors recommend bilateral supraomohyoid neck dissections as a biopsy technique for:

1. Tumors greater than 1.5 cm in dimension.
2. Tumors of the commissure or upper lip.
3. Recurrent tumors.
4. Tumors with aggressive and infiltrative pathologic patterns.
5. Palpable lymph nodes in unreliable patients.

Reconstruction

As a guide to functional adequacy, the reconstructed oral opening should be innervated, mobile, and large enough to admit a spoon. For small oral commissures, hinged dentures can sometimes be made. Defects of less than 2 cm can usually be closed primarily. Many confusing and complicated methods are described in the literature for reconstruction of lip defects.[240] The prototype is the two-stage "lip switch" (Estlander-Abbé) flap (Fig. 20–18A). The Karapandzic flap is a technically simple and versatile local innervated myocutaneous advancement flap,[241,242] widely applicable for reconstruction of defects of a wide range of sizes of both upper and lower lips (Fig. 20–18E). Bilateral nasolabial[243] and hair-bearing flaps have also been described for total lip reconstruction.[244]

Cancer of the Gums (Gingivae and Alveolar Ridges)

SCC of the gums is another relatively favorable site for cancer in the oral cavity. Tumors of this site comprise 10% of oral carcinomas in Western countries and occur in elderly patients. In India, this site is much more frequently involved, and more than 70% occur in patients less than 50 years old. Women without a history of tobacco usage are more prone to develop SCC of the gums than cancers in other mouth sites.[23] Patients with cancer of the gums associated with leukoplakia are at greater risk to develop another primary tumor in the mouth.[23]

The premolar and molar regions are favored sites. They rarely involve the anterior third of the dental arch. Edentulous areas are preferential sites. The mandibular alveolar ridge is involved in 80% of cases; the maxillary alveolar ridge in 20%.

Ninety-five percent are well-differentiated SCC. Six percent of minor salivary gland tumors of the oral cavity occur on the gums. Most of the rare primary basal cell carcinomas in the oral cavity occur on the gums.

Patients present with complaints of poorly fitting dentures, loosening of the teeth, pain, and ulceration. In these situations, confusion of SCC with benign inflammatory disease is common, and the diagnosis may be delayed because of lack of awareness on the part of the examining physician. The initial diagnosis is frequently made after dental extractions, as is another entity that must be included in the differential diagnosis: metastatic tumors *to* the mandible (bone marrow), which frequently present through a dental extraction socket. A nonhealing dental extraction site should be biopsied.

Initially, tumors appear as flat, elongated, friable ulcers on the alveolar ridge. More rarely, nodular plaque-like, papillary exophytic, or fungating forms are seen. Because the alveolar mucosa is thin, tumors readily invade underlying bone and can extend along the periodontal membrane, sulci, FOM, palate, and buccal mucosa. In edentulous mandibles where the alveolar ridge has been resorbed, the inferior alveolar nerve frequently lies unroofed directly beneath involved mucosa (see Fig. 20–5E and F).

Thirty-five percent of patients have cervical metastases in the submandibular area. Mandibular primary cancers have a greater tendency to metastasize than do maxillary primary cancers.

Treatment

Survival is similar for tumors of both alveolar ridges, with an overall 5-year rate of 50%. Survival decreases as the tumor stage increases: 73% 5-year determinate survival for stage I and 17% for stage III. Small primary tumors are more easily cured, with 80% cures reported for tumors less than 3 cm.[245] Advanced lesions with bone destruction or cervical metastases are best treated by radical surgery and adjunctive RT.

Incisions providing access to the alveolar ridges and other oral cavity sites are shown in Figure 20–19. A lower lip-splitting incision (Fig. 20–19A) sacrifices the mental nerve ipsilaterally, and a visor flap may tran-

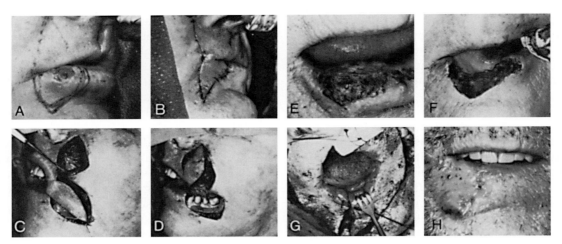

Fig. 20–18. A to D. Two patients with carcinoma of the lower lateral lip border. Reconstructed with Estlander flap after total resection. E to H. A third patient, with carcinoma resected and repaired with a Karapandzic flap. (Courtesy of Dr. GJ Spector.)

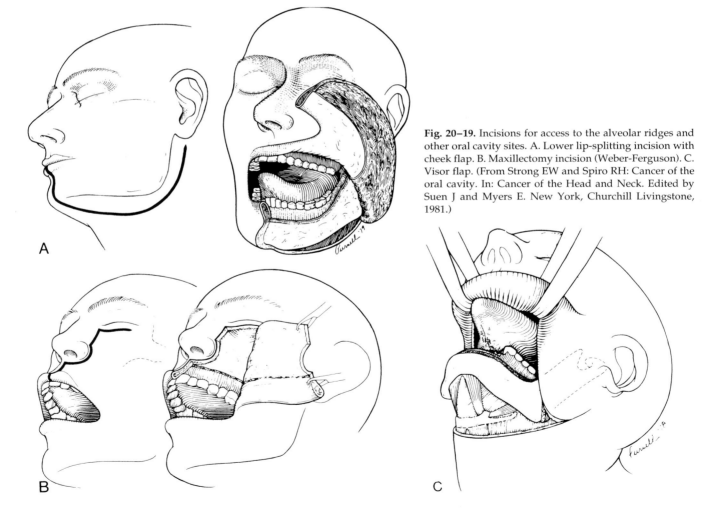

Fig. 20–19. Incisions for access to the alveolar ridges and other oral cavity sites. A. Lower lip-splitting incision with cheek flap. B. Maxillectomy incision (Weber-Ferguson). C. Visor flap. (From Strong EW and Spiro RH: Cancer of the oral cavity. In: Cancer of the Head and Neck. Edited by Suen J and Myers E. New York, Churchill Livingstone, 1981.)

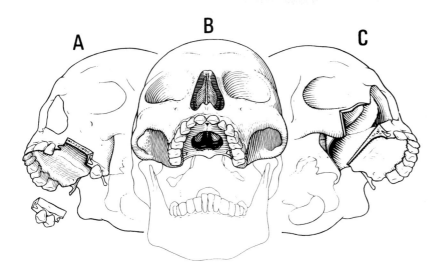

Fig. 20–20. Types of excision for alveolar ridge and palatal cancers. A. Maxillary alveolectomy. B. Partial palatectomy. C. Subtotal maxillectomy. (From Strong EW and Spiro RH: Cancer of the oral cavity. In: Cancer of the Head and Neck. Edited by Suen J and Myers E. New York, Churchill Livingstone, 1981.)

sect the nerves bilaterally (Fig. 20–19C). In the latter situation, one must try to preserve motor capability of the lower lip by sparing the marginal branches of the facial nerve because an immobile and insensate lower lip is a severe functional handicap, leading to oral crippling with drooling and interference with mastication.

The standard operation for a cancer located in the maxillary alveolus with minor extension onto the hard palate is a partial horizontal maxillectomy (Fig. 20–20A). A coronal CT can help to define bone erosion of the hard palate, although bone erosion by cancer is seldom seen in previously untreated patients. In a partial horizontal maxillectomy, the alveolar ridge is removed with a variable portion of hard palate over a distance adequate to remove the tumor with a 1-cm margin of normal tissue. This can be performed transorally for a small lesion. Exposure can be enhanced, if necessary, by a midface "degloving" approach,[246] using an incision made in the gingivolabial sulcus at a point that constitutes an adequate margin for the tumor, although I prefer not to undermine widely in an area of cancer, to decrease the risk of implantive cancer cells over a wider area[107] (as has been seen once at our institution with a midface degloving approach). A maxillary antrostomy widened by removing the anterior face of the maxilla allows visualization to ascertain whether the floor of the sinus is also involved. Larger tumors may require a subtotal maxillectomy (Fig. 20–20C) performed through a lateral rhinotomy incision with an upper lip-splitting extension (see Fig. 20–19B). A prosthetic obturator is frequently used to rehabilitate the defect.

The standard operation for cancer located in the mandibular alveolus is a partial horizontal mandibulectomy (Fig. 20–21G) (marginal or rim resection, alveolectomy) by way of a transoral approach with exposure enhanced as necessary by a lower lip-splitting incision with a cheek flap (see Fig. 20–19A).

Cancer of the Buccal Mucosa

Cancers of the buccal mucosa comprise 10% of intraoral carcinomas in Western countries and 50 to 70% of oral cancers in Southeast Asia and the Indian subcontinent. These cancers are generally asymptomatic until ulceration or infection leads to cheek swelling and pain. Trismus results from neoplastic infiltration of the masseter muscle. Most patients have extensive local disease, and 30 to 50% have cervical metastases at presentation. The first nodes involved are in the submandibular area.

Most tumors are well-differentiated SCCs: exophytic, ulceroinfiltrative, and verrucous types, in decreasing order of frequency. The buccal mucosa is the most common intraoral site for verrucous carcinoma, which is usually associated with leukoplakia. The most common location is opposite the lower third molar (Fig. 20–22). Other rare tumors that occur in this location are salivary gland tumors, melanomas, lymphomas, fibrosarcomas, malignant schwannomas, and hemangiomas.[247] SCC of Stensen's (parotid) duct may present as a lesion in the buccal mucosa.[248] Adenocarcinoma and mucoepidermoid carcinomas have also been reported in this location.

Advanced buccal squamous cell tumors tend to invade deeply and involve adjacent structures including the buccal fat pad (Bichat's pad), cheek skin, mandible, infratemporal fossa, parotid gland, anterior tonsillar pillars, soft palate, alveolar ridges, retromolar trigone, labial commissure, and lips. In one series, contiguous structures were involved in 17% of T1 lesions and 85% of T3 or T4 lesions.[247] Anteriorly located tumors have a better prognosis than those in the posterior third of the buccal mucosa. Neoplasms located at the commissures, along the occlusal line (where the upper and lower teeth meet), or in the retromolar areas tend to be aggressive. Deep penetration of local tissues is asso-

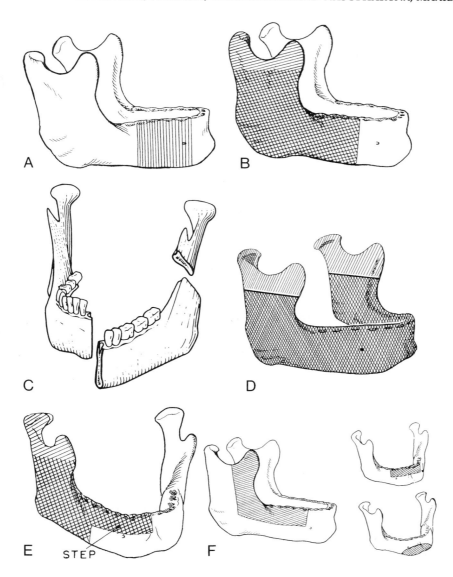

Fig. 20–21. Types of mandibulectomy. A. Segmental resection. B to D. Total or subtotal segmental resection. E. Partial and step segmental resection. F. Marginal resection. *(continued)*

ciated with invasion of regional lymphatics and cervical metastatic disease.

Treatment

The overall 5-year determinate cure rate is 40%. Survival depends on stage: in stage I it is 77%, and in stage IV, 18%.[247] These tumors tend to recur locally because multicentric foci are common: 40% in 1 series.[249] Salvage of initial treatment failures is poor: 10 to 15%.

Smaller lesions (T1 or T2) may be treated with RT or simple excision. The laser is convenient for excision of lesions suitable for a transoral approach. The parotid duct generally does not become obstructed if transected after either laser or "cold knife" excision, provided it is not included in a suture line.

RT as a curative modality is best applied as a combination of external beam and interstitial implants. A 50% 3-year NED (no evidence of disease) survival using RT alone has been reported for T1 or T2 lesions.

RT is unlikely to be curative for invasive or large lesions, and combination therapy is recommended for this situation.

The extent of surgery varies from local resection with mucosal flap or skin-dermal graft resurfacing for T1 or T2 lesions to radical excision. Through-and-through excisions with marginal or segmental mandibulectomy, partial maxillectomy, or combinations of both are sometimes necessary for large lesions.

Reconstruction

Closure of full-thickness defects is difficult and has been traditionally attempted with local-regional flaps such as forehead, tongue, cervical skin, and deltopectoral, usually with imperfect cosmetic and functional results (Fig. 20–23). (A caution should be mentioned with respect to undermining and transposing local flaps from adjacent "uninvolved" areas: because removal of every cancer cell at the primary site can never

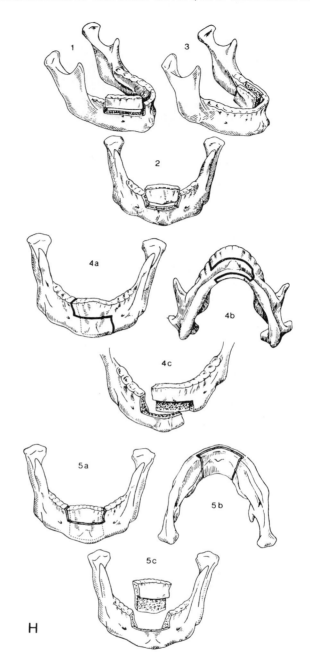

Fig. 20–21. *(continued)* G and H. Modifications of marginal resection of the mandible. (A, B, D, E, and F, from Martin H: Surgery of Head and Neck Tumors. New York, Harper & Row, 1964; C and G, from Strong EW and Spiro RH: Cancer of the oral cavity. In: Cancer of the Head and Neck. Edited by Suen J and Myers E. New York, Churchill Livingstone, 1981; H, from Flynn MB, Moore C: Am J Surg *128*:491, 1974.)

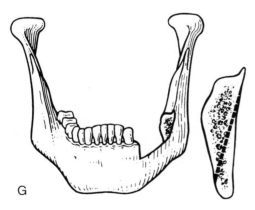

be guaranteed, subclinical disease as well as implantation from the tumor bed can grow rapidly in adjacent tissue with disastrous results.[107]) Pectoralis myocutaneous and myofascial flaps surfaced on both sides with split-thickness skin grafts (see subsequent text) are common reconstructive options. Free flap transfers probably achieve the best cosmetic results in skilled hands.

Cancer of the Palate

In Western countries, cancer of the palate is the rarest site for SCC of the oral cavity, comprising less than 5%. As mentioned previously, the incidence is much higher in countries where reverse smoking is practiced. In the hard palate, the ratio of glandular to squamous cell tumors is 3 or 4:1. This preponderance of salivary tumors (usually submucosal) is not seen in the soft palate. Other tumor types reported in the palate are lymphoma, plasmacytoma, malignant melanoma, Ewing's sarcoma, myxosarcoma, and undifferentiated tumors. Plasmacytoma not infrequently presents on the alveolar ridge. These rare types of tumors are generally associated with poor survival.[250]

Of note in the differential diagnosis is that maxillary sinus cancers can present intraorally, as can nasal can-

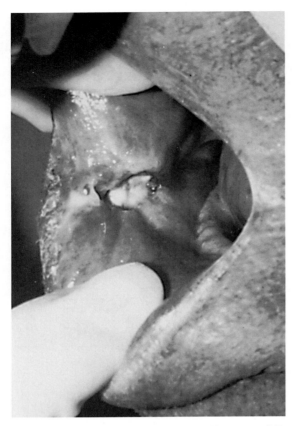

Fig. 20–22. Cancers of the buccal mucosa. (Courtesy of Dr. GJ Spector.)

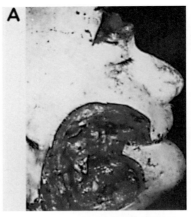

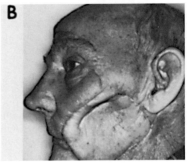

Fig. 20–23. A. Resection of large buccal carcinoma involving the mandible and floor of the mouth. B. Reconstruction of a similar defect with a lined forehead flap. (Courtesy of Dr. GJ Spector.)

cers (Fig. 20–24). With respect to differential diagnosis, several types of "benign metastasizing" lesions have been reported on the palate. Follicular lymphoid hyperplasia can recur after local excision and can involve ipsilateral neck and buccal lymph nodes. The usual presentation is of a slow-growing mass of the hard palate that simulates nodular lymphoma or Mikulicz' disease. Local excision is the treatment of choice. Malignant sialadenoma papilliferum may present as an intraoral papillary tumor of the soft palate. It arises from the minor salivary gland excretory ducts of the palate.[251]

SCC occurs more frequently on the soft palate (70%) than on the hard palate (30%).[252] Soft palate tumors are generally considered tumors of the oropharynx (see subsequent text). Cancers of the soft palate tend to metastasize bilaterally or contralaterally to cervical lymph nodes more frequently than those on the hard palate (40% versus 15%). Some series show a similar incidence for both sites of about 35%.[253]

Signs and symptoms include swelling on the roof of the mouth, pain, ulceration, and ill-fitting dentures. Early tumors are frequently asymptomatic. Several cancers of the hard and soft palate are illustrated in Figure 20–25.

Tumors of the palate tend to grow laterally and

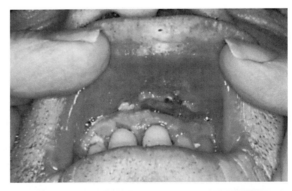

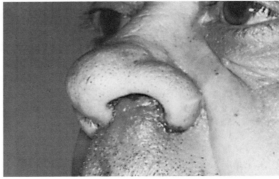

Fig. 20–24. Nasal cancer presenting intraorally. (Courtesy of Dr. GJ Spector.)

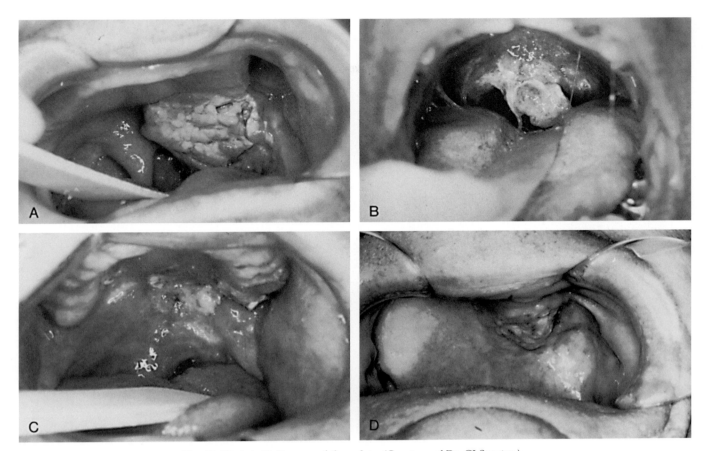

Fig. 20–25. A to D. Cancers of the palate. (Courtesy of Dr. GJ Spector.)

show little tendency for deep invasion. Extensive tumors seldom perforate the nasal cavities. Areas of extension from palatal tumors include the maxillary antrum, pterygoid muscles, root of the tongue, skin of the neck or cheek, tonsil, and pharynx. Palatal cancers also have access to nerves at the skull base and thence to the brain by way of the foramen rotundum, foramen ovale, and orbital fissures. CT and MR imaging are used to evaluate invasion of the base of skull, pterygomaxillary space, lymph nodes, and venous sinuses. Traditionally, one sees virtually no survivors when tumor extends to these areas, at least partly because, in the past, such tumor extensions were considered unresectable if they destroyed the pterygoid plates, petrous pyramid, base of the skull, or eustachian tube, or if they penetrated the posterior wall of the maxillary sinus.

Treatment
With advances in skull base surgery, however, the contraindications cited previously may no longer be absolute. Techniques originally developed for neuro-otologic procedures are now used more adequately to encompass head and neck cancers extending cephalad and posteriorly.[254,255] Such adjunctive techniques require special training and skill, and data are inade-

quate at this point to define the utility of this type of surgery in the context of SCC. Whether the increased risk of such operations (actually minimal in experienced hands, especially when procedures are extradural) is balanced by a survival advantage to the patient or an increased ability to control local-regional disease remains to be seen. Certainly, without such radical surgery, the prognosis is virtually hopeless.

Extensive disease requiring skull base operations also mandates postoperative RT. Skull base surgery also has applications for tumors in the oropharynx and maxillary sinus, to provide a cephalad and posterior margin on tumors extending beyond the traditional limits of standard operations (Fig. 20–26).

Surgical treatment is preferred for SCC of the hard palate because of the proximity of bone and the traditional belief that RT is less suitable for lesions involving bone, although this dogma has been challenged.[145] Surgery is tailored to the size and extent of the lesion. Traditional operations include transoral excision (alveolectomy) and partial or subtotal maxillectomy (usually horizontal) (see Fig. 20–20). The greater palatine nerve should be submitted for frozen section, and the greater palatine foramen and pterygoid canal should be resected when nerve involvement is demonstrated. This situation might well mandate skull base surgery

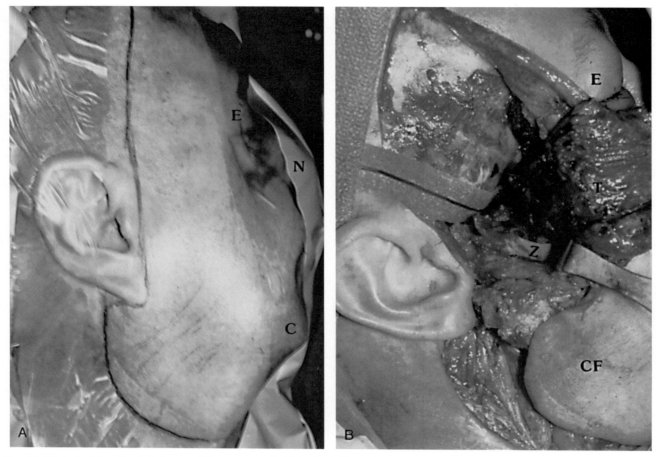

Fig. 20–26. A. Incisions for infratemporal fossa approach (right face). E, Eyelid; N, nose; C, chin. B. Exposure of infratemporal fossa. Z, Zygoma; CF, cheek flap; T, temporalis muscle; E, eyelid. (Courtesy of Dr. JP Leonetti.)

in the contemporary context. The overall cure rate for SCC of the palate has been about 40%.

Cancers of the soft palate are typically diffuse mucosal lesions and tend to be radiosensitive. Unless the lesion is bulky over an extensive area, RT with curative intent is preferred. This is effective in controlling local disease in suitable cases and avoids morbidity pursuant to full-thickness soft palate surgical defects.

Reconstruction

Small mucosal defects of the palate heal by secondary intention. On rare occasions in the past, tongue or nasolabial flaps[243] were used. Both such flaps require a second operation under local anesthesia to release the pedicle and are inconvenient during the interim. Larger palate defects are managed with prosthetic obturators. These decrease nasal regurgitation and improve speech quality and deglutition, but normalization of functions related to velopharyngeal competence is seldom complete.

Cancer of the Floor of the Mouth

In the oral cavity, SCCs occur in the FOM and tongue most frequently. FOM cancers are usually asymptom-

atic, but patients may complain of a lump, discomfort, increased salivation or drooling, limitation of tongue motion, or speech difficulty with advanced tumors. Local pain and referred otalgia are late symptoms. The neural pathways for referred otalgia in tumors of various sites of the oral cavity, oropharynx, and hypopharynx are shown in Figure 20–27. Anatomic relationships of the FOM are shown in Figure 20–28. Representative T1 and T4 FOM cancers are illustrated in Figure 20–29.

These cancers are usually well differentiated; they may be exophytic, papillary, or ulcerative, and they can invade Wharton's duct, although the substance of the submandibular gland is rarely infiltrated. They spread anteroposteriorly and laterally. The loose submucosal tissue of the submental and submandibular space facilitates deep extension. In one study of 700 patients, about 25% of FOM cancers were confined to the FOM, and 75% extended to involve more than one adjacent structure at the time of diagnosis. Forty percent of these tumors crossed the midline, 15% invaded bone, and only 25% were less than 2 cm at presentation.[256] This series reported a compilation accumulated over decades in the first half of this century, during

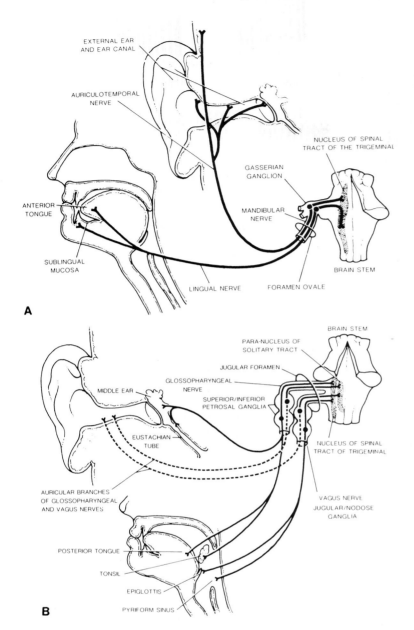

Fig. 20–27. Neural pathways for referred otalgia. A. From floor of mouth and anterior tongue. B. From posterior tongue, oropharynx, and pharynx. (From Lingeman RE and Singer MI: Evaluation of the patient with head and neck cancer. In: Cancer of the Head and Neck. Edited by Suen J and Myers E. New York, Churchill Livingstone, 1981.)

which time proportionately more tumors were diagnosed in an advanced stage than currently.

The lymphatic drainage of the FOM and anterior tongue is shown in Figure 20–30. The incidence and location of neck metastases associated with primary tumors of the FOM as compiled from the literature is seen in Tables 20–5 and 20–6. Half of the initially palpable lymph nodes occur in areas I and II (see Fig. 20–12). About 10% of patients have lymphadenopathy in regions III or IV without palpable nodes higher in the neck, however.

Treatment
Infiltrative lesions, regardless of surface dimension, require more radical treatment than superficial tumors.

Deep biopsies in areas of nodularity and induration allow assessment of vertical growth. Superficial or microinvasive T2 lesions behave similarly to T1 lesions and are amenable to wide local excision. T2 lesions with a nodular-invasive vertical growth pattern frequently recur locally, and 44% had regional metastases in one series.[257] Many clinicians believe that elective treatment of the neck is warranted for invasive T3 lesions; however, prophylactic neck treatment for superficial T1 to T3 lesions is generally not thought to be indicated.

Transoral wide local excision is the standard surgical treatment for small FOM tumors involving only soft tissue. The laser is convenient in this context, as discussed previously. The excision bed is left open to

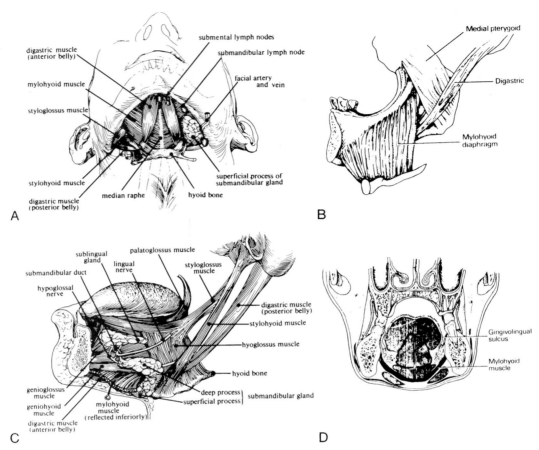

Fig. 20–28. Anatomic relationships of the floor of mouth. (A and C, from Vidic B and Melloni BJ: Otolaryngol Clin North Am *12*:8, 1979; B and D, from Barron JN and Saad MN (eds): Operative Plastic and Reconstructive Surgery. New York, Churchill Livingstone, 1980.)

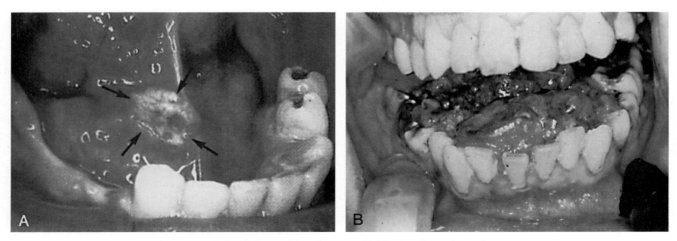

Fig. 20–29. A. Small floor-of-mouth cancer. B. Massive floor-of-mouth cancer.

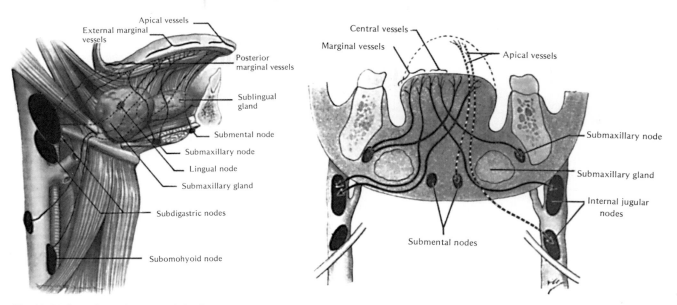

Fig. 20–30. Lymphatic drainage of the floor of mouth and anterior tongue. (From Rouvière H: Anatomie des lymphatiques de l'homme. Paris, Masson, 1932.)

heal secondarily by reepithelialization, and the submandibular gland ducts usually stay open to the surface, as opposed to the scarring that generally follows surgery performed with electrocautery or knife. (In the latter context, subsequent submandibular gland obstruction is problematic and may mandate gland excision to rule out recurrent cancer if conservative management of sialadenitis fails.) Tracheostomy is rarely necessary with laser resection.

The standard surgical approach to moderate-sized invasive FOM lesions is the "pull-through" operation[258] (Fig. 20–31). This approach is also suitable for some lesions with an epicenter in the tongue. The excision typically includes sublingual glands, extrinsic muscles of the tongue, and FOM diaphragm; the inferior limit of resection is at the level of the hyoid bone (which is not removed unless necessary to adhere an adequate cancer margin).

A pull-through operation can be performed through a horizontal upper neck incision with the neck flaps elevated to expose the inferior aspect of the mandible. Access to and closure of a pull-through procedure are facilitated by including the anterior mandibular alveolus (rim section) and inner periosteum with the primary resection en bloc. The "pull-through" designation refers to the procedure by which the anterior mandible and chin skin are left intact without incisions or mandibulotomy. The illustrations in Figure 20–32 show how wide exposure to the oral cavity and the oropharynx is afforded without the need to split the mandible. A "pull-through" approach can similarly be used for cancers located more posteriorly in the oral cavity and oropharynx (see later).

The indications for preservation of the mandible ad-

jacent to FOM tumors are not clearly defined. Principles relevant to excision of bone in conjunction with excision of oral cavity cancer are discussed previously. In the absence of flagrant, radiologically demonstrable bone invasion, a reasonable alternative to full-thickness anterior segmental resection between the mandibular angles is removal of the inner table of the mandible in continuity with requisite soft tissue, which can also be performed in the manner of a pull-through (Fig. 20–33). An anterior marginal mandibulectomy in continuity with the inner table of the mandible leaves the inferior outer cortex intact for continuity and chin projection (Fig. 20–33G), especially important within the mandibular arch.[90] The indications for including the inner table of the mandible are *absence* of gross bone erosion or a pitted surface when the periosteum is stripped from the inner surface intraoperatively (Fig. 20–33D). This is not a reliable sign of cancer invasion in previously irradiated patients.

A lateralized FOM tumor that requires segmental bony excision can be encompassed with a composite-type resection (see Fig. 20–37).

Advanced, neglected FOM tumors (fortunately now rare in the United States) can penetrate the anterior mandible bicortically and involve the chin skin (see Fig. 20–29B). This situation requires through-and-through anterior segmental resection between the mandibular angles, as well as appropriate intraoral soft tissue excision, which may include total glossectomy (Fig. 20–34). This is discussed further in the subsequent section on tongue cancer.

The defect pursuant to anterior bone resection, the "Andy Gump" deformity, is the most difficult head and neck cancer defect to reconstruct (Fig. 20–35), and

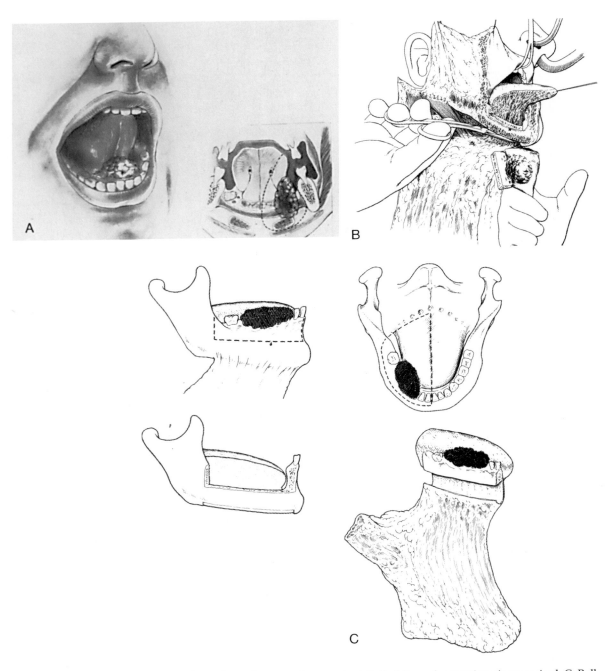

Fig. 20–31. A. Transoral approach to floor of mouth cancer; tissue excised. B. Pull-through operation; tissue excised. C. Pull-through operation; intraoperative maneuvers. (A, from Novack AJ: Otolaryngol Clin North Am *Oct*:578, 1969; B and C, from Barbosa JF (ed): Surgical Treatment of Head and Neck Tumors. New York, Grune & Stratton, 1974.)

maneuvers to avoid creating it include completely "degloving" the symphysis (including periosteum circumferentially) while leaving a 1-cm rim inferiorly to support a myocutaneous flap. Although the bone may later necrose, it usually persists long enough to provide an adequate framework for soft tissue that can maintain the anterior arch configuration and oral competence caused by scarring. Various types of mandibulectomy are shown in Figure 20–21.

Reconstruction

Reconstruction of various-sized soft tissue or bony defects in the oral cavity is discussed subsequently.

Cancer of the Tongue

Tongue cancer is treacherous. One can still find statements in the literature such as "no lethal disease is easier to cure than oral cancer less than 1 cm in diame-

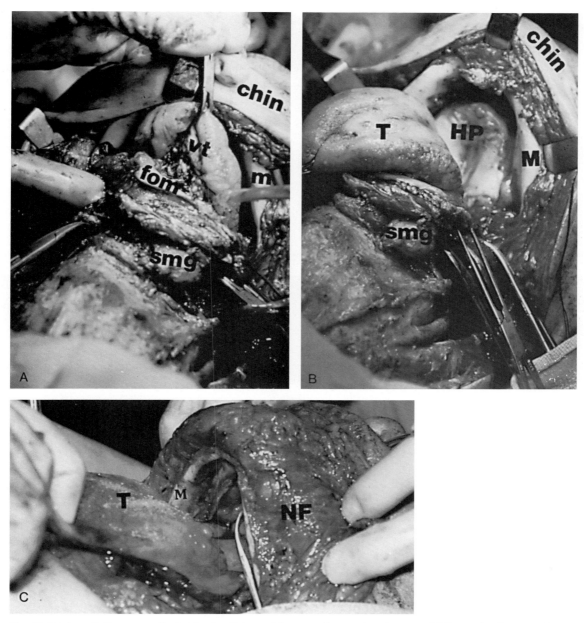

Fig. 20–32. A to C. Exposure afforded by ''pull-through'' approach to oral cavity. m or M, Lower border mandible; T, tongue; NF, neck flap turned up over chin; fom, floor of mouth; smg, submandibular gland; HP, hard palate; vt, ventral tongue.

ter.''[48] This is not always true. Because of the lack of natural barriers to spread at the primary site and the significant incidence of neck metastases even with small primary cancers (frequently bilateral and of delayed onset, and possibly enhanced by the muscular activity at the primary site pumping cancer cells into the regional lymphatics), local-regional disease is difficult to control.

Two major tongue sites are divided by the circumvallate papillae: the anterior two thirds (oral tongue, mobile tongue) and the posterior third (base of

tongue). The base of the tongue is generally classified as a site in the oropharynx because of a suggestion of different biologic behavior from the anterior two thirds in the oral cavity; however, this may be an artifact, as discussed previously. Both tongue sites are discussed in this section.

Tongue cancers constitute 20 to 50% of all oral cavity carcinomas. In Western countries, approximately 75% are located anteriorly and 25% in the base of the tongue. The ratio is reversed in Asia because of regional smoking habits. Ninety-seven percent of oral

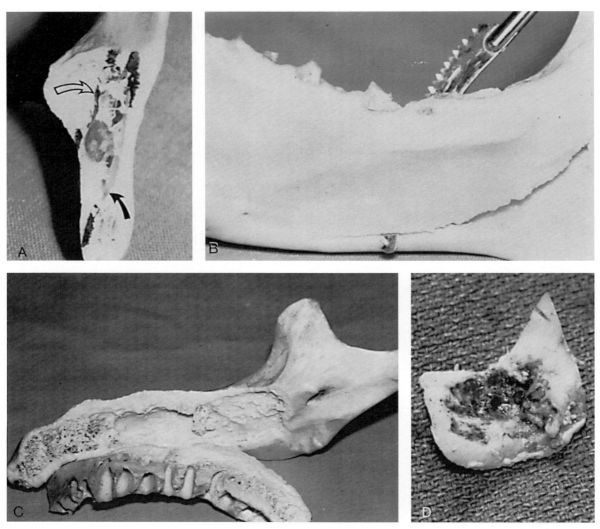

Fig. 20–33. A. Mandible cross-section. Angles for marginal (rim) resection (open arrow) and for inner-table mandibulectomy (solid arrow). B. Inner-table mandibulectomy: making bone cut with reciprocating side-cutting "banana" saw blade. C. Completed bone cut, inner-table mandibulectomy. D. Excised bone. Note pitted surface. *(continued)*

tongue cancers are SCCs. Most are moderately well differentiated. Adenocarcinoma and sarcomas (1 to 2%) are rare.

The most common location of SCC of the oral tongue is along the lateral borders of the middle third and ventral surface (Figs. 20–14B and 20–36). Cancers of the tip and dorsum are uncommon. Most tumors are larger than 2 cm at diagnosis, and 25 to 50% have extended beyond the oral tongue to involve adjacent areas, especially the FOM and alveolar ridge. Symptoms are few. Pain and dysphagia occur late. A frequent comment from patients who present with large tumors is "it didn't hurt, so I didn't think it was anything bad"—an example of denial and cancerophobia. Pain may result from neural invasion or tumor ulceration. Tongue tethering and asymmetry on protrusion indicate deep muscle fixation or hypoglossal nerve involvement (rare). Altered articulation may result.

The incidence of cervical metastases is compiled in Tables 20–5 and 20–6. Metastases occur most frequently in the subdigastric, submandibular, and midjugular areas; however, skip metastases are not uncommon. The middle third and tip of the tongue have bilateral lymphatic drainage and contralateral metastases may be found in the absence of ipsilateral disease. Neck disease is emerging as a significant cause of mortality in patients with small tongue cancers.[129]

Treatment

ANTERIOR TWO THIRDS OF THE TONGUE. The surgical principles for excision of tongue cancers involving only soft tissue are similar to those described in the previous section for FOM cancers—transoral wide excision or pull-through operations. The adequate margin for tongue cancers has not been scientifically defined. The

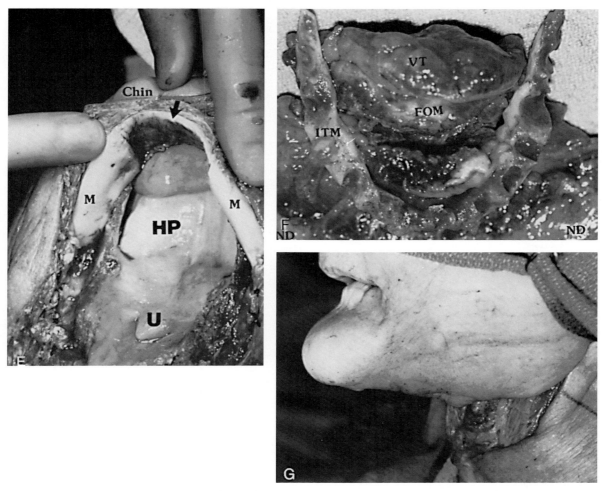

Fig. 20–33. *(continued)* E. View from below, inner-table mandibulectomy. Defect (arrow) and preserved mandible. HP, Hard palate; U, uvula; M, lower border of mandible. F. Specimen, floor of mouth (FOM) resection with inner-table mandibulectomy (ITM). VT, Ventral tongue; ND, neck dissections. G. Maintenance of chin projection after inner-table plus marginal mandibulectomy.

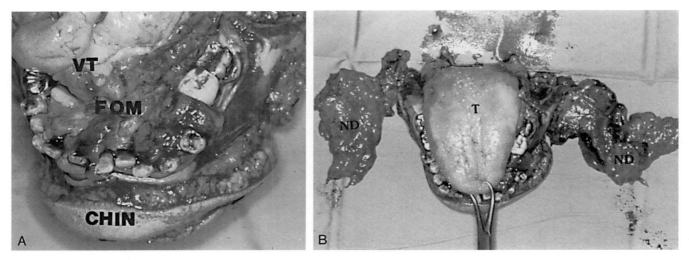

Fig. 20–34. A. Massive floor of mouth (FOM) cancer penetrating anterior mandible. VT, Ventral tongue. B. Specimen, subtotal mandibulectomy, total glossectomy (T), bilateral neck dissections (ND).

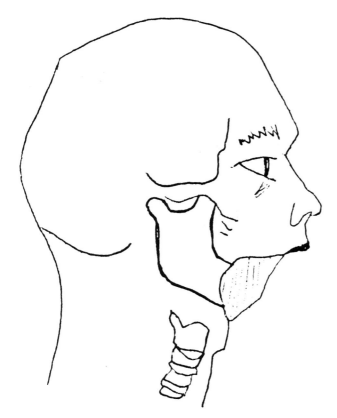

Fig. 20–35. "Andy Gump" deformity.

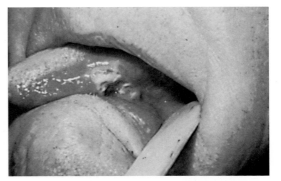

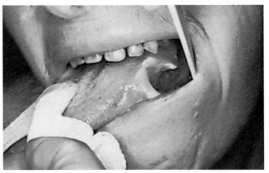

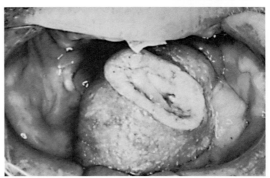

Fig. 20–36. Tongue cancers. (Courtesy of Dr. GJ Spector.)

recommendations of Harrison[64] and others have been discussed previously.

For tongue cancers, wide local excision refers to a lesser excision than hemiglossectomy. Hemiglossectomy removes half the tongue, with the midline raphe as the medial margin. Subtotal glossectomy removes more tissue than hemiglossectomy, but is less extensive than total glossectomy. Total glossectomy removes the entire anterior two thirds of the tongue and the base (see subsequent section).

When surgery is the only treatment, one sees an increase in local recurrence with increasing size of the primary tumor: 20% with lesions less than 4 cm and 50% with larger lesions.[259] One series, however, reported a 30% local recurrence rate with T1 to T3, N0 lesions, demonstrating that local recurrence is independent of primary tumor size.[260] Johnson and associates showed a 30 to 50% local recurrence rate for T1 tumors treated with wide local excision. Such statistics emphasize the treacherous nature of tongue cancer.[261]

For large tumors invading bone, (usually recurrent) because the hemimandible is relatively expendable, composite resection is recommended to ensure more adequate clearance of the soft tissue, rather than attempting to preserve the outer table of the mandible laterally. In this situation, a lateral inner-table mandibulectomy procedure with pull-through is technically difficult, unnecessary, and potentially dangerous with respect to tumor recurrence. In previously untreated patients, however, lateralized tumors of the oropharynx or the base of the tongue often do not penetrate beyond the plane of the paratonsillar space and can be removed with a soft tissue pull-through. Alternatively, a posterior "marginal" rim resection by cheek-flap exposure can often adequately encompass a tumor that abuts or involves the retromolar trigone-pterygoid area. This leaves the inferior aspect of the mandible intact for jaw continuity.

Composite (monoblock, "commando" jaw-neck, or jaw-tongue-neck) resection (Fig. 20–37) involves a hemimandibulectomy with an ipsilateral neck dissection and, in view of the other resection options just discussed, is one I usually use for patients with recurrent disease or massive cancers with an epicenter at the maxillary tuberosity (skull base). The bone is typically resected just anterior to the mental foramen and at the

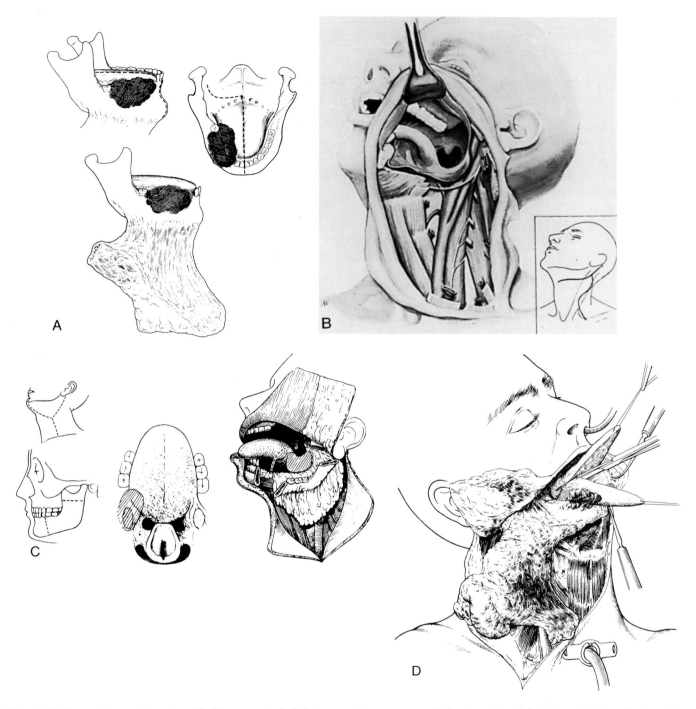

Fig. 20–37. Composite resection. A and B. Tissues excised. C. Intraoperative maneuvers. D. Postoperative defect. (A and C, from Barbosa JF (ed): Surgical Treatment of Head and Neck Tumors. New York, Grune & Stratton, 1974; B, from Daly JF: Otolaryngol Clin North Am *Oct*:600, 1969; D, from Shumrick D and Gluckman JL: Cancer of the oropharynx. In: Cancer of the Head and Neck. Edited by Suen J and Myers E. New York, Churchill Livingstone, 1981.)

notch between the coronoid and condylar process to encompass the inferior dental canal and its contents. The adjacent medial soft tissue removed encompasses the tumor with an adequate margin of normal tissue and typically includes some tongue, lateral FOM, and sometimes oropharynx tissue. "Incontinuity" neck dis-

section is not essential, except in cases with direct extension of tumor between the primary site and the neck.

For many years, starting in the 1940s, the composite resection was the standard operation ("one operation fits all") for cancer of the oral cavity and oropharynx.

The jaw was removed regardless of oncologic need to facilitate primary closure. This is no longer necessary or acceptable with modern reconstructive techniques (see subsequent text).

With or without reconstruction, patients function well after this type of operation if at least half the tongue is retained. Speech is readily understandable, and a nearly soft diet is usually tolerated by mouth. The cosmetic deformity is acceptable, especially with soft tissue reconstruction (see Fig. 20–59). Bony reconstruction is not necessary after lateral mandibulectomy. (Mandibulectomy refers to removing a portion of bone that is not replaced, whereas mandibulotomy refers to transecting the mandible to allow exposure without removing any bone. The bone segments are later reapproximated.)

BASE OF TONGUE TUMORS. Primary SCCs of the base of the tongue are relatively rare, although the area is frequently involved by extension from tumors in adjacent sites. Involvement of perineural, vascular, and lymphatic structures is frequent. Lymphomas of Waldeyer's ring and minor salivary gland tumors should also be considered in the differential diagnosis.

Because the base of the tongue is almost devoid of pain fibers, these tumors are usually asymptomatic, and almost 75% of such tumors involve adjacent structures at presentation. Tumors of the base of the tongue may extend to involve the oral tongue, tonsillar area, vallecula, epiglottis, preepiglottic space, and hypopharyngeal wall. Referred otalgia may be a presenting complaint because of involvement of the sensory branches of the glossopharyngeal nerve or lingual nerve (see Fig. 20–27), and large lesions may produce a sore throat, which increases during deglutition, coughing, or tongue protrusion. A "hot potato" voice results from the gurgling of pooled secretions or tongue tethering and tumor bulk. The tongue should be examined during protrusion for decreased mobility and deviation. Trismus results from invasion of the pterygoid muscles. Tumors in this location frequently have a submucosal component, and delayed diagnosis is common when the patient initially presents to nonspecialists. The typical history is of prolonged treatment with antibiotics without resolution of symptoms, usually for weeks or months.

The biologic behavior of tumors of the base of the tongue is stated to be more similar to those of the oropharynx than to those of the oral cavity. SCCs of the base of the tongue are generally considered highly anaplastic, invasive, and widely metastatic. The concept that tumors of the base of the tongue are unusually aggressive lesions may be a misconception. Diagnosis is typically delayed, and the tumor is usually at an advanced stage at presentation because of the obscure nature of symptoms and relative inaccessibility of the area to examination.[118] Careful palpation of the base

of tongue should be routine during *any* head and neck examination.

The incidence of cervical metastases is presented in Tables 20–5 and 20–6.

Lesions in the base of tongue can seldom be approached transorally. Median or labiomandibular glossotomy is described as an acceptable approach for benign tumors in the base of the tongue (or for lingual thyroid requiring excision) but should not be used for epidermoid cancers (Fig. 20–38C). This method results in scarring and tethering of the tongue and FOM and severely inhibits the oral phase of swallowing. A wide

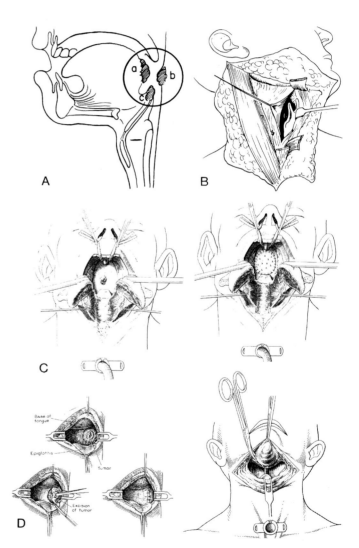

Fig. 20–38. Approaches to the pharynx. A. Tumor sites (a, b and c) accessible by median labiomandibular glossotomy, lateral or transhyoid pharyngotomy. B. Lateral pharyngotomy. C. Median labiomandibular glossotomy. D. Transhyoid pharyngotomy. (A and B, from Shumrick D and Gluckman JL: Cancer of the oropharynx. In: Cancer of the Head and Neck. Edited by Suenn J and Myers E. New York, Churchill Livingstone, 1981; C and D (right), from Barbosa JF (ed): Surgical Treatment of Head and Neck Tumors. New York, Grune & Stratton, 1974; D (left), from Martin H: Surgery of Head and Neck Tumors. New York, Harper & Row, 1964.)

local excision operation may be performed by means of a transcervical pull-through and may interfere with swallowing if it alters the hyomandibular complex. This may have little adverse effect on swallowing if the hyoid is preserved (at least the contralateral half), if one hypoglossal nerve can be preserved and the patient is physiologically sound and motivated to cooperate in the rehabilitation. Primary closure of such a defect is usually possible by retrodisplacing the anterior tongue.

Such an approach often yields adequate exposure without the need to perform mandibulotomy with paralingual extension—the mandibular "swing" approach[262,263] (Figs. 20–39 and 20–40), although this approach is preferred by some surgeons. Mandibular "swing" is performed through a lower lip-splitting incision, which is frequently depicted as vertical through the lower lip and curving in a chin crease around the mental protuberance. A straight midline incision through the lip and chin, continued laterally in the upper neck, is more cosmetically acceptable (Fig. 20–40). This operation incises the lateral FOM (without transecting the hypoglossal nerve and sometimes preserving the lingual nerve with oral cavity tumors, Fig. 20–40B) to allow exposure to the oropharynx area (Fig. 20–40C). The tissue is reapproximated primarily at the

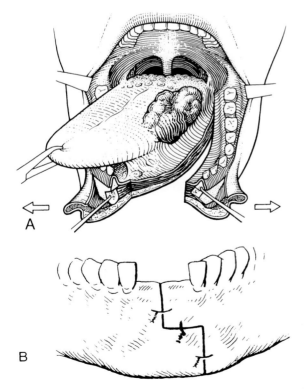

Fig. 20–39. A. Median mandibulotomy with paralingual extension ("mandibular swing") operation. B. Rewiring of median mandibulotomy. (From Strong EW and Spiro RH: Cancer of the oral cavity. In: Cancer of the Head and Neck. Edited by Suen J and Myers E. New York, Churchill Livingstone, 1981.)

end of the procedure, and the mandibulotomy is plated or wired (Figs. 20–39 and 20–40A).

The defect resulting from resection of relatively small lateralized tumors of the base of the tongue through this approach can usually be closed primarily by reapproximating the posterior tongue and residual tissue in the vallecula. Methods of securing the anterior (stepped, "V"-shaped, straight) mandibulotomy are varied.[264] Wires frequently lack the necessary stability to ensure bony union. This is often manifested as a self-healing transient fistula in the submental area, although occasional nonunion results with persistent mobility. A more reliable method of reapproximating the mandibulotomy is application of lag screws or a metal bone plate (see subsequent text), although plates are difficult to mold to the symphyseal area. A small reconstruction plate is probably preferable for this purpose. Miniplates are inadequate to stabilize the anterior mandibulotomy.

Operations providing wide access decrease the incidence of local recurrence. One series reported a local recurrence rate of 36% using the transhyoid and lateral pharyngotomy approaches (see Figs. 20–38B and D), 33% with local excision, and 20% using composite resection.[265] Results with mandibular "swing" approach have been reported by Spiro and colleagues.[262] Tumors of the base of the tongue that extend laterally or recur after irradiation or prior surgery are probably best handled with a composite resection approach.

The need for adjunctive laryngeal excisions—subtotal supraglottic laryngectomy (SSL) or total laryngectomy—can influence the amount of tongue that needs to be resected. Tumors of the base of the tongue can invade the preepiglottic space and, conversely, supraglottic tumors of the larynx can extend into the vallecula and involve the base of the tongue. This latter situation can sometimes be handled by "extended SSL" if the anterior resection margin would be at or posterior to the circumvallate papillae. Because successful deglutition after SSL depends mainly on the action of the base of the tongue, in one series all patients who had an extended SSL of this sort eventually required completion total laryngectomy to facilitate deglutition.[266] With modern reconstructive techniques, a pectoralis myofascial flap can be placed in an extended SSL defect to replace tissue lost from the base of the tongue, and properly selected patients can be well rehabilitated with restoration of essentially normal swallowing and preservation of the glottic larynx.

Some lesions could be anatomically encompassed by a combination of total glossectomy and SSL, but this operation is incompatible with regaining the ability to swallow by mouth, even with reconstruction using a bulky pectoralis myocutaneous flap. The patient is able to vocalize, but the speech is generally not articulate enough to warrant the trade-off of a feeding gastros-

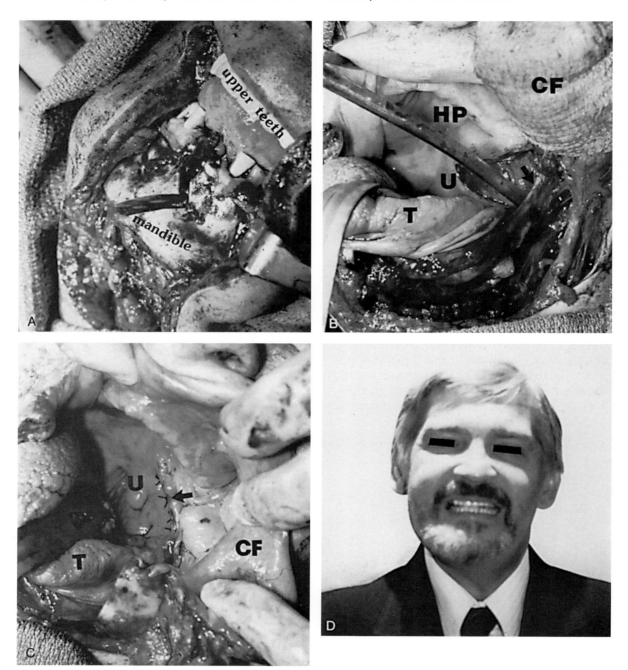

Fig. 20–40. Mandibular "swing" operation. A. Stepped "V" osteotomy at anterior midline. B. Exposure to oral cavity and oropharynx. Lingual nerve preserved (arrow). T, Tongue; CF, cheek flap; U, uvula; HP, hard palate. C. Primary closure of oropharynx defect (sutures). D. Cosmetic result. Mandibulotomy stabilized with lag screw.

tomy. Therefore, the operation performed should be total glossectomy combined with total laryngectomy.

TOTAL GLOSSECTOMY. The necessity for total glossectomy depends on both the extent of tumor in the substance of the tongue and the tumor's relationship with the innervation and blood supply to the tongue. Total glossectomy may be required in three situations: (1) for massive tumors of the oral tongue (Fig. 20–41); (2) for tumors involving both sides of the base of the

tongue, excision of which would require a margin anterior to the circumvallate papillae; and (3) for massive FOM tumors that involve the ventral surface of the tongue and extend deeply in the FOM diaphragm area to involve the submental area (see Figs. 20–29B and 20–34).

The lingual arteries and hypoglossal nerves enter the base of tongue in the suprahyoid area. Even if excision of a tumor of the base of the tongue would allow

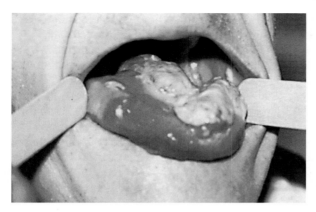

Fig. 20–41. Lesion requiring total glossectomy. Massive involvement of entire oral tongue.

the anterior two thirds to be preserved, if the blood supply will be sacrificed bilaterally, the remaining oral tongue will necrose, and if both hypoglossal nerves are sacrificed, the tongue will be immobile and its preservation will be functionally pointless and may compromise the cancer operation. Large tumors of the FOM or the base of the tongue can extend posteriorly or anteriorly, respectively, and because of the relatively small anteroposterior distance between the lingual surface of the epiglottis and the hyoid bone, cancer growth can easily permeate this area.

Intraoperative palpation under general anesthesia should be bimanual; palpation in the hyoid area allows assessment of the extent of tumor in the vallecula and preepiglottic space. CT can sometimes be helpful in this regard also.

It can be difficult to assess the exact extent of tongue cancers in either the anterior or base area if the tumors have a submucosal component. During endoscopic staging, the tongue should be pulled straight forward with a towel clip through the tip, and a finger should be slid down the midline raphe from anterior to posterior. This gives the palpator the most accurate impression of whether the tumor crosses the midline. Errors in this assessment can result from palpation with the tongue pulled to one side. The usual mistake is to think that both sides of the base of the tongue are involved, when actually the tumor does not cross the midline.

Endoscopic examination sometimes gives the surgeon occasionally the false impression that the tumor is too massive to be removed with anything less than total glossectomy, because anatomically the tongue is constricted at the base between nonyielding structures (the mandibular angles). Normal lateral base of tongue can therefore be compressed against the tumor, which feels as though it crosses the midline. Consequently, tongue tumors should be approached in the manner of a partial glossectomy, although permission is obtained for a total glossectomy if necessary. Tongue tethering is a good clinical indicator that frequently

correlates with the need for total glossectomy. If the goal of removing all gross tumor with an adequate normal margin can be achieved, subtotal glossectomy will be rewarded by a more favorable result to the patient.

The issue of function after total glossectomy is complex. In earlier decades, whenever a patient required total glossectomy, a total laryngectomy was also performed because, in the absence of reconstruction, patients tended to develop intractable aspiration pneumonia with its lethal consequences. Even if the larynx was retained, completion total laryngectomy was generally required. With modern reconstructive techniques, specifically using a bulky pectoralis myocutaneous flap in the area of the missing tongue, retention of the larynx can be considered in selected patients who are in good enough physiologic condition to tolerate some degree of aspiration and who are motivated to attempt to relearn swallowing. A significant number of patients who require total glossectomy have already adjusted to the postoperative situation because of tongue fixation and tethering from progressive cancer growth, and such patients often have less difficulty than would be expected with postoperative swallowing rehabilitation. After total glossectomy, the patient has no separation between the oral and pharyngeal phases of swallowing, and the mouth acts as a passive conduit because the lack of a mobile tongue substitute eliminates the ability to control and propel the bolus into the posterior oral cavity. Feedings are usually performed with a special syringe filled with a liquid or blenderized diet directed into the posterior oral cavity before the swallow.

Many surgeons believe that ancillary surgical procedures are necessary to decrease aspiration when the larynx is retained in patients undergoing total glossectomy. Maneuvers that have been suggested include suspending the larynx from the mandible[267] and protecting the laryngeal inlet by manipulating the residual supraglottic tissue. Krespi and Sisson favor tacking the epiglottis to the posterior pharyngeal wall (which usually pulls away),[268] and Biller, Lawson, and Baek unfurl and resuture the supraglottic tissues along the area of the aryepiglottic margins into a conical configuration to protect the glottic chink.[269] A permanent tracheostomy tube is necessary for respiration with these modifications, and this can in itself tether laryngeal elevation and interfere with swallowing. An occasional patient is able to eat by mouth and can be decannulated if the larynx is not oversewn or suspended, although a feeding gastrostomy is generally placed at the time of ablative surgery because it is anticipated that swallowing retraining will be lengthy. My preference is to suspend the larynx under the tongue base replacement by "circling" the thyroid cartilage to the hyoid uni- or bilaterally, if that bone can be preserved (method of R.W. Bastian, MD).

After total glossectomy, speech is intelligible to family members, close acquaintances, and head and neck cancer surgeons. Speech is sometimes surprisingly good, but inevitable deficits in articulation occur because of the lack of a mobile tongue substitute.

These severe functional consequences after total glossectomy raise ethical questions in the minds of some surgeons as to whether this operation should be performed. In selected cases, it certainly seems warranted because 25% of patients with advanced primary cancers have no evidence of cervical metastatic disease, and "cure" may be achieved with aggressive treatment of the primary tumor.[270]

The frequent bilaterality of cervical metastatic disease favors the elective treatment of N0 necks in all patients with primary cancers of the base of the tongue, with the possible exception of T1 tumors. In one series, 34% of patients with occult ipsilateral metastases developed contralateral metastases.[271]

Alternatives to total glossectomy, allegedly with equally good results, include a combination of external beam RT with interstitial implants[272] and simultaneous chemoradiotherapy.[273]

Cancer of the Oropharynx

Sites in the oropharynx (see Table 20–1) are described as occupying four walls: anterior, lateral, posterior, and superior. The lateral wall houses the tonsil, the tonsillar fossa, and the tonsillar (faucial) pillars. The anterior pillar is called the palatoglossal arch, and the posterior pillar is called the palatopharyngeal arch. The posterior wall of the oropharynx is described along with the anatomy of the pharyngeal wall (see subsequent text). The superior wall is composed of the inferior surface of the soft palate and the uvula. The oropharynx constitutes the interface between the oral cavity and the pharynx, and tumors have an intermediate prognosis with respect to controllability.

Histologically, more than 90% of tumors of the oropharynx are SCC. "Lymphoepitheliomas" occur in 3 to 5%. These represent poorly differentiated, nonkeratinizing epidermoid carcinomas in a lymphocytic stroma. "Transitional cell carcinoma" is an epidermoid carcinoma without keratinization that clinically behaves as an undifferentiated tumor. Tumors of the faucial arch tend to be well differentiated. Tumors of the tonsil are generally poorly differentiated and are said to be exquisitely radiosensitive. They occur relatively more frequently in nonsmoking and nondrinking women than SCCs in other sites. In smokers, tumor laterality may be attributable to holding the cigarette and inhaling preferentially on one side of the mouth.

At presentation, only 5 to 20% of tumors are confined to the tonsil. Most frequently, extension involves the ipsilateral soft palate to the uvula and the ipsilateral base of the tongue. Other sites of extension for massive tumors include the lateral pharyngeal wall, retromolar trigone area, pterygoid muscles, nasopharynx, mandible, and buccal mucosa. Tumors are superficial in 20% of patients. Deep invasion of muscle, yielding trismus, occurs in 15%. At presentation, tumors less than 2 cm are rare (5%), and 60% of tumors are greater than 4 cm. Tumors cross the midline rarely, in 10% of patients.[274]

Tumors are relatively asymptomatic until they are large because the only sensory fibers to this area are from the glossopharyngeal nerve. Pain occurs when mucosa is involved. The presenting symptoms are referred otalgia, sore throat, sensation of a foreign body, and a lump in the neck representing metastatic spread to cervical nodes. Bleeding, trismus, and dysphagia are associated with advanced disease. Trismus reflects either deep invasion of the pterygoid muscles (sometimes also seen on CT) or irritation from mucosal ulceration. Regardless of the cause, when mouth opening is limited, one cannot assume that general anesthesia will relax it, and a local tracheostomy is frequently required to ensure the airway as the initial step at staging endoscopy.

Small tonsillar tumors have a red, granular, friable surface and may be hidden at the lower pole behind the anterior pillar in tonsillar crypts or the glossotonsillar sulcus. The usual SCC can appear exophytic, flat and spreading, or ulceroinfiltrative. Exophytic tumors tend to be more highly differentiated than ulceroinfiltrative types. The tumors may invade deeply to produce a submucosal mass with little or no surface ulceration. Clinical examination must include palpation of the tonsil (comparison with the contralateral side is frequently helpful) and adjacent areas (especially the base of the tongue), and evaluation of tongue mobility on protrusion.

A unilaterally enlarged tonsil in an adult currently evokes a differential diagnosis that includes neoplastic, granulomatous, and infectious entities (Fig. 20–42). SCC (the most common cancer in smokers) is generally exophytic but can present submucosally, although this

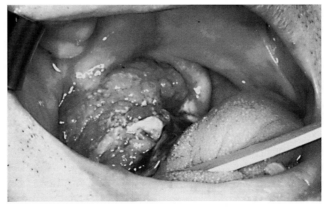

Fig. 20–42. Large tonsil cancer. (Courtesy of Dr. GJ Spector.)

is more typical of lymphoma of the tonsil, which is a more likely diagnosis in nonsmokers. The lymphoid tissue of Waldeyer's ring (nasopharynx, tonsil, and base of the tongue) are common sites for primary lymphomas of the head and neck. Although lymphomas are usually submucosal, they can be exophytic and ulcerative. Therefore, SCC or lymphoma of the tonsil can have an identical appearance and can only be definitively diagnosed by biopsy. Lymphoma of the tonsil can be confused with poorly differentiated SCC or granulomatous inflammatory tissue if only a small portion is taken for biopsy. Whenever a pathology report of "undifferentiated carcinoma" is returned, the surgeon should realize that lymphoma must be ruled out, and this can be done only by obtaining a large amount of tissue devoid of crush artifact. In the tonsil, this might include a tonsillectomy as excisional biopsy. The specimen should be submitted "fresh" to the pathologist, so lymphoma markers and gene rearrangement studies can be done.

The differential diagnosis also includes metastases *to* the tonsil, which arise by way of hematogenous dissemination, primarily from the kidney. Metastatic renal cell carcinoma is extremely vascular, and uncontrollable hemorrhage can result from biopsy in the clinic. Granulomatous entities such as sarcoidosis can also cause unilateral tonsillar enlargement. The first manifestations of AIDS can also appear in the head and neck, most commonly with either cervical adenopathy or oropharyngeal Kaposi's sarcoma[275]—violaceous unilateral tonsillar lesions. Appropriate precautions must be taken when obtaining tissue from patients with this suspected diagnosis.[276] Many homosexual patients are so literate with respect to their risks that they frequently announce their own diagnosis (e.g., "Kaposi's sarcoma in my tonsil"). This level of awareness is not typical of those who have the disease because of intravenous drug abuse or from receiving blood transfusions before 1985.

Anatomic relationships of the oropharynx and pharyngeal space are shown in Figure 20–43. Tonsillar lymphatic drainage is efferent from the superior and inferior poles of the tonsil (Fig. 20–44). Lymphatic vessels penetrate the superior constrictor muscle and pass to the upper deep jugular and subdigastric ("tonsillar") ipsilateral lymph nodes. Posterior triangle metastases occur in 10% of patients. Bilateral metastasis is associated with extension of the primary tumor into the base of the tongue or soft palate, which are midline structures with bilateral lymphatic drainage. The literature states that trismus, dysphagia, pharyngeal wall invasion, and extension across the midline are associated with poor survival because such signs and symptoms represent deep invasion and favor cervical metastasis (in addition, such massive tumors are sometimes not operated on). Tumor extension into the base of the tongue is ominous; in older retrospective series, twice

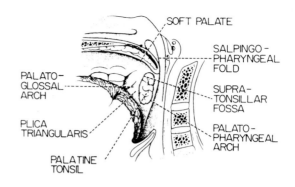

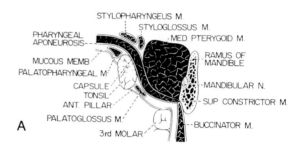

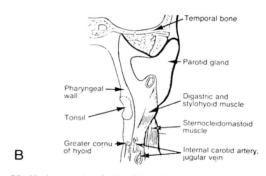

Fig. 20–43. Anatomic relationships of the oropharynx and parapharyngeal space. A. Oropharynx anatomy. B. Parapharyngeal space anatomy. (A, from Daly JF: Otolaryngol Clin North Am *Oct*:596, 1969; B, from Lawson VG, et al: J Otolaryngol *8*:247, 1979.)

as many patients survived when the tongue was not involved.

The incidence of cervical metastases is listed in Tables 20–5 and 20–6. Occult metastases are frequent, upgrading 50% of clinical stage II patients to stage III. Clinical evaluation of neck metastases from tonsil primaries has a false-positive rate of 10% and a false-negative rate of 45 to 50%.[2]

An interesting feature is that *cystic* neck metastases, representing central necrosis in positive lymph nodes, are especially frequent with tonsillar SCCs, even if the primary tumor is occult,[101,277] although they have also been reported from primaries of the lip, tongue, FOM, retromolar trigone, and gingiva. Cystic neck metastases can be mistaken for "cancer in branchiogenic cysts," which can also appear first in the elderly.

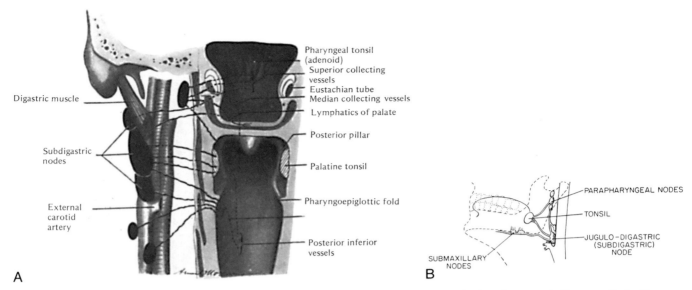

Fig. 20–44. A and B. Lymphatic drainage of the oropharynx. (A, from Rouvière J: Anatomie des lymphatiques de l'homme. Paris, Masson, 1932; B, from Shumrick D and Gluckman JL: Cancer of the oropharynx. In: Cancer of the Head and Neck. Edited by Suen J and Myers E. New York, Churchill Livingstone, 1981.)

"Branchiogenic carcinoma" implies a primary cancer in the neck arising from an embryonic rest, not associated with cancer elsewhere in the head and neck. The existence of this entity has seldom, if ever, been compellingly proved, although many articles refer to it.[278] Because cystic neck metastases can be the initial presentation, followed as late as 11 years subsequently by the appearance of tonsillar cancer, the patient should be continually surveyed for later development of a primary tumor in the tonsil or elsewhere in the head and neck. Performing an ipsilateral tonsillectomy sometimes identifies the occult primary tumor (if the specimen is serially sectioned), which then spares the patient wide-field RT to "unknown primary parts" with attendant xerostomia.

Surgery
Because of the radiosensitivity of tumors in the oropharynx and the difficulty of obturating defects in the soft palate with complete restoration of velopharyngeal competence, extensive *surface* lesions of the tonsil and soft palate should be considered for RT with curative intent.

Most of the surgical approaches appropriate for tumors in the oropharynx have already been described. As with other sites, choosing the appropriate operation to fit the extent of disease requires considerable experience and clinical judgment.

Transoral excision of carcinoma of the tonsil has been discredited because of results such as those reported in one series,[279] in which a local recurrence rate of 23% was observed after osteotomy (for small lesions); local recurrence rates were 41% after composite resection and 63% following transoral excision. If sur-

gery is appropriately tailored to the size of the tumor and the correct approach is chosen, local recurrence rates should be comparable. The problem arises when too large a tumor is approached with too small an operation. Inadequate exposure invites incomplete cancer excision. The "occasional" head and neck surgeon is best advised to err on the side of radicality.

Many tonsil cancers, however, do not extend beyond the capsule of the tonsil, which is the normal plane of tonsillectomy, although they may be bulky and involve adjacent mucosa of the tonsillar pillars and retromolar trigone. This type of mobile, circumscribed lesion (no trismus) can often be adequately excised with transoral laser excision in carefully selected patients (see Fig. 20–15). Tumors suitable for this approach are generally T1 or T2 (and a few T3 lesions) in size. Underlying bone should not be exposed (i.e., the pterygoid muscles and periosteum remain in situ). The individual anatomy of the patient may preclude transoral laser excision even though the tumor extent might be suitable. This should be assessed under general anesthesia with Crowe-Davis mouth gag exposure.

If exposure is a problem, a pull-thru operation, cheek-flap, or mandibular "swing" approach is generally adequate. The last approach (see previous section) allows access to primary tumors in the oral cavity and oropharynx when normal tissue exists in the FOM between the tumor and the mandible.[262,263] When tumors in the oropharynx are excised by this route, the lingual nerve is generally sacrificed in the excision, whereas this is not always necessary for tumors in the oral cavity.

Composite resection is the traditional approach to

cancers in the oropharynx. The "garden variety" tonsil tumor for which this approach is used is generally of T3 or T4 size and involves the tonsillar fossa, pillars, and soft palate unilaterally, has extension into the base of the tongue and posterior FOM, and is inseparable from the inner aspect of the mandibular ramus, although gross bone erosion may not be seen. Mandibular "swing" is not an acceptable approach for this type of tumor because of the proximity to the mandible. This type of defect is generally reconstructed with a pectoralis flap (see later). The myocutaneous form is suitable for use in thin or cachectic individuals in whom maximum bulk is required. In patients who are not malnourished and who are corpulent, the myofascial form without the subcutaneous paddle can subserve structure and function better. The patient's subcutaneous tissue in the cheek and neck provide adequate thickness in combination with the myofascial flap, and this avoids too much bulk in the reconstructed oropharynx, which can interfere with swallowing. A mandibular reconstruction plate can maintain continuity if the condyle is left in situ. Mandibular prostheses with a condylar head have been associated with middle cranial fossa erosion and complications.

Cancer of the Posterior Pharyngeal Wall

Although SCC in *any* head and neck site can be difficult to control locally, cancer growth in the posterior pharyngeal wall has traditionally been considered one of the worst sites (along with sinus cancer metastatic to neck nodes and cervical esophageal cancer). Whereas the end point for reporting local-regional control for most head and neck cancer sites is 2 to 3 years, pharyngeal cancer control rates are sometimes reported at 1 year because 85 to 90% of relapses occur within that period, and patients usually die in 2 years. The problem in such patients has historically been failure to control local disease and second primary cancers rather than neck disease or DMs.

Most patients have been treated with full-course RT, even though most cancers of the posterior pharyngeal wall are large at presentation and are therefore unlikely to be (and have not been) cured by RT alone. With single-modality RT, the disease is never controlled in 30 to 60% of patients. Because of the lack of facile ablative and reconstructive techniques for this area in the past, few patients have been operated on as part of their treatment. Basically, most patients in recorded series have received only palliative treatment, and the outcome reflects this.

In patients who have had surgery as part of their treatment, the operation typically performed is total laryngopharyngectomy (TLP). Although the larynx is seldom involved with cancer, it is removed primarily to allow closure of the defect, usually with gastric pull-up. Experience with a personal series of 67 patients

with primary pharyngeal wall cancers managed over the past 10 years proves that aggressive initial larynx-sparing surgery followed by aggressive RT can, in fact, control local-regional disease in 85% of patients and can result in long-term survival comparable to or even better than that seen with SCC in other head and neck sites. Therefore, aggressive local-regional treatment is eminently worthwhile in these patients, and they apparently do *not* have an intrinsically hopeless prognosis or endogenously lethal "natural history."

General Features

The staging system for cancer of the pharynx is strange. The posterior pharyngeal wall extends from the base of skull to the esophageal inlet, thereby traversing three zones: the nasopharynx, oropharynx, and hypopharynx. Unique features and differing biologic behavior of nasopharynx cancers put them in a separate category. The pharyngeal mucosa proper is spoken of as having lateral and posterior walls. For practical purposes, however, the lateral pharyngeal wall does not exist, but is occupied by the tonsillar fossa and pillars at the oropharynx level and by the lateral wall of the piriform sinus in the hypopharynx. Therefore, we are speaking mainly of tumors that arise between the level of the junction of the hard and soft palates superiorly and the esophageal inlet inferiorly that involve the posterior pharyngeal wall. With the current staging system, if the bulk of the tumor occupies the oropharynx, the tumor is classified on the basis of size dimension, whereas if the epicenter is in the hypopharynx (extending from the level of the floor of the vallecula to the level of the cricoarytenoid joints), the tumor is classified by hypopharyngeal staging: by the number of sites or extension of the tumor (see Table 20–2).

The literature states that tumors of the pharynx comprise 15% of hypopharyngeal tumors and tend to be multicentric in time and space. Heavy drinkers seem especially prone to develop SCC in this site. Whereas a 15% incidence of multiple primary tumors is seen in most sites of SCC of the head and neck, the incidence is 50% with tumors in the posterior pharyngeal wall.

The primary tumor is frequently advanced at diagnosis because it arises in a silent area.[280] The patient may present with referred otalgia, a sore throat, "hot potato" voice, or a neck mass. This site is associated with a 50% incidence of palpable cervical metastases at presentation, increasing to 75% later in the course, a 15% incidence of DM, and involvement of the retropharyngeal lymph nodes in 25 to 40% of cases. In some older series, 40% of patients presented with bilateral lymphadenopathy because of the midline location of the primary tumor.

Patients may not present until weight loss results from nearly total pharyngeal obstruction. Airway problems are rare. The tumors are typically described as having an exophytic surface with an endophytic

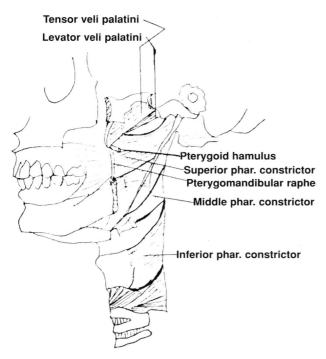

Fig. 20–45. Anatomic relationships of the pharyngeal constrictor muscles.

component involving the underlying pharyngeal constrictor muscle (Fig. 20–45). Cancers of the pharynx are allegedly associated with significant submucosal spread beyond the visible and palpable margins of the tumor,[281] as well as with satellite or "skip" lesions in the adjacent mucosa. The prevertebral fascia is variously described as being penetrated seldom or frequently. Mobility can be assessed by finger palpation at endoscopy. Some articles in the older literature mention frequent spread to the posterior tonsillar pillar, soft palate, nasopharynx, cervical esophagus, and piriform fossa. In my experience, tumors of the posterior phayngeal wall seem to be restricted to the posterior mucosa of the oropharynx and hypopharynx and to be limited by the prevertebral fascia posteriorly. Inferiorly, the tumors have not been seen to extend below the level of the cricopharyngeus and seldom involve even the extrinsic larynx (and rarely the endolarynx) (Fig. 20–46).

Treatment
Treatment results reported in the literature are so poor that they are hardly worth mentioning. The best overall 5-year survival rate is 20 to 30% (40% with stages I and II and 10% with stage IV). The 5-year survival rate is 50% for patients with clinically negative lymph nodes and small primary tumors and 10 to 20% for those with positive lymph nodes, for the reasons alluded to earlier.

Single-modality therapy is inadequate to control

any but the smallest lesions. In one series of 15 patients staged T1 to T3, N0, almost 50% were NED at 3 years after full-course RT.[282] Single-modality RT is ineffectual for advanced tumors. The study by Pene and colleagues gives typical results in a large series.[283] Half of the patients treated achieved no local control, and one third of the patients with initial control had recurrences within 1 year at the primary site or in the neck. In 50% of the patients with 4-cm primary tumors, death occurred within 6 months. Only 25% of the patients survived more than 1 year, and 75% died of local disease. In this study, there were *no* T1, N0 5-year survivors.

With respect to RT with curative intent, one report appears promising. A combination of brachytherapy ([125]I "seeds" inserted into the tumor with a Mick gun) and megavoltage external beam RT was used in sequence for pharyngeal wall tumors of all sizes,[284] with an 85% control rate. This phenomenally good result has not been confirmed with additional patients. My results with larynx-sparing surgery followed by RT show equivalent local-regional control in a larger group of patients.

With respect to single-modality surgery, a series of 94 patients undergoing surgery alone showed a 30% control rate at 2 years that was increased to 40% with salvage therapy.[285]

In respect to planned combined therapy, 41 patients treated with low-dose preoperative RT followed by surgery demonstrated 47% control of the tumor in the head and neck, a significant postoperative wound-

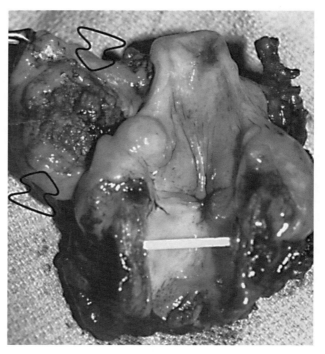

Fig. 20–46. Pharyngeal wall cancer (arrows) suitable for larynx-sparing partial pharyngectomy. Note uninvolved larynx.

healing complication rate, and difficulties with reconstruction.[286,287] These authors suggested that, in the future, aggressive planned surgery followed by RT should be evaluated, with the availability of new reconstructive techniques. The former series (surgery followed by RT) of 19 patients (17 of whom had TLP) showed that 15 of 19 were dead at 5 years, with 6 failures in the head and neck. A high incidence of DM was noted in this series (37%).

SURGICAL APPROACHES. Several ablative approaches are available.

Transoral laser excision, in my opinion, can be considered only for tumors that are fully exposable with the Crowe-Davis mouth gag and freely mobile whose in respect to the prevertebral fascia and the margins of those that can be brought into range of laser handpiece use.

Any procedure that interferes with laryngeal elevation, that is, that transects the suprahyoid muscles, adds to the absolute swallowing disability pursuant to any excisional surgery of the pharyngeal constrictors and should therefore not be used. This includes transhyoid pharyngotomy and medial labiomandibular glossotomy approaches. Although both afford excellent exposure, interference with the suprahyoid musculature (as well as scarring of the tongue and FOM with the latter procedure) imposes an additional deglutition problem on the patient that can be avoided with other routes.

A *lateral* approach such as lateral pharyngotomy (with or without mandibular "swing" for enhanced exposure of tumors with an epicenter in the upper oropharynx) has fewer swallowing consequences and is much better tolerated. The hypoglossal and lingual nerves are preserved.

Cricopharyngeal myotomy can be performed to facilitate swallowing, although its utility has not been scientifically proven (a multi-institutional study report is in preparation). If this larynx-sparing procedure is performed, one must avoid damage to the recurrent laryngeal nerve. An alternative posterior approach has also been reported.[288]

This is useful for any pharyngeal cancer operation (or for any in the oral cavity or oropharynx, too) because it allows a transcervical approach to be extended through the lower lip to increase exposure by cheek-flap or mandibulotomy if necessary.

The issue of whether the larynx should be saved during surgery for pharyngeal cancer has not been formally addressed in the literature. Trotter (a pioneer in pharyngeal cancer surgery) commented in 1931, "I should not feel able to record as a true success the cure of pharyngeal carcinoma done at the expense of laryngectomy."[289] Ogura and colleagues reasoned that, because the lymphatic drainage of the pharynx is toward the lateral cervical nodes, not toward the larynx, and because the larynx is involved only in advanced cases because of local invasion or retrograde tumor spread, one should obtain as good an oncologic result by saving the larynx as by sacrificing it.[290] The surgeon must assess whether or not larynx-sparing pharyngeal cancer operations show recurrences in the vicinity of the retained larynx. This information is not available in the literature because so few patients have had larynx-sparing surgery as part of their treatment. It is not acceptable to remove the larynx simply to aid reconstruction if the patient's swallowing mechanism can be adequately rehabilitated otherwise.

An occasional tumor massively involves the larynx and pharynx and mandates TLP with its inherent reconstructive problems, but large tumor size is not an absolute contraindication to a larynx-sparing approach. The surgeon should procure at least a 1-cm margin of normal tissue beyond the apparent limits of the visible and palpable tumor and some authors (e.g., Ogura and associates[290]) believe that a 2-cm margin is more adequate. Thus, except for small primary tumors, the majority of the pharyngeal wall is resected.

Larynx-sparing surgery of the pharynx requires meticulous attention to detail on the part of the surgeon, and this is a classic example in which "anatomic and physiological knowledge of the part in question is necessary to allow the surgeon access with the least disturbance and to enable him to carry out his task with as little effect on function as may be."[289] Specifically, attention is directed to saving all possible structures that may assist swallowing (suprahyoid muscles, superior laryngeal nerve bundle, recurrent laryngeal nerve). The ipsilateral lobe of the thyroid gland can be retracted posteriorly and preserved, allowing access for lateral pharyngotomy. Larynx-sparing pharyngeal surgery can also be useful in carefully selected patients with recurrent cancers of the pharyngeal wall when the original extent of the tumor is accurately known.

Retropharyngeal Lymph Nodes

With pharyngeal cancers, an additional feature is important: the problem of retropharyngeal lymph nodes. The pharynx is drained by a lymphatic network (see Fig. 20–7): superiorly in the retropharyngeal chain to the node of Rouvière near the base of skull, laterally to the jugular chain and posterior triangle lymph nodes, and anteriorly through the thyrohyoid membrane. According to Ballantyne,[110] the retropharyngeal lymph nodes may be involved with 30 to 40% of primary pharyngeal cancers, and when they are involved, the prognosis is especially grave. Involvement of these lymph nodes can be suspected clinically based on a syndrome of pain and stiffness in the neck. The pain radiates to the ipsilateral eye and forehead and can be increased by flexion or extension of the neck. Involvement of these lymph nodes should be sought on the patient's preoperative CT (see Fig. 20–11).

In the adult cancer patient, a single lateral retropharyngeal lymph node is adjacent to the styloid process and the internal carotid artery at the skull base. This area is not encompassed in a standard neck dissection, and exposure for surgical removal is afforded by TLP, by neck dissection with mandibular "swing" approach, by composite resection, or transcervically. Dissection of positive retropharyngeal lymph nodes is technically difficult and can theoretically result in exsanguinating hemorrhage intraoperatively (not seen in my series). If the lymph node is positive, however, this must be attempted (preferably by an experienced head and neck cancer surgeon) because no other treatment modality is curative. Elective dissection of retropharyngeal lymph nodes has been recommended, but postoperative RT is a welcome alternative for presumed microscopic disease. Of note is the proximity of the superior cervical ganglion, which has the appearance of a lymph node at the base of the skull and should not be mistakenly resected. One can differentiate by the egress of the cervical sympathetic chain from its inferior aspect.

Adequate aggressive postoperative RT that covers the base of skull (similar to the treatment plan for nasopharyngeal carcinoma) is part of the treatment with curative intent for patients who have had surgery.

Reconstruction

Historically, the lack of a reliable reconstructive method resulted in the overall preference for RT. In the rare instances in which larynx-sparing surgery was performed, there was inadequate tissue for closure, and the patient was left with a large lateral pharyngostome for which reconstruction would subsequently be attempted with local neck flaps, which were unreliable multistaged procedures (if the patient had not already died of exsanguination from an exposed carotid artery or tumor recurrence).

A TLP defect is usually reconstructed (Fig. 20–47) with stomach pull-up or jejunal interposition, although functional results are far from perfect.[291–295]

My preferred method uses mucosa preserved from the usually uninvolved larynx (pyriforms and postcricord) with or without a medially based longus colli muscle flap uni- or bilaterally to reconstitute the circumference of the pharynx. Because tumors of the posterior pharyngeal wall do not involve the esophagus, this reconstruction method eliminates the need for (and morbidity of) visceral interposition. TLP may be necessary to excise adequately the occasional massive posterior pharyngeal wall with an epicenter abutting the skull base.

In reconstruction of larynx-sparing pharyngectomy defects, the mucosal margins are tacked to the prevertebral fascia. If it is intact, there is no need for skin or dermal graft coverage. Flap reconstruction is necessary if the prevertebral fascia has been penetrated by tumor (which is rare), and excision requires removal of the underlying longus colli muscle layer (in this situation, the anterior spinal ligaments constitute the deep margin of the defect and must be protected with soft tissue bulk) or if the patient has a large lateral pharyngeal defect.

The pectoralis myofascial flap[296] is ideal because its thickness approximates that of the tissue removed (pharyngeal constrictor layer). The flap is brought in through lateral exposure and is sutured to the residual mucosal margins. It is then tubed on itself to form a new lateral pharyngeal wall. It also provides protection for the carotid artery when sutured to the prevertebral fascia medial to the artery (see subsequent text). Naturally, the flap is adynamic and does not reconstitute pharyngeal constrictor *function.* That such a defect can be reliably closed without wound-healing complications is, however, an advantage that facilitates radical larynx-sparing surgery as the first step in the management of these patients.

Postoperative Swallowing Function

If one were to attempt to devise a treatment plan that would maximally impair swallowing, radical larynx-sparing surgery of the pharynx followed by postoperative high-dose RT would be the plan. The addition of high-dose postoperative RT completely dries out the UADT mucosa—an added insult to the swallowing mechanism. As indicated previously, the surgical approach can increase or decrease the disability. Patients who undergo this type of treatment, however, should be informed that they may never swallow again by mouth, and a feeding gastrostomy is generally placed at the time of the ablative surgery (after removal of the primary tumor[10]).

Expert swallowing therapy helps rehabilitate the patient, but the results of cinefluorography may frighten the swallowing therapist who is not familiar with rehabilitation of head and neck cancer patients. One must not convey hopelessness with respect to swallowing outcome to the patient, whose instincts and motivation can compensate for remarkable anatomic defects. Favorable physiologic condition and motivation on the part of the patient are essential, and these factors enter into selection of patients for larynx-sparing operations. It is helpful to decannulate the patient or to replace the tracheostomy tube with an Olympic button before swallowing retraining begins.

Liquids are the easiest food substances for patients to handle after this type of surgery, and therapeutic maneuvers that enhance swallow retraining include repeated swallows after a single bolus. As swallowing ability progresses, liquid and solid swallows can be alternated.[297] Teaching the "supraglottic swallow" maneuver is an important adjunct (see Chap. 33). (Because of the absence of the efferent arc of the swallowing reflex—the pharyngeal muscles—thermal stimula-

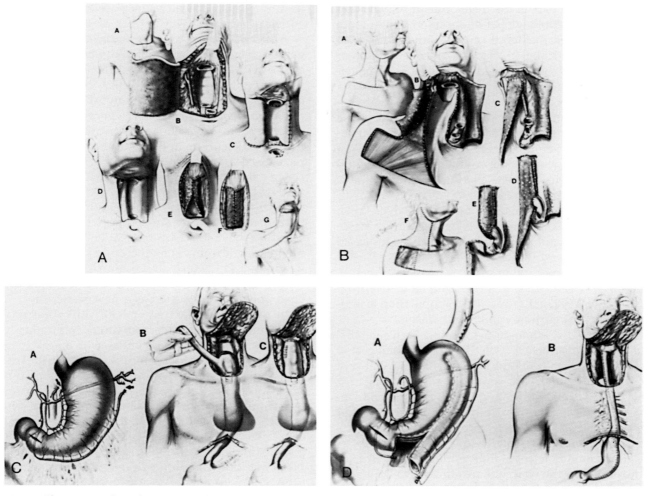

Fig. 20–47. Pharyngoesophageal reconstruction. A. Combination of cervical skin (Wookie) and lateral-based chest flaps. B. Deltopectoral flap. C and D. Gastric pull-ups. (From Silver C: Am J Surg *132*:428, 1976.)

tion to enhance the swallow reflex is unlikely to be helpful.)

Many patients in my series eat totally or "recreationally" by mouth.

Nasopharyngeal Carcinoma

Etiopathogenesis

Epidemiologic data suggest three factors in the etiology of nasopharyngeal carcinoma (NPC): Epstein-Barr virus (EBV),[298] a genetically determined susceptibility,[117,299,300] and environmental factors that vary among populations.[301–323] NPC is unique among other head and neck cancers because of marked differences in geographic distribution and its association with EBV. Genetic associations with several blood types and histocompatibility antigens have been noted (HLA-A2, HLA-B17, HLA-BW16).

Although NPC constitutes less than 1% of all malignant diseases in North America, Western Europe, and Japan (incidence 0.1 to 1.7 of 100,000 population per year) and comprises only 3% of all head and neck tumors in North America, it is very common in southeast China, Taiwan, Singapore, and Malaysia. In certain areas of China, NPC is the most common cancer, comprising 18% of all cancers in Hong Kong and 30% in Canton ("Kwangtung tumor") with an incidence of 150 of 100,000 population; a risk 118 times higher in native Chinese than in North American whites. An intermediate risk is reported in the Mediterranean basin (5 to 9 of 100,000), North Africa, and the Arctic (Greenland, Alaska) as well as in southern Chinese born in Western areas such as Australia, Hawaii, and California (7.3 times the risk in Chinese persons born in America versus native white). The risk appears to lower in second-generation than in first-generation Chinese-Americans, implicating environmental factors in addition to genetic components, although genetic differences among subpopulations within China are also a possible explanation for differences in rates among emigrants.[299]

Largely unidentified environmental factors are believed to play a part in the development of NPC and to explain its curious global distribution. Ho noted a particularly high incidence of NPC among the boat people of Hong Kong,[302,323] in whom consumption of salted fish in early childhood—possibly in combination with vitamin deficiency—has been considered a likely risk factor because of the presence of carcinogenic dimethylnitrosamines in salted fish. Ho points out that if an environmental factor is an essential cofactor in NPC, then the cancer is easily preventable if the factor is known. (If the southern Chinese would stop feeding their children salted fish, this hypothesis could be tested in 20 to 30 years.)

Among the numerous risk factors that have been linked to the development of NPC are chronic nasopharyngeal irritation from smoking and exposure to industrial dust and formaldehyde (a more prominent risk factor among whites than among Chinese). Among North American patients with NPC, the prognosis of the Alaskan Eskimo native population is unusually poor, for currently unknown reasons.[303]

VIROLOGY. An etiologic association between EBV and *undifferentiated* NPC (UNPC) was first suggested in 1966 (based on serologic studies showing that sera from patients with UNPC contained antibodies against EBV-infected cell lines,[304] and later by the demonstration of EBV DNA within UNPC cells by nucleic acid hybridization.[305] EBV is a herpes virus that infects human B lymphocytes and is the causative agent of infectious mononucleosis. Infected B lymphocytes are transformed by the virus but are efficiently eliminated in immunocompetent hosts, mainly by cytotoxic T lymphocytes that recognize virus-coated surface antigens such as latent membrane protein. Up to 90% of adults carry latent EBV in the nasopharynx and bone marrow.

Currently, the presence of EBV can be detected with both in situ hybridization and polymerase chain reaction techniques. The virus has been detected in metastatic as well as primary lesions.[306] Such tests have demonstrated an association of EBV with NPC worldwide.

Serologic studies are useful in the diagnosis of UNPC, with which they are positive 90% of the time but not for the better-differentiated keratinizing SCC of the nasopharynx. The most specific serologic test is the IgA antibody response to EBV-induced viral capsid antigen (VCA) and the IgG antibody response to early antigen (EA/d). Anti-VCA and anti-EA/d titers are also related to total tumor burden; antibody titers progressively increase with advancing disease stage and are commonly lower in treated long-term survivors than in untreated patients. In some areas of China, the anti-VCA test is used to detect UNPC in mass screening programs.[307] In Kwangtung province, 60,000 residents were tested, and a subset of 6000 apparently

healthy people showed an increased titer. Of these, 48 patients had occult NPC.

Antibody response to EBV-induced membrane antigen is measured by the antibody-dependent cellular cytotoxicity assay (ADCC), which has been correlated with prognosis in several studies.[303,308,309] In studies on North American patients, low ADCC titers at presentation were associated with a poor prognosis; recurrence tended to develop after treatment in such patients, and increases in titer after treatment portended recurrence—usually in the form of DMs—which preceded clinically detectable disease. Conversely, patients who presented with high ADCC titers typically had a good response to treatment and remained free of recurrence. Thus, it was proposed that ADCC tests could help define a high-risk patient population who might benefit from chemotherapy or immunotherapy in addition to RT early in the course of treatment, but the ADCC assay is not widely performed and has not been universally accepted as a prognosticator.

In the primary lesions of NPC, EBV presumably passes into epithelial cells from tumor-infiltrating lymphocytes with cytotoxic potential, which heavily infiltrate the tumors. Although the role of EBV in the pathogenesis of NPC remains unclear, the virus may be a prerequisite for or may play a facultative role in development of the tumor, which may represent EBV-initiated clonal expansion of a single infected progenitor cell.[298] The maintenance of episomal viral genomes in primary and metastatic NPC lesions suggests that EBV plays a critical role in oncogenic transformation and growth. Environmental factors geographically related to areas of endemic UNPC may be significant in the reactivation of persistent EBV genomic material. Gene transfer studies have shown that expression of a latent membrane protein, representing the presence of EBV viral genes and expressed in NPC cells, in a human epithelial cell line can impair the ability of cells to undergo terminal differentiation. Thus, EBV infection may result in a persistent population of relatively undifferentiated epithelial cells that may be at risk for secondary oncogenic mutations.[310,311]

HISTOLOGY. The nasopharynx is lined with stratified squamous epithelium, ciliated pseudostratified columnar (respiratory) epithelium, and intermediate (transitional) epithelium, and carcinoma can arise in any of these epithelial types. Focal squamous cell metaplasia increases with age and chronic infection but does not appear to be a prerequisite for the development of cancer.

The histologic classification of NPC has been changed several times, leading to confusion. Before 1991, NPC was classified by the World Health Organization (WHO) into three histologic categories,[312] all of which can be identified as SCC by electron microscopy: keratinizing SCC (WHO type I); nonkeratinizing SCC, which resembles transitional cell carcinoma of the bladder (WHO type II); and undifferentiated carcinoma (WHO type III), which contained the subcategories "lymphoepithelioma" and anaplastic carcinoma. The descriptive term "lymphoepithelioma" (no longer used) consisted of anaplastic carcinoma cells surrounded by a prominent lymphocytic infiltrate with the neoplastic epithelial cells present either as well-defined, cohesive cell nests (Regaud pattern) or as isolated cells within a dense lymphocytic infiltrate (Schmincke pattern).[368]

Clinically, two types of NPC can be defined by their natural history; keratinizing versus nonkeratinizing or poorly differentiated carcinomas. This biologic distinction leads to the separation of WHO type I versus the combined WHO types II and III, respectively. The latter category is associated with EBV and the poorly differentiated variety comprises most cases of NPC in the orient. Thus, the newest WHO categorization of NPC (1991) now includes only two major types: (1) keratinizing SCC; and (2) nonkeratinizing carcinoma with two subcategories: differentiated and undifferentiated.[312]

Prognostication has been related to the histologic subtype of NPC. In general, the prognosis for nonkeratinizing and undifferentiated varieties is better (because the tumors are radiosensitive or radiocurable and chemosensitive) than for keratinizing SCCs, which are more likely to recur or persist in the nasopharynx after radiation therapy. UNPC (lymphoepithelioma) has a short overall natural history, however, with 80% of DMs diagnosed within 2 years of the first symptoms. Distant failure (pulmonary, skeletal) is linked to the presence of bulky cervical lymph node disease and is far more frequent with undifferentiated carcinoma than with SCC. The N3 subgroup has the worst prognosis, with 5-year survival below 15%.

These competing factors are demonstrated in one series,[313] which showed that although patients with "lymphoepitheliomas" had a higher 5-year survival than those with SCC, no difference was noted in ultimate local control, disease-free survival, or 10-year survival. The longer 5-year survival was thought to be related to slower regrowth of lymphoepitheliomas (longer median time to local recurrence), but patients with lymphoepitheliomas were more likely to develop late DMs.

The differential diagnosis of UNPC should include large cell lymphoma, and the possibility of metastatic nasopharyngeal carcinoma should be considered in adults with enlarged cervical lymph nodes that resemble Hodgkin's disease histopathologically. Immunophenotypic studies can easily resolve this diagnostic dilemma if the possibility of metastatic NPC is considered.[314]

Patterns of Cancer Spread

PRIMARY TUMOR. Several articles are recommended that illustrate how malignant lesions appear and spread in the nasopharynx with radiographic examples and anatomic drawings.[315,316,363] In 1911, Trotter noted that nasopharyngeal tumors spread mostly submucosally without marked projection in the nasal cavity, and that once suspicions were aroused, digital examination made the diagnosis by detecting the presence of a hard nodular infiltration of the tissues around the eustachian tube orifice—confirmed by biopsy.[317]

The primary tumor in the nasopharynx is often small, submucosal, and difficult to detect: clinically "occult." In Kwangtung province, 6000 apparently healthy patients had an increased anti-EBV titer (of 60,000 residents tested); 130 had nasopharyngeal biopsy performed with a flexible endoscope at 6 sites (bilaterally in the roof, pharyngeal recess, and posterior wall). Eleven biopsies in 7 patients were positive in asymptomatic patients with normal-appearing nasopharynges: 2 at the roof, 7 in the pharyngeal recess, and 2 in the posterior wall.[307]

Tumors arising at the skull base can invade the bone directly or may infiltrate along structures proceeding through foramina and fissures such as nerves and vessels extending between the extracranial and intracranial spaces (Fig. 20–48A to D). The primary tumor in the nasopharynx can spread by direct continuity in five directions; anteriorly, posteriorly, laterally, inferiorly, or superiorly. Lateral spread is either through the pharyngobasilar fascia or along the pharyngotympanic tube, where it passes through the sinus of Morgagni to involve the parapharyngeal space. If spread is into the prestyloid parapharyngeal space, the third division of the trigeminal nerve may be involved, with metastases spreading to the skull base (foramen ovale) and thence intracranially. If spread is to the poststyloid parapharyngeal space, cranial nerves IV through XII and the sympathetic trunk may be affected. Base of skull erosion can occur at the sphenoid sinus, clivus, retro-occipital fissure, petrous portion of the temporal bone, or along the greater wing of the sphenoid.

Perineural spread intracranially can occur through the foramen lacerum, foramen spinosum, foramen ovale, hypoglossal canal, jugular foramen, and carotid canal.[318] Parasellar spread can compromise the optic nerve. Spread directly through the foramen lacerum or through the sphenoid sinus can result in tumor invasion of the cavernous sinus, encroachment on sympathetic nerves, and involvement of cranial nerves VI, IV, and III (listed in order of most common involvement). Cephalad extension may also involve the pterygoid canal and the vidian nerve. Posterior spread through the pharyngobasilar fascia can involve the retropharyngeal space, and if extension continues into the prevertebral space, destruction of the lateral articular process of the atlas can result. Rarely, one sees infiltration of the prevertebral fascia and the cervical spine.

In one report of CT findings on NPC with skull base

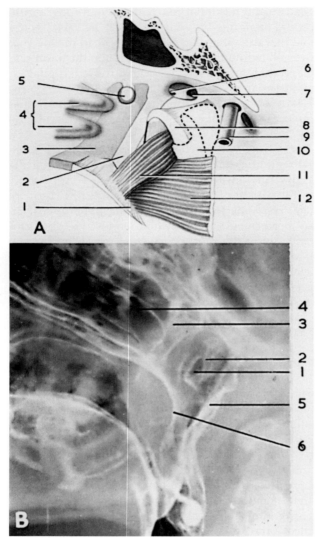

A. 1. Soft palate.
    2. Medial pterygoid plate.
    3. Palatine bone.
    4. Turbinates.
    5. Spheno-palatine foramen.
    6. Vidian canal.
    7. Carotid canal. ⎫
    8. Eustachian tube. ⎬ Seen through for. lac. med.
    9. Internal carotid artery.
   10. Fossa of Rosenmuller.
   11. Levator palati muscle.
   12. Superior constrictor muscle.
B. Radiograph of Barium in a normal nasopharynx for comparison
    1. Eustachian opening.
    2. Eustachian cushion.
    3. Pterygopalatine fossa.
    4. Turbinates.
    5. Fossa of Rosenmuller.
    6. Levator palati and soft palate.

Fig. 20–48. Pathways of spread of nasopharyngeal carcinoma: anatomic aspects.

and intracranial involvement,[319] anterior extension was seen most frequently, with posterolateral extension the second most common route of spread. Extension through foramina was noted in only 3 of 29 cases (histology-dependent; adenoid cystic carcinoma has a propensity for perineural extension). CT has shown that lateral and posterolateral extension can occur early in the course of the disease. In fact, the propensity for early extension into the paranasopharyngeal spaces and extension into the infratemporal fossa at the styloid base is so characteristic of NPC that it helps to differentiate this tumor from malignant tumors that extend to involve the nasopharynx secondarily.

Involvement of a variety of paranasopharyngeal structures was related to local control and survival in a recent report.[320] The sinus of Morgagni, through which the levator palatini muscle passes into the pharyngeal recess (the preferred site for development of NPC), appears to be an important "pathway of least resistance"

(Fig. 20–48A and B) which allows early tumor spread into the paranasopharyngeal space; a prevertebral route of tumor extension into the nasal fossa or oropharynx; and erosion of the skull base. In Sham and Choy's multivariate analysis, cranial nerve palsy, oropharyngeal involvement, and paranasopharyngeal extension were significant factors with respect to local tumor control, whereas erosion of the skull base, intracranial extension of tumor, and involvement of the nasal fossa were not.

CRANIAL NERVE INVOLVEMENT. Cranial nerve deficits and erosion of the base of skull are findings in about 25% of patients with NPC. Cranial nerve abnormalities noted in the literature include abnormalities of cranial nerves III, IV, V, VI, IX, X, and XII and Horner's syndrome, with abnormalities of cranial nerves V and VI by far the most common (Fig. 20–49 and Table 20–9). Cranial nerve deficits can resolve with definitive RT, and long-term disease-free survival can be achieved in

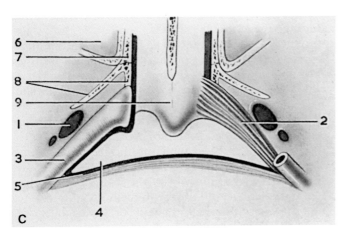

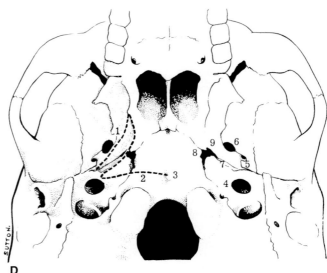

The fossa of Rosenmuller seen from above (after Prentiss):

1. Foramen ovale.
2. Levator palati muscle.
3. Eustachian tube.
4. Fossa of Rosenmuller.
5. Internal lamina of the pharyngeal fascia.
6. Antrum.
7. Palatine bone.
8. Internal and external pterygoid laminae.
9. Soft palate.

The attachments of the pharyngeal fascia to the base of the skull:

1. External lamina (the pharyngeal portion of the buccopharyngeal fascia).
2. Internal lamina (pharyngo-basilar fascia).
3. Pharyngeal tubercle.
4. Carotid canal.
5. Spine of sphenoid.
6. Foramen ovale.
7. Petrosphenoidal fissure.
8. Foramen lacerum medium.
9. Scaphoid fossa.

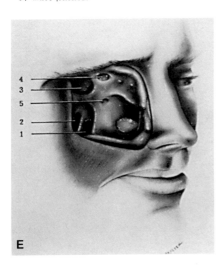

Nasal fossa exposed after removal of right upper jaw, orbit, septum and left nasal wall to show the possible pathways of spread of neoplasm from the nasopharynx:

1. Eustachian opening.
2. The fossa of Rosenmuller.
3. Sphenoidal sinus opening.
4. Posterior ethmoidal cell opening, leading to apex of opposite orbit.
5. Spheno-palatine foramen.

Fig. 20–48. (*continued*) Pathways of spread of nasopharyngeal carcinoma: anatomic aspects. A to C. Anatomy of fossa of Rosenmueller. for. lac. med = Foramen lacerum medium. D. Base of skull bony anatomy. E. Base of skull anatomy: cut-away view.

some patients. One study showed a 94% overall response rate (in a series of 18 patients) after definitive RT: 62% with complete recovery and 32% with partial recovery. The magnitude of response depended on the cranial nerve involved and the pretreatment duration of the abnormality. All responses except one occurred within 1 month after the completion of therapy; deficits that persisted longer than 2 months after the end of radiation did not resolve completely; however, partial responses were obtained in some. The onset of new or

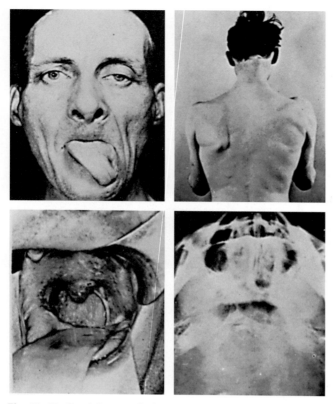

Fig. 20–49. Cranial nerve findings related to tumor in the naso-pharynx.

recurrent cranial nerve deficits after improvement was an indication of recurrent tumor in all 7 cases in which it occurred. The actuarial 5-year disease-free survival for the group of patients who presented with cranial findings was 31%.[321]

LYMPHATIC METASTASIS. The first-echelon lymphatic drainage from the nasopharyngeal mucosa is to the retropharyngeal nodes of Rouvière adjacent to the carotid canal just medial to the styloid process at the skull base (Fig. 20–50A). This area is involved in 70 to 90% of infiltrative malignant lesions of the nasopharynx, usually diffusely and often bilaterally.[322]

Ho's work,[301,302,323] which is the basis of his neck stage classification (see later), suggests that NPC is distinct from other primary head and neck cancers in having a predictable and orderly development of cervical metastases, with spread usually occurring down the cervical chain from the high internal jugular lymph nodes caudally to the supraclavicular fossa. This sequence was substantiated by a prospective study in Hong Kong.[324] At presentation, cervical metastases were present in 75% of 271 patients and were bilateral in 40%. The subdigastric and upper jugular group was involved in more than 95% of patients, with progressively less frequent involvement of lower nodal groups. Similarly, the largest lymph nodes appeared in the upper neck and the two lower neck levels (Ho's neck stage classification[302]; Table 20–10) were involved in only 4% of cases in the absence of involvement of

TABLE 20–9. Cranial Nerve Syndromes in Relation to Nasopharyngeal Tumours (After Godtfredsen)

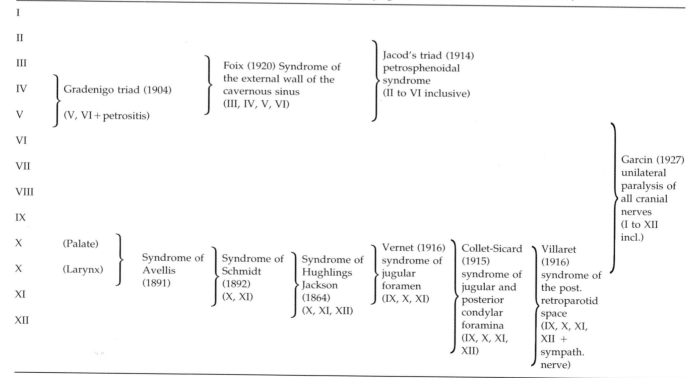

I

II

III

IV   Gradenigo triad (1904)   Foix (1920) Syndrome of the external wall of the cavernous sinus (III, IV, V, VI)   Jacod's triad (1914) petrosphenoidal syndrome (II to VI inclusive)

V   (V, VI + petrositis)

VI

VII

VIII

IX

X   (Palate)

X   (Larynx)   Syndrome of Avellis (1891)   Syndrome of Schmidt (1892) (X, XI)   Syndrome of Hughlings Jackson (1864) (X, XI, XII)   Vernet (1916) syndrome of jugular foramen (IX, X, XI)   Collet-Sicard (1915) syndrome of jugular and posterior condylar foramina (IX, X, XI, XII)   Villaret (1916) syndrome of the post. retroparotid space (IX, X, XI, XII + sympath. nerve)   Garcin (1927) unilateral paralysis of all cranial nerves (I to XII incl.)

XI

XII

Syndrome of Tapia (1906), hemiparalysis of Larynx and tongue (X + XII); Trotter's triad (1911), ipsilateral temporofacial neuralgia, palatal paralysis and deafness (V + X). (Modified from Lederman M: Cancer of the Nasopharynx: Its Natural History and Treatment. Springfield, IL, Charles C Thomas, 1961, p 35.)

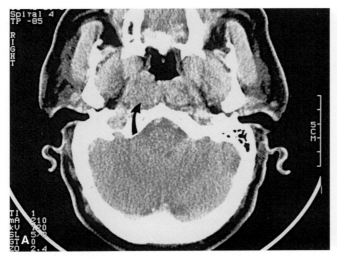 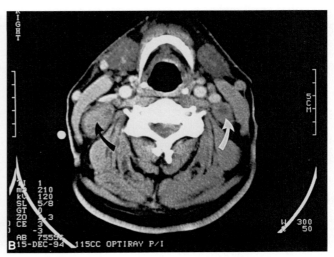

Fig. 20–50. CT findings in a patients with nasopharyngeal carcinoma. A. Increased soft tissue density at the primary site associated with a probable retropharyngeal lymph node on the right (arrow). B. Bilateral cervical lymphadenopathy is typical (arrows) and in this patient is associated with necrosis.

the upper ipsilateral neck; the contralateral side of the neck was extensively involved in these patients.

DISTANT METASTASES. Systematically disseminated cancer is a major limiting factor to overall improvement in cure rate in patients with NPC and is predicted by the presence of bulky cervical metastases.[1,325] The lung is the most common site of metastases, followed by bone. Because of the unique location of the primary tumor, DMs may also develop by direct vascular invasion of Batson's paravertebral venous plexus.

In one study, the pattern of distant failure in 759 patients with stage I to IV NPC was studied in Asia.[326] Although in the aggregate literature, N status most closely predicts the eventual development of DMs (usually within 2 years of presentation), in this report N stage, T stage, and nodal characteristics (size and degree of fixation) were found to be significant prognosticators of the development of systemic disease. A high incidence of distant failure was noted in patients with T3, N3, or bulky or fixed neck lymph node involvement. Contralateral neck involvement was found to be of no significance.

Despite the high degree of awareness of NPC in Asian communities, only 9% of 5037 patients in a recent series were diagnosed while disease was still confined within the nasopharynx.[327] The rest had locally advanced tumors associated with bone erosion and cranial nerve palsies, and the majority of patients (75%) also presented with overt lymphatic metastases, including 27% with spread to the supraclavicular level. Six percent of the patients presented with DMs.

Diagnosis

Diagnosis of NPC is based on history and physical examination, imaging studies (CT or MR), biopsy at the primary site, or fine-needle aspiration of a neck mass and serologic testing for EBV. The polymerase chain reaction can be applied to fine-needle aspiration specimens to identify EBV genomes with DNA amplification. This is particularly useful in identifying an occult primary tumor location in some patients with "unknown primary" neck lymph nodes.[306]

SIGNS AND SYMPTOMS. Trotter gave a classic description of the presentation of NPC in 1911.[317] He emphasized hearing loss of the "Eustachian tube type," which may be relieved temporarily by insufflation of the middle ear. Pain is typical in the second and third divisions of the trigeminal nerve (often mistaken for trigeminal neuralgia) especially in young adult males. The palate is asymmetric at rest because of tumor involvement of the levator palati muscle (see Fig. 20–49). Enlargement of "cervical glands" is common (Figs. 20–50B and 20–51).

Serous otitis media is one of the earliest presenting signs of NPC. Middle ear effusion results from eustachian tube obstruction because of presence of the primary tumor in the nasopharynx (see Fig. 20–50A). Other common findings are purulent, bloody rhinorrhea, frank epistaxis, cranial nerve palsy due to invasion of the parapharyngeal space and cranial cavity by tumor,[315,320] and metastatic cervical lymphadenopathy. The majority of patients present with a neck mass. Pain, epistaxis, trismus, and cervical adenopathy are associated with malignancy. Other symptoms are nasal obstruction, conductive hearing loss, tinnitus, and headache.

The differential diagnosis of a tumor in the nasopharynx includes infectious mononucleosis (which can resemble lymphoma microscopically) and lymphoma, especially Hodgkin's disease.[328]

RADIOLOGY. Intracranial tumor extension and parapharyngeal involvement were poorly assessable in the

TABLE 20–10. Comparison of Nasopharyngeal Carcinoma Staging Systems

Staging System		T		N		M		Stage
AJC*	TIS:	carcinoma in situ		Standard AJC Neck Staging	MX:	not assessed	I:	T1 N0 M0
	T1:	tumor confined to one site of nasopharynx or no tumor visible (positive biopsy only)			M0:	no (known) distant metastasis	II:	T2 N0 M0
	T2:	tumor involving two sites (both posterosuperior and lateral walls)			M1:	distant metastasis present. Specify sites: pulmonary, osseous, hepatic, brain, lymph nodes, bone marrow, pleura, skin, eye, other	III:	T3 N0 M0
	T3:	extension of tumor into nasal cavity or oropharynx						T1 or T2 or T3, N1, M0
	T4:	tumor invasion of skull or cranial nerve involvement, or both					IV:	T4, N0 or N1, M0
								Any T, N2 or N3, M0
								Any T, any N, M1
Ho†	T1:	T1 tumor confined to nasopharynx (space behind choanal orifices and nasal septum and above posterior margin of soft palate in resting position)	0:	N0 none palpable (nodes thought to be benign excluded)	0:	M0 no evidence of distant metastasis	I:	A tumor confined to nasopharyngeal mucosa (T1, N0, M0)
	2:	T2 tumor extended to nasal fossa, oropharynx, or adjacent muscles or nerves below base of skull	1:	N1 node(s) wholly in upper cervical level bounded below by skin crease extending laterally and backward from or just below thyroid notch (laryngeal eminence)	1:	M distant metastasis present	II:	B tumor extended to nasal fossa, oropharynx, or adjacent muscles or nerves below base of skull (T2) and or N1 involvement
	3:	T3 tumor extended beyond T2 limits and subclassified as follows:	2:	N2 node(s) palpable between crease and supraclavicular fossa, upper limit being line joining upper margin of sternal end of clavical and apex of angle formed by lateral surface of neck and superior margin of trapezius			III:	tumor extended beyond T2 limits or bone involvement (T3) and or N2 involvement
	4:	T3a bone involvement below base of skull (floor of sphenoid sinus is included in this category)	3:	N3 node(s) palpable in supraclavicular fossa and or skin involvement in form of carcinoma en cuirasse or satellite nodules above clavicles			IV:	C N3 involvement, irrespective of primary tumor
	5:	T3b involvement of base of skull					V:	D hematogenous metastasis and/or involvement of skin or lymph node(s) below clavicles (M)
	6:	T3c involvement of cranial nerve(s)						
	7:	T3d involvement of orbits, laryngopharynx (hypopharynx), or infratemporal fossa						
UICC‡	0:	no evidence of primary tumor	0:	no evidence of regional lymph node involvement	0:	no evidence of distant metastases	I:	T1 N0 M0
	1:	tumor confined to one site (including tumor identified from positive biopsy)	1:	evidence of involvement of movable homolateral regional lymph nodes	1:	evidence of distant metastasis	II:	T2 N0 M0
	2:	tumor involving two sites	2:	evidence of involvement of movable contralateral or bilateral regional lymph nodes	8:	minimum requirements to assess presence of distant metastases cannot be met	III:	T3 N0 M0
	3:	tumor with extension to nasal cavity and or oropharynx	3:	evidence of involvement of fixed regional lymph nodes				T1 or T2 or T3, N1, M0
	4:	tumor with extension to base of skull and/or involving cranial nerves	8:	minimum requirements to assess regional lymph nodes cannot be met			IV:	T4, N0 or N1, M0
	5:	preinvasive carcinoma (carcinoma in situ)						Any T, N2 or N3, M0
	8:	minimum requirements to assess primary tumor cannot be met						Any T, any N, M1

* Data from American Joint Committee for Cancer (AJCC) Staging and End-Results Reporting: Manual for Staging of Cancer. Chicago, AJCC, 1977.
† Data from Ho JH: Stage classification of nasopharyngeal carcinoma: a review. IARC Sci Pub 20:99, 1978.
‡ Data from Harmer MH (ed): TNM Classification of Malignant Tumours. 3rd ed. Geneva, International Union Against Cancer, 1978.

pre-CT era.[329] Newer imaging methods have contributed to earlier recognition of failure and more appropriate choices and methods of salvage treatment as well as influencing initial and retreatment radiation technique, such as giving a posterolateral boost for extensive parapharyngeal space involvement.[319] Gadolinium-enhanced MR imaging has the potential to detect perineural extension along nerves at the skull base.[318] Although single photon emission CT (SPECT) using the tumor-seeking agent technetium-99m dimercaptosuccinate acid does localize in some neck metastases in patients with NPC, it is currently not a reliable imaging agent to detect the primary tumor.[330]

Classification Systems

That several staging systems have been used for NPC contributes to confusion, nonuniform end-result reporting, and difficulties in interpreting results of pa-

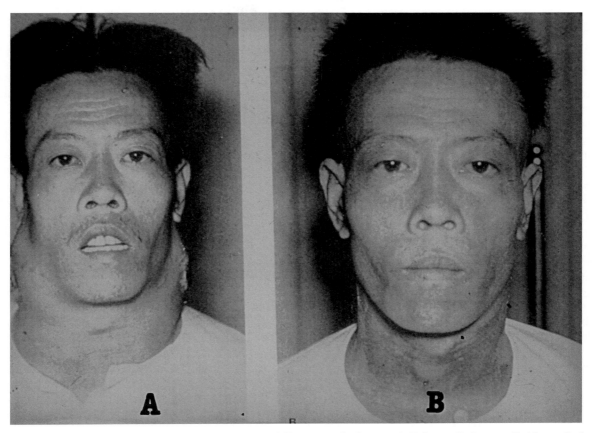

Fig. 20–51. Response of massive cervical lymphadenopathy to full-course radiotherapy. A. Before radiotherapy. B. After radiotherapy.

tient treatment series. A TNM system is used by the American Joint Committee on Cancer (AJCC)[362] and the International Union Against Cancer (UICC).[364] A separate system was proposed by Ho.[302] The Neel-Taylor[303,309] system includes additional biologic factors. These systems are compared in Table 20–10.[309,367] In general, the non-TNM staging systems are considered to predict the risk of death better than the TNM system.

PROBLEMS IN STAGING THE PRIMARY TUMOR. The TNM systems uses the number of nasopharyngeal regions involved, and this can be difficult to determine on physical examination. A primary tumor may be submucosal and invisible, with the diagnosis established only by biopsy.

The UICC classification[364] considers bone involvement but not involvement of cranial nerves, although the latter implies invasion of the cranial cavity and an intuitively graver prognosis than bone involvement. Lateral and posterior extension to the paranasopharyngeal space is ignored in all staging systems, although its importance has been emphasized.[320]

PROBLEMS IN NECK STAGING. Ho's system for staging cervical metastases differs from the AJCC and UICC staging systems, which previously emphasized contralateral and bilateral neck lymph node involvement but now rank size of lymph nodes as the most important

variable. Ho's system divides the neck into three levels, and the level of nodal involvement on either side of the neck is the sole criterion used in staging; the lowest level of the neck which is involved by tumor is noted.[301] The Ho classification of N stage has been found to be superior to others in that it discriminates even among patient groups stratified by the size of the lymph nodes,[324] although this system has not been widely used internationally.

The separate system of Neel evolved from a prospective collaborative study of North American patients with NPC. A prognostic score was derived from a complex analysis of many variables, including immunologic ones. Five factors were considered important determinants of survival: (1) the presence of 7 or more symptoms (nasal, ear, throat, neck, cranial nerve, weight loss, duration of symptoms, number of symptoms); (2) nodes in the lower neck or supraclavicular region; (3) histologic WHO type I; (4) extensive tumor in the nasopharynx; and (5) symptoms present for less than 2 months before presentation. Patients with WHO type I tumors had a significantly higher death rate than those with either WHO type II or III (an outmoded histologic classification, as discussed earlier).

Patients with high ADCC titers had significantly lower death rates than those with low titers. Because

ADCC measurements are not commercially available, this is primarily of academic interest. Changes in VCA or EA anti-EBV titers would probably provide another clue to prognosis but only after diagnosis and treatment,[309] and the new staging system would require prospective study at other institutions to determine its worldwide relevance. Regional extent and involvement of cranial nerves were important prognostic variables, but involvement of the skull bone itself did not necessarily reflect a bad prognosis. Ho's system of neck staging was the most relevant because no significant difference was noted in survival among patients with uni- or bilateral nodes, and size and fixation of nodes was not important either.

Treatment Results

OVERVIEW. NPC has traditionally been treated with full-course RT because many tumors are radiosensitive (see Fig. 20–51) and radiocurable and because surgical resection has historically been considered anatomically unfeasible. The standard RT regimen uses external beam delivered in the range of 60 to 76 Gy. Intracavitary brachytherapy boosts are sometimes delivered, in addition. When treated with appropriate radiation sources, doses, and techniques, only 10 to 20% of patient deaths are due to isolated local failure. Patients typically undergo radical neck dissection 4 to 8 weeks after the end of radiation if regression of lymph nodes is incomplete. The role of adjuvant chemotherapy is currently controversial (see later).

The major current challenges in the treatment of patients with NPC are (1) a high incidence of local failure with tumors of advanced T stage (T4) with evidence of bone destruction or cranial nerve involvement and (2) a high incidence of DM—currently incurable—which is predicted by bulky cervical node disease and results in less than 20% 5-year survival.

Overall 5-year survival in aggregate for SCC of the nasopharynx ranges from 25 to 65%, and in the few series with long-term results, 10-year survival ranges from 20 to 55%. As with most other head and neck cancer sites, results are more favorable in early-stage disease (small primary tumors with absent or minimal neck disease) than in advanced disease; for patients with stage I or II disease, the 5-year survival rate can be as high as 93%, but it drops to about 40% for stage III and IV disease.[331] In patients with advanced nodal disease (N3), the majority succumb to DMs.

Improvements in treatment results over the decades have been attributed to use of megavoltage rather than orthovoltage radiation, increase in total dose of external irradiation, boosting by intracavitary sources, increase in target volume, prophylactic neck irradiation in lymph node-negative patients, improvement in technical accuracy, hyperfractionation, improved assessment of local extent by advanced imaging techniques, and addition of adjuvant chemotherapy. Al-

most all claims of improved treatment results are based on comparison with historical data, however, and in the absence of prospective randomized trials (rarely conducted in Asia because of limited resources or in the West because of insufficient patient numbers), none of these factors can be considered scientifically compelling.

Current treatment controversies in the treatment of NPC include the need for elective RT to the N0 neck, reirradiation at the primary site, surgery for recurrent or persistent cancer at the primary site and in the neck, and the role of chemotherapy. Chemotherapy has been studied as an induction protocol and as simultaneous chemoradiotherapy for advanced (stage III and IV) NPC. The role of surgery consists of salvage attempts at the primary site or neck dissection for persistent or recurrent disease after RT with curative intent.

REPRESENTATIVE SERIES. As with most other sites of head and neck cancer, reports in the literature of overall survival and local control rates vary and are difficult to interpret because of treatment, which is nonstandard with respect to fields and doses of radical radiation, the use of different staging and histologic classification systems, and the inclusion of nonepithelial malignancies in some series. Large series consisting of more than 1000 patients have been reported only from Asian centers, and such reports provide the best information on the etiopathogenesis of this disease. The authors often acknowledge that they are "service departments" with limited resources, however, and different fractionation schedules have been used over time with pursuant variability in the area treated, total dose, regimen, and so forth.

A recent series gives a typical picture of treatment results from a top-level North American institution representing adequate treatment and evolving technology[332]; a retrospective analysis of 143 patients with NPC treated with definitive irradiation from 1956 to 1986. Histologically, the group consisted of 17 keratinizing SCCs, 20 nonkeratinizing SCCs, 60 SCCs "not otherwise specified," 30 undifferentiated carcinomas, and 16 "lymphoepitheliomas." The patients were treated with a combination of cobalt-60, 4 to 6 MV x-rays, and 18 to 25 MV x-rays to the primary tumor and the upper neck excluding the spinal cord at 40 to 45 Gy, to total doses of 60 to 70 Gy. The local failure rate increased with the size of the primary tumor: 15% for T1 and 60% for T4. Failure in the neck increased in direct proportion to the volume of neck disease: 18% for N0 and 33% for N2 or N3 lymphadenopathy. The incidence of DMs correlated with the extent of cervical lymphadenopathy: 16% for N0 or N1 versus 40% for N2 or N3. The actuarial 10-year disease-free survival rate was 55 to 60% for T1 to T3, N0 or N1 tumors, and decreased to 35% for T4, N0 or N1, and further to 20% for T4, N2 or N3 tumor stages. The overall 10-year survival rate was about 40% for patients with T1 or T2,

N0 or N1 tumors and only 10% for patients with T4 lesions.

A dose-response relationship was noted in control of the primary tumor, with 80% of tumors controlled in patients who received 66 to 70 Gy, and 100% control in those with T1 to T3 tumors who received over 70 Gy. Local tumor control did not rise above 55% for T4 lesions, however, even with doses over 70 Gy. Simulation proved important in enhancing local tumor control by more accurately identifying the extent of anatomy to be radiated and allowing more accurate dose delivery planning.

Complications in this series included osteoradionecrosis of the mandible in two patients and soft tissue necrosis requiring surgical repair in two others. Brain necrosis was seen in two patients and osteomyelitis of the cervical spine occurred in one patient with diabetes mellitus. Carotid rupture and pharyngeal hemorrhage occurred in four patients undergoing radical neck dissection for persistent nodal disease with fatal outcome.

NPC is typically seen in a bimodal age distribution, but few reports address treatment results in children, specifically. A recent retrospective analysis of 40 children and adolescents with NPC (32 "lymphoepithelioma," 8 SCC) included 23 patients with primary tumors confined to the nasopharynx with the remainder extending beyond the nasopharynx, and with palpable cervical lymphadenopathy present in 31. No DMs were identified at presentation. All patients were treated with primary RT, and some had chemotherapy in addition. Ten of the patients are alive 5 to 30 years from the time of diagnosis, with a median follow-up of 10 years.[333]

Management of Neck Disease

The two controversies in this area concern (1) whether the N0 neck should be electively irradiated and (2) the appropriate management of persistent or recurrent cancer in the neck.

The need to include the regional lymphatics bilaterally (both entire heminecks) in the primary treatment of stage I patients remains controversial. The literature, in aggregate, shows that few patients die with uncontrolled neck disease as the only site of failure and that neck recurrence can be successfully salvaged with additional treatment. Neck disease as a site of treatment failure is insignificant in comparison with the currently incurable higher incidence of hematogenous dissemination. Nevertheless, elective neck irradiation to the N0 neck is strongly advocated by many authors because of the high incidence (62 to 85%) of occult lymph node involvement even for T1 tumors,[334] the universal experience of low regional relapse rates following such treatment, and the low morbidity of the treatment. The exact impact of elective neck irradiation on the final outcome has never been extensively tested in controlled trials, however, and conflicting results showing a lack of significant benefit have also been published. A concern of those who recommend elective treatment to the neck is the possibility that occult untreated cancer foci in lymph nodes could contribute to the high incidence of DMs. Tumor biology studies show that hematogenous and lymphatic metastases occur simultaneously, however, usually by the time the primary tumor is detectable, rather than occurring in a cascade phenomenon consistent with the halstedian paradigm.[1]

Ho performed a randomized study on the value of elective neck irradiation for stage I NPC and showed that, although patients receiving this treatment had a lower incidence of overt lymph node metastases (5% versus 25%), those who did develop such nodes without elective RT could be salvaged with additional therapeutic irradiation with comparable 5-year actuarial survival and disease-free rates.[302] He concluded that elective neck irradiation could be safely withheld if the patient could be closely observed, provided the first-echelon lymphatic drainage area (retropharyngeal lymph nodes) was adequately covered within the primary target volume. Additional support for withholding elective neck irradiation appears in other recent reports.[335–338] If elected, prophylactic irradiation to the neck should be given to at least one level beyond the clinical extent of disease. For patients with N0 necks, this would mean prophylactic irradiation of only the upper neck.[324,337]

TREATMENT OF PERSISTENT OR RECURRENT NECK DISEASE. Persistent or recurrent neck disease (about 18% incidence overall) can be treated by additional radiation or surgery. Reirradiation of neck recurrences is probably inferior to surgery (with or without additional radiation), although these treatments have not been directly compared.

Primary, radical RT should deliver booster doses to the site of bulky nodal disease and should include portals that cover the whole neck, including the supraclavicular fossa.[338] Because of suboptimal control with additional RT compared with surgical treatment and the possibility of RT-related complications from the high dose, surgery is generally recommended as the treatment of choice for persistence or recurrence of neck lymph node disease after primary RT for NPC.

The extent of surgical resection, that is, local excision with or without additional radiation versus radical neck dissection has been debated in the literature. Because cervical lymph nodes in NPC are often large at presentation (60 to 90% of patients initially) and because operations in a previously treated field must be wider than in untreated patients, radical neck dissection is the procedure of choice for recurrent or persistent neck disease after RT. A lesser operation might be acceptable before RT. ,

Wei reported a 5-year regional control rate of 65% and corresponding survival of 37% (with a median follow-up of 3 years) following 71 salvage radical neck dissections (1981 to 1989).[307] Careful histologic study on 43 of these neck dissection specimens showed a 5 to 10% false-positive rate; histologic examination revealed only keratin granulomas without cancer. Extracapsular spread was found in 70% of the neck dissection specimens, present as dissociated tumor clusters diffusely infiltrating the soft tissue in 35%, and close to the spinal accessory nerve in 28%. More disease was evident histologically than clinically in 73% of cases; 59 positive lymph nodes were seen clinically, 117 intraoperatively, and 294 histologically. Therefore, Wei concluded that radical neck dissection was the *minimum* salvage operation acceptable. In Wei's study, the probability of control of neck disease with radical neck dissection was 66% at 5 years; limited by node "fixation."[339]

Although salvage neck lymph node "lumpectomy" has been recommended by some,[340] based on Wei's findings of extracapsular extension of nodal disease and adherence to surrounding structures at operation in 35% of patients, a wider-field operation is more likely to achieve durable control of multiple lymph node involvement, which is typical in NPC.[340a]

The significant incidence of false-negative fine-needle aspiration (5 to 30%) means that the clinician must often proceed with a radical neck dissection based on clinical grounds alone. Surgery in the management of neck lymph node recurrence is a relatively safe procedure,[339,341,342] especially when augmented by use of a vascularized regional flap to aid neck wound-healing whenever important structures (carotid artery) are at risk. Thus, radical neck dissection is also useful for palliation of persistent neck disease even in patients who also have simultaneous DMs, if not otherwise contraindicated.

The addition of brachytherapy with iridium wire implantation after salvage radical neck dissection is associated with a higher complication rate (carotid rupture) and has not been shown to be of additional benefit compared with surgery alone.[338] If brachytherapy is used, the neck should probably be protected with a pectoralis (myofascial) flap covered with skin graft[296] or a deltopectoral flap to decrease the likelihood of complications. Brachytherapy is generally considered only in patients with extensive extranodal extension or when resection margins are microscopically positive and has not proved useful for gross residual disease.[213,340,343]

Management of Persistent or Recurrent Disease in the Nasopharynx

Locally persistent or recurrent NPC may be due to intrinsic radioresistance of the primary tumor, insufficient dose, or a "geographic miss" during the initial therapy. The diagnosis of persistent cancer following the end of RT probably requires biopsy because neither CT nor MR can distinguish post-therapy fibrosis-radiation edema-infection from residual tumor.[344] Because some tumors regress slowly and various types of dysplasia can be noted following the end of RT, additional treatment is indicated only if cancer is documented on biopsy 8 to 10 weeks following treatment.[325,345]

Persistent or recurrent disease at the primary site can be treated with additional radiation (megavoltage or brachytherapy) or surgery. The goal of retreatment at the primary site is basically palliative, with cure achieved in only a few cases. Aggressive initial RT results in local failures in 5 to 30% of cases. Surgery is usually not appropriate because of the inaccessibility of the recurrent lesion although attempts are being reported using skull base techniques (see later). Chemotherapy alone does not produce durable responses.

High doses of reirradiation are required for worthwhile symptomatic relief or possible cure, and this carries with it a risk of severe late effects in previously irradiated normal tissue. Complications of RT (primary or reirradiation) include radiation myelitis, brain stem necrosis, bone necrosis of the skull base and mandible, radiation damage to cranial nerves IX, X, XI, and XII with paralysis, rupture of the carotid artery after salvage neck dissection, symptomatic hypothalamic-pituitary dysfunction (hyperprolactinemia, hypothyroidism, panhypopituitarism), temporomandibular joint dysfunction, and conductive hearing loss.

Improvements in diagnostic imaging help localize the full extent of the primary tumor and assist by allowing portals to be better defined and higher doses delivered. Improved radiation techniques now limit the amount of brain and other normal tissues in the initial treatment fields, which can decrease the rate of severe complications pursuant to (expert) retreatment. Three-dimensional treatment planning (conformal RT) should further increase the safety of this approach at the few institutions where this technology is available.

Several options exist for radiation treatment of recurrent primary disease; radiation boosts can include high-dose external beam radiation through reduced portals with or without brachytherapy (afterloading intracavitary cesium or interstitial gold-192 or ^{125}I). Additional radiation doses should be in the range of 60 to 70 Gy to be effective, and reirradiation appears to be more effective for T1 or T2 rather than for larger lesions. Using brachytherapy as part of all of the source for reirradiation can decrease the high incidence of significant damage to neuroendocrine and soft tissues that accompanies reirradiation with external beam therapy and can serve as an adjunctive method to additional external beam radiation or surgery to decrease the morbidity of each. Brachytherapy has the advantage of giving a high radiation dose to tumor with a much lower dose to adjacent normal tissue. This allows additional radiation to be given to an area that has previously received full-course RT.

The benefit of a booster dose to residual primary cancer was confirmed in a prospective randomized trial initiated in 1980.[346] The local recurrence rate was similar (6%) in boosted patients to the rate in those who had no residual tumor (4%) and was much less than in those with positive residual disease who were observed and received no additional treatment (36%).

Results of retreatment of 53 patients with local persistent or recurrent NPC treated with megavoltage RT from 1954 to 1989 was reported.[313] The median dose (megavoltage with or without brachytherapy) was 112 Gy. Overall 5-year actuarial local control, disease-free survival, and overall survival rates were 35%, 18% and 21%, respectively. The rate of complications increased significantly with doses over 100 Gy, and 8 patients developed severe complications from retreatment of which 5 were fatal (2 brain, 1 spinal cord, 2 lower cranial nerves). In patients treated with a combination of external beam and intracavitary cesium, 7 of 9 achieved local control with a follow-up of 7 to 102 months, and none had a severe complication. Five-year actuarial, local control, and disease-free survival in that subgroup was 67%, 44%, and 60% respectively. The actuarial incidence of severe complications at 5-years was 17%.

Brachytherapy (gold grains, intracavitary cesium) delivery is complicated by difficult anatomic logistics. One trend is to afford better exposure for placement of interstitial radiation sources by invasive surgery such as a palatal split approach.[347] Between 1986 and 1991, Wei's group[307] used this approach in 43 *small* primary recurrences of 2 cm or less. With a median follow-up of 39 months, 9 of the evaluable patients have had recurrences and 32 have not. Complications include headaches, dislodged seeds, and palatal fistulas. A lateral rhinotomy approach or a maxillary "swinging trap-door" has also been used to enhance exposure for placement of brachytherapy sources.[348] Often, as much recurrent or persistent tumor is removed as possible at the same time. Because little residual soft tissue may remain to hold interstitial sources in place, a mold fashioned to conform to the cavity can be used to retain the radiation sources.

Wei's[307] approach to *large* recurrences (greater than 2 cm) is to use a "maxillary swing" approach. Between 1989 and 1994, 21 patients were treated surgically for primary recurrences, with curative intent in 18 and palliative intent in 3. With a median follow-up of 18 months, recurrences have been reported in 4 patients. Two carotid ruptures occurred (in patients who had had additional brachytherapy, which has since been discontinued). Reconstruction uses a free graft obtained from turbinate mucosa.

SURGERY. Surgery for recurrent NPC has been investigated at several institutions during the past decade. Although seemingly a recent development enhanced by technology, Trotter reported an operation in 1911 similar to those used today, "the osteoplastic resection of the upper jaw," which exposed the nasopharynx through a bone flap in the upper jaw. "The operation, although formidable in appearance, is easy to carry out, is not dangerous in itself, and leaves no deformity." Despite recent advances in surgical access to the skull base, the complexity of the anatomy and the intimate proximity of vital structures (carotid artery and optic nerve) often make it impossible to obtain a satisfactory resection with traditionally adequate margins (see later).

Surgery for NPC is difficult because of the proximity of important structures: carotid, cerebral, and vertebral arteries, brain, spinal cord, cavernous sinus, and cranial nerves. Surgery is additionally complicated by wound-healing problems when carried out in previously radiated patients. Operative fields reached by conventional approaches through the palate[365] and maxillary sinus may be appropriate for limited tumors, but they are too narrow to remove extensive tumors, and various combined approaches have been used including a lateral transparotid approach, infratemporal fossa, transpalatine, transmandibular-transpterygoid,[349] and transmaxillary (facial translocation-maxillary swing); these are types of "craniofacial disassembly." During such surgery, important structures are isolated and protected. Goals of surgery are achieving an oncologically sound resection, uncomplicated wound-healing, restoration of critical barriers to infection by various types of vascularized flaps (galeal-pericranial, temporalis muscle, free flaps) as well as functional and aesthetic restoration. Osteotomies can be repositioned with titanium microplates, which will not interfere with MR scanning postoperatively.

Anecdotal treatment results using these heroic measures include long-term survival in 2 of 5 patients in the series of Yumoto and colleagues at 50 and 68 months, and a 5-year survival rate of 44% in 9 patients reoperated for primary recurrence in the series of Tu and associates.[340]

Stereotactic radiosurgery (gamma knife[111]) is also a new alternative. At this point, stereotactic radiosurgery, brachytherapy, and salvage surgery are considered primarily in the palliation of symptoms, and it is unlikely that many cures will result.

A related issue in the management of patients with NPC is whether pressure-equalizing (P-E) tubes should be placed for serous otitis media, which can result from the disease process or from treatment. Historically, in Hong Kong P-E tubes were routinely placed before RT. Better hearing results are noted up to 1½ years but are counterbalanced by complications including persistent tympanic membrane perforations and otorrhea (in 15 of 32 patients). Hearing results appear to be the same after 1½ years, presumably because of ossicular fixation or other causes. Wei's conclusion[307] is that it is not necessary to place grommets uniformly before treatment, but to do so after RT if abnormal hearing persists. A report from New Zealand also recommends conservative management of effusions in patients with NPC because of troublesome tympanic membrane perforations and otorrhea in patients with tubes.[350]

CHEMOTHERAPY. In addition to being radiosensitive, undifferentiated NPC is also chemosensitive to platinum-based regimens, and the role of chemotherapy for NPC is being actively investigated. Systemic chemotherapy has been used in a variety of ways in an attempt to increase local control and survival: in neoadjuvant and adjuvant settings, and concomitantly with radiation, as well as in alternating chemoradiotherapy regimens (which have shown efficacy in other rapidly growing tumors such as non-Hodgkin's lymphoma and small cell lung cancer). As for other sites of head and neck cancer, the efficacy of induction chemotherapy is less convincing than the possible benefit of concomitant chemoradiation in improving disease-free and overall survival and in reducing the incidence of DMs. When compared with historical controls of single-modality therapy (RT), however, no randomized trial has confirmed the utility of adding chemotherapy to the standard best treatment for NPC.[351–354,366] A randomized, phase III study (Southwest Oncology Group Protocol 8892) of RT with or without concurrent cisplatin in patients with NPC is in progress.

The combination of chemotherapy with altered fractionation RT for NPC (alternating chemoradiotherapy) appears promising.[355] An unusually high degree of local control of 89% (minimum 4-year follow-up) was seen above the clavicles, particularly encouraging because the majority of patients had advanced local-regional disease (93% N3 and 50% T4). Four-year estimated survival was 52%. Half of the patients developed DMs.

FUTURE DIRECTIONS. As with other sites of head and neck cancer, aggressive surgical resection, altered-fractionation RT, stereotactic radiosurgery, simultaneous chemoradiotherapy and biologic response modifiers are said to hold hope for future improvement in survival of patients with NPC.

Experimental work is underway to investigate the cellular and molecular structure of NPC cells, antigens, the release of cytokines, the interaction between malignant cells and those of the immune response, and to define further NPC pathogenesis, development, and possible markers for treatment.[357] Currently, heterogeneity for a variety of subcellular products such as cytokines and other gene products are being described in animal models and cell lines.[358] Differences in molecular genetic profiles[359] between primary tumor and metastases are also noted. The variable expression of inflammatory cytokines and other substances makes it unlikely that they will be useful to monitor a clinical response to therapy, at this point.[360]

Various biologic response modifiers are also being used in experimental clinical trials. Recently, interferon γ was tried in a series of 13 patients who were refractory to conventional chemotherapy. Unfortunately, there were no objective responses, and interferon γ was unable to induce antitumor activity alone in these heavily pretreated patients.[361] To improve survival results, the need exists for effective adjuvant systemic chemotherapy to eradicate microscopic systemic disease, which is currently lacking.

RECONSTRUCTION OF HEAD AND NECK CANCER DEFECTS

Before any reconstruction is effected, the surgeons change gowns and gloves, and clean instruments are used. A surgical tradition also includes irrigating the wound profusely with water, which is hypotonic and theoretically lyses free-floating tumor cells.

Head and neck cancer surgery causes both soft tissue and bony defects. The initially limited reconstructive armamentarium of the head and neck surgeon has expanded over the years and now includes a plethora of options. Both the ablation and the reconstruction must be carried out with a view to optimal reconstruction of function as well as appearance. According to McConnel,[369] in the past, the major rehabilitative concern of head and neck surgeons was to close the wound, and function was the secondary concern. To make decisions, postoperative function must be *quantitated*. Only by analyzing functional results can data be obtained to enable the surgeon to make the best reconstructive decisions. Thus, attention is now being directed (correctly) to quantitative assessment of how the patient functions after various reconstructive techniques.[370,371]

Historical Overview

The current state of head and neck cancer reconstruction can be appreciated only by relating it to developments that have gone before. Myocutaneous and "free" flaps are the standard of reconstruction and represent the culmination of many decades of development, which has been agonizing for both patient and surgeon. Moreover, not every head and neck cancer defect requires the magnitude of soft tissue reconstruction available with these methods, and familiarity with other reconstruction options such as local flaps is vital to the versatility of the head and neck cancer surgeon.

Major head and neck cancer ablations were life-threatening procedures before the late 1940s, and defects were frequently left unreconstructed or closed primarily, often with severe consequences to function and appearance. Such management led to ethical questions as to whether the "cure" was better than the disease, and head and neck cancer surgery developed the reputation of being brutal and mutilating. This perception has persisted and has led to the preference for nonsurgical treatment modalities, possibly to the detriment of cancer control, because most patients cured of solid cancers have had surgery as part of their initial treatment.

Major head and neck cancer surgery was undertaken more frequently starting in the 1940s, with the advent of antibiotics, blood transfusion methods, and more modern surgical techniques and support. Hayes Martin's "Commando" procedure became the "one-operation-fits-all" standard for excising cancers of the oral cavity and oropharynx. This included hemimandibulectomy with excision of involved intraoral soft tissue in the tonsil, FOM, and tongue area, in continuity with a radical neck dissection. The operation derived its name not from the fact that patients looked postoperatively as though they had walked through a mine field, but because at the time (in the 1940s), Commando units were being used in the European war theater, and their missions required special courage and daring. To undergo a head and neck cancer resection of this magnitude during this era also required special courage and daring on the part of both patient and surgeon. We now use the term "composite resection," which is less terrifying for patient and surgeon.

The usual method of closure at this time was reapproximation of the residual intraoral soft tissues, or "primary closure." Usually, residual tongue was sutured to the buccal mucosa, and the hemimandible was removed (regardless of oncologic need) to facilitate such closure. Although the result was cosmetically suboptimal, these patients could function reasonably well in respect to intelligibility of speech and swallowing by mouth. In fact, some studies indicate that this method of closure is functionally superior to some of the "fancy" reconstructive methods now available.

Whereas the lateral "Commando" procedure with primary closure could excise cancer and rehabilitate the patient adequately, segmental resection of the *anterior* mandible could not be similarly reconstructed, and ablations in this area resulted in the undesirable "Andy Gump" deformity (see Fig. 20–35), named after the contemporary cartoon character who had no face below his mustache. Excisions of tissue in this area (typically segmental mandible between the angles with or without chin skin, adjacent FOM, and sometimes even total glossectomy) interfere with the hyomandibular complex and rendered the patients oral cripples who frequently needed feeding gastrostomies and permanent tracheostomies. Persistent drooling and an unacceptable cosmetic appearance separated the patients from their families and society, causing an ethical dilemma with respect to the validity of the treatment undertaken.[372,373]

In this early era, such large soft tissue defects of the oral cavity and oropharynx were reconstructed by "waltzing" tubed pedicle flaps from distant sites to the head and neck. For example, a rolled tube of skin and subcutaneous tissue might be created on the abdomen (attached at the proximal and distal ends). After several weeks, the ingrowth of blood vessels would support viability of the flap as it was moved up toward the recipient site, usually in several additional stages, in the manner of an inchworm. Depending on the length of flap available, it might be rotated from the abdomen to the chest and then directly to the neck, or it might require an intermediate transit out to the arm and finally to the neck. This time-consuming, multistage type of reconstruction provided relatively little soft tissue, and cosmetic and functional results were poor. Usually, the patient stayed in the hospital during reconstruction and succumbed to local-regional cancer recurrence during the interim.

A major revolution in head and neck cancer reconstruction came about in 1965: the *deltopectoral flap (DP)* of Bakamjian[374] (Figs. 20–52 and 20–56A). It could be used without an initial "delay" (see subsequent text), although this enhanced its blood supply. Although the flap was still a two- to three-stage procedure, the stages were much less time-consuming, and the flap was predictably successful because it was left attached to a reliable blood supply (internal mammary perforators). The nature of the recipient bed in the head and neck in radiated and malnourished patients had previously

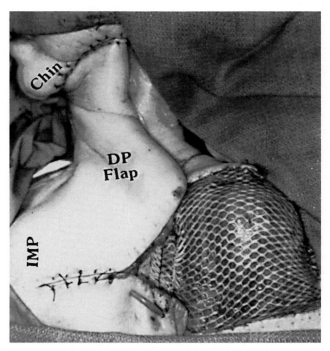

Fig. 20–52. Deltopectoral (DP) flap closure of fistula. IMP, Territory of internal mammary perforators. Meshed skin graft over shoulder donor site.

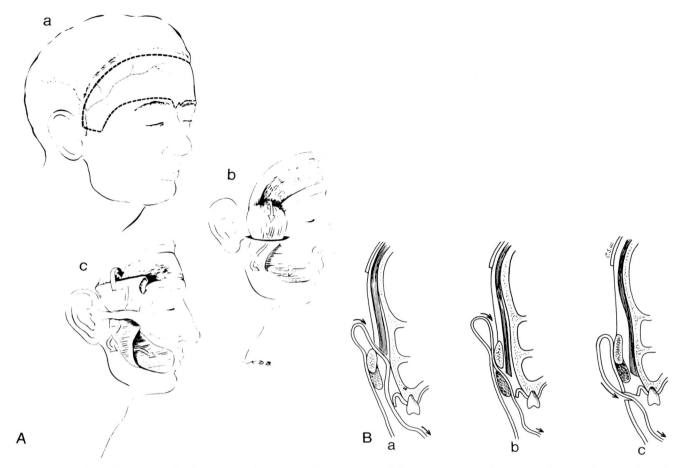

Fig. 20–53. Forehead flaps. A. a, Blood supply; b, elevation; and c, passage to defect site. B. Routes for passing flap to defect site. (A, from Sharzer LA, et al: Clin Plast Surg 3:503, 1976; B, from Matz G and Stankiewicz J: Application of the forehead flap for reconstruction of the floor of mouth. In: Controversy in Otolaryngology. Edited by Snow JB. Philadelphia, WB Saunders, 1980.)

doomed to failure reconstruction with most local flaps. A "random" portion of the DP flap extended out over the deltoid area enhancing length, and the flap was versatile for reconstructing many defects in the mouth and throat (see Fig. 20–47B),[375] as well as for repairing complications of previous treatment such as fistulas or nonhealing planned "controlled" pharyngostomies (see Fig. 20–66B and C).

The forehead flap (supplied by the temporal vessels) was also frequently used during the 1960s and 1970s (Fig. 20–53). It required a delay and left a cosmetic deformity that in this modern era would be considered unacceptable, but was valuable for lining intraoral defects in the buccal mucosa and FOM. It could also be lined with a skin graft for repair of full-thickness defects (cheek, pharynx) (Figs. 20–54 and 20–55).

Similar flaps from the back and shoulder consisting of skin and subcutaneous tissue were also used (Fig. 20–56B to D). The prototype of the omocervical,[376] deltoscapular,[377] and extended shoulder flaps was the "nape of neck flap" originally used by Mutter in the

1840s for reconstructing neck burn contractures or congenital malformations. The blood supply to this flap is extremely unreliable, and nape-of-neck flaps usually had to be "delayed" two or three times before use.

The flaps described previously currently comprise a secondary armamentarium for the head and neck surgeon when the first-line flaps (described later) have been used already, typically in patients who survive one or more ablative operations and develop multiple primary or recurrent cancers.

In the late 1970s, myocutaneous flaps were applied to reconstruction of head and neck cancer defects.[378] They had previously been used by plastic surgeons for reconstruction of defects in other areas such as chest wall and decubitus ulcers. Initially, myocutaneous flaps for head and neck cancer reconstruction were obtained from three muscle territories: pectoralis major, sternocleidomastoid, and trapezius[379] (Fig. 20–57). Within a few years, it became obvious that the vascularity of the sternocleidomastoid myocutaneous flap[380] was unreliable (possibly because it was not a true myocutaneous flap, as a result of the intervening platysma muscle) and that the trapezius flap was awkward with respect to intraoperative patient positioning.

The pectoralis major myocutaneous flap emerged as the "workhorse" for head and neck cancer reconstruction and revolutionized the field. It provides a large amount of well-vascularized soft tissue bulk and allows reconstruction to be completed at the time of ablation in one stage.

"Free" flaps[381] transfer tissue detached from a distant site such as the groin, dorsum of foot, forearm, or more recently abdomen and scapula and require microvascular anastomosis of a donor and recipient artery and vein, which is time-consuming and requires special expertise. Free flaps enjoyed a flurry of interest in the late 1970s, but the need for microvascular expertise and the popularity of the pectoralis myocutaneous flap decreased this enthusiasm. The ethics of adding extra time to lengthy ablative procedures in the usually frail head and neck cancer patient were questioned.

Interest in free-flap technology was revived in the middle to late 1980s by the impressive work of Ian Taylor of Australia on reconstruction of the jaws with revascularized groin flaps (bone and soft tissue). Since that time, this technology has mushroomed and is once again assuming a significant role in reconstruction of

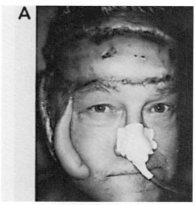

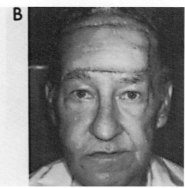

Fig. 20–55. Lined forehead flap (A) delivered through a cheek stab incision to line floor of mouth, mandible, retromolar trigone and cheek. Flap returned (B). (Courtesy of Dr. GJ Spector.)

head and neck cancer defects. Many academic departments now have either a head and neck surgeon who specializes in this technology or ancillary help from a similar person in the plastic surgery department because proficiency in these techniques requires a full-time commitment. The surgeon must be ready to take the patient back to the operating room at any time of the day or night, if flap viability comes into question, for an attempted emergency salvage procedure. It is stated that "when you have a hammer, everything is a nail," and departments that have a microvascular surgeon tend to use this type of flap reconstruction to maintain the surgeon's expertise, whereas when this technology is not available, myocutaneous flaps are generally used.

Types of Flaps for Soft Tissue Reconstruction

Flaps for soft tissue reconstruction are defined as "random," "axial," or "free" by their blood supply (see Fig. 20–56). *Random flaps* (intraoral rotation-advancement flaps of mucosa and tongue) derive nutrition from local unnamed vessels such as the dermal-subdermal plexus in the skin and are therefore severely restricted with respect to size. *Axial flaps* have a recognizable, usually named, arteriovenous circulation (deltopectoral flap,

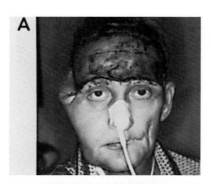

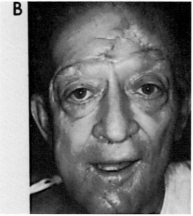

Fig. 20–54. Forehead flap (A) used to reconstruct the entire floor of mouth (B). Note the forehead scarring at the donor site. Flap is delivered to defect subcutaneously over the zygoma. (Courtesy of Dr. GJ Spector.)

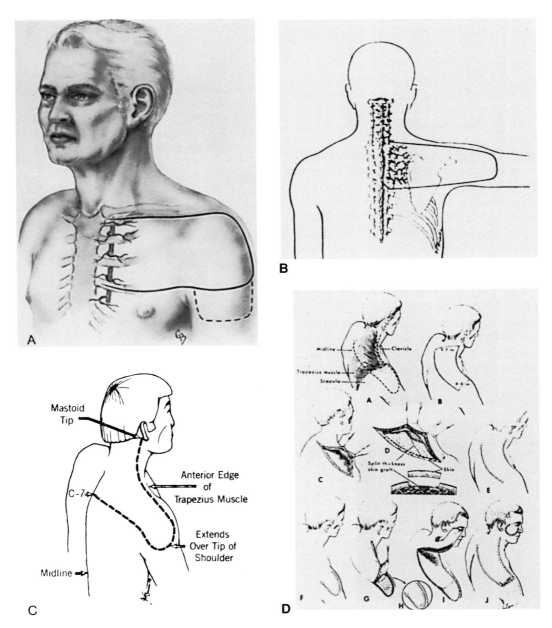

Fig. 20–56. Regional flaps for head and neck reconstruction. A. Deltopectoral flap. B. Deltoscapular flap C. Omocervical flap. D. Extended shoulder flap. (A, from Litton WB and Krause CJ: Otolaryngol Clin North Am 5:317, 1972; B, from Smith CJ: Arch Otolaryngol 104:391, 1978; C, from Gilmore B and Olson N: Arch Otolaryngol 105:589, 1979; D, from Chretien PB, et al: Am J Surg 118:754, 1969.)

forehead flap), and a specific length-to-width ratio (usually 3:1) is required for their survival. An axial flap may include a "random" extension to increase the amount of skin available, and survival of the random portion is increased by "staging" or "delaying" the flap (see later). Standard axial flaps are composed of skin and underlying subcutaneous tissue (fat) and include the underlying fascia to incorporate the blood supply from fasciocutaneous perforating vessels.

The term "*pedicle flap*" is also used, implying attachment of the flap to its blood supply for some period of time. The DP flap is an example. Typically, three

"stages" are required. The first stage is the "delay," in which the flap margins are incised down to the underlying muscle along three edges of the flap (the edges not in the vicinity of the supplying vessels—internal mammary perforators) and the flap, including its underlying fascia, is elevated from the pectoralis muscle. The flap is then replaced, the bed is drained, and the edges are sutured. The purpose of this first stage "delay" is to enhance the blood supply coming to the flap from its named vessels, which is facilitated by transecting the blood vessels along the other three surfaces. This is usually performed 10 to 14 days before

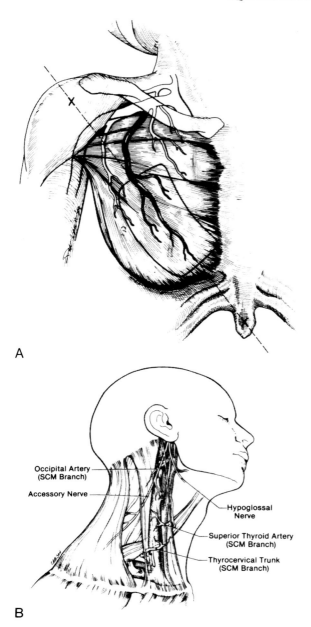

A

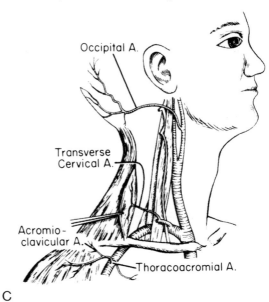

Fig. 20–57. Myocutaneous flap. A. Anatomy and vascular supply of pectoralis major flap, (1) superior thoracic artery, (2) pectoralis branch of thoracoacromial artery, (3) lateral thoracic artery. B. Vascular supply to sternocleidomastoid flap. C. Vascular supply to trapezius flap. (A, from Sharzer LA, et al: Clin Plast Surg 3:495, 1976; B, from Larson DL and Goepfert H: Plast Reconstr Surg 70:328, 1982; C, from Panje WR: Head Neck Surg 2:206, 1980.)

B

C

the use of the flap because the "delay" phenomenon is short-lived. The blood supply to some of these flaps is adequate to support flap transfer reliably without preliminary "delay" (DP but not nape-of-neck flaps).

The second stage takes place at the time of cancer excision. The flap is elevated, and the distal portion is sutured into the defect with the proximal end still left attached to its vascular supply (see Fig. 20–52). This condition is allowed to persist until the distal portion of the flap has presumably obtained a blood supply by ingrowth of vessels from the recipient bed. When this blood supply is adequate, the distal portion of the flap will not blanch when the pedicle is constricted with a tourniquet, and the flap can be "taken down." At the third stage, the portion of the flap not used in

the reconstruction (between the origin of the vascular supply and the recipient bed) is either returned to the donor site or is transected and discarded.

An *"island" pedicle flap* can be created in which the middle portion of the flap can be deepithelialized and tunneled into the defect under neck skin flaps, thereby eliminating the need for the third (and sometimes the first) stage.

Soft Tissue Reconstruction

The head and neck surgeon should be able to tailor the reconstruction to the size of the defect and the nature of the recipient bed and should always have two or three reconstructive options in mind for each patient, designed to fit various magnitudes of excision defect and as backup in the event of unforeseen intraoperative problems. Flap failure can result from improper design (for example, length-to-width ratios in axial flaps), tension at the suture line or at the pedicle base, hematoma and edema, venous stasis, spasm of feeding vessels, infection, and a technical error such as transecting the vessels to the flap.

Small defects in the oral cavity and oropharynx do not always require reconstruction with myocutaneous or free flaps, all other things being equal. This would be "long run for a short slide" and could use up a flap that may be necessary later in these patients who are prone to develop recurrences and multiple primary tumors. A small defect in a heavily pretreated patient who may also be malnourished or a diabetic may, however, require flap reconstruction, which brings its own blood supply into the area to ensure healing, rather than because of the size of the defect.

In previously treated patients with small defects of the oral cavity and oropharynx, a variety of reconstructive options are available (Fig. 20–57). Primary closure can be considered (Fig. 20–57A). This is typically used for partial glossectomy defects and has the theoretic disadvantage of burying the margin in the substance of the tongue. The application of skin and dermal grafts to the cut surface is preferred by some surgeons.[381a] These free grafts can be anchored to the recipient bed with "quilting sutures"[382] (Fig. 20–57B). This manner of resurfacing defects, however, contributes to wound contracture and scarring, which can mask early recurrent cancer. If the defect has been created with a laser (see previous text), partial closure or allowing the surface to heal by reepithelialization (see Fig. 20–15A) is preferable to applying a graft that does not "take" well over a lasered bed in animal models.[163] Figure 20–58 shows the vascular supply to flaps used in head and neck surgery; Figure 20–59 shows closure of tongue and FOM defects.

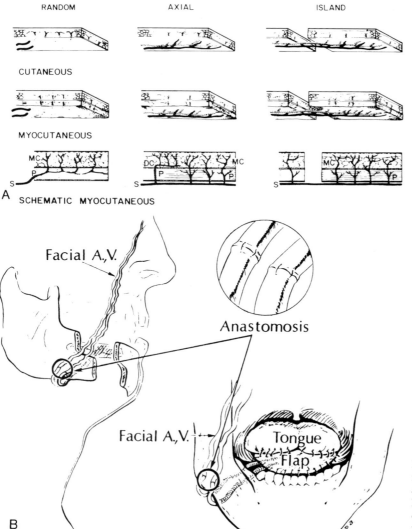

Fig. 20–58. Vascular supply to flaps used in head and neck reconstruction. A. Blood supply to random, axial, and island flaps. S, Segmental vessel; P, perforator; MC, musculocutaneous vessel. B. Representative microvascular anastomosis for a "free" flap. (A, from Ariyan S and Cuono AB: Head Neck Surg 2:321, 1980; B, from Sharzer LA, et al: Clin Plast Surg 3:507, 1976.)

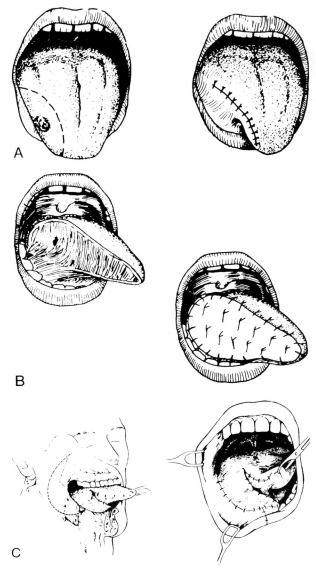

Fig. 20–59. A to C. Closure of tongue and floor of mouth defects. (A and B, from Barron JN and Saad MN (eds): Operative Plastic and Reconstructive Surgery. New York, Churchill Livingstone, 1981; C, from Papaioannon AN and Farr HW: Surg Gynecol Obstet *122*:809, 1966.)

Dermal[383] or skin graft[384] "pouches" can be constructed to line composite resection defects and restore function well (Fig. 20–60). The pouch is created by suturing the graft to the mucosal margins of the intraoral defect (usually lateral tongue, oropharynx, and buccal mucosa; Fig. 20–60A) and to itself anteriorly and inferiorly (Fig. 20–60B). The pouch extends down to the level of the hyoid bone (Fig. 20–60C). It is packed with a large bolus of Betadine-soaked cotton balls and aromatic Peruvian balsam for olfactory aesthetics wrapped in Xerofoam gauze, which distends the cheek flap for 10 days. The bolus is removed, and over time the pouch contracts upward, leaving a normally posi-

tioned sulcus in the lateral and posterior floor of mouth.

A variety of tongue flaps can be used to reconstruct small oral cavity defects.[385–388] The hemitongue flap is especially useful to resurface a defect of the alveolar ridge or anterolateral FOM (see Fig. 20–59C). An anteriorly or posteriorly based digastric flap may also be available to "plug" small defects communicating between the oral cavity and neck, such as after transoral (laser) excision of FOM cancers in combination with a neck dissection. Depending on the extent of excision, a masseter muscle flap is sometimes available for reconstruction of the oropharynx.[389] Nasolabial flaps can be used for FOM reconstruction (Fig. 20–61), but these flaps tend to pull away from the recipient bed.[243] This is a two-stage procedure unless it is used as an island pedicle flap. The platyma myocutaneous flap is another option for FOM reconstruction if neck surgery has not been performed.[390,391] This seldom-used flap is technically challenging and somewhat unreliable.

At the opposite end of the size spectrum, reconstruction of the TLP defect is discussed previously in the section on pharyngeal cancer (see Fig. 20–47). Stomach pull-up operations require a special team to perform the abdominal and transthoracic portion and can be associated with life-threatening postoperative complications (including hypoparathyroidism), especially in previously irradiated patients. The functional result is not perfect, and patients frequently have difficulty with gastric dilatation and regurgitation. Jejunal interpositions require the expertise of a microvascular team and are also associated with postoperative dysphagia. Lee and Lore[392] described a method of reconstructing the TLP defect that is accessible to the head and neck surgeon: partial tubing of a myocutaneous flap against the intact prevertebral fascia or against a dermal or skin graft if this fascia has been resected. The pectoralis flap is brought into a defect under the neck skin flaps and is left permanently attached to its blood supply (thoracoacromial vessels). Flap death (which is rare) is usually a result of venous stasis rather than arterial anemia. The vascular pedicle can be compromised by constricting or compressing it, as with placement within an intact mandible, a too-tight pressure dressing, or circumferential tracheotomy ties. This is circumvented by sewing the tracheotomy tube to the peristomal skin. A loose bulky dressing helps support the weight of the flap. The skin portion of the paddle frequently becomes mucosa-like over time (Fig. 20–62B and C).

In addition to bringing a reliable blood supply into the frequently compromised recipient bed, the pectoralis myocutaneous or myofascial flap has the additional advantage that the muscle pedicle can be used to protect the carotid artery. For this function to be subserved, however, a portion of the muscle must be anchored between the mucosal suture line and the ca-

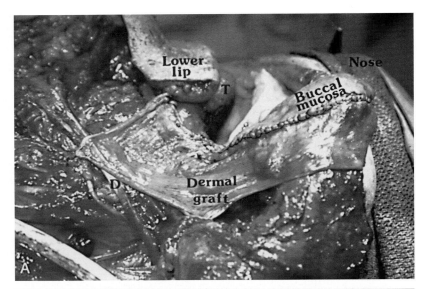

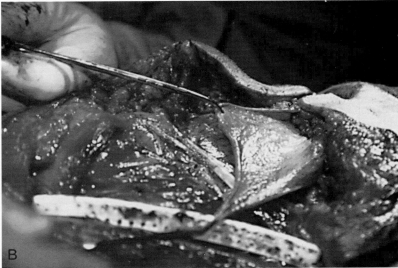

Fig. 20–60. A to C. Dermal pouch reconstruction of hemimandibulectomy defect. A. Dermal graft sutured to mucosal margins. T, Tongue; N, nose; D, digastric muscle; XII, hypoglossal nerve. B. Dermal graft folded and sutured anteriorly and inferiorly to itself. C. Completed pouch packed with bolster extends toward hyoid level.

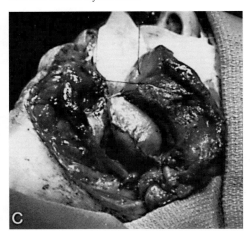

rotid artery, that is, medial to the carotid. A second layer to adjacent bony structures or muscle tendons helps to support the weight of the myocutaneous flap. Myocutaneous flaps have been combined and modified in a variety of ingenious ways. Combinations of two myocutaneous flaps have been used for internal and external resurfacing of full-thickness deficits—a "knotty problem" in head and neck cancer reconstruction.

Myocutaneous flaps, which can be bulky in corpulent or mesomorphic individuals, have a role in reconstruction of major soft tissue defects in the oral cavity and oropharynx, such as after total glossectomy or in reconstructing the composite resection in cachectic individuals, in whom maximum soft tissue replacement is necessary. The bulk of a tubed myocutaneous flap can be a problem in some individuals, however, and the "thin" pectoralis *myofascial flap* addresses this problem.[296] The "thin" pectoralis flap uses only the muscle with its intact fascia (Fig. 20–63B) and is approximately half the thickness of the myocutaneous flap (Fig. 20–63A). For this reason, it reconstitutes structure and function in many head and neck defects better than standard myocutaneous flap, especially FOM (Fig. 20–63C) and larynx-sparing pharyngectomy defects. If necessary, a skin graft can be placed on the muscle for single- or double-sided lining. The thin myofascial pectoralis flap is developed through an incision on the chest wall along the lower limb of the deltopectoral flap. No chest wall deformity results (Fig. 20–63E) because a subcutaneous and cutaneous paddle is not transposed, and the territory of the deltopectoral flap is preserved for future use.

The free radial forearm flap[393] and rectus abdominis free flap[394] have had more widespread use in FOM reconstruction because they are thin; however, the myofascial flap is a simple alternative. Similarly, its use for posterior pharyngeal wall defects (when the larynx

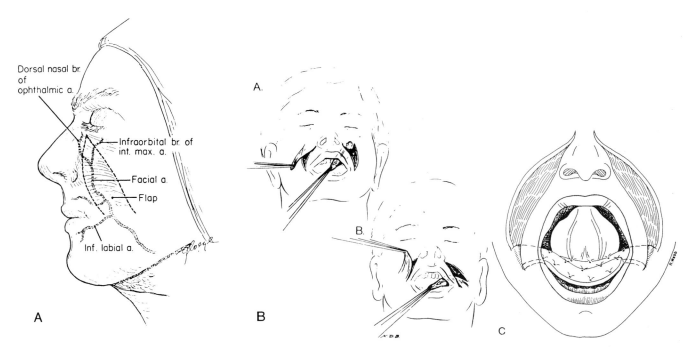

Fig. 20–61. Nasolabial flaps. A. Dual vascular supply of the nasolabial flap. B. (A) Superiorly based flap, (B) Inferiorly based flap. C. Flap insert for floor of mouth reconstruction. (A, from Gewirtz HS, et al: Am J Surg *136*:510, 1978; B, From Sharzer LA, et al: Plast Reconstr Surg *3*:499, 1976; C, from Matz G and Standiewics J: Application of the forehead flap for reconstruction of the floor of the mouth. In: Controversy in Otolaryngology. Edited by Snow JB. Philadelphia, WB Saunders, 1980.)

is preserved) reconstitutes the normal thickness of the tissue excised and obviates the need for free flap reconstructing or performing a total laryngopharyngectomy "simply" to facilitate reconstruction.

The pectoralis myofascial flap tends to contract, however, and it works best if a rigid support (bony margin) is included in its circumference to counteract this tendency. For example, the myofascial flap is not suitable for extended total laryngectomy or total laryngectomy defects unless compensatory bougienage is started as soon as healing is complete to prevent total stenosis of the lumen. The patient passes a large, red rubber Maloney dilator into the pharynx for 20 minutes to dilate the reconstructed pharyngoesophageal segment passively. Use of this dilator two or three times a week is adequate.

Tissue expanders are used to advantage to enhance the amount of soft tissue available for reconstruction of some defects (mainly traumatic or congenital) and may find applicability in cancer work in the future.[395]

Reconstruction of Bony Defects
Mandibular excisions that are less than segmental (full-thickness) do not require bone reconstruction and are convered with local tissue or appropriate flaps, or they are obturated with a denture or prosthesis. Examples include marginal (rim) resections and removal of one cortical plate.

Bone reconstruction of lateral hemimandibulectomy is seldom indicated or undertaken. Lateral segmental

loss of the mandible (hemimandibulectomy as in complete resection) is tolerated without significant functional or cosmetic defects when reconstructed with appropriate soft tissue (pouch of flap) (Fig. 20–64).

A full-thickness anterior arch defect between the mandibular angles is the most necessary and difficult to reconstruct. Many reconstructive options have been suggested and used over the years, indicating the lack of suitability of any individual technique.

Suggested methods have included use of alloplasts, bone homografts (free bone grafts), solid or particulate autogenous bone grafts, irradiated frozen or autoclaved autogenous mandible, and cadaver mandible hollowed out and packed with cancellous bone and marrow from the patients's iliac crest. Myocutaneous flaps have been raised with attached bone (clavicle, rib, scapula) as osteomyocutaneous flaps, but these compound flaps are not reliable because the bone lacks its own blood supply and tends to shear off the soft tissue. Problems associated with these methods are bone resorption, loosening of implants, and infection from intraoral soft tissue breakdown.

With respect to alloplastic materials, the use of metal reconstruction plates is controversial (see general references). The main problem is exposure of the metal plate, either intaorally or through the skin externally, which can necessitate removal of the prosthesis and secondary reconstruction. The keys to avoiding this problem lie in underprojecting rather than overprojecting the reconstruction plate and completely wrapping

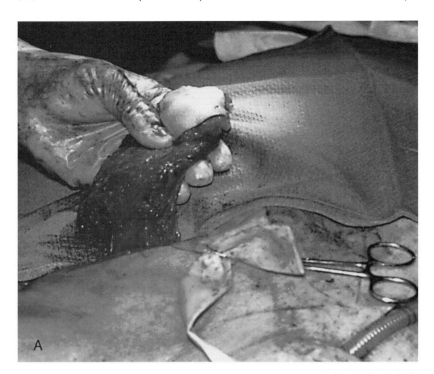

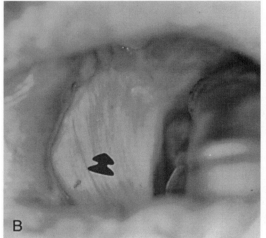

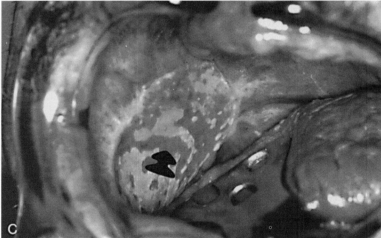

Fig. 20–62. A. Standard pectoralis myocutaneous flap, raised off chest. B. Pectoralis myocutaneous flap used for intraoral reconstruction. Arrow, Center of flap. C. Same flap as in B several months later, "mucosalized."

the metal replacement bar in bulky soft tissue flaps. The best results are reported by Gullane and Holmes.[396] Postoperative radiation distribution is apparently not significantly altered by having a metal plate in the field.[397]

In the past 5 years, a new era of anterior mandibular arch reconstruction has begun with more common use of revascularized bone grafts. Microvascular free tissue transfer of well-vascularized bone is the best method of reconstituting segmental anterior mandibular defects. Compound flaps including both soft tissue and bone can be developed and placed into the defect and reanastomosed through recipient vessels with microvascular technique at the time of ablative surgery. Considerable expertise and artistry are required for this type

of mandibular reconstruction; however, optimistic reports are beginning to appear in the literature.[398]

Heretofore, cosmesis, avoidance of the oral crippling of the "Andy Gump" deformity with respect to handling secretions, and enabling a soft diet to be taken by mouth were the major objectives of anterior arch bone reconstruction because even successfully reconstructed mandibles were generally unable to support a denture or the stress of chewing. Now mere reconstruction of mandibular continuity is no longer the end point of patient rehabilitation. Rather, goals of mandibular reconstruction include restoration of occlusal relationships, lower face contour, oral continence, and establishment of a denture-bearing surface. The technology developed in Scandanavia of osseointegration

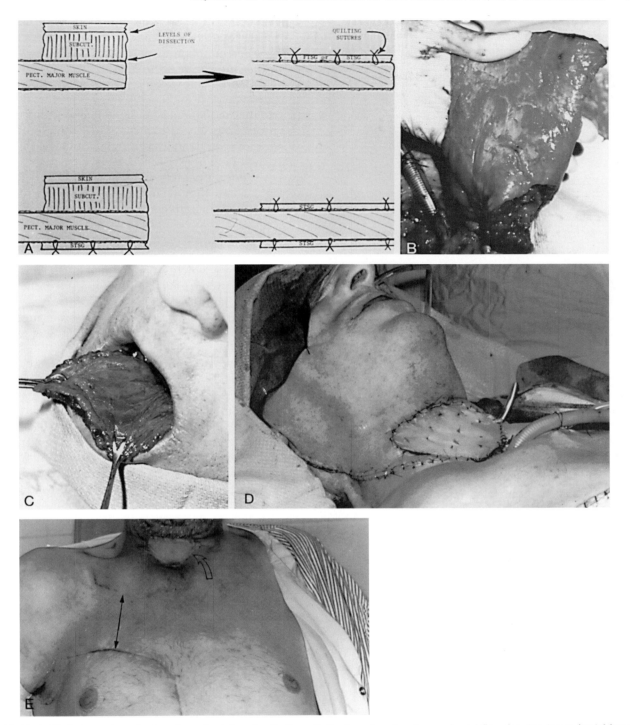

Fig. 20–63. A. Variations of standard and myofascial pectoralis flaps. B. Surface of pectoralis myofascial flap showing intact fascial layer. C. Pectoralis myofascial (thin) flap used for floor of mouth reconstruction. D. Double-lined pectoralis myofascial flap for full-thickness defect, covered externally with quilted split-thickness skin graft. E. Double-lined pectoralis myofascial flap at neck (curved arrow). Chest incision spares deltopectoral flap territory (between double-headed arrows).

of implants allows metal pegs to be incorporated over time into reconstructed revascularized mandibles that can anchor a prosthesis.[399–401] This can apparently be stable enough to allow functional chewing.[402]

With the wide spectrum of reconstructive options available to the head and neck cancer surgeon, as de-

scribed previously, considerations other than the size of the defect and nature of the tissue removed can enter into the reconstruction choice. The extent of the resection should never be dictated or compromised by the reconstructive method planned. Another general principle is that reconstruction should not increase patient

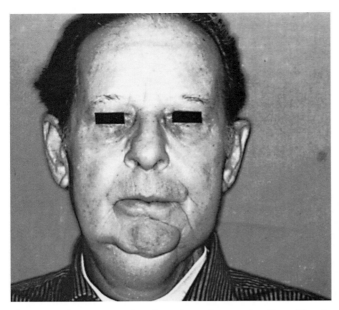

Fig. 20–64. Appearance after dermal pouch reconstruction of hemimandibulectomy defect (patient's left side).

morbidity or mortality (a consideration with time-consuming free flap methods). Complicated reconstructions should be avoided when simpler ones or a prosthesis (for hard or soft palate defects) would suffice.

To some extent, the job requirements, sports preferences, and handedness of the patient can also be considered, for example, when a pectoralis flap from either side would be equally suitable. If the patient is a young construction worker or avid golfer, the reconstructive surgeon should consider options other than the routine pectoralis flap. Such considerations may seem frivolous in comparison with the objective of achieving oncologic cure. As emphasized often in this chapter, however, the ultimate curability of these patients is limited, and therefore a primary treatment goal is optimal patient rehabilitation in respect to job and recreational activities. A major goal for the future of head and neck reconstruction is creating innervated flaps that are sensate and mobile.[403]

COMPLICATIONS OF THERAPY

The following sections detail considerations in the preoperative, intraoperative, and postoperative periods to allow both avoidance and timely recognition of evolving complications.

Preoperative Assessment

For patients referred for management of recurrent disease who have been initially treated elsewhere with surgery or radiation, the treatment manager must obtain all relevant data. This information includes RT port films, operative reports, and either repeat biopsy of the lesion or obtaining of the actual pathology slides from the outside institution. A written or telephone report is inadequate to confirm the diagnosis. Knowing the radiation dose and area covered is frequently valuable to the surgeon intraoperatively in deciding on the appropriate extent of excision. For example, if additional radiation (usually brachytherapy) can be delivered, the extent of excision may not have to be as wide as when additional RT is not possible.

Patient and tumor factors should be well enough evaluated preoperatively that the planned procedure generally will be the one that is carried out. It is prudent, however, to have a spectrum of ablative and reconstructive options available, of which the patient is aware and for which he or she has given consent. In other words, the patient should be aware of the smallest and the largest ablative and reconstructive procedure that may be necessary. This does not mean that a patient with a T1 cancer of the tongue should be signed up for a possible composite resection or total glossectomy. An example of a borderline situation is when planned transoral laser excision of an oropharynx cancer is found inappropriate once the patient is under general anesthesia, and pull-through procedure must be carried out. Moreover, a tumor abutting the mandible may be amenable to pull-through excision including the inner periosteum of the mandible; however, intraoperative bone-pitting, as discussed previously (see Fig. 20–33), may mandate removal of a portion of the mandible. When situations such as these are anticipated, no need exists to abort the procedure or to obtain permission for a larger operation from the family members, which would indicate inadequate preparation on the part of the surgeon.

Similarly, in patients who have undergone previous surgery elsewhere, exact knowledge of which structures have been removed and retained is absolutely necessary. Information from operative notes should be augmented by careful clinical examination of the patient, including all cranial nerves. For example, if a hypoglossal nerve is paralyzed on one side and surgery is needed in the vicinity of the opposite nerve, an immobile, functionless tongue may result if the contralateral hypoglossal nerve is damaged or sacrificed.[404] The patient should be aware of such a significant possibility. One must also determine the presence and patency of the internal jugular veins ultrasonically because, if a second jugular vein is to be sacrificed, appropriate fluid restriction[209] will have to be observed intraoperatively. Before performing a second (contralateral) neck dissection in a patient, one must determine whether both phrenic nerves are operating, either by fluoroscopy of the diaphragm (the most accurate method) or by obtaining an inspiratory and expiratory chest radiograph, because damage to both phrenic nerves is a disastrous complication.

Patients with cancer of the mouth and throat are frequently malnourished and have frequently had considerable weight loss during the preceding 6 months. Alcoholism and painful intraoral lesions can aggravate cancer dysphagia. Assessment of the albumin, total protein, and transferring levels preoperatively can help to assess the profundity of the derangement. The resulting catabolic state with negative nitrogen balance should be corrected preoperatively, if time allows, to decrease wound healing complications postoperatively (nasogastric feedings or hyperalimentation). If the treatment goal is palliation, several weeks can usually be spared to optimize the patient's nutritional status. In previously untreated patients, however, when such a delay may alter the magnitude of surgery as the cancer grows (requiring sacrifice of more anatomy and function), the luxury of waiting is not possible.[405,406] Nutritional repletion of a cancer patient is controversial because some studies indicate that nutrients may preferentially feed the tumor.[407]

Placing a large-bore nasogastric tube directly against a tumor in the oropharynx and pharynx can erode and inflame the area and seed cancer over a larger area. Assessment of the true margins of the cancer intraoperatively can be difficult, and this leads to sacrifice of the tissue that might not otherwise have been necessary. To obviate these problems, either a small feeding tube (Dobhoff type) or a feeding gastrostomy should be considered.

A preoperative loss of 15% of the patient's body weight, or 20 pounds, a hemoglobin of less than 10, total protein of less than 3.5, diabetes mellitus, cardiovascular disease, and chronic obstructive pulmonary disease place the patient at high risk of postoperative healing complications. Cardiopulmonary status should be optimized by cessation of smoking, vigorous pulmonary hygiene, diuresis, and digitalization when indicated. Alcoholics may have a clotting diathesis, which can lead to hematomas in the operative bed or gastrointestinal problems. Coagulopathies should be corrected before surgery, and appropriate medications should be used postoperatively (H_2 blockers) to decrease the gastrointestinal bleeding tendency. Prophylaxis against delirium tremens is particularly necessary because, in the postoperative period, they are still associated with a 50% mortality rate.

Intraoperative Complications

The surgeon is responsible for everything that happens in the operating room. In patients with head and neck cancer, management of the airway is crucial, and discussion between the surgeon and the anesthesiologist should always precede intubation. Intubation and extubation are the most dangerous times of the operation,

during which the patient can die if not managed properly. Clinical judgment is particularly necessary in deciding whether the airway can be maintained and intubated after the patient is paralyzed, or whether a tracheostomy under local anesthesia is necessary first. In a marginal situation, "breathing the patient down" so spontaneous respiration is maintained is safer than using an agent that paralyzes the respiratory muscles. "High-tech" apparatus and monitoring do not substitute for close patient observation at these critical times. Machines may not register a problem when one exists. For example, a carbon dioxide monitor may indicate that the patient is ventilating adequately through the endotracheal tube, whereas clinical sounds may indicate an esophageal intubation or that the cuff is no longer below the vocal cords (vocalization).

According to the literature of the 1970s, surgical mortality (death within 30 days of surgery) was 1 to 3% for major head and neck operations. Patients undergoing laryngopharyngeal procedures tended to die of pulmonary causes (pneumonia, pneumothorax, empyema), whereas patients undergoing jaw, tongue, and neck surgery died more often of cardiovascular problems (arrhythmia, myocardial infarction, pulmonary embolism, stroke, deep vein thrombophlebitis). Intraoperative compression boots can be used to decrease the incidence of deep vein thrombosis. The incidence of postoperative complications is related directly to the duration of surgery. Prolonged procedures are followed by an increased incidence of wound infections and other problems.

Intraoperative air embolism can result from sucking of air into holes in large veins. This may not be recognized and can result in cardiac arrest when enough air accumulates in the pulmonary artery to block outflow. Diagnosis and management of this condition are discussed by Hybels.[408]

Pneumothorax can result from injury to the apex of the pleura during tracheostomy or neck dissection. Postoperative chest radiography is routine in the recovery room. In general, patients should be sterilely draped to a level below the second intercostal space anteriorly so, if a pneumothorax occurs intraoperatively, a catheter can be immediately inserted to evacuate air under tension. An occasional substitute for traditional management is the Heimlich tube, which is the size of a large catheter and is useful only if no air has to be evacuated from the pleural cavity.

Leakage of air, causing subcutaneous or mediastinal emphysema, can occur intraoperatively or postoperatively and is related to trapping of air at the tracheostomy site. This can be avoided if the soft tissue around the tracheostomy is not closed too tightly, and it is not recommended that packing be used to stop bleeding at the tracheostomy site. Bleeding should be controlled as it is encountered during the tracheostomy procedure. Crepitance can indicate the extremely serious complication of a dislodged tracheostomy tube whose lumen is no longer in the trachea but is lying in the soft tissue of the neck. Continued positive-pressure ventilation in this situation can cause bilateral pneumothoraces, which can be quickly fatal if not recognized.

A chyle fistula can result intraoperatively from damage to the thoracic duct or to the major lymphatic duct on the right side of the neck. The thoracic duct can extend as high as 6 cm above the clavicle on the left side. The major lymphatic channels in the lower neck can be avoided by making the lower limit of dissection approximately two fingerbreadths above the clavicle. Injury is recognized by the egress of milky fluid. If this complication is recognized intraoperatively, control of the leaking vessel is required. Use of the operating microscope is helpful in identifying the site of injury and confirming its closure. Ligation should not be attempted because the tear in the lymphatic vessel propagates with manipulation. Ligaclips are convenient in "trapping" the site of leakage. If long enough, the stump of the sternocleidomastoid can be sutured over the area of the leak to the deep cervical fascia (taking care to avoid the phrenic nerve) to tamponade the leak further. Some surgeons prefer using an open drainage system with a pressure dressing postoperatively in this situation, whereas others use closed suction drainage. Additional discussion is presented in the section of this chapter on postoperative complications. References on chylothorax can be found in the report by Gullane and Marsh.[409]

The head and neck cancer surgeon must be aware of the functional consequences of sacrificing the various cranial and sensory nerves encountered in the head and neck. Although any of the nerves encountered in the neck can be sacrificed if involved with tumor, deficits of varying significance result. Transection of the lingual nerve results in numbness in the ipsilateral side of the tongue. Swallowing difficulties occur with transection of the vagus,[410] both hypoglossal nerves,[404] or, to a lesser extent, the glossopharyngeal nerve. High-level vagus lesions (the main trunk and the pharyngeal and laryngeal branches) result in unilateral palatal and pharyngeal paralysis, supraglottic anesthesia, and ipsilateral glottic paralysis.[410] If sacrifice of the vagus nerve is necessary, cricopharyngeal myotomy may facilitate swallowing.

Preservation of the recurrent laryngeal nerves is important because the resultant aspiration can aggravate other types of swallowing defects imposed by ablative surgery in the mouth and throat. Loss of one hypoglossal nerve is not crippling unless large amounts of adjacent structures are removed. Resection of both hypoglossal nerves leaves the residual portion of the tongue immobile, a consequence to be avoided except when total glossectomy is performed.[404,410] In some situations, when one desires that the hemitongue not move to ensure adjacent flap immobility, the hypoglossal

nerve can be crushed with a clamp intraoperatively. Function returns over time.

Transection of the marginal branch of the facial nerve leads to lip asymmetry because of elevation of the ipsilateral lower lip because the nerve innervates a depressor. Damage to mental nerves results in lip numbness. The combination of both these injuries is serious, especially if bilateral, resulting in a paralyzed numb lower lip with pursuant oral incompetence and drooling.

Injury to the phrenic nerve causes paralysis (elevation) of the hemidiaphragm. Injury to the cervical sympathetic nerves, which lie behind the carotid artery, results in Horner's syndrome. The superior cervical ganglion, although generally lying below the deep cervical fascia, is sometimes large, protrudes lateral to the carotid artery above the bifurcation, and can be mistaken for a lymph node at the level of C2 or higher.[411] The differentiation can be made by identifying egress of the cervical sympathetic chain from its inferior pole.

Transection of the spinal accessory nerve can cause a shoulder droop with painful immobilization if a "frozen shoulder" occurs, and this is the major morbidity of a radical neck dissection. Overlap in the nerve distribution of the spinal accessory nerve accounts for the finding that, in some cases in which the nerve was apparently transected, this deficit is not seen postoperatively.[203] This problem must be resolved with physical therapy before permanent disability occurs. Attempting to preserve the spinal accessory nerve whenever possible is appropriate. When the nerve must be sacrificed, grafting between the stumps with the greater auricular nerve is recommended by some surgeons.

Resection of the superficial sensory nerves (cervical plexus), an inevitable consequence of incisions used in head and neck surgery, causes skin numbness and may become the patient's major postoperative complaint. Preserving major branches such as the greater auricular nerve can help somewhat in this regard. Overlapping innervation of these nerves allows sensation to return over time, although this generally requires several months.

Resection of the brachial plexus is contraindicated in head and neck cancer surgery because tumor penetration of the deep cervical fascia generally indicates incurable disease. If some of the nerve roots are damaged, motor deficits resulting from injury to the brachial plexus may only be partial because of overlapping trunks.

As with any type of surgery, gentle handling of the tissues and anatomic bloodless dissection techniques are recommended. Needless to say, the surgeon must be able to handle any cardiopulmonary arrest situation that occurs intraoperatively and to administer drugs if necessary. The surgeon should not rely on the anesthesia personnel present to handle such situations.

Post-Treatment Complications

Postoperative Complications

Wound infection is said to be the most common minor complication. Operations that invade the digestive tract are, by definition, contaminated but not necessarily infected. Intraoral pathogens can infect cervical wounds when the operation includes a suture line in the mucosa of the UADT. Prophylactic antibiotics are routinely used when the mouth or pharynx is entered and are generally continued for 24 to 48 hours after major resections,[394,412,413] The usual microorganisms are staphylococci and streptococci. Penicillins or cephalosporins are appropriate antibiotics. If an infection arises, culture and sensitivity allow appropriate alteration of the antibiotic regimen. Culturing the contents of closed drainage systems just before their removal can expedite identification of unusual microorganisms.

In the context of major head and neck cancer surgery, a "wound infection" should be considered a manifestation of an underlying problem such as necrosis of a reconstructive flap or a fistula rather than simple infection of the skin at the suture line, until proved otherwise. A problem in the cervical area is heralded by induration, erythema, and tenderness on *gentle* palpation.

Flap elevation results from fluid accumulation (blood, serum, chyle) under the neck flaps. The telltale sign of an underlying hematoma is bruising of the cervical skin flap. This leads to wound infection and skin necrosis because the flap must seat against the underlying tissue bed to be revascularized. Delayed adherence of the neck skin flaps to the underlying tissue bed also predisposes to infection and significant scar formation in the subcutaneous tissues, which can compromise examination for recurrent disease. Fluid accumulations result from malfunctioning drainage systems or inadequate hemostasis. Some surgeons prefer to use closed suction drainage systems without dressings because this allows continuous wound observation. Such drainage systems are generally placed to self-suction rather than wall suction to avoid excess suctioning against mucosal suture lines. Because the reservoirs of these systems can easily become unstoppered when the patient moves and may lose their suction without being noticed, however, other surgeons prefer to use a pressure dressing as a "back-up" to closed suction drainage. Using an open drainage system (Penrose drain) with a pressure dressing is also possible, but these drains tend to become exposed and contaminated and are outmoded.

The surgeon must recognize fluid accumulations quickly so that they can be evacuated because they can compromise the viability of the neck skin flaps and the blood supply to reconstructive flaps by exerting local pressure.

Hematomas occurring in the first 24 hours are treated by returning the patient to the operating room expeditiously, opening the wound, removing clots, irrigating the area, ligating the bleeding source if evident (rarely), and inserting a new suction drainage system. Delayed accumulations are treated more conservatively with repeated aspiration or placement of a Penrose drain and pressure dressing.

The problem of intraoperative chyle fistulas is discussed in the previous section on intraoperative complications. Delayed chyle fistulas can also be detected when tube feedings are started. A milky fluid appears in the drainage system, and the volume may reach 1500 ml per day. The fat-laden chyle stimulates a local inflammatory reaction, violaceous discoloration of the skin, and woody induration. Changes in the diet are made to eliminate fat that passes through the lacteals to the thoracic duct. Feeding the patient medium-chain triglyceride solution (Portagen) directs fat into the portal system and away from the lymphatics. Local management is controversial. Some surgeons prefer to remove suction drainage and to place a straight open drainage system with a pressure dressing. Others prefer to continue suction drainage. Delayed chyle fistulas are usually self-limited and resolve in 2 to 3 weeks. Recalcitrant cases are returned to the operating room for control with the aid of the operating microscope. Transthoracic ligation is another theoretic option that is fortunately seldom needed because many contemporary thoracic surgeons are unfamiliar with the method. If a chyle fistula occurs in the neck, a chest radiograph should be made sequentially to rule out accumulation of chylothorax, which can compromise respiratory function.[409]

Wound necrosis is associated with wound infection, preoperative radiation, nutritional deficiency, tension at the closure, hematoma, and thinning of cervical flaps.

Incisions that respect the blood supply to the cervical skin should be used,[414] although if scars from previous surgery exist on the skin of the neck and face, additional incisions are planned to incorporate them. As seen in Figure 20–65, the major blood supply to the neck skin comes in vertically from the face and the lower neck, and an incision should be used that does not horizontally transect the blood supply high and low in the neck. For that reason, the MacFee[415] incision (Fig. 20–65B) should theoretically result in the most compromise; however, many surgeons use this incision with good results.

Flap (reconstructive or cervical skin) necrosis (Fig. 20–66) can cause a fulminant neck infection, necessitating returning the patient to the operating room for immediate debridement to prevent sepsis. Necrosis of cervical skin is particularly critical when exposure of the carotid artery can occur (after neck dissection). If a dermal graft or other type of protection (levator scapulae flap) has been placed over the carotid bulb intra-

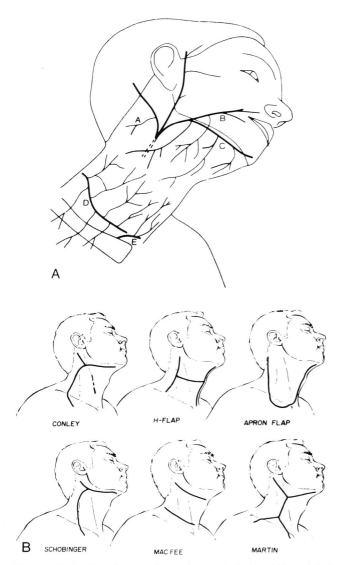

Fig. 20–65. A. Vascular supply to the cervical skin, (A) occipital branch of sternomastoid artery, (B) facial artery, (C) submental branch of facial artery, (D) transverse cervical artery, (E) suprascapular artery. B. Types of neck incisions. (A, from Freeland AP and Rogers JH: Laryngoscope *85:*720, 1975; B, from Reed GF and Rabuzzi DD: Otolaryngol Clin North Am *Oct:*548, 1969.)

operatively, the overlying skin defect usually reepithelializes. Necrotic areas can be debrided and resurfaced with skin grafts or regional unirradiated pedicle flaps, which bring new blood supply to the area.

Impending loss of the skin paddle of a myocutaneous flap can generally be managed conservatively. If the flap pulls away from a suture line because of excess weight (e.g., in the anterior FOM), it can sometimes be resutured to the alveolar mucosa and heal uneventfully. In the event that the paddle of a myocutaneous flap is lost, the underlying muscle frequently remains intact, and the area of flap loss is allowed to demarcate naturally. Separation is facilitated by debridement and frequent cleansing and irrigation with a

peroxide-based mouthwash (Peridex has a long-acting residual effect on the tissue to which it is applied) or a dental irrigation apparatus (Waterpik). If healing by secondary intention after major flap loss will significantly delay planned postoperative RT, more expeditious treatment may be indicated. A second operation with placement of a new flap should be undertaken as soon as the decision is made.

Fistulas in cancer surgery of the mouth and throat represent breakdown of the mucosal suture line, resulting in accumulation of saliva under the neck skin flaps and eventual external communication. Factors predisposing to orocutaneous or pharyngocutaneous fistulas include poor patient nutrition, inadequate suturing at the site of tumor excision, lack of a multilayered closure, surgery in a previously radiated field, poor blood supply, flap necrosis, and diabetes mellitus. Seventy to eighty percent of fistulas appear within 3 weeks of surgery. The weakest day of the suture line is postoperative day 6 in previously untreated patients. This is related to the number of fibroblasts in the wound. Earlier presentation indicates a mechanical fault in the closure. Delayed presentation results from recurrent cancer (until proved otherwise) or radionecrosis of tissue.

Fistulas are detected by smell, vision, and palpation. The neck flaps become thick and red, and pressure elicits pain. After major cancer surgery in the mouth and throat, dehiscence usually occurs at the posterosuperior aspect of the suture line where the tension is greatest or at trifurcation points. The presence of a fistula can be confirmed by having the patient swallow methylene blue dye, which will extrude if a hole exists in the neck flap. Alternatively, a radiopaque dye can be swallowed to demonstrate the fistula. If dye is used to confirm a suspected fistula, a water-soluble radiopaque dye (Gastrografin) should be used that will not persist in the tissue if it leaks out into the neck. Barium is water-insoluble and tends to persist in the neck and can aggravate or cause infectious problems as a foreign body contaminated by saliva, but it is the dye of choice in a patient in whom severe aspiration is a problem; pneumonia resulting from barium aspiration is more easily cleared than pneumonia resulting from aspiration of a water-soluble dye.

Methods of preventing fistulas include the time-honored creation of a "planned" orostoma or pharyngostoma at the time of surgery in high-risk wounds. A hole is deliberately created between the mucosa and the cervical skin. This theoretically removes tension from the suture line during healing and creates a controlled situation rather than allowing spontaneous wound breakdown and development of an uncontrolled fistula. In the types of wounds in which this is considered necessary, however, frequently a planned pharyngostoma undergoes additional breakdown. Traditional techniques for creating planned stomas

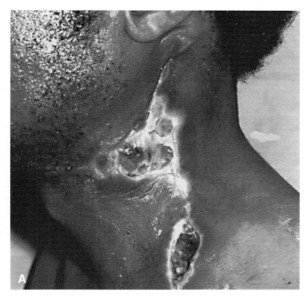

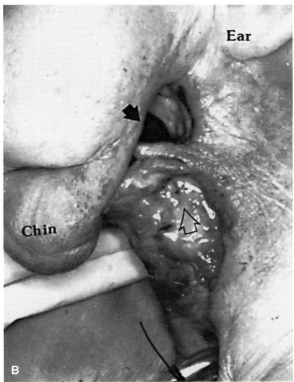

Fig. 20–66. A. Neck flap necrosis along Schobinger incision. B. Orocutaneous fistula (solid arrow) and neck flap necrosis (open arrow). C. Pharyngocutaneous fistula (clamp) and bilateral neck flap necrosis (arrows) in a radiated diabetic. (B, courtesy of Dr. J Ogura.)

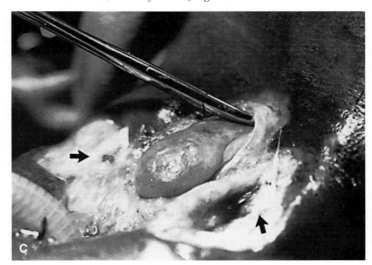

and closing unplanned fistulas are well summarized in the literature.[416,417]

Fistulas are dangerous because they allow saliva to drain through the lateral neck over the carotid artery, which can rupture. Therefore, the basic principle of conservative fistula management is of "medializing" the fistula to redirect salivary flow away from the lateral neck to the anterior midline, where there are no vital structures traditionally, a dependent opening near the anterior midline of the neck is created in the subplatysmal plane, packing is placed to the likely site

of the fistula, and a pressure dressing is used to compress the lateral neck. Oral rest is instituted using tube feedings or hyperalimentation. A cuffed tracheostomy tube is necessary to decrease aspiration because the fistula lies near the tracheostomy.

A newer method, used at our institution (method of R.W. Bastian, MD), is to deliberately place a question drain intraoperatively along the point of the suture line most likely to breakdown. If this occurs, these "control drains" are already in position and can be progressively shortened and replaced over time to allow the fistulous tract to heal. Although contrary to traditional dogma, this method works well, and patients can be discharged with "control draws" in place to have their fistulas managed as outpatients, a procedure that decreases hospitalization time and expense.

Spontaneous closure of the majority of fistulas occurs within 1 month with traditional local wound care. Characteristics that favor spontaneous closure include lack of residual tumor or previous radiation, minimal necrosis of overlying skin, and a long, narrow tract. Once a skin-lined tract is formed, the opening tends to persist, and this coaptation must be disrupted. Using silver nitrate sticks on the edge of the tract is one method of encouraging continued contracture of the fistula.

A more contemporary antifistula prophylactic method is reinforcement of a tenuous closure with a regional flap from an unirradiated source to bring blood supply into the wound. In cases in which a myocutaneous flap is used in the reconstruction, this function is already subserved. Some surgeons use a myofascial pectoralis flap to reinforce a suture line that does not have such a flap as part of its reconstruction. Fibrin glue can also be placed over tenuous suture lines in high-risk patients and, in a small personal series, has reduced the incidence of postlaryngectomy fistulas from 50 to 10%.[418] In high-risk patients, evidence indicates that metronidazole is a particularly good antibiotic and has some prophylactic effect in preventing postoperative fistula formation.[419]

Local wound care to a neck with a wound healing problem from any of the causes previously discussed typically consists of appropriately frequent dressing changes and irrigation of the wound with half-strength peroxide or Peridex. Silvadene cream is an invaluable adjunct in healing of wounds with massive wound breakdown and infection. This substance acts as a nonspecific bactericidal agent and enhances formation of granulation tissue, which aids in wound healing. Hyperbaric oxygen treatments (see subsequent text) foster angiogenesis and wound-healing. A biopsy should rule out recurrent tumor before this modality is applied.

Vascular Complications

The most dreaded of these is carotid artery rupture, and its overall incidence in the head and neck literature is about 3%. Predisposing factors include cervical flap necrosis, the presence of oropharyngocutaneous fistulas, positive margins at the primary site, and recurrent tumor in the neck. Vascular ruptures have been reported in patients treated with RT alone[420] who have never had surgery.

Ruptures typically occur because of exposure and desiccation of the artery, rather than from tumor invasion, because SCCs of the head and neck seldom invade arterial walls. Large veins in the neck are commonly invaded by tumor but rarely rupture because of slow infiltration with embolic occlusion of the low pressure vessel.

The most common site of hemorrhage is at the carotid bulb. Most patients have had prodromal (sentinel or herald) bleeding during the preceding 48 hours.[421] Bleeding can present externally or intraorally. This allows preparation for elective carotid ligation by achieving hemodynamic stabilization of the patient.

Prophylactic steps at the time of primary surgery designed to decrease this complication include preserving the adventitia and vasa vasorum at the carotid bulb from which the carotid artery receives 80% of its blood supply. Covering the carotid bulb with a dermal graft or levator scapulae muscle flap is also recommended if the operation creates a mucosal suture line, although several studies have shown no difference in the incidence of carotid rupture whether carotid protection was used or not. Eventual carotid rupture has been shown to correlate primarily with the presence of positive margins at the primary site, presumably because this is the precursor of uncontrolled local-regional disease and necrotic tumor in the neck.[422] Surgical options in controlling acute or impending carotid rupture have been discussed in the literature (see previous references).

Stabilization of the patient before carotid ligation or neuroradiologic embolization is the major predictor of a favorable neurologic outcome. The mortality rate in elective carotid ligation is 0 to 17%. Neurologic complications occur in 0 to 40%. Emergent treatment is associated with a mortality of 40 to 75% (average 50%) and a neurologic complication rate of 10 to 90%, which is related to inability to stabilize the patient because of the emergent nature of the rupture. Hypotension and hypovolemia are the most important factors leading to major cerebral complications and death. Major neurologic complications after emergency ligation include coma and stroke (hemiplegia or monoplegia). Ligation of the carotid artery on the side opposite the patient's "handedness" can result in aphasia. Neurologic sequelae are commonly seen, either immediately postoperatively or within the first 48 hours when a clot flips off the ligated distal stump and lodges in the cerebral circulation. The carotid artery should not be simply ligated but controlled and transected above and below the point of rupture, so pulsations from the proximal stump are not transmitted to the distal area, which favors dislodgement of the clot. Depending on the location and extent of recurrent cancer in the neck, this may not be technically possible. A conservative alternative is transfemoral balloon occlusion of the carotid performed by a neuroradiologist.[229] This procedure itself is sometimes associated with stroke and is generally temporizing measure only because tumor neovascularization can cause rebleeding.

Other reported vascular complications include arteriovenous fistulas and thrombosis of the internal carotid artery.[423] A rupture of the innominate artery can result from an improperly fitting tracheostomy tube that erodes the anterior tracheal wall or from prolonged intubation with an overinflated cuff, resulting in tracheomalacia.

In uncontrollable local-regional disease with an impending fatal outcome, major vascular ruptures can be a quick and painless way for the patient to die, and whether or not to intervene in such situations should be decided in consultation by the surgeon, the patient's family, and the patient.

Complications of Chemotherapy

Preoperative chemotherapy in previously untreated patients does not seem to increase healing problems after surgery, but surgery following combined chemoradiation is fraught with complications.[178] The complications of chemotherapy are related to the systemic toxic effects of the various agents used and are summarized in the literature.[112] The agents typically used for neoadjuvant therapy of SCC of the head and neck have potential toxic effects on the lungs, kidneys, and bone marrow. Physicians involved in the care of these patients should be aware of these clinical signs that warn of impending toxic problems. For example, development of painful oral ulcers during infusion of 5-fluorouracil (5-FU) can be a manifestation of neutropenia, which can result in fulminate sepsis (especially in diabetic or immunocompromised patients), progressing to a rapidly fatal outcome despite heroic measures. If this clinical sign develops, the 5-FU drip should be turned off immediately.

Complications of Radiation Therapy

Radiation to the mouth and throat results in progressive mucositis, which becomes symptomatic (to a varying extent among individuals) about 3 weeks into the treatment. This subsides during the month following the end of treatment (which usually lasts 6 to 6 1/2 weeks). Patients undergoing high-dose RT to the oropharyngeal mucosa generally lose about 10 pounds during the treatment because of painful dysphagia and loss of taste. Conservative measures to palliate this temporary condition include use of topical anesthetic solutions and mild systemic analgesics and frequent oral irrigations with a mixture of salt water and baking soda, which help dissolve the stringy saliva that forms and keeps the oral lining as normal as it can be during treatment. Use of cigarettes, alcohol, and other irritants (mouthwashes) should be discouraged. Elderly debilitated patients may require tube feedings during this period to supplement their nutrition. Patients must be encouraged to maintain their weight during treatments, and this can be facilitated by having the patient eat small meals frequently during the day.

A profoundly dry mouth occurs when all the major salivary glands are included in the radiation ports and is one of the major sources of morbidity after radiation to the head and neck. The dry mouth persists for the rest of the patient's life because the salivary glands do not regenerate. Many patients complain bitterly of the unpleasant sensation and must constantly carry water with them. Artificial saliva preparations generally offer only short-term relief. Planning treatment to leave one parotid gland out of the RT port greatly reduces this problem.

Delayed cerebral and neurovascular complications, including stroke and peripheral and cranial neuropathies (optic, hypoglossal, oculomotor, abducens, recurrent laryngeal, brachial plexus) have been reported after RT without surgery, presumably from progressive constrictive fibrosis superimposed on underlying arterial disease.[424,425]

The most dreaded complication following radiation is *radionecrosis* of the oral tissues. Osteoradionecrosis has a specific definition. It represents exposure of nonviable irradiated bone that fails to heal without intervention. True bone necrosis is almost always associated with overlying soft tissue necrosis; however, minor soft tissue necrosis manifesting as breakdown early in the postradiation course can heal without intervention, and regenerative capacities are often sufficient to cover viable bone. Therefore, not all exposed bone represents osteoradionecrosis. Major changes in conceptualizing the pathophysiology of this condition and recommendations for its treatment are based primarily on the elegant and scientifically compelling experimental and clinical work of oral surgeon Robert Marx and his associates. The reader is encouraged to read the original article on the topic.[144]

The traditional view of radionecrosis is as follows; irradiation leads to thickening of the intimal lining of blood vessels, producing edema, endarteritis, hyalinization, thrombosis, and finally, fibrosis. The reduced blood supply decreases resistance to infection and superimposed xerostomia, mucositis, cariogenic flora, periodontal breakdown, and altered saliva composition are aggravating factors. RT to the mouth reduces intraoral secretions and induces soft tissue atrophy and bone necrosis. The mandible is more susceptible than the maxilla because of its limited vascular supply. Trauma to the bone or overlying soft tissue resulting from periodontal or dental disease, denture sores, or oral surgery results in inadequate healing, infection, and sepsis. The response to the injury varies from spontaneous sequestration (involucrum formation), with exfoliation of small segments of alveolar bone, to total destruction of large segments of bone with or without pathologic fractures.

The incidence of osteoradionecrosis has been reported at 3 to 40%, and the risk of mandibular necrosis increases in direct proportion to the dose of the radiation. Spontaneous osteoradionecrosis is unlikely at doses lower than 60 Gy. Modern RT using megavoltage techniques has a lower coefficient of bone absorption and has decreased the incidence of osteoradionecrosis to the range of 3 to 10%. The risk of osteoradionecrosis is said to increase for tumors overlying or adjacent to bone.

Patients with osteoradionecrosis have deep, boring pain, trismus, and ulceration of soft tissue with a foul-smelling discharge and exposed bone. Bone chips may extrude intraorally or externally through orocutaneous sinus tracts. Radiographs are not accurate indicators of the extent of osteoradionecrosis, and that which is clinically apparent is generally the "tip of the iceberg."

Traditional goals and treatment of osteoradionecrosis include relief of pain, maintenance of function, and preservation of appearance. Conservative management has been the mainstay, and a "hands-off" approach in respect to surgical procedures of involved mandible is the dogma. Control of infection with antibiotics and local irrigation methods to optimize oral hygiene and judicious debridement of necrotic tissue are permissible. This type of management results in chronic pain and oral hygiene problems for the patient.

The new view of osteoradionecrosis as enunciated by Marx is as follows. Facial bone osteoradionecrosis is a pathologic process now conceived of as a radiation-induced wound-healing defect. Radiation leads to development of hypovascular-hypocellular-hypoxic tissue, which can be followed by trauma-induced or *spontaneous* tissue breakdown and, finally, a nonhealing wound. All irradiated patients have underlying radiation tissue injury consisting of progressive vascular damage causing endarteritis, thrombosis, and fibrosis. The diminishment of microvascular circulation is unending, and no evidence indicates spontaneous microvascular revascularization with time. Loss of microvascular content first begins about 6 months after radiation and progressively worsens with time, as does fibrosis. Hypovascularity and fibrosis are the end stage of radiation tissue injury, provided frank necrosis does not supervene.

Another major difference in conceptualization is that two different forms of osteoradionecrosis exist, spontaneous and trauma-induced, which have entirely different time courses and radiation pathogenesis. The spontaneous form represents a greater outright cell kill of normal tissue elements, and the involved tissues progress directly into the stage of necrosis, usually within the first 2 years. Spontaneous osteoradionecrosis represents an injury so severe that the effects of radiation overwhelm the repair capacity, and this form of the disorder is associated with implant sources and neutron beam and high-dose external beam radiation. Almost all cases of spontaneous osteoradionecrosis first appear between 6 and 24 months after radiation treatment.

Trauma-induced osteoradionecrosis represents a mixture of cell death and cell injury. The initial radiation tissue injury is far less than that associated with spontaneous osteoradionecrosis, and most patients do not cross over into radiation necrosis unless trauma occurs. Recovery of the tissues is greater in this context and accounts for the finding that not every tooth removed or biopsy performed in irradiated tissue produces osteoradionecrosis. Trauma-induced osteoradionecrosis has a bimodal incidence, with the first peak developing in the first 3 months after RT and related to surgical insult either shortly before or during the delivery of radiation, and a second rise at about 2 years, peaking at 5 years and maintained for many years. The potential for osteoradionecrosis does not decrease over time.

Marx's studies have shown that the severity of osteoradionecrosis correlates with the type of radiation delivered (neutrons, implant), the total dose (particularly when it is greater than 70 Gy), the dosage regimen (hyper- or accelerated fractionation), and the concomitant therapy (surgery, chemotherapy, hyperthermia), but not with anatomic location. Virtually every portion of the mandible can be involved, either alone or as an extension from other regions. Severe radiation tissue injury is indicated by the clinical signs of induration of tissue, mucosal radiation telangiectasias, loss of facial hair growth, cutaneous atrophy, cutaneous flaking and keratinization, profound xerostomia, and profound taste loss.

On the basis of new information, the dogma that irradiated tissue gradually revascularizes over time is incorrect, and the teaching to defer surgical procedures (particularly tooth removal) in irradiated tissue for as long as possible to take advantage of this anticipated but unproved event is erroneous. Similarly, the philosophy that dentures should not be placed for 6 to 12 months after RT does not make sense pathophysiologically. In fact, after the first 6 months, the longer after radiation one waits, the less vascularity and tissue perfusion are present, and the greater are fibrosis and the risk of osteoradionecrosis. Because the longevity of patients with head and neck SCC is limited, denture rehabilitation should be expeditious to optimize the quality of life.

Marx's recommendations for avoiding osteoradionecrosis include deferring radiation treatment for 21 days after tissue wounding (e.g., after initial tooth extractions or surgery) and avoiding tissue wounding during the radiation course. The tissue is in the most favorable physiologic state to cope with a surgical wound after RT is completed and the patient has recovered from the mucositis-dermatitis reaction. Even at this time, and certainly at others, strong consideration should be given to the adjunctive use of hyperbaric oxygen before wounding.

Hyperbaric oxygen amplifies angiogenesis in radiated tissue.[425a] During this form of treatment, 100%

oxygen is delivered in a compression or diving chamber at 2.4 atm. Each "dive" lasts about 90 minutes. Although hyperbaric oxygen enhances leukocyte function by increasing tissue oxygen tension, it does not resurrect dead infected bone. The control of infection is the result of aggressive debridement by the surgeon. Marx's current recommendation is for 20 hyperbaric treatments before elective oral surgery and 20 before surgery to correct problems related to flagrant osteoradionecrosis, followed by 10 sessions after the most extensive surgical procedure in the treatment plan.

Concern about the permissive effect of the high oxygen tension associated with hyperbaric oxygen on cancer growth remains problematic. It is traditional to perform a biopsy of the area of tissue breakdown to "rule out" cancer, but this is inaccurate because of the focal nature of recurrent or persistent subclinical cancer. In one animal study, no permissive effect was seen.[426] In a more recent report, Syrian hamsters developed fewer but larger DMBA-induced SCCs of the cheek pouch when hyperbaric oxygen was given concurrently with the chemical carcinogen. This was interpreted by the authors to indicate that hyperbaric oxygen has a suppressive effect on carcinogenesis during the induction period but a stimulatory effect during tumor proliferation.[427] Clinically, patients have occasionally been irradiated in a hyperbaric environment to counteract the radioresistance of the hypoxic tumor core, but the effect of this variable on tumor response is difficult to assess in the absence of a randomized prospective study format. The issue remains unresolved at this time.

Marx also directs attention to the finding that many irradiated patients are treated as "dental lepers" because of the practitioner's fear of initiating osteoradionecrosis. In fact, providing comprehensive competent dental care to irradiated patients is critical because avoiding deterioration of the dentition from radiation caries and periodontal disease is necessary to prevent osteoradionecrosis. In fact, as the wounding agent and precursor to osteoradionecrosis, periodontal disease may be more injurious than tooth removal, and control of periodontal disease on a regular basis by a specialist is recommended, in addition to intensive use of fluoride by the patient. The latter is not a predictable preventive measure, however, because of some patients' noncompliance and frequent lifelong habit patterns of poor plaque control.

Reviews of the traditional management of oral sequelae of radiation appear in the literature.[428–430] Conservation of healthy teeth has been shown to be a viable option to full-mouth extraction, contingent on the patient's reliability. With vigorous lifelong oral hygiene, the incidence of osteoradionecrosis can be decreased when teeth are conserved, as opposed to after full-mouth extraction.[431]

The traditional philosophy that surgical removal of major portions of radionecrotic bone should be held in reserve and used only as a "last-ditch attempt" is changing. This philosophy has led to protracted painful conditions that frequently compromise the quality of life in patients with head and neck cancer, whose longevity is frequently limited. This is therefore not consistent with the goal of optimizing function during the remainder of the patient's sometimes short life. Established osteoradionecrosis does not heal with hyperbaric treatments alone, although these are a necessary prerequisite before surgical removal of necrotic bone because of promotion of vascular proliferation and inhibition of intraoral anaerobic bacterial colonization.[425a]

Unrelenting pain is traditionally considered the most important indicator of the need for surgery. Dogma states that the mandibular symphysis is rarely involved because it is generally shielded from radiation, although Marx's anatomic studies are at odds with this conclusion. Most osteoradionecrosis of the mandible occurs laterally.[432] Pathologic fracture dictates hemimandibulectomy with appropriate soft tissue plate reconstruction using a vascularized flap, which additionally helps wound healing.

The extent of surgical management of osteoradionecrosis is dictated by two basic principles: (1) the necrotic bone must be removed until healthy bleeding bone is encountered; and (2) the defect must be covered with adequate soft tissue, preferably with a blood supply that has not been compromised by radiation. With adjunctive hyperbaric oxygen coverage, relatively small operations appropriate to the extent of necrosis anticipated can be planned at the initial stage, such as alveolectomy with inner-table mandibulectomy and coverage by local soft tissue. A transoral route is sometimes adequate.[433] Residual dead bone and inadequate soft tissue coverage will declare themselves, and additional surgery may be necessary. For anterior segmental problems, Marx has had good results with cadaver mandible packed with cancellous bone and particulate marrow from the patient's iliac crest and augmented with soft tissue flaps such as pectoralis myocutaneous flaps.

Follow-Up

One broad category of complications that can arise after any of the treatments cited is development of recurrent disease. Specific follow-up methods are well prescribed for patients with head and neck cancer with the goal of detecting early recurrent local disease, disease in the neck, multiple primary tumors, or DMs. The patients are generally seen once a month for the first 2 years, once every 2 months for the third year, and once every 3 months for the fourth year. Only when 5 years have elapsed do visits occur at 6-month intervals. Chest radiographs are obtained to look for second primary tumors and metastatic disease twice a year, and a complete set of laboratory data should be evaluated yearly.[201]

The surgeon is traditionally the "captain of the ship," even for patients whose treatment does not include surgery. Multidisciplinary treatment protocols must be closely supervised to ensure that the planned treatment is completed. The surgeon typically sees patients undergoing RT every 2 weeks to monitor the development of complications. Similarly, the surgeon should see patients undergoing chemotherapy before each cycle to help the medical oncologists (who are not as able to examine the anatomy of the UADT) to assess the patient's response or lack of response. Changes in the initial plan may occasionally be required, depending on how the patient and the cancer are responding to the treatment.

Patients who have undergone neck irradiation are susceptible to hypothyroidism. Pretreatment levels of thyroid hormones (and antibodies, ideally) should be checked. After treatment, thyroid-stimulating hormone (TSH) levels should be obtained every 3 months for the first 3 years and semiannually thereafter. All patients who develop elevated TSH levels should receive thyroid replacement.[434] Thyroid replacement therapy should be started at a low dose (0.05 mg Synthroid per day) and advanced slowly in patients with a history of cardiac disease to avoid arrhythmias and congestive heart failure.

An elevated calcium level should be investigated. Hypercalcemia can result from dissolution of bone by tumor metastases or from pseudohyperparathyroidism as a paraneoplastic syndrome associated with various nonendocrine tumors. SCCs of the head and neck, particularly those in the oral cavity and oropharynx, are associated with elaboration of parathyroid hormone or similar substances in 3 to 25% of patients.[435,436] Such hypercalcemia is typically seen in advanced disease. Hypercalcemia, hypophosphatemia, and increased parathyroid hormone in the absence of significant bone metastases are typical of pseudohyperparathyroidism.

Metastatic bone disease is associated with parathormone suppression, low serum chloride, and metabolic alkalosis. A radiographic bone survey, bone scan, and bone biopsy can evaluate metastases as a source of hypercalcemia. Osteoblastic bone metastases rarely produce hypercalcemia, but commonly raise the serum alkaline phosphatase level.

The presence of bone metastases does not exclude parathyroid or ectopic parathormone secretion by the tumor as the source of hypercalcemia. Persistence of hypercalcemia after local tumor control suggests that the parathyroid glands are the source of increased parathormone or that clinically undetectable metastases are present. If hypercalcemia persists longer than 3 to 6 months and the patient does not have evidence of recurrent or metastatic cancer, primary hyperparathyroidism should be considered.

A syndrome of inappropriate secretion of antidiuretic hormone (SIADH) can also be seen in patients with head and neck cancer.[437]

Hypomagnesemia should be monitored in patients who have had chemotherapy, and audiograms (before each cycle of drugs) should be taken to look for high-frequency sensorineural hearing loss if cisplatin is used. If progressive, this may be a contraindication to further chemotherapy.

During follow-up, changes in the patient's general appearance and demeanor should be noted. Weight loss is always of concern as a possible indicator of the development of metastatic disease. The patient should always be questioned about signs and symptoms, including otalgia, odynophagia, and head pain (lateralized forehead pain, retro-orbital, which suggests development of disease at the skull base), and new "lumps and bumps" anywhere in the body (dermal metastases can present in any location).

The general topic of complications of head and neck surgery and specifically those pursuant to therapy for malignant disease in the mouth and throat is the subject of a now classic book,[438] which is recommended to the reader. Rehabilitation of swallowing and other disorders after major head and neck surgery is enjoying increased interest and investigation and is the subject of several reviews by interdisciplinary team members.[439–441]

SUGGESTED READINGS

1. Collins SL: Controversies in the Management of Cancer in the Neck. In: Comprehensive Management of Head and Neck Tumors. Edited by Thawley SE and Panje WR. Philadelphia, WB Saunders, 1987, p 1386. (Second edition is in press for 1996.)
2. Ali S, Tiwari RM, and Snow GB: False positive and false negative neck nodes. Head Neck Surg 8:78, 1985.
3. Fisher B, et al: The contribution of recent NSABP clinical trials of primary breast cancer therapy to understanding of tumor biology: an overview of findings. Cancer 46:1009, 1980.
4. Fisher B: Cancer surgery: a commentary. Cancer Treat Rev 68: 31, 1984.
5. Fidler IJ: Recent concepts of cancer metastasis and their implications for therapy. Cancer Treat Rev 68:193, 1984.
6. Bundgaard T, Wildt J, and Elbrond O: Oral squamous cell cancer in non-users of tobacco and alcohol. Clin Otolaryngol 19: 320, 1994.
7. Spitz MR, et al: Squamous cell carcinoma of the upper aerodigestive tract: a case comparison analysis. Cancer 61:203, 1988.
8. Hurt RD, et al: A comprehensive model for the treatment of nicotine dependance in a medical setting. Med Clin North Am 76:495, 1992.
9. Garfinkel L: Perspectives on cancer prevention. CA Cancer J Clin 45:5, 1995.
10. Greenwald P, et al: Chemoprevention. CA Cancer J Clin 45:31, 1995.
11. Devries N, Van Zandwijk N, and Pastorino U: The Euroscan Study: a progress report. Am J Otolaryngol 14:62, 1993.

12. Blot WJ, et al: Smoking and drinking in relation to oral and pharyngeal cancer. Cancer Res 48:3282, 1988.

13. Mashberg A, Garfinkel L, and Harris S: Alcohol as a primary risk factor in oral squamous carcinoma. Cancer 31:146, 1981.

14. Bailey B: Smokeless tobacco: the fight goes on. Bull Am Acad Otol Head Neck Surg 8:4, 1989.

15. Schaefer SD, et al: Patterns of use and incidence of smokeless tobacco consumption in school-age children. Arch Otolaryngol Head Neck Surg 111:639, 1985.

16. Winn D, et al: Snuff dipping and oral cancer among women in the southern United States. N Engl J Med 304:345, 1981.

17. Wood NK: Smokeless tobacco and oral cancer: a summary. IL Dent J 57:334, 1988.

18. Tewfik HH, et al: Di George syndrome associated with multiple squamous cell carcinomas. Arch Otorhinolaryngol 103:105, 1977.

19. Lee YW and Gisser SP: Squamous cell carcinoma of the tongue in a nine-year renal transplant survivor. Cancer 41:4, 1978.

20. Shillitoe ET, et al: Neutralizing antibody to HSV Type I in patient with oral cancer. Cancer 49:2315, 1982.

21. Bottomley WK: Physiology of the oral mucosa. Otolaryngol Clin North Am 12:15, 1979.

22. Stram JR: Topographical histology of the oral cavity. Otolaryngol Clin North Am 5:201, 1972.

23. Pindborg JJ: Oral Cancer and Precancer. London, John Wright and Sons, 1980.

24. Silverman S, et al: Malignant transformation and natural history of oral leukoplakia in 57,518 industrial workers of Gujarat, India. Cancer 38:1790, 1976.

25. Waldron CA and Shaefer WG: Leukoplakia revisited: a clinicopathological study of 3256 oral leukoplakias. Cancer 36:1386, 1975.

26. Mashberg A, et al: A study of the appearance of early asymptomatic oral squamous cell carcinoma. Cancer 32:1436, 1973.

27. Mashberg A and Myers H: Anatomical site and size of 222 early asymptomatic oral squamous cell carcinomas. Cancer 37:2149, 1976.

28. Fulling HJ: Cancer development in oral lichen planus. Arch Dermatol 108:667, 1973.

29. Reddy CRRM, et al: Changes in the ducts of the glands of the hard palate in reverse smokers. Cancer 30:231, 1972.

30. Pindborg JJ: Atlas of Diseases of the Oral Mucosa. 4th Ed. Philadelphia, WB Saunders, 1985.

31. Raslan WF, et al: Basaloid squamous cell carcinoma of the head and neck: a clinicopathologic and flow cytometric study of 10 new cases with review of the English literature. Am J Otolaryngol 15:204, 1994.

32. Bauer WC: Varieties of squamous carcinoma: biological behavior. Front Radiat Ther Oncol 9:164, 1974.

33. Lichtiger B, et al: Spindle-cell variant of squamous carcinoma: a light and electron microscope study of 13 cases. Cancer 26:1311, 1970.

34. Leventon GS and Evans HL: Sarcomatoid squamous cell carcinoma of the mucous membranes of the head and neck: a clinicopathologic study of 20 cases. Cancer 48:994, 1981.

35. Friedel W, et al: Pseudosarcomas of the pharynx and larynx. Arch Otolaryngol Head Neck Surg 102:286, 1976.

36. Takagi M, et al: Adenoid squamous cell carcinoma of the oral mucosa: report of two autopsy cases. Cancer 40:2250, 1977.

37. Ackerman LV: Verrucous carcinoma of the oral cavity. Surgery 23:670, 1989.

38. Dische S, et al: Cell proliferation and differentiation in squamous cancer. Radiother Oncol 15:19, 1989.

39. McClure DL, Gullane PJ, and Slinger RP: Verrucous carcinoma: changing concepts in management. J Otolaryngol 13:7, 1984.

40. Batsakis JG, et al: The pathology of head and neck tumors: verrucous carcinoma. Part 15. Head Neck Surg 5:29, 1982.

41. Proffitt SD, Spooner TR, and Kosek JC: Origin of undifferentiated neoplasm from verrucous epidermal carcinoma of oral cavity following radiation. Cancer 26:389, 1970.

42. McDonald JS, Crissman JD, and Gluckman JL: Verrucous carcinoma of the oral cavity. Head Neck Surg 5:22, 1982.

43. Perez CA, et al: Anaplastic transformation in verrucous carcinoma of the oral cavity after radiation therapy. Radiology 86:108, 1966.

44. Medina JE, Dichtel W, and Luna MA: Verrucous-squamous carcinomas of the oral cavity: a clinicopathologic study of 104 cases. Arch Otolaryngol Head Neck Surg 110:437, 1984.

45. Nair MK, et al: Oral verrucous carcinoma treatment with radiotherapy. Cancer 61:458, 1988.

46. Strong MS, Vaughn CW, and Incze JS: Toluidine blue and the management of carcinomas of the oral cavity. Arch Otolaryngol Head Neck Surg 87:527, 1968.

47. Mashberg A: Final evaluation of tolonium chloride rinse for screening of high-risk patients with asymptomatic squamous carcinoma. J Am Dent Assoc 106:319, 1983.

48. Mashberg A and Barsa P: Screening for oral and oropharyngeal squamous carcinoma. Cancer 34:262, 1984.

49. Bouquot JE, Weiland LH, and Kurland LT: Metastases to and from the upper aerodigestive tract in the population of Rochester, Minnesota 1935 to 1984. Head Neck Surg 11:212, 1989.

50. Slaughter DP, Southwick HW, and Smejkal W: "Field cancerization" in oral stratified squamous epithelium: clinical implications of multicentric origin. Cancer 6:963, 1953.

51. Maisel RH and Vermeersch H: Panendoscopy for second primaries in head and neck cancer. Ann Otol Rhinol Laryngol 90:460, 1981.

52. Larson JT, Adams GL, and Fattah HA: Survival statistics for multiple primaries in head and neck cancer. Otolaryngol Head Neck Surg 103:14, 1990.

52. Reynolds RD, et al: Lung cancer as a second primary. Cancer 42:2887, 1978.

53. Haughey BH, Arfken CL, and Gates GA: Meta-analysis of second malignant tumors in head and neck cancer: the case for an endoscopic screening protocol. Ann Otol Rhinol Laryngol 101:105, 1992.

53a. Johnson JT, et al: Significance of positive bronchial cytology and presence of squamous cell carcinoma of the upper aerodigestive tract. Ann Otol Rhinol Laryngol 90:454, 1981.

54. Marchetta FC, et al: Multiple malignancies in patients with head and neck cancer. Am J Surg 110:711, 1971.

55. Friedman M, Toriumi DM, and Strorigl T: Effects of therapeutic radiation on the development of multiple primary tumors of the head and neck. Head Neck Surg 10:548, 1988.

56. Boddie AW, et al: Head and neck cancer developing in patients with pre-existing reticuloendothelial malignancies. Laryngoscope 87:2090, 1977.

57. Vikram B: Changing patterns of failure in advanced head and neck cancer. Arch Otolaryngol Head Neck Surg 110:564, 1984.

58. Goepfert H: Are we making any progress? Arch Otolaryngol Head Neck Surg 110:562, 1984.

59. Viadana E: The metastatic spread of head and neck tumors in man: an autopsy study of 371 cases. Z Krebsforsch 83:293, 1975.

60. Bhatia R and Bahadur S: Distant metastasis in malignancies of the head and neck. J Laryngol Otol 101:925, 1987.

61. Papac RJ: Distant metastases from head and neck cancer. Cancer 53:342, 1984.

62. Mazer TM, et al: Resection of pulmonary metastases from squamous cell carcinoma of the head and neck. Am J Surg 156:238, 1988.

63. Noyek AM: Bone scanning in otolaryngology. Laryngoscope 89:1, 1979.

63a. Finley RK III, et al: Results of surgical resection of pulmonary metastases of squamous cell carcinoma of the head and neck. Am J Surg 164:594, 1992.

64. Harrison DFN: The questionable value of total glossectomy. Head Neck Surg 6:632, 1983.

65. Carter RL, et al: Direct bone invasion in squamous carcinomas of the head and neck: pathological and clinical implications. Clin Otolaryngol 5:107, 1980.

66. McGregor AD and MacDonald DG: Reactive changes in the mandible in the presence of squamous cell carcinoma. Head Neck Surg 10:378, 1988.

67. McGregor AD and MacDonald DG: Patterns of spread of squamous cell carcinoma within the mandible. Head Neck Surg 11:457, 1989.

68. Davidson TM, et al: Mohs for head and neck mucosal cancer: report on 111 patients. Laryngoscope 98:1078, 1988.

69. Scanlon EF: The role of the fifth circulation in cancer dissemination. Am J Surg 138:474, 1979.

70. Batsakis JG: The pathology of head and neck tumors. X. The occult primary and metastases to the head and neck. Head Neck Surg 3:409, 1981.

71. Hora JS: Preoperative radiation therapy as an adjunctive measure to radical neck dissection: a histopathologic study. Laryngoscope 79:1921, 1969.

72. Skolnick EM, et al: Preoperative radiation of the larynx: analysis of serial secretions. Ann Otol Rhinol Laryngol 79:1033, 1970.

73. Norris CM Jr, et al: Pathology of surgery after induction chemotherapy: an analysis of resectability and local regional control. Laryngoscope 96:292, 1986.

74. Jakobsson PA, et al: Histologic classification and grading of malignancy in carcinoma of the larynx. Acta Radiol 12:1, 1973.

75. Lee JG: Detection of residual carcinoma of the oral cavity, oropharynx, hypopharynx and larynx: a study of surgical margins. Trans Am Acad Ophthalmol Otolaryngol 79:49, 1974.

76. Sultan MR and Coleman JJ III: Oncologic and functional considerations of total glossectomy. Am J Surg 198:297, 1989.

77. Ballantyne AJ, McCarter AB, and Ibanez ML: The extension of cancer of the head and neck through peripheral nerves. Am J Surg 106:651, 1963.

78. Trobe JD, et al: Intracranial spread of squamous cell carcinoma along the trigeminal nerve. Arch Ophthalmol 100:608, 1982.

79. Carter RL, et al: Perineural spread in squamous cell carcinomas of the head and neck: a clinicopathological study. Clin Otolaryngol 4:271, 1980.

80. Carter RL, Pittam MR, and Tanner NSB: Pain and dysphagia in patients with squamous cell carcinoma of the head and neck: the role of perineural spread. J R Soc Med 75:598, 1982.

81. Southam JC: The extension of squamous carcinoma along the inferior dental neurovascular bundle. Br J Oral Surg 7:137, 1970.

82. Larson DL, et al: Perineural lymphatics: myth or fact? Am J Surg 112:488, 1966.

83. Batsakis JG: Invasion of the microcirculation in head and neck cancer. Arch Otol Rhinol Laryngol 93:646, 1984.

84. Close LG, et al: Microvascular invasion and survival in cancer of the oral cavity and oropharynx. Arch Otolaryngol Head Neck Surg 115:1304, 1989.

85. Carter RL, et al: Patterns and mechanisms of bone invasion by squamous carcinomas of the head and neck. Am J Surg 146:451, 1983.

86. O'Brien CJ, et al: Invasion of the mandible by squamous cell carcinoma of the oral cavity and oropharynx. Head Neck Surg 8:247, 1986.

87. Huang CC, et al: Collagenase and protease activities in head and neck tumors. Otolaryngol Head Neck Surg 88:749, 1980.

88. Marchetta FC, Sako K, and Badillo J: Periosteal lymphatics of the mandible and intraoral carcinoma. Am J Surg 108:505, 1964.

89. Marchetta FC, Sako K, and Murphy JB: The periosteum of the mandible and intraoral cancer. Am J Surg 122:711, 1971.

90. Collins SL and Saunders VW Jr: Excision of selected intraoral cancers by use of sagittal inner table mandibulectomy. Otolaryngol Head Neck Surg 97:558, 1987.

91. Sugarbaker EV: Cancer metastasis: a product of tumor-host interaction. Curr Probl Cancer 3:1, 1979.

92. Spiro RH and Strong EW: Discontinuous partial glossectomy and radical neck dissection in selected patients with epidermoid carcinoma of the mobile tongue. Am J Surg 123:544, 1973.

93. Lindberg RD: Distribution of cervical lymph node metastasis from squamous cell carcinoma of the upper respiratory and digestive tracts. Cancer 29:1446, 1972.

94. Fisch UP, et al: Cervical lymphatic system as visualized by lymphography. Ann Otol Rhinol Laryngol 13:869, 1964.

95. Sharpe DT: The pattern of lymph node metastases in intraoral squamous cell carcinoma. Br J Plast Surg 34:97, 1981.

96. Fiend CR and Cole RM: Contralateral spread of head and neck cancer. Am J Surg 118:660, 1969.

97. Martin H and Morfit H: Cervical lymph node metastasis as the first symptom of cancer. Surg Gynecol Obstet 78:133, 1944.

98. Frable WJ and Frable MAS: Thin-needle aspiration biopsy: the diagnosis of head and neck tumors revisited. Cancer 43:1541, 1979.

99. Silverman CL, et al: Treatment of epidermoid and less differentiated carcinoma from occult primaries presenting in cervical lymph nodes. Laryngoscope 93:645, 1983.

100. McGuirt WF and McCabe BG: Significance of node biopsy before definitive treatment of cervical metastatic carcinoma. Laryngoscope 88:594, 1978.

101. Cinberg JL, et al: Cervical cysts: cancer until proven otherwise? Laryngoscope 92:27, 1982.

102. Riggins RS and Ketcham AS: Effect of incisional biopsy on the development of experimental tumor metastasis. J Surg Res 5:200, 1965.

103. Razack M, et al: Influence of initial neck node biopsy on the incidence of recurrence in the neck and survival in patients who subsequently undergo curative resectional surgery. J Surg Oncol 9:347, 1977.

103a. Ellis ER, et al: Incisional or excisional neck-node biopsy before definitive radiotherapy, alone or followed by neck dissection. Head and Neck Surg 13:177, 1991.

104. Jesse RH and Neff LE: Metastatic carcinoma in cervical nodes with an unknown primary lesion. Am J Surg 112:547, 1966.

105. Robinson LD, et al: Head and neck malignancies in children: an age-incidence study. Laryngoscope 98:11, 1988.

106. Harris AH and Smith RR: Operative wound seeding with tumor cells: its role in recurrences of head and neck cancer. Ann Surg 151:330, 1960.

107. Collins, SL: Decreasing the risk of implanting cancer cells intraoperatively. Laryngoscope 103:825, 1993.

108. Der Hagopian RP, et al: Inflammatory oncotoxis. JAMA 240:374, 1978.

109. Papay FA, et al: Evaluation of syncope from head and neck cancer. Laryngoscope 99:382, 1989.

110. Ballantyne AJ: Significance of retropharyngeal nodes in cancer of the head and neck. Am J Surg 108:500, 1964.

111. Larson DA, Loeffler JS, and Flickinger J: Radiobiology of radiosurgery. Int J Radiat Onc Biol Phys 25:557, 1993.

112. Creekmore SP, Collins SL, and Leipzig B: Medical therapy for head and neck cancer. In: Pharmacology in Otolaryngology—Head and Neck Surgery. Edited by Collins SL. Washington, DC, American Academy of Otolaryngoly—Head and Neck Surgery Foundation, 1987.

113. Cherny NI and Portenoy RK: The management of cancer pains. CA Cancer J Clin 44:262, 1994.

114. Olsen KD and Creagan ET: Pain management in advanced cancer of the head and neck. Am J Otolaryngol 12:154, 1991.

115. Grond S, et al: Validation of World Health Organization guidelines for pain relief in head and neck cancer: a prospective study. Ann Otol Rhinol Laryngol 102:342, 1993.

116. Piccirillo JF: Purposes, problems and proposals for progress in cancer staging. Arch Otolaryngol Head Neck Surg 121:145, 1995.

117. Copper MP, et al: Role of genetic factors in the etiology of squamous cell carcinoma of the head and neck. Arch Otolaryngol Head Neck Surg 121:157, 1995.

118. Leipzig B, et al: Carcinoma of the anterior tongue. Ann Otol Rhinol Laryngol 91:94, 1982.

119. Shear M, Hawkins DM, and Farr HW: The prediction of lymph node metastases from oral squamous cell carcinoma. Cancer 37:1901, 1976.

120. Kennedy KA, et al: The hypoxic tumor cell: a target for selective cancer chemotherapy. Biochem Pharmacol 29:1, 1980.

121. Moulder JE and Rockwell S: Tumor hypoxia: its impact on cancer therapy. Cancer Metastasis Rev 5:313, 1987.

122. Sartorelli AC: Therapeutic attack on hypoxic cells of solid tumors. Cancer Res 48:775, 1988.

123. Nathanson A, et al: Evaluation of some prognostic factors in small squamous cell carcinoma of the mobile tongue: a multicenter study in Sweden. Head Neck 11:387, 1989.

124. Crissman JD, et al: Prognostic value of histopathologic parameters in squamous cell carcinoma of the oropharynx. Cancer 54:2995, 1984.

125. Yamamoto E, Miyakawa A, and Kohama G-I: Mode of invasion and lymph node metastasis in squamous cell carcinoma of the oral cavity. Head Neck Surg 6:938, 1984.

126. Breslow A: Thickness, cross-sectional area and depth of invasion in the prognosis of cutaneous melanoma. Ann Surg 172:902, 1970.

127. Mohit-Tabatabai MA, et al: Relationship of thickness of floor of mouth stage I and II cancers to regional metastasis. Am J Surg 152:351, 1986.

128. Spiro RH, et al: Predictive value of tumor thickness in squamous carcinoma confined to tongue and floor of mouth. Am J Surg 152:345, 1986.

129. Fakih AR, et al: Elective vs therapeutic neck dissection in early carcinoma of the oral tongue. Am J Surg 158:309, 1989.

130. Johnson JT, et al: The extracapsular spread of tumors in cervical node metastasis. Arch Otolaryngol Head Neck Surg 107:725, 1981.

131. Sessions DG: Surgical pathology of cancer of the larynx and hypopharynx. Laryngoscope 86:814, 1976.

132. Vandenbrouck C, et al: Elective vs therapeutic radical neck dissection in epidermoid carcinoma of the oral cavity: results of a randomized clinical trial. Cancer 46:386, 1980.

133. Cachin Y, et al: Nodal metastasis from carcinomas of the oropharynx. Otolaryngol Clin North Am 12:145, 1979.

134. Benninger MS, et al: Squamous cell carcinoma of the head and neck in patients 40 years of age and younger. Laryngoscope 98:531, 1988.

135. Cusumano RJ and Persky MS: Squamous cell carcinoma of the oral cavity and oropharynx in young adults. Head Neck Surg 10:229, 1988.

136. Johnston WD and Ballantyne AJ: Prognostic effect of tobacco and alcohol use in patients with oral tongue cancer. Am J Surg 134:444, 1977.

137. Loré JM Jr: Dabbling in head and neck oncology (a plea for added qualifications). Arch Otolaryngol Head Neck Surg 113:1165, 1987.

138. Harrison DFN: Down with the dabblers (Letter). Arch Otolaryngol Head Neck Surg 114:809, 1988.

139. Lucente FE: Treatment of head-and-neck carcinoma with noncurative intent. Am J Otolaryngol 15:99, 1994.

140. Callery CD, Spiro RH, and Strong EW: Changing trends in management of squamous carcinoma of the tongue. Am J Surg 148:449, 1984.

141. Mendenhall WM, et al: Radiotherapy after excisional biopsy of carcinoma of the oral tongue and floor of mouth. Head Neck Surg 11:129, 1989.

142. Collins SL: CO_2 laser surgery for cancer in the oral cavity, oropharynx and pharynx. In: Lasers in Head and Neck Surgery. Edited by Weisberger ED. New York, Igaku-Shoin, 1990.

143. Boice JD: Cancer following medical irradiation. Cancer 47:1081, 1981.

144. Marx RE and Johnson RP: Studies in the radiobiology of osteoradionecrosis and their clinical significance. Oral Surg Oral Med Oral Pathol 64:379, 1987.

145. Million RR: The myth regarding bone or cartilage involvement by cancer and the likelihood of cure by radiation therapy. Head Neck 11:30, 1989.

146. Pierequin B, et al: The place of implantation in tongue and floor of mouth cancer. JAMA 215:961, 1971.

147. Fee W, et al: Intraoperative iodine^{125} implants: their use in large tumors of the neck attached to the carotid artery. Arch Otolaryngol Head Neck Surg 109:727, 1983.

148. Vikram B, et al: I^{125} implants in head and neck cancer. Cancer 51:310, 1980.

149. Parsons JT, Mendenhall WM, and Cassisi NJ: Hyperfractionation for head and neck cancer. Int J Radiat Oncol Biol Physiol 14:649, 1988.

150. Wang CC: The enigma of accelerated hyperfractionated radiation therapy for head and neck cancer. Int J Radiat Oncol Biol Phys 14:209, 1988.

151. Weichselbaum R: Cellular and molecular aspects of human tumor radio resistance. In: Important Advances in Oncology 1991. Edited by de Vita VT, Hellman S, and Rosenberg SA. Philadelphia, JB Lippincott, 1991, p 73.

152. Byers RM, et al: The prognostic and therapeutic value of frozen section determination in the surgical treatment of squamous carcinoma of the head and neck. Am J Surg 136:525, 1978.

153. Looser KG, Shah JP, and Strong EW: The significance of positive margins in surgically resected epidermoid carcinomas. Head Neck Surg 1:107, 1978.

154. Chen TY, Emrich LJ, and Driscoll DL: The clinical significance of pathological findings in surgically resected margins of the primary tumor in head and neck carcinoma. Int J Radiat Oncol Biol Phys 13:833, 1987.

155. Vikram B, et al: Elective postoperative radiation therapy in Stage III and IV epidermoid carcinoma of the head and neck. Am J Surg 146:580, 1980.

156. Scholl P, Byers RM, and Batsakis JG: Microscopic cut-through of cancer in the surgical treatment of squamous carcinoma of the tongue: prognostic and therapeutic implications. Am J Surg 152:354, 1986.

157. Schramm VL, et al: Surgical management of early epidermoid carcinoma of the anterior floor of the mouth. Laryngoscope 90:207, 1980.

158. King GD: Transoral resection for cancer of the oral cavity. Otolaryngol Clin North Am 5:321, 1972.

159. Oosterhuis JW, et al: The viability of cells in the waste products of CO_2 laser evaporation of Cloudman mouse melanomas. Cancer 49:61, 1982.

160. Nezhat C, et al: Smoke from laser surgery: is there a hazard? Lasers Surg Med 7:376, 1987.

161. Strong MS, et al: Transoral management of localized carcinoma of the oral cavity using the CO_2 laser. Laryngoscope 89:897, 1979.

162. Guerry TL, Silverman S, and Dedo HH: Carbon dioxide laser resection of superficial oral carcinoma: indications, technique and results. Ann Otol Rhinol Laryngol 95:547, 1986.

163. Fisher SE, et al: A comparative histological study of wound healing following CO_2 laser and conventional surgical excision of canine buccal mucosa. Arch Oral Biol 28:287, 1983.

164. Nagorsky MJ and Sessions DG: Laser resection for early oral cavity cancer: results and complications. Ann Otol Rhinol Laryngol 96:556, 1987.

165. Marcial VA, et al: Does preoperative irradiation increase the rate of surgical complications in carcinoma of the head and neck? Cancer 49:1297, 1982.

166. Vikram B: The importance of the time interval between surgery and postoperative radiation therapy in the combined management of head and neck cancer. Int J Radiat Oncol Biol Phys 5: 1837, 1979.

167. Schiff PB, et al: Impact of the time interval between surgery and postoperative radiotherapy on locoregional control in advanced head and neck cancer. J Surg Oncol 43:203, 1990.

168. Schuller DE, et al: Symposium. Adjuvant cancer therapy of head and neck tumors: increased survival with surgery alone versus combination therapy. Laryngoscope 89:582, 1979.

169. Panje WR, Smith B, and McCabe BF: Epidermoid carcinoma of the floor of mouth: surgical therapy vs radiation therapy. Otolaryngol Head Neck Surg 88:714, 1980.

170. Suen JY, et al: Evaluation of the effectiveness of postoperative radiation therapy for the control of local disease. Am J Surg 140:577, 1980.

171. De Santo LW, et al: Neck dissection and combined treatment: study of effectiveness. Arch Otolaryngol Head Neck Surg 111: 366, 1985.

172. Kramer S, Gelber RD, and Snow JB: Combined radiation therapy and surgery in the management of advanced head and neck cancer: final report of study 73–03 of the Radiation Therapy Oncology Group. Head Neck Surg 10:19, 1987.

173. Jesse RH, et al: The efficacy of combining radiation therapy with a surgical procedure in patients with cervical metastasis from squamous cancer of the oropharynx and hypopharynx. Cancer 35:1163, 1975.

174. Head and Neck Contracts Program: Adjuvant chemotherapy for advanced head and neck squamous carcinoma: final report of the head and neck contract program. Cancer 60:301, 1987.

175. Schuller DE, et al: Preoperative chemotherapy in advanced resectable head and neck cancer: final report of the Southwest Oncology Group. Laryngoscope 98:1205, 1988.

176. Wolf GT, et al: Induction chemotherapy plus radiation compared with surgery plus radiation in patients with advanced laryngeal cancer. VA Laryngeal Cancer Study Group. N Engl J Med 324:1685, 1991.

177. Laramore GE, et al: Adjuvant chemotherapy for resectable squamous cell carcinomas of the head and neck: report of Intergroup Study 0034. Int J Radiat Oncol Biol Phys 23:705, 1992.

178. Sassler AM, Esclamado RM, and Wolf GT: Surgery after organ preservation therapy: analysis of wound complications. Arch Otolaryngol Head Neck Surg 121:162, 1995.

179. Slotman GJ, et al: The incidence of metastasis after multimodality therapy of cancer of the head and neck. Cancer 54:2009, 1984.

180. Tashiro H, et al: Late occurring recurrence of oral cancer after combined treatment with bleomycin and radiation therapy. Cancer 61:2412, 1988.

181. Taylor SG IV: Why has so much chemotherapy done so little in head and neck cancer? J Clin Oncol 5:1, 1987.

182. Tannock IF: Neoadjuvant chemotherapy in head and neck cancer: no way to preserve a larynx. J Clin Oncol 10:343, 1992.

183. Vokes EE and Weichselbaum RR: Concomitant chemoradiotherapy: rationale and clinical experience in patients with solid tumors. J Clin Oncol 8:911, 1990.

184. Snow GB and Clark JR (eds): Multimodality Therapy for Head and Neck Cancer. New York, Thieme, 1992.

185. Collins SL: Controversies in multimodality therapy for head and neck cancer. In: Comprehensive Management of Head and Neck Tumors. 2nd Ed. Edited by Thawley SE and Panje WR. Philadelphia, WB Saunders, 1995.

186. Schneider JJ, et al: Control by irradiation alone of nonfixed clinically positive lymph nodes from squamous cell carcinoma of the oral cavity, oropharynx, supraglottic larynx and hypopharynx. Am J Roentgenol 123:42, 1975.

187. Fletcher GH: Elective irradiation of subclinical disease in cancers of head and neck. Cancer 29:1450, 1972.

188. Fletcher GH: Subclinical disease. Cancer 33:1274, 1984.

189. Mendenhall WM, et al: Elective neck irradiation in squamous cell carcinoma of the head and neck. Head Neck Surg 3:15, 1980.

190. De Santo LW, et al: Neck dissection: is it worthwhile? Laryngoscope 92:502, 1982.

191. Robbins KT, et al: Standardizing neck dissection terminology. Arch Otolaryngol Head Neck Surg 117:601, 1991.

192. Bocca E, et al: Functional neck dissection: evaluation and review of 843 cases. Laryngoscope 94:942, 1984.

193. Conley JJ: Radical neck dissection. Laryngoscope 85:1344, 1975.

194. Calearo C and Teatini G: Functional neck dissection: anatomical grounds, surgical technique, clinical observations. Ann Otol Rhinolaryngol 92:215, 1983.

195. Gavilan J, Gavilan C, and Herranz J: Functional neck dissection: three decades of controversy. Ann Otol Rhinol Laryngol 101: 339, 1992.

196. Spiro JD, Spiro RD, and Shah JP: Critical assessment of supraomohyoid neck dissection. Am J Surg 156:286, 1988.

197. Jesse RH, et al: Cancer of the oral cavity: is elective neck dissection beneficial? Am J Surg 120:505, 1970.

198. Jesse RH, et al: Radical or modified neck dissection: a therapeutic dilemma. Am J Surg 136:516, 1978.

199. Spiro RH, and Strong EW: Epidermoid carcinoma of the oral cavity and oropharynx: elective versus therapeutic radical neck dissection as treatment. Arch Surg 107:302, 1973.

200. Lee JG, and Krause CJ: Radical neck dissection: elective, therapeutic and secondary. Arch Otolaryngol Head Neck Surg 101: 656, 1975.

201. Marchant FE, et al: Current national trends in the post-treatment follow-up of patients with squamous cell carcinoma of the head and neck. Am J Otolaryngol 14:88, 1993.

202. Fialka V and Venzenz K: Investigations into shoulder function after radical neck dissection. J Craniomaxillofac Surg 16:143, 1988.

203. Soo K-C, et al: Anatomy of the accessory nerve and its contributions in the neck. Head Neck Surg 9:111, 1986.

204. Medina JE, and Byers RM: Supraomohyoid neck dissection: rationale, indications and surgical technique. Head Neck Surg 11: 111, 1989.

205. Byers RM, Wolf PF, and Ballantyne AJ: Rationale for elective modified neck dissection. Head Neck Surg 10:160, 1988.

206. Byers RM: Modified neck dissection: a study of 927 cases from 1970 to 1980. Am J Surg 150:414, 1985.

207. Donegan JO, et al: The role of suprahyoid neck dissection in the management of cancer of the tongue and floor of the mouth. Head Neck Surg 4:209, 1982.

208. Ballantyne AJ and Jackson GL: Synchronous bilateral neck dissection. Am J Surg 144:452, 1982.

209. McQuarrie DG, et al: A physiologic approach to the problems of simultaneous bilateral neck dissection. Am J Surg 134:455, 1977.

210. Baffi R, et al: Nonsimultaneous bilateral radical neck dissection. Head Neck Surg 2:272, 1980.

211. Smith PG and Collins SL: Repair of head and neck defects with "thin" and double-lined pectoralis flaps. Arch Otolaryngol Head Neck Surg 110:468, 1984.

212. Marks JE, Imanzahrai A, and Collins SL: Iodine-125 seed implants after neck dissection and carotid peel for head and neck cancer in cervical lymph nodes. Endocuriether Hypertherm Oncol 8:195, 1992.

213. Emami B, et al: Reirradiation of recurrent head and neck cancers. Laryngoscope 97:85, 1987.

214. Conley JJ: The meaning of life-threatening disease in the area of the head and neck. Acta Otolaryngol (Stockh) 99:201, 1985.

215. Conley JJ: Have I performed the right operation? Arch Otolaryngol Head Neck Surg 112:385, 1986.

216. Frank HA and Davidson TM: Ethical dilemmas in head and neck cancer. Head Neck Surg 11:22, 1989.

217. O'Dwyer TP, et al: Percutaneous feeding gastrostomy in patients with head and neck tumors: a five year review. Laryngoscope *100*:29, 1990.

217a. Meuer MF and Kenady DE: Metastatic head and neck cancer in a percutaneous gastrostomy site. Head Neck Surg *15*:70, 1993.

218. Neal HB, et al: Cryosurgery for the treatment of cancer. Laryngoscope *90(suppl)*:23, 1980.

219. Chambers RG: Treatment of advanced cancer of the head and neck: don't give up. Am J Surg *140*:478, 1980.

220. Tucker HM, et al: Massive surgery for palliation in malignancy of the head and neck. Laryngoscope *83*:1635, 1973.

221. McGuirt WF and Davis SP III: Demographic portrayal and outcome analysis of head and neck cancer surgery in the elderly. Arch Otolaryngol Head Neck Surg *121*:150, 1995.

222. Snyderman CH and d'Amico F: Outcome of carotid artery resection for neoplastic disease: a meta-analysis Am J Otolaryngol *13*:373, 1992.

223. Konno A, et al: Analysis of factors affecting complications of carotid ligation. Ann Otol Rhinol Laryngol *90*:222, 1981.

224. Matas R: Testing the efficacy of the collateral circulation. JAMA *63*:1441, 1914.

225. Gee W, et al: Measurement of collateral cerebral hemispheric blood pressure by ocular plethysmography. Am J Surg *130*:121, 1975.

226. De Vries EJ, et al: Elective resection of the internal carotid artery without reconstruction. Laryngoscope *98*:960, 1988.

227. Erba SM, et al: Balloon test occlusion of the internal carotid artery with xenon/CT cerebral blood flow mapping. Am J Neuroradiol *9*:533, 1988.

228. De Vries EJ, et al: A new method to predict safe resection of the internal carotid artery. Laryngoscope *100*:85, 1990.

229. Zimmerman MC, et al: Treatment of impending carotid rupture with detachable balloon embolization. Arch Otolaryngol Head Neck Surg *113*:1169, 1987.

230. Butcher RB II: Malignant potential of keratoacanthoma. Laryngoscope *89*:1092, 1979.

231. Baker SR and Krause CJ: Carcinoma of the lip. Laryngoscope *90*:19, 1980.

232. Harris JP and Penn I: Immunosuppression and the development of malignancies of the upper airway and related structures. Laryngoscope *91*:520, 1981.

233. Sack JG and Ford CN: Metastatic squamous cell carcinoma of the lip. Arch Otolaryngol Head Neck Surg *104*:282, 1978.

234. Fazekas-May M, Sullivan M, and Collins SL: Recurrent squamous cell carcinoma of the lower lip. Head and Neck Surg *11*:188, 1989.

235. Heller JS and Shah JP: Carcinoma of the lip. Am J Surg *138*:600, 1979.

236. Pigneux J, et al: The place of interstitial therapy using ¹⁹²iridium in the management of carcinoma of the lip. Cancer *43*:1073, 1979.

237. Calhoun KH: Reconstruction of small and medium-sized defects of the lower lip. Am J Otolaryngol *13*:16, 1992.

238. Barbosa JF: Tumors of the lip. In: Surgical Treatment of Head and Neck Tumors. Edited by Barbosa JF. New York, Grune & Stratton, 1974.

239. Marshall KA and Edgerton MT: Indications for neck dissection in carcinoma of the lip. Am J Surg *133*:216, 1977.

240. Converse JM and Wood-Smith D: Techniques for the repair of defects of the lips and cheeks. In: Reconstructive Plastic Surgery. Vol 3. Edited by Converse JM. Philadelphia, WB Saunders, 1977.

241. Karapandzic M: Reconstruction of lip defects by local arterial flaps. Br J Plast Surg *29*:93, 1974.

242. Smith PG, Muntz HR, and Thawley SE: Local myocutaneous advancement flaps. Arch Otolaryngol Head Neck Surg *108*:714, 1982.

243. Gewirtz HS, et al: Use of the nasolabial flap for reconstruction of the floor of mouth. Am J Surg *136*:508, 1978.

244. Wilson JPS and Walker EP: Reconstruction of the lower lip. Head Neck Surg *4*:29, 1981.

245. Cady B and Catlin D: Epidermoid carcinoma of the gum: a 20-year survey. Cancer *23*:551, 1969.

246. Paavolainen M and Malmberg H: Sublabial approach to the nasal and paranasal cavities using nasal pyramid osteotomy and septal transection. Laryngoscope *96*:106, 1989.

247. Bloom ND and Spiro RH: Carcinoma of the cheek mucosa. Am J Surg *140*:556, 1980.

248. Vigorita VJ, et al: Squamous cell carcinoma of Stensen't duct. Head Neck Surg *2*:513, 1980.

249. Conley JJ and Sadoyama JA: Squamous cell carcinoma of the buccal mucosa: a review of 90 cases. Arch Otolaryngol Head Neck Surg *97*:330, 1973.

250. Chung CK, et al: Radiation therapy in the management of primary malignancies of the hard palate. Laryngoscope *90*:576, 1980.

251. Solomon MP, et al: Intraoral papillary squamous cell tumor of the soft palate with features of sialadenoma papilliferum. Cancer *42*:1859, 1978.

252. Fee WR Jr, et al: Squamous cell carcinoma of the soft palate. Arch Otolaryngol Head Neck Surg *105*:710, 1979.

253. Evans JF and Shah JP: Epidermoid carcinoma of the palate. Am J Surg *142*:451, 1981.

254. Krespi YP and Sisson GA: Skull base surgery in composite resection. Arch Otolaryngol Head Neck Surg *108*:681, 1982.

255. Close LG, Mickey BE, and Anderson RG: Resection of upper aerodigestive tract tumors involving the middle cranial fossa. Laryngoscope *95*:908, 1985.

256. Harrold CC: Management of cancer of the floor of mouth. Am J Surg *122*:487, 1971.

257. Crissman JD, et al: Squamous cell carcinoma of the floor of mouth. Head Neck Surg *3*:2, 1980.

258. Kremen AK: Cancer of the tongue: a surgical technique for a primary combined en bloc resection of tongue, floor of mouth and cervical lymphatics. Surgery *30*:227, 1951.

259. Spiro RH and Strong EW: Epidermoid carcinoma of the mobile tongue: treatment by partial glossectomy alone. Am J Surg *122*:707, 1971.

260. Lee JG and Litton WB: Symposium on malignancy. II. Occult regional metastasis: carcinoma of the oral tongue. Laryngoscope *82*:1273, 1972.

261. Johnson JT, et al: Management of T1 carcinoma of the anterior aspect of the tongue. Arch Otolaryngol *106*:249, 1980.

262. Spiro RH, et al: Mandibulotomy approach to oropharynx tumors. Am J Surg *150*:466, 1985.

263. McGregor IA and McDonald DG: Mandibular osteotomy in the approach to the oral cavity. Head Neck Surg *5*:457, 1983.

264. Cohen JI, Marentette LJ, and Maisel RH: The mandibular swing: stabilization of the midline mandibular osteotomy. Laryngoscope *98*:1139, 1988.

265. Whicker JH, et al: Surgical treatment of squamous cell carcinoma of the base of the tongue. Laryngoscope *82*:1853, 1972.

266. DuPont JB, et al: Surgical treatment of advanced carcinomas of the base of tongue. Am J Surg *136*:501, 1978.

267. Hillel AD and Goode RL: Lateral larynx suspension: a new procedure to minimize swallowing disorders following tongue base resection. Laryngoscope *93*:26, 1983.

268. Krespi YP and Sisson GA: Reconstruction after total or subtotal glossectomy. Am J Surg *146*:488, 1983.

269. Biller HF, Lawson W, and Baek SJ: Total glossectomy: a technique of reconstruction, eliminating laryngectomy. Arch Otolaryngol Head Neck Surg *109*:69, 1983.

270. Myers EN: The role of total glossectomy in the management of cancer of the oral cavity. Otolaryngol Clin North Am *5*:343, 1972.

271. Sessions DG, et al: Total glossectomy for advanced carcinoma of the base of the tongue. Laryngoscope 39:39, 1973.

272. Harrison LB, et al: Base-of-tongue cancer treated with external beam irradiation plus brachytherapy: oncologic and functional outcome. Radiology 184:267, 1992.

273. Taylor SG IV: Personal communication, 1995.

274. Terez JJ and Farr HW: Carcinoma of the tonsillar fossa. Surg Gynecol Obstet 125:581, 1967.

275. Goldberg AN: Kaposi's sarcoma of the head and neck in acquired immunodeficiency syndrome. Am J Otolaryngol 14:5, 1993.

276. Sooy CD, et al: The risk for infection: report of an in-process study. Laryngoscope 97:430, 1987.

277. Micheau C, et al: Cystic metastases in the neck revealing occult carcinoma of the tonsil. Cancer 33:228, 1974.

278. Khafif RA, Prichep R, and Minkowitz S: Primary branchiogenic carcinoma. Head Neck Surg 11:153, 1989.

279. Barrs DM, et al: Squamous cell carcinoma of the tonsil and tongue-base region. Arch Otolaryngol 105:479, 1979.

280. Collins SL: Avoiding delay and misdiagnosis of head and neck cancer: rare tumors with common symptoms. Compr Ther 21: 59, 1995.

281. Harrison DFN: Pathology of hypopharynx cancer in relation to surgical management. J Laryngol Otol 84:349, 1970.

282. Wang CC: Radiotherapy management of carcinoma of the posterior pharyngeal wall. Cancer 27:894, 1971.

283. Pene F, et al: A retrospective study of 131 cases of carcinoma of the posterior pharyngeal wall. Cancer 42:2490, 1978.

284. Son YH and Kucinski BM: Therapeutic concept of brachytherapy/megavoltage in sequence for pharyngeal wall cancers. Cancer 59:1268, 1987.

285. Guillamondegui OM: Surgical treatment of squamous cell carcinoma of the pharyngeal walls. Am J Surg 136:474, 1978.

286. Marks JE, et al: Pharyngeal wall cancer: an analysis of treatment results, complications and patterns of failure. Int J Radiat Oncol Biol Phys 4:587, 1978.

287. Marks JE, Smith PG, and Sessions DG: Pharyngeal wall cancer: a reappraisal after comparison of treatment methods. Arch Otolaryngol Head Neck Surg 111:79, 1985.

288. Mladick RA, et al: Cricopharyngeal myotomy: application and technique in major oropharyngeal resections. Arch Surg 102:1, 1971.

289. Trotter W: Some principles in the surgery of the pharynx. Lancet 2:833, 1931.

290. Ogura JH, et al: Partial pharyngectomy and neck dissection for posterior hypopharyngeal cancer: immediate reconstruction with preservation of voice. Laryngoscope 70:1523, 1960.

291. McConnel FMS, et al: Manofluorography of deglutition after total laryngopharyngectomy. Proc R Soc Lond 81:346, 1988.

292. Maniglia AJ, et al: Tracheogastric puncture for vocal rehabilitation following total pharyngolaryngoesophagectomy. Head Neck Surg 11:524, 1989.

293. Zeismann M, Boyd B, and Manktelow RT: Speaking jejunum after laryngopharyngectomy with neoglottic and neopharyngeal reconstruction. Am J Surg 158:321, 1989.

294. Harrison DFN and Thompson AE: Pharyngolaryngoesophagectomy with pharyngogastric anastomosis for cancer of the hypopharynx: review of 101 operations. Head Neck Surg 8:418, 1986.

295. Flynn MB, Banis J, and Acland R: Reconstruction with free bowel autografts after pharyngoesophageal or laryngopharyngoesophageal resection. Am J Surg 158:333, 1989.

296. Smith PG and Collins SL: Repair of head and neck defects with "thin" and double-lined pectoralis flaps. Arch Otolaryngol Head Neck Surg 110:468, 1984.

297. McConnel FMS, et al: Analysis of pressure generation and bolus transit during pharyngeal swallowing. Laryngoscope 98:71, 1988.

298. Gaffey MJ and Weiss LM: Viral oncogenesis: Epstein-Barr virus. Am J Otolaryngol 11:375, 1990.

299. Buell P: The effect of migration on the risk of nasopharyngeal cancer among Chinese. Cancer Res 34:1189, 1974.

300. Papavasilou C, Pavlatou M, and Pappas J: Nasopharyngeal cancer in patients under the age of 30 years. Cancer 40:2312, 1977.

301. Ho JHC: The natural history and treatment of nasopharyngeal carcinoma. In: Oncology. Vol 4. Edited by Lee-Clark R, Cumley RW, McKay JE, and Copeland M. Chicago, Year Book, 1970, p 1.

302. Ho JHC: Stage classification of nasopharyngeal carcinoma: a review. In: Nasopharyngeal Carcinoma: Etiology and Control. Edited by DeThe G and Ito Y. IARC Scientific Publication No. 20. Lyon, International Agency for Research on Cancer, 1978, p 99.

303. Neel III HB and Taylor WF: New staging system for nasopharyngeal carcinoma: long-term outcome. Arch Otolaryngol Head Neck Surg 115:1293, 1989.

304. Old LJ, et al: Precipitating antibody in human serum to an antigen present in cultured Burkett's lymphoma cells. Proc Natl Acad Sci USA 56:1699, 1966.

305. zur Hausen H, et al: EBV DNA and biopsies of Burkett tumors and anaplastic carcinomas of the nasopharynx. Nature 228: 1056, 1970.

306. Feinmesser R, et al: Diagnosis of nasopharyngeal carcinoma by DNA amplification of tissue obtained by fine-needle aspiration. N Engl J Med 326:17, 1992.

307. Wei WI: Eugene Myers Lecture: nasopharyngeal carcinoma. Otolaryngol Head Neck Surg, in press.

308. Neel III HB, et al: Application of Epstein-Barr virus serology to the diagnosis and staging of North American patients with nasopharyngeal carcinoma. Otolaryngol Head Neck Surg 91: 255, 1983.

309. Neel III HB, Taylor WF, and Pearson GR: Prognostic determinants and a new view of staging for patients with nasopharyngeal carcinoma. Ann Otol 94:529, 1985.

310. Dawson CW, Rickinson AB, and Young LS: Epstein-Barr virus latent membrane protein inhibits human epithelial cell differentiation. Nature 344:777, 1990.

311. Desuiky S, Voelkerding K, and Gilbert-Barness E: Pathological case of the month: nasopharyngeal carcinoma. Am J Dis Child 147:75, 1993.

312. Geneva, 1991, International Histological Classification of Tumors: Histological typing of oral and oropharyngeal tumors. WHO Abstract, Scandinavian Society for Head and Neck Oncology. Clin Otolaryngol 19:172, 1994.

313. Pryzant RM, Wendt CD, Delclos L, and Peters LJ: Retreatment of nasopharyngeal carcinoma in 53 patients. Int J Radiat Oncol Biol Phys 22:941, 1992.

314. Zarate-Osorno A, Jaffe ES, and Medeiros LJ: Metastatic nasopharyngeal carcinoma initially presenting as cervical lymphadenopathy: a report of two cases that resembled Hodgkin's disease. Arch Pathol Lab Med 116:862, 1992.

315. Sham JS, Chung YK, and Choy D: Cranial nerve involvement and base of skull erosion in nasopharyngeal carcinoma. Cancer 68:422, 1991.

316. Ruprecht A and Dolan KD: The nasopharynx in oral and maxillofacial radiology. II. Malignant lesions. Oral Surg Oral Med Oral Path 75:106, 1993.

317. Trotter W: On certian clinically obscure malignant tumours of the naso-pharyngeal wall. Br Med J 2:1057, 1911.

318. Mineura K, Kowada M, and Tomura N: Perineural extension of nasopharyngeal carcinoma into the posterior cranial fossa detected by magnetic resonance imaging: clinical Imaging 15: 172, 1991.

319. Miura T, et al: Computed tomographic findings of nasopharyngeal carcinoma with skull base and intracranial involvement. Cancer 65:29, 1990.

320. Sham JST and Choy B: The prognostic value of paranasopharyngeal extension of nasopharyngeal carcinoma on local control and short-term survival. Head Neck Surg *13*:298, 1991.

321. Stillwagon GB, et al: Response of cranial nerve abnormalities in nasopharyngeal carcinoma to radiation therapy. Cancer *57*:2272, 1986.

322. Jing JS: Tumors of the nasopharynx. Radiol Clin North Am *8*:323, 1970.

323. Ho HJC: Epidemiologic and clinical study of nasopharyngeal carcinoma. Int J Radiat Biol Phys *4*:181, 1978.

324. Sham JST, Cho ID, and Wei WI: Nasopharyngeal carcinoma: orderly neck node spread. Int J Radiat Oncol Biol Phys *19*:929, 1990a.

325. Sham JST, et al: Nasopharyngeal carcinoma: pattern of tumor regression after radiotherapy. Cancer *64*:216, 1990.

326. Sham JST and Choy B: Prognostic factors of nasopharyngeal carcinoma: a review of 759 patients. Br J Radiol *63*:51, 1990.

327. Lee AWM, et al: Retrospective analysis of 5037 patients with nasopharyngeal carcinoma treated during 1976 to 1985: overall survival and patterns of failure. Int J Radiat Oncol Biol Phys *23*:261, 1992.

328. Hopping SB, Goodman ML, Keller JD, and Montgomery WW: Nasopharyngeal masses in adults: Geneva, World Health Organization. Ann Otol Rhinol Laryngol *92*:137, 1983.

329. Ho JHC: Radiologic diagnosis of nasopharyneal cancer. JAMA *220*:396, 1972.

330. Kao SH, et al: The detection of nasopharynx carcinoma on Technetium-99m (V) dimercaptosuccinate acid SPECT imaging. Clin Nucl Med *4*:321, 1993.

331. Neel III HB: Nasopharyngeal carcinoma. Otol Clin North Am *18*:479, 1985.

332. Perez CA, et al: Carcinoma of the nasopharynx: factors affecting prognosis. Int J Radiat Oncol Biol Phys *23*:271, 1992.

333. Barrios NJ: Childhood nasopharyngeal carcinoma. J LA State Med Soc *145*:151, 1993.

334. Mancuso AA, Harnsburger HR, Muraki AS, and Stevens MH: Computed tomography of cervical and retropharyngeal lymph nodes: normal anatomy, variants of normal, and applications in staging head and neck cancer. Part II: Pathology, radiology *148*:715, 1983.

335. Lee WM, Sham JST, Poon YF, and Ho JHC: Treatment of stage I nasopharyngeal carcinoma: analysis of the pattern of relapse and the results of withholding elective neck irradiation. Int J eRadiat Oncol Biol Phys *17*:1183, 1989.

336. Mestre M and Modig H: Radiotherapy of nasopharyngeal carcinoma: is prophylactic neck irradiation necessary? (Abstract.) Scandinavian Society for Head and Neck Oncology. Clin Otolaryngol *19*:172, 1994.

337. Sham JST, Choy B, and Choi PHK: Nasopharyngeal carcinoma: the significance of neck node involvement in relation to the pattern of distant failure. Br J Radiol *63*:108, 1990.

338. Sham JST and Choy B: Nasopharyngeal carcinoma treatment of neck node recurrence by radiotherapy. Australas Radiol *33*:370, 1991.

339. Wei WI, et al: Efficacy of radical neck dissection for the control of cervical metastases after radiotherapy for nasopharyngeal carcinoma. Am J Surg *160*:439, 1990.

340. Tu GY, Hu YH, Xu GZ, and Yu M: Salvage surgery for nasopharyngeal carcinoma. Arch Otolaryngol Head Neck Surg *114*:328, 1988.

340a. Wei WI, et al: Pathological basis of surgery in the management of postradiotherapy cervical metastasis in nasopharyngeal carcinoma. Arch Otolaryngol Head Neck Surg *118*:923, 1992.

341. Ho YH, Chan M, Tsao SY, and Lee LY: Treatment of residual and recurrent cervical metastases from nasopharyngeal carcinoma. Ann Acad Med Singapore *17*:22, 1988.

342. Tung WWK and Teo PML: Patterns of failure after radical neck dissection for recurrent nasopharyngeal carcinoma. Am J Surg *164*:599, 1992.

343. Wang CC. Re-irradiation for recurrent nasopharyngeal carcinoma: treatment techniques and results. Int J Radiat Oncol Biol Phys *13*:952, 1987.

344. Gong QY, Zheng GJ, and Zhu HY: MRI differentiation of recurrent nasopharyngeal carcinoma from post-radiation fibrosis. Comput Med Image Graph *15*:423, 1991.

345. Nicholls JM, et al: Radiation therapy for nasopharyngeal carcinoma: histological appearances and patterns of tumor regression. Hum Pathol *23*:742, 1992.

346. Yan JH, et al: Management of local residual primary lesion of nasopharyngeal carcinoma. II. Results of prospective randomized trial on booster dose. Int J Radiat Oncol Biol Phys *18*:295, 1990.

347. Harrison LB, et al: Nasopharyngeal brachytherapy with access via a transpalatal flap. Am J Surg *164*:173, 1992.

348. Russell JD, Bleach NR, Glaser M, and Cheesman AD: Brachytherapy for recurrent nasopharyngeal and nasoethmoidal tumours. J Laryngol Otol *107*:115, 1993.

349. Yumoto E, Okamura H, and Yanigihara N: Transmandibular transpterygoid approach to the nasopharynx, parapharyngeal space, and skull base. Ann Otol Rhinol Laryngol *101*:383, 1992.

350. Morton RP, Woollons AC, and McIvor NP: Nasopharyngeal carcinoma and middle ear effusion: natural history and the effect of ventilation tubes. Clin Otolaryngol *19*:529, 1994.

351. Tannock I, et al: Sequential chemotherapy and radiation for nasopharyngeal cancer: absence of long-term benefit despite a high rate of tumor response to chemotherapy. J Clin Oncol *5*:629, 1987.

352. Al-Sarraf M, Pajak TF, and Cooper JS: Chemoradiotherapy in patients with locally advanced nasopharyngeal carcinoma: a Radiation Therapy Oncology Group study. J Clin Oncol *8*:1342, 1990.

353. Peters LJ, et al: Acute and late toxicity associated with sequential platinum-containing chemotherapy regimens and radiation therapy in the treatment of carcinoma of the nasopharynx. Int J Radiat Oncol Biol Phys *14*:623, 1988.

354. Choi KN, et al: Locally advanced paranasal sinus and nasopharynx tumors treated with hyperfractionated radiation and concomitant infusions with cisplatin. Cancer *67*:2745, 1991.

355. Azli N, et al: Alternating chemoradiotherapy with cis-platin and 5-fluorouracil plus bleomycin by continuous infusion for locally advanced undifferentiated carcinoma nasopharyngeal type. Eur J Cancer *28A*:1792, 1992.

357. Rousselet G, et al: Structure and regulation of the blas-2/CD23 antigen in epithelial cells from nasopharyngeal carcinoma. Int Immunol *2*:1159, 1990.

358. Mahé Y, et al: Heterogeneity among human nasopharyngeal carcinoma cell lines for inflammatory cytokine mRNA expression levels. Biochem Biophys Res Commun *27*:121, 1992.

359. Cheng DS, et al: DNA content in nasopharyngeal carcinoma. Am J Otolaryngol *11*:393, 1990.

360. Shu MM, Ko JY, and Cheng YL: Elevated levels of interleukin-2 receptor and tumor necrosis factor in nasopharyngeal carcinoma. Arch Otolaryngol Head Neck Surg *117*:1257, 1991.

361. Mahjoubi R, et al: Phase II trial of recombinant interferon gamma in refractory undifferentiated carcinoma of the nasopharynx. Head Neck Surg *15*:115, 1993.

362. American Joint Committee on Cancer: Manual for Staging of Cancer. 4th Ed. Philadelphia, JB Lippincott, 1992.

363. Fletcher GH and Million RR: Malignant tumors of the nasopharynx. Am J Roentgenol Radiat Ther *93*:44, 1965.

364. International Union Against Cancer TNM Classification of Malignant Tumors. 4th Ed. New York, Springer-Verlag, 1987.

365. Fee Jr WE, Gilmer PA, and Goffinet BR: Surgical management of recurrent nasopharyngeal carcinoma after radiation failure at the primary site. Laryngoscope *98*:1220, 1988.

366. Pannik I, Pain ED, and Cummings B: Sequential chemotherapy and radiation for nasopharyngeal cancer: absence of long-term benefit despite a high rate of tumor response to chemotherapy. J Clin Oncol 5:629, 1987.

367. Wei WI: A comparison of clinical staging systems in nasopharyngeal carcinoma. Clin Oncol 10:225, 1984.

368. Yeh S: A histological classification of carcinoma in the nasopharynx with a critical review as to the existence of lymphoepitheliomas. Cancer 15:895, 1962.

369. McConnel FMS: Treatment of posterior wall carcinoma. Otolaryngol Head Neck Surg 94:287, 1986.

370. Teichgraber J, Bowman J, and Goepfert H: New test series for the functional evaluation of oral cavity cancer. Head Neck Surg 8:9, 1985.

371. Doberneck RC and Antoine JE: Deglutition after resection of oral, larynx and pharynx cancers (functional analysis system). Surgery 75:87, 1974.

372. Conley JJ: Swallowing dysfunction associated with radical surgery of the head and neck. Arch Surg 80:602, 1960.

373. Conley JJ and Seaman W: Function in the crippled laryngopharynx. Ann Otol Rhinol Laryngol 72:441, 1963.

374. Bakamjian VY: A two-stage method for pharyngoesophageal reconstruction with a primary pectoral skin flap. Plast Reconstr Surg 36:173, 1965.

375. Sofferman RA: Unusual uses of the deltopectoral flap. Laryngoscope 89:1326, 1979.

376. Gilmore BB and Olson NR: The omocervical flap. Arch Otolaryngol Head Neck Surg 105:589, 1979.

377. Smith CJ: The deltoscapular flap. Arch Otolaryngol 104:390, 1978.

378. Ariyan S and Cuono CB: Myocutaneous flaps for head and neck reconstruction. Head Neck Surg 2:321, 1980.

379. Panje WR: Myocutaneous trapezius flap. Head Neck Surg 2:206, 1980.

380. Sasaki CT: The sternocleidomastoid myocutaneous flap. Arch Otolaryngol Head Neck Surg 106:74, 1980.

381. Shestak KC, Myers EN, and Ramasastry SS: Vascularized free-tissue transfer in head and neck surgery. Am J Otolaryngol 14:148, 1993.

381a. Schramm VL, Johnson JT, and Myers EN: Skin grafts and flaps in oral cavity construction. Arch Otolaryngol Head Neck Surg 109:175, 1983.

382. McGregor IA and McGrowther DA: Skin-graft reconstruction in carcinoma of the tongue. Head Neck Surg 1:47, 1978.

383. La Ferriere KA, et al: Composite resection and reconstruction for oral cavity and oropharynx cancer: a functional approach. Arch Otolaryngol Head Neck Surg 106:103, 1980.

384. Schramm VL and Myers EN: Skin graft reconstruction following composite resection. Laryngoscope 91:1737, 1980.

385. Conley JJ, et al: The use of tongue flaps in head and neck surgery. Surgery 41:745, 1957.

386. Sharzer LA, et al: Intraoral reconstruction in head and neck cancer surgery. Clin Plast Surg 3:495, 1976.

387. Druck NS and Lurton J: Repair of anterior floor of mouth defects: the island pedicle tongue flap. Laryngoscope 88:1372, 1978.

388. Komisar A and Lawson W: A compendium of intraoral flaps. Head Neck Surg 8:91, 1985.

389. Tiwari R and Snow GB: Repair of intraoral defects with masseter flap after cancer surgery. Head Neck Surg 10:530, 1988.

390. Conley JJ, Lanier DM, and Tinsley P: Platysma myocutaneous flap revisited. Arch Otolaryngol Head Neck Surg 112:711, 1986.

391. Cannon CR, et al: Reconstruction of the oral cavity using the platysma myocutaneous flap. Arch Otolaryngol Head Neck Surg 108:491, 1982.

392. Lee KY and Loré JM Jr: Two modifications of the pectoralis major myocutaneous flap (PMMF). Laryngoscope 96:363, 1986.

393. Soutar DS, et al: The radial forearm flap: a versatile method for intraoral reconstruction. Br J Plast Surg 36:1, 1983.

394. Meland NB, et al: Experience with 80 rectus abdominis free-tissue transfers. Plast Reconstr Surg 83:481, 1979.

395. Antonyshyn O, et al: Tissue expansion in head and neck reconstruction. Plast Reconstr Surg 82:58, 1988.

396. Gullane PJ and Holmes H: Mandibular reconstruction: new concepts. Arch Otolaryngol Head Neck Surg 112:714, 1986.

397. Castillo MH, Button TM, and Doerr R: Effects of radiation therapy on mandibular reconstruction plates. Am J Surg 156:261, 1988.

398. Urken ML, et al: The internal oblique iliac crest osseomyocutaneous free flap in oromandibular reconstruction: a report of 20 cases. Arch Otolaryngol Head Neck Surg 115:339, 1989.

399. Tjellstrom A: Osseointegrated systems and their applications in the head and neck. In: Advances in Otolaryngology—Head Neck Surg. Vol 3. Edited by Myers EN. Chicago, Year Book, 1989, p 39.

400. Hellems S, and Olofsson J: Titanium-coated hollow screw and reconstruction plate system (THORP) in mandibular reconstruction. J Craniomaxillofac Surg 16:173, 1988.

401. Sanger JR, Head MD, and Matloub MS: Enhancement of rehabilitation by use of implantable adjuncts with vascularized bone grafts for mandibular reconstruction. Am J Surg 156:243, 1988.

402. Urken ML, et al: Primary placement of osseointegrated implants in microvascular mandibular reconstruction. Otolaryngol Head Neck Surg 101:56, 1989.

403. Conley JJ, Sachs ME, and Parke RB: The new tongue. Otolaryngol Head Neck Surg 90:58, 1982.

404. Rontal E and Rontal M: Lesions of the hypoglossal nerve: diagnosis, treatment and rehabilitation. Laryngoscope 92:927, 1982.

405. Brookes GB: Nutritional status: a prognosticator in head and neck cancer. Otolaryngol Head Neck Surg 93:69, 1985.

406. Williams EF III and Meguid MM: Nutritional concepts and considerations in head and neck surgery. Head Neck Surg 11:393, 1989.

407. Shaw JHF, Humberstone DA, and Holdaway C: Weight loss in head and neck cancer: malnutrition or tumour effect? Aust NZ J Surg 58:505, 1988.

408. Hybels RL: Venous air embolism in head and neck surgery. Laryngoscope 90:946, 1980.

409. Gullane PJ and Marsh AS: Bilateral spontaneous chylothorax presenting as a neck mass. J Otolaryngol 13:255, 1984.

410. Rontal M and Rontal E: Lesions of the vagus nerve: diagnosis, treatment and rehabilitation. Laryngoscope 87:72, 1977.

411. Collins SL: The cervical sympathetics in surgery of the neck. Otolaryngol Head Neck Surg 105:544, 1991.

412. Johnson JT and Yu W: Antibiotic use during major head and neck surgery. Ann Surg 207:108, 1988.

413. Jones TR, et al: Efficacy of antibiotic mouthwash in contaminated head and neck surgery. Am J Surg 158:324, 1989.

414. Freeland AD and Rogers JH: The vascular supply of the cervical skin with reference to incision planning. Laryngoscope 85:714, 1975.

415. MacFee WF: Transverse incisions for neck dissection. Ann Surg 151:279, 1960.

416. Myers EN: The management of pharyngocutaneous fistula. Arch Otolaryngol Head Neck Surg 95:10, 1972.

417. Bellinger CG: Classification of pharyngostomas: a guideline for closure. Plast Reconstr Surg 47:54, 1971.

418. Mamikunian C, Collins SL, and Matz GJ: Decreasing fistulas in radiated head and neck cancer patients with autologous fibrin seal. Submitted for publication.

419. Innes AJ, et al: The role of metronidazole in the prevention of fistulas following total laryngectomy. Clin Oncol 6:71, 1980.

420. Fajardo LF and Lee A: Rupture of major vessels after radiation. Cancer 36:904, 1975.

421. Stell PM: Catastrophic hemorrhage after major neck surgery. Br J Surg 56:525, 1969.

422. Gall AM, et al: Complications following surgery for cancer of the larynx and hypopharynx. Cancer 39:624, 1977.

423. Miller DR and Bergstrom L: Vascular complications of head and neck surgery. Arch Otolaryngol Head Neck Surg 100:136, 1974.

424. Conomy JP and Kellermyer RW: Delayed cerebrovascular consequences of therapeutic radiation. Cancer 36:1702, 1975.

425. Cheng VST and Schulz MD: Unilateral hypoglossal nerve atrophy as a late complication of radiation therapy of head and neck carcinoma: a report of four cases and a review of the literature on peripheral and cranial nerve damage after radiation therapy. Cancer 35:1537, 1975.

425a.Hart GB and Mainous EG: The treatment of radiation necrosis with hyperbaric oxygen. Cancer 37:2580, 1976.

426. Feder B Jr, et al: The effect of hyperbaric oxygen on pulmonary metastasis in C3H mice. Radiology 90:1181, 1968.

427. McMillan T, et al: The effect of hyperbaric oxygen on oral mucosal carcinoma. Laryngoscope 99:241, 1989.

428. Beumer J III, et al: Radiation therapy of the oral cavity: Sequelae and management. Parts I and II. Head Neck Surg 1:301, 1979.

429. Carl W, et al: Oral care of patients irradiated for cancer of the head and neck. Cancer 30:448, 1972.

430. Carl R, et al: Dental management and prosthetic rehabilitation of patients with head and neck cancer. Head Neck Surg 3:27, 1980.

431. Bedwinek JM, et al: Osteonecrosis in patients treated with definitive radiation therapy for squamous cell carcinoma of the oral cavity and naso- and oropharynx. Radiology 11:665, 1976.

432. Bras J, de Jonge HKT, and van Merkesteyn JPR: Osteoradionecrosis of the mandible: pathogenesis. Am J Otolaryngol 11:244, 1990.

433. Klein JC: Transoral mandibulectomy in advanced osteoradionecrosis. Head Neck Surg 2:160, 1979.

434. Tami TA, et al: Thyroid dysfunction after radiotherapy in head and neck cancer patients. Am J Otolaryngol 13:357, 1992.

435. Goodwin WJ and Chandler JR: Hypercalcemia in epidermoid carcinoma of the head and neck. Am J Surg 132:444, 1976.

436. Minotti Am, Kountakis SE, and Stiernberg CM: Paraneoplastic syndromes in patients with head and neck cancer. Am J Otolaryngol 15:336, 1994.

437. Talmi YP, Hoffman HT, and McCabe BF: Syndrome of inappropriate secretion of arginine vasopressin in patients with cancer of the head and neck. Ann Otol Rhinol Laryngol 101:946, 1992.

438. Conley JJ (ed): Complications of Head and Neck Surgery. Philadelphia, WB Saunders, 1979.

439. Olson ML and Shedd DP: Disability and rehabilitation in head and neck cancer patients after treatment. Head Neck Surg 1:52, 1978.

440. Summers GW: Physiological problems following ablative surgery of the head and neck. Otolaryngol Clin North Am 7:217, 1974.

441. Logemann JA: Evaluation and Treatment of Swallowing Disorders. San Diego, College-Hill Press, 1983.

FURTHER SUGGESTED READINGS

General

Sessions DG, et al (eds): Atlas of Access and Reconstruction in Head and Neck Surgery. St. Louis, Mosby-Year Book, 1992.

Gingiva

Lerheim TA, Kolbenstvedt A, and Lien HH: Carcinoma of the maxillary gingiva: occurrence of jaw destruction. Scand J Dent Res 92:235, 1984.

Martin HE: Cancer of the gums: Am J Surg 54:769, 1941.

Nathanson A, et al: Prognosis of squamous cell carcinoma of the gums. Acta Otolaryngol (Stockh) 15:301, 1973.

Soo KC, Spiro RH, and King W: Squamous carcinoma of the gums. Am J Surg 156:281, 1988.

Buccal Mucosa

Vegers JW, Snow GB, and Waal IV. Squamous cell carcinoma of the buccal mucosa. Arch Otolaryngol 97:220, 1973

Palate

Esche BA, et al: Interstitial and external radiation therapy in carcinoma of the soft palate and uvula. Int J Radiat Oncol Biol Phys 15:619, 1988.

Ildstad ST, Bigelow ME, and Remensynder JP: Squamous cell carcinoma of the alveolar ridge and palate: a 15-year survey. Ann Surg 199:445, 1984.

Jacques DJ: Epidermoid carcinoma of the palate. Otolaryngol Clin North Am 12:125, 1979.

Konrad HR, Canalis RF, and Calcaterra TC: Epidermoid carcinoma of the palate. Arch Otolaryngol Head Neck Surg 104:208, 1978.

Russ JE, Applebaum EL, and Sisson GA: Squamous cell carcinoma of the palate. Laryngoscope 87:1151, 1977.

Floor of Mouth

Flynn MB, et al: Selection of treatment in squamous carcinoma of the floor of mouth. Am J Surg 126:477, 1973.

Fu KK, Lichter A, and Gallente M: Cancer of the floor of mouth: analysis of treatment results and the sites and causes of failure. Int J Radiat Oncol Biol Phys 1:829, 1976.

Guillamondequi OM, et al: Carcinoma of the anterior floor of mouth: selective choice of treatment and analysis of failures. Am J Surg 140:560, 1980.

Harrold CC Jr: Management of cancer of the floor of mouth. Am J Surg 122:487, 1971.

Martin HE and Sugarbaker EL: Cancer of the floor of mouth. Surg Gynecol Obstet 71:347, 1940.

Schramm VL, et al: Surgical management of early epidermoid carcinoma of the anterior floor of mouth. Laryngoscope 90:207, 1980.

Tongue

Bradfield JS and Scruggs RP: Carcinoma of the mobile tongue: incidence of cervical metastases in early lesions relative to method of primary treatment. Laryngoscope 93:1332, 1983.

Donaldson RC, Skelly M, and Paletta F: Total glossectomy for cancer. Am J Surg 116:585, 1969.

Dupont JB, et al: Surgical treatment of advanced carcinoma of the base of tongue. Am J Surg 136:501, 1978

Effron MS, et al: Advanced carcinoma of the tongue. Arch Otolaryngol Head Neck Surg 107:694, 1981.

Gilbert HE, et al: Carcinoma of the oral tongue and floor of mouth: 15 years experience with linear acceleration therapy. Cancer 35:1517, 1975.

Johnson JT, et al: Management of T1 carcinoma of the anterior aspect of the tongue. Arch Otolaryngol Head Neck Surg 106:249, 1980.

Keyserlingk JR, et al: Recent experience with reconstructive surgery following major glossectomy. Arch Otolaryngol Head Neck Surg 115:331, 1989.

Kothary PM, Paymaster JC, and Potdar GG: Radical total glossectomy. Br J Surg 61:209, 1974.

Marks JE, et al: Carcinoma of the oral tongue: a study of patient selection and treatment results. Laryngoscope 91:1548, 1981.

Martin H: The history of lingual cancer. Am J Surg 48:703, 1940.

Martin H, Munster H, and Sugarbaker ED: Cancer of the tongue. Arch Surg 41:888, 1946.

Parsons JT, Million R, and Cassisi NJ: Carcinoma of the base of tongue: results of radical irradiation with surgery reserved for irradiation failure. Laryngoscope 92:689, 1982.

Rollo J, et al: Squamous carcinoma of the base of tongue. Cancer 47: 333, 1980.

White D and Byers RM: What is the preferred initial method of treatment of squamous carcinoma of the tongue? Am J Surg 140: 553, 1980.

Whitehurst JO and Droulias CA: Surgical treatment of squamous cell carcinoma of the oral tongue: factors influencing survival. Arch Otolaryngol Head Neck Surg 103:212, 1977.

Oropharynx

Barrs DM, et al: Squamous cell carcinoma of the tonsil and tongue-base region. Arch Otolaryngol Head Neck Surg 105:479, 1979.

Jesse RH and Sugarbaker EV: Squamous carcinoma of the oropharynx: why we fail. Am J Surg 132:435, 1976.

Kaplan R, et al: Carcinoma of the tonsil: results of radical irradiation with surgery reserved for radiation failure. Laryngoscope 87: 600, 1977.

Maltz R, et al: Carcinoma of the tonsil: results of combined therapy. Laryngoscope 84:2172, 1974.

Perez CA, et al: Carcinoma of the tonsil: sequential comparison of four treatment modalities. Radiology 94:649, 1970.

Quenelle DJ, et al: Tonsil carcinoma: treatment results. Laryngoscope 89:1842, 1979.

Rolander TL, et al: Carcinoma of the tonsil: a planned combined therapy approach. Laryngoscope 81:1199, 1971.

Shumrick DA and Quenelle DJ: Malignant disease of the tonsillar region, retromolar trigone and buccal mucosa. Otolaryngol Clin North Am 12:115, 1979.

Whicker JH, et al: Surgical treatment of squamous cell carcinoma of the tonsil. Laryngoscope 84:90, 1974.

Pharynx

Ballantyne AJ: Principles of surgical management of cancer of the pharyngeal walls. Cancer 20:633, 1967.

Beekhuis GJ and Croushore JE: Surgical approach to neoplasms of the mesopharynx. Laryngoscope 73:519, 1963.

Cunningham MP and Catlin D: Cancer of the pharyngeal wall. Cancer 20:1859, 1967.

Harris PF, et al: Lateral pharyngotomy approach for lesions of the base of tongue, pharynx and larynx. South Med J 61:1276, 1968.

McNeill R: Surgical management of carcinoma of the posterior pharyngeal wall. Head Neck Surg 3:389, 1981.

Orton HB: Lateral transthyroid pharyngotomy: Trotter's operation for malignant disease of the pharynx. Arch Otolaryngol 12:320, 1930.

Trotter W: Operations for malignant disease of the pharynx. Br J Surg 16:82, 1928.

Trotter W: Principles and techniques of the operative treatment of malignant disease of the mouth and pharynx. Lancet 1:1075, 1913.

Wilkins SA: Carcinoma of the posterior pharyngeal wall. Am J Surg 122:477, 1971.

Nasopharynx

Lederman M: Cancer of the Nasopharynx: Its Natural History and Treatment. Springfield, IL, Charles C Thomas, 1961.

Van Hassett CA and Gibb AG: Nasopharyngeal Carcinoma. Hong Kong, Chinese University Press, 1991.

Neck

Beahrs OH and Barber KW: The value of radical dissection of structures of the neck in the management of carcinoma of the lip, mouth and pharynx. Arch Surg 85:49, 1962.

Crile GC: Excision of cancer of the head and neck with special reference to the plan of dissection based on one hundred and thirty two operations. JAMA 47:1780, 1906.

Jesse RH, et al: Cancer of the oral cavity: is elective neck dissection beneficial? Am J Surg 120:505, 1970.

21 Diagnosis and Treatment of Facial Fractures

Jonathan M. Sykes and Paul J. Donald

The successful management of the patient with facial injuries and fractures requires a multisystem approach. Initial attention should be devoted to establishing a secure airway and to maintaining hemodynamic stability.[1] After the patient's condition has been stabilized, careful physical and radiographic examination of the cervical spine must be performed to rule out cervical spine injury. At this point, a systematic evaluation of other important systems is performed.

Treatment of the patient with facial trauma should include a thorough history and physical examination to determine the location and extent of all injuries.[2] Both soft tissue and bony injuries should be assessed, and a treatment plan should be established. The goals of treatment should be the restoration of function and appearance. The premorbid form and function of dental, skeletal, and soft tissues should be reestablished if possible.

The goal of treatment of patients with craniomaxillofacial injuries should be reconstitution of all injured regions.[3] Attention must be paid to both soft tissue and skeletal injuries. If the initial injury involves skin or mucosal lacerations, attempts should be made to utilize these lacerations when possible. If no epithelial injury is present, approaches to fractures should attempt to maximize exposure, while minimizing scarring and risk to adjacent neurovascular structures.

Treatment of the patient with a facial fracture includes stabilization of the patient's condition, establishment of a secure airway, accurate diagnosis of all fractures, and careful reduction and fixation of fracture segments. Accurate diagnosis of facial fractures depends on a careful history, physical examination, and appropriate radiologic studies. The diagnosis should be strongly suspected after the physical examination, which should include inspection of the facial contour, the dental occlusion, and a complete neurologic exami-

nation. All facial bones should be palpated to evaluate symmetry and contour. Radiologic examination should be used to confirm suspected skeletal fractures.

After fracture diagnosis is completed, a systematic treatment plan is established. Surgical treatment of facial fractures involves adequate exposure, meticulous reduction, and stable fracture fixation. Surgical approaches should utilize transmucosal incisions or incisions that are camouflaged in relaxed skin tension lines (RSTL) or at junctions of facial aesthetic units.[4] Of course, the incisions and approach chosen must not compromise the basic principle of providing adequate exposure for diagnosis and treatment of the given fracture. After exposing the facial fracture, meticulous reduction must be performed and maintained until the fracture can be adequately fixated. Precise reduction is imperative when rigid fixation is utilized. Fixation techniques should allow for complete bone healing with reconstitution of all facial buttresses. The facial skeleton should be reconstituted in three dimensions: height (superior-inferior), width (lateral-medial), and depth or projection (anterior-posterior).

Repair of soft tissue injuries is often as important as fracture treatment in the complete restoration of the patient with craniomaxillofacial injuries. This is especially true in the periorbital region, where injuries such as telecanthus, enophthalmos, and diplopia often accompany the skeletal injury. Complete treatment of facial injuries requires attention to these soft tissue injuries and accurate reattachment of soft tissue fascial layers after fracture repair.

The basic principles of diagnosis and initial treatment of patients with facial fractures are listed in Table 21–1. The principles of fracture repair are listed in Table 21–2. Adherence to these basic principles will maximize function and appearance.

The key to proper fracture reduction is the restora-

TABLE 21–1. Principles of Diagnosis and Initial Treatment of Facial Fractures

Establishment and securing of airway
Control of bleeding
Detailed history
Careful physical examination
Radiologic studies

TABLE 21–2. Principles of Fracture Repair

Repair of both skeletal and soft tissue injuries
Use of lacerations when possible
Use of mucosal incisions when possible
Exposure of all fractures adequately for fracture reduction
Reduction of all fractures
Stabilization of fractures
Fixation of all fractures adequately to allow bone healing

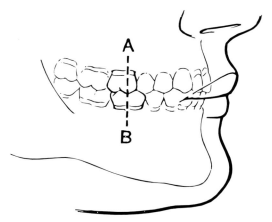

Fig. 21–2. Class I occlusion. A. Mesial buccal cusp of first molar. B. Buccal intercuspal groove of mandibular first molar. (From Donald PJ: The Surgical Management of Structural Facial Dysharmony: A Self-Instructional Package No. 85100. Washington, D.C., American Academy of Otolaryngology—Head and Neck Surgery, 1985, p 13.)

tion of the patient's premorbid occlusion. The understanding of dental occlusion is an essential element in the management of facial fractures.

DENTAL OCCLUSION

Dental occlusion, simply stated, is the relationship of the maxillary with the mandibular teeth. The most important functional relationship is that of their cutting and grinding surfaces. This relationship largely depends on the relative position of the teeth and their angulation to one another. In 1899, Angle described three basic types of occlusion.[5] Certain subtypes of this system, as well as other classifications of occlusion, have been devised, sometimes adding to the confusion rather than clarifying the problem. In the Angle system, the reference point is the relationship of the first

maxillary molar tooth with the mandibular molar tooth below it. Each molar commonly has four grinding surfaces, called cusps. The cusps adjacent to the tongue are called lingual, and those adjacent to the cheek, buccal. Those cusps situated toward the oropharynx in the posterior aspect of the oral cavity are described as distal, and those located more anteriorly are mesial (Fig. 21–1).

Class I occlusion is the ideal form (Fig. 21–2). In this type, the mesial buccal cusp of the first maxillary molar fits in the groove on the lateral or buccal surface of the first mandibular molar tooth. The buccal cusps of the maxillary teeth overlap the buccal surfaces of the mandibular molars.

In class II occlusion, the mesial buccal cusp of the

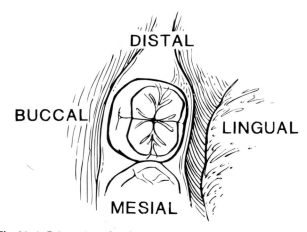

Fig. 21–1. Orientation of molar cusp. (From Donald PJ: The Surgical Management of Structural Facial Dysharmony: A Self-Instructional Package No. 85100. Washington, D.C., American Academy of Otolaryngology—Head and Neck Surgery, 1985, p 12.)

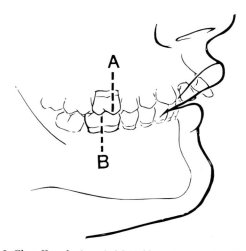

Fig. 21–3. Class II occlusion. A. Mesial buccal cusp of first molar. B. Buccal intercuspal groove of mandibular first molar. (From Donald PJ: The Surgical Management of Structural Facial Dysharmony: A Self-Instructional Package No. 85100. Washington, D.C., American Academy of Otolaryngology—Head and Neck Surgery, 1985, p 14.)

first maxillary molar is mesial, or in front of the buccal groove of the first mandibular molar (Fig. 21–3). It may be over the mandibular molar's mesial cusp, or even between it and the second premolar (bicuspid). In class III occlusion, the reverse of class II is seen. The mesial buccal cusp of the first maxillary molar now sits over the corresponding mandibular molar's distal cusp, or between it and the second molar (Fig. 21–4).

Usually, these relationships are maintained in the remaining teeth as progression toward the anterior aspect of the dental arches occurs. In class II and III occlusion, this results in aberrations in the relationship of the incisor teeth that are reflected in characteristic facial deformities.

In class II, the mesial or anterior relationship of the maxillary teeth may result in a protrusion of the upper incisors beyond the lower. Not only does one see a jutting forward of these upper central teeth, a condition called overjet, but often the lower incisors bite more deeply toward the palate, a condition called overbite (Fig. 21–5). The profile this condition produces is described as the "buck tooth" or "weak chin" look. This look is caricatured in cartoons by such characters as Andy Gump and Sad Sack. If this condition comes about through the lack of mandibular development with a backward positioning of the lower jaw, it is called retrognathia. The set-back chin often prevents the upper lip from completely covering the upper incisor teeth. Lack of lip protection of the upper incisors caused by lip procumbency renders them more vulnerable to injury; fractured incisors are not an uncommon finding in this group.

In class III occlusion, the abnormal distal relationship of the maxillary molars, most commonly brought about by an abnormally protrusive mandible, trans-

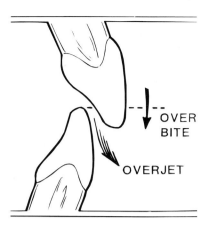

Fig. 21–5. Cuspal relationships of central maxillary incisor with central mandibular incisor. Direction of overbite and overjet are indicated (arrows). (From Donald PJ: The Surgical Management of Structural Facial Dysharmony: A Self-Instructional Package No. 85100. Washington, D.C., American Academy of Otolaryngology—Head and Neck Surgery, 1985, p 16.)

lates into a position of the maxillary incisors behind or distal to the mandibular incisors. This produces a so-called bulldog or Dick Tracy profile. The overbite results in the biting of the upper incisors into the gingival lingual sulcus below. The malocclusion is often so severe that the patient has an extremely difficult time chewing solid food. Often the occlusion of two or three cuspal pairs is all that is possible. In edentulous patients, it is often exceedingly difficult to fit them with a denture.

The opposite of the closed bite of overbite deformities may be seen in both class II and class III types of malocclusion. This so-called open bite deformity produces a marked functional disturbance and is extremely unsightly. Even though the molar teeth are in some form of apposition, the anterior teeth never meet.

Both class II and III malocclusions may come about from discrepancies in development of either the mandible or the maxilla. Class II may arise from an underdeveloped mandible or from an abnormally protuberant maxilla. Similarly, a class III bite may come about as the result of a large, overdeveloped mandible or a retruded or retroplaced maxilla. Retrognathia is classically used to describe a class II type of occlusion, and prognathism, the class III type.

In addition to aberrations in the anteroposterior relationship of the dentition are deformities involving malposition in a medial and lateral direction, as well as abnormalities involving a lateral tilt of the occlusal plane. The maxillary molar teeth, instead of having their buccal cusps positioned lateral to the buccal face of the opposing mandibular molars, may be biting end to end or even over the lingual cusps of these latter teeth (Fig. 21–6). This is called a lingual crossbite deformity. If both arches are symmetric, the maxillary molars of the opposing side will be put into a more buccal relationship with the opposing mandibular teeth, thereby creating a buccal crossbite on this particular side. Because an abnormality in the arch configuration of either or both of the dental arches is often present,

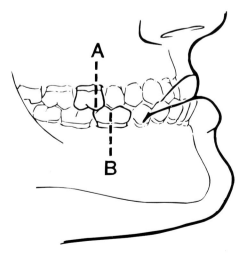

Fig. 21–4. Class III occlusion. A. Mesial buccal cusp of first molar. B. Buccal intercuspal groove of mandibular first molar. (From Donald PJ: The Surgical Management of Structural Facial Dysharmony: A Self-Instructional Package No. 85100. Washington, D.C., American Academy of Otolaryngology—Head and Neck Surgery, 1985, p 15.)

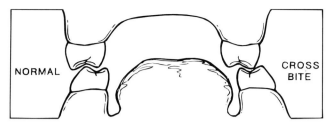

Fig. 21–6. Coronal view of oral cavity showing normal relationship (left) with maxillary buccal cusp related to buccal surface of underlying molar. Example of lingual crossbite is shown (right). (From Donald PJ: The Surgical Management of Structural Facial Dysharmony: A Self-Instructional Package No. 85100. Washington, D.C., American Academy of Otolaryngology—Head and Neck Surgery, 1985, p 16.)

it is not uncommon to have a crossbite on one side with a fairly normal occlusal relationship on the other. For instance, a narrow maxillary arch coupled with a fairly normal mandibular arch, such as that seen in Crouzon's disease, produces a bilateral lingual crossbite. As asymmetric mandibular arch, such as that seen in hemimandibular hypoplasia, often produces a buccal crossbite on one side and normal occlusion on the other. In patients with hypoplasia, the plane of the bite is commonly abnormal as well. These patients commonly have a diagonal bite, so when they bite down on a tongue blade placed laterally across the teeth, the blade tilts at an angle that is oblique to the horizontal plane (Fig. 21–7). Of course, it is not uncommon to see a combination of many of these occlusal abnormalities in any given patient.

PREOPERATIVE AND PERIOPERATIVE MANAGEMENT

Paramount in the management of facial fracture patients is control of the airway. Mandibular and maxillary fractures are often accompanied by lacerations, contusion, and hematomas within the upper airway. This is especially true of maxillary fractures, which are often accompanied by lacerations, contusions, and hematomas within the upper airway. In addition to the edema and suffusion of blood into the soft tissues of the oral cavity and pharynx are certain characteristics of these fractures that predispose the airway to compromise. In the Le Fort fractures of the maxilla, the pterygoid muscles tend to pull the disattached maxillary fragment toward their insertion on the mandible. This results in a posteroinferior displacement of bone that further narrows the airway.

Similarly, bilateral body fractures of the mandible may produce upper airway compromise by posteroinferior displacement of the anterior segment brought about by contraction of the geniohyoid, digastric, and geniohyoid muscles.

Airway control may necessitate tracheostomy. Forward traction on the anterior segment of a displaced bilateral body fracture of the mandible often relieves obstruction. Endotracheal intubation, especially through the nose, is an excellent alternative and provides an airway until the fracture has undergone fixation. Endotracheal intubation in maxillary fractures is often followed by tracheostomy. The endonasal route is dangerous in the presence of possible cranial floor fractures. Cerebrospinal fluid (CSF) leaks may be manifest at the time of initial fracture evaluation or may remain occult. Only careful scrutiny of the radiographs may lead to the diagnosis. Because high-quality films may not be present when the patient is first seen and the airway is compromised, the oral route of intubation or tracheostomy is preferred.

Because establishing premorbid occlusion is the primary goal of facial fracture reduction and fixation, an oral tube cannot be placed for delivery of anesthesia at the time of surgery. In mandibular fractures, a nasal tube is generally placed, and in Le Fort fractures, a tracheostomy is usually done. If the maxillary fracture is not too comminuted, or if the Le Fort is I type and the patient is cooperative and compliant, consideration of interosseous plate fixation without intermaxillary fixation may be entertained. Nasotracheal intubation may then be done, and intubation is maintained overnight or for a few days until swelling abates. In most cases, however, tracheostomy is done and discontinued at about the fifth to seventh postoperative day.

Antibiotic therapy for the prophylaxis of infection is controversial in facial fracture management. Indeed, antibiotics may be considered therapeutic because of the frequency of wound contamination. Studies of efficacy are conflicting. A prior argument would favor the institution of antibacterial prophylaxis on the basis of exposure to infectious elements during the fracturing process. Compound wounds expose facial bones to the environment. Virtually all mandibular fractures in the

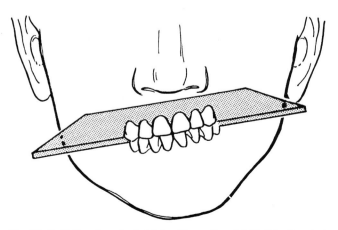

Fig. 21–7. Obliquely oriented bite. (From Donald PJ: The Surgical Management of Structural Facial Dysharmony: A Self-Instructional Package No. 85100. Washington, D.C., American Academy of Otolaryngology—Head and Neck Surgery, 1985, p 17.)

tooth-bearing aspect of the mandible and maxilla are compound because they fracture into either the oral cavity proper or into the periodontal ligament. In addition, this patient population not uncommonly has poor dentition. Carious teeth provide a bacteria-laden reservoir. A well-controlled study by Chole and Yee showed a statistically significant decrement in infection rate in patients with facial fractures who were given prophylactic antibiotics preoperatively, intraoperatively, and for a short period postoperatively.[6] The antibiotic coverage must include gram-positive cocci as well as anaerobic bacteria. Combinations such as nafcillin and metronidazole provide such coverage. In the Chole and Yee study, cefazolin sodium was used.[6] Therapy should be initiated when the patient is first seen and continued for 10 to 14 days.

Data for maxillary fractures are less clear. Even if a CSF leak supervenes, some centers do not use prophylactic antibiotics. Mathog and associates argued the importance of treatment in maxillary fractures because of the communication with the nose and paranasal sinuses.[7] External contamination and stasis of blood and secretions within these cavities set the stage for infection. In addition, foreign materials such as wires, plates, and screws are placed in the wound and increase the potential for infection by acting as foreign bodies.

FRACTURES OF THE MANDIBLE

Anatomy

The mandible is the largest and strongest of the facial bones.[8] This single, horseshoe-shaped bone has a horizontal, tooth-bearing portion and two vertical edentulous portions, which articulate with the skull bilaterally. The central symphyseal-parasymphyseal region is the thickest portion and is bounded by the two mental foramina (Fig. 21–8). Each mental foramen can be found by dropping a vertical line from the midpupil. These foramina can also be approximated by a vertical line just distal to the lower canine teeth (Fig. 21–9).

The body of the mandible is bounded by the canine line (medially) and the anterior border of the masseter muscle (laterally). The symphyseal and body are the tooth-bearing regions of the mandible. The angle of the mandible is located between the body and ramus. The angle region is nontooth bearing, triangular, and bounded by the anterior border of the masseter muscle (anteriorly), the posterior attachment of the masseter (posteriorly), and the oblique line (superiorly). The ramus of the mandible is vertically oriented and extends from the body (anteriorly or mesially) to the coronoid region and the condylar region (distally).

The mandible articulates with the skull at the temporomandibular joint. This joint is composed of the condylar process of the mandible and the glenoid fossa of the temporal bone. The temporomandibular joint is a hinge joint, lined with fibrocartilage in the adult. The condylar region is composed of a condylar head and fragile neck, which represents the weakest portion of the mandible. The coronoid region is located above the ramus anteriorly, and this region is protected by the insertion of the temporalis muscle.

Classification

Fractures of the mandible may be classified according to specific characteristics and anatomic location (Fig. 21–10). A fracture is considered simple when both the external skin and oral mucosa are intact, or compound (open) when a laceration in the skin or intraoral mucosa is present. If the fracture is incomplete and involves only one cortex, it is termed greenstick. The comminuted mandible fracture is one with several fragments of bone.

Mandibular fractures are most commonly characterized by anatomic location (see Fig. 21–9). The most

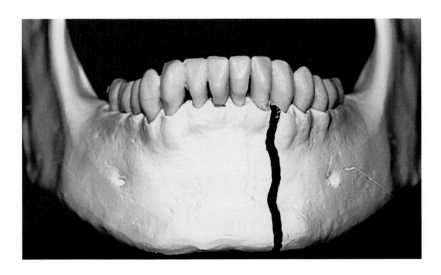

Fig. 21–8. Symphyseal and parasymphyseal region of the mandible. A vertical line is drawn in the left parasymphyseal region representing a common area for anterior fracture. The two mental foramina bound the symphyseal and parasymphyseal region.

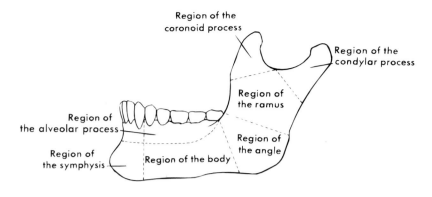

Fig. 21–9. Schematic diagram of the regions of the mandible. The canine line can be seen to distinguish the parasymphyseal region from the body of the mandible. (From Dingman RO and Natvig P: Surgery of Facial Fractures. Philadelphia, WB Saunders, 1969, p 144.)

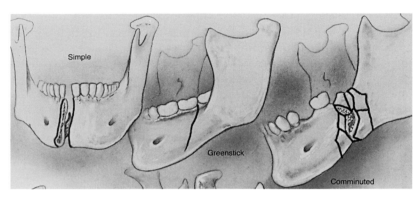

Fig. 21–10. Classification facial fractures according to the characteristics of the fracture. (From Mathog RH: Atlas of Craniofacial Trauma. Philadelphia, WB Saunders, 1992, p 26.)

frequent location of fractures of the mandible is the condylar-subcondylar region. Other common sites include the body and mandibular angle. The coronoid process is rarely involved. Fractures of the alveolar ridge include the occlusal surface of a part of the mandible but do not include the inferior cortical surface (Fig. 21–11).

Diagnosis

Any history of previous trauma or any prior orthodontic work should be known. The patient should be asked

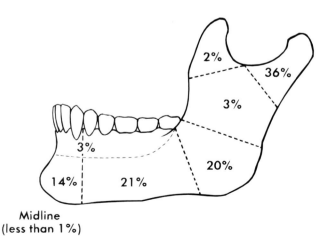

Fig. 21–11. Schematic diagram of fractures of the mandible according to the incidence of fracture. (From Dingman RO and Natvig P: Surgery of Facial Fractures. Philadelphia, WB Saunders, 1969, p 144.)

about associated symptoms such as numbness, difficulty opening the mouth, and malocclusion.[8] The patient should also be questioned about symptoms that could relate to other facial fractures.

Physical examination usually reveals malocclusion, palpable step-offs in the mandible, and tenderness. Examination of the teeth often shows broken or missing teeth and intraoral mucosal lacerations. Anesthesia or hypesthesia of the lower lip and teeth may result from injury to the inferior alveolar or mental nerves.

Mandibular radiographs usually demonstrate the extent and location of the fracture. Panoramic roentgenograms (Panorex) improve visualization of fractures of the ramus, angle, and body of the mandible. This x-ray study can distort and limit the view of the symphyseal-parasymphyseal region.[9] Dental occlusal views can assist in the diagnosis of greenstick fractures involving the occlusal surface of the mandible.

The cornerstone of facial fracture repair is still intermaxillary fixation. This method of repair entails the ligation of the teeth of each arch to those that oppose it. According to Dingman and Natvig, ligation of teeth to each other dates back to the time of Hippocrates.[10] The ancients advised fixing the teeth to one another with gold wire or linen thread.[10] The concept of support of the fractured jaw by a barrel-type bandage was first described by the Greek physician Soranos of Ephesus in the second century A.D.[11] These first methods appeared to rely on healing resulting from the wiring of adjacent teeth in the same arch. Interarch fixation for mandibular fractures was first suggested in the thirteenth century by William of Saliceto, who practiced in Bologna and Verona. He used waxed, twisted silk threads and bound "the injured to the uninjured jaw." It remained for Gilmer in 1887 to be the first to propose actual rigid interdental and intermaxillary fixation, which he accomplished with iron wire.[12]

Intermaxillary fixation began by separately wiring each individual tooth of the maxillary and mandibular arches and then connecting these wires one by one as the teeth were brought into occlusion. From this method, certain modifications were made and evolved into the method we know today. The most significant contribution was the development of the arch bar. Grunell Hammond in 1871 may have described the first arch bar, a firm metal wire that went around the lingual and buccal surfaces of the teeth. Sauer in 1884 used a circumferential gold wire with a spring attachment.[11] These evolved into the Erich and Jelanko arch bars we recognize today. The Erich bar, the one most commonly used, is a malleable metal bar that easily adapts to the buccal surfaces of the teeth and has hooks to which intermaxillary wires or rubber bands can be attached. The Jelanko bar is rigid and difficult to accommodate to the dental arches. Only the application of eyelet wires and the Erich arch bar will be described.

Eyelet Wires

The eyelet wire is best used for subcondylar fractures, greenstick fractures, and favorably aligned noncomminuted mandibular fractures in patients who are cooperative and compliant. The eyelet wire may also be used as temporary fixation until definitive fixation is done. The wire is constructed by taking a half length of No. 26 gauge wire, bending it in half, and twisting in a small loop.

The idea of the eyelet wire is to capture two independent teeth on each side of a mandibular fracture and then fix these to two adjacent pairs of maxillary teeth. The ends of the wire are directed from the buccal side through the interdental space below the contact point and close to the gum between the pair of mandibular teeth distal to the fracture. Each wire is brought around the neck of each tooth, and the end of one is passed through the loop and twisted to its mate at a comfortable distance from the loop (Fig. 21–12). The two teeth are now captured by the wire ligature. Care is taken to be sure the wire is pushed below the embrasure of each tooth and cinched around the tooth neck. The pair of teeth mesial to the fracture line are now ligated in the same way. Similar wires are placed in the same fashion around the maxillary teeth that occlude with the opposing wired mandibular teeth. A pair of mandibular and maxillary teeth are captured with eyelet wires on the opposite side of the arch for additional stabilization. The patient is placed in pre-

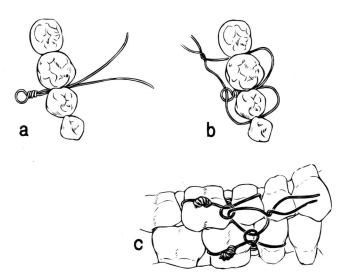

Fig. 21–12. Technique of placing eyelet wires for intermaxillary fixation. (From Bernstein L: Fractures of the mandible. Otolaryngol Clin North Am, 380, 1969.)

morbid occlusion, and each loop on the mandibular side is individually wired to the loop above. The fracture is now fixed, and the wires checked on a weekly basis. Occasionally, the interloop wires may loosen or break and may need tightening or replacement. The eyelet wire itself may also come loose and require tightening. Wires are removed at 3 weeks for subcondylar fractures and 6 weeks for others.

Arch Bars

Erich arch bars generally come in a roll. The correct length of bar for each arch is measured by placing one end of the bar on the most distal tooth in the arch on which it is to be fixed. The bar is bent around to the space between the central incisors. This length is now doubled and the bar cut from the roll. Adjustments are made for missing molar teeth. If significant gaps of two or more teeth are present, the gap can be filled in with a pad of cold cure acrylic pressed into the bar.

Once trimmed to length, the bar is carefully contoured to the teeth by hand. Great care is taken to shape the distal ends to fit around the last teeth in the arch, so the bar will not dig into the cheek. Each bar is placed over the buccal surfaces of the teeth and wired into position with the hooks facing away from the occlusal surface.

The best teeth for securing the bar are the molars and premolars. The canine has the longest root but has a shape that is not conducive to retention of a wire. The incisor teeth, because of their peg-like configuration, holds the wire even more poorly. If enough teeth are present in the arch, the four incisor teeth of each arch are left unligated. For purposes of orientation, the application of the arch bar to the maxillary teeth will be

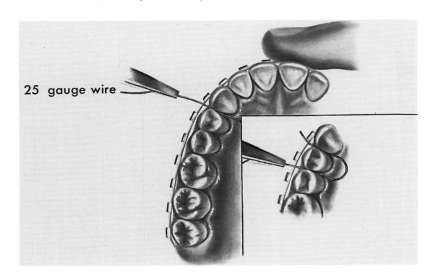

25 gauge wire

Fig. 21–13. The wiring of an arch bar to the teeth (see text). (From Chayra GA, et al: Comparison of panoramic and standard radiographs for the diagnosis of mandible fractures. J Oral Maxillofac Surg 44:126, 1986.)

described first. A 6-inch piece of prestretched 26-gauge wire is passed through the interdental space anteriorly above the bar, looped around the tooth, and then passed through the next interdental space below the bar (Fig. 21–13). Care is taken to prevent injury to the interdental papilla; however, in patients with periodontal disease, this may be unavoidable. The two ends are twisted together with forceps while a periosteal elevator holds the wire at the level of the neck of the tooth (Fig. 21–14). The wire is twisted until tight. The resulting knot is turned into a tight loop and placed away from the lug on the arch bar. Its end is twisted away from the cheek. The molar and premolar teeth are all ligated to the arch bar using the anterior wire above the bar and the posterior below formula-

tion. All the wires are twisted in a clockwise direction (Fig. 21–14). This convention helps in tightening loose wires during follow-up.

Special attention is spent in securing the canine tooth. Its long root embedded in thick bone makes it the key anchor for the bar. Because of its unfavorable shape, adaptation of the wire ligature enhances its holding ability. The wire is placed above the bar, both anteriorly and posteriorly to the tooth, and then looped around the anterior aspect of the bar (Fig. 21–15).

Once bars have been placed on both upper and lower teeth, they are secured to one another either with wire or elastics (Fig. 21–16). Dental wax may be placed on a protrusive edge that irritates the soft tissues. The patient is also given a stick of wax and instructed how to apply it to irritating wires or lugs. All patients are

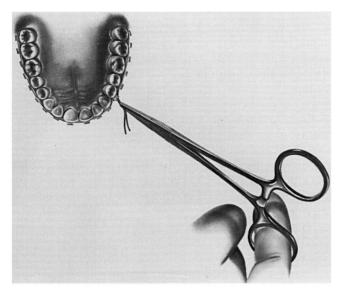

Fig. 21–14. Wire twisting to lock arch bar into position. (From Chayra GA, et al: Comparison of panoramic and standard radiographs for the diagnosis of mandible fractures. J Oral Maxillofac Surg 44:126, 1986.)

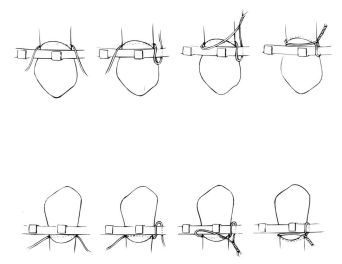

Fig. 21–15. The special adaptation for wiring a canine tooth. (From Chayra GA, et al: Comparison of panoramic and standard radiographs for the diagnosis of mandible fractures. J Oral Maxillofac Surg 44:119, 1986.)

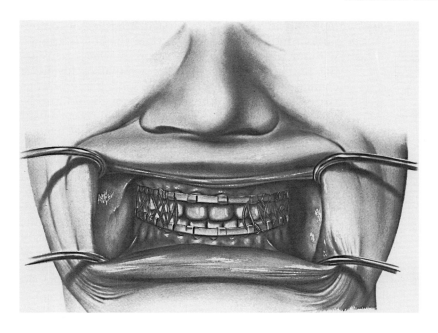

Fig. 21–16. Maxillary and mandibular arch bars applied and intermaxillary wires in place. (From Chayra GA, et al: Comparison of panoramic and standard radiographs for the diagnosis of mandible fractures. J Oral Maxillofac Surg 44:129, 1986.)

followed on a weekly basis to check for bar stability and tightness of the interarch wires. Loose wires are tightened and broken wires replaced. Additionally, careful attention is paid to dental hygiene and nutrition. Already carious dentition, a condition not uncommon in patients with facial fractures, is usually the reflection of past neglect. Careful and insistent instruction in proper brushing technique and the use of a "water pick" type of device are essential features in the follow-up regimen. Dental caries can lead to the formation of dental abscess during the healing phase, which may, in turn, result in osteomyelitis of the jaw.

Nutritional advice is important. The average weight loss in our patient population following intermaxillary fixation is 15 lb. A booklet on dental hygiene and nutrition is supplied to each patient, with instruction on brushing technique and diets that can be employed while in fixation. Of course, only food of a consistency that can be sucked in the free space around the back of the teeth can be used. Balanced high-calorie supplements such as Ensure-plus and Sustacal can be used to augment caloric intake. These products come in both a liquid and pudding form and are quite palatable.

Surgical Approaches

Intraoral approaches have the advantages of scar camouflage and more direct approach to fracture reduction and fixation. Intraoral approaches require more elaborate instrumentation to allow for precise fracture fixation, however. In that intraoral incisions allow less direct visualization of fractures, adequate exposure and accurate reduction through this approach require an experienced surgeon. Extraoral approaches have the advantage of increased exposure and increased visual-

ization in the region of the posterior part of the body, angle, and ramus. External exposure requires a cervical incision and involves potential risk to the marginal mandibular branch of the facial nerve, however.

The incision and approach chosen for a given fracture of the mandible depend on several factors. These include the location and type of the fracture as well as the available instrumentation and technology and, most important, the surgeon's comfort with the given approach. The choice for simple fractures of the symphyseal and parasymphyseal region is intraoral. Simple, linear posterior fractures may be approached intraorally, whereas more comminuted fractures or fractures with significant bone loss usually require an extraoral approach. The approach chosen should allow adequate exposure to diagnose, reduce, and immobilize the given fracture.

The symphyseal and parasymphyseal regions of the mandible are easily approached through either an intraoral or an extraoral route. The intraoral incision is made from canine tooth to canine tooth, leaving an adequate mucosal cuff for closure of the incision (Fig. 21–17). Subperiosteal dissection is made, identifying and preserving the mental nerves. The symphyseal and parasymphyseal regions are also easily approached through an external submental incision oriented in RSTL. Reapproximation of the mentalis muscle must be carefully performed to prevent postoperative ptosis of the soft tissues of the chin.

The approach to mandibular fractures posterior to the mental foramina depends on the surgeon's experience and the degree of fracture.[12] Intraoral approaches to the body and angle are best performed by making a gingivobuccal incision immediately adjacent to the fracture. Repair of posterior mandibular fractures re-

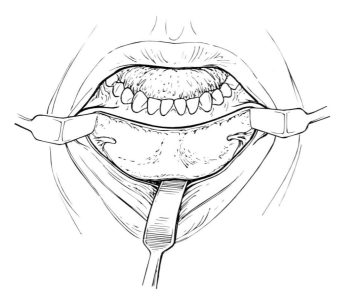

Fig. 21–17. Schematic diagram of intraoral approach to symphyseal and parasymphyseal fractures. The dissection is subperiosteal and isolates and preserves the neurovascular pedicles from the mental foramina.

quires surgical experience and advanced technology to achieve fracture reduction and fixation. Fracture fixation is achieved by a transbuccal system placed through transcutaneous facial stab incisions (Fig. 21–18). The extraoral approach to fractures of the mandibular body, angle, or ramus is made through a transcervical incision two fingers breadths below the angle of the mandible. Care is taken to elevate the marginal mandibular branch of the facial nerve to prevent injury. This approach is preferred when the patient has significant comminution of the fracture or bone loss. In each of these cases, a larger reconstruction plate may be required for repair. The external approach allows greater exposure for placement of larger reconstruction plates.

Treatment

As instrumentation and technology have progressed, treatment of mandibular fractures has evolved, but the goals have not changed. These goals include anatomic and functional stability of the mandible. Reduction and stabilization of any mandibular fracture should result in pain-free function of the mandible without any eventual changes in the temporomandibular joint.

The strength of any bony fixation must be adequate to overcome any forces that will act on the repaired bone during function.[13] As previously mentioned, former techniques utilized skeletal fixation with interosseous wiring.[14,15] This method allows the bone to heal indirectly. Skeletal fixation is rarely used today. The only theoretic advantage of skeletal fixation for repair of mandibular fractures is the possibility of increased

flexibility in cases with significant bone loss or comminution. In these situations, if rigid fixation is applied without proper restoration of pre-morbid occlusion, the result can be either poor eventual occlusion or change in the temporomandibular joint. If interosseous wiring is used, intermaxillary fixation should also be used for approximately 6 weeks for stable bone repair.

The rationale for the use of rigid internal fixation for repair of mandibular fractures is well documented.[14–16] This includes the clinically proved decrease in mouth opening seen 6 months after release of intermaxillary fixation.[17–20] Additional experimental and clinical evidence against skeletal fixation includes muscle atrophy[20] and histologic changes in the temporomandibular joint[21] after prolonged periods of intermaxillary fixation. Although an increased rate of infection has not been conclusively shown with intermaxillary fixation and interosseous wiring, the increased bone movement with nonrigid fixation makes this a theoretic consideration. As knowledge and technology have progressed, rigid internal fixation has become the standard in most centers for treatment of mandibular fractures. This allows active use of the facial skeleton during the bone healing phase. Use of this type of bone repair requires surgical experience, advanced technology, and patient compliance. Direct bone healing can only be achieved with rigid fixation. If properly applied, stable rigid fixation of the mandible obviates the need for intermaxillary fixation.

Rigid fixation of the mandible can be performed by a variety of methods. The fracture is usually first reduced and the teeth put into premorbid occlusion by placing the patient in intermaxillary fixation. The fractures are then directly approached (with intermaxillary fixation in place), and anatomic fragment reduction is obtained. Rigid fixation is then performed. This can be accomplished with an inferior mandibular fracture plate (2.4 to 2.7 mm) and a superior monocortical two-hole tension band. Fixation can also be achieved with two miniplates (2.0 mm). In either case, screws placed to attach superiorly located plates should spare all tooth roots and be monocortical only. Another means to achieve stable rigid fixation is the placement of lag screw fixation.[22] This method employs a basic principle of wood working and applies compression across the fracture line with maximal direct bone healing (Fig. 21–19). This technique requires adequate exposure and subperiosteal undermining to allow placement of long screws that engage sufficient bone for fixation.

If rigid fixation is stable, the patient may be taken out of intermaxillary fixation and allowed to function. Of course, this decision is based on the stability of the rigid fixation and on the individual patient's compliance. If either the fixation stability or patient compliance is in question, the patient may be left in intermaxillary fixation for up to 6 weeks.

The method employed to repair any mandibular fracture is based on the surgeon's experience, the loca-

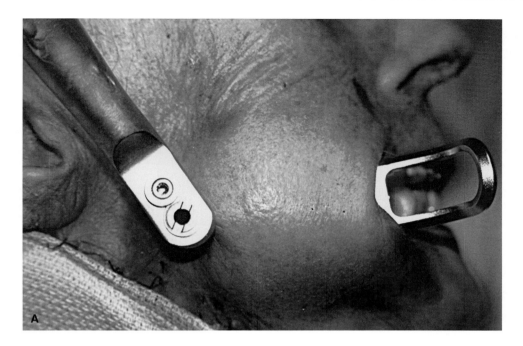

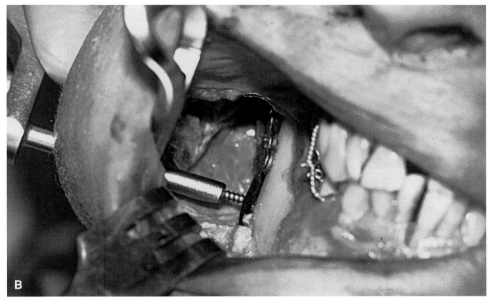

Fig. 21–18. A. Lateral view of cadaver showing the use of the transcutaneous-transbuccal system for approach for posterior fractures of the mandible. A stab wound incision has been used to insert the transbuccal system. B. Intraoral view showing utilization of the transbuccal system to place a plate and screws for fixation of a fracture of the angle of the mandible.

tion and extent of the fracture, and the ability to expose the fracture well enough to provide fixation. Simple anterior fractures may be repaired with many techniques, whereas more comminuted posterior fractures may limit the fixation methods. If the lag screw technique is used, increased exposure may be necessary to fixate a fracture. The fracture technique chosen should allow stable bone healing and overcome the forces of tension and compression on the mandible.

DENTAL INJURY

Injury to the dentition is a common accompaniment to fractures of the mandible and maxilla. A simple chip-

ping of the teeth that does not extend to the dentin can be managed by the dentist by simply grinding the occlusal surface smooth. Such injuries are usually unaccompanied by pain. Larger fractures of the tooth substance expose the dentin or pulp and are painful. It is important to dress the tooth immediately with a dental compound that not only protects the tooth, but also alleviates the discomfort. A simple mixture of zinc oxide and eugenol done with a metal spatula or a glass plate forms a sticky compound with the consistency of putty that hardens when wet by the saliva. Eugenol helps to soothe the pain. Other proprietary compounds such as Dycal may be used. Later, the dentist can restore the tooth with a crown. In the case of fracturing

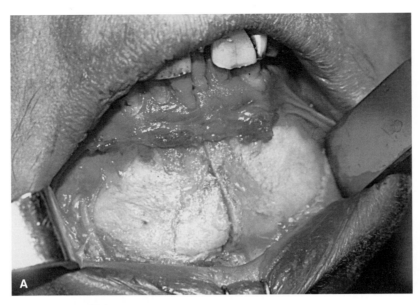

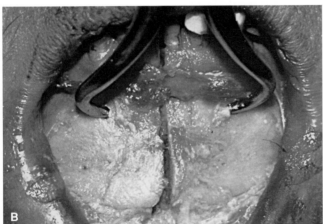

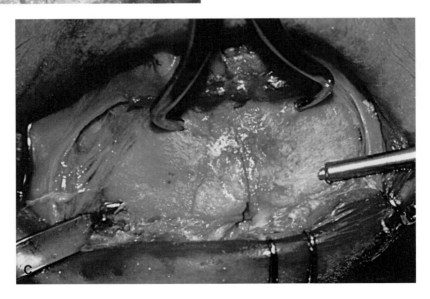

Fig. 21–19. A. Intraoral approach to repair a symphyseal fracture of the mandible on a cadaver. B. Placement of small drill holes and a towel clip for reduction of a symphyseal fracture. C. Placement of lag screw for fixation of a symphyseal fracture. Note that the towel clip is left in place to maintain fracture reduction while the lag screws are placed.

of a slab of a tooth face in a vertical direction, especially from the incisors, the tooth can be repaired by bonding.

Avulsion of the crown at the gum line is managed either by the extraction of the root or by application of a dressing until the tooth can later be restored with a crown. If the dentition is neglected and carious, then extraction is the best solution.

Dental fractures that occur through the root present a special problem. Root fractures seriously jeopardize the viability of the tooth. If the soft tissue of the pulp is sufficiently traumatized, the tooth will die. Once the pulp undergoes necrosis, the stage is set for the development of a root abscess. This may occur a short time after the injury or may be delayed for years. If such an abscess were to occur during intermaxillary fixation, an osteomyelitis and even a nonunion could occur.

The management of a tooth in the line of fracture is controversial. Some guidelines do exist that may be of help. If the tooth is carious and the root is fractured, then the tooth should be removed. If a carious tooth has a fracture through the periodontal ligament, but the root is intact, extraction should be seriously entertained. If the tooth is healthy, the vital consideration is the importance of the tooth in the stability of the fracture. This is especially cogent in the circumstance of the erupted third molar tooth that lies in an unfavorably aligned fracture of the mandibular angle. In such a fracture, the line extends obliquely from anterior to posterior as it proceeds from the occlusal surface to the inferior border of the mandible. If the molar is in the distal fagment, its occlusion with the maxillary third molar above it will preclude its displacement. If this molar is extracted, then the pull of the medial pterygoid and masseter will displace the distal fragment upward. The wisdom tooth, being the most poorly calcified in the mouth, is the most susceptible of all to caries. One should probably remove a carious or impacted third molar in such a circumstance and achieve fixation by an open technique.

Any dental trauma can cause pulp necrosis, even without a root fracture. It is important to follow-up patients after facial fractures with vitality testing of the teeth. Once viability is lost, then a root canal procedure should be done to prevent abscess and tooth loss.

The final consideration is that of avulsed teeth. Such teeth should be immediately replaced in the avulsion socket and fixed by wires to the adjacent teeth for splinting. Many such teeth later become nonvital and require a root canal. Most are retained, however, and their preservation helps greatly in the maintenance of dental arch integrity.

ZYGOMATICOMAXILLARY COMPLEX FRACTURES

Anatomy

The zygoma is one of the seven bones comprising the orbit and is located in the anteriolateral region of the orbit.[23] The zygoma has four sutures lines, with the temporal, frontal, maxillary, and sphenoid bones. The temporalis and masseter muscles arise on this bone. Additionally, more superficial muscles of facial expression (zygomaticus major and minor) also arise on its surface. The infraorbital foramen is a small opening at the articulation of the zygoma and maxilla approximately 7 mm from the infraorbital rim. The infraorbital nerve, a branch of the second division of the trigeminal nerve, exits from this foramen and supplies sensation to the cheek, the lateral aspect of the nose, and the ipsilateral upper teeth and lip. Zygomaticomaxillary complex (ZMC) fractures often damage this nerve and result in anesthesia or hypoesthesia of the supplied region.

The lateral canthal tendon attaches to the orbit just medial to the lateral orbital rim at Whitnall's tubercle. ZMC fractures may result in detachment of the lateral canthal tendon and suspensory ligaments of the globe and cause downward displacement of the globe. The orbital floor is primarily composed of portions of the zygoma and maxillary bones. Fractures of the orbital floor (orbital blowout) usually occur along the infraorbital groove and canal. These blowout fractures may result in herniation and entrapment of orbital contents into the fracture line and maxillary sinus below. Entrapped orbital contents may include orbital fat and the inferior rectus muscle, causing enophthalmos and diplopia, respectively.

Diagnosis

ZMC fractures may be associated with a variety of symptoms and signs (Table 21–3). Symptoms include pain, diplopia, numbness in the distribution of the infraorbital nerve, epistaxis, and trismus. Signs vary according to the type and severity of fracture. If the fracture involves only the floor of the orbit (pure "blowout" fracture), signs may include diplopia, enophthalmos, and hypoesthesia. If the fracture involves the entire ZMC, a cosmetic deformity including flattening of the malar eminence and ectropion of the lower eyelid may also occur. Other signs include epistaxis, trismus, subconjunctival hemorrhage, periorbital swelling, hyphoxia, and reduced visual acuity. Because

TABLE 21–3. Symptoms and Signs of Zygoma Fractures

Symptoms	Signs
Pain	Infraorbital tenderness
Double vision	Diplopia
Numbness	Hypoesthesia: cheek, upper teeth
Epistaxis	Malar flattening
	Hypoophthalmus/Enophthalmos
Trismus	Subconjunctival hemorrhage
Cosmetic deformity	

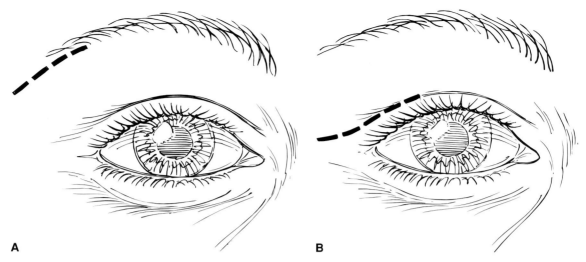

Fig. 21–20. A. Schematic diagram of a lateral brow incision for approach to the frontozygomatic suture line. B. Schematic diagram of a right extended upper blepharoplasty incision for approach to the frontozygomatic suture line.

of the risk of associated intraocular injury, all patients should have ophthalmologic consultation.[23]

Radiologic confirmation of ZMC fractures is obtained with standard Waters, Caldwell, Towne, and submental vertex views. Fractures of the zygomatic arch may be seen on the submental vertex view. Other views may show fractures at the frontozygomatic suture, infraorbital rim, and the zygomaticomaxillary buttress. Isolated blowout fractures of the floor of the orbit may show a dehiscence in the orbital floor and

an air-fluid level in the maxillary sinus. Computed tomography is usually indicated to determine the extent of the fracture.[24] It can delineate the degree of infraorbital injury and show whether other midface fractures are present.

Surgical Approaches

Treatment of ZMC fractures usually requires multiple incisions. The frontozygomatic suture line may be ap-

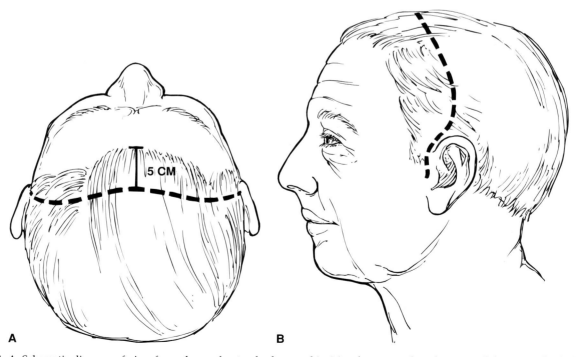

Fig. 21–21. A. Schematic diagram of view from above of a standard coronal incision for approach to fractures of the upper third of the facial skeleton. Note that the incision is approximately 5 cm behind the hairline. B. Schematic diagram of the lateral view of the coronal incision. The incision is carried down into the preauricular crease for added exposure.

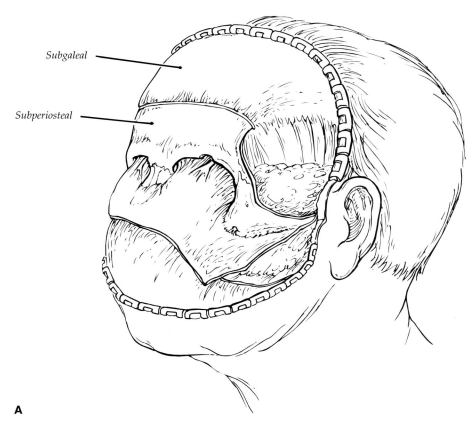

Subgaleal

Subperiosteal

A

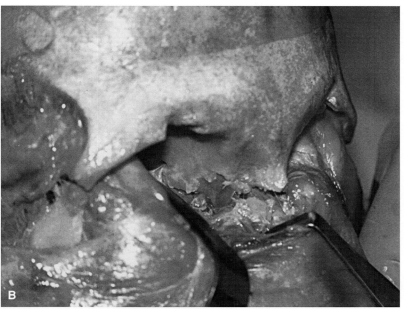

B

Fig. 21–22. A. Schematic diagram of an extended coronal approach of the upper facial skeleton. Note that this approach is initially subgaleal and becomes subperiosteal at the temporal line. This approach gives good exposure to the frontozygomatic suture line, the zygomatic arch, and the nasofrontal suture line. B. Right oblique view on a cadaver showing the extended approach to the supraorbital rim and nasofrontal suture line after the supraorbital neurovascular bundles have been carefully dissected from their foramina and retracted inferiorly.

proached through a lateral brow incision (Fig. 21–20), an extended upper eyelid blepharoplasty incision, or a coronal incision (Figs. 21–21 and 21–22). The coronal incision can facilitate exposure of the entire supraorbital rim, the nasofrontal region, the frontozygomatic suture, and the zygomatic arch. The initial dissection is in the subgaleal plane and converts to the subperiosteal plane at the temporal line. To improve exposure, dissection of the supraorbital neurovascular pedicles may be necessary. This may require removal of a small amount of bone surrounding the supraorbital foramina. The lateral brow, extended blepharoplasty, or coronal incision allows exposure of the supraorbital rim and lateral orbital rim and provides access to elevate fractures of the zygomatic arch. The incision chosen depends on the location and extent of the fractures.

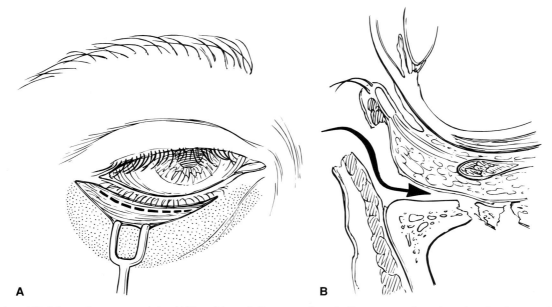

Fig. 21–23. A and B. Schematic anteroposterior (AP) and lateral diagrams of a subciliary approach to the infraorbital rim and orbital floor. The dotted line on the AP view represents the incision in the orbicularis oculi muscle, which is somewhat inferior to the cutaneous incision. This stair step contributes to the prevention of postoperative ectropion.

The infraorbital rim and orbital floor may be approached by an infraorbital rim incision, subciliary incision (Fig. 21–23), or transconjunctival incision (Fig. 21–24). The transconjunctival incision has become the preferred approach because it provides complete exposure through a camouflaged incision.[25] This approach utilizes a lateral canthotomy and cantholysis to optimize exposure. The transconjunctival-lateral canthot-

omy approach must be meticulously performed and reapproximated to prevent blunting of the lateral canthus and postoperative lower eyelid malposition. Last, the zygomaticomaxillary buttress may be approached through a gingivobuccal incision. This incision may be required to diagnose and reduce fully a complex fracture.

The incision or combination of incisions used to

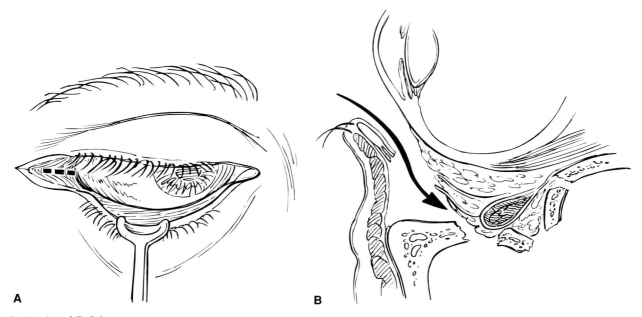

Fig. 21–24. A and B. Schematic anteroposterior (AP) and lateral diagram of a transconjunctival approach to the infraorbital rim and orbital floor. The AP view shows the transconjunctival incision and the lateral canthotomy already performed. The dotted line indicates the area for inferior cantholysis to improve exposure.

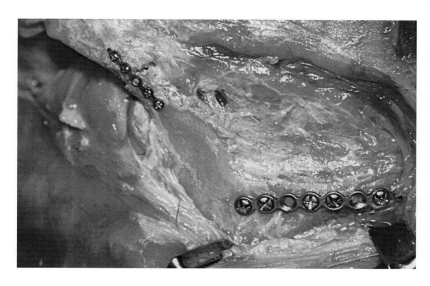

Fig. 21–25. Microplate fixation of a fracture of the left frontozygomatic suture line and the left zygomatic arch. This is done through a coronal approach.

treat a given fracture depends on the type and exact location of the fracture. Successful treatment requires adequate exposure and accurate diagnosis. The incisions must allow for complete exposure of the orbital floor for repair.

Treatment

Reduction must reestablish the three-dimensional anatomy. Fixation must be adequate to maintain the fracture fragments in their anatomic position during bone healing. Displacement of the ZMC may be minimal, moderate, or severe. If displacement is minimal, no fixation or fixation at only one place may be required to produce a stable result.[26] If displacement is moderate, two-point fixation is usually required. In fractures with severe displacement or in those associated with comminution, fixation at the lateral orbital rim and at the zygomaticomaxillary buttress is required. Open reduction and fixation of the zygomatic arch may be required in these cases. Additionally, fixation of comminuted fragments of the zygomatic body may be necessary.

Fixation of fragments of ZMC fractures may be accomplished with interosseous wires or with plate fixation (Fig. 21–25). True rigid stabilization requires plate fixation at the zygomaticomaxillary buttress and the frontozygomatic suture and is usually performed with miniplate (2.0 mm) or low profile (1.5 to 1.7 mm) miniplate fixation. Stabilization of the infraorbital rim is performed with microplate (1.0 to 1.2 mm) fixation (Fig. 21–26).

Exploration of the orbit is indicated in patients with significant enophthalmos or any diplopia (Fig. 21–27).[27] Orbital exploration is also indicated for any injury to the infraorbital nerve or any severe displace-

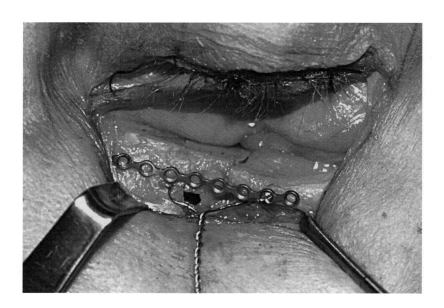

Fig. 21–26. Microplate fixation of a fracture of the infraorbital rim. Note that a single interosseous wire has been placed to assist in reduction of the fracture while plating is performed.

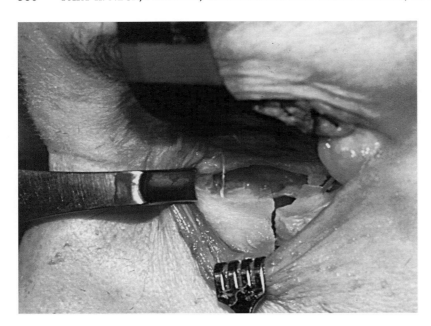

Fig. 21–27. Transconjunctival approach to the infraorbital rim and orbital floor. Note that the fracture in infraorbital rim extends into the orbital floor where a defect is present in the bone with herniation of intraorbital contents.

ment of the ZMC. Repair of enophthalmos acutely is usually more successful than late repair, because precise correction of this defect as a late sequela is difficult. Orbital exploration for diplopia only is controversial, but replacement of entrapped orbital contents at the time of repair clearly affords the best chance for full function of extraocular muscles and restoration of orbital volume. Repair of orbital contour and volume may be achieved with only reduction of fragments themselves if no bone is missing. If significant bone loss of the orbital floor is present, reconstruction can be achieved with septal cartilage, maxillary or cranial bone, or orbital reconstruction plates. Autologous materials are usually preferred over alloplasts.

FRACTURES OF THE MIDFACE

Fractures of the midface require considerable force. They usually result from severe blunt trauma and are much less frequent than isolated nasal, zygomatic, or mandibular fractures. In 1901, Rene Le Fort applied severe blunt trauma to cadaver heads to determine the characteristics of the most common midfacial fractures.[28,29]

The Le Fort I fracture involves separation of the lower maxilla from the rest of the face (Fig. 21–28). This fracture traverses the pyriform apertures, the lower nasal septum, the lateral and posterior walls of the maxillary sinuses, and the pterygoid plates. It may occur in isolation or in association with other complex midfacial fractures (Le Fort II or III).

The Le Fort II fracture begins at one maxillary buttress, traverses the inferior orbit, and separates the nasal bones from the skull. This series of fractures extends through the perpendicular plate of the ethmoid medially and through the posterior walls of the maxillary sinuses. This fracture is often associated with a nasal, nasoethmoid fracture, or other midfacial injury, such as a zygomaticomaxillary fracture.

The Le Fort III fracture involves separation of the cranium and the facial skeleton. This fracture traverses the lateral and medial orbital walls, the nasofrontal area, and the upper nasal septum. The zygomatic arches are also fractured bilaterally. Craniofacial separation is completed by posterior fracture of the orbits and pterygoid plates. It is usually associated with other midfacial fractures.

Surgical Approaches

Incisions used to approach midfacial fractures are varied according to the specific location of the fracture. Isolated Le Fort I fractures are usually approached by an extended sublabial incision (Figs. 21–29 and 21–30). This incision allows exposure of the zygomaticomaxillary buttresses and pyriform apertures bilaterally. If the fracture involves the infraorbital rim (Le Fort II), a transconjunctival-lateral canthotomy or subciliary incision is usually used to expose these fracture sites. If a Le Fort II fracture is more extensive and greater exposure to the nasoethmoid complex is required, an external Lynch incision or extended coronal incision may be used. The frontozygomatic suture line may be approached by a coronal, brow, or extended upper blepharoplasty (supratarsal) incision. The coronal incision has the advantage of providing exposure to the zygomatic arch and the nasoethmoid region. This obviates the need for a Lynch incision for nasoethmoid exposure.

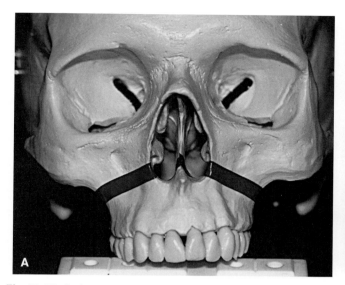
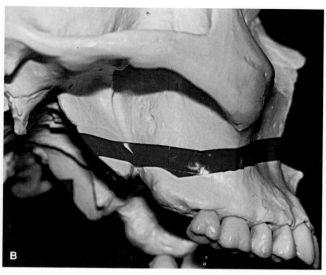

Fig. 21–28. A. Anteroposterior view of the upper facial skeleton. A tape has been placed in the area of a Le Fort I fracture traversing the pyriform aperture and the inferior nasal septum. B. Lateral view of a Le Fort I fracture crossing the pterygoid plates.

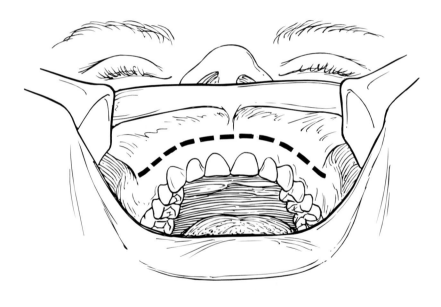

Fig. 21–29. Schematic diagram of a sublabial incision for approach to midfacial fractures.

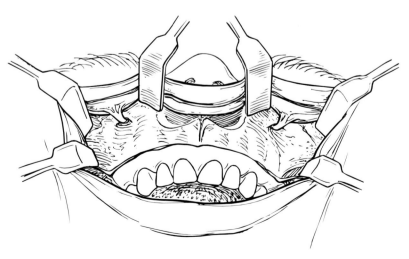

Fig. 21–30. Schematic diagram of subperiosteal dissection through a sublabial incision exposing the infraorbital nerves.

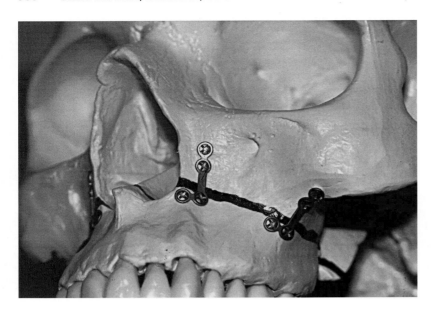

Fig. 21–31. Miniplate fixation of a Le Fort I fracture. Note the stabilization of the nasomaxillary and zygomaticomaxillary buttresses.

The incisions used depend on the location and extent of the fractures. Most Le Fort fractures do not manifest as the original description, but are combinations of complex fractures of the midface and require knowledge of multiple surgical approaches.

Treatment

Surgical treatment of midfacial fractures requires accurate diagnosis and precise reduction. All areas of fracture should be determined by physical examination and radiographic imaging, and these areas should be fully exposed surgically.

In patients with dentition, arch bars and intermaxillary fixation are initially applied to reestablish pretraumatic occlusion. In patients in whom midfacial fractures are displaced, disimpaction of fractures may be required before placement of intermaxillary fixation. In edentulous patients, a splint or denture containing an arch bar is fixed to the mandible or maxilla to reestablish appropriate skeletal relationships. This is performed with circummandibular (mandible) circumpyriform or circumzygomatic (maxilla) wires. The maxillary (palatal) splint may also be fixed to the palate with two transpalatal screws. In any case, splints or dentures are placed to reestablish the occlusal and skeletal relationship.

After the occlusal relationship is reestablished, all fractures sites are fully exposed. The facial skeleton should then be reconstituted in three dimensions:

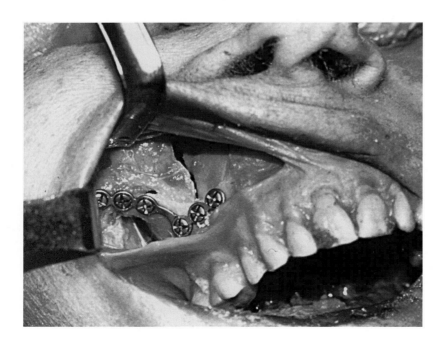

Fig. 21–32. Intraoral approach of a right hemi-Le Fort fracture showing miniplate fixation of the zygomaticomaxillary buttress.

height, width, and depth.[30,31] Careful attention should be paid to reestablishing all important facial buttresses. In particular, the vertical zygomaticomaxillary and nasomaxillary buttresses should be carefully reduced and fixated to reestablish vertical facial height (Figs. 21–31 and 21–32). All rigid fixation should be applied with sufficient stability to counteract any forces that could disrupt bone repair during healing. If rigid fixation is considered stable and if the patient is compliant, intermaxillary fixation may be removed at the conclusion of the operation or within the first 1 to 2 weeks after the operation. If the stability of rigid fixation is in question (i.e., with bone comminution or bone loss), intermaxillary fixation should be left in place for up to 6 to 8 weeks. This will help maintain the occlusion while bone healing occurs.

In some patients with midfacial fractures, bone comminution or bone loss prevents proper reestablishment of facial buttresses. Loss of vertical height with midfacial shortening can result. When this condition is recognized, immediate bone grafting is indicated.[32] Grafting is usually best performed by harvest of split calvarial bone grafts. These endochondral grafts have good viability and stabilize fixation in cases with significant bone loss. In these patients, intermaxillary fixation usually should remain in place for at least 6 weeks.

In summary, treatment of facial fractures requires a multisystem approach. All bony and soft tissue injuries should be diagnosed and reconstitution of all tissue layers should be performed, if possible. The advancement of technology has enabled rigid fixation to become the standard of care for the fixation of most facial fractures. More precise stability and fixation of fractures have become possible, and intermaxillary fixation is used less frequently. Well-planned incisions minimize scarring. Adequate exposure, precise reduction, and stable fixation remain the hallmarks of treatment of facial fractures.

SUGGESTED READINGS

1. Mathog RH: Atlas of Craniofacial Trauma. Philadelphia, WB Saunders, 1992, p 3.
2. Dingman RO: General principles. In: Surgery of Facial Fractures. Philadelphia, WB Saunders, 1964, p 43.
3. Sykes JM and Donald PJ: In: Reconstruction of the Head and Neck. Edited by Meyerhoff WL and Rice D. Philadelphia, WB Saunders, 1992, p 923.
4. Sykes JM and Murakami C: Principles of local flaps in head and neck reconstruction. Operative Tech Otolaryngol Head Neck Surg 4:2, 1993.
5. Angle EH: Classification of malocclusion. Dent Cosmos 41:248, 1899.
6. Chole RA and Yee J: Antibiotic prophylaxis for facial fractures: a prospective randomized trial. Arch Otolaryngol Head Neck Surg 105:1055, 1987.
7. Mathog RH, Crane LR, and Nowak GS: Antimicrobial therapy following head and neck trauma. In: Antibiotic Therapy in Head and Neck Surgery. Edited by Johnson JT. New York, Marcel Dekker, 1987, p 31.
8. Dingman RO: The mandible. In: Surgery of Facial Fractures. Philadelphia, WB Saunders, 1964, p 133.
9. Chayra GA, et al: Comparison of panoramic and standard radiographs for the diagnosis of mandible fractures. J Oral Maxillofac Surg 44:677, 1986.
10. Dingman RO and Natvig P: Occlusion and intermaxillary fixation. In: Surgery of Facial Fractures. Philadelphia, WB Saunders, 1964, p 114.
11. Hoffman-Axthelm W: The treatment of mandibular fractures and dislocations: an historical perspective. In: Oral and Maxillofacial Traumatology. Vol I. Edited by Kruger E and Schilli W. Chicago, Quintessence Books, 1982, p 17.
12. Gilmer TL: A case of fracture of the lower jaw with remarks on the treatment. Arch Dent 4:388, 1887.
13. Kellman R and Marentette L: Atlas of Craniomaxillofacial Fixation. New York, Raven Press, 1995, p 71.
14. Kellman R: Repair of mandibular fractures via compression plating and more traditional techniques: a comparison of results. Laryngoscope 94:1560, 1984.
15. Freihofer HM and Sailer HF: Experiences with intraoral wiring of mandibular fractures. J Maxillofac Surg 1:248, 1973.
16. Larsen OD and Nielsen A: Mandibular fractures: II. A follow-up study of 229 patients. Scand J Plast Reconstr Surg 10:219, 1976.
17. Perren SM: Physical and Biological aspects of fracture healing with special reference to internal fixation. Clin Orthop 138:175, 1979.
18. Reitzik M and Schoorl W: Bone repair in the mandible: a histologic and biometric comparison between rigid and semirigid fixation. J Oral Maxillofac Surg 41:215, 1983.
19. Rahn BA: Theoretical considerations in rigid fixation of facial bones. Clin Plast Surg 16:21, 1989.
20. Amaratunga NA: Mouth opening after release of maxillomandibular fixation in fracture patients. J Oral Maxillofac Surg 45:383, 1987.
21. Ellis E and Carlson DS: The effects of mandibular immobilization on the masticatory system: a review. Clin Plast Surg 16:133, 1989.
22. Glineburg RW, Laskin DM, and Blaustein DI: The effects of immobilization of the primate temporomandibular joint: a histological and histochemical study. J Oral Maxillofac Surg 40:3, 1982.
23. Zide BM and Jelks GW: Surgical Anatomy of the Orbit. New York, Raven Press, New York, NY, 1985, p 1.
24. Binder P: Evaluation of the eye following periorbital trauma. Head Neck Surg 1:134, 1978.
25. Fujii N and Yamshiro M: Classification of malar complex fractures using computed tomography. J Oral Maxillofac Surg 41:562, 1983.
26. Appling WD, Patrinely JR, and Salzer TA: Transconjunctival approach vs. subciliary skin-muscle flap approach for orbital fracture repair. Arch Otolaryngol Head Neck Surg 119:1000, 1993.
27. Eisele D and Duckert L: Single point stabilization of zygomatic fractures with minicompression plates. Arch Otolaryngol Head Neck Surg 113:267, 1987.
28. Kellman R and Marentette L: Zygomatic "tripod" fractures. In: Atlas of Craniomaxillofacial Fixation. New York, Raven Press, 1995, p 288.
29. Le Fort R: Étude experimentale sur les fractures de la machoire superieure. Rev Chir Paris 23:208, 1901.
30. Stanley RB: Reconstruction of the midfacial vertical dimension following Le Fort fractures. Arch Otolaryngol Head Neck Surg 110:571, 1984.
31. Manson P, Hoopes J, and Su C: Structural pillars of the facial skeleton: An approach to the management of Le Fort fractures. Plast Reconstr Surg 66:54, 1980.
32. Manson PN, et al: Midface fractures: advantages of immediate extended open reduction and bone grafting. Plast Reconstr Surg 76:1, 1985.

22 Salivary Glands

William R. Carroll and Gregory T. Wolf

The major salivary glands include the parotid gland, submandibular gland, and sublingual glands. Numerous minor salivary glands are located within the mucous membrane of the lip, tongue, hard and soft palate, buccal mucosa, pharyngeal walls, larynx, nose, and paranasal sinuses. In this chapter, the anatomy, physiology, and major disease processes of the major and minor salivary glands are considered.

ANATOMY

Parotid Gland

The parotid gland is located subcutaneously in the space between the ramus of the mandible and the external auditory canal and mastoid tip. Anteriorly, the gland overlies part of the masseter muscle, and posteriorly, the gland overlies a portion of the sternocleidomastoid muscle. The deep, medial portion of the gland lies adjacent to the parapharyngeal space. The styloid process is immediately adjacent to the deep portion of the gland, and the carotid artery and internal jugular veins lie just medially and posteriorly. The parotid gland fascia is an extension of the superficial layer of the deep cervical fascia, which splits to envelop the gland. Inferiorly, the condensation of the fascial envelope suspended between the styloid process and the mandible is termed the stylomandibular ligament. The stylomandibular ligament separates the inferior portion of the parotid gland from the posterior portion of the submandibular gland. The parotid duct (Stensen's duct) exits the superficial part of the gland anteriorly and passes across the masseter muscle at a vertical location halfway between the zygoma and the oral commissure. Once the duct reaches the anterior portion of the masseter muscle, it turns medially to pierce the buccinator muscle and enters the buccal mucosa of the oral cavity opposite the upper second molar tooth. Because the parotid gland is encapsulated relatively late during embryogenesis, lymph nodes may be found just inside or outside the parotid gland fascia. These lymph nodes drain the scalp, forehead, eye, cheek, and oral commissure.

The parotid gland is innervated by parasympathetic fibers originating in the glossopharyngeal nerve. These fibers leave the ninth nerve by means of its tympanic branch and mingle on the promontory of the cochlea in the tympanic plexus. These fibers then leave the middle ear as part the lesser petrosal nerve, which exits the skull and joins the otic ganglion just outside the foramen ovale. The parasympathetic fibers then join the auriculotemporal nerve, which originates from the mandibular division of the trigeminal nerve. The auriculotemporal nerve enters the parotid gland along its superior and medial border. The facial nerve is the dominant consideration in surgery of the parotid gland. As the nerve exits the stylomastoid foramen, it enters the posterior and medial portion of the gland prior to its primary division at the pes anserinus and subsequent secondary divisions into the five facial and cervical branches. Numerous variations in the branching pattern of the facial nerve have been described, and detailing these variations is beyond the scope of this chapter.[1]

The parotid gland is often referred to as consisting of superficial and deep lobes. Some have suggested that the facial nerve lies in a true cleavage plane between these two lobes, which are essentially folded over the facial nerve. Most anatomists, however, conclude that no true anatomic division occurs. The terms superficial lobe and deep lobe simply refer to the presence of tissue both medial and lateral to the facial nerve. The nerve itself lies within the substance of the gland and is not simply folded within the gland. A detailed understanding of the location of the main trunk of the facial nerve and of the location of the main facial branches is essential for safe surgical procedures involving the parotid gland.

Submandibular Gland

The submandibular gland is located within the submandibular triangle of the neck and occupies most of the volume of that triangle. The submandibular gland is covered with a fascial capsule that originates from the superficial layer of the deep cervical fascia, which splits to envelop the gland. A condensation of this fascia, the stylomandibular ligament, separates the posterior portion of the submandibular gland from the parotid gland. The anterior border of the submandibular gland is folded over the posterior border of the mylohyoid muscle. Thus, the submandibular gland has components both superficial and deep to the mylohyoid muscle. The facial artery arises from the external carotid artery and joins the posterior border of the submandibular gland after coursing superior to the posterior belly of the digastric muscle. The facial artery indents the posterior and superior border of the gland and usually gives off two to three dominant arterial branches to the gland. The duct of the submandibular gland runs anteriorly along the lateral surface of the hyoglossus and genioglossus muscles. The lingual nerve is also on the medial surface of the gland and initially is located superior to the submandibular duct. As these two structures course anteriorly, however, the lingual nerve loops around the submandibular duct before entering the tongue. The submandibular duct assumes a submucosal position near the anterior floor of the mouth and is located medial to the sublingual gland. The duct drains at a papule adjacent to the frenulum of the tongue in the anterior part of the floor of mouth (Wharton's duct). The hypoglossal nerve runs between the medial portion of the submandibular gland and the hyoglossus muscle.

The nerve supply to the submandibular gland is primarily parasympathetic and consists of fibers originating in the seventh cranial nerve (CN VII). As the facial nerve descends in the mastoid, it gives origin to the chorda tympani nerve, which traverses the middle ear and enters the infratemporal fossa. The chorda tympani joins the lingual nerve (a branch of the mandibular division of the trigeminal nerve) just below the foramen ovale. The parasympathetic fibers then run with the lingual nerve to the submandibular ganglion, which is suspended from the lingual nerve just superior to the submandibular gland. These parasympathetic fibers are also distributed from the submandibular ganglion to the sublingual gland within the floor of the mouth.

Sublingual Glands

The sublingual glands are located submucosally in the floor of the mouth. They are positioned between the mandible on their lateral surface and the hyoglossus and genioglossus muscles on their medial surface. The

2 sublingual glands nearly meet in the midline. Most sublingual glands have no single dominant duct. Rather, approximately 12 smaller ducts pass into the mucosa of the floor of the mouth. The sublingual glands are innervated by parasympathetic fibers of the chorda tympani. These fibers arrive at the sublingual glands by the route described previously.

Minor Salivary Glands

Small unnamed salivary glands are widespread in the oral cavity and pharynx. These are both mucus- and serous-secreting glands, each of which has its own duct draining into the mucous membranes. These glands are most prominent in the oral cavity and are located in the hard and soft palate, lips, buccal mucosa, floor of mouth, and tongue. Small mucus-secreting glands can also be found in the larynx, hypopharynx, nasopharynx, nose, and paranasal sinuses. Disorders or diseases involving the major salivary glands may also be found within the minor salivary glands.

HISTOLOGY

On a microscopic level, the salivary glands are composed of an acinus, a secretory tubule, and a collecting duct (Fig. 22–1). The acinar cells are responsible for producing the secretions. The tubules and duct function in resorption of water and electrolytes. The acinar cells within the parotid gland are primarily serous. The acinar cells in the sublingual glands are mostly mucus-producing cells. The submandibular gland contains both serous- and mucus-producing acinar cells. The minor salivary glands similarly can contain both mucous and serous acinar cells. Myoepithelial cells surround the acini and contract on stimulation to help expel the secretions. Neoplasms of the salivary glands arise from different histologic components of the secretory apparatus, as discussed in greater detail later in this chapter.

PHYSIOLOGY

The saliva produced by the salivary glands has several functions, including initial digestion of food, lubrication of food, protection of dental structures, control of oral cavity bacterial counts, and immune system function (secretory antibodies). On stimulation, the acinar cells of the salivary glands produce a transudate of fluids, and they actively excrete proteins and other organic substances. The salivary flow results from excretion of stored saliva, as well as production and secretion of newly formed saliva. Normal saliva typically includes 99% water, electrolytes, and organic compounds including proteins, urea, lipids, and amino

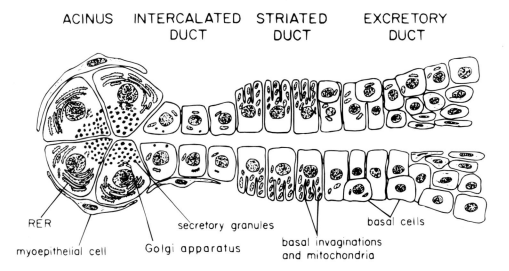

ACINUS   INTERCALATED   STRIATED   EXCRETORY
                DUCT   DUCT   DUCT

RER   myoepithelial cell   Golgi apparatus   secretory granules   basal invaginations and mitochondria   basal cells

Fig. 22–1. Schematic of the salivary gland acinus and duct system. RER, Rough endoplasmic reticulum.

acids.[2] Included with the protein portion of saliva are amylase, albumin, IgA, and lysozyme. Although the parotid glands are the largest of the salivary glands, the submandibular glands account for roughly 70% of the total volume of saliva produced in a 24-hour period. The parotid glands are responsible for approximately 25% of the total saliva, and the sublingual and minor salivary glands produce the remainder.[2] A baseline secretion of saliva occurs to lubricate the oral cavity and pharynx. The major salivary glands secrete primarily in response to reflex stimuli. On recognition of the appropriate stimuli, the afferent fibers signal the superior and inferior salivatory nuclei of the brain stem, which, in turn, stimulate nerve fibers of CN VII and IX, as outlined previously. Parasympathetic stimulation is propagated to the end organ, and saliva is produced.

PATHOLOGY

Hormonal and Metabolic Disorders

Endocrine and metabolic disorders alter the volume of saliva produced by the salivary glands or may produce noninflammatory enlargement of the salivary glands.

Sialadenosis is a chronic, noninflammatory enlargement of the salivary glands that is often associated with malnutrition. Primary protein malnutrition is a common cause, but in the United States, malnutrition secondary to alcoholism is probably more often responsible for sialadenosis. Chronic vitamin deficiencies such as beriberi, pellagra, and vitamin A deficiency have also been associated with parotid gland enlargement. Hepatic cirrhosis is often accompanied by salivary gland enlargement and should be considered in the differential diagnosis of parotid hypertrophy of unknown origin.

Endocrine Disorders

Salivary gland enlargement has been reported with almost all the endocrine abnormalities. Chronic benign swelling of the salivary glands can be seen during the latter half of pregnancy and often resolves following delivery. The parotid gland enlargement seen in diabetes is the most common salivary gland abnormality in association with an endocrine disorder. Hypothyroidism and Cushing's disease may also result in salivary gland enlargement or sialadenitis. Finally, any disorder that produces a neuropathy of the peripheral autonomic nervous system is probably capable of causing salivary gland enlargement.

Drug Effects

Many drugs inhibit salivary gland secretions. These include the anticholinergic agents such as atropine, sympathomimetic drugs such as pseudoephedrine, and antidepressant agents including amitriptyline, imipramine, and dibenzepin. The phenothiazines may have atropine-like side effects and cause salivary gland enlargement. Other drugs associated with enlargement of the salivary glands include methyldopa, isoproterenol, hydrochlorothiazide, and phenylbutazone. For many years, it was assumed that the parasympathomimetic agents such as pilocarpine produced side effects that would preclude use in chronic hyposalivation. Recently, a large, placebo-controlled study has demonstrated efficacy for orally administered pilocarpine in relieving the symptoms of radiation-induced stomatitis in patients with head and neck cancer.[3] The study demonstrated that, for most patients, the gastrointestinal, genitourinary, and cardiac side effects of oral pilocarpine were minimal. Although symptomatic improvement was evident with oral pilocarpine, significant quantitative changes in salivary flow were less apparent in treated patients, and the eventual role of pilocarpine in treating xerostomia remains to be defined.

Inflammatory Disorders

Inflammatory disorders of the salivary glands may occur as a component of systemic disease or as a disease process isolated to the salivary gland itself. Inflammatory disease processes may be infectious, autoimmune, or idiopathic.

Systemic Inflammatory Diseases Affecting the Salivary Glands

Viral Infections

MUMPS. Mumps is a disease of viral origin most commonly occurring in pediatric age groups. Typical symptoms include fever, malaise, and headache, followed by tenderness and enlargement of the parotid glands. As the parotid glands enlarge, trismus and dysphagia may develop. Typically, the disease involves the parotid glands primarily, but the submandibular and sublingual glands may be involved on occasion. The disease is usually self-limited and uncomplicated. The swelling of the glands characteristically subsides within 2 weeks. Serious sequelae include orchitis, sensorineural hearing loss, aseptic meningitis, and encephalitis. To prevent these more serious complications, mumps virus vaccine is recommended for all children as part of the mumps, measles, rubella (MMR) vaccination.

CYTOMEGALOVIRUS. Cytomegalovirus (CMV) is part of the herpesvirus family. Infection with this virus causes identifiable cellular changes in the lungs, gastrointestinal tract, liver, and adrenal glands, as well as the salivary glands. Distinctive intranuclear inclusions within affected cells are characteristic of the infection. CMV infection of newborns may lead to mental and physical retardation and hepatosplenomegaly. By the age of 70 years, the majority of Americans are exposed to CMV and are seropositive. Immunocompromised individuals may experience a serious and potentially fatal infection on first exposure to CMV.

Sjögren's Syndrome

Sjögren's syndrome is an autoimmune disease, the symptoms and signs of which were first described by Hadden in 1883. Sjögren was a Swedish ophthalmologist who published a paper on keratoconjunctivitis sicca and elaborated on the systemic nature of the disease, including polyarthritis, dry mouth, and elevated sedimentation rates.[4] Sjögren's syndrome has more recently been classified as primary or secondary. In the former, the disease involves the exocrine glands alone. In the latter, the autoimmune disorder also includes a collagen vascular disease such as rheumatoid arthritis,

lupus, progressive systemic sclerosis, or dermatomyositis. Approximately half the patients with Sjögren's syndrome have the primary form.

For many patients, the course is self-limited. In others, the disease may be progressive and result in multiorgan involvement, including biliary cirrhosis, interstitial fibrosis of the lungs, interstitial nephritis, and peripheral neuropathy. The development of malignant lymphomas in patients with Sjögren's syndrome occurs at a significantly higher rate than in the general population.

Salivary gland involvement in Sjögren's syndrome is often bilateral and diffuse. The parotid or submandibular glands may be involved, and the swelling occurring in the glands may be episodic and fluctuating. The patients typically complain of dry mouth, which may be manifest as difficulty in swallowing, speaking, or wearing dentures or as an increase in dental caries. Biopsy of minor salivary glands of the lip or of the tail of major salivary glands reveals a lymphocytic infiltrate with acinar atrophy, as discussed later. As this process progresses, epimyoepithelial islands existing in a widespread lymphocytic infiltrate may be found.

The salivary gland enlargement associated with Sjögren's syndrome is typically painless, firm, and bilateral. The enlargement may be asymmetric, however. Asymmetric enlargement or rapid enlargement of one gland should raise the suspicion of a newly developed lymphoma.

Benign Lymphoepithelial Lesion

The benign lymphoepithelial lesion is the histologic lesion appearing in the salivary glands in patients with Sjögren's syndrome; however, the benign lymphoepithelial lesion may also be found in patients with no evidence of Sjögren's syndrome. These lesions were previously referred to as Mikulicz's disease and were characterized by enlargement of the salivary and lacrimal glands. The benign lymphoepithelial lesion typically appears as a firm, asymptomatic swelling in the parotid gland. The parotid gland is involved in approximately 80% of cases, and approximately 80% of the patients are female.[5]

Benign lymphoepithelial lesions have also been associated with an increased risk of lymphoma. The risk of developing lymphoma is approximately 40 times higher than in the general population.[6] Once the diagnosis of a benign lymphoepithelial lesion has been established, a search for the coexistence of Sjögren's syndrome should begin.

Human Immunodeficiency Virus

Patients infected with the human immunodeficiency virus (HIV) may develop a spectrum of salivary gland disorders, including diffuse infiltrative lymphocytosis syndrome (DILS), benign lymphoepithelial lesion, lymphoepithelial cysts, and malignant salivary gland tumors, including lymphoma, Kaposi's sarcoma, and adenoid cystic carcinoma. DILS is characterized by salivary gland enlargement associated with xerostomia and xerophthalmia. The salivary enlargement and the accompanying symptoms may resemble those of Sjögren's syndrome, but the autoantibodies commonly found in Sjögren's syndrome are lacking.[7]

Lymphoepithelial cysts are distinct from the lymphoepithelial lesions listed previously. Lymphoepithelial cysts are often seen as a manifestation of HIV infection. These lesions frequently involve the parotid gland and may be unilateral or bilateral. These lesions often arise within lymphoid tissue deposits within the salivary glands. The association of lymphoepithelial cysts with HIV infection is strong enough that, if this diagnosis is rendered on the basis of a needle biopsy, testing for HIV infection should be initiated.[8]

Clinically, parotid gland enlargement in patients with HIV infection is usually diffuse and symmetric. The parotid glands are involved more frequently than the submandibular glands. This salivary gland enlargement may coexist with generalized or regional lymphadenopathy. In rapidly enlarging salivary glands, the possibility of lymphoma should be considered. The disfigurement produced by salivary gland enlargement has led many HIV-infected individuals to seek surgical therapy.

Sarcoidosis

The salivary glands are involved in fewer than 10% of cases of sarcoidosis. Parotid gland involvement is more common than involvement of the other salivary glands. Heerfordt's syndrome or uveoparotid fever may result from sarcoidosis and includes uveitis, lacrimal and salivary gland inflammation, and facial paralysis. Corticosteroids are used for advanced ocular and pulmonary forms of sarcoidosis. The diagnosis is confirmed by biopsy revealing noncaseating granulomas. Usually, the disease is self-limited, and, even without treatment, the facial paralysis commonly resolves.

Wegener's Granulomatosis

Wegener's granulomatosis is a systemic disorder often involving the respiratory tract from the nose to the lungs, as well as the kidneys. The classic histologic findings include necrotizing granulomas with vasculitis of small and medium-sized arteries. A characteristic autoantibody, antineutrophil cytoplasmic antibody (ANCA), can be detected in the serum and has allowed recognition of earlier and more limited forms of Wegener's granulomatosis.

Clinically, salivary gland enlargement may accompany the nasal and sinus symptoms of early Wegener's granulomatosis. The process can involve either the parotid or the submandibular glands. Treatment options include immunosuppressive therapy with prednisone and cyclophosphamide, or trimethoprim-sulfamethoxazole for more limited cases.[9]

Granulomatous Diseases

Mycobacterial Sialadenitis

In the pediatric age group, infections caused by atypical mycobacteria are more common than infections resulting from Mycobacterium tuberculosis. These microorganisms often gain access to the salivary glands through a lesion in the oral cavity and manifest as an enlarging mass. Infections with atypical mycobacteria are also being seen with increasing frequency in patients suffering from immunodeficiency disorders. These microorganisms are often resistant to multiple antituberculous antibiotics. Surgical treatment is often sufficient, consisting either of excision or of incision and curettage.

Pulmonary tuberculosis may also involve the salivary glands as a secondary site. The submandibular and sublingual glands are more frequently involved than the parotid gland. These cases are more effectively treated with antituberculous antibiotics.

Actinomycosis

Actinomycosis commonly involves the head and neck. Direct infection of the salivary glands is rare, however, and often originates via extension into the salivary glands from an adjacent site. Typically, one notes a firm, indurated mass over the site of infection. Later in the course, a draining fistula forms that produces a purulent exudate containing yellow "sulfur" granules. Extended treatment with penicillin is typically curative.

Cat-scratch Disease

Like actinomycosis, cat-scratch disease does not often directly involve the salivary glands. The periglandular and intraglandular lymph nodes may, however, become involved. The microorganism causing cat-scratch disease is a pleomorphic gram-negative bacillus. The disease typically involves children and young adults. The initial lesion is a papule or pustule near the site of inoculation of the skin, which heals. Approximately 2 weeks later, tender lymphadenopathy follows. This lymphadenopathy frequently involves the head and neck. Primary involvement of the salivary glands is rare. The adenopathy typically resolves spontaneously over 2 to 3 months. No antibiotic has been found to be effective against the infection. Node biopsy or debridement may be required for diagnostic purposes.

Other Granulomatous Diseases

Syphilis may affect the salivary glands during any stage of the disease process. The diagnosis can be established on the basis of serology and response to treatment. Excisional biopsy to establish the diagnosis may occasionally be necessary.

Systemic fungal infections may involve the salivary glands. These infections typically produce granulomatous inflammation and may present as an enlarging mass in the submandibular or parotid area. Fungal infections often involve lymphoid tissues in and around the salivary glands. Systemic antifungal antibiotics may be required for treatment. Rarely, a fungal infection may become invasive in an immunocompromised host and may require aggressive surgical debridement as well as systemic antibiotics.

Toxoplasmosis is a parasitic disease thought to be transferred to humans through undercooked meat or contact with cat feces. The infection causes necrotizing granulomatous inflammation within lymph nodes in and around the salivary glands. A disseminated form of the disease involving multiple organ systems can also affect immunocompromised hosts. Antibiotic therapy includes pyrimethamine and trisulfapyrimidine.[10]

Inflammatory Disease Isolated to the Salivary Glands

Acute Suppurative Sialadenitis

Acute bacterial sialadenitis most frequently involves the parotid gland. Elderly adults are affected most often. The site of entry of the bacteria is retrograde transmission from the oral cavity along the salivary duct. This process occurs in most patients; however, the bacteria are usually flushed from the duct system by high salivary flow rates. In postoperative patients who may be dehydrated from blood loss, fluid shifts, or volume depletion, salivary flow rates may be diminished, and the opportunity for acute sialadenitis is enhanced. The organisms most commonly causing acute sialadenitis include penicillinase-producing varieties of Staphylococcus aureus, pneumococcus, group A streptococcus, and Haemophilus influenza. Treatment involves hydration, massage of the affected gland, and antibiotic therapy directed at the microorganisms cultured from the purulent exudate.

Symptoms of acute bacterial sialadenitis include rapid onset of pain, swelling, induration, and fever. Occasionally, the infection may coalesce and form an abscess that responds poorly to systemic antibiotics. Because improvement with appropriate antibiotics is typically rapid, if a patient with findings of acute suppurative sialadenitis has not improved after 48 to 72 hours of antibiotic therapy, or if pitting edema over the affected gland develops, the presence of an abscess should be considered. Incision and drainage of the abscessed gland may be necessary.

The inflammatory process stimulated by bacterial sialadenitis may cause replacement of gland parynchema, fibrosis, and ductal ectasia. These changes may result in reduced salivary flow rates and may leave the gland at higher risk of recurrent suppurative infection.

Chronic Sialadenitis

A salivary gland in which salivary flow rates are chronically diminished or in which dilation or stenosis of the ductal system occurs is predisposed to chronic sialadenitis. Similarly, patients with poor oral hygiene and immunosuppressive disorders are more susceptible. Clinically, one notes recurrent swelling and tenderness of the affected gland that may be associated with eating. The swelling and discomfort may resolve shortly after eating, or the patient may have a more protracted bacterial infection that again requires antibiotic therapy and aggressive hydration. During an acute episode, purulence may be produced from the duct orifice. Often, however, secretions are simply decreased. An attempt to identify a stone or stricture within the salivary duct should be made. The process may wax and wane, with disease-free intervals lasting from several weeks to several months. Conservative treatment usually quiets the inflammation. If the inflammation recurs frequently, however, surgical excision of the gland may be ultimately required. A total parotidectomy or submandibular gland excision is usually recommended in this instance. Other treatment options popular in the past included repeated dilation of the duct, ligation of the duct, tympanic neurectomy, and gland irradiation.

Benign Parotid Neoplasms

Pleomorphic Adenoma

Pleomorphic adenoma is the most common of all salivary gland neoplasms. These lesions are also called benign mixed tumor and are most frequently found in the parotid gland where they comprise 80% of the benign tumors. Pleomorphic adenomas contain both mesenchymal and epithelial cell lines. The tumors are typically encapsulated, but, on close microscopic examination, have pseudopod extensions into the surrounding tissues. Treatment of pleomorphic adenomas requires wide local excision including a cuff of normal salivary gland tissue. When simple enucleation is attempted, recurrence rates are approximately 30%. Because most of these lesions occur in the parotid gland, a superficial parotidectomy is typically the minimal operation required for resection of these lesions. Within the parotid gland, most pleomorphic adenomas arise in the superficial lobe. The 10% that arise in the deep lobe of the parotid gland may manifest as a parapharyngeal space mass with medial displacement of the tonsil and intra-oral swelling.

Warthin's Tumor

Warthin's tumor is named for the University of Michigan pathologist who first reported two cases in the

United States. The tumor had been identified earlier in Europe by Hildebrad, but the pathogenesis of the lesion was unclear. Warthin coined the term papillary cystadenoma lymphomatosum. This tumor occurs next in frequency following the pleomorphic adenoma. Warthin's tumor typically involves the lower pole of the parotid glands. It rarely occurs in any of the other salivary glands. Elderly men are most commonly affected. The tumor is bilateral in 10% of cases. Microscopically, the tumor contains a double layer of papillary epithelium that forms cystic spaces in a background of lymphoid tissue. The most popular etiologic theory suggests that Warthin's tumor arises in salivary ducts that are trapped within intraparotid lymph nodes. Complete surgical excision is the accepted treatment for Warthin's tumors. In an elderly, debilitated patient, a fine-needle aspirate characteristic of Warthin's tumor coupled with consistent clinical findings may be grounds for expectant, nonsurgical management.

Monomorphic Adenomas

Monomorphic adenomas arise from the ductal epithelium of the salivary glands. The monomorphic adenomas include basal cell adenoma, clear cell adenoma, and glycogen-rich adenoma, among other less common tumors. Basal cell adenomas, the most common type of monomorphic adenomas, are most frequently found in the minor salivary glands of the upper lip. The parotid gland is the most common major salivary gland giving rise to basal cell adenomas. Investigators have suggested that adenoid cystic carcinomas represent a malignant form of basal cell adenomas. These two tumors must be distinguished by the pathologist to ensure proper treatment. Treatment involves wide excision with a cuff of surrounding salivary gland parynchema or surrounding soft tissue.

Oncocytomas

Oncocytomas comprise less than 1% of all salivary gland neoplasms. These tumors are typically found in the superficial lobe of the parotid gland. The oncocytes concentrate technetium-99m pertechnetate in radioisotope scans. This tumor and Warthin's tumor, which also contains oncocytes, may appear as a "hot" nodule on a radionuclide scan. Malignant oncocytomas have been reported. Their histologic appearance is very similar, and they are often distinguishable only by their biologic behavior. Treatment of oncocytomas includes wide excision with a cuff of normal surrounding soft tissue. Because they most commonly occur in the parotid gland, these tumors typically require a superficial parotidectomy with facial nerve preservation.

Malignant Neoplasms

When the salivary glands are considered in aggregate, benign tumors are more common than their malignant

TABLE 22–1. Histologic Types of Salivary Gland Tumors in 2807 Patients

	No. of Patients	Percentage (%)
Benign		
Pleomorphic adenoma	1274	45.4
Warthin's tumor	183	6.5
Benign cyst	29	1.0
Lymphoepithelial lesion	17	0.6
Onocytoma	20	0.7
Monomorphic adenoma	6	0.2
Malignant		
Mucoepidermoid carcinoma	439	15.7
Adenoid cystic carcinoma	281	10.0
Adenocarcinoma	225	8.0
Malignant mixed tumor	161	5.7
Acinic cell carcinoma	84	3.0
Epidermoid carcinoma	53	1.9
Other (anaplastic, etc.)	35	1.3
Total	2807	100.0

(Adapted from Spiro RM: Salivary neoplasms: overview of a 35-year experience with 2,807 patients. Head Neck Surg 8:177, 1986.)

counterparts. In the sublingual glands and minor salivary glands, however, the ratios are reversed. The commonly encountered salivary gland malignant tumors by site are listed in Table 22–1. Spiro reviewed a total of 2807 salivary gland tumors.[11] Of this total, 1278 (45%) were malignant. In a compilation of over 7000 salivary gland neoplasms reported in the medical literature, 78% of parotid neoplasms were found to be benign, 54% of submandibular gland neoplasms were benign, and 35% of minor salivary gland neoplasms were benign.[12] The presentation of malignant salivary gland tumors is variable, depending on site and histologic features. Facial nerve paralysis is uncommon and generally indicates a malignant lesion. Tumors of the deep lobe of the parotid gland may produce dysphagia, earache, or trismus. When the parapharyngeal space is invaded, CN IX, X, XI, or XII may be involved. The usual presentation of submandibular gland tumors is painless swelling below the mandible.

Mucoepidermoid Carcinoma

Mucoepidermoid carcinoma is the most common malignant salivary gland tumor, comprising one fourth to one third of the total number of salivary malignant tumors in most series. Roughly half of all mucoepidermoid carcinomas occur in the parotid gland, with the majority of the remainder occurring in minor salivary glands. Mucoepidermoid carcinomas appear to arise from the excretory and intercalated ducts of the salivary glands. As the name implies, mucoepidermoid carcinomas contain both mucus-secreting and epidermoid cells. Histologic grading as low grade or high grade has been helpful in predicting biologic behavior. The low-grade tumors have prominent cystic structures with mature cellular elements. Neural invasion is uncommon. Low-grade tumors are characterized by a slow growth rate, a low recurrence rate after complete surgical excision (about 15%), and rare metastatic spread. High-grade mucoepidermoid carcinomas, on the other hand, are characterized by sheets of solid cells displaying a noticeable degree of atypia. High-grade mucoepidermoid carcinomas are aggressive. The local recurrence rate following surgery approaches 60%. Nodal metastases may develop in 40 to 70% of patients, and 30% of patients develop distant metastases. For low-grade mucoepidermoid carcinomas, treatment usually consists of wide surgical excision. Neck dissection or adjuvant irradiation is used only when clinically evident metastases are detected or when direct invasion of bone, nerve, or other extraglandular structures has occurred. High-grade mucoepidermoid carcinomas are treated more like squamous cell carcinomas. Wide excision, combined with regional node dissection and often including adjuvant radiation therapy, is commonplace. The issue of facial nerve preservation in high-grade mucoepidermoid carcinomas is a source of controversy. Some surgeons only sacrifice the facial nerve when it is directly involved with tumor, whereas others routinely sacrifice the facial nerve in an attempt to gain a wide surgical margin. No one recommends preserving a nerve that is clearly invaded by tumor.

Low-grade mucoepidermoid carcinomas have 5-year survival rates in the 80 to 95% range. Five-year survival rates for high-grade tumors are more typically 30 to 50%.[11]

Adenoid Cystic Carcinoma

Adenoid cystic carcinoma is the next most common malignant tumor of the salivary glands. It is the most common malignant tumor in the submandibular gland and the minor salivary glands, comprising 30 to 40% of the malignant tumors identified in those locations. Adenoid cystic carcinoma often manifests with pain in association with a salivary gland mass. Its course is slow but relentless, and survival figures are quoted in terms of 10- to 20-year follow-up, rather than 5-year follow-up. Perineural invasion is frequently seen in patients with adenoid cystic carcinoma and allows distant extension along perineural lymphatic vessels, which frustrates attempt at local control. Although local control is the major problem in treatment of this tumor, the lesion does have the capacity for distant metastasis, and 40% of patients ultimately develop regional and/or distant metastases. Treatment of adenoid cystic carcinoma includes wide local excision and therapeutic lymph node dissections. Elective lymph node dissections are typically not recommended. Recently, neutron-beam radiation has been shown to be effective in controlling adenoid cystic carcinomas that were surgically incurable. The role of adjuvant neutron irradiation following surgical excision is being investigated.[13]

Adenocarcinoma

Adenocarcinomas constitute approximately 10 to 15% of all malignant salivary gland carcinomas. Only mucoepidermoid carcinomas and adenoid cystic carcinomas are more common. The majority of cases of adenocarcinoma occur in the parotid gland, where the majority are high-grade tumors, followed by the minor salivary glands, and then the submandibular gland. These tumors typically occur as a mass in the parotid region or a submucosal intraoral mass. Adenocarcinomas arising in the nose and paranasal sinuses probably originate from minor salivary gland tissue as well. Surgery is the primary mode of treatment for adenocarcinomas of the salivary glands. The issue of elective regional lymph node resection is disputed. If lymph nodes are palpable in the regional lymph node groups, lymphadenectomy certainly should be performed. Adenocarcinomas may be less sensitive to radiation therapy than other types of carcinomas. The high-grade adenocarcinomas are typically treated with adjuvant radiation therapy, however, in an attempt to improve local control rates.

In a large series of adenocarcinomas of the salivary glands, local recurrences were detected in 51% of patients, cervical metastases in 27% of patients, and distant metastases in 26% of patients.[14] Five-year survival rates may be inadequate when considering adenocarcinoma of the salivary glands. Ten- and 15-year curves have demonstrated decreasing survival rates beyond 5 years. The most accurate predictor of outcome is clinical stage at presentation. Patients with large tumors and nodal metastases had a significantly poorer prognosis than those with smaller, localized lesions.[15]

Acinic Cell Carcinoma

Most acinic cell carcinomas arise in the parotid gland. They are rare tumors, comprising roughly 1 to 3% of all salivary gland tumors. At one time, acinic cell carcinoma was referred to as acinic cell tumor, illustrating the difficulty that pathologists have had with predicting clinical behavior based on histologic appearance. A subset of acinic cell carcinomas behaves aggressively. Recent research studies suggest that tumors with high proliferative rates may be associated with early recurrence and biologic "aggressiveness." Acinic cell carcinomas arise from the acinar cells of the salivary unit. The tumors typically appear as a mass in the parotid gland. Occasionally, the mass may grow quickly and may involve the facial nerve or produce pain. The tumors are bilateral in 3% of cases.[16] Treatment of acinic cell carcinoma has centered on wide surgical excision. Lymph node dissection should only be performed when clinically detectable nodes are present. Survival rates are comparable with those of low-grade mucoepidermoid carcinoma. Late, distant, and regional metastases may be seen.

Carcinoma Ex-Pleomorphic Adenoma and Malignant Mixed Tumors

Carcinoma ex-pleomorphic adenoma is a malignant neoplasm that arises from a previously benign pleomorphic adenoma. In contrast, true malignant mixed tumors arise de novo and are rare, constituting only 2 to 5% of all malignant salivary gland tumors. Carcinoma ex-pleomorphic adenoma is by far the more common of the two. The malignant tumor developing in a carcinoma ex-pleomorphic adenoma arises within the epithelial component. The risk of malignant transformation increases with time: 0.6% for adenomas of less than 5-years' duration and 1.4% for adenomas present for more than 15 years.[17] In contrast, in a malignant mixed tumor, both the epithelial and mesenchymal components are malignant. In a long-standing pleomorphic adenoma, malignant transformation is usually marked by rapid growth and possible development of pain and ulceration. Aggressive surgical resection with adjuvant radiation therapy is recommended for either carcinoma ex-pleomorphic adenoma or malignant mixed tumor. Both are aggressive neoplasms with relatively high rates of nodal and distant metastases. The prognosis is poor.

Squamous Cell Carcinoma

Primary squamous cell carcinoma of the salivary gland is rare; however, given the rich lymphatic network that penetrates the parotid gland, squamous carcinomas of the skin of the forehead, temple, or ear may metastasize to this region. Such primary sites must be excluded before the diagnosis of primary squamous carcinoma of the parotid can be made. About 50% of patients with primary squamous carcinoma ultimately develop positive regional nodes.

STAGING. Recently, the American Joint Committee on Cancer (AJCC) and the Union Internationale Contre le Cancer (UICC) have agreed to changes in the staging system for salivary gland tumors to bring the two schema into agreement. The T-stage criteria are listed in Table 22–2. The N- and M-stage criteria are the same as for the more common head and neck squamous cell carcinomas.

TREATMENT. Overall treatment recommendations for malignant salivary gland tumors can be summarized based on histologic features and tumor size. For patients with resectable early stage T1/T2 salivary gland cancer, surgery is the primary form of treatment. Low-grade mucoepidermoid carcinomas are generally treated with local excision. Such tumors arising in the parotid gland are treated with total parotidectomy with preservation of the facial nerve. Early-stage, high-grade tumors of all other histologic types are treated with surgical resection plus dissection of the regional lymph nodes. Such tumors arising in the parotid require total parotidectomy, but usually the facial nerve can be spared. Patients with clinically positive neck

TABLE 22–2. Staging of Primary Salivary Gland Tumors According to the American Joint Committee on Cancer, 1988

T Stage

Tx	Primary tumor cannot be assessed
T0	No evidence of primary tumor
T1	Tumor less than or equal to 2 cm in greatest diameter
T2	Greatest diameter of tumor more than 2 cm but less than 4 cm
T3	Greatest diameter of tumor more than 4 cm but less than 6 cm
T4	Tumor more than 6 cm in greatest diameter

Subdivisions

The foregoing categories are subdivided into (a) no local extension or (b) local extension. Local extension is defined as clinical or macroscopic evidence of tumor invading the skin, soft tissues of the neck, bone, or nerve

Stage Grouping

Stage I	T1a	N0	M0
	T2a	N0	M0
Stage II	T1b	N0	M0
	T2b	N0	M0
	T3a	N0	M0
Stage III	T3b	N0	M0
	T4a	N0	M0
	Any T	N1	M0 (excluding T4b)
Stage IV	T4b	Any N	M0
	Any T	N2 or N3	M0
	Any T	Any N	M1

(From Robbins KT (ed): Pocket Guide to Neck Dissection Classification and TNM Staging of Head and Neck Cancer. Alexandria, VA, American Academy of Otorhinolaryngology—Head and Neck Surgery, 1991, p 26.)

lymph nodes should have a radical neck dissection on the involved side.

In the past, patients with T3 or T4 parotid disease required radical parotidectomy with sacrifice of the facial nerve. More recently, nerve-sparing surgery has been used, followed by radiotherapy. For many years, salivary gland tumors were thought to be resistant to conventional photon irradiation, but investigators now recognize that this treatment can be effective when given in a postoperative setting to eradicate subclinical disease. Postoperative radiation therapy is indicated when (1) tumor grade is high, including any histologic type except low-grade mucoepidermoid carcinoma, or is metastatic squamous carcinoma, regardless of the surgical margins, (2) the surgical margins are close or microscopically positive, including most tumors involving the deep lobe of the parotid gland regardless of the grade, (3) resection has been performed for recurrent disease regardless of the histologic features or margin status, (4) tumor has invaded skin, bone, nerve, or extraparotid tissue, (5) regional nodes are confirmed as positive on neck dissection, and (6) gross residual or unresectable disease is present.[18]

Doses given to the primary resection site are in the range of 5500 to 6500 cGy, depending on the postsurgical tumor status. In patients with low-grade mucoepidermoid carcinomas, it is generally not necessary to treat the neck lymph nodes in the elective situation. For other histologic types, neck nodal drainage is generally treated with doses of about 5000 cGy. In the case of adenoid cystic carcinomas, the radiation fields must include the courses of the adjacent cranial nerves because perineural spread is common.

For patients with large, inoperable salivary gland cancers, fast neutron radiotherapy is an alternative treatment. A randomized clinical trial was performed comparing neutron irradiation and photon irradiation in patients with large, inoperable lesions.[19] The tumor clearance rate at the primary site was 85% for the neutron group versus 33% for the photon group. Review of nonrandomized trials showed the local or regional control rate to be 60 to 70% with definitive neutron radiation and only 24% with definitive photon radiation.[20]

Control of local and regional disease is only a part of the problem, because the incidence of distant metastases varies, depending on histologic type, ranging from a high of over 40% for adenoid cystic carcinomas to a low of less that 10% for mucoepidermoid carcinomas.[21] The role of chemotherapy in the treatment of malignant salivary gland tumors is still under development. The more rapidly growing subtypes that more closely resemble squamous carcinoma in their biologic and clinical behavior tend to respond to drugs effective against squamous carcinoma. Several single-agent studies have been conducted in salivary gland cancers. Promising results have been achieved with *cis*-platin, methotrexate, doxorubicin, and 5-fluorouracil. *Cis*-platin alone or in combination with other agents has been evaluated in over 130 patients and has yielded response rates in the range of 17 to 100%.

IMAGING

Procedures for imaging the salivary glands have evolved considerably over the past few years. Plain radiography, sialography, radionuclide scanning, ultrasonography, computed tomography (CT) scanning, and magnetic resonance (MR) imaging have all been employed to image the salivary glands. In practice, however, only the last two modalities are used with any frequency at our institution at this time. The other techniques are discussed briefly, because they are still often referenced in the medical literature.

Plain Radiography

Salivary calculi can be detected within the ducts of the major salivary glands on occasion using plain radiographs. Salivary duct stones occur much more commonly in the submandibular duct and, in this location, often contain calcium and are radiopaque. These stones are often palpable, but their presence may be confirmed using radiographs. Stones in the parotid ductal system are most often translucent and smaller and are less frequently detected by plain radiographs.

Contrast Sialography

The injection of radiopaque contrast material into the salivary gland ductal system is used to detect calculi and also to detect chronic inflammatory changes within the ductal systems. Among the changes seen are dilation of the terminal ducts and acini, strictures within the ductal system, and cyst formation. In the past, sialography was used to define parotid gland masses, and specific sialographic criteria were used to determine whether a particular mass had benign or malignant characteristics. This use of this technique has basically been replaced by CT and MR scanning.

Radionuclide Scanning: Technetium Pertechnetate

This study is most commonly used for characterizing masses within the parotid and submandibular glands. It was also used in the past for assessment of physiologic function. As mentioned earlier in this chapter, Warthin's tumor and oncocytomas concentrate the radioisotope. Most other salivary neoplasms do not, and they leave a "cold spot" on images of the salivary glands.

Computed Tomography

CT has largely replaced other imaging studies for salivary masses. CT scans delineate solid from cystic masses and can detect masses as small as 1 cm within the substance of the salivary glands. The anatomic delineation of a mass involving any of the salivary glands can be well defined by CT scanning. Benign masses within the parotid glands often have smooth, clearly defined borders on CT scans. Aggressive and infiltrative malignant neoplasms often have diffuse borders and may show evidence of adjacent bone destruction or invasion of adjacent tissues.

In a large retrospective study of 110 sequentially resected parotid masses, CT scans, along with other imaging techniques, were compared with final histologic features. The CT characteristics emerging from this study included the following: (1) for tumors with well-defined borders, homogenous appearance, and high-signal density, the diagnosis was more likely a benign tumor or a low-grade malignant tumor; (2) ill-defined tumor borders, heterogeneous appearance, and high density were more consistent with a high-grade malignant tumor; and (3) ill-defined borders, heterogeneous appearance, and mixed-signal density were more consistent with an inflammatory process such as benign lymphoepithelial lesion or sialodenitis.[22]

Magnetic Resonance Imaging

MR imaging is especially useful for detecting small lesions within the substance of the salivary glands. Often, these lesions are isointense on CT scans, making them difficult to delineate clearly. Because the MR image registers proton content rather than absolute tissue density, tissues that would appear isointense on x-ray studies are often clearly delineated by MR imaging. Even in early comparisons with CT scanning, neoplasms within the salivary glands could be delineated more clearly by MR imaging.[23]

Benign tumors as seen on MR imaging typically have low T1 signal intensities and high T2 signal intensities. Malignant tumors may demonstrate less signal intensity on T2-weighted images, but are often enhanced with gadolinium.[24] Infiltration of adjacent structures by a mass demonstrated on MR imaging has been a consistent predictor in distinguishing benign from malignant processes within the gland. Among benign tumors in the parotid gland, pleomorphic adenomas typically have a homogenous appearance with enhancement after contrast injection, whereas Warthin's tumors have demonstrated varying areas of signal intensity within the mass and are not enhanced after contrast injection.[25]

SUGGESTED READINGS

1. Hollingshead WH: Anatomy for Surgeons. 3rd Ed. Vol I: The Head and Neck. Philadelphia, Harper & Row, 1982.
2. Mandel ID: Sialochemistry in diseases and clinical situations affecting the salivary glands. Crit Rev Clin Lab Sci 12:321, 1980.
3. Johnson JT, et al: Oral pilocarpine for post-irradiation xerostomia in patients with head and neck cancer. N Engl J Med 329:390, 1993.
4. Rice DM: Diseases of the salivary glands, non-neoplastic. In: Head and Neck Surgery: Otolaryngology. Edited by Bailey BJ. Philadelphia, JB Lippincott, 1993, p 478.
5. Gleason MJ, Kossen RA, and Bennett MH: Benign epithelial lesion, a less than benign disease. Clin Otolaryngol 11:47, 1986.
6. Seifert, G: Tumor-like lesions of the salivary glands: the new WHO classification. Pathol Res Pract 188:836, 1992.
7. Rosenberg ZS, et al: Spectrum of salivary gland disease in HIV-infected patients: characterization with gallium 67 citrates imaging. Radiology 184:761, 1992.
8. Elliott J and Ortell YC: Lymphoepithelial cysts of the salivary glands. Am J Clin Pathol 93:39, 1990.
9. Specks U, et al: Salivary gland involvement in Wegener's granulomatosis. Arch Otolaryngol Head Neck Surg 117:218, 1991.
10. Rafaty FM: Cervical adenopathy secondary to toxoplasmosis. Arch Otolaryngol Head Neck Surg 103:547, 1977.
11. Spiro RH: Salivary neoplasms: overview of a 35-year experience with 2,807 patients. Head Neck Surg 8:177, 1986.
12. Spiro RH and Spiro JD: Cancer of the salivary glands. In: Cancer of the Head and Neck. 2nd Ed. Edited by Myers EN and Suen JY. New York, Churchill Livingstone, 1989, p 646.
13. Koh WJ, et al: Fast neutron radiation for inoperable and recurrent salivary gland cancers. Am J Clin Oncol 12:316, 1989.
14. Spiro RH, Huvos, and Strong EW: Adenocarcinoma of salivary origin: a clinical pathologic study of 204 patients. Am J Surg 144:423, 1982.
15. AuClair PL and Ellis GL: Adenocarcinoma, not otherwise specified. In: Surgical Pathology of the Salivary Glands. Edited by Ellis G, AuClair P, and Gnepp DR. Philadelphia, WB Saunders, 1991.
16. Eisele DW and Johns ME: Salivary gland neoplasms. In: Head and Neck Surgery: Otolaryngology. Edited by Bailey B. Philadelphia, JB Lippincott, 1993.
17. Bjorklund A and Eneroth CM: Management of parotid gland neoplasms. Am J Otolaryngol 1:155, 1980.
18. Tapley ND: Irradiation treatment of malignant tumors of the salivary glands. Ear Nose Throat J 56:110, 1977.
19. Griffin TW, et al: Neutron vs. photon irradiation of inoperable salivary gland tumors: results of an RTOG-MRC cooperative randomized study. Int J Radiat Oncol Biol Phys 15:1085, 1988.
20. Griffin TW, et al: Predicting the response of head and neck cancers to radiation therapy with a multivariate system: an analysis of the RTOG head and neck registry. Int J Radiat Oncol Biol Phys 10:481, 1984.
21. Johns ME and Kaplan MJ: Malignant neoplasms. In: Otolaryngology Head and Neck Surgery. Edited by Cummings CW, et al. St. Louis, CV Mosby, 1986, p 1049.
22. Byrne MN, Spector JG, Garvin CF, and Gado MH: Preoperative assessment of parotid masses: a comparative evaluation of radiologic techniques to histopathologic diagnosis. Laryngoscope 99:284, 1989.
23. Rice DH and Becker T: Magnetic resonance imaging of the salivary glands: a comparison with computed tomographic scanning. Arch Otolaryngol Head Neck Surg 113:78, 1987.
24. Som PM and Biller HF: High grade malignancies in the parotid gland: identification with MR imaging. Radiology 171:823, 1989.
25. Joe VQ and Westesson PL: Tumors of the parotid gland: MR imaging characteristics of various histologic types. AJR Am J Roentgenol 163:433, 1994.

23 Diseases of the Thyroid Gland

Robert A. Hendrix

The thyroid gland (thyroeides, from Greek meaning shield-like) is a brownish-red, highly vascular, ductless gland situated anteriorly in the visceral compartment of the neck at the level of the fifth, sixth, and seventh cervical and first thoracic vertebrae. The normal adult gland weighing 20 to 25 g is slightly larger in women. It enlarges further during puberty, menstruation, and pregnancy. It consists of right and left cone-shaped lobes 5 cm in length, connected by a narrow region of gland termed the isthmus. The base of each lobe lies on a level with the fourth or fifth tracheal ring, with the apex oriented laterally and superiorly to the level of the oblique line of the thyroid cartilage. The pyramidal lobe is a variable tail of thyroid tissue trailing superiorly from a paramedian attachment to the isthmus. A true capsule of fibrous connective tissue contains the parenchyma and sends fine septa between lobules of the thyroid gland.

PHYSIOLOGY

The thyroid gland contains two types of functioning endocrine cells of different origins. The follicular cells secrete L-thyroxine (T4) and 3,5,3'-triiodo-L-thyronine (T3), which influence a wide range of metabolic processes. The parafollicular cells or C-cells influence calcium metabolism by secretion of calcitonin.

The lumina of follicles of the thyroid contain thyroglobulin as a colloid. This glycoprotein is produced only by follicular cells. Production of active thyroid hormone begins with energy-dependent uptake and transport of extracellular iodide across the follicular cell membrane. Following oxidation of iodide and repeated iodinations of tyrosine residues on newly synthesized thyroglobulin at the cell-colloid interface, T3 and T4 are produced and stored in the follicular lumen bound to thyroglobulin.

Liberation of active thyroid hormone requires up-take of colloid droplets from the lumen by pinocytosis and transport through the follicular cell with hydrolysis of thyroglobulin and release of free T3 and T4. Thus, normal secretion of thyroid hormone requires not only an adequate rate of hormone synthesis, but also the capacity to hydrolyze thyroglobulin to liberate thyroxine.

The follicles secrete only 20% of serum T3; dehalogenation of circulating T4 produces the remainder. The concentration of unbound T3 is about 10 times greater than unbound T4 because of different affinities for thyroid-binding globulin and other plasma proteins. Nonetheless, plasma proteins reversibly bind almost all the serum T3 and T4, leaving only 0.3% of T3 and 0.03% of T4 (or one tenth the level of T3) free to act on receptor sites.

The metabolic effects and the regulation of thyroid hormone depend solely on the concentration of free or unbound T4 and T3 in plasma. Approximately one third of the T4 is deiodinated to T3, and **T3 is three times more potent than T4.** Thus, T4 exerts most of its metabolic effects through its conversion to T3. The weaker binding of T3 to plasma protein carriers may also contribute to the more rapid onset and shorter duration of its action.

Thyrotropin (thyroid-stimulating hormone, TSH) is a glycoprotein secreted by basophilic (thyrotropin) cells of the anterior pituitary gland. TSH mediates suprathyroid regulation of thyroid hormone secretion. TSH acts to increase all aspects of follicular cell metabolism, including synthesis of hormone and thyroglobulin, and hormone secretion. Hypothalamic secretion of thyrotropin-releasing hormone (TRH) controls TSH secretion. Free thyroid hormones in serum exert negative feedback at the level of the pituitary by inhibiting TSH secretion and antagonizing TRH by decreasing the number of receptors on the thyrotropin cell.

At the level of the thyroid gland, iodine depletion enhances the responsiveness to TSH, whereas iodine enrichment inhibits the TSH response. The biosynthesis and secretion of T3 and T4 can be affected, not only by deficiency of dietary iodide, but also by drugs such as lithium, propylthiouracil, sulfonamides, phenytoin, and nitrophenols.

Deiodination of approximately 40% of T4 produces inactive 3,3′,5′-triiodo-L-thyronine or reverse T3 (rT3). Certain conditions (e.g., starvation) increase the T4 conversion to rT3, thereby requiring occasional measurement of rT3.

LABORATORY ASSESSMENT OF THYROID FUNCTION

Serum Tests Related to Thyroid Hormone

The most widely used serum assays of thyroid hormone are the T4 radioimmunoassay (RIA) and T3 uptake of resin. T4 RIA, as a measure of total serum thyroxine, has a normal range of 5 to 13 mg/dl.

States of altered thyroxine-binding affect available thyroid hormone. Adequate assessment requires T4 RIA measurement in combination with the T3 uptake of resin as an indirect measure of thyroxine-binding protein. The T3 uptake of resin test is performed by incubating serum with radioactive, labeled T4 or T3 in the presence of insoluble particles of resin or charcoal that absorb any labeled hormone not bound by serum protein. After removal of the serum, the percentage of radioactive hormone not taken up by serum proteins is measured in the precipitate. The result varies inversely with the concentration of unoccupied sites on serum protein carriers of thyroid hormone. T3 uptake of resin may vary in certain conditions such as pregnancy, when the T4 is increased and T3 uptake is low because of increased thyroid-binding globulin.

The "free" thyroxine determination (FT4) measures the metabolically effective fraction of circulating T4. FT4 provides the best assay of thyroid hormones in regard to function because it is not affected by thyroid-binding globulin. FT4 may be estimated from the more commonly available free thyroxine index (FTI), equal to the product of the T4 and the T3 uptake of resin. This calculation is used to correct for abnormalities of thyroxine binding. Nonetheless, this is unnecessary if the free T4 test is available.

Thyroxine-binding globulin (TBG-RIA) is a direct and specific test for thyroxine-binding abnormalities and is unaffected by changes in other serum proteins.

T3 assessments made by RIA can be valuable in the diagnosis of thyrotoxicosis with normal T4 values (T3 thyrotoxicosis) and in some cases of toxic nodular goiter.

The measurement of serum TSH concentration by RIA is useful to evaluate hyperfunction of the thyroid gland. This, however, is not a useful assay to evaluate hypothyroidism because most assays cannot distinguish between normal and abnormally low levels of TSH.

Direct Tests of Function

The most commonly used direct test of gland function is the thyroid radioactive iodine uptake (RAIU). Historically, the RAIU involved in vivo administration of iodine-131(^{131}I), but ^{123}I has become the agent of choice because of lower radiation dosages. ^{123}I is administered orally in capsule form 24 hours before measurement of thyroid accumulation of ^{123}I. The RAIU is also used in the thyroid suppression test, in which the RAIU is repeated after 7 days of daily administration of T3. A decrease in the RAIU is evidence of the presence of thyroid suppression. This is of value in the assessment of glandular hyperfunction. Similarly, the thyrotropin stimulation test (RAIU performed following TSH administration) is useful to differentiate primary thyroid insufficiency from thyroid hypofunction caused by pituitary hypofunction.

IMAGING OF THE THYROID GLAND

Closely related to the RAIU is the thyroid scintiscan by gamma camera 24 hours after administration of ^{123}I. To evaluate metastatic thyroid cancer or a substernal thyroid, ^{131}I should be used to overcome photon attenuation by bone.

The thyroid also concentrates monovalent ions such as sodium technetium-99m (^{99m}Tc) pertechnetate. Because ^{99m}Tc has a short half-life and is not organically bound, its presence in the thyroid is only transient. Thus, if radioactive iodine uptake is blocked or contraindicated, ^{99m}Tc, at a dose of approximately 5 mCi, may be administered intravenously, with a scan performed at 20 minutes. Either technique adequately assesses thyroid enlargement or cold nodules. Increased sensitivity to the planar ^{99m}Tc scan has been recently reported using single-photon emission tomography (SPECT) for preoperative localization of occult medullary carcinoma of the thyroid gland.[1]

B-mode (two-dimensional) ultrasonography is a useful adjunctive tool for the evaluation of thyroid masses.[2] This method is particularly recommended in children or pregnant women, in whom radioactive isotopes are undesirable. The chief role of this modality is to distinguish between two cystic and solid lesions, particularly in goiter.

Computed tomography (CT) and magnetic resonance (MR) imaging are useful to evaluate thyroid anatomy and relationships with adjacent structures, particularly in preoperative planning. CT scan with iodinated contrast interferes with performance of the radioactive iodide uptake and scan for up to 6 weeks.

Thyroid scans and RAIU should therefore be performed before CT with contrast.

Positron emission tomography (PET) is a promising modality for investigation of thyroid lesions. Measuring uptake of [^{18}F]-2-deoxy-2-fluoro-D-glucose (FDG) in thyroid nodules, increased uptake was seen in malignant lesions, distinguishing benign from malignant disease in each of 19 cases.[3] Further evaluation of this imaging modality in larger series provides an important future research direction.

ASPIRATION BIOPSY CYTOLOGY

Aspiration biopsy cytology (ABC) of thyroid nodules is a valuable technique for cytopathologic evaluation. This office procedure requires a 10-ml syringe with a fine needle (21 or 22 gauge) passed through alcohol-prepared skin to a palpable nodule or area of interest in the thyroid during continuous aspiration. The specimen may be smeared on a slide and fixed immediately or submitted in appropriate media (e.g., carbowax) for later examination. The validity of this technique depends largely on the expertise and experience of the individual cytopathologist. Reportedly, sensitivity ranges from 75 to 93.5%, and specificity from 75 to 100%.[4,5] The gross appearance of aspirated fluid often yields diagnostic information: crystal-clear fluid is suggestive of a parathyroid cyst; yellow fluid is suggestive of a transudate; chocolate, green, or turbid fluid suggests degeneration; and bloody fluid from a palpable mass can suggest a rapidly growing vascularized tumor or aspiration of a vessel. Complications of this procedure include hematoma formation, recurrent laryngeal nerve injury, and a low risk of infection.

EMBRYOLOGY

The parafollicular cells of the thyroid gland are part of the amine precursor uptake and decarboxylation (APUD) cell population, which are derived from neuroectoderm or neural crest cells.

The primordium of thyroid follicles arises from endoderm in the floor of the pharynx between the first and second pharyngeal pouches. This area evaginates to form a median diverticulum by the end of the fourth week. It grows caudally as a tubular thyroglossal duct through the midline of the primordium of the hyoid bone, eventually to bifurcate and develop into the isthmus, pyramidal lobe, and lateral lobes of the thyroid gland. The foramen cecum marks the site of origin of the thyroglossal duct, often identified in examination of the dorsum of the tongue. Maldevelopment of the thyroglossal duct can result in midline cervical ectopic thyroid or even lingual thyroid. Lingual thyroid is an irregular base-of-tongue mass that may interfere with aerodigestive function as it increases in size. Remnants of the thyroglossal duct that persist can give rise to midline cysts. Because of the developmental course of the thyroid gland, effective surgical extirpation requires complete excision of the cyst and any tract up to the foramen cecum including the central portion of the hyoid bone (Sistrunk procedure).

The fetal thyroid begins to collect and organify iodine by about 10 weeks of gestation. Adequate fetal thyroid function becomes necessary because maternal-fetal transfer of T3 and T4 is minimal. By the end of the first trimester, colloid follicles are visible, and both T4 and TSH are detectable in the fetal blood. Fetal thyroid function increases in the second trimester because of increasing thyroid secretion and also because of the increase in plasma of TBG. Further, an increase in fetal TSH occurs as the fetal hypothalamus matures and produces TRH. Maternal TRH crosses the placenta and may contribute to the fetal pituitary activity, but otherwise, the fetal pituitary-thyroid axis is a functional unit distinct from the mother.

DISORDERS OF THE THYROID GLAND

Goiter

Goiter (from Latin guttur, meaning throat) is an enlargement of the thyroid gland resulting in swelling of the front of the neck. The term struma (from Latin struere, to build) is occasionally applied to describe this condition. A diffusely enlarged thyroid gland becomes palpable when the volume of the gland is doubled, and a visible goiter is usually at least three times the normal thyroid mass of 20 g.

Simple (Nontoxic) Goiter
During puberty and pregnancy, the thyroid gland normally undergoes a diffuse enlargement. This is related in part to increased estrogens and subsequent increase in TBG. Colloid goiter can thus arise and is typified histologically by large colloid spaces and flattened follicular epithelium. This condition is usually self-limited and rarely requires treatment.

The term endemic goiter is applicable when 10% or more of the population has generalized or localized thyroid enlargement. It generally reflects a dietary deficiency of iodide particular to a geographic region, causing insufficient thyroid hormone secretion. Five percent of the world's population have goiter or associated disorders (cretinism, impairment of growth and mental development, etc.). Of these, 75% live in less developed countries where iodine deficiency is prevalent.[6] Twenty-five percent of goiters occur in more developed countries. These so-called ''sporadic goiters'' arise largely from iodine-sufficient conditions including autoimmune thyroiditis, hypo- or hyperthyroidism, and thyroid carcinoma. Histologically, endemic goiter is identical with colloid goiter.

Nodular Goiter

The cause of nodular goiter is poorly understood but may be related to varying levels of TSH over a lifetime. The percentage of individuals with nodular goiter increases with advancing age. Histologically normal parenchyma is interspersed between nodules of varying size and consistency. Nodules smaller than 2 cm are rarely noticed by patients, although with quick growth or painful cystic hemorrhage, the patient may seek attention. Large multinodular goiters are usually asymptomatic. They can, however, cause compression of neck structures resulting in dysphagia, cough, or respiratory distress or a feeling of constriction in the throat.

Medical therapy is indicated if a goiter is a cosmetic problem or if it becomes symptomatic because of compression and displacement of vital structures. Exogenous thyroid hormone is given to suppress TSH secretion. Radioiodine is usually effective for more extensive cases.

Substernal goiter can develop from downward growth of the thyroid gland into the superior mediastinum. This can potentially cause serious symptoms from compression of tracheal or venous and arterial structures. Substernal goiter not responsive to thyroid hormone suppression is generally managed by thyroidectomy, usually through a standard cervical incision.

Thyroid cancer has reportedly been found in 4 to 17% of patients with multinodular goiter; however, this likely represents bias in selection of patients for surgery. The incidence of carcinoma is probably closer to 0.2%. For multinodular goiters with behavior or findings suggestive of malignancy, evaluation by fine-needle aspiration biopsy cytology may be useful. In the event of sudden, continued growth of a hard nodule, whole goiter progression, symptoms related to compression or displacement, or severe cosmetic deformity despite medical treatment, a subtotal thyroidectomy is appropriate.

Hypothyroidism

Hypothyroidism results from insufficient thyroid hormone secretion. In adults, this appears as myxedema characterized by weakness, lethargy, nonpitting edema, coarse, dry skin, and possibly hearing loss. Hypothyroidism is present in approximately 1 in 5000 neonates, although cretinism may not become evident until after several months of extrauterine life. This may arise from inadequate iodide intake in the maternal diet, thyroid agenesis, or administration of propylthiouracil or radioactive iodide during pregnancy. In infants, hypothyroidism causes cretinism with lethargy, stunted growth, mental retardation, and hearing loss.

Hypothyroidism is not in itself an indication for thyroidectomy, but it can arise from surgical or medical intervention. In particular, surgical extirpation of a lingual thyroid or a thyroglossal duct cyst without a preoperative thyroid scan may unexpectedly remove all functioning thyroid tissue. Patients at high risk for myxedema coma require effective teaching regarding the signs and symptoms of hypothyroidism as well as annual thyroid function tests (including serum TSH).[7]

Thyrotoxicosis

Thyrotoxicosis is the clinical and physiologic response of the tissues to an excess supply of active thyroid hormone. Causes of this syndrome fall into one of three main categories. The most important category includes diseases in which the gland sustains overproduction of thyroid hormone. This can arise in the presence of an unregulated thyroid stimulator of extrapituitary origin, as in Graves' disease or in patients who develop hyperthyroidism in association with Hashimoto's thyroiditis.[8] Rarely, excessive secretion of TSH from a pituitary tumor causes thyrotoxicosis.

The second category involves the development of thyrotoxic states secondary to subacute (de Quervain's) thyroiditis or in the syndrome of chronic thyroiditis with spontaneously resolving thyrotoxicosis. In the presence of an inflammatory process, preformed hormone leaks from the gland in excess. The gland, however, fails to produce new hormone because of the suppression of TSH by feedback inhibition—this process is therefore self-limited. This often results in a transient insufficiency of thyroid hormones.

The third category is unusual and arises when a source of excess hormone arises from other than the thyroid gland, as in the case of a community-acquired outbreak of transient thyrotoxicosis arising from ingestion of ground beef contaminated with bovine thyroid gland.[9] Rarely, functioning metastatic follicular carcinoma can account for thyrotoxicosis. Up to 25% of patients with multinodular goiter may develop Jod-Basedow disease, which is thyroxicosis in response to the use of exogenous iodine (e.g., radiographic contrast dye or iodide expectorants). This disorder is self-limited and is treated principally by discontinuing iodide use.

Hyperthyroidism

If sustained hyperfunction of the thyroid gland leads to thyrotoxicosis, the condition is properly termed hyperthyroidism. Thus, not all thyrotoxic states are associated with hyperthyroidism. In true hyperthyroidism, an increased radioactive iodine uptake is found. In contrast, nonhyperthyroid thyrotoxic states have a decreased RAIU. Furthermore, in conditions with sustained hyperfunction of the thyroid gland, the use of treatments to decrease hormone synthesis (antithyroid agents, surgery, or radioiodine) is appropriate. In the absence of a true hyperthyroid state, however, these are inappropriate and ineffective methods for treatment of thyrotoxicosis. Young patients more commonly develop thyrotoxicosis from Graves' disease, whereas older patients develop toxic nodular goiter.

Graves' Disease

Graves' disease is a relatively common disorder of unknown origin consisting of a triad of hyperthyroidism with diffuse goiter, ophthalmopathy, and dermopathy. All aspects of the triad need not appear together. Graves' disease is more frequent in women and has a definite familial predisposition. The basic disorder is a disruption of homeostatic mechanisms caused by the presence of an abnormal thyroid stimulator in the plasma. This long-acting thyroid stimulator (LATS) is present in the IgG class of immunoglobulins. LATS, however, does not appear to be the antibody responsible for ophthalmopathy. Thus, Graves' disease appears to be an autoimmune process in which an antibody to the thyroid TSH receptor is produced by the patient's own lymphocytes.

The symptoms of Graves' disease include nervousness and tremors with mood swings, tachycardia, hypertension, diarrhea, insomnia, and heat intolerance, particularly in younger patients. In older patients, weakness, dyspnea, and even cardiac failure can arise. Thyrotoxicosis may lead to degeneration of skeletal muscle fibers, enlarged heart, fatty infiltration and fibrosis of the liver, and bony decalcification.

Ocular signs include a characteristic stare with infrequent blinking and lid lag due to sympathetic overstimulation. In contrast to the infiltrative ophthalmopathy, these findings subside when thyrotoxicosis is treated. The ophthalmopathy of Graves' disease is caused by an inflammatory infiltrate of the orbit that spares the globe. Edema and inflammation of the muscles, with infiltration by lymphocytes, mast cells, and plasma cells, account for the increased volume of orbital contents and proptosis. Eventually, muscle fibers degenerate and fibrose.

The dermopathy of Graves' disease is characterized by a thickened dermis caused by a lymphocytic infiltration.

In the triad of Graves' disease, diffuse toxic goiter is the most common presentation. In a severe case, Graves' disease is a straightforward diagnosis. Increased radioactive iodide uptake, serum T4 RIA, and T3 resin uptake serve more as baseline than diagnostic aids.

The treatment of hyperthyroidism in Graves' disease has two approaches, both of which are directed to limit thyroid hormone production by the gland. The first approach uses antithyroid agents to blockade hor-

mone synthesis chemically. The second approach is ablation of thyroid tissue either by surgery or by means of radioactive iodine.

A trial of antithyroid therapy is desirable in children and patients under 40, including pregnant women, but it may also be employed in older patients. This includes propylthiouracil or methimazole. Propylthiouracil is preferred in pregnancy because it has less transference across the placenta. Furthermore, the drug is not excreted in breast milk. Iodide inhibits release of hormones from the thyroid gland in hyperfunction. This is useful in treatment of thyrotoxic crisis, although the response is often incomplete and transient. Large doses of glucocorticoids such as dexamethasone help to reduce the serum T4 concentration and can contribute to management of thyrotoxicosis as well as oculopathy.

In the past, a major cause of mortality in Graves' disease was thyroid storm, characterized by hyperthermia, tachycardia, hypertension, profuse sweating, intense irritability, extreme anxiety, and eventual prostration with irreversible hypotension and death.[7] This phenomenon represents an acute adrenergic crisis caused by thyroid hormone augmentation of the effects of catecholamines, particularly by induction of additional myocardial catecholamine receptors. Treatment with sympatholytic drugs including reserpine, guanethidine, and β-adrenergic blockers (propranolol), as well as oxygen, intravenous glucose, iodide, and adrenal steroids, has brought this serious problem under control for the surgeon.

Surgical ablation of the thyroid gland in Graves' disease is recommended in patients who have relapse or recurrence after drug therapy, in patients with a large goiter or drug toxicity, and in patients who fail to follow a medical regimen or fail to return for periodic examinations.

Though a radioiodide has no known carcinogenic effects as a β emitter in adults treated for hyperthyroidism, many physicians prefer to reserve therapy for patients over 30 years of age who are unlikely to bear children. Hypothyroidism occurs with insidious onset in 40 to 70% during the 10-year period following treatment with [131]I. Patients treated for Grave's disease are particularly vulnerable to serious complications of myxedema. Some clinicians recommend treatment with large doses of ^{131}I followed by permanent physiologic replacement with exogenous thyroid hormone. In younger patients or in those for whom radioiodide is contraindicated, a subtotal thyroidectomy can be performed as described in a later section of this chapter. Surgical patients must attain a stable euthyroid through antithyroid agents before any operation.

Toxic Adenoma

Thyrotoxicosis caused by thyroid hormone secreted by an autonomous follicular adenoma is termed toxic adenoma. This can follow a long period of euthyroid function in which suppression of normal gland balances the hyperfunctioning adenoma. Radioiodide is generally an effective treatment, often sparing the normal remaining gland, which has low uptake of iodide. Thyroid lobectomy is appropriate for patients at risk, as discussed later in this chapter in relation to the solitary nodule.

Toxic Multinodular Goiter

Toxic multinodular goiter (Plummer's disease) is a disease of aging that arises in a simple (nontoxic) goiter of long standing. The development of thyrotoxicosis with slow progression of multinodular goiter is usually caused by an autonomous functioning adenoma. Approximately 10% of solitary palpable nodules have autonomous function. In multinodular goiters over 100 g, two thirds have autonomous secretion of thyroid hormone. Treatment is primarily medical, consisting of antithyroid drugs (propylthiouracil or methimazole), sympatholytic therapy, and radioiodide. In the absence of symptoms caused by mass effects of goiter, surgery is reserved for toxicity not controlled medically.

Thyroiditis

Rarely, the thyroid gland may have a bacterial infection. Of much greater significance are the inflammatory diseases of the thyroid that do not become manifest in the acute phase. Among these is subacute (de Quervain's granulomatous) thyroiditis, a febrile disease in which the thyroid becomes acutely congested, edematous, and mildly tender, often after an upper respiratory infection. The disease is characterized by repeated remissions and exacerbations over several months without hypothyroidism or evidence of stimulating antibodies. Thyroid microsomal and thyroglobulin antibodies, however, do appear in low titers in subacute thyroiditis. Histologically, an inflammatory infiltrate with large, multinucleated giant cells containing vesicles of colloid suggests a foreign body reaction. This condition is not treated by a surgical procedure.

Hashimoto's disease (struma lymphomatosum) is the most common type of thyroiditis. This goitrous form of autoimmune thyroiditis and its variant, lymphocytic thyroiditis, appears mostly in women as a symmetric, rubbery enlargement of the gland. Although microsomal and thyroglobulin antibodies are present, tissue damage appears to be cell-mediated. Histologically, a lymphocytic infiltrate tending to form lymphoid follicles with plasma cells is seen. Follicles are progressively compressed and distorted into fused masses of cells without a colloid space. Follicular cells may eventually be transformed into Hürthle cells, which appear as nests of large pink cells with abundant granular cytoplasm packed with mitochondria. Al-

though this condition is associated with mild thyrotoxicosis in the early stages because of release of stored hormone from damaged follicles, most patients have depressed thyroid function (RAIU low to normal). In the later and chronic stage, hypothyroidism commonly develops. Fine-needle aspiration biopsy cytology can assist in the diagnosis. Open biopsy or procedures to alleviate compression of the trachea or esophagus are sometimes necessary.

Riedel's struma (invasive fibrous thyroiditis) is a rare presentation of thyroiditis characterized by irreversible, profound hypothyroidism and a stony hard, irregular, fibrous gland. Symptoms can include cough, dyspnea, and difficulty in swallowing. Replacement thyroid hormone is the principal treatment.

Management of Thyroid Neoplasia

Solitary Nodule of the Thyroid

The most common indication for thyroidectomy (50% of cases) in the United States is the presence of a solitary thyroid nodule, defined as a discrete mass, greater than or equal to 1 cm in diameter, discovered by palpation of a thyroid gland otherwise of normal size and consistency. Solitary nodules occur in fewer than 5% of the population and are most often found in patients 30 to 50 years of age, with a fourfold increase in frequency in women. It is important to distinguish clinically between the solitary nodule and a multinodular thyroid gland because the latter has a low incidence of malignancy. One series reports spontaneous disappearance as the most common outcome for an untreated, long-standing nodule (38.3%); on the other hand, 13% of nodules in this series were enlarging. Needle biopsy demonstrated malignancy in 26.3% of enlarging nodules, compared with 6.4% of nodules that were of stable size.[10] The most common cause of solitary thyroid nodules in children and adolescents is follicular adenoma, although malignancy is reported in 25.5% of cold nodules.[11] Neck mass is the most common presenting symptom of papillary or follicular thyroid carcinoma in patients under 20 years of age.[12]

The evaluation of patients with thyroid nodules should include an assessment of laryngeal motor function, serum thyroid hormone levels, radioactive iodide uptake, and scintiscan. If a hot nodule is demonstrated by ^{99m}Tc scanning, reexamination with radioiodide is recommended. Ultrasonography to differentiate between cystic and solid thyroid nodules is accurate in 82 to 95% of cases. Fine-needle aspiration biopsy cytology often provides an accurate diagnosis and is used by some practitioners to treat cystic lesions. The reported incidence of carcinoma in solitary nodules ranges from 1.3 to 20.3%.

The series with the highest yield of carcinomas on thyroidectomy had stringent selection of patients based on risk factors. Thus, using known risk factors, patients with solitary nodules at increased risk for malignancy can be identified and selected for surgical procedures.[13] Increased risk is found in the following situations:

1. Thyroid nodules associated with vocal cord paralysis (infrequently, benign nodules can cause paresis or paralysis by compression—this is usually alleviated by excision of the mass).[14]
2. Solitary nodules in men.
3. Solitary nodules in patients under 20 years old or over 50 years old.
4. Solitary nodules in patients with a history of head and neck irradiation.
5. Palpable lower or midcervical lymph nodes and apparently normal thyroid glands in young patients.
6. Functioning or cold nodules on scintiscan or radionuclide uptake outside the thyroid gland.
7. Solid or partially cystic lesions by ultrasonography.
8. Recurrent cystic lesions following needle aspiration.
9. Abnormal cytologic findings on needle aspiration biopsy.
10. Solitary nodules that fail to disappear in response to thyroid hormone suppression therapy.
11. Solitary nodules that show diffuse calcification radiographically.

In patients with chronic thyroid disease, high-risk patients who are candidates for surgery may be identified by the following criteria:

1. Multinodular goiter containing cold nodules that enlarge in response to suppression with thyroid hormone.
2. Rapidly enlarging nodules in chronic goiters with or without suppression.
3. Goiters with vocal cord paralysis.
4. A history of head and neck irradiation.
5. A history of neoplasm of the thyroid gland.

Thyroid adenomas are benign, encapsulated neoplasms with a glandular cellular structure. These lesions may be classified as follicular adenoma, Hürthle cell, and papillary adenomas. If a "hot" or hyperfunctioning adenoma is demonstrated by technetium scan and this finding persists on a thyroid suppression test, this lesion can be treated with radioactive iodide. Benign teratoma can also occur in the thyroid gland.

Malignant Lesions

Malignant tumors of the thyroid include: papillary adenocarcinoma, follicular adenocarcinoma, Hürthle cell carcinoma, medullary carcinoma, and undifferentiated carcinomas (small cell carcinoma and giant cell carci-

noma). Various miscellaneous malignant lesions include lymphoma, sarcoma, and teratoma.

Papillary Adenocarcinoma

Thyroid carcinomas comprise approximately 1% of all malignant tumors in the United States. Of these, 60 to 70% are papillary carcinomas. These account for 80 to 90% of radiation-induced thyroid carcinomas. Dietary iodine in childhood is also regarded as an etiologic factor. Approximately 25% of papillary carcinomas are occult, discovered incidentally at surgery, and of questionable clinical significance. The peak incidence is in the third and forth decades, with a threefold increase in frequency in women.

Thyroglossal duct cysts are second in incidence only to enlarged cervical lymph nodes as the cause of pediatric neck masses. One percent of thyroglossal duct cysts are malignant, and 81.7% of these are papillary carcinomas.[15]

Although two thirds of papillary thyroid carcinomas have follicular elements, their behavior is determined by the papillary aspect. These are unencapsulated tumors that tend to invade lymphatic vessels as well as normal surrounding thyroid parenchyma directly. Multicentricity of the primary neoplasm is a common feature, seen in 20 to 80% of patients.

This lesion generally has a prolonged course, and the overall mortality is estimated at 10% or less. The patient's age at diagnosis is the most important prognostic factor. The prognosis is excellent in children and young adults, even in the presence of advanced primary disease or lymph node metastases.[16] Despite the good prognosis, almost 50% of patients who die of papillary carcinoma do so because of local invasion.

Various surgical procedures have been recommended, ranging from subtotal lobectomy to total thyroidectomy. Microscopic disease in the contralateral lobe has been reported in 8 to 88% of cases by various investigators. Total ipsilateral lobectomy, isthmusectomy, and subtotal contralateral lobectomy probably comprise the most common procedure for papillary carcinoma confined to the thyroid gland. For more extensive disease, aggressive management of the primary and cervical node disease by surgery, followed at 6 weeks by thyroid scan and ^{131}I administration, improves survival.

With the application of excellent surgical skills, a complete extirpation of the thyroid gland can be performed without recurrent laryngeal nerve injury or the reported 2% incidence of permanent hypoparathyroidism. Recurrent neck disease must be treated by neck dissection. The concept of "node plucking" is controversial.[17]

Follicular Carcinoma

Follicular carcinoma accounts for approximately one of five thyroid cancers, peaking in the fifth decade of life, with a 3:1 female preponderance. Like papillary carcinoma, it is well-differentiated, despite a worse prognosis. These tumors can be encapsulated, or they can manifest with vascular invasion. Distant metastases, especially to lung and bone, are found commonly. Of deaths from follicular carcinoma, 75% arise from distant metastases.

For patients under 40 years of age with encapsulated follicular carcinoma, isthmusectomy and lobectomy are performed, with total thyroidectomy reserved for patients over 40 years old. Some surgeons prefer to perform total thyroidectomy for all patients because follicular carcinoma, like papillary carcinoma, can undergo late anaplastic transformation. For invasive follicular carcinoma, total thyroidectomy is recommended, followed by ablative radioiodine, because of the potential for distant metastases. In the presence of palpable lymph nodes in the neck, modified radical neck dissection is recommended with preservation of the eleventh cranial nerve and the sternocleidomastoid muscle. Some surgeons do remove the ipsilateral internal jugular vein.

A major difficulty is distinguishing between follicular adenoma and follicular carcinoma. In up to one third of cases, a frozen-section diagnosis of follicular adenoma is changed to follicular carcinoma. The extent of resection with indeterminate lesions must take this into account with consideration of prognostic factors such as the patient's age and sex and the size of the lesion.[18]

Thallium-201 scintigraphy with serum thyroglobulin provides a basis for follow-up of well-differentiated thyroid cancer. Moderate elevations in thyroglobulin may be due to inadequate thyroid suppression therapy and may require assessment by careful assay of TSH levels. Patients with elevated thyroglobulin levels despite adequate suppression therapy following definitive treatment of a well-differentiated carcinoma are at increased risk of recurrence.[19]

Hürthle Cell Carcinoma
The Hürthle cell observed in thyroid gland atrophy of Hashimoto's disease is a benign entity. Hürthle cells occur in clusters as a degenerative transformation of the follicular cells. Hürthle cell carcinoma can occur as a malignant thyroid neoplasm composed of this cell type, however. This is sometimes classified as a variant of follicular carcinoma. This disease behaves clinically as an intermediate between low-grade and angioinvasive follicular carcinoma. It is difficult to confirm malignancy of a Hürthle cell mass on a pathologic basis alone; therefore, any isolated nodule should be considered malignant on clinical grounds.

Treatment of Hürthle cell carcinoma involves at least an isthmusectomy and lobectomy.[20] If Hürthle cell carcinoma appears as a solitary thyroid nodule exceeding 2.0 cm or if it is bilateral, total thyroidectomy

is recommended. Radical neck dissection is further recommended in the event of cervical nodal metastases.

Medullary Carcinoma With Amyloid Stroma
Medullary carcinoma accounts for 5 to 10% of thyroid carcinomas. Lesions are capable of local invasion, spread to regional lymphatic vessels, or distant metastases. They are derived from C-cells of the thyroid gland and are capable of producing calcitonin.

Multiple endocrine neoplasia type I (MEN-I) is characterized by parathyroid chief cell hyperplasia with pancreatic islet cell and pituitary adenomas.[21] Two further familial syndromes, multiple endocrine neoplasia type IIa (MEN-IIa) and the rarer type IIb (MEN-IIb), were found in association with medullary carcinoma of the thyroid after its first description in 1959.[22,23]

MEN-IIa (Sipple's syndrome) is manifested by medullary thyroid carcinoma with associated pheochromocytoma and parathyroid hyperplasia. MEN-IIb is characterized by medullary carcinoma of the thyroid, pheochromocytoma and multiple mucosal neuromas, ganglioneuromatosis, and a Marfan's habitus. Further, a familial non-MEN (FN-MEN) is recognized in which hereditary medullary carcinoma of the thyroid occurs without associated endocrinopathy. Each of these clinical syndromes, MEN-IIa, MEN-IIb, and FN-MEN, is inherited as an autosomal dominant trait. Kindred should be screened by detection of increased serum calcitonin, either basally or following pentagastrin stimulation. Patients with medullary carcinoma or C-cell hyperplasia as a premalignant precursor require prompt and thorough surgical intervention because this malignant lesion is biologically aggressive, with onset at a young age.[24] Children with MEN-IIb should be studied shortly after birth, and those with MEN-IIa should be evaluated by the age of 1 year.[25]

The basis for these familial syndromes associated with medullary carcinoma lies in the common embryologic origin of the parafollicular cell and the adrenal medullary cell. Both are members of the APUD cell population, derived from neural crest cells. The presence of abnormal (nondiploid) DNA as determined by flow cytometric analysis of nuclear suspensions appears to be associated with a worse prognosis in sporadic and familial medullary thyroid carcinoma.[26]

Though papillary thyroid carcinoma is not a characteristic of MEN-II, the diseases have associated genes. The ret proto-oncogene (RET), which has been demonstrated to be rearranged in papillary cancer, has been mapped near the predisposition locus for MEN-II, with apparent tight linkage between loci. RET is expressed in medullary thyroid carcinoma and pheochromocytoma, making it a candidate gene for MEN-II. The variations in expression of the MEN-II syndrome may be due to structural alteration of several contiguous genes in the MEN-II chromosomal region.[27] Techniques of molecular biology will likely provide the means to assess and control this form of malignant disease in the foreseeable future.

Medullary carcinoma does not take up radioiodide, so this treatment is not recommended. Because of the propensity of medullary carcinoma for local microvascular invasion, late recurrence (up to 20 years after treatment), and metastatic disease, aggressive surgical intervention is recommended. Furthermore, external ionizing radiation and chemotherapy are of limited value. A total thyroidectomy is generally recommended because of the high incidence of bilaterality, especially in familial syndromes. Most clinicians favor a radical neck dissection on the side of the primary neoplasm with a modified neck dissection on the contralateral side in the event of bilateral thyroid gland involvement. The incidence of bilateral disease in the gland or neck is especially high in the familial disease. Attention to family history and evaluation for other endocrinopathies are imperative. As with the other well-differentiated adenocarcinomas, medullary carcinomas can eventually degenerate to anaplastic carcinoma.

Anaplastic Carcinoma

Anaplastic carcinoma, largely a disease of the elderly, accounts for less than 10% of malignant thyroid tumors. This disease has shown a threefold to fourfold decline in incidence internationally over the past 45 years, relating inversely to the increase in extirpative thyroid procedures.[28] Foci of differentiated thyroid cancer are commonly observed, suggesting a degenerative origin, based on "clonal evolution." Up to 20% of patients have a history of a previously treated well-differentiated carcinoma of the thyroid.

Anaplastic carcinoma is an often rapidly fatal, aggressive, enlarging, bulky mass that distorts the anterior neck and often obstructs the aerodigestive tract. In many cases, the patient undergoes biopsy by needle aspiration or open biopsy, and the neoplasm is deemed inoperable. Palliative radiation therapy and chemotherapy may prolong life.[29] Patients with the small cell type may have a slightly longer survival than those with large cell anaplastic carcinoma.

Other Malignant Lesions

Sarcomas comprise less than 1% of malignant tumors of the thyroid. They have a poor prognosis despite aggressive surgical intervention. All varieties of lymphoma arise in the thyroid gland, most frequently non-Hodgkin's lymphoma. This lesion may appear as a rapidly enlarging goiter in an elderly person, producing obstructive symptoms. Treatment usually involves lobectomy or total thyroidectomy followed by external beam radiation. A wide range of thyroid neoplasms representing metastases from distant sites has been reported.

SURGICAL ANATOMY

Relations

In the medial aspect, the thyroid gland is deep to the sternohyoid and underlying sternothyroid (strap) muscles. Inferiorly, the sternocleidomastoid muscle overlaps the strap muscles, whereas more superiorly it overlaps the lateral most extent of the thyroid gland. The anterior surface of the thyroid gland faces the pretracheal layer of the deep cervical fascia, which extends around posteriorly to envelop the trachea, esophagus, and recurrent laryngeal nerve.

The deep or medial surface of the thyroid gland is adapted to the larynx and trachea. At the superior pole of each lateral lobe, the medial surface is in contact with the inferior pharyngeal constrictor and the posterior portion of the cricothyroid muscle. The medial aspect of the thyroid gland is also intimately related to the parathyroid glands and the recurrent laryngeal nerves. The correct level of dissection for dorsal mobilization is anatomically defined as lying anterior to the lamella that covers the vessel and nerve containing plane of the neck.[30] On occasion, the gland may extend posterior to the trachea. Appreciation of these relations contributes to surgical technique and understanding of the symptoms of thyroid masses.

Suspension of the Thyroid Gland

The thyroid gland is suspended in the neck from the cricoid and thyroid cartilage by two ligaments: the anterior suspensory ligament and the surgically more important posterior suspensory (Berry's) ligament.

The anterior suspensory ligament attaches the superior border of the isthmus and superomedial aspect of each lateral lobe to the cricoid cartilage and cricothyroid muscle.

The posterior suspensory (Berry's) ligament is distinct from the anterior suspensory ligament and becomes a pedicle for the thyroid gland in the course of thyroid lobectomy. Berry's ligament extends from the medial and deep portions of each lateral lobe of the thyroid to the lateral surface of the cricoid cartilage as well as the posterior lateral aspect of the first and second tracheal rings. It is an important surgical landmark because the recurrent laryngeal nerve passes either deep to this ligament or between leaves of the ligament in its cephalic course. The recurrent laryngeal nerve often divides into two branches inferior to this ligament; therefore, all branches must be visualized to avoid injury. Furthermore, a portion of the lateral thyroid lobe extends deep to the ligament. In some patients, the ligament may actually be embedded in glandular tissue, demanding meticulous surgical dissection.

An occasional anomaly observed is a unilateral or

paired bilateral muscle, the levator glandulae thyroideae muscle, inserting into the thyroid gland and originating from the hyoid bone.

Blood Supply

The blood flow to the thyroid gland is on the order of 100 ml/min, reflecting the importance of thyroid hormone to whole body metabolism. The thyroid gland receives this abundant blood supply through paired inferior thyroid arteries as well as an occasional unpaired thyroidea ima artery of variable size (Fig. 23–1).

The dominant artery to the thyroid is usually the inferior thyroid artery, although it can be of variable origin and relationship. Typically, it ascends along the medial side of the anterior scalene muscle behind the prevertebral fascia. Thereafter, it loops down onto the anterior surface of the longus colli to pass behind the common carotid artery in variable relation to the middle cervical ganglion of the sympathetic trunk. Medial to this point, it penetrates the prevertebral fascia and, in variable relationship to the recurrent laryngeal

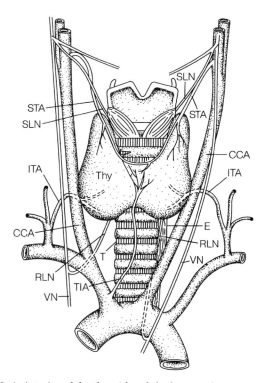

Fig. 23–1. Arteries of the thyroid and the laryngeal nerves, anterior view. Dissection of the recurrent laryngeal nerve (RLN) begins in the triangle bounded by the trachea (T), the common carotid artery (CCA), and the thyroid gland (Thy). Branches of the inferior thyroid artery (ITA) can run close to the recurrent nerve. The esophagus (E) runs somewhat to the left of the trachea. The superior thyroid artery (STA) is closely related to the external branch of the superior laryngeal nerve (SLN). The vagus nerve (VN) courses parallel to the carotid artery. The thyroid ima artery is labeled TIA.

nerve, divides into a dominant upper branch to just below the midportion of the lateral thyroid lobe and a lower branch to the inferior border of the lobe. Small branches of the inferior thyroid artery cross deep to Berry's ligament and along its inferior edge, where clamping for hemostasis may injure the recurrent laryngeal nerve. Duplication of the inferior thyroid artery has been observed; in this case, both inferior thyroid arteries arise from the subclavian artery on one side. In the occasional absence of an inferior thyroid artery, the thyroid ima artery may replace it, or it may be simply an accessory vessel. Most commonly, the thyroid ima arises from the innominate (brachiocephalic) artery.

The superior thyroid artery is the first anterior branch of the external carotid artery, although it can arise from the bulb of the common carotid artery. In its descent toward the apex of the thyroid lobe, the artery is closely related to the course of the external branch of the superior laryngeal nerve. This nerve is therefore a potential source of complication in thyroid surgery. On approach to the gland, the superior thyroid artery divides into an anterior and a posterior branch. The anterior branch runs close to the medial aspect of the lobe and across the isthmus superiorly, often anastomosing with the superior thyroid artery from the opposite side. The course of the superior thyroid artery is the most constant of the arteries to the thyroid gland.

Venous drainage of the thyroid gland is by two or three pairs of veins that anastomose freely in the gland. These vessels are named by location: superior, middle, and inferior thyroid veins (Fig. 23–2).

The superior thyroid vein emerges from the upper portion of the thyroid gland and accompanies the superior thyroid artery to empty into the internal jugular vein or lower end of the common facial vein at the level of the carotid bifurcation.

The middle thyroid vein is variable in presence and size and arises from the lateral surface of the thyroid, crossing in front of the common carotid artery to drain into the internal jugular vein. It may be torn in dissecting the gland from the carotid sheath. The middle thyroid vein is present in roughly 50% of patients.

The inferior thyroid vein drains the lower portion of the gland to the brachiocephalic vein of the same side. The inferior thyroid veins form the plexus thyroideus impar, a rich anastomosis in front of the trachea, which can produce troublesome bleeding in a tracheostomy. Occasionally, the inferior thyroid veins join inferiorly to drain by way of a common trunk to the left brachiocephalic vein—this is referred to as a thyroidea ima vein.

Neural Input

Neural fibers reach the thyroid gland from the superior cervical ganglion of the sympathetic trunk and the su-

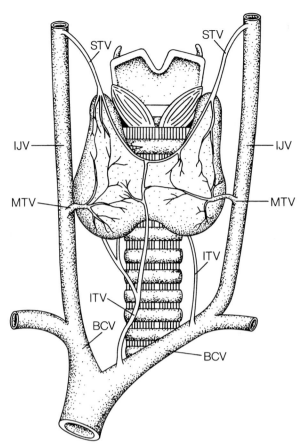

Fig. 23–2. Venous drainage of the thyroid gland, anterior view. The superior thyroid vein (STV) closely approximates the course of the superior thyroid artery. The middle thyroid vein (MTV) occurs variably, draining into the internal jugular vein (IJV). The inferior thyroid veins (ITV) drain into either of the branchiocephalic veins (BCV).

perior laryngeal branch of the vagus. It is generally accepted, however, that these nerves are related functionally to blood vessels only, and not directly to the function of glandular tissue.

Lymphatics

Lymphatic drainage of the thyroid is chiefly by inferior and superior lymphatic vessels accompanying the arterial blood supply. The isthmus is mostly drained by inferior lymphatic channels, as are the lower portions of the lateral lobes. The lower channels then distribute to the lower deep cervical nodes, the supraclavicular nodes, and the pretracheal and paratracheal nodes, as well as the prelaryngeal nodes just above the isthmus. The Delphian node is a median prelaryngeal node often palpable in the presence of thyroid disease. Drainage also occurs to the brachiocephalic lymph nodes, which are related to the thymus in the superior mediastinum. Lymph vessels from the thyroid gland may enter into the thoracic duct directly. Superior lymphatic channels drain the superior and medial surfaces

of the lateral lobes as well as the superior surface of the isthmus. The upper channels empty into the upper deep cervical lymph nodes.

SURGICAL TECHNIQUES

Total Thyroid Lobectomy and Isthmusectomy

The patient is placed in a supine position on a shoulder roll with hyperextension of the neck. A transverse incision is made through skin and platysma muscle in the anterior neck approximately 3 cm above the sternal notch and extended laterally as necessary. Hereafter, meticulous hemostasis should be maintained throughout the procedure. By subplatysmal dissection, skin flaps are developed vertically from the sternoclavicular border to the eminence of the thyroid cartilage and laterally from the midline to the anterior border of the sternocleidomastoid muscle. The strap muscles, sternohyoid and sternothyroid, are divided vertically in the midline; dissection progresses in the plane of the pretracheal fascia, allowing retraction of the strap muscles to expose the true capsule of the isthmus and entire lateral lobe on the superficial surface. Superiorly and laterally, this requires dissection underneath the sternocleidomastoid muscle. The middle thyroid vein, if present, may be divided and ligated at the lateral border of the gland at this time. Dissection of the deep surface of the thyroid gland begins inferiorly and laterally with exposure of the main trunk of the recurrent laryngeal nerve. This is bounded by a triangle consisting of the trachea and esophagus medially, the common carotid artery laterally, and the inferior border of the thyroid lobe superiorly. The apex of this triangle faces inferiorly, and blunt dissection begins at this area. The recurrent laryngeal nerve is at a depth at or just anterior to the tracheoesophageal sulcus and may lie in the sulcus or several centimeters lateral to it. Occasionally, the right laryngeal nerve enters the triangle laterally from behind the common carotid and passes superiorly and medially in an oblique course. Because the esophagus lies to the left of midline, the left recurrent laryngeal nerve may be close to the esophagus.

The parathyroid glands should now be identified. They appear as vascular, brownish fat. Whereas the inferior parathyroid glands have a variable location, the superior parathyroid glands are located more consistently at the midportion of the deep surface of the thyroid lobe. As the dissection progresses, the inferior thyroid vein is divided and ligated. With the recurrent laryngeal nerve identified, the inferior thyroid artery is now divided and ligated close to the gland to avoid damaging the blood supply to the parathyroid gland.

The isthmus is now transected on the contralateral side and oversewn with a running 0-silk suture. The anterior suspensory ligament is transected, freeing the

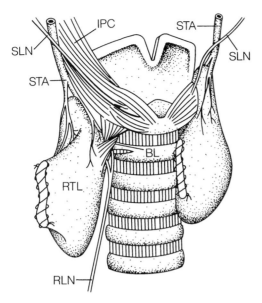

Fig. 23–3. Total thyroid lobectomy and isthmusectomy, oblique view. The right thyroid lobe (RTL) and isthmus are under traction laterally and inferiorly, which tends to separate the superior thyroid artery (STA) from the external branch of the superior laryngeal nerve (SLN). Note the relation of the superior pole of the lateral lobe to the inferior pharyngeal constrictor (IPC). The recurrent laryngeal nerve (RLN) often branches as it runs deep to or through the postero-lateral suspensory (Berry's) ligament (BL).

superior border of the isthmus and superior pole medially from the cricoid cartilage. With the course of the recurrent laryngeal nerve exposed nearly to the superior border of the thyroid lobe, the posterior suspensory ligament is identified by lateral retraction of the lobe. The recurrent laryngeal nerve runs between leaves of this ligament or deep to it (Fig. 23–3). As with dissection of the facial nerve, the recurrent laryngeal nerve should be exposed and in full view when dividing any tissue.[31] The posterior ligament is sharply transected close to the trachea and cricoid cartilage. The gland may be adherent in this area, and a postoperative scan often reveals uptake from residual gland.

The parathyroid glands may be superficial to the recurrent laryngeal nerve in the plane of dissection or even attached or contained by the thyroid capsule; therefore, it is prudent to examine the capsule after removal of the thyroid lobe. Parathyroid glands may appear as dark tissue suggestive of a subcapsular hematoma. Parathyroid tissue sinks in saline, which provides an intraoperative means to test suspect tissue. Frozen section of a small portion of the tissue in question should be used to confirm the presence of a parathyroid gland. If a parathyroid gland is removed, reimplantation, as described later, is recommended.

At this point, the superior thyroid artery and vein should be skeletonized by blunt dissection while held on tension with slight downward traction of the thyroid lobe. The veins and arteries should be ligated sep-

arately with free ligatures to avoid superior laryngeal nerve injury and arteriovenous fistula. It is possible to find thymus tissue attached to the superior pole of the thyroid gland. The lateral lobe and isthmus are then removed from the surgical field.

In certain situations, the recurrent laryngeal nerve is appropriately sacrificed. These situations include ipsilateral vocal cord paralysis with reasonable certainty of malignant disease grossly invading the nerve, so the patient's life would be compromised by preserving the nerve.

Assuming that the parathyroid glands have either been preserved or reimplanted, the wound is closed in layers, with good cosmetic technique. Suction drainage of the surgical field is practiced by most surgeons, usually through a separate stab incision. Postoperative management without drainage of the surgical field has been reported in large numbers without evidence of increased risk, however.[32,33] Some surgeons perform flexible fiberoptic endoscopy in the operating room immediately following extubation to document intact laryngeal motor function.

Technique for Reimplantation of Parathyroid Tissue

Parathyroid glands removed inadvertently should be cleaned carefully in saline and diced into small pieces measuring approximately 1×1 mm.[34] Up to 40 pieces of parathyroid grafting material may be obtained by this technique. The parathyroid gland may be implanted into the sternocleidomastoid muscle[35] or into the volar surface of the previously prepared and draped nondominant forearm. Small pieces of parathyroid tissue can be implanted into the brachial, radialis, or flexor muscle group, closing the overlying muscle and fascia with interrupted suture of 5–0 mersilene to prevent extrusion and further to serve as a marker for the implantation site. Bleeding in the implantation site should be carefully avoided. The total surface area of the parathyroid transplantation site is generally 5×5 cm. This is closed in standard fashion. In the immediate postoperative period, parathyroid hormone levels can be undetectable but generally recover to preoperative levels within about 2 weeks.[36]

COMPLICATIONS OF THYROID SURGERY

Complications of thyroid surgery are best avoided by a thorough working knowledge of the anatomy and embryology of the visceral compartment of the neck, careful preoperative planning, and excellent surgical technique.[37] Although numerous reports advocate subtotal thyroidectomy, we recommend total lobectomy (uni- or bilateral) in most situations. Although improved local control of disease is achieved with more radical procedures, no convincing evidence of improved survival exists.[38] General anesthesia is most commonly utilized, and it is important for the otolaryngologist to be present at induction to secure an airway by emergency open bronchoscopy or tracheostomy if patient has respiratory embarrassment due to large goiter. A trend exists toward increased use of local anesthesia and outpatient surgery for thyroid procedures. No significant difference is found in the rate of major complications for hemithyroidectomy performed under local anesthesia as compared with general anesthesia.[39]

Thyroid operations including total thyroidectomy have been performed in large numbers as outpatient or short-stay procedures in several centers in the United States and Europe. Extensive perioperative patient teaching is required for the layperson to recognize and react properly to the symptoms and signs of surgical complications. More complex procedures such as reoperation, neck dissection, and sternal splits are more safely managed on an inpatient basis.[40]

Good exposure is an absolute necessity. Collar incisions allow the best cosmetic result for the exposure needed. In some cases, exposure is improved by division of the strap muscles approximately halfway between the hyoid bone and the sternum. This avoids injury to their innervation from the ansa cervicalis. Early in the operation, the trachea should be exposed caudal to the isthmus so emergency access to the airway can be obtained in the event of obstruction.

Exposure of the recurrent laryngeal nerve is mandatory when a lateralized procedure is performed. The nerve should be preserved from the thoracic inlet to its entry into the larynx at the cricothyroid membrane. Unilateral laryngeal nerve injury is reported in 2.3% of cases, largely because of lack of nerve identification.[41] One must remember that at least 1 in 400 cases may not have a recurrent nerve. An anomalous inferior laryngeal nerve occurs almost always on the right and is always associated with an anomalous retroesophageal subclavian artery, that is, a right subclavian artery arising from the left descending aorta. In these cases, the inferior laryngeal nerve passes directly from the vagus to the larynx. Digital subtraction angiography can confirm this anomaly and is recommended in any reoperation on the right side of the thyroid, especially if the nerve was not identified in the previous surgery.[42]

If reoperation is required within 2 weeks, anatomic landmarks will be obliterated because of the inflammatory response. Blunt dissection should be used, although if the reoperation is months to years later, fibrosis often requires sharp dissection. Operating away from the primary site of surgery is recommended. The risk of morbidity is roughly doubled in a second thyroidectomy procedure.

Hemorrhage is usually not a problem. The thyroid ima artery is divided and ligated first, and then the middle thyroid artery if it is present. The inferior thyroid artery is best divided near the capsule of the gland to prevent injury to the sympathetic trunk (with a resultant Horner's syndrome) and to preserve blood supply to the parathyroid glands. On the left, the thoracic duct can be injured, with resulting chylous fistula. The safest way to divide the superior laryngeal artery and vein is with careful downward traction and skeletonization of the vessels. Caution is advisable if retraction stretches or places pressure on the carotid artery because this has been associated with embolic occlusion of the retinal artery.[43]

Infection occurs in less than 1% of thyroidectomies; however, suction drainage is traditionally recommended to prevent hematoma. Some surgeons have experienced no increased risk by not placing drains or using drainage only in select cases.[32,33] Tracheostomy may be necessary because of tracheal malacia or injury to the recurrent laryngeal nerves. If necessary, a suture can be placed in the second tracheal ring and brought out through the wound as a quick guide to the anterior tracheal wall. Rarely, pneumothorax can occur, and a postoperative chest radiograph is recommended.

Postoperative hemorrhage occurs in fewer than 1% of patients. The resulting hematoma remains in the midline below the strap muscles, creating an increasing pressure and causing collapse of the airway and respiratory embarrassment. In this event, the wound must be opened immediately "wherever you are." Thereafter, the patient can return to the operating room for reexploration, control of the bleeding vessel, and repeat closure of the wound. Subsequently, edema of the airway can be expected and may require tracheostomy. Tracheotomy may also be necessary in the presence of marked tracheal malacia secondary to large goiter, or during incomplete resection of cancer and anticipated postoperative radiation therapy, as in patients with anaplastic carcinoma. The need for elective tracheostomy to prevent postoperative airway obstruction occurs in fewer than 1% of patients.

The parathyroid glands should be looked for and protected when found. In one fourth of thyroidectomies, the patient has a transient mild decrease in serum calcium, which is generally asymptomatic. Transient hypocalcemia can be severe in 8% of patients over the first 96 hours postoperatively.[44] This is probably caused by trauma to the glands and blood supply. Permanent hypoparathyroidism occurs in up to 8% after total thyroidectomy.[41]

Tetany with hypocalcemia can be treated with calcium gluconate intravenously or calcium carbonate orally in patients without achlorhydria. In patients with achlorhydria, calcium lactate in water and, often, vitamin D are required. Myxedema can occur in 4 to 6 weeks after a thyroidectomy, particularly if the gland has been totally ablated. Hashimoto's disease also progresses to hypothyroidism eventually. This can be treated with a variety of drugs for thyroid replacement. Some of these include 2 to 3 g of desiccated thyroid extract, up to 0.2 mg of tetraiodinated sodium levothyroxine (Synthroid), or 25 to 75 µg of triiodinated liothyronine sodium (Cytomel) as needed.

The greatest cause of death in the past was thyroid storm, which can now be effectively controlled. The mortality rate of thyroidectomy today is approximately 0.1%.

SUGGESTED READINGS

1. Udelsman R, et al: Preoperative localization of occult medullary carcinoma of the thyroid gland with single-photon emission tomography dimercaptosuccinic acid. Surgery *114*:1083, 1993.
2. Rosen IB, Walfish PG, and Miskin M: The ultrasound of thyroid masses. Surg Clin North Am *59*:19, 1979.
3. Bloom AD, Adler LP, and Shuck JM: Determination of malignancy of thyroid nodules with positron emission tomography. Surgery *114*:728, 1993.
4. Bouvet M, et al: Surgical management of the thyroid nodule: patient selection based on the results of fine-needle aspiration cytology. Laryngoscope *102*:1353, 1992.
5. Bapat RD, et al: Analysis of 105 uninodular goiters. J Postgrad Med *68*:60, 1992.
6. Gaitan E, Nelson NC, and Poole GV: Endemic goiter and endemic thyroid disorders. World J Surg *15*:205, 1991.
7. Gavin LA: Thyroid crises. Med Clin North Am *75*:179, 1991.
8. Roitt IM, Doniach D, Campbell RN, and Hudson RV: Autoantibodies in Hashimoto's disease (lymphadenoid goitre). Lancet *2*:820, 1956.
9. Kinney JS, et al: Community outbreak of thyrotoxicosis: epidemiology, immunogenetic characteristics, and long term outcome. Am J Med *84*:10, 1988.
10. Kuma K, et al: Outcome of long standing solitary thyroid nodules. World J Surg *16*:583, 1992.
11. Hung W, et al: Solitary thyroid nodules in 71 children and adolescents. J Pediatr Surg *27*: 1407, 1992.
12. Frankenthaler RA, Sellin RV, Cangir A, Goepfert H: Lymph node metastasis from papillary-follicular thyroid carcinoma in young patients. Am J Surg *160*:341, 1990.
13. Lawson W and Biller HF: The solitary thyroid nodule: diagnosis and management of malignant disease. Am J Otolaryngol *4*:43, 1983.
14. Habashi S: Benign thyroid adenoma causing recurrent laryngeal nerve palsy in a child. J Laryngol Otol *105*:141, 1991.
15. Weiss SD and Orlich CC: Primary papillary carcinoma of a thyroglossal duct cyst: report of a case and literature review. Br J Surg *78*:87, 1991.
16. Cady B: Papillary carcinoma of the thyroid. Semin Surg Oncol *7*:81, 1991.
17. Nicolosi A, et al: The role of node-picking lymphadenectomy in the treatment of differentiated carcinoma of the thyroid. Minerva Chir *48*:459, 1993.
18. Shaha AR, DiMaio T, Webber C, and Jaffe BM: Intraoperative decision making during thyroid surgery based on the results of preoperative needle biopsy and frozen section. Surgery *108*:964, 1990.
19. Black EG and Sheppard MC: Serum thyroglobulin measurements in thyroid cancer: evaluation of "false" positive results. Clin Endocrinol (Oxf) *35*:519, 1991.
20. McLeod MK and Thompson NW: Hürthle cell neoplasms of the thyroid. Otolaryngol Clin North Am *23*:441, 1990.
21. Wermer P: Endocrine adenomatosis and peptic ulcer in a large kindred. Am J Med *35*:205, 1963.
22. Block MA, et al: Familial medullary carcinoma of the thyroid. Ann Surg *166*:403, 1967.
23. Sipple JH: The association of pheochromocytoma with carcinoma of the thyroid gland. Am J Med *31*:163, 1961.
24. Decker RA, et al: Evaluation of children with multiple endocrine neoplasia type IIb following thyroidectomy. J Pediatr Surg *25*:939, 1990.
25. Telander RL, et al: Medullary carcinoma in children: results of early detection and surgery. Arch Surg *124*:841, 1989.
26. Jay ID, et al: Prognostic significance of nondiploid DNA determined by flow cytometry in sporadic and familial medullary thyroid carcinoma. Surgery *108*:972, 1990.
27. Decker RA: Expression of papillary thyroid carcinoma in multiple endocrine neoplasia type 2A. Surgery *114*:1059, 1993.
28. Lampertico P: Anaplastic (sarcomatoid) carcinoma of the thyroid gland. Semin Diagn Pathol *10*:159, 1993.
29. Ekman ET, Lundell G, Tennvall J, and Wallin G: Chemotherapy and multimodality treatment in thyroid carcinoma. Otolaryngol Clin North Am *23*:523, 1990.
30. Gemsenjager E: Significance of the limiting lamella in struma surgery. Helv Chir Acta *59*:815, 1993.
31. Loré JM: Surgery of the thyroid gland. Otolaryngol Clin North Am *13*:69, 1980.
32. Shaha AR and Jaffe BM: Selective use of drains in thyroid surgery. J Surg Oncol *52*:241, 1993.
33. Ariyanayagam DC, et al: Thyroid surgery without drainage: 15 years of clinical experience. J R Coll Surg Edinb *38*:69, 1993.
34. Wells SA, et al: Transplantation of the parathyroid glands in man: clinical indications and results. Surgery *78*:34, 1975.
35. Shaha AR, Burnett C, and Jaffe BM: Parathyroid autotransplantation during thyroid surgery. J Surg Oncol *46*:21, 1991.
36. Funahashi H, et al: Our technique of parathyroid autotransplantation in operation for papillary thyroid carcinoma. Surgery *114*:92, 1993.
37. Loré JM Jr: Complications in management of thyroid cancer. Semin Surg Oncol *7*:120, 1991.
38. Staunton MD and Bourne H: Thyroid cancer in the 1980s: a decade of change. Ann Acad Med Singapore *22*:613, 1993.
39. Hochman M and Fee WE: Thyroidectomy under local anesthesia. Arch Otolaryngol Head Neck Surg *117*:405, 1991.
40. Lo-Gerfo P, Gates R, and Gazetas P: Outpatient and short-stay thyroid surgery. Head Neck *13*:97, 1991.
41. Herranz-Gonzalez J, Gavilan J, Matinez-Vidal J, and Gavilan C: Complications following thyroid surgery. Arch Otolaryngol Head Neck Surg *117*:516, 1991.
42. Campbell RP, Serpell JW, and Young AE: Non-recurrent laryngeal nerves: the role of digital subtraction angiography to identify subjects. Aust N Z J Surg *61*:358, 1991.
43. Kihara S, et al: Branch retinal artery occlusion following thyroidectomy for papillary carcinoma of the thyroid: report of a case. Surg Today *23*:750, 1993.
44. Bourrel C, et al: Transient hypocalcemia after thyroidectomy. Ann Otol Rhinol Laryngol *102*:496, 1993.

III THE LARYNX

John J. Ballenger

24 Development of the Human Larynx

Ronan O'Rahilly and Fabiola Müller

Prenatal life is divided into embryonic and fetal periods. The embryonic period, which comprises the first 8 weeks, is subdivided into 23 developmental stages, the details of which have been described elsewhere.[1] A summary of the developing respiratory system in relation to staging was published by O'Rahilly and Boyden,[2] and many further details were provided by O'Rahilly and Müller.[3] Since the classic study of the larynx by Soulié and Bardier,[4] the development of this organ has been investigated by, among others, O'Rahilly and Tucker,[5] and Müller, O'Rahilly and Tucker.[6,7] Many references to the earlier literature can be found in these publications.

Although the details of the developing larynx have been identified stage by stage, their relationship with the developing pharyngeal arches and pouches remains obscure. It is known that the hyoid bone is derived from the cartilaginous elements of pharyngeal arches 2 and 3, and the thyroid and other cartilages of the larynx are believed to be associated with the more caudally situated arches.

EMBRYONIC PERIOD

The larynx may in a certain sense be considered as a diverticulum of the (future laryngo) pharynx, with which (except for a temporary embryonic closure) it communicates throughout life.

3 to 4 Weeks

At 3 weeks, when the embryo is only about 3 mm long (stage 10), a median pharyngeal groove (internally) and ridge (externally) are discernible, and the groove includes the laryngotracheal sulcus. Within a few days (stage 12), the "lung bud" appears as a respiratory diverticulum that projects from the digestive tube. The mesenchyme and epithelium between the respiratory and digestive primordia are termed the tracheoesophageal septum. The rostralmost limit of the septum is known as the separation point, and, contrary to most accounts, it remains at a constant level from 4 to 7 weeks. The idea that the tracheoesophageal septum grows in a caudorostral direction is a myth that is still being promulgated. Right and left lung buds are soon detectable (stage 13), and the trachea becomes visible in the more advanced specimens. The bifurcation point of the trachea soon begins to descend.

4 to 6 Weeks

At about 32 to 33 days (stages 14 and 15), the future larynx begins its differentiation. The lateral epithelial walls become apposed in the median plane, thereby forming what is known as the epithelial lamina. This bilaminar plate is situated between the arytenoid swellings, behind which the pharyngeal lumen still communicates with the trachea (pharyngoinfraglottic duct or canal). The hypopharyngeal (formerly called hypobranchial) eminence does not represent the epiglottis, which is identifiable a little later.

By 5 weeks, the hyoid condensation begins to appear, and by 6 weeks the cricoid can be identified in mesenchyme (Fig. 24–1). This is followed by the appearance of a cartilaginous cricoid center, or possibly of bilateral centers.

The larynx is clearly definable by 6 weeks (stage 17) (Fig. 24–1B). At this time, or a few days earlier, the front portion of the epithelial lamina can be regarded as its vestibular part. Lateral expansions of this portion soon form the embryonic vestibule (coronal or transverse cleft, Fig. 24–1B). The laryngeal cavity is now T-shaped in transverse section, but the transverse cleft that constitutes the embryonic vestibule corresponds to only a portion of the adult vestibule, which also includes the median cleft.

The appearance of the epithelial lamina at 6 weeks

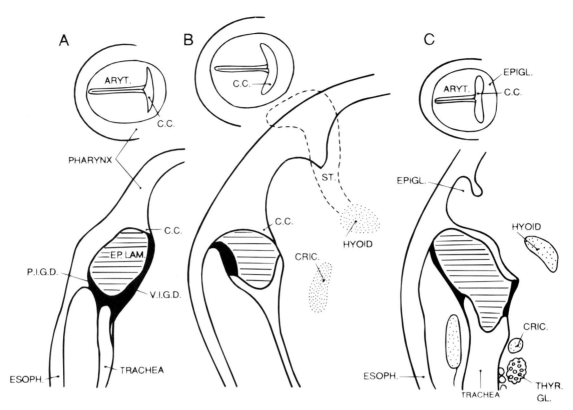

Fig. 24–1. Development of the epithelial lamina and the first skeletal elements of the larynx in stages 16 to 21 (37 to 52 days). The upper row shows the larynx as seen from above, and the lower row provides median sections at the corresponding stages (16, 17, and 21). ARYT, Arytenoid swelling; C.C., coronal cleft; CRIC, cricoid condensation; EPIGL, epiglottis; EP. LAM., epithelial lamina; ESOPH, esophagus; P.I.G.D., pharyngoinfraglottic duct; ST, styloid process; THYR GL, thyroid gland; V.I.G.D., vestibuloinfraglottic duct.

(stage 18) resembles type 1 congenital atresia, which may be essentially a persistence of the embryonic condition.[3] The rostral end of the tracheal lumen is believed to represent the future infraglottic cavity. A tendency for the vestibule and the trachea to communicate with each other (vestibuloinfraglottic duct or canal) is characteristic. Laryngeal muscles are beginning to develop, but the existence of one or two common sphincters initially is doubtful. The hyoid condensation is undergoing chondrification, and condensations for the thyroid laminae begin to appear.

7 to 8 Weeks

The pharyngoinfraglottic duct is largely, if not entirely, open in most embryos, and the track of the vestibuloinfraglottic duct is visible (Fig. 24–1C). The ventricles of the larynx begin to appear as right and left laterally projecting epithelial buds. The right and left leaves of the epithelial lamina are beginning to separate, but, at the end of the embryonic period (stage 23), areas of fusion generally persist rostrally and caudally. The pharyngeal lumen, however, is continuous with the infraglottic cavity and hence with the trachea. Cavitation is beginning in the ventricles.

By the end of the embryonic period (stage 23, Fig. 24–2), the hyoid cartilage consists of the body and greater horns, the lesser horns being distinct nodules separated from the styloid processes. The cartilaginous thyroid laminae, which may show a foramen, are united below by mesenchyme (''copula''). The superior horns may or may not be continuous with the laminae and arise from the greater horns of the hyoid. The cricoid cartilage is a continuous ring that comprises an arch and a lamina. Each arytenoid cartilage possesses a cartilaginous muscular process and a mesenchymal vocal process.

Most of the major laryngeal muscles (cricothyroid, posterior and lateral cricoarytenoid, thyroarytenoid, transverse arytenoid) are now present (although not yet striated), and their innervation follows the adult pattern closely.[6] Motor fibers penetrate the muscles. The vocalis muscle is beginning to differentiate.

The laryngeal cavity now comprises (as in the adult) the vestibule, the ventricles and the part between them, and the infraglottic cavity. The ventricles are not at the level of the future glottis, which lies more caudally. The sensory innervation is well established, although most fibers do not yet reach the epithelium. In the laryngopharynx, however, receptors are present.[7]

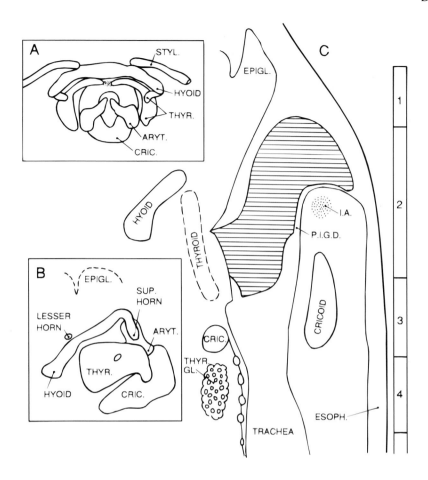

Fig. 24–2. Larynx at the end of the embryonic period (8 weeks), showing reconstructions of three embryos of stage 23. A. Skeletal elements from above. B. Lateral view of skeleton. Note the foramen in the thyroid cartilage, through which nerve fibers of the external laryngeal nerve and an artery may enter; the opening can be found as a variation in the adult. The hyoid is remarkably ventral with regard to the thyroid cartilage. C. Median section. The numbers 1 to 4 indicate vertebral levels. STYL, styloid process; ARYT, arytenoid cartilage; CRIC, cricoid cartilage; EPIGL, epiglottis; ESOPH, esophagus; I.A., interarytenoid muscle; P.I.G.D., pharyngoinfraglottic duct; THYR, thyroid cartilage; THYR GL, thyroid gland.

FETAL PERIOD

Much information concerning the fetal larynx is available in Soulié and Bardier.[4]

During trimester 1 (Fig. 24–3A), the larynx increases in size from about 3 to 7 mm. The thyroid laminae become fused, and the cricothyroid membrane develops. The vocal ligaments begin to form early (33 mm), and the ventricular ligaments and the glottis become increasingly apparent. The ventricles acquire their saccules. The cricoarytenoid joints undergo cavitation, in which they are followed by the cricothyroid joints. By 90 mm, the laryngeal cavity has its adult form.[4]

During trimester 2 (Fig. 24–3C), the larynx increases in size from about 8 to 15 mm. The thyroid cartilage becomes a single structure. The epiglottis begins to chondrify. The hyoid cartilage commences ossification. The corniculate and cuneiform cartilages develop. The joints acquire ligaments. Glands become well developed. Elastic fibers have been detected in the epiglottis.[8]

During trimester 3, the larynx increases in size to about 15 to 20 mm, and the inlet is about 5 mm in diameter. Laryngeal connective tissue compartments in trimesters 2 and 3 were studied by Tucker and Smith.[9]

Measurements of the larynx can be found in Soulié and Bardier (embryonic and fetal),[4] Peter and associates (infantile and child's),[10] Eckenhoff (infantile),[11] Kahane (prepubertal and pubertal),[12] and Schild (fetal and infantile).[13] The larynx, as indicated by the tip of the epiglottis, the hyoid, and the lower border of the cricoid, descends from embryonic and fetal life to adulthood (Fig. 24–4). Vertebral levels are available in Magriples and Laitman,[14] Noback (fetal, infantile,

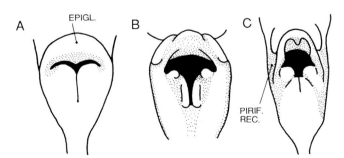

Fig. 24–3. Dorsal view of the prenatal larynx at (A) 32 mm (8 weeks), (B) 55 mm (10 weeks), and (C) 160 mm (18 weeks). Note the appearance of the corniculate tubercles, the aryepiglottic folds, and the piriform recess (PIRIF. REC.). (Based on Soulié A and Bardier E: Recherches sur le développement du larynx chez l'homme. J Anat Physiol 43:137, 1907.)

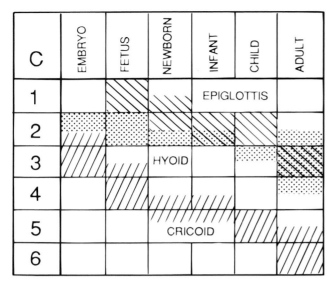

Fig. 24–4. Graph showing the prenatal and postnatal descent of the epiglottis (left-to-right shading), hyoid (stippled), and cricoid (right-to-left shading) with reference to cervical vertebrae 1 to 6.

child's),[15] Roche and Barkla (child's),[16] and O'Rahilly and Müller (embryonic).[3] The infantile larynx has been described by Tucker[17] and Wilson,[18] and detailed views have been provided by Bosma.[19]

Ossification in the thyroid cartilage frequently begins from about 20 years onward in the posterior border of each lamina. It would be imprudent, however, to attempt to estimate age from the extent of the ossific process.[20]

CONGENITAL ANOMALIES

Only some congenital anomalies of the larynx are currently amenable to interpretation in developmental terms.

Posterior laryngeal cleft probably develops during separation of the trachea and esophagus at 4 weeks (stage 13), as suggested by the frequent association with tracheoesophageal fistula. Hence the subsequent skeletal anomaly (split cricoid) that develops in infraglottic types would in all likelihood be secondary, perhaps similar to that formed during the genesis of spina bifida cystica. Moreover, the occurrence of bilateral chondrific centers in the normal cricoid primordium has yet to be established.

Congenital laryngeal atresia probably arises between 6 and 10 postovulatory weeks, the more extensive examples representing embryonic stages and the less severe forms being fetal. A combination of supraglottic and infraglottic atresia resembles closely the normal appearance of the larynx at 6 weeks (stage 18) and may be basically a persistence of the embryonic condition. At this time, when the embryo is about 15 mm in

length, the epithelial lamina has reached its full expansion (see Fig. 24–1C). Atresia that is either purely infraglottic or largely glottic probably arises early during the fetal period, when the epithelial lamina has failed to undergo further reorganization.

Congenital laryngeal webs, situated ventrally and extending dorsally to a variable degree, are also thought to result probably from a localized failure of splitting of the epithelial lamina into two walls, most likely early in the fetal period.

Congenital subglottic stenosis may also be associated with the persistence of the epithelial lamina, but some instances seem to be produced by deformities of the cricoid cartilage.

Congenital laryngeal cysts are usually in the region of the saccule and may indicate disturbed development in fetal life.

Some laryngeal anomalies are part of a more widespread disturbance. Thus, congenital webs may be accompanied by subglottic stenosis, and structures far removed are affected in some instances, such as anomalies of the limbs. Similarly, cleft larynx may be associated with a congenital cardiac defect or cleft lip and palate and has been considered a median developmental field defect that can occur in causally different syndromes.

SUGGESTED READINGS

1. O'Rahilly R and Müller F: Developmental Stages in Human Embryos, including a Revision of Streeter's "Horizons" and a Survey of the Carnegie Collection. Washington DC, Carnegie Institution of Washington, 1987.
2. O'Rahilly R and Boyden EA: The timing and sequence of events in the development of the human respiratory system during the embryonic period proper. Z Anat Entwicklungsges 141:237, 1973.
3. O'Rahilly R and Müller F: Respiratory and alimentary relations in staged human embryos: new embryological data and congenital anomalies. Ann Otol Rhinol Laryngol 93:421, 1984.
4. Soulié A and Bardier F: Recherches sur le développement du larynx chez l'homme. J Anat Physiol 43:137, 1907.
5. O'Rahilly R and Tucker JA: The early development of the larynx in staged human embryos. Part I: Embryos of the first five weeks (to stage 15). Ann Otol Rhinol Laryngol 82:1, 1973.
6. Müller F, O'Rahilly R, and Tucker JA: The human larynx at the end of the embryonic period proper. I. The laryngeal and infrahyoid muscles and their innervation. Acta Otolaryngol (Stockh) 91:323, 1981.
7. Müller F, O'Rahilly R, and Tucker JA: The human larynx at the end of the embryonic period proper. 2. The laryngeal cavity and the innervation of its lining. Ann Otol Rhinol Laryngol 94:607, 1985.
8. Patzelt V: Über die menschliche Epiglottis und die Entwicklung des Epithels in den Nachbargebieten. Z Anat Entwicklungsges 70:1, 1924.
9. Tucker GF and Smith HR: A histological demonstration of the development of laryngeal connective tissue compartments. Trans Am Acad Ophthalmol Otolaryngol 66:308, 1962.
10. Peter K, Wetzel G, and Heiderich F (eds): Handbuch der Anatomie des Kindes. 2 vols. Munich, Bergmann, 1938.

11. Eckenhoff JF: Some anatomic considerations of the infant larynx influencing endotracheal anesthesia. Anesthesiology *12*:401, 1951.

12. Kahane JC: A morphological study of the human prepubertal and pubertal larynx. Am J Anat *151*:11, 1978.

13. Schild JA: Relationship of laryngeal dimensions to body size and gestational age in premature neonates and small infants. Laryngoscope *94*:1284, 1984.

14. Magriples U and Laitman JT: Developmental change in the position of the fetal human larynx. Am J Phys Anthropol *72*:463, 1987.

15. Noback GJ: The developmental topography of the larynx, tra-chea and lungs in the fetus, new-born, infant and child. Am J Dis Child *26*:515, 1923.

16. Roche AF and Barkla DH: The level of the larynx during child-hood. Ann Otol Rhinol Laryngol *74*:645, 1965.

17. Tucker G: The infant larynx: direct laryngoscopic observation. JAMA *99*:1899, 1932.

18. Wilson TG: Some observations on the anatomy of the infantile larynx. Acta Otolaryngol (Stock) *43*:95, 1953.

19. Bosma JF: Anatomy of the Infant Head. Baltimore, Johns Hopkins University Press, 1986.

20. Keen JA and Wainwright J: Ossification of the thyroid, cricoid and arytenoid cartilages. S Afr J Lab Clin Med *4*:83, 1958.

25 Anatomy and Physiology of the Larynx

Clarence T. Sasaki, Brian P. Driscoll, and Carol Gracco

The larynx essentially serves as an elaborate sphincter to the lower airway. In certain animals this sphincter has been modified for vocal production. The classic study of the comparative anatomy of the larynx by Negus allows prioritization of the three functions of the larynx.[1] These three functions, in order of priority, are (1) protection of the lower airway, (2) respiration, and (3) phonation. The precise sphincteric action of the larynx allows the air and food passages to share a common pathway, and this common pathway affords human beings the complex muscular movements needed for effective vocal communication. We are most clearly reminded of the sphincteric nature of the larynx in the occasional patient with intractable aspiration requiring surgical intervention as a means of separating the food and air passages. Thus, in many ways our clinical experiences serve to confirm Negus' original phylogenic observations.

ANATOMY

Thyroid Cartilage

As its name implies (thyeros, shield, in Greek), the thyroid cartilage is a shield-shaped structure that serves to protect the internal anatomy of the larynx.[2–7] It is the largest cartilage of the larynx and is composed of two wings, the alae and laminae. The alae are fused in the midline and open posteriorly (Fig. 25–1). In the male the alae fuse at about 90 degrees, making a laryngeal prominence or Adam's apple. In the female, this prominence is absent because of the more oblique fusion angle of 120 degrees. Superiorly, the fusion of the alae is deficient, accounting for the thyroid notch. Each ala posteriorly has a superior and inferior horn or cornu. The inferior cornu articulates with a facet on the cricoid cartilage to form the cricothyroid joint. This synovial joint allows rotation of the cricoid cartilage. This rotation varies the tension placed on the vocal folds. The superior cornu is attached to the greater cornu of the hyoid bone by way of the lateral thyrohyoid ligament. This ligament sometimes contains small triticeal cartilages. The two lateral thyrohyoid ligaments along with the median thyrohyoid ligament are condensations of the thyrohyoid membrane; these structures attach the hyoid bone to the thyroid cartilage. At the attachment of the superior cornu to the alae of the thyroid, a protuberance called the superior tubercle is found. About 1 cm anterior and superior to this tubercle, the superior laryngeal artery and the internal branch of the superior laryngeal nerve and associated lymphatic vessels pierce the membrane to supply the supraglottic larynx. At this point transcutaneous anesthesia of the internal branch can be performed. Running obliquely from the superior tubercle to the inferior tubercle (along the inferior margin of the thyroid cartilage) is a ridge called the oblique line that serves as the attachment point for the thyrohyoid, sternothyroid, and inferior constrictor muscles.

The relationship of the surface anatomy with internal laryngeal anatomy merits consideration. Most important is the level of the true vocal cords in relation to the thyroid cartilage. An understanding of this relationship is crucial to performing supraglottic laryngectomy and phonosurgery (thyroplasty type I). In this regard, the midline vertical distance from the thyroid notch to inferior border of the thyroid cartilage is about 20 mm in males and 15.5 mm in females. The anterior commissure is found at the midpoint between these landmarks. The posterior extent of the vocal cords is anterior to the oblique line and found in the middle third of this line.[8]

The thyroid cartilage is lined by a thick layer of perichondrium on all surfaces except the inner surface at the anterior commissure. At this point are attached five ligaments that form the scaffolding for the corresponding laryngeal folds. From superior to inferior, they are the median thyroepiglottic ligament (median thyrohy-

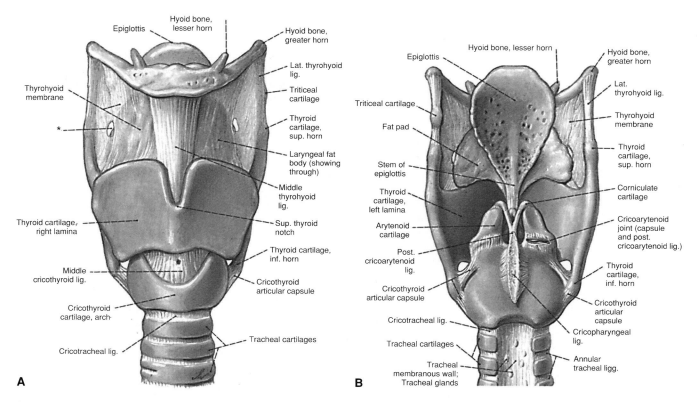

Fig. 25–1. A. Anterior view of the cartilages and ligaments of the larynx and hyoid bone. B. Posterior view of the cartilages, ligaments, and articulations of the larynx and hyoid. (From Staubesand J and Taylor AN: Sobotta: Atlas of Human Anatomy. 11th Ed. Vol 1. Baltimore, Urban & Schwarzenberg, 1990.)

oid fold), bilateral vestibular ligaments (vestibular folds or false cords), and the bilateral vocal ligaments (vocal folds). The attachments of these ligaments penetrate the inner perichondrium, forming Broyle's ligament. This ligament contains blood vessels and lymphatic vessels and constitutes an important barrier to the spread of laryngeal neoplasms.

Cricoid Cartilage

As its name (krikos, ring, in Greek) implies, the cricoid cartilage is a complete ring.[2–7] It is the only supporting structure that completely encircles the airway and serves as the major support for the functioning larynx. Its shape is classically described as that of a signet ring, with the anterior arch measuring 3 mm in height and the posterior lamina about 20 to 30 mm in height. Its inferior border is nearly horizontal and is attached to the first tracheal cartilage by the cricotracheal ligament.

On the posterior surface of the cricoid, the posterior cricoarytenoid muscles are attached in depressions that are separated by a midline vertical ridge. These muscles are the only abductors of the vocal folds. Attached to this midline vertical ridge are two fasciculi of longitudinal fibers of the esophagus. Housed on the superior surface of the posterior cricoid lamina are the paired arytenoid cartilages.

Posterior to anterior, the superior portion of the cricoid lamina slopes steeply downward to form the anterior cricoid arch. In the midline, between the superior portion of the arch and the inferior border of the thyroid cartilage, is the cricothyroid membrane. This structure must be incised during an emergency cricothyrotomy.

Arytenoid Cartilages

The arytenoids are paired cartilages that articulate with the posterosuperior portion of the cricoid cartilage.[2–7] Movement of these cartilages and their attached vocal folds allows the larynx its often diverse and complex functions. Each arytenoid is roughly pyramidal, giving it a base, an apex, and three sides. The base of the arytenoid provides the articular facet as well as the muscular and vocal processes. The cricoarytenoid joint is a synovial joint with complex movements that are debated. It appears, however, that the most important movement of the joint is a rocking motion of the cartilage around the long axis of its facet. Laterally the base forms a broad muscular process, and anteriorly it forms the thinner vocal process. The anterolateral surface receives the vestibular ligament as well as the thyroarytenoid and vocalis muscles. The posterior surface receives muscular attachments, and to the medial surface is attached the prominent posterior cricoarytenoid ligament. Sitting at the apex of the arytenoid is the corniculate cartilage.

Corniculate and Cuneiform Cartilages

The corniculate and cuneiform cartilages are small, paired, and fibroelastic.[3,9] The corniculate, or cartilage of Santorini, is housed on the apex of the arytenoid cartilage. The cuneiform, or cartilage of Wrisberg, when present, is lateral to the corniculate cartilages and is embedded in the aryepiglottic fold. Although some investigators believe that these cartilages are vestigial, they do appear to add rigidity to the aryepiglottic fold. This rigidity augments the important rampart function of these folds, thus diverting swallowed matter laterally away from the larynx into the pyriform sinuses.

Epiglottis

The epiglottis is a leaf-shaped elastic fibrocartilage that functions mainly as a backstop against the entrance of swallowed matter into the laryngeal aditus.[2–7] During swallowing, the larynx is raised anterosuperiorly. This action pushes the epiglottis against the base of tongue posteriorly displacing it over the laryngeal aditus. The epiglottis has two anterior attachments. Superiorly it is attached to the hyoid bone by the hyoepiglottic ligament. Inferiorly at the stem or petiole it is attached to the inner surface of the thyroid cartilage just above the anterior commissure by the thyroepiglottic ligament. The surface of the epiglottic cartilage is multiply pitted and filled with mucus glands; these pits potentially allow the spread of cancer from one surface of the epiglottis to the other.

The epiglottis may arbitrarily be divided into a suprahyoid and an infrahyoid portion. The suprahyoid portion is free on both its laryngeal and lingual surfaces, with the laryngeal mucosal surface more adherent than the lingual. As the mucosa of the laryngeal surface is reflected back onto the base of tongue, three folds result: two lateral glossoepiglottic folds and a median glossoepiglottic fold. The two depressions formed by these folds are known as the valleculae (depression, in Latin). The infrahyoid portion is free only on its laryngeal or posterior surface. This surface contains a small protuberance known as the tubercle. Between the anterior surface and the thyrohyoid membrane and the thyroid cartilage exists the fat pad of the preepiglottic space. Attached laterally is the quadrangular membrane extending to the arytenoid and corniculate cartilages constituting the aryepiglottic folds.

Ossification of Laryngeal Cartilages

Clinicians have long recognized that incomplete ossification of the laryngeal cartilages can be mistaken for a foreign body on plain roentgenograms of the neck.[5,10] This particularly applies to ossification of the superior and inferior cornua of the thyroid cartilage and linear ossification of the posterior portion of the cricoid. Thus, the need for understanding the normal ossification pattern of the larynx is self-evident. Only those structures composed of hyaline cartilage undergo ossification, that is, the thyroid, cricoid and arytenoid cartilages. The hyoid bone is completely ossified at 2 years of age and is generally not a point of radiographic confusion.

The thyroid cartilage undergoes ossification in the male about age 20 and in the female a few years later. Ossification begins posterioinferiorly on the lamina. It then extends anteriorly on the inferior border and superiorly at the posterior border. At this time, nuclei of ossification can be seen in the inferior and superior cornua.

The cricoid and arytenoid cartilages undergo ossification later than the thyroid cartilage. Ossification of the cricoid cartilage generally begins at the inferior border, although the superior margin of the quadrate lamina may be an early site of ossification.

Neoplastic invasion of the laryngeal cartilages generally takes place in the ossified portion of the cartilage.[11] The incomplete ossification pattern may make it difficult to appreciate small areas of invasion.

Elastic Tissue

The elastic tissue of the larynx consists of two main parts: (1) the quadrangular membrane of the supraglottic larynx; and (2) the thicker conus elasticus and vocal ligaments of the glottic and infraglottic larynx.[2–7]

The quadrangular membrane attaches anteriorly to the lateral margin of the epiglottis and curves posteriorly to attach to the arytenoid and corniculate cartilages. This structure and the overlying mucosa constitute the aryepiglottic folds. These folds form part of the medial wall of the pyriform sinus. The inferior edge of the quadrangular membrane constitutes the vestibular ligament.

The conus elasticus is a thicker elastic structure than the quadrangular membrane. It attaches inferiorly at the superior border of the cricoid cartilage. It then projects upward and medial to its superior attachments, the anterior commissure of the thyroid cartilage and the vocal process of the arytenoid. Between these superior attachments, the conus thickens to form the vocal ligament. Anteriorly, the conus forms the cricothyroid membrane, and in the midline, this membrane condenses to form the cricothyroid ligament (Figs. 25–1 to 25–4).

Muscles

Extrinsic Muscles

The extrinsic muscles of the larynx are those muscles of the laryngohyoid complex that serve to raise, lower,

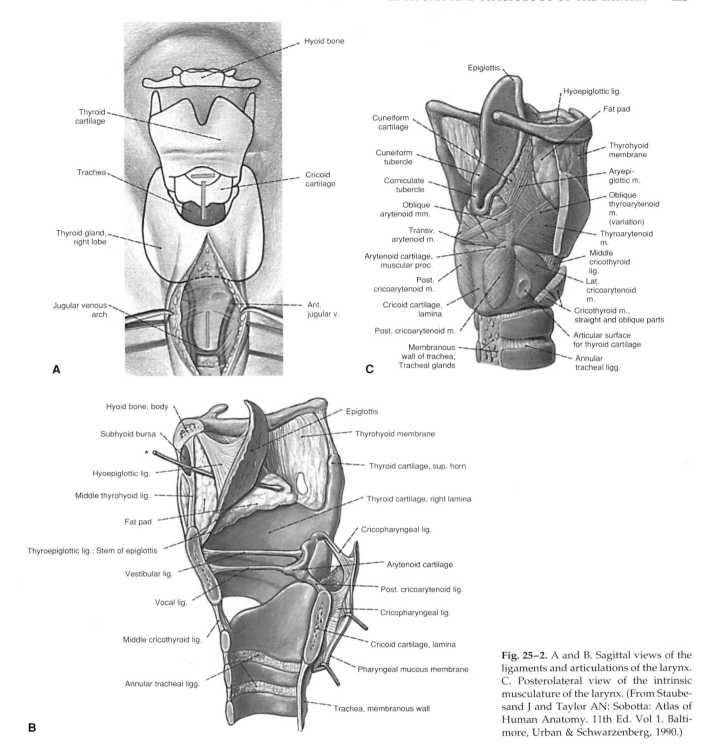

Fig. 25–2. A and B. Sagittal views of the ligaments and articulations of the larynx. C. Posterolateral view of the intrinsic musculature of the larynx. (From Staubesand J and Taylor AN: Sobotta: Atlas of Human Anatomy. 11th Ed. Vol 1. Baltimore, Urban & Schwarzenberg, 1990.)

or stabilize the larynx.[2–7,12] Those muscles that elevate the larynx are the thyrohyoid, stylohyoid, digastric, geniohyoid, mylohyoid, and stylopharyngeal. These muscles are important in the elevation and anterior displacement of the larynx during swallowing. They also help to suspend the larynx, via the hyoid bone, from the skull base and mandible. The principal de-pressors of the larynx are the omohyoid, sternothyroid, and sternohyoid. These muscles displace the larynx downward during inspiration. The middle constrictor, inferior constrictor, and cricopharyngeus muscles are also important extrinsic laryngeal muscles. The proper function of these muscles is crucial to the precisely timed swallowing reflex.

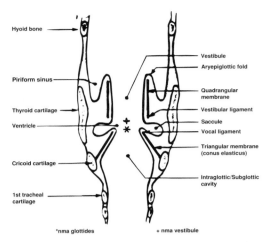

Fig. 25–3. Coronal section of the larynx, demonstrating the internal cavity and its subdivisions. Note the valve-like nature of the true and false vocal folds. (From Cooper MH: Anatomy of the larynx. In: Neurologic Disorders of the Larynx. Edited by Blitzer A, et al. New York, Thieme, 1992.)

Intrinsic Muscles

The intrinsic muscles of the larynx are those muscles that are anatomically restricted to the larynx proper. They modify the size of the glottic opening along with the length and tension on the vocal folds. They consist of multiple adductors but only a single abductor. With the exception of the interarytenoid, the intrinsic muscles are paired, and these paired muscles act synchronously (Fig. 25–5).

Cricothyroid Muscle

The cricothyroid muscle is located on the external surface of the laryngeal cartilages. It is classically described as consisting of two bellies. The straight portion or pars recta attaches from the lateral portion of the anterior arch of the cricoid to the inferior border of the thyroid. As its name implies, this muscle belly runs in a fairly vertical direction. The second belly, the pars obliqua, also attaches from the anterolateral border of the cricoid arch but travels obliquely upward to insert on the anterior portion of the inferior cornu. When the right and left cricothyroid muscles contract, they rotate the cricoid at the cricothyroid joint. This action brings the anterior arch of the cricoid superiorly toward the inferior border of the thyroid laminae while displacing the posterior cricoid lamina (and the arytenoid cartilages) inferiorly. This inferior displacement increases the distance between the vocal processes and the anterior commissure, the result of this action is to lower, stretch, and thin the vocal folds while bringing them into a paramedian position.

The stretching of the vocal fold also sharpens the edge of the vocal fold and passively stiffens the component layers of the vocal folds (Fig. 25–6). Biomechanically this translates into a higher fundamental frequency produced by the vocal folds.

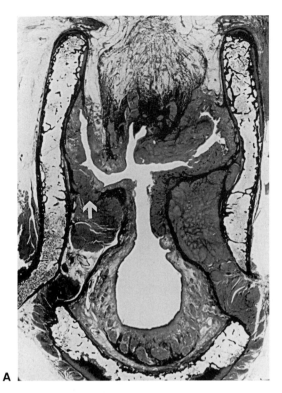

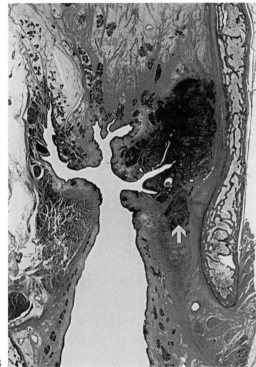

Fig. 25–4. A. The thyroglottic membrane may be naturally dehiscent (arrow). B. Dehiscence in the thyroglottic membrane can allow transglottic cancer to extend inferiorly along the paraglottic space (arrow). (Courtesy of Dr. John A. Kirchner.)

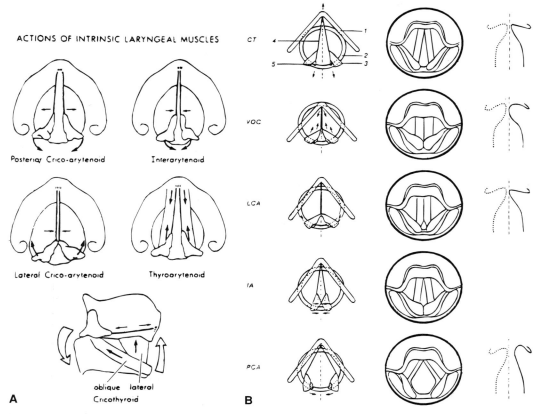

Fig. 25–5. A. The intrinsic muscles of the larynx and their actions. Heavy arrows indicate the direction of muscle action; fine arrows indicate the motion of vocal ligaments; open arrows indicate the motion of cricoid and thyroid cartilages. (From Ballenger JJ (Ed): Diseases of the Nose, Throat, Ear, Head, and Neck. 13th Ed. Philadelphia, Lea & Febiger, 1985.) B. Schematic presentation of the function of the laryngeal muscles. The left column shows the location of the cartilages and the edge of the vocal folds when the laryngeal muscles are activated individually. The arrow indicates the direction of the force exerted. 1, Thyroid cartilage; 2, cricoid cartilage; 3, arytenoid cartilage; 4, vocal ligament; 5, posterior cricoarytenoid ligament. The middle column shows views from above. The right column presents contours of frontal sections at the middle of the membranous portion of the vocal fold. The dotted line shows a control, where no muscle is activated. (From Hirano M: Clinical Examination of Voice. New York, Springer, 1981.)

Posterior Cricoarytenoid Muscle

This muscle is the sole abductor of the vocal folds. It is seated in a depression on the posterior surface of the cricoid lamina, and its fibers run obliquely superior and lateral to attach onto the muscular process of the arytenoid cartilage. Contraction of these fibers brings the muscular process medially, posteriorly, and inferiorly while laterally rotating and elevating the vocal process. This action abducts, elongates, and thins the vocal folds while causing the vocal fold edge to be rounded. The stretching of the vocal fold leads to passive stiffening of its layers.

Lateral Cricoarytenoid Muscle

This muscle is the main antagonist of the posterior cricoarytenoid. It attaches along the superior border of the cricoid cartilage and then sends its fibers posteriorly to insert on the anterior portion of the muscular process. Contraction of this muscle brings the muscular process anterolaterally while adducting and lowering the vocal process. This results in adduction, elonga-

tion, and thinning of the vocal folds. The edge of the vocal fold becomes sharper, and its component layers are passively stiffened.

Interarytenoid/Aryepiglottic Muscle

The interarytenoid is the only unpaired intrinsic muscle, consisting of two types of muscle fibers. The bulk of the muscle consists of transverse fibers passing from the posterior surface of one arytenoid cartilage to the posterior surface of the other. This muscle contracts to bring together the arytenoid cartilages, thus assisting in closing the posterior portion of the glottis. This does not significantly affect the mechanical properties of the vocal folds. Along with these transverse fibers are oblique fibers. These oblique fibers pass from the posterior portion of the arytenoid on one side to the apex of the arytenoid on the other side, thus crossing in the midline. Some fibers insert at the apex, whereas others travel along the quadrangular membrane. These fibers contract to narrow the laryngeal aditus. Those fibers

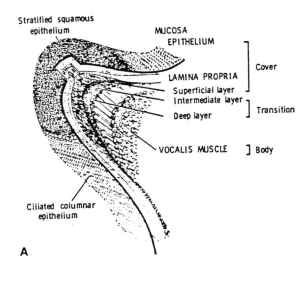

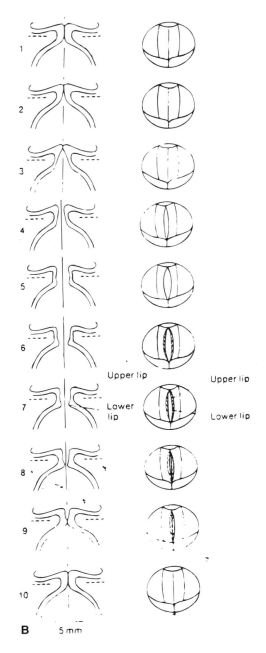

Fig. 25–6. A. Schematic illustration showing the layered structure of the adult vocal fold. (From Hirano M: Phonosurgery: basic and clinical investigations. Otologia (Fukuoka) *21*:239, 1975.) B. Coronal section showing the movement of the vocal folds during one vibratory cycle. (From Hirano M: Clinical Examination of Voice. New York, Springer, 1981.)

traveling along the quadrangular membrane (thus the aryepiglottic fold) constitute the aryepiglottic muscle.

Thyroarytenoid Muscle

This muscle is classically divided into the thyroarytenoid internus and externus. These have similar attachments, but the internus lies deep or internal to the externus. In addition, the internus is better developed than the externus.

The thyroarytenoid externus arises from the anterior commissure and inserts onto the lateral surface of the arytenoid cartilage. It contracts to bring the vocal process and anterior commissure closer to each other,

thus adducting the vocal folds. It also contracts to adduct the false vocal cords. The externus sends a few slips of muscle fibers onto the quadrangular membrane to establish the thyroepiglottic muscle. This muscle, like the aryepiglottic muscle, acts to narrow the laryngeal inlet.

The thyroarytenoid internus or vocalis muscle attaches at the anterior commissure and inserts onto the vocal process, sending a few slips of muscle fiber below the vocal ligament onto the conus elasticus. It contracts to adduct, shorten, thicken, and lower the vocal fold while rounding its edge. The body (muscle) of the vocal fold is actively stiffened while the cover is passively slackened.

Internal Anatomy

The internal anatomy of the larynx consists of three compartments separated by two folds[2-7] (see Fig. 25–3). The three compartments are the vestibule, the ventricle, and the infraglottic cavity. The false and true vocal folds separate the foregoing compartments. These mucosa-lined compartments demarcate two spaces of importance: the preepiglottic space and the paraglottic space.

Vestibule

A laryngoscopic view of the larynx reveals the vestibule as that portion of the larynx from the tip of the epiglottis to the false or vestibular folds. Thus, the vestibule is bounded by the epiglottis anteriorly, the aryepiglottic folds laterally, and the arytenoid and corniculate cartilages with the interarytenoid muscle posteriorly. In the laryngoscopic view, the anterior commissure is frequently hidden by the protuberance of the epiglottis known as the tubercle. The vestibular folds as previously discussed are formed by mucosa overlying the vestibular ligament (inferior border of the quadrangular membrane). The submucosa of the ventricle contains numerous seromucinous glands. The secretions produced by these exocrine glands provide both mechanical and immune (lysozyme) protection for the vocal folds.[13]

Ventricle

The ventricle or sinus of Morgagni is the small space between the false and true vocal folds. The ventricle is often hidden during laryngoscopic examination of the larynx unless exposed by lateralization of the false vocal fold. At the anterior end of the ventricle is a diverticulum known as the laryngeal saccule. The saccule (of Hilton) is lined with mucus glands that are thought to lubricate the vocal folds. Fibers of the thyroarytenoid muscle line the walls of the saccule and are thought to contract to express mucus from the saccule. The size of the saccule is variable, although it seldom extends above the superior border of the thyroid cartilage. Abnormal dilatation of the saccule results in an air-filled laryngocele that should be distinguished from a mucocele of the saccule (saccular cyst), which lacks free communication with the ventricle and thus is not air-filled.[14] The vocal folds that form the inferior boundary of the ventricle are described in more detail later in this chapter.

Infraglottic Cavity

The infraglottic cavity extends from the glottis down to the inferior border of the cricoid cartilage. Its lateral boundary is formed by the conus elasticus and walls of the cricoid cartilage.

Pyriform Sinus

Although the pyriform sinus is anatomically part of the hypopharynx, an understanding of the anatomy of the pyriform sinus and its relationship with the larynx is essential. The pyriform sinus is a gutter formed by the aryepiglottic fold, arytenoid, and superior cricoid medially and the thyrohyoid membrane and internal surface of the thyroid lamina laterally. Superiorly, it begins at the lateral glossoepiglottic fold. Inferiorly, the apex of the sinus blends with the esophageal inlet at about the superior border of the cricoid (Fig. 25–7). Thus, invasion of the apex by cancer implies the necessity of removing a portion of cricoid if conservation laryngectomy is planned.

Two important markings are seen within the pyriform sinus. Anteriorly in the floor of the sinus, a small fold marks the course of the superior laryngeal nerve. This submucosal course of the nerve makes it possible to anesthetize the nerve in the pyriform sinus topically. The second, more variable landmark is the protrusion made into the sinus from the superior cornu of the thyroid cartilage. This smooth protrusion, which is usually seen in the elderly, should not be confused with neoplasm.

Mucosa

The mucosa of the larynx is of two types, ciliated pseudostratified columnar cell (respiratory) epithelium and squamous cell epithelium. Much of the larynx is surfaced by respiratory epithelium, although the superior epiglottis, upper aryepiglottic folds, and the free edges of the vocal folds are surfaced by squamous cell epithelium. Beneath this covering epithelium is a variable basement membrane, and separating these two is a layer of loose fibrous stroma. This loose fibrous layer is absent on the true vocal folds, as well as on the laryngeal (posterior) surface of the epiglottis. The absence of this layer on the posterior surface of the epiglottis accounts for the more intense swelling of the lingual (anterior) surface of the epiglottis in inflammatory conditions of the larynx.

Preepiglottic Space

The preepiglottic space, as its name implies, lies anterior to the epiglottis, which serves as its posterior boundary. Superiorly, it is bounded by the hyoepiglottic ligament and mucosa of the vallecula and, inferiorly, by the thyroepiglottic ligament. The anterior boundaries are the thyrohyoid membrane and the inner surface of the thyroid lamina. Laterally, the preepiglottic space opens in the paraglottic space. Cancer on the infrahyoid portion of the epiglottis can penetrate this structure and gain access to the preepiglottic space.

Paraglottic Space

The paraglottic space, as its name implies, lies on each side of the glottis. This space lies above and below

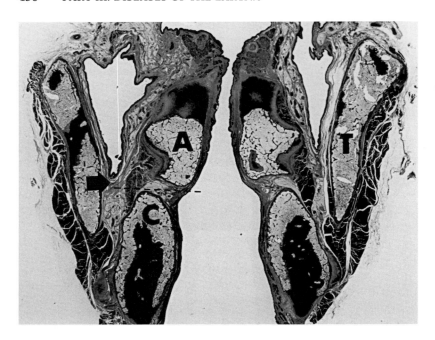

Fig. 25–7. Coronal section through the human larynx demonstrating the relationship of the cricoid cartilage (C) with the apex of the pyriform sinus (arrow). A, Arytenoid cartilage; T, thyroid cartilage. (Courtesy of Dr. John A. Kirchner.)

the true and false vocal folds and is important in the transglottic and extralaryngeal spread of tumors. Medially, the space is bounded by the quadrangular membrane, the ventricle and the conus elasticus. Laterally, it is bounded by the perichondrium of the thyroid lamina and the cricothyroid membrane. Anterosuperiorly, the space opens in the posterior portion of the preepiglottic space. The mucosa of the pyriform sinus forms the posterior boundary. The relationships of this paraglottic space make it important in considering the spread of laryngeal cancer. Supraglottic cancer invading into this space may quickly extend extralaryngeally.

Vocal Folds

The anatomy of the vocal folds is complex and is thus considered separately. The vocal fold is considered the structure between the vocal process of the arytenoid and the anterior commissure. The vocal folds and the slit between them (rima glottidis) constitute the glottis. The glottis can be divided by a horizontal line between the tips of the vocal processes. This imaginary line divides the glottis into an intermembranous portion and a intercartilaginous portion. The anterior-to-posterior (length) ratio of the intermembranous portion to the intercartilaginous is 3:2; however, the ratio of cross-sectional areas defined by them is 2:3. Thus, because of its more rectangular shape, the intercartilaginous portion is larger. Some have called this the respiratory portion of the rima.[3,15] The membranous or vibratory portion of the vocal folds consists of three well-defined structural layers. From superficial to deep they are the epithelium, the lamina propria (three layers), and the vocalis muscle. Hirano divides these layers according

to a body-cover concept[15] (see Fig. 25–6A). The cover consists of the overlying epithelium and the gelatinous superficial layer of the lamina propria. The body consists of the vocalis muscle, which he likens to thick rubber bands. Between these exists a transitional zone composed of the intermediate (elastic) and deep (collagenous) layers of the lamina propria. According to this concept, the vocal folds consist of a multilayered vibrator with increasing stiffness from the cover to the body. Thus, the cover is responsible for most of the vibratory action of the vocal folds. At the anterior and posterior ends of the vocal folds are an anterior and a posterior macula flava, respectively. They are essentially a thickening of the intermediate (elastic) layer of the lamina propria. These are thought to function as "cushions" protecting the ends of the vocal folds from vibratory damage. The same body-cover concept does not apply to the larynx of children because of the more homogenous nature of the lamina propria. Not until nearly the end of adolescence does the lamina mature into its adult form. In the senile larynx, the elastic layer and the vocalis muscle tend to atrophy while the collagenous layer thickens. The cover becomes thickened and edematous secondary to changes in the superficial layer of the lamina, although the epithelium itself changes little.

The shape of the true and false vocal folds carries biomechanical significance. When seen in coronal section, both appear as valve-like structures with the leaflets of the false folds pointing inferiorly and those of the true folds pointing superiorly (see Fig. 25–3). Thus, the false folds passively impede egress of air, whereas the true folds impede its ingress. Working with cadaver larynges, Brunton and Cash demonstrated that the false folds offer a resistance equaling 30 mm Hg to the egress of air from below,[16] whereas the true folds offered a resistance equaling 140 mm Hg to the ingress of air from above. Both structures offered little resistance to the opposite flow of air; that is, they act as one-way valves.

Vessels

Arteries and Veins

The arterial supply to the larynx consists of the superior and inferior laryngeal arteries.[2–7] After the superior thyroid artery branches off the external carotid artery, it courses lateral to the laryngohyoid complex and gives off the superior laryngeal artery at approximately the level of the hyoid bone. This artery then runs anteromedially with the internal branch of the superior laryngeal nerve to enter the thyrohyoid membrane inferior to the nerve. It then enters the submucosa of the pyriform sinus and is distributed to intralaryngeal structures. The superior thyroid artery also gives off a cricothyroid branch that courses horizontally below the thyroid cartilage. The inferior laryngeal artery is a branch of the inferior thyroid artery that comes off the thyrocervical trunk branching from the subclavian artery. After coursing posterior to the cricothyroid joint with the recurrent laryngeal nerve, the artery enters the larynx by passing through a gap in the inferior constrictor muscle known as the Killian-Jamieson area. The artery is then distributed to the remainder of the internal larynx, making multiple anastomoses with the superior laryngeal artery. The venous supply parallels the arterial supply.

Lymphatics

An appreciation of the lymphatics of the larynx is prerequisite to understanding the spread of cancer of the larynx, as well as the operative procedures so designed to eradicate the disease.[2–7,17] The lymphatics of the larynx are divided into superficial (intramucosal) and deep (submucosal) groups. The deep network is further divided into right and left halves, with little communication between them. These two halves can be further divided into supraglottic, glottic, and subglottic, with special consideration given to the ventricle in the supraglottic region. Although the superficial network is richly anastomotic throughout the larynx, the deep network is important in the spread of cancer and is given further consideration.

The drainage of the supraglottic structures (aryepiglottic folds and false cords) follows the superior laryngeal and superior thyroid vessels. Thus, the lymphatics flow from the pyriform sinus through the thyrohyoid membrane to end primarily in the deep jugular chain around the carotid bifurcation. The epiglottis is a midline structure, and thus its lymphatic drainage is bilateral.

The lymphatic drainage of the ventricle is different from the other supraglottic structures. Dye injected into the ventricle enters the paraglottic space and is quickly spread by the lymphatic system through the cricothyroid membrane and also into the ipsilateral lobe of the thyroid (justifying its resection in laryngectomy).

The true vocal folds are devoid of lymphatics, accounting for the high curability of cancer localized to this structure.

The subglottic larynx has two lymphatic drainage systems. One system follows the inferior thyroid vessels to end in the lower portion of the deep jugular chain as well as the subclavian, paratracheal, and tracheoesophageal chains. The other system pierces the cricothyroid membrane. This system appears to receive lymphatics from both sides of the larynx and disseminate bilaterally to the middle deep cervical nodes as well as the prelaryngeal (Delphian) nodes.

PHYSIOLOGY

As previously stated, the three functions of the larynx, in order of priority, are (1) protection of the lower airway, (2) respiration, and (3) phonation.[1] Flawless performance of these functions requires an intact neuromuscular system to respond to both volitional and reflex signals presented to the larynx.

Innervation

The pattern of innervation to and from the larynx, as well as the type and distribution of its receptors, determines the functional capabilities of the larynx. The larynx is innervated by the superior and inferior laryngeal nerves. The superior laryngeal nerve leaves the nodose ganglion to pass between the carotid artery and the laryngohyoid complex. It divides into a larger internal and a smaller external branch. The internal branch pierces the thyrohyoid membrane with the superior laryngeal artery and becomes the sensory supply to the ipsilateral supraglottic larynx, whereas the external branch innervates the cricothyroid and inferior constrictor muscles. The inferior laryngeal nerve originates from the recurrent laryngeal nerve and runs in the tracheoesophageal groove. It enters the larynx posterior to the cricothyroid joint and classically divides into an anterior adductor and a posterior abductor branch. This branching is variable, however, as is the muscular innervation from the branches.[3]

The receptors of the larynx can be divided into mucosal, articular, and myotatic. These receptors mediate much of the reflex activity of the larynx. The mucosal receptors respond to such stimuli as touch, mucosal deformation (mechanoreceptors), and liquids. The articular receptors are located in the joint capsule and respond to deformation of the capsule. The myotatic receptors respond to muscular stretch and appear to be most abundant in the vocalis muscle.[18]

Afferent System

The internal branch of the superior laryngeal nerve supplies sensory innervation to the mucosa of the ipsilateral supraglottic larynx as well as the cricoarytenoid joint and thyroepiglottic ligament. The inferior laryngeal nerve supplies the mucosa below the glottis as well as muscle spindles of intrinsic muscles. The external branch of the superior laryngeal nerve contains afferent fibers from the cricothyroid joint and from deep muscle receptors. The majority of sensory receptors are at the laryngeal inlet, with the greatest density occurring on the laryngeal surface of the epiglottis. This sensory distribution facilies the supraglottic larynx in its role to prevent foreign material from penetrating into the larynx.[9] The supraglottic larynx also has chemical and thermal sensors. In this regard, the water receptors of the epiglottis appear to play a role in the production of prolonged apnea. When stimulated, they lead to a slowing of respiration with an increase in tidal volume. This same response does not occur with saline. Investigators believe that the receptors may be responding to the washout of chloride ions.[18] Theoretically, this may be the mechanism by which cold-steam mist assists the child with croup (slowing and deepening breathing, thus decreasing turbulent flow).[19] Interestingly, this response is more potent early in life. This apneic response has also been implicated in sudden infant death syndrome.[18] The vocal folds also have touch receptors that are more abundant posteriorly than anteriorly. The afferent impulses generated are delivered to the tractus solitarius through the ganglion nodosum.

Efferent System

The motor innervation is primarily through the inferior laryngeal nerve. This nerve innervates all the intrinsic muscles of the larynx except the cricothyroid, which is innervated by the external branch of the superior laryngeal nerve. Each nerve is responsible for the muscles on the ipsilateral side of the larynx, with the exception of the interarytenoid muscle. Thus, the only unpaired muscle of the larynx receives its innervation from both inferior laryngeal nerves. Injury to the recurrent laryngeal nerve leaves the injured cord in the paramedian position, resulting from the adductor effect of the intact cricothyroid. Unilateral injury to the superior laryngeal nerve causes the posterior glottic opening to rotate to the paralyzed side bowing the paralyzed cord.[3,9] These changes in the larynx can be seen on indirect laryngoscopy.

Neurophysiology of Protective Function

The glottic closure reflex is a polysynaptic reflex that allows the larynx to protect the lower airway from pen-

etration and aspiration. When exaggerated, however, this reflex accounts for the production of laryngospasm. Protective closure of the larynx occurs in three tiers.

In the first tier, the laryngeal inlet is contracted by collapsing the aryepiglottic folds medially. The anterior and posterior gaps are filled by the epiglottic tubercle and the arytenoid cartilages, respectively. In the second tier, the false vocal folds are brought together. The final and most important tier occurs at the level of the true vocal folds. Because the valvular action of the true vocal folds resists ingress of material, these folds offer the most important level of protection. The thyroarytenoid or slips from this muscle contract at each level of closure. This muscle is one of the fastest contracting of all striated muscles in the body. Classically, the afferent limb of this reflex occurs through stimulation of touch, chemical receptors, or thermal receptors in the supraglottic larynx.[20]

Laryngospasm occurs when stimulation of the superior laryngeal nerve leads to a prolonged adductor response. This response is maintained well after the initiating stimulus is removed, and section of the superior laryngeal nerves abolishes the response. Clinically, this response is typically seen in the setting of endotracheal intubation/extubation or after manipulation of the airway, especially if blood has contaminated the laryngeal inlet. The response is dampened in patients who have received barbiturates and in patients with hypercapnia, positive intrathoracic pressure, and severe hypoxia.[21]

Although not classically considered part of the protective reflex, reflex swallowing from stimulation of the superior laryngeal nerve may have protective functions. Reflex swallowing occurs with application of hypotonic fluids to the supraglottic larynx, particularly the laryngeal surface of the epiglottis, the glottis, and the internal larynx. Although this is not the normal mechanism initiating swallowing, it may serve to protect the larynx against fluid that enters the laryngeal inlet.[18]

Neurophysiology of Respiratory Function

It is intuitive that if the larynx is the sphincter to the lower airway, for respiration to occur the sphincter needs to be actively opened during inspiration. Moreover, the opening of the folds must be synchronous with, but slightly precede, the decent of the diaphragm. Through the work of many individuals this observation is well supported.[9,22,23] The respiratory center of the medulla, with the help of higher central nervous system and peripheral input, maintains eupneic respiration. It drives the synchronous opening of the glottis and decent of the diaphragm during inspiration. The opening of the glottis is primarily through the action of the posterior cricoarytenoid. In hyperpneic conditions, however, the cricothyroid contracts rhythmically with the posterior cricoarytenoid.[22,23] The contraction of both these muscles increases the glottic opening. During phonation, the cricothyroid lengthens and passively adducts the vocal folds. During respiration, however, when the cricothyroid is contracted in concert with the posterior cricoarytenoid, the effect is the lengthening of the open glottis, thus increasing the cross-sectional area for airflow. Understanding the role the cricothyroid plays as an accessory muscle of inspiration underlies the rationale for superior laryngeal nerve section in the face of bilateral recurrent laryngeal nerve paralysis. Bilateral paralysis produces dyspnea, which leads to cricothyroid contraction, further adducting the paralyzed folds. Unilateral superior laryngeal nerve (external branch) section reduces glottic resistance by preventing its full adduction.

The rhythmicity of the phrenic and posterior cricoarytenoid can be increased by hypercapnia and ventilatory obstruction. It is lessened by hypocapnia. The effect on ventilatory resistance and posterior cricoarytenoid activity has been extensively studied in the canine model. In this model, when ventilatory resistance is eliminated, so is the reflex abductor activity of the posterior cricoarytenoid. The afferent limb of this reflex is thought to reside within the ascending vagus nerve, and the end-organ receptors are believed to be located within the thorax, although their precise location is unknown. The longer abductor activity is lost, the more difficult it is to reestablish.[24] This is the rationale for downsizing tracheotomy tubes (thus gradually increasing ventilatory load) prior to decannulation.

The role of the larynx in controlling expiration must also be considered. The control of respiratory rate primarily occurs through variation of the expiatory phase. The time of expiration depends on the ventilatory resistance produced by the glottis. As discussed previously, the cricothyroid muscle contracting with the posterior cricoarytenoid gives the maximal glottic opening and hence the lowest ventilatory resistance. In this regard, cricothyroid contraction during expiration occurs when the critical subglottic pressure change of 30 cm H_2O/sec is exceeded and continues as long as positive subglottic pressure is maintained. As expected, this threshold for activation is reduced in hypercapnia (allowing for quicker expiration and a faster respiratory rate) and is increased in hypocapnia.[25]

Neurophysiology of Phonation

The complex mechanisms of phonatory control coordinate central and peripheral components. Electromyographic investigations of the control of peripheral neuromuscular systems involved in phonation have demonstrated specific intrinsic and extrinsic muscle function in human primates. Central mechanisms are less well understood and often rely on animal models, which may only infer function in unique phonatory systems of the human.

As a general model, the larynx as a system must respond to central commands from linguistic and motor centers. Signals are relayed to the motor cortex in the precentral gyrus and then to motor nuclei in the brain stem and the spinal cord. These signals are transmitted to the respiratory, laryngeal, and articulatory muscles responsible for speech and voice production. These messages are influenced by the extrapyramidal system including the cerebral cortex, cerebellum, and basal ganglia, exerting fine control of respiration, phonation, and articulation.[12]

Specific connectivity and the central control of brain stem motoneurons responsible for voluntary control of phonation remain illusive. Laryngeal reflexes that are key to the coordination of respiration, phonation, and deglutition are understood primarily from research focused on respiration and deglutition.[18] Further, central projections to laryngeal mechanisms are not consistent across species and may differ from nonhuman primates to humans as well. The nucleus tractus solitarii, periaqueductal gray, parabrachial nucleus, locus caeruleus, and ventromedial nucleus of the thalamus are all areas anatomically associated with the laryngeal system.[18] Figure 25–8 illustrates branching of the superior laryngeal nerve with central connectivity and projections of the nucleus tractus solitarii cells. Specific mechanisms of control are not well defined, however. In some cases, the central terminations of specific sensory receptors and the origin of the motoneuron fibers are known, as in somatotopic organization for the face and limbs. To date, studies of the role of the cerebral cortex in phonation in primates reveal no such individual muscle representation or somatotopic mapping of the laryngeal system.[18]

The role of peripheral mechanisms in phonatory control has been studied more successfully using electromyography, air flow, and pressure studies in the vocal tract, as well as imaging techniques that allow observation of the vocal tract during phonatory postures. Phonation takes place in concert with upper articulators, the lip, tongue, jaw, and velum.

Mechanical tissue deformation and, in particular, the pull of the upper articulators on the larynx via the laryngeal-hyoid complex necessarily influence the phonatory environment. For example, Figure 25–9 illustrates vocal tract shaping for four distinct vowels. Note the apparent pull of the tongue high and forward for production of /i/, in contrast to posterior and low posture for /a/. The consequent constriction or, conversely, the opening of the posterior pharynx plays a key role in the acoustics of sound produced for each of these postures and are known influences on laryngeal posturing for phonation.[26]

Electromyographic studies of specific muscle function indicate firing rates uniquely suited for fine con-

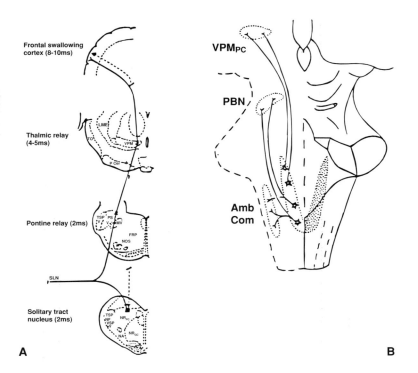

A

B

Fig. 25–8. A. Schematic illustration of fibers of the superior laryngeal nerve dividing into two branches, one going to the nucleus tractus solitarius (NTS), the other to the parabrachial nuclei, where synapses are made with cells projecting to the thalamus. (From Car A, Jean A, and Roman C: A pontine primary relay for ascending projections of the superior laryngeal nerve. Exp Brain Res 22:197, 1975.) B. Schematic illustration of the projection of NTS cells. Rostral cells project directly to the thalamus, whereas more caudal cells project to the nucleus ambiguus and parabrachial nuclei. (From Beckstead RM, Morse JR, and Rorgren R: The nucleus of the solitary tract in the monkey: projections to the thalamus and brain stem nuclei. J Comp Neurol 190:259, 1980.

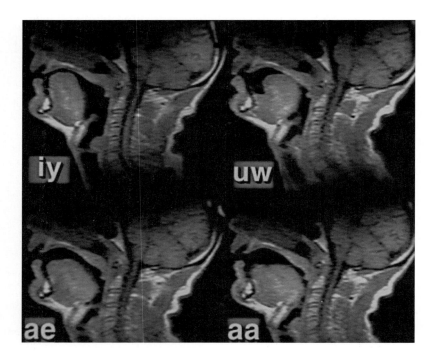

Fig. 25–9. Magnetic resonance images of the vocal tract during sustained production of four vowels illustrate contrast in shape as viewed in sagittal section. (Courtesy of C. Gracco.)

TABLE 25–1. Contraction Times in Milliseconds for Laryngeal Muscles by Species

Muscle	Subject		
	Dog	*Cat*	*Human*
Thyroarytenoid	14 (3)	21 (7)	35 (4)
	12.5 (6)	25 (5)	—
Posterior Cricoarytenoid	30 (3)	22 (7)	—
	44 (8)		
Lateral Cricoarytenoid	16 (3)	19 (9)	—
Cricothyroid	35 (3)	44 (7)	35 (4)

Number in parentheses are references, which are listed in the Suggested Readings list.

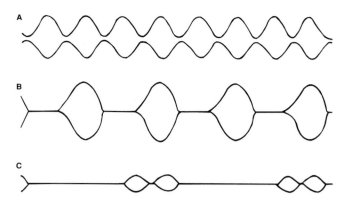

Fig. 25–10. Typical vibratory patterns of normal vocal folds. A. Falsetto. B. Modal voice. C. Vocal fry. (Adapted from Hirano M: Clinical Examination of Voice. New York, Springer, 1981.)

trol of laryngeal function, as summarized in Table 25–1. Further, the high innervation ratio for human laryngeal muscles, estimated at 100 to 200 cells per motor unit,[27] makes laryngeal muscles capable of a great degree of precise control, as required for adjustment of speaking frequency and intensity.

Intrinsic and extrinsic musculatures, described previously in this chapter, influence specific action of laryngeal muscles during phonatory shaping of the glottis in sound production, as described by Hirano[12] (see Fig. 25–5). Table 25–2 summarizes the influence of each of these muscles on the shape and tension of the glottis during phonation.

The laryngeal muscles start to contract about 100 to 200 msec before the onset of phonation.[28] Further, the most important muscle in varying the phonation style (from hypotense to hypertense) is the thyroarytenoid muscle.[29] The frequency of vibration depends on the following: (1) vibratory mass of both vocal folds; (2) anterior to posterior tension; (3) functional damping at high pitch; and (4) subglottic pressure. In this regard, Gay and associates showed that in chest register the cricothyroid and vocalis, with a possible contribution of the posterior cricoarytenoid, most consistently control changes in fundamental frequency.[30]

Lovquist and others later described electromyographic recordings obtained from four intrinsic laryngeal muscles with simultaneous transillumination and acoustic signals.[31] The vocalis and lateral cricoarytenoid muscles were observed to participate in the control of both articulation and phonation. The interarytenoid muscle appeared to be involved only in articulatory adjustments. Activity in the cricothyroid was primarily related to changes in fundamental frequency. This muscle also showed an increase in activity for voiceless sounds. In addition, the vocalis muscle appeared to participate in glottal adduction without complete closure in voiceless clustered sounds with the lateral cricoarytenoid, and the interarytenoid playing no particular roles. Studies such as these underscore the complex interactive nature of laryngeal musculature in phonatory/articulatory interaction.

In considering the phonatory process, a variety of factors necessarily contribute to the acoustic product, as defined in Table 25–3. The psychoacoustic parameters of pitch, loudness, quality, and fluctuation are correlated with acoustic qualities of fundamental frequency, amplitude, wave form, and acoustic spectrum. High-speed photography and observation of vocal-fold vibration via videostroboscopic endoscopy reveal much about the behavior of the glottis during phonation. The vibratory patterns of the vocal folds are thus characterized by fundamental period symmetry, periodicity, uniformity, glottal closure, amplitude, mu-

TABLE 25–2. Characteristic Functions of the Laryngeal Muscles in Vocal Fold Adjustments

	CT	VOC	LCA	IA	PCA
Position	Paramedial	*Adduct*	*Adduct*	*Adduct*	*Abduct*
Level	Lower	Lower	*Lower*	0	*Elevate*
Length	*Elongate*	*Shorten*	Elongate	(Shorten)	*Elongate*
Thickness	*Thin*	*Thicken*	Thin	(Thicken)	Thin
Edge	*Sharpen*	*Round*	Sharpen	0	Round
Muscle (body)	*Stiffen*	*Stiffen*	Stiffen	(Slacken)	Stiffen
Mucosa (cover and transition)	*Stiffen*	*Slacken*	Stiffen	(Slacken)	Stiffen

0, no effect; (   ), slightly; italics, markedly; CT, cricothyroid muscle; VOC, vocalis muscle; LCA, lateral cricoarytenoid muscle; IA, interarytenoid muscle; PCA, posterior cricoarytenoid muscle.

(Adapted from Hirano M: Clinical Examination of Voice. New York, Springer, 1981.)

TABLE 25–3. Parameters in the Peripheral Process of the Production and Perception of Voice

| Level | Parameters that Regulate Vibratory Pattern of Vocal Fold | | Parameters that Specify Vibratory Pattern | Parameters that Specify Sound Generated | |
	Physiological	*Physical*	*Physical*	*Acoustic*	*Psychoacoustic*

Parameters	Neuromuscular control
	  Respiratory muscles
	  Laryngeal muscles
	  Articulatory muscles
		Primary
		  Expiratory force
		  Vocal fold
		    Position
		    Shape & size
		    Elasticity
		    Viscosity
		  State of vocal tract
		Secondary
		  Pressure drop across glottis
		  Volume velocity
		  Glottal impedance
			Fundamental period
			Symmetry
			Periodicity
			Uniformity
			Glottal closures
			Amplitude
			Mucosal wave
			Speed of excursion
			Glottal area wave form
				Fundamental frequency
				Amplitude (intensity)
				Wave form
				Acoustic spectrum
				Fluctuation
					Pitch
					Loudness
					Quality
					Fluctuation

(Adapted from Hirano M: Clinical Examination of Voice. New York, Springer, 1981.)

cosal wave, speed of excursion, and glottal area wave form.

The vibrations of the vocal folds are passive phenomena and represent the basis of the aerodynamic theory of sound production. Vibration of the vocal folds changes DC air flow into AC airflow, converting aerodynamic energy to acoustic energy. The mucosal wave produced by these vibrations has been captured on ultrahigh-speed photography by Hirano.[12] The vibratory cycle is described as having three phases: opening, closing, and closed. The duration of phase determines voice type (Fig. 25–10). By convention, the cycle is described as beginning with the vocal folds closed. Frames 1 to 5 (see Fig. 25–6B) represent the opening phase. During this phase, subglottic pressure increases, forcing the vocal folds apart from an inferior to superior direction until the glottis opens, letting air escape and thus releasing subglottic pressure. As the elastic recoil of the vocal folds forces them back together, that portion of the vocal fold that was the last to open (superior portion) is the last to close. Thus, the vocal folds close from inferior to superior (frames 6 to 8). The folds then remain closed until the subglottic pressure builds up enough to force them open again. Anatomically, the movement of the mucosal wave depends on the soft and complaint lamina propria and a healthy layered structure.

The coordination of higher cortical centers interacts with specific musculature in the vocal tract to produce acoustic products recognized as speech. The laryngeal contribution to this product continues to be revealed in basic studies of phonation as an interactive process.

SUGGESTED READINGS

1. Negus VE: The Comparative Anatomy and Physiology of the Larynx. London, Heinemann, 1949.
2. Maue WM and Dickinson DR: Cartilages and ligaments of the adult larynx. Arch Otolaryngol *94*:432, 1971.
3. Hollinshead WH: Anatomy for Surgeons. Vol 1: The Head and Neck. 3rd Ed. Philadelphia, JB Lippincott, 1982.
4. Spector GJ: Anatomy of the larynx. In: Diseases of the Nose, Throat, Ear, Head and Neck. 13th Ed. Edited by Ballenger JJ. Philadelphia, Lea & Febiger, 1985.
5. Petcu LG and Sasaki CT: Laryngeal anatomy and physiology. In: Diseases of the Nose, Throat, Ear, Head and Neck. 14th Ed. Edited by Ballenger JJ. Philadelphia, Lea & Febiger, 1991.
6. Hast MH: Anatomy of the Larynx. In: Otolaryngology. Vol 3. Edited by English GM. Philadelphia, JB Lippincott, 1993.
7. Fink BR and Demerest RJ: Laryngeal Biomechanics. Cambridge, MA, Harvard University Press, 1978.
8. Meiteles LZ, Pi-Tang L, and Wenk EJ: An anatomic study of the external laryngeal framework with surgical implications. Otolaryngol Head Neck Surg *106*:235, 1992.
9. Sasaki CT: Physiology of the larynx. In: Otolaryngology. Vol 4. Edited by English GM. Philadelphia, JB Lippincott, 1993.
10. Chamberlain WE and Young BR: Ossification (so-called "calcification") of normal laryngeal cartilages mistaken for foreign body. Am J Roentgen Radium Ther *33*:441, 1935.
11. Kirchner JA: Fifteenth Daniel C. Baker, Jr, Memorial Lecture: What have whole organ sections contributed to the treatment of laryngeal cancer? Ann Otol Rhinol Laryngol *98*:661, 1989.
12. Hirano M: Clinical Examination of Voice. New York, Springer, 1981.
13. Gracco C and Kahane JC: Age-related changes in the vestibular folds of the human larynx: a histoporhometric study. J Voice *3*:204, 1989.
14. Holinger LD: Pharyngoceles, laryngoceles, and saccular cysts. In: Otolaryngology. Vol 3. Edited by English GM. Philadelphia, JB Lippincott, 1993.
15. Hirano M: Phonosurgical anatomy of the larynx. In: Phonosurgery: Assessment and Surgical Management of Voice Disorders. Edited by Ford CN and Bless DM. New York, Raven Press, 1991.
16. Brunton TL and Cash T: The valvular action of the larynx. J Anat Physiol *17*:363, 1883.
17. Johner CH: The lymphatics of the larynx. Otolaryngol Clin North Am *3*:439, 1970.
18. Garrett DJ and Larson CR: Neurology of the laryngeal system. In: Phonosurgery: Assessment and Surgical Management of Voice Disorders. Edited by Ford CN and Bless DM. New York, Raven Press, 1991.
19. Sasaki CT and Suzuki M: The respiratory mechanism of aerosol

inhalation in treatment of partial airway obstruction. Pediatrics *59*:689, 1977.

20. Sasaki CT and Suzuki M: Laryngeal reflexes in cat, dog and man. Arch Otolaryngol *102*:400, 1976.

21. Suzuki M and Sasaki CT: Laryngeal spasm: neurophysiologic redefinition. Ann Otol Rhinol Laryngol *86*:150, 1977.

22. Suzuki M and Kirchner JA: The posterior cricoarytenoid as an inspiratory muscle. Ann Otol Rhinol Laryngol *78*:849, 1969.

23. Suzuki M, Kirchner JA, and Murakami Y: The cricothyroid a respiratory muscle. Ann Otol Rhinol Laryngol *79*:1, 1970.

24. Sasaki CT, Hiroyuki F, and Kirchner JA: Laryngeal abductor activity in response to varying ventilatory resistance. Trans Am Acad Ophthalmol Otolaryngol *77*:403, 1973.

25. Sasaki CT: Electrophysiology of the larynx. In: Neurologic Disorders of the Larynx. Edited by Blitzer A, et al. New York, Thieme Medical Publishers, 1992.

26. Gracco C: Vocal Tract Imaging. New York, Biomedical Communications, 1994.

27. Kempster GB, Larson CR, and Distler MK: Effects of electrical stimulation of cricothyroid and thyroarytenoid muscles on voice fundamental frequency J Voice *2*:221, 1988.

28. Buchthal F and Faaborg-Anderson K: Electromyography of laryngeal and respiratory muscles: correlation with phonation and respiration. Ann Otol Rhinol Laryngol *73*:118, 1964.

29. Hirano M, Koike Y, and Joyner J: Style of phonation: an electromyographic investigation of some laryngeal muscles. Arch Otolaryngol *89*:902, 1969.

30. Gay T, et al: Electromyography of the intrinsic laryngeal muscles during phonation. Ann Otol *81*:401, 1972.

31. Lovqvist A, McGarr N, and Honda K: Laryngeal muscles and articulatory control. J Acoust Soc Am *76*: 951, 1984.

26 Disorders of Voice, Speech, and Language

Fred D. Minifie, G. Paul Moore, and Douglas M. Hicks

Disorders of oral communication comprise some of the most vexing problems faced by the physician because these disorders can have a large influence on the vocational, social, and emotional adjustment of the patient. When a patient experiences a significant communication disorder, it is likely that a whole series of sequelae will be activated. This chapter addresses disorders of voice, speech, and language. Emphasis on these disorders is appropriate in a book dealing with the diseases and disorders of the nose, throat, ears, head, and neck because these are the structures used in oral communication. Whether the underlying causes are congenital, learned, or the consequence of disease, trauma, or stress, disorders of communication cause the patient or parent great distress. Physicians, particularly otolaryngologists, usually are the first persons approached when the voice sounds abnormal, speech is difficult to understand, language is delayed, or stuttering is present. Adult speakers and singers, both professional and nonprofessional, also often visit the otolaryngologist first when aphonia, hoarseness, or some other voice or speech problem occurs. In addition to providing appropriate management of the medical problems that may be present, the conscientious physician will refer the patient to a speech-language pathologist, or other specialist, when possible. Many otolaryngologists are properly reluctant to provide rehabilitation for communicative disorders beyond the treatment of disease because they believe they are not qualified. Patients, however, inevitably seek answers to questions about communication disorders, and while attempting to be helpful, the physician often finds it necessary to play the role of a part-time speech-language pathologist and counselor. Consequently, the otolaryngologist must understand communication disorders, not only for consultation with patients, but also as an aid in selecting an appropriate surgical procedure, deciding on other appropriate treatments, or referral. The concerned physician must also consider the significance and potential consequences of therapy to provide the greatest possible benefit to the patient. Functional familiarity with the communication process is essential to fulfill this responsibility. The need for real understanding of communication disorders is also essential to help the physician avoid offering casual, insupportable comments about communication disorders and innocent but incorrect advice. Efforts to remedy speech defects have been made for hundreds of years, and many myths and half-truths are still believed.

Oral communication is composed of a sequence of events containing thinking, symbolization, speaking, transmission of the sound, hearing, listening, and perceiving. Impairment of any of the mechanisms in this sequence—the nervous system, the organs used in the production of voice and speech, and the auditory mechanism—may cause a communicative disorder that becomes the concern of the otolaryngologist, speech-language pathologist, and audiologist.

This chapter is organized around three major categories of communication disorders: disorders of voice, speech, and language. Each category is discussed separately. Communication disorders stemming from hearing impairments are discussed in Chapters 44 and 58.

VOICE DISORDERS

Normal Voice Production

Voiced sound during speech production may be called "phonation." Depending on the length, tension, and thickness adjustments of the vocal folds, the tone produced by normal vibrating vocal folds can vary in frequency (perceived as variations of the pitch of the voice), intensity (loudness), duration, or quality. Although such parameters can contribute to changes in intonation and stress during speech production and speech perception, it is fair to say that vocal sound, as it emerges from the larynx, has little or no intrinsic linguistic character.

Pitch

The pitch of the sound produced is directly related to the frequency at which the pulses are released through the glottic aperture, a rate determined primarily by the mass and elasticity of the vocal folds in relation to their length. Large folds produce a lower pitch than smaller folds because the greater mass causes them to vibrate more slowly. This is why adults have lower vocal pitches than do infants and young children; vocal pitch is directly related to the size of the vocal folds. Each talker also has the ability to change the frequency of vocal fold vibration, however. When the folds in any normal larynx are shortened, their cross-section becomes larger and the myoelasticity is reduced. Such folds tend to move more slowly. Conversely, when the vocal folds are elongated, they become thinner and their elasticity is increased. As a result, when the airstream pushes tightened and thinned vocal folds apart, they return to their approximated positions more quickly. This reaction results in increased frequency of vocal fold vibration (higher pitch). Frequency of vibration may also be altered by isotonic tension in the muscles of the vocal folds. This type of contraction increases the stiffness of the folds and consequently causes them to vibrate more rapidly.

Loudness

Loudness of the voice is related to the sound pressure created by the released pulsations of air through the glottis; that is, sound pressure is directly proportional to the volume-velocity of the air flow in the glottis. By increasing the thickness and stiffness of the vocal folds, increased resistance can be offered to the flow of air from the lung, and the folds can remain closed for a longer percentage of time during each cycle of vibration. The longer closed period allows greater subglottal air pressure to build up—necessary to overcome the increased resistance offered by the folds. With the increased subglottal driving pressure, on opening of the glottis increased volume velocities of air flow occur. Moreover, because the increased stiffness and thickness of the vocal folds have markedly increased the elasticity of the vocalis and internal thyroarytenoid muscles, they snap back to midline with increased velocity. The rapidly changing volume-velocity of the escaping train of pressure pulses increases the amplitude of the sound waves generated, causing greater excursions of the tympanic membrane in the ear of a listener and a sensation of louder sound. The increased air pressure for loud sound production is acquired through a delicate balance between greater resistance at the glottis and a stronger driving force provided by the subglottal air pressure.

Quality

The quality of voice is determined by both vocal fold vibration and resonance. The phonatory aspect includes the manner of air pulse release related to the vibratory pattern of the vocal folds. The opening, closing, and closed phases of the glottal cycle can vary in relation to each other. For example, laryngeal lesions can influence the pattern of movement of the vocal folds, independently and in combination, as discussed later in this chapter. These factors can influence the number and relative intensity of the harmonic partials composing the complex vocal sound and, consequently, the quality of the voice. Modification of the sound as it travels through the pharynx, mouth, and nose (resonance) results from selective emphasis and damping of the overtones and other partials in the complex sound generated in the larynx.

The contribution of voice to the normal communication process is demonstrated succinctly by its absence; speech without phonation is whispering. In whispered speech, the vocal folds do not vibrate, there is no phonation, and the voice is aphonic. When this condition is present, the speaker can produce speech and language but has no vocal pitch in the musical sense, and the sound is a relatively weak noise composed of breath sounds produced when the air becomes turbulent as it rushes past the irregularities that jut from the walls of the respiratory tract (the true and false vocal folds). This turbulent air noise is a sound source that is acted on by the resonances of the mouth, pharynx, and nose much as resonance occurs when vocal sound arises at the glottis. When the vocal folds vibrate, vocal sound occurs that has pitch and many of the distinguishing vocal qualities that identify individual voices, whereas in whisper they are absent.

Causes of Voice Disorders

Voice disorders always have causes. Something must be abnormal or atypical in the way in which the vocal folds function to produce disordered voice. A clinical appreciation of the features of vocal fold vibration can begin with the concept of an ideal larynx. In such an organ, the two vocal folds would have the same dimensions, they would move symmetrically and regularly, and each vibratory cycle would include three phases: glottal opening, glottal closing, and closed glottis. The vocal sound from this ideal larynx would be judged "excellent;" it would be smooth and free of all hoarseness, have an appropriate pitch range for the age and gender of the talker, and would be capable of wide pitch and loudness variation. When the vibration of the vocal folds varies from the ideal, the characteristics of the voice also vary from the ideal—the extent of vocal difference depending on the type and amount of alteration in the vibratory pattern.

The assumption that no two faces are exactly alike is commonly accepted. Observation of living and dissected larynges leads to the parallel assumption that no two larynges are exactly alike. Each larynx reflects its uniqueness in its behavioral physiology. Many larynges are capable of producing sound that is classified as "normal," that is, is judged in a particular culture to be within the accepted ranges of pitch, loudness, and quality found in the majority of individuals of the same age and sex.

Abnormal vocal fold vibration takes many forms, most of them not visible to the unaided eye. Ultra slow-motion films and, to a limited degree, stroboscopy have revealed that one fold may move faster than the other; one may have a greater lateral excursion; vibration may be limited to one vocal fold; there may be no glottal closure or incomplete glottal closure; closure may occur at a paramedian position; vibratory patterns may be dissimilar at different regions along one or both folds; and the vibratory periods and amplitudes may be randomly variable in consecutive glottal openings. Acoustic indicators of such patterns may include pitch period perturbations (jitter), amplitude perturbations (shimmer), decreased signal-to-noise ratio (more glottal noise), altered fundamental frequency (F0), increased standard deviations of F0, and many others. The potential complexity of vibratory patterns resulting from combinations of these cyclic abnormalities and sequential irregularities is almost endless. Accordingly, if hoarseness in its various forms can be presumed to result from abnormal vocal fold vibration, its origin should be found in one or more of the deviations that have been mentioned.[1]

As deviations from that "ideal" become greater, the acoustic properties of voice can be expected to reflect the differences in vocal fold vibration; however, only laryngeal deviations that cause randomly irregular vocal fold vibration, or that interfere with glottal closure, adversely affect the sounds produced. Voice disorders can be classified as pitch disorders, loudness disorders, voice quality disorders, and those with mixed symptoms.

Pitch Disorders

Pitch disorders are present when the voice is consistently higher or lower (in relation to the musical scale) than would be expected for a particular individual of a given gender and age, or when the sound is tremulous, monotonous, or bizarre, such as when the pitch patterns do not convey the ideas expressed. An involuntary, high-pitched voice in males does not necessarily interfere with communication, and if it were produced by a woman, it would probably not be considered un-

pleasant. A similar example could be provided for women with low-pitched voices. The "voice disorder," therefore, is not the sound itself, which may be quite appropriate for the size and shape of the larynx that produced it, but the inappropriateness of the sound to the circumstances (the age and gender of the talker).

Functional Pitch Problems

In contrast to the foregoing example, high-pitched male voices frequently have functional origins. Verdolini has described mutational falsetto as "the continued use of a high-pitched (falsetto) voice by a postpubertal male, without any apparent physical basis. For some patients, psychological conflict is implied as a basis for the disorder. In other patients, the disorder may simply reflect a learned pattern."[2] To tell a person with this type of voice that he has nothing wrong with his larynx and that he should go home and speak normally may reassure him, but it does not help him, and usually it serves only to increase his frustration. He is already speaking "normally" and needs to be taught how to phonate in a way that is "abnormal" for him. Most of these patients respond readily to voice therapy and adopt the new voice after a brief period of self-consciousness. Those with normal structure who voluntarily maintain the high pitch reflect an abnormal self-image and should be referred to a psychiatrist or clinical psychologist.

Another form of functional pitch problem is ventricular phonation wherein the talker produces a low-pitched, gravelly voice through vibration of the false vocal folds. This type of phonation most often develops as a compensatory mechanism.

Organic High-Pitch Problems

Although most abnormally high-pitched voices are probably caused by functional problems, cases with organic causes are not uncommon and may be classified into four categories. Causes of high-pitched voices include underdeveloped larynx, laryngeal web, structural asymmetry, and swelling in the anterior commissure.

UNDERDEVELOPED LARYNX. The underdeveloped larynx has small vocal folds that vibrate more rapidly than larger folds and consequently create a high pitch. The small larynx may accompany a general structural retardation or may be part of a hereditary familial body size. The clinician should be particularly sensitive to genetic syndrome effects from various forms of dwarfism, short neck, an abnormality associated with syndromes of short stature, and other possible syndromic effects when an underdeveloped larynx is observed.[3] The larynx may also fail to develop as a result of hormonal imbalance, which is usually revealed in simultaneous retardation of other secondary sex characteristics.

LARYNGEAL WEB. Another organic cause of the high-pitched voice is laryngeal web, which may be congenital or cicatricial. When this structure is small enough not to interfere with breathing or when it does not contribute to stridor, it may go undetected until the voice is observed as abnormal. A web need not extend far along the borders of the vocal folds to create a voice problem. Its effect is to shorten the free portions of the folds and thereby to produce faster vibration and a resulting higher pitch. The vocal tone in children with webs resembles falsetto and tends to be weak. Hoarseness may be present also, accompanied by the audible evidence of vocal strain, particularly in men who have attempted to force a lower pitch.

STRUCTURAL ASYMMETRY. A third organic cause of chronic high pitch is abnormal approximation of the vocal folds. In this condition a structural asymmetry may cause the vocal process of one arytenoid cartilage to slide on top of, or below, its opposite member such that posterior parts of the membranous folds are pressed together, thereby effectively shortening their vibrating portions. The adjustment approximates that which is often observed in the male larynx when a high-pitched, falsetto voice is produced.

SWELLING AT THE ANTERIOR COMMISSURE. A fourth condition, and one that may be overlooked or ignored as the cause of excessively high pitch, is enlargement of the glottal margin of one or both vocal folds adjacent to the anterior commissure. A localized protrusion no more than 1 mm high and 2 mm long on the glottal margin is sufficient to shorten the vibrating length of the folds and to produce a higher than normal pitch. This lesion can be seen only when the anterior commissure is visualized, while the folds are widely abducted. During adduction, the protruding areas are compressed into the underlying tissue and create the illusion of a prominent commissural attachment without significance. The location of the offending lesion at the anterior attachment where the folds converge enables it to modify the vibratory pattern more extensively than it would if it were located more posteriorly. When a protruding mass is located where it is not pinched between the vocal folds, it usually does not shorten the vibrators and consequently does not raise vocal pitch; instead, it often causes a lower pitch accompanied by hoarseness or breathiness.

Organic Low-Pitch Problems

Defects of vocal pitch encompass the abnormally low voice as well as the deviations of high pitch discussed in the preceding paragraphs. Excessively low pitch in both men and women is usually associated with organic change; however, functional disorders are observed in persons who attempt to speak at a pitch below that which is optimum for the structures involved. The most common organic origins of low-pitched voices are Reinke's edema, virilization, glottalization or "vocal fry," and tremulousness.

REINKE'S EDEMA. Verdolini suggests that "Reinke's edema involves the widespread accumulation of fluid or swelling, usually in both vocal folds, in the layer of tissue right below the vocal fold epithelium. Although the causes for this edema are not entirely clear, some clinicians think that chronic exposure to irritants such as smoke may play a role in the development of the condition. The most obvious effect of Reinke's edema on voice typically is a extremely low speaking pitch (due to the increased mass of the folds) and loss of the ability to produce high notes. The voice is also described as raspy."[2,4]

VIRILIZATION. An abnormally low pitch or masculine type of voice in a woman is as distressing to the woman possessing it as is high pitch in the male, for the same kinds of psychosocial reasons. Virilization of the female voice after hormone therapy in young women has been reported with increasing frequency.[5,6] Recovery of normal pitch in these patients does not occur with interruption of medication, and at present no specific counteragent seems to exist. The larynges of women with virilized voices appear to be normal in all aspects except perhaps for some general enlargement of the vocal folds toward their glottal margins. This observation, however, must be considered tentative at this time because the involved larynges have been seen only after the condition has developed; consequently, the premorbid appearance cannot be described. Furthermore, the effects of compensatory vocal adjustments on the size and condition of the structures are not known.

GLOTTALIZATION OR "VOCAL FRY." A form of excessively low pitch characterized by a low-frequency popping or ticking sound is referred to as vocal fry or glottalization. It is produced normally when only a little breath pressure is exerted against the vocal folds, such as during the ending of a phrase or when glottal resistance to breath flow is high. This low-pitched voice is adopted occasionally by adolescent boys and young men in an effort to sound "more masculine." Although glottalization is often functional, it also has organic causes. Edematous swelling of the vocal folds from whatever cause is frequently associated with this voice. Other alterations of the vocal folds, such as dry mucosa following irradiation therapy and the absence of a flexible covering membrane, may be present also.

TREMULOUSNESS. Vocal pitch deviation such as persistent tremulousness, and its opposite, extreme monotony, are rare in young persons and are usually considered psychogenic. In older individuals, however, these vocal characteristics may be symptomatic of deterioration or injury to the nervous system.[7] In instances of brain stem involvement, the vocal changes may appear among the early symptoms and consequently deserve careful consideration in the diagnosis.[8,9] On the other hand, when either tremulousness or monotony develops as a secondary symptom, other impairments are usually so prominent that the voice, as an entity, is relatively unimportant as a priority in therapy.[10,11] One of the most common diseases of the extrapyramidal system of the brain is Parkinson's disease, in which chemical deficiencies (specifically a lack of dopamine) produces a generalized movement disorder characterized by small movements (hypokinesia) and slow movements (bradykinesia) that impose low-frequency variations on voice production.[2,12]

Loudness Disorders

Disorders of loudness may also be classified into categories that parallel those used with pitch deviations; some are functional and some are organic. The voice may be too loud or not loud enough in relation to the place and circumstances, or there may be loudness variations that are not appropriate for conveying the meaning of the utterance. Moreover, any generalized swelling of the glottal margins that improves approximation without stiffening the folds contributes to glottal closure and sound generation. This fact is illustrated by patients whose voices become louder when they have laryngitis or mild edema.

Functional Loudness Problems

PERSONAL ADJUSTMENT. Atypical loudness is often an indicator of such personality types as the overly aggressive, the shy, and the socially insecure. Voices may be too loud or too soft depending on the personality. Fortunately, these adjustment problems are amenable to counseling procedures by a speech-language pathologist or clinical psychologist. Voice improvement is usually enhanced by direct training of voice production along with the counseling.

ENVIRONMENTAL STRESS. Some persons are required to speak loudly in their occupations. This vocal requirement often creates laryngeal trauma, subsequent changes in the vocal organs, and consequent voice disorders. Excessively loud speaking, or loud cheering at sports events, is recognized as one of the principal types of vocal abuse and a difficult problem to manage when the basic occupational conditions persist. Voices can be trained to meet most requirements, however, if the patient is willing to learn how to use the voice. An adjunct to voice training and a substitute when circumstances are not conducive to such therapy is the use of a speech aid. Small, portable amplifying systems consisting of a clip-on microphone, amplifier, and loud speaker are available, and when used properly, can provide adequate loudness of voice in noisy environments. The focal problem with the occupational voice disorder, when work requires daily vocal abuse, is the lack of opportunity to recover from traumatic effects and to institute a period of training to prepare the voice for unusual demands. Such patients benefit from periods of complete vocal rest (silence) before participat-

ing in vocal retraining therapy. Ideally, it is helpful to the professional speaker, as well as to workers in noisy environments, to acquire "big voices" during therapy. Fortunately, amplification can satisfy the job needs and reduce vocal abuse for some patients.

Organic Loudness Problems

PARALYSIS OR PARESIS. When a slowness, weakness, or absence of complete glottal closure occurs, the voice is weak and breathy. The basic causes are as follows: impaired neural control from cerebral cortex lesions (stroke) or peripheral factors such as local trauma (including surgery), viruses, and heart disease (the relation to heart disease is that the same nerve that partially innervates the heart also innervates the left side of the larynx); myasthenia gravis; arthritis; and general debility from anemia or other diseases. In the larynx, peripheral paralyses and pareses usually affect only one vocal fold. The unaffected vocal fold usually compensates to some degree by crossing the midline of the glottal space to achieve closure during phonation.[2] When the disease and organic conditions permit, direct therapy for voice improvement often produces good results. Suggestions about therapy are presented later in this chapter.

BOWED VOCAL FOLDS. This muscular deformation stems from long-term heavy use of the voice, particularly in elderly patients. Patients produce a weak voice because of an impaired ability to develop closure of the glottis during voicing.

SULCUS VOCALIS. A groove parallel to the vocal fold margin may be present in one or both vocal folds as a result of congenital or possibly developmental causes. Although this condition is not well understood because data are limited, the weak voice may result from an inability to achieve adduction of the vocal fold along its entire length.[2]

HEARING IMPAIRMENT. When a loss of hearing is sufficient to cause the individual to speak more loudly than circumstances warrant, the hearing problem is usually evident, and the offending vocal symptoms (similar to those described previously under the topic of functional loudness problems) are approached through treatment of the hearing loss.

Voice Quality Disorders

Voice quality disorders are the most common and complex vocal problems. They encompass resonance and phonatory components, which may be mixed in various ways, and are complicated further by changes in the degree of severity from moment to moment. The several phonatory deviations can be placed along an auditory continuum extending from aphonia to hoarseness with such intervening and intermixing qualities as breathiness and harshness. In this chapter phonatory disorders are presented under four headings: aphonia, breathiness, harshness, hoarseness and spasmodic dysphonia. Authors reporting in the medical literature tend to classify all voice disorders under the headings aphonia and hoarseness. These terms are useful but not adequate for a discussion of the variety of existing phonatory defects. Because many of the physiologic factors related to phonatory problems are known, one can enlarge the classifications and differentiate among the disorders on a physiologic basis. That is, certain voice defects can be associated with specific, atypical vocal fold movement, which can, in turn, be related to types of laryngeal disorder.

Aphonia and Its Causes

Aphonia, the absence of phonated sound, is revealed as a whispered voice, which indicates that the vocal folds are not vibrating. One should be careful not to confuse aphonia with elective mutism, in which the patient has the potential to phonate but simply chooses not to speak. Aphonia exists when the folds do not approximate sufficiently to be activated by the airstream or when the folds themselves are not capable of vibrating even when approximated. The underlying causal factors include lateral positioning of the arytenoid cartilages with the associated open glottis, massive intrusion of some neoplasm, atrophy or absence of vocal fold tissue, excessively stiff folds, or nonflexible mucosal covering of the folds. Aphonia is often a functional disorder of psychogenic origin, most commonly conversion aphonia/dysphonia. Treatment of such disorders must be sensitive to the underlying psychogenic bases of the disorders. Aphonia can also result from organic disease. The associated organic diseases range from paralyses and other neural impairments to various tumors, inflammatory disease, scarring, and other localized laryngeal lesions. Aphonia may be present continuously, but is more frequently intermittent. Intermittent aphonia varies considerably, sometimes even within the speech of a single patient. Some persons whisper most of the time; others may be aphonic momentarily within words or parts of sentences. These differences in vocal symptoms arising from the same larynx are caused frequently by variations in air flow.

Breathiness

Chronic breathiness can be recognized by excessively audible breath-flow noise that is accompanied by a relatively low vocal loudness level (a low vocal signal-to-noise ratio). The problem is common and varies from scarcely discernible levels of breathiness in the voice to the almost aphonic. The vocal folds vibrate during the production of a breathy voice, but do not impede the air flow sufficiently to allow much increase in subglottal pressure. Air flows alternately more and less, but is not completely interrupted during the vibratory cycle. Several organic conditions modify the glottal

configuration sufficiently to create incomplete glottal closure associated with a breathy voice. Muscular tension dysphonia (simultaneous contraction of laryngeal adductor and abductors) can create incomplete closure during each glottal cycle and produce breathy voice.[6] Moreover, various conditions of paralysis (unilateral or bilateral) as well as growths protruding into the glottal space (these include discrete mass lesions such as nodules, sessile polyps, peduncular polyps, cysts, papilomas, keratosis, leukoplakias, cancers, contact ulcers, and edema) can prevent the glottal borders from touching firmly during the vibratory cycle. Even complete closure of the muscular borders of the glottis can be associated with a breathy voice if glottal resistance is markedly reduced, for example, when flaccid vocal folds result from a lower motor neuron disease such as myasthenia gravis, or in the presence of hypokinetic neurologic disorders such as Parkinson's disease, or if a chronic posterior glottal chink (intercartilaginous portion) is observed.[13]

In many respects the causes of a breathy voice are similar to, or may be the same as, those of aphonia. This fact stresses the observation that the voice is not a reliable indicator of the type or extent of laryngeal impairment or disease. At any given moment, the degree of vocal fold approximation that can be achieved is influenced by the vowel sound produced,[14] the vocal effort used by the talker,[15,16] and the muscle tension in the larynx. These factors can determine whether the voice is aphonic, breathy, or hoarse. Although many attempts have been made to identify laryngeal disease based on acoustic measurements of the vocal signal-to-noise ratio, particularly by investigators in Japan, such measures appear to be more related to perceived levels of breathiness than to specific diseases of the larynx.[17–21]

Breathy voice has been associated traditionally and sometimes exclusively with the availability of breath. This association is not valid apart from a consideration of the concurrent condition of the larynx. Breath supply may be expressed in two ways: the amount of air available and the force with which it is expelled. Observation reveals that a reduced air supply, such as that resulting from the removal of one lung, is not in itself a cause of breathiness. Substantial clinical evidence also indicates that reduced breath pressure alone is not a cause of breathiness. If low pressure produced the defect, a person with a normal voice would necessarily have a breathy voice whenever he or she uttered a tone of low intensity. Many persons with low vital capacity have normal voices.

Harshness

Harshness is a physiologic opposite of breathiness. The basic cause of the breathy voice has been described as the failure of the vocal folds to close the glottis completely during the vibratory sequence. When the opposite condition exists, that is, when the vocal folds remain in contact for a disproportionately long time in the vibratory cycle, a voice quality known as harshness results. This vocal problem is usually functional. Harshness is accompanied by increased air pressure and tighter glottal closure. When the harsh voice is produced loudly, as it is sometimes by hyperactive, aggressive individuals, the speech is staccato and the listener perceives hyperactive contraction in the entire respiratory, phonatory, and articulatory musculature. This behavior is called hyperfunctional voice production. Organic causes of harshness include edematous vocal folds, neoplasms, and any other structural alteration that may prolong the closed phase of the vibratory cycle.

Hoarseness

Hoarseness and harshness are often confused with each other, partly because both terms are imprecise. Hoarseness varies from mild to severe and is so common in the population as the result of acute upper respiratory infections that it evokes little concern unless it is severe or chronic. The differentiating, audible feature of hoarseness is a roughness that results from random variations in the periodicity of the glottal waveform (these pitch period perturbations are called "jitter") and/or random variations in the intensity of consecutive sound waves (amplitude perturbations are called "shimmer"). Such variations may contribute to, or be accompanied by, noise in the phonation. Consequently, it is understandable that the perceptual conditions of hoarseness and breathiness often coexist.

Normal musical sound, whether produced by a musical instrument or the larynx, results from repetitive vibrations that are similar to each other in time and intensity or that vary progressively as pitch or intensity shifts upward or downward. Physical conditions that cause the random aperiodicity probably result from a combination of transient and interference factors, and may include any disease or condition in the larynx that changes the size, stiffness, or surface characteristics of one or both vocal folds (laryngitis or any of the discrete mass lesions, e.g., nodules, polyps, cysts, papilomas) or that causes excessive squeezing of one fold against the other (e.g., pressed phonation by a patient with contact ulcers). Any of these factors may create the conditions for hoarseness. Enlargements caused by tumor or edema, reductions resulting from surgery or atrophy, flaccidity subsequent to neural involvement, and functional hypercontraction of the adductor muscles represent the kinds of changes to which reference has been made. Moreover, under certain circumstances, swollen tissue or secretions above or on the vocal folds may be set into more or less independent vibration and may thereby create hoarse or rough sounds. Vocal sound is generated by the motions of the folds in conjunction with the breath stream that activates them, and that any condition that alters their regular, repetitive, synchronous vibration, causing randomly timed or randomly intense pressure pulses, creates the voice quality called hoarseness. Descriptions of the many laryngeal diseases and anomalies potentially related to hoarseness occupy much of this volume. The possible effects of some of these conditions are summarized in a later section of this chapter, on voice therapy.

Spasmodic Dysphonia

The term spasmodic dysphonia (sometimes called spastic dysphonia) designates one of the most handicapping of communication disorders. It is probably an organic movement disorder of unknown cause. It prevents or seriously limits the person from holding positions in which speaking is required. The problem originates in the larynx and is heard most frequently as a sudden, momentary interruption of the voice caused by brief, spasmodic glottal closure. In some patients, instead of closing, the glottis spasmodically opens to allow the air to escape as in a whisper.[22] The closure form of the disorder is often referred to as adductor spasmodic dysphonia and the open form as abductor spasmodic dysphonia.[23] In addition to these symptoms, some patients describe difficulty with breathing in the adductor type. Also, as patients attempt to "speak through" the spasmodic closure, the voice may be described as "squeezed," "effortful," or "struggle strained." Occasionally, when a vowel sound is prolonged as in singing, a prominent intermittent pulsing occurs, suggesting a tremor. The adductor form is more common than the abductor, but both may be heard in a single patient. The spasmodic episodes occur most frequently on vowel sounds, particularly at the beginning of words. The abductor form is most prominent on vowels that follow unvoiced fricative sounds. Almost without exception, persons with spasmodic dysphonia can whisper normally without interruption in the flow of speech. Superficially, spasmodic dysphonia resembles stuttering, but significant differences exist between these disorders. One of the puzzling features of this type of dysphonia is that the severity and type of symptoms can vary within as well as among patients. Inconsistency of symptoms undoubtedly contributes to the traditional assumption that spasmodic dysphonia is psychogenic.[24,25] Indeed it may be, but research evidence indicates the possibility of a neural etiologic component.[26-28] A discussion of the several theories is not appropriate here, but may be explored through references at the end of the chapter.[29-32] Differing concepts are mentioned simply because the neurogenic theory has led to surgical therapeutic procedures that have been more successful in treating the adductor type than other approaches.[33] The tenacious persistence of spasmodic dysphonia has caused patients to seek help from psychiatry, clinical psychology, speech therapy, hypnosis, drugs of many varieties, and bizarre remedies of every type, all unsuccessfully.[34]

The observed freedom from spasmodic dysphonia during whispering, and almost complete fluency by patients when they produce a breathy voice, demonstrates that the spasmodic adductory speech symptom is absent when glottal closure does not occur. Short-term clinical relief of the dysphonia can be achieved by chemically blocking one recurrent laryngeal nerve to create a temporary unilateral vocal fold paralysis. This injection procedure is also useful in diagnosis because it demonstrates the effect of a unilateral paralysis on the speech symptoms. When the injected anesthetic results in immediate elimination of both the tight glottal closure and the symptoms of spasmodic dysphonia, the diagnosis of the disorder is strongly supported. The resulting voice is not normal, however, although useful for communication purposes.

Patients with spasmodic dysphonia who seek assistance usually have had the disorder for many years and have become frustrated with the uniform lack of assistance from various therapies. They are generally eager to prolong the fluent speaking they experience during the nerve block and request some way to accomplish that end. The three options available are: (1) the creation of a permanent unilateral paralysis by sectioning of one of the recurrent laryngeal nerves, a therapy that has become widely used;[35–37] (2) the establishment of a temporary unilateral paralysis by crushing one recurrent laryngeal nerve;[38] and (3) the production of another temporary laryngeal nerve paralysis by the injection of botulinum toxin.[39] The crushing and toxin procedures are usually followed in 3 to 6 months by the return to pretreatment function. The underlying rationalization for the temporary paralysis procedures is that, if spasmodic dysphonia is psychogenic, the fluent speech practiced during the period of paralysis should persist after recovery from the paralysis. Unfortunately, the speech symptoms tend to recur with return of function. When unilateral paralysis is permanent after section of one recurrent nerve, the voice is almost always normally fluent for at least the first year, but as time passes, more and more patients report recurrence of their symptoms.[40–42] The several reported failures signal the need for increased caution with the surgical approach and careful assessment of the conditions associated with the occurrences.[43] In contrast, some patients are known to have maintained normal fluency for more than 10 years. These varying results lead to the speculation that spasmodic dysphonia symptoms are probably the result of multiple causes.

The abductor type of spasmodic dysphonia is not helped by intentional unilateral vocal fold paralysis. This procedure simply exaggerates the undesired glottal opening. Patients with this problem report considerable variation in symptoms, with the disorder worsening with anxiety and worry.[44] Psychiatry, clinical psychology, speech-language pathology, medicine, and many exotic approaches have been as unsuccessful with this form of spasmodic dysphonia as with the adductor form. Unfortunately, no known temporary alleviation of the abductor symptoms parallels the anesthetic blocking of one recurrent laryngeal nerve used with the adductor form of the disorder. There is substantial evidence of neurogenic disorder with the abductor as well as the adductor form of the dysphonia. Support for neural involvement has been found in electromyography,[45] electroencephalography,[46] magnetic resonance imaging,[47] auditory brain stem response,[48] and various clinical neurologic tests.

Resonance and Resonance Disorders

When the shapes and adjustments of the resonance spaces do not conform to the customary configurations, resonance disorders are apt to be present. The two most common resonance defects are too much nasal resonance (hypernasality) and insufficient nasal resonance (hyponasality). The first is caused by incomplete closure of the nasopharyngeal valve, or by an opening in the structures separating the oral and nasal spaces, and the second is caused by blockage of the nasal passageway. The incomplete closure results from one or more of five possible causes: (1) congenital deformity, such as cleft palate, submucous cleft, excessively deep pharynx, or short palate; (2) paralysis of pharyngeal or palatal muscles; (3) destructive disease; (4) surgical procedure in which adenoidal tissue vital to velopharyngeal closure has been removed; and (5) imitation of hypernasal speech. The second general condition, blockage of the nasal passageway, causes denasality (cold-in-the-head speech), which also results from one or more of five causes: (1) growths such as adenoid tissue, papillomas, polyps, and nasal spurs; (2) hypertrophy resulting from chronic disease; (3) swollen mucosa associated with allergies; (4) trauma to the nose; and (5) imitation. A blockage situated anteriorly in the nasal passageway may contribute to hypernasality instead of hyponasality because the posterior nasal areas act as resonators if an opening is present at the velopharyngeal valve. This form of hypernasality can be demonstrated by pinching the nose closed and trying to speak "through the nose." A resonance disorder identified as muffled quality or "hot potato speech" is often difficult to identify because it is similar to some rural dialects. It results from space-occupying lesions such as masses of lymph tissue or tumors in the vallecula between the epiglottis and the base of the tongue. Confusion with dialects occurs because some speakers habitually retract the base of the tongue into the pharynx on sounds that customarily do not use that adjustment.

Combined Sources of Voice Quality Disorders

The two separate sources of voice quality disorders, the larynx and resonance cavities, are capable of functioning independently; consequently, quality deviations can be generated in either one separately or in both concurrently. This condition provides the means by which many combinations of phonatory and resonance problems may be produced simultaneously and presents a basis for the variety of known voice quality disorders. The potential array of vocal problems may be compounded by the simultaneous presence of both organic and functional deviations. It is apparent that vocal disorders deserve careful evaluation and diagnosis; it is equally clear that vocal rehabilitation may require more than one type of therapy.

Summary of Conditions Affecting Laryngeal Health and Function

To stress the need for careful and complete medical evaluation and treatment of the individual who has a voice disorder is probably redundant. Otolaryngologists, particularly, are aware that voice problems are among humankind's most subtle disorders; they reflect certain aspects of the patient's thinking, behavior, health, and diseases. Voice problems require definitive evaluation and deserve careful treatment. The range of causal factors suggested in the preceding section indicates the array of causes that may be found in the medical literature. These causes of voice disorders may be arbitrarily grouped into the following nine categories:

1. Structural modifications that result from misuse of the voice, such as thickened vocal fold tissue, myasthenia laryngis, vocal nodules, and contact ulcer. Furthermore, vocal abuse combined with infection may cause such chronic conditions as laryngitis, corditis with hypertrophic and hyperplastic laryngitis, and atrophic laryngitis.
2. Anxiety, emotional turmoil, frustration, and similar psychologic problems that cause excessive contraction of the laryngeal, thoracic, and associated musculature during speech, but which do not cause observable organic disease.
3. Diseases and growths, including infections not related to vocal abuse; paralyses of central, peripheral, and myopathic origin; cysts; and both benign and malignant tumors.
4. Mechanical and chemical irritants affecting the mucosa: fumes, irritating vapors and gases, dry air, dusts, allergens, caustic fluids, and stomach reflux.
5. Substances causing noninflammatory edema, such as internal medicaments, mechanical compression of venous blood flow, glandular imbalance, and allergy.
6. Irradiation therapy, antihistamines, and other medications that cause drying of the mucosa.
7. Congenital anomalies.
8. Destruction of laryngeal tissue by surgery, trauma, or disease.
9. Systemic disorders leading to chronic fatigue, such as anemia, metabolic disturbances, malnutrition, and inadequate rest, can also affect the voice adversely, but vocal symptoms are rarely linked with such factors in the literature on voice disorders. This is unfortunate because, on the one hand, the vocal sound may be a revealing diagnostic clue to a specific disease or a generalized condition and, on the other hand, the treatment of the fundamental problem is basic to any direct voice therapy.

Therapy for Voice Disorders

The long history of medicine has demonstrated that medical and surgical treatment may eliminate some types of voice disorders, but such treatment cannot always restore normal function. Nonmedical rehabilitative measures may be necessary to help compensate for altered anatomic and physiologic conditions, and re-educative procedures are usually indicated in the treatment of habitual or functional disorders. The preceding descriptions of voice disorders and their causes have indicated the potential complexity of voice problems. Rehabilitative measures used in the management of such problems follow the approved convention of adapting the therapy to the specific patient and the disorder. Because this presentation must play a relatively minor role in a volume on otorhinolaryngology, however, the suggestions for therapy have been limited to basic or universal recommendations that can be used by the physician who cannot devote much time to vocal rehabilitation. When greater depth is needed, one should refer to detailed books and extensive reports in the periodical literature to support systematic therapy. The purpose of this volume is best served by directing the physician's attention to the following four aspects of diagnosis and voice therapy: (1) conditions affecting the patient's general health and the function of the larynx; (2) the environment; (3) the psychologic adjustment; and (4) the voice.

Environmental Factors
A program of voice therapy that does not recognize the demands of the environment on the communication needs of the patient is incomplete and may be doomed to failure. The person who must talk more or less continuously in a noisy environment may develop detrimental vocal habits and may also abuse the larynx and create tissue changes. Parallel situations exist in recreational activities in which the individual competes or fights vocally and in which yelling is the method of discipline or instruction. In some families, excessive and harmful use of the voice is so common or so subtle that the persons involved are not aware of the excess

and do not associate the behavior with the voice problem. Therapy for a voice disorder that is generated and nourished within an environment often encompasses complex personal management problems. Frequently, the patient cannot move to another job or otherwise modify his or her living situation; when such changes can be made, however, the restoration of the voice is simplified. When the environmental conditions cannot be altered, the voice therapy must include a review of the situation with the patient, or with the parents if children are involved, to provide insight and a rationale for adjustment to the environment. The physician, as well as the speech clinician, recognizes the incredible difficulty that may be present in these suggestions concerning environmental adjustment, but to ignore the patient's work setting, recreation routines, and living patterns is to invite failure.

Psychologic Factors

An individual's attitude toward self and the environment is reflected in such vocal elements as the rate of speech, choice of words, vocal pitch, the loudness of voice, and vocal quality.[49] These factors often indicate the degree of poise, anxieties, emotional states, feelings of friendship or hostility, and belief about acceptance or rejection. When these concepts cause the individual to use an unpleasant, inadequate, or defective voice, any successful modification of the problem must include a consideration of the person's concepts about self, environment, and speech. Often the factors influencing vocal behavior are not deep-seated or abnormal. The boy who attempts to emulate a movie hero or the adolescent who forces his pitch to an abnormally low level to "sound more masculine" usually changes quickly when the situation is discussed with him and his behavior is described. In our western culture, the low-pitched male voice seems to be identified strongly with concepts of masculinity, and unless the young man realizes that a tenor voice is just as masculine as a bass one, he is apt to develop detrimental vocal habits that will be carried into adulthood. Children as well as adults sometimes use loud voices or rough-sounding, hoarse voices to dominate, to control, or to compete in their family or social groups. The chronic laryngeal changes that may result have been mentioned earlier. The focus of attention here is that the attitudes and needs of the individual that led to vocal nodules or thickened vocal fold tissue must be considered in any program of vocal rehabilitation. Individuals occasionally demonstrate overwhelming anxieties in such vocal disorders as hysterical aphonia, intermittent dysphonia, and tremulousness. In these conditions, psychiatric assistance is usually desirable, and if any work on the voice is recommended, it is carried on as a supporting activity in close cooperation with the psychiatrist. The preceding paragraphs have suggested that psychogenic factors of many degrees of severity may cause voice disorders. It follows that successful vocal rehabilitation must include appropriate psychotherapeutic procedures when indicated.

Direct Voice Therapy

Two general types of instruction relate specifically to direct voice therapy: the first can be classified as "recovery," the second as "training." Recovery procedures presume a need for healing, for a return of the structures to normal. They are based on the premise that the vocal organs will restore themselves if abusive behavior is discontinued. Recommendations commonly given to achieve these goals include complete vocal silence for a week or two (or sometimes longer) with no whispering; limited vocal use in which speaking is allowed only when absolutely necessary; reduced vocal intensity; elimination of all singing; limitation of physical exercises and activities that cause the breath to be impounded by the closure of the glottis; and avoidance of coughing and clearing of the throat whenever possible. These recommendations are essentially passive. Although they may be desirable early in therapy, they have little or no effect on improvement of voice production. For example, if a phonatory voice disorder has been caused by habitual vocal abuse and if recovery procedures have allowed the larynx to become more normal, the resumption of habitual patterns of phonation ordinarily causes a relapse. To be successful with these patients, voice therapy must include a period of training that modifies previous habit patterns and replaces them with more efficient phonatory behavior. Direct training procedures vary widely, underscoring that art and science coexist in voice therapy. Agreement appears to be considerable, however, about the general objectives of the methods used. The following suggestions are intended to be used as general guides by the otolaryngologist or other physician when he or she is unable to refer the patient to a speech-language pathologist or vocal specialist. These recommendations are not presumed to provide a program of voice therapy.

Analysis of the Voice Problem

Defective voices are usually not consistently abnormal in the same degree under all circumstances. A voice that is hoarse at a low pitch may be completely clear in falsetto. The excellence of vocal sound may vary during the production of different vowels, and the characteristics of vocal defects often change with loudness or vocal effort. The individual who provides voice therapy must know the capacities and limitations of the patient's voice because this information not only provides diagnostic data but also determines the pattern of rehabilitation. Therapy begins with an assessment of what the patient can do; one cannot practice something one cannot do. To determine the dimensions of a voice disorder, the clinician should evaluate systematically and individually the pitch, loudness, and quality characteristics of the voice. The patient should be asked to sing a vowel, such as /a/, up and down a musical scale to the limits of the individual's range. It may be necessary to provide a tone to imitate, because many patients with voice disorders have poor pitch discrimination. The adequacy of the pitch range should be noted, as well as any changes in vocal quality that occur at different positions on the scale. This procedure should be repeated at various vocal loudness levels with at least two other vowel sounds: /i/ and /u/. The patient should also be required to read a few paragraphs of simple material to reveal typical vocal habits. Generous samples of the patient's vocal production should be recorded during the evaluation process. Recordings are essential for objective listening to the voice, and they serve as a basis for determining improvement or regression during the course of therapy. The vocal evaluation should answer the following questions: Is the pitch of the voice that the patient uses in conversation and while reading aloud normal for a person of that age, sex, and size? Are any unusual inflections or atypical pitch variations present? Is the pitch range satisfactory, such as a minimum of five to six tones? Can the patient match the pitch of a given tone and voluntarily go up and down a scale? Is the loudness of the voice appropriate to the circumstances? Does the patient have any evidence of a hearing loss? Is the quality of the voice predominantly normal? Is it aphonic? Breathy? Harsh? Mildly hoarse? Severely hoarse? Does the quality change when the pitch is high or low? Does the speaker appear to be using too much or too little effort during speaking? Does too much sound seem to come out through the nose? Does too little sound pass through the nose on the /m/, /n/, and /ng/ sounds? Is there any tremulousness? Is the speech commensurate with the socioeconomic background of the patient? Under what conditions of pitch, vowel sounds, and loudness levels does the subject produce the best vocal sound?

Patient's Evaluation of the Voice Problem

Two basic premises support the concept that one must evaluate one's own voice problem if one wishes to modify it. First, an individual does not hear one's own voice as others hear it; second, the clearer and more specific a goal or task can be made, the faster it will be reached. The corollary to these concepts is that, unless an individual can recognize the voice problem and can form a clear concept of the improved vocal sound that one wishes to produce, remedial efforts will be relatively ineffective. The process by which a person evaluates his or her own voice is systematic listening, sometimes called "ear training." The most efficient approach is through tape recording (or digital recording on a computer). Samples of the patient's voice should be recorded at appropriate intervals during therapy,

and these should be studied carefully with frequent comparison of the vocal features in the several recordings. The clinician should choose one vocal element at a time for special attention and must avoid both discouraging and overwhelming the patient with the re-educative task. This purposeful listening requires great clinical skill to make it meaningful and to keep the patient motivated. Inexperienced listeners do not hear many of the elements of vocal sound, particularly their own, until they are instructed; this is the function of the clinician. The temptation to send the patient home to listen to voice recording as a therapeutic measure should be resisted until one is assured that the patient can identify specific faults. Another aspect of evaluative listening is detailed analytic study of the vocal characteristics of other persons with both good and poor voices. This type of exercise improves the patient's ability to identify specific vocal features and augments efforts to modify voice production through imitation and experimental variations.

Voice Therapy

IMITATION AND EXPERIMENTATION. Soon after learning to hear specific flaws in the voice, the patient should be encouraged to experiment with voice production in an effort to modify specific faults and also to develop greater control over the voice. It is often helpful to use computer software that permits two voice samples to be displayed at once.[50] One channel can display a previously recorded voice sample, or the clinician's live voice sample, and the other displays the patient's efforts to match the model.

RELAXATION. In voice disorders in which vocal abuse is present, the patient usually has excessive tension in the muscles of the larynx as well as elsewhere throughout the body. Unless this tension can be controlled, vocal therapy cannot progress. The patient needs to relax. The term relaxation commonly has two meanings: it may refer to the absence of muscle contraction, or it may signify coordination in which the opposing sets of muscles exert just enough reciprocal tension on each other to accomplish a desired movement with perfect control. Both types of relaxation can be, and sometimes must be, learned for the successful alleviation of a voice disorder. Learning to relax involves both muscle training, which can be approached directly through exercise, and emotional control, which is managed through modification of attitudes, anxiety, worry, and comparable problems. Relaxed control of phonation is difficult to achieve if the patient is in chronic mental turmoil. The efficient, coordinated type of movement so desirable in phonation is based on the ability to relax voluntarily and incorporates the capacity to produce the optimum voice as determined through evaluative listening.

PITCH ADJUSTMENT. Many persons, particularly men, attempt to use a vocal pitch lower than normal for their laryngeal structures. This behavior not only produces an unpleasant voice but also traumatizes the laryngeal structures. If this vocal tendency is observed, its inadequacy should be explained and assurance provided that a more normal pitch will supply a satisfactory masculine image. Subsequently, direct instruction can be given to establish a habitual pitch that averages four or five musical notes above the lowest tone that the patient can produce. An average shift of as little as one tone upward "feels" much higher to the speaker and causes reluctance to accept the change. Furthermore, the speaker is usually surprised to discover little change in the recording and is startled when the average listener does not recognize a change of as much as several tones in the speaking pitch.

SPEECH ARTICULATION IN PATIENTS WITH VOICE DISORDERS. Although articulatory disorders are discussed later in this chapter, a close relationship exists between disorders of articulation and certain voice problems that need attention in a discussion of voice therapy. Two types of phonatory problems are effectively treated through the management of articulation. One of these is observed when generalized excessive muscle tension is chronic during speaking, and the other is found in indistinct speech caused by imprecise or inaccurate movements of the lips and tongue. Where excessive muscle tension exists, mouth opening is usually minimal; talking is of the "clenched jaw" variety; and the vocal sound may be hoarse, harsh, or hypernasal. Easier, more efficient speaking usually accompanies increased opening of the mouth, reduction of rate, and relaxation of the muscles of the head and neck. When imprecise, inaccurate, or lax speech exists, the tongue and lips do not make firm contact with their opposing structures; that is, movements are often incomplete in a phonetic sense. The speech is frequently called "slurred" or "careless." Actually, the atypical sounds are usually learned in an environment where such speech is typical. When speakers with these habits are requested to talk so that they can be more easily understood, they attempt to comply by speaking more loudly and by increasing laryngeal and respiratory muscle contraction. Training in more appropriate production of speech sounds usually increases intelligibility and reduces the detrimental, excessive effort.

VOCAL PRACTICE. If the physician finds it necessary or desirable to direct the vocal practice of a patient, the focus should be on the use of a quiet voice. More specifically, practice sessions of 5 to 10 minutes should be advised in which vowel sounds are prolonged gently at various pitches, and short selections from magazine stories and other sources are read aloud. If the subject has experimented successfully with various voice qualities and is able to relax adequately, such practice will prove beneficial. If the patient uses detrimental vocal behavior when reading aloud, however, this practice should be postponed. Vocal practice requires patience and constancy. Patients are often disturbed when they are told that they may not detect much improvement in 3 months or more and that 6 months may be required to achieve some skill in the use of new vocal habits. Persons preparing their voices for singing or acting accept the concept of lengthy training, but those correcting voice defects seem to expect a magical change. Consequently, one of the most difficult and important aspects of voice therapy is motivation of the patient.

Laryngeal Cancer and Vocal Rehabilitation

Hoarseness, laryngeal cancer, and speech rehabilitation are intimately related. The sound of the voice is often the first evidence of disease and consequently is important in diagnosis. The choice of medical treatment for the disease, whether it be irradiation, chemotherapy, partial laryngectomy, total laryngectomy, or combinations of these procedures, influences the type and amount of speech therapy to be used after control of the disease. Although cancer in the larynx may not influence the voice, in more than half of the patients, hoarseness is present and is accompanied frequently by pitch change and reduction of loudness. A retrospective study of 260 laryngeal carcinomas by Lowry and others reported that, "Hoarseness was the predominant symptom in all four stages of glottic and supraglottic lesions."[51] In 1974, the American Cancer Society anticipated 9500 new cases of laryngeal cancer for that year, 8300 expected in men and 1200 in women.[52] In 1981, the Society estimated a total of 10,700 new cases with 9000 in men and 1700 in women. In 1988 the estimate was 12,200 new cases, with 9900 in men and 2300 in women.[53] The estimated new cases in 1994 total 12,500: 9800 men and 2700 women. These data have not been adjusted to general population growth. There appears to be little or no real change in the proportion of cases in the general population over the 20-year period, but the female-to-male ratio has increased from 0.144 in 1974, to 0.188 in 1981, 0.232 in 1988, and 0.276 in 1994.[54] A report by Gates and associates in 1982 revealed that "of 103 people with clinical diagnosis of laryngeal cancer studied by the authors, 53 eventually were treated by total laryngectomy and, in some cases, radical neck dissection (43 cases), preoperative radiation therapy (15 cases), postoperative radiation therapy (29 cases), and postoperative chemotherapy (7 cases)."[55] The implication of these reports is that in approximately half of the patients, laryngeal cancer will be treated by total laryngectomy. Subtotal laryngectomy and irradiation will be used with the other half, only a relatively small number of whom will require extensive vocal rehabilitation. Training in communication skills is almost always desirable for patients who have had a total laryngectomy.

Presurgical Considerations

The presurgical management of the person who must have the larynx removed is extremely important in the total therapy and should be handled with great care. Most laryngeal surgeons have developed effective procedures for informing and advising their patients about the surgery and its sequelae. A study by Snidecor of approximately 150 laryngectomees, however, indicated that presurgical management could be improved.[56] Of the patients studied, 85% believed that they had been counseled well and at the right time, but the majority of these patients also stated that they would have benefited from more specific counseling for themselves and their spouses about the operation, the postsurgical physical conditions, and the impending speech impairments. Only 53% learned from their surgeons about the kinds of devices available for replacement of voice. The remainder obtained their information from other laryngectomees, speech-language pathologists, and the American Cancer Society. At the time when the diagnosis of laryngeal cancer was reported to the patients, about three fourths of them were accompanied by their spouses, which was considered helpful and desirable, but more than half of the spouses were "shocked, anxious, and deeply concerned."[56] The same study confirmed what most laryngologists know: that patients who have been told they have cancer and need surgery are filled with anxiety and many fears. They fear the cancer and the possibility of death, the surgery, the loss of voice and its consequences, and they are distressed about the potential effects of vocal impairment on their work, family life, and social relationships. Such fears and anxieties are to be expected, but the sensitive counselor who acknowledges such feelings and whose experience allows anticipation of the postsurgical conditions can often reduce the patient's apprehension. The importance of patient attitudes and their improvement as part of the counseling of patients was revealed also in a study by Gates and associates.[57] In their analysis of factors related to success or failure in rehabilitation these investigators stated: "Factors that correlated with successful rehabilitation were less postoperative radiotherapy, more vigor, greater imaginativeness, independence and self-assuredness, and absence of denial."[58] The latter four factors are amenable to counseling and reflect the importance of this process in both the pre- and postsurgical periods.

Presurgical Speech Training

Some laryngeal surgeons regularly introduce a skilled laryngectomized speaker to the patient before surgery. Others believe this practice to be unwise. Gates and associates state that " . . . a preoperative visit by a laryngectomee is not associated with success in learning esophageal speech or in rehabilitation and in fact, is statistically significantly correlated with a poorer outcome."[57]

Reliable estimates on the prevalence of presurgical speech training are not available, but few speech-language pathologists currently seem to advise this practice. Perhaps the most satisfactory way to plan for postsurgical speech in the presurgical period and to handle the many questions about work, family, and social relationships is to introduce a mature speech-language pathologist who has had extensive experience with laryngectomized persons. The speech-language pathologist's function is to encourage and to motivate the patient to make plans for the postsurgical period. The speech-language pathologist does not promise fluent speech or that the learning will be easy. (According to Gardner,[59] approximately 30% of laryngectomized patients do not learn to speak well with esophageal speech.) The speech-language pathologist expresses with confidence, however, the opinion that verbal communication is usually possible with esophageal speech, a tracheoesophageal prosthesis, or an artificial larynx.

Early Postsurgical Period

Within a few days after surgery, the patient begins to assess the new condition. The patient is relieved that the operation is successfully past and is glad to be alive, but discovers new problems and fears to add to those that linger. The patient is bothered by breathing and coughing through the stoma and is dismayed by the reality of voicelessness. Attempts to whisper are frustrating. During convalescence, anxieties often grow about employment, personal appearance, family relationships, and association with friends. If the patient or the patient's associates have impaired hearing, communication becomes doubly difficult. The inability to talk leads to depression and withdrawal from social situations, a condition that becomes progressively more difficult to reverse. The distinction between vocal tone production and speech sound formation is clearly illustrated by the laryngectomized person. Without the larynx (voice generator), the patient can simply mouth the words. The removal of the larynx usually leaves the articulatory mechanism intact. Consequently, when the patient substitutes some other sound for the missing laryngeal tones, speech is possible. The options open to the laryngectomized person to develop a new voice are discussed later in this chapter. If the person who loses the larynx could resume talking immediately after the laryngectomy, concern would be no greater than that associated with any other major surgery. Unfortunately, when the means of communication is disrupted, the patient feels isolated and at a great disadvantage. The early restoration of the ability to communicate is apparently a major consideration in successful rehabilitation. Every possible effort should be made while the patient is still in the hospital to establish communication by computer, writing, picture boards, signing, or the use of an artificial larynx. In addition, plans should be made during this period for instruction at home. This program should include direct work with the patient. Of equal importance is instruction of the spouse and other family members. Because individuals vary greatly in their ability to understand alaryngeal speech, the problem listeners in the family group should be identified and taught to comprehend. Some of the instruction will include speech reading skills and the use of hearing aids where indicated.[60]

Hospital care of laryngectomees, whether in the immediate postsurgical period or at some later admission for any reason, deserves special attention from all service levels. The inability of the patient to communicate creates serious problems, especially when specialized nursing care is not available. Many horror stories have been related by laryngectomized persons, ranging from aides splashing water into the stoma during bathing, and application of oxygen to the nose, to failure to open a plugged stoma. The International Association of Laryngectomees recommends that every hospitalized laryngectomee be identified by a special "warning" sign at the bed and on the patient's chart, and that the care providers be given specific instructions.[61]

Restoring Speech Communication Following Laryngectomy

It is a truism that any form of substitute voice is inferior to that produced normally. Similarly, any usable speech is superior to mutism, whispering, writing, or signing. Clinicians must search for the best substitute voice sources in relation to the needs and capacities of the individual patient. Because structural adjustments above the larynx regulate the acoustic filtering of the laryngeal sound source, they are primarily responsible for creating the sounds of spoken language. Thus, any complex sound that can be put into the upper airway can be substituted for the laryngeal sound source and molded into speech. The need to restore speech to the laryngectomized patient has enabled engineers, surgeons, speech-language pathologists, and others to devise various means for producing sound that can substitute for the normal voice.

ENGINEERING APPROACH. The engineering approach involves the development of artificial sound generators. These can be separated into two general types according to the driving force used in the production of sound. One kind is powered by the breath stream, the other by electricity from batteries.

BREATH-ACTIVATED INSTRUMENTS. The various forms of breath-activated instruments have three elements in common: (1) a flexible tube that conveys the breath from the tracheal stoma to a small capsule held in one hand; (2) the capsule, which contains a reed or membrane that is vibrated by the breath, thereby generating

the sound; and (3) a second, smaller tube that carries the sound from the capsule into the mouth, where it is articulated into speech. Breath-powered, hand-held artificial larynges are inexpensive and offer the patient an early means of talking with little or no special instruction. The speech sound can be relatively loud, phrasing and sentence length are normal, and speech is intelligible, even though it has a monotonous pitch. Unfortunately, the disadvantages attending the use of these simple instruments are substantial; consequently, few of them are currently in use. The problems can be listed as follows: moisture from the exhaled breath condenses relatively quickly at the vibrator, causing malfunction and the necessity of draining or drying it; the tube conveying air from the stoma to the vibrator becomes congested with mucus from the trachea, causing both hygienic and aesthetic problems; saliva seeps into the sound-conducting tube, contributing to vibrator problems and necessitating frequent changes and washing of the tube to keep it clean. Because the unit is held by one hand, it interferes with two-handed activities; furthermore, because it must be transported by the user and kept readily available for speaking, it becomes a nuisance.

ELECTRICAL ARTIFICIAL LARYNGES. Two major types of electrical instruments are in common use. In one, the sound is generated by a battery-powered buzzer, about the size of a hearing aid phone, that is held in the hand and from which the sound travels by way of a tube into the mouth. The sound is formed into speech by articulatory movements as it is with the breath-powered unit. The second type of instrument has several forms, but basically it is a hand-held unit, about the size of a two-cell flashlight, that transmits a buzzer type of sound through the tissues of the neck into the pharynx, mouth, and nose, where the sound is articulated into speech in the customary manner. The vibrating element of these units is a disc that is placed against the skin of the neck. It is activated by a battery and controlled by a switch similar to that on a flashlight. Battery-powered artificial larynges share with the breath-activated units such advantages as low cost, early and easy restoration of speech, and good intelligibility. The electrical tissue-vibrating instruments have the additional positive features of freedom from hygienic problems, moisture condensation, and instrument care that accompany the breath-powered units. On the negative side, electrical artificial larynges require one hand for operation and must be carried continuously by the user. Furthermore, the vibrating disc models generate a field noise that is transmitted directly to the surrounding air, where it competes with the sound that comes from the speaker's mouth. The ambient noise and the monotonous speech sound produce an artificial, machine-like utterance. Breathing and phrasing are interrelated in normal speech. When the basic sound is produced more or less continuously, as with the electrical instruments, utterance tends to become "mechanical." Experienced users of these units, however, learn to start and stop the sound to approximate the appropriate phrasing of the sentences.

SURGICAL APPROACH. Surgical efforts to produce substitute vocal sound have extended over many years and can be classified into three forms.

TRACHEOESOPHAGEAL SHUNTS. A primary surgical approach to the construction of a substitute sound source is the formation of a tracheoesophageal shunt.[62,63] Basically, the shunt is a small channel extending from the upper, posterior wall of the trachea through the anterior wall of the esophagus. When the tracheal stoma is closed with a finger, exhaled air passes through the shunt into the esophagus, where it vibrates the pharyngoesophageal sphincter or other esophageal tissue to create a sound. At least four advantageous features are associated with the surgical creation of a shunt for the production of voice. When the air resistance in the shunt is relatively small, the manner of speaking is almost effortless; the voice is produced on the exhalation of pulmonary air as in ordinary speaking; phrases and pauses occur at linguistically appropriate places; occasionally, slight pitch variation is achieved, and little training in the use of the method is needed. The Blom-Singer and Panje prostheses are comfortable, reliable, and relatively unobtrusive.[64] Detailed descriptions of these prostheses and the procedures for placing them are presented in Chapter 32. Additional information appears in the literature.[65,66] The major limitation, from a speech standpoint, is that a finger must be used to close the tracheal stoma whenever sound is produced unless the patient is able to wear a tracheostoma valve.[67] Vocal intensity is usually reduced from that of normal speech, and the prosthesis must be removed, cleaned, and reinserted. The new prostheses have greatly reduced problems of leakage, infection, and stenosis.[68] Patients must be selected carefully and motivated to want to improve their speech, and each must be capable of managing the hygienic care of the prosthesis as well as having the dexterity to remove and replace it.

CONSTRUCTION OF A PSEUDOGLOTTIS. Theoretically, the ideal solution to the loss of voice through the removal of the larynx would be the construction of a living tissue substitute that would produce sound and have no detrimental sequelae. In this approach the surgeon constructs a pseudoglottis at approximately the location of the original larynx. Muscle and cartilage that can be spared are formed into an airway continuous with the trachea. At the junction with the pharynx or esophagus, a vibrator "buttonhole" is formed that can generate a sound when the breath is exhaled through it. Some success has been achieved through this approach by highly skilled surgeons with carefully selected patients. Unfortunately, the pseudoglottis is

usually not a liquid-tight valve. Fluids leak from the pharynx or esophagus into the trachea, leading to pneumonia and other diseases. In patients with whom the procedure has been successful, the voice has been good. When a tracheal stoma has been maintained, however, the patient has the disadvantage of using a finger to cover the opening to divert the airstream.

COMBINED SURGICAL AND ARTIFICIAL DEVICES. In this approach, an artificial, breath-powered sound-generating reed is mounted in a small box and is activated by air conducted through a tube from the tracheal stoma to the box. The sound is discharged through a second tube that extends from the generator to a surgically created fistula that passes through the skin and deeper structures at the side of the neck into the pharynx. The small enclosure containing the sound source lies on the patient's chest just below the stoma.[69] The surgical creation of a fistula into the pharynx, permitting the connection of an external, artificial sound source, appeals to some laryngectomized persons, particularly those who have been unable to learn esophageal speech and who do not want to use one of the hand-held artificial larynges. Advantages of the surgical fistula and attached mechanical device include the capacity to produce highly intelligible, fluent speech with customary phrasing and the utterance of sentences of normal length. Both hands are freed for normal activity. The disadvantages of this system are (1) the obvious aesthetics, the hygienic and clothing annoyances caused by a device attached at both the tracheal stoma and the fistula; (2) the special surgical procedure that is necessary to create the fistula; (3) occasional rupture of a neck artery when the fistula is located incorrectly; (4) the hygienic care of the fistula and instrument; and (5) the need to insert a stopper into the fistula to prevent leakage when the tube that passes through the fistula is removed for sleeping or other reasons.

ESOPHAGEAL SPEECH APPROACH. The third approach to speech recovery for laryngectomees is the development of esophageal speech. This procedure allows the patient to control and to refine the natural eructation sound as the basis for speech. The advantages of esophageal speech are that (1) natural physiologic structures and functions are used, thereby obviating the need for an artificial device; (2) both hands are free for normal activities during speech; and (3) the good esophageal speaker presents a relatively normal appearance and speaking manner. The disadvantages of esophageal speech are that (1) it is often difficult to learn, and frequently 3 months or more are required to achieve fluency; (2) phrasing is usually changed, so fewer words than normal are uttered in a sequence without pause for phonatory air; and (3) the voice lacks sufficient loudness to be heard easily over common environmental noise. All the substitute methods of creating voice except the battery-powered, disc-type artificial larynges encounter maximal problems when the patient eats. Swallowing food and the stimulation of salivary secretion complicate speaking and frequently embarrass the patient in social situations. Esophageal voice production and the artificial larynges with oral tubes are probably more adversely affected while eating than with the other methods discussed.

The air used in ordinary eructation comes from the stomach, and the sound usually does not result from voluntary acquisition and expulsion of air. Many persons, however, can learn to take air into the esophagus and expel it without allowing it to reach the stomach. In this method, air in the esophagus is put under slight pressure by respiratory movements and escapes in vibratory pulses through the sphincter mechanism at the upper end of the esophagus. This organ does not produce sound as effectively as the larynx, but its phonation function is similar, and it is subject to considerable regulation. The ability to control the air charge and consequently the moment of sound production is the primary problem in learning esophageal speech. Before air can be expelled from the esophagus, it must be taken in. If it is allowed to enter the stomach, it cannot be returned readily for voice; consequently, the air charge must not be swallowed in the sense that water is swallowed. Instead, it must either be "inhaled" or "injected" into the esophagus. Experience proves that either of these procedures is serviceable, for each has been used by good esophageal speakers. Indeed, many of these speakers use both methods interchangeably.

INHALATION METHOD. If the esophagus were held open as the trachea is, the ordinary respiratory expansion of the thorax would draw air into the esophagus as readily as into the lungs. Many laryngectomized persons can learn to relax the upper esophageal sphincter at the moment of inhalation and thereby allow air to be pulled into the esophagus. In the initial stages of learning this procedure, however, before the laryngectomee is able to relax the esophageal valve readily, he or she can facilitate the intake of air by momentarily covering the stoma with a finger. This action suddenly decreases the pressure in the thorax, causing the air in the pharynx to be drawn into the esophagus. As soon as the air has been taken in, it can be expelled by increasing the thoracic pressure, as in exhalation. This return flow is interrupted intermittently by the vibration of the tissues of the pseudoglottis, thereby producing sound.

INJECTION METHOD. The "injection" method of putting air into the esophagus uses a different principle from that used in the inhalation procedure just described. In "injection," the air is forced, pumped, or squeezed from the mouth and pharynx into the esophagus. Injection is accomplished by closing the lips and the velopharyngeal valve to provide an airtight oropharyngeal area while simultaneously thrusting the back of the tongue upward from the /d/ position. This movement

pumps the air out of the mouth (oral cavity) into the pharynx, and because it is not permitted to escape through the nose and no longer has access to the larynx and trachea, it passes into the esophagus. Squeezing the air from the mouth into the esophagus can also be achieved by compressing the lips and buccal spaces as in making a /b/ sound and simultaneously lifting the mandible.

Several manuals and instructional booklets are also available through local cancer societies. It is often necessary for the person working with a laryngectomee to help with suggestions about everyday hygiene and appearance. The instructor should be able to advise on such items as care of the tracheal tube and prostheses, cleanliness, coverings for the stoma, suitable neckwear for men and women, precautions related to bathing, difficulties of speaking while eating, and similar personal problems. The clinician should also be able to help the laryngectomee join a "Lost Cord Club" for instruction, practice, and recreation. Addresses can be obtained from the International Association of Laryngectomees listed at the end of the references or from a local cancer society.

SELECTING A METHOD OF SPEECH REHABILITATION. The welfare of the patient is, of course, the first consideration in the rehabilitation process. The laryngologist, speech-language pathologist, and others involved in restoration of communication should assess the patient's needs and potential for rehabilitation as early as possible, preferably while the patient is still in the hospital. If the team determines that a shunt with a Blom-Singer or Panje prosthesis is appropriate, the steps toward spoken communication are clearly evident. When surgery is not indicated, attention can be given immediately to the use of an artificial larynx. Subsequently, when healing and the effects of postsurgical irradiation have progressed satisfactorily, esophageal speech instruction can be introduced. Most clinicans agree that good esophageal speech is more desirable than speech with artificial devices. The rehabilitation team, however, can determine when or whether such instruction should be introduced. If the decision is made to use an artificial larynx, either temporarily or permanently, the patient should be taught how to manipulate it most effectively and how to care for it.[70] Manufacturers customarily include printed instructions, but usually these need to be supplemented by demonstration and personal experimentation.

DISORDERS OF SPEECH

Speech-language pathologists recognize that substantial segments of the adult population as well as the younger groups have serious speech, language, and voice disorders, the problems that involve otolaryngologists most directly. Prevalence of speech and language disorders in children is high, with a gradual decline through adolescence. It appears safe to estimate that at least 5% of school-age children (up to age 17) have significant speech impairment, although this estimate is considered extremely conservative by most professionals. Some researchers have reported a prevalence as high as 10% for certain samples of children.[71] Most of these difficulties in children involve functional articulation disorders; faulty language formulation and dysfluency (stuttering) comprise the remainder. The presence of communication problems appears to stabilize during adulthood and tends to increase after the age of 40 years. In addition, there seems to be a higher percentage of disorders in men than women. Fewer disorders are assumed to occur within this group than among children. The ever-increasing size of our geriatric population, however, with its associated communication disorders, may require us to change that assumption. In addition, many neurogenic speech and language disorders, unlike stuttering and many articulatory disorders, develop in adulthood.

Speech and language disorders can be divided into three major categories. First and most common are the *articulation disorders.* These problems involve the production of defective speech sounds and sound combinations that may be distorted, omitted, substituted, or added as accessory sounds. Sometimes articulatory disorders are the result of neurogenic disorders, the dysarthrias. A second type of disorder is the *impairment of speech fluency,* called *stuttering* or *stammering.* Dysfluent behavior is characterized by repetition of sounds, syllables, words, or phrases; sound prolongations; atypical pauses (hesitations); word substitution; or use of word fillers. A third category is variously labeled *language impairment, linguistic disability,* or *faulty symbolization,* which refers to disorders in both expression of thought through verbal language and its comprehension. The category includes various disorders, ranging from delayed/deviant language development to neurogenic disorders known as aphasia.

Some concept of the complexity of communicative disorders is revealed in this three-part classification. Therapy is equally complex in all of them because both organic and functional causes are present in all the problems. Communicative problems that can be diagnosed as functional result from the faulty behavior of normal organs of speech and are causally related to psychologic, environmental, and habit-strength factors and to intelligence. The organic defects result from malfunction of one or more parts of an impaired speech-producing mechanism, which encompasses the nervous, muscular, skeletal, glandular, and circulatory systems.

Normal Speech Development in Children

The normal acquisition of speech may be expected to follow much the same pattern as the motor, adaptive, and personal-social behavior of the child. As in all other types of learned behavior, speaking depends on the process of maturation. A "speech readiness period" extends from birth to the fifth year of life, when the child acquires the ability to develop speech as a method of communication. This capacity, however, represents the cumulative learning of many bits and pieces of language that begin within the first few weeks of life.[72] Although endowed by nature with the capability of learning language, it appears that a child learns to talk only because people in the immediate environment speak to each other and to the infant. For example, Kuhl has shown that in the first few months of life, infants are capable of perceptually differentiating a wide variety of speech sound contrasts,[73] giving children the capability of learning any of the languages of the world. By 6 months of age, however, children have already begun to lose some of the capability of perceptually differentiating among sound contrasts that are not used by talkers within their immediate language environment.[74] Moreover, by 6 months of age infants show an enhanced ability to distinguish perceptually those sounds used by talkers within their native language environment.[75] Infants and young children are typically "bathed in language" by their caregivers during the first months of life. Such stimulation, often called motherese, serves to nurture proper language development.[76] This potential for language-learning is graphically highlighted by cases of abandoned, nonstimulated children who manifest severe language impairments. Before the child can learn to use oral symbols as a form of social behavior, he or she normally lives through a series of prelinguistic overlapping stages of sound production. The child's physical, emotional, and intellectual needs are served and expressed in each stage.[77] Furthermore, the emergence of speech in the "normal" child serves as an excellent index of physical, intellectual, and emotional status. From a body systems perspective, the general sequence of speech development involves attaining proficiency with breath control, then laryngeal control, and finally articulatory control.[78] The development of speech can be classified into a sequence of five stages, each of which has distinctive characteristics that blend cumulatively.

The Cry

The first stage is crying, which includes both the undifferentiated and differentiated cry. During the first month or two, the cry does not differentiate sensations of hunger or pain, heat, cold, or other kinds of discomfort. Differentiated crying appears within the first few months, and the mother soon learns to interpret variations in the cry as signals of immediate needs or desires.[79]

Babbling

In the second stage, babbling, the infant does not abandon differentiated crying, but usually by the third or fourth month produces a variety of sounds at random, and may appear to be "listening" as well as responding to sounds in the environment. Most of these are "cooing" sounds that are like vowels. Prosodic features (pitch, stress, duration) begin to develop. Later the child begins to use the lips and tongue to make consonant-like sounds that combine with those vowels, producing what we call babbling.[80] Because the child's sensory feedback loop (primarily auditory) is beginning to develop now, the child's babbling becomes progressively imitative of the prosodic and phonemic aspects of the input (adult) language. Children at 3 to 10 months of age progressively play with adult forms of speech.

Reduplicated Babbling

Reduplicated babbling (repeated syllables like pa, pa, pa, ba, ba, ba, ku, ku, ku, etc.) begins during the second 6 months. At first, the sounds produced are carried over from babbling, but later the infant appears to be responding more selectively to the sounds of others, as well as to those just produced. Reduplicated babbling appears to be a good index of normal development. Virtually all normal hearing children produce reduplicated babbling before 12 months of age, whereas children with significant hearing impairments rarely do.[81] The speech development of the congenitally deaf child differs from that of the child with normal hearing beyond the babbling stage. The deaf child does not continue babbling for as long as the hearing child, and speech development usually follows a different pattern from that of a hearing child.

Echolalia

Echolalia, the name given to the fourth stage, begins somewhere around the ninth to tenth month, when the baby repeats sounds heard in the environment. The infant seems to produce sounds that are pleasurable and repeats sounds that another individual produces. This is the stage in which the infant demonstrates that speech and language comprehension are emerging. Up to this stage the baby has been acquiring an inventory of sound complexes that later will be used in learning to speak and in developing a vocabulary. The ages at which children typically master the sounds of English are shown in Table 26–1.[82]

Intentional Speech

The fifth stage is the acquisition of speech as a practical tool for communication. Before entering this final but ever-expanding stage, the child must have established a functional understanding of conventionalized speech patterns. Providing meaningful time sequences for the mastery of speech sounds is difficult because many factors influence and regulate their acquisition. Girls generally surpass boys in learning speech sounds and tend to be accelerated in articulation skill from about

TABLE 26–1. Guidelines of Normal Acquisition of Consonant

Sounds	Customary Articulation: 50% of Children (yr)	Customary Articulation: 90% of Children (yr)
p, m, h, n, w, b	1.5	3.0
k, g, d	2.0	4.0
t, ng	2.0	6.0
f, y	2.5	4.0
r, l	3.0	6.0
s	3.0	8.0
ch, sh	3.5	7.0
z	3.5	8.0
j	4.0	7.0
v	4.0	8.0
th	4.5	8.0
zh	6.0	8.0+

(Adapted from Sander E: When are speech sounds learned? J Speech Hear Disord 37: 55, 1972.)

$4\frac{1}{2}$ years on. Girls normally approximate mature articulation by the age of 7, whereas boys usually take an additional year to reach the same degree of proficiency. Whereas development of articulation skills is nearly complete for most normal children by age 8 years, subtle performance differences still exist for several years. Research evidence emphasizes that the accuracy of speech motor control continues to improve until age 11 or 12 years, at which point adult-like articulation performance is achieved.[83] In general, research indicates that the average child of 36 months should have acquired a vocabulary of approximately 1000 words and should be using short, meaningful sentences. Errors in the articulation will probably occur; nevertheless, 80 to 90% of conversational speech should be intelligible to an interested listener. If a child is not speaking acceptably by the age of 7 years, it may be because of any one or a combination of the following: (1) defective hearing; (2) poor motor coordination; (3) physical defects; (4) poor speech models in the family environment; (5) insufficient language stimulation; (6) mental retardation; or (7) emotional disturbance. As Table 26–1 highlights, however, occasional difficulty with later developing sounds should not prompt undue concern by parent, clinician, or physician.

Since the mid-1970s, a major shift has occurred regarding the theory behind speech sound development. Rather than tracking the developmental timetable of individual speech sounds, contemporary researchers investigate the emergence and disappearance of phonologic processes (e.g., cluster reduction, unstressed syllable deletion, stop for fricative substitutions, etc.).[84,85] A detailed discussion of the chronology of phonologic processes is beyond the scope of this chapter, but developmental charts and graphs are available to the interested reader.[78,86,87]

Articulation Disorders

Disorders of speech articulation may be described as faulty or atypical production of sounds in the spoken language. These problems encompass many kinds of articulatory defects, both functional and organic, and constitute the most frequent type of speech disorder observed within the population.

Functional Articulation Disorders

When a disorder is designated functional, it does not necessarily indicate a simple problem. The cause of an articulatory disorder that appears to be functional may be partially or entirely lost in the acquisition of speech. Although some functional articulation disorders are truly psychogenic, most represent problems stemming from faulty learning, and/or habits of misuse. Because successful therapy may depend on discovering causal factors, however, one must explore certain aspects of the individual's physical and social development. Habit-strength is a learning theory concept that relates to the automaticity of both appropriate and inappropriate behavior. Applied to speech, habits can account for the persistence of a problem and the resistance to its successful treatment.

The child's mental age or intelligence must also be considered when articulation is being evaluated. Intelligence, reflected in cognitive functioning, underlies one's ability to learn. Because learning is fundamental to speech and language acquisition, intelligence factors can influence speech performance. It is not surprising, then, that numerous studies have demonstrated that children of low mentality produce more articulation errors than children of normal intelligence. Moreover, children with severe articulation defects frequently have depressed scores in reading and spelling, which may help to explain their low scores on verbal intelligence tests.

The word delay implies normal sound development as a reference, and impairment of this type is manifested as (1) a delay in onset, (2) slowness of development, and/or (3) termination of development before the average adult skills are achieved.[78,88] Furthermore, delay assumes that between the onset and termination of a particular child's development, the course of events will follow the developmental sequence observed with children who are acquiring speech normally.[89]

Answers to the following questions may supply useful insight into the problems: Did the child follow a normal pattern in sitting, walking, eating, talking, and using the toilet? Did the child have any periods of extreme illness or temporary hearing loss? Did the child have extended absences from the family environment? Did emotional conflicts arise between the mother and father or between the parents and the child? Did any undue penalties and frustrations occur that may have been associated with the speech readiness period? Did or do persons in the environment have similar speech problems that could have been imitated?

In summary, a child with a delay profile demonstrates performance similar to that of a normal but younger speaker. In contrast, deviant speech refers to an articulation profile unlike that of a normally developing child, even a younger one.[78] Although both appropriate and delayed characteristics may still be present in the speech of these children, the deviant speaker's articulation reveals unique error patterns that cannot be accounted for on the basis of a "delayed" concept.

The traditional way of describing the nature of articulation disorders is in terms of the following four classic error types:

SUBSTITUTIONS. One standard sound is substituted for another in the initial, medial, or final position within the word. For example, the sound w is frequently substituted for r, producing *wed* for *red*; t or d may replace th, and *mother* becomes *mudder* and *something* changes to *someting*; th may substitute for s, and *miss* becomes *mith*. The most frequently misarticulated sounds are often those that are mastered later in the course of speech development /s, z, r, l, th, ch, sh, zh/.

OMISSIONS. Sounds are omitted in a word and are not replaced by a substitute. The child may produce *tep* for *step*, *air* for *where*, or *daw* for *dog*.

DISTORTIONS. The target sounds are produced, but are modified so that the perceptual result is inaccurate. A distortion might be considered a special case of substitution error, in that a standard sound is replaced by a nonstandard sound. The /s/ and /z/ are among the most misarticulated speech sounds because adjustments of the tongue, teeth, and bite relationships during normal growth and development during the preschool and primary years are so exacting that minor deviations easily occur. The distortion of one or more of the sibilant consonants /s, z, sh, zh/ is called lisping.

ADDITIONS. Extra sounds are added that are not part of the word: examples are *warsh* for *wash* or *plass* for *pass*. Additions are not as common as substitutions, omissions, and distortions.

Organic Articulation Disorders in Children

Many speech-language pathologists now approach the subject of organic articulation disorders cautiously. Bernthal and Bankson state, "Although individuals with oral structural deviations frequently experience articulation problems, the relationship between structural deficits and articulation skills is not very predictable. The literature cites many instances of individuals with structural anomalies who have developed appropriate compensatory gestures to produce acoustically acceptable speech. Why some individuals are able to compensate for relatively gross abnormalities and others are unable to compensate for lesser deficits has not been resolved."[90]

These observations clearly emphasize that the relationship between oral structure and articulation proficiency is neither simple nor automatic. The remarkable compensatory potential of the oral-peripheral mechanism seems to account for the clinically observed inconsistencies in speakers whose performance is relatively better than would be expected from the individual's structural status. In general, structural deviations can affect articulation by interfering with articulatory contact points, breath stream flow (force and direction), oral breath pressure, and oral-nasal cavity coupling. Disorders such as cleft lip and palate can involve all these aspects, whereas the normal loss of front teeth in a growing child might create involvement of only the first two factors. As Carrell points out, a good rule of thumb is to "consider any structural deviation a possible cause of misarticulation provided the nature of the speech defect is consistent with the deviation."[91]

STRUCTURAL AND SYNDROME-RELATED SPEECH DISORDERS. Many structural deviations (e.g., clefts of the lip and/or palate) are associated with speech, hearing, and language disorders. The physician should be sensitive to the possibility that structural anomalies concomitant to speech disorders can result from dysmorphologies of genetic origin, commonly referred to as syndromes, or a "pattern of things that run together."[3] When multiple dysmorphologies appear in the same patient, consultation with a medical geneticist is prudent, to determine whether evaluation and treatment of the family as well as the patient is necessary. Shprintzen identifies some syndromic patterns commonly associated with language and speech disorders. Contiguous gene disorders give rise to Prader-Willi, Beckwith-Wiedemann, velo-cardial-facial, and Rubinstein-Taybi syndromes.[3] Mechanically induced syndromes that cause deformations from tearing or mutilation of the embryo include sequences in which multiple anomalies stem from a single factor. Such sequences that result in speech and language disorders include ADAM sequence (amniotic deformations, adhesions, and mutilations—the cranio-facial complex and limbs are particularly susceptible to amniotic adhesions resulting in cleft lip, facial clefts, and anencephaly), Pierre Robin syndrome (micrognathia, large u-shaped cleft palate, and upper airway obstruction), and Stickler syndrome (clefting of palate, micrognathia, and perhaps Robin sequence). Other teratogenic disorders are associated with multiple anomalies. Examples include the effects of thalidomide, German measles virus, and fetal alcohol syndrome. Myotonic dystrophy (Steinert syndrome), neurologic diseases associated with lysosomal storage diseases (Hunter syndrome), cleft of the larynx (Opitz syndrome), and vocal chord atrophy (due to Werner syn-

drome) all can have specific consequences on the voice and speech production capabilities of the patient. Although a discussion of these syndromes is well beyond the scope of this chapter, interested readers should consult the excellent references provided.[3,92–94]

TONGUE-TIE (ANKYLOGLOSSIA). Parents frequently take children with articulatory defects to physicians to determine whether or not the child is "tongue-tied." The term "tongue-tied" (ankyloglossia) is used when the lingual frenum appears to be abnormally short or taut, restricting the movement of the tongue so it cannot move upward to the alveolar ridge. Although this condition is known to exist, its interference with articulation is considered comparatively rare. McEvery and Gaines examined 1000 children who had a short frenum and found only four with articulatory defects.[95] They recommended that the frenum not be clipped because of possible infection, hemorrhage, and residual scar tissue. A more recent study confirmed the minimal relationship between ankyloglossia and articulation disorders,[96] finding that an individual who presents a tongue-tie and an associated articulatory problem can usually be successfully re-educated without surgical removal or clipping of the frenum. The exception is when the tip of the tongue is almost completely immobilized. Even in these cases, however, surgical intervention does not independently remedy the speech problem. The freedom of the tongue that results from clipping the frenum provides a potential for improvement, but the tongue habits that have developed will persist during speaking until the individual has been retrained.

DENTAL ABNORMALITIES AND TONGUE THRUST. Normally, the teeth serve an important function in the production of speech sounds. Research and clinical observations have indicated, however, that many individuals with dental abnormalities are able to make compensatory adjustments that produce acceptable speech. Professional debate related to the developmental nature of swallowing (normal and abnormal), the impact of tongue thrust on dentition and articulation, and the efficacy of speech and/or myofunctional therapy has created an ongoing controversy that is still unresolved. Review of the various positions in the literature led Bernthal and Bankson to the following conclusions:[90]

1. Currently, no data support the existence of a distinct clinical entity sometimes referred to as "tongue thrust." Behavior so identified is probably "normal," especially in preadolescent children.
2. Speech sound errors, particularly sibilant distortions, are present in greater number in those who evidence reverse swallow patterns than in those who do not.
3. The speech-language pathologist should focus on

the correction of speech sound errors. On the basis of developmental data, techniques designed to change swallow patterns as part of an overall remediation program appear ill-advised before a client has reached adolescence.

Treatment of Articulation Disorders in Children

The complexity of speech production requires awareness of many factors that could influence speech sound learning / monitoring / modification / and performance. One must evaluate the articulation problem in terms of (1) the degree of sound variation, (2) the consistency of misarticulation, (3) the effect of the disorder on intelligibility, and (4) the total number of sounds affected. This clinical strategy naturally results in capturing an essential component of any treatment plan; it must be prescriptive. The goal in treating articulation disorders is to identify and correct defective sounds. Most treatment is directed at improving performance accuracy and consistency. The four general steps of remediation are (1) training the speaker's perceptual skills (phonologic process or sound identification and discrimination), (2) establishing the new response (correct sound production), (3) strengthening and generalizing the correct sound production or phonologic process to connected speech levels, and (4) carrying over the new response to conversational speech both within and outside of the clinical setting. The last three stages are really designed to habituate the new response.[78] Although the steps are straightforward, the complexity of the behavior and the clinical process dictate that treatment be guided by a professional speech-language pathologist rather than by the client or parents attempting a self-improvement program. Additionally, the parents should guard against continually correcting the child in speech production. When proper therapy for articulatory problems is administered, the prognosis is good.

Disorders of Speech Motor Control

"Neuromotor speech disorders are disturbances of movement of the speech production system that result in someone being imperfectly understood or creating the impression that something is unusual or bizarre about his or her speech pattern."[97] The two major types of neuromotor speech disorders are dysarthria and apraxia.

Dysarthria

Dysarthria may be defined as a defect of articulation resulting from a lesion in the central or peripheral nervous system, which directly regulates the muscles used for speaking. It involves an impairment in the control and execution of speech movements because of muscle weakness, slowness, incoordination, or altered muscle tone.[97] Depending on the type of damage to the neuro-

muscular control system, dysarthria can result in impaired respiration, phonation, articulation, resonance, and prosodic aspects of speech. Largely through the work of Darley and his colleagues at Mayo Clinic in the 1970s differential diagnosis of types of dysarthrias can be made.[98] Table 26–2 presents a list of recognizable dysarthria types along with the neurologic conditions or level of brain damage associated with them. Dysarthrias associated with Parkinson's disease[7,9,11–13,99,100] and amyotrophic lateral sclerosis.[10,101–105] have probably received more research attention during the past 5 years than other types of speech disorders.

Apraxia

In contrast, apraxia of speech represents an impairment in the programming of speech movements in the absence of muscle impairments associated with dysarthria.[97] Apraxia is considered to involve damage to the speech programming area of the brain in the left frontal lobe (Broca's area).[106] With both conditions, dysarthria and apraxia, articulation proficiency of the speaker is adversely affected. As would be expected, the degree to which speech intelligibility is compromised depends on the type and severity of the underlying neuromuscular impairment. Darley and associates suggest that a comparison of dysarthria and apraxia of speech reveals distinctive performance profiles.[98] According to their extensive study of these clinical entities at the Mayo Clinic, the "most characteristic error made by dysarthric patients is imprecise production of consonants, usually in the form of distortions and omissions." These are considered errors of "simplification." In contrast, the patient demonstrating apraxia of speech reveals errors of "complication," and relatively few simplification errors. These complication errors include "substitutions of other phonemes, often unrelated substitutions, as well as additions of phonemes, repetitions of phonemes, and prolongations of phonemes."

Treatment of the Motor Speech Disorders

Although distinctive articulation profiles can be described for both motor speech disorders, differential diagnosis between these two clinical entities is usually difficult to make with confidence. The prognosis for improvement with therapy for both of these motor speech disorders should be guarded, but judgment varies with the type and severity of the underlying neuromuscular impairment. Because patients with either disorder may benefit from a formal, structured remediation program, rehabilitation should be provided. According to Darley and associates,[98] any treatment program should incorporate five fundamental principles: (1) the patient must be assisted to develop functional compensation from the healthy body systems; (2) the patient must develop the perspective that speech production must now become a highly con-

TABLE 26–2. Types of Dysarthria

Dysarthria Type	Neurogenic Condition or Level of Damage	Speech Deviations
Flaccid	Brain stem, lower motor neuron	Hyponasality, breathiness, poor articulation
Spastic	Bilateral, motor strip	Strained-strangled voice, low pitch, poor articulation
Ataxic	Cerebellum	Irregular speech and syllable repetition
Hypokinetic	Basal ganglia, parkinsonism	Reduced loudness, rushes of speech
Hyperkinetic	Many levels of extrapyramidal motor system	Unsteady rate, pitch, loudness; sudden or slow variations in speech or voice; stoppages; tics; grunts

scious, deliberate effort; (3) the patient must develop the ability to monitor speech performance continuously; (4) remediation must begin as soon as possible because waiting is not beneficial; and (5) the patient must receive continued support and reassurance. In an attempt to enumerate various treatment options with neurogenic speech disorders, LaPointe and Katz included medical (alleviate cause), behavioral (modify neuromuscular and aerodynamic events), palliative (make the behavior, as well as the reaction to it, more moderate), and alternate mode (implement alternative communication systems) intervention strategies.[107] Typically, the speech-language pathologist uses one or all of the final three options, in conjunction with the appropriate medical intervention.

Disorders of Fluency (Stuttering)

The terms stuttering and stammering are synonymous, although the term stuttering is preferred in the United States. Stuttering is one of the most enigmatic speech disorders encountered by the speech-language pathologist. This phenomenon is difficult to define because "no two stutterers are alike" and no single stutterer is the same from one time to the next. A workable definition of stuttering that has been acceptable to all speech-language pathologists has not yet been formulated. Wingate,[108] however, has provided professional personnel with a useful description of the disorder that enumerates behaviors common to all stutterers and indicates kinds of accessory behaviors shown only by some.

"I. (a) Disruption in the fluency of verbal expression, which is (b) characterized by involuntary, audible or silent, repetitions or prolongations in the utterance of short speech elements, namely: sounds, syllables, and words of one syllable. These disruptions (c) usually occur frequently or are marked in character and (d) are not readily controllable. II. Sometimes the disruptions are (e) accompanied by accessory activities involving the speech apparatus, related or unrelated body structures, or stereotyped speech utterances. These activities give the appearance of being speech-related struggles. III. Also, there are not infrequently (f) indications or report of the presence of an emotional state, ranging from a general condition of 'excitement'

or 'tension' to more specific emotions of a negative nature such as fear, embarrassment, irritation, or the like. (g) The immediate source of stuttering is some incoordination expressed in the peripheral speech mechanism; the ultimate cause is presently unknown and may be complex or compound."

Although no conclusive prevalence figures currently exist, it has been estimated that stuttering has its highest occurrence in the preschool years (above 4%), declining thereafter to an unstable value of less than 1%. This declining pattern appears to relate to two factors, successful therapy and spontaneous recovery. Research has confirmed the clinical observation that stuttering is more common among boys than girls in a ratio of approximately 3:1.[109] The literature presents a variety of theories regarding the origin of stuttering; unfortunately, none represent professional consensus. Based on extensive case study, Van Riper concludes that one cannot determine or account for the onset of stuttering in terms of the conditions surrounding it for the vast majority of cases studied soon after onset.[110] At a basic physiology level, however, Van Riper states that it seems reasonable to attribute stuttering to the "difficulty some children are bound to experience in mastering the synchronized timing of the motor coordinations required for speech." We can concur with this conclusion, particularly in light of the emerging research evidence that differences in speech physiology do exist between stutterers and nonstutterers.[109–111] In fact, research into the nature of stutterers' *fluent* utterances indicates subtle motoric differences (not auditorily perceptible) that suggest some underlying difficulty with motor control and timing.[112–114] Substantial agreement exists on the general "facts" regarding the onset and development of stuttering. The typical onset occurs during the preschool years, usually 1 or 2 years after the child first learns to speak (onset is rare in adulthood). The onset is usually gradual and is most often characterized by an excessive amount of repetitive speech (sounds or syllables), usually without tension or effort. Although the exact nature of development varies among stutterers, virtually all demonstrate a change of behavior as long as the disorder persists. The initial speech characteristics of part-word repetitions is often supplemented with sound prolongations and hesitations, usually associated with increasing struggle and avoidance behavior. Reactions by listeners, important "others," and the stutterer tend to create fear, anxiety, and self-doubt. These observations tend to confirm the accuracy and utility of Wingate's "definition" presented earlier. Moreover, stability of these behaviors is not observed to occur until the advanced stage of the disorder. Until that time, the severity of stuttering has been described as cyclic, changing from better to worse with no apparent logic. Despite differences in severity and symptom profile, clear evidence indicates that as long as the disorder persists, the stutterer must face exposure of the disability to an ever-growing number of situations that come with social and professional growth in adulthood. Stuttering is truly a disorder of social living, not just a speech impediment.

Research regarding the development of speech and language skills makes it clear that most children experience periods of "normal nonfluency" during their early years that look and sound similar to the behaviors described as onset characteristics of stuttering. The number and duration of such episodes vary among children, but their occurrence does *not* automatically confirm the existence of stuttering. Therefore, great caution should be exercised to avoid the unnecessary stigmatizing effect of labeling a child's nonfluencies as clinically significant (stuttering) when they could be variations of *normal* speech development. Although differentiation between normal nonfluencies and those reflective of incipient stuttering is difficult, research has generated behavior guidelines to assist the speech-language pathologist in making these clinical distinctions.[110,115,116] Almost all stutterers have periods of relative freedom from hesitancies, repetitions, blocks, or prolongations. The stutterer can usually sing or speak in unison without disruption in the flow of speech and usually has no difficulty when speaking aloud to one's self or to a pet. The degree of communicative stress in a speaking situation appears to govern the degree of stuttering severity.

Common Questions About Stuttering

What is primary stuttering? This term is sometimes used to describe a child's speech when it is marked by effortless repetitions or prolongations of words, phrases, or syllables without an awareness on the child's part that these mannerisms are different or abnormal. Johnson states that "practically all stutterers are originally diagnosed (regarded as 'stutterers,' 'not talking right,' or 'having difficulty saying words,' and so forth) by . . . their parents, more often than not the mother being the first to become concerned."[117] Is stuttering hereditary? No clear evidence supports the view that stuttering is a characteristic that can be transmitted, in a biologic sense, from one generation to another. Does stuttering run in families? The research studies pertaining to the families of stutterers and nonstutter-

ers indicate that, to a limited extent, stuttering does tend to run in families. The reason appears to involve tradition more than heredity. When parents have had a background of experience with stuttering, they appear to react to the speech imperfections of their children differently from parents who are unfamiliar with the condition. The parents with stuttering in their background may be so conditioned in attitude, policies, and concern that they view their child's normal speech imperfections as stuttering. Does confused laterality (handedness) cause stuttering? The basic concept of this theory gained popular acceptance in the 1920s and 1930s. The belief was that stutterers were individuals who lacked adequate margins of unilateral dominance for the purpose of speech. Research and clinical observation have pointed out, however, that changing a child's handedness per se does not cause stuttering, but rather the environmental influences, such as the emotional tone involved in the change, might do so. Is stuttering caused by imitation? Parents are frequently concerned about the possibility of a child becoming a stutterer if their child associates with a stuttering child. Imitation in and of itself does not cause stuttering. If this were true, the incidence of stuttering would be considerably higher than currently reported. Children have been exposed to stuttering for years in public and private schools, and no "epidemic" has ever been recorded.

Why do more boys stutter than girls? Studies have shown that male stutterers outnumber female stutterers by about 3 to 1. From a physical standpoint, the sex ratio might reflect a less stable neuromuscular control system for speech in boys, at least during the early years of development.

Treatment of Stuttering

Parents of a young child who demonstrates minor hesitations and repetitions in speech must remain unemotional about these speech patterns to prevent the development of undue awareness and concern on the part of the child. Being an attentive, thoughtful listener is the best response. The young child with incipient stuttering should not be subjected to direct speech therapy or any type of therapy related to speech production. According to Shames,[118] the family is a critical factor in dealing with the young child because "the family can either reinforce or counteract the efforts of the speech-language pathologist." The advanced, or secondary stutterer, should seek the assistance of a qualified speech-language pathologist. The stutterer or the family should be warned against treatment employing unethical procedures, such as gimmicks, devices, pills, or the guarantee of a "cure for stuttering." The treatment should always be conducted by individuals who have had academic training and experience in the areas of speech-language pathology, clinical psychology, or psychiatry. A multitude of different therapy strategies are currently available, and each reflects a theoretic view of the cause and nature of stuttering. Recent theories and treatment strategies have centered on fluency disorders as a motor speech disorder. In general, however, clinical management of stuttering involves changing the stutterer's attitude, the method of talking, and/or the environment. The advanced or secondary stutterer must perceive the need for therapy. Frequently, the family of the secondary stutterer is also in need of appropriate treatment.

DISORDERS OF SYMBOLIZATION (LANGUAGE)

Language may be defined as an organized symbolic representation of thought and action used as a means of communication on an abstract level by human beings. Therefore, preceding the act of speaking is the process of symbolization, which involves the comprehension and formulation of language. When this process is disturbed, the result may be classified as a communication disorder that is manifested in the inability or limited ability to use linguistic symbols as a means of oral communication. This difficulty is common to many different types of children (including children with "specific language impairment," children with aphasia, mentally retarded children, children with autistic-like characteristics, and hearing-impaired children) and markedly influences normal language acquisition. Language disorders are also central to the adult aphasic patient.

Children with Specific Language Impairment

Children with specific language impairment generally have a disorder profile limited to the area of language. The particular difficulty may be in some or all of the following components of language: (1) lexicon (the concepts and labels of our vocabulary); (2) syntax (word order); (3) morphology (word forms); (4) semantics (word meaning); and (5) pragmatics (use of language in social contexts). According to Leonard's description of children with specific language impairment, "the most notable feature of these children's language is that the large majority of the linguistic features reflected in their speech are slow to emerge and to develop."[119] This is descriptive of a delay profile. Although no consensus exists on the causes underlying the problems of this group of children, causes most often cited are perceptual difficulties, cognitive development problems, environmental and personal interaction difficulties, and brain damage.

In many respects, language intervention is similar to that used for other disorders of communication. A prescriptive program, based on comprehensive language testing, should be directed to the necessary area of oral language production and/or comprehension.

Children with Acquired Aphasia

The general term aphasia (dysphasia) refers to the difficulty experienced in the comprehension (receptive-sensory) and use of linguistic symbols (expressive-motor) in verbal communication. A useful operational definition, presented by Myklebust,[120] is as follows:

"Childhood aphasia refers to one or more significant deficits in essential processes as they relate to facility in use of auditory language. Children having this disability demonstrate a discrepancy between expected and actual achievement in one or more of the following functions: auditory perception, auditory memory, integration, comprehension, expression. The deficits referred to are not the result of sensory, motor, intellectual, or emotional impairment, or of the lack of opportunity to learn. They are assumed to derive from dysfunctions in the brain, though the evidence for such dysfunctioning may be mainly behavioral, rather than neurological, in nature."

Leonard emphasized that children with acquired aphasia differ from other language-disordered children in that they have an initial period of normal language development.[119] They then lose that ability, usually because of some known brain damage caused by either illness or trauma. The most prominent disorder feature has been described as a noticeable reduction in the amount of speech generated, sometimes approaching mutism.[121] Apraxia of speech and word-retrieval problems are not uncommon; however, comprehension deficits are less severe. In general, language recovery is usually more rapid and complete than for adult aphasics, particularly when focusing on production-side symptoms. The age of damage onset and the location of the lesion are the two critical factors that dictate the impairment profile and the prognosis. For example, if the damage occurs before age 9 and is limited to one cerebral hemisphere, the child often demonstrates normal or near-normal language development and performance. In general, the best prognosis is associated with a discrete lesion of late onset, whereas the worst prognosis emerges with a widespread lesion early in life. Parents frequently seek professional assistance after their child has been "diagnosed" erroneously as mentally retarded, deaf, or emotionally disturbed. The child may appear mentally retarded because of poor performance on standardized intelligence tests; the label deaf may be applied because of an inability to use verbal symbols that require hearing for response. The emotionally disturbed classification may seem appropriate because of exhibited behavioral problems, yet more inclusive evaluation of all the data usually differentiates the several problems and identifies the aphasic child. Diagnosing aphasia in children is a complex process requiring the united efforts of many specialists, including the neurologist, pediatrician, psychologist, otologist, audiologist, speech-language pathologist, and educational consultant. Only through the combined efforts of these specialists, using a systematic, diagnostic approach, will the child be led to a more prescriptive type of educational training.

Because many aphasic children recover quickly after head injury or illness, the role of the speech-language pathologist and other professionals may be minimal. When residual deficits persist, however, a formal remediation program appears justified.[122] Holland and Reinmuth remind us that for an unfortunate minority of these children the prognosis is not good.[123] Extensive residual problems require intensive, specialized, interdisciplinary remediation available only through special rehabilitation centers or special schools. In those settings, "restitution of linguistic, cognitive and physical skills is the primary goal." The diagnosis and prescribed training program for the aphasic child would be woefully incomplete if the emotional factors of the family environment were not considered. The family may protect or shield the child excessively or else coerce or reject the child. The presence of an aphasic child in the family unit may be deeply disturbing; the situation requires a thorough appraisal of both the family structure and the need for therapeutic counseling.

Aphasia (Dysphasia) in Adults

Aphasia is associated with cortical disturbances or lesions resulting from vascular impairment (thrombosis, embolism, hemorrhage), tumors, degenerative and infectious disease, and trauma. Holland and Reinmuth state that aphasia is a general term applied to different but related syndromes that impair the ability to formulate, retrieve, and/or decode the symbols of language.[123] As a common adult disorder of communication, it disrupts speech and verbal output, comprehension of speech, and reading and writing skills. The onset of aphasia is usually abrupt and typically occurs in adults with no previous speech or language difficulty. According to Holland and Reinmuth, most syndromes of aphasia share several concepts:

1. Aphasic symptoms are not bizarre, but rather are extreme extensions of language problems demonstrated daily by normal speakers (i.e., losing one's train of thought, forgetting how to spell a word, not understanding a spoken word or concept).
2. All aphasics have some fundamental difficulty with both comprehension and word retrieval, regardless of the presence of other deficits.
3. A continuum of severity is seen within each syndrome.

The linguistic disturbances of the aphasic have been classified in numerous ways that reflect the clinical experience of the classifiers and their concepts of cortical function related to language. These classifications have attempted also to recognize the major types and specific forms of language disturbance. One classification system currently in wide use is the one developed by a Boston-based group of professionals that highlights fluent versus nonfluent types.[124,125] The six options are summarized by Boone as follows:[71]

1. Broca's or motor aphasia: marked reduction in speech output; common oral-verbal apraxia; relatively good speech comprehension; word-retrieval problem; writing performance matching output.
2. Transcortical motor aphasia: rare type with significant struggle in producing an utterance; telegraphic speech common; relatively good speech comprehension; impaired-writing skills.
3. Anomic aphasia: word-retrieval problems predominant for both speech and writing; nearly normal comprehension for speech and reading.
4. Wernicke's or jargon aphasia: significant comprehension deficit for speech and reading; fluent but jargon-like verbal output; writing paralleling speech patterns.
5. Conduction aphasia: nearly normal comprehension for speech and reading; marked deficit in speech repetition; fluent speech output with numerous sound and word errors.
6. Global aphasia: most severe and most common type; profound problems with both verbal output and comprehension; poor reading and writing functions.

The emotional language of the adult aphasic is usually better than propositional language. The patient may find it easier to swear, to count, or to use other forms of automatic speech or nonpropositional forms of speech but is at a loss when requested to develop this emotional language into abstract or propositional language situations. The patient experiences difficulty in combining simple linguistic symbols into more complex linguistic units. The patient is not without words, but rather cannot quickly command the response appropriate to the situation. Boone emphasizes that the brain damage (regardless of its cause) can produce other deficits or symptoms.[71] These include hemiplegia (gross motor paralysis), hemianopsia (visual field defect), intellectual deficits, seizures, dysarthria (motor speech impairment), and apraxia (inability to execute voluntary movement).

Prognosis for the recovery of the aphasic patient must be based on many factors, including the site and extent of lesion, general health, attitude toward self and environment, age and educational attainment, vocation and avocations, and family attitude, and degree of cooperation. Assuming that these and other factors are relatively positive, considerable recovery may be expected from the overall linguistic and physical impairments. Spontaneous improvement may be noted during the first few months after the onset without structured training. This may give false hope to the patient and family for additional recovery without seeking professional assistance. Depending on the degree of involvement, the family, with the physician's guidance, should enlist the services of a physical therapist, occupational therapist, speech-language pathologist, psychologist, and vocational counselor in formulating a personalized rehabilitation program. Ideally, the adult aphasic should be started on a program of rehabilitation as soon after the traumatic episode as possible.

SUGGESTED READINGS

1. Ludlow CL: Research needs for the assessment of phonatory function. In: Proceedings of the Conference on the Assessment of Vocal Pathology. Edited by Ludlow C and Hart MO. ASHA Reports No. 11. Rockville, MD, American Speech-Language-Hearing Association, 1981.
2. Verdolini K: Voice disorders. In: Diagnosis in Speech-Language Pathology. Edited by Tomblin JB, Morris HL, and Spriestersbach DC. San Diego, Singular Publishing Group, 1994.
3. Shprintzen RJ: Syndrome delineation and communicative impairment. In: Introduction to Communication Sciences and Disorders. Edited by Minifie F. San Diego, Singular Publishing Group, 1994.
4. Bastian RW, Keidar AK, and Verdolini-Marston K: Simple vocal tasks for detecting vocal fold swelling. J Voice 4:172, 1990.
5. Damste PH: Virilization of the voice due to anabolic steroids. Folia Phoniatr (Basel) 16:10, 1964.
6. Damste PH: Voice change in adult women caused by virilizing agents. J Speech Hear Disord 32:126, 1967.
7. Ramig LA, et al: Acoustic analysis of voice in amyotrophic lateral sclerosis. J Speech Hear Disord 55:2, 1990.
8. Hanson K, Gerratt B, and Ward R: Cinegraphic observations of laryngeal function in Parkinson's disease. Laryngoscope 94:348, 1984.
9. Coutryman MA, Ramig LA, and Pawlas AA: Speech and voice deficits in Parkinsonism plus syndromes: Can they be treated? National Center for Voice and Speech status progress report. J Med Speech Lang Pathol 2:211, 1994.
10. Ramig LO, Scherer RC, Titze I, and Ringel S: Acoustic characteristics of voice in amyotrophic lateral sclerosis: a longitudinal study. Ann Otol Rhinol Laryngol 97:164, 1988.
11. King JB, Ramig LO, Lemke JH, and Horii Y: Parkinson's disease: longitudinal changes in acoustic parameters of phonation. J Med Speech Lang Pathol (in press).
12. Strand E and Yorkston K: Description and classification of dysarthric individuals: toward a new taxonomy. In: Clinical Dysarthria. Edited by Till J, Beukelman D, and Yorkston K. Baltimore, Paul Brookes, 1994.
13. Ramig LO: Speech therapy for Parkinson's disease. In: Therapy of Parkinson's Disease. Edited by Koller W and Paulson G. New York, Marcel Dekker, 1994.
14. Orlikoff RF and Huang ZD: Influence of vowel production on acoustic and electroglottographic perturbation measures. American Speech-Language-Hearing Convention, 1991.
15. Huang ZD, Minifie FD, and Lin XS: Measures of vocal function
16. Huang ZD, Minifie FD, and Lin XS: Effects of vocal effort level on acoustic perturbation measures. In: Proceedings of Conference on Standardization of Acoustic Measures of Voice, National Institute on Deafness and Other Communication Disorders and NCVS. Denver, National Center for Voice and Speech, 1994.
17. Koike Y: Application of some acoustic measures for the evaluation of laryngeal dysfunction. Studia Phonol 7:17, 1973.
18. Yoshida M: Study on perceptive and acoustic classification of pathological voices. Pract Otol (Kyoto) 72:249, 1979.
19. Sawashima M and Hirano M: Clinical evaluation of voice disorders. Ann Bull Res Inst Logoped Phoniatr (University of Tokyo) 15:164, 1981.
20. Yumoto E, Gould WJ, and Baer T: Harmonics-to-noise ratio as an index to harshness. J Acoust Soc Am 71:1544, 1982.
21. Yumoto E, Sasaki Y, and Okamura H: Harmonics-to-noise ratio and psychophysical measurement of the degree of hoarseness. J Speech Hear Res 27:2, 1984.
22. Zwitman DH: Bilateral cord dysfunctions: abduction type spastic dysphonia. J Speech Hear Disord 44:373, 1979.
23. Freeman F, Cannito M, and Finitzo-Hieber T: Classification of spasmodic dysphonia by perceptual-acoustic means. In: Spastic Dysphonia: State of the Art 1984. Edited by Gates GA. New York, Voice Foundation, 1985.
24. Brodnitz FS: Spastic dysphonia. Ann Otolaryngol 85:210, 1975.
25. Spiegel H: Psychiatric aspects of spasmodic dysphonia. In: Spastic Dysphonia: State of the Art 1984. Edited by Gates GA. New York, Voice Foundation, 1985.
26. Aronson AE, Brown JP, Litin EM, and Pearson JS: Spastic dysphonia: I. voice, neurologic and psychiatric aspects. J Speech Hear Disord 33:203, 1968.
27. Feldman M, Nixon J, Finitzo-Hieber T, and Freeman F: Abnormal parasympathetic vagal function in patients with spasmodic dysphonia. Ann Intern Med 100:491, 1984.
28. Dedo HH, Townsend JJ, and Izdebski K: Current evidence for the organic etiology of spastic dysphonia. Otolaryngology 86:875, 1978.
29. Izdebski K and Shipp T: Model of spastic dysphonia. In: Spastic Dysphonia: State of the Art 1984. Edited by Gates GA. New York, Voice Foundation, 1985.
30. Fink M: Neurobiology of spastic disorders. In: Spastic Dysphonia: State of the Art 1984. Edited by Gates GA. New York, Voice Foundation, 1985.
31. Malmgran L: Neuromuscular anatomy of the larynx. In: Spastic Dysphonia: State of the Art 1984. Edited by Gates GA. New York, Voice Foundation, 1985.
32. Bochino JV and Tucker HM: Recurrent laryngeal nerve pathology in spasmodic dysphonia. Lanyngoscope 88:1274, 1978.
33. Dedo HH and Shipp T: Spastic Dysphonia: A Surgical and Voice Therapy Treatment Program. Houston, TX, College-Hill Press, 1980.
34. Freeman F, Cannito M, Finitzo-Hieber T, and Ross E: Spasmodic dysphonia: myths and facts. In: Speech News. Edited by Rosenfield D. Houston, TX, Baylor College of Medicine, 1984.
35. Dedo HH: Recurrent laryngeal nerve section for spastic dysphonia. Ann Otol Rhinol Laryngol 85:451, 1976.
36. Barton TT: Treatment of spastic dysphonia by recurrent laryngeal nerve section. Laryngoscope 89:244, 1979.
37. Levine HL, et al: Recurrent laryngeal nerve section for spasmodic dysphonia. Ann Otol Rhinol Laryngol 88:527, 1979.
38. Biller HF, Som MI, and Lawson W: Laryngeal nerve crush for spastic dysphonia. Ann Otol Rhinol Laryngol 88:531, 1979.
39. Miller R, Woodson G, and Jankovic J: Botulinum toxin injection of the vocal fold for spasmodic dysphonia. Arch Otolaryngol Head Neck Surg 113:603, 1987.
40. Dedo HH: Intermediate results of 306 recurrent laryngeal nerve sections for spastic dysphonia. Laryngoscope 93:1, 1983.

41. Aronson A and DeSanto L: Adductor spasmodic dysphonia: three years after recurrent nerve section. Laryngoscope 93:9, 1983.

42. Wilson FB, Oldring DJ, and Mueller K: Recurrent laryngeal nerve dissection: A case report involving return of spastic dysphonia after initial surgery. J Speech Hear Disord 41:315, 1976.

43. Fritzell B, et al: Experiences with recurrent laryngeal nerve section for spastic dysphonia. In: Phoniatric and Logopedic Progress Report No. 3. Stockholm, Department of Logopedics and Phoniatrics, Huddinge University Hospital, Karolinska Institute, 1981.

44. Hartman DE and Aronson AE: Clinical investigations of intermittent breathy dysphonia. J Speech Hear Disord 46:428, 1981.

45. Blitzer A: Electromyographic findings in spastic dysphonia. In: Spastic Dysphonia: State of the Art 1984. Edited by Gates GA. New York, Voice Foundation, 1985.

46. Robe E, Brumlik J, and Moore P: A study of spastic dysphonia: neurologic and electroencephalographic abnormalities. Laryngoscope 70:219, 1960.

47. Schaefer S, et al: Magnetic resonance imaging findings and correlations in spasmodic dysphonia patients. Ann Otol Rhinol Laryngol 94:595, 1985.

48. Finitzo-Hieber T, et al: Auditory brain stem response abnormalities in adductor spasmodic dysphonia. Am J Otolaryngol 3:26, 1982.

49. Boone DR and McFarland S: The Voice and Voice Therapy. Englewood Cliffs, NJ, Prentice-Hall, 1990.

50. Huang ZD, Minifie FD, and Lin XS: Dr. Speech Science. Software produced by Tiger Electronics, Seattle, WA, 1994.

51. Lowry LD, Marks JE, and Powell WJ: 260 Laryngeal carcinomas. Arch Otolaryngol 98:147, 1973.

52. Silverberg E: Cancer statistics, 1981. Reprinted by American Cancer Society from CA Cancer J Clin 37:13, 1981.

53. Anonymous: Cancer Facts and Figures. New York, American Cancer Society, 1988.

54. Anonymous: Cancer Facts and Figures. Atlanta, GA, American Cancer Society.

55. Gates GA, et al: Current state of laryngectomee rehabilitation: I. Results of therapy. Am J Otolaryngol 3:1, 1982.

56. Snidecore JC: The family of the laryngectomee. In: The Family as Supportive Personnel in Speech and Hearing Remediation. Proceedings of a Postgraduate Short Course, University of California, Santa Barbara, United States Department of Health, Education and Welfare, 1971, p 12.

57. Gates GA, Ryan W, and Lauder E: Current status of laryngectomee rehabilitation: IV. Attitudes about laryngectomee rehabilitation should change. Am J Otolaryngol 3:2, 1982.

58. Gates GA, Ryan W, Cantu E, and Hearne E: Current status of laryngectomee rehabilitation: II. Causes of failure. Am J Otolaryngol 3:1, 1982.

59. Gardner WH: Laryngectomee speech and rehabilitation. Springfield, IL, Charles C Thomas, 1971.

60. Ryan W, Gates GA, Cantu E, and Hearne E: Current status of laryngectomee rehabilitation: III. Understanding of esophageal speech. Am J Otolaryngol 3:2, 1982.

61. Anonymous: Ignorance of laryngectomee care confirmed by medical authorities. IAL News 27, 1982.

62. Singer M and Blom E: An endoscopic technique for restoration of voice after laryngectomy. Ann Otol Rhinol Laryngol 89:529, 1980.

63. Zwitman DH and Calcaterra TC: Phonation using the tracheaesophageal shunt after total laryngectomy. J Speech Hear Disord 38:368, 1973.

64. Weinberg B: Airway resistance to the voice button. Arch Otolaryngol 108:498, 1982.

65. Singer M, Blom E, and Hamaker R: Further experience with voice restoration after total laryngectomy. Ann Otol Rhinol Laryngol 90:4898, 1981.

66. Singer M and Blom E: A selective myotomy for voice restoration after total laryngectomy. Arch Otolaryngol 107:670, 1981.

67. Blom E, Singer M, and Hamaker R: Tracheostoma valve for postlaryngectomy voice rehabilitation. Ann Otol Rhinol Laryngol 91:576, 1982.

68. Andrews J, et al: Major complications following tracheoesophageal puncture for voice rehabilitation. Laryngoscope 97:562, 1987.

69. Sisson G, McConnell FM, Logemann JA, and Yeh S: Voice rehabilitation after laryngectomy. Arch Otolaryngol 101:178, 1975.

70. Lauder E: The laryngectomee and the artificial larynx: a second look. J Speech Hear Disord 35:62, 1970.

71. Boone D: Human Communication and Its Disorders. Englewood Cliffs, NJ, Prentice-Hall, 1987.

72. Eimas PD, Siqueland ER, Jusczyk P, and Vigorito J: Speech perception in infants. Science 171:303, 1971.

73. Kuhl PK: Speech perception. In: Introduction to Communication Sciences and Disorders. Edited by Minifie FD. San Diego, Singular Publishing Group, 1994.

74. Werker JF and Tees RC: Cross-language speech perception: evidence for perceptual reorganization during the first year of life. Infant Behav Dev 7:49, 1984.

75. Kuhl PK, et al: Linguistic experience alters phonetic perception in infants by 6 months of age. Science 255:606, 1992.

76. Greiser DL and Kuhl PK: Maternal speech to infants in a tonal language: support for universal prosodic features in Motherese. Dev Psychol 24:14, 1988.

77. Bloom L: Language development. In: Introduction to Communication Sciences and Disorders. Edited by Minifie FD. San Diego, Singular Publishing Group, 1994.

78. Stone JR and Stoel-Gammon C: Phonological development and disorders in children. In: Introduction to Communication Sciences and Disorders. Edited by Minifie FD. San Diego, Singular Publishing Group, 1994.

79. Lewis MM: How Children Learn to Speak. New York, Basic Books, 1957.

80. Locke JL: Phonological Acquisition and Change. New York, Academic Press, 1983.

81. Oller DK and Eilers RE: The role of audition in infant babbling. Child Dev 59:441, 1988.

82. Sander E: When are speech sounds learned? J Speech Hear Disord 37:55, 1972.

83. Kent RD: Anatomical and neuromuscular maturation of the speech mechanism: evidence from acoustic studies. J Speech Hear Res 19:421, 1976.

84. Ingram D: Phonological Disability in Children. London, Edward Arnold, 1976.

85. Dyson AT: Phonetic inventories of 2- and 3-year-old children. J Speech Hear Disord 53:89, 1988.

86. Crary MA and Fokes J: Phonological processes in apraxia of speech: a systemic simplification of articulatory performance. Aphasia Apraxia Agnosia 4:1, 1980.

87. Grumwell P: Clinical Phonology. 2nd Ed. Baltimore, Williams & Wilkins, 1987.

88. Smit AB: Speech sound disorders. In: Diagnosis in Speech-Language Pathology. Edited by Tomblin JB, Morris HL, and Spriestersbach DC. San Diego, Singular Publishing Group, 1994.

89. Stoel-Gammon C and Dunn C: Normal and Disordered Phonology in Children. Austin, TX, Pro-Ed, 1985.

90. Bernthal JE and Bankson NW: Articulation and Phonological Disorders. 2nd Ed. Englewood Cliffs, NJ, Prentice-Hall, 1988.

91. Carrell J: Disorders of Articulation. Englewood Cliffs, NJ, Prentice-Hall, 1968.

92. Cohen MM, Jr: The Child with Multiple Birth Defects. New York, Raven Press, 1982.

93. Fraser FC: The genetics of cleft lip and cleft palate. Am J Hum Genet 22:336, 1970.

94. Siegel-Sadewitz VL and Shprintzen RJ: The relationship of communication disorders to syndrome identification. J Speech Hear Disord *47*:338, 1982.

95. McEvery ET and Gaines FP: Tongue-tie in infants and children. J Pediatr *18*:252, 1941.

96. Fletcher S and Meldrum J: Lingual function and relative length of the lingual frenulum. J Speech Hear Res *11*:328, 1968.

97. LaPointe LL: Neurogenic disorders of communication. In: Introduction to Communication Sciences and Disorders. Edited by Minifie FD. San Diego, Singular Publishing Group, 1994.

98. Darley F, Aronson A, and Brown J: Motor Speech Disorders. Philadelphia, WB Saunders, 1975.

99. Hartelius L and Svensson P: Speech and swallowing symptoms associated with Parkinson's disease and multiple sclerosis. Folia Phoniatr (Basel) *146*:9, 1991.

100. Yorkston KM, Hammon VL, Beukelman DR, and Traynor CD: The effect of rate on the intelligibility and naturalness of dysarthric speech. J Speech Hear Disord *55*:550, 1990.

101. Hartelius L, Nord L, and Buder EH: Acoustic analysis of dysarthria associated with multiple sclerosis. Clin Linguist Phonet *8*:143, 1994.

102. Kent RD, et al: Quantitative description of the dysarthria in women with amyotrophic lateral sclerosis. J Speech Hear Res *35*:723, 1992.

103. Kent RD, et al: Impairment of speech intelligibility in men with amyotrophic lateral sclerosis. J Speech Hear Disord *55*:721, 1990.

104. Kent RD, et al: Speech deterioration in amyotrophic lateral sclerosis: a case study. J Speech Hear Res *34*:1269, 1991.

105. Weismer G, Martin R, Kent RD, and Kent JF: Formant trajectory characteristics of males with amyotrophic lateral sclerosis. J Acoust Soc Am *91*:1085, 1992.

106. Kent RD: Neurological bases of communication disorders. In: Introduction to Communication Sciences and Disorders. Edited by Minifie FD. San Diego, Singular Publishing Group, 1994.

107. LaPointe L and Katz RC: Neurogenic disorders of speech. In: Human Communication Disorders. 4th Ed. Edited by Shames G, Wiig E, and Secord WB. Columbus, OH, Charles E. Merrill, 1994.

108. Wingate M: A standard definition of stuttering. J Speech Hear Disord *29*:484, 1964.

109. Prins D: Fluency and stuttering. In: Introduction to Communi- cation Sciences and Disorders. Edited by Minifie FD. San Diego, Singular Publishing Group, 1994.

110. Van Riper C: The Nature of Stuttering. 2nd Ed. Englewood Cliffs, NJ, Prentice-Hall, 1982.

111. Starkweather CW: Fluency and Stuttering. Englewood Cliffs, NJ, Prentice-Hall, 1987.

112. Hillman R and Gilbert H: Voice onset times for voiceless stop consonants in fluent reading of stutterers and nonstutterers. J Acoust Soc Am *61*:610, 1977.

113. Metz D, Conture E, and Caruso A: Voice onset time, frication and aspiration during stutterers fluent speech. J Speech Hear Res *22*:649, 1979.

114. Zimmerman G: Articulatory dynamics of fluent utterances of stutterers and nonstutterers. J Speech Hear Res *23*:95, 1980.

115. Ingham RJ: Stuttering and Behavior Therapy. San Diego, College Hill Press, 1984.

116. Adams M: A clinical strategy for differentiating the normal nonfluent child and the incipient stutterer. J Fluency Disord *2*:141, 1977.

117. Johnson W: People in Quandaries. New York, Harper and Row, 1946.

118. Shames G: Disorders and fluency. In: Human Communication Disorders. 3rd Ed. Edited by Shames G and Wiig W. Columbus, OH, Charles E. Merrill, 1990.

119. Leonard L: Early language development and language disorders. In: Human Communication Disorders. 2nd Ed. Edited by Shames G and Wiig E. Columbus, OH, Charles E. Merrill, 1986.

120. Myklebust H: Childhood aphasia: An evolving concept. In: Handbook of Speech Pathology and Audiology. Edited by Travis LE. Englewood Cliffs, NJ, Prentice-Hall, 1971.

121. Chase R: Neurological aspects of language disorders in children. In: Principles of Childhood Language Disabilities. Edited by Irwin J and Marge M. Englewood Cliffs, NJ, Prentice-Hall, 1972.

122. Wood NE: Delayed Speech and Language Development. Englewood Cliffs, NJ, Prentice Hall, 1964.

123. Holland A and Reinmuth O: Asphasia in adults. In: Human Communication Disorders. 2nd Ed. Edited by Shames G and Wiig E. Columbus, OH, Charles E. Merrill, 1986.

124. Benson D and Geschwind N: The aphasias and related disturbances. In: Clinical Neurology. Vol 1. Edited by Baker A and Baker L. Hagerstown MD, Harper and Row, 1976.

125. Goodglass H and Kaplan E: The Assessment of Aphasia and Related Disorders. 2nd Ed. Philadelphia, Lea & Febiger, 1983.

27 Airway Control and Laryngotracheal Stenosis

Ellis M. Arjmand and J. Gershon Spector

The techniques used for airway management in adult and pediatric patients continue to evolve. In the first section of this chapter, standard techniques of intubation, cricothyrotomy, and tracheostomy are reviewed. The procedure of percutaneous tracheostomy is also discussed. The second section of this chapter addresses the problems of laryngeal and tracheal stenosis. Standard techniques for airway recontruction in adult patients are reviewed, as are recent reports of the application of these techniques. Rapid advances in the techniques used for airway reconstruction in children have occurred, and a review of these techniques is provided.

AIRWAY CONTROL

Control of the airway to provide oxygenation and hygiene of the tracheobronchial tree, or to maintain and assist respiration, is the basis of all treatment of respiratory insufficiency. This control is obtained by intubation or tracheostomy. The relative merits of each procedure have been controversial (Fig. 27–1).

Historical Background

The earliest recorded evidence of artificial resuscitation is in the Old Testament, involving mouth-to-mouth respiration by Elijah to revive a child who was probably suffering from heat stroke. The Rigveda, a Hindu text circa 2000 B.C., describes spontaneous healing of a tracheostomy incision. Asclepiades, in 100 B.C., described an incision to improve a compromised airway. Hippocrates condemned tracheotomy because of the fear of carotid artery damage. He knew that laceration or ligation of the carotid vessels could cause death (carotid is derived from the Greek karotides, meaning

sleep). Aretaeus of Cappadocia, in the first century A.D., did not advocate tracheotomy to avoid suffocation caused by infection. He noted that secondary wound infections at the operative site produced complications, increased dyspnea, cough, and death. Antyllus, in the second century A.D., disapproved of tracheotomy in severe laryngotracheobronchitis, saying that the operation was not effective because the disease was below the operative site. With obstructive adenoidal, tonsillar, and oral disease, however, he advocated a tracheotomy between two tracheal rings (in the tracheal membrane). He also advocated a horizontal incision to avoid cartilage damage. This was the first modern tracheotomy. Galen, about 20 years later (A.D. 131) described the anatomy of the larynx (including the six paired intralaryngeal muscles and three cartilages), the trachea (including the cartilages, membranes, and flail posterior wall), and the esophagus (including the sphincters). He was the first to localize voice production to the larynx, to describe the adductors and abductors of the larynx, and to define the innervation of the larynx (Galen's anastomosis was the arborization of the superior and recurrent laryngeal nerves posteriorly). He also described respiration, noting the humidification, temperature regulation, and particulate filtering that the supralaryngeal compartments provide. The Hebrew Babylonian Talmud, in the fourth and fifth centuries A.D., advocated a longitudinal incision as safer than a transverse incision in tracheotomy. By the end of the fifth century A.D., tracheotomies were well recognized in India (e.g., the Hindu text Susruta). Brasavola, in 1546, published the first account of tracheotomy for tonsillar obstruction. Sanctorius (1561 to 1636) used a trocar and cannula. The latter was left in place for 3 days. Habicot (1550 to 1624) performed four tracheotomies for disease and aspiration of foreign bodies. George Martine (1702 to 1743) developed the

466

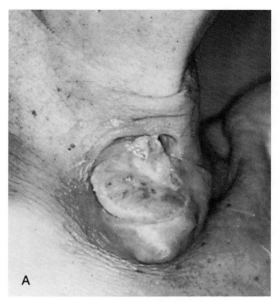

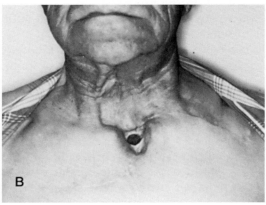

Fig. 27–1. A. Adenocarcinoma of thyroid gland invading the larynx and trachea causing respiratory distress and hypoventilation. This required intubation while awake and immediate resection with a sternal split and mediastinal dissection. B. Postoperative sternal tracheostomy. This case demonstrates the need for multiple approaches to obstructive hypoventilation. (Courtesy of Dr. G.J. Spector.)

double-cannula tracheotomy tube. The inner cannula was to be removed for cleansing and the outer cannula left in place. Lorenz Heister (1718) coined the term tracheotomy. The procedure gained wide acceptance in Europe. In 1921, Jackson defined the factors leading to tracheotomy complications. He also advocated a low tracheotomy (in the second and third tracheal rings), as opposed to a high tracheotomy (cricothyrotomy).

Clinical Evaluation

A complete history and physical examination are mandatory before airway management and control. The most common symptoms for upper airway obstruction include hoarseness or voice change, dyspnea and stridor, dysphagia, pain, restlessness, cough, drooling, and progressive aggravation of symptoms. The rapid-

ity of symptom progression has a direct bearing on final outcome. Physical findings include airway bleeding, subcutaneous emphysema, palpable laryngotracheal fractures, and generalized labored respiration with cyanosis, suprasternal and intercostal retraction, and the inability to move air into the lungs. Diagnostic assessment must utilize direct, indirect, or fiberoptic laryngoscopy, evaluation of blood gases, and radiologic studies. Radiologic studies should generally include a chest x-ray film; soft tissue or tomographic assessment of the neck, cervical airway, and cervical spine; specialized radiography of the face; barium swallow; and arteriography when needed. Pulmonary function tests are valuable in evaluating the nature of the obstruction. In many acute obstructions, these parameters are not available, and speed is required to maintain the airway to keep the patient alive.

The goal of the surgeon is to provide the most facile control of the airway with the lowest potential for injury. To achieve this goal, the surgeon must (1) accurately assess the nature and the level of the obstruction and establish airway control below the lowest level of the obstruction; (2) be cognizant of the general status of the patient and the presence of other associated injuries, such as cervical spine trauma, vascular injury, pulmonary status, sepsis, and penetrating visceral injuries; (3) select the simplest and least traumatic method for airway control, bearing in mind that any method of airway control has the potential for injury and complications, and the limitations imposed by personal experience, equipment available, and the team assembled for resuscitation are of paramount importance; and (4) be aware of the specific goals to be achieved, that is, airway control in obstruction, secretional control and hygiene, assisted mechanical ventilation, assisted respiration in unconscious or individuals with central nervous system (CNS) injury, conversion from one mode of airway control to another (endotracheal to tracheotomy), and control of the airway as prevention for potential obstruction (as with some head and neck oncologic procedures).

Many therapeutic options are available today. Basically, these procedures are divided into two groups: endoluminal and transluminal. All have their intrinsic value and their specific problems or complications. Moreover, at times it may be wise to observe the patient and provide medical support before airway intervention. It is best to use constant observation and monitoring, such as in an intensive care unit. Medical support usually involves respiratory therapy service personnel, who provide oxygenation and humidification. In addition, as indicated, one may use antibiotics and corticosteroids. Endoluminal airways include the nasopharyngeal airway, oral airway, transoral intubation, and nasal intubation. The transluminal procedures include transcricothyroid or transtracheal needle ventilation (usually with larger than 16-gauge plastic sheathed needles or plastic catheters), cricothyrotomy, tracheotomy, and tracheostomy.

Control of the Airway

Jackson noted that, in his day, all medical graduates were taught "that there were two kinds of tracheostomy, high and low, the low operation being more difficult and the high operation very easy."[1] He analyzed 200 patients with chronic laryngeal stenosis and noted that, in 158 (79%), the primary cause was a high tracheotomy and improper postoperative care. He defined the offending factors as a high incision, improper large cannulae, poor postoperative care, improper surgical technique, and splitting of the cricoid cartilage. Jackson stated that it is "improper to divide the cricoid cartilage, the only complete ring in the trachea." In addition, he reasoned that stenosis was caused by pressure necrosis from a large cannula in the narrowest part of the airway and that the subglottis in children was susceptible to edema and the loss of the cricoid support. He advocated the use of the low tracheotomy and transection of the thyroid isthmus. In his lifetime, Jackson saw the incidence of laryngeal stenosis drop from 75 to 25% and finally to 2%. He also advocated the conversion of all high tracheotomies to low tracheotomies as soon as possible.

The use of cricothyroidotomy, especially in cardiothoracic operative cases, has been advocated. This allows greater distance between the sternotomy site (sterile) and the airway control (contaminated). In addition, the procedure can be performed quickly, with fewer instruments, and in patients with difficult exposure (kyphoscoliosis). Brantigan and Grow reviewed 655 cases of cricothyroidotomy and reported a complication rate of 6.1%.[2] Complications included bleeding, infection, subcutaneous emphysema, voice changes, persistent cutaneous fistula, and laryngeal stenosis (1.8%). They reasoned that the low incidence of complication was because today cricothyroidotomies are performed for respiratory failure, airway hygiene, and mechanical ventilation, rather than for infections. Boyd and associates reported a 9% complication rate in 105 cricothyroidotomies.[3] The 2% subglottic stenoses in this series were in patients with prolonged endotracheal intubation. The conclusion was that endotracheal tubes in place for more than 7 days should be converted to standard tracheotomies. Sise and colleagues noted a higher incidence of subglottic stenosis in children and adolescents.[4]

A few factors appear to predispose patients to subglottic stenosis. These include (1) prolonged previous endotracheal intubation, (2) bilateral vocal cord paralysis, (3) acute laryngeal trauma, (4) subglottic inflammatory disease or granulation tissue, (5) large cannulae (i.e., the average cricothyroid membrane is 9 mm and the average diameter of a cannula is 10 or more mm

[Shiley No. 4 cannula is 8.5 mm], leading to pressure necrosis), (6) pediatric and adolescent patients, and (7) mechanically assisted ventilation (shearing forces cause necrosis of subglottis and cricoid ring).

Other complications produce no life-threatening emergencies. These include a high incidence of voice changes. This is primarily noted in high tones and is caused by limitation of vocal cord motion and anterior commissure scarring.

Animal studies have demonstrated that cricoid transection in dogs is associated with subglottic scarring.[5] Minimal trauma, however, was noted to the subglottis in dogs when the mucosa was damaged but the cricoid was intact.[6] The use of antibiotics reduced subglottic granulation tissue. On the other hand, Nelson noted an appreciable degree of stenosis in 5 of 6 dogs cannulated through the cricothyroid membrane for 10 days.[7-9] Stauffer and associates,[10] in a prospective study using laryngeal and tracheal tomograms and a criterion of 10% reduction in the transverse air column, noted a high rate of complications of endotracheal intubation (62%), of which 9% developed stenosis.

The conclusion, therefore, is that all methods for airway access have the potential for complications. Beatrous analyzed 1000 consecutive cases of tracheotomy and found no stenosis.[11] Arola and Anttinen,[12] in 812 cases, had 1.1% tracheal stenosis, but none following low-pressure, high-volume cuffs. Furthermore, the post-tracheotomy strictures are usually located in the cervical trachea and are easily correctable, but cricothyroidotomy produces complicated repair problems occasionally requiring cricoid and tracheal resections and laryngeal repairs. Mortality rates from laryngeal stenosis range from 3 to 18%.

Endotracheal Intubation

Endotracheal intubation is the fastest method of establishing the airway. It may be performed transnasally or transorally. Intubation is indicated as a prelude to tracheostomy or to maintain the airway when the clinician believes that the respiratory problem is likely to be temporary. Whenever possible, the procedure should precede tracheostomy, especially in infants and children. The advantages of intubation are as follows:

1. It provides immediate control of the airway.
2. A hasty and traumatic tracheostomy is avoided.
3. A general anesthetic may be given for the tracheostomy.
4. The complication of pneumothorax, occurring during tracheostomy performed on a patient exerting marked ventilatory effort, is avoided.

Although intubation is an appropriate technique for airway control in progressive upper airway obstruction, deteriorating pulmonary dynamics, secretional hygiene, neuromuscular paralysis or fatigue, and loss of the respiratory drive, a few relative contraindications to aggressive intubation exist. These include the following: (1) the presence of laryngeal or upper airway acute trauma (intubation may aggravate the injury and/or be difficult in locating the lumen); (2) cervical spinal fractures (hyperextension of the neck may destabilize the fracture and produce or aggravate the neurologic defects); (3) oral and nasal trauma, which may preclude proper intubation because of blood, secretion, tissues, and unstable facial fractures; and (4) any instance in which an adequate endolaryngeal or tracheal lumen cannot be visualized or established. Several specific disadvantages to prolonged intubation are discussed later in this chapter.

TECHNIQUE. The larynx is exposed with a laryngoscope, and an endotracheal tube or bronchoscope is inserted. Under emergency conditions, the tube should be inserted orally. Many patients requiring intubation are unconscious or semicomatose and require no anesthesia. Although no evidence indicates that lack of anesthesia increases the incidence of vasovagal reflex and cardiac arrest, when possible, it is wise to attempt improving oxygenation before intubation.

If the patient is conscious, local anesthesia may be obtained by topical application by way of the pharynx and piriform sinus or injection of the internal laryngeal nerves.

COMPLICATIONS. The presence of a tube in the larynx for a long period may produce mucosal ulceration, granulation tissue formation, subglottic edema, and, finally, laryngeal and tracheal stenosis. The complications of intubation have been reviewed and categorized by Benjamin,[13] whose recommendations are based on clinical observation in over 700 pediatric and adult patients. Factors noted to contribute to intubation trauma include underlying laryngeal abnormalities, traumatic or repeated intubation, gastroesophageal reflux, impairment of mucociliary clearance, and prolonged intubation. Endoscopic assessment to assess for airway trauma is recommended after 5 to 7 days of intubation in adults or after 1 to 2 weeks of intubation in children. The timing of endoscopy in infants is not based on the duration of intubation, but rather endoscopy is recommended after failed extubation. Intubation changes are categorized as follows: (1) early nonspecific changes (hyperemia or superficial ulceration); (2) edema; (3) ulceration with exposed perichondrium or cartilage; (4) granulation tissue; and (5) miscellaneous (arytenoid dislocation, damage to the muscles, or vocal cord laceration).

A tracheostomy should be performed if exposed cartilage or widespread subglottic ulceration is seen. In adults, tracheostomy should also be considered if the duration of intubation exceeds 1 week. The need for tracheostomy is more urgent if secretions are excessive and problematic, because tracheobronchial hygiene is more effective with a tracheostomy in place. An endotracheal tube may be of more value in infants and small children in whom the high incidence of acute complications associated with tracheostomy outweighs the disadvantages of intubation. Here again, however, the tube obstruction is a major problem; the nasotracheal tube may require frequent replacement.

Cricothyrotomy

In certain situations, an airway may be obtained by opening the trachea through the cricothyroid membrane. The procedure was described by Vicq d'Azur in 1805. The advantage of this procedure is that the cricothyroid membrane is directly under the skin and subcutaneous tissue, and a minimum amount of equipment and dissection is necessary to establish an airway rapidly.

The numerous disadvantages of the procedure limit its usefulness. The cricothyroid space is relatively narrow, and often is not wide enough to allow insertion of a tracheostomy tube of adequate caliber without damage to the cricoid cartilage. This is particularly true in pediatric patients. Any injury to the cricoid cartilage may be followed by perichondritis and subsequent laryngeal stenosis. Incision of the cricothyroid membrane may damage the conus elasticus, producing permanent voice changes. The cricothyroid arteries enter the cricothyroid space near the midline and may be the source of considerable bleeding during the procedure.

The major complication of cricothyrotomy is laryngeal stenosis. The longer a tube is left in place in the cricothyroid membrane, the greater the chance of perichondritis, granulation tissue formation, and eventual stenosis of the laryngeal lumen. Complications of cricothyrotomy were reviewed in a previous section of this chapter.

INDICATIONS. When endotracheal intubation is not possible, either tracheostomy or cricothyrotomy may be necessary to relieve respiratory obstruction. Generally, tracheostomy is the better procedure, but under certain emergency circumstances, cricothyrotomy may be the most expedient method of establishing an airway to avoid asphyxia and death of the patient. The indications for cricothyrotomy include the following:

1. Lack of equipment and instruments to perform endotracheal intubation or tracheostomy for relief of severe respiratory obstruction.
2. The need to establish an airway by nonmedically trained personnel.
3. The need to establish an airway in the presence of an obstructing neoplasm of the larynx, so the entire site of the cricothyrotomy may be excised at the time of definitive surgery.
4. The need to establish an airway in cardiopulmonary postoperative cases at a site distant from the chest incision to avoid cross-contamination and infection. This is basically used for short-term airway control.

5. Complete airway obstruction that is acute and requires immediate airway control. Cricothyrotomy is the quickest access to the airway before tracheotomy.

TECHNIQUE. The cricothyroid space is identified by extending the patient's head and palpating the prominent arch of the cricoid cartilage, which is 2 to 3 cm below the prominent V-notch of the thyroid cartilage in the average adult. A small horizontal incision is made with any sharp instrument just above the upper border of the cricoid cartilage. This exposes the cricothyroid membrane, which is punctured in the midline. The puncture wound is enlarged laterally by inserting a thin, blunt instrument into the wound and using blunt force to avoid hemorrhage from the cricothyroid artery. If a tube is not available, the airway is maintained by spreading the cricoid and thyroid cartilages apart, using a knife handle or other thin instrument. Placing the incision through the cricothyroid membrane nearer the cricoid cartilage can usually avoid hemorrhage from the cricothyroid arteries.

Puncturing the cricothyroid space using a large hypodermic needle (No. 16) may be attempted in extreme situations, but the airway is inadequate unless more than one needle is used.

POSTOPERATIVE CARE. An ordinary small tracheostomy tube (No. 6) should be inserted through the cricothyrotomy as soon as it is available. As soon as the patient's condition is stabilized, the cricothyrotomy should be converted to a tracheostomy through a separate lower incision. If at all possible, conversion should be performed within 24 hours or, at the most, 48 hours.

Tracheostomy: Adult

Tracheostomy consists of making an opening in the anterior wall of the trachea for purposes of establishing an airway.

INDICATIONS. Tracheostomy may be necessary for therapeutic purposes or it may be performed as an elective procedure. Elective tracheostomy may be necessary when respiratory problems are anticipated in the postoperative period in patients subjected to major head, neck, or thoracic operations or in patients with chronic pulmonary insufficiency. Rarely, it may be indicated in patients in whom orotracheal intubation is difficult or impossible for purposes of inducing general anesthesia. Tracheostomy should also be performed as a preliminary measure in operations for oropharyngeal or laryngeal neoplasms to avoid unnecessary manipulation of the tumor. A tracheotomy should be considered for airway control whenever prolonged airway intubation is anticipated.

Therapeutic tracheostomy is indicated in any case of respiratory insufficiency caused by alveolar hypoventilation to bypass obstruction, to remove secretions, or to provide for the use of mechanical ventilation.

Whenever possible, therapeutic tracheostomy should be preceded by endotracheal intubation. Although endotracheal intubation provides relief of the immediate airway problem, tracheostomy should be performed secondarily when prolonged airway care is anticipated because of the following:

1. Secretion removal is much easier through a tracheostomy tube, and tubal obstruction is less likely to occur.
2. It is extremely difficult for a patient to swallow around an endotracheal tube.
3. An endotracheal tube is difficult to clean in situ, and tube replacement necessitates repeated laryngoscopy.
4. Prolonged endolaryngeal intubation produces mucosal ulceration, which may eventually lead to the development of granulomas, adhesions, and laryngeal stenosis.
5. A tracheostomy causes less stimulation of the cough reflex, which may be important in some neurologic and postoperative patients.
6. A tracheostomy allows speech in conscious patients.

A contraindication to tracheostomy is in the patient with obstructing carcinoma of the larynx. Some evidence indicates that tracheostomy performed more than 48 hours before a definitive surgical procedure leads to an increased incidence of stomal recurrence. It is extremely difficult to excise widely a low tracheostomy site at the time of laryngectomy. Therefore, a temporary airway should be provided by endoscopic removal of sufficient tumor or cricothyrotomy.

TIMING. The conscious patient with upper respiratory obstruction usually manifests obvious signs of acute hypoxemia. These signs include rising pulse and respiratory rates, restlessness, confusion, and decreased air entry. Under such circumstances, the patient becomes exhausted in maintaining adequate blood gas levels before arterial O_2 desaturation occurs, that is, pO_2 falls to 40 mm Hg. When desaturation occurs, rapid circulatory and respiratory decompensation develops, and death becomes imminent. Therefore, the signs of desaturation, including cyanosis, coma, and hypotension, are late indications of insufficiency and may preclude resuscitation. Generally, when a patient presents with respiratory obstruction with signs of increasing hypoxemia, a tracheostomy is warranted.

In the unconscious patient with respiratory insufficiency, the clinical signs of hypoxemia may be less obvious, but because of the loss of protective mechanisms, a tracheostomy is indicated considerably earlier.

When the onset of respiratory insufficiency is slow, the signs of hypoxemia are minimal, and the manifestations of hypercapnia are more obvious. Headache, diz-

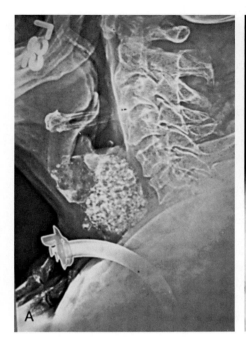
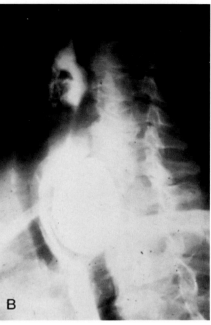

Fig. 27–2. A. Xeroradiogram of laryngeal chondrosarcoma. The stippled pattern is characteristic. Gradual, progressive, well compensated hypoventilation, requiring preoperative tracheotomy. B. Barium swallow of tracheal obstruction secondary to large Zenker's diverticulum. (Courtesy of Dr. G.J. Spector.)

ziness, sweating, and flushing are early symptoms and signs. Later, twitching, confusion, and coma may develop. In many instances, these patients are given O_2, which may produce transient improvement but may worsen the CO_2 retention. Therefore, in this situation, serial blood gas studies are of great help in determining a need for assisted ventilation. Generally, if a patient is unable to maintain an O_2 saturation of 85% or reduce pCO_2 below 50 mm Hg when breathing 50% O_2, a tracheostomy is indicated (Fig. 27–2).

FUNCTION. In addition to bypassing an upper airway obstruction, a tracheostomy has several other functions, which include the following:

1. Decreasing the amount of dead space in the tracheobronchial tree, usually 70 to 100 ml. The decrease in dead space may vary from 10 to 50%, depending on the individual's physiologic dead space.
2. Reducing resistance to airflow, which in turn reduces the force required to move air. This will result in increased total compliance and more effective alveolar ventilation, provided the tracheostomy opening is large enough (at least a No. 7 tube).
3. Providing protection against aspiration.
4. Enabling the patient to swallow without reflex apnea, which is important in patients with respiratory insufficiency.
5. Providing access to the trachea for cleaning.
6. Providing a pathway to deliver medication and humidification to the tracheobronchial tree, with or without intermittent positive pressure breathing.

7. Decreasing the power of the cough and thereby preventing peripheral displacement of secretions by the high negative intrathoracic pressure associated with the inspiratory phase normal cough.

TECHNIQUE. The technique of tracheostomy is dictated to some extent by the circumstances necessitating the operation. The important point is to obtain an airway as rapidly and efficiently as possible while avoiding injury to the larynx, trachea, and adjacent structures.

Whenever possible, endotracheal intubation should be performed before therapeutic tracheostomy. Intubation may be accomplished without anesthesia, if necessary. If intubation is not possible, ventilation and oxygenation by means of a bag and mask are valuable adjuncts to the procedure. If the airway is under control, a more orderly and less traumatic tracheostomy can be performed.

The patient should be positioned on his or her back with a pillow well under the shoulders to allow maximal extension of the neck. This is a difficult position for conscious patients with respiratory distress to maintain, and it may be necessary to hold patients in position.

Anesthesia for tracheostomy is unnecessary in unconscious patients. A local anesthetic is usually all that is necessary in conscious patients. A general anesthetic may be used if an endotracheal tube is in position, but is contraindicated if intubation has not been performed. Local anesthesia is obtained by infiltrating the skin in the line of the incision and depositing the agent in the deeper midline tissues to the level of the anterior tracheal wall. Lidocaine (Xylocaine), 1%, with epinephrine 1:150,000, is a satisfactory agent.

The skin incision is determined by the circumstances. When the tracheostomy is combined with a head and neck procedure, the incision is placed in accordance with the dictates of the proposed procedure. When tracheostomy is performed as an individual procedure, a horizontal or vertical skin incision may be used. The horizontal incision is made 5 cm long, approximately two finger-breadths above the sternal notch. When the situation is urgent and help is unavailable, a 4-cm vertical midline incision may be used to obtain rapid access with a minimum of dissection and bleeding.

The skin incision is deepened until the strap muscles are encountered (Fig. 27–3). At this point, the trachea should be palpated to ascertain its location and to avoid dissecting lateral to it. The strap muscles are separated vertically in the midline and are retracted laterally. This procedure exposes the pretracheal fascia, which covers the trachea and the thyroid isthmus. Numerous veins descend in the fascia from the thyroid, but if the incision stays in a midline vertical plane, most of the veins can be avoided. The thyroid isthmus is almost always above the level of the third tracheal ring. It is usually possible to retract the isthmus superiorly with a small blunt retractor to expose the trachea. Transection of the thyroid isthmus is seldom necessary; thus, the bleeding and delay so often encountered when this is done are avoided. An exceptionally wide isthmus must be divided between clamps, and a suture

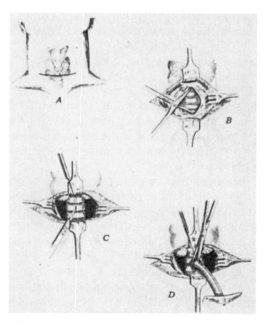

Fig. 27–3. Tracheostomy. A. A horizontal skin incision is made about 3 cm above the sternum. B. Blunt midline dissection is used to expose the anterior tracheal wall. C. The thyroid isthmus is retracted superiorly and a hook is inserted into the second tracheal ring. A vertical incision is made through the third and fourth rings. D. A hemostat is inserted into the trachea to spread the incision and permit insertion of the tracheostomy.

ligature is used to ligate the cut margins. A few drops of 4% lidocaine injected into the trachea at this point help to lessen the severe coughing initiated by insertion of the tracheostomy tube.

The trachea should be fixed by inserting a hook in the anterior wall between the first and second ring, pulling the trachea in an upward and outward direction. The anterior wall of the trachea is incised vertically, dividing two to three rings. The tracheal incision should never extend above the second tracheal ring, to prevent the tracheostomy tube from impinging on the cricoid cartilage and producing perichondritis. Cartilage should not be removed from the anterior tracheal wall because an unnecessarily large tracheal defect is left after extubation, which is often the site of bothersome granulations and delayed healing. Some clinicians, however, recommend creating an inferiorly based U-shaped anterior tracheal wall flap, which is then sutured to the inferior aspect of the skin incision. This procedure allows for easy replacement of the tube should it become dislodged in the early postoperative period. The tracheal incision is spread with a Trousseau dilator or large hemostat, and the tube is inserted, taking care not to injure the posterior tracheal wall. The cuff should be checked after insertion by inflation to determine whether the cuff has been damaged during insertion.

As soon as the tube is inserted, patients frequently have a bout of violent coughing, and some patients may become apneic because of loss of hypoxic respiratory drive. This should be anticipated and ventilation instituted if necessary.

Care should be used in the selection of the tracheostomy tube. In recent years, the use of the standard silver tube of the Holinger and Jackson type has largely been abandoned in favor of the silicone or Portex type of tube. The reasons for this change are reduction of trauma to tracheal walls, elimination of an inner cannula, and economy. The length of the tracheostomy tube is also important, and it is often necessary to adjust the length for an individual. This is easily accomplished by trimming a silicone tube, but is impossible with a metal tube. A custom-made tube of specified size may also be used. The diameter of the tube is selected so the largest tube that fits comfortably is used. This is approximately three quarters of the diameter of the trachea. In the average woman, a No. 6 (30 French) or No. 7 (33 French) suffices, and in men, a No. 7 or No. 8 (36 French) is used. A cuffed tube may be necessary when aspiration is a problem or when a positive pressure respirator is required. The low-pressure cuffed tubes now available should be used, but the cuffs should still be deflated at regular intervals.

The skin incision should not be sutured or dressed tightly because this may lead to the development of subcutaneous emphysema, pneumomediastinum, and pneumothorax. A small gauze pad may be placed between the flange of the tube and the skin of the neck.

Percutaneous tracheostomy has been proposed as an alternative to the technique described here. Most references to this procedure are found in the nonotolaryngologic literature. Two methods are described, one involving the use of graded dilators,[14] and the other involving the use of a speculum-like "tracheotome."[15] In either case, the procedure begins with a small external incision, which may be placed below the first tracheal ring[14] or in the suprasternal notch.[15] A tracheostomy tube with an inner diameter of 7 to 8 mm may be placed after dilation of the tract. Advocates of this technique report that it is safe, fast, easy to learn, and may be performed at the bedside rather than in the operating room.[14–16] Some investigators report that the complication rate with the tracheotome system is comparable to that of conventional tracheostomy,[16] but others have reported that the complication rate with the tracheotome system is higher than that with either the graded dilators or conventional tracheotomy.[17] Unfortunately, these conclusions are based on experience with a relatively small number of patients, and long-term results with these techniques are not yet available.

Tracheostomy: Pediatric

Because of the size and consistency of the trachea in pediatric patients, some special points should be noted. Tracheostomy in all cases should be done only after a bronchoscope, endotracheal tube, or catheter has been inserted to provide an airway and some rigidity to the trachea. This facilitates dissection and identification of the trachea. It is easy, in these small patients, to carry dissection too deeply and lateral to the trachea, with resulting damage to the recurrent laryngeal nerve, the common carotid artery, or apex of the pleura. Caution must be used when the tracheal wall is being incised not to insert the knife too deeply and lacerate the posterior wall. A bronchoscope in the trachea helps to avoid this complication.

A vertical skin incision is used. Care must be taken to identify the hyoid bone, thyroid cartilage, and cricoid cartilage by palpation. Before the anterior tracheal wall is incised, silk retraction sutures are placed in either side of the midline. These sutures should not enter the tracheal lumen. The dermis at the margin of the skin incision is then sutured to the anterior wall of the trachea on either side of the incision using absorbable suture material. This reduces the potential for the development of granulation tissue by minimizing the exposure of raw tissue along the tracheostomy tract. A vertical tracheostomy incision is also used (Fig. 27–4). The trachea should be inspected after the tube is inserted to guard against infolding of the cut ends of the tracheal rings, which may contribute to tube displacement and obstruction at the time of decannulation (Fig. 27–5). After the tube has been placed, the silk

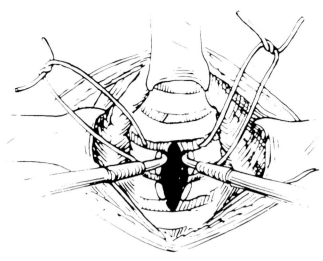

Fig. 27–4. Pediatric tracheostomy. Retraction sutures are used routinely. The dermis may be sutured to the anterior wall of the trachea, to allow for rapid healing of the stoma.

retraction sutures are marked and taped to the chest wall.

Difficulty may be encountered in obtaining a proper fit of the tracheostomy tube. The tube that is too long may ride on the carina or slip into one bronchus, causing atelectasis of the opposite lung. If the curvature is too sharp, the tube may compress the trachea at the upper margin of the tracheal incision, while the lower

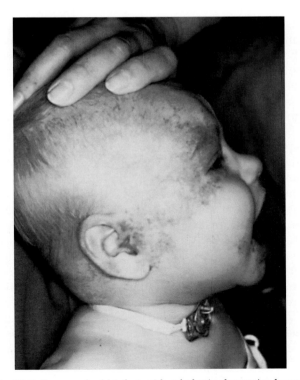

Fig. 27–5. Four-week-old infant with subglottic obstructive hemangiomata requiring tracheotomy. Note the generalized hemangiomata of the face, scalp, and lips. (Courtesy of Dr. G.J. Spector.)

TABLE 27–1. Tracheostomy Tube Sizes

Age	Outside Diameter (mm)	Diameter of Respirator Cannula (mm)
Premature	4.5	4.5 to 5.0
Newborn to 3 months	4.5 to 5.0	5.0 to 5.5
3 to 6 months	5.0 to 5.5	5.5
6 to 12 months	5.0 to 5.5	5.5 to 6.0
1 to 2 years	5.5 to 6.0	5.5 to 6.0
3 years	5.5 to 6.0	6.0 to 6.5

end of the tube rides on the anterior tracheal wall, whereas an excessively obtuse curve may cause ulceration of the posterior tracheal wall and esophagus. Because of these difficulties in infants, postoperative roentgenograms of the neck and chest should be obtained routinely.

A Silastic tube is preferable for use in infants and children. It is flexible, can be cut to appropriate length, and allows a greater movement of air because of the absence of an inner cannula. Suggested tracheostomy tubes for various age children are listed in Table 27–1.

Postoperative Tracheostomy Care
The most important part of the tracheostomy operation is postoperative care, which requires diligence and patience. Many patients, especially children, still die because of inadequate postoperative care.

A tracheostomy tube in a fresh tracheostomy should be left in place for 3 to 5 days before it is changed. By this time, a permanent tract will exist, and there is little danger that one will be unable to reinsert the tube. Changing a tube before this time may result in loss of the tracheal opening into the neck wound, with disastrous consequences. A tracheostomy tube in an infant should not be changed for the first time without a bronchoscope on hand.

Special humidification of inspired air is necessary to prevent tracheitis and crust formation. A room with Walton humidifiers or a tracheal collar with nebulized moisture provides adequate humidification. In addition to atmospheric humidification, 3 or 4 drops of hypotonic saline solution or Ringer's lactate solution should be dropped into the tube every 3 to 4 hours. After several days, the necessity for additional humidity decreases, and it may eventually be discontinued. Patients with thick, copious secretions may require a mucolytic agent to help liquefy secretions for suction removal.

A suction machine is an absolute necessity for tracheostomy care. Sterile rubber catheters with two distal openings with Y-connectors should be available and should be used only in the trachea. Two openings are necessary to prevent the catheter from being sucked against the tracheal wall. A Y-connector allows the catheter to be inserted into the trachea without suction

being exerted, and only during withdrawal is the open end of the Y occluded and suction applied. Suction should be maintained only for 15 seconds or less because it is possible to precipitate hypoxia and cardiac arrest by prolonged suctioning. Suctioning must be done often, especially during the first few days after tracheostomy, because of the increase in tracheobronchial secretions secondary to tracheal irritation.

Children with a need for prolonged tracheostomy maintenance may be cared for at home. This requires careful education of the parents in the use of sterile suctioning technique, humidification, and changing of tracheostomy tubes. A nurse or other practitioner should be specifically trained to prepare the parents for home tracheostomy care. Home health care providers should also be used as needed in the early period of home tracheostomy care. The mortality associated with prolonged pediatric tracheostomy should be reduced as improvements are made in the home care of these patients.

Complications of Tracheostomy
Complications are numerous, but most can be avoided if the operation is carefully performed and if postoperative care is diligent. They may occur at any time postoperatively but can be roughly divided into immediate, intermediate, and late complications, as outlined in Table 27–2.

IMMEDIATE COMPLICATIONS. Immediate complications of tracheostomy include those present at the termination of the operation. When tracheostomy is performed on a patient with a history of chronic hypoxia, the first one or two breaths after the tube is inserted

TABLE 27–2. Complications of Tracheostomy

Immediate
1. Apnea due to loss of hypoxic stimulation of respiration
2. Hemorrhage
3. Surgical injury of neighboring structures, i.e., esophagus, recurrent laryngeal nerve, and cupula of the pleura
4. Pneumothorax and pneumomediastinum
5. Injury of the cricoid cartilage (high tracheostomy)

Intermediate
1. Tracheitis and tracheobronchitis
2. Tracheal erosion and hemorrhage
3. Hypercapnia
4. Atelectasis
5. Displacement of the tracheostomy tube
6. Obstruction of the tracheostomy tube
7. Subcutaneous emphysema
8. Aspiration and lung abscess

Late
1. Persistent tracheocutaneous fistula
2. Stenosis of the larynx or trachea
3. Tracheal granulations
4. Tracheomalacia
5. Difficult decannulation
6. Tracheoesophageal fistula
7. Problems with the tracheostomy scar

may be followed by cessation of respiration. This is caused by physiologic denervation of the peripheral chemoreceptors by the sudden increase of pO_2; because hypoxia may be largely responsible for respiratory drive in these patients, apnea results. Some form of ventilatory assistance is necessary until enough CO_2 is removed to allow a return of sensitivity of central chemoreceptors.

Hemorrhage is a frequent postoperative problem because patients requiring tracheostomy are often hypotensive, and bleeding does not occur until arterial blood pressure is restored or venous pressure is increased by the coughing associated with insertion of the tube.

Patients with sudden respiratory obstruction manifest markedly increased respiratory effort. If tracheostomy is performed in this situation before a temporary endotracheal airway is inserted, air may be sucked into the mediastinum. This may produce circulatory embarrassment, or the air may rupture into a pleural space to produce a simple or tension pneumothorax. Pneumothorax also occurs secondary to laceration of the apex of the pleural space. This injury is most common in children because of the relatively higher position of the pleura in relation to the trachea. A roentgenogram of the chest should be obtained after any difficult tracheostomy and after tracheostomy in a child for early diagnosis of this complication.

Surgical injury of adjacent structures during tracheostomy is usually caused by carrying dissection lateral and deep to the trachea. The trachea can be easily recognized by palpation in the adult, but difficulty may be encountered in children. This can be avoided by inserting a rigid endotracheal airway. Injury to the cricoid cartilage is caused by performance of high tracheostomy, an operation for which no clinical justification exists. Inadvertent performance of high tracheostomy can be avoided if the tracheostomy tube is inserted below the level of the thyroid isthmus.

INTERMEDIATE COMPLICATIONS. Intermediate complications develop during the first few hours or days after tracheostomy. Some degree of tracheitis and tracheobronchitis occurs in all patients because of by-passing of the upper respiratory tract air conditioning. This is particularly severe in infants, and necrotizing tracheobronchitis is a frequent cause of death after tracheostomy in these small patients. Careful attention to humidification, humidifiers, nebulizers with a tracheal collar or a croup tent, and endotracheal instillation of fluid prevent this complication. The use of high concentrations of O_2 has a drying effect on the tracheal mucosa and is best avoided; when it is necessary, a nebulizer must always be used.

Improper fit of a tracheostomy tube is a source of many complications, but careful preoperative selection of a tube followed by postoperative roentgenographic

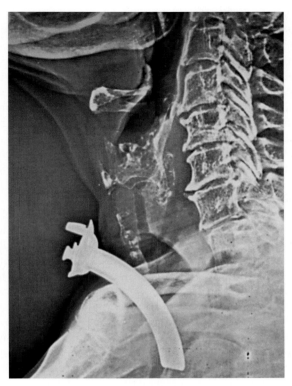

Fig. 27–6. Soft tissue film of traumatic subglottic stenosis. Tracheotomy is anterior to the trachea in the superior mediastinum, compressing the anterior tracheal wall.

evaluation is necessary for prevention (Fig. 27–6). Tubes of excessive length may impinge on the anterior wall of the trachea or the carina, producing partial tracheal obstruction, as well as ulceration and possible rupture of the innominate artery. The tube may extend down one bronchus with resultant atelectasis of the opposite lung. Too short a tube may predispose to displacement of the tube out of the trachea, especially when the neck is flexed in obese individuals or small children.

Obstruction of the tracheostomy tube by a mucus plug or blood clot is caused by lack of care. If suctioning does not relieve obstructive symptoms, changing of the tube is indicated. Equipment to reestablish an airway should be kept in the room of a patient with a fresh tracheostomy.

Subcutaneous emphysema is caused by suturing the incision tightly or packing the wound around the tracheostomy tube. It may also follow insertion of the tube through a small hole in the pretracheal fascia, which then fits snugly around the tube. The emphysema is usually localized in the neck and upper chest but may involve the whole body. If allowed to progress, it may lead to pneumomediastinum and pneumothorax. Any constricting force around the tube between the skin and trachea must be removed to prevent progression. Insertion of a chest tube with an underwater seal may be necessary if pneumothorax develops.

When tracheostomy is performed on patients with alveolar hypoventilation secondary to decreased respiratory effort, secretional obstruction, or chronic pulmonary insufficiency, the improvement in alveolar oxygenation may be enough to relieve hypoxemia, especially if O_2 is administered; however, no associated improvement in the respiratory minute volume may occur, and hypercapnia may persist. In fact, because the hypoxic stimulus of respiration has been removed, hypoventilation may worsen and hypercapnia increase, producing clinical deterioration. Ventilation must be assisted until enough CO_2 is blown off to restore normal respiratory stimulation.

LATE COMPLICATIONS. Late complications of tracheostomy are most frequent when the tube has been left in place for a prolonged period. Persistent tracheocutaneous fistula is caused by epithelialization of the cannula tract. The epithelium must be removed and the wound closed in layers to obtain permanent closure.

Stenosis of the larynx follows injury and perichondritis of the cricoid cartilage. Tracheal stenosis is most common in children and most often follows excision of cartilage from the anterior tracheal wall. Exuberant granulations may develop on the anterior tracheal wall as a result of delayed epithelialization when the patient has a large defect in the anterior tracheal wall and may cause obstruction and bleeding.

Localized tracheomalacia following tracheostomy usually involves the area immediately superior to the tracheal opening. It may be associated with the use of a tracheostomy tube that is too large and sharply angled, causing the tube to impinge on the tracheal ring above the tracheostomy, pushing posteriorly and causing loss of its rigidity. This may be avoided by using a more flexible tube of Teflon or Silastic when necessary. Tracheomalacia may delay decannulation in children.

The use of a vertical skin incision is the most frequent cause of unsightly scar formation. The duration of tracheostomy is also important in scarring, which is lessened by early removal of the tube. Vertical contracture and widening of a hypertrophic scar require a Z-plasty for repair. Other scar problems may occur, including adherence of the skin to the trachea, which may affect swallowing, or formation of a depressed scar. In these cases, the old tracheostomy wound must be revised and closed with careful approximation of tissue layers.

Tracheoesophageal fistula may be a complication of inadvertent incision of the posterior tracheal wall or ulceration secondary to tubal trauma. Tracheal ulceration is most frequent when cuffed tracheostomy tubes are used for prolonged periods. When the use of a cuffed tube is necessary, the cuff should be inspected for symmetry of inflation, because uneven inflation may cause the end of the tube to press on one of the tracheal walls, causing an ulcer and perhaps a fistula. The balloon should be deflated at least once an hour to help prevent mucosal necrosis. Once a fistula is present, spontaneous closure is unlikely, and operative obliteration of the tract will be necessary.

Decannulation

A tracheostomy tube should be left in place no longer than necessary, especially in children. Removal as soon as it is expedient helps to reduce the incidence of tracheobronchitis, tracheal ulceration, tracheal stenosis, tracheomalacia, and persistent tracheocutaneous fistula.

As soon as the patient's condition permits, the size of the tracheostomy tube should be reduced to a size that allows air to bypass the tube and pass into the upper respiratory tract. This helps to avoid physiologic dependence on a large tube because of decreased respiratory resistance. The tube is then plugged, and the adequacy of the airway, as well as the ability to swallow and handle secretions, is determined. When tubal occlusion has been tolerated for 8 to 12 hours, the tube is removed and the tracheocutaneous fistula is taped shut. Bronchoscopy should always be performed before decannulation in the pediatric patient, and any suprastomal granulation tissue must be removed. Immediately after decannulation, the patient must be closely observed, and means for reestablishing the airway must be at hand.

Difficulty with decannulation is a frequent problem in children and may be secondary to both psychic and organic factors. Children have poorly developed respiratory habits that are readily altered by tracheostomy. Children become rapidly accustomed to the reduction in airway resistance associated with the operation, and they are loath to resume the increased respiratory effort required for the use of the normal airway. Tracheostomy also causes a breakdown in the apneic reflex associated with deglutition, and this may cause aspiration by some small children when the tube is first removed, thus instilling a fear of choking.

The tracheal lumen of small children may measure 10 mm in diameter, but because of the membranous posterior wall, collapse to a diameter of 5 mm or less during expiration is frequent. Therefore, the mucosal edema always present with the tracheostomy may result in considerable compromise of the lumen, producing anatomic obstruction.

In addition to the unavoidable problems of tracheostomy in children, errors in procedure and care may be a source of further difficulty in decannulation. These include the use of too large or too sharply curved tubes, excision of tracheal cartilage, recurrent nerve paralysis, and unnecessary prolongation of intubation, which are causes of tracheomalacia, granulation tissue formation, and edema.

When symptoms of respiratory obstruction develop after tubal removal, a thorough investigation should be undertaken to determine the cause. This investigation should include inspiratory and expiratory roentgenograms of the larynx and trachea to note collapse, the presence of granulations, or stenosis. Direct laryngoscopy and tracheoscopy are indicated to assess vocal cord mobility and to inspect the tracheal lumen for granulations, infractured cartilage, or collapse of the lumen.

Treatment is directed at the cause, if one is present. Surgical removal of granulations and bits of loose cartilage is accomplished by direct laryngoscopy. Stenosis must also be corrected surgically. Tracheomalacia involving the area immediately above the tracheostomy site may be improved by using a better-fitting metal tube or constructing an individual flexible tube of synthetic material to relieve pressure on the cartilage and permit return of rigidity. In some cases, it may be necessary to wait for tracheal growth and increased rigidity before decannulation is accomplished.

When no organic cause of obstructive symptoms is obvious, decannulation may be carried out by gradual reduction of cannula size. The use of an indwelling, pliable, plastic nasotracheal tube may be helpful in difficult cases to approximate more closely the normal airway resistance and to provide support for the healing trachea. The tube may be left in place for several days if it is adequately fixed to prevent displacement. This helps the child readjust to the increased respiratory effort required to resume use of the normal respiratory tract while still allowing normal deglutition. Finally, waiting may be the only answer in decannulating some children, and the use of a valved or fenestrated tube permits the use and development of normal speech mechanisms.

Tracheal Fenestration

When the problem of handling secretions is likely to be permanent, because of either the nature of the secretions or irreversible changes in pulmonary function, creation of a permanent tracheal fenestra may be indicated. This allows the use of a tracheostomy tube to be discontinued, thus avoiding the problems associated with continuous wearing of an intratracheal tube. The disadvantages of a tube are that it requires changing, irritates the trachea, and may result in ulceration or squamous metaplasia of the epithelium with loss of ciliary function. In addition, an open tube permits air escape during phonation unless it is occluded each time, whereas a valved tube must be removed every time tracheal suctioning is required.

The fenestra may be constructed so it is covered by an operculum, which, when fixed with a piece of adhesive, obliterates the opening when it is not in use. Moreover, normal speech is possible without the necessity of occluding a tube.

INDICATIONS. The main indication for this procedure is removal of secretions from the tracheobronchial tree. The procedure is most useful in patients with chronic pulmonary insufficiency and chronic lung disease with secretional obstruction. Evidence in the literature indicates that tracheostomy is specifically contraindicated in cystic fibrosis because it diminishes the effectiveness of the cough. It certainly is not practiced in patients with cystic fibrosis today. Other indications include CNS disorders that require assistance with respiration and airway hygiene, neuromuscular diseases that inhibit the movement of the rib cage and diaphragm, and sleep apnea syndromes.

Tracheal fenestration has been advocated in the treatment of chronic pulmonary insufficiency because of an anticipated improvement in alveolar ventilation. This is not borne out by clinical experience, however. The operation is of value, nevertheless, for patients with pulmonary insufficiency who are subject to recurrent attacks of bronchitis with secretion accumulation, which induce respiratory crises. In this situation, the fenestra provides for tracheobronchial hygiene and facilitates the use of intermittent positive pressure breathing or other types of assisted respiration when indicated. This procedure is rarely indicated in the pediatric patient.

TECHNIQUES. Two standard methods are used to produce lined, collapsible, permanent tracheostoma. The first method is basically a double "Z" plasty in the anterior cervical skin. This produces two flaps, which can line the tracheal opening. The cutaneous skin interdigitates with the anterior tracheal wall opening. Care must be taken not to excise or damage anterior tracheal wall cartilage. The end result is the production of an elliptical opening in the trachea. The resultant tracheostoma has tissue tension forces that tend to separate and keep the lumen open; that is, the vector of the tissue tension forces caused by scar contracture are dispersed at oblique angles to the tracheostomal opening. This prevents tracheostomal stenosis and allows for early extubation.

The second method is the use of two horizontal sliding advancement flaps to line the tracheostoma. We never excise the anterior tracheal wall, but create a trap-door opening of two tracheal rings based inferiorly. The use of an inferior tracheal flap provides added rigid protection to the superior mediastinal structures such as the innominate vessels, carotid arteries, and aorta. The superior mediastinal structures have a tendency to be eroded by prosthetic devices, that is, endotracheal tubes, tracheotomy cannulae, and so on, especially when attached to mechanical ventilators, which create significant shearing forces (Fig. 27–7).

The patient is placed in the usual tracheotomy position with the neck extended. Local anesthesia is used. The appropriate incisions are made in the anterior cervical skin, that is, either "Z" plasties or horizontal incisions. Our flaps are usually based one or two fingerbreadths above the clavicles. The skin flaps are mobilized. The underlying soft tissues are excised to remove excess fat and connective tissue to the level of

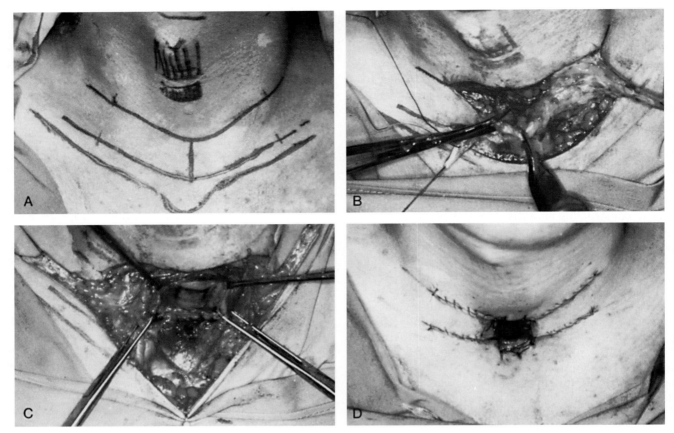

Fig. 27–7. Tracheal fenestration. A. Outlined in methylene blue are the major cartilages (hyoid, thyroid, and cricoid), above and superior border of the clavicle, and sternum below. Two horizontal laterally based skin flaps are in the center of the photograph. B. Flap elevation and fat removal in the subcutaneous layers. Upper and lower flaps are undermined. C. An inferiorly based tracheal flap (two rings) is made. Note that lateral tracheal walls are left intact. D. The skin flap edges are sutured to the cut tracheal wall raw edges.

the superficial layer of the deep cervical fascia. Therefore, the subcutaneous fat and fascia are excised. Occasionally, some muscles need to be released. The thyroid isthmus is cross-clamped, ligated, and excised. The anterior tracheal wall is isolated and carefully preserved. An inferiorly based flap, approximately 1.5 × 1.0 cm, including the third and fourth tracheal rings, is created. The posterior and lateral tracheal walls are preserved. The skin flaps are approximated to the cut margins of the tracheostoma using Vicryl 3–0 sutures. The superior and lateral skin flaps are made intentionally redundant to form an operculum. When wound healing is complete, the patient is able to occlude the fenestra by neck flexion, taping, or finger pressure. This permits relatively normal speech in the intermittent periods. We place a tracheostomy tube with a cuff in the immediate postoperative period in case of mild bleeding. The tube is removed on the third postoperative day.

LARYNGOTRACHEAL STENOSIS

Anatomy

The adult trachea is 10 to 13 cm long (average 11 cm) and 17 to 24 mm in diameter and extends from the inferior border of the cricoid cartilage to the carinal spur. The first tracheal cartilage is partly inset in the lower border of the cricoid cartilage. The cervical trachea is 6 to 7 cm long and the thoracic trachea is 5 to 6 cm long. There are 14 to 20 tracheal cartilages (average width 4 mm), all incomplete posteriorly, or about 2 per cm of trachea. A transverse smooth muscle in the posterior wall of the trachea ("party wall" of the trachea and esophagus) can constrict the lumen minimally and is countered to some extent by the outward spring of the cartilages. The balance between these tensions and the intra- and extraluminal pressures accounts for the tracheal shape and luminal size. Inspiration causes luminal enlargement, most dramatically reflected in the posterior wall. On inspiration the lumen is circular, and on expiration it is crescent shaped.

In young adults, the trachea is mobile and lies within the supple cervical and mediastinal fascial sheaths (pretracheal fascia). During hyperextension of the neck, more than 50% of the trachea lies in the cervical region. On flexion, the trachea can be accommodated almost entirely in the thorax. The carina may lie at the level of the fourth through the seventh thoracic vertebra. Aging causes limitation of tracheal motion, an increase in the intrathoracic location, and less flexibility of the tracheal walls. In the elderly, the cartilages are generally calcified.

The tracheal blood supply is segmental. The upper trachea is supplied by branches of the inferior thyroid artery, the lower trachea by branches of the bronchial arteries with contributions from the subclavian, supreme intercostal, internal thoracic, and innominate arteries.[18–19] These vessels branch anteriorly to the trachea and posteriorly to the esophagus. They arrive at the trachea through lateral pedicles, and posterior to the esophagus they form fine longitudinal anastomoses. Intercartilaginous arteries run transversely, branching into submucosal capillaries. There the vessels travel circumferentially anteriorly between the cartilages and linearly in the posterior "party wall." Close dissection on the external surface can devitalize the anterior and lateral tracheal walls. Intraluminally, the most susceptible area to pressure necrosis is the mucosa overlying a tracheal ring.

The trachea has a pseudostratified, ciliated columnar epithelium interspersed with submucosal tubuloacinar glands and goblet cells. The cilia beat at more than 1000 times per minute and move the mucus blanket 1 to 1.5 cm per minute. Mucosal repair occurs at a rate of 1 mm per 24 hours and is caused by migration of the subepithelial marginal cells. Infection, necrosis, and foreign bodies inhibit mucosal repair. The tracheal cartilages do not regenerate when injured, but heal by calcification or fibrosis.

The recurrent laryngeal nerves lie in the tracheoesophageal grooves and pass medial to the inferior cornua of the thyroid cartilage. The right nerve approaches the trachea at a sharper angle than the left.

The thyroid gland is intimately adherent to the trachea at the second and third tracheal rings. The innominate artery crosses the trachea at its midpoint as it leaves the right side of the aorta and mediastinum. The aorta lies anterior to the carina and crosses the left main stem bronchus. Lymph nodes surround the trachea. These are the left and right paratracheal nodes, the subcarinal nodes, and the tracheobronchial nodes. The lymphatic drainage is segmental and regional.

Classification

Congenital airway malformations are discussed in detail elsewhere in this text, as are inflammatory, neoplastic, and idiopathic diseases causing airway obstruction (see Chap. 28). For completeness, however, an overview of congenital and acquired causes of airway compromise is included here.

Congenital Malformations

Congenital malformations may be divided into two pathologic subgroups. Primary or intrinsic malformations are caused by maldevelopment of the trachea itself. Secondary or extrinsic malformations are secondary to extratracheal malformations, which compress the tracheal airway.[20]

The trachea and primary bronchii form at 9 weeks in utero as a ventral outgrowth of the primitive foregut (tracheal epithelium and glands). The surrounding mesoderm differentiates into cartilage, muscles, vessels, and connective tissue. The growth is not tubular but forms a laryngotracheal groove, which runs caudad to the pharyngeal pouches lengthwise. Damage to these primordial tissues can cause stenosis. Congenital subglottic stenosis can be caused by cartilage agenesis, congenitally small cricoid annulus, or failure of luminal canalization. Tracheal agenesis is generally caused by mesenchymal failure, which leads to a failure of luminal development below the cricoid and bronchial maldevelopment from the midesophagus region. Atresia is characterized by a membranous or cartilaginous stenosis at the junction of the larynx and trachea. Intrinsic stenosis of the trachea is divided into three types, depending on the extent and form. Cantrell and Guild distinguish among these types: (1) generalized hypoplasia—diffuse tracheal narrowing; (2) fusiform stenosis—narrowest part at the carina; and (3) segmental stenosis—selective areas of fibrosis and tracheal cartilage agenesis.[21] Holinger and associates noted that the intrinsic stenosis is most frequently secondary to a fibrous membranous circular web.[22–24] The tracheal lumen has a characteristic hourglass shape. In addition, other malformations include aplasia of the membranous wall, fibrous tracheal rings, cartilaginous rings, cartilage duplication, or wegs. The tracheal orifice in a tracheoesophageal fistula is usually above the carina or left main stem bronchus.[25] These fistulas are caused by faulty development of the tracheoesophageal septum. Other causes of obstruction are tracheal bronchi or aberrant take-off of the right main stem bronchus.

Tracheomalacia causes stenosis by the absence or deformity of the tracheal cartilages. This may be segmental or diffuse. It is associated with other malformations, such as, auricular cartilage, genitourinary, and cardiac defects. Segmental cartilaginous malformations are more common in the cervical or carinal regions.[24] In addition, cartilaginous segments may be fused to each other or may be completely annular with union of the free ends. A rare malformation is tracheomegaly, which is associated with respiratory tract dyskinesia, cystic fibrosis, and generalized dilatation of the bronchi. Tracheal diverticuli are rare. They usually arise from the posterolateral wall and are asymptomatic. Tracheoceles are diverticula that do not communicate with the lumen. Most diverticula and tracheoceles occur in the "party wall."

Extrinsic tracheal compression is a less common cause of congenital tracheal stenosis (10% of cases). In this group, vascular compressions constitute the largest entity.[26-29] The ventral aorta gives rise to the innominate arteries. The descent of the heart into the thorax draws the vessels caudad. The degeneration of the dorsal or retroesophageal connections and of the right aortic arch breaks the vascular ring that surrounds the mediastinal viscera. Maldevelopment of the vascular structures can cause tracheal compression because of

a double aortic arch, aberrant right subclavian artery, right aortic arch with a left ductus or ligamentum arteriosum, displaced innominate arteries, and anomalous left pulmonary artery. Other anomalies include dextroposition of the left common carotid artery, incomplete vascular rings, anomalous azygous vein, anomalous vena cava, etc. The double arch and aberrant innominate artery malformations are most common. On bron-

TABLE 27–3. Classification of Tracheal Obstruction

I. Developmental
  A. Primary Tracheal Malformations
    1. Agenesis or aplasia
    2. Atresia
    3. Segmental cartilage hypoplasia
    4. Intrinsic tracheal stenosis
    5. Congenital subglottic stenosis
    6. Tracheomegaly
    7. Tracheal diverticula
    8. Tracheal bronchi and bifurcation anomalies
    9. Congenital tumors—hamartoma, angiomata
    10. Tracheoesophageal malformations
  B. Secondary Tracheal Compression
    1. Aortic arch anomalies—most common
      a. left innominate artery
      b. right-sided left common carotid artery
      c. double aorta—vascular ring
      d. right-sided aorta
      e. aberrant ductus arteriosus
      f. aberrant subclavian artery
      g. persistent arterial ligaments
      h. anomalous azygos vein, vena cava, or pulmonary artery
    2. Esophageal anomalies
      a. megaesophagus
      b. Tracheoesophageal fistula
      c. atresia
    3. Thymic cysts and remnants
    4. Ectopic thyroidal tissue
      a. intratracheal goiter
      b. congenital mediastinal goiter
      c. myxedema
    5. Mediastinal cysts and tumors
      a. teratoma
      b. cystic hygroma
      c. lymphangioma
      d. cysts—hilum, paratracheal, intrapericardial and retrosternal
II. Inflammatory
  A. Primary
    1. Granulomatous tuberculosis, sarcoid, scleroma
    2. Luetic
    3. Bacterial—diphtheria
    4. Fungal—histoplasmosis
  B. Secondary
    1. Mediastinitis
    2. Thyroiditis
    3. Perforated viscus—esophageal perforation
III. Traumatic
  A. External Trauma
    1. Blunt neck injuries
    2. Blunt chest injuries
    3. Penetrating neck injuries
    4. Postoperative

  B. Internal Trauma
    1. Postintubational
    2. Post-tracheostomy
    3. Cuff injuries
    4. Foreign bodies
    5. Chemical injuries
    6. Physical injuries
IV. Neoplastic
  A. Benign Tracheal Tumors
    1. Papilloma
    2. Fibroma
    3. Chondroma
    4. Glandular tumors
  B. Malignant Tracheal Tumors
    1. Squamous cell carcinoma
    2. Adenoid cystic carcinoma
    3. Mucoepidermoid carcinoma
    4. Undifferentiated or oat cell carcinoma
    5. Chondrosarcoma
    6. Lymphosarcoma
    7. Lymphoma
  C. Malignant Extratracheal Tumors
    1. Invasive thyroid adenocarcinoma
    2. Metastatic tumors to mediastinum and hilum
    3. Primary mediastinal tumors
    4. Esophageal carcinomas
    5. Thymic malignancies
  D. Benign Extratracheal Tumors
    1. Neck—goiter
    2. Mediastinal—substernal goiter, thymoma
    3. Tuberculosis
    4. Sarcoidosis
V. Mechanical
  A. Obesity
  B. Pickwickian syndrome
  C. Micrognathia—Pierre Robin syndrome
  D. Secretional obstruction
    1. Severe CNS injuries
    2. Tracheitis sicca
    3. Bronchiolitis
    4. Broncholiths
    5. Bronchiectasis
    6. Immobile cilia syndrome
VI. Idiopathic
  A. Tracheopathia osteoplastica
  B. Relapsing polychondritis
  C. Amyloidosis
  D. Tracheomalacia
  E. Eosinophilic granulomatosis

choscopy, an anterior tracheal pulsatile indentation implies an aberrant innominate artery, a posterior esophageal pulsatile compression, an aberrant right subclavian artery, and bilateral pulsatile indentations a vascular ring. Angiography is required for confirmation. Because tracheal compression occurs during vascular development, tracheal indentations persist even after vascular release.

Tracheal obstruction caused by extrinsic masses in the neck and mediastinum result from compression of the noncalcified flexible tracheal cartilages. Esophageal compression can be of two types: prolapse of the posterior membranous tracheal wall or compression by a distended bulk of a megaesophagus or esophageal achalasia.[30] These are associated with overspill aspiration. Thyroid compression can be caused by three types of disorders: intratracheal thyroid, cervical thyroid goiters, and mediastinal thyroid tumors.[31] Other paratracheal congenital masses are listed in Table 27–3.

Acquired Diseases

Malignant tracheal tumors are rare, occurring at the rate of 2.7 cases per million people per year.[32–33] The two major types of malignant lesions are squamous cell carcinoma and adenoid cystic carcinoma.[34–36] The

major presenting symptoms occur in the following sequence: dyspnea, hemoptysis, cough, wheezing, dysphagia, hoarseness, stridor, and pneumonia. Dyspnea, wheezing, and stridor are the presenting symptoms in 89% of the patients[37,38] (Fig. 27–8).

Benign tracheal tumors can originate from the epithelial lining (papilloma), connective tissues (fibroma, fibromyoma, chondroma, osteoma, osteochondroma) and glandular elements (adenoma).[39] The most frequent tumors are papillomas, which account for 56% of all tracheal tumors in children. The next most common lesion is the fibroma.

Chronic inflammatory disease may also cause tracheal stenosis. Tuberculosis (Mycobacterium tuberculosis) is well known to produce chronic cicatricial sequelae in the pulmonary system. Negus reviewed 1255 tuberculous autopsies and found a 10.4% incidence of tracheobronchial disease.[40] The ulcerative and nonulcerative forms of tuberculosis have a predilection for the posterior tracheal wall, the tips of the tracheal cartilage rings, and the intercartilaginous spaces. The larynx may also be affected, usually in association with pulmonary disease. Tracheal involvement implies advanced pulmonary disease. Few patients survive such advanced disease. The treatment of tuberculosis is

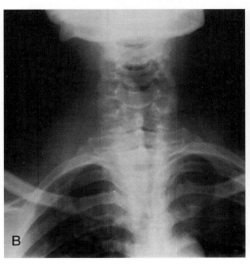

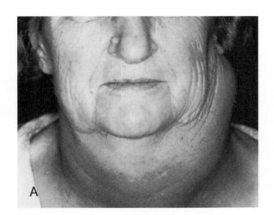

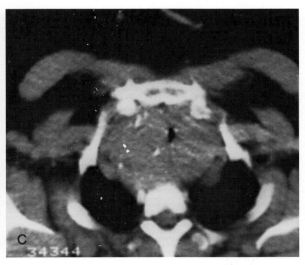

Fig. 27–8. Large goiter, present for many years. A. Note that patient is in no significant distress. B. Neck x-ray study denotes trachea deviation with substernal extension. C. CT scan demonstrates the substernal goiter extent and tracheal compression circumferentially.

medical, but the tracheal stenosis is corrected surgically.

Scleroma (Klebsiella rhinoscleromatis or Frisch bacillus) can cause tracheal lesions in 3% of the cases. These are secondary to laryngeal involvement. The obstruction is treated by intubation, dilatation, or resection. During medical management, dilatation and indwelling endotracheal stents are mainstays of tracheal therapy.[41]

Diphtheria (Corynebacterium diphtheriae) may involve the trachea and bronchi in 10% of the cases. The thick, grayish, patchy membrane, which bleeds on stripping, can form casts of the entire airway. The patient may asphyxiate from the laryngotracheal membrane, vocal cord paralysis (usually late stages or delayed), tracheal casts, or cicatricial tracheal stenosis.

Other causes of tracheal stenosis should also be remembered. Syphilis (Treponema pallidum) is a rare cause of tracheitis. The tracheitis can be caused by tracheal gummas or extension and compression from an aortic luetic aneurysm. Laryngeal syphilis may cause pseudoepithelial hyperplasia; chronic inflammation may lead to scarring and laryngeal stenosis. Histoplasmosis (Histoplasma capsulatum) generally causes mediastinal tracheal compression because of fibrosis or enlargement of mediastinal lymph nodes.[42] Tracheopathia osteoplastica is a disease of unknown cause marked by cartilaginous and osseous formations within the submucosa of the tracheobronchial tree. Its course is generally benign. Relapsing polychondritis and other collagen diseases can cause rare tracheomalacia and collapse. Eosinophilic granulomatosis has been described in the trachea as a lytic lesion of the tracheal rings. Amyloidosis can occur as a solitary nodule obstructing the trachea,[43,44] or it may occur in single or multiple sites in the larynx. Only about one dozen primary amyloid tumors of the trachea have been reported in the literature. Secondary amyloidoses are most often associated with tracheal, mediastinal, or pulmonary malignant diseases; lymphomas; or diseases of the reticuloendothelial system. Another form is the diffuse tracheobronchial amyloidosis of unknown etiology.[45] These lesions appear as pale lilac-blue nodules under the mucosa. They may cause narrowing and rigidity of the tracheobronchial tree. Sarcoidosis and Wegener's granulomatosis may involve the larynx, but the trachea is rarely involved. Radiation may cause tracheitis sicca, secretional obstruction, fibrosis, and rarely stenosis. Chemical tracheal stenoses caused by lye or acid ingestion are rare. More common are injuries caused by steam, irritant gases, burning gases, or hot air from fires. In children, one must always suspect inhalation of foreign bodies. These injuries may persist over long periods of time. They can cause mucosal ulceration and secondary proliferative granulation or cicatricial stenosis. Other causes of intermittent stenosis are laryngotracheal infections, angioneurotic edema, or drug sensitivity.

Traumatic Tracheostenosis

Many classifications of tracheal stenosis have been proposed (Table 27–3), based on different pathophysiologic parameters. Pearson divides the stenosis into an exogenous and endogenous group based on the mechanism of injury.[46] McComb,[47] considering only cicatricial stenosis of the trachea, distinguishes among four groups: short annular stenosis, tubular cervical stenosis, tubular thoracic stenosis, and tracheostomal stenosis. Post-tracheostomy stenosis may be classified as stomal, suprastomal,[48] intermediate, or distal (Fig. 27–9). Stomal and suprastomal stenosis has accounted for 90% of the cases. A useful classification is that of Montgomery,[49] who classifies cervical tracheal stenosis after tracheostomy based on the location and pathophysiology of the injury. He has four subgroups: above tracheostomy, at tracheostomy, just below tracheostomy, and distal to tracheostomy tube (Fig. 27–10). This concept is important because 90% of obstructions are caused by intubation or tracheostomy injuries (Fig. 27–11). Meyer and Flemming classified stenosis into functional stenosis (tracheomalacia), cicatricial stenosis (partial loss of substance), and defects created after tumor resection.[48] This classification is based on two concepts: the length

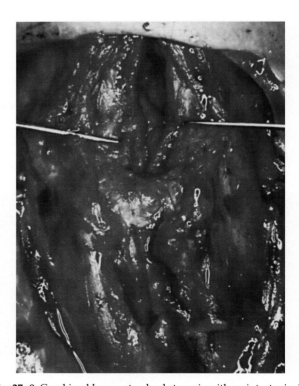

Fig. 27–9. Combined laryngotracheal stenosis with an intact cricoid. The nerve hooks demonstrate laryngeal component of stenosis. Below the intact cricoid is a collapsed trachea with intraluminal granulation. This is a complication of prolonged intubation with a large endotracheal tube and an improperly high tracheostomy.

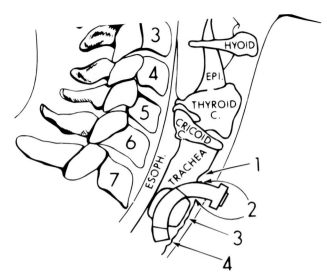

Fig. 27–10. Four types of post-tracheostomy tracheal injuries: (1) above tracheotomy, (2) at tracheotomy, (3) below tracheotomy, and (4) distal to tracheotomy.

of the stenosis and the thickness of the tracheal wall or lumen that is lost. We have used computed tomography to delineate pediatric subglottic and tracheal stenosis as mucosal defects, supporting cartilaginous defects, and combined stenosis.[50] From a surgical point of view, it appears that the following parameters are important: the length of the stenosis, the location of the defect, the thickness of the stenosis (does it involve mucosa, submucosa, or cartilaginous framework or is it a combined defect?), the age of the patient (older patients can undergo smaller resections), and the nature of the injury (e.g., cuff injuries are annular, suprastomal and tracheal cannula tip injuries involve the

anterior wall, and intubational injuries involve mostly the mucosa and submucosa). In general, the incidence of tracheal stenosis, based on location of the lesion, decreases as one moves inferiorly from the larynx. The most common lesions, listed in a decreasing order of incidence, are laryngotracheal, subglottic, suprastomal, stomal, infrastomal, high retrosternal, and low retrosternal.

POSTINTUBATIONAL STENOSIS. Florange and associates classified four types of endotracheal tube injuries: type I, superficial mucosal ulceration; type II, submucosal and perichondreal damage; type III, cartilaginous necrosis with venous and lymphatic engorgement and with cartilaginous or membranous inflammation; and type IV, tracheal necrosis and fistulization[51] (Fig. 27–12). The major positive correlation is the relative size of the outer diameter of the endotracheal tube to the size of the tracheal lumen; that is, the diameter of the endotracheal tube is too large for the tracheal lumen. Lesser factors are traumatic or forceful intubation, duration of intubation, persistent tubal motion (mechanical respirators), and the use of corticosteroids. The endotracheal tube causes mucosal trauma, pressure necrosis of the submucosa, occlusion or thrombosis of the tracheal vasculature, and avascular necrosis of the tracheal cartilages. These are followed by sepsis caused by retention of purulent secretions because the

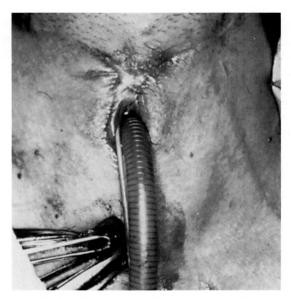

Fig. 27–11. High tracheostomy resulting in laryngotracheal stenosis, necrosis for cricoid ring, and subglottic stenosis.

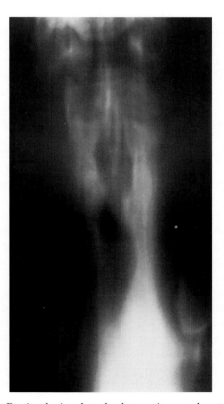

Fig. 27–12. Postintubational tracheal stenosis secondary to improperly inflated cuff. Note granulation tissue subglottically and necrosis of the right tracheal wall.

ciliary motion of the tracheal lining is locally damaged and the mucous blanket remains stationary. In severe cases, perforation, fistulization, and mediastinitis are seen. The posterior wall that is most flaccid is less easily damaged (this is not true if a high-pressure cuff is used). Thus, tracheoesophageal fistulas are less common than cartilaginous (a more rigid framework) damage.

Benjamin has recently reported his observations on post-intubational laryngeal injuries.[13] His findings are reviewed earlier in this chapter, in the discussion of complications of endotracheal intubation.

Endotracheal cuff injuries generally cause circumferential stenosis because of the equal distribution of the intraluminal pressure by the self-adjusting flexible cuff. Unlike primary mucosal injury of the endotracheal tube, cuff injuries initially cause vascular occlusion. Arteriolar pressure in the tracheal mucosa is 40 mm Hg. Inflation of the cuff to the point of a seal can cause pressure necrosis and tracheal wall distortion (the posterior tracheal wall is flexible). Moreover, secretions tend to pool above the cuff. The tube is fixed in place, but the movement of the head and breathing cause tracheal motion, resulting in shearing forces between the cuff and the tracheal wall. In fact, tracheal stenoses tend to occur slightly higher than the cuff, indicating that the most dangerous area for stenosis is the interface between the tube and the cuff. Grillo and Cooper noted that symptoms start at 10 to 42 days after extubation.[52,53] An attempt to avoid this injury has been made by the use of low-pressure cuffs and double-cuff systems. The latter are used to alternate the location of the cuff pressures in the tracheal wall lumen. The shearing forces between the two cuffs, however, characteristically cause the stenosis at the interface of the two cuffs. The soft low-pressure cuffs, on the other hand, tend to be overinflated and may protrude over the endotracheal lumen, causing airway obstruction. Today we use atraumatic, compliant, low-pressure, and pressure-absorbent (reservoir chamber) cuffs. Examples of these are made by such companies as Shiley and Bivona.

Other traumatic variables that should be considered are the sterilization procedures (gas sterilization can produce ethylene oxides, polyvinyl chloride, alkylating agents, and hydrolytic products, which are toxic to the tracheal mucosa); traumatic suctioning (the vacuum invaginates the mucosa into the catheter and causes hemorrhagic lesions); patient positioning and ventilation assistance (agitated patients and respirators tend to create shearing forces between the trachea and endotracheal tube).

POST-TRACHEOTOMY STENOSIS. The incidence of tracheal stenosis has increased because of the increased use of endotracheal intubation and tracheostomy.[54–57] Tracheostomy is used primarily for alleviation of airway obstruction, for airway hygiene for secretional

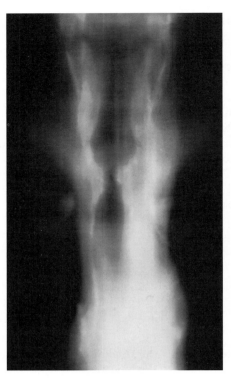

Fig. 27–13. Post-tracheotomy tracheal stenosis at the fenestration site. The tracheal lumen is filled with granulation tissue.

clearance and, with assisted ventilation, for treatment of respiratory insufficiency. Tracheotomy can cause four types of tracheal stenosis (Fig. 27–13). These have been described by Montgomery.[49]

POST-TRAUMATIC STENOSIS. The chin and sternum protect the trachea from external trauma. Extension of the head exposes the trachea to anteroposterior blunt trauma (vehicular accidents).[58,59] Penetrating tracheal injuries are usually oblique or lateral to the neck.[60] The tracheal injury varies with the size, shape, site of impact, and force of impact of the offending object. Blunt objects usually buckle the anterior tracheal wall and bow the lateral walls. These in-fracture the cartilage or produce minimal injuries. High-velocity blunt cervical injuries such as the front seat passenger automobile injury to the extended neck by the dashboard may cause cricotracheal avulsion, partial or complete. The first tracheal ring usually remains attached to the larynx because of its subcricoid insertion. There may be tracheal separation with retraction of the distal segment into the mediastinum. The esophagus, recurrent laryngeal nerves, and larynx are frequently injured. Lack of dyspnea in tracheal avulsion can be misleading because the pretracheal fascia may form a rigid temporary airway. On the other hand, an extended neck striking a wire or rope at high velocities (motorcycle accidents) can result in clean tracheal transection. The patient may have no associated external neck wound.

Less frequently, blunt chest trauma causes tracheal

avulsion or stenosis.[61] When the trachea is injured, however, it can become manifest in two different ways. Compression of the trachea between the sternum and thoracic vertebral bodies can cause longitudinal tears at the cartilaginous and membranous junctions. If these are associated with high-velocity injuries, rapid extension of the neck will increase the shearing forces at points of relative fixation such as the carina (most common), bronchi, esophagus, or aorta. If the glottis is closed at the time of tracheal compression (breath holding) and the trachea is filled with air under pressure, a blunt injury can cause a blow-out with rupture and separation of the trachea within the mediastinum. This generally leads to massive distal stenosis. Persistent coughing, subcutaneous emphysema, xiphisternal crepitation (Hamman's sign), dyspnea, cyanosis, loss of suprasternal curvature, ecchymosis, hemoptysis, and pneumothorax lead to a suspicion of substernal tracheal laceration.

Penetrating tracheal injuries are usually secondary to gunshot wounds that enter the visceral compartment from a lateral or oblique direction. These are limited high-velocity injuries. Usually, two or three tracheal rings are damaged. The major problem is the associated secondary sepsis and chondritis. Major injuries to neck vessels and esophagus are common. Lacerations by sharp objects (knives) are usually anteroposterior injuries. Premeditated injuries are associated with major vascular injuries (primarily lacerated internal jugular veins). If the patient can be resuscitated, repair is fairly simple. Occasionally, one or both recurrent nerves are damaged.

Diagnostic Assessment and Evaluation

History and Physical Examination

Patients with chronic upper airway obstruction manifest slow, deep breathing to decrease the work of respiration. In the acute phase, the breathing is rapid and shallow. The voice changes and becomes weak and breathy. The tidal volume is increased, but the lung volume and FEV_1 remain normal. The chest radiograph may also remain normal. The patient may demonstrate stridor over the trachea. This is especially true on inspiration after prolonged intubation. Occasionally, the patient may have rhonchi or low-pitched groaning or whistling over the trachea, especially with increased retention of secretions. These are more common in inspiration. The expiratory phase of respiration, however, is prolonged. The obstructive disease does not respond to bronchodilators (i.e., the expiratory phase does not change with medications) but is markedly improved with assisted respiration or tracheostomy.

The patient complains of dyspnea or a conscious sensation of breathlessness. This is mediated from the muscle receptors in the chest wall and chemoreceptors of the carotid and aortic bodies by way of the glossopharyngeal and vagus nerves to the CNS respiratory center and then to the higher consciousness centers of the cortex. The maximal breathing capacity is reduced, and the respiratory rate is less than 12 per minute. Many patients have a persistent cough. This may be a weak short cough with severe tracheal obstruction, a brassy cough with aortic aneurysm compression, a dry persistent cough with a foreign body (in the acute phase with a large foreign body it may be associated with asphyxia or a tracheal clap), a dry unproductive cough with breathlessness in chronic tracheal obstruction, or hemoptysis with tissue expectoration with tracheal tumors. Patients may have fever in the presence of associated tracheobronchial or pulmonary aspiration or infection (pneumonia). Persistent coughing leads to generalized chest wall and muscle pain. In chronic disease, cyanosis may occur secondary to higher levels of reduced hemoglobin in the dermal subpapillary venous plexus. The severity and duration of the obstruction determine the symptom complex at presentation.

Upper airway obstruction has various clinical signs. These are divided into tracheal, laryngeal, and soft tissue signs. Fixation of the larynx on upward motion during respiration or swallowing is a sign of paratracheal or mediastinal disease. A laryngeal tug with each heartbeat is a sign of compression of the trachea by a vascular ring or aortic aneurysm. Laryngeal tactile fremitus during phonation or respiration denotes tracheal obstruction.

The trachea may be deviated or displaced sideways. In atelectasis, it is displaced to the side of the lesion on inspiration. In pneumothorax, it is displaced to the opposite side on expiration. The suprasternal notch may be shallow or eliminated with superior mediastinal masses or deepened by anterior lesions, such as thyroid carcinomas. Fluctuation in the suprasternal notch may imply esophageal dilation, as in achalasia.

Soft tissue signs include palpable paratracheal and supraclavicular metastatic lymph nodes. Persistent venous distension in the neck veins is a sign of increased venous pressure secondary to chronic coughing and respiratory effort or cor pulmonale. Crepitation in the neck indicates mediastinal emphysema or a ruptured viscus. Ecchymosis denotes neck and mediastinal bleeding. Normally, during Valsalva and Mueller (the opposite of Valsalva) maneuvers, one notes a corresponding bulging or retraction of the supraclavicular soft tissues. These are absent in patients with tracheal stenosis. Percussion may denote a widened mediastinum. d'Espine's sign indicates tubular breathing over the thoracic spine or anterior chest wall with tracheal obstruction. Of course, the stridor generally remains the same during inspiration and expiration, especially when the glottis is open. The latter is pathognomonic for tracheal stenosis.

Other observations include a prolongation of the forced vital capacity (greater than 6 seconds), increase in functional residual capacity, increase in airway resistance, and decrease in the FEV_1 (forced expiratory volume during the first second of expiration).

Diagnostic Testing

Radiologic tests are required to reveal the location, extent or composition of the stenosis.[37,38,62,63] Overpenetrated, lateral soft tissue neck films or xeroradiograms are excellent to demonstrate the tracheal air column. Tomograms delineate the site, type, and composition of the stenosis.[50] They are particularly helpful in delineating mucosal cicatricial stenosis from injuries to the cartilaginous framework and the length of the stenosis. The use of computed tomography in the coronal plane has allowed the precise delineation of the stenosis, its composition, and its length. Fluoroscopy is useful in delineating dynamic functional obstructions, such as tracheomalacia and sternal retraction with tracheal collapse. Contrast studies producing tracheograms are rarely used because they may lead to airway compromise and poor pulmonary hygiene. Esophagoscopy and esophageal contrast studies are used if one suspects esophageal laceration or concomitant penetrating injury.

Pulmonary function tests and flow-volume loop studies (Fig. 27–14) may be useful in identifying the level of the obstruction. Endoscopy is reserved for tracheal assessment before definitive therapy. Flexible fiberoptic bronchoscopy has facilitated the evaluation and has decreased the risk of preoperative and postoperative manipulation. Fiberoptic bronchoscopy is performed under topical or local anesthesia, with general anesthesia standby. One must delineate the superior border of the stenosis as related to cardinal landmarks such as vocal cords and cricoid or tracheostomy orifices. The inferior border can be delineated by the previous radiologic studies and at exploration.

Rigid bronchoscopy is useful for emergency treatment of patients with tracheal obstruction. The bronchoscope may be insinuated past the obstruction and the distal airway suctioned and maintained. Then a careful tracheostomy is performed over the bronchoscope. A biopsy may also be taken at this time. The view of the obstruction is better than with a flexible bronchoscope, even if the latter is passed through an endotracheal tube.

Surgical Repairs: Adult

Epithelial Cicatrization

Defects involving loss of tracheal epithelium without concomitant structural defects, such as cartilaginous suprastructural loss, may be handled endoscopically. Acute lesions resulting in granulomas or granulation tissue within the airway can be resected endoscopically. CO_2 laser excision may be preferred to manual or mechanical excision because it reduces the need for tracheostomy. The use of corticosteroids is widespread, although it has not been shown to be of benefit in controlled studies. Nevertheless, we use systemic corticosteroids, which are tapered over a period of 1 to 2 weeks.

Chronic cicatrization is the result of excessive circumferential loss of mucosa. If, after repeated excisions, the stenosis is not relieved, we proceed to an open procedure. The latter usually involves a vertical or castellated incision[64] in the anterior tracheal wall. This is preceded by a low tracheostomy and a careful dissection to avoid devitalizing the tracheal cartilages. The pretracheal fascia and lateral tracheal vascular pedicles are not separated. The cicatricial stenosis is resected carefully, and a silicone or Portex stent lined with oral mucosa or dermis is inserted. The stent is fixed by passing guide wires attached to cutaneous buttons. The edges are carefully approximated with absorbable sutures (4–0 Vicryl). The tracheal cartilages are closed primarily and reinforced by the pretracheal fascia or strap muscles. The stent is removed at 4 to 6 weeks endoscopically. We prefer to use a stent separate from the tracheostomy tube and to lower the tracheostomy below the level of the stenosis. If this is not possible, a Montgomery T-tube is used as the mold for the grafting tissue.[65]

Dilatation has largely been abandoned as ineffective. To dilate a moving functional organ and lyse adhesions indiscriminately is illogical. This creates more trauma and causes progression of the stenosis. The

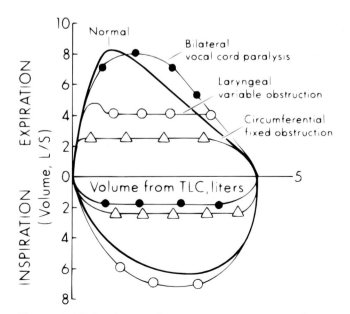

Fig. 27–14. Air flow loop studies on various upper airway obstructive lesions. Note that various lesions can be delineated by the inspiratory and expiratory flow curves.

main problem is a loss of surface epithelium and not the cicatrization.

Composite Anterior Wall Defects

Acute crushing anterior tracheal wall injuries without massive tissue loss are repaired with minimal debridement and careful approximation. After a preliminary tracheostomy, the repaired area is stented for 2 to 3 weeks. This maintains the tracheal lumen while the tracheal wall integrity is reconstituted. In these cases we do not use corticosteroids, but maintain the patients on systemic antibiotics. On stent removal, mild granulation tissue is carefully resected endoscopically with a CO_2 laser. We avoid diathermycoagulation.

Suprastomal stenosis is a result of traumatic, improper, or high tracheotomy with buckling or fracture of the cartilage and subglottic edema. These stenoses become manifest late after extubation. Generally, the patient has no associated tissue loss. The best approach is to lower the tracheostomy orifice by means of a horizontal (apron) incision. The buckled or subluxed cartilage is fixed in its shape by fibrosis. A vertical incision is used to open the trachea. Occasionally, partial lateral cartilaginous releasing incisions are used to mobilize the anterior tracheal wall. A careful approximation over a stent, using extraluminal 4–0 Vicryl sutures, is instituted. If the anterior wall cartilage is missing, it may be reconstituted by a hyoid bone or septal or auricular cartilaginous graft (Fig. 27–15). Occasionally, suturing the strap muscles and fascia over the defect and placing traction sutures (tracheopexy) is all that is necessary. If a graft is required, we prefer to use a separate stent and tracheostomy cannula (Fig. 27–16). If inadequate space is available, we use the Montgomery T-tube (Fig. 27–17). If mucosal defects are present, the stents are lined with dermis or oral buccal mucosal grafts.

Tracheostomal and infrastomal anterior wall stenoses are handled in a fashion similar to that discussed

previously, except the tracheostoma may not be lowered. In such cases, we use the T-tube (the largest size that will fill the lumen).[66] Again, the cartilages are released from their fibrosis and reapproximated. Grafting is used when epithelium is missing. This is the usual case because of the invariable intraluminal granuloma. Lateral tracheopexy sutures are applied to the tracheal wall and are sutured to the clavicular periosteum. An anterior tracheal wall gap is not approximated but covered by the inner investing strap muscle fascia (sternohyoid muscle). The stent is left in place for 4 to 12 weeks. Removal of the stent is followed by a tracheal tube, which may be fenestrated and of a smaller diameter (No. 6 or 5). Intraluminal granulation is removed with a CO_2 laser.

Composite Circumferential Defects

The method of repair of these defects varies with the level of the stenosis. In general, lower tracheal stenosis is repaired using the technique of resection and anastomosis; higher tracheal and subglottic defects are repaired using either augmentation grafting or resection and anastomosis.

Most recent reports of the repair of higher tracheal and subglottic stenosis are based on experience with variations of the resection and anastomosis procedure. These reports make reference to the early work of Ogura and Roper,[67] Gerwat and Bryce,[68] and Pearson and colleagues.[69] Grillo successfully decannulated 16 of 18 patients with low subglottic and upper tracheal stenosis.[70] Resection with primary laryngotracheal anastomosis was used for each patient. The technique varied slightly for true circumferential stenosis, as compared with anterolateral stenosis. Some patients were extubated immediately, whereas others had a tracheostomy in the perioperative period. Grillo and associates subsequently reported their experience over the next 10 years, with a total of 80 patients.[71] Most had postintubational stenosis. Thirty-one of these patients had extended cricoid resection resulting from circumferential stenosis. Overall, 74 of the 80 patients were decannulated, with satisfactory or better results. Of 35 patients with idiopathic laryngotracheal stenosis, 32 were successfully decannulated. Only 1 patient had progression of the stenosis to the lower trachea.[72]

Other investigators have reported similar results. Macchiarini and associates used tracheal resection and anastomosis to treat 26 adult patients with postintubational subglottic stenosis.[73] A partial cricoidectomy was also performed. The stenosis treated in this series extended up to 1 cm below the true vocal cords. Good results were reported in 96%. Bisson and associates performed 200 tracheal sleeve resections and primary anastomosis.[74] Twenty-one patients also had a partial cricoid resection. Overall, 88% were eventually decannulated. The results were equally good for the patients who also had some degree of subglottic stenosis. Paris

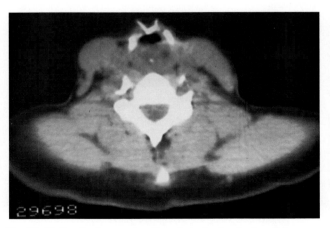

Fig. 27–15. Tracheal reconstruction. Anterior tracheal wall is reconstituted with a hyoid bone graft.

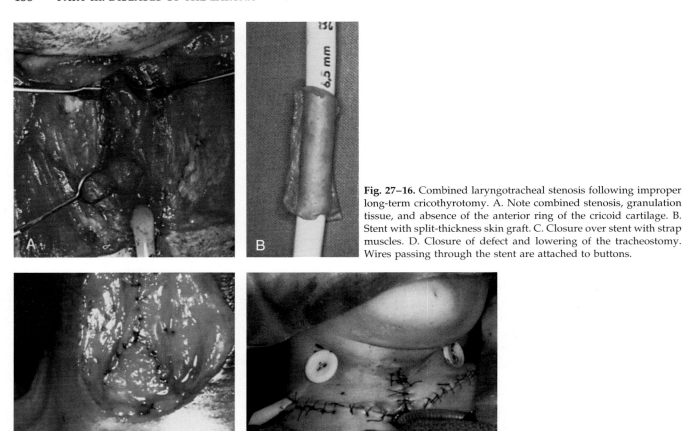

Fig. 27–16. Combined laryngotracheal stenosis following improper long-term cricothyrotomy. A. Note combined stenosis, granulation tissue, and absence of the anterior ring of the cricoid cartilage. B. Stent with split-thickness skin graft. C. Closure over stent with strap muscles. D. Closure of defect and lowering of the tracheostomy. Wires passing through the stent are attached to buttons.

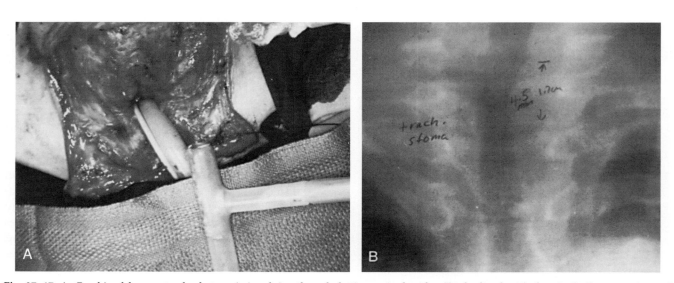

Fig. 27–17. A. Combined laryngotracheal stenosis involving the subglottis repaired with a T-tube lined with dermis. B. Postoperative and postextubational result.

and associates used a variety of procedures in treating 54 patients with tracheal stenosis and 27 patients with laryngotracheal stenosis.[75] Of the patients with laryngotracheal stenosis, anteroposterior grafting was performed in some, and resection with anastomosis was performed in others. A mortality rate of 9% was reported; 97% of the survivors were decannulated. Reintervention was more common in patients with laryngotracheal involvement than in those with tracheal involvement alone, however.

A special note should be made of a recent series in which circumferential tracheal resection with anastomosis was combined with laryngofissure for laryngeal reconstruction.[76] A stent was used in each case. Thirteen of 15 patients were successfully decannulated. Finally, although most of the experience cited previously has been with cricotracheal resection and anastomosis, anteroposterior cricoid division with augmentation grafting has been used successfully in treating subglottic and glottic stenosis in adults. These techniques are similar to those reported in the extensive literature on pediatric laryngotracheal reconstruction, which is reviewed later in this chapter. In a series of 21 tracheostomy-dependent adult patients with subglottic stenosis, but without tracheal stenosis, anterior and posterior cricoid division with costal cartilage augmentation grafting was performed.[77] Postoperative stenting was used for 3 to 4 weeks. Sixteen of 21 patients were successfully decannulated. Better success was reported in patients with isolated subglottic stenosis than in those who also had glottic stenosis.

The surgical techniques described in the following paragraphs are similar to those reported in the papers cited previously. The treatment of acute tracheal transection is reviewed first, followed by some principles used in the repair of chronic tracheal stenosis. Alternative techniques for total cervical tracheal reconstruction are also reviewed.

Acute tracheal transection is best treated by immediate control of the airway and patient stabilization. With the tracheostomy in place, and with the patient under general anesthesia, an endotracheal tube is inserted orally into the distal tracheal segment. Usually one or two tracheal rings remain attached to the cricoid cartilage. One or both recurrent nerves may have been damaged. The proximal and distal tracheal segments are mobilized. The distal segment is elevated by traction sutures from the mediastinum to the cervical area, and a primary anastomosis, around the endotracheal tube, is performed with extraluminal 2–0 Vicryl sutures. If mucosal damage is minimal, the endotracheal tube is left in place for 2 to 3 days. The patient is decannulated in the operating room. Most of the time, a subanastomotic tracheostomy is performed to maintain the airway and to decompress the suture line. We generally use bilateral tracheopexy sutures to reduce traction

on the tracheal anastomosis (Fig. 27–18). Complete chronic tracheal stenosis is best corrected by resection and end-to-end anastomosis. In young adults, a 3-cm defect can be closed without tracheal or laryngeal release. An accurate mucosal approximation is paramount.

We use three tracheal lengthening procedures. The most common is the suprahyoid laryngeal release, the second is the infrahyoid laryngeal release, and the third is incision in a stepladder fashion of alternating lateral annular tracheal (intercartilaginous) ligaments. The tracheal lumen is not entered. The first two methods can gain 5 cm and the third method 1 to 1.5 cm of tracheal length. Excessive tracheal mobilization within the visceral fascia should be avoided lest cartilage and vascular damage and devitalization occur. The end-to-end anastomosis is achieved with extraluminal synthetic absorbable sutures over an endotracheal tube, which may be left in place for 2 to 3 days. Occasionally, a T-tube or stent with tracheostomy is used. These devices are to be avoided if possible because they may damage the mucosa and the anastomotic site. We use these only when grafting is required. Tracheopexy sutures are used for support and to delineate the trachea in case of an emergency airway leak or obstruction.

Whenever mucosal continuity is present, we endeavor to maintain it. Thus, on many occasions we use an anterior wedge excision and primary anastomosis because the posterior mucosa of the trachea is generally intact. The anterolateral walls of the trachea are repaired extraluminally. Additional support may be obtained from the surrounding soft tissues. These repairs are more common with stomal and infrastomal stenosis. Partial cricoid resection is performed when the stenosis extends to the subglottic region. The technique varies with the degree of posterior stenosis.[67-70] Recent results have been encouraging.[71-75]

Another method to be considered is total cervical tracheal reconstruction. Complete cervical tracheal loss is uncommon. A successful repair that consistently gives satisfactory results is still elusive. The use of prosthetics has been universally unfavorable. Most techniques use cervical or pectoral flaps for reconstructing a lined lumen. Montgomery uses a horizontal cervical trapdoor flap that may be stented with rib cartilage.[78] This is a two-stage procedure. Fleming uses bipedicled deltopectoral flaps.[79] McComb uses bipedicled thoracic flaps.[47] Grillo uses horizontal cervical flaps reinforced with wires.[80] Rethi used a tubed pedicle flap.[81] Basically, all these techniques use a similar concept, which is, first, create a posterior wall or gutter and, second, cover this fissure anteriorly. The superior and inferior borders of the flaps are sutured to the edges of the remaining trachea. These techniques do not fulfill the reconstructive criteria discussed previously, and the results are unpredictable.

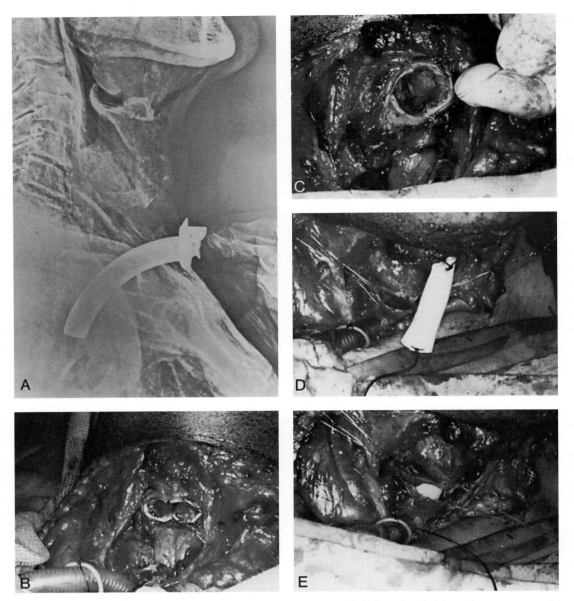

Fig. 27–18. Tracheal transection following automobile accident. A. Xeroradiogram of the lateral neck. Note subcutaneous emphysema, loss of laryngeal and tracheal air column, and tracheal cannula in place in distal tracheal stump. B. At operation, the upper tracheal stump is crushed. C. Undersurfaces of the tracheolaryngeal stump. Note the undersurface of the vocal cords. Also, the right recurrent nerve is intact. The tracheal ring is reconstituted with 4–0 braided wire. D. The lower tracheal stump is elevated from the chest into the neck with wire trachea sutures and stabilized to the sternum and clavicles. The tracheostomy is below the anastomosis site. Because there is little mucosal damage, a stent without skin is placed into the lumen. The two cut edges of the trachea are sutured together, starting posteriorly and progressing laterally on both sides. The anterior deficit is closed last. E. The stent is in place. The trachea is about to be closed. Note that, if the trachea had not been crushed, this defect would have been closed without stenting or grafting.

Complications

Complications of tracheal reconstruction can be divided into early and delayed problems.

EARLY COMPLICATIONS. The most common early complication is pooling of secretions with resultant pulmonary atelectasis. Occasionally, this follows intraoperative aspiration of blood or other secretions or the introduction of a long tracheostomy tube inserted into one main stem bronchus.

Laryngeal edema can be caused by the endotracheal intubation or a long stent that compresses the subglottis or glottis, or it can occur when laryngotracheal procedures are used. This is treated by the use of corticosteroids (inhaled topical corticosteroids) and racemic epinephrine.

Apnea may follow surgery when air or O_2 is used following tracheostomy. Because, in patients with chronic upper airway obstruction, CO_2 frequently is the main respiratory drive, O_2 therapy physiologically denervates the chemoreceptor respiratory drive.

Hypotension may result from a decrease in CO_2 retention following tracheostomy. CO_2 mediates (by way of the CNS) increased cardiac output, high blood flow, increased peripheral resistance, and hypertension.

Hemorrhage can occur during or immediately after operation because of damage to the anterior jugular vein, the inferior thyroid veins, the innominate artery, the internal jugular veins, or the aortic arch and its branches. Delayed bleeding is usually secondary to thyroid isthmus bleeding.

Injury to the recurrent laryngeal nerves is a major concern, especially in post-traumatic cicatricial paratracheal stenosis.

Pneumothorax and pneumomediastinum are major concerns because patients in respiratory distress may have a high-rising pleura that can be perforated during the operation. These complications may be manifest as shock, subcutaneous emphysema, and deteriorating respiratory functions. An underwater sealed chest tube is required.

Tracheoesophageal fistula is an unusual complication that may be caused by improper surgical technique or necrosis secondary to an excessively large tracheostomy tube or stent.

Subcutaneous emphysema can occur from air leakage around a tracheostomy tube that is packed too tightly. One must, however, suspect the most dreaded complication of this kind of operation, separation of the suture line or partial tracheal separation. This is most often caused by excessive tension on the suture line or damage to the tracheal blood supply (avascular necrosis). In the immediate postoperative period, it signifies a surgical error. This complication requires immediate reoperation with insertion of a T-tube or a tracheostomy. The repair is usually delayed until reduction of the inflammation and the beginning of fibrosis occur. After stenting, delayed operation is used for late stenosis.

DELAYED COMPLICATIONS. Pneumonia is a delayed complication that occurs at the end of the first postoperative week. It is associated with poor tracheal hygiene, atelectasis, use of contaminated suction tips, or poor sterility techniques (nosocomial infection).

Aerophagia (air swallowing) can cause abdominal distension, pulmonary atelectasis, diaphragmatic elevation, and respiratory distress. It is most common in young children. Treatment is to decompress the stomach with a nasogastric tube and adjust the tracheotomy tube to one that is slightly smaller.

A disturbing but common problem is tracheal tube dislocation into the anterior mediastinum, resulting in respiratory distress and occasionally death. It is our policy to have a physician change the tracheostomy tube until the stoma is mature (lined with skin) and to suture the initial tracheostomy tube to the cervical skin.

Delayed respiratory distress can occur secondary to inspissated secretional obstruction of the tracheal tube lumen, tracheal crusting (tracheitis sicca), bleeding, granulation tissue (tip granuloma), overinflation of the soft tracheal cuff, or improper tracheal tube curvature (occlusion along the anterior tracheal wall).

Dysphagia is usually temporary because of postoperative pain, aspiration, vagal nerve paralysis, or the use of a large tracheal tube with esophageal compression by tracheal cuff.

Difficulty in decannulation can occur after prolonged tracheal intubation. It is best treated by gradual decrease in tracheal tube size to a No. 4 tube, then progressive plugging of the tube until it is tolerated for 12 hours or more.

Persistent tracheocutaneous fistula implies that the tract is lined by skin. This requires surgical closure a few weeks after decannulation. Occasionally, these tracts have intratracheal inflammation and granulomas, which must be removed before closure.

A worrisome complication is persistent granulation tissue at the anastomotic suture line. This may lead to partial stenosis. These complications are handled bronchoscopically with minimal trauma and the CO_2 laser. Nebulized corticosteroids are used, as well as systemic corticosteroids, for a 2-week period. The stenoses are handled conservatively by rigid bronchoscopic dilatation. True restenosis requires resection. This is usually delayed for 4 to 6 months after the original procedure. This time period allows more rigid fibrosis and decreases the incidence of inflammation of the tracheal walls. Staged resections with mediastinal tracheostomas are to be avoided. The key feature is to make the initial resection work by eliminating tension, maintaining careful tissue approximation, using extraluminal absorbable synthetic polymeric sutures, and conserving as much tissue as possible during the initial definitive procedure.

Surgical Repairs: Pediatric

A great deal of activity has occurred in recent years in the field of pediatric laryngotracheal reconstruction. Endoscopic procedures have been used for the management of laryngotracheal stenosis when the stenosis is composed of soft tissue and cartilagenous support has not been lost.[82,83] Care must be taken to avoid worsening a circumferential stenosis with repeated attempts at endoscopic scar excision, including the use of the CO_2 laser. Open procedures for pediatric laryngotracheal reconstruction have advanced greatly over the past 2 decades, with the popularization of augmentation grafting[84,85] and anterior cricoid decompression.[86] Open reconstructive procedures are discussed in this section.

Subglottic Stenosis

ANTERIOR CRICOID SPLIT. The anterior cricoid split procedure is advocated as an alternative to tracheostomy in neonates who have failed repeated attempts at extubation.[86] A 10-year experience with this technique was published by Cotton and associates,[87] and a further update was provided by the same group in 1991.[88] Patients with other airway lesions that would prevent extubation were excluded for consideration for the anterior cricoid split; such conditions include severe laryngomalacia, laryngeal clefts, supraglottic webs, vocal cord paralysis, and choanal atresia. The authors also recommend delaying the procedure until the infant weighs at least 1500 g. The surgical procedure involves an anterior midline incision of the cricoid cartilage, caudal thyroid cartilage, and the first two tracheal rings. A nasotracheal tube is used as a stent for 1 to 2 weeks postoperatively. Tight closure of the skin incision is avoided, to prevent the development of subcutaneous emphysema (Fig. 27–19).

An overall success rate of approximately 70% was reported. In the case of a failed anterior cricoid split, some authors have recommended a repeat anterior cricoid split, rather than a tracheostomy with subsequent laryngotracheal reconstruction.[89] This recommendation is based on experience with a relatively small number of patients, however. Finally, some investigators have reported a better experience (higher success rate with fewer complications) with immediate costal cartilage grafting for anterior augmentation than with the use of the anterior cricoid split alone.[90] All patients in this series had acquired subglottic stenosis.

SINGLE-STAGE REPAIRS. Repairs in which augmentation grafting is used may be performed without prolonged stent placement, although endotracheal intubation is used in the first week postoperatively. Lusk and associates[91] and Seid and colleagues[92] independently

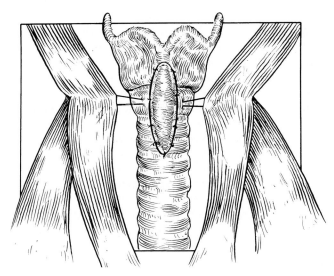

Fig. 27–20. Auricular cartilage grafts may be used for anterior augmentation. The natural curvature of the conchal cartilage is advantageous in reconstructing the anterior wall. (Courtesy of Dr. Rodney P. Lusk.)

reported their results using costal cartilage grafts for single-stage repairs in 1991. Lusk and associates performed anterior grafting, without posterior cricoid split or grafting, in 19 pediatric and adult patients. Eighteen of 19 were successfully extubated. Seid and associates treated 13 patients using a similar technique; 12 were successfully extubated. The single failure was in a patient with grade IV stenosis. Lusk and colleagues subsequently reported a modification of their technique for single-stage reconstruction, using auricular cartilage grafts, rather than costal cartilage grafts.[93] Twenty-three patients were treated, some of whom had failed anterior cricoid split procedures. Seventeen were successfully extubated. The authors advocated the use of auricular cartilage for laryngotracheal reconstruction in patients with mild to moderate subglottic stenosis or in those whose anterior cricoid split had failed. The length of the graft may be a limitation in some cases (Fig. 27–20).

When posterior stenosis is also present, anteroposterior grafting with costal cartilage may also be performed as a single-stage procedure. The published experience with this technique, although promising, is limited.[94]

STAGED REPAIRS. In general, staged repairs using prolonged stenting are applied to more severe cases of laryngotracheal stenosis. Numerous authors have documented their experience with augmentation using cartilage grafts, and some others have used the technique of resection and anastomosis.

A thorough review of the history of laryngotracheal reconstruction was published in 1991 by Cotton.[95] The viability of posterior cartilage grafts was established in the same report, and 59 of 61 pediatric patients who

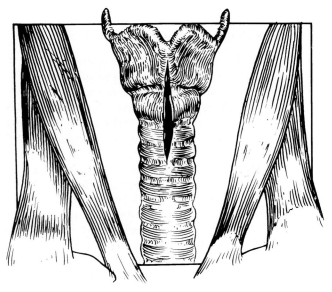

Fig. 27–19. Anterior cricoid split (anterior cricoid decompression). Lateralization of the cricoid segments aids in the widening of the subglottis. (Courtesy of Dr. Rodney P. Lusk.)

were treated with anterior and posterior grafting were decannulated. Aboulker stents were used in all patients. Zalzal reported similar results in a group of 41 pediatric patients treated with anterior and posterior grafting and Aboulker stent placement; 90% of the patients were decannulated after one procedure.[96] Two patients died, however, and the voice quality was reported to be disappointing.

Good success with decannulation has also been reported in a series in which some patients had anterior grafting alone. Maddolozzo and Holinger reported that 80% of 20 patients with congenital or acquired subglottic stenosis were decannulated after costal cartilage grafting and Aboulker stent placement.[97] Smith and Catlin treated 19 patients with grade II or grade III stenosis; 95% of these patients were decannulated.[98] Only 6 of 8 patients with grade IV stenosis were decannulated, however, and some of these patients required more than one procedure. The authors recommend counseling that patients with grade IV stenosis will more likely require multiple procedures. Other investigators also report that decannulation is less likely in patients with more severe stenosis. In a series of 108 patients, some of whom were treated with a castellated incision laryngotracheoplasty and others with augmentation grafting, 83% were ultimately decannulated.[99] Only 50% of the patients with grade IV stenosis were decannulated, however.

In a comparison between costal cartilage graft laryngotracheal reconstruction and castellated incision laryngotracheoplasty, the decannulation rates were found to be similar for each group. The complication rate was higher in patients treated with the castellated incision laryngotracheoplasty, however, and the time to decannulation was longer[100] (Fig. 27–21).

Monnier and associates used a different surgical approach to the problem of congenital and postintubational subglottic stenosis in infants and children.[101] The patients all had grade III or grade IV stenosis. The technique of resection and thyrotracheal anastomosis was used. The recurrent laryngeal nerves were identified bilaterally, and the cricoid cartilage was resected anteriorly. A rubber-silicone or a T-tube stent was used routinely. One single-stage procedure was performed. The stents were removed after 10 days. Ninety-three percent (14 of 15) of the patients were decannulated between 2 and 6 months after undergoing a single surgical procedure. Normal tracheal growth was seen in follow-up for as long as 5 years. Wiatrak and Cotton treated 8 patients with tracheal stenosis from blunt trauma or papillomatosis using tracheal resection and anastomosis.[102] Lower subglottic involvement was minimal. All 6 trauma patients were decannulated, and 1 patient with papillomatosis was decannulated.

Tracheal Stenosis

Long-segment tracheal stenosis is a less common problem than subglottic stenosis. As is the case for subglot-

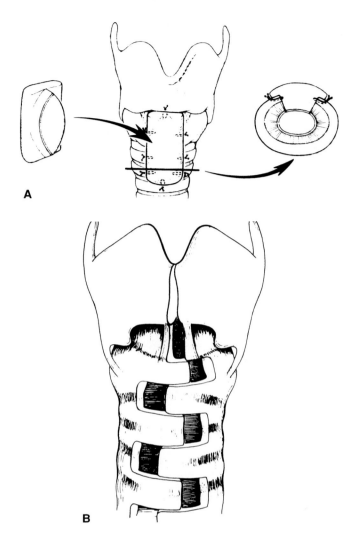

Fig. 27–21. Costal cartilage graft laryngotracheal reconstruction (A) and castellated incision laryngotracheoplasty (B). (Courtesy of Dr. Rodney P. Lusk.)

tic stenosis, repair can be achieved either through augmentation grafting or by resection and anastomosis.

Early references to augmentation grafting for tracheal stenosis include the use of both costal cartilage[103] and pericardium.[104] Current reports indicate that most such repairs are performed with the use of cardiopulmonary bypass. Postoperative intubation of 1 to 2 weeks is used, and long-term stenting is not common. Multiple postreconstructive bronchoscopies with dilation and removal of granulation tissue are often required. Even in the presence of complete tracheal rings to the level of the carina, decannulation rates of approximately 80% have been reported with the use of pericardial patching.[105] Other investigators have noted a preference for rigid graft material, such as costal cartilage.[106] The postoperative problem of tracheomalacia is thought by some to be worse if pericardium is used.[107]

The repair of tracheal stenosis using resection and anastomosis is technically similar to that reported in adults.[108–110] As much as 50% of the infant trachea can be resected with primary anastomosis.[111] A review by Weber and associates reported on 62 pediatric cases of acquired subglottic and tracheal stenosis.[112] Of 12 patients treated with the technique of resection and anastomosis, 10 were decannulated. The success rate is thus similar to that reported with the use of augmentation grafting.

SUGGESTED READINGS

1. Jackson C: High tracheostomy and other errors: the chief causes of chronic laryngeal stenosis. Surg Gynecol Obstet 32:392, 1921.
2. Brantigan GO and Grow JB: Cricothyroidotomy: elective use in respiratory problems requiring tracheotomy. J Thorac Cardiovasc Surg 71:72, 1976.
3. Boyd AD, et al: A clinical evaluation of cricothyroidotomy. Surg Gynecol Obstet 149:365, 1979.
4. Sise MJ, et al: Cricothyroidotomy for long-term tracheal access: a prospective analysis of morbidity and mortality in 76 patients. Ann Surg 200:13, 1984.
5. Romita MC, Colvin SB, and Boyd AD: Cricothyroidotomy: its healing and complications. Surg Forum 28:174, 1977.
6. Loopman CF, Feld RA, and Coulthard SW: Effects of antibiotics and injury of cricoid cartilage in cricothyroidotomy. Surg Forum 30:507, 1979.
7. Nelson TG: Tracheotomy: a clinical and experimental study. Part III. Am Surg 23:841, 1957.
8. Nelson TG: Tracheotomy: a clinical and experimental study. Part I. Am Surg 23:66, 1957.
9. Nelson TG: Tracheotomy: a clinical and experimental study. Part II. Am Surg 23:750, 1957.
10. Stauffer JL, Olson DE, and Petty TL: Complications and consequences of endotracheal intubation and tracheotomy: a prospective study of 150 critically ill adult patients. Am J Med 70:65, 1981.
11. Beatrous WP: Tracheostomy (tracheotomy): its expanded indications and its present status. Based on an analysis of 1000 consecutive operations and a review of the recent literature. Laryngoscope 78:3, 1968.
12. Arola MK and Anttinen J: Post-mortem finding of tracheal injury after cuffed intubation and tracheostomy: a clinical and histopathological study. Acta Anesthaesiol Scand 23:57, 1979.
13. Benjamin B: Prolonged intubation injuries of the larynx: endoscopic diagnosis, classification, and treatment. Ann Otol Rhinol Laryngol Suppl 15:160, 1993.
14. Ciaglia P and Graniero KD: Percutaneous dilatational tracheostomy: results and long-term follow-up. Chest 101:464, 1992.
15. Schachner A, et al: Percutaneous tracheostomy: a new method. Crit Care Med 17:1052, 1989.
16. Ivatury R, et al: Percutaneous tracheostomy after trauma and critical illness. J Trauma 32:133, 1992.
17. Leinhardt DJ, et al: Appraisal of percutaneous tracheostomy. Br J Surg 79:255, 1992.
18. Miura T and Grillo HC: The contribution of the inferior thyroid artery to the blood supply of the human trachea. Surg Gynecol Obstet 123:99, 1966.
19. Salassa JR, Pearson BW, and Payne WS: Gross and microscopical blood supply of the trachea. Ann Thorac Surg 24:100, 1977.
20. Dietzsch HJ: Angeborene Fehlbildungen der Trachea und Bronchien als ursache cheonischrezidivievierender Lungenerkrankungen. Kinderarzt Prax 32:11, 1964.
21. Cantrell JR and Guild HG: Congenital stenosis of the trachea. Am J Surg 22:297, 1964.
22. Holinger PH, Johnston KC, and Basinger CE: Benign stenosis of the trachea. Ann Otol Rhinol Laryngol 59:837, 1950.
23. Holinger PH, et al: Congenital malformations of the trachea. Ann Otol Rhinol Laryngol 61:1159, 1952.
24. Holinger PH: Clinical aspects of congenital anomalies of the larynx, trachea, bronchi and esophagus. J Laryngol Otol 75:1, 1961.
25. Pettersson G: Inhibited separation of larynx and the upper part of trachea from esophagus in a newborn: report of a case successfully operated upon. Acta Chir Scand 110:250, 1955–1956.
26. Fearon B and Shortreed R: Tracheobronchial compression by congenital cardiovascular anomalies in children. Ann Otol Rhinol Laryngol 72:949, 1963.
27. Maurseth R: Tracheal stenosis caused by compression from the innominate artery. Ann Radiol 9:287, 1966.
28. Mournier-Kuhn P: Le syndrome tracheal et les compressions mediastinales. Ann Otolaryngol (Paris) 69:385, 1952.
29. Edwards FR: Vascular compression of the trachea and esophagus. Thorax 14:187, 1959.
30. Maier HC: Tracheal compression from bronchiogenic cyst in esophageal wall. Am J Dis Child 80:423, 1950.
31. Bruckner H: Die trachealstenose durch: Struma beim Kinde. Beitr Klin Chir 181:507, 1951.
32. Rostom AY and Morgan RL: Results of treating primary tumors of the trachea by irradiation. Thorax 33:387, 1978.
33. McCafferty GJ, Parker LS, and Suggit SC: Primary malignant disease of the trachea. J Laryngol Otol 78:441, 1964.
34. Houston HE, Payne WS, Harrison EG Jr, and Olsen AM: Primary cancers of the trachea. Arch Surg 99:132, 1969.
35. Hajdu SI, et al: Carcinoma of the trachea: clinicopathologic study of 41 cases. Cancer 25:1448, 1970.
36. Grillo HC: Tumors of the cervical trachea. In: Cancer of the Head and Neck. Edited by Suen JY and Myers EN. New York, Churchill Livingstone, 1981, p 500.
37. Weber AL and Grillo HC: Tracheal tumors: radiological, clinical and pathological evaluation. Adv Otorhinolaryngol 24:170, 1978.
38. Weber AL and Grillo HC: A radiological, clinical and pathological evaluation of 84 cases. Radiol Clin North Am 16:227, 1978.
39. Weber AL, et al: Cartilaginous tumors of the larynx and trachea. Radiol Clin North Am 16:261, 1978.
40. Negus VE, cited in Thomson S, Negus VE, and Bateman GH: Diseases of the Nose and Throat: A Textbook for Students and Practitioners. 6th Ed. London, Cassell, 1955, p 885.
41. Tapia-Acuna R: Endoscopy of the air passages with special reference to scleroma. Ann Otol Rhinol Laryngol 82:765, 1973.
42. Greenwood MF and Holland P: Tracheal obstruction secondary to histoplasma mediastinal granuloma. Chest 62:642, 1972.
43. Holinger PH, Johnston KC, and Delgado A: Amyloid tumor of the larynx and trachea. Arch Otolaryngol 70:555, 1959.
44. Stark DB and McDonald JR: Amyloid "tumors" of the larynx, trachea and bronchi: a histologic study of fifteen cases. Am J Clin Pathol 18:778, 1948.
45. Attwood HD, Price CG, and Riddell RJ: Airway diffuse tracheobronchial amyloidosis. Thorax 27:620, 1972.
46. Pearson HW: Trachea: tracheal stenosis. In: Scientific Foundations of Otolaryngology. Edited by Hinchcliffe R and Harrison D. London, William Heinemann, 1976.
47. McComb H: Treatment of tracheal stenosis: Plast Reconstr Surg 39:43, 1967.
48. Meyer R and Flemming I: Reconstructive Surgery of the Trachea. New York, Thieme, 1982, p 25.
49. Montgomery WW: Surgery of the Upper Respiratory System. Vol 2. Philadelphia, Lea & Febiger, 1973.
50. Faw K, Muntz H, Siegel M, and Spector G: Computed tomography in the evaluation of acquired stenosis in the neonate. Laryngoscope 92:100, 1982.

51. Florange W, Muller J, and Forster E: Morphologie de la nécrose trachéale après trachéotomie et utilisation d'une prothèse respiratoire. Anesth Analg 22:693, 1965.

52. Grillo HC: Surgical approaches to the trachea. Surg Gynecol Obstet 129:347, 1969.

53. Cooper JD and Grillo HC: The evolution of tracheal injury due to ventilatory assistance through cuffed tubes: a pathologic study. Am Surg 169:334, 1969.

54. Murphy DA, MacLean LD, and Dobell AR: Tracheal stenosis as a complication of tracheostomy. Ann Thorac Surg 2:44, 1966.

55. Pearson FG, et al: The reconstruction of circumferential tracheal defects with a porous prosthesis. J Thorac Cardiovasc Surg 55:605, 1968.

56. Pearson FG, Goldberg M, and Da Silva AJ: A prospective study of tracheal injury complicating tracheostomy with a cuffed tube. Ann Otol Rhinol Laryngol 77:867, 1968.

57. Johnston JB, Wright JS, and Hercus V: Tracheal stenosis following tracheostomy: a conservative approach to treatment. J Thorac Cardiovasc Surg 53:206, 1967.

58. Curtin JW, Holinger PH, and Greeley PW: Blunt trauma to the larynx and upper trachea: immediate treatment, complications and late reconstructive procedures. J Trauma 6:493, 1966.

59. Nahum AM and Siegel AW: Biodynamics of injury to the larynx in automobile collisions. Ann Otol Rhinol Laryngol 76:781, 1967.

60. Lemay SR Jr: Penetrating wounds of the larynx and cervical trachea. Arch Otolaryngol 94:558, 1971.

61. Shaw RR, Paulson DL, and Kee JL Jr: Traumatic tracheal rupture. J Thorac Cardiovasc Surg 42:281, 1961.

62. Momose KJ and MacMillan AS Jr: Roentgenologic investigations of the larynx and trachea. Radiol Clin North Am 16:321, 1978.

63. James AE, MacMillan AS Jr, Eaton SB, and Grillo HC: Roentgenology of tracheal stenosis resulting from cuffed tracheostomy tubes. Am J Roentgenol 109:455, 1970.

64. Evans JNG: Laryngotracheoplasty. Otolaryngol Clin North Am 10:119, 1977.

65. Montgomery WW: T-tube tracheal stent. Arch Otolaryngol 82:320, 1965.

66. Westaby S and Sheperd MP: Palliation of intrathoracic tracheal compression with a Silastic tracheobronchial stent. Thorax 38:314, 1983.

67. Ogura JH and Roper CL: Surgical correction of traumatic stenosis of larynx and pharynx. Laryngoscope 72:468, 1962.

68. Gerwat J and Bryce DP: The management of subglottic laryngeal stenosis by resection and direct anastomosis. Laryngoscope 84:940, 1974.

69. Pearson FG, Cooper JD, Nelems JM, and van Nostrand AWP: Primary tracheal anastomosis after resection of the cricoid cartilage with preservation of the recurrent laryngeal nerves. J Thorac Cardiovasc Surg 70:806, 1975.

70. Grillo HC: Primary reconstruction of airway after resection of subglottic laryngeal and upper tracheal stenosis. Ann Thorac Surg 33:3, 1982.

71. Grillo HC, Mathisen DJ, and Wain JC: Laryngotracheal resection and reconstruction for subglottic stenosis. Ann Thorac Surg 53:53, 1992

72. Grillo HC, Mark EJ, Mathisen DJ, and Wain JC: Idiopathic laryngotracheal stenosis and its management. Ann Thorac Surg 56:80, 1993.

73. Macchiarini P, et al: Laryngotracheal resection and reconstruction for postintubation subglottic stenosis. Eur J Cardiothorac Surg 7:300, 1993.

74. Bisson A, et al: Tracheal sleeve resection for iatrogenic stenosis. J Thorac Cariovasc Surg 104:882, 1992.

75. Paris F, et al: Management of non-tumoral tracheal stenosis in 112 patients. Eur J Cardiothorac Surg 4:265, 1990.

76. Maddaus MA, Toth JL, Gullane PJ, and Pearson FG: Subglottic tracheal resection and synchronous laryngeal reconstruction. J Thorac Cardiovasc Surg 104:1443, 1992.

77. McCaffrey TV: Management of subglottic stenosis in the adult. Ann Otol Rhinol Laryngol 100:90, 1991.

78. Montgomery WW: Reconstruction of the cervical trachea. Am Otol 73:1, 1964.

79. Fleming IK: Behandlung der tracheal Stenosen. Berlin, Habil-Schrift, 1970.

80. Grillo HC: Circumferential resection and reconstruction of the mediastinal and cervical trachea. Am Surg 162:374, 1965.

81. Rethi A: Behandlungsmoglichkeiter der Stenosen der oberen luftwege. HNO 18:193, 1970.

82. Simpson GT, et al: Predicted factors of success or failure in the endoscopic management of laryngeal and tracheal stenosis. Ann Otol Rhinol Laryngol 91:384, 1982.

83. Holinger LD: Treatment of severe subglottic stenosis without tracheotomy. Ann Otol Rhinol Laryngol 91:407, 1982.

84. Fearon B and Cotton RT: Surgical correction of subglottic stenosis of the larynx. Ann Otol Rhinol Laryngol 81:508, 1972.

85. Fearon B and Cotton RT: Surgical correction of subglottic stenosis of the larynx in infants and children: progress report. Ann Otol Rhinol Laryngol 83:428, 1974.

86. Cotton RT and Seid AB: Management of the extubation problem in the premature child: anterior cricoid split as an alternative to tracheotomy. Ann Otol Rhinol Laryngol 89:508, 1980.

87. Cotton RT, Myer CM, Bratcher GO, and Fitton CM: Anterior cricoid split, 1977–1987. Arch Otolaryngol Head Neck Surg 114:1300, 1988.

88. Silver FM, Myer CM, and Cotton RT: Anterior cricoid split. Am J Otolaryngol 12:343, 1991.

89. Ochi JW, Seid AB, and Pransky SM: An approach to the failed cricoid split operation. Int J Pediatr Otorhinolaryngol 14:229, 1987.

90. Richardson MA and Inglis AF: A comparison of anterior cricoid split with and without costal cartilage graft for acquired subglottic stenosis. Int J Pediatr Otorhinolaryngol 22:187, 1991.

91. Lusk RP, Gray S, and Muntz HR: Single-stage laryngotracheal reconstruction. Arch Otolaryngol Head Neck Surg 117:171, 1991.

92. Seid AB, Pransky SM, and Kearns DB: One-stage laryngotracheoplasty. Arch Otolaryngol Head Neck Surg 117:408, 1991.

93. Lusk RP, Kang DR, and Muntz HR: Auricular cartilage grafts in laryngotracheal reconstruction. Ann Otol Rhinol Laryngol 102:247, 1993.

94. Stenson K, Berkowitz R, McDonald T, and Gruber B: Experience with one-stage laryngotracheal reconstruction. Int J Pediatr Otorhinolaryngol 27:55, 1993.

95. Cotton RT: The problem of pediatric laryngotracheal stenosis: a clinical and experimental study on the efficacy of autogenous cartilage grafts placed between the vertically divided halves of the posterior lamina of the cricoid cartilage. Laryngoscope 101(suppl 56):1, 1991.

96. Zalzal GH: Treatment of laryngotracheal stenosis with anterior and posterior cartilage grafts. Arch Otolaryngol Head Neck Surg 119:82, 1993.

97. Maddolozzo J and Holinger LD: Laryngotracheal reconstruction for subglottic stenosis in children. Ann Otol Rhinol Laryngol 96:665, 1987.

98. Smith RJ and Catlin FI: Laryngotracheal stenosis: a 5-year review. Head Neck 13:140, 1991.

99. Ochi JW, Evans JN, and Bailey CM: Pediatric airway reconstruction at Great Ormond Street: a ten-year review. Ann Otol Rhinol Laryngol 101:465, 1992.

100. Muntz HR and Lusk RP: A comparison of the cartilagenous rib graft and Evans-Todd laryngotracheoplasties for subglottic stenosis. Laryngoscope 100:415, 1990.

101. Monnier P, Savary M, and Chapuis G: Partial cricoid resection with primary tracheal anastomosis for subglottic stenosis in infants and children. Laryngoscope 103:1273, 1993.

102. Wiatrak BJ and Cotton RT: Anastomosis of the cervical trachea in children. Arch Otolaryngol Head Neck Surg *118:*58, 1992.

103. Kimura K, et al: Tracheoplasty for congenital stenosis of the entire trachea. J Pediatr Surg *17:*869, 1982.

104. Idriss FA, et al: Tracheoplasty with pericardial patch for extensive tracheal stenosis in infants and children. J Thorac Cardiovasc Surg *88:*527, 1984.

105. Cosentino CM, et al: Pericardial patch tracheoplasty for severe tracheal stenosis in children: intermediate results. J Pediatr Surg *26:* 879, 1991.

106. Van Meter CH, Lusk RM, Muntz H, and Spray TL: Tracheoplasty for congenital long-segment intrathoracic tracheal stenosis. Am Surg *57:*157, 1991.

107. Laing MR, Albert DM, Quinney RE, and Bailey CM: Tracheal stenosis in infants and young children. J Laryngol Otol *104:*229, 1990.

108. Alstrup P and Sorensen HR: Resection of acquired tracheal stenosis in childhood. J Thorac Cardiovasc Surg *87:*547, 1984.

109. Halsband H: Long-distance resection of the trachea with primary anastomosis in small children. Prog Pediatr Surg *21:*76, 1987.

110. Jonas RA: Invited letter concerning: tracheal operations in infancy. J Thorac Cardiovasc Surg *100:*316, 1990.

111. Mattingly WT, Berlin RP, and Todd EP: Surgical repair of congenital tracheal stenosis in an infant. J Thorac Cardiovasc Surg *81:*738, 1981.

112. Weber TR, Connors RH, and Tracy TF: Acquired tracheal stenosis in infants and children. J Thorac Cardiovasc Surg *102:*29, 1991.

FURTHER SUGGESTED READINGS

Historical Background

Brock AJ (Ed and Trans): Galen. London, Loeb Classical Library, 1916.

Dionis P: Cours d'opérations de chirurgie. Paris, L d'Houry, 1751.

Frost EAM: Tracing the tracheostomy. Ann Otol Rhinol Laryngol *85:*618, 1976.

Goodall EW: The story of tracheotomy. Br J Child Dis *31:*167, 1934.

Jackson C: High tracheotomy and other errors: the chief cause of chronic laryngeal stenosis. Surg Gynecol Obstet *32:*392, 1923.

Martine G: Phil Trans R Soc, 448, 1730.

The Seven Books of Paulus Aegineta. London, Adams, 1846–1847, p 30.

Stevenson RS and Guthrie D: History of Otolaryngology. Edinburgh, E&S Livingstone, 1949, pp 17, 31.

Wright J: A History of Laryngology and Rhinology. Philadelphia, Lea & Febiger, 1914, p 65.

Control of the Airway

Andrews MJ and Pearson FG: An analysis of 59 cases of tracheal stenosis with cuffed tubes and assisted ventilation with special reference to diagnosis and treatment. Br J Surg *60:*208, 1973.

Ardran GM and Caust LJ: Delayed decannulation after tracheostomy in infants. J Laryngol Otol *77:*555, 1963.

Brantigan CO and Grow JB: Subglottic stenosis after cricothyroidotomy. Surgery *91:*217, 1982.

Brantigan CO and Grow JB: Cricothyroidotomy revisited again. Ear Nose Throat J *59:*289, 1980.

Caparosa RJ and Zavatsky AB: Practical aspects of the cricothyroid space. L-Scope *67:*577, 1957.

Carden ET: Letter to the editor. Plast Reconstr Surg *67:*99, 1981.

Cotton RT: Pediatric laryngotracheal stenosis. Pediatr Surg *19:*699, 1984.

Gleeson MJ: Cricothyroidotomy: a satisfactory alternative to tracheostomy? (Editorial) Clin Otolaryngol *9:*1, 1984.

Griesz H, Qvarnstrom O, and Willen R: Elective cricothyroidotomy: A clinical and histopathologic study. Crit Care Med *10:*387, 1982.

Grillo HC: Primary reconstruction of the airway after resection of subglottic laryngeal and upper tracheal stenosis. Ann Thorac Surg *33:*3, 1981.

Grillo HC: Reconstruction of the trachea: experience in 100 consecutive cases. Thorax *28:*667, 1973.

Harley HRS: Laryngotracheal complications of tracheostomy or endotracheal intubation with assisted respiration. Thorax *26:*493, 1971.

Kennedy TL: Epiglottic reconstruction of laryngeal stenosis secondary to cricothyroidostomy. Laryngoscope *90:*1130, 1980.

Kress TD and Balasubramaniam S: Cricothyroidotomy. Ann Emerg Med *11:*197, 1982.

Lawrence GD: Personal communication, cited by Brantigan and Grow.

Lindholm GE and Grenvik A: Flexible fibreoptic bronchoscopy and intubation in intensive care. In: Recent Advances in Intensive Therapy. Edited by Ledingham R. Edinburgh, Livingstone, 1977.

McDowell DE: Cricothyroidostomy for airway access. South Med J *75:*282, 1982.

McGill J, Clinton JE, and Ruiz E: Cricothyroidotomy in the emergency department. Ann Emerg Med *11:*361, 1982.

Mitchell SA: Cricothyroidotomy revisited. Ear Nose Throat J *58:*54, 1979.

Morain WD: Cricothyroidotomy in head and neck surgery. Plast Reconstr Surg *65:*424, 1979.

Nahum AM: Early Management of Acute Trauma. St. Louis, CV Mosby, 1966.

Nicholas TH and Ruimer GF: Emergency airway: a plan of action. JAMA *174:*1930, 1960.

O'Connor JV, Reddy K, Ergin MA, and Griepp RG: Cricothyroidotomy for prolonged ventilatory support after cardiac operations. Ann Thorac Surg *39:*353, 1985.

Pearson FG, Goldberg M, and DaSilva AJ: A prospective study of tracheal injury complicating tracheostomy with a cuffed tube. Ann Otol Rhinol Laryngol *79:*867, 1968.

Pierce WS, Tyers FO, and Wardhausen JA: Effective isolation of a tracheostomy for a median sternotomy wound. J Thorac Cardiovasc Surg *66:*841, 1973.

Ruke DS, Williams GV, and Proud GO: Emergency airway by cricothyroid puncture or tracheotomy. Trans Am Acad Ophthalmol Otol *13:*182, 1960.

Schecter WP and Wilson RS: Management of upper airway obstruction in the intensive care unit. Crit Care Med *9:*577, 1981.

Taylor PA and Towey RM: The bronchofiberscope as an aid to endotracheal intubation. Br J Anaesth *44:*611, 1926.

Ward PH, Canalis R, Fee W, and Smith G: Composite hyoid sternohyoid muscle grafts in humans. Arch Otolaryngol Head Neck Surg *103:*531, 1977.

Weymuller EA and Cummings CW: Cricothyroidotomy: the impact of antecedent endotracheal intubation. Ann Otol Rhinol Laryngol *91:*437, 1982.

Wong MD, Kashima H, Finnegan DA, and Jafek BW: Vascularized hyoid interposition for subglottic and upper tracheal stenosis. Ann Otol Rhinol Laryngol *87:*491, 1978.

Tracheal Stenosis

Areola MK, Inberg MV, Puhakka H: Tracheal stenosis after tracheostomy and after cuffed orotracheal intubation. Acta Chir Scand *147:*183, 1981.

Barclay RS, McSwan N, and Welsh TM: Tracheal reconstruction without the use of grafts. Thorax *12:*177, 1957.

Bjork VO and Rodriguez LE: Reconstruction of the trachea and its bifurcation: an experimental study. J Thorac Surg *35:*596, 1958.

Bryce DP and Lawson VG: The "through" method of laryngotracheal reconstruction. Ann Otol Rhinol Laryngol 76:793, 1967.

Bryce D: The surgical management of laryngotracheal injury. J Laryngol Otol 86:547, 1972.

Cantrell JR and Folse JR: The repair of circumferential defects of the trachea by direct anastomosis: experimental evaluation. J Thorac Cardiovasc Surg 42:589, 1961.

Cotton R: Management of subglottic stenosis in infancy and childhood: a review of a consecutive series of cases managed by surgical reconstruction. Ann Otol Rhinol Laryngol 87:649, 1978.

Dedo HH and Fishman NH: Laryngeal release and sleeve resection for tracheal stenosis. Ann Otol Rhinol Laryngol 78:285, 1969.

Eschapasse H: Les tumeurs trachéales primitives: traitement chirurgical. Rev Fr Mal Respir 2:425, 1974.

Evans JN: Laryngotracheoplasty. Otolaryngol Clin North Am 10:119, 1977.

Fishman AP: Pulmonary Diseases and Disorders. St. Louis, McGraw-Hill, 1980.

Gluck T and Zeller A: Die prophylaktische Resektion der Trachea. Arch Klin Chir 26:427, 1891.

Greenberg SD: Tracheal homografts in dogs. Arch Otolaryngol 67:577, 1958.

Greenberg SD and Williams RK: Tracheal prostheses. Arch Otolaryngol 75:335, 1962.

Grillo HC, Bendixen HH, and Gephert T: Resection of the carina and lower trachea. Ann Surg 158:889, 1963.

Grillo HC: The management of tracheal stenosis following assisted respiration. J Thorac Cardiovasc Surg 57:52, 1969.

Grillo HC: Tracheal reconstruction: indication and techniques. Arch Otolaryngol 96:31, 1972.

Grillo HC: Tracheal anatomy and surgical approaches. In: Textbook of General Thoracic Surgery 2nd Ed. Edited by Shields TW. Philadelphia, Lea & Febiger, 1983, p 341.

Grillo HC: Tracheal surgery. Scand J Thor Cardiovasc Surg 17:67, 1983.

Juvenelle A and Citret G: Transplantation de la bronche souche et résection de la bifunction trachéale: une étude experimentale sur le chien. J Chir (Paris) 67:666, 1951.

Koenig F: Zur Deckung von Defecten in der vorderen Trachealwand. Berl Klin Wochenschr 33:1129, 1896.

Kuster E: Vorstellung eines Patienten bei welchem der halbe Kehlkopf extirpiert worden ist. Zentralbl Chir 13:95, 1884.

Michaelson E, Solomon R, Maun L, and Ramirez J: Experiments in tracheal reconstruction. J Thorac Cardiovasc Surg 41:748, 1961.

Moghissi K: Tracheal reconstruction with a prosthesis of Marlex mesh and pericardium. J Thorac Cardiovasc Surg 69:499, 1975.

Montgomery WW: Suprahyoid release for tracheal anastomosis. Arch Otolaryngol Head Neck Surg 99:255, 1974.

Natellis F: Osservazioni sull'uso della placenta per la riparazione di perdite di sostanza dell'albero bronchiale. Arch Ital Chir 75:463, 1952.

Neville WE, Bolanowski PJ, and Soltanzadeh H: Prosthetic reconstruction of the trachea and carina. J Thorac Cardiovasc Surg 72:525, 1976.

Ogura JH and Powers WE: Functional restitution of traumatic stenosis of the larynx and pharynx. Laryngoscope 74:1081, 1964.

Ogura JH, Heeneman H, and Spector GJ: Laryngotracheal trauma: diagnosis and treatment. Can J Otolaryngol 2:112, 1973.

Ogura JH and Spector GJ: Reconstructive surgery of the larynx and laryngeal part of pharynx: experimental aspects and their clinical application. In: Scientific Foundations of Otolaryngology. Edited by Hinchcliffe R and Harrison D. London, William Heinemann, 1976.

Pearson FG and Andrews MJ: Detection and management of tracheal stenosis following cuffed tube tracheostomy. Ann Thorac Surg 12:359, 1971.

Pearson FG: Techniques in surgery of the trachea. In: Surgery of the Lung. The Coventry Conference: Proceedings of a Conference Held at the Postgraduate Medical Centre, Coventry. Edited by Smith RE and Williams WG. London, Butterworth, 1974, p 91.

Perelman MI and Koroleva N: Surgery of the trachea. World J Surg 4:583, 1980.

Rob CG and Bateman GH: Reconstruction of the trachea and cervical oesophagus; preliminary report. Br J Surg 37:202, 1950.

Som ML and Klein SH: Primary anastomosis of the trachea after resection of a wide segment: an experimental study. J Mount Sinai Hosp 25:211, 1958.

Spector GJ: Respiratory insufficiency, tracheostenosis, and airway control. In: Diseases of the Nose, Throat, Ear, Head, and Neck. 14th Ed. Edited by Ballenger JJ. Philadelphia, Lea & Febiger, 1991.

Taffel M: The repair of tracheal and bronchial defects with free facial grafts. Surgery 8:56, 1940.

Uhlschmid G: Die experimentelle tracheal-Verlangerung. Langenbecks Arch Chir 331:255, 1972.

Voena G and Maritano M: Sostituzione della trachea cervicale con tubi di Dacron (studio sperimentale nel cane). Minerva Otolaryngol 11:143, 1961.

von Mangoldt F: Die Einpflanzung von Rippenknorpel in den Kehlkopf zur Heilung schwerer Stenosen und and Defecte, und Heilung der Sattelnase durch Knorpelubertragung. Verh Dtsch Ges Chir 49:460, 1900.

Waddell WR and Cannon B: A technic for subtotal excision of the trachea and establishment of sternal tracheostomy. Ann Surg 149:1, 1959.

28 Congenital Anomalies of the Larynx

Rodney P. Lusk

Congenital lesions of the larynx are relatively rare; however, in their laryngeal laboratory, Chen and Holinger found congenital laryngeal lesions in 33 of 115 specimens.[1] Of all the anomalies noted, the most common deformity is of the cricoid cartilage. The lesions develop during respiratory differentiation, which occurs during the fourth to tenth weeks of gestation. The clinical manifestations of laryngeal lesions fall into three broad categories:

1. *Respiratory distress* may range from complete obstruction with no air movement to minor types of stridor. The characteristics of the stridor are variable and depend on the site and degree of the obstruction. Most laryngeal lesions produce stridor during the inspiratory phase. The reason for this is found in Bernoulli's principle, which states that when a fluid or a gas is in motion, the pressure exerted on the wall of the airway decreases as the velocity of the gas increases. A well-known example is the wing of an airplane, shown in Figure 28–1. When the site of the obstruction is in an area not firmly fixed or supported, such as the supraglottis or larynx, as the air rushes into the airway, it produces a relatively negative pressure, which tends to close the airway (Fig. 28–2). The harder the child breathes in, the faster the flow and the greater the created negative pressure, with the net effect of further decreasing the airway lumen. The negative pressure generated during inspiration also causes supraclavicular and sternal retractions and nasal flare.
2. *Dysphonia* may be caused by laryngeal lesions that interfere with vocalization, with voice quality ranging from complete aphonia to hoarseness.
3. *Failure of the larynx to close the airway* during swallowing may cause feeding difficulties, with aspiration, cyanosis, or respiratory compromise.

Although this chapter deals only with laryngeal lesions, any airway lesion may result in stridor, tachycardia, tachypnea, cyanosis, or restlessness. When evaluating patients with these signs, a history and examination of the entire airway should be performed. The history and physical examination are the most important diagnostic tools. Radiographic imaging (plain films, computed tomography, and magnetic resonance imaging) and laryngoscopy (direct and indirect) are important adjuncts and are discussed in each section.

LARYNGOMALACIA

Laryngomalacia is a condition in which the laryngeal inlet collapses on inspiration, causing stridor. The terminology is confusing, with congenital laryngeal stridor,[2] congenital laryngeal obstruction,[3] congenital stridor of infants,[4] and inspiratory laryngeal collapse[5] all used synonymously. The term laryngomalacia, introduced by Jackson and Jackson in 1942,[6] is most frequently used. Some physicians confuse this entity with tracheomalacia, which is altogether another disease.

Incidence and Etiology

Laryngomalacia is the most common cause of stridor in the newborn. In some children, it may be an autosomal dominant lesion.[7] Hawkins and Clark evaluated 453 patients with the flexible fiberscope and found 84 with primary and 29 with secondary laryngomalacia.[8] Nussbaum and Maggi found that 68% of 297 children with laryngomalacia had other respiratory disorders, as noted with flexible bronchoscopy.[9] Therefore, their recommendation was that all "symptomatic" children be evaluated by bronchoscopy. The disadvantage of using a flexible scope is that it does not accurately assess the subglottis. The incidence noted by other authors has ranged from 50 to 75% in patients with congenital la-

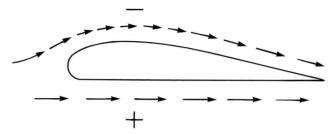

Fig. 28–1. For a wing to produce lift, the air pressure on the top of the wing must be less than the pressure on the bottom. According to Bernoulli's principle, this can occur only when the velocity of the air is greater over the top of the wing, which is accomplished by increasing its upper curvature.

ryngeal lesions[10–12] to 59.8% of all patients presenting with stridor.[10] In 10%[5] to 15%[13] of patients, the laryngomalacia is severe, with surgical intervention warranted. Deaths have been described in patients with severe disease.[14,15]

Signs and Symptoms

The most common symptoms produced by laryngomalacia are inspiratory stridor, feeding problems, and gastric reflux. The inspiratory stridor worsens with increased respiratory effort, such as crying or feeding, and in the supine position. The symptoms begin shortly after birth in most patients,[16] increase in severity until 8 months of age, plateau at 9 months, and steadily improve thereafter.[5,17,18] The mean duration

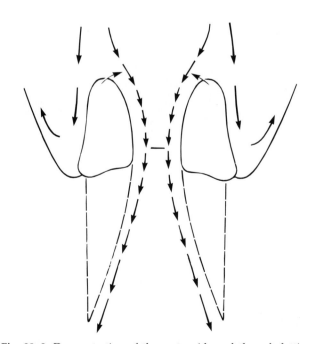

Fig. 28–2. Demonstration of the arytenoids and the subglottis as compared to an air foil. Note as the velocity of the air flow increases in the glottis, it creates negative pressure in the airway pulling the cuneiform cartilages and aryepiglottic folds into the airway.

of stridor is 4 years 2 months.[19] No correlation exists between the duration of stridor and the severity or time of onset.[16]

Two theories have been proposed to account for the narrowing of the laryngeal inlet. The first is that a neuromuscular abnormality, by not allowing proper support of the supraglottis, causes increased flaccidity.[20] Kelemen suggested that the cause is ineffective dilators of the supraglottis,[21] but dissections by Belmont and Grundfast showed the dual insertion of the palatopharyngeus, lateral glossoepiglottic, and stylopharyngeal muscles, which could dilate the laryngeal inlet.[20] The incidence of neuromuscular disorders appears to be higher in children with laryngomalacia.[17] Reports of higher incidence of mental retardation in these patients[17] have not been substantiated.[16,20,22]

The other proposed mechanism is anatomic, with the narrowing resulting from (1) a flaccid epiglottis that folds against the posterior laryngeal wall or into the airway, (2) a long, tubular epiglottis that curls on itself, or (3) short and redundant aryepiglottic folds with varying sizes of cuneiform cartilage that rotate medially into the airway (Figs. 28–3 and 28–4).[23] The ω-shaped epiglottis is not thought to be a significant factor because it occurs in 30 to 50% of patients,[3,24–26] most of whom do not have stridor.

Feeding problems are frequent. Radiographic evidence of gastric reflux occurs in 80% and regurgitation in 40%[20] past 3 months of age. In the study by Zalzal and associates, 5 of 21 patients presented with feeding problems.[27] Some investigators believe that feeding problems are secondary to the high negative pressures generated during inspiration. Aspiration pneumonitis has been reported in 7% of children with laryngomalacia.[20] The mechanism for this is unclear but may be associated with the negative pressure and feeding problems.

Obstructive sleep apnea (23%) and central apnea (10%) have also been noted.[20,28] Cor pulmonale can develop secondary to laryngomalacia.[27]

Diagnosis

The diagnosis is most frequently based on the symptoms and signs, flexible laryngoscopy, and lateral radiographs of the neck and chest to rule out subglottic lesions. Hawkins and Clark have shown flexible laryngoscopy to be effective, even in neonates.[8] Sixty-five percent of their patients were younger than 6 months. The advantage of using the flexible scope with an awake patient is that the dynamics of the supraglottis can readily be appreciated. The disadvantage is that the milder forms of laryngomalacia may be missed if the child is crying. The flexible scope can also be used to diagnose other glottic lesions such as vocal cord paralysis. Although the laryngoscope has been the time-honored method of diagnosis, when the blade is placed

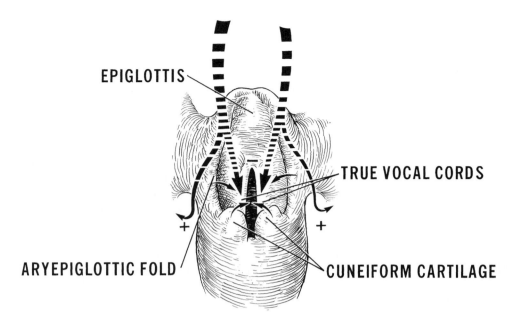

EPIGLOTTIS

TRUE VOCAL CORDS

ARYEPIGLOTTIC FOLD

CUNEIFORM CARTILAGE

Fig. 28–3. The airflow through the larynx creates a relative negative pressure and pulls the aryepiglottic folds and cuneiform cartilage into the airway.

in the vallecula, it may splint the epiglottis and prevent prolapse of the supraglottis into the airway. Many surgeons believe that if the symptoms and the results of the flexible scope examination are compatible with laryngomalacia, and if the child is thriving, no further workup is needed. If symptoms are not compatible with laryngomalacia or if the patient fails to thrive, however, direct laryngoscopy and bronchoscopy should be done to rule out secondary lesions. The flexible scope should not take the place of rigid endoscopy, especially if a second subgottic lesion is suspected. If dysphagia is present, the patient should have a barium swallow examination and rigid endoscopy to rule out concomitant lesions.

Treatment

Expectant observation is sufficient in most cases. The small percentage of patients (10 to 15%) with failure to thrive or more than one lesion may require surgical intervention. The airway has traditionally been managed through a tracheostomy. This procedure is not to be taken lightly because the risks are significant.

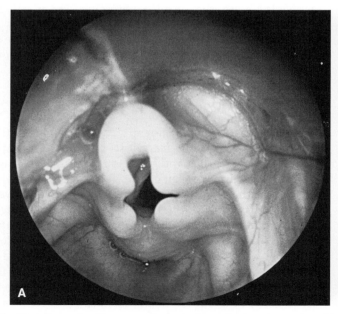
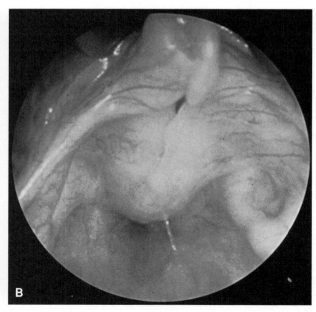

Fig. 28–4. Example of laryngomalacia. A. Supraglottis at beginning of inspiration. B. Complete collapse of the supraglottis toward the end of inspiration. (Courtesy of Dr. G.B. Healy, Boston Children's Hospital, Boston.)

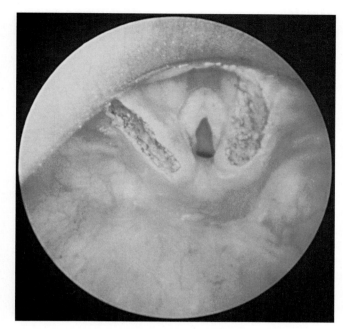

Fig. 28–5. Example of supraglottoplasty with the laser. Note the sparing of the posterior commissure.

Children in poor social environments may require prolonged hospitalization.

Iglauer,[29] in 1922, was the first to alter the supraglottis surgically in laryngomalacia. Schwartz,[5] in 1944, removed a V-shaped wedge from an epiglottis with good results. Fearon and Ellis,[30] in 1971, successfully treated a patient by suturing the epiglottis to the base of the tongue. In that same year, hyomandibulopexy was advocated in France.[31,32] Templer and colleagues,[33] in 1981, performed a supraglottectomy in an adult for long-standing stridor and obstructive sleep apnea secondary to laryngomalacia. Lane and associates,[34] in 1984, excised the tips of the arytenoids, edematous mucosa, a portion of the corniculate cartilages, and a portion of the aryepiglottic fold with microcupped forceps and Bellucci scissors. Seid and colleagues successfully treated three patients with the laser in 1985.[35] Since then, numerous case reports have appeared in the literature.[28] Zalzal and associates trimmed the lateral edges of the epiglottis, aryepiglottic folds, and the corniculate cartilages with microlaryngeal scissors.[27] Solomons and Prescott recommended trimming the supraglottis and performing an anterior epiglottopexy.[24]

Holinger and Konior prefer the term supraglottoplasty to describe the surgical procedures for removing the flaccid supraglottic tissues.[23] These investigators used the laser to remove a portion of the cuneiform cartilage and the aryepiglottic folds (Fig. 28–5). Care must be taken not to excise or traumatize the strip of mucosa between the arytenoids in the posterior glottis. Holinger and Konior believe that prophylactic antibiotics should be used, and most patients may be extu-

bated in the immediate postoperative period but should be observed overnight in the intensive care unit.[23]

BIFID AND ABSENT EPIGLOTTIS

Incidence

These rare lesions can be associated with stridor and aspiration. In the only thorough review of the world literature, Montreuil found only five clearly documented cases.[36] Since then, an additional six cases have been reported.[37–39]

Signs and Symptoms

Patients have presented with respiratory distress secondary to rotation of the two halves of the epiglottis into the airway. The incidence of multiple congenital anomalies is high. A 44% incidence of polydactyly has been reported.[40] Graham and colleagues have reported three cases of hypopituitarism.[38]

Diagnosis

The only means of diagnosing a bifid epiglottis is with flexible or direct laryngoscopy (Fig. 28–6). Because of the high incidence of associated airway lesions, direct laryngoscopy is suggested for all patients.

Treatment

If the airway distress is significant, a tracheostomy is warranted. Montreuil amputated the epiglottis with

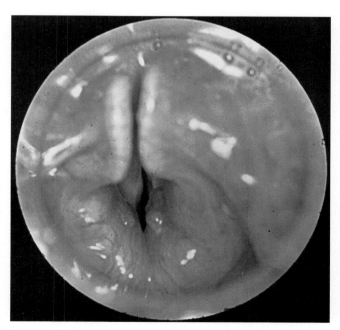

Fig. 28–6. Bifid epiglottis. (Courtesy of Dr. L.D. Holinger, Children's Memorial Hospital, Chicago.)

good results.[36] Healy and associates performed a tracheostomy in two patients, and in time the epiglottis matured and both patients were decannulated without surgical intervention on the epiglottis.[40]

ATRESIA

Atresia occurs when the laryngeal opening fails to develop and an obstruction is created at or near the glottis.

Incidence and Etiology

Congenital laryngeal atresia is a rare lesion, with only 51 cases reported in the world literature in 1987.[41] It is thought to be the rarest laryngeal lesion, accounting for only 1 of 846 congenital lesions evaluated by Holinger and colleagues,[11,42] and none of 433 congenital lesions evaluated by Fearon and Ellis.[30] The lesion is thought to arise from the premature arrest of normal vigorous epithelial ingrowth into the larynx during the 14th to 17th stages of embryonic development.[43] In the embryonic larynx, a pharyngoglottic duct divides the larynx into an anterior (membranous) portion and a posterior (cartilaginous) portion.[44]

Signs and Symptoms

At delivery, the child makes strong respiratory efforts but does not move air, cry, or manifest any stridor. The child becomes markedly cyanotic when the umbilical cord is clamped. Most of these children die at birth unless an emergency tracheostomy is performed. Some children survive if they have a large tracheoesophageal fistula and if the esophagus is intubated. Not infrequently, a pharyngotracheal duct is present in the larynx. This should not be confused with a tracheoesophageal fistula, which is located much lower.

Diagnosis

The diagnosis is most frequently made at autopsy. With the increased use of ultrasound, the diagnosis of laryngeal atresia can be made before birth by noting enlarged edematous lungs, compressed fetal heart, severe ascites, and fetal hydrops.[45-47] Smith and Bain outlined three types of laryngeal atresia deformities;[48] these investigators indicated that these types are not absolute but are gradations of a continuous spectrum. Type 1 involves the supraglottic and infraglottic larynx with fused arytenoids, an absent vestibule, and a deformed cricoid. Type 2 involves only the cricoid (subglottic area) with normal arytenoids, vestibule, and vocal cords. Type 3 involves a fused glottis with a nor-

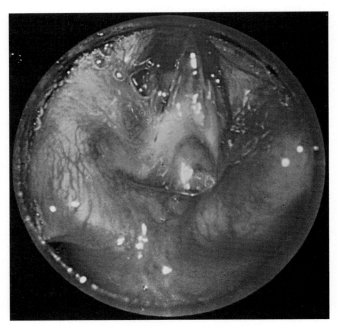

Fig. 28–7. Type 3 laryngeal atresia. (Courtesy of Dr. L.D. Holinger, Children's Memorial Hospital, Chicago.)

mal vestibule and cricoid (Fig. 28–7). The subglottic lesions have been found to be cartilaginous or membranous.[43]

Treatment

The patient will not survive unless an emergency tracheostomy is performed or the patient is ventilated through a tracheoesophageal fistula. Tracheoesophageal fistulas are frequently associated with this condition and usually arise at the tracheal bifurcation[48,49] (Fig. 28–8). Of the four known survivors, three had the membranous type 3 lesion, and one had a type 2 lesion and a tracheoesophageal fistula, which allowed ventilation until a tracheostomy could be performed. In one

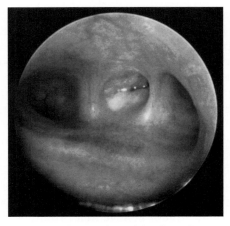

Fig. 28–8. Tracheoesophageal fistula at the carina.

report, a patient who had an atresia, without a fistula, was resuscitated with an 18-gauge intravenous cannula into the trachea.[50]

WEBS

Laryngeal webs occur in the glottis. Rarely, webs extend from the epiglottis to the lateral or posterior aspects of the hypopharynx and can result in significant airway compromise.[51] Holinger and associates described a patient with simultaneous supraglottic and laryngeal webs.[52] Most webs are located anteriorly and extend a varying length toward the arytenoids. The webs vary in thickness from a thin structure to one that is thicker and more difficult to eradicate. Benjamin and Mair described a rare type known as a congenital interarytenoid web, which limits the abduction of the arytenoids.[53]

Incidence

Congenital laryngeal webs are uncommon, occurring in 5% of all congenital laryngeal lesions.[42,54] Acquired lesions are more common than congenital lesions, in a 60:40 ratio.[55] Associated anomalies are frequently seen, especially higher in the airway.[54,56,57] Posterior glottic webs occur in only 1 to 4% of patients.[55]

Signs and Symptoms

Symptoms of laryngeal webs are present at birth in 75% of patients and within 1 year in all patients.[57] The types of symptoms depend on the severity of the web. Many children are asymptomatic until they are stressed, have an infection, or are intubated for a surgical procedure.

Vocal dysfunction is the most frequent symptom and was noted in 47 of 51 patients evaluated by Cohen.[56] The severity of the dysphonia is not necessarily indicative of the severity of the web. Cohen reported on 11 patients who complained of aphonia, 16 with weak or whispery voices, 7 with husky voices, and 4 with some hoarseness.

The second most common symptom is airway obstruction, and the severity is directly proportional to the degree of obstruction. The compromise may be so severe that stridor cannot be produced because of limited air movement through the larynx. If stridor is present, it will occur in both inspiratory and expiratory phases, and if stridor is severe, the airway must be secured with intubation or a tracheostomy. Forty percent of Cohen's patients required a tracheostomy.[56]

Croup rarely occurs in children younger than 6 months. Cohen reported 15 of 51 children with a significant history of recurrent croup,[56] of whom 7 required

tracheostomy, 9 presented with pneumonia, and 6 had tracheobronchitis.

Diagnosis

The only way to make the correct diagnosis is by direct laryngoscopy under general anesthesia. The flexible scope may also have a role, but experience in using it in patients with laryngeal webs is limited. Lateral radiographs of the neck may allow assessment of the width of the web.

Cohen has divided laryngeal webs into four types, based on their appearance and an estimation of the degree of airway obstruction.[56] Type 1 is uniform in thickness, with no subglottic extension, with the true vocal cords clearly visible in the web, and compromises less than 35% of the airway (Fig. 28–9). Hoarseness is usually only slight. Type 2 is slightly thicker, with a significantly thicker anterior component that may extend into the subglottis. The web restricts the airway by 35 to 50% and usually causes little airway distress unless the patient has an acute infection or is traumatized during intubation (Fig. 28–10). The voice is usually husky. Type 3 is a thick web that is solid anteriorly with the true vocal cords not well delineated. The web restricts the airway by 50 to 75%, and one notes marked vocal dysfunction, with a weak and whispery voice. Type 4 is a uniformly thick, solid web occluding 75 to 90% of the airway (Fig. 28–11). Respiratory obstruction is severe, and the patient is almost always aphonic.

Treatment

Approximately 60% of patients require surgical intervention.[57] Some webs are not repaired because the pa-

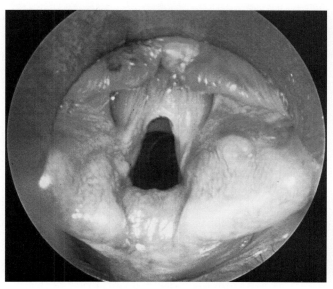

Fig. 28–9. Type 1 laryngeal web.

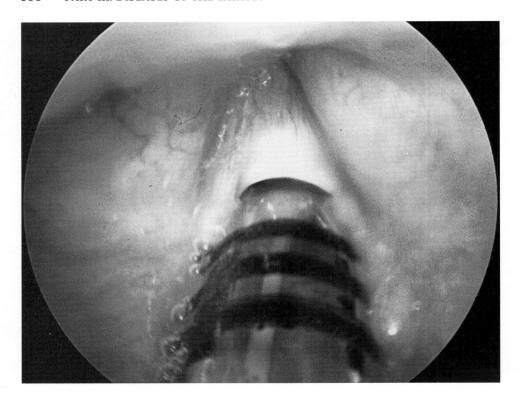

Fig. 28–10. Type 2 laryngeal web that is intubated. This patient will likely be symptomatic after extubation.

tients succumb to other systemic complications. Of all patients with laryngeal webs, 30 to 40% require a tracheostomy.[56,57] The type of lesion dictates the surgical approach. In general, the thinner webs are easier to treat; the more severe webs are resistant to surgical management. It is difficult to obtain a crisp anterior

commissure, and even if one is obtained, this does not ensure a good voice.

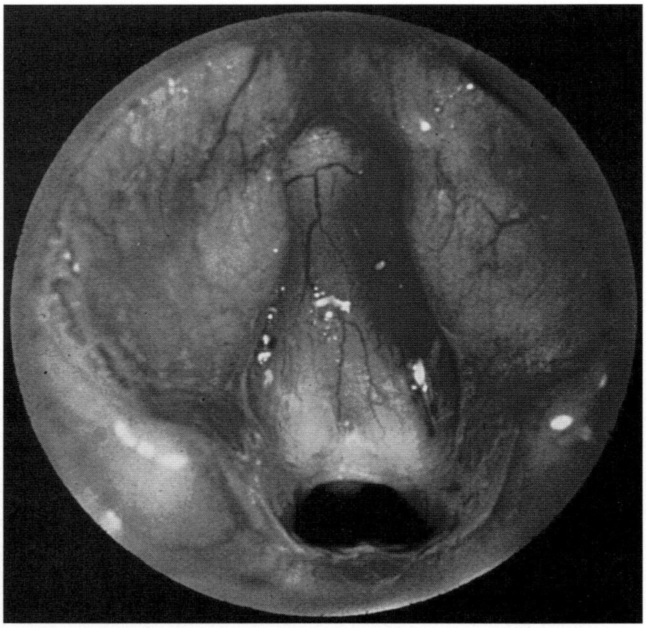

Type 1 lesions are not life-threatening. Many do not require surgery, but if surgery is performed, dilations or excisions with a knife, scissors, or laser is effective. Type 2 lesions require treatment, but not in childhood. Multiple procedures are necessary for excising small portions of the web in multiple steps. Corticosteroids and antibiotics decrease the amount of scarring, and speech therapy may be necessary to maximize phonation. Type 3 lesions frequently require tracheostomy to establish the airway. The child may develop progressive airway distress because of increased airway demands, trauma from intubation, or infection. These lesions may require multiple excisions and frequently necessitate the placement of a keel.[58,59] McGuirt and associates described a method using the laser to develop flaps of the web and reported near normal results in all patients.[55] Type 4 lesions all require a tracheostomy and excision of the web with placement of a keel. Because they are tracheostomy dependent, these patients should be monitored with apnea monitors. Most surgeons would resect the web and place the keel through a laryngofissure. The airway results are good, but the voice is poor.[56]

SACCULAR CYSTS AND LARYNGOCELES

Laryngoceles and laryngeal saccular cysts are thought to arise from the laryngeal or saccular appendage[60–64]

Fig. 28–11. Type 4 laryngeal web. (Courtesy of Dr. L.D. Holinger, Children's Memorial Hospital, Chicago.)

or from retention cysts resulting from obstruction of mucus gland ducts.[65] Hilton detailed the anatomy of the saccular appendage in 1837. Morgagni incompletely described the saccule, and Galen also had mentioned it previously.[66] The appendage arises from the anterior ventricle, extends superiorly, and curves slightly posteriorly deep to the false vocal cords and aryepiglottic folds. The orifice opens into the ventricle and measures only 0.5 to 1 mm. The ventriculosaccular fold probably serves to help store mucus and direct it posteromedially to lubricate the vocal cords.[67] In the adult, the appendage extends as high as the superior border of the thyroid cartilage. Broyles found that 75% of the saccules measured 6 to 8 mm in length, 25% measured more than 10 mm, and 7% measured more than 15 mm.[68] In the fetus, 25% extend as high as the thyrohyoid membrane.[66] The type of lesion that develops is based on the size of the saccule, whether there is free communication with the laryngeal lumen, and whether there is inflammation within the sac. DeSanto and colleagues believe that the differentiating factor between the development of a cyst or a laryngocele is the patency of the ventricle.[66,69]

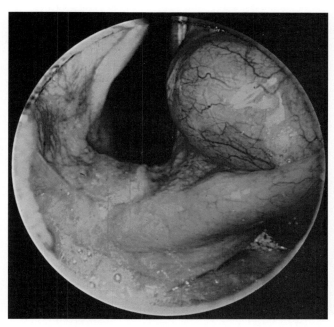

Fig. 28–12. Lateral saccular cyst. (Courtesy of Dr. L.D. Holinger, Children's Memorial Hospital, Chicago.)

Saccular Cysts

Incidence
Laryngeal saccular cysts are most likely to become manifest in infancy.[66] Congenital laryngeal cysts are rare, but the awareness of their possibility is important because almost 50% of these cysts are diagnosed at autopsy after the infant has asphyxiated.[70] In 1967, Suehs and Powell found 27 reported cases of congenital laryngeal cysts.[70]

Signs and Symptoms
Forty percent of congenital laryngeal cysts are discovered within a few hours of birth, and 95% of the children have symptoms before 6 months of age.[71] The most frequent symptom is stridor (90%), which is primarily inspiratory, although it may be biphasic.[67] The stridor improves in some infants during extension of the head. The cry has been reported as feeble, muffled, shrill, hoarse, or normal.[42,70] Dyspnea, apnea, and cyanosis have been noted in 55% of patients.[71] The associated feeding problems are similar to those in esophageal atresia or tracheoesophageal fistula without atresia and lead to failure to thrive in a large number of patients.[70,71]

Diagnosis
Chest and lateral neck radiographs, barium swallow, and computed tomographic scan are useful preoperative evaluations of the stridor, but they are not diagnostic.[67,72] Hemangiomas, for example, can cause identical findings, although these lesions appear most frequently in the subglottis. The only way to make the

diagnosis definitive is with direct laryngoscopy.[71] Cotton and Richardson suggested that at the time of endoscopy one should have a large-bore needle, a tracheostomy tray, and an appropriate-size rigid bronchoscope available.[73] The cysts are typically divided into lateral wall saccular cysts and anterior saccular cysts. Lateral saccular cysts are most frequently located in the aryepiglottic fold, epiglottis, or lateral wall of the larynx[70,71] (Fig. 28–12). Anterior saccular cysts extend medially and posteriorly between the true and false vocal cords and directly into the laryngeal lumen[71,72] (Fig. 28–13). They are most frequently sessile but may be pedunculated. Mitchell and associates reported four subglottic cysts in patients who had previously been intubated and considered the cysts to be probably secondary to intubation.[71]

Treatment
Treatment of laryngeal cysts may require emergency tracheostomy.[67,74,75] Mitchell and associates noted that 20% of their patients required emergency intervention.[71] In the infant, the cysts should be treated primarily with endoscopic deroofing or aspiration. Suehs and Powell recommended endoscopic incision and drainage as needed.[70] Holinger and colleagues thought that smaller anterior saccular cysts could be effectively treated with cup forceps removal (excision biopsy) at the time of direct laryngoscopy.[67] These investigators would not attempt endoscopic dissection of the entire sac. Aspiration has also been recommended, but the incidence of recurrence is high.[67,76] Mitchell and associates reported successful treatment of 7 of 17 patients

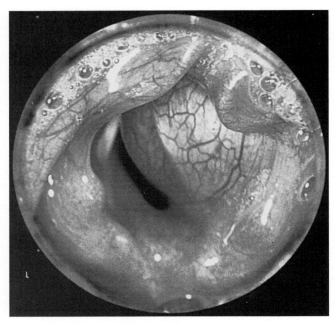

Fig. 28–13. Anterior saccular cyst. (Courtesy of Dr. L.D. Holinger, Children's Memorial Hospital, Chicago.)

with deroofing or marsupialization.[71] A second deroofing was required in 6 of the 7 recurrences. The remaining failure was treated with total excision through a laryngofissure.

Laryngoceles

Incidence

As of 1977, 300 laryngoceles had been recorded in the world literature. They may occur in infants and children,[77] and they cause airway obstruction.[78] The presence of laryngoceles in this age group appears to be rare, however. Laryngoceles are much more common in adults and appear most commonly in the fifth decade.[77] Holinger and Braw reported on 12 patients with congenital laryngocele in infancy.[42] Baker and associates found an increased incidence of laryngoceles in laryngeal cancer and suggested that obstruction of the saccule by the carcinoma was a factor in developing laryngoceles.[79]

Signs and Symptoms

Laryngoceles are symptomatic only when they are filled with air or fluid, so the symptoms may be intermittent. Because the laryngocele may rapidly inflate and deflate, several radiographs may be necessary to document the lesion. A fluid-filled laryngocele may be difficult to differentiate from a cyst. If it becomes infected, it fills with mucopus and is called a laryngopyocele.

Diagnosis

The definitive diagnosis is made with direct laryngoscopy, but because the symptoms are intermittent, more

than one examination may be necessary. Laryngoceles originate from the ventricle and bulge out between the true and false vocal cords or dissect posteriorly into the arytenoid and aryepiglottic fold. In general, three types have been described: internal, external, and mixed;[77] however, this classification is artificial. The internal type is limited to the larynx, whereas the external type extends into the neck through the isthmus of the thyrohyoid membrane. The mixed type involves both internal and external cysts and is the most common. Laryngoceles should be diagnosed with direct laryngoscopy when they are symptomatic, in addition to radiographic findings. Trapnell has emphasized that the radiographic appearance of a large saccule does not warrant the diagnosis of a laryngocele.[80]

Treatment

Only symptomatic lesions require treatment. DeSanto preferred the external approach;[66] however, most of his experience was in adults. The procedure described by Yarington and Frazer provides adequate exposure for resection.[81] Holinger and associates emphasized that true laryngoceles are rare in children and should be treated endoscopically by deroofing with cup forceps.[67] On occasion, the laryngocele can be aspirated and a more orderly resection can be performed at a later date.[82] The laser is also an alternative.

LARYNGEAL CLEFTS

Congenital laryngotracheoesophageal cleft is characterized by a deficiency in the separation between the esophagus and the trachea or larynx. Clefts of the larynx alone are less common.[83]

Incidence

Most clefts occur through the posterior glottis; however, ventral or rare anterior clefts have been reported.[84–86] Clefts may be classified into three broad categories. Type I is called the laryngeal cleft and is found only in the posterior glottis. Type II and type III involve the trachea in addition to the larynx (Fig. 28–14). Type II extends down to but not beyond the sixth tracheal ring, and type III can extend to the carina. As of 1983, 85 well-documented cases of clefts have been reported in the world literature.[87] Finlay observed a family in which 2 of 5 children developed a cleft larynx.[88] Other investigators have reported similar examples.[89–91] The inheritance pattern is almost always autosomal dominant.[91] Posterior glottic clefts have been associated with tracheal agenesis, as well as many other congenital anomalies.[87]

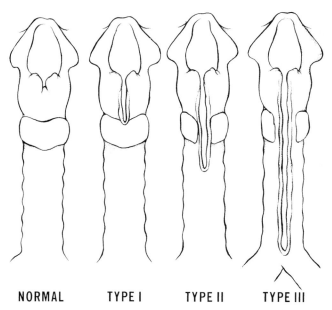

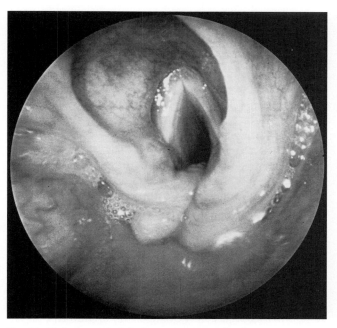

Fig. 28–14. Classification of laryngeal and tracheoesophageal clefts as proposed by Evans.

Fig. 28–15. Laryngeal cleft demonstrating redundant mucosa prolapsing into the larynx on inspiration.

Signs and Symptoms

In the world literature, 35 of 85 patients had type I clefts, 36 of 85 had type II clefts, and 14 of 85 had type III clefts. The following manifestations, in order of frequency, are associated with laryngotracheoesophageal clefts: aspiration and cyanosis (53%), postpartum asphyxia (33%), increased mucus production (23%), recurrent pneumonia (16%), voiceless crying (16%), stridor, (10%) and impaired swallowing (5%).[87] The simultaneous occurrence of increased saliva production, low, soundless, or hurried crying, and stridor should lead to the suspicion of a cleft. The inspiratory stridor is produced by the collapse of redundant mucosa around the cleft and from the intrusion of the arytenoid into the airway.[93,94] Cohen reported that the stridor may be expiratory because of aspirated secretions.[83] One sees a frequent combination of posterior laryngeal clefts and tracheoesophageal fistulas.

Diagnosis

Occult posterior laryngeal clefts have been diagnosed with magnetic resonance imaging.[95] A laryngeal cleft is frequently demonstrated by an esophagram with water-soluble contrast medium[96] or is suggested by aspiration pneumonia on a chest radiograph. The most important diagnostic test, however, is direct laryngoscopy. If one does not specifically look for the entity, it frequently escapes detection.[97] When the larynx is examined, redundant mucosa in the posterior cleft is usually the first clue to the defect (Fig. 28–15). On inspiration, this redundant mucosa may rotate into the airway. The cleft can best be demonstrated by placing a laryngoscope, such as a Dedo or Jako, into the supraglottis and examining the posterior glottis. If a posterior laryngeal cleft is present, this maneuver will clearly demonstrate the lesion and its extent (Fig. 28–16). The posterior glottis can also be palpated with a spatula or a similar thin instrument to demonstrate the defect. Some authors find microlaryngoscopy helpful.[93] Some clefts are submucous, and diagnosis is made only on laryngeal sections.[98,99] The clinical significance of submucous clefts is unknown.

There is a high incidence of associated esophageal lesions and tracheoesophageal fistulas, for which careful examination must be made.[83,93,98,100]

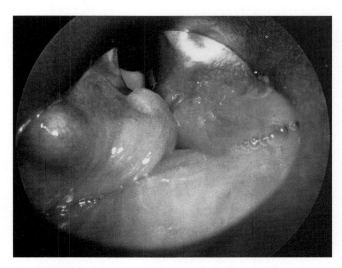

Fig. 28–16. Jako laryngoscope inserted into the posterior commissure, demonstrating the laryngeal cleft.

Treatment

The prognosis for a patient with this lesion is not favorable. In the review presented by Roth and colleagues,[87] 24 patients died before surgical intervention; of patients with type III clefts, 13 of 14 died; of those with type II clefts, 13 of 31 died; and of those with type I, 13 of 30 died. Almost two thirds of the deceased patients had other severe malformations. Clefts were repaired in 48 patients, 13 of whom died. A tracheostomy was performed in 50% of all patients. The first successful operative correction of the defect in the larynx was achieved by Petterson.[101]

Three surgical approaches to the posterior aspect of the larynx have been described: (1) minor (type I clefts) can be repaired endoscopically;[102,103] (2) lateral pharyngotomy has been used frequently, especially for the smaller laryngeal clefts;[87,93] the major disadvantage of this approach lies in the danger of injuring the recurrent nerve; the exposure is limited, and it is difficult to obtain a good layered closure; and (3) anterior laryngofissure does not risk the recurrent laryngeal nerve and has been used in neonates.[83,87,94,104–106] Evans reported better exposure and a better two-layer closure in type II and III clefts with a laryngofissure[93] (Fig. 28–17). A disturbance of the laryngeal growth appears unlikely. Intraoperative airway management has been a problem in repairing these lesions. Ahmad and associates solved the problem by using a bifurcated endotracheal tube.[107] Geiduschek and colleagues reported the use of extracorporeal membrane oxygenation for extensive cleft repair.[108] We have used bypass to repair long-segment tracheal stenosis.

Cotton and Schreiber have noted that, after repair of posterior clefts, the patient may have continued esophageal reflux and aspiration of gastric contents.[109]

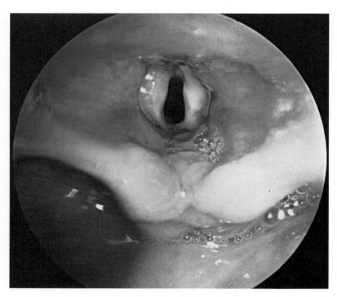

Fig. 28–17. Type I cleft repaired through a laryngofissure.

When this occurs, these investigators recommend a high gastric section with a double gastrostomy to minimize the chance of aspiration of gastric contents. Robie and associates reported that of 170 clefts repaired, 19 required revision surgery.[106]

VOCAL CORD PARALYSIS

Vocal cord paralysis can be categorized into congenital and acquired lesions. One or both of the true vocal cords may be involved, and bilateral vocal cord paralysis is more frequent.[110–112] Apnea is frequently seen in bilateral vocal cord paralysis.[113–115] Congenital lesions are frequently associated with central nervous system lesions, including hydrocephalus, meningomyelocele, Arnold-Chiari malformation, meningocele, encephalocele, cerebral agenesis, nucleus ambiguus dysgenesis, neuromuscular disorders, and myasthenia gravis.[116,117] Arnold-Chiari is the most frequent malformation and is likely a contributing factor in most cases.[118]

Incidence and Etiology

Estimates of the frequency of vocal cord paralysis range from 1.5 to 23%;[112,119,120] according to some authors, it ranks second in frequency among all congenital laryngeal lesions.[116] Holinger and associates found that congenital lesions were more frequent than acquired.[117] The acquired group can be further categorized into traumatic, infectious, or neoplastic. Traumatic lesions are most frequent secondary to stretching of the recurrent nerve during vaginal delivery or surgical trauma in management of bronchogenic cysts, tracheoesophageal fistulas, or patent ductus arteriosus.[116] Infectious diseases such as whooping cough, encephalitis, poliomyelitis, diphtheria, rabies, tetanus, syphilis, and botulism are now rarely seen but can cause vocal cord paralysis.[115] Tumors of the brain and spinal column are also rare but can cause unilateral or bilateral vocal cord paralysis.

The pathophysiology of bilateral vocal cord paralysis is unclear, but the condition may result from (1) compression of the vagus nerve in its course through the foramen magnum, (2) traction of the cervical rootlets of the vagus nerve by the caudal displacement of the brain stem, or (3) brain stem dysgenesis.[121,122] Most authors favor the compression theory because, with timely decompression of hydrocephalus or the Arnold-Chiari malformation, the vocal cords regain function. Familial bilateral cord paralysis[123–125] and persistent apnea after tracheostomy[113] appear to be most appropriately explained by the dysgenesis theory. Probably, more than one lesion can cause vocal cord paralysis.

Laryngeal lesions such as subglottis stenosis, laryngomalacia, and posterior laryngeal clefts have also been associated with, but do not cause, vocal cord paralysis.[110]

Signs and Symptoms

Any of the three laryngeal functions of respiration, voice production, and deglutition can be affected by vocal cord paralysis. With unilateral vocal cord paralysis, the voice is breathy and weak, but the patient has an adequate airway unless stressed. Stridor, weak cry, and some degree of respiratory distress can be seen in all patients with bilateral vocal cord paralysis.[122] Dedo noted that, if *both* the recurrent and superior laryngeal nerves are paralyzed, the vocal cords will be in the intermediate position and the airway then will frequently be sufficient to allow adequate ventilation.[116,121] If the recurrent nerve only is paralyzed, the vocal cord will be in the paramedian position, resulting in an inadequate airway.

Stridor is the most frequent presenting symptom of bilateral vocal cord paralysis,[117] and its onset may be sudden.[122] Older children suppress laughing and coughing because of the increased respiratory demand. The airway becomes narrower and there will be an increase in stridor, the development of nasal flaring, restlessness, and the use of accessory respiratory muscles, with an indrawing of the sternum and epigastrium. The stridor may progress to cyanosis, apnea, and respiratory and cardiac arrest if not recognized and treated.

Aspiration and dysphagia are frequently noted in patients with bilateral vocal cord paralysis.[121] Pneumonia may first be apparent when signs of increasing cranial pressure appear.

Diagnosis

The diagnosis is made by flexible laryngoscopy or direct laryngoscopy. Vocal cord mobility may be difficult to examine in an infant, and the intermediate versus paramedian position may be impossible to assess.

Treatment

Once the diagnosis of vocal cord paralysis is made, the airway should be secured if the patient has significant airway distress. The airway is best established with intubation, followed by a full workup to ascertain the cause of the vocal cord paralysis. One must look specifically for associated findings of meningomyelocele, Arnold-Chiari malformation, and hydrocephalus.[117] If the compression of the nerve is relieved within 24 hours, the vocal cords will regain function within 2 weeks;[117,122] otherwise, vocal cord function may not return for a year and a half, if at all. If intervention has been timely, the larynx should be examined periodically to assess vocal cord function. If the patient shows no evidence of function within 1 to 2 weeks, a tracheostomy should be performed to relieve the airway distress,[115] but central apnea may continue even with appropriate early decompression.[113] Once the tracheostomy is in place, periodic examinations will be necessary to assess vocal cord function.

Approximately 50% of children with bilateral vocal cord paralysis require tracheostomy.[110,117,122] Bluestone and colleagues noted a 50% mortality rate secondary to shunt failure or infection in patients with Arnold-Chiari malformation.[122] Of those who survive, 25 to 48% can be decannulated.[110,121]

SUBGLOTTIC LESIONS

The principal subglottic lesions are stenoses and hemangiomas.

Stenosis

Stenoses of the subglottic area can be divided into cartilaginous stenoses, which are usually congenital, and acquired membranous or soft tissue stenoses.

Incidence and Etiology

A stenosis is considered to be congenital when the patient has no history of endotracheal intubation or trauma. The normal subglottic lumen is 4.5 to 5.5 mm in a full-term neonate and 3.5 mm in a premature neonate. We do not know in how many infants extubation fails because of congenitally small cricoid cartilages.

Congenital subglottic stenosis is the third most common congenital abnormality. Cricoid cartilage deformities are usually congenital and consist of abnormal shapes and sizes. The cricoid cartilage may have a normal shape but be small or hypoplastic. It may also be elliptical, flattened, or otherwise distorted. The first tracheal ring can also be trapped under the cricoid cartilage resulting in a narrowed subglottis. The primary causes of acquired or membranous subglottic stenosis (Fig. 28–18) in children are (1) external injury from blunt trauma or a high tracheostomy and (2) internal injury from prolonged intubation and chemical or thermal burns. External injuries are rare in infants. Internal trauma, secondary to prolonged intubation, is thought to account for approximately 90% of acquired subglottic stenosis.[126,127] The incidence of stenoses after intubation ranges from 0.9 to 8.3%.[128–131] The stenoses most frequently occur in the subglottis because (1) the cricoid cartilage is a complete circular ring without any "give" for edema, (2) the edema can accumulate rapidly in the loose areolar tissue of the subglottis, (3) the pseudostratified, ciliated columnar respiratory epithelium is delicate and easily traumatized, and (4) the narrowest portion of the upper airway is in the subglottis and is therefore the most likely to be traumatized.[127]

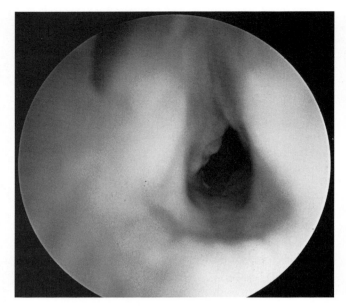

Fig. 28–18. Membranous subglottic stenosis.

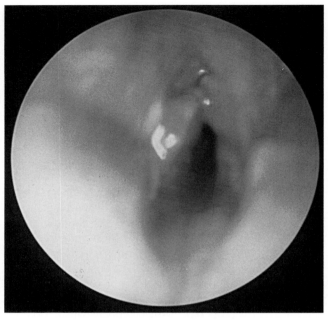

Fig. 28–19. Ulcerated right vocal process.

The pathophysiology of acquired subglottic stenoses is well described. The endotracheal tube causes pressure necrosis of the respiratory epithelium. Edema and superficial ulceration begin, and the normal ciliary flow is interrupted. As the ulcer deepens, secondary infection of the areolar tissue and perichondrium begin. Chondritis may eventually occur, with necrosis and collapse of the cricoid cartilage. Benjamin characterized the traumatic lesions formed in the larynx with prolonged intubation.[132] He noted that, in the acute phase, one sees formation of posterolateral ulcerations at the vocal processes ("ulcerated troughs") (Fig. 28–19), and usually one sees an "intact median strip" of mucosa and an "annular ulceration" of mucosa in the subglottis. "Tongues of granulation tissue" (Fig. 28–20) form anterior and posterior to the ulceration, and frequently one sees generalized inflammation and edema of the ventricle that results in ventricular protrusions. The long-term complications of these lesions are characterized as posterior glottic synechiae, "healed furrows," posterior subglottic and glottic stenoses (Fig. 28–21), "healed fibrous nodules," submucosal mucous gland hyperplasia with ductal cysts, and submucosal fibrosis and stenosis. The scar tissue forms in the subglottis and limits the airway.[133–137] Healing is inhibited in part by poor blood supply in the subglottis and constant motion of the larynx.

Neonates tolerate prolonged intubation better than adults. The reasons for this are unclear, but more pliable cartilage[133] and the higher position in the neck[135] have been suggested as considerations.

Certain factors can increase the chances of developing subglottic stenosis. An oversized endotracheal tube or a tube of appropriate size in a patient with a small cricoid cartilage can increase the mucosal pressure and

result in a deep ulceration. Primary intubation can traumatize the subglottis. In children, an endotracheal tube that allows a leak at pressure less than 20 cm H_2O should be chosen. Reintubation,[133,138] shearing motion of the tube on movement of the head,[139] and superimposed local or systemic bacterial infections[134] increase the risk. Gastroesophageal reflux can increase the inflammation and tissue trauma. Nasogastric tubes and endotracheal tubes have been noted to cause pressure necrosis of the cricoid[134] and increase the risk of reflux.

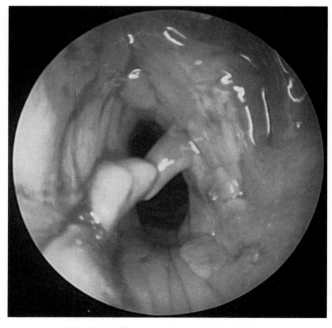

Fig. 28–20. Tongues of granulation tissue.

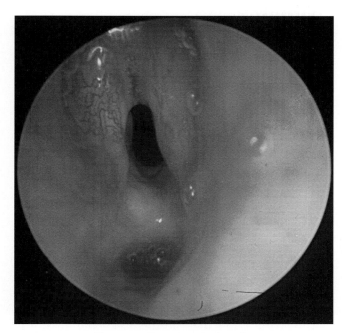

Fig. 28–21. Posterior glottic web.

Systemic factors such as immunodeficiency, anemia, neutropenia, toxicity, hypoxia, dehydration, and poor perfusion increase the risk of developing mucosal ulceration and subsequent scar formation.

Signs and Symptoms

In the intubated neonate, evidence of subglottic stenosis may not manifest until the patient is ready for extubation. If a subglottic ulcer is present, the airway may be compromised immediately or edema may accumulate over a few hours. In some patients, symptoms do not develop until 2 to 4 weeks after intubation. If the patient has mild to moderate congenital subglottic stenosis, symptoms may not appear until an infection of the upper respiratory tract causes additional narrowing and respiratory distress.

If the stenosis is congenital, the only manifestation may be prolonged or recurrent croup. A common dictum is that "there is no such thing as croup under one year of age." As respiratory demands increase, the infant may become symptomatic.[73]

The main symptoms and signs relate to airway, voice, and feeding. Stridor is the primary sign and is biphasic, with the inspiratory phase always louder. With progressive narrowing of the airway, respiratory distress ensues. If the vocal cords are affected, hoarseness, abnormal cry, and aphonia will indicate that an anterior web is present. Dysphagia and aspiration pneumonia can occur.

Diagnosis

Soft tissue radiographs of the lateral neck may demonstrate subglottic narrowing. Xeroradiography demonstrates the tissue-air interface better and is believed by many to be the best method for evaluating chronic airway problems.[140–142] Computed tomographic scans do not give adequate additional information.

Direct laryngoscopy is the most important diagnostic step in assessing the thickness and length of the stenosis and involvement of the larynx. Flexible fiberoptic laryngoscopy is most useful in assessing vocal cord function.[140] Because the flexible scope provides only a limited view of the posterior glottis and subglottis, rigid endoscopy is necessary to assess the size and patency of the lumen. The airway may be sized with the bronchoscope or endotracheal tubes. Storz-Hopkins optical telescopes are especially important in visualizing the extent of the stenosis in the subglottis. Because of the wide-angle view, estimating the actual dimensions of the lumen is difficult. Often the narrowing is so great that only the telescope can be used.

Treatment

Congenital subglottic stenosis that is mild and causing mild symptoms and signs can be treated expectantly. Some patients outgrow their lesions and are unlikely to need surgical correction.[143] Treatment must be individualized.

Tracheostomy is required in fewer than half of patients with congenital subglottic stenosis.[133] Normal growth and development may allow decannulation within 2 to 5 years.

The *anterior cricoid split* was initially devised to treat acquired subglottic stenosis,[144] and it was later applied to patients with the congenital form.[145,146] This procedure breaks the cartilaginous cricoid ring anteriorly to allow expansion of the subglottis. It is used in patients who have confirmed stenosis and failed extubation but do not require airway support and have mature lungs with oxygen requirements less than 35%. The procedure involves making a vertical incision through the lower third of the thyroid cartilage, the cricoid cartilage, and the first two tracheal rings. Many of the cricoid rings spring open, and the endotracheal tubes are readily seen through the incision. Others do not open to any significant degree. Some surgeons have recommended placement of auricular or rib grafts at the time of the decompression.[147–149] The patient is left intubated with an endotracheal tube one size bigger for 5 to 7 days and reexamined at the time of extubation. Corticosteroids are usually administered 3 to 5 days before planned extubation.

In weighing the advantages of endoscopic and open procedures, the surgeon must take into account the extent of the scarring and the expertise required. The goal of any surgical procedure is to extubate or decannulate the patient by repairing the stenosis with minimal effect on the voice.

Dilatation is useful if the ulceration is still present and granulation tissue is forming. It is most appropriately used with immature scar or submucosal fibrosis. Gentle dilation is performed with a round, smooth instrument usually in conjunction with corticosteroid injection.[150] Aggressive dilatation with corticosteroid injection can induce additional trauma and cause significant necrosis of the cartilage.

The use of *corticosteroids* is controversial. They tend to decrease scar formation through their anti-inflammatory action and by delay of collagen synthesis. They may be used systemically or injected locally. Corticosteroids have not been successfully used to treat mature scar in the subglottis.

A variety of methods for *endoscopic correction* of subglottic stenosis have been suggested, including microcauterization,[151] cryosurgery[152,153] serial electrosurgical resection,[154,155] and carbon dioxide laser.[127,156] The carbon dioxide laser appears to be the current modality of choice.[135,156–161] The laser can only be used to resect membranous stenosis, and the procedure has to be performed in stages. The more aggressively the laser is used, the less the likelihood of a successful outcome and the greater the risk of inducing additional scarring. Cotton and Manoukian identified several factors associated with poor results: (1) circumferential scarring; (2) scar tissue greater than 1 cm in length; (3) scar in the posterior commissure; (4) severe bacterial infection of the trachea after a tracheostomy; (5) exposure of the perichondrium or cartilage with the laser; (6) combined laryngotracheal stenosis; (7) failure of previous endoscopic procedures; and (8) previous loss of cartilaginous framework.[162] Prophylactic systemic antibiotic therapy is recommended for endoscopic procedures. Adequate exposure of the subglottis is necessary. The subglottiscope designed by Healy is useful if the patient does not have a tracheostomy in place. Supraglottic jet ventilation provides the best exposure. Thin webs are most appropriately treated with the laser.

The *open procedures* have been traditionally used for the more severe lesions. Surgeons are increasingly using single-stage reconstruction.[147,163] This allows for more rapid correction of the problem and is perhaps more cost effective. The *hyoid interposition* was first reported by Looper.[164] Bennett also reported the use of a hyoid bone graft for the treatment of subglottic stenosis.[165] Bone resorption was a problem, which led to the development of pedicle hyoid-sternohyoid myoosseous flaps.[166–168]

The anterior cricoid split with endotracheal tube stenting has been recommended for treatment of milder forms of stenosis. The standard reconstruction has been with autogenous costal cartilage.[169–171] Because of its abundance, costal cartilage is a better material to use than thyroid cartilage, hyoid bone, or muscle pedicle.

The *costal cartilage reconstruction* has been the standard method for subglottic reconstruction for the past several years. The fifth or sixth cartilaginous rib or cos-

tal margin cartilage is harvested. One incision can be used to harvest two ribs, but this is seldom necessary. The perichondrium is left on the lateral surface of the rib, with incisions through it along the superior and inferior borders, and stripped from the medial surface. Some surgeons use the rib stripper on small double-prong hooks and a Freer elevator. The incision in the neck is usually a U-shaped flap through the tracheostoma or a horizontal incision over the cricoid if a tracheostomy is not in place. The larynx and trachea are exposed, and a midline incision is made through the length of the stenosis. If the stenosis is severe, the lumen can be first identified with a 25-gauge needle under endoscopic visualization. When only an anterior graft is used, the incision usually extends from the tracheal rings through the cricoid and the lower third of the larynx. If a posterior graft and stent are required, a full laryngofissure will be necessary. The intraluminal scar and mucosa are incised strictly in the midline. This is best performed by first marking the lumen transtracheally with a 25-gauge needle. Once the airway is open, the scar is not removed. The length of the trachea and larynx to be reconstructed is measured, and the rib graft is designed to fit the defect. The graft is elliptical, with the perichondrium toward the lumen. The rib is not thinned, and care is taken to shape the cartilage to be as wide as possible, with a lip or shelf to prevent the graft from falling into the airway (Fig. 28–22).

In patients with greater subglottic stenosis, a posterior graft is needed, and the posterior cricoid lamina is divided in the midline to, but not through, the hypopharyngeal mucosa. In complete stenosis, a four-quadrant split has been recommended.[172] The cricoid is separated to a distance of approximately 1 mm per year of age up to 10 mm between the two halves.[162] An appropriate wedge of rib with the perichondrium facing the lumen is sutured into the posterior cricoid cleft. If a posterior graft has been performed, a stent will be required to maintain the lumen postoperatively. The current stent of choice is the Aboulker-styled Teflon

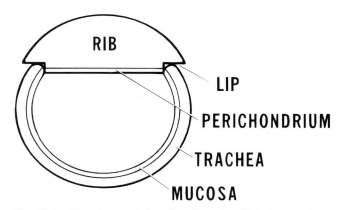

Fig. 28–22. Drawing depicting the rib graft, which has not been thinned, and a lip to prevent collapse into the lumen.

stent, which is round. Unfortunately, it can cause significant blunting, trauma, and granulation tissue formation at the anterior commissure.

Once the posterior cricoid graft is positioned, the stent is placed and the anterior tracheal wall is closed. Usually, posterior and anterior grafts are used concomitantly. When a stent is used, it first must be positioned in the airway with the tracheostomy in place. The best method of securing the tracheostomy to the stent is with wire, as described by Cotton and Manoukian.[162] Placement must be checked endoscopically. The stent should come to the level of the false vocal cords. If necessary, the stent length should be revised to hold the proper position. The rib is sutured into place with 4–0 Vicryl or polydioxanone suture, taking care to go through the cartilage and not allowing the suture to be exposed intraluminally. If suture is located in the lumen, granulation tissue and chronic infection will result. The neck wound is closed in layers. The stent is left in place for a variable length of time based on the surgeon's judgment and the severity of the stenosis.

Recently, auricular cartilage has been used as a graft material.[147,148] It is useful because it is malleable; its curved shape allows for greater anterioposterior dimensions than available with the rib graft (Fig. 28–23). The auricular cartilage graft has not been used extensively with staged reconstructions.

Results of successful decannulation depend in part on the severity of the stenosis. The ultimate outcome of grade 1 is 92% successful, that of grade 2 is 85% successful, that of grade 3 is 70% successful and, that of grade 4 is 36% successful.

Subglottic Hemangioma

Incidence and Etiology

Congenital subglottic hemangiomas are relatively rare lesions and develop primarily in the submucosa. Fifty percent are associated with cutaneous hemangiomas. No correlation exists between the size of the cutaneous lesion and the size of the laryngeal lesion.[173] A 2:1 female preponderance is recognized.

Signs and Symptoms

The subglottic hemangioma develops in a typical growth pattern, with increasing size usually causing symptoms in the first 8 weeks of life. Almost all these lesions will become manifest before 6 months of age. Some lesions extend into the perichondrium and tracheal rings and beyond the trachea. Variable and fluctuant respiratory distress usually progresses to persistent distress. The stridor is more prominent on inspiration but is present during expiration. The voice is altered to a varying degree, depending on the involvement of the larynx. Altered cry, hoarseness, barking cough, and failure to thrive are the other frequently noted manifestations. Recurrent croup is the most frequent erroneous diagnosis.

Diagnosis

Lateral radiographic studies suggest a subglottic abnormality consistent with hemangioma. This is not diagnostic, however, and the diagnosis can only be made endoscopically (Fig. 28–24). The appearance of these lesions is characteristic and can be made by the experienced endoscopist without a biopsy. The lesion is ses-

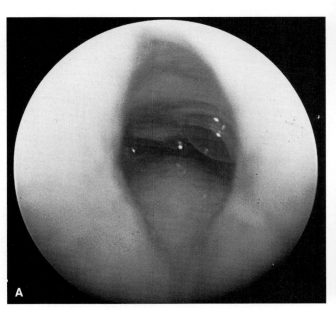
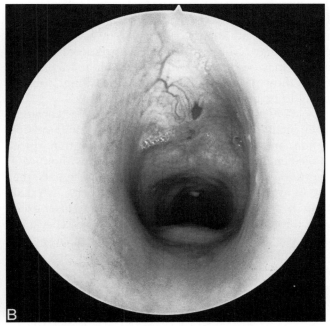

Fig. 28–23. Preoperative (A) and postoperative (B) photographs after a laryngotracheoplasty with auricular cartilage.

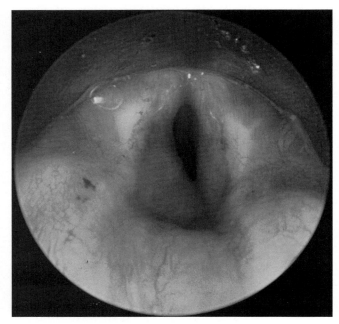

Fig. 28–24. Subglottic hemangioma.

sile, fairly firm but compressible; pink, red, or bluish; and poorly defined. The vessels are rarely, if ever, cavernous. If a biopsy is performed, the bleeding is usually not profuse, but the airway must be maintained, most frequently with a tracheostomy. The lesion is usually unilateral or asymmetric. Multiple hemangiomas of the airway have been reported.[174] A thorough workup of the possible extent of the hemangioma in the mediastinum is recommended.

Treatment

If the airway distress is significant at the time of diagnosis, immediate airway control will be necessary. Endoscopy may compromise the airway. If necessary, the airway may be secured with extubation or a tracheostomy. If the patient is intubated, tracheostomy is more likely to be required.

A wide range of treatments have been advocated. They include the following: tracheostomy with observation and awaiting spontaneous resolution; prolonged endotracheal intubation, with and without corticosteroid injection; injection of sclerosing agents; the use of systemic corticosteroids; cryosurgery; external beam irradiation; gold seed irradiation; and laser excision. Prospective studies are not available. The judicious use of a laser to excise the lesion in stages, with the patient's airway protected by a tracheostomy when necessary, appears to be the treatment favored by most surgeons. External beam irradiation has been reported to have a cure rate of 93%, but the threat of radiation-induced malignant tumors of the thyroid gland strictly limits its use. Gold seeds are the treatment favored

by Benjamin.[173] Unrecognized or mistreated subglottic hemangiomas have a high mortality rate.

SUGGESTED READINGS

1. Chen JC and Holinger LD: Congenital laryngeal lesions: pathology study using serial macrosections and review of the literature (review). Pediatr Pathol *14*:301, 1994.
2. Thomson JM: On infantile respiratory spasm (congenital laryngeal stridor). Edinburgh Med J *38*:205, 1892.
3. Sutherland GA and Lack HM: Congenital laryngeal obstruction. Lancet *2*:653, 1897.
4. Thomson JM and Turner AL: On the causation of congenital stridor of infants. Br Med J *2*:1561, 1900.
5. Schwartz L: Congenital laryngeal stridor (inspiratory laryngeal collapse): new theory as to its underlying cause and the desirability of a change in terminology. Arch Otolaryngol *39*:403, 1944.
6. Jackson C and Jackson CL: Diseases and Injuries of the Larynx. New York, Macmillian, 1942, p 63.
7. Ford GR, Irving RM, Jones NS, and Bailey CM: ENT manifestations of Fraser syndrome. J Laryngol Otol *106*:1, 1992.
8. Hawkins DB and Clark RW: Flexible laryngoscopy in neonates, infants, and young children. Ann Otol Rhinol Laryngol *96*:81, 1987.
9. Nussbaum E and Maggi JC: Laryngomalacia in children. Chest *98*:942, 1990.
10. Holinger LD: Etiology of stridor in the neonate, infant and child. Ann Otol Rhinol Laryngol *89*:397, 1980.
11. Holinger PH, Johnson KC, and Schiller F: Congenital anomalies of the larynx. Ann Otol Rhinol Laryngol *63*:581, 1954.
12. Evans JNG: Laryngotracheoplasty. Otolaryngol Clin North Am *10*:119, 1977.
13. Nussbaum E: Flexible fiberoptic bronchoscopy and laryngoscopy in children under 2 years of age. Crit Care Med *10*:770, 1982.
14. Reardon TJ: Congenital laryngeal stridor. Am J Med Sci *134*: 242, 1907.
15. Blackader AD and Muckleston HS: Inspiratory stridor and dyspnea in infants. Arch Pediatr *26*:401, 1909.
16. McSwiney PF, Cavanagh NP, and Languth P: Outcome in congenital stridor (laryngomalacia). Arch Dis Child *52*:215, 1977.
17. Apley J: The infant with stridor: a follow-up survey of 80 cases. Arch Dis Child *28*:423, 1953.
18. Holinger PH and Johnston KC: The infant with respiratory stridor. Pediatr Clin North Am *2*:403, 1955.
19. Smith GJ and Cooper DM: Laryngomalacia and inspiratory obstruction in later childhood. Arch Dis Child *56*:345, 1981.
20. Belmont JR and Grundfast K: Congenital laryngeal stridor (laryngomalacia): etiologic factors and associated disorders. Ann Otol Rhinol Laryngol *93*:430, 1984.
21. Kelemen G: Congenital laryngeal stridor. Arch Otolaryngol *58*: 245, 1953.
22. Phelan PD, Gilliam FL, Stocks JG, and Williams HE: The clinical and physiological manifestations of the "infantile larynx": natural history and relationship to mental retardation. Aust Pediatr *7*:135, 1971.
23. Holinger LD and Konior RJ: Surgical management of severe laryngomalacia. Laryngoscope *99*:136, 1989.
24. Solomons NB and Prescott CA: Laryngomalacia: a review and the surgical management for severe cases. Int J Pediatr Otorhinolaryngol *13*:31, 1987.
25. Cotton RT and Richardson MA: Pediatric Otolaryngology. Philadelphia, WB Saunders, 1983, p 1216.
26. Ferguson CF: Congenital abnormalities of the infant larynx. Otolaryngol Clin North Am *3*:185, 1970.

27. Zalzal GH, Anon JB, and Cotton RT: Epiglottoplasty for the treatment of laryngomalacia. Ann Otol Rhinol Laryngol 96:72, 1987.

28. Katin LI and Tucker JA: Laser supraarytenoidectomy for laryngomalacia with apnea. Trans Penn Acad Ophthalmol Otolaryngol 42:985, 1990.

29. Iglauer S: Epiglottidectomy for the relief of congenital laryngeal stridor, with report of a case. Laryngoscope 32:56, 1922.

30. Fearon B and Ellis D: The management of long term airway problems in infants and children. Ann Otol Rhinol Laryngol 80:669, 1971.

31. Narcy P, Bobin S, and Contencin P: Anomalies laryngies du nouveau-né àpropos de 687 observations. Ann Otolaryngol Chir Cervicofac 101:363, 1984.

32. Cagnol C, Garcin M, and Unal D: Un cas de stridor larynge congenital grave laoite pan hyomandibulopexie. J Fr Otorhinolaryngol 20:625, 1971.

33. Templer J, Hast M, Thomas JR, and Davis WE: Congenital laryngeal stridor secondary to flaccid epiglottis, anomalous accessory cartilages and redundant aryepiglottic folds. Laryngoscope 91:394, 1981.

34. Lane RW, Weider DJ, and Steinem C: Laryngomalacia: a review and case report of surgical treatment with resolution of pectus excavatum. Arch Otolaryngol Head Neck Surg 110:546, 1984.

35. Seid AB, Park SM, Kearns MJ, and Gugenheim S: Laser division of the aryepiglottic folds for severe laryngomalacia. Int J Pediatr 10:153, 1985.

36. Montreuil F: Bifid epiglottis: report of a case. Laryngoscope 59:194, 1949.

37. DelMonico ML and Haar JG: Bifid epiglottis: report of a case. Arch Otolaryngol 96:178, 1972.

38. Graham JM, et al: Bifid epiglottis, hand anomalies, and congenital hypopituitarism (letter). Lancet 2:443 1985.

39. Tobeck A: Halbseitige Aplasie der Epiglottis. Z Laryngol Rhinol Otol 28:502, 1949.

40. Healy GB, Holt GP, and Tucker JA: Bifid epiglottis: a rare laryngeal anomaly. Laryngoscope 86:1459, 1976.

41. Gatti WM, MacDonald E, and Orfei E: Congenital laryngeal atresia. Laryngoscope 97:966, 1987.

42. Holinger PH and Braw WT: Congenital webs, cysts, laryngoceles and other anomalies of the larynx. Ann Otol Rhinol Laryngol 76:744, 1967.

43. Woo P and Karmody CS: Congenital laryngeal atresia: histopathologic study of two cases. Ann Otol Rhinol Laryngol 92:391, 1983.

44. McIlwain JC: The posterior glottis (review). J Otolaryngol 20(suppl 2):1, 1991.

45. Dolkart LA, Reimers FT, Wertheimer IS, and Wilson BO: Prenatal diagnosis of laryngeal atresia. J Ultrasound Med 11:496, 1992.

46. Watson WJ, et al: Prenatal diagnosis of laryngeal atresia. Am J Obstet Gynecol 163:1456, 1990.

47. Garel C, et al: Laryngeal ultrasonography in infants and children: anatomical correlation with fetal preparations. Pediatr Radiol 20:241, 1990.

48. Smith II and Bain AD: Congenital atresia of the larynx. Ann Otol Rhinol Laryngol 74:338, 1965.

49. Peison B, Levitzky E, and Sprowls JJ: Tracheoesophageal fistula associated with tracheal atresia and malformation of the larynx. J Pediatr Surg 5:464, 1970.

50. Nakayama DK, et al: Pulmonary function studies in a newborn with congenital laryngeal atresia. J Pediatr Surg 26:210, 1991.

51. Gerson CR, Tansek K, and Tucker GF: Pharyngolaryngeal web: report of a new anomaly. Ann Otol Rhinol Laryngol 92:331, 1983.

52. Holinger LD, Wong HW, and Hemenway WG: Simultaneous glottic and supraglottic laryngeal webs: report of a case. Arch Otolaryngol 101:496, 1975.

53. Benjamin B and Mair EA: Congenital interarytenoid web (review). Arch Otolaryngol Head Neck Surg 117:1118, 1991.

54. McHugh HE and Loch WE: Congenital webs of the larynx. Laryngoscope 52:43, 1942.

55. McGuirt WF, Salmon J, and Blalock D: Normal speech for patients with laryngeal webs: an achievable goal. Laryngoscope 94:1176, 1984.

56. Cohen SR: Congenital glottic webs in children: a retrospective review of 51 patients. Ann Otol Rhinol Laryngol Suppl 121:2, 1985.

57. Benjamin B: Chevalier Jackson Lecture: congenital laryngeal webs. Ann Otol Rhinol Laryngol 92:317, 1983.

58. Parker DA and Das Gu: An endoscopic Silastic keel for anterior glottic webs. J Laryngol Otol 101:1055, 1987.

59. Mouney DF and Lyons GD: Fixation of laryngeal stents. Laryngoscope 95:905, 1985.

60. Laff HI: Cysts in the ventricular area of the larynx. Laryngoscope 63:227, 1953.

61. Davidson JI: Congenital cyst of the larynx. Lancet 2:508, 1943.

62. Ahlen G and Ranstrom S: Congenital laryngeal cysts in early infancy. Acta Otolaryngol 32:483, 1944.

63. Beautyman W, Haidak GL, and Taylor M: Laryngopyocele: report of a fatal case. N Engl J Med 260:1025, 1959.

64. Horowitz S: Laryngoceles. J Laryngol Otol 65:724, 1951.

65. Hockmuth LN and Martin SJ: An obstructing laryngeal cyst in a newborn. Conn Med 26:691, 1962.

66. DeSanto LW: Laryngocele, laryngeal mucocele, large saccules, and laryngeal saccular cysts: a developmental spectrum. Laryngoscope 84:1291, 1974.

67. Holinger LD, Barnes DR, Smid LJ, and Holinger PH: Laryngocele and saccular cysts. Ann Otol Rhinol Laryngol 87:675, 1978.

68. Broyles EN: Anatomical observations concerning the laryngeal appendix. Ann Otol Rhinol Laryngol 68:461, 1959.

69. DeSanto LW, Devine KD, and Weiland LH: Cysts of larynx: classification. Laryngoscope 80:145, 1970.

70. Suehs OW and Powell DB: Congenital cyst of the larynx in infants. Laryngoscope 77:654, 1967.

71. Mitchell DB, Irwin BC, Bailey CM, and Evans JN: Cysts of the infant larynx. J Laryngol Otol 101:833, 1987.

72. Shackelford GD and McAlister WH: Congenital laryngeal cyst. Am J Roentgenol Radium Ther Nucl Med 114:289, 1972.

73. Cotton RT and Richardson MA: Congenital laryngeal anomalies. Otolaryngol Clin North Am 14:203, 1981.

74. English GM and DeBlanc GB: Laryngocele: a case presenting with acute airway obstruction. Laryngoscope 78:386, 1968.

75. Ferguson GB: Laryngocele. Laryngoscope 77:1368, 1967.

76. Donegan JO, et al: Internal laryngocele and saccular cysts in children. Ann Otol Rhinol Laryngol 89:409, 1980.

77. Canalis RF, Maxwell DS, and Hemenway WG: Laryngocele: an updated review. J Otolaryngol 6:191, 1977.

78. Chu L, Gussack GS, Orr JB, and Hood D: Neonatal laryngoceles: a cause for airway obstruction (review). Arch Otolaryngol Head Neck Surg 120:454, 1994.

79. Baker HL, Baker SR, and McClatchey KD: Manifestations and management of laryngoceles. Head Neck Surg 4:450, 1982.

80. Trapnell DH: The radiological diagnosis of laryngoceles. Clin Radiol 13:68, 1962.

81. Yarington CT and Frazer JP: An approach to the internal laryngocele and other submucosal lesions of the larynx. Ann Otol Rhinol Laryngol 75:956, 1966.

82. Thomas DM and Madden GJ: Bilateral laryngoceles. Ear Nose Throat J 72:819, 1993.

83. Cohen SR: Cleft larynx: a report of seven cases. Ann Otol Rhinol Laryngol 84:747, 1975.

84. Cohen SR and Thompson JW: Ventral cleft of the larynx: a rare congenital laryngeal defect (review). Ann Otol Rhinol Laryngol 99:281, 1990.

85. Decreton SJ and Clement PA: Comparative study of standard

X-ray of the maxillary sinus and sinusoscopy in children. Rhinology *19:*155, 1981.

86. Pattisapu JV and Parent AD: Subdural empyemas in children. Pediatr Neurosci 13:251, 1987.

87. Roth B, Rose KG, Benz-Bohm G, and Gunther H: Laryngo-tracheo-oesophageal cleft: clinical features, diagnosis and therapy. Eur J Pediatr *140:*41, 1983.

88. Finlay HV: Familial congenital stridor. Arch Dis Child 24:219, 1949.

89. Forrester RM and Cohen SJ: Esophageal atresia associated with an anorectal anomaly and probable laryngeal fissure in three siblings. J Pediatr Surg 6:674, 1970.

90. Zachary RB and Emery JL: Failure of separation of larynx and trachea from the esophagus: persistent esophagotracea. Surgery 49:525, 1961.

91. Phelan HC, Stocks JG, Williams HE, and Danks DM: Familial occurrence of congenital laryngeal clefts. Arch Dis Child *48:*275, 1973.

92. Holinger LD, Volk MS, and Tucker GF: Congenital laryngeal anomalies associated with tracheal agenesis. Ann Otol Rhinol Laryngol 96:505, 1987.

93. Evans JN: Management of the cleft larynx and tracheoesophageal clefts. Ann Otol Rhinol Laryngol 94:627, 1985.

94. Jahrsdoerfer RA, Kirchner JA, and Thaler SU: Cleft larynx. Arch Otolaryngol *86:*108, 1967.

95. Garel C, et al: Contribution of MR in the diagnosis of ''occult'' posterior laryngeal cleft. Int J Pediatr Otorhinolaryngol 24:177, 1992.

96. Delahunty JE and Cherry J: Congenital laryngeal cleft. Ann Otol Rhinol Laryngol *78:*96, 1969.

97. Corbally MT, et al: Laryngo-tracheo-oesophageal cleft: a plea for early diagnosis. Eur J Pediatr Surg 3:241, 1993.

98. Holinger LD, Tansek KM, and Tucker GF: Cleft larynx with airway obstruction. Ann Otol Rhinol Laryngol 94:622, 1985.

99. Tucker GF and Maddalozzo J: ''Occult'' posterior laryngeal cleft. Laryngoscope *97:*701, 1987.

100. Tyler DC: Laryngeal cleft: report of eight patients and a review of the literature. Am J Med Genet 21:61, 1985.

101. Petterson G: Inhibited separation of larynx and the upper part of trachea from oesophagus in a newborn. Acta Chir Scand *110:*250, 1955.

102. Koltai PJ, Morgan D, and Evans JN: Endoscopic repair of supraglottic laryngeal clefts. Arch Otolaryngol Head Neck Surg *117:*273, 1991.

103. Nuutinen J, Karja J, and Karjalainen P: Measurements of impaired mucociliary activity in children. Eur J Respir Dis Suppl 128:454, 1983.

104. Pettit PN, Butcher RB, Bethea MC, and Danks DM: Surgical correction of complete tracheoesophageal cleft. Laryngoscope 89:804, 1979.

105. Froehlich P, et al: Cleft larynx: management and one-stage surgical repair by anterior translaryngotracheal approach in two children. Int J Pediatr Otorhinolaryngol 27:73, 1993.

106. Robie DK, et al: Operative strategy for recurrent laryngeal cleft: a case report and review of the literature (review). J Pediatr Surg 26:971, 1991.

107. Ahmad R, Horwitz PE, Sami KA, and Rabeeah A: A bifurcated endobronchial tube in the management of laryngotracheo-oesophageal cleft repair (published erratum appears in Br J Anaesth 72:371, 1994). Br J Anaesth 70:696, 1993.

108. Geiduschek JM, et al: Repair of a laryngotracheoesophageal cleft in an infant by means of extracorporeal membrane oxygenation. Ann Otol Rhinol Laryngol 102:827, 1993.

109. Cotton RT and Schreiber JT: Management of laryngotracheo-esophageal cleft. Ann Otol Rhinol Laryngol 90:401, 1981.

110. Cohen SR, Geller KA, Birns JW, and Thompson JW: Laryngeal paralysis in children: a long-term retrospective study. Ann Otol Rhinol Laryngol 91:417, 1982.

111. Swift AC and Rogers J: Vocal cord paralysis in children. J Laryngol Otol 101:169, 1987.

112. Phelan PD: ''Oscopy'' in children: laryngoscopy and bronchoscopy. Aust Fam Physician 8:853, 1979.

113. Hoffman JH, Hendrick EB, and Humphreys RP: Manifestations and management of Arnold-Chiari malformation in patients with myelomeningocele. Childs Brain 1:255, 1975.

114. Krieger AJ, Detwiler JS, and Trooskin SZ: Respiratory function in infants with Arnold-Chiari malformation. Laryngoscope *86:*86:718, 1976.

115. Cavanagh F: Vocal palsies in children. J Laryngol Otol 69:399, 1955.

116. Dedo DD: Pediatric vocal cord paralysis. Laryngoscope 89:1378, 1979.

117. Holinger LD, Holinger PC, and Holinger PH: Etiology of bilateral abductor vocal cord paralysis: a review of 389 cases. Ann Otol Rhinol Laryngol 85:428, 1976.

118. Gardner E, O'Rahilly R, and Prolo D: The Dandy-Walker and Arnold-Chiari malformations. Arch Neurol 32:395, 1975.

119. Mackenzie IJ, Kerr AI, and Cowan DL: A review of endoscopies of the respiratory tract and oesophagus in a children's hospital. Health Bull (Edinb) 42:78, 1984.

120. Richardson MA and Cotton RT: Anatomic abnormalities of the pediatric airway. Ear Nose Throat J 64:47, 1985.

121. Holinger PC, Holinger LD, Reichert TJ, and Holinger PH: Respiratory obstruction and apnea in infants with bilateral abductor vocal cord paralysis, meningomyelocele, hydrocephalus, and Arnold-Chiari malformation. J Pediatr 92:368, 1978.

122. Bluestone CD, Delerme AN, and Samuelson GH: Airway obstruction due to vocal cord paralysis in infants with hydrocephalus and meningomyelocele. Ann Otol Rhinol Laryngol 81:778, 1972.

123. Gacek RR: Hereditary abductor vocal cord paralysis. Ann Otol Rhinol Laryngol 85:90, 1976.

124. Watters GV and Fitch N: Familial laryngeal abductor paralysis and psychomotor retardation. Clin Genet 4:429, 1973.

125. Plott D: Congenital laryngeal-abductor paralysis due to nucleus ambiguus dysgenesis in three brothers. N Engl J Med 27:593, 1964.

126. Cotton RT and Evans JN: Laryngotracheal reconstruction in children: five-year follow-up. Ann Otol Rhinol Laryngol 90:516, 1981.

127. Holinger LD: Treatment of severe subglottic stenosis without tracheotomy: a preliminary report. Ann Otol Rhinol Laryngol 91:407, 1982.

128. Hawkins DB: Hyaline membrane disease of the neonate prolonged intubation in management: effects on the larynx. Laryngoscope 88:201, 1978.

129. Papsidero MJ and Pashley NR: Acquired stenosis of the upper airway in neonates: an increasing problem. Ann Otol Rhinol Laryngol 89:512, 1980.

130. Parkin JL, Stevens MH, and Jung DL: Acquired and congenital subglottic stenosis in the infant. Ann Otol Rhinol Laryngol *85:*573, 1976.

131. Whited RE: A prospective study of laryngotracheal sequelae in long-term intubation. Laryngoscope 94:367, 1984.

132. Benjamin B: Prolonged intubation injuries of the larynx: endoscopic diagnosis, classification, and treatment. Ann Otol Rhinol Laryngol Suppl 160:1, 1993.

133. Holinger PH, Kutnick SL, Schild JA, and Holinger LD: Subglottic stenosis in infants and children. Ann Otol Rhinol Laryngol 85:591, 1976.

134. Sasaki CT, Horiuchi M, and Koss N: Traheostomy-related subglottic stenosis: bacteriologic pathogenesis. Laryngoscope 89:857, 1979.

135. Healy GB: An experimental model for the endoscopic correction of subglottic stenosis with clinical applications. Laryngoscope 92:1103, 1982.

136. Cotton RT, Silver P, and Nuwayhid NS: Chronic laryngeal and tracheal stenosis. In: Otolaryngology. Edited by Paparella MM and Shumrick DA. Philadelphia, WB Saunders, 1980, p 2931.

137. Fee WE and Willson GG: Tracheoesophageal space abscess. Laryngoscope 89:377, 1979.

138. Lindholm CE: Prolonged endotracheal intubation, a valuable alternative to tracheostomy. Bronches 18:398, 1968.

139. Pashley NR: Risk factors and prediction of outcome in acquired subglottic stenosis in children. Int J Pediatr Otorhinolaryngol 4:1, 1982.

140. McMillan WG and Duvall AJ: Congenital subglottic stenosis. Arch Otolaryngol 87:272, 1968.

141. Marshak G and Grundfast KM: Subglottic stenosis. Pediatr Clin North Am 28:941, 1981.

142. Noyek AM: Xeroradiography in the assessment of the pediatric larynx and trachea. J Otolaryngol 5:468, 1976.

143. Cotton RT: Management of subglottic stenosis in infancy and childhood: review of a consecutive series of cases managed by surgical reconstruction. Ann Otol Rhinol Laryngol 87:649, 1978.

144. Cotton RT and Seid AB: Management of the extubation problem in the premature child: anterior cricoid split as an alternative to tracheotomy. Ann Otol Rhinol Laryngol 89:508, 1980.

145. Cotton RT: Prevention and management of laryngeal stenosis in infants and children. J Pediatr Surg 20:845, 1985.

146. Holinger LD, Stankiewicz JA, and Livingston GL: Anterior cricoid split: the Chicago experience with an alternative to tracheotomy. Laryngoscope 97:19, 1987.

147. Lusk RP, Gray SD, and Muntz HR: Single-stage laryngotracheal reconstruction. Arch Otolaryngol Head Neck Surg 117:171, 1991.

148. Lusk RP, Muntz HR, and Kang DR: Auricular cartilage grafts in laryngotracheal reconstruction. Ann Otol Rhinol Laryngol 102:247, 1993.

149. Richardson MA and Inglis AF: A comparison of anterior cricoid split with and without costal cartilage graft for acquired subglottic stenosis. Int J Pediatr Otorhinolaryngol 22:187, 1991.

150. Otherson HB: Steroid therapy for tracheal stenosis in children. Ann Thorac Surg 17:254, 1974.

151. Kirchner FR and Toledo PS: Microcauterization in otolaryngology. Arch Otolaryngol 99:198, 1974.

152. Rodgers BM and Talbert JL: Clinical applications of endotracheal cryotherapy. J Pediatr Surg 13:662, 1978.

153. Strome M and Donahoe PK: Advances in management of laryngeal and subglottic stenosis. J Pediatr Surg 17:591, 1982.

154. Downing TP and Johnson DG: Excision of subglottic stenosis with the urethral resectoscope. J Pediatr Surg 14:252, 1979.

155. Johnson DG and Stewart DR: Management of acquired tracheal obstructions in infancy. J Pediatr Surg 10:709, 1975.

156. Simpson GT, et al: Predictive factors of success or failure in the endoscopic management of laryngeal and tracheal stenosis. Ann Otol Rhinol Laryngol 91:384, 1982.

157. Friedman EM, Healy GB, and McGill TJ: Carbon dioxide laser management of subglottic and tracheal stenosis. Otolaryngol Clin North Am 16:871, 1983.

158. Healy GB, McGill T, Simpson GT, and Strong MS: The use of the carbon dioxide laser in the pediatric airway. J Pediatr Surg 14:735, 1979.

159. Koufman JA, Thompson JN, and Kohut RI: Endoscopic management of subglottic stenosis with the CO_2 surgical laser. Otolaryngol Head Neck Surg 89:215, 1981.

160. Lyons CD, Owens R, Lousteau RJ, and Trail ML: Carbon dioxide laser treatment of laryngeal stenosis. Arch Otolaryngol 106:255, 1980.

161. Strong MS, Healy GB, Vaughan CW, and Fried MP: Endoscopic management of laryngeal stenosis. Otolaryngol Clin North Am 12:797, 1979.

162. Cotton RT and Manoukian JJ: Glottic and subglottic stenosis. In: Otolaryngology—Head and Neck Surgery. Edited by Cummings CW, et al. St. Louis, CV Mosby, 1986, p 2159.

163. Seid AB, Pransky SM, and Kearns DB: One-stage laryngotracheoplasty. Arch Otolaryngol Head Neck Surg 117:408, 1991.

164. Looper EA: The use of hyoid bone as graft in laryngeal stenosis. Arch Otolaryngol 28:106, 1938.

165. Bennett T: Laryngeal strictures. South Med J 53:1101, 1960.

166. Finnegan DA, Wong ML, and Kashima HK: Hyoid autograft repair of chronic subglottic stenosis. Ann Otol Rhinol Laryngol 84:643, 1975.

167. Thawley SE and Ogura JH: Panel discussion: the management of advanced laryngotracheal stenosis. Use of the hyoid graft for treatment of laryngotracheal stenosis. Laryngoscope 91:226, 1981.

168. Ward PH: Composite hyoid sternohyoid muscle grafts in humans: its use in reconstruction of subglottic stenosis and the anterior tracheal wall. Arch Otolaryngol Head Neck Surg 103:531, 1977.

169. Cotton RT: Pediatric laryngotracheal stenosis. J Pediatr Surg 19:699, 1984.

170. Fearon B and Cinnamond M: Surgical correction of subglottic stenosis of the larynx: clinical results of the Fearon-Cotton operation. J Otolaryngol 5:475, 1976.

171. Fearon B and Cotton RT: Surgical correction of subglottic stenosis of the larynx in infants and children: progress report. Ann Otol Rhinol Laryngol 83:428, 1974.

172. Anonymous: Lateral cricoid cuts as an adjunctive measure to enlarge the stenotic subglottic airway: an anatomic study. Int J Pediatr Otorhinolaryngol 18:129, 1989.

173. Benjamin B: Congenital disorders. In: Otolaryngology—Head and Neck Surgery. Edited by Cummings CW, et al. St. Louis, CV Mosby, 1986, p 2329.

174. Wooley AL and Lusk RP: Multiple vascular lesions of an infant's airway. Otolaryngol Head Neck Surg 111:305, 1994.

29 Laryngeal Trauma

Hugh F. Biller, Juan Moscoso, and Ira Sanders

BLUNT LARYNGEAL TRAUMA

Blunt laryngeal trauma is relatively uncommon. Its incidence has been estimated at 1 patient per every 14,000 to 42,000 emergency department visits. This low incidence is explained by the flexibility and elasticity of the laryngeal cartilages and the protection offered by the mandible, sternum, and cervical spine. Anteriorly directed forces, however, can compress the larynx against the cervical vertebrae, resulting in tearing of endolaryngeal soft tissues and fracture or dislocation of laryngeal cartilage. High-speed motor vehicle accidents are the most common cause of blunt laryngeal injuries. During rapid deceleration, the unrestrained body is pushed forward and the neck strikes the steering wheel or dashboard. Laryngeal trauma is also encountered as a result of physical confrontation in an increasingly violent society and, less commonly, as a result of sporting injuries or "clothesline" accidents—hitting a horizontal object while riding a bicycle, horse, or snowmobile. Because of their relative infrequency and their association with other life-threatening injuries, laryngeal injuries often go unrecognized. This is unfortunate, because glottic insufficiency, aspiration and laryngeal stenosis are the end result of delayed or inappropriate treatment of laryngeal injuries.

Injury to the larynx is followed by distinctive signs and symptoms. The distensibility of the submucosal tissue of the larynx, particularly in the supraglottic portions, permits the accumulation of fluid or blood; therefore, laryngeal edema or hematoma typically involves the aryepiglottic folds and false vocal cords. Because fluid or blood accumulations may be rapid, symptoms of laryngeal obstruction may appear abruptly.

The mucosal lining of the larynx and pharynx is easily torn by traumatic forces, and this may be followed by the rapid appearance of subcutaneous emphysema (Fig. 29–1). Interruption of the mucosal barrier also allows contamination of the deep tissues of the neck and can result in cellulitis, abscess, and perhaps fistulous tracts.

Widely varying fractures and dislocations of the laryngeal cartilages and joints can occur and tend to be more severe in the less resilient, calcified cartilages of older individuals. Perichondrial injury often leads to subperichondrial hematoma with devascularization and necrosis of hyaline cartilage. If the area is contaminated by communication with the laryngeal lumen, perichondritis and chondritis may follow.

Laryngeal wounds are usually secondarily infected, and epithelization is often delayed, with the result that excessive granulation and fibrous tissue are laid down. This scarring can alter laryngeal function permanently, and loss of patency may develop secondary to relatively minor injuries. Prompt management of laryngeal injuries is mandatory to prevent the sequelae of healing by secondary intention. Differences of opinion persist with regard to multiple aspects of management, however, including (1) indications for surgery, (2) timing of surgical intervention, and (3) need and duration of stenting of the endolarynx.

DIAGNOSIS

All patients sustaining anterior cervical injury should be carefully examined to rule out the presence of significant laryngeal trauma. The following symptoms are suggestive of derangement of laryngeal integrity:

1. Increasing airway obstruction with dyspnea and stridor.
2. Dysphonia or aphonia.
3. Cough.
4. Hemoptysis and hematemesis.
5. Neck pain.
6. Dysphagia and odynophagia.

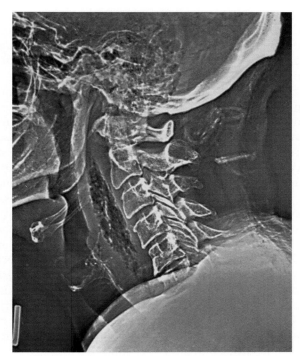

Fig. 29–1. Xeroradiogram following blunt neck trauma. Note air in the prevertebral compartment. (Courtesy of Dr. G.J. Spector.)

Distinctive clinical signs indicating laryngeal injuries are as follows:

1. Loss of normal cartilaginous landmarks.
2. Laryngeal tenderness.
3. Bony crepitus.
4. Subcutaneous emphysema.
5. Open neck wound.

Frequently, a laryngeal injury is only one of multiple injuries resulting from an automobile accident. Unfortunately, in many such situations, a tracheostomy is performed, but no further thought is given to the larynx until the time arrives for decannulation, when the presence of dysphonia, aphonia, or persistent obstruction is noted. By this time, it is usually too late to perform a definitive, simple repair, and one must accept the less desirable results of delayed repair. Therefore, laryngeal trauma must be considered in any patient requiring tracheostomy who has a history of possible neck trauma.

After the patient's airway is stabilized, the initial step in diagnosis is the physical examination. The physical examination should include palpation of the neck, feeling for cervical emphysema, soft tissue swelling, loss of the normal laryngeal contours, and crepitus. The most important part of the physical examination is laryngoscopy. Direct examination of the endolarynx should assess vocal cord mobility, the presence of mucosal edema, hematomas or tears, exposed cartilage, or dislocated arytenoid cartilages. In recent years, fiberoptic nasopharyngoscopy has replaced mirror examination as a diagnostic tool because of improved visualization and its ease of use in patients unable to cooperate with the examination.

RADIOLOGIC EVALUATION

Radiologic evaluation should be performed only after the patient's airway is stabilized. If cervical spinal injury is suspected, cervical spinal films must be obtained before moving the patient's head. In patients with suspected laryngeal injuries, computed tomography (CT) has replaced the use of laryngeal tomography or laryngograms. All patients in whom the diagnosis of laryngeal trauma is entertained should undergo a neck CT scan. Although the decision for surgical exploration is usually based on clinical findings, CT scanning can be helpful when surgical indications are in doubt. In severe cases, CT can aid in preoperative planning and in patient counseling when resection of large amounts of laryngeal tissue is likely. Three-dimensional CT has been found to be an useful adjunct in the evaluation of laryngeal trauma. It enables one to identify abnormalities overlooked on two-dimensional CT scanning alone, as well as distinguishing between cartilaginous fractures and anatomic variants. Chest films should be obtained to rule out associated chest trauma or pneumothorax. Gastrograffin swallow may also be needed to rule out esophageal tears.

INITIAL TREATMENT

Initial management of the patient with laryngeal trauma involves establishing a patent airway. The means of achieving this should be individualized, based on (1) the status of the cervical spine, (2) the skills of the available personnel, and (3) the severity of the injury. The least traumatic method is the preferred means of securing the airway. Elective endotracheal intubation can often be performed in even severe laryngeal injuries, provided it is done by an experienced clinician under direct vision. Tracheostomy under local anesthesia should be performed when the airway is deteriorating rapidly, when cervical spinal fracture is suspected or confirmed, and when experienced personnel are not available to perform an elective orotracheal intubation. Blind intubation is contraindicated because it may cause false passages, it may increase laryngeal damage, and it may precipitate the abrupt loss of an already tenuous airway. Before any attempt at intubation is made, a bronchoscope and the material and personnel required for an immediate tracheostomy must be at hand. In tenuous cases, the patient's neck should be prepared and anesthetized for tracheostomy before the attempt at intubation. The surgeon should participate in the intubation, to obtain a direct view of the larynx before the endotracheal tube obscures the field.

PRINCIPLES OF TREATMENT OF ACUTE LARYNGEAL FRACTURES AND INJURIES

Nonoperative management is reserved for patients in whom uneventful healing of the injured larynx can be expected to occur without alteration of laryngeal function. It consists of (1) voice rest, (2) 24 hours of close observation, (3) head elevation, and (4) humidification of inspired air. Anecdotal evidence suggests the use of corticosteroids to reduce the inflammatory response and prevent the progression of edema. Because swelling may worsen in the days following an injury, a systematic schedule of frequent clinical reevaluation is critical. Conservative management is indicated in the treatment of patients with minimal soft tissue swelling or hematomas not requiring airway control (Fig. 29–2).

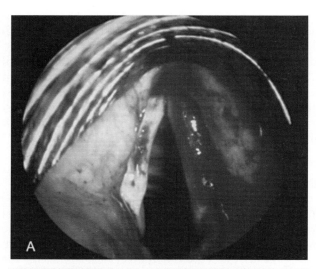

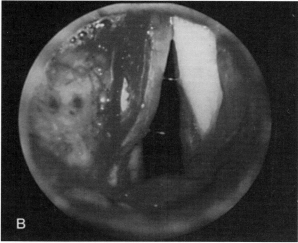

Fig. 29–2. Glottic trauma. A. Post-traumatic intubation hematoma of right vocal cord. B. Blunt trauma causing hematoma of left vocal cord and ventricle. (Courtesy of Dr. J.H. Ogura.)

Edema and hematoma usually resolve spontaneously and completely in the absence of other injury. Patients with minor mucosal avulsions or lacerations that spare the free edge of the vocal cord or anterior commissure are also managed conservatively.

Surgical exploration of the larynx is indicated in any patient with a neck injury with airway obstruction, extensive disruption of endolaryngeal soft tissues, bare cartilage in the laryngeal lumen, thyroid cartilage fracture, cricoid collapse, or cervical emphysema. Direct laryngoscopy and open esophagoscopy are performed to evaluate the extent of endolaryngeal disruption and to rule out cricoarytenoid dislocation and mucosal tears of the hypopharynx or esophagus. Operative treatment of laryngeal injuries is carried out as soon as the patient's overall medical condition allows it. Wounds open to the laryngeal lumen or external neck must be explored within 24 hours to minimize the risk of infection and to allow primary closure. The best chance for restoring the phonatory and sphincteric functions of the larynx is obtained when closed laryngeal fractures are explored within 48 hours of injury. Delaying surgical treatment beyond this time is associated with a deterioration of laryngeal function.

Exploration is performed through a horizontal incision at the level of the previous tracheostomy incision to minimize scarring of the anterior neck. An apron flap is elevated superiorly to expose the desired portion of the larynx, and the presence of a fracture is confirmed by direct palpation. Depending on the injury, the larynx is entered through the thyrohyoid membrane, a midline thyrotomy, or a thyroid cartilage fracture within 2 to 3 mm of the thyroid notch. Mucosal tears should be meticulously repaired with absorbable suture, with the knots placed outside the lumen. Large defects can be closed by the advancement of pyriform sinus mucosa or the placement of grafts bolstered by a laryngeal stent. Extensive damage to soft tissue in the supraglottic region is best treated by excision to prevent supraglottic stenosis. This may include amputation of the epiglottis. Lesions involving the anterior commissure (i.e., midline glottic injuries) with foreshortening of the anteroposterior glottic axis are treated with a midline thyrotomy and keel. Avulsed vocal ligaments must be sutured to the thyroid alae. Arytenoid dislocations are replaced on the cricoid cartilage.

Laryngeal cartilage fractures, like any other fractures, must be reduced and immobilized. Even minimally displaced thyroid cartilage fractures have the potential to disrupt multiple parameters of vocal function. Small, isolated cartilage fragments devoid of perichondrium are debrided. Historically, wire suture has been the material of choice to immobilize reduced laryngeal cartilage fractures. The use of titanium miniplates to achieve fixation of laryngeal fractures has been advocated recently by Woo. Miniplates can be bent in three dimensions, allowing for a superior restoration of the proper geometry of displaced cartilaginous segments. Once secured to cartilage with screws, rigid fixation is maintained in all dimensions, to allow primary healing of the fracture.

The use of laryngeal stents remains controversial. Internal splinting of the larynx should be done in most comminuted laryngeal cartilage fractures when fixation with wire sutures or miniplates does not afford rigid immobilization. Their use is also indicated in the presence of extensive endolaryngeal soft tissue injury, particularly if mucosal grafting is required, or when the injury disrupts the anterior commissure. In these patients, the risk of chronic stenosis outweighs the disadvantages of a stent. A rubber finger-cot, filled with Ivalon sponge, or a Silastic, Portex, or silicone laryngeal mold may be used. These molds do not cause as much epithelial injury as do firmer stents. The stent is usually inserted through a thyrotomy or infrahyoid laryngotomy and is fixed above and below the glottis by wire sutures passed through the skin. The stent is fixed in a position so the upper end is at the level of the aryepiglottic folds and the lower end is just above the tracheostomy site. It should be left in place for 2 to 6 weeks, depending on the site or type of injury.

Antibiotic therapy is probably indicated in most cases because the fractures are compound and there is a high incidence of local infection and perichondritis, which contribute to delayed healing, formation of excessive granulation tissue, and stenosis. In the absence of obvious infection, corticosteroid therapy may be of value in retarding granulation tissue formation and later fibrosis. Antireflux therapy with H_2 blockers is also indicated because acid reflux may potentiate the tendency toward granulation tissue formation and stenosis.

DISLOCATION OF THE CRICOTHYROID JOINT

Disturbance of the cricothyroid articulation may follow any trauma to the anterior neck and may be unilateral or bilateral. The inferior cornu of the thyroid cartilage is usually displaced posteriorly in relation to the cricoid cartilage. This may produce a deficiency in the tensor mechanism of the vocal cord on the side of the injury; moreover, the recurrent laryngeal nerve may be injured in its position just behind the joint, causing vocal cord paralysis. The injury may result in temporary or permanent disarticulation or the luxation may become recurrent, in which case it reoccurs with swallowing or yawning.

Cricothyroid dislocation may follow minor trauma, and the presence of the deformity is often undetected. At the time of injury, the patient usually has pain in the neck, which may radiate to the ear. A snapping

sensation may be felt in the neck. In patients without vocal cord paralysis, some change in voice is noted, but with vocal cord paralysis, hoarseness, weakness of the voice, and aspiration on swallowing may be present. Usually, aspiration is temporary, and the voice undergoes considerable spontaneous improvement.

Diagnosis is difficult, but dislocation may be suspected when the patient can voluntarily dislocate the joint or when the patient has vocal cord paralysis associated with minor neck trauma. Examination of the larynx may disclose some bowing and lack of tension or paralysis of the vocal cord on the affected side. CT of the larynx may demonstrate a fracture through the inferior cornu of the thyroid cartilage or dislocation of the joint, if the cartilages are well calcified.

Only patients with persistent vocal cord paralysis, persistent dysphonia, or recurrent dislocation require treatment. Paralysis of the vocal cord, with this injury, is often temporary, and spontaneous return of function usually occurs in 3 to 4 weeks. Paralysis lasting more than 6 to 8 weeks is unlikely to resolve spontaneously. The patient should be observed during this period, and then consideration should be given to decompression of the recurrent laryngeal nerve if no return of function is evident. Electromyographic studies of the paralyzed vocal cord may be helpful in determining the need for decompression.

Patients with persistent vocal cord paralysis or bothersome, habitual dislocation may benefit from resection of the inferior cornu of the thyroid cartilage. Many patients with persistent vocal cord paralysis have only physiologic block (neuropraxia) to nerve conduction, and decompression of the nerve by excision of the cornu permits a rapid return of function. The prognosis for return of function of a vocal cord paralyzed for more than 9 months is poor.

When dysphonia is a serious complaint and decompression is not feasible, improvement in voice may be obtained by the intrachordal injection of Teflon paste. This procedure is usually delayed 9 to 12 months to make sure that paralysis is permanent.

DISLOCATION OF THE CRICOARYTENOID JOINT

Dislocation of the cricoarytenoid joint may be caused by internal or external trauma. Blunt injury to the neck may precipitate dislocation of the arytenoid by pressure from a medially displaced thyroid ala or by compression against the cervical vertebrae. In such cases, injury to other parts of the larynx is often present. Endoscopic procedures can also cause this injury (Fig. 29–3). Dislocation may occur if the end of the esophagoscope catches on an arytenoid cartilage, or if extreme force is exerted on the vocal cord while a bronchoscope or endotracheal tube is being passed,

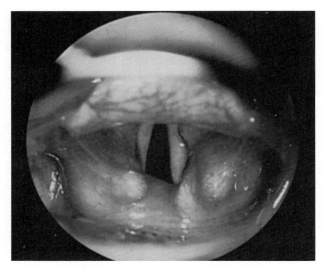

Fig. 29–3. Right arytenoid cartilage dislocation after a traumatic intubation. (Courtesy of Dr. G.J. Spector.)

which pulls the arytenoid anteromedially. The arytenoid may be dislocated anteriorly or posteriorly, but anterior dislocation is more frequent. Dislocations are rarely bilateral.

The symptoms include hoarseness, pain, and, if edema is severe, dyspnea and stridor. Dysphagia, odynophagia, and aspiration also occur.

Indirect laryngoscopy may disclose edema involving the arytenoid area and aryepiglottic fold, which obscures the vocal process and vocal cord. In the absence of edema or after it subsides, the arytenoid will be seen to be tipped forward and rotated medially, whereas the vocal cord is bowed, flaccid, and immobilized in an intermediate position. The posterior portion of the vocal cord may be hidden by the arytenoid and corniculate cartilages, which are tipped forward. This deformity may permit the superior surface of the cricoid lamina to be seen as a small shelf posterior to the mound of the arytenoid. When the patient is asked to phonate, the vocal cords do not completely approximate, and the displaced arytenoid may move farther anteriorly unless it is fixed by scar tissue.

Direct laryngoscopy should be performed, and in addition to visual inspection, the dislocated arytenoid should be palpated with a laryngeal spatula to test its mobility. A key feature in visualizing a dislocated arytenoid is the position of the muscular process. In anterior dislocations, this process tips forward into the glottic lumen at the posterior commissure. Posterior dislocation forces the muscular process posterolaterally, and the body of the arytenoid and vocal process are turned to the glottic lumen. A dislocated arytenoid does not have the same mobility as an arytenoid in normal position. In long-standing cases of arytenoid dislocation, however, the arytenoid becomes fixed by scar tissue and joint arthrodesis. This also occurs in

long-standing cases of paralysis of neurogenic origin; passive mobility tests are of little diagnostic value in older injuries. CT scanning has been useful in identifying arytenoid subluxation in patients in whom physical findings on indirect laryngoscopy are obscured by edema or hematoma. The radiographic image of a dislocated arytenoid typically reveals anteromedial and inferior displacement of the arytenoid body. Electromyographic studies used to demonstrate the existence of normal innervation of the muscles are of little benefit.

At the time of acute injury, tracheostomy may be necessary because of edema. After the edema has subsided, it may be possible to reduce the arytenoid by direct manual manipulation with a laryngeal spatula. Pressure is exerted on the lateral surface of the vocal process and the body of the arytenoid to lift and push the cartilage in a medioposterior direction into its normal relation to the cricoid cartilage. In some patients, reduction can be effected by inserting an anterior commissure laryngoscope well into the larynx and exerting pressure in an anterior direction while depending on the tension of the vocal cord to pull the arytenoid into position. The posterior surface of the laryngoscope forces the superior tip of the arytenoid posteriorly to aid in the reduction. Occasionally, postreduction fixation of the arytenoid is possible by a brief period (2 weeks) of laryngeal stenting. Usually, reduction is possible only when the patient is seen within 14 days of injury.

When reduction is not possible, disability may persist because of severe dysphonia and dysphagia caused by an incompetent glottis. These problems may be eliminated by performance of a "reverse King operation," intracordal injection of Teflon paste, or pinning of the arytenoid medially. Vocal cord medialization via a laryngeal framework procedure is another option for management of long-standing arytenoid dislocation. Its use avoids the potential disadvantages of Teflon paste injection and does not require tracheostomy or laryngofissure.

FRACTURES OF THE HYOID BONE

This injury may occur as an isolated result of neck trauma or in association with fractures of the other laryngeal cartilages. The fracture may involve any part of the hyoid bone, but it generally occurs in the central body area because of the resiliency of the cornua. Isolated fracture of the hyoid is more common in women. At the time of acute injury, the patient has pain and swelling over the upper anterior aspect of the neck, and bony crepitus may be noted on palpation of the neck and swallowing. The patient usually has odynophagia, dysphagia, and pain on protrusion of the tongue and may also complain of the grating of the fracture fragments. The fracture can usually be seen on soft tissue roentgenograms of the larynx. CT should be performed to rule out the presence of other cartilaginous injuries. Indirect and direct laryngoscopic examinations are necessary to rule out an associated avulsion of the epiglottis.

If a fracture of the hyoid bone is an isolated injury, no treatment is necessary. If such fractures are found during exploration for other reasons, however, they can be immobilized and approximated by direct interosseous wiring using No. 28 stainless steel wire. Because of the intimate relation of the hyoid bone to the muscles of deglutition, delayed union or nonunion of fractures is common. This may cause persistent discomfort associated with deglutition. In cases of symptomatic nonunion, the area of the fracture may be excised to separate the fragments.

SUPRAGLOTTIC INJURY

These injuries generally result in horizontal fractures of the upper part of the thyroid alae with loss of the prominence of the thyroid notch (Fig. 29–4). Disruption of the attachment of the epiglottis causes it to be displaced superiorly and posteriorly, which may cause inspiratory stridor and obstruction. As a result of rupture of the hyoepiglottic ligament, a false passage may be created anterior to the epiglottis; this may empty into the laryngeal cavity at a lower level or may pass anterior to the thyroid cartilage into the lower neck and cause cervical emphysema.

On examination, any of the manifestations of acute laryngeal injury may be present, but some are peculiar to supraglottic injury: (1) a normal, but muffled, voice in the face of increasing airway obstruction; (2) signs of coughing and aspiration on attempting to eat or swallow liquids; (3) appearance of food or liquid at the tracheostomy opening without coughing or choking, indicating an extralaryngeal fistula; and (4) flattening of the upper neck contour and inability to palpate the thyroid notch.

Indirect laryngoscopy is extremely important in these patients, both to assess vocal cord motion and to achieve a realistic assessment of the location of the epiglottis. Fistula tracts into the preepiglottic space may be difficult to demonstrate, and therefore the valleculae and vestibula must be carefully inspected by direct laryngoscopy. Cineradiography studies may be necessary to detect the presence and site of a sinus or fistula. Aqueous contrast should be used for such studies, and barium should not be given to these patients. CT scanning will delineate the cartilaginous fractures.

In isolated supraglottic injuries, the larynx is entered by the anterior pharyngotomy approach. Minor mucosal lacerations are repaired, and, if the epiglottis is

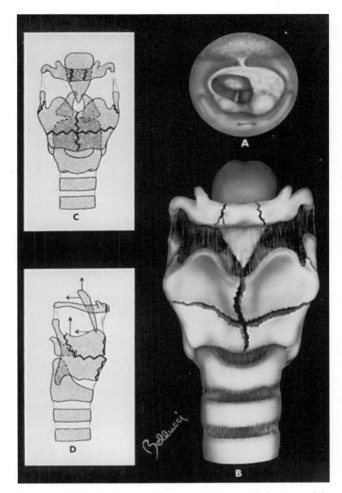

Fig. 29–4. Supraglottic type of laryngeal injury with fracture of the thyroid alae and posterior displacement of the epiglottis. A. This may be followed by supraglottic stenosis in untreated cases. B and C. Cartilage injury. D. Displacement of epiglottis and arytenoid. (Courtesy of Dr. G.J. Spector.)

avulsed from its attachment, it is excised. In severe injuries, the fractured thyroid segments are usually removed along with the false vocal cords and epiglottis. Closure is the same as after supraglottic resection for neoplasm.

This aggressive approach is dictated by the nature of supraglottic injuries. They are often associated with contamination and infection, and healing begins with production of granulation tissue and ends with fibrosis and scar contracture. The epiglottis becomes fixed in a posterior position by scarring. Moreover, fixation of the arytenoids may occur secondary to the healing process. The end result in an untreated injury is supraglottic laryngeal stenosis.

If the patient has vocal cord paralysis or glottic injury, supraglottic resection should not be performed because of the high incidence of intractable aspiration. In these patients, the larynx is entered through a midline thyrotomy, the epiglottis is excised, and the supraglottic area is reconstructed and stented.

GLOTTIC INJURIES

With this injury, the thyroid cartilage is fractured in the region of attachment of the true vocal cords. The fractures may be vertical, transverse, or cruciate (Figs. 29–5 and 29–6). The severity can vary from minor, nondisplaced fractures to severely comminuted fractures exposed externally. Associated injuries may include mucosal lacerations, avulsion of the vocal ligaments off the thyroid cartilage, and arytenoid dislocations.

Patients usually demonstrate marked alteration of the voice and some degree of laryngeal obstruction. Physical examination may demonstrate cervical emphysema, and the cartilage deformity may be palpated through the ecchymotic skin of the anterior aspect of the neck.

On indirect examination, edema, hematoma, and mucosal tears are commonly seen. Foreshortening of the anteroposterior diameter of the glottic chink may be observed, although this may become apparent only after edema subsides. Laceration or avulsion of a vocal cord, with exposure of pieces of fractured cartilage, may be seen as well as displacement of one or both arytenoids or vocal cord paralysis due to nerve injury.

Laryngograms are often more consistent in outlining alterations in the endolaryngeal configuration and in demonstrating fistula or sinus formation than direct laryngoscopy. CT scanning delineates the fragments of the fractured thyroid cartilage and their relative locations.

In the presence of such an injury, a thyrotomy should be done carefully in the midline so the interior of the larynx may be explored. Mucosal tears should be carefully sutured with fine chromic catgut. The epiglottis may be sutured forward to the hyoid bone and thyroid cartilage if it has been only slightly avulsed; otherwise, it should be excised. Dislocated arytenoid

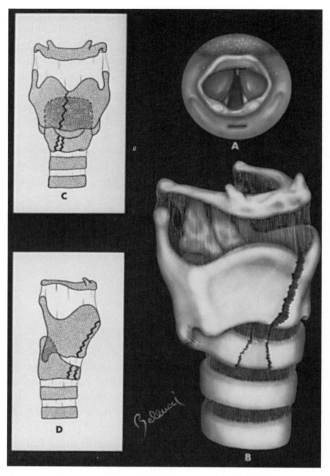

Fig. 29–6. Glottic type of laryngeal injury with vertical fracture of the thyroid ala and displacement of cartilage into the laryngeal lumen (A). B, C, and D. Cartilages fractured and displaced. (Courtesy of Dr. G.J. Spector.)

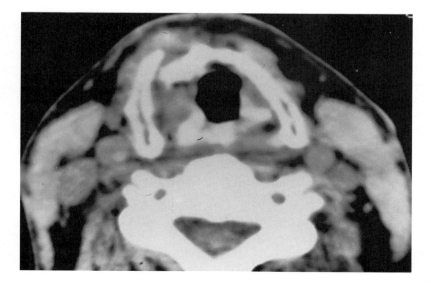

Fig. 29–5. CT scan demonstrating fracture of the thyroid alae.

cartilages should be replaced in their correct relation to the cricoid cartilage. No attempt is made to remove or fixate these cartilages. Sufficient stabilization can be obtained by closure of mucosal tears that accompany cartilage fragment dislocation. When primary closure of mucosal surfaces is not possible because of tissue loss, advancement flaps of pyriform sinus mucosa can be utilized to cover bare cartilage. This is preferable to the use of skin grafts, which may contract excessively during healing. If bilateral vocal cord paralysis secondary to nerve injury is present, it should not be corrected at that time. Frequently, the function of one or both paralyzed vocal cords returns in 3 to 4 months.

Fractures of the thyroid cartilage should be elevated and aligned and approximated with fine No. 32 stainless steel wire, or miniplates as described previously. Loose pieces of cartilage should be removed because they only act as foreign bodies in an already contaminated wound. The vocal ligaments should be sutured to their normal locations on the thyroid alae.

INFRAGLOTTIC INJURIES

These injuries are characterized by crushing of the cricoid cartilage and are usually associated with tracheal damage. Occasionally, the injury is limited to the upper trachea, which may be completely avulsed from its attachment to the cricoid cartilage and may retract into the upper mediastinum (Fig. 29–7).

These severe injuries are associated with airway distress, dysphonia, odynophagia, and hemoptysis. The airway distress may be delayed 4 to 6 hours after injury, when sudden airway compromise occurs. The cricoid prominence is lost to palpation. The subglottic lumen is foreshortened, and the arytenoid cartilages are generally dislocated. The patient usually has an associated subglottic hematoma. Vocal cord paralysis, often bilateral, frequently accompanies this injury as a result of disturbance of the cricothyroid joints and injury to the recurrent laryngeal nerves (Fig. 29–8).

Tracheotomy is generally indicated immediately in these patients. Many such patients have no obvious injury to the thyroid cartilage, and thyrotomy may not be necessary if the site of injury can be adequately examined and reduced through the cricothyroid space or the tracheostomy wound. Depression or comminution of the anterior cricoid arch can usually be stabilized by wiring. If the anterior arch is comminuted beyond repair, a pedicled hyoid bone graft can be inserted, or the trachea can be directly sutured to the thyroid cartilage. Alternatively, a laryngotracheal trough may be created after debridement of devitalized anterior cricoid and tracheal cartilage by suturing the cervical skin to the remnants of the tracheal and infraglottic mucosa. A Montgomery T-tube of appropriate size is then inserted, and a planned, staged reconstruction of the anterior cricoid and tracheal wall is performed with buried Marlex on titanium mesh. Bilateral vocal cord paralysis is usually present in patients with severe cricoid injuries because of severe recurrent nerve injury. When the possibility of neural recovery appears slight, unilateral arytenoidopexy should be performed when the cricoid is repaired. A stent should always be inserted in patients with this injury. If a thyrotomy has not been done, a stent is inserted through the mouth and is pulled into the larynx from below.

Separation of the trachea from the cricoid cartilage or separation of the upper tracheal rings occurs frequently with this injury, and care must be taken to reapproximate these structures. The mucosa should be approximated with fine catgut, and No. 32 wire sutures should be used to approximate the cartilages. Patients should keep the head flexed for 2 weeks.

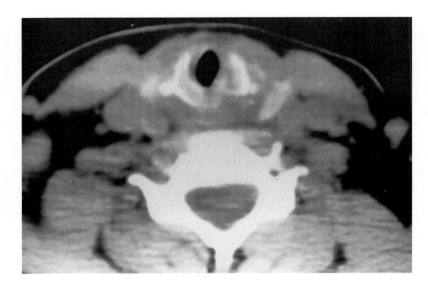

Fig. 29–7. CT scan demonstrating a fracture of the cricoid cartilage.

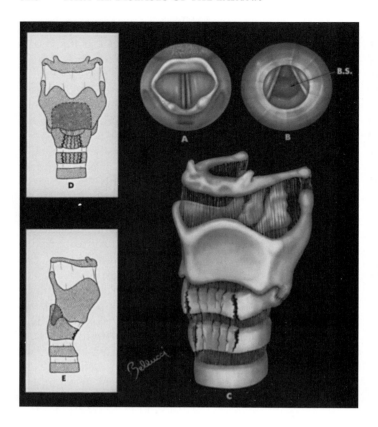

Fig. 29–8. Crushing injury of the larynx with fracture of the cricoid cartilage and upper tracheal ring, accompanied by bilateral vocal cord paralysis (A) and infraglottic stenosis (B). C, D, and E. Cartilages fractured and displaced. B.S., Blind sac. (Courtesy of Dr. G.J. Spector.)

MISSILE INJURIES TO THE LARYNX

Gunshot wounds to the larynx, particularly high-velocity rifle wounds, are unusual, but are encountered with increasing regularity in the civilian population because of the intensifying of urban violence. In patients who survive their injuries, destruction of laryngeal cartilage and soft tissue may be so extensive that effective reconstruction—maintaining an airway, providing an acceptable voice, and restoring sphincteric capability to prevent aspiration—may prove impossible.

Initial management consists of establishing an airway, usually via tracheotomy. Early surgical intervention may be required to address concomitant vascular or pharyngeal injuries. Definitive management of the laryngeal injuries is complicated by the unpredictable viability of tissue traumatized by a high-kinetic-energy missile. In these instances, surgical intervention is best delayed to allow the full extent of devitalized tissue to become evident. Regardless of the timing of the operation, the same surgical principles discussed previously regarding the management of blunt laryngeal injuries are applicable. The surgeon's policy should be one of conservation of all viable laryngeal structures. Stenting is nearly always required because of instability, comminution, and massive disruption of endolaryngeal soft tissues. In some instances, the impact damage is so severe that partial, or even total, laryngectomy is necessary.

IATROGENIC LARYNGEAL INJURIES

High Tracheostomy

Iatrogenic injury is the most common cause of chronic laryngeal stenosis and typically occurs in the management of acute airway obstruction when the tracheostomy tube is inserted through the cricothyroid membrane or the cricoid cartilage. The injury is most common in children because the cricoid cartilage is often difficult to distinguish from a tracheal ring. The injury itself would not be harmful if the tracheostomy tube were removed within 24 hours. In the rush of an emergency tracheostomy, however, the tube position is often ignored until too late. Many elective cricothyroidotomies are still performed in adults undergoing cardiothoracic surgery in an attempt to decrease the possibility of sternal wound contamination.

If the tracheostomy has been especially traumatic, one may see fragmentation of the arch of the cricoid cartilage. The major source of trouble, however, is secondary perichondritis of the cricoid, which contributes to significant, and at times irreversible, airway stenosis. This is associated with the appearance of infected granulation tissue about 48 hours after operation, and, later, healing by fibrosis and circumferential scarring of the infraglottic airway. Factors contributing to the development of perichondritis in patients undergoing cricothyrotomy include (1) advanced age, (2) diabetes mellitus, (3) antecedent endotracheal intubation in excess of 1 week, and (4) preexisting laryngotracheal inflammation.

Signs and symptoms of laryngeal obstruction are not usually evident until the time for decannulation arrives. Even then, symptoms of laryngeal obstruction may not appear for several weeks. In many instances, the voice may be good.

Indirect and direct laryngoscopy may disclose exuberant granulation in the infraglottic area in an injury 10 to 14 days old. Later, granulation is replaced by firm scar tissue, which may completely occlude the laryngeal lumen.

Diagnosis of a high tracheostomy in the immediate postoperative period is highly important. If the flange of a tracheostomy tube, after a new tracheostomy, rests in the center of the neck, suspicion of a misplaced tracheostomy should be aroused. If the tracheostomy tube can be easily seen just below the vocal cords by mirror examination, it is too high. A lateral radiograph of the neck may indicate a high tracheostomy, and such an radiograph should be taken postoperatively in all children with a tracheostomy.

The primary *treatment* is removal and replacement of the tube at a lower level. If this is done within 24 to 48 hours, no further treatment is necessary unless the cricoid cartilage has been badly damaged. In injuries over 10 days old, chronic stenosis usually develops despite use of a stent because of the diffuse perichondritis.

If the diagnosis is made more than 48 hours and less than 10 days after injury, repair, without residual deformity, can still be performed by insertion of an intralaryngeal stent. The stent can be placed by pulling it down into the larynx from the lowered tracheostomy site under laryngoscopic guidance. If granulations are present, they should be removed before the silicone stent is inserted. Occasionally, the intraluminal adhesions and granulations can be removed with a carbon dioxide laser bronchoscope under direct vision. The stent should be left in place for 4 weeks. During this time, any perichondritis should be treated vigorously with antibiotics. Corticosteroid preparations may be used in selected patients to retard granulations.

Intubation Injuries

Endotracheal intubation injuries may occur acutely as a result of the act of intubation itself, or they may be a delayed result of the presence of the endotracheal tube. Acute intubation injuries occur most commonly during emergencies and in patients in whom visualization of the larynx is difficult. These injuries include mucosal edema, abrasions and lacerations, vocal cord hematomas, and arytenoid dislocations. Less common complications include perforation of the pyriform sinus and avulsion of the epiglottis. Complications related to the presence of the endotracheal tube include intubation granuloma, ankylosis of the cricoarytenoid joints, vocal cord paralysis, and subglottic stenosis. Most of these conditions are addressed in other chapters.

Mucosal abrasions that are clinically significant may occur in either the anterior or posterior aspect of the glottis. Anteriorly, the traumatic insertion of the endotracheal tube may denude both vocal cords simultaneously. On healing, these regions may adhere to each other and form an anterior glottic web. Webs are treated by surgical lysis and placement of a laryngeal keel.

Damage to the posterior glottic area may occur, either on endotracheal tube insertion or over time as a result of pressure necrosis of mucosa (Fig. 29–9). One area that is especially susceptible is the medial aspect of the vocal process, where thin mucosa overlies rigid arytenoid cartilage. Women are more susceptible to this injury because of their smaller laryngeal size. Other factors that cause this injury include the use of large endotracheal tubes, excessive tube motion, and the presence of diabetes mellitus. The altered immune function in patients with diabetes along with microangiopathy contributes to poor wound healing and a greater susceptibility to infection.

In many cases of mucosal injury, reepithelialization is prevented by irritation from continued laryngeal function, and infection and granulation tissue forms. This lesion is called a traumatic granuloma.

Traumatic granulomas usually appear about 3 weeks after endolaryngeal injury. Symptoms include

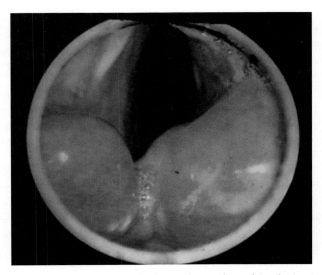

Fig. 29–9. Bilateral arytenoid edema after prolonged intubation in cardiac surgical procedure. (Courtesy of Dr. G.J. Spector.)

hoarseness and pain on swallowing or talking that may radiate to the ear. Indirect laryngoscopy demonstrates a dark red, sessile mass between the arytenoids. Over time, the lesion becomes paler and usually involutes; however, it may become pedunculated and persist. Treatment in the early stages involves voice rest, corticosteroids, and antibiotics. Surgical removal for symptomatic relief is indicated when the mature pedunculated granuloma is present, and usually such treatment is curative.

Traumatic granulomas must be distinguished from contact granuloma. The latter occurs in men because of excessive adducting force in the vocal cords during phonation. The lesion is sessile, often pale from the beginning, and associated with an ulcer on the opposite vocal process. The contact granuloma tends to recur after surgical removal and rarely undergoes spontaneous involution.

Injury Associated with Indwelling Nasogastric Tubes

More and more patients who undergo radical head and neck surgery require prolonged feeding through an indwelling nasogastric tube. The tube must pass posterior to the cricoid lamina, and with constant swallowing and phonatory movements, trauma to the postcricoid mucosa is a frequent complication. Generally, polyethylene tubes cause less difficulty than rubber nasogastric tubes.

Mucosal ulceration in the postcricoid area is the most common lesion, and if it persists, infection of the cricoid cartilage and perichondrium may develop. This may progress to diffuse perichondritis and chondrial necrosis, with possible stenosis of the infraglottic area and hypopharynx. Occasionally, one may see esophagolaryngeal or esophagotracheal fistulas. Rarely, esophageal erosion and death occur.

The patient complains of a sharp pain localized to the lower neck and made much worse by swallowing. Pain may radiate to the ear. If perichondritis develops, cough and signs of laryngeal destruction will be present, as well as pain and tenderness over the larynx.

Indirect laryngoscopy may reveal the superior margin of the ulcer in the postarytenoid area, or an area of erythema and edema is visible at this point. The presence of an ulcer is confirmed by hypopharyngoscopy.

A necrotic ulcer of the body of the arytenoid may be associated with gastroesophageal reflux with or without a hiatal hernia. This may be exacerbated by an indwelling nasogastric tube. Treatment is conservative (namely, to reduce the reflux and neutralize the acidity).

Removal of the nasogastric tube is mandatory. All oral feedings should be withheld until the ulcer is healed. Antibiotics are indicated for infection. Mouth care is important, and frequent use of astringent and antiseptic mouthwashes is helpful.

If a prolonged delay in the reestablishment of oral feeding is anticipated, a cervical esophagostomy or gastrostomy should be performed. When delayed healing or prolonged reconstructive procedures are anticipated after a head and neck operation that precluded normal deglutition, the performance of an elective gastrostomy preoperatively is advisable.

LARYNGEAL BURNS

Thermal Burns

Burns of the laryngeal mucosa occur after inhalation of hot gases or smoke and are a common injury in fire fighters. They may also be secondary to the ingestion of excessively hot food or liquid.

As with external burns, the patient may have first-, second-, and third-degree burns. Third-degree burns are uncommon because the period of contact is usually short. First- and second-degree burns cause supraglottic edema with respiratory obstruction.

Hoarseness, pain, stridor, and respiratory obstruction may be present. Indirect laryngoscopy reveals the false vocal cords to be red, swollen, and edematous. Patches of grayish exudate may cover the areas of second-degree burns. The true vocal cords, if involved, are usually burned over the anterior two thirds, with redness and swelling occurring in this area.

Emergency tracheostomy may be necessary for edematous obstruction of the larynx and pulmonary hygiene. The edema, however, usually subsides rapidly. Adequate humidification and complete voice rest are indicated. Healing is usually prompt, and the complication of chronic stenosis is rare with this type of burn.

Chemical Burns

Many corrosive chemicals may cause burns by ingestion or inhalation, but sodium hydroxide is the most common offender. Potassium hydroxide, Lysol, and chlorine bleach are other commonly ingested corrosive agents; however, burns secondary to the last two are usually not severe. Burns of the larynx are most often secondary to lye ingestion and are associated with hypopharyngeal and esophageal burns.

Burns may be first, second, or third degree. The burned areas of the larynx may include the epiglottis, the aryepiglottic folds, the arytenoid cartilages, and the postcricoid area. Third-degree burns are not uncommon and are associated with full-thickness loss of mucosa. Ulceration and infection develop secondary to the burns and are followed by granulation tissue formation and fibrosis. Cicatricial stenosis of the supraglottic portion of the larynx may be the end result because of adhesions between the false vocal cords or adherence of the epiglottis to the posterior pharyngeal wall. Postcricoid burns may be associated with perichondritis and destruction of the cricoid cartilage.

The patient usually has a history of chemical ingestion, and burns are seen in the mouth and oropharynx. A burn of the larynx or hypopharynx without burns in the mouth is uncommon. In patients with severe burns, respiratory obstruction may develop secondary to edema and may appear within an hour after the burn.

Indirect laryngoscopy may disclose only redness and edema of the supraglottic structures. With severe burns, however, actual charring may occur, with a gray-black membranous exudate covering the involved areas. The epiglottis may be denuded of epithelium and may appear white in contrast to the surrounding black areas. Cervical esophagoscopy is necessary to detect postcricoid burns.

These burns are treated in association with hypopharyngeal and esophageal burns. Attempts to neutralize the caustic substance are usually a waste of time by the time the patient, usually a child, is seen. The introduction of substances such as vinegar, lemon juice, and sodium bicarbonate invites aspiration and the risk of aspiration pneumonia because of altered sphincter function. Vomiting should not be induced because it may subject the esophagus to a second exposure to the corrosive agent. After the airway is controlled, by tracheostomy if necessary, every effort must be made to prevent laryngeal stenosis. Broad-spectrum antibiotics and corticosteroids are given in adequate doses to retard infection and fibrosis. Insertion of a silicone stent in the supraglottic area may be of value in preventing stenosis because most of the burning is usually around the superior margins of the laryngeal vestibule.

Patients with postcricoid burns must be watched for the development of perichondritis. The use of nasogastric tubes for feeding such patients is contraindicated, and a gastrostomy tube should be inserted for this purpose. Chronic supraglottic laryngeal stenosis may be the end result despite preventive efforts.

IRRADIATION INJURY OF THE LARYNX

The diagnosis of carcinoma of the larynx has improved in recent years, with the result that more early lesions of the true vocal cords are being treated by irradiation. Because therapy must be delivered through overlapping ports on each side of the neck, the possibility of a "hot spot" near the anterior commissure exists. This area may receive a dose far in excess of the estimated tumor dose. Moreover, the Ca^{++} ions in the thyroid cartilage have the effect of increasing the effect dose

in the cartilage itself. The result of gamma irradiation overdose is avascular necrosis of cartilage, which may be complicated by perichondritis if the cartilage becomes secondarily infected. Other etiologic factors in addition to overdose include therapy by insufficiently trained personnel, errors in dosimetry, and poor calibration of machines. Individual tissue response to therapy is also variable, and some patients develop severe complications with relatively small doses of gamma irradiation.

Pathology

The initial effects of irradiation involve the surface epithelium. The ciliated epithelium ceases to function, and a loss of epithelial glands occurs. The result is mucositis with a dry, granular mucosa, areas of epithelial loss, and patches of exudate. This is called laryngitis sicca and is generally associated with mucositis. Edema of subepithelial tissue develops secondary to venous and lymphatic obstruction.

When a tissue dose exceeds 1000 to 1400 cGy, irreversible vascular injury occurs because of endothelial proliferation and subintimal fibrosis. These changes cause obstruction of arterioles, small veins, and lymphatics that tends to progress over several years.

Injury to cartilage is secondary to injury of the chondrocytes and progresses slowly unless secondary infection develops. Secondary infection causes perichondritis, cartilage necrosis, and chronic laryngeal stenosis.

Clinical Manifestations

Most patients receiving irradiation to the area of the larynx experience difficulty with hoarseness, sore throat, dryness, and coughing because of mucositis developing toward the end of the course of therapy. These symptoms usually subside after termination of therapy. Some patients may develop considerable edema of the larynx, which may precipitate obstruction; the edema generally disappears but may persist for months or years. Persistent edema after radiation therapy may indicate viable tumor deep in the region.

In the most acute phase, the laryngeal mucosa is bright red and granular; a variable amount of translucent edema may be present in the arytenoid region. Thick, tenacious, greenish secretions are seen lying on the mucosa.

Chronic Radiation Injury

Cancericidal doses of irradiation destroy the seromucous glands, and many patients complain of cough, dryness, hoarseness, and difficulty in clearing secretions.

Irradiation also alters the blood and lymphatic supply of the larynx. Obstruction of arterioles causes a decrease in the blood supply to the already poorly supplied cartilage; thus, chondrial necrosis and secondary infection may develop. Laryngeal biopsy in the postirradiation larynx may precipitate perichondritis. Therefore, biopsy must be performed with extreme discrimination and care to avoid exposure of cartilage. Because the vascular supply to the cartilage is precarious, exposure of the cartilage to infection often leads to perichondritis and chondral necrosis. The onset of perichondritis and chondral necrosis is marked by fever, pain, tenderness, dysphonia, and increasing laryngeal obstruction. Examination of the larynx discloses redness, edema, purulent secretion, and usually impaired mobility of the true vocal cords.

Persistent laryngeal edema may be a problem after radiation therapy. This may be worsened by lymphatic obstruction secondary to radical neck dissection. Dysphonia is the usual symptom, although obstructive symptoms are frequent. The visible portions of the larynx are involved by a pale, translucent edema, and the overlying mucosa is thin, dry, and atrophic.

If perichondritis is suspected, a trial of conservative therapy is indicated before direct laryngoscopy and biopsy are performed. Soft tissue roentgenograms may indicate cartilage destruction, in which case a biopsy may be performed because some surgical procedure will be necessary whatever the diagnosis. When direct laryngoscopy is performed, the tissues should be palpated with a spatula for induration or fluctuation, and any purulent material expressed should be cultured. Biopsies should be small and precise to avoid complication and to obtain maximum assurance of the presence or absence of recrudescent carcinoma. Usually, a deep or double biopsy in the edematous area is needed to obtain a positive specimen for tumor.

Treatment

Acute radiation injury does not necessitate specific therapy, but empiric treatment for subjective complaints, such as the use of bland gargles, humidification, analgesics, and cough suppressants, is helpful.

Treatment of chronic injuries should be as conservative as possible. No surgical procedure should be attempted until infection is brought under control by antibiotic therapy. Cultures should be obtained and the appropriate antibiotic given in large doses. Mouth and pharyngeal care is important, and frequent saline irrigations are indicated, in addition to the use of weak solutions of sodium perborate or hydrogen peroxide as a mouthwash and gargle three times a day. Absolute voice rest is necessary. A tracheostomy is useful to control obstruction.

In the presence of noninfective obstructive edema, administration of a corticosteroid such as prednisone, 5 mg four times daily, may be helpful. Corticosteroids should not be used in the presence of an acute infection.

When the diagnosis of perichondritis and chondral necrosis is made and the presence of carcinoma has been ruled out, preservation of the larynx should be attempted. Loose, dead pieces of cartilage may be removed endoscopically when present in the laryngeal lumen or in a laryngeal-cutaneous fistula. Abscesses must be drained to prevent endolaryngeal rupture and aspiration of pus.

When acute infection is controlled, surgical debridement may be indicated. Surgery on the neck of such a patient, however, practically always leads to sloughing of soft tissues and poor healing, which should be anticipated. At surgery, skin and soft tissue exhibiting marked radiation changes and poor vitality should be excised. Any necrotic cartilage must be removed, but perichondrium and mucosa should be preserved if laryngeal function is to be retained. During this period, it may be necessary to support the larynx with an endolaryngeal stent. The wounds should be left open until healthy granulations appear, unless the surgeon believes that further necrosis is unlikely and additional blood supply from a transposed tissue flap would be more advantageous. In most of these patients, definitive surgery is followed by a tissue defect, which must be repaired by transposed pedicle flaps. Repair by pedicle flaps may be immediate or delayed. The pedicle flaps bring additional blood supply to the involved areas. Hyperbaric oxygen has been demonstrated to successfully increase oxygen partial pressures in tissues with radiation-induced microvascular insufficiency. This, in turn, allows renewed fibroblastic activity, which serves as a framework for capillary ingrowth and neovascularization. Documentation of efficacy of this method is now sufficient to recommend its administration in all patients with severe laryngeal radionecrosis. During hyperbaric oxygen treatment, the patient breathes 100% oxygen while sitting in a chamber compressed to 2.0 ATA (atmosphere absolute) with air. Most patients experience an amelioration of symptoms and a resolution of laryngeal obstruction following 35 to 40 treatments. Retreatment is possible if symptoms recur. On rare occasions, laryngectomy may be the only appropriate procedure.

SUGGESTED READINGS

Alexander FW: Micropathology of radiation reaction in the larynx. Ann Otol Rhinol Laryngol 72:831, 1963.

Bennett T: Laryngeal trauma. Laryngoscope 70:793, 1960.

Bent III JP, et al: Acute laryngeal trauma: a review of 77 patients. Otolaryngol Head Neck Surg 109:441, 1993.

Bergstrom J, et al: On the pathogenesis of laryngeal injuries following prolonged intubation. Acta Otolaryngol 55:342, 1962.

Ferguson BJ, Hudson WR, and Farmer JC: Hyperbaric oxygen therapy for laryngeal radionecrosis. Ann Otol Rhinol Laryngol 96:1, 1987.

Fitz-Hugh GS, et al: Injuries of the larynx and cervical trauma. Ann Otol Rhinol Laryngol 71:419, 1962.

Gard MA and Cruikshank LF: Factors influencing the incidence of sore throat following endotracheal intubation. Can Med Assoc J 84:662, 1961.

Harrison DFN: Bullet wounds of the larynx and trachea. Arch Otolaryngol 110:203, 1984.

Hoffman HT, et al: Arytenoid subluxation: diagnosis and treatment. Ann Otol Rhinol Laryngol 100:1, 1991.

Holinger PH and Loeb WJ: Feeding tube stenosis of the larynx. Surg Gynecol Obstet 83:253, 1946.

Inglauer S and Molt WF: Severe injury to the larynx resulting from indwelling duodenal tube. Ann Otol Rhinol Laryngol 48:886, 1939.

Jackson C: High tracheostomy and other errors, the chief causes of chronic laryngeal stenosis. Surg Gynecol Obstet 32:392, 1921.

Knight JS: Cricothyroid dislocation. Laryngoscope 70:1256, 1960.

Kuriloff DB, et al: Laryngotracheal injury following cricothyroidotomy. Laryngoscope 99:125, 1989.

Lu AT, et al: The pathology of laryngotracheal complications: lesions of the larynx and trachea after intubation anesthesia. Arch Otolaryngol 74:323, 1961.

Lyons MB, et al: Adhesives in larynx repair. Laryngoscope 99:376, 1989.

Meglin AJ, Biedringmaier JF, and Mirvis SE: Three-dimensional computerized tomography in the evaluation of laryngeal injury. Laryngoscope 101:202, 1991.

Miles WK, Olson NR, and Rodriguez A: Acute treatment of experimental laryngeal fractures. Ann Otol Rhinol Laryngol 80:710, 1971.

Montgomery WW: The surgical management of supraglottic and subglottic stenosis. Ann Otol Rhinol Laryngol 76:786, 1967.

Myerson MC: Granulomatous polyp of the larynx following intratracheal intubation. Arch Otolaryngol 62:182, 1955.

Ogura JH and Powers WE: Surgical correction of the traumatic stenosis of the larynx and pharynx. Laryngoscope 72:468, 1962.

Ogura JH, et al: Laryngotracheal trauma: Diagnosis and treatment. Can J Ophthalmol 2:112, 1973.

Pennington J: Glottic and supraglottic laryngeal injury and stenosis from external trauma. Laryngoscope 74:317, 1964.

Rush BF Jr: Repair of the injured larynx following destruction of the cricoid cartilage. Surg Gynecol Obstet 112:507, 1961.

Schaefer SD: The treatment of acute external laryngeal injuries. Arch Otolaryngol Head Neck Surg 117:35, 1991.

Shaw R, et al: Traumatic tracheal rupture. J Thorac Cardiovasc Surg 42:281, 1961.

Stanley RB Jr, et al: Phonatory effects of thyroid cartilage fractures. Ann Otol Rhinol Laryngol 96:493, 1987.

Warren S: Histopathology of lesions due to irradiation. Physiol Rev 24:225, 1944.

Woo P: Laryngeal framework reconstruction with miniplates. Ann Otol Rhinol Laryngol 99:772, 1990.

30 Infectious and Inflammatory Diseases of the Larynx

James A. Koufman

The majority of patients with disorders of the larynx and voice suffer from infectious and noninfectious inflammatory conditions. The term *inflammation* implies a local response to tissue injury, characterized by capillary dilation and leukocyte infiltration. The typical signs and symptoms of inflammation are swelling, redness, and, sometimes, discomfort or pain. The term *laryngitis* is synonymous with laryngeal inflammation, although not with hoarseness. Laryngitis (laryngeal inflammation) may result from infection by an invading microorganism or from irritative, traumatic, metabolic, allergic, autoimmune, or idiopathic causes.

Acute and chronic laryngitis are common, and the causes (differential diagnoses) in pediatric and in adult patients are different. In infants and children, for example, the most common cause of laryngitis is acute infection, whereas in adults, laryngitis generally tends to have a chronic, noninfectious cause.

Within the last decade, gastroesophageal reflux has been discovered to be a far more important cause of laryngeal inflammation than was previously recognized. In addition, primarily because of the acquired immunodeficiency syndrome (AIDS) epidemic, infecting microorganisms that were rarely encountered just a few years ago are reemerging. Thus, the physician must again become familiar with the clinical manifestations of infection by a wide spectrum of microorganisms.

Laryngeal inflammatory disorders are unusual in that often more than one causative factor or condition can be identified. For example, patients with Reinke's edema are frequently smokers who also misuse their voices and have gastroesophageal reflux. Such patients may also develop laryngeal carcinoma (Fig. 30–1).

Each of the underlying causes must be identified and corrected if treatment is to be successful. As more has been learned about the larynx, about environmental influences, and about the effects of systemic disorders on the larynx, imprecise diagnostic terms, such as "nonspecific laryngitis," have appropriately begun to disappear from the otolaryngologic literature.

The differential diagnosis of the infectious and noninfectious causes of laryngitis is shown in Table 30–1.

GASTROESOPHAGEAL (LARYNGOPHARYNGEAL) REFLUX DISEASE

Investigators have estimated that 10% of Americans have heartburn on a daily basis, and an additional 30 to 50% have it less frequently.[1] Of all the causes of laryngeal inflammation, gastroesophageal reflux disease (GER, GERD) is the most common cause, and as many as 10 to 50% of patients with laryngeal complaints have a GER-related underlying cause.[2]

The term *reflux* literally means "back flow." Reflux of stomach contents into the esophagus is common, and many patients with GERD have symptoms such as heartburn and regurgitation of acid and digestive enzymes. When refluxed material escapes the esophagus and enters the laryngopharynx above, the event is termed *laryngopharyngeal reflux* (LPR). Although the terms *gastroesophageal reflux* and *laryngopharyngeal reflux* are often used interchangeably, the latter is more specific.

LPR affects both children and adults and may be associated with an acute, chronic, or intermittent pattern of laryngitis, with or without granuloma formation. Indeed, LPR has also been implicated in the development of laryngeal carcinoma and stenosis, recurrent laryngospasm, and cricoarytenoid fixation, as well as many other conditions, including globus pharyngeus, cervical dysphagia, and subglottic stenosis.[2–9]

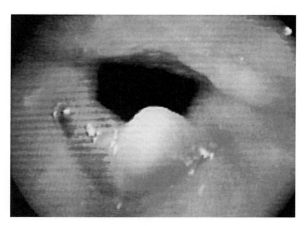

Fig. 30–1. Laryngeal inflammation may be multifactorial. The larynx shown is that of a 65-year-old female smoker who also has reflux laryngitis and hypothyroidism. The larynx is diffusely erythematous and edematous, and there is massive Reinke's edema (polypoid degeneration) of the true vocal cords. In addition, the white area on the left cord is an early squamous cell carcinoma.

The symptoms of LPR are different from the GER-associated symptoms of heartburn, regurgitation, and esophagitis. Patients with reflux laryngitis present with hoarseness, but almost two thirds deny ever having heartburn.[2,5] Other throat symptoms, such as globus pharyngeus (a sensation of a lump in the throat), dysphagia, chronic throat clearing, and cough, are often associated with LPR.[5] Gastroenterologists call reflux patients who deny having gastrointestinal symptoms "atypical refluxers," but these patients are typical of those encountered by the otolaryngologist.[10] The symptoms and laryngeal conditions that have been reported to be associated with LPR are summarized in Table 30–2, and the differences between the typical patient with reflux laryngitis and the typical patient with reflux esophagitis are summarized in Table 30–3.

Laryngeal Findings

When the larynx of a patient with reflux laryngitis is examined, one of four patterns is encountered: (1) "posterior laryngitis," that is, red arytenoids with piled-up interarytenoid mucosa; (2) diffuse edema, Reinke's space edema, and mucosal thickening without significant erythema; (3) diffuse erythema with granular, friable mucosa; or (4) vocal-process or other discrete granulomas, with or without associated laryngeal edema and erythema.

Diagnosis

Ambulatory 24-hour double-probe pH monitoring (pH-metry) is the current standard for the diagnosis of reflux in otolaryngologic patients.[2,11,12] The first probe is placed 5 cm above the lower esophageal sphincter. The second probe is placed in the hypopharynx, be-

TABLE 30–1. Inflammatory Disorders of the Larynx

Gastroesophageal (laryngopharyngeal) reflux disease
Pediatric laryngitis
  Acute (viral or bacterial) infections
    Laryngotracheitis (croup)
    Supraglottitis (epiglottitis)
    Diphtheria
  Noninfectious causes
    Spasmodic croup
    Traumatic laryngitis
Acute laryngeal infections of adults
  Viral laryngitis
    Common upper respiratory infection
    Laryngotracheitis
    Herpes simplex infection
  Bacterial laryngitis
    Supraglottitis
    Laryngeal abscess
    Gonorrhea
Chronic (granulomatous) diseases
  Bacterial diseases
    Tuberculosis
    Leprosy
    Scleroma
    Actinomycosis
    Tularemia
    Glanders
  Spirochetal disease (syphilis)
  Mycotic diseases (fungal)
    Candidiasis
    Blastomycosis
    Histoplasmosis
    Coccidioidomycosis
    Aspergillosis
    Sporotrichosis
  Idiopathic disease
    Sarcoidosis
    Wegener's granulomatosis
Allergic, immune, and idiopathic disorders
  Hypersensitivity reactions
    Angioedema
    Stevens-Johnson syndrome
  Immune and idiopathic disorders
    Infections of the immunocompromised host
    Rheumatoid arthritis
    Systemic lupus erythematosus
    Cicatricial pemphigoid
    Relapsing polychondritis
    Sjögren's syndrome
    Amyloidosis
Miscellaneous inflammatory conditions
  Parasitic infections
    Trichinosis
    Leishmaniasis
    Schistosomiasis
    Syngamus laryngeus
  Inhalation laryngitis
    Acute (thermal) injury
    Pollution and inhalant allergy
    Carcinogens
  Radiation injury
    Radiation laryngitis
    Radionecrosis
  Vocal abuse and misuse syndromes
    Vocal cord hemorrhage
    Muscle tension dysphonias
    Contact ulcer and granuloma

TABLE 30–2. Symptoms and Laryngeal Conditions Associated with Gastroesophageal Reflux Disease

Symptoms
    Chronic dysphonia
    Intermittent dysphonia
    Vocal fatigue
    Voice breaks
    Chronic throat clearing
    Excessive throat mucus
    "Postnasal drip"
    Chronic cough
    Dysphagia
    Globus
Conditions
    Reflux laryngitis
    Subglottic stenosis
    Carcinoma of the larynx
    Endotracheal intubation injury
    Contact ulcers and granulomas
    Posterior glottic stenosis
    Arytenoid fixation
    Paroxysmal laryngospasm
    Sudden infant death syndrome
    Globus pharyngeus
    Vocal nodules
    Polypoid degeneration
    Laryngomalacia
    Pachydermia laryngitis
    Recurrent leukoplakia

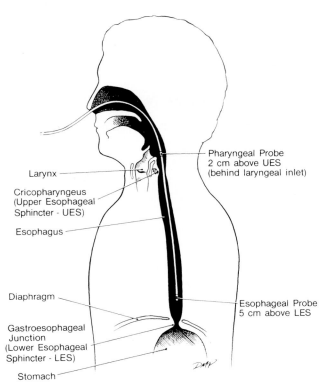

Fig. 30–2. Technique of ambulatory 24-hour double-probe pH monitoring. The distal probe is placed 5 cm above the lower esophageal sphincter (LES), and the proximal (pharyngeal) probe is placed 2 cm above the upper esophageal sphincter (UES).

TABLE 30–3. Differences Between the Patient with Esophagitis and the Patient with Reflux Laryngitis

	Esophagitis	Reflux Laryngitis
Symptoms		
Heartburn and/or regurgitation	Yes	No
Hoarseness, dysphagia, globus	No	Yes
Findings		
Endoscopic esophagitis	Yes	No
Laryngeal inflammation	No	Yes
Diagnostic yield (abnormality)		
Esophageal biopsy (inflammation)	Yes	No
Abnormal esophageal radiography	Yes	Sometimes
Esophageal pH monitoring	Yes	Yes
Pharyngeal pH monitoring	No	Yes
Pattern of reflux		
Supine (nocturnal)	Yes	Sometimes
Upright (awake)	Sometimes	Yes
Response to treatment		
Dietary/life-style modification	Yes	Sometimes
Rate of success with H_2 blockers*	85%	65%
Rate of success with omeprazole*	99%	99%

* Assuming adequate dosage and duration of therapy.

hind the laryngeal inlet (Fig. 30–2). This technique is highly sensitive and specific for LPR, and it also delineates each patient's reflux pattern so treatment can be customized.

pH-metry has been available for many years, and standards (normal values) have been established in many laboratories.[2,13] In general, the most important parameter is considered to be the percentage of time that the pH is less than 4, and this measurement is usually recorded for time in the *upright position*, time in the *supine position*, and the *total time* of the study. For the upright period, the upper limit of normal is approximately 8.0%, and for the supine period, it is approximately 2.5%.[13]

The (second) pharyngeal probe is invaluable in patients with reflux laryngitis, because it is placed behind the larynx just above the cricopharyngeus, and thus reflux recorded by it is diagnostic of laryngopharyngeal reflux (Fig. 30–3). In addition, without the second probe, LPR is underdiagnosed in approximately one third of patients with reflux laryngitis.

One should also obtain a barium swallow/esophagogram in patients with reflux laryngitis because this test allows assessment of the integrity of the esophageal lining.[14] Although this barium study is not a sensitive test for diagnosing GERD, it may demonstrate significant abnormalities that might otherwise be missed.

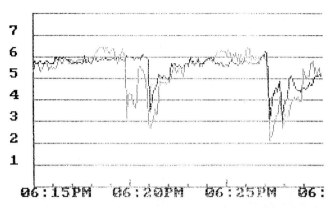

Fig. 30–3. Example of an abnormal double-probe pH study. The light tracing is the esophageal pH, and the darker tracing is the pharyngeal pH. Three pharyngeal reflux episodes (pH < 4) are demonstrated at 6:21, 6:27, and 6:28. Note that the pH in the esophageal probe tracing drops just before each pH drop in pharyngeal probe.

In a series of 128 patients, the results of a barium study revealed that 18% had esophagitis, 14% had a lower esophageal ring, and 3% had a peptic stricture.[2]

Treatment

Three levels of antireflux treatment are recognized: *level I*, dietary and life-style modification plus antacids; *level II*, level I plus use of an H_2 blocker (such as cimetidine, ranitidine, or famotidine); and *level III*, antireflux surgery (e.g., fundoplication) or omeprazole therapy. The details of each of the three levels are listed in Table 30–4.

Clinical experience with patients with reflux laryngitis indicates that treatment must be individualized, with the level of treatment depending on the severity of the patient's condition. For many patients with reflux laryngitis, level I or level II treatment is appropriate initial therapy, but both forms will fail in up to 35% of patients.[2,12,15] If level II treatment fails, level III treatment with the proton pump inhibitor omeprazole may be indicated. In addition, for patients with severe reflux laryngitis, initial treatment with omeprazole may be indicated.

At present, omeprazole is by far the most effective antireflux medication available, because, unlike the H_2 blockers, it usually accomplishes total acid suppression (when administered in a dose of 20 mg twice daily).[15,16] Figure 30–4 shows the larynx of a patient before and after treatment with omeprazole. Unfortunately, omeprazole still is not recommended for use in children or as long-term treatment in adults—hence the need for fundoplication in some patients.

Potentially Life-Threatening Manifestations of Reflux Disease

Paroxysmal Laryngospasm

Laryngospasm is an uncommon complaint, but patients who experience this frightening symptom usu-

TABLE 30–4. Treatment ("Levels") for Reflux Laryngitis

LEVEL I: Antireflux therapy [ART]
  Dietary modification
    No eating or drinking within 3 hours of bedtime
    Avoidance of overeating or reclining right after meals
    No fried food; low-fat diet
    Avoidance of coffee, tea, chocolate, mints, and soda pop
    Avoidance of other caffeine-containing foods and beverages
    Avoidance of alcohol, especially in the evening
    Avoidance of other foods that cause problems
  Life-style modification
    Elevation of the head of the bed 4 to 6 inches
    Avoidance of tight-fitting clothing or belts
    Avoidance of tobacco
  Liquid antacids four times daily (1 tablespoon 1 hour after each meal and at bedtime)
LEVEL II: Medication plus ART
  Level I above
  Initial treatment
    Ranitidine, 150 mg twice daily, or
      An equivalent dose of another H_2 blocker
        Prokinetic agent (e.g., cisapride) used as an adjunct
  Escalation for treatment failures
    Ranitidine, 150 to 300 mg four times daily or
    An equivalent dose of another H_2 blocker
LEVEL III: Proton pump inhibitors or antireflux surgery
  Level I above (minus antacids)
  Omeprazole, 20 mg twice daily (first thing in the morning and at 5 PM; the duration of "initial" treatment should be 6 months; large patients may require larger doses)
  Fundoplication

ally are able to describe the "event" in vivid detail. If the clinician mimics severe inspiratory stridor, the patient will confirm that the breathing pattern during attacks was, indeed, similar. Laryngospasm is often paroxysmal, and it usually occurs without warning. In some patients, the attacks awake them from sleep, and in others, the attacks occur during the day. The attacks may have a predictable pattern, such as, occurring after meals or during exercise, and some patients are aware of a relationship between GER and the attacks (others are not). Loughlin and I studied a series of 12 patients with recurrent paroxysmal laryngospasm, 11 of whom had documented LPR by pH-metry, and all of whom responded to treatment with omeprazole by a cessation of laryngospastic episodes.

Laryngeal Stenosis

Excluding trauma, LPR is the primary cause of laryngeal stenosis, including subglottic stenosis and posterior laryngeal stenosis;[2–4,9] pH-metry-documented GER has been found in 92% of cases.[2] Treatment with omeprazole or fundoplication results in subsequent decannulation of most patients with such stenosis, in some cases without surgery.[2,9]

The traditional dichotomy between mature and immature stenoses probably represents an oversimplification. *Immature* implies that massive edema and granulation tissue are present and that the inflammatory

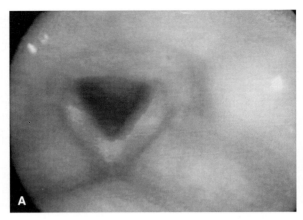
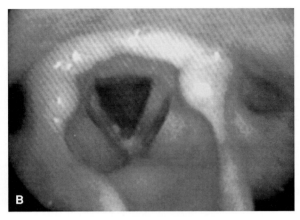

Fig. 30–4. Fiberoptic laryngoscopic view of reflux laryngitis before and after treatment. A. Reflux laryngitis, before treatment. Note that there is diffuse laryngeal edema, but very little mucosal erythema. This is common. B. Same patient after one month of treatment with antireflux therapy (omeprazole), showing an almost normal larynx. She does have small asymmetrical vocal nodules that could not be appreciated prior to antireflux treatment (due to the amount of edema).

process is ongoing; *mature* implies that acute inflammation has resolved and that the stenosis is composed of mature fibrous tissue with thin (normal) overlying epithelium. Surgical attempts to correct immature stenoses usually fail unless the LPR is controlled. Conversely, mature stenoses usually can be corrected surgically. In reality, however, many cases are neither mature nor immature, but somewhere in between. The same also may be true of many acquired laryngeal webs.

pH-Metry and antireflux therapy should be used in all patients with laryngeal stenosis. As the data base grows, this admonition probably will become dogma. Meanwhile, treatment with omeprazole or fundoplication should be considered adjuncts to surgical therapy.

Laryngeal Carcinoma

The risk factors for the development of laryngeal carcinoma include GERD.[6,7] I reported a series of 31 consecutive patients with laryngeal carcinoma in whom abnormal reflux was documented in 84%, but only 58% were active smokers.[2] The relationship between GERD and malignant degeneration remains unproved, but the available pH-metry data suggest that most patients who develop laryngeal malignant disease both smoke and have GERD. In addition, apparently premalignant lesions may resolve with appropriate antireflux therapy.[2]

The previously identified risk factors for laryngeal carcinoma—tobacco and ethanol—also strongly predispose to reflux. Tobacco and alcohol adversely influence almost all the body's antireflux mechanisms; they delay gastric emptying, decrease lower esophageal sphincter pressure and esophageal motility, decrease mucosal resistance, and increase secretion of gastric acid. Routine pH-metry, followed by omeprazole treatment, is recommended for all patients with laryngeal neoplasia, with or without other risk factors for the development of carcinoma of the larynx. Figure 30–5 shows an example of a reflux-induced laryngeal carcinoma in a lifetime nonsmoker.

Laryngopharyngeal Reflux Disease in Infants and Children

LPR is ubiquitous and pernicious in pediatric otolaryngologic patients. The diagnosis may be particularly difficult to make because infants and children rarely complain of heartburn or other reflux symptoms. LPR has been clearly associated with the development of childhood laryngeal and tracheal stenosis, as well as with reactive airway disorders (laryngospasm, asthma, sudden infant death syndrome, laryngomalacia, bron-

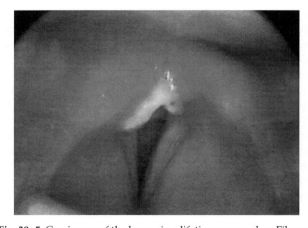

Fig. 30–5. Carcinoma of the larynx in a lifetime nonsmoker. Fiberoptic laryngoscopic appearance of a "reflux-induced" carcinoma of the larynx in a 70-year-old life-time nonsmoker. He had no other risk factors. Biopsy confirmed that the lesion was microinvasive squamous cell carcinoma. The lesion has an unusual (interarytenoid) location for laryngeal carcinoma, and the larynx shows other signs of reflux laryngitis. The patient had a grossly abnormal pH study.

chopulmonary dysplasia, and aspiration pneumonia).[8,9,17,18]

A high index of suspicion is necessary for the diagnosis of LPR to be considered; currently, only prolonged pH-metry is diagnostic. Other tests, such as barium esophagography, radionuclide scanning, and the lipid-laden macrophage test, lack sufficient sensitivity and/or specificity to be of value in the majority of cases.

PEDIATRIC LARYNGITIS

Pediatric patients with laryngeal inflammation and edema present with one or more of the following symptoms: dysphonia, odynophonia, cough, dysphagia, odynophagia, stridor, and dyspnea.

Airway obstruction from inflammatory laryngeal edema is more common in children than in adults, because of the small size of the pediatric larynx. Equivalent amounts of mucosal swelling may result in critical narrowing and obstruction in a child, while causing only minimal symptoms in an adult. Table 30–5 shows the effects of 1 mm of edema on the cross-sectional (subglottic) area of a small neonate, an average child, and an adult male. The magnitude of the difference between the effect in each explains why laryngeal inflammation is more often a life-threatening illness requiring airway management in infants and children than it is in adults.

Laryngotracheitis ("Croup")

Viral laryngotracheitis is the most common laryngeal inflammatory disorder of childhood. Usually, this condition is self-limited, occurs in children under the age of 3 years, and has a seasonal peak, with most cases occurring during the winter. Typically, for several days before presentation, the child's history is compatible with that of a viral upper respiratory infection—rhinitis, cough, and low-grade fever. When symptoms of hoarseness, dyspnea, stridor, and a barking cough develop, the diagnosis of laryngotracheitis is made. The characteristic cough gives laryngotracheitis its common name, "croup." Rhinovirus, parainfluenza virus, respiratory syncytial virus, and adenovirus have all been implicated. Less common causes of laryngotracheitis are influenza, measles, mumps, pertussis, and chickenpox[19] (see Chap. 3).

When airway obstruction is caused by laryngotracheitis, the stridor is characteristically inspiratory, or biphasic. Whereas the diagnosis of laryngotracheitis is generally based on the history, examination of the larynx, although not necessary, shows erythematous and edematous mucosa with normal vocal cord mobility. Radiographs, which reveal a narrowing of the subglottic lumen, the "steeple sign," may be used to differentiate this condition from supraglottitis (discussed later) (Fig. 30–6).

The need for inpatient hospitalization depends on the degree of airway obstruction. Treatment is aimed at decreasing laryngeal edema and preventing stasis and crusting of secretions within the airway. Therapy usually includes hydration, humidification of inspired air, and treatments with nebulized racemic epinephrine. Antipyretics, decongestants, and parenteral corticosteroids are often administered. Although the value of corticosteroids remains controversial, many experienced clinicians use them because they believe that the anti-inflammatory effect can obviate the need for intubation when the airway is marginally adequate. Artificial airway support, such as by intubation, is necessary in a relatively small proportion of patients with laryngotracheitis. When needed, however, intubation should be carried out by experienced personnel, preferably in the operating room, where maximum airway control can be achieved.

Endoscopy with cultures of the airway surfaces and secretions should be considered for patients with atypical or severe laryngotracheitis, particularly those who cannot be extubated successfully. Secondary bacterial infection of the airway ("membranous croup") is more serious and is usually attended by high temperature spikes and exudative, purulent drainage. Radiographically, the lumen of the upper airway appears narrowed, shaggy, and irregular. The microorganisms most commonly involved are Haemophilus influenzae, pneumococcus, and hemolytic streptococci. Antibiotic therapy is indicated and is directed at the causative microorganisms.

Supraglottitis ("Epiglottitis")

Acute supraglottitis is a life-threatening infection of the supraglottic larynx most often caused by Haemophilus influenzae type B. It is a true medical emergency. Children aged 2 to 4 years are the most frequently affected

TABLE 30–5. The Effect of One Millimeter of Edema on the Cross-Sectional Area of the Subglottic Larynx in the Neonate, Child, and Adult (Area = πr^{2}*)

	Neonate	Child	Adult
"Normal"			
Subglottic diameter (mm)	4	8	14
Subglottic radius (mm)	2	4	7
Subglottic area (mm^2)	12	48	147
Effect of 1 mm of edema			
Subglottic diameter (mm)	2	6	12
Subglottic radius (mm)	1	3	6
Subglottic area (mm^2)	3	27	108
Percentage of reduction of airway area	75%	44%	27%

* For the sake of simplicity, for these calculations $\pi = 3$

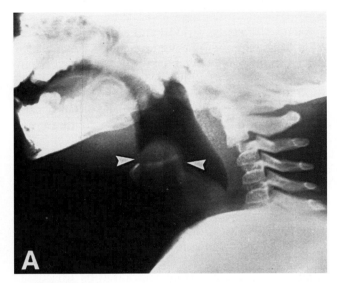

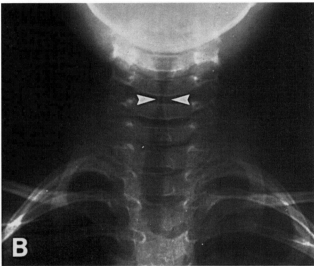

Fig. 30–6. Radiographic appearance of supraglottitis (epiglottitis) and laryngotracheitis ("croup"). A. Lateral radiograph of the neck of a child with supraglottitis. Note the haziness of the supraglottis, the thickening of the epiglottis (the "thumb sign") (arrows), and the dilation of the hypopharynx. B. Anteroposterior radiograph of the neck of a child with laryngotracheitis. Note the narrowing of the subglottic lumen (the "steeple sign") (arrows).

group, and cases are more frequent in the winter and spring. The illness begins rapidly over 2 to 6 hours with the onset of fever, sore throat, and inspiratory stridor. The voice tends to be muffled, and the patient has no "barky" cough, as in croup. As the supraglottic structures become more edematous, airway obstruction develops.

The child is generally ill-appearing, stridulous, sitting upright, and drooling, because swallowing is painful. The diagnosis is usually based purely on the history and clinical findings. Examination of the epiglottis (in the hospital emergency department) may precipitate airway obstruction and thus is not recom-

mended. Lateral soft tissue radiographs may reveal the classic "thumb" sign of the edematous epiglottis with a dilated hypopharynx (Fig. 30–6). Occasionally, the epiglottis itself is not enlarged, but the supraglottic region still appears hazy and indistinct because of edema of other supraglottic structures. In severe cases, treatment should not be delayed to obtain radiographs. If radiographs are deemed necessary, the study should be carried out in the presence of personnel capable of intubating the patient immediately should airway obstruction occur.

The child with suspected epiglottitis should be taken to the operating room immediately to establish the diagnosis and secure an airway. The child is transported to the operating room by the parents, an otolaryngologist, and an anesthesiologist. Direct laryngoscopy usually shows the epiglottis to be swollen and "cherry red," as are the aryepiglottic folds and the false vocal cords. The true vocal cords and subglottis typically appear to be normal or only minimally involved.

Treatment is directed at airway maintenance and then toward providing antimicrobial and supportive care. Drawing blood, starting intravenous lines, obtaining a rectal temperature, or otherwise disturbing the patient should be postponed until the airway is secured.

After the child is anesthetized and the diagnosis is made, the child should be orally intubated to secure the airway. The oral endotracheal tube can then be converted to a nasotracheal tube, with direct visualization of the glottis as the orotracheal tube is removed. Instruments necessary for rigid bronchoscopy and tracheotomy should be available and ready in the operating room in case the airway is lost before intubation.[20] In institutions without a highly skilled pediatric intensive care staff available around the clock, a tracheotomy may be preferable to endotracheal intubation, because it is easier to secure and to reestablish if the tube is inadvertently dislodged.[21]

Cultures of the epiglottis and blood are obtained after the airway is secured. Empirically, antimicrobial therapy is initiated against Haemophilus influenzae and classically consists of ampicillin and chloramphenicol. Cefuroxime and other second- and third-generation cephalosporin antibiotics are now considered equally effective. Extubation is usually possible after 48 to 72 hours, when the edema has subsided sufficiently to allow an air leak around the endotracheal tube. Transnasal fiberoptic laryngoscopy is the most reliable and most commonly employed technique to ensure resolution of the edema before extubation.

Haemophilus influenzae type B polysaccharide vaccine has been available since 1985 for children over 18 months of age. The recent development of polysaccharide-protein conjugate vaccines has made possible the immunization of children beginning at 2 months of

TABLE 30–6. Some of the Distinguishing Characteristics of Laryngotracheitis ("Croup") and Supraglottitis ("Epiglottitis")

Feature	Croup	Epiglottitis
Age	Less than 3 years	Over 3 years
Onset	Gradual (days)	Rapid (hours)
Cough	"Barky"	None
Posture	Supine	Sitting
Drooling	No	Yes
Radiograph	"Steeple sign," narrowed subglottis	"Thumb sign," enlarged epiglottis, dilated hypopharynx
Cause	Viral	Bacterial
Treatment	Supportive (croup tent, corticosteroids)	Airway management (intubation or tracheotomy) and antibiotics

age. One hopes that provision of this immunologic protection will cause epiglottitis to become a rare disease.

Differentiating acute epiglottitis from laryngotracheitis is not always easy, but it is of paramount importance. Some of the differentiating signs and symptoms are shown in Table 30–6, and the radiographic findings of the two conditions are demonstrated by Figure 30–6.

Diphtheria

Worldwide, diphtheria is an uncommon laryngeal infection, although a report from India suggests that outbreaks still occur there.[22] Laryngeal diphtheria is caused by Corynebacterium diphtheriae and generally affects children over the age of 5 years. A febrile illness of slow onset associated with sore throat and hoarseness is then followed by progressive airway obstruction.

The microorganism causes an inflammatory response in the mucous membranes, which results in a thick, grayish-green, plaque-like membranous exudate over the tonsils, pharynx, and laryngeal structures. Characteristically, the exudate is difficult to dislodge and bleeds when removed. The diagnosis requires that the clinician have a high index of suspicion confirmed by observing the typical oropharyngeal findings. Cultures and smears are obtained for confirmation.

Treatment consists of establishing a safe airway via a tracheotomy (intubation is contraindicated because it may dislodge a portion of the plaque and cause airway obstruction) and administering diphtheria antitoxins and penicillin or erythromycin to eradicate the microorganisms. Mortality results largely from the neuropathies that develop secondary to the diphtheria toxin. Even in the patient immunized against diphtheria, the disease may occur, but is usually mild.

Spasmodic Croup

Spasmodic croup, or "false croup," is a noninfectious form of laryngeal inflammation associated with a mild, chronic-intermittent, croup-like pattern. Spasmodic croup generally affects children 1 to 4 years of age, and it may be associated with a mild respiratory tract infection, but not with a febrile illness. An affected child generally wakes at night with a "barky" cough, stridor, and mild dyspnea of sudden onset. Nocturnal attacks may occur as isolated events or may recur over 2 to 3 nights, but generally the child is asymptomatic during the day.

Typically, each episode subsides spontaneously, within a few hours. Examination may show mildly erythematous laryngeal mucosa, with boggy mucosal edema present in the subglottis. Humidified oxygen is generally recommended as the principal treatment.

Because of the pattern of the affliction, allergy was once assumed to be the underlying cause of spasmodic croup. Now, although the cause of spasmodic croup remains unknown, evidence suggests that GER may frequently be the cause.[8] When spasmodic croup is suspected, 24-hour pH monitoring may be diagnostic.

Traumatic Laryngitis

Traumatic laryngitis is most commonly caused by vocal abuse, such as excessive shouting or yelling, but it also can result from persistent coughing, inhalation of toxic fumes, or direct endolaryngeal injury. Such patients present with varying degrees of hoarseness and odynophonia. The mucosa of the true vocal cords is hyperemic from dilated vessels present on the superior and free surfaces of the cords. Edema within Reinke's space develops, and submucosal hemorrhage may occur. This form of laryngitis is self-limited, and it subsides within a few days when treated with voice conservation and humidification.

Vocal nodules may become chronic in children who continually abuse their voices. Nevertheless, for two reasons, surgical treatment is rarely indicated. First, it is difficult to modify the vocal behaviors of such children, and when such nodules are removed, they usually promptly recur. Second, the nodules resolve spontaneously in most children before puberty. One notable exception is in female cheerleaders.

ACUTE LARYNGEAL INFECTIONS OF ADULTS

Viral Laryngitis

Laryngitis Due to Viral Upper Respiratory Infection
Acute viral laryngitis in adults is common, and it is generally less serious than in children because of the

larger adult airway, which is able to accommodate more swelling without compromise of the airway. The typical type of "acute laryngitis" seen in adults is almost always viral. Influenza and parainfluenza viruses, rhinoviruses, and adenoviruses are the most common causative agents, although many other viruses have been implicated. Adult patients with viral laryngitis do not usually seek medical attention unless they are professional voice users, in which case, the laryngitis may be of great significance to the patient's ability to earn a living. Such patients present with symptoms of a generalized viral syndrome (low-grade fever, malaise, rhinitis) and hoarseness. The dysphonia is characterized by voice breaks, episodic aphonia, and a lowering of pitch. Often, a hoarse cough is present.

Characteristically, the laryngeal mucosa is diffusely erythematous and edematous, especially over the true vocal cords. The disease is self-limited and is best treated symptomatically with humidification, voice rest, hydration, cough suppressants, and expectorants. Antibiotic treatment is not usually necessary. In the professional vocalist, corticosteroids are sometimes used to reduce the vocal-fold edema, particularly during the recovery phase. The physician's administration of such anti-inflammatory medications does not imply that the vocalist with laryngitis can or should perform, however.

Laryngotracheitis
Adult "infectious croup" is uncommon; when it does occur it is similar to the laryngotracheitis seen in children. The viral prodrome lasts 1 to 7 days, followed by the development of a "barking" cough and, sometimes, inspiratory stridor. Throat cultures are usually negative.

On fiberoptic laryngoscopy, adults with laryngotracheitis demonstrate subglottic edema and erythema. A large proportion of adults with this syndrome are reported to require airway intervention.[23]

Herpes Simplex
Herpes simplex infection is ubiquitous, may affect any age group, and, uncommonly, may infect the larynx. Most cases of herpetic laryngitis have been reported in young or debilitated patients. At the time of delivery, a neonate passing through the birth canal may contract genital herpes from a mother with active disease. Subsequent herpes infection in the infant may involve the upper airway and, if the larynx is involved, may cause acute airway obstruction.[24] Therefore, when a child develops stridor in the neonatal period, herpetic infection should be one of the diagnoses considered. Today, laryngeal herpes is most commonly seen in the immunocompromised patient, although herpetic epiglottic infection, causing airway obstruction in otherwise healthy adults, has been reported.[25]

Herpes infection should be suspected whenever a patient presents with a painful vesicular mucosal eruption. After the vesicles rupture, ulceration and tissue necrosis may occur, and the surrounding inflammatory response may be intense. The diagnosis of a primary herpetic infection may be made by serologic testing; however, swab, culture, and polymerase chain reaction detection of viral DNA are the most reliable diagnostic tests. Symptomatic treatment depends on the site of involvement; topical or systemic acyclovir, a specific antiherpetic medication, may hasten recovery.

Bacterial Laryngeal Infections

Bacterial laryngitis may develop secondary to purulent rhinosinusitis or tracheobronchitis and generally is less commonly diagnosed in adults than in children. Supraglottic involvement, as in pediatric patients, is the most common form of bacterial laryngitis.

Supraglottitis in the Adult
In adults, supraglottitis is manifested by fever, sore throat, a muffled voice, dysphagia, and odynophagia. The onset of symptoms before presentation is typically longer than that seen in children (usually more than 24 hours). The diagnosis of supraglottitis is made by observing the swollen, bright-red epiglottis and/or supraglottic structures by fiberoptic laryngoscopy or by noting the presence of a swollen epiglottis and dilated hypopharynx on a lateral neck radiograph.

Haemophilus influenzae is still the most common causative microorganism in adults, but Streptococcus pneumoniae, Staphylococcus aureus, and β-hemolytic streptococcus are also commonly found. In contrast to pediatric patients with supraglottitis, only about half of adult patients with supraglottitis require airway intervention, although all must be hospitalized in an intensive care setting.[26] Conservative measures include oxygenation, humidification, hydration, corticosteroids, and intravenous antibiotics.

In adults, there appear to be two relatively useful clinical predictors of the need to establish an airway. Patients who present to the emergency room less than 8 hours after the onset of a sore throat and patients who are drooling at presentation (in preference to swallowing because of severe odynophagia) almost always require airway intervention.[27]

Laryngeal Abscess
Laryngeal abscess is a complication of perichondritis and a recognized sequela of bacterial laryngeal infection. It is more common in adults than in children, even though epiglottic abscess occurs most often as a complication of supraglottitis. Often the adult patient who develops a laryngeal abscess has a preexisting, predisposing laryngeal condition, such as prior irradiation for cancer.

In the preantibiotic era, typhoid fever was a frequent

cause, and it was usually fatal. Other less frequently associated infections include measles, scarlet fever, erysipelas, gonorrhea, syphilis, tuberculosis, and diphtheria. Laryngeal abscess also may be a complication of prolonged nasogastric or endotracheal intubation.[28]

Symptoms of laryngeal abscess are similar to those of supraglottitis. Localizing tenderness to palpation over the laryngeal framework is its hallmark. Fluctuance in the anterior neck, although uncommon, denotes necrosis of the thyroid cartilage. The diagnosis of laryngeal abscess may be made by computed tomographic scanning of the larynx and by fiberoptic or direct laryngoscopy; however, no current radiographic method accurately predicts the condition of the laryngeal cartilages, unless, of course, widespread destruction is obvious.

When abscess is suspected and the patient's airway is marginal, a tracheotomy should be performed under local anesthesia before direct laryngoscopy. If the airway is uncompromised, direct laryngoscopy, with laser-assisted incision and drainage of the abscess, may suffice as initial treatment. Granular mucosa should be removed, and an attempt should be made to determine whether necrotic cartilage is exposed within the endolarynx. Infection of the laryngeal framework can lead to severe laryngeal stenosis.

Gram stain and bacteriologic cultures of the abscess contents or necrotic debris should be obtained routinely, and the results should influence the choice of antibiotic. In cases not complicated by necrotic cartilage, conservative management is usually successful. When necrotic cartilage is present, the combination of surgical debridement, prolonged parenteral antibiotic therapy, and hyperbaric oxygen therapy may enhance recovery and preserve laryngeal function. When all other alternatives have failed, laryngectomy may be considered.

Gonorrhea

Gonorrhea is a sexually transmitted genital, and sometimes oropharyngeal, infection caused by the bacterium Neisseria gonorrhoeae. The genital infection may be asymptomatic, so carriers can unknowingly infect their sexual partners. Pharyngeal gonorrhea is transmitted by orogenital contact and is manifested as a diffuse and severe exudative pharyngitis that may directly or indirectly involve the larynx. The infection may produce a pseudomembranous inflammation, which may be confused with diphtheria and streptococcal pharyngitis. Diagnosis is made by culture and identification of N. gonorrhoeae from swabs of the pharynx (and of the genitalia). Most cases of laryngopharyngeal gonorrhea are treated with a single intramuscular dose of ceftriaxone or with a course of oral cefixime.

CHRONIC INFECTIONS (GRANULOMATOUS DISEASES)

Granulomatous infections, such as tuberculosis and syphilis, were recognized in antiquity and continued to be common afflictions throughout the world in the preantibiotic era. During the twentieth century, these conditions appeared to be on the wane, and some had all but disappeared until recently. With the advent of effective anticancer chemotherapy, organ transplantation, and AIDS, it was discovered that the microorganisms causing many of the granulomatous diseases may thrive in the immunocompromized host.

Granulomas are nodular histopathologic lesions characterized by a central mass of epithelioid cells and giant cells surrounded by lymphocytes and other inflammatory cells. Central necrosis (caseation) is seen in many granulomatous conditions and is conspicuously absent in others. A (noncaseating) sarcoid granuloma is shown in Figure 30–7.

Unlike children, adults have many chronic forms of granulomatous laryngitis, and these may go unrecognized for many years. Chronic granulomatous conditions involving the larynx may be due to numerous types of microorganisms (bacteria, spirochetes, fungi, viruses), to an autoimmune process, or to an idiopathic cause. Although not included in this section, some parasitic infections also may cause laryngeal granulomas.

In the larynx, granulomatous lesions may appear as smooth, diffuse swellings of the affected tissues, diffuse "cobblestone mucosa," well-defined, discrete nodules, or an ulcerating inflammatory mass. Sometimes, granulomatous diseases mimic laryngeal carcinoma, so the need for biopsy is obvious. Even when the suspicion of malignancy is low, however, biopsy is frequently necessary to make a diagnosis. Some of the distinguishing features of the most common laryngeal granulomatous conditions are shown in Table 30–7.

Granulomatous Diseases Caused by Bacteria

Tuberculosis

At the end of the nineteenth century, laryngeal tuberculosis was common, occurring in approximately half of patients with advanced pulmonary disease. With the discovery of effective antituberculous drugs, the incidence of both pulmonary and laryngeal tuberculosis rapidly declined. Nevertheless, tuberculosis laryngitis remains one of the most common granulomatous diseases of the larynx, and today, it is frequently unassociated with advanced active pulmonary disease. In 1993, Ramadan and associates reported on 16 patients with laryngeal tuberculosis, only 5 of whom had active cavitary lung disease.[29]

Patients with laryngeal tuberculosis commonly

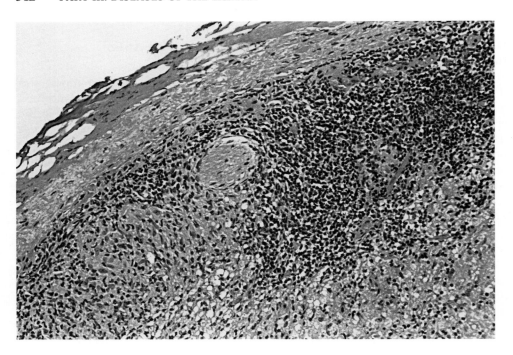

Fig. 30–7. Histologic appearance of a sarcoid granuloma. Low-power (100×) photomicrograph of a biopsy of the epiglottis in a patient with sarcoidosis showing a granuloma with an intense round-cell infiltrate but no caseation. Although no giant cells are seen here, they are sometimes present in sarcoid granulomas.

present in their third to fourth decade of life with varying symptoms, including hoarseness, odynophagia, otalgia, and odynophonia. Respiratory obstruction may develop in later stages of the disease, and approximately one quarter of patients with laryngeal tuberculosis have airway obstruction at the time of their initial presentation.

Laryngeal examination may reveal diffuse edema and hyperemic, hypertrophic mucosa involving the posterior third of the larynx, or the process may be diffuse, nodular, and ulcerative. In the nodular, ulcerative (later) stages, tuberculosis may easily be confused with laryngeal carcinoma. It is a misconception that interarytenoid (posterior commissure) involvement, alone, is the most commonly observed pattern.[30] In the modern era, the true vocal cords appear to be the most commonly involved site.[31]

TABLE 30–7. Some Distinguishing Characteristics of Granulomatous Conditions that Affect the Larynx

Tuberculosis	Posterior third of larynx involved
Leprosy	Supraglottic involvement
Scleroma	Catarrhal stage; Mikulicz's cells
Actinomycosis	Draining sinuses; sulfur granules
Syphilis	Painless ulcers; + syphilis serology
Candidiasis	Leukoplakia-like lesions; identifiable on Gram stain
Blastomycosis	Painless ulcers; microabscesses
Histoplasmosis	Anterior laryngeal involvement; pseudocarcinoma
Coccidioidomycosis	Painless abscesses; spores seen on histology
Sarcoidosis	Supraglottic swelling, nodules, granulomas
Wegener's granulomatosis	Subglottic involvement; necrotizing vasculitis; pulmonary and/or renal involvement

The diagnosis is made by demonstrating typical caseating granulomas and acid-fast microorganisms by smear and/or culture. Treatment with antituberculous drugs usually resolves both the pulmonary and the laryngeal disease. If tuberculous laryngitis is left untreated, cicatricial laryngeal stenosis with vocal cord fixation may develop, necessitating surgical correction or tracheotomy.

Leprosy (Hansen's disease)

Laryngeal leprosy, caused by infection by Mycobacterium leprae, is rare in the United States, but it is still endemic in many parts of the developing world. In 1988, the World Health Organization estimated that over 12 million persons were infected in Asia and Africa, approximately one third of them in India.[32]

The larynx is involved in approximately half of patients with leprosy, and it most consistently involves the epiglottis. As the disease progresses to involve the glottis, hoarseness develops, and later destruction of the cartilaginous laryngeal framework may occur, as well as lepromatous nerve involvement, which may cause laryngeal paralysis.[33,34] With lepromatous laryngitis, odynophagia, odynophonia, and referred otalgia are uncommon, but they do occur.

In patients with lepromatous leprosy, direct laryngoscopy typically reveals a nodular, edematous supraglottis with ulceration. Diagnosis is made by biopsy, which reveals a chronic inflammatory cell infiltrate with foamy leprous cells that contain the bacillus Mycobacterium leprae (Hansen's bacillus). Nasal smears for the intracellular microorganisms also may be diagnostic. Treatment consists of the long-term use of diaminodiphenylsulfone (Dapsone) in combination with other antileprosy drugs. Tracheotomy may be required if laryngeal stenosis develops.

Scleroma

Scleroma, previously also called "rhinoscleroma" because of its predilection for the nose, is a chronic infection caused by Klebsiella rhinoscleromatis. Scleroma remains endemic today in Europe, Mexico, Central America, South America, and Egypt. Most cases found in the United States are in immigrants.[35-37]

The disease primarily involves the mucosa and submucosa of the nasal cavity, but it may also involve the larynx, especially the subglottic region and the trachea. Laryngeal involvement has been reported in approximately 15 to 80% of cases.[38]

The disease has three distinct stages: (1) *the catarrhal stage,* characterized by persistent purulent rhinorrhea, with nasal crusting and obstruction; (2) *the granulomatous stage,* characterized by small, painless granulomatous nodules within the upper respiratory tract, including the larynx; and (3) *the sclerotic stage,* in which the glottis and subglottis are usually involved and hoarseness and respiratory obstruction may develop. The progression through these three stages usually takes many years.

The diagnosis is made by isolating the microorganism from the tissues, although positive complement fixation and agglutination tests are highly suggestive. Foamy vacuolated histiocytes (Mikulicz's cells) and bloated plasma cells with red birefringent inclusions (Russell's bodies) are seen histologically.

Treatment consists of intravenous aminoglycosides, tetracycline, or cephalosporins. Laryngeal dilatation, endoscopic resection, and tracheotomy may be required during the sclerotic phase. Untreated rhinoscleroma may cause death from airway obstruction.

Actinomycosis

Cervicofacial actinomycosis is a chronic suppurative disease caused by the anaerobic bacteria Actinomyces bovis or Actinomyces israelii. Initial involvement of the cervical or mandibular region leads first to pararyngeal and then to laryngeal disease. Pain is the most common initial manifestation, followed by hoarseness, cough, and, eventually, airway obstruction.

The larynx appears diffusely erythematous and swollen with draining sinuses; its consistency is firm and woody.[39] Diagnosis is made by identifying the typical "sulfur granules" in biopsy material and by culturing the microorganism. Long-term therapy with penicillin or tetracycline is effective. Stenosis and laryngeal fixation secondary to deep ulcerations and chondritis may develop if the disease is left untreated. Laryngeal dilatation, arytenoidectomy, or tracheotomy may be required.

Nocardia species of the Actinomyces family are soil saprophytes that are widely distributed throughout the world. Nocardia may infect humans by inhalation or through a break in the skin. Nocardiosis is characterized by diffuse microabscesses, which, on histologic examination, show a neutrophilic predominance; sulfur granules are atypical. Aerodigestive tract involvement is common. The diagnosis is made by culture and isolation of the nocardia microorganism, and treatment is with systemic sulfisoxazole.

Tularemia

Tularemia, also called "rabbit fever" and "deer fly fever," is caused by the bacteria Francisella tularensis. It is found only in the northern hemispheres of Europe and Asia and in North America. Most cases occur from contact with rabbits or squirrels, but many other wild and domesticated animals have been reported to carry the disease. Transmission to humans can also occur by a bite from a tick or a deer fly, which are the intermediate hosts and insect vectors.

In humans, the most common portal of entry is the skin or mucous membranes. Headache, myalgia, and malaise are common symptoms. Oropharyngeal tularemia, which occurs in approximately 1% of cases, produces an intense exudative pharyngitis associated with lymphadenopathy.[40] Diagnosis is made by serologic tests, because the microorganisms are difficult to identify on culture or histologic examination. Treatment is with streptomycin or gentamicin for 7 to 10 days.

Glanders

At one time, glanders was "the plague of horses," and secondarily, it affected humans. Today, glanders is rare around the world, but it still occurs in Asia, Africa, and South America. The disease is caused by infection by the bacterial microorganism, Pseudomonas mallei. Transmission is still by contact with an infected horse or by inhalation or inoculation of contaminated material, and infected humans are almost exclusively horse handlers.[41]

Infection by inoculation of broken skin causes systemic infection characterized by fever, malaise, prostration, pneumonia, and lymphadenopathy. Truly systemic (septicemic) involvement may be fatal. Infection by inhalation produces an intense, ulcerative mucopurulent granulomatous reaction in the mucous membranes of the aerodigestive tract and pneumonia. Treatment is with sulfonamides.

Granulomatous Diseases Caused by Spirochetes

Syphilis is a sexually transmitted spirochetal infection caused by Treponema pallidum. Syphilitic chancres do not usually involve the larynx, and most commonly, the larynx becomes involved during the secondary and tertiary stages. Tertiary syphilis may not develop until years after the initial infection, however. Diffuse erythematous papules, painless superficial ulcers, and cervical lymphadenopathy are seen during the secondary stage and generally clear without treatment within several weeks. Gumma formation during the tertiary stage can lead to laryngeal fibrosis, chondritis, and stenosis.

The typical laryngeal findings are diffuse erythema and edema, with necrotic ulcers that mimic carcinoma or tuberculous laryngitis. Serologic tests for syphilis are diagnostic, and a lumbar puncture should be performed to rule out central nervous system involvement. Penicillin is the treatment of choice.[42]

Although rare, congenital syphilitic laryngitis can occur in infants born to mothers with syphilis. This diagnosis should be considered in the differential diagnosis of neonates with laryngeal stenosis. Treatment should be instituted if one finds serologic evidence of active disease.[43]

Mycotic (Fungal) Granulomatous Diseases

Candidiasis

Although laryngeal candidiasis (usually infection by Candida albicans) is infrequently reported, its occurrence is not rare in laryngologic practice. Laryngeal candidiasis rarely occurs in the absence of identifiable (local and/or systemic) predisposing factors, but it does sometimes occur in reasonably healthy patients who are not severely immunocompromised.

Among the risk factors for development of laryngeal candidiasis are the use of corticosteroids and broad-spectrum antibiotics, diabetes, burns, alcoholism, endotracheal intubation, and previous (viral or bacterial) laryngeal infection. "Candida laryngotracheitis," for example, may occur as a complication of treatment in previously healthy children hospitalized for laryngotracheitis and treated with systemic corticosteroids and broad-spectrum antibiotics.[44]

Cases of laryngeal candida infection may occur in ambulatory patients as well. A relatively benign, isolated form of laryngeal candidiasis (without the involvement of any other contiguous anatomic structures) occurs in some patients who use corticosteroid inhalers. Typically, such patients have used them on a daily basis for years. (The most common indication for the chronic use of corticosteroid inhalers is asthma.) This form of isolated laryngeal candidiasis has a distinctive appearance: intense, diffuse laryngeal erythema with an irregular, friable, white exudate (occurring most notably on the true vocal cords). The infection is superficial, and no ulceration or necrosis is seen (Fig. 30–8). Patients with this particular condition usually complain of hoarseness, but no other symptoms. The diagnosis is usually made on the basis of the history and clinical findings. A 2-week course of treatment with nystatin (swish and swallow) or an oral antifungal agent, such as ketoconazole or fluconazole,

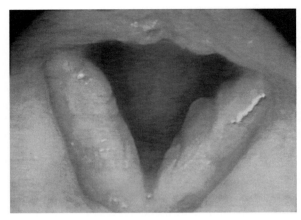

Fig. 30–8. Candidiasis of the larynx. Fiberoptic appearance of the larynx of a 45-year-old woman with life-long asthma, who had been using corticosteroid inhalers for many years. This appearance is different from that usually seen in immunocompromised patients, the latter group having a more invasive, necrotizing form of candidiasis.

is effective for most patients with this type of candida laryngitis; however, in some cases, treatment must be continued for several weeks to eradicate the disease.

Severe immunosuppression (due to chemotherapy or AIDS) (see Chap. 5) is more often associated with the development of invasive laryngeal candidiasis, and as expected in such patients, the infection is often more serious and sometimes can be life-threatening because of bleeding or airway obstruction. In the immunocompromised patient, laryngeal candidiasis may be due to local aerodigestive tract infection, which can subsequently give rise to widespread systemic candidiasis. The converse, secondary involvement of the larynx by disseminated candidiasis, is uncommon. Infection is rarely confined to the larynx, however, but usually involves adjacent areas of the airway and esophagus as well.

Sometimes the esophagus is involved, but, initially, not the larynx. When a patient presents with dysphagia and barium esophagography suggests candida esophagitis, the clinician should suspect that the patient has AIDS. Indeed, aerodigestive-tract candidiasis may be the first presenting manifestation of full-blown AIDS.

Invasive candida laryngitis in the immunocompromised host produces painful, ulcerative lesions and deep tissue necrosis and it may progress rapidly. In addition to hoarseness, patients with this type of infection complain of sore throat, dysphagia, and odynophagia. For the diagnosis to be made, it must be suspected. Unlike other fungi, candida species can easily be identified on the Gram stain.[45] Confirmation of the diagnosis is made by the histopathology and culture of biopsy tissue samples. Invasive laryngeal candidiasis is treated with parenteral amphotericin B and, when necessary, airway support.[46]

Blastomycosis

North American blastomycosis is a chronic pulmonary infection caused by the fungus Blastomyces dermatitidis, with laryngeal involvement in 2 to 5% of cases.[45,47] The microorganism is generally found in damp areas where decaying wood is present. Its distribution in the United States and Canada is concentrated around the Great Lakes and along the Mississippi, Ohio, and Saint Lawrence rivers. Primary laryngeal blastomycosis has been reported.[48]

Patients typically present with multiorgan systemic involvement; severe hoarseness and cough occur when the larynx is involved. The microorganism produces erythematous, granular, mucosal lesions in the larynx, which progress to small, painless abscesses and ulcerations. Histologically, caseous necrosis with abundant acute inflammatory cells and microabscesses are seen, as well as giant cells in the surrounding tissue. Pseudo-epitheliomatous hyperplasia is a characteristic change seen in the epithelial layer. The fungus in yeast form may be seen in the region of the microabscesses and is periodic acid-Schiff (PAS)-positive. Treatment is with long-term oral itraconazole, with amphotericin B reserved for severe or recalcitrant cases. In the absence of treatment, progressive fibrosis with vocal cord fixation develops, as do pharyngocutaneous fistulas.

Histoplasmosis

Histoplasmosis is a systemic mycotic disease caused by Histoplasma capsulatum, and it may involve the larynx and tongue. Nodular superficial granulomas that may ulcerate and become painful involve the anterior portions of the larynx and epiglottis. Histologic examination shows granulation tissue composed of plasma cells, microorganism-laden macrophages, lymphocytes, and giant cells, which may be confused with the granulation tissue of carcinoma or tuberculosis. Diagnosis is made by culture and the complement fixation test.

Amphotericin B is the treatment of choice. Laryngeal stenosis may develop when extensive ulceration leads to chondritis. In this instance, laryngeal dilatation, arytenoidectomy, or tracheotomy may be required to provide a safe airway.

Coccidioidomycosis

Coccidioidomycosis, also called "desert fever" (or "San Joaquin Valley fever" in the United States), is caused by the microorganism Coccidioides immitis, which is found in desert soil. It is primarily a pulmonary fungal infection endemic to the southwestern United States, Mexico, and central South America. Reportedly, 60% of people with this infection are asymptomatic; 40% develop a flu-like illness; and among those, 0.5% develop a systemic, disseminated, more severe form of the disease. Patients with the disseminated form may develop hoarseness, cough, and airway obstruction from laryngeal coccidioidomycosis.[49] Disseminated extrapulmonary disease is far more common in males and in the black population.[50]

Laryngeal disease usually develops during the acute phase of the primary infection; however, laryngeal involvement can develop in patients who have had granulomatous lung disease for months or years. In addition to the laryngeal findings of intense, diffuse laryngeal erythema (with or without focal ulceration), most patients with C. immitis infection have cervical lymphadenopathy. Histologic study reveals caseating granulomas with multinucleated giant cells and pathognomonic, double-walled endospores. The diagnosis is made by serologic testing and biopsy of affected tissue. Treatment is with amphotericin B. When death occurs, it is usually due to meningeal involvement.

Aspergillosis

Aspergillosis is generally an infection of immunocompromised patients, and respiratory tract involvement is common. When the larynx is involved, patients complain of hoarseness, dysphagia, and sometimes, symptoms of airway obstruction.

In the immunocompromised patient, aspergillus infection is usually necrotizing, invasive, and associated with a poor prognosis. Despite aggressive antifungal treatment with amphotericin B and attempted wide surgical excision (including laryngectomy), most such patients with this infection die of progressive disease.[51]

Sporotrichosis

Sporotrichosis, an uncommon fungal infection of the skin or airway, is caused by Sporothrix schenckii and occurs worldwide. The causative fungus is most commonly found in sphagnum moss and wood. People who work with wood usually get the cutaneous form of sporotrichosis, whereas most cases of laryngeal sporotrichosis occur in people working with the moss.[52]

The more common cutaneous form of sporotrichosis causes granulomas in the subcutaneous layer of the skin and in regional lymph nodes. If the mucous membranes of the upper airway are damaged or abraded for any reason, inhalation of the fungus may result in laryngopharyngeal infection. Hoarseness and cough are the most common symptoms, and the lesions appear granulomatous. Diagnosis is made by biopsy and by culturing the microorganism. Oral potassium iodide is sufficient treatment for patients with superficial involvement; deep tissue involvement requires a course of amphotericin B therapy.[53]

Idiopathic Granulomatous Diseases

Sarcoidosis

Sarcoidosis is a slowly progressive, rarely fatal, systemic granulomatous disease of unknown cause; it afflicts blacks 10 times more commonly than whites. The lungs and skin are most commonly involved, and laryngeal sarcoid occurs in 1 to 5% of cases.[54,55] When the skin of the nasal rim is affected, upper respiratory sarcoid involvement is seen in approximately 75% of cases.[56] Rarely, the larynx is involved without clinical or radiographic evidence of lung involvement.[57]

Laryngeal sarcoid usually involves the supraglottic larynx and sometimes involves the subglottis, but typically it spares the true vocal cords. Characteristically, the entire supraglottis appears pale pink and massively edematous, sometimes obscuring visualization of the vocal cords. The ''turban-like'' appearance of the epiglottis is virtually pathognomonic.[54] Less commonly, some patients with laryngeal sarcoidosis present with a few discrete, sometimes hemorrhagic, nodules (up to 1 cm in diameter) on the epiglottis or other supraglottic structures.

Laryngeal sarcoidosis is a diagnosis of exclusion, based primarily on finding noncaseating granulomas and diffuse edema with miliary nodules involving mainly the supraglottic structures and on excluding tuberculosis and other fungal diseases. Patients may present with hoarseness and varying degrees of airway obstruction; however, ulcerative lesions and pain are rare. Figure 30–7 shows the typical histopathologic features.

The use of systemic and intralesional corticosteroids generally results in improvement or apparent resolution of the lesions. In severe cases, however, endoscopic dilatation and laser resection of involved supraglottic tissues, or tracheotomy, may be necessary.

Wegener's Granulomatosis

Wegener's granulomatosis is a systemic disease of unknown origin characterized by necrotizing granuloma with vasculitis involving the upper respiratory tract, lungs, and kidneys. On presentation, laryngeal involvement may resemble acute laryngitis, but the eventual development of granulomatous ulcers throughout the larynx may lead the clinician to suspect the diagnosis. Subglottic stenosis occurs in approximately 20% of cases and can lead to significant airway obstruction, requiring tracheotomy and surgical correction of the stenosis.[58] Diagnosis is based on typical histologic findings of necrotizing granulomas and vasculitis. The anticytoplasmic autoantibody test (C-ANCA) has recently been shown to be highly specific for Wegener's granulomatosis. Recommended treatment includes corticosteroids and cyclophosphamide.

ALLERGIC, IMMUNE, AND IDIOPATHIC DISORDERS

Hypersensitivity Reactions

The term *hypersensitivity* implies an overzealous response of the immune system to an antigenic stimulus. Hypersensitivity reactions include conditions such as allergic rhinitis, contact dermatitis, and urticaria, but these conditions do not produce life-threatening, obstructive edema within the airway (see Chaps. 4 and 8).

Anaphylaxis, an acute and profoundly life-threatening immunologic allergic response, is made up of a triad of clinical manifestations: (1) flushing, pruritus, and/or urticaria; (2) airway obstruction (angioedema, laryngospasm, and/or bronchospasm); and (3) circulatory collapse (shock).

Angioedema

Angioedema, which may occur with or without anaphylaxis, is an acute, allergic, histamine-mediated, inflammatory reaction characterized by acute vascular dilation and capillary permeability. This reaction can occur in many parts of the body; when the airway is acutely affected, the condition is potentially life-threatening. Oral and laryngopharyngeal structures are frequently affected.

In susceptible patients, angioedema can be precipitated by medications (e.g., penicillin, aspirin, other nonsteroidal anti-inflammatory drugs, and angiotensin-converting enzyme inhibitors), by food additives and preservatives, and by blood transfusions, infections, or insect bites. In addition, the condition may be associated with a coexisting connective tissue disorder.[59]

Hereditary angioedema is an autosomally dominant inherited deficiency of C1 esterase inhibitor that leads to recurrent attacks of mucocutaneous edema. An acquired form of C1 esterase deficiency has also been reported in patients with angioedema who have occult lymphoma.

Diagnosis is made primarily from the history, although the offending agent may not be readily apparent. Patients present with edema that may involve the face, oral cavity, oropharynx, or larynx. The onset is rapid and may be associated with pruritus. Hoarseness is common when the larynx is involved.

Treatment of both types of angioedema must be prompt and aggressive. Epinephrine, corticosteroids, antihistamines, and aminophylline are the mainstays of therapy. If progressive airway obstruction develops, intubation or tracheotomy may be required. Chronic ''pretreatment'' of hereditary angioedema with danazol appears to elevate levels of functional C1 esterase inhibitor and to help prevent recurrent episodes.

Stevens-Johnson Syndrome

Stevens-Johnson syndrome is a mucocutaneous hypersensitivity reaction (at the severe end of the erythema multiforme spectrum), usually triggered by medications, such as sulfonamides, phenobarbital, and carbamazepine. It is an acute febrile illness characterized by conjunctivitis, rash, and severe oropharyngeal mucositis. The mucosal and skin lesions rapidly progress to formation of bullae and desquamation of the skin in sheets. The most severe form of this syndrome is called toxic epidermal necrolysis, and this variant may involve the larynx.[60] Diagnosis is made by biopsy, and treatment is primarily supportive removal of the offending agent and tracheotomy when the airway is compromised. If death occurs, it usually is due to sepsis from bacterial superinfection.

Immune and Idiopathic Disorders

Infections of the Immunocompromised Host

Immunocompromised patients, whether immunocompromised from diabetes, long-term corticosteroid therapy, chemotherapy, or AIDS, are at risk to develop opportunistic infections of the aerodigestive tract. The most commonly reported opportunistic infections that affect the larynx are shown in Table 30–8. Of those listed, laryngeal candidiasis, tuberculosis, and herpes infections are the most commonly encountered in patients with AIDS (see Chap. 5).

When any immunocompromised patient develops even slight hoarseness, dysphagia, or odynophagia, the otolaryngologist should suspect infection of the laryngopharynx. Even microorganisms that are usually considered indolent may aggressively invade tissue and cause acute inflammation, massive tissue destruction, and rapid obstruction of the airway. When new throat symptoms arise in the immunocompromised patient, the clinician should perform an examination promptly, and if evidence of infection is present, the clinician should aggressively attempt to obtain material for culture and for histologic examination.

Rheumatoid Arthritis

Rheumatoid arthritis is a systemic autoimmune disorder that can affect any organ in the body. Its most common manifestation is symmetric polyarthritis, but it

TABLE 30–8. Common Laryngeal Infections of the Immunocompromised Host

Viral infections
   Herpes simplex
   Herpes zoster
   Cytomegalovirus
   Papova (papilloma)
   Toxoplasmosis
Bacterial infections
   Tuberculosis
   Atypical mycobacterium
   Actinomycosis
Fungal infections
   Candidiasis
   Aspergillosis
   Histoplasmosis
   Coccidioidomycosis

also can cause inflammation in nonjoint structures, vasculitis, and pulmonary changes.[61] Rheumatoid arthritis may affect the larynx both directly and indirectly.

First, rheumatoid involvement of the cricoarytenoid joints may cause hoarseness or airway obstruction. At postmortem examination, up to 87% of patients with rheumatoid arthritis have cricoarytenoid joint changes, but, based on laryngoscopy, only 17 to 33% of such patients have clinical signs of laryngeal involvement, namely, posterior laryngeal inflammation and decreased arytenoid mobility.[62]

Second, rheumatoid nodules may occur anywhere in the larynx or within the substance of the vocal cord itself, leading to hoarseness. The gross appearance of rheumatoid laryngeal nodules is variable. They may appear as white submucosal nodules, as ulcerated friable polypoid lesions, or as ill-defined masses deep within the substance of the vocal cords. Occasionally, unsuspected rheumatoid nodules are discovered during direct laryngoscopy by palpation of the nodule within the vocal cord.

Histologically, these lesions show a central area of fibrinoid necrosis surrounded by histiocytes, plasma cells, and lymphocytes. They can be highly vascularized and hyalinized; they may have a fibrous capsule. Frequently, rheumatoid nodules of the larynx are misdiagnosed as pyogenic granulomas.[63]

Third, rheumatoid arthritis, like other collagen vascular diseases, often involves the esophagus, causing esophageal dysmotility and reflux disease. Thus, patients with rheumatoid arthritis may have reflux laryngitis, but whether such reflux contributes to the arytenoid fixation is unknown.

The choice of treatment for rheumatoid airway obstruction secondary to arytenoid fixation depends on the patient's overall medical condition. Because surgical rehabilitation of arytenoid function is not possible, endoscopic arytenoidectomy is usually the treatment of choice. This procedure leaves the patient with an adequate airway and a somewhat breathy, dysphonic voice. Sometimes, the rheumatoid arthritis so severely affects the neck that endoscopic exposure of the larynx is not possible. In such patients, an open surgical procedure, or simply a tracheotomy, may be performed.

Because rheumatoid nodules of the larynx frequently lie within the substance of the vocal cord and may be inflamed, the vocal cord may be scarred after their removal. As a consequence, most patients with this type of rheumatoid involvement of the larynx have persistent hoarseness following nodule removal.

Systemic Lupus Erythematosus

Lupus is a systemic, autoimmune disease. It affects women more commonly than men, and it usually appears in the second and third decades of life. Patients with this condition may have autoantibodies to a variety of different tissues, and head and neck manifestations are common. Although the most common manifestations of lupus are arthritis, malar rash, and photosensitivity, up to 40% of patients have mucosal lesions of the aerodigestive tract as well.

The lesions may be varied, including petechiae, ulcerations, or raised nonulcerated lesions with erythematous borders. The palate and nose are commonly involved. Painless nasal septal perforations may also occur. The larynx may be involved by these mucosal lesions or, on occasion, by cricoarytenoid arthritis.[61]

Laryngeal involvement usually occurs at times of acute exacerbation of the systemic disease. Airway compromise is uncommon, but it does occur. Biopsy reveals a mononuclear cell infiltrate. Positive fluorescent antinuclear antibody tests are important for diagnosis and are a key part of the American Rheumatism Association criteria. Corticosteroids and symptomatic measures are the treatment.

Cicatricial Pemphigoid

Pemphigus and pemphigoid are idiopathic, autoimmune epithelial disorders. Several clinical variations are recognized: however, in common, they share subepithelial bullous inflammation. The primary distinctions between the two entities are the clinical patterns and the histologic features. In pemphigus, one sees suprabasilar separation (cantholysis), and in pemphigoid, the bullae are subepidermal. Clinical variations, that is, the manifestations and sites of involvement, are believed to be the result of autoimmunity to distinct basement membrane antigens. Pemphigus and pemphigoid also may be associated with systemic lupus erythematosus. Of this group of uncommon bullous diseases, only cicatricial pemphigoid appears to involve the larynx with any frequency (9 to 20% of cases).

Cicatricial pemphigoid is a painful, unremitting, chronic inflammatory, vesiculobullous disease. Cicatricial scar formation may occur at any site of involvement, including the nose, nasopharynx, pharynx, larynx, and esophagus. Cicatricial pemphigoid affects women twice as often as men, and most patients are over 50 years of age. The oral cavity and eyes are most commonly involved; the aerodigestive tract is sometimes involved. The largest series reported in the otolaryngology literature contained 13 (9%) of 142 patients with laryngeal involvement, 3 of whom required airway intervention.[64] All 13 had involvement of other areas of the aerodigestive tract as well, but isolated laryngeal involvement has been reported. The primary symptom of laryngeal pemphigoid is severe odynophagia, and the most common findings are ulcers of the epiglottis and aryepiglottic folds.

Diagnosis depends on biopsy, which shows inflammatory subepithelial bullae surrounded by a mixed cellular inflammatory infiltrate. Immunofluorescent studies usually reveal linear deposition of immunoglobulins (IgG and IgM) along the basement membrane.[64] Long-term treatment is with the systemic corticosteroids and/or immunosuppressive therapy. Intralesional corticosteroids are ineffective. Stenoses of the larynx and other sites require surgical correction.

Relapsing Polychondritis

Relapsing polychondritis is a rare, idiopathic, generally progressive, autoimmune disease that causes inflammation of cartilage. It can mimic rheumatoid arthritis, and it sometimes occurs in patients with other autoimmune diseases, such as Sjögren's syndrome, systemic lupus erythematosus, and psoriatic and rheumatoid arthritis.

Relapsing polychondritis occurs in all age groups, having a bell-shaped age distribution and a peak incidence in the fourth decade. Although only 10% of patients present with respiratory tract involvement (larynx and trachea), more than 50% eventually develop such involvement, and 20% require tracheotomy. Of the 20 to 30% of patients who eventually die of the disease, most die of respiratory complications.[65]

This disease is characterized by episodes of inflammation with subsequent destruction of the cartilage of the ears, nose, and larynx. Arthritis involving the large joints is also common. Laryngeal involvement is manifested by hoarseness, dyspnea, stridor, cough, and, sometimes, pain and hemoptysis.

On examination of the larynx, severe glottic and subglottic edema and inflammation are seen. No laboratory test is diagnostic, although patients with active disease usually have an elevated erythrocyte sedimentation rate. Relapsing polychondritis is therefore a clinical diagnosis confirmed by cartilage biopsy, although most patients with this disorder also have autoantibodies to type II collagen.

Initially, most patients present with bilateral involvement of the ear cartilage. Typically, the ears suddenly become red, swollen, and tender. With or without treatment, the condition may subside within 5 to 10 days. The next most common sites of involvement are the nose and the costal cartilages; the eye can also be involved.

Histologically, the normal cartilage is replaced by an eosinophilic material, and acute and chronic infiltrates of lymphocytes and plasma cells are present. The usual basophilic appearance of the cartilage matrix is lost, lacunae are interrupted, and fibrous tissue replaces cartilage. As the disease progresses, fibrosis and chondronecrosis become marked.

Treatment includes corticosteroids, and tracheotomy may be necessary in the later stages of the disease. Corticosteroid and immunosuppressive medications are used for patients with severe, recalcitrant, or rapidly progressive disease, especially when the larynx or other airway structures are involved.

Sjögren's Syndrome

Sjögren's syndrome is an idiopathic autoimmune disorder characterized by the clinical triad of xerostomia (dry mouth), conjunctivitis sicca (dry eyes), and rheumatoid arthritis. Patients with Sjögren's syndrome have a high incidence of lymphoma. A "limited" form of the disease, occurring without the arthritis, is called "sicca syndrome."

Although the cause (or causes) of these syndromes is unknown, both the limited and the full-blown forms have in common autoantibodies to glandular tissue in the eyes, nose, oral cavity, and laryngopharynx. In addition to the lacrimal glands and the major salivary glands, minor salivary and seromucinous glands are usually affected throughout the aerodigestive tract.

The diagnosis is made clinically using Schirmer's test to document the dryness of the eyes and by salivary gland biopsy. In the major salivary glands, the histologic picture demonstrates (1) an intense lymphoid infiltrate, especially in periductal areas, (2) glandular atrophy, and (3) myoepithelial hyperplasia. Although the salivary glands are affected, biopsy of a major salivary gland is rarely necessary. Instead, biopsy of minor salivary gland tissue (lip biopsy) is usually sufficient to make the diagnosis.

The seromucinous glands of the larynx may be involved, leading to inflammation of the larynx similar to that seen in the salivary glands. Clinically, this involvement produces edema, erythema, dryness, crusting, and hence, chronic hoarseness. Laryngeal Sjögren's syndrome, however, does not occur in isolation.[66]

In some cases, the mucosa of the posterior commissure appears so hypertrophic that the clinician must consider the possibility of tumor. The appearance of the larynx in Sjögren's syndrome is shown in Figure 30–9; intense erythema and hypertrophy of the posterior commissure can be seen, as well as dry, tenacious mucus between the vocal cords.

Biopsies of the larynx reveal histologic findings similar to those seen in the salivary glands. In addition, patients with Sjögren's syndrome often have impaired esophageal function and GER. Treatment is symptomatic, and antireflux and anti-inflammatory medications are sometimes prescribed.

Amyloidosis

Amyloidosis is a dysproteinemia in which a characteristic, amorphous, eosinophilic substance is deposited in the tissues of various organs. Amyloidosis is classified as being either "systemic" or "localized." The systemic types are familial, primary (with or without myeloma), and secondary (usually associated with chronic inflammatory disease). Primary amyloidosis has a 5-year survival of only 20%, with patients dying of renal, central nervous system, or cardiac involvement.[67] The "localized" type of amyloidosis rarely

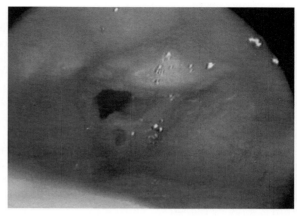

Fig. 30–9. Sjögren's syndrome of the larynx. Fiberoptic appearance of the larynx of a patient with long-standing Sjögren's syndrome. The larynx appears diffusely edematous and erythematous, and the interarytenoid area is so hypertrophic that it gives the appearance of a mass. (A biopsy of this area showed findings similar to those seen in the minor salivary glands of patients with Sjögren's syndrome.) Also, there is tenacious, inspissated mucus on the vocal cords.

causes death and is the type that most commonly involves the larynx (on rare occasions, the larynx may become involved by primary or secondary systemic amyloidosis). In other words, most cases of laryngeal amyloidosis occur in isolation, although simultaneous involvement of the trachea, and to a lesser extent, the bronchi, occurs in about one third of those cases.

On laryngoscopy, amyloidosis appears as diffuse mucosal thickening or as subepithelial nodules, localized mainly to the anterior subglottis. Patients are usually asymptomatic until the deposits involve the vocal cords or critically narrow the airway. When amyloidosis is suspected, biopsy specimens should be stained with Congo red, which, when viewed with polarized light, shows a pathognomonic apple-green birefringence.

Laryngeal amyloidosis usually has a benign course. Symptomatic cases are best treated by endoscopic carbon dioxide laser excision of the lesions; laryngeal dilatation and tracheotomy are rarely necessary.[68]

MISCELLANEOUS INFLAMMATORY CONDITIONS

Parasitic Infections

Trichinosis

Trichinosis in humans is caused by ingesting meat contaminated with the helminthic organism Trichinella spiralis. Trichinosis is relatively common worldwide. In the past, contaminated pork was the most common source of infection, but today, in the United States at least, most cases are caused by eating feral meat, such as bear or wild boar.

Humans are particularly susceptible to trichinosis infection. Soon after ingestion, the larvae penetrate the intestinal wall, where copulation and multiplication occur. The next generation of larvae then enter the blood, are distributed throughout the body, and finally enter and grow in skeletal muscle. The muscles of the diaphragm, eyes, tongue, chest, shoulders, and calves are often affected. Laryngeal involvement is uncommon.

In tissue, the larvae elicit an eosinophilic and lymphocytic inflammatory response. The severity of the clinical manifestations depends on the location and the density of the larvae. The first symptoms occur within 2 days of ingestion. During the initial stage of infection, diarrhea, nausea, and malaise are common. During the muscle-invasion stage (lasting 1 to 6 weeks), fever, weakness, skin rash, myalgia, muscle tenderness, and facial and periorbital edema are usually present. Some cases are complicated by urticaria, splinter hemorrhages, and angioedema. The primary symptom of laryngeal involvement is hoarseness. Trichinosis should be suspected by the history and by eosinophilia. Diagnosis can be made by serologic testing and by muscle biopsy. Treatment is with a 7-day course of thiabendazole.

Leishmaniasis

Leishmaniasis, although uncommon in the United States, is indigenous throughout the rest of the world. It is estimated that there are 12 million cases worldwide. The organism infects rodents and dogs, and transmission to humans is usually from an animal, although the bite of an intermediate host, the sandfly, may cause the disease as well. Although several clinical forms of the disease are known, the mucocutaneous form, caused by Leishmania braziliensis and L. mexicana, most commonly involves the airway. Espundia, the form caused by L. mexicana, is endemic in south-central Texas.

Usually, one or more skin lesions on the lower extremity begin as sores that slowly enlarge and ulcerate over a period of months. These untreated lesions seldom ever heal. Months or years later, metastatic lesions appear on the lips and nose and in the pharynx. Leishmaniasis involves the larynx in approximately one third of cases.[69]

Fever, anemia, weight loss, and hoarseness are common symptoms. As time passes, extensive soft tissue destruction may lead to grotesque facial disfiguration and to progression of the laryngeal disease as well. Examination of the larynx may reveal a localized, polypoid, inflammatory lesion, or diffuse, granular, spongy mucosa throughout the larynx, and the lesions may be ulcerated. With this type, airway obstruction may occur. These lesions are often mistaken for laryngeal cancer, tuberculosis, histoplasmosis, or blastomycosis.

Biopsy reveals a chronic granulomatous pattern, with a predominance of lymphocytic and histiocytic cells. The diagnosis can be made by identification of the parasite in biopsy specimens, but, in some cases, the parasites may be difficult to find. A specific agglutination test for leishmaniasis and the leishmaniasis skin test are diagnostic. The mucocutaneous form of leishmaniasis should be treated with antimonial agents for at least 30 days.

Schistosomiasis

Endemic in the tropics and subtropics, schistosomiasis ("bilharziasis" in Egypt) is widespread in 72 countries of the world, and it infects an estimated 5% of the world's population—200 million people. It is the most prevalent helminthic infection in the world.

Three schistosome species are parasitic in humans: Schistosoma mansoni, S. japonicum, and S. haematobium. S. mansoni and S. japonicum inhabit the mesenteric veins; the eggs are found along the wall of the intestine and in the liver and are passed in the feces. S. haematobium invades the veins of the pelvic plexus, and the eggs are passed in the urine. "Ectopic" lesions occur in 18% of cases and may be found in any part of the body. How the parasite reaches other parts of the body, outside the gastrointestinal and urinary tracts, is unknown.

Humans contract schistosomiasis from water infested by cercariae, the microscopic infective stage. Cercariae penetrate the intact skin and "schistosomules" form in the skin. After several days, the schistosomules migrate to the lungs and portal veins, where the male and female species mate. Weeks later, depending on the species and the time of transit, eggs are deposited in the infected organs.

To complete the life cycle, organisms excreted by humans must contaminate water, because the snail is the intermediate host. The cercariae grow in the soft tissue of the snail, and after 1 to 2 months they are released back into the water, whence they can again enter the human body, thus completing the organism's life cycle.

Schistosomiasis in the aerodigestive tract is characterized by intense inflammatory granulomas around deposits of schistosome eggs. Granulomas may be as small as a pin head or as large as an orange. Histologically, coagulation necrosis occurs around the egg deposits, and eosinophils, plasma cells, and lymphocytes predominate in the cellular response.[70]

Patients with laryngeal schistosome granulomas present with hoarseness. The laryngeal lesion has the appearance of a pink-gray, cauliflower-like granuloma, with surrounding inflammation. Ipsilateral paralysis may be present.[70,71] The degree of surrounding fibrosis is determined by the egg density and the duration of the infection.

Diagnosis may be suspected by the histologic examination; however, confirmation of the diagnosis is made by identification of parasitic ova in the urine or feces. Treatment is with antihelminthic medication (praziquantel or oxamniquine).

Syngamus laryngeus

Syngamus laryngeus is a unique "gapeworm" indigenous to Brazil, Puerto Rico, Martinique, Trinidad, British Guiana, the West Indies, and the Philippines. It invades the upper respiratory tract of cattle, water buffalo, and (rarely) humans. Transmission to humans is believed to be through consumption of contaminated vegetables. Once ingested, the adult worms migrate to the larynx and upper trachea and firmly attach themselves to those mucosal surfaces.

The primary symptoms of S. laryngeus infestation are cough, a foreign body sensation in the throat, and, occasionally, hemoptysis. The diagnosis may be suspected if the patient coughs up worms in copula, or if they are seen on laryngoscopy. Removal of the worms by direct laryngoscopy is the only known treatment.[72]

Inhalation Laryngitis

When nebulized, radiolabeled, acidic fog is inhaled and scanned, the density of aerosol deposit in the larynx is greater than in any other site in the aerodigestive tract.[73] The size and anatomic configuration of the larynx (having the narrowest and most convoluted lumen of the upper airway) may explain this phenomenon. Perhaps for this reason, the larynx is especially susceptible to the effects of tobacco smoke, dust, and other air-borne environmental contaminants. Table 30–9 lists some of the commonly reported substances associated with acute and chronic inhalation injuries of the larynx.

Acute (Thermal) Injury

Thermal and toxic injuries of the airway are often seen in patients with facial burns. In this regard, thermal injury usually plays a greater role than chemical injury in the larynx. Intense heat produces intense vasodilation, capillary permeability, massive edema, and thus, airway obstruction. The edema usually peaks 8 to 24 hours following injury, and resolves within 4 to 5 days.

The severity of "permanent" damage depends on the severity of the burn. Complete laryngeal stenosis can occur. Treatment consists of providing humidified oxygen and maintaining the airway. In most cases, corticosteroids and antibiotics should be avoided. Weeks after the acute injury has resolved, laryngeal dilation and surgical procedures to reestablish the airway, if necessary, may be performed.

Pollution and Inhalant Allergy

The common clinical manifestations of allergy to inhalants are well known: sneezing, watery rhinorrhea, and

TABLE 30–9. Causes of Inhalation Laryngitis (substances associated with acute and chronic laryngeal inflammation)

Acute inhalation injury
Steam
Hot dry gasses
Smoke
Common allergens
Dust
Animal dander
Formaldehyde (plus the list of pollutants below)
Pollutants
Dust
Ozone
Ammonia
Chlorine
Nitrous oxide
Hydrogen disulfide
Sulfur dioxide
Carbon monoxide
Sulfuric acid
Hydrochloric acid
Kerosene (heaters)
Insecticides
Pesticides
Known Carcinogens
Tobacco
Asbestos
Radon
Nickel
Sulfuric acid
Isopropyl oils
Mustard gas

nasal congestion and obstruction. The most common offending allergens are dust, pollen, molds, and chemicals. Allergic reactions of the larynx, similar to those seen in the nose, are uncommon. The diagnosis is made by the history, by the clinical findings, and by intradermal skin testing. Treatment should consist of removal of the offending allergen(s), if possible, and desensitization. Corticosteroid inhalers are ineffective in laryngeal allergy and should be avoided.

Carcinogens

Tobacco and several other carcinogens cause chronic inflammation of the larynx (Table 30–9). These substances can cause mucosal thickening, submucosal edema, hyperkeratosis, dysplasia, and, eventually, carcinoma. In the larynx, leukoplakia, pachydermia, and Reinke's edema (polypoid degeneration) should be viewed as precursors to the development of carcinoma.

Leukoplakia, which means "white plaque," is histologically hyperkeratosis. This is a typical metaplastic response of epithelium to chronic irritation, regardless of the cause. When the laryngeal mucosa becomes diffusely thickened (and also usually diffusely hyperkeratotic) to the point of narrowing the lumen of the endolarynx, the condition is termed "pachydermia laryngis." Pachydermia ("thick skin") is frequently found in the larynges of patients who have smoked cigarettes for many years.

Reinke's edema also results from chronic laryngeal irritation over many years. It is almost always bilateral, and although it occurs most frequently in elderly female smokers, it is also seen is nonsmoking patients with LPR and hypothyroidism.

Leukoplakia, pachydermia, and Reinke's edema may improve with cessation of smoking and antireflux therapy (when the patient has LPR), but often patients with these lesions require surgical treatment.

Radiation Injury

Radiation Laryngitis

Radiation therapy for early laryngeal carcinoma, as well as for tumors in other head and neck sites, may deliver significant radiation doses to normal laryngeal tissue. The initial effects produce an intense inflammatory response, characterized by increased capillary permeability, edema, neutrophilic infiltration, vascular thrombosis, and obliteration of lymphatic channels.

Patients undergoing radiation treatment complain of a globus sensation, dysphagia, odynophagia, dysphonia, and odynophonia. On laryngeal examination, the larynx appears red and swollen, and a fibrinous exudate may be present. Symptoms tend to worsen as the treatment progresses; they are worst at the completion of treatment, and they gradually abate thereafter.[74]

Late tissue sequelae consist of degenerative changes and fibrosis in adipose, connective, and glandular tissues, and a pronounced obliterative endarteritis of small blood vessels. These changes may take place over a period of years, and the symptoms of many patients worsen with time.

Atrophy of glandular elements of the larynx leads to "laryngitis sicca," a dry larynx. This, in turn, increases the susceptibility of the larynx to infection, and to damage from LPR. Patients often complain about the effects of dryness, including hoarseness, crusting, globus, and cough. Treatment is symptomatic, consisting of hydration, administration of expectorants, and environmental humidification.

Radionecrosis

Like laryngitis sicca, radionecrosis is a late complication of laryngeal irradiation and the result of ischemia of the cartilaginous framework. Patients with laryngeal radionecrosis usually present with dysphagia, weight loss, fetor oris (foul breath), severe dysphonia, impaired vocal fold mobility, and relative airway obstruction, the last three depending on the amount and location of swelling. Massive edema of the larynx with airway obstruction is not uncommon.

When a patient presents after radiation therapy with increasing symptoms and laryngeal edema, the clinician must determine the cause or causes. The differential diagnosis of laryngeal radionecrosis also includes tumor recurrence and reflux. Which of these, known as "the three R's" (radionecrosis, recurrence, reflux), has caused the patient's increasing symptoms determines the treatment. Each patient must be evaluated for each of the three possibilities.

Computed tomographic scanning of the larynx may reveal tumor recurrence; however, unless destruction is massive, scans are notoriously unreliable for evaluating the integrity of the laryngeal cartilages. Tumor recurrence is usually treated by surgical salvage, and reflux is usually treated with omeprazole.

Treatment for radionecrosis should be individualized. In some cases, necrotic cartilage and soft tissue can be removed through an endoscopic approach. Often, however, an open surgical procedure is needed. The larynx then may be "stented" for 2 to 4 weeks. If the necrotic sequestration has been adequately removed, the larynx may heal in a satisfactory manner, even if much of the cartilaginous framework is resected. When available, hyperbaric oxygen treatment may be of significant benefit, completely obviating the need for surgery in selected cases.[75] Laryngectomy should be a last resort and should be considered only when all conservative measures have failed.

Vocal Abuse and Misuse Syndromes

Vocal Cord Hemorrhage

Screaming and other forms of vocal abuse can lead to acute submucosal hemorrhage of the vocal cords. By history, such hemorrhage occurs abruptly and produces severe dysphonia. On examination, the appearance of hematoma is unmistakable. Voice rest is the usual treatment, although some laryngologists recommend surgical drainage in selected cases.

Muscle Tension Dysphonias

Muscle tension dysphonia is a generic term for any "functional" voice disorder caused by chronic vocal abuse or misuse. Patients with vocal nodules, contact ulcers, and granulomas, or the Bogart-Bacall syndrome[76] all fit into this category, as do patients with psychogenic voice disorders[75] (see Chap. 10).

Muscle tension dysphonias are common in professional voice users, and they are frequently initiated or complicated by reflux laryngitis. These disorders can produce traumatic laryngitis; however, the "secondary" histopathologic lesions that sometimes result may resolve spontaneously when the underlying problem is corrected. Treatment with voice therapy and, when appropriate, antireflux therapy, often successfully resolves the problem.

Sometimes, surgical removal of the lesions is necessary. In general, vocal process granulomas and immature vocal nodules do not require surgery, but submucosal cysts and vascular (red, "angiomalike") nodules do.

Contact Ulcers and Granulomas

Anatomically, only a thin layer of mucosa and perichondrium overlies the cartilaginous vocal processes, so ulceration of a vocal process can occur from a variety of insults, including vocal abuse, coughing, viral infection, GER, and endotracheal intubation.[78–80] Because of the shape of the larynx, endotracheal tubes reside in the posterior commissure and thus have contact with the vocal processes. Examination of 99 postintubation laryngeal specimens obtained at autopsy showed that those intubated for less than 12 hours demonstrated pale, oval areas on the mucosa of the vocal processes, which under microscopic examination revealed complete or focal loss of surface epithelium, whereas those intubated for 12 to 48 hours almost uniformly demonstrated ulcerations of the vocal processes.[81]

Granulomas of the vocal process are five times more common than ulcers. Chronic ulcers of the vocal processes are uncommon, because most either heal or go on to form granulomas.[82] The most common sequence of granuloma formation is as follows. First, the mucosa overlying the vocal process is acutely damaged. Then, because of continued trauma, such as throat clearing, cough, or reflux, ulceration may occur. Next, as the ulcer attempts to heal, secondary infection and/or reflux perpetuates the inflammation, and a granuloma forms.

As recently as 25 years ago, contact ulcers and granulomas were believed to be exclusively caused by vocal abuse, and consequently, prolonged periods of voice rest were prescribed. Such treatment was, however, usually unsuccessful. Today, regardless of the inciting cause, patients with these lesions should initially be treated with "voice modification" (not voice rest) to reduce continual vocal process trauma and antireflux therapy (preferably with omeprazole). This regimen will result in healing in the majority of cases within 6 months.

Although surgical removal of a vocal process granuloma is seldom indicated, in three instances it should be considered: (1) when the clinician is concerned about the possibility of carcinoma; (2) when the lesion has matured and taken on the appearance of a fibroepithelial polyp; and (3) when the airway is obstructed. The carbon dioxide surgical laser is useful in removing granulomas.[82] Finally, in carefully selected patients, if traumatic vocal behaviors persist and cannot be corrected, a "one-time" botulinum toxin injection may be used "to put the larynx to rest" long enough for recalcitrant granulomas to heal.

SUGGESTED READINGS

1. Castell DO, Wu WC, and Ott DJ (eds): Gastro-esophageal Reflux Disease: Pathogenesis, Diagnosis, Therapy. Mt. Kisco, NY, Futura, 1985, p 325, 1985.
2. Koufman JA: The otolaryngologic manifestations of gastroesophageal reflux disease (GERD). Laryngoscope 101(suppl 53): 1, 1991.
3. Bain WM, et al: Head and neck manifestations of gastroesophageal reflux. Laryngoscope 93:175, 1983.
4. Little FB, et al: Effect of gastric acid on the pathogenesis of subglottic stenosis. Ann Otol Rhinol Laryngol 94:516, 1985.
5. Ossakow SJ, et al: Esophageal reflux and dysmotility as the basis for persistent cervical symptoms. Ann Otol Rhinol Laryngol 96: 387, 1987.
6. Ward PH and Hanson DG: Reflux as an etiological factor of carcinoma of the laryngopharynx. Laryngoscope 98:1195, 1988.
7. Morrison MD: Is chronic gastroesophageal reflux a causative factor in glottic carcinoma? Otolaryngol Head Neck Surg 99:370, 1988.
8. Burton DM, et al: Pediatric airway manifestations of gastroesophageal reflux. Ann Otol Rhinol Laryngol 101:742, 1992.
9. Jindal JR, et al: Gastroesophageal reflux as a likely cause of "idiopathic" subglottic stenosis. Ann Otol Rhinol Laryngol 103:186, 1994.
10. Wiener GJ, et al: Chronic hoarseness secondary to gastroesophageal reflux disease: documentation with 24-H ambulatory pH monitoring. Am J Gastroenterol 84:1503, 1989.
11. Richter JE (ed): Ambulatory Esophageal pH Monitoring: Practical Approach and Clinical Applications. Tokyo, Igaku-Shoin, 1991.
12. Frank M and Komisar A: Ambulatory pH monitoring in the management of reflux. Ann Otol Rhinol Laryngol 102:243, 1993.
13. Richter JE, et al: Normal 24-hour pH values: Influence of study center, pH electrode, age, and gender. Dig Dis Sci 37:849, 1992.
14. Ott DJ, et al: The role of diagnostic imaging in evaluating gastroesophageal reflux disease. Postgrad Radiol 6:3, 1986.
15. Kamel PL, Hanson D, and Kahrilas PJ: Omeprazole for the treatment of posterior laryngitis. Am J Med 96:321, 1994.
16. Wolfe MM and Soll AH: The physiology of gastric acid secretion. N Engl J Med 319:1707, 1988.
17. Contencin P and Narcy P: Gastropharyngeal reflux in infants and children: a pharyngeal pH monitoring study. Arch Otolaryngol 118:1028, 1992.
18. Wetmore RF: Effect of acid on the larynx of the maturing rabbit and their possible significance to the sudden infant death syndrome. Laryngoscope 103:1242, 1993.
19. Cressman WR and Meyer CM, III: Diagnosis and management of croup and epiglottitis. Pediatr Clin North Am 41:265, 1994.
20. Crockett DM, Healy GB, McGill TJ, and Friedman EM: Airway management of acute supraglottitis at the Children's Hospital, Boston: 1980–1985. Ann Otol Rhinol Laryngol 97:114, 1988.
21. Cantrell RW, Bell RA, and Morioka WT: Acute epiglottitis: intubation versus tracheotomy. Laryngoscope 88:994, 1978.
22. Havaldar PV: Diphtheria in the eighties: experience in a south Indian district hospital. J Indian Med Assoc 90:155, 1992.
23. Deeb ZE and Einhorn KH: Infectious adult croup. Laryngoscope 100:455, 1990.
24. Nadel S, et al: Upper airway obstruction in association with perinatally acquired herpes simplex virus. J Pediatr 120:127, 1992.
25. D'Angelo AJ, et al: Adult supraglottis due to herpes simplex virus. J Otolaryngol 19:179, 1990.
26. Murrage KJ, Janzen VD, and Ruby RR: Epiglottitis: adult and pediatric comparisons. J Otolaryngol 17:194, 1988.
27. Deeb ZE, Yenson AC, and DeFries HO: Acute epiglottitis in the adult. Laryngoscope 95:289, 1985.

28. Souliere CR and Kirchner JA: Laryngeal perichondritis and abscess. Arch Otolaryngol 111:481, 1985.

29. Ramadan HH, Tarazi AE, and Baroudy FM: Laryngeal tuberculosis: presentation of 16 cases and a review of the literature. J Otolaryngol 22:39, 1993.

30. Soda A, et al: Tuberculosis of the larynx: clinical aspects in 19 patients. Laryngoscope 99:1147, 1989.

31. Bailey CM and Windle-Taylor PC: Tuberculosis laryngitis: a series of 37 patients. Laryngoscope 91:93, 1981.

32. Soni NK: Leprosy of the larynx. J Laryngol Otol 106:518, 1992.

33. Younus M: Leprosy in ENT. J Laryngol Otol 100:1437, 1986.

34. Flanagan PM and McIlwain JC: Tuberculosis of the larynx in a lepromatous patient. J Laryngol Otol 107:845, 1993.

35. Holinger PH, Gelman HK, and Wolfe CK, Jr: Rhinoscleroma of the lower respiratory tract. Laryngoscope 87:1, 1977.

36. Stiernberg CM and Clark WD: Rhinoscleroma: a diagnostic challenge. Laryngoscope 93:866, 1983.

37. Jay J, Green RP, and Lucente FE: Isolated laryngeal rhinoscleroma. Otolaryngol Head Neck Surg 93:669, 1985.

38. Alfaro-Monge JM, Fernandez-Espinosa J, and Soda-Morhy A: Scleroma of the lower respiratory tract: case report and review of the literature. J Laryngol Otol 108:161, 1994.

39. Nelson EG and Tybor AG: Actinomycosis of the larynx. Ear Nose Throat J 71:356, 1992.

40. Everett ED and Templer JW: Oropharyngeal tularemia. Arch Otolaryngol 106:237, 1980.

41. Wilkinson L: Glanders: medicine and veterinary medicine in common pursuit of a contagious disease. Med Hist 25:363, 1981.

42. Musher DM: Syphilis, neurosyphilis, penicillin, and AIDS. J Infect Dis 163:1201, 1991.

43. McNulty JS and Fassett RL: Syphilis: an otolaryngologic perspective. Laryngoscope 91:889, 1981.

44. Burton DM, Seid AB, Kearns DB, and Pransky SM: Candida laryngotracheitis: a complication of combined steroid and antibiotic usage in croup. Int J Pediatr Otorhinolaryngol 23:171, 1992.

45. Vrabec DP: Fungal infections of the larynx. Otolaryngol Clin North Am 26:1091, 1993.

46. Tashjian LS and Peacock JE, Jr: Laryngeal candidiasis: report of seven cases and review of the literature. Arch Otolaryngol 110:806, 1984.

47. Reder PA and Neel HB, III: Blastomycosis in otolaryngology: review of a large series. Laryngoscope 103:53, 1993.

48. Lester CF, Conrad FG, and Atwell RJ: Primary laryngeal blastomycosis: review of the literature and presentation of a case. Am J Med 24:305, 1958.

49. Boyle JO, Coulthard SW, and Mandel RM: Laryngeal involvement in disseminated coccidioidomycosis. Arch Otolaryngol Head Neck Surg 117:433, 1991.

50. Ward PH, Berci G, Morledge D, and Schwartz H: Coccidioidomycosis of the larynx in infants and adults. Ann Otol 86:655, 1977.

51. Bolivar R, et al: Aspergillus epiglottis. Cancer 51:367, 1983.

52. Remington PL, et al: Sporotrichosis in Wisconsin. Wis Med J 82:25, 1983.

53. Agger WA and Seager GM: Granulomas of the vocal cords caused by Sporothrix schenckii. Laryngoscope 95:595, 1985.

54. Neel HB III and McDonald TJ: Laryngeal sarcoidosis: report of 13 patients. Ann Otol Rhinol Laryngol 91:359, 1982.

55. Gallivan GJ and Landis JN: Sarcoidosis of the larynx: preserving and restoring airway and professional voice. J Voice 7:81, 1993.

56. Jorizzo JL, et al: Sarcoidosis of the upper respiratory tract in patients with nasal rim lesions: a pilot study. J Am Acad Dermatol 22:439, 1990.

57. Bower JS, Belen JE, Weg JG, and Dantzer DR: Manifestations and treatment of laryngeal sarcoidosis. Am Rev Respir Dis 122:325, 1980.

58. Lebovics RS, et al: The management of subglottic stenosis in patients with Wegener's granulomatosis. Laryngoscope 102:1341, 1992.

59. Werber JL and Pincus RL: Oropharyngeal angioedema associated with the use of angiotensin-converting enzyme inhibitors. Otolaryngol Head Neck Surg 101:96, 1989.

60. Wahle D, Beste DJ, and Conley SF: Laryngeal involvement in toxic epidermal necrolysis. Otolaryngol Head Neck Surg 107:796, 1992.

61. Campbell SM, Montanaro A, and Bardana EJ: Head and neck manifestations of autoimmune disease. Am J Otolaryngol 4:187, 1983.

62. Jurik AG, Pedersen U, and Nrgård A: Rheumatoid arthritis of the cricoarytenoid joints: a case of laryngeal obstruction due to acute and chronic joint changes. Laryngoscope 95:846, 1985.

63. Friedman BA and Rice DH: Rheumatoid nodules of the larynx. Arch Otolaryngol 101:361, 1975.

64. Hanson RD, Olsen KD, and Rogers RS III: Upper aerodigestive tract manifestations of cicatricial pemphigoid. Ann Otol Rhinol Laryngol 97:493, 1988.

65. McAdam LP, O'Hanlan MA, Bluestone C, and Pearson CM: Relapsing polychrondritis: prospective study of 23 patients and a review of the literature. Medicine 55:193, 1976.

66. Barrs DM, McDonald TJ, and Duffy J: Sjögren's syndrome involving the larynx: report of a case. J Laryngol Otol 93:933, 1979.

67. Gertz MA and Kyle RA: Primary systemic amyloidosis: a diagnostic primer. Mayo Clin Proc 64:1505, 1989.

68. Lewis JE, Olsen KD, Kurtin PJ, and Kyle RA: Laryngeal amyloidosis: a clinicopathologic and immunohisto-chemical review. Otolaryngol Head Neck Surg 106:372, 1992.

69. Marsden PD: Mucosal leishmaniasis ("espundia" Escomel, 1911). Trans R Soc Trop Med Hyg 80:859, 1986.

70. Toppozada HH: Laryngeal bilharzia. J Laryngol Otol 99:1039, 1985.

71. Manni HJ, Lema PN, van Raalte JA, and Westerbeek GF: Schistosomiasis in otorhinolaryngology: review of the literature and case report. J Laryngol Otol 97:1177, 1983.

72. Weinstein L and Molavi A: Syngamus laryngeus infection (syngamosis) with chronic cough. Ann Intern Med 74:577, 1971.

73. Bowes SM, III, Laube BL, Links JM, and Frank R: Regional disposition of inhaled fog droplets: preliminary observations. Environ Health Perspect 79:151, 1989.

74. Chandler JR: Radiation fibrosis and necrosis of the larynx. Ann Otol Rhinol Laryngol 88:509, 1979.

75. Ferguson BJ, Hudson WR, and Farmer JC, Jr: Hyperbaric oxygen therapy for laryngeal radionecrosis. Ann Otol Rhinol Laryngol 96:1, 1987.

76. Koufman JA and Blalock PD: Vocal fatigue and dysphonia in the professional voice user: Bogart-Bacall syndrome. Laryngoscope 98:493, 1988.

77. Koufman JA and Blalock PD: Functional voice disorders. Otolaryngol Clin North Am 24:1059, 1991.

78. Feder RJ and Mitchell MJ: Hyperfunctional, hyperacidic, and intubation granulomas. Arch Otolaryngol 110:582, 1984.

79. Cherry J and Margulies SI: Contact ulcer of the larynx. Laryngoscope 78:1937, 1968.

80. Delahunty JE and Cherry J: Experimentally produced vocal cord granulomas. Laryngoscope 78:1941, 1968.

81. Donnelly WH: Histopathology of endotracheal intubation: an autopsy study of 99 cases. Arch Pathol 88:511, 1969.

82. Koufman JA: Contact ulcer and granuloma of the larynx. In: Current Therapy in Otolaryngology—Head and Neck Surgery. 5th Ed. Edited by Gates GA. St. Louis, CV Mosby, 1994, p 456.

FURTHER SUGGESTED READINGS

Baugh R and Gilmore BB Jr: Infectious croup: a critical review. Otolaryngol Head Neck Surg 95:40, 1986.

Caldarelli DD, Friedberg SA, and Harris AA: Medical and surgical aspects of the granulomatous diseases of the larynx. Otolaryngol Clin North Am 12:767, 1979.

Cann CI, Fried MP, and Rothman KJ: Epidemiology of squamous cell cancer of the head and neck. Otolaryngol Clin North Am 18:367, 1985.

Klinkenberg-Knol EC: Recent Advances in the Diagnosis and Management of Gastro-oesophageal Reflux Disease: The Role of Omeprazole in Clinical Practice. Amsterdam, VU University Press, 1990.

Lucente FE: Impact of the acquired immunodeficiency syndrome epidemic on the practice of laryngology. Ann Otol Rhinol Laryngol 102(suppl 161):1, 1993.

Pillsbury HC and Sasaki CT: Granulomatous diseases of the larynx. Otolaryngol Clin North Am 15:539, 1982.

Richtsmeier WJ and Johns ME: Bacterial causes of granulomatous disease. Otolaryngol Clin North Am 15:473, 1982.

Sataloff RT: The impact of pollution on the voice. Otolaryngol Head Neck Surg 106:701, 1992.

31 Neurogenic and Functional Disorders of the Larynx

Christy L. Ludlow, Carol Gracco, Clarence Sasaki, Valerie Asher, and Steve Salzer

Normal speech requires the complex integration of peripheral and central motor control mechanisms. The voice component of speech requires (1) neural control of the intrinsic and extrinsic laryngeal muscles to shape the glottis and (2) a steady stream of air flow from the respiratory system to support regular, symmetric, and synchronous vibration of the vocal folds. Thus, the neural components of the respiratory and phonatory mechanism must work in concert to produce normal phonation during speech.

The larynx does not function in isolation from other structures in the vocal tract. Muscles contributing shape to the pharynx and oral cavity, specifically those that control the tongue, lip, and jaw, have dramatic effects on the mechanism of laryngeal tension and overall vocal tract posture. In normal speech, the vocal tract takes on distinct postures, providing characteristic shaping for specific sounds.

Valving mechanisms including the glottis, velum, tongue, lips, and jaw also provide posture and shape to the vocal tract resulting in characteristic distribution of sound energy into formants. This distribution of energy is responsible for distinctly different sounds. A simple example is illustrated in Figure 31–1. Sagittal sections show specific vocal tract configuration for production of /i/, /a/, /aw/, and /u/. In the vowel /i/, posture of the tongue high and forward exerts anterior tension from the tip to base of tongue. Close coupling with the hyoid bone and suspended thyroid cartilage distribute elements of tension to extrinsic and intrinsic laryngeal musculature that may be affected by tilt of the thyroid cartilage. For the vowel /i/, the pharyngeal cavity is large, making conditions for air flow different than for production of /a/, which is characterized by constricted pharyngeal cavity in part because of the low and posterior placement of the tongue muscula-

ture. This can set the stage for turbulence in the airway, particularly in the face of neurogenic disorders, which may place further constriction on this portion of the pharyngeal cavity. The acoustic product is thus affected indirectly by changes in constriction and air pressures in the pharynx and oral cavity.

Peripheral and central neurogenic diseases may produce changes in the acoustic product or vocal output by changing the configuration of the vocal tract. Functional voice disorders, idiopathic or of known cause, can present movement abnormalities similar to those found in neurogenic disorders. Vocal tract tension or movement due to voluntary or involuntary muscle contractions is altered by nervous system injury and/or functional abnormalities. The origins may be traumatic, neoplastic, vascular, infectious, degenerative, or idiopathic. It follows that such vocal disorders do not exist in isolation. They are often presented in conjunction with disease processes that may alter lip, tongue, and jaw control as well as other motor systems.

The diagnostic process must also take into account the body's capacity for reorganization and compensation, meaning that the degree of motor impairment may not be reflected in the perceived severity of deviation in speech. Perceptual voice parameters such as pitch, loudness, vocal quality, and the degree of consistency or variability in each of these may help to characterize neurogenic and functional voice disorders. Quantification of characteristics of such disorders may be useful based on a variety of instrumental techniques.[1–4] Computer-assisted mathematic quantification of the acoustic product is a valuable diagnostic adjunct to the perceptual parameterization of voice.[5] Measures based on pressure and flow transduction during phonation provide information about the functional relationship between the respiratory and phona-

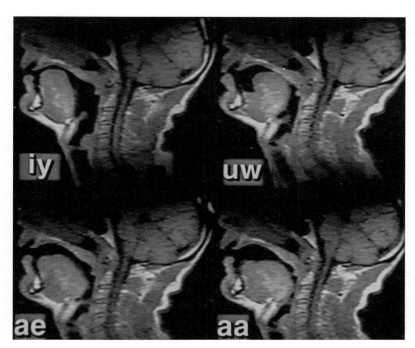

Fig. 31–1. Sagittal sections from magnetic resonance images of the vocal tract illustrate vocal tract shape during production of four vowels. (Adapted from Baer T, Gore JC, Gracco LC, and Nye PW: Analysis of vocal tract shape and dimensions using magnetic resonance imaging: vowels. J Acoust Soc Am *90*:799, 1993.)

tory systems. Further, the use of diagnostic imaging techniques including fiberoptic videoendoscopic examination has made possible the observation of laryngeal and pharyngeal movement. Stroboscopic examination is useful in assessing the vibratory characteristics of the vocal folds.[4] High-speed photography, ultrasound, videofluoroscopy, and magnetic resonance (MR) are other imaging tools that have value in the diagnostic protocol.[6–11] Use of electromyography (EMG) accompanied by magnetic stimulation of the laryngeal nerve may be valuable in differentiating peripheral and central neurogenic dysfunction.[12] The goal of instrumental and perceptual techniques has been to characterize vocal fold movement control in terms of timing, speed, and accuracy of movement of vocal tract structures and to quantify these parameters as they may relate to and be useful for documentation of the status and progression of disease for therapeutic purposes.

NEUROGENIC VOICE DISORDERS

Dysphonia or voice disorder may be the first sign of neurogenic disease, with the upper articulator symptoms or dysarthria following as the disease progresses. "Flaccid, spastic, ataxic, hypokinetic, and hyperkinetic dysarthrias sound different because physiologically and anatomically dissimilar regions of the nervous system are damaged in each type, producing different muscular pathophysiology."[13]

Functionally, neurogenic disorders resulting in dysphonia may be divided into the following four categories:

1. Consistent neurogenic voice disorders characterized by vocal quality loudness or pitch deviations that are constant during speech and sustained vowel production: flaccid dysarthria, associated with lower motor neuron disease; and spastic dysarthria, associated with upper motor neuron disease.
2. Arhythmically fluctuating neurogenic voice disorders, which cause unpredictable, irregular quality, loudness, and pitch variation during speech. Sustained vowel production may accentuate irregularities. Ataxic, choreic, and dystonic dysphonias each display this type of irregularity.
3. Rhythmically fluctuating neurogenic voice disorders, including palatopharyngolaryngeal myoclonus and essential voice tremor. These dysphonias are marked by dysphonia that fluctuates in a regular or rhythmic way. Paroxysmal neurogenic voice disorders exhibit bursts of dysphonic voice, as in Gilles de la Tourette syndrome.
4. Neurogenic voice disorders associated with loss of volitional phonation, including apraxia of phonation or loss of volitional control over respiration and phonation, akinetic mutism.

Characteristic categories of voice deficit such as the aforementioned not only share similar presentation of voice symptoms, but have similar site of lesion as well.[13]

Upper Motor Neuron Disease

Parkinson's Disease
Upper motor neuron diseases with characteristic voice components include Parkinson's disease and related

TABLE 31–1. Classification of Parkinsonism

Parkinson's disease
Postencephalitic parkinsonism
Iatrogenic parkinsonism
Parkinsonism occurring as part of multiple system atrophy
    Striatonigral degeneration
    Olivopontocerebellar atrophy
    Progressive supranuclear palsy
    Parkinsonism with Alzheimer's disease
Symptomatic parkinsonism
Pseudoparkinsonism
    Arteriosclerotic
    Post-traumatic
    Endocrinopathy
    Metabolic or toxic disorder

(From Duvoisin RC: The cause of Parkinson's disease. In: International Medical Reviews. vol 2: Movement Disorders. Edited by Fahn S and Marsden CD. London, Butterworth, 1982.)

syndromes. Parkinsonism is defined as a pathophysiologic state reflecting failure of the nigrostriatal dopaminergic neuronal system as a result of degeneration or destruction of the substantia nigra by various morbid processes or caused by pharmacologic agents depleting neuronal dopamine, inhibiting its synthesis, or blocking the striatal dopamine receptors.[14] The basal ganglia, a portion of the extrapyramidal motor system, modulates nerve impulses via the thalamus to the cortex, which, in turn, controls the lower motor neurons. Hence, damage to the basal ganglia can release inhibition of nerve impulses affecting the lower motor neurons, resulting in rigidity and reduced rate of movement.

Although parkinsonism can be described as a syndrome of diverse origin, distinct syndromes are recognized from clinical features, secondary or associated manifestations, laboratory findings, and postmortem study, although differentiation is often difficult. See Table 31–1 for a summary classification of parkinsonism.

Although Parkinson's disease occasionally occurs in families of the same generation, incidence in identical twins is as low as 5 to 7%, suggesting little genetic predisposition. Onset is typically in the sixties or later, but the disease may appear as early as the middle thirties, with some cases reported as early as 15 years.[14]

Reduced loudness and breathy vocal quality may be the hallmark of voice disorders in early Parkinson's disease. Essential features include fading voice quality into breathiness in contextual speech. The patient may have difficulty with production of glottal stops or sound generated at the glottis dependent on laryngeal resistance and with voice onset after voiceless consonants such as /s/. There may be reduced range and speed of vocal fold movement, particularly on the more affected side. Distinctions between voiceless and voiced sounds become reduced with impaired ability to produce glottal stops to mark word boundaries and a tendency to maintain sounds as all voiced or all voiceless.[15–17] In later stages of the disease, the patient may be unable to produce phonation even with instruction. In advanced disease, severe "on-off" drug-related phenomena may occur, during which patients may experience breathy voice followed by periods of propulsive speech with strained quality. Vocal fold imaging studies in Parkinson's disease illustrate glottic gap and bowing of the vocal folds,[18] often associated with breathiness and reduced loudness (Fig. 31–2).

Asymmetries have also been demonstrated in vocal

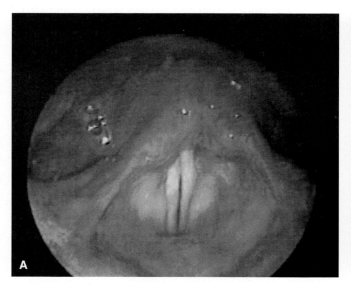 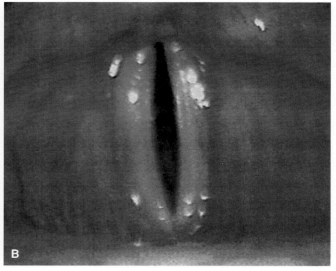

Fig. 31–2. Videostroboscopic endoscopic view of the vocal folds during phonatory closure in an individual with Parkinson's disease. A. Note the difference in apparent level of the two vocal folds in the posterior commissure. B. Characteristic bowing typically seen in geriatric individuals and Parkinson's disease may indicate reduced air flow and resistance or structural changes weakening the vocal fold margin. (From Gracco LC, Marek K, and Sasaki C: Vocal tract function in parkinsonian dysarthria. Laryngoscope, in press.)

fold closure, as well as thinning of the mucosa and appearance of aging of the vocal folds.

Patients with postencelphalitic Parkinson's disease are known to show little difference in vegetative, deep, and speech breathing and air wastage before speaking. Vocal intensity studies in parkinsonism fail to prove habitually lower intensity levels, although this is often reported. Patients do present louder voicing on demand, but few show the ability to monitor and alter phonatory intensity spontaneously.

In addition to neuropharmacologic management, the most effective form of voice treatment in Parkinson's disease includes vocal strengthening exercises. Compared to more traditional articulation therapy alone, vocal strengthening shows overall improvement in intelligibility. Focus on upper articulator (lip, tongue, and jaw) movement produces little in the way of increased intelligibility for this population.[19]

Progressive Supranuclear Palsy

Progressive Supranuclear Palsy (PSP) is a rare degenerative neurologic disorder. Clinically, PSP is characterized by supranuclear ophthalmoplegia, frequently accompanied by complaints of falling backwards, nuchal dystonia in extension, moderate axial dystonia, pseudobulbar palsy, difficulty in swallowing, dysarthria, bradykinesia, masked facies, nonspecific changes in personality, lability, sleep disturbance, and performance decrements on various neuropsychologic tasks. PSP may be differentiated from Parkinson's disease in that supranuclear ophthalmoplegia is characteristic of PSP and is not present in Parkinson's disease. Similarly, the tremor present in parkinsonism is typically absent in PSP. Patients with PSP may have voice symptoms similar to those in parkinsonism, with the possible exception of vocal tremor. Hypophonia is present, with unilaterally reduced vocal fold range and speed of movement. The associated dysarthria may include palilalia and oral motor rigidity.[20]

Multiple Systems Atrophy

Multiple systems atrophy represents a group of degenerative movement disorders with lesions in the cerebellum, brain stem, and basal ganglia.[21] Three groups of clinically varied patients are recognized within this category. Depending on the degree of system involvement, the voice may be affected in various ways: (1) spinocerebellar degeneration (olivopontocerebellar atrophy, or OPCA); (2) progressive autonomic failure (Shy-Drager syndrome); and (3) atypical parkinsonism (striatonigral degeneration).[22,23] These are rare movement disorders, with the exception of OPCA.

In OPCA, characterized by progressive cerebellar ataxia, coordination of the laryngeal muscles is affected as in ataxic dysarthria. One sees loss of muscle coordination (dyssynergia); loss of ability to gauge range of motion (dysmetria) and tremor may be present during voluntary movement (intention tremor). The degree of laryngeal impairment depends on the severity of ataxia. Dysphonia may take one of several forms: sudden bursts of loudness, irregular increases in pitch and loudness, or coarse voice tremor.[13]

In Shy-Drager syndrome, clinical symptoms of Parkinson's disease are present, along with progressive autonomic dysfunction. Voice may be affected as the vocal folds may show reduced range and speed of abduction. Speech may be slowed with reduction in intensity and absence of glottal stops with poor voicing contrasts and a tendency for laryngospasm. The most prominent feature is airway compromise from bilateral abductor paresis usually requiring a tracheostomy in the late stages of the disease.[13,24]

Striatonigral degeneration is characterized by parkinsonian bradykinesia, rigidity, and tremor but typically has no symptoms of autonomic dysfunction. Patients with this syndrome tend to show severe voice deficits with marked reduction in intensity levels of phonation. Many patients become completely aphonic in the end stages of this disease process.

Voice treatment for these syndromes largely depends on the stage of disease and may include compensatory strategies as well as supportive nonverbal communication alternatives in end stages. Treatment is necessarily linked to residual level of function. In the case of Parkinson's disease, however, evidence suggests that early intervention may reduce the symptoms of voice deficit in early and later stages of the disease.[19]

Pseudobulbar Palsy

Pseudobulbar palsy results from supranuclear lesions above the level of the nucleus of cranial nerve X. They include lesions of the corticobulbar tracts bilaterally, vascular and degenerative lesions involving the motor cortical areas bilaterally, vascular lesions and tumors of the internal capsule or brain stem, degenerative lesions involving the entire corticobulbar tract system, and infections. Dysphonia associated with these types of lesions is characterized by strained-strangled, harsh voice, likely the result of hyperadduction of true and false vocal folds. This is thought to be the result of release of inhibition of excitatory nerve impulses transmitted to vagal nuclei. There are also reports of breathy voice with vocal fold asymmetry.[13]

Multiple Sclerosis

Multiple Sclerosis (MS) is a progressive demyelinating disorder, having sensory and motor impairments of the limb, cognitive problems, and tremor. It is likely one of the most common causes of ataxia; however, patients with MS usually have evidence of central nervous system disease outside the cerebellum and its pathways.[25] For example, optic nerve and corticospinal tract involvement are usually present. Dysarthria, tremor, and decomposition of movement are frequently associated with gait and limb ataxia in MS.

Essential features include staccato speech and harsh voice quality with intermittent hyperadduction of the vocal folds. Spasticity and tremor may affect all or some regions of the vocal tract, thereby reducing speech intelligibility and making speech effortful. Breathy voice and vocal fold asymmetry are predominant findings. Depending on the systems involved, voicing may or may not be affected in some stages of this disease. Given the predominant ataxia that may influence speech motor systems, voicing is characteristic of other ataxic dysarthrias (see the section of this chapter on cerebellar degeneration).

Myoclonus

Myoclonus is defined as a sudden, brief, shock-like involuntary movement caused by active muscular contractions.[26] The distribution may be focal, multifocal, or generalized, with the presentation spontaneous, active, and stimulus-sensitive. The source of the neural discharge may be cortical, brain stem, or spinal. Obeso[26] and associates described four main pathophysiologic categories of myoclonus, as discussed in the following paragraphs.

CORTICAL MYOCLONUS. In this disorder, the abnormal activity originates in the sensory-motor cortex and is transmitted down the spinal cord through the pyramidal tract.

SUBCORTICAL MYOCLONUS. These forms of myoclonus arise in structures located between the cerebral cortex and the spinal cord, including reticular reflex myoclonus, which originates in the brain stem and is characterized by jerks produced by eternal stimuli.

CORTICAL-SUBCORTICAL MYOCLONUS. This disorder results from either an abnormal cortical discharge spreading by corticoreticulospinal pathways and giving rise to generalized myoclonus or a subcortical focus producing its effect by the motor cortex-pyramidal tract.

SPINAL MYOCLONUS. This disorder results from abnormal overactivity of spinal neurons.

PALATAL MYOCLONUS. In this focal myoclonus, movements of the palate occur unilaterally or bilaterally at 1.5 to 3 Hz and frequently are accompanied by synchronous movements of adjacent muscles such as the extraocular muscles, tongue, larynx, face, neck, or diaphragm.[27] When the soft palate is involved, abrupt, rhythmic, anteroposterior, and vertical movements are present during speech and at rest. Pharyngeal muscle contractions can open and close the eustachian tube, thereby producing a bruit or clicking sound transmitted by the tympanic membrane and sometimes heard by others. Movements are often present during sleep and may occur without the patient's knowledge. Myoclonus may be idiopathic or may be seen in association with stroke, MS, tumors, trauma, or metabolic

encephalopathy.[28–30] Dubinsky and Hallett demonstrated increased metabolism on positron emission tomographic (PET) scan in the medulla in these patients.[31] This is consistent with implication of the inferior olivary nuclei in the origin of palatal myoclonus.[32] When the pharynx and larynx are involved, rhythmic adductor movements of the vocal folds and gross upward and downward movements of the larynx cause momentary and rhythmic phonatory interruptions. Because of the brevity of movement, voicing deficits are not often perceived during connected speech but may be apparent on vowel prolongation.

Lower Motor Neuron Disorders

Amyotrophic Lateral Sclerosis

Amyotrophic lateral sclerosis (ALS), a motor neuron disease, may produce a mixed dysarthria because of primarily upper motor neuron involvement and some lower motor neuron involvement, particularly in the late stages of the disease (flaccid-spastic paralysis). ALS is a degenerative disease of the corticobulbar tracts and lower motor neuron nuclei. The speech and voice symptoms may vary depending on the predominance of spastic or flaccid components. Flaccid symptoms present with hypoadduction of one or both vocal folds and pooling of saliva in the pyriform sinuses on laryngeal examination. Voicing is characterized by breathy, hypernasal quality with reduced intensity range. A "wet" phonation is the result of poor management of secretions due to flaccidity. If spastic components prevail, voicing will be strained and harsh because of hyperadduction of the true and false vocal folds. A mixed form of dysphonia may result in voicing characterized by both flaccid and spastic components.

ALS occurs in the fifth to seventh decade of life and may present with primarily pyramidal tract signs or lower motor neuron signs of progressive muscular atrophy. Fasciculations are more common in the pyramidal tract form. When the disease affects the brain stem rather than the spinal cord, it may progress more rapidly. Speech symptoms are considered to be the first signs in the bulbar type.[33] Facial muscle weakness, palatal weakness, and lip, tongue, and jaw weakness with tongue fasciculations are predominant and cause poor speech intelligibility. Voicing is weak and breathy because of flaccidity of the vocal folds.

Myasthenia Gravis

Myasthenia gravis is a disorder of acetylcholine transfer at the myoneural junction, characterized by weakness and fatigability of striated muscle. Muscle contraction, dependent on stimulation of the motor end plate by acetylcholine, is weakened or reduced by the reduction of acetylcholine receptors. This disorder causes a flaccid dysphonia, characterized by breathy, weak phonation. Intensity range is reduced, and sustained effort causes progressive weakness. Although this disorder may affect phonation (larynx), resonation (velum), and articulation (lip, tongue, and jaw), these systems may be affected separately or serially as the disease progresses. The larynx is less frequently affected, whereas the extraocular muscles are usually the first affected. This and other early disorders of neurogenic origin may present with reduced movement range and speed of the vocal folds on laryngoscopic examination and are often mistaken for psychogenic voice disorders. Flaccid dysphonia may be an early symptom of neurogenic disease.[33]

Wallenberg Syndrome

Occlusion of the posterior inferior cerebellar artery may produce infarction of the lateral medulla, resulting in Wallenberg syndrome, also known as lateral medullary syndrome. The medial and descending vestibular nuclei are usually included in the zone of infarction consisting of a wedge of the dorsolateral medulla just posterior to the olive. This syndrome is marked by dysarthria and dysphagia, ipsilateral impairment of pain and temperature sensation on the face, and contralateral loss of pain and temperature in the trunk and extremities. Major symptoms include vertigo, nausea, vomiting, intractible hiccupping, ipsilateral facial pain, and diplopia. Unilateral vocal fold paralysis and flaccid dysphonia occur when the nucleus ambiguus or corticobulbar tracts leading to it are affected.[34]

Postpolio Syndrome

Of the 250,000 survivors of the poliomyelitis epidemics, approximately 25% experience progressive muscle weakness known as postpolio syndrome (PPS). Postpolio patients who complain of swallowing difficulties are at risk for laryngeal dysfunction. This syndrome is characterized by the new onset of progressive muscle weakness, fatigue, and pain. This may occur 30 to 40 years after the initial infection with polio. Electrodiagnosis of neuronal dropout or axonal loss in these patients is consistent with neurogenic change. Patients with previous bulbar symtoms show evidence of neurogenic change. The progressive nature of this disease is variable; however, if the disease leads to progressive weakness, patients with vocal fold paralysis and with EMG evidence of contralateral vocal fold involvement may be at high risk for bilateral vocal fold paralysis and subsequent acute respiratory distress. Patients with active swallowing complaints require thorough laryngeal and voice assessment to evaluate the coexistent laryngeal pathologic process in addition to appropriate therapy.[35]

Disorders of the Peripheral Nervous System

Because the tenth cranial nerve contains sensory and motor fibers that supply the larynx, central and periph-

eral lesions affecting pathways of this nerve have varied effects on phonation. The vagus nerve (CN X) is the longest cranial nerve and also innervates the pharynx, palate, trachea, bronchi, lungs, heart, external ear, and parts of the gastrointestinal tract. Originating in the medulla, cranial nerves IX, X, and XI traverse the cranial cavity through the jugular foramen, enlarging here to form the jugular ganglion. On exiting the jugular foramen, another enlargement becomes the nodose ganglion. The jugular and nodose ganglia are considered sensory ganglia, each containing cell bodies of sensory fibers contained in the vagus nerve.

The vagus nerve passes down the neck close to the carotid artery within the carotid sheath. The left vagus nerve crosses to the left of the arch of the aorta and angles down and back to pass behind the left pulmonary artery. The right vagus crosses over the subclavian artery. Both sides continue behind the heart to supply the remaining structures in the thorax and abdomen.

On exiting the skull, each vagus nerve branches to form pharyngeal, superior, and recurrent laryngeal nerves. The pharyngeal nerve supplies the pharynx and muscles of the soft palate, with the exception of the tensor veli palatini (CN V) (Fig. 31–3). The superior laryngeal nerves (SLNs) arise from the vagus nerves near the caudal end of the nodose ganglia. Coursing deep to the carotid arteries, the nerves split, forming internal and external branches. The internal branch of the SLN passes by the larynx through the thyrohyoid membrane. The internal branch supplies sensory receptors above the level of the glottis. Parasympathetic secretomotor fibers that supply seromucinous glands above the level of the vocal folds are also innervated by the internal branch of the SLN. The external branch of the SLN supplies motor function to the cricothyroid muscle.

Recurrent laryngeal nerves (RLNs) contain sensory and motor fibers that travel within each vagus nerve, branching from the vagus into the thorax to form the RLN. The left RLN originates from the left vagus nerve, passing superficial to the aortic arch, and loops under and passes behind, then traveling up to the trachea and the larynx. The right RLN arises from the right vagus nerve, passing superficial to the subclavian artery. It then loops around the subclavian artery, passing up the trachea to the larynx. The RLNs enter the larynx after passing deep to the thyroid gland and inferior constrictor, then passing behind the inferior cornu of the thyroid cartilage.[36] Considered mixed nerves, the RLNs supply all the intrinsic laryngeal muscles except the cricothyroid. Sensory fibers supply receptors below the level of the vocal folds.

The RLNs and external branches of the SLNs supply motor innervation to the laryngeal muscles, providing support for fine control, as described in Table 31–2. The conduction velocity is high, and the innervation

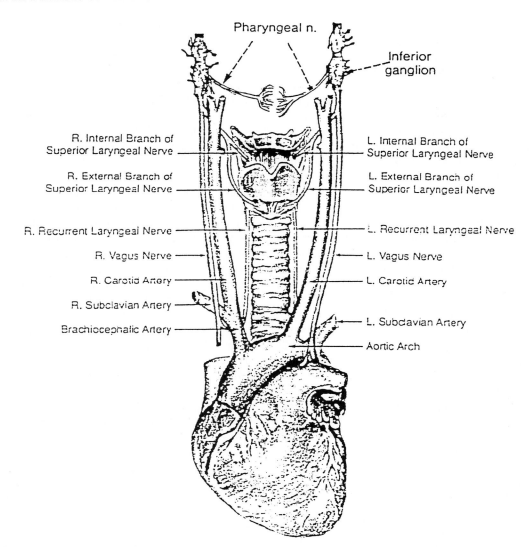

Fig. 31–3. Peripheral components of the laryngeal nervous system. (Adapted from Garrett JD and Larson CR: Neurology of the Laryngeal system. In: Phonosurgery. Edited by Ford CN and Bless DM. New York, Raven Press, 1991, p 43.)

ratio per motor unit is low, estimated at 100 to 200 cells per motor unit. This suggests a smaller innervation ratio than the hand, indicating a finer degree of contraction and the ability to control precisely phonatory parameters such as fundamental frequency (Fig. 31–4).[36,37]

Lesions of the tenth cranial nerve at any point along its pathway from the nucleus ambiguus in the brain

TABLE 31–2. Characteristic Functions of the Laryngeal Muscles in Vocal Fold Adjustments

	CT	VOC	LCA	IA	PCA
Position	Paramed	*Adduct*	*Adduct*	*Adduct*	*Abduct*
Level	Lower	Lower	*Lower*	0	*Elevate*
Length	*Elongate*	*Shorten*	Elongate	(Shorten)	*Elongate*
Thickness	*Thin*	*Thicken*	Thin	(Thicken)	Thin
Edge	*Sharpen*	*Round*	Sharpen	0	Round
Muscle (body)	*Stiffen*	*Stiffen*	Stiffen	(Slacken)	Stiffen
Mucosa (cover and transition)	*Stiffen*	*Slacken*	Stiffen	(Slacken)	Stiffen

0, no effect; ( ), slightly; italics, markedly. CT, cricothyroid muscle; VOC, vocalis muscle; LCA, lateral cricoarytenoid muscle; IA, interarytenoid muscle; PCA, posterior cricoarytenoid muscle.

(From Hirano M: Clinical Examination of Voice. New York, Springer-Verlag, 1981.)

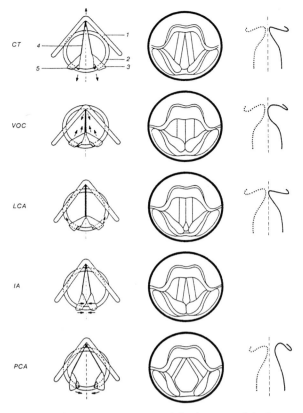

Fig. 31–4. A schematic presentation of the function of the laryngeal muscles. The left column shows the location of the cartilages and the edge of the vocal folds when the laryngeal muscles are activated individually. The arrow indicates the direction of the force exerted; 1, the thyroid cartilage; 2, the cricoid cartilage; 3, the arytenoid cartilage; 4, the vocal ligament; 5, the posterior cricoaryenoid ligament. The middle column shows views from above. The right column presents contours of frontal sections at the middle of the membranous portion of the vocal fold. The dotted line shows a control where no muscle is activated. CT, Cricothyroid muscle; VOC, vocalis muscle; LCA, lateral cricoarytenoid muscle; IA, interarytenoid muscle; PCA, posterior cricoarytenoid muscle. (From Hirano M: Clinical Examination of Voice. New York, Springer, 1981.)

stem to the musculature cause paresis or paralysis of the laryngeal muscles as well as dysphonia or aphonia. The extent of weakness and the degree of dysphonia depend on the location of the lesion along this pathway. Lesions at this level may be vascular, such as hemorrhage, thrombosis, or arteriovenous malformations, or traumatic. Primary or metastatic lesions may also be implicated. Other causes include congenital defects of bone such as the Arnold-Chiari malformation; inflammation, as in poliomyelitis and Guillain-Barré syndrome; neurodegenerative disease, such as ALS; metabolic abnormalities as in myasthenia gravis; neurotoxicity due to metal (arsenic) or botulinum or tetanus toxin poisoning; and others including MS, diphtheria, and tetany. The effects of neurogenic lesions in various locations are summarized in Table 31–3.

Evaluation of Vocal Cord Paralysis

Clinical evaluation of vocal fold paralysis includes diagnostic procedures to determine the cause of the voice disorder, the degree of phonatory deficit, and the prognosis and to establish therapeutic recommendations, which may involve surgery or behavioral treatment. The most effective treatment plan often includes a multidisciplinary approach, using complementary techniques. Some patients who present with vocal fold paralysis may require medialization surgery. To optimize the surgical effects on phonation, however, voice therapy is often recommended pre- and postoperatively to help the patient learn to use the "new vocal instrument." Some diagnostic measures are designed to measure the degree and nature of vocal impairment to determine appropriate intervention. Monitoring the patient's progress throughout treatment is essential to successful outcome. For example, because phonosurgery does not always result in a normal voice, the speech-language pathologist or laryngologist must decide whether difficulties in ease of phonation are structurally or behaviorally based. This is best accomplished with a combination of instrumental and perceptual tests. The importance of adequate visualization of the larynx during phonation and respiration cannot be underscored. These observations are easily made using videostroboscopic endoscopy, which allows viewing of the vibratory characteristics of the vocal folds, as well as opening and closing gestures. A description of vibratory characteristics of the vocal folds should include basic information about the (1) symmetry of bilateral movements, (2) regularity, (3) glottal closure, (4) amplitude, (5) mucosal wave, (6) extent of nonvibratory portions, and (7) the opening-closing pattern.[38]

In addition to visualization of the larynx, subjective perceptual assessment and acoustic objective measures are useful in documenting progress and success of treatment. The degree of impairment is necessarily reflected in the nature and degree of control available to the patient. Measures of frequency and intensity characteristics of phonation should include mean, range fluctuation, extent, and periodicity. Frequency is the correlate of pitch, measured in Hertz. Intensity, measured in decibels, is percieved as loudness level. The range in each of these parameters indicates the limits of laryngeal movement dynamics available to the subject. Instrumental assessment of these factors, as well as noise and harmonic structure in the voice signal, is now available in a variety of computer-based systems designed specifically for voice analysis. Some measure of the irregularity in frequency and intensity, or perturbation, analysis may be useful in monitoring vocal performance.[1] Jitter refers to cycle-to-cycle variation in time or period of vibration (frequency). Shimmer refers to variation in amplitude from cycle to cycle. Harmon-

TABLE 31–3. Effects of Neurogenic Lesions

Level of Lesion	Effect on Vocal Folds		Effect on Phonation		Effect on Soft Palate		Effect on Nasal Resonation	Associated Signs
	Unilateral Lesion	Bilateral Lesions	Unilateral Lesion	Bilateral Lesions	Unilateral Lesion	Bilateral Lesions		
I. Above origin of pharyngeal, superior laryngeal, and recurrent laryngeal nerves	One vocal fold fixed in abducted position	Both vocal folds fixed in abducted position	Breathy, moderate, reduced loudness and pitch	Extremely breathy to whispered (aphonia)	One side low, immobile	Both sides low, immobile	Hypernasality, nasal emission	Glottal coup and cough absent, weak, or mushy; difficulty in swallowing; nasal regurgitation of food; aspiration of secretions; pharyngeal paralysis
II. Above origin of superior laryngeal and recurrent laryngeal nerves but below origin of pharyngeal nerve	Same as above	Same as above	Same as above	Same as above	None	None	None	Same as above, except no pharyngeal paralysis or difficulty in swallowing
III. Superior laryngeal nerve	Both vocal folds able to adduct, affected vocal fold shorter, asymmetric shift of epiglottis and anterior larynx toward intact side on phonation	Absence of tilt of thyroid on cricoid cartilage, inability to view full length of vocal folds because of epiglottic overhang, vocal folds bowed	Breathy, hoarse	Breathy, hoarse, reduced loudness, restricted pitch range	None	None	None	None
IV. Recurrent laryngeal nerve	One vocal fold fixed in paramedian position	Both vocal folds fixed in paramedian position	Breathy, hoarse, reduced loudness, diplophonia (not in all cases)	Breathy, hoarse, reduced loudness	None	None	None	Unilateral: Marginal airway, weak cough. Bilateral: Severe difficulty on inhaling for life purposes, inhalatory stridor, tracheostomy often necessary
V. Myoneural junction (myasthenia gravis)	Not applicable	Restriction of adductor-abductor movements	Not applicable	Breathy, hoarse, reduced loudness; symptoms worsen with sustained speaking	Not applicable	Both sides low, immobile	Hypernasality, nasal emission; symptoms worsen with sustained speaking	Difficulty in swallowing, nasal regurgitation of food, inhalatory stridor, articulation defects

(From Darley FL, Aronson AE, and Brown JR: Motor Speech Disorders. Philadelphia, WB Saunders, 1975.)

ics-to-noise ratio is often used to assess the degree of harmonic structure compared to the noise present during phonation. These values are thought to reflect asymmetries in mass, neural control, tension, and biomechanical characteristics of the vocal fold.[39,40]

Some measure of airflow or volume velocity is useful in determining how rapidly the air passes through the glottis. Mean airflow may be obtained from averaged measures over several glottal cycles. Mean airflow rates are useful in documenting change following phonosurgery, especially in RLN paralysis, because preoperative airflow is high. These measures may be made using a spirometer, pneumotachograph, or hot-wire anemometer.[1,2]

Subglottal pressure is important for vocal fold vibration and intensity changes and may vary with levels of each. Subglottal pressure may be measured indirectly by a pressure transducer placed in the oral cavity. During production of sound "p" requiring lip closure, the vocal tract is a closed tube with equal pressure throughout. Pressure measured in the oral cavity reflects pressure beneath the glottis. In a related measure, glottal resistance is calculated by dividing subglottal pressure by mean airflow. Glottal resistance increases with vocal intensity and is thought to be low in cases of RLN paralysis. These and other quantifiable measures are currently routinely used in the evaluation of voice deficits including vocal fold paralysis. The acquisition of perceptual and objective data is key in the treatment program of patients with neurogenic voice disorders.[2,4,5]

EMG evaluation is a useful adjunct in the assessment of neuromuscular disorders and is often used in prognostic judgements about patients with those disorders. Electrical silence, fibrillation potentials, polyphasic potentials, high-amplitude potentials, and percentage of normal potentials are the basis for interpretation of such examinations. EMG may be useful in differentiating peripheral from central paralysis and functional disorders or arytenoid fixation (Table 31–4)[2,41,42]

Others have suggested the use of neuromyographic assessment that involves the direct stimulation of a laryngeal nerve in conjunction with the use of EMG to monitor resulting muscle activity.[43] During this examination, the contraction of laryngeal muscles is monitored with EMG while the skin surface is stimulated in the area of the SLN. This produces a short latency response that is brain stem-mediated and effected by the RLN nerve to the thyroarytenoid muscle. This method is thought to be one means of obtaining an early estimate of the type and degree of laryngeal nerve injury. Compared with standard EMG, this technique may offer some advantage in monitoring the reinnervation of paralyzed laryngeal muscles following different reinnervation techniques.[41,43,44]

Phonosurgery for Vocal Fold Paralysis

The larynx has evolved to accomplish various tasks. The glottic larynx must remain closed for airway protection during swallowing,[45–47] must be patent for respiration, and must oscillate for vocalization. Neither of the first two vital functions can be compromised in surgery aimed at improving phonation. Successful application of phonosurgery requires not only an un-

TABLE 31–4. Electromyographic (EMG) Patterns in Relation to the Duration of Vocal Fold Paralysis

Muscle	Duration EMG	−2W	2W–1M	1M–2M	2M–3M	3M–6M	6M–12M	12M +	Total
VOC	S	0	3	1	1	2	3	6	16
	F	1	3	11	5	6	0	5	31
	P	0	0	0	1	4	2	0	7
	H	0	0	1	0	0	0	0	1
	N or n	3	3	15	2	5	4	3	35
	Total	4	9	28	9	17	9	14	90
LCA	S	1	2	0	0	3	2	3	11
	F	1	6	7	7	8	0	4	33
	P	0	0	0	3	6	5	1	15
	H	0	0	1	0	1	1	0	3
	N or n	2	8	25	5	9	6	13	68
	Total	4	16	33	15	27	14	21	130
PCA	S	0	2	0	0	3	2	6	13
	F	0	5	11	7	4	0	4	31
	P	0	0	0	1	0	3	0	4
	H	0	0	1	0	0	0	0	1
	N or n	2	3	14	4	5	7	9	44
	Total	2	10	26	12	12	12	19	93

W, weeks of paralysis; M, months of paralysis; S, electrical silence; F, fibrillation potential; P, polyphasic potential; H, high amplitude potential; n, normal potential (reduced in number); N, normal potential. When two or more different patterns were observed within a given muscle, the categorization in this table was made according to the following rule: F + S → F, P + x → P (x: any pattern), H + x → H, n + S and/or F → n, N + S and/or F → N.

(From Hirano M: Clinical Examination of Voice. New York, Springer-Verlag, 1981.)

derstanding of what the larynx does, but also of what it does not do. Optimal speech requires effective and coordinated function of the central nervous system, auditory system, muscles of respiration, lungs, nasal system, pharynx, mouth, teeth, sinuses, tongue, and larynx.

The vocal fold is a multilayered structure. The mechanical relationships between these layers determine the vibratory properties of the vocal fold and thus the quality of the phonation produced. Any proposed phonosurgery must take into account not only the effect on the position of the vocal fold as a whole, but also the effect on the mechanical relationships between its layers. This becomes particularly important in the selection of locations for vocal fold injections aimed at augmentation.

The vocal fold consists of the thyroarytenoid muscle with its covering of mucosa. The mucosa has two principal layers, epithelium and lamina propria. At the medial edge of the vocal fold, the lamina propria has three layers: superficial, intermediate, and deep. The movement of the vocal folds during phonation can be artificially divided into two types: (1) the gross shutter-like opening and closing of the vocal folds called postural movement; and (2) the cyclic movement of the mucosa on the surface of the vocal folds.

In addition to the gross inward and outward motion of the vocal folds that occurs with each cycle, the mucosa at the edge of the vocal folds undergoes characteristic cyclic changes in shape. Just before glottic opening, the edges of the vocal folds are sharp and meet along their superior border. As the vocal folds move apart, their edges flatten. As the folds start to move together, their inferior edges protrude briefly and then recede as the superior edges advance and meet before the start of the next vibratory cycle.

A theory of vocal fold motion that more closely approximates observation describes the vocal folds in three functional layers: (1) the cover, which consists of the epithelium and the superficial layer of the lamina propria, or Reinke's space; (2) the vocal ligamant, which consists of the confluence of the intermediate and deep layers of the lamina propria; and (3) the vocalis muscle. The cover is the most compliant layer and vibrates most during phonation. Scarring within this layer must be avoided because it can severely disturb the mucosal wave and thus the quality of the voice.

Perioperative Management

Numerous disease processes can negatively influence the results of phonosurgery. Because phonosurgery is elective, these conditions must be treated before surgery is performed. Preoperatively, all patients should discontinue tobacco use. Many patients benefit from an appropriate program of aerobic or vocal exercise. It is also important to optimize management of nutrition, diabetes, pulmonary disease, especially in patients

with chronic obstructive pulmonary disease (COPD), chronic allergy, and esophageal reflux. The benefits of the most technically suberb phonosurgery are likely to elude patients with either (1) inability to sustain phonation because of active COPD, vocal edema due to chronic allergy and smoking, or continued damage to the larynx due to persistent reflux or (2) a postoperative wound infection due to uncontrolled diabetes and poor nutrition. Postoperatively, some surgeons recommend a short period of voice rest (less than 1 week). Although this is probably not harmful, the benefit from complete vocal rest is not proved. Although whispering can be damaging and is not indicated after any phonosurgery, modified voice rest is recommended following surgery. This indicates a period of time during which extended speaking without adequate rest and loud phonation are avoided.

Unilateral Paralysis

Phonosurgical techniques include injections to augment the paralyzed vocal fold,[48-50] reinnervation of paralyzed portions of the larynx, denervation of dysfunctional portions, and deliberate alterations in the laryngeal framework.[51] Regardless of procedure, one must minimize damage to the normal mechanical properties of the vocal folds.

Before phonosurgery is done, a careful search must be made for the primary cause of the dysfunction. Failure to adduct a vocal fold may be due to surgical damage to the RLN, such as during thyroid or cancer surgery, or it may result from invasion of the nerve by tumor, from neuromuscular disorders, or from trauma to the glottis. Medializing the vocal fold of a patient without identifying the cancer invading the RLN is not appropriate. Procedures that are appropriate to perform while waiting for recovery and compensation include medialization thyroplasty and fat injection, which have less chance of causing permanent damage. Voice and swallowing therapy should be initiated during this period. For patients with known unresectable disease, such as advanced cancer invading the RLN, time should not be wasted, and phonosurgery, if desired, should proceed at once.

Surgery for Glottic Incompetence

Glottic closure is essential not only for phonation, but also for airway protection. Procedures to correct glottic insufficiency are of three major types: (1) reinnervation; (2) medialization; and (3) augmentation. Reinnervation techniques include nerve and nerve muscle pedicle transfer. In medialization, the inner perichondrium of the thyroid lamina is included in the tissues that are advanced. Augmentation only advances tissues medial to the inner perichondrium. Medialization procedures include those such as the Isshiki thyroplasty, which reshape the laryngeal framework. Examples of augmentation include injection of materials into or behind the vocal fold. With all techniques, a delicate balance must be reached: providing sufficient glottic closure for phonation and airway protection while leaving sufficient opening to allow respiration.

AUGMENTATION. Vocal fold injection places material within or behind the vocal fold to move it medially or to smooth its medial edge. It is usually performed under direct laryngoscopy with the patient awake to allow for intraoperative assessment of results. Topical 4% cocaine anesthesia is sufficient for most patients. Injection is accomplished with a Bruening syringe, which delivers about 0.2 ml of material with each click of its racheted piston. The injection must be in the plane of the vocal fold, and the vocal fold must advance evenly. One or two injection sites are usually sufficient.

Teflon paste is currently the preferred nonabsorbable susbstance for the treatment of unilateral adductor paralysis in patients with unresectable disease. Because a foreign material is introduced, granulomas and scarring can occur. In any case, the mechanical properties of the vocal folds may be altered. As a result, following Teflon injection, the voice may not return to its premorbid baseline. Teflon should be injected deep and lateral to the thyroarytenoid muscle to prevent extrusion and to minimize alteration of the mechanical properties of the vocal fold layers. Teflon injection in the anterior third of the vocal fold is rarely necessary and may compromise glottic closure. Rubbing the edge of the vocal fold with the shaft of the needle can help to distribute the Teflon evenly. This must be done at the initial procedure before encapsulation occurs. Inflammation following Teflon injection is usual. As this resolves, the results should approximate those observed intraoperatively. If postoperative evaluation reveals persistent undercorrection, repeat injection is possible. Although overcorrection may require tracheostomy, it can be treated with laser debulking, but phonation results are usually poor because of vocal fold scarring.

Disadvantages of Teflon are related to its irreversible nature, potential interference with mucosal wave if injected superficialy, paste migration (Fig. 31–5), and, most important, exclusion of future motor recovery.

Collagen injection is a preferred technique for correction of gaps caused by vocal fold atrophy and other small defects. Collagen should be injected superficially, into the deep layer of the lamina propria, to prevent rapid reabsorption. If this rule is followed, the correction present after 3 months tends to persist. Over time, collagen has a softening effect on the tissues, so reinjection at a later date is usually easy. This is especially useful when correcting a deficit in an area of dense scar tissue.

Gelfoam paste can be injected when only temporary results are desired. An effect lasting 6 weeks to 3 months is typical. Although scarring and deformation of the vocal fold can occur, this material is usually ab-

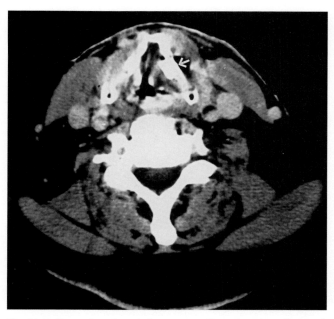

Fig. 31–5. Coronal section of a larynx revealing migration of injected teflon (arrow). (Courtesy of Dr. John A. Kirchner.)

sorbed, so no permanent damage is done if normal function returns to the vocal fold.

Autologous fat may prove to be an excellent substance for injection. It must be carefully harvested to prevent fat cell destruction and is injected into the vocalis muscle. Atrophy of the injected fat may prove a problem.

Vocal fold injection is a simple technique but is not without pitfalls. The ideal material for injection has not yet been found. Nonetheless, vocal fold injection can provide marked benefit for patients with glottic insufficiency causing aspiration, weak or absent cough, short maximum phonation time, breathy voice, insufficient loudness, and limited pitch range.[52–57]

MEDIALIZATION. Laryngeal framework surgery provides methods to medialize, separate, shorten, or lengthen the vocal folds. These techniques, referred to a thyroplasties type I through IV, respectively, were popularized by Isshiki and bear his name. The lateral compression test is useful for preoperative assessment of these patients if the laryngeal framework remains cartilagenous. In this maeuver, the examiner uses the thumb and forefinger to compress the thyroid ala medially while the patient sustains a vowel sound. Subjective and objective measures (i.e., maximum phonation time, videostroboscopy, acoustic analysis) of change, if any, are noted. If improvement is noted with the lateral compression test, then thyroplasty 1 (T-I) is almost always sucessful. T-I may still be successful even if no improvement is noted on manual compression, especially in older patients with ossified, inflexible thyroid cartilages.

Like vocal fold injection, thyroplasty is best per-

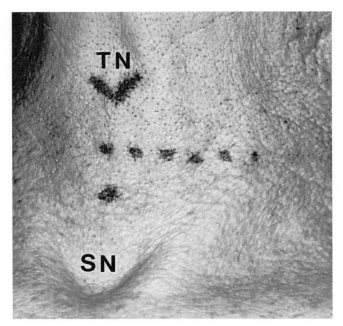

Fig. 31–6. Proposed horizontal skin incision overlying the middle left thyroid ala. TN, Thyroid notch; SN, sternal notch.

formed with the patient awake to allow intraoperative monitoring of results. The patient is placed supine on the operating room table. Intraoperative flexible fiberoptic laryngoscopy is used to verify the side of paralysis.

The entire procedure is accomplished under local anesthesia consisting of 0.5% lidocaine and 1:200,000 epinephrine. A 3- to 4-cm transverse incision is made along a skin crease overlying the involved thyroid ala

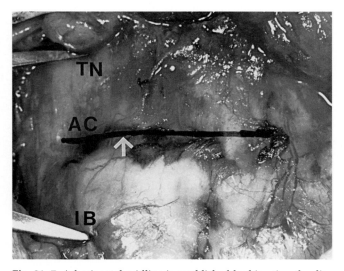

Fig. 31–7. A horizontal midline is established by bisecting the distance between the thyroid notch (TN) and the inferior border (IB) of the thyroid cartilage. The arrow identifies a point on the horizontal midline 5 mm lateral to the external position of the anterior commissure (AC).

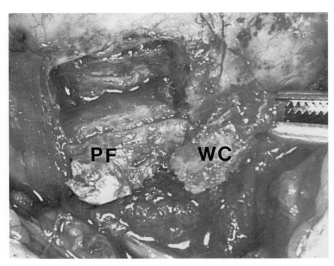

Fig. 31–8. An inferiorly based perichondrial flap (PF) is elevated, and a window of cartilage (WC) is removed.

from a point on the anterior cervical midline extending laterally (Fig. 31–6). Superior and inferior subplatysmal flaps are raised, and the dissection is carried through the strap muscles to the outer perichondrium of the thyroid cartilage ala.

Using a caliper, a horizontal midline of the thyroid ala is determined (Fig. 31–7). The size of the alar window for men measures 5 × 10 mm and 4 × 8 mm for women. The window is carefully positioned below the horizontal midline 5 mm from the anterior commissure (arrow).

An inferiorly based perichondrial flap is raised according to the calculated window dimensions (Fig. 31–8). The cartilage window is cut with a side-cutting bur (Brasseler US 700 84 shank cross-cut, tapered, fissure bur). Care is taken to avoid violating the inner alar perichondrium. The cartilage window is then removed, and the inner perichondrium is elevated from the medial surface of the thyroid cartilage using a Woodson elevator. Too high an elevation from the horizontal midline may lead to perforation at the laryngeal ventricle. A Silastic prosthesis is placed into the alar window (Fig. 31–9). With medial pressure applied to the prosthesis, the surgeon has the ability to adjust the depth of medialization to achieve maximum phonation time. When optimum medialization has been established, the prosthesis is scored flush with the outer perichondrium and is cut across with a scalpel to result in an embedded edge.

The inferior perichondrial flap is sutured back to its anatomic position with interrupted 5–0 nylon sutures (Fig. 31–10). The wound is closed in a two-layer fashion over a quarter-inch Penrose drain. Figure 31–11 demonstrates the medialized vocal fold seen on axial computed tomography (CT).

Advantages of T-I over Teflon injection include easy

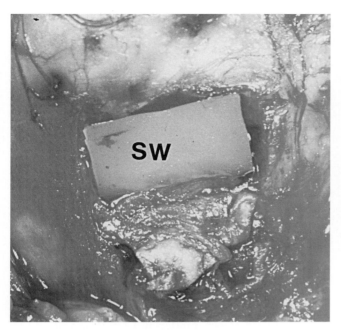

Fig. 31–9. A Silastic wedge (SW) is inserted to medialize the affected vocal fold.

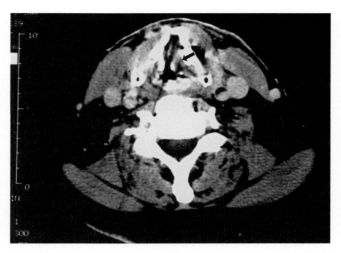

Fig. 31–11. Computed tomographic scan demonstrates a medialized vocal fold (arrow).

intraoperative adjustability and a degree of reversibility with 24 to 48 hours. Furthermore, in patients who may spontaneously recover neuromuscular function, corrective surgery can be performed before the usual 6- to 8-month waiting period. Moreover, because no surgery is performed directly on the vocal folds, their mechanical properties remain largely unaltered. T-I allows the medialization of the entire fold rather than an isolated or uneven segment often observed following many injection techniques.[58–69]

Following successful T-I, an immediate improve-

ment is seen both in breathiness and maximum phonation time. Over time, reductions in voice strain are also common. Long-term changes up to 4 years following T-I in 5 patients demonstrate a durable efficacy (Table 31–5).

REINNERVATION. Reinnervation techniques succeed to the degree that they can reproduce these normal characteristics.[67–75] A major problem following crush, transection, and reanastomosis, or severe stretch injury to the RLN is synkinesis. Following such injuries, regenerating adductor nerve fibers may reach abductor muscles and vice versa. This may lead to inappropriate, uncoordinated movements. Adduction may occur during inspiration or abduction during attempted phonation. More likely, however, the vocal fold may be immobile in a paramedian position because of simultaneous opposing abductor and adductor action. EMG combined with videostroboscopy of fiberoptic laryngoscopy is useful in examining motion control abnormalities.

Bilateral Vocal Fold Paralysis

Patients with bilateral vocal fold paralysis usually require treatment because of loss of abductor function

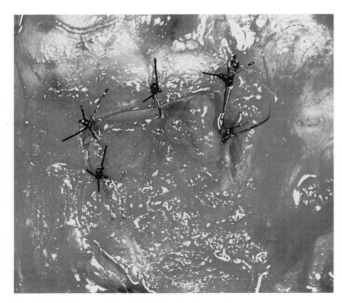

Fig. 31–10. The perichondrial flap is returned.

TABLE 31–5. Prethyroplasty Type I and Post-thyroplasty Type I Group Means (and standard deviations) for Voice Fo, Intensity, and MPT

		Prethyroplasty (N = 5)	Postthyroplasty (N = 5)
Fo (Hz)	$\overline{X}$	135.1	191.4*
	SD	(23.7)	(39.2)
Intensity (dB)	$\overline{X}$	49.8	43.6*
	SD	(7.7)	(6.5)
MPT (s)	$\overline{X}$	5.7	9.8†
	SD	(2.9)	(3.3)

* $p < 0.01$ (two-tailed).
† $p < 0.05$ (one-tailed).

leading to airway obstruction. Not only is the glottic chink narrowed by the resting position of the vocal folds, but also, with inspiration, the Bernoulli effect causes the folds to move medially as the velocity of the airflow increases. Surgical treatment of this problem usually involves one of three strategies: (1) bypassing the site of obstruction; (2) increasing the caliber of the airway; (3) or attempting to restore abductor function. In weighing treatment options, points to consider include effectiveness, preservation of vocal quality, and possible complications.

TRACHEOSTOMY. Tracheostomy bypasses the site of obstruction, providing immediate, effective treatment. Although long-term tracheostomy may be less appealing than other treatments, it often plays a role in the treatment of acute bilateral vocal fold paralysis by stabilizing the patient. When quick recovery of function is expected, it may be possible to avoid operation altogether with the use of continuous positive airway pressure to splint the airway.[76] In other cases, tracheostomy may be useful as an interim treatment, allowing other techniques to be performed under less pressing circumstances.

INCREASING AIRWAY CALIBER. Techniques for enlarging the airway usually involve lateralization of one of the vocal folds and/or the removal of tissue, particularly from the posterior glottis. Work by Hirano and colleagues has shown that the posterior glottis accounts for 50 to 65% of the area of the total glottis.[77] Thus, enlarging the posterior glottis has a greater effect on the airway while preserving vocal quality. These techniques have been applied using both transcervical and endoscopic approaches.

TRANSCERVICAL APPROACHES. Chevalier Jackson used the midline thyrotomy to resect the vocal fold and ventricle in 1922, resulting in a satisfactory airway but a poor-quality voice.[78] Subsequent techniques that used a laryngofissure included cordopexy,[79] submucous resection of the vocal fold,[80] and arytenoidectomy with cordopexy.[81] Later, this approach was used to perform arytenoidectomy alone,[82] without lateralization, which was successful in expanding the airway while preserving voice.[83] In 1946, Woodman[84] modified a lateral open approach used by King[85] and Kelly[86] to perform arytenoidectomy, avoiding laryngofissure. While the arytenoid was excised, the vocal process was preserved and used to lateralize the cord by suturing it to the lesser cornu of the thyroid cartilage.

ENDOSCOPIC APPROACHES. Thornell introduced the endoscopic arytenoidectomy in 1948.[87] Good results have been reported with this procedure, and it has been widely used. El Chazly and associates reported better airway results when posterior cordectomy was added to arytenoidectomy, although vocal quality was reportedly impaired.[88] Problems with hemostasis during traditional endoscopic arytenoidectomy were overcome with the introduction of the carbon dioxide laser

arytenoidectomy by Ossoff and colleagues in 1984.[89] They reported a success rate of 86% for this procedure, which includes vaporization of a portion of the vocalis muscle as well as the arytenoid.[90] In contrast, a procedure that involves vaporization of only the medial portion of the arytenoid has been described in patients with more moderate airway compromise.[91] This procedure is reportedly superior in preserving voice and can be done as a staged bilateral procedure if necessary. Rontal and Rontal also reported preservation of arytenoid mass by resecting the vocal process alone but also cutting the interarytenoid muscle at its point of attachment to the arytenoid.[92]

Some endoscopic techniques do not involve arytenoidectomy. Kirchner described a procedure in which he resected a portion of the thyroarytenoid muscle and then lateralized the vocal fold with temporary sutures.[93] Success has also been reported for endoscopic lateralization with permanent sutures without any tissue resection.[94] Other techniques have made use of the carbon dioxide laser. Linder and Lindholm described using the laser to reduce the bulk of the vocal fold laterally, followed by fibrin glue to maintain it in the lateral position.[95] The laser has also been used to remove a portion of the posterior vocal fold,[96] most recently by Dennis and Kashima, who created a crescent-shaped 3.5- to 4-mm defect anterior to the vocal process.[97] Even less tissue was removed with the subsequent development of transverse cordotomy, in which the incision anterior to the vocal process leads to the development of a wedge-shaped defect as the thyroarytenoid muscle retracts.[98]

RESTORATION OF FUNCTION. The techniques described previously often involve a trade-off between airway and vocal quality. Thus, the ideal treatment of bilateral vocal fold paralysis remains restoration of function with reinnervation. Direct repair of the injured RLN did not lead to satisfactory results; vocal fold motion tended to be uncoordinated and synkinetic.[99–101] Better results were obtained in animals with selective reinnervation of the laryngeal abductor muscle, the posterior cricoarytenoid (PCA).[102] Use of a cable graft directly to the PCA was not successful in humans, however.[103] A more successful procedure has been the use of a nerve-muscle pedicle based on the ansa hypoglossi to reinnervate the PCA.[104] In 1989, Tucker reported a long-term success rate of 74% with more than 200 patients with bilateral vocal fold paralysis, with success based on the rate of decannulation.[105,106] Other centers have not been able to achieve such good results with this method, however. Another strategy for restoring function in bilateral RLN paralysis involves the use of electrical pacing devices.[107] Such devices have not yet been tested in humans, however.

In summary, tracheostomy and endoscopic procedures, particularly those that make use of the carbon dioxide laser, are the mainstays of treatment for bilateral vocal fold paralysis. Because of the trade-off often involved between airway and vocal quality, however, much research continues to focus on the development of techniques to restore function to the larynx.

Laryngeal Paralysis and Aspiration

Vocal fold paralysis alone, whether unilateral or bilateral, rarely results in aspiration. When vocal fold paralysis occurs in conjunction with other motor or sensory dysfunction, however, the combination may significantly impair the protective function of the larynx, leading to aspiration. Neurogenic causes of aspiration may include cerebrovascular accidents, degenerative diseases, neuromuscular disorders, peripheral nerve disorders, intracranial neoplasms, and anoxic or traumatic brain injury.[108]

Evaluation of the patient with aspiration begins with a thorough history and physical examination and requires multidisciplinary evaluation.[109] The history should elicit information about symptoms of any associated neurogenic disorder as well as information about respiratory symptoms that may indicate the degree of severity of aspiration. Physical examination should include visualization of the larynx. Other testing should include chest radiography and modified barium swallow,[45] using contrast material of different consistencies performed under the supervision of a speech-language pathologist.

Nonsurgical management of the patient with aspiration usually consists of discontinuing oral intake and providing alternative methods of alimentation. Enteral alimentation is preferable and may be provided with a nasogastric feeding tube. For long-term feeding, however, gastrostomy or jejunostomy may be performed. Attention should also be given to pulmonary toilet. Tracheostomy may be helpful in caring for patients with copious secretions; however, the presence of a tracheostomy may also contribute to problems with aspiration.[46,47]

Specific surgical treatment of the patient with significant aspiration and vocal fold paralysis includes a variety of procedures to medialize the vocal fold discussed elsewhere in this chapter.[47,48] In patients in whom recovery of function is expected, procedures that are temporary or reversible are indicated, such as Gelfoam paste injection[49,50] or thyroplasty.[51]

Other surgical techniques are not specifically directed at treatment of vocal fold dysfunction; rather, they involve separation of the upper digestive tract from the upper respiratory tract. Unfortunately, patients undergoing such procedures frequently lose the ability to phonate and may also require permanent tracheostomy. Such procedures can be performed with low morbidity, however, and some of these procedures are at least theoretically reversible should function return.

Narrow-field laryngectomy remains the oldest and one of the most effective surgical treatments of aspiration. Tracheoesophageal puncture can be used to restore phonation. Reluctance to sacrifice an otherwise normal larynx has led to the development of other procedures to close the larynx. Montgomery described a glottic closure technique in which the true and false vocal cords were approximated.[110] Closure was improved by Sasaki and associates with the interposition of a sternohyoid muscle flap.[111] This procedure was extremely effective but did not permit phonation, which was sometimes possible with supraglottic laryngeal closure methods. Since first being described in 1972,[112] the epiglottic flap closure technique has undergone certain modifications, including intentionally leaving an opening posteriorly to permit phonation.[113] Successful reversal of this procedure has been reported by an endoscopic approach.[114] Biller and colleagues have also described a supraglottic closure technique, vertical laryngoplasty, intended for use in patients undergoing total glossectomy.[115] This method also permits speech.

Efforts to devise a procedure that is completely reversible have led to the development of different endolaryngeal stents. Weisberger and Huebsch used a solid Silastic stent in conjunction with a tracheostomy,[116] whereas Eliachar and Nguyen devised vented silicone stents that permit phonation.[117] Advantages of stenting include the use of the endoscopic approach and ease of reversibility. Successful control of aspiration has not been uniform, however, and long-term use of stents carries the risk of endolaryngeal injury, limiting their utility.

Tracheoesophageal diversion was developed by Lindeman with the goal of controlling aspiration definitively while preserving the larynx and RLNs and thus the potential for reversal.[118] In this procedure, the trachea is divided at the level of the fourth or fifth ring. The proximal trachea is anastomosed to the esophagus, whereas the distal trachea is anastomosed to the skin. Thus, aspirated secretions are diverted back into the gastrointestinal tract. This procedure is not possible in patients who have previously undergone high tracheostomy. In the modified laryngotracheal separation procedure, the proximal segment is instead closed as a blind pouch.[119] Both techniques have provided good control of aspiration, and both have been successfully reversed.[120,121]

Because no current method is completely satisfactory, investigations continue in an attempt to find a safe, effective means of controlling aspiration without disrupting respiratory or phonatory function. One possibility for the future may be implantable electronic systems now being developed in animals that can produce tight glottic closure during swallow.[122]

FUNCTIONAL VOICE DISORDERS

The term functional voice disorders has been used to designate voice disorders that are thought to be (1) of unknown origin, that is, idiopathic, (2) due to misuse of the larynx for voice production (abnormal patterns used for voice production), or (3) psychogenic, resulting from psychologic difficulties interfering with voice production.

Often, the term functional voice disorder is used when a patient's voice disorder cannot be diagnosed as the result of a disease process, a structural abnormality, or a neurogenic disorder. These disorders, therefore, are by definition, voice production disorders of unknown origin. Many have distinctive symptom patterns allowing their recognition as separate disorders and respond differently to treatment, however. Some of these disorders, such as essential voice tremor and adductor spasmodic dysphonia, are thought to be focal laryngeal dystonias,[123] that is, neurogenic disorders possibly due to basal ganglia dysfunction. No studies have demonstrated neural dysfunctions that could be used for diagnosis in all patients having these voice production disorders, however.[124–127] Therefore, the identification of these disorders continues to be by voice production characteristics alone,[128] as is the case for the other voice function disorders.[129–131] Because diagnosis is based on behavioral characteristics, consensus is not available regarding their diagnosis even among the large, well-recognized voice centers. Because of the efficacy of botulinum toxin injection for controlling symptoms in adductor spasmodic dysphonia, diagnosis has become important for determining whether such treatment is warranted.

Idiopathic Disorders

In this group of voice disorders, volitional control of vocal fold movement during the specific types of movement is affected, such as speaking in the spasmodic dysphonias and respiration in paradoxic vocal fold movement.

Spasmodic Dysphonias

The spasmodic dysphonias include[128] either adductor spasmodic dysphonia (excessive or uncontrolled closing of the vocal folds), abductor or breathy spasmodic dysphonia (prolonged or excessive vocal fold opening for voiceless sounds extending into vowels),[132] or vocal fold tremor (most evident during prolonged vowels).[133] These problems may be manifested by involuntary changes in pitch control (pitch breaks) or the inability to maintain voicing during speech without having intermittent glottal catches (voice breaks due to adductions) or breathy breaks due to uncontrolled vocal fold abductions. Often, the problem first appears with a specific task,[134] gesture, or posturing of the larynx, such as vowel production during speech, and then it may progress to interfere with other tasks or postures such as singing and speaking using falsetto. In mild to moderate forms of spasmodic dysphonia, patients may

have uncontrolled spasms affecting the speaking voice, but they can have normal singing and falsetto phonation.

Onset usually follows an upper respiratory infection, laryngeal injury, a period of excessive voice use, or occupational or emotional stress.[135] Increased effort is one of the major patient complaints as well as loss of control and an increased difficulty with prolonged voice use and practice or stress. Usually, patients are between 30 and 50 years of age, and at least 60% of those affected are women. Puzzling to both the patients and professionals are the following characteristics of these disorders:

1. They are specific to a particular task, gesture, or posture of the larynx.
2. They are action induced, that is they appear only with voluntary movement and are not usually apparent either at rest or during less skilled or slow movements.
3. They become worse with prolonged speaking, practice, or performance.
4. Onset is usually gradual, often following some upper respiratory infection, inflammation, or stressful event.
5. Reflexive and emotional aspects of function are unaffected, such as coughing and laughter.
6. In professional voice users, they may appear with heavy professional schedules, new performance demands, or following injury.

Sometimes, during the early stages of the disorder, some degree of vocal fold asymmetry is apparent, suggesting injury within the first months.[136–138] With time, this asymmetry often disappears, but the disorder remains.

These disorders affect voluntary motor control. Movement abnormalities occur when the patient attempts specific gestures such as phonation of vowels in adductor spasmodic dysphonia, voiceless consonants (such as s, h, f, t, k) followed by vowels in abductor spasmodic dysphonia, or a particular part of the pitch range in vocal tremor.

No information is available on the origin of these disorders. Sometimes they occur in persons with a family history of dystonia.[123] In clinics specializing in voice disorders, however, few patients with spasmodic dysphonia have a positive family history of dystonia.

DIAGNOSIS AND ASSESSMENT. Because these movement disorders affect the larynx, diagnosis depends on observing the vocal folds during movement and production of the affected task, speaking. In addition, the larynx must be visualized to rule out other disorders that could account for the symptoms. Fiberoptic nasolaryngoscopy allows the voice team, usually an otolaryngologist, a speech-language pathologist, and a neurologist to rule out vocal fold nodules, polyps, carcinoma, cysts, contact ulcers, inflammation (laryngitis), and vocal fold paralysis. A neurologic examination is necessary to rule out ALS, Parkinson's disease, and supranuclear palsy, which can all produce similar vocal fold movement abnormalities.[139] Some patients may also have concomitant focal dystonias such as writer's cramp or blepharospasm, which can be successfully managed by a neurologist. Many patients may have some degree of laryngeal tremor in addition to spasmodic hyperadduction or hyperabduction. These patients are usually included as a subtype of the spasmodic dysphonias[140–142] and may have a more severe disorder.[124]

Extensive history taking, a trial of voice therapy, and a psychosocial interview are needed to rule out psychogenic dysphonia.[143–145] Often, a patient has developed several reactions to poor speaking control by the time of professional diagnosis, and these reactions confound the ability to differentiate idiopathic spasmodic dysphonia from psychogenic disorders through history and interview. For example, many patients no longer use the telephone and avoid social gatherings as a result of their disorder.

TASKS TO BE EXAMINED DURING FIBEROPTIC LARYNGOSCOPY. Both speech and nonspeech tasks must be sampled to identify (1) movement control abnormalities during vocal fold abduction (opening) and adduction (closing) in speech and (2) normal movement during nonspeech activities such as respiration, sniffing, and throat clearing. This is in contrast to paradoxic vocal fold movement disorder, in which vocal fold abnormalities only appear during inspiration. Movement characteristics seen during fiberoptic examination are described in Table 31–6.

Further, these movements are often useful when examining many of the neurogenic disorders that affect vocal fold movement, altering either the symmetry of vocal fold movement during both adduction and abduction or the range of motion. Usually, stroboscopy is not helpful; in patients with tremor or spasms during prolonged vowels, the phonatory cycle is not regular enough for tracking, and the mucosal wave cannot be seen. In patients with muscular tension dysphonia, the constant hoarseness similarly interferes with tracking.

SPEECH TESTING. Voice symptoms should be compared during three tasks to discriminate among adductor spasmodic dysphonia, abductor spasmodic dysphonia, and vocal tremor.

1. Prolonged vowel phonation usually manifests tremor if it is present; prolonged vowel production is affected only in the more severe forms of adductor and abductor spasmodic dysphonia.
2. Production of sentences in which all the sounds are voiced, such as "We mow our lawn all year" and "We eat eels everyday," are usually most difficult and demonstrate frequent breaks or voice arrest in adductor spasmodic dysphonia.
3. Production of sentences with voiceless consonants (s, t, p, k, h), "She speaks pleasingly," "Keep Tom at the party," "When he comes home we'll feed him," are usually most difficult in abductor spasmodic dysphonia. Sentences with predominantly voiced sounds are much easier to produce and smoother for these patients.

ELECTROMYOGRAPHY. The laryngeal muscle activation abnormalities that can produce problems of vocal motor control differ greatly among patients and can account for the wide variety of symptoms manifested.[124,146] The laryngeal muscles should be examined to determine which muscles contain spasms concurrent with a patient's voice symptoms. In adductor spasmodic dysphonia,[147,148] the thyroarytenoid is that most often considered to be affected. In abductor spasmodic dysphonia,[132] spasms can be seen in the cricothyroid in some patients, in the posterior cricoarytenoid in others, or in combinations of either of these muscles with the strap muscles such as the sternothyroid. In some patients with abductor spasmodic dysphonia, however, the voice symptoms are associated with reduced activation in the thyroarytenoid muscles. In vocal tremor, a variety of muscles can be involved.[149] Most often, the thyroarytenoid is affected, but other muscles including the strap muscles can be affected, including the thyrohyoid, the sternothyroid, and in some patients with abductor tremor, either the cricothyroid or the posterior cricoarytenoid, or both.

By using a concentric EMG electrode connected to an amplifier with a dual-channel storage oscilloscope and slow sweep speed, quick identification can be made of the muscles having spasms during voice breaks. EMG techniques are described in greater detail elsewhere.[12,150–152]

For the thyroarytenoid and interarytenoid muscles, speech items to be examined for spasmodic bursts concurrent with voice and pitch breaks include prolonged ee, repeated ee and all voiced sentences such as "We mow our lawn all year." For the cricothyroid, posterior cricoarytenoid, thyrohyoid, and sternothyroid, speech items to be examined include "see-see-see," "pea-pea-pea," "he-he-he," "Kathy took a potato," and "Keep Tom at the party." The occurrence of bursts of muscle activity during speech preceding voice and pitch breaks is the basis for the name designating spasmodic dysphonia.[148,153]

TREATMENT. In the last 10 years, the following treatments have been used for managing symptoms in adductor spasmodic dysphonia.

VOICE THERAPY. This can assist the patient in learning to alter the abnormal pattern of movements so the spasmodic abnormalities are not elicited when the patient proceeds to speak. This therapy is most successful in milder cases and frequently does not have long-lasting effects, but it has the advantage of not causing injury.

TABLE 31–6. Movement Characteristics Observed During Fiberoptic Laryngoscopy in Various Types of Functional Voice Disorders

Task	Movement Examined	Adductor SD	Abductor SD	Tremor Adductor	Tremor Abductor	Paradoxical Vocal Fold Movement Disorder	Muscular Tension Dysphonia
Deep inhalation	Abduction range	Normal abduction	May be increased	Normal	May have tremor	Vocal fold adduction	Normal
Prolonged vowel "ee"	Adduction for voice	Normal or intermittent hyper-adductions	Normal	Repetitive hyper-adductions (5 Hz)	Repetitive abductions (5 Hz)	Normal	Constant hyper-adduction
Throat clear 3 times	Adduction	Normal	Normal	Normal	Normal	Normal	Normal
Whisper	Vocal fold partial abduction	May have hyper-adduction	May have increased abduction	Normal	May have tremor	Normal	May have constant adduction
Whistling	Vocal fold abduction and adduction	Normal	Normal	Normal	Normal	Normal	Normal
Repeated and quick sniffs	Speed of abduction	Normal	May be increased in range	Normal	May have tremor on abduction	Adduction on sniff	Normal
Alternating between sniff and vowel "ee"	Speed and range of abduction and adduction	Intermittent hyper-adduction on vowel	Normal	Tremor on vowel	Tremor on vowel	May have hyper-adduction on sniff	Constant hyper-adduction on vowel
Rapid repetition of vowel "ee" 6 times	Phonation offset due to glottal stop	Prolonged glottal stops	Normal	Tremor on vowel	Tremor on vowel	Normal	Constant hyper-adduction with antero-posterior squeeze
Rapid repetition of "see" 6 times	Speed of abduction and adduction	Normal or intermittent adductions on vowel	Prolonged abductions during "s"	Adductor tremor on vowel	Abductor tremor on vowel	Normal	Constant hyper-adduction
Ascending and descending glides	Controlled lengthening and shortening of folds	Normal or intermittent adductions on low end	Normal	Adductor tremor on low end	Abductor tremor	Normal	Constant hyper-adduction
Sentences: "We eat eels everyday"	Glottal stops in sentences	Prolonged glottal stops	Normal	Adductor tremor	Abductor tremor	Normal	Constant hyper-adduction
"The waves were rolling along"	Constant voicing in sentences	Intermittent spasms in vowels	Normal	Adductor tremor	Abductor tremor	Normal	Constant hyper-adduction
"He will keep the keys"	Voiceless consonants in sentences	Normal	Prolonged voiceless consonants "he," "k"	Adductor tremor	Abductor tremor	Normal	Constant hyper-adduction

When uncertain of the diagnosis of a patient's voice disorder, a trial of voice therapy is recommended. Usually within three sessions, a speech-language pathologist will report whether voice therapy might be beneficial for a patient.

INHALATION VOICE THERAPY. This therapeutic technique of speaking on inhalation is sometimes helpful in mild to moderate cases; it may not have long-lasting effects, and it may not produce a normal voice. This technique is difficult for some patients to learn, given that they often have respiratory control problems as well.

RECURRENT LARYNGEAL NERVE SECTION. This procedure has dramatic initial results but has a return of symptoms in 60% of cases,[154] causes long-standing unilateral vocal fold paralysis, and sometimes has respiratory complications.[155]

THYROPLASTY, ISSHIKI TYPE 3. This surgical approach pushes the thyroid keel posteriorly, thus shortening and adducting the vocal folds.[156] In most cases, this can be detrimental to the voice and results in pitch lowering. This surgery cannot be easily reversed because of the long-term effects of fibrosis and scarring. Because other more successful approaches are available, it is not recommended for patients with adductor spasmodic dysphonia.

BOTULINUM TOXIN. This approach was developed in 1987[157] and has been evaluated using unilateral or bilateral thyroarytenoid injection in adductor spasmodic dysphonia.[158–160] The results seem excellent, with restoration of normal voice in 70% of patients for up to 3 months, followed by gradual symptom return within 4 to 5 months. Because the effect is temporary, this regimen can be used on a trial basis in certain muscles in a particular patient. At 3-month intervals, injections can be administered in different muscle combinations to identify the correct muscles and dosage to be used for a particular patient.

The most commonly used method of injection is the percutaneous EMG-guided approach through the cricothyroid membrane.[159] The injection needle is Teflon coated except for the bared tip, which serves as a monopolar EMG electrode when the bared hub is connected to a physiologic amplifier. This allows monitoring for a characteristic physiologic signal to determine that the needle tip is located in muscle before injecting. Because the monopolar electrode has a large recording field and may pick up signals from any of the laryngeal adductor muscles in the region, however, such monitoring is not necessarily specific for the targeted thyroarytenoid muscles.[12]

To approach the thyroarytenoid percutaneously, the needle is passed through the cricothyroid membrane and is angled superiorly and slightly laterally to approximate the mediolateral aspect of the vocalis portion of the thyroarytenoid muscle.[150] The needle tip can easily be placed more posteriorly than intended, however, medial to the lateral cricoarytenoid muscle and mediosuperior to the cricothyroid muscle.[161] This can be seen in coronal sections of the adult human larynx.[162] From this, it is apparent that posteriorly placed injections may denervate portions of the lateral cricoarytenoid and cricothyroid muscles, in addition to the thyroarytenoid either by direct injection of these muscles or by diffusion across fascial planes.[163] This could account for the variability in response that is often seen (1) among patients and (2) in the same patient from consecutive EMG-guided injections several

months apart, even though the same technique and dosages are used.

Two approaches have been used, either large, unilateral injections producing unilateral vocal fold paralysis[164] or small, bilateral injections not altering the range of vocal fold movement on either side.[165] The advantage of the unilateral injection technique is that muscles on only one side of the larynx are affected by botulinum toxin. The long-term effects of repeated-needle insertion and repeated denervation by botulinum toxin on laryngeal muscles are as yet unknown. Muscle biopsies in blepharospasm patients treated repeatedly with botulinum toxin injection have demonstrated significant muscle scarring and atrophy.[166–168] Similar changes in both thyroarytenoid muscles could have long-term effects on airway protection. The disadvantages of the unilateral injection approach are that a large dose of toxin must be administered and immobility of the injected fold often results.[164]

The advantage of the bilateral approach is that much smaller doses of botulinum toxin can be used, reducing the cost. Further, effective symptom control can be obtained without any observable change in range of motion. Partial denervation seems to be effective in reducing the degree of hyperadduction, resulting in less interference with phonation. The disadvantages are that injections and needle insertions are performed on both sides of the larynx. With repeated injections every 4 to 6 months over many years, damage might result to both sides of the larynx, reducing airway closure and protection during swallowing. Another difficulty with the bilateral approach is that if symptom control is not obtained with the usual dosage of 2.5 U on each side, further bilateral injections have the risk of causing bilateral adductor paralysis. With unilateral injections, repeated injection at higher dosages can be administered without danger of aspiration.

Other injection techniques that use visualization of the vocal folds rather than EMG to guide placement of the injection needle are the indirect laryngoscopic peroral method[169] and the transcartilaginous method.[170] The availability of the flexible fiberoptic nasolaryngoscope with a working channel has made possible an endoscopic method of injecting the thyroarytenoid muscle using a flexible catheter needle.[171] The usual dosages used by each technique are presented in Table 31–7.

Within 5 days of botulinum toxin injection into the thyroarytenoid muscle, the numbers of breaks in phonation on vowels are reduced, the presence of voice roughness or hoarseness is reduced on spectrographic analyses, and speech rate is increased.[164] Patients' subjective reports include a reduction in speech effort and tension, reduced numbers of breaks, and greater voice control.[172] Two major side effects are reported, breathiness and swallowing difficulties. These side ef-

TABLE 31–7. Dosages Used for Unilateral and Bilateral Injection of the Thyroarytenoid Muscle in Adductor Spasmodic Dysphonia

Unilateral/Bilateral	EMG Guided[159] (U)	Injection Technique Peroral[169] (U)	Transcartilagenous[170] (U)	Endoscopic[171] (U)
Unilateral	15[164]	2.5		6
Bilateral	2.5 each[165]	2.5 +3 opposite	2 each	2 each
Totals	5	5.5	4	4

Superscript numbers refer to references in the Suggested Readings list of this chapter.

fects do not occur in all patients, but they can be significant in males following bilateral injections.[172]

Caution should be exercised in the use of botulinum toxin, particularly in undiagnosed patients with functional voice disorders. In such patients, the injections should be as small as possible (see Table 31–7) and combined with voice training. The injections should only be in those muscles demonstrated to be affected through a thorough EMG study during patient performance of affected and unaffected tasks.

Although botulinum toxin injections have been employed in abductor spasmodic dysphonia in both the cricothyroid muscles[132] and the posterior cricoarytenoid,[173] only a proportion of patients are helped, and the duration of benefit is reduced.[172]

The effects of vocal tremor on voice production can also be reduced by botulinum toxin injection.[172] In those patients with tremor affecting only the vocal folds and involving just the thyroarytenoid muscles, this treatment can be as effective as in adductor spasmodic dysphonia. However, many patients with this disorder have involvement of the strap muscles[149] and have limited benefit even when these additional muscles are injected.

Paradoxic Vocal Fold Movement

Paradoxic vocal fold movement is the adduction of the vocal folds during the inspiratory phase of respiration producing either a complete stoppage of air or stridor. These patients have normal vocal fold movement during speech, however, and often can inspire during and between phrases while speaking. Several different categories of patients with these disorders have been recognized: (1) as an idiopathic focal dystonia, or part of Meige syndrome (oral facial dyskinesia[174]); (2) associated with or masquerading as asthma[175]; (3) exercise-induced stridor[176]; (4) psychogenic[177,178]; and (5) associated with gastroesophageal reflux.[179]

These movement disorders are rare but have become increasingly recognized in the last 5 years. Most of these patients were previously diagnosed as having psychogenic disorders,[175,177,178,180,181] although it is becoming apparent that some are not.[174,182] The first presentation of this as a focal laryngeal dystonia specific to inspiration suggested that in some pa-

tients this was not psychogenic, but rather due to involuntary spasmodic bursts in the thyroarytenoid muscle.[174] Patients with a focal dystonia report that the symptoms are not present during sleep, but the symptoms are almost always present during the daytime, when they may become exacerbated by exercise and stress. Treatment with botulinum toxin is difficult because swallowing problems can be experienced as a result.[183] Some success has been reported in selected cases not responsive to speech therapy, psychotherapy, and pharmacotherapy.[174,184]

Patients with Meige syndrome, an oral facial dyskinesia, can develop pharyngeal spasms producing intermittent airway obstruction, either because of pharyngeal constriction or obstruction at the epiglottis. Often, the cricopharyngeus muscle is overly active in these patients. Again, the symptoms are absent during sleep and are almost always present during the day, but they are exacerbated by stress.

Patients with chronic asthma can have laryngeal vocal fold adduction during asthmatic attacks.[176,182] Whether this is due to psychologic overlay, whether it is a learned response, or whether it is a dystonic abnormality is unknown, however. Exercise-induced asthma has also been reported to have a laryngeal adduction component.[176]

Most cases on paradoxic vocal fold dysfunction causing stridor or episodes of airway obstruction have been reported as psychogenic.[175,177,178,180,181] In these patients, the symptoms abate following psychotherapy and speech therapy.

Koufman suggested that gastroesophageal reflux is a common cause of paroxysmal laryngospasms.[179] He reported on 12 patients who presented with intermittent, sudden-onset, noisy obstructed breathing that some patients termed choking episodes. These attacks of stridor often occurred following a meal, after the start of exercise, or after bending over. Sometimes they occurred at night. Some patients had them up to twice a day; other patients had them much less frequently, only a few a year. These attacks usually only lasted a few minutes. All complained of symptoms of reflux such as a lump in the throat, chronic throat clearing, cough, intermittent hoarseness, and difficulty in swallowing. He reported that all responded well to lifestyle modification and omeprazole, 20 mg twice daily.

Disorders of Misuse

Disorders of misuse are often thought of as psychogenic; however, these disorders are best conceptualized as disorders of muscle misuse.[130]

Muscular Tension Dysphonia

This disorder complex was first described by Morrison and his colleagues,[185,186] as dysphonia resulting from increased muscular tension in the larynx and neck associated with (1) palpably increased phonatory muscle tension in the paralaryngeal and suprahyoid muscles, (2) elevation of the larynx in the neck on increasing vocal pitch, (3) an open posterior glottic chink between the arytenoid cartilages on phonation, and (4) variable degrees of mucosal changes such as vocal nodules or chronic laryngitis. Morrison later named this "laryngeal isometric" to denote the high level of generalized muscle tension in all the laryngeal muscles.[130] These patients often have a high level of anxiety and may have learned an abnormal pattern of laryngeal muscle use. Aronson includes these patients as psychogenic voice disorders and recommends laryngeal maneuvering, progressive relaxation, and voice training going through several stages from simple to more complex voice production.[128]

Other variants of vocal misuse due to muscle tension include lateral to medial hypercontraction, which produces a tense harsh voice with high laryngeal resistance. This posture of the larynx may be triggered by an infection or chronic reflux and is often associated with erythema or diffuse thickening of the mucosa. These poor vocal habits can be reversed by therapy working directly on changing vocal posture and technique. Fiberoptic videotaping can be an instructive feedback tool.

Supraglottic hyperconstriction is a third variant of muscular tension. Hyperadduction of the ventricular folds along with the vocal folds produces a squeaky voice with a great deal of effort. Rarely, phonation is produced at the ventricular folds, but most often both the vocal folds and ventricular folds are involved in voice production.

Anteroposterior supraglottic contraction produces a "pinhole" type larynx in the most severe form with no voice, or an anteroposterior shortening in milder forms that results in a rough, hoarse, low-pitched voice.

The cause of these misuse disorders is unknown; rarely are these patients' voice production abnormalities helped by psychologic counseling. Usually, they respond to voice reeducation and life-management counseling to change their patterns of voice use.

The distinction between these patients and adductor spasmodic dysphonia is the degree to which the abnormal laryngeal posture is used consistently for voice production (see Table 31–6). In muscular tension dysphonia and other variants of vocal misuse, the abnormal vocal fold positioning seen on fiberoptic videoendoscopy is consistent regardless of the type of speech. In the spasmodic dysphonias, the abnormalities are intermittent, depending on the voicing gesture required and contain irregular rapid adductor or abductor movements causing intermittent voice breaks. In benign essential tremor, these intermittent voice breaks are regular, usually around 5 Hz. In some of the more extreme forms of spasmodic dysphonia or muscular tension dysphonia, however, the differentiation can be difficult because the spasmodic involuntary movement abnormalities may be difficult to identify when patients have extreme muscular tension. Whenever a possibility of either diagnosis exists, a trial of voice therapy by a speech-language pathologist experienced in treatment of these disorders is recommended, before considering botulinum toxin. If botulinum toxin is used, a combined regimen of voice therapy following injection can be helpful in training patients to eliminate those abnormal postures that may be contributing to their voice disorder in addition to the spasmodic involuntary movements.

Voice Fatigue Syndrome

This disorder is only diagnosed after other disorders have been excluded, including myasthenia gravis, Parkinson's disease, ALS, muscle atrophy associated with aging, Epstein-Barr virus, and sulcus vocalis. When a misuse disorder is present, patients use excessive muscular tension in one muscle group that interferes with voice production for extended periods. Often, patients must use their voice for authority or change their use for special demands such as classroom teaching. The patient then complains about the loss of voice and fatigue by the end of the day. Fiberoptic videotaping can be beneficial in retraining normal voice production. Voice fatigue can also be associated with aging, when an apparent loss of muscle bulk can become apparent. If neurogenic disease can be excluded, then a regimen of increased physical exercise can often be beneficial in increasing voice function.

Abnormal Loudness

This can be identified as a misuse disorder when patients have increased and excessive loudness, often when they have experienced a rapid diminution in their hearing or that of a family member. These patients may have assumed abnormal voice production patterns with excessive tension similar to the variants of muscular tension dysphonia.

Abnormal Pitch

The continuation of a high pitch sometimes remains in males following pubescent voice change. This can also be referred to as puberphonia or mutational falsetto. The misuse of a tense elongated vocal fold position during voicing can be seen. Often, when this condition continues into adulthood, it is difficult to reverse because the misuse has become part of the voicing gesture. Laryngeal maneuvering can sometimes be successful in reducing the abnormal posturing.[128] The combination of an initial treatment with botulinum toxin into the cricothyroid muscles in association with voice retraining can be beneficial in patients with the most resistant form.

False Vocal Fold Phonation (Dysphonia Plicae Ventricularis)

This was described earlier in this chapter as a variant of muscular tension dysphonia associated with excessive lateral approximation. Phonation involving only the ventricular folds is extremely rare and usually occurs following injury to the true vocal folds caused by vocal fold paralysis, intubation injury, radiation, vocal fold atrophy, or operations for carcinoma. In most functional cases, hyperadduction of both the glottis and ventricular folds are involved. When this condition occurs with functional vocal folds, it is best treated using fiberoptic videoendoscopy to demonstrate gestures such as throat clear, humming, and sighing, when glottal phonation is most likely to be independent of ventricular adduction.

Psychogenic Voice Disorders

These voice disorders are related to psychologic processes in the patient resulting in inappropriate use of a normal vocal mechanism for speech communication. A psychogenic origin should be considered only when all other possible structural, neurogenic, or functional voice disorders have been excluded. Sometimes patients can have a psychologic history similar to that usually found in patients with a psychogenic voice disorder, but they have an unrelated voice disorder, for example, resulting from a neurogenic disorder. Many of the other functional disorders, such as the spasmodic dysphonias, were considered psychogenic voice disorders until recently. Only the behavioral characteristics are available for differentiating among these disorders.[140,141,187–190] In general, psychogenic voice disorders do not produce chronic habitual abuse or overuse of the peripheral vocal mechanism and rarely produce secondary peripheral tissue abnormalities. Sometimes, the abnormal voice production can be intermittent, with normal periods of voice production.

At least five different types of psychogenic voice disorders can be identified: conversion reaction dysphonia, malingering dysphonia, psychogenic dysphonia, elective mutism, and psychologic overlay. Conversion reaction dysphonia is most commonly found in patients who are experiencing a strong emotional reaction to a traumatic experience or chronic depression. In malingering dysphonia, the patient is attempting to feign a voice disorder for secondary gain. Psychogenic

dysphonias are those in patients not meeting the criteria for a conversion reaction dysphonia.[191] Elective mutism occurs most frequently in young children in response to traumatic events. Psychologic overlay occurs when a patient with another voice disorder has symptom exaggeration, usually to draw attention to the disorder or for some other secondary gain.

Patients with vocal misuse are sometimes classified as having psychogenic voice disorders. In disorders of vocal misuse, however, successful management can include vocal retraining alone. In psychogenic voice disorders, management is most successful when vocal retraining, psychologic or psychiatric counseling, and life-situation change are simultaneously employed. Otherwise, voice symptoms return intermittently.

Most psychogenic dysphonias are hypofunctional vocal behaviors, but they may also appear as hyperfunctional behaviors or as a variable mix of the two.

Conversion Reaction Dysphonia

The essential feature of conversion reaction dysphonia is the experience of severe psychologic or emotional trauma that is closely associated in time with the onset of the dysphonia.[191] The traumatic experience may be concrete and easily identified, such as the loss of a loved one or the experience of a direct threat to the patient or a loved one, or it may be more subtle and difficult to identify, such as the experience of psychologic or physical abuse, or the patient's fear of losing a loved one.

Voice quality in conversion reaction dysphonia is typically, but not exclusively, hypofunctional, or aphonic.[192] Sometimes, the voice can be tremorous as well.[193] Laryngeal function for vegetative purposes, such as for swallowing or coughing, is within normal limits. Fiberoptic evaluation of the larynx is remarkable for lack of vocal fold adduction during attempts to produce voicing for speech without evidence of vocal fold paresis, paralysis, arytenoid fixation, or other movement difficulties. Vocal fold adductions for coughing and Valsalva maneuver are within normal limits.

In some cases, conversion reaction dysphonia occurs as hyperfunctional dysphonia and may accompany complaints regarding inconsistent, mild respiratory distress. Voice quality in those patients may be strained and effortful. Conversion disorders most frequently affect women in their twenties and thirties, but they can occur at any time after the development of speech, more commonly in adults than in children. Onset is usually sudden, following the experience or perception of psychologic trauma. Vocal symptoms appear in their final form, rather than gradually increasing in severity. The patient's ability to work and socialize may be seriously impaired.

Because diagnosis requires the confirmation of a sudden onset of vocal symptoms closely associated with the experience of an event that may have caused severe psychologic trauma, the patient's history, provided either by the patient or others in the patient's environment, is essential.[128,143,145] In some cases, the patient is aware of the event and talks about it freely. Sometimes, however, extensive interview and counseling may be required before the patient may be willing or able to talk about the event directly. Interviews with close relatives or friends may be important in these patients, along with referrals for professional psychologic evaluation and counseling.

In hypofunctional cases, weak, breathy voice quality with complete or near complete absence of vocal fold contact or vibratory activity is common. In hyperfunction, however, vocal fold tension is increased such that vocal fold vibration for speech is difficult or impossible to achieve. Such tension is frequently associated with palpable tension in the extrinsic laryngeal muscles.[128,130] In some cases, symptoms may be more noticeable during formal testing situations than during informal communication.

Malingering Dysphonia

Although the presentation is similar to conversion reaction dysphonia in symptoms, malingering dysphonia involves conscious intent on the part of the patient to simulate a voice disorder for some gain, often financial or emotional. The patient may be pursuing a medical malpractice suit, an injury or accident case, a legal redress against an employer, or special disability assistance. Other agendas may be less concrete, although no less motivating for the patient, such as attempting to avoid communication with an individual or attempting to avoid an experience that the patient considers objectionable. A carefully obtained, complete patient history and interview are the most useful tools for distinguishing a malingering dysphonia from conversion reaction dysphonia.

Voice quality in malingering dysphonia is usually hypofunctional or aphonic for speech communication purposes, although it may be hyperfunctional or variable. Voice quality associated with vegetative functions such as coughing or throat clearing is usually normal. No evidence of laryngeal physiologic abnormality is present. Cognitive distracters, such as counting backwards in sevens or reading difficult material, are often important in eliciting voice production inconsistencies.

Psychogenic Dysphonia

In most psychogenic dysphonias, patients exhibit inconsistent voice symptoms such as intermittent aphonia, abnormal vocal pitch, or periods of severe or markedly abnormal voice interspersed with periods of normal voice. These symptoms may be in reaction to psychosocial stresses in the intermediate or distant past. Symptoms range from a noticeable voice abnormality in pitch, stuttering-like voice breaks, to complete aphonia disrupting all attempts to communicate. Often, patients express a lack of responsibility for their voice problem and poor insight into their voice difficulties. These patients usually have a history of frequent somatic complaints and are unable to take responsibility for their life situations. They may respond to symptom-oriented voice therapy early in the course or may become resistant to voice therapy and require psychosocial management. They often become dependent on others for communication; in fact, the voice abnormalities may be used unconsciously by the patient to avoid certain social or occupational situations that they find stressful.[193]

Diagnosis may depend on identifying significant psychosocial trauma or physical or sexual abuse, a dissociative personality, or a history of frequent somatizations. An inconsistency of the voice symptoms is often noted by others in the patient's environment. Often, the voice symptoms become less exaggerated during distraction such as reading difficult material orally, counting backwards, or during examinations such as fiberoptic nasolaryngoscopy. The disorder is more often seen in females who are unable to control their environment.

In aphonia, the patient does not adduct vocal folds for speech but has normal Valsalva maneuver and throat clearing. Although patients may have secondary gains from their disorder, they are usually unconscious of the secondary gain. Symptoms may range from periods of intermittently abnormal pitch or hoarseness with strained voice to a consistent aphonia with an absence of voice fold adduction only for speech.

Elective Mutism

Although rare, this usually appears in young children immediately following a traumatic event or in extreme anger. It is characterized by a complete withholding of oral communication in the presence of normal laryngeal structure and function and language skills. It frequently occurs with psychosocial problems relating to the family situation (abuse or conflicts within the family or with the community). This condition appears most often in the preschool or kindergarten child, and the child becomes mute on entering school. It may occur at other times during the school-age years in response to traumatic events, and it sometimes occurs in adults. Without intervention, the disorder can persist for several years. The withholding of vocal communication is related to issues of control, emotional disengagement, manipulation, secondary gain, and low self-esteem and indicates maladaptive psychosocial development. The family may have a history of frequent somatizations, hostility toward school or community, and disturbed interpersonal relationships.

The child may be described as shy, cooperative, and attentive in class. Normal results are obtained on receptive language tests. Reading and writing and other school-related abilities are normal, as are the structure and function of the larynx. The parents may minimize the problem, suggesting that no difficulty exists at home and the child does not like to talk at school. The child may have a continuous and consistent refusal to talk in almost all situations (e.g., school, school bus, playground) but demonstrates the ability to comprehend spoken language and to read and speak appropriately when not observed. A team approach including voice therapy and psychosocial counseling and intervention is beneficial.

Psychogenic Overlay

Frequently, patients have complex voice disorders; they may develop emotional complaints as the result of having a voice disorder that may make it appear psychogenic in origin,[187,194] or they may either consciously or unconsciously exaggerate their symptoms to draw attention to themselves, to receive sympathy, or receive further secondary gains from their voice disorder. Treatment is most effective by combining appropriate treatment of the primary voice disorder (phonosurgery, voice therapy, pharmacotherapy) with counseling to emphasize the advantages of recovery.

In conclusion, because of the complexity and diagnostic uncertainty of most of the functional voice disorders, diagnostic caution must be exercised. Usually, the disorder is not acute or life-threatening, except in the case of acute airway obstruction in paradoxic vocal fold adduction for breathing. Therefore, a trial of voice therapy is often warranted before embarking on phonosurgery, botulinum toxin therapy, pharmacotherapy, or psychologic counseling.

SUGGESTED READINGS

1. Baken JR: Clinical Measurement of Speech and Voice. Boston, Little, Brown, 1987.
2. Hirano M: Clinical Examination of Voice. New York, Springer, 1981.
3. Yanagihara N: Significance of harmonic changes and noise components in hoarseness. J Hear Speech Res 10:531, 1967
4. Bless DM, Hirano M, and Feder R: Videostroboscopic examination of the larynx. Ear Nose Throat J 66(special issue):289, 1987.
5. Ramig LA, Cherer RC, Titze IR, and Ringel SP: Acoustic analysis of voice patients with neurological disease: rationale and preliminary data. Ann Otol Rhinol Laryngol 97:164, 1988.
6. Sonies BC, et al: Ultrasonic visualization of tongue motion during speech. J Acoust Soc Am 70:683, 1981.
7. Stone M, Faber A, Raphael LJ, and Shawker TH: Cross-sectional tongue shape and linguopalatal contact patterns in [s], [S], and [l]. J Phonet 20:253, 1992.
8. Stone M, Morish K, Sonies B, and Shawker T: Tongue curvature: a model of shape during vowel production. Folia Phoniatr 39:302, 1987.
9. Stone M and Shawker T: An ultrasound examination of tongue movement during swallowing. Dysphagia 1:78, 1986.
10. Stone M, Shawker T, Talbot T, and Rich A: Cross-sectional

11. Baer T, Gore JC, Gracco LC, and Nye PW: Analysis of vocal tract shape and dimensions using magnetic resonance imaging: vowels. J Acoust Soc Am 90:799, 1991.
12. Ludlow CL: Neurophysiological assessment of patients with vocal motor control disorders. In: Assessment of Speech and Voice Production: Research and Clinical Applications. Edited by Cooper JA. Bethesda, MD, NIDCD Monograph, 1991, p 161.
13. Darley FL, Aronson AE, and Brown JR: Motor Speech Disorders. Philadelphia, WB Saunders, 1975.
14. Duvoisin RC: The cause of Parkinson's disease. In: Movement Disorders. Vol 2. Edited by Fahn S and Marsden CD. London, Butterworth, 1982.
15. Forest K, Weismer G, and Turner GS: Kinematic, acoustic and perceptual analyses of connected speech produced by parkinsonian and normal geriatric adults. J Acoust Soc Am 85:2608, 1989.
16. Logemann JA, Fisher HB, and Bocshes B: Frequency and co-occurrence of vocal tract dysfunction in the speech of a large sample of Parkinson's patients. J Speech Hear Disord 434:47, 1978.
17. Connor MP, Ludlow CL, and Schulz GM: Stop consonant production in isolated and repeated syllables in Parkinson's disease. Neurophsychologia 27:829, 1989.
18. Hanson DB, Gerratt BR, and Ward PH: Cinegraphic observations of laryngeal function in Parkinson's disease. Laryngoscope 94:348, 1984.
19. Ramig LO: Speech therapy for patients with Parkinson's disease. In: Therapy of Parkinson's Disease. Edited by Koller W and Pulson G. New York, Marcel Dekker, 1994.
20. Steele JC, Richardson JC, and Olszewski J: Arch Neurol 10:333, 1964.
21. Jankovic J and Tolosa E: Parkinson's Disease and Movement Disorders. Baltimore, Williams & Wilkins, 1993.
22. Oppenheimer DR: Diseases of the basal ganglia, cerebellum and motor neurons. In: Greenfields' Neuropathology. Edited by Adam JH, Corsellis JAN, and Duchen LW. London, Edward Arnold, 1984, p 700.
23. Harding AE: Commentary: olivopontocerebellar atrophy is not a useful concept. In: Movement Disorders. Vol 2. Edited by Marsden CD and Fahn S. London, Butterworth, 1987, p 269.
24. Hanson DG, Ludlow CL, and Bassich CJ: Vocal fold paresis and Shy-Drager syndrome. Ann Otol Rhinol Laryngol 92:85, 1983.
25. Lechtenberg R: Multiple Sclerosis Fact Book. Philadelphia, FA Davis, 1983.
26. Obeso JA, Artieda J, and Marsden CD: Different clinical presentations of myoclonus in Parkinson's disease and movement disorders. Edited by Jankovic J and Tolosa E. Baltimore, Williams & Wilkins, 1984, p 315.
27. Lapresle J: Palatal myoclonus. Adv Neurol 43:265, 1986.
28. Marsden CD, Hallet M, and Fahn S: The nosology and pathophysiology of myoclonus. In: Movement Disorders. Edited by Marsden CD and Fahn S. London, Butterworth, 1982, p 196.
29. Jankovic J and Pardon R: Segmental myoclonus: clinical and pharmacologic study. Arch Neurol 43:1025, 1986.
30. Dubinsky R and Hallett M: Palatal myoclonus and facial involvement of other types of myoclonus. In: Facial Dyskinesias. Edited by Jankovic J and Tolosa E. New York, Raven Press, 1988, p 263.
31. Dubinsky R, et al: Increased glucose metabolism in the medulla of patients with palatal myoclonus. Neurology 41:557, 1991.
32. Deuschl GA, Ebner A, Hanners R, Luching CH: Differences of cortical activation in spontaneous and reflex myoclonus. Electroencephalogr Clin Neurophysiol 80:326, 1991.
33. Rose FC (ed): Motor Neuron Disease. New York, Grune and Stratton, 1977.
34. Goodhart SP and Davison C: Syndrome of the posterior inferior

and anterior inferior cerebellar arteries and their branches. Arch Neurol Psychiatr *35*:501, 1936.

35. Driscoll BP, et al: Laryngeal function in postpolio patients. Laryngoscope *105*:35, 1995.

36. Garrett JD and Larson CR: Neurology of the laryngeal system. In: Phonosurgery: Assessment and Surgical Management of Voice Disorders. Edited by Ford CN and Bless DM. New York, Raven Press, 1991, p 43.

37. Martensson A: The functional organization of the intrinsic laryngeal muscles. Ann NY Acad Sci *2*:381, 1968.

38. Hirano M and Bless DM: Videostroboscopic Examination of the Larynx. San Diego, Singular Publishing, 1993.

39. Schutte H and Seidner W: Recommendation by the union of European Phoniatricians (WEP): standardizing voice measurement/phonetography. Folia Phoniatr *35*:286, 1983.

40. Baer T: Vocal jitter: a neuromuscular explanation. Transcripts of the Eighth Symposium: Care of the Professional Voice. Edited by Lawrence V. Vol I, Part II. New York, Voice Foundation, 1979, p 19.

41. Kotby MN, et al: Electromyography and neurography in neurolaryngology. J Voice *5*:316, 1991.

42. Blair RL, Berry H, and Briant TDR: Laryngeal electromyography: techniques and application. Otolaryngol Clin North Am *2*:325, 1978.

43. Thumfart F: From larynx to vocal ability: new electrophysiological data. Acta Otolaryngol (Stockh) *105*:425, 1988.

44. Ford CN and Bless DM (eds): Phonosurgery: Assessment and Surgical Management of Voice Disorders. New York, Raven Press, 1991.

45. Logemann JA: Treatment for aspiration related to dysphagia: an overview. Dysphagia *1*:34, 1986.

46. Sasaki CT: The effect of tracheostomy on the laryngeal closure reflex. Laryngoscope *87*:1428, 1977.

47. Nash M: Swallowing problems in the tracheotomized patient. Otolaryngol Clin North Am *21*:702, 1988.

48. Lewy RB: Glottic rehabilitation with Teflon injection: the return of voice, cough, and laughter. Acta Otolaryngol *58*:214, 1964.

49. Rontal E: Vocal cord injection in the treatment of acute and chronic aspiration. Laryngoscope *86*:625, 1976.

50. Schramm VL, May M, and Lavorato AS: Gelfoam paste injection for vocal cord paralysis: temporary rehabilitation of glottic incompetence. Laryngoscope *88*:1268, 1978.

51. Isshiki N, Okamura H, and Ishikawa T: Thyroplasty type I (lateral compression) for dysphonia due to vocal cord paralysis or atrophy. Acta Otolaryngol *80*:465, 1975.

52. Rubin HJ: Pitfalls in treatment of dysphonias by intracordal injection of synthetics. Laryngoscope *75*:1381, 1965.

53. Ellis JC, McCaffrey TV, DeSanto LW, and Reiman HV: Migration of Teflon after vocal cord injection. Otolaryngol Head Neck Surg *96*:63, 1987.

54. Schramm VL, May M, and Lavorato AS: Gelfoam paste injection for vocal cord paralysis: temporary rehabilitation of glottic incompetence. Laryngoscope *88*:1268, 1978.

55. Dedo HH, Urrea RD, and Lawson L: Intracordal injection of Teflon in the treatment of 135 patients with dysphonia. Ann Otol Rhinol Laryngol *82*:661, 1973.

56. Hurst WB: Percutaneous injection of a vocal cord with Teflon. J Laryngol Otol *86*:663, 1972.

57. Ward PH, Hanson DG, and Abemayor E: Transcutaneous Teflon injection. Laryngology *75*:380, 1966.

58. Isshiki N, Morita H, Okamura H, and Hiramoto M: Thyroplasty as a new phonosurgical technique. Acta Otolaryngol (Stockh) *78*:451, 1974.

59. Koufman JA: Laryngoplasty for vocal cord medialization: an alternative to Teflon. Laryngoscope *96*:726, 1986.

60. Meurman Y: Operative mediofixation of the vocal cord in complete unilateral paralysis. Arch Otolaryngol Head Neck Surg *55*:544, 1952.

61. Waltner JG: Surgical rehabilitation of voice following laryngofissure. Arch Otolaryngol Head Neck Surg *67*:99, 1958.

62. Ophein O: Unilateral paralysis of the vocal cord: operative treatment. Acta Otolaryngol (Stockh) *45*:226, 1955.

63. Sawashima M, Totsuke G, Kobayashi T, and Hirose H: Reconstructive surgery for hoarseness due to unilateral vocal cord paralysis. Arch Otolaryngol Head Neck Surg *87*:289, 1968.

64. Kamer FM and Som ML: Correction of the traumatically abducted vocal cord. Arch Otolaryngol Head Neck Surg *95*:6, 1972.

65. Smith GW: Aphonia due to vocal cord paralysis corrected by medial positioning of the affected vocal cord with a cartilage autograft. Can J Otolaryngol *1*:295, 1972.

66. Sasaki CT, Leder SA, and Petar L: Immediate and long term vocal change following Isshiki thyroplasty. Laryngoscope *100*:848, 1990.

67. Crumley RL: Update of laryngeal reinnervation concepts and options in surgery of the larynx. In: Surgery of the Larynx. Edited by Bailey BJ and Biller HF. Philadelphia, WB Saunders, 1985.

68. Rice DH: Laryngeal reinnervation. Laryngoscope *92*:1049, 1982.

69. Crumley RL: Selective reinnervation of vocal cord adductors in unilateral vocal cord paralysis. Ann Otol Rhinol Laryngol *93*:351, 1984.

70. Hengerer AS and Tucker HM: Restoration of abduction in the paralyzed canine vocal cord. Arch Otolaryngol (Stockh) *97*:247, 1973.

71. Tucker HM: Human laryngeal reinnervation. Laryngoscope *86*:769, 1976.

72. Tucker HM: Human laryngeal reinnervation: long-term experience with the nerve-muscle pedicle technique. Laryngoscope *88*:598, 1978.

73. Applebaum EL, Allen GW, and Sisson GA: Human laryngeal reinnervation: the Northwestern experience. Laryngoscope *89*:1784, 1979.

74. May M and Beery Q: Muscle-nerve pedicle laryngeal reinnervation. Laryngoscope *96*:1196, 1986.

75. Neal DG, Cummings CW, and Sutton D: Delayed reinnervation of unilateral vocal cord paralysis in dogs. Otolaryngol Head Neck Surg *89*:608, 1981.

76. Zitsch R: Continuous positive airway pressure: use in bilateral vocal cord paralysis. Arch Otolaryngol *118*:875, 1992.

77. Hirano M, Kurita S, Kiyokawa K, and Sato K: Posterior glottis: morphologic study in excised human larynges. Ann Otol Rhinol Laryngol *96*:576, 1986

78. Jackson C: Ventriculocordectomy: a new operation for the cure of goitrous glottic stenosis. Arch Surg *4*:257, 1922.

79. Moore J: Operative procedures in the treatment of stenosis of the larynx caused by bilateral paralysis of the abductor muscles. Proc R Soc Med *16*:32, 1923.

80. Hoover WB: Bilateral abductor paralysis, operative treatment of submucous resection of the vocal cord. Arch Otolaryngol *15*:337, 1932.

81. Lore J: A suggested operative procedure for the relief of stenosis in double abductor paralysis: an anatomic study. Ann Otol Rhinol Laryngol *45*:679, 1936.

82. Helmus C: Microsurgical thyrotomy and arytenoidectomy for bilateral recurrent laryngeal nerve paralysis. Laryngoscope *32*:491, 1972.

83. Singer MI, Hamaker RC, and Miller SM: Restoration of the airway following bilateral recurrent laryngeal nerve paralysis. Laryngoscope *95*:1204, 1985.

84. Woodman D: A modification of the extralaryngeal approach to arytenoidectomy for bilateral abductor paralysis. Arch Otolaryngol Head Neck Surg *43*:63, 1946.

85. King BT: A new and function-restoring operation for bilateral abductor cord paralysis. JAMA *112*:814, 1939.

86. Kelly JD: Surgical treatment of bilateral paralysis of the abductor muscles. Arch Otolaryngol Head Neck Surg *33*:293, 1941.

87. Thornell WC: Intralaryngeal approach for arytenoidectomy in bilateral abductor vocal cord paralysis. Arch Otolaryngol 47:505, 1948.

88. El Chazly M, Rifai M, and El Ezz AA: Arytenoidectomy and posterior cordectomy for bilateral abductor paralysis. J Laryngol Otol 105:454, 1991.

89. Ossoff RH, et al: Endoscopic laser arytenoidectomy for the treatment of bilateral vocal cord paralysis. Laryngoscope 94:1293, 1984.

90. Ossoff RH et al: Endoscopic laser arytenoidectomy revisited. Ann Otol Rhinol Laryngol 99:764, 1990.

91. Crumley RL: Endoscopic laser medial arytenoidectomy for airway management in bilateral laryngeal paralysis. Ann Otol Rhinol Laryngol 102:81, 1993.

92. Rontal M and Rontal E: Use of laryngeal muscular tenotomy for bilateral midline vocal cord fixation. Ann Otol Rhinol Laryngol 103:583, 1994.

93. Kirchner FR: Endoscopic lateralization of the vocal cords. Laryngoscope 89:1779, 1979.

94. Geterud A, Ejnell H, Stenborg R, and Bake B: Long-term results with a simple surgical treatment of bilateral vocal cord paralysis. Laryngoscope 100:1005, 1990.

95. Linder A and Lindholm CE: Vocal fold lateralization using carbon dioxide laser and fibrin glue. J Laryngol Otol 106:226, 1992.

96. Prasad U: CO_2 surgical laser in the management of bilateral vocal cord paralysis. J Laryngol Otol 99:891, 1985.

97. Dennis DP and Kashima H: Carbon dioxide laser posterior cordectomy for treatment of bilateral vocal cord paralysis. Ann Otol Rhinol Laryngol 98:930, 1989.

98. Kashima H: Bilateral vocal fold motion impairment: pathophysiology and management by transverse cordotomy. Ann Otol Rhinol Laryngol 100:717, 1991.

99. Doyle PJ, Brummet RE, and Everts EC: Results of surgical section and repair of the recurrent laryngeal nerve. Laryngoscope 77:1245, 1967.

100. Gordon JH and McCabe BF: The effect of accurate neurorrhaphy on reinnervation and return of laryngeal function. Laryngoscope 78:236, 1968.

101. Dedo HH: Electromyographic and visual evaluation of recurrent laryngeal nerve anastomosis in dogs. Ann Otol Rhinol Laryngol 80:664, 1971.

102. Crumley RL: Experiments in laryngeal reinnervation. Laryngoscope 92(suppl 30):1, 1982.

103. Rice DH: Laryngeal reinnervation. Laryngoscope 92:1049, 1982.

104. Crumley RL: Phrenic nerve graft for bilateral vocal cord paralysis. Laryngoscope 93:425, 1983.

105. Tucker HM: Human laryngeal reinnervation. Laryngoscope 86:769, 1976.

106. Tucker HM: Long-term results of nerve-muscle pedicle reinnervation for laryngeal paralysis. Ann Otol Rhinol Laryngol 98:674, 1989.

107. Zealear DL, et al: Technical approach for reanimation of the chronically denervated larynx by means of functional electrical stimulation. Ann Otol Rhinol Laryngol 103:705, 1994.

108. Eisele DW: Chronic aspiration. In: Otolaryngology—Head and Neck Surgery. Edited by Cummings CW, et al. St. Louis, CV Mosby, 1993.

109. Martens L, Cameron T, and Simonsen M: Effects of a multidisciplinary management program on neurologically impaired patients with dysphagia. Dysphagia 5:147, 1990.

110. Montgomery WW: Surgery to prevent aspiration. Otolaryngol Head Neck Surg 101:679, 1975.

111. Sasaki CT, et al: Surgical closure of the larynx for aspiration. Arch Otolaryngol Head Neck Surg 106:422, 1980.

112. Habal MB and Murray JE: Surgical treatment of life-endangering chronic aspiration pneumonia: use of an epiglottic flap to the arytenoids. Plast Reconstr Surg 49:305, 1972.

113. Vecchione TR, Habal MB, and Murray JE: Further experiences with the arytenoid-epiglottic flap for chronic aspiration pneumonia. Plast Reconstr Surg 55:318, 1975.

114. Strome M and Fried MP: Rehabilitative surgery for aspiration: a clinical analysis. Arch Otolaryngol Head Neck Surg 109:809, 1983.

115. Biller HF, Lawson W, and Baek SML: Total glossectomy: a technique of reconstruction eliminating laryngectomy. Arch Otolaryngol 109:69, 1983.

116. Weisberger C and Huebsch SA: Endoscopic: treatment of aspiration using a laryngeal stent. Otolaryngol Head Neck Surg 90:215, 1982.

117. Eliachar I and Nguyen D: Laryngotracheal stent for internal support and control of aspiration without loss of phonation. Otolaryngol Head Neck Surg 103:837, 1990.

118. Lindeman RC: Diverting the paralyzed larynx: a reversible procedure for intractable aspiration. Laryngoscope 85:157, 1975.

119. Lindeman RC, Yarington CT, and Sutton D: Clinical experience with the tracheoesophageal anastomosis for intractable aspiration. Ann Otol Rhinol Laryngol 85:609, 1976.

120. Eisele DW, et al: The tracheoesophageal diversion and laryngotracheal separation procedures for treatment of intractable aspiration. Am J Surg 157:230, 1989.

121. Snyderman CH and Johnson JT: Laryngotracheal separation for intractable aspiration. Ann Otol Rhinol Laryngol 97:466, 1988.

122. Broniatowski M: Dynamic control of the larynx and future perspectives in the management of deglutitive aspiration. Dysphagia 8:334, 1993.

123. Blitzer A, Brin MF, Fahn S, and Lovelace RE: Clinical and laboratory characteristics of focal laryngeal dystonia: study of 110 cases. Laryngoscope 98:636, 1988.

124. Schaefer SD: Neuropathology of spasmodic dysphonia. Laryngoscope 93:1183, 1983.

125. Schaefer SD, et al: Magnetic resonance imaging findings and correlations in spasmodic dysphonia patients. Ann Otol Rhinol Laryngol 94:595, 1985.

126. Finitzo-Hieber T, et al: Auditory brainstem response abnormalities in adductor spasmodic dysphonia. Am J Otolaryngol 3:26, 1981.

127. Pool KD, et al: Heterogeneity in spasmodic dysphonia. Arch Neurol 48:305, 1991.

128. Aronson AE: Clinical Voice Disorders: An Interdisciplinary Approach. New York, Thieme-Stratton, 1980.

129. Colton RH and Casper JK: Understanding Voice Problems: A Physiological Perspective for Diagnosis and Treatment. Baltimore, Williams & Wilkins, 1990, p 73.

130. Morrison M, et al: The Management of Voice Disorders. San Diego, Singular Publishing, 1994, p 50.

131. Boone DR and McFarlane SC: The Voice and Voice Therapy. 5th Ed. Englewood Cliffs, NJ, Prentice-Hall, 1994, p 66.

132. Ludlow CL, Naunton RF, Terada S, and Anderson BJ: Successful treatment of selected cases of abductor spasmodic dysphonia using botulinum toxin injection. Otolaryngol Head Neck Surg 104:849, 1991.

133. Ludlow CL, Bassich CJ, Connor NP, and Coulter DC: Phonatory characteristics of vocal fold tremor. J Phonet 14:509, 1986.

134. Rosenbaum F and Jankovic J: Task specific focal tremor and dystonia: categorization of occupational movement disorders. Neurology 38:522, 1988.

135. Izdebski K, Dedo HH, and Boles L: Spastic dysphonia: a patient profile of 200 cases. Am J Otolaryngol 5:7, 1984.

136. Blitzer A, et al: Electromyographic findings in focal laryngeal dystonia (spastic dysphonia). Ann Otol Rhinol Laryngol 94:591, 1985.

137. Lieberman JA and Reife R: Spastic dysphonia and denervation signs in a young man with tardive dyskinesia. Br J Psychiatry 154:105, 1989.

138. Dedo HH, Townsend JJ, and Izdebski K: Current evidence for the organic etiology of spastic dysphonia. Otolaryngol Head Neck Surg 86:875, 1978.

139. Hartman DE: Neurogenic dysphonia. Ann Otol Rhinol Laryngol 93:57, 1984.

140. Aronson AE, Brown JR, Litin EM, and Pearson JS: Spastic dysphonia: II. Comparison with essential (voice) tremor and other neurologic and psychogenic dysphonias. J Speech Hear Disord 33:219, 1968.

141. Aronson AE, Brown JR, Litin EM, and Pearson JS: Spastic dysphonia. I. Voice, neurologic, and psychiatric aspects. J Speech Hear Disord 33:203, 1968.

142. Aronson AE and Hartman DE: Adductor spastic dysphonia as a sign of essential (voice) tremor. J Speech Hear Disord 46:52, 1981.

143. Aronson AE, Peterson HW, and Litin EM: Psychiatric symptomatology in functional dysphonia and aphonia. J Speech Hear Disord 31:115, 1966.

144. Sapir S and Aronson AE: The relationship between psychopathology and speech and language disorders in neurologic patients. J Speech Hear Disord 55:503, 1990.

145. Aronson AE: Importance of the psychosocial interview in the diagnosis and treatment of "functional" voice disorders. J Voice 4:287, 1990.

146. Watson BC, et al: Laryngeal electromyographic activity in adductor and abductor spasmodic dysphonia. J Speech Hear Res 34:473, 1991.

147. Ludlow CL, Baker M, Naunton RF, and Hallett M: Intrinsic laryngeal muscle activation in spasmodic dysphonia. In: Motor Disturbances. Edited by Benecke R, Conrad B, and Marsden CD. Orlando, FL, Academic Press, 1988, p 119.

148. Ludlow CL, et al: The pathophysiology of spasmodic dysphonia and its modification by botulinum toxin. In: Motor Disturbances. Edited by Berardelli A, Benecke R, Manfredi M, and Marsden CD. Orlando, FL, Academic Press, 1990, p 274.

149. Koda J and Ludlow CL: An evaluation of laryngeal muscle activation in patients with voice tremor. Ann Otol Rhinol Laryngol 107:684, 1992.

150. Hirano M and Ohala J: Use of hooked-wire electrodes for electromyography of the intrinsic laryngeal muscles. J Speech Hear Res 12:362, 1969.

151. Fujita M, Ludlow CL, Woodson GE, and Naunton RF: A new surface electrode for recording from the posterior cricoarytenoid muscle. Laryngoscope 99:316, 1989.

152. Lovelace RE, Blitzer A, and Ludlow CL: Clinical laryngeal electromyography. In: Neurological Disorders of the Larynx. Edited by Blitzer A et al. New York, Thieme Publishers, 1992, p 66.

153. Shipp T, Izdebski K, Reed C, and Morrissey P: Intrinsic laryngeal muscle activity in a spastic dysphonic patient. J Speech Hear Disord 50:54, 1985.

154. Aronson AE and Desanto LW: Adductor spasmodic dysphonia: three years after recurrent nerve section. Laryngoscope 93:1, 1983.

155. Salassa JR, Desanto LW, and Aronson AE: Respiratory distress after recurrent laryngeal nerve section for spastic dysphonia. Laryngoscope 92:240, 1982.

156. Tucker HM: Laryngeal framework surgery in the management of spasmodic dysphonia: preliminary report. Ann Otol Rhinol Laryngol 98:52, 1989.

157. Miller RH, Woodson GE, and Jankovic J: Botulinum toxin injection of the vocal fold for spasmodic dysphonia. Arch Otolaryngol Head Neck Surg 113:603, 1987.

158. Ludlow CL: Treatment of speech and voice disorders with botulinum toxin. JAMA 264:2671, 1990.

159. Consensus Statement: Clinical Use of Botulinum Toxin. NIH Consensus Development Conference Consensus Statement. Vol 8. Bethesda, MD, National Institutes of Health, 1990, p 1.

160. Blitzer A and Brin MF: Laryngeal dystonia: a series with botulinum toxin therapy. Ann Otol Rhinol Laryngol 100:85, 1991.

161. Ludlow CL, et al: Limitations of laryngeal electromyography and magnetic stimulation for assessing laryngeal muscle control. Ann Otol Rhinol Laryngol 103:16, 1994.

162. Hirano M and Sato K: Histological Color Atlas of the Human Larynx. San Diego, Singular Publishing, 1993, p 48.

163. George EF, et al: Quantitative mapping of the effect of botulinum toxin injections in the thyroarytenoid muscle. Ann Otol Rhinol Laryngol 101:888, 1992.

164. Ludlow CL, et al: Effects of botulinum toxin injections on speech in adductor spasmodic dysphonia. Neurology 38:1220, 1988.

165. Blitzer A, Brin MF, Fahn S, and Lovelace RE: Localized injections of botulinum toxin for the treatment of focal laryngeal dystonia (spastic dysphonia). Laryngoscope 98:193, 1988.

166. Alfieri G, et al: Structural changes in extraocular muscle treated with botulinum toxin (BT) in man. Mov Disord 5:72, 1990.

167. Wojno T, Campbell P, and Wright J: Orbicularis muscle pathology after botulinum toxin injection. Ophthalmol Plast Reconstr Surg 2:7174, 1986.

168. Borodic GE and Ferrante R: Effects of repeated botulinum toxin injections on orbicularis oculi muscle. J Clin Neuroophthalmol 12:121, 1992.

169. Ford CN, Bless DM, and Lowery JD: Indirect laryngoscopic approach for injection of botulinum toxin in spasmodic dysphonia. Otolaryngol Head Neck Surg 103:1:752, 1990.

170. Green DC, Berke GS, Ward PH, and Gerratt BR: Point-touch technique of botulinum toxin injection for the treatment of spasmodic dysphonia. Ann Otol Rhinol Laryngol 101:883, 1992.

171. Rhew K, Fiedler D, and Ludlow CL: Technique for injection of botulinum toxin through the flexible nasolaryngoscope. Otolaryngol Head Neck Surg 111:787, 1995.

172. Ludlow CL, Bagley JA, Yin SG, and Koda J: A comparison of different injection techniques in the treatment of spasmodic dysphonia with botulinum toxin. J Voice 6:380, 1992.

173. Blitzer A, et al: Abductor laryngeal dystonia: a series treated with botulinum toxin. Laryngoscope 102:163, 1992.

174. Marion MH, Klap P, Perrin A, and Cohen M: Stridor and focal laryngeal dystonia. Lancet 339:457, 1992.

175. Christopher KL, et al: Vocal-cord dysfunction presenting as asthma. N Engl J Med 306:1566, 1983.

176. Hurbis CG and Schild JA: Laryngeal changes during exercise and exercise-induced asthma. Ann Otol Rhinol Laryngol 100:34, 1991.

177. Cormier Y, Camus P, and Desmeules M: Non-organic acute upper airway obstruction. Am Rev Respir Dis 121:147, 1980.

178. Craig T, et al: Vocal cord dysfunction during wartime. Milit Med 157:614, 1992.

179. Koufman JA: Gastroesophageal reflux and voice disorders. In: Diagnosis and Treatment of Voice Disorders. Edited by Gould WJ, Rubin JS, Korovin G, and Sataloff R. New York, Igaku-Shoin, 1994.

180. Brown TM, Merritt WD, and Evans DL: Psychogenic vocal cord dysfunction masquerading as asthma. J Nerv Ment Dis 176:308, 1988.

181. Caraon P and O'Toole C: Vocal cord dysfunction presenting as asthma. Ir Med J 84:98, 1991.

182. Hayes JP, Nolan MT, Brennan N, and Fitzgerald MX: Three cases of paradoxical vocal cord adduction followed up over a 10 year period. Chest 104:678, 1993.

183. Lew MF, et al: Adductor laryngeal breathing dystonia in a patient with lubag (X-linked dystonia-parkinsonism) syndrome. Mov Disord 9:318, 1994.

184. Grillone GA, et al: Treatment of adductor laryngeal breathing dystonia with botulinum toxin type A. Laryngoscope 24:30, 1994.

185. Morrison MD, et al: Muscular tension dysphonia. J Otolaryngol 12:302, 1983.

186. Belisle G and Morrison MD: Anatomic correlation for muscle tension dysphonia. J Otolaryngol 12:319, 1983.

187. Cannito MP: Emotional considerations in spasmodic dysphonia: psychometric quantification. J Commun Dis 24:313, 1991.

188. Chevrie-Muller C, Arabia-Guidet C, and Pfauwadel MC: Can one recover from spasmodic dysphonia? Br J Dis Commun 22: 117, 1987.

189. Elias A, Raven R, Butxher P, and Littlejohns DW: Speech therapy for psychogenic voice disorder: a survey of current practice and training. Br J Dis Commun 24:61, 1989.

190. Ginsberg VI, Wallach JJ, Srain JJ, and Biller HF: Defining the psychiatric role in spastic dysphonia. Gen Hosp Psychiatry 10: 132, 1988.

191. Diagnostic and Statistical Manual of Mental Disorders. Revised (DSM-III-R). 3rd Ed. Washington, DC, American Psychiatric Association, 1987.

192. Kinzl J, Biebl W, and Rauchegger H: Functional aphonia: a conversion symptom as defensive mechanism against anxiety. Psychother Psychosom 49:31, 1988.

193. Koller WC and Huber SJ: Tremor disorders of aging: diagnosis and management. Geriatrics 44:33, 1989.

194. Murry T, Cannito MP, and Woodson GE: Spasmodic dysphonia: emotional status and botulinum toxin. Arch Otolaryngol Head Neck Surg 120:310, 1994.

32 Tumors of the Larynx and Laryngopharynx

Paul F. Castellanos, J. Gershon Spector, and Timothy N. Kaiser

BENIGN TUMORS

Benign tumors are described collectively because of the relative rarity of these tumors as compared with malignant neoplasms in the same areas. Benign tumors occur in the following rough order of frequency: papilloma, chondroma, neurofibroma, leiomyoma, angiofibroma, myoblastoma, myoma, hemangioma, and chemodectoma. Vocal nodules, cysts, and laryngoceles, as well as lesions denoted by older terms such as "fibroma of the cord," varix, and angioma, are not neoplasms and are discussed elsewhere in this text.

Diagnosis and Treatment

Papillomas
Papillomas usually appear as single or multiple warty excrescences of the true vocal fold (Fig. 32–1). They may also be located over the supraglottis. Less frequently, they are found in the infraglottic region (see Chap. 30).

Neuroendocrine and Neurogenic Tumors
Neuroendocrine cells, derivatives of the neural crest, have been demonstrated in the larynx.[1,2] These mainly produce two types of tumors: carcinoids and paragangliomas (glomus tumors). Laryngeal tumors of neural origin are rare and mostly arise in the region of the superior laryngeal nerve (supraglottis).[3] The larynx is the locus of chief and Kulchitsky cells or paraganglia that are associated with the superior and recurrent laryngeal nerves. Carcinoid tumors are discussed later in this chapter.

PARAGANGLIOMAS. Chemodectomas arise from the "paraganglia," along the vagus nerve. These are paired structures along the internal branch of the superior laryngeal nerve and the posterior branch of the recurrent laryngeal nerve (i.e., along sensory nerve branches and around Galen's anastomosis). On rare occasions, paragangliomas are found in the anterior cricothyroid membrane. Multiple tumors are found in some patients. Laryngeal lesions are most commonly associated with carotid body tumors.[4] Since the original descriptions by Andrews[5] and Blanchard and Saunders[6] in 1955, about 50 cases have been reported. Almost all reported cases conform to the theory that these tumors arise from (near) the superior laryngeal nerve. No age or sex predilection has been reported. The symptoms are nonspecific. Tumors may have an hourglass shape with components within and outside the larynx. On laryngeal examination, one sees a rounded, red, mucosally covered mass with a hyperemic, vascularized overlying mucosa. These tumors may appear similar to laryngoceles, and a computed tomographic (CT) or magnetic resonance (MR) examination may be needed to differentiate them. These are best treated by conservative procedures. When the tumors are large, preoperative tumor embolization may be required. Metastases have been reported, but they are rare.[7] An unusual symptom of the tumor has been reported by Ali and associates,[8] consisting of pain that radiates to the ipsilateral ear and is aggravated by swallowing.

NEURILEMMOMA. Neurilemmomas (schwannomas) arise from Schwann cells and occur most frequently in the head and neck region. Laryngeal lesions were first described by Suchanek in 1925.[9] Over 100 cases have been reported.[10] Neurilemmomas arise most often from the superior laryngeal nerves and are found in the aryepiglottic folds (Fig. 32–2A). The symptoms are nonspecific and vague. These tumors are yellowish, well encapsulated, pedunculated, and covered with mucosa that hangs from the aryepiglottic folds. There is a slightly higher female predisposition, and most tumors occur in the fifth to sixth decades of life. Most

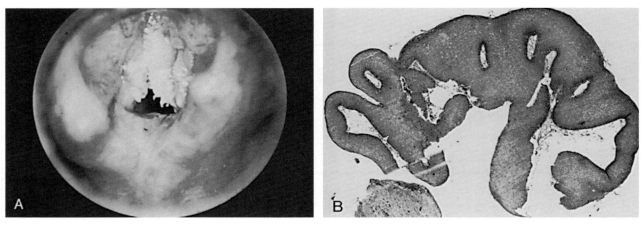

Fig. 32–1. A. Endoscopic view of laryngeal papilloma. B Histologic appearance of pedunculated papilloma. ×40, hematoxylin and eosin stain.

can be removed by means of endoscopic procedures. Large tumors can be removed through a lateral pharyngotomy. Only one case of malignant schwannoma of the larynx has been reported.[11]

NEUROFIBROMA. A neurofibroma is a rare tumor with a combination of neural axonal or dendritic fibers and Schwann cell elements. It usually appears in the extrinsic portion of the larynx. As with chemodectomas, diagnosis by means of laryngoscopy may be difficult because of the large quantity of material needed for pathologic examination.

Most often, neurofibromas are associated with von Recklinghausen's neurofibromatosis, an autosomal dominant trait. In 1930, Colledge described the first laryngeal lesion, and to date about two dozen cases have appeared in the literature.[12] Most lesions occur in children or adolescents. The usual symptom is stridor. The tumors are lobular and nodular, and they are covered by mucosa. They occur most often in the supraglottis and can spread extensively because they are not encapsulated. They can be best removed by a lateral pharyngotomy approach. Surgical cure usually results in some form of paresis, either sensory or motor.[13,14]

Granular Cell Myoblastoma

This tumor was first described by Abrikosoff in 1926.[15] "Myoblastoma" is a misnomer because the tumor was first assumed to originate from striated muscle, but it is now recognized to be of neural derivation. Although these tumors may arise anywhere, 50% arise in the head and neck region, with 35% in the tongue and 10% in the larynx. Synchronous tumors are common. In the larynx, over 150 cases have been reported. Granular particles seen on electron microscopy are found on histochemical analysis to consist of myelin-like protein

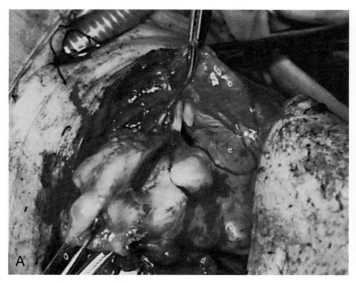

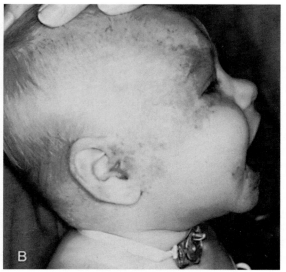

Fig. 32–2. A. Subtotal supraglottic laryngectomy for a schwannoma of the aryepiglottic fold on the left side. Note that epiglottis is saved and vocal folds are free of tumor. B. Male infant with subglottic congenital hemangioma and facial and mucosal capillary hemangiomas.

particles, remnants of nerve fibers, and S-100 proteins.[15-17] Multiple synchronous primary tumors have been described.[18]

These tumors have no sexual predilection and are found in both adolescence and middle age, but most commonly in the fourth to fifth decades. They usually arise at the junction of the vocal ligaments and vocal process of the arytenoid cartilage, within the vocalis muscle, and they appear as a bulging in the posterior vocal fold. Rarely, they occur in the supraglottis and subglottis. Small lesions can be removed endoscopically, whereas larger lesions may require a midline thyrotomy exposure. These lesions are not encapsulated and infiltrate the surrounding musculature. They appear grayish on excision.[19,20]

Vascular Tumors

HEMANGIOMAS. Angiomas appear as simple (capillary) or cavernous hemangiomas of the pharynx or larynx. The most common symptom produced by these masses is bleeding, which may be severe. On physical examination, these lesions appear as bluish masses, and when exophytic they may resemble a "bag of blue worms." Biopsy of such a lesion is generally not indicated in an uncontrolled setting. Because of the profuse bleeding that may be produced by these tumors, excision is best handled by suspension laryngoscopy if they are small, or by lateral pharyngotomy to provide for adequate vascular control if they are large.

Cavernous hemangiomas usually occur in the false vocal folds, and capillary hemangiomas can occur in the supraglottis or vocal folds. Congenital hemangiomas are found in infants, generally in the subglottic region (Fig. 32–2B). First described by Phillips and Ruh in 1913,[21] and clearly defined by Sweetser in 1921,[22] these lesions are now considered a distinct entity. The lesion is twice as common in boys. Most cavernous hemangiomas cause stridor and shortness of breath in the first weeks of life. An association with capillary hemangiomas of the skin and oral mucosa is present in 50% of patients. About 5% of patients have other congenital anomalies, and over 70% of these lesions arise in the posterior wall of the larynx or trachea. Treatment is outlined in Chapter 9.[23-25]

LYMPHANGIOMA. Lymphangiomas are generally associated with cystic hygromas in infancy. Isolated lesions are rare. Their most common location is in the supraglottis and the hypopharynx, producing inspiratory stridor and airway compromise. Supraglottic extensions usually involve the vallecula, epiglottis, false vocal folds, and aryepiglottic folds.[26-28]

HEMANGIOPERICYTOMA. Hemangiopericytomas arise from the pericytes in the vascular wall. Most of these tumors are benign and arise in the supraglottis. They affect older patients of both sexes. They are usually pedicled and bleed easily.[29]

Myogenic Tumors

LEIOMYOMA. Leiomyomas of the larynx are rare. Approximately 15 cases have been described. These tumors are found on the false vocal folds, aryepiglottic folds, and ventricles, in adults. Some lesions are pedicled and mucosally covered.[30] A vascular form called angioleiomyoma has been described in older men. Leiomyomas are usually found in the vestibular and aryepiglottic folds, deep to the mucosa and arising from the vocalis muscle. They may be associated with lancinating pain. Bleeding may be profuse on partial endoscopic excision.[31,32]

MYOMA AND MYOBLASTOMA. Myomas and myoblastomas are benign tumors that originate over the arytenoid areas. They appear as red, smooth excrescences of the larynx. Both should be treated by transoral excision, or by a pharyngotomy approach if they are located deeper in the soft tissues or have broad bases in the larynx or pharynx.

SQUAMOUS CELL CARCINOMA

Because the natural histories of cancer of the larynx and the laryngopharynx differ significantly, and because the ultimate outcome for the patient often depends on the initial therapy, patients with these diseases are best handled by those thoroughly familiar with accurate assessment of the primary lesion. Cancer of the larynx is a highly curable disease, whereas cancer of the laryngopharynx is less curable because of its aggressive nature and relatively late presentation.[33] In most instances, the treatment of cancer of the pharynx and larynx incorporates therapeutic modalities that yield as much physiologic preservation of the organ as possible without compromising cure rates. Thus, it is no longer valid that treatment for these disorders is restricted either to radiation therapy or total laryngectomy or laryngopharyngectomy.

At present, the treatment of cancer of the larynx and pharynx can be divided into four methods: (1) curative radiotherapy; (2) a primary surgical procedure involving some form of conservation technique or a total laryngectomy; (3) a combination of preoperative or postoperative radiation with a conservation procedure or total laryngectomy; or (4) chemotherapeutic, hyperthermic, or photoradiative techniques for the treatment of recurrent or advanced tumors that do not respond to radiation therapy and are not amenable to surgical treatment.

Much new information has been obtained during the past two decades from detailed studies of cancers arising from the pharynx and larynx. Because of certain anatomic, physiologic, and pathologic information obtained from these studies, a change in the types of surgical procedures used to treat them has taken place. Better understanding of the physiology of deglutition and of the ability of the larynx and pharynx to compensate and to adapt has resulted in an attempt to preserve more function in the pharynx and larynx that remain after curative procedure. Continued improvements in surgical technique for tumors restricted in anatomic location in the pharynx and larynx have led to further applications in situations previously considered to be treated adequately only by total laryngectomy. Five factors have accounted for this change of attitude:

1. The addition of routine neck dissection to the treatment of certain forms of cancer of the pharynx and larynx has yielded better cure rates than those obtained with total laryngectomy and watchful waiting for possible metastasis to occur.
2. A review of the pathologic material from a homogeneous series of cases treated in one manner has allowed a study of the relationship between primary lesions and nodal metastases.
3. The development of CT and MR imaging has provided critical diagnostic tools for separating lesions into various zones, which can then be handled differently.
4. Cure rates in patients on whom conservation of function surgery is performed are as good as those in patients with the same lesion previously treated by total laryngectomy.
5. Present-day radiotherapeutic techniques yield excellent results for certain tumors. The value of radiotherapy as a postoperative therapeutic measure combined with radical surgery has been reflected in the decrease in early failure rates.

Additional factors, fast becoming more important, are the apparent increase in cure rates of other types of cancers treated with conservative surgery and adjuvant chemotherapy and the attempt to apply such techniques to head and neck tumors.

Incidence

The incidence of laryngeal carcinoma compared with that of carcinomas of all organs is relatively low. The incidence is comparable to that of cancer of the mouth (11,700 cases per year) and thyroid (10,600 cases per year), but only one tenth as high as that of lung cancer (149,000 cases per year), according to data from the National Cancer Institute Surveillance, Epidemiology, and End Results Program, 1977 to 1981.

Laryngeal cancer comprises 2 to 5% of all malignant diseases diagnosed annually worldwide. For instance, absolute data available from the former German Democratic Republic (1972) show 59,113 new cancers reported, of which 507 in men and 41 in women were in the larynx. Thus, the ratio of laryngeal carcinomas to all other carcinomas is 1:54 in men and 1:775 in women.[34] Only a slight increase in incidence has been noted in the past 30 years.

In heavily industrialized areas, the incidence appears to be slightly higher, from 6 to 8%. In the Connecticut Tumor Registry, carcinoma of the larynx comprises approximately 12% of all tumors diagnosed. Approximately 10,000 men and 2300 women were expected to be diagnosed with new laryngeal cancers in the United States in 1989. About 3000 men and 700 women were expected to die of their disease in 1989. In the United States, the predicted mortality for laryngeal carcinomas was approximately 32% in 1986, according to the American Cancer Society. At the time of diagnosis, both men and women had regional disease in approximately 25% of cases. Approximately 8 to 10% had distant metastases, and the remainder had only local disease.

The greatest incidence of laryngeal cancer occurs in the fifth, sixth, and seventh decades (more than 80% of all tumors). The largest number of lesions occur in the sixth decade (approximately 40%), with the average age for the occurrence of laryngeal carcinoma appearing to be approximately 59 years. In Scandinavian countries, several age peaks are frequently seen in men, usually at 60 to 65 years, 66 to 69 years, and 55 to 59 years. Norway also notes a high incidence in older men, from 70 to 74 years of age, but Sweden has a relatively flat occurrence rate from age 54 to 74 years.[35] In general, worldwide, the incidence of laryngeal cancer is highest in men aged 55 to 65 years. In age-corrected data, the incidence continues to rise until age 75. Laryngeal cancer in adolescents and children is rare and tends to be papillary-lymphocytic and nonkeratinizing.

The frequency in women varies in different regions. The male-to-female ratio varies from 5 to 20:1 (with the exception of postcricoid carcinomas, which are found more frequently in women). This disparity between sexes appears to have decreased in the past decade. In the United States, DeRienzo and associates examined the tumor registries at the Ben Taub General Hospital and found, in a comparison between 15-year periods from 1959 to 1973 and 1974 to 1988, that the ratio of male to female incidence of laryngeal cancer dropped from 5.6:1 to 4.5:1.[36] Wynder and associates noted a decrease in this ratio from 14.9:1 to 4.6:1 and an increase in the incidence of supraglottic lesions in women.[37] This finding was further supported by a British study by Robin in 1991.[38]

Laryngeal and laryngopharyngeal cancers have remained the most common malignant tumors of the head and neck despite increases in tumors of the oral cavity and oropharynx in the past two decades. Increases have also occurred in laryngeal cancer incidence rates in many countries since the 1940s,[39,40] although this increase in incidence rate is not uniform throughout the world. For instance, in Italy, incidence and mortality have doubled.[41] Similar findings have been observed in Scandinavian countries, Connecticut,

Uruguay, and Puerto Rico.[42–44] Countries or regions with a high incidence of laryngeal carcinoma as calculated per 100,000 persons per year include Uruguay and Poland (5.5 to 7.8 men, 0.3 to 0.8 women), Croatia (6.2), Connecticut (6.1), Ohio (6.7), and the former German Democratic Republic (6.4). Six highly industrialized regions in the United States have an incidence of 7.5 per 100,000.[45–48] Lower incidences for laryngeal carcinomas are reported in Japan (0.59), Singapore (1.9), Syria (2.0), Armenia (2.6), and Australia (1.9).[49–51] Most studies show that inhabitants of the most industrialized cities have an incidence of laryngeal carcinoma 2 to 3 times higher than that of rural inhabitants.[52] In Europe, higher incidence of laryngeal cancer is reported in Finland and the former Yugoslavia, 6.7 and 6.5 cases per 100,000, respectively, or 1.5% of all tumors.

The current record for the highest incidence of laryngeal cancer is found in northern Thailand (Chaing Mai province), which has a rate of 18.4 per 100,000 in males and 3.4 per 100,000 in females. This high incidence is presumed to be caused by the prevalence of smoking a particularly dangerous type of cigar.[53]

Older literature indicates a higher incidence of laryngeal cancer in Asian and Indian populations. Apparently, laryngeal cancer is more common in Africa, in white or urbanized black populations, whereas nasopharyngeal and oral cancers appear to be more common in nonurbanized tribal communities, as discussed at the Centennial Conference on Laryngeal Cancer in Toronto in 1974.

Religious groups that forbid drinking of ethanol and smoking have a low incidence of laryngeal cancer (e.g., Mormons, Seventh-Day Adventists, Parsi), as do certain other racial groups (e.g., North American Jews and North and South American Indians).

Tumor incidence at different locations in the larynx is variable. In Belgrade, in the former Yugoslavia, 60% of tumors occur in the supraglottic larynx, whereas in Scandinavia, this site accounts for only approximately 15% of tumors. Other regions report supraglottic cancers ranging from 11% (Sweden) to 22% (Finland) to 35% (Germany). In Japan, England, and most of Asia, the proportion of supraglottic to glottic cancers is approximately equal, and in other areas (Tunisia, Chile) the proportion of supraglottic cancers is higher in women. In Italy, approximately half of the tumors are supraglottic, and the population is generally younger, as opposed to carcinoma of the glottis and hypopharynx, which occurs in older populations. In the Chicago Cooperative Study of 682 cancers, 40% were noted to be glottic tumors. In France, 66% of tumors were glottic. In the Barnes Hospital (St. Louis, MO) experience with over 1600 patients, we have noted approximately 60% glottic tumors, 30% supraglottic, and 10% marginal.

Survival rates for laryngeal cancer have been in-

creasing. In 1960 to 1963, the relative 5-year survival rate for patients diagnosed with laryngeal cancer was 53% overall. In 1979 to 1984, this rate rose to 66%, although in black Americans it remained at about 55%. Long-term (10-year) relative survival rates have remained at about 50% for quite some time.

Second Primary Malignant Tumor

The incidence of multiple synchronous primary carcinomas in patients with laryngeal cancer is approximately 1%. The incidence of metachronous primary tumors is approximately 5 to 10%. Kleinsasser and associates reported a 10% incidence of second malignant tumors in 496 patients with laryngeal cancer.[30] Furthermore, the incidences were three times more common in supraglottic than glottic carcinomas.[54] Wagenfeld and associates noted secondary tumors in 12% of patients with laryngeal cancer and in 19% of those with supraglottic cancer.[55,56] Boysen and Loven found an annual second malignant neoplasm rate of 3.5% overall for head and neck carcinoma that was only 2.1% for laryngeal carcinoma; they acknowledged the findings by other authors that supraglottic cancers were as much as 3-fold more likely to be followed by a second malignant neoplasm than purely glottic tumors.[57] Laryngeal carcinoma may be the index cancer for multiple malignant tumors in other organ systems.[58] The most frequent concomitant tumor, however, is bronchial carcinoma, following laryngeal cancer with an incidence of 7 to 15%. When patients have double carcinomas, 10% occur synchronously, 30% within 1 year, 30% within 5 years, and the rest within 20 years. This is related to the duration and degree of smoking and continuation of smoking after definitive therapy.[59]

Savary and associates reported the incidence of second primary cancers in the population of head and neck cancer patients as a whole to be as high as 1:3 (cumulative 5-year risk).[60] They also found the cumulative risk of a third malignant tumor to be 1:2. Although patients with nonlaryngeal malignant tumors tended to have other upper aerodigestive tract tumors, those with laryngeal cancers had a higher percentage of pulmonary cancers. Eighty percent of patients with second primary tumors tended to have carcinoma in situ or T1 disease, and their treatment program was modified in five of six patients when a second tumor was discovered.

The diagnostic benefit of a yearly chest radiograph is therefore easy to understand, although the effect on survival may not support this as standard practice. Engelen and associates reported the diagnosis of a malignant lung tumor in 12.4% of patients being followed-up for laryngeal cancer.[61] They also noted that 69% of these patients were asymptomatic when diagnosed with lung neoplasia by routine chest radiograph, and their survival time was significantly longer than that of patients whose lung cancers were diagnosed after the onset of symptoms. This difference, however, was negligible when the symptom prodrome was taken into account.

Causes

Numerous animal studies have indicated the clear contribution of both ethanol and smoking to laryngeal cancer. The relationship between tobacco smoking and carcinoma of the larynx has been most thoroughly investigated. The reports of these studies, some dating back to the 1940s, remove any reasonable doubt about the causal relationship between tobacco consumption and carcinoma of the larynx.[62-64] It appears that nicotine is not carcinogenic, but that the residual tars, which contain polycyclic aromatic hydrocarbons, are.

The earlier one begins to smoke, and the more one smokes, the higher the incidence of laryngeal carcinoma.[65,66] Using filters that absorb n-nitrosamines, using low-tar tobaccos, and stopping smoking reduce the risk of cancer.[67] Generally, 88 to 98% of patients with laryngeal cancers have been smokers at one time, with over 50% smoking more than 20 cigarettes per day. Furthermore, vocal fold cancer is almost exclusively found in smokers. Smokers of more than 2 packs per day have a 13 times higher risk of dying of laryngeal cancer, and this risk increases even more in the sixth and seventh decades of life.[68] This risk was found to be as high as 16 times higher in the Tuyns report of smokers in Europe.[38]

Alcohol has been proposed as a cocarcinogen. Boyle and associates reviewed the molecular biology of alleged cancer-causing or cancer-promoting agents such as alcohol and tobacco, diet, oral hygiene, and other factors that may predispose to the development of malignancy.[69] It appears that alcohol and smoking potentiate each other,[70] although how this occurs is not clear. Blot reviewed the epidemiologic data implicating ethanol use in carcinogenesis in the head and neck as well as elsewhere in the body.[71] The incidence of cancer of the larynx is higher among alcoholics than in nondrinkers.[72,73] The current suspected causes in alcoholics are a deficiency of riboflavin and other vitamins, changes in immunoglobulin and other immune molecule levels, poor nutrition, cirrhosis, and other vitamin deficiency. For smokers who are alcoholics, the increase in incidence of laryngeal cancer is 25 to 50 times.

Although most patients with laryngopharyngeal cancer smoke, an increase in smoking has been noted in the United States with a lesser concomitant increase in the number of laryngeal cancers. The United States Surgeon General's report on smoking and health in the past specifically stated a definite correlation between heavy smoking and laryngeal cancer. More recent researchers, including Auerback and associates in 1970,[74] have shown that metaplasia and malignant change in human laryngeal epithelium develop in proportion to the quantity of tobacco smoke exposure, especially with cigarettes. These changes appear to be reversible. Other experimenters have noted that organic amines and polycyclic hydrocarbons can produce laryngeal tumors in animals.

Some evidence also implicates a hereditary predisposition to formation of laryngeal cancers. For example, in animals, Syrian hamsters can be inbred to increase their rate of formation of cancers when exposed to smoke.[75] Some evidence suggests that patients with carcinomas have a high level of arylhydrocarbon hydroxylase, which hydroxylates polycyclic aromatic hydrocarbons to epoxides. This enzyme may have differing activities in persons with differing susceptibilities to formation of cancer on exposure to smoke.[76] Several reviews have noted a 7 to 15% association of laryngeal carcinomas with tumors in other family members. In Japan, 56.1% of laryngeal cancer patients have relatives with gastric carcinoma, lung cancer, or laryngeal cancer.[50] Although pedigree data demonstrating clusters of affected relatives suggest that some squamous cell cancers of the head and neck result from an interaction between environmental factors and genetic predisposition, no genetic marker has been described. One study demonstrated that, in 83 patients with head and neck carcinoma diagnosed before age 40 years, 30% denied using tobacco, compared with only 9% of the controls (P less than 0.05). The 5-year disease-free survival rate of the young adults who did not use tobacco was 66%, compared with 86% for their matched control group with a history of smoking. These differences were most significant in young adults with stage II disease. The growth and progression of head and neck cancer in these young adults is characterized by tobacco use patterns; a family history of head and neck cancer in 5 of 17 young adults who did not use tobacco raises the issue of an inherent genetic determinant. Another study found that, when fibroblasts were cultured from 30 patients with biopsy-proved oropharyngeal and laryngeal squamous cell cancer, 43% had significantly elevated (7 to 12%) hyperdiploidy, compared with about 2% for controls.[77] Six of the 7 clinically affected women had hyperdiploidy, a proportion significantly greater than that of the men.

Recent studies have also implicated herpes simplex infections as predisposing to laryngeal cancer. These patients have an elevated carcinoembryonic antigen level; they have antibodies to herpes simplex and positive reactions to are dinitrofluorobenzene. One supposition is that these patients may have a cellular immune suppression, which leads to their predisposition to the formation of cancers. A series of 22 squamous cell carcinomas of the oral cavity, pharynx, and larynx was studied by conventional light microscopy and a method to identify the presence of human papillomavirus (HPV) DNA.[78] HPV DNA was found in 8 of 22 carcinomas (36%, 2 of 4 G1 tumors, 5 of 11 G2 tumors, 1 of 7 G3 tumors). HPV DNA was not observed in normal mucosal tissues. The capsid antigen was also isolated by Kashima and associates in 14 of 20 tumor specimens removed from patients with laryngeal cancer.[79] These findings provide evidence for the presence of HPV infections in tumors of the upper respiratory and digestive tract. Brandwein and colleagues have suggested that the presence of HPV DNA in a laryngeal tumor "may portend a worse prognosis."[80] Prospective studies now have to clarify the biologic importance of HPV infections in this group of human cancers.

A major recent advance in cancer research has been in the field of oncogenes. Oncogenes are genes with a proved cancer association and appear to be particularly implicated in cellular regulation and proliferation. The oncogenic potential of specific cellular genes has now been recognized, and this has influenced current thinking concerning the initiation of carcinogenesis. An excellent pair of reviews was published in *Current Opinion in Oncology* by Schantz and Carter in 1993.[81,82]

Laryngoceles, enlargements of the ventricles, are found in about 2% of healthy older adults and in 18% of patients with carcinomas of the larynx (see Fig. 32–10). Marschick, in 1927, first reported this association.[83] Today, 16% of laryngeal carcinomas are associated with laryngoceles (see Fig. 32–11) or prolapsing ventricular mucosa, and 7% of laryngoceles are associated with laryngeal carcinoma.[84,85] In older men, elongation of the laryngeal ventricles is a common concomitant of aging. The specific role of an oncogene is still incompletely understood, but research with one particular oncogene (ras) has demonstrated that it can be involved in more than one stage of multistep carcinogenesis. New techniques are being developed and evaluated to determine the expression of specific oncogenes in normal and neoplastic tissues, with a view to using them in future diagnostic immunohistopathologic methods. The tumor suppressor protein p53 has received an enormous amount of attention in the recent past for its relation to carcinogenesis. It has been detected by multiple groups in about 60% of laryngeal carcinomas. It has also been detected in premalignant lesions and may therefore represent an early change in the protein manifestation of carcinogenesis.[81,82,86] The DNA content and density has also be studied by several groups and has been found to be directly correlated to the length of the posttreatment disease-free interval in patients with laryngeal carcinoma.[87,88] Future prospects of this research field are being examined for possible implications in cancer therapy.

Other causative factors implicated in laryngeal carcinoma include anatomic malformations, ionizing radiation, Plummer-Vinson syndrome, chemicals, physical factors, and environmental exposure.[89] Another surface epithelial malformation found occasionally at the free edge of the vocal fold, known as sulcus vocalis,

has also been found to be associated with an increased incidence of carcinoma of the larynx.[90]

Ionizing radiation as a cause of induction of laryngeal carcinoma was first proposed in the 1930s by von Eicken and Soerusen.[91] Occupational exposure to alpha particles in pitchblende workers induced laryngeal cancers.[92] Radioactive iodine used in therapeutic doses (for example in Graves' disease), has also been implicated.[93] External beam irradiation, used for a variety of diseases in the past (thyrotoxicosis, malignant skin diseases, mycoses, or scrofula), has apparently induced laryngeal carcinomas as well. Reports have documented the malignant degeneration of juvenile laryngeal papillomatosis after external radiation. Some have speculated that metachronous carcinomas occurring many years after primary irradiation to head and neck tumors were irradiation-induced.[94,95]

Patterson-Kelly-Brown or Plummer-Vinson syndrome (sideropenic dysplasia with atropic gastritis, glossitis, and achlorhydria) is associated with postcricoid carcinoma.[96] Middle-aged and older women are affected in 95% of cases. The syndrome appears to be determined by exogenous factors and is more common in northern latitudes.[97] Iron deficiency has been implicated because the incidence has dropped with the introduction of iron and multivitamins into diets of the populations affected.[98] Various studies estimate that up to 30% of women with this syndrome develop postcricoid carcinoma.[99]

Various environmental factors have been implicated in laryngeal carcinoma. These include steam and heat inhalation, thermal burns, organic chemical compounds (polycyclic aromatic hydrocarbons, nitrosamines) that are produced in coal, iron, and rubber industries; insecticides (benzopyrenes); alkylating substances produced in mustard gas factories; chemical fumes (vinyl chloride, formaldehyde); fibers in textile manufacturing and the leather industry; nickel and chromate mining; and asbestosis.[100–106]

Pathology

About 95 to 98% of all malignant neoplasms of the larynx are squamous cell carcinomas; they vary in degree of cellular differentiation. True vocal fold cancers are generally well differentiated (Fig. 32–3). Lesions involving the hypopharynx, pyriform sinus, and aryepiglottic fold are less well differentiated (Fig. 32–4). Roels has written an excellent review of the various histologic studies used to evaluate tumors of the larynx including benign disease.[107]

Hyperkeratosis is often associated with carcinoma in situ and invasive carcinoma, but the incidence of isolated hyperkeratosis becoming invasive cancer appears to be low (3%). Hyperkeratosis usually involves the true vocal folds and is related to smoking or trauma. At times, the lesion may appear white or gray;

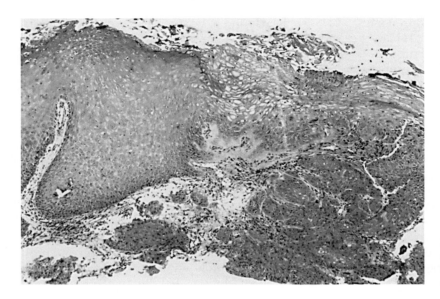

Fig. 32–3. Well-differentiated invasive keratinizing squamous cell carcinoma. ×90, hematoxylin and eosin stain. Note the junction between invasive and in situ lesions. (Courtesy of Dr. W. Bauer.)

in such instances, the term "leukoplakia" is used (Fig. 32–5). Histologically, cellular atypia may be present. Treatment is usually conservative and consists of microexcision of mucosa or, in more extensive cases, stripping of the true vocal folds. Cessation of smoking is imperative.

Carcinoma in situ is indistinguishable grossly from hyperkeratosis or carcinoma. Characteristically, the surface vasculature of the vocal folds becomes engorged and hyperemic, and the vessels assume a tortuous or U-shaped appearance. Any area of the larynx may be involved, but characteristically carcinoma in situ is confined to the true vocal fold. It may be an isolated lesion, but it is more commonly associated with invasive cancer. One may assume that, if left untreated, carcinoma in situ will progress to invasive car-

cinoma. Treatment should be conservative; microexcision or stripping of the entire lesion from the vocal fold is adequate therapy. Close follow-up examinations are necessary, and repeated removals for recurrences are indicated. Irradiation is generally not indicated. Lubsen and Kalter published a detailed review of the histopathologic features of premalignant lesions and compared various grading scales and methods of histologic preparation.[108] Immunohistochemistry and its role in the generation of diagnosis in unusual tumors of the larynx were well reviewed by Carter in 1993.[82] He included an extensive section on the benefits to diagnosis and perhaps prognosis of staining for the presence of the various *oncogenes* as well as the expression of proteins such as that generated by the *p53* nuclear phosphoprotein.

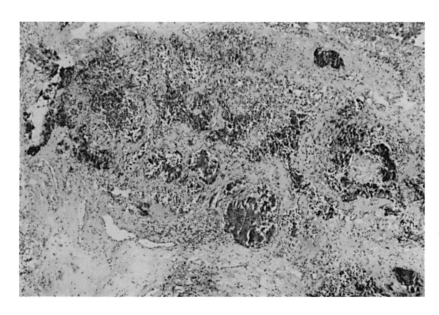

Fig. 32–4. Poorly differentiated squamous cell carcinoma of the supraglottis. ×90, hematoxylin and eosin stain.

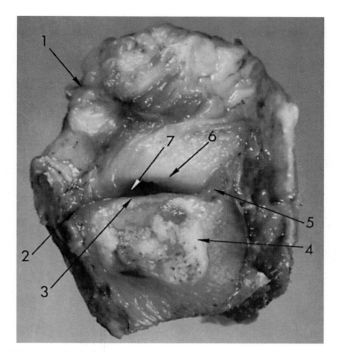

Fig. 32–5. Right hemilaryngectomy specimen with well-differentiated squamous cell carcinoma surrounded by areas of leukoplakia (4) in the subglottis. Anatomic points of interest include epiglottic petiole (1), anterior commissure (2), vocal fold (3), muscular process of the arytenoid (5), false vocal fold (6), and laryngeal ventricle (7).

Cytology

The technique of fine-needle aspiration was first described for use in the diagnosis of malignant tumors of the head and neck by Martin in 1930.[109] Since then, the technique has been shown to be both safe and effective in providing a diagnosis in the hands of skilled clinicians and cytologists. No significant incidence of needle track seeding has been described. The limits of the procedure are met in the context of difficult cellular patterns to interpret such as lymphoma or in the diagnosis of recurrent tumor in patients who have undergone radiation or surgery. In this setting, inflammatory or cytotoxic effects may make the diagnosis of malignancy difficult. Abram and associates reported a series of fine-needle aspiration studies performed in patients suspected of having recurrent disease after radiotherapy or chemotherapy or surgery followed by radiotherapy.[110] Although the incidence of false-negative studies was higher in patients previously treated, no false-positive results were reported. Several patients required more than one fine-needle aspiration, and several required open biopsy for ultimate diagnosis based on clinical suspicion. The authors likened this to the same clinical problem in the physical diagnosis of malignancy, in which previous treatment may make the palpation of recurrent disease more difficult, if not impossible. These investigators emphasized that a positive diagnosis by an experienced cytologist was a basis for treatment.

Classification of Tumor Sites (Fig. 32–6)

Glottic Tumors

Glottic tumors are those that involve the true vocal folds. The inferior limit of the glottis is generally considered to be approximately 10 mm below the level of the free margin of the cord. The 10-mm designation represents the inferior limit of intrinsic muscles of the vocal fold. The superior margin is the laryngeal ventricle. A glottic lesion therefore may involve one or both cords, may extend subglottically for 10 mm (this has recently been extended to almost 20 mm), and may involve the anterior or posterior commissure or vocal process of the arytenoid cartilage.

Supraglottic Tumors

Supraglottic cancers are those confined to an area extending from the free border of the laryngeal epiglottis to and including the false vocal folds and laryngeal ventricles.

Marginal Tumors

Aryepiglottic fold lesions exhibit biologic behavior similar to that of pyriform sinus lesions and therefore are classified as marginal lesions and not as supraglottic lesions.

Infraglottic Tumors

Infraglottic cancers extend or arise more than 10 mm below the free margins of the true vocal fold and may extend to or past the inferior border of the cricoid cartilage.

Transglottic Tumors

Transglottic cancers are those that cross the ventricle from the supraglottis to involve the true and false vocal folds or that involve the glottis and extend subglottically more than 10 mm, or both.

Superior Hypopharyngeal Tumors

Cancers of the superior hypopharynx involve the vallecular surface of the epiglottis, vallecula, or base of the tongue, posterior to the circumvallate papillae. The lateral borders of this zone are the glossoepiglottic folds.

Inferior Hypopharyngeal (Pyriform Sinus) Tumors

Inferior hypopharyngeal tumors are confined to an area bounded superiorly by the glossoepiglottic fold, inferiorly by the apex of the pyriform sinus, laterally by the thyroid cartilage, and medially by the aryepiglottic fold and the arytenoid. The posterior medial limit is determined by a vertical line directed posteriorly from the arytenoid at midabduction. This area is encased

CLASSIFICATION

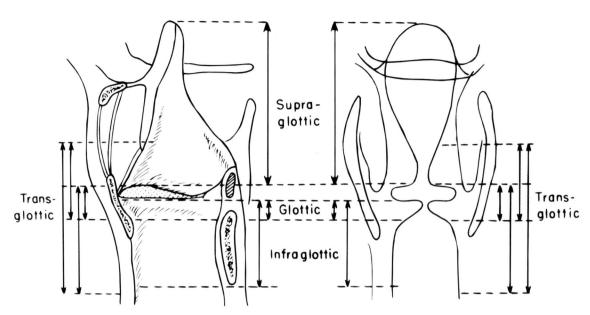

Fig. 32–6. Schematic representation of the anatomic classification of laryngeal tumors.

three quarters of the way around by laryngeal cartilage.

Posterior hypopharyngeal wall tumors are those in the zone between a posteriorly projected line from the superior margin of the base of the tongue to the level of the arytenoids and medial to each lateral wall of the pyriform sinus. Tumors in this area are rare and often involve the glossoepiglottic fold. Their metastatic behavior pattern is similar to that of superior hypopharynx tumors, and they are included in this classification for statistical consideration.

The postcricoid region is considered part of the inferior hypopharynx. This region includes the mucosal coverage of the cricoid region in the hypopharyngeal surface. The American Joint Committee on Cancer (AJCC) divides the inferior hypopharynx into three compartments, that is, the posterior hypopharyngeal wall, the pyriform sinus, and the postcricoid area.

Symptoms and Signs

Dysphonia
Hoarseness is the cardinal symptom of laryngeal carcinoma. It is caused by any condition that interferes with normal phonatory function of the larynx. As vocal folds approximate for phonation, they vibrate as air passes through the larynx. The tone quality is variously affected by the size of the glottic chink, the bulk of the vocal folds, the sharpness of the vocal fold edges, the rapidity and symmetry of cordal vibration, the tension of the cords, and the ability of the cordal mucosa to vibrate freely. In cancer of the larynx, the vocal folds

fail to perform properly because of vocal fold irregularities, tight attachment of the mucosal surface to the underlying submucosa; occlusion or narrowing of the glottic chink, invasion of the vocalis muscles, cricoarytenoid joints, and ligaments; and rarely, neural invasion. Hoarseness alters the quality of the voice to one that is rough, grating, harsh, discordant, and lower in pitch than usual. Rarely, aphonia is caused by pain, total laryngeal airway obstruction, or complete paralysis.

Of patients with vocal fold carcinomas who eventually came to therapy, 51% have been hoarse for 3 months or longer, and 30% have been hoarse for at least 12 months before consultation with a physician.[111,112]

The temporal relation of hoarseness to the laryngeal tumor depends on the location of the lesion. When the tumor arises on the true vocal folds, hoarseness is an early and persistent symptom. When tumors arise in the adjacent regions, in the laryngeal ventricles, under the surface of the ventricular folds, or in the inferior border of the true vocal folds, hoarseness develops only later. Time is required for tumor invasion and fixation of the true vocal fold and the cricoarytenoid joint and for tumor bulk to increase in size to occlude the airway significantly. In tumors arising in the supraglottis and subglottis, hoarseness may be a late symptom or may not develop at all. In the latter cases, the first symptoms may be vague and subjective, such as discomfort, a tickling sensation, or a lump in the throat that is sometimes misdiagnosed as globus hystericus.

Tumors arising in the hypopharynx rarely produce hoarseness unless they are extensive. Tumors in the superior hypopharynx (vallecular) alter the voice quality late in the course of the disease. This occurs when deep structures such as strap muscles, intrinsic and extrinsic laryngeal muscles, or tongue muscles are involved. The resultant fixation and pain produce a muffled "hot-potato" voice. The inferior hypopharynx alters the voice late in the course of the disease, when the intrinsic larynx is compromised by arytenoid fixation or vocal fold invasion.

Any patient who is hoarse for longer than 2 weeks should have careful inspection of the larynx.

Dyspnea and Stridor

Dyspnea and stridor are late findings caused by airway obstruction and may be present with any laryngeal lesion. They are caused by compromise of the airway because of tumor bulk, accumulation of debris and secretions, or vocal fold fixation. Generally, patients with large supraglottic tumors have inspiratory stridor; those with subglottic tumors have expiratory stridor; and patients with glottic or transglottic tumors have both. The gradual obstruction is well compensated by the patient. Acute airway obstruction, however, may be precipitated by secondary edema, infections, or instrumentation. Characteristically, the dyspnea is aggravated by exertion and anxiety; that is, the harder the patient tries to breathe, the less air is inspired. The reason is mechanical because fast, in-rushing air has a closing effect on the glottis (Bernoulli effect). Generally, dyspnea and stridor are ominous prognostic signs. Stertor is the sound produced during inspiration by the supraglottic larynx and pharynx that is colloquially known as snoring. It may be the a sign of a mass lesion in someone who describes the new onset of this problem without an accompanying weight gain.

Pain

Sore throat is a frequent complaint in patients with superior hypopharyngeal, epiglottic, or pyriform cancer. This may vary from a scratching sensation to a sharp pain. If the pain is of the stabbing type and is accentuated by deglutition, involvement of deep structures such as the muscles of the base of the tongue and hypopharynx, or invasion of the laryngeal skeleton, is most probable.

Referred pain, usually to the ipsilateral ear, is mediated by the tenth nerve and is more characteristic of the pyriform, base of the tongue, and vallecular lesions. This pain is lancinating, of short duration, and sharp.

Dysphagia

Dysphagia (difficulty in swallowing) is characteristic of cancers of the base of the tongue and supraglottic, superior hypopharynx, and pyriform sinus cancers. It is the most common complaint in postcricoid carcinomas. Many patients may complain of fullness in the throat, irritations or scratching sensations, and changes in swallowing habits (such as frequent clearing of mucus from the throat and preference for warm liquids). True odynophagia (pain in swallowing), however, denotes advanced carcinomas involving extralaryngeal structures, particularly those about the pharynx, base of the tongue, postcricoid, and superior esophagopharyngeal inlet.

Cough

Cough, a rare symptom with glottic cancers, usually develops in hypopharyngeal involvement with overflow of secretions and fluids into the larynx, attempted clearing of the throat to eliminate discomfort, or anesthesia of the larynx caused by tumor involvement of the supraglottic area (superior laryngeal nerves).

Other Late Findings

Hemoptysis is seen most frequently with infraglottic tumors and large, fungating supraglottic tumors or any tumors that cause persistent coughing. It can be a presenting symptom, but on closer questioning, other symptoms are usually elicited.

Weight loss is an ominous symptom that indicates extralaryngeal tumor extension or distant metastasis. It generally denotes obstruction of the food passageway or odynophagia caused by deep muscle invasion.

Halitosis is present in many patients because of generalized poor oral and dental hygiene or necrosis of large, fungating tumors. Occasionally, patients cough up the tissue specimen.

Swelling in the neck may be the presenting complaint. Usually, this is caused by an enlarged cervical lymph node and should be considered metastatic cancer. A primary lesion should be searched for and identified. Areas where occult primary lesions occur should undergo biopsy. These include the nasopharynx, tongue, tonsil, and pyriform sinus. Incisional biopsy of the cervical node (which we do not advocate), if performed, should be done in a manner that will not complicate future case management. Fine-needle aspiration of cervical node masses is an acceptable procedure in the presence of a competent pathologist. Generally, laryngeal tumors presenting with a "lump in the neck" are extensive lesions.

Tenderness of the larynx is a late sign of ominous significance because of the suppurative complication of tumors that invade the thyroid cartilage and perichondrium.

Gross Morphology

Supraglottic Tumors

The gross appearance of squamous cell cancer of the larynx varies greatly with time and location. Supraglottic tumors are often fungating, with heaped-up edges and multiple areas of central ulceration. These are infiltrating tumors with spreading peripheries (Fig.

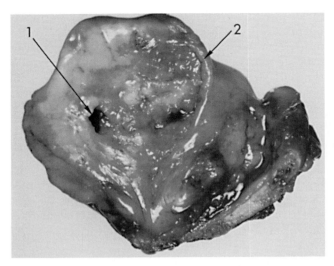

Fig. 32–7. Specimen from a subtotal supraglottic laryngectomy demonstrating gross appearance of the tumor. Note infiltrating and spreading margins (2), and central area of necrosis with epiglottic foraminal invasion of the cartilage (1).

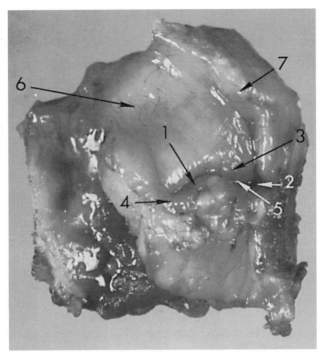

Fig. 32–8. Left hemilaryngectomy specimen with glottic carcinoma invading the ventricle and subglottis (1). Anterior commissure (2), false cord (3), vocal process of arytenoid (4), laryngeal ventricle (5), aryepiglottic fold (6), and epiglottic petiole (7). Note vascularity and heaped-up appearance of the tumor.

32–7). Often, at initial examination, the usual appearance of the larynx is greatly distorted by a bulky, ulcerated lesion that has eroded the epiglottis and bleeds easily on palpation.

Glottic Tumors

Glottic tumors have a slight irregular thickening and roughening of the mucosal surface in early cases. This is usually surrounded by an area of hyperemia and increased vascularity. An early finding is tortuosity and engorgement of the vessels along the long axis of the vocal fold. Instead of a linear appearance, the vessels form irregular and aberrant loops. The characteristic lesion has a whitish "cauliflower" appearance that is friable to palpation (Fig. 32–8). In other cases, it appears as a whitish or red area of superficial ulceration (see Fig. 32–5). Patients with larger lesions may have impairment of vocal fold motion or extension above and below the true vocal fold. These tumors are generally surrounded by areas of hyperkeratosis or whitish plaques (see Fig. 32–5). Glottic lesions tend to be proliferative rather than ulcerating (Fig. 32–9).

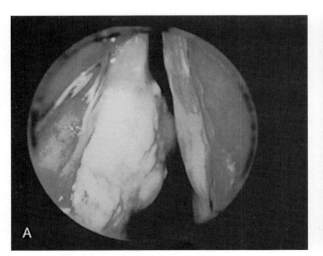

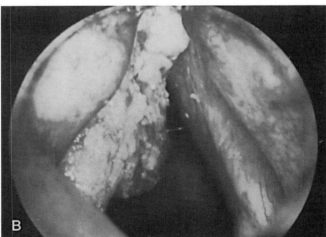

Fig. 32–9. Two endoscopic examples of glottic carcinoma. A. Hyperkeratotic lesion with posterior and subglottic extension. B. Entire vocal fold involvement with anterior commissure and subglottic extension. Note hyperkeratosis and ulceration.

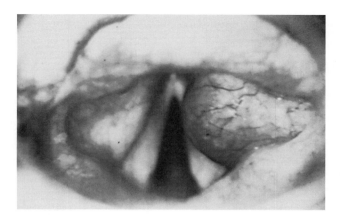

Fig. 32–10. Endoscopic view of internal laryngocele.

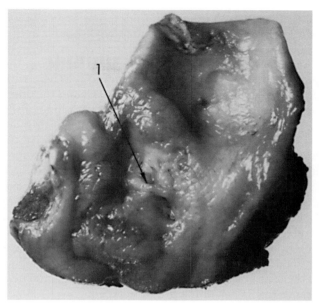

Fig. 32–12. Specimen from a partial laryngopharyngectomy denoting pyriform fossa squamous cell carcinoma (1). Note the bulky, fleshy, nonulcerated appearance with elevated margins.

Subglottic Tumors

Subglottic tumors are more flattened and have superficial ulceration. They have diffuse margins that fade into the surrounding mucosa. They tend to be raised over a broad area, but are not usually fungating. They appear whitish or red and generally do not have much accumulated debris.

Marginal Lesions

Marginal lesions are proliferative and tend to be fungating, with small central ulcerations and heaped-up margins. They are not as ragged looking as supraglottic tumors. Smooth swellings of one or both aryepiglottic folds may be laryngoceles (Figs. 32–10 and 32–11). They are occasionally inflamed and symptomatic (e.g., pain and tenderness) if they become infected, then known as laryngopyoceles.

Pyriform Sinus Tumors

Pyriform sinus tumors are large, bulky tumors that are not frequently ulcerated. They have heaped-up margins and are dark red with a fleshy appearance (Fig. 32–12).

Carcinoma in Situ

Carcinoma in situ occurs mainly on the true vocal folds and appears as a whitish hyperkeratotic area.

Diagnosis

Physical Examination

To avoid the common pitfall of incomplete examination of the larynx, the clinician must establish a stan-

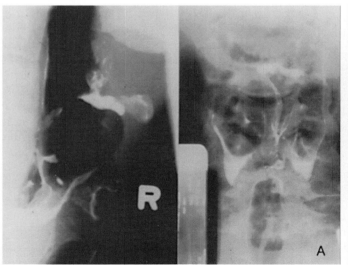

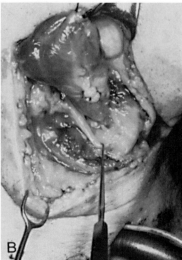

Fig. 32–11. Combined internal and external laryngocele. A. Laryngogram in the anteroposterior and lateral views. B. Supraglottic excision of the same laryngocele.

dard routine of examination that allows visualization of all parts of the larynx and must be thorough in this examination. *Palpation* and examination of the neck should be methodic. It is best to begin by facing the patient and observing for neck asymmetry. Then, with one hand (usually the left) on the occiput and the other on the larynx, the clinician palpates the midline of the neck in flexed and extended positions and during the act of swallowing. The cartilages of the laryngeal framework can be palpated to (1) detect abnormalities in texture and form, (2) test mobility and physiologic crepitus, (3) note fullness in the cricothyroid and thyrohyoid membranes, (4) examine for any widening of laryngeal cartilage, and (5) accurately localize areas of tenderness. This examination is repeated bimanually. The thyroid gland and suprasternal notch are also examined. Having the patient swallow during this part of the examination lifts the gland lobes and pretracheal tissues to further the depth of detection.

Then the examiner goes behind the patient and palpates the lateral aspects of the neck, that is, the anterior and posterior triangles. This is done while the patient's neck is in erect, extended, and flexed (the best) positions. Careful palpation along the carotid sheath, submandibular triangle, parotid gland, and eleventh cranial nerve (posterior triangle) is essential, because these are the lymph node-bearing areas. Bilateral simultaneous palpation of the carotid arteries or palpation that is too vigorous is not recommended and can result in syncope or even cerebrovascular accident. If lymph nodes are palpable, they must be described according to size (direct measurement), location, mobility (to test for fixation), and tenderness. These are then drawn on a prestamped diagram in the patient's chart.

Precise examination of the oral cavity, oropharynx, nasopharynx, and base of the tongue is essential in all patients with supraglottic lesions, especially when immobility is present on mirror examination in supraglottic tumors. This suggests submucosal extension with the vallecula and intrinsic musculature of the tongue.

If large neck lymph nodes, fixed to the underlying tissues, are present, auscultation of the carotid artery above and below the mass is mandatory. Lack of pulsation of the superficial temporal artery, facial artery, or occipital vessels, and observation of superficial localized venous engorgement, may denote vascular occlusion. This finding is unusual.

Some nonspecific signs occur late in the course of laryngeal cancer:

1. Broadening of the larynx on palpation is a significant sign of advanced disease and denotes tumor extension to the thyroid cartilage and extensive invasion of the larynx.
2. Tenderness of larynx to palpation denotes tumor invasion of inner perichondrium and cartilage or

laryngeal chondritis secondary to tumor invasion.
3. Loss of crepitation on side-to-side movement of the larynx implies postcricoid tumor invasion or tumor extension and edema between the larynx and inferior hypopharynx or esophagus. This sensation is caused by the rolling of the thyroid lamina cornua over the irregular surface of the vertebral bodies through supple and uninflamed tissues. The absence of this physiologic crepitus is sometimes a variant of normal and is not pathognomonic of neoplasia.
4. Fullness of cricothyroid membrane to palpation denotes subglottic and usually extralaryngeal tumor extension.
5. Fullness in the thyrohyoid membrane implies tumor invasion of the preepiglottic space, base of the epiglottis, and probable extralaryngeal tumor extension.
6. Digital palpation of the base of the tongue may demonstrate induration. In such cases, with supraglottic tumors, there is usually submucosal tumor extension into the vallecula and base of the tongue.

Endoscopy

INDIRECT LARYNGOSCOPY.

MIRROR. As with all intraoral examinations, the examiner should wear protective eyeglasses and gloves, as well as a mask, because he or she is vulnerable to infections transmitted by bodily fluids. For indirect laryngoscopy, a No. 4 to No. 6 laryngeal mirror is warmed (over alcohol flame or other heat source) to prevent fogging. The temperature of the mirror is checked on the back of the hand or the cheek of the examiner. Sitting or standing, the examiner faces the patient with the examiner's head at the same level as the patient's head. The patient is instructed to sit straight up with the chin slightly protruded. Holding folded gauze, the examiner grasps the patient's tongue with the thumb on top and the third finger underneath. The examiner's index finger is used to elevate the patient's upper lip. The mirror is placed into the patient's oropharynx to elevate the uvula but not touch the back or sides of the oropharynx or the base of the tongue. If there is persistent gagging, the patient's throat may be sprayed with 4% lidocaine solution, and the examination resumed after 1 to 2 minutes.

Using a head mirror and the source of illumination behind of the patient, the examiner proceeds to visualize the larynx at rest, during respiration, and during vocalization. The examiner systematically observes the symmetry, motion, and surface architecture of the base of the tongue, lateral and posterior hypopharyngeal walls, vallecula, epiglottis, aryepiglottic folds, arytenoids, pyriform sinuses, false vocal folds, true vocal folds, subglottis, first through fifth tracheal rings, and introitus of the esophagus.

The interpretation of the reflected image must be borne in mind. The angulation of the mirror foreshortens the ventral axis (shortens the vocal folds by about one third). The anterior and posterior areas are reversed, but the right and left sides of the patient remain the same. Depth perception distortion occurs in which the larynx is farther away than it seems by mirror examination. The ventricular bands and epiglottis may hide vital laryngeal areas, that is, the laryngeal ventricle or anterior commissure.

Once the lesion is visualized, it can be drawn on a prestamped diagram of the area and placed in the patient's records.

TELESCOPIC, RIGID. For rigid telescopic laryngoscopy, a rigid laryngeal telescope is treated (usually with defogging agent) to prevent fogging. The examiner's head should be at the same level as the patient's head. The patient is instructed to sit straight up with the chin slightly protruded. Holding folded gauze, the examiner grasps the patient's tongue with the thumb on top and the third finger underneath. The examiner's index finger is used to elevate the patient's upper lip. The telescope is placed into the patient's oropharynx to elevate the uvula but not touch the back or sides of the oropharynx or the base of the tongue. If there is persistent gagging, the patient's throat may be sprayed with 4% lidocaine solution, and the examination resumed after 1 or 2 minutes. At this point, the examination is carried out as for indirect laryngoscopy. With the proper instruments and sufficient skill, however, biopsy and removal of small benign lesions of the vocal folds can be performed in the office or in the operating suite under local anesthesia.

TELESCOPIC, FLEXIBLE. Flexible fiberoptic telescopic laryngoscopy can be performed in the office or at the bedside of a hospitalized patient. After careful inspection and choice of the more patent of the two nasal passages, a brief pulse of atomized oxymetazoline or phenylephrine can be administered to enlarge the aperture further and to facilitate the examination. Once the passage is open, a small amount of 2% lidocaine is sprayed in the side about to be traversed and is allowed to act for several seconds to 1 minute. If residual sensitivity is detected, a second application can be administered, or 4% lidocaine can be used. Although much stronger solutions are available, such as 10% lidocaine or sprays intended for oral or pharyngeal topical anesthesia, they should be avoided because in high concentration or in orally intended vehicles, these agents cause severe burning and tearing. In new patients, this irritation unnecessarily strains the usually tenuous trust the patients may have, anticipating the feeling of this "lighted tube" in their nose and throat.

The fiberoptic telescope is guided into position, under the examiner's constant vision, into the naso-pharynx. The scope tip is then turned inferiorly, and the scope is pushed past the palate and uvula, at which time the larynx is seen. At this point, the examination is carried out in the same manner as for the mirror or rigid telescope.

The skilled clinician will truly benefit fully from this technology. This is particularly the case when making some of the more difficult diagnoses of laryngeal function or superficial tumor extension. The diagnosis of true vocal fold paralysis, and even more so, of true vocal fold paresis can be difficult to make and is important to establish. If the patient can be convinced by soothing coaching not to swallow, to breath in a slow measured rhythm, and to remain calm, the endoscopist can pass the tip of the endoscope well into the introitus of the larynx and gain the view necessary to observe the vocal fold motion associated with the respiratory cycle, that is, adduction with expiration and abduction with inspiration. These motions are usually not obscured by the mass effect of the flexion of the bilaterally innervated interarytenoideus muscle, believed by some to be the most common reason that the diagnosis of true vocal fold paralysis is missed. When the anesthesia of the nose is carefully limited, the diagnosis of high vagal nerve based paralysis or superior laryngeal nerve injury can be accurately made. The scope can be used to touch the superior surface of the affected true vocal fold gently and prove anesthesia. If the subglottis or trachea is in need of examination, the topical anesthesia can be combined with transoral drip anesthesia directly on the larynx, or percutaneously delivered through the cricothyroid membrane. From 1 to 2 ml of 1 or 2% plain lidocaine is administered with a 27-gauge needle 1 ml at a time; the patients is instructed to take a deep breath and to cough just as the medication is being delivered. This reliably provides adequate anesthesia to examine the whole of the trachea without the risk of laryngospasm or patient discomfort. Care must be taken to ensure an intraluminal location by aspirating air before administering the medication. The clinician should, of course, always be ready for any airway or cardiovascular emergency in the office whenever performing such endoscopic procedures using potentially cardiotoxic medications.

DIRECT LARYNGOSCOPY. Direct laryngoscopy can be performed under three types of anesthesia: topical, regional block, and general. The patient must be completely relaxed and confident in the ability of the surgeon performing the procedure. The patient lies supine with the neck extended; the head must not be flexed or suspended. With topical anesthesia, 2% lidocaine is sprayed into the oropharynx, hypopharynx, and larynx with a Lukens syringe, and pyriform sinuses are anesthetized with curved forceps holding cotton moistened with 4% lidocaine. Local anesthetics can be administered by syringe using 2% lidocaine injected in the midline and intraluminally by way of the thyrohyoid membrane, or by laterally injecting the superior laryngeal nerves at the level medial to the superior cornu of the thyroid cartilage. Direct laryngoscopy is performed under general anesthesia using a No. 6 endotracheal tube and a Jackson laryngoscope or an anterior commissure laryngoscope. Employing suspension microlaryngoscopy using a vallecular scope such as a Lindholm laryngoscope can be of great value for magnified inspection of the larynx and hypopharynx. A systemic routine examination is performed of all anatomic areas in the larynx, hypopharynx, and esophageal introitus. The lesion can be measured with a ruler in millimeters.

When partial laryngeal surgery procedures are to be used, just obtaining a tissue diagnosis is insufficient. One must assess accurately the full extent of the tumor. Vocal fold mobility is determined by indirect laryngoscopy and is confirmed by direct laryngoscopy. This is achieved during general anesthesia by decreasing the anesthetic and stimulating the larynx.

A generous biopsy is taken of the tumor bulk. If one has questions concerning tumor extent, multiple biopsies are taken. Ruling out interarytenoid or postcricoid involvement is crucial to performing a successful vertical hemilaryngectomy. Ruling out penetration of a supraglottic tumor into the true vocal folds is essential to a successful subtotal supraglottic laryngectomy (SSL).

From time to time, various authors have suggested triple endoscopy at the time of direct laryngoscopy to detect synchronous primary lesion of other head and neck sites. The multicentric occurrence of tumors of the upper aerodigestive tract has been well described, with an incidence ranging from 5 to 16%. Detection of a synchronous primary tumor at the time of initial workup is crucial for both management and final outcome. Some investigators consider routine panendoscopy essential, although routine esophagoscopy and bronchoscopy with bronchial washings in the absence of specific symptoms appear to have minimal benefit and high cost.[113] In a study of 140 consecutive patients with primary squamous cell carcinoma of the head and neck who were seen over 3 years, detailed history, thorough head and neck examination, routine chest radiograph, and barium swallow when indicated were sufficient to identify 18 patients (13%) with a second primary tumor in the upper aerodigestive tract.[114] (See the previous section of this chapter on second primary tumors.)

Radiographic Evaluation

Multiple radiologic modalities are available for the head and neck surgeon investigating the extent of a laryngeal tumor. Plain radiographs of the larynx and chest are the least informative but are good screening examinations. Laminography visualizes tissue bulk, asymmetry, cartilage invasion, and intraluminal masses of the larynx. Its most important function in the past was to delineate thyroid cartilage destruction and tumor size accurately. Xerography has been applied to the study of the larynx, and some reports indicate that it is 97% accurate in diagnosing subglottic extension of tumor and 73% accurate in delineating thyroid cartilage destruction (Fig. 32–13). Laryngogra-

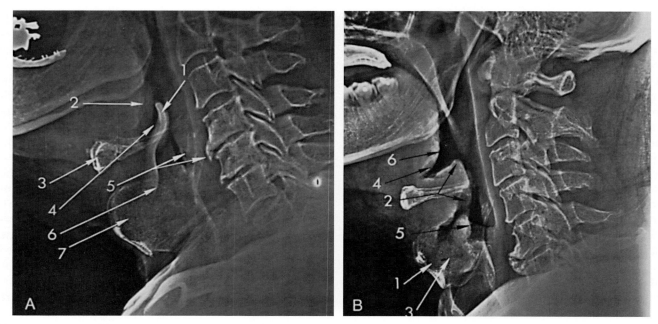

Fig. 32–13. A. Normal larynx demonstrated by xeroradiography. Epiglottis (1), base of tongue (2), hyoid body (3), vallecula (4), aryepiglottic folds (5), petiole of the epiglottis (6), thyroid lamina (7). B. Xeroradiography of supraglottic carcinoma involving the epiglottis (2) and aryepiglottic folds (5). The base of the tongue (6), vallecula (4), thyroid lamina (1), and laryngeal ventricle (3) are normal.

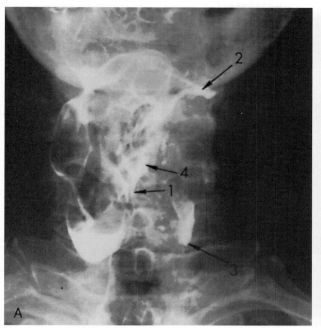
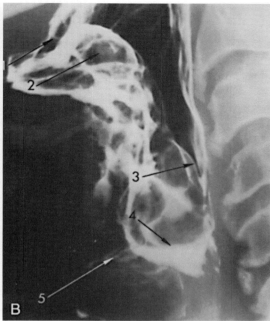

Fig. 32–14. Laryngogram of a supraglottic carcinoma. A. Anteroposterior view demonstrating filling defect of the pyriform sinus. Note the level of the vocal fold (1), bulging false cord (4), lateral vallecula (2), and patent pyriform sinus apex (3). B. Lateral view of the same lesion denoting epiglottic tumor (2), vallecular invasion (1), aryepiglottic fold (3), and pyriform sinus (4) filled with tumor. Laryngeal ventricle is free of disease (5).

phy, using aqueous propyliodone (Dionosil), is an accurate radiographic method to determine the full extent of lesions in two specific situations: (1) subglottic tumor extension, and (2) assessment of anterior commissure when large bulky lesions of the false vocal fold fix the epiglottis (Fig. 32–14). Most of these older techniques are used little today in the United States. Recent studies of the use of CT and MR scanning indicate that these techniques are extremely helpful in evaluating thyroid cartilage invasion, tumor size, and extension to adjacent structures. These methods of study are the current standard for radiographic evaluation of laryngeal lesions (Fig. 32–15).

Thallium chloride has been used for tumor imaging in patients with head and neck cancer.[115] Technetium-99m (v) dimercaptosuccinic acid has also been used as an imaging agent for head and neck squamous carcinoma with some success.[116] Neither method has achieved wide use.

Radiolabeled antibodies to tumor-associated antigens may also be used to image tumors.[117] In one pilot study, antibody against epidermal growth factor receptor (EGFR-1) was used to delineate tumors in patients with squamous cell carcinomas of the head and neck. Positive images of large tumors (greater than 3 cm in diameter) were obtained in 8 of 11 patients after intravenous administration of indium-labeled EGFR-1. Two patients gave equivocal results, and negative scans were obtained from the patient with the smallest tumor (1 cm in diameter). No false-positive images

were reported. The success of this study in delineating relatively large squamous carcinomas indicates that the antibody should be evaluated in patients with smaller tumors to establish the limits of detection of the technique.

Ultrasonography
Diagnostic ultrasound has become established in head and neck surgery. Modern equipment allows high-resolution imaging of neck tissue masses, cervical vessels, and lymph nodes. The major advantage of B-mode sonography is its ability to detect neoplasms in solid scarred neck tissue, commonly seen in patients who have undergone radical neck surgery or radical radiotherapy. Postoperative or radiogenic edema, tumor recurrence, and lymph node involvement can be differentiated.[118] Inflammatory and neoplastic lymph node diseases detected by echography must be differentiated by biopsy. This technology has demonstrated substantial use in the guidance of the fine-needle aspiration of these masses, which are difficult to palpate.[119] B-mode sonography is an important instrument in the follow-up examination of head and neck tumors for early detection of tumor recurrence or tumor persistence.[118]

Serologic Examination
Serologic markers of head and neck cancer have been investigated. In one study,[120] tumor markers in the serum were determined to evaluate their possible use-

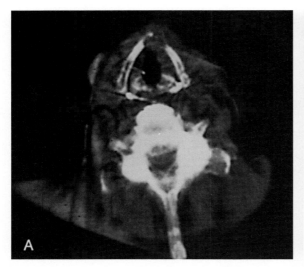 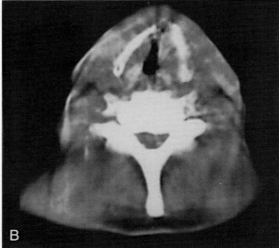

Fig. 32–15. Computed tomographic scans of two vocal fold tumors. A. Anterior commissure and cartilage invasion. B. Left vocal fold carcinoma with vocalis muscle, anterior commissure, and thyroid cartilage invasion.

fulness as parameters for monitoring therapy as well as for early detection of cancer. Patients with primary tumors (n = 101) were distributed into two groups, TI-II and TIII-IV, according to the Union Internationale contre le Cancer (UICC) classification of 1978 and were investigated together with a group of known recurrences (n = 105). Fifty age-matched healthy individuals served as controls. Substances investigated were β_2-microglobulin (β_2-M), immunoglobulin E (IgE), ferritin, N-acetyl neuraminic acid (sialic acid, NANA), and phosphohexose-isomerase (PHI). The results led to the conclusion that, in particular, IgE, NANA and (with some reservations) ferritin should be further investigated. These biologic serum markers may be useful in serial determination with special regard to their possible relevance for cancer treatment.

Tumor Staging
To describe accurately the location and extent of tumors and areas of metastasis, laryngeal lesions at different sites are staged according to the AJCC tumor, node, metastasis (TNM) classification (Table 32–1; see also Chap. 20).

The present system of classification of a cancer patient is based solely on tumor morphology. The TNM system classifies cancers based on the extent of anatomic spread. Despite its excellence in describing a tumor's size and extent of anatomic spread, the TNM system does not account for the clinical biology of the cancer. The clinical biology refers to functional aspects of the tumor as reflected in the severity of cancer-related symptoms. Another important aspect of the clinical biology of the cancer is the comorbidity of the patient.

Piccirillo and associates developed a staging system for patients with cancer of the larynx that combined

descriptions of the patient with descriptions of the tumor.[121] Severity of cancer-related symptoms were combined with comorbidity to create an intermediary three-category functional severity index. The 5-year survival rate overall was 66% (127 of 193) and within functional severity classes were 83% (89 of 107), 58% (34 of 59), and 15% (4 of 27). The functional severity index was then combined with the TNM system to create the clinical severity index. Survival rates within stages of the clinical severity index were 88% (53 of 60), 80% (24 of 30), 63% (38 of 60), and 28% (12 of 43). When compared with the TNM system alone, the clinical severity index achieved statistically significant better prognostication. These results suggest that the inclusion of clinical variables in a formal staging system can greatly improve prognostic accuracy. This significant advancement of the standard TNM system is necessary to assess the patient as a whole and not just on the basis of the size and location of tumor tissue.

Differential Diagnosis
Carcinoma of the larynx can be confused with other lesions of the larynx on clinical examination. The most important test of differentiation is an adequate biopsy specimen examined by a competent pathologist.

In the glottis, a general predilection exists for cancers to develop on the anterior two thirds of the length of the vocal fold and the anterior commissure, arytenoids, and vocal folds (reddening and thickening). Generalized edema affects the aryepiglottic folds and epiglottis, which may be ragged and necrotic. Lupus erythematosus of the larynx appears as an area of irregular raised nodules, scattered ulcers with irregular shaggy borders, scars of healed ulcers, and epiglottic notching (Fig. 32–16).

Syphilis of the larynx has protean manifestations

TABLE 32–1. TNM Classification

Primary Tumor			Nodal involvement		
TX	Tumor not assessable by rules		NX	Nodes cannot be assessed	
T0	No evidence of primary tumor		N0	No clinically positive node	
T1S	Carcinoma in situ		N1	Single clinically positive homolateral node 3 cm or less in diameter	
Supraglottis					
T1	Tumor confined to site of origin with normal mobility		N2	Single clinically positive homolateral node more than 2 cm and less than 6 cm in diameter or multiple clinically positive homolateral no more than 6 cm in diameter	
T2	Tumor involving adjacent supraglottic site(s) and glottis				
T3	Tumor limited to larynx with fixation and/or extension to cricoid area, medial wall of pyriform sinus, or preepiglottis		N2a	Single clinically positive homolateral node more than 3 cm and less than 6 cm in diameter	
T4	Massive tumor extending beyond the larynx to involve oropharynx tissues of neck, or destruction of thyroid cartilage		N2b	Multiple clinically positive homolateral nodes, none more than 6 cm in diameter	
Glottis			N2c	Contralateral nodes	
T1	Tumor confined to vocal fold(s) with normal mobility (including involvement of anterior or posterior commissures)		N3	Clinically positive node greater than 6 cm	
			Distant Metastasis		
T1a	Tumor confined to one vocal fold with normal motion		MX	Not assessed	
T1b	Tumor extending to both vocal folds with normal motion		M0	No (known) distant metastasis	
			M1	Distant metastasis present; specify sites	
T2	Supraglottic and/or subglottic extension of tumor with normal fold mobility		**Histopathology**		
			Predominant cancer is squamous cell carcinoma		
T3	Tumor confined to larynx with vocal fold fixation		**Grade**		
T4	Massive tumor with thyroid cartilage destruction and/or extension to the confines of the larynx		GX	Differentiation not available	
			G1	Well differentiated	
Subglottis			G2	Moderately differentiated	
T1	Tumor confined to the subglottic region		G3	Poorly differentiated	
T2	Tumor extension to vocal folds with normal or impaired fold		G4	Undifferentiated	
			Stage Grouping		
T3	Tumor confined to larynx with vocal fold fixation		Stage I	T1N0M0	
T4	Massive tumor with cartilage destruction and/or extension beyond the larynx, or both		Stage II	T2N0M0	
			Stage III	T3N0M0	
				T1 or T2 or T3 N1 M0	
			Stage IV	Any T4	
				Any T N2 or N3 M0	
				Any T Any N M1	

(Modified from American Joint Committee on Cancer: Manual for Staging of Cancer. 4th ed. Philadelphia, JB Lippincott, 1992.)

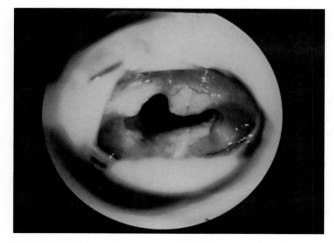

Fig. 32–16. Indirect mirror examination of epiglottic notching caused by lupus erythematosus.

ranging from edema and mucopurulent exudate (early stages) to ulcers and gummas (late stages) on the epiglottis. The ulcers are superficial with hyperemic undermined edges, irregular borders, and a granulating but necrotic bed. Syphilis affects the epiglottis, laryngeal ventricles, arytenoids, and interarytenoid space most commonly.

Benign tumors such as polyps, organizing hematomas, vocal nodules, contact ulcers, and traumatic or postintubational polyps can be differentiated readily because of their location, smooth outer surface, and sessile or pedunculated appearance. Carcinomas generally have a roughened surface and are rarely pedunculated. Even though polyps are rarely malignant, complete histologic study of all polyps is necessary. Papillomas have a roughened surface and pinkish color, but they are diffuse or multiple at different locations.

Rarer conditions that can simulate laryngeal cancer include ventricular prolapse, blastomycosis, scleroma, amyloid disease, neurofibroma, chondroma, and lymphomas. These can be ruled out by biopsy and histopathologic interpretation. Blastomycosis can be mistaken for laryngeal carcinoma because of a reaction histologically termed pseudoepitheliomatous hyperplasia. Several disorders of the upper aerodigestive tract can cause this histologic picture and should be excluded if any equivocal features are noted in the pathologic report. Histoplasmosis can also give the outward appearance of laryngeal carcinoma and must be distinguished from cancer as well as from tuberculosis.[122] Laryngeal tuberculosis can have an appearance that is grossly identical to cancer but on biopsy is identified by the likely presence of acid-fast bacilli.[123] It should be suspected whenever an abnormal chest radiograph is encountered or the constitutional symptoms of tuberculosis are reported in a review of systems.

Certain chronic diseases are difficult to differentiate clinically from early carcinomas. Leukoplakia, keratosis, pachydermia laryngitis sicca, and chronic laryngitis can produce suspicious clinical pictures. These are more generalized endolaryngeal conditions and must be examined and observed frequently. Some may be precancerous.

Treatment

Surgery

CONSERVATION SURGERY OF THE LARYNX. Conservation surgery of the larynx has as its aim the removal of the malignancy with preservation of deglutition, respiration, and phonation. The principles of conservation surgery demand that it be performed with precision. Factors that determine the modality of choice include the precise location of the lesion, immediate areas of extension, feasibility of total resection, and possibility of functional surgical restoration, coupled with the highest possible cure rate. The results of indirect and direct laryngoscopy, laryngograms, and CT and MR scans must be correlated to determine the maximal excision that is consistent with complete tumor resection and with reconstitution of function. Conservation techniques can be combined with en bloc neck dissection.

Conservation surgery in selected cases of glottic, supraglottic, pyriform sinus, hypopharynx, and base-of-tongue lesions can be performed without compromising survival.

PATIENT SELECTION. The selection of candidates for conservation surgery is based on assessment of the tumor and the general medical status of the patient. The first point is discussed in the next sections. Patient selection is based on many imprecise factors, the most important of which are the surgeon's personal experience and judgment. Although no absolute rules exist, some factors can be listed:

1. The patient's general medical state is evaluated. For older patients with cerebral deterioration, disorientation, or generalized debility, conservation surgery may not be the proper choice of treatment.
2. The patient must have the willpower and ability for reeducation of deglutition. The patient must be able to follow directions and instructions for rehabilitation. Patients with poor cardiovascular status may not be able to withstand the longer operative time, protracted convalescence, and rehabilitation needed to achieve success.
3. Excellent pulmonary function tests are a must for conservation surgery. The patient should be able to cough and expand the lungs and must have good compliance and chest motion because aspiration is frequently encountered early on relearning how to swallow. Controlled deglutition requires adequate control of the rib cage, plosive forces for cough, and lung expansion to avoid persistent aspiration and pneumonia. Generally, patients who cannot climb two flights of stairs or blow out a candle at 1 foot are not candidates for conservation surgery. Occasionally, when pulmonary function is marginal, rehabilitation and exercises are used before surgical intervention is undertaken.

When the patient's age is evaluated, chronologic age is not as pertinent as "functional" age. For instance, patients in their seventies and in otherwise poor physical condition are probably better treated by total laryngectomy or irradiation. The patient's reliability, occupation, and general life style as well as the local medical facilities play an important part in the surgeon's judgment. Experience is often the best judge of the correct choice of therapy. The major questions that should be answered are: "What is the procedure with the highest possible cure rate and least disability, and what is best for the patient?"

PROCEDURE SELECTION. The principles of conservation surgery of the larynx demand that it be precise. The tumor is visualized by direct laryngoscopy, it is measured and staged, and it is drawn on a prestamped schematic diagram of the larynx. The boundaries of the tumor are delineated by multiple biopsies. The location, size, and areas of spread are then evaluated in comparison with the anatomic regions that are free of tumor. The latter are needed to restore normal laryngeal function. The selection of the particular surgical procedure includes the precise delineation of the lesion, the immediate area of extension, the feasibility of total resection, the ability for functional surgical restoration, and the highest possible cure rate.

The three major classes of conservation procedures are the vertical, horizontal, and oblique lines of resection. The prototype for the vertical resection is the hem-

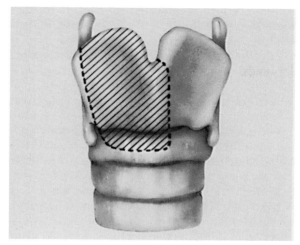

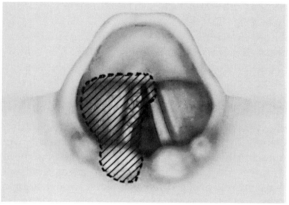

Fig. 32–17. Schematic representation of hemilaryngectomy. A vertical resection; the shaded areas denote resection region.

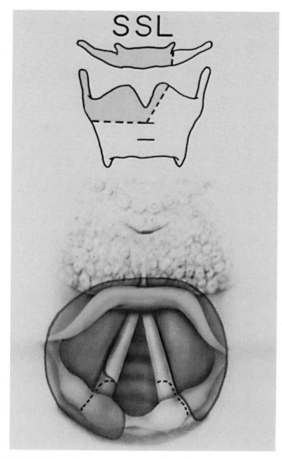

Fig. 32–18. Schematic representation of a subtotal supraglottic laryngectomy (SSL). A horizontal resection; the shaded areas represent resection regions.

ilaryngectomy (Fig. 32–17); for the horizontal resection, it is the SSL (Fig. 32–18); and for the oblique resection, it is the partial laryngopharyngectomy (PLP) (Fig. 32–19). With various technical modifications, approximately 20 to 30 different procedures for conservation laryngeal surgery are performed.

GLOTTIC TUMORS. Resection of glottic lesions can be accomplished by hemilaryngectomy, anterior commissure resection, or frontoanterior or frontolateral partial laryngectomy. These subperichondrial vertical resections of the larynx are followed by immediate reconstruction (Fig. 32–20).

Vertical partial laryngectomy (cordectomy by means of laryngofissure) is one of the oldest procedures for treatment of laryngeal carcinoma. It was originally described by Brauers in 1834. Von Bruns, in 1878, performed 15 operations, with one cure. Today, cordectomy has been replaced by partial hemilaryngectomy as the procedure of choice for vocal fold carcinomas and as a primary modality of therapy for radiation failures. The modern hemilaryngectomy was originally described by Billroth and Gluck and was later modified by Hautant.[124]

Lesions of the true vocal fold, with involvement of

the anterior commissure or vocal process, or extension less than 2 cm subglottically, are treated by one of the vertical hemilaryngectomy procedures.

Lesions involving both vocal folds and anterior commissure are treated by a frontolateral, frontoanterior, or anterior commissure resection, as indicated by lesion location (Fig. 32–21).

The minimal resection is a cordectomy with a strip of cartilage including the anterior commissure.[125] Decortication of areas adjacent to the tumor, where carcinoma in situ or microinvasion is suspected, can be performed under frozen-sectional control.

Surgical variations of the hemilaryngectomy approach are many. The structures that may be removed are the entire arytenoid, one third of the opposite vocal fold, and a partial section of the cricoid cartilage. In the event that more than one third of the remaining vocal fold is removed together with the commissure, the opposite arytenoid should not be removed, and a McNaught Keel can be used (Fig. 32–22). Many other variations exist, including frontolateral, frontoanterior, bilateral thyrotomy, intrathyroid subperichondrial, and anterior commissure resections.

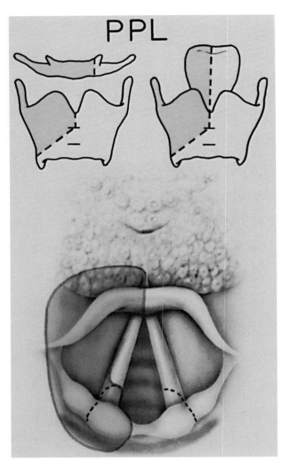

Fig. 32–19. Schematic representation of a partial laryngopharyngectomy (PLP). An oblique resection; the shaded areas represent resection regions.

A Kambic epiglottic reconstruction may be used for large resections if the patient has only a single functioning arytenoid. This procedure uses a flap of epiglottis as a pedunculated graft to close the hemilaryngectomy defect (Fig. 32–23).

If the arytenoid is to be removed, the glottis is reconstructed by a variety of procedures, the most common of which is a pedicled muscular graft using thyrohyoid and omohyoid muscles, free cartilage grafts (Figs. 32–24 and 32–25). Teflon injection has been used to fine-tune the repair of voice quality. Delayed changes in the location of the Teflon and the granulomatous reaction to the material make it less than ideal.

SUPRAGLOTTIC TUMORS. When the supraglottis needs to be resected, a horizontal SSL[126] is performed in continuity with en bloc neck dissection. SSL procedures probably originated with Trotter, 1920, who described a lateral transhyoid pharyngotomy, and Huet, who in 1938 described the hyothyroepiglottectomy. Alonso, in 1947,[126] described a two-stage procedure for supraglottic resection, which was converted by Ogura in 1958 into the one-stage procedure most frequently used today (Fig. 32–26).

This procedure is indicated for cancers of the epiglottis, false vocal folds, and aryepiglottic folds. The procedure may be extended to include one arytenoid cartilage, the vallecula, and the base of the tongue. Extralaryngeal tumor spread, cartilage destruction, subglottic tumor extension, and pyriform apex involvement are contraindications to this technique. At least one normal functional arytenoid and vocal fold must be present. The other partially resected vocal fold may be reconstituted in the midline to the cricoid cartilage (reverse King procedure) or adducted toward the midline in a variety of other ways: muscle flaps, free cartilage grafts, or in-fracturing the thyroid ala to form a new fixed cord. The last technique is most useful in the three-quarter laryngectomy, one of the most extensive "conservation" glottectomy procedures. A primary hypopharyngeal perichondrial closure is then performed (Fig. 32–27).

Three-quarter laryngectomy is a combination of the supraglottic and hemilaryngectomies, for tumor involving the supraglottis and glottis on the same side of the larynx. This technique was originally described by Ogura (see the discussion in Dedo[127]). Tumors of the lateral epiglottis and those of the false vocal fold that extend posteriorly to the aryepiglottic folds and inferiorly to the glottis are the most frequent tumors treated by this technique. Lesions of the aryepiglottic fold, false vocal fold, and marginal areas that extend to the ventricle and glottis, as well as some transglottic tumors, can also be encompassed by this method. The defect is reconstructed by transposition or infracture of the superior cornu of the thyroid cartilage or posterior border of the thyroid ala, which is pedicled on the inferior pharyngeal constrictor muscle to form a pseudocord. This pseudocord then apposes the mobile vocal fold on the opposite side (Fig. 32–28).

SUPERIOR HYPOPHARYNX TUMORS. For tumors involving the superior hypopharynx, base of tongue (posterior to circumvallate papillae), and vallecula, an extended horizontal supraglottic subtotal laryngectomy can be performed. In these patients, mucosal approximation may not be possible, but closure of the laryngeal perichondrium to the anterior base of the tongue can be accomplished (Fig. 32–29).

INFERIOR HYPOPHARYNX TUMORS. For lesions involving the pyriform sinus and the lateral and posterior hypopharyngeal wall, an oblique PLP is performed (Fig. 32–30). This is not applicable to lesions that involve the pyriform apex, invade cartilage, extend beyond the laryngopharynx, involve the glottis or subglottic larynx, or extend beyond the paralaryngeal space (Fig. 32–31).

Primary reconstruction is performed at the time of resection. Split-thickness skin grafts over prevertebral muscle flaps can be used in conjunction with a stent to reconstruct the hypopharynx. This produces adequate results; however, fistula rates of 18 to 32% are reported. Therefore, pedicled flaps (pectoralis major or latissi-

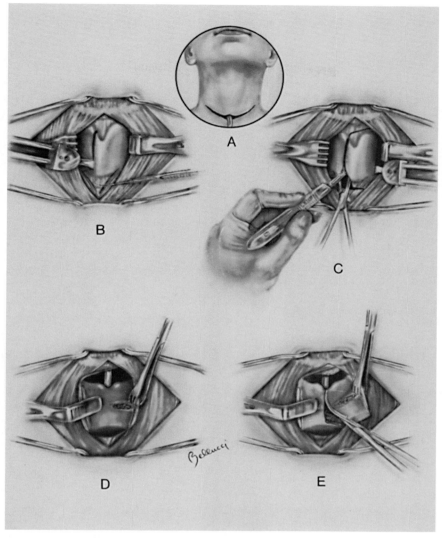

Fig. 32–20. Hemilaryngectomy technique. A. Horizontal skin incision and preliminary tracheotomy. B. Following perichondrial elevation, an anterior vertical cartilaginous incision is made. C. Posterior cartilaginous incision. D. Larynx is opened in the midline anteriorly. E. The hemilarynx is exposed and the tumor removed. This is followed by immediate reconstruction.

mus dorsi myocutaneous flaps) are used routinely to close the defect. Although the pectoralis major myocutaneous pedicle flap is still the "workhorse" for reconstruction in head and neck surgical oncology, it is lacking in the distance that it can be extended and is considered too bulky by some surgeons for many applications. Many medical centers around the world are basing their postablative surgical reconstruction programs on the use of distant tissue transfer using microvascular anastomoses to local vessels.[128–130] The advantages include the benefit of tissues that have a minimum of bulk and a substantial ease in contouring. This is particularly valuable in the reconstruction of the pharynx and hypopharynx. A method for the reconstruction of the pharynx with an emphasis on restoring a vibratory segment for tracheoesophageal speech following total laryngopharyngectomy was

published by Haughey and associates in 1995.[131] Of the 12 patients presented in the series, 11 achieved intelligible speech.

REHABILITATION. The cricopharyngeal myotomy is one of the most effective measures for rehabilitation of a functioning pharynx.[127,132,133] Myotomy, however, may not completely control aspiration in patients unless they have a competent glottis.[134–136] The selection of patients has been based purely on the location and extent of the lesion, which often includes parts of the larynx. This location, of course, should be determined preoperatively by direct laryngoscopy and radiographic studies. Observations by Singer and associates indicate that pharyngeal plexus neurectomy may be as effective as myotomy to release the cricopharyngeus and inferior constrictor.[172a]

NEAR-TOTAL LARYNGECTOMY. Subtotal or near-total

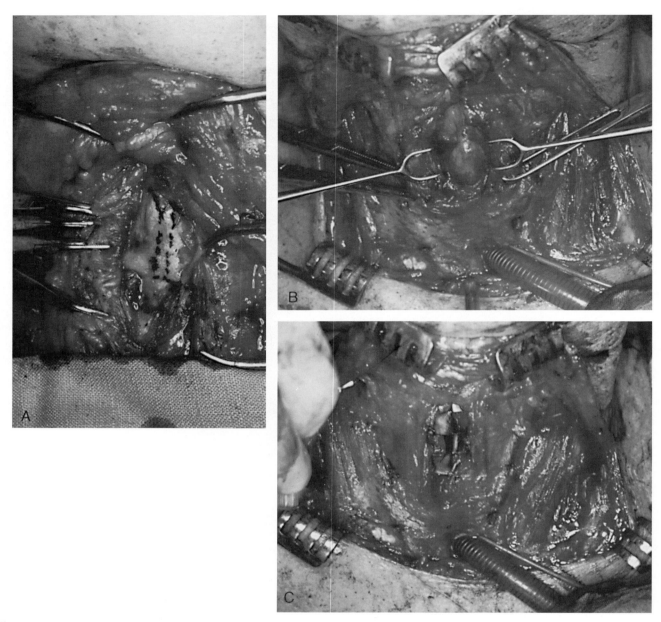

Fig. 32–21. Anterior commissure resection. A. Marked cartilagenous incision. B. Resultant defect corrected by a keel. C. Today, Silastic keels are used and removed endoscopically.

laryngectomy is used in patients to preserve some phonation. Most experience with procedures so classified has been limited and unpredictable. At least one functioning arytenoid must be present, and there must be less than 2 cm of subglottic tumor extension. Some of the procedures also may fall into the "three-quarter laryngectomy" category.

The earliest procedures similar to those in use today were "window resections," described by Patterson in 1932.[137] In these procedures, the thyroid alae were opened as two panel doors and closed following tumor extirpation. Norris described the extended frontolateral laryngectomy in 1958.[138] Moser, in 1961, described

a horizontal glottic resection including a strip of thyroid alar cartilage.[139] The epiglottis was used to resurface the anterior defect. Pleet and associates, in 1977, used the superior thyroid cartilage edge and false cords; these were folded and sutured to the cricoid to close the defect.[140] Calearo and Teatini, in 1978, performed a horizontal glottic-subglottic laryngectomy and reconstructed the defect by a superior thyrocricoidpexy.[141] These were based on studies by Majer and Reeder in 1958[142] and Labayle in 1973.[143] Hofman Saquez extended this to the first three tracheal rings and sutured the false vocal folds and epiglottis to the trachea (thyrotracheopexy).[144]

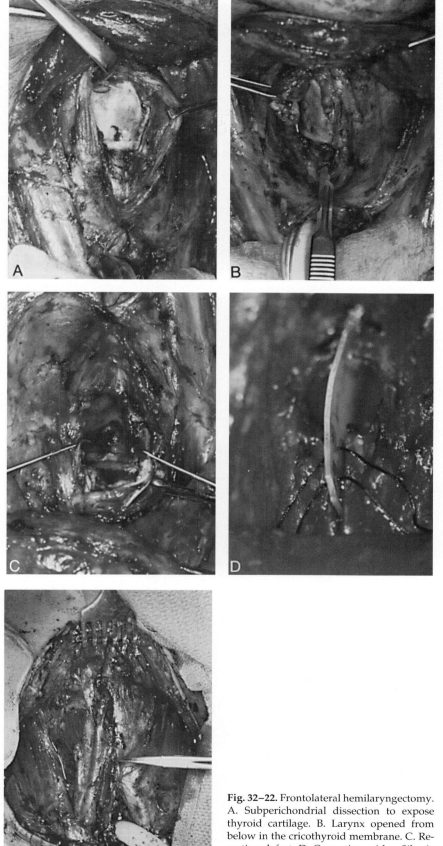

Fig. 32–22. Frontolateral hemilaryngectomy. A. Subperichondrial dissection to expose thyroid cartilage. B. Larynx opened from below in the cricothyroid membrane. C. Resection defect. D. Correction with a Silastic keel after cord elongation. E. The strap muscles and perichondrium are closed in layers.

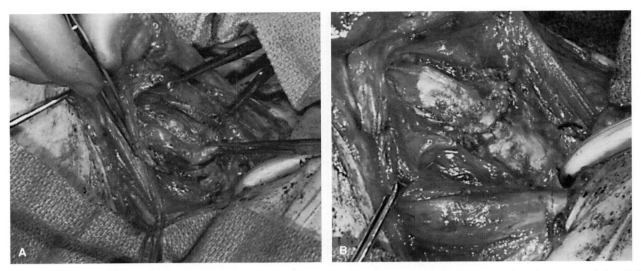

Fig. 32–23. Anterior epiglottoplasty for larger glottic resections. A. The dissected epiglottis is pulled down to close the anterior defect. B. The base of the free epiglottis is sutured to the cephalic portion of the cricoid with extraluminal sutures.

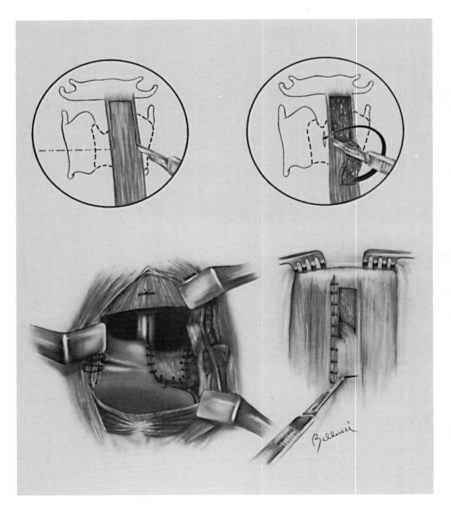

Fig. 32–24. Schematic representation of a sterno-thyroid muscle flap laryngoplasty. Upper left, outline of the muscle flap. Upper right, invaginating the muscle flap into the laryngeal lumen. Lower left, mucosal coverage of the muscle. Lower right, the larynx is closed with layered perichondrium and strap muscles.

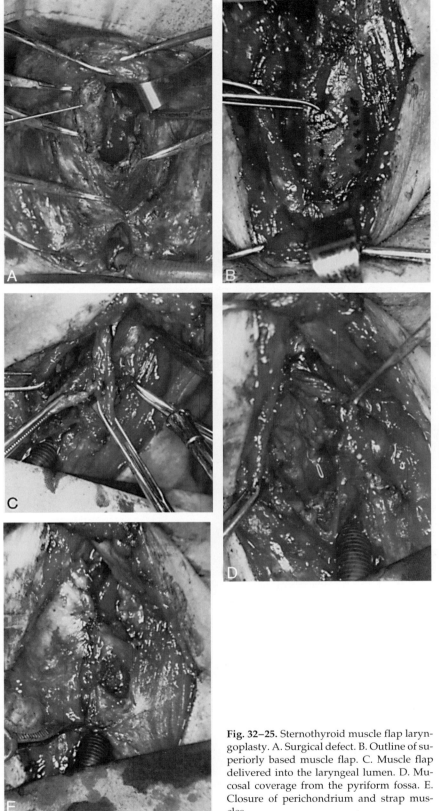

Fig. 32–25. Sternothyroid muscle flap laryngoplasty. A. Surgical defect. B. Outline of superiorly based muscle flap. C. Muscle flap delivered into the laryngeal lumen. D. Mucosal coverage from the pyriform fossa. E. Closure of perichondrium and strap muscles.

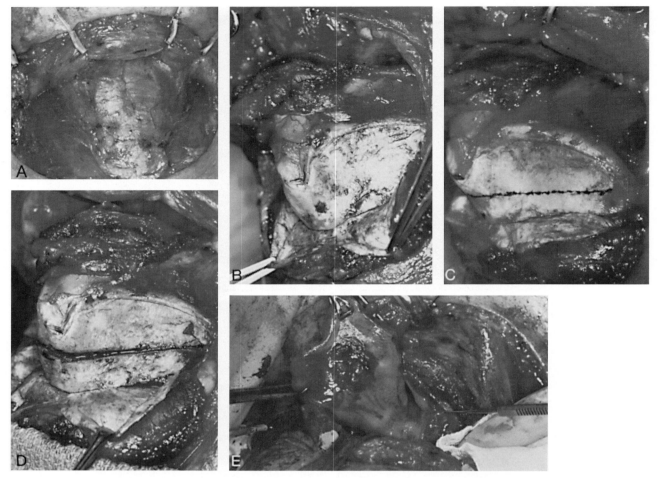

Fig. 32–26. Subtotal supraglottic laryngectomy includes the following steps: A. Anterior neck exposure. B. Perichondrial elevation. C. Horizontal subperichondrial incision outlined. D. Incision completed with oscillating saw. E. Resection of the supraglottis with direct vocal fold visualization.

Foderl, in 1899, first fixed the hyoid bone directly to the trachea using the epiglottis for reconstruction.[145] Serafin modified this method for hyotracheopexy by "laryngealizing" the trachea under and forward relative to the hyoid to avoid aspiration.[146] The free portion of the epiglottis or redundant mucosa was preserved as a flap over the open tracheal stump. Staffieri and Calearo modified this to create a small opening in a flap on the tracheal stump.[146a] He claimed that 100% of his patients could speak and 98% could swallow, but 60% continued to require a tracheotomy. Other investigators report considerable aspiration.[147] Mozolewski and associates created arytenoid shunts using the arytenoids and mucosal flaps from the pharyngeal wall.[148] Weisberger and Lingeman used this method to preserve speech after total glossectomy.[149] Pearson, in 1981, extended the procedure to allow only a portion of one arytenoid to remain, creating a tract from laryngeal remnants that is capped by an arytenoid and a tube created from hypopharyngeal mucosa.[150]

Multiple other modifications of these techniques have been tried, with mixed results with regard to aspiration, recurrence, and phonatory function.[143,151,152]

For these procedures to be even marginally successful, at least one functional arytenoid must remain. Postoperatively, the main problem is aspiration. Approximately 60% of patients can be decannulated in some series, although the reported numbers are small. With other voice restoration procedures available (Singer-Blom, Panje, Montgomery tubes), these procedures seem to have limited indications.

WIDE-FIELD TOTAL LARYNGECTOMY. Wide-field laryngectomy, rather than narrow-field laryngectomy, is considered the method of choice when total removal of the larynx is required. Total laryngectomy is reserved for the following situations: lesions involving both vocal folds with fixation; large transglottic carcinomas; cancer of the vocal fold with subglottic extension of more than 2 cm; extralaryngeal cancer; interarytenoid cancer; cancer extending to the cricopharyngeus, preepiglottic space, or postcricoid areas; or with laryngeal cartilage destruction.

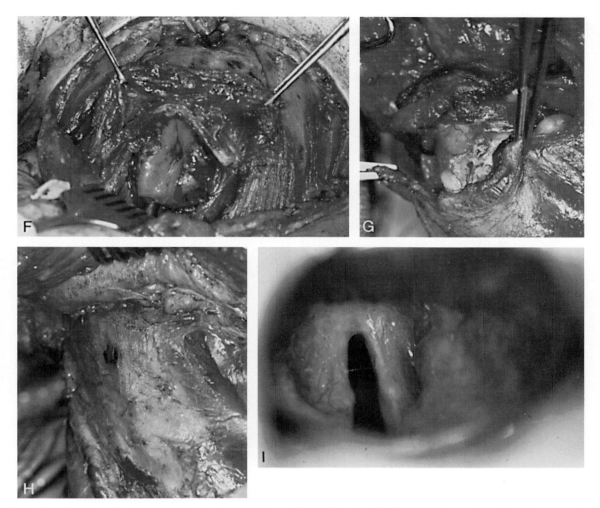

Fig. 32–26. *(continued)* F. Anesthesia lightened to test vocal fold mobility (adduction). G. Strap muscles and perichondrium are elevated and H. Sutured to the base of the tongue. I. Indirect laryngoscopy of vocal fold mobility after subtotal supraglottic laryngectomy.

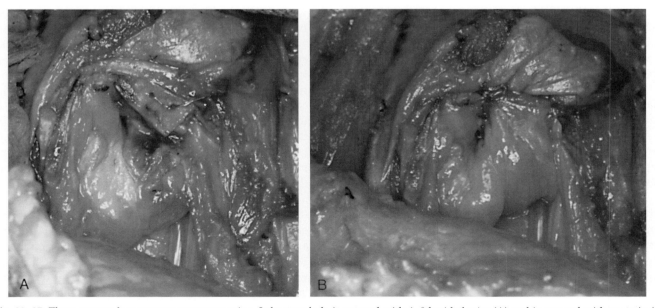

Fig. 32–27. Three-quarter laryngectomy reconstruction. Infractured ala is sutured with 4–0 braided wire (A) and is covered with postcricoid mucosa (B).

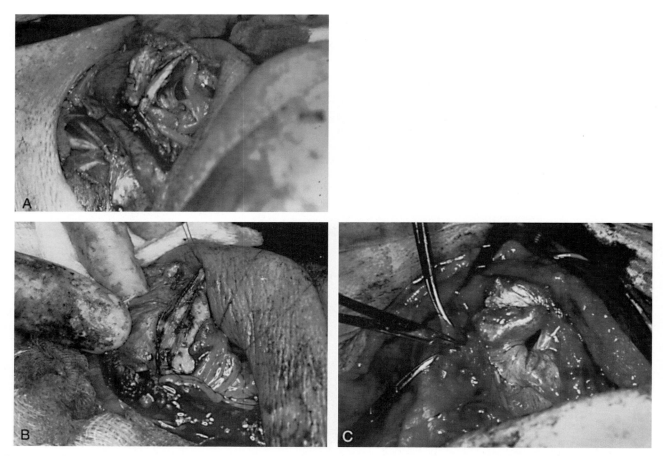

Fig. 32–28. Three-quarter laryngectomy after resection of an entire vocal fold. A. Defect (note preservation of superior thyroid cornu) B. Infracture of superior thyroid cornu to form fixed pseudocord and C. Coverage with postcricoid mucosa. Note abduction of the right functional vocal fold.

Billroth, in 1873, first successfully performed a total laryngectomy for cure. This was soon followed by reports from Gussenbauer in 1874 and Langenbeck in 1875. Today numerous methods are used. We generally use an apron flap based on a U-shaped incision, and perform a wide-field laryngectomy, often combined with a neck dissection.

NECK DISSECTION. Mackenzie (1990) and Crile (1906) laid the foundation for radical neck dissection for carcinomas of the head and neck. Their concept stressed early total extirpation of the entire "lymphatic organ" with its tributaries and glands, whether the latter were apparently diseased or not, as the only possible safeguard against local recurrence and metastasis.

The absolute contraindications to neck dissection for the possible cure of head and neck cancer are few. No operation should be considered if evidence of distant metastasis exists, if the primary lesion cannot be controlled, or if the patient has bony invasion of the cervical vertebrae or base of the skull. No medical contraindications exist to cancer surgery.

TREATMENT CLASSIFICATIONS OF NECK DISSECTION. Primary therapeutic neck dissection specifies the surgical removal of clinically evident lymph node metastases, which are noted at initial examination, in continuity with the primary malignant tumor. This can be combined with preoperative or postoperative irradiation.

Secondary or delayed therapeutic neck dissection specifies the surgical removal of clinically evident lymph node metastases noted on follow-up examination or after the primary lesion has been treated. This can be combined with preoperative or postoperative irradiation and chemotherapy. Most often, this dissection is performed for contralateral lymph node metastasis after the ipsilateral neck nodes have been removed or in patients who need bilateral neck dissections that are staged.

Elective or prophylactic neck dissection indicates an operation performed in the absence of clinically apparent lymph node metastasis. The argument for and against elective ("prophylactic") neck dissection has been raging among head and neck surgeons for many years, but a well-controlled, definitive study is still lacking. As a result, the decision for such surgery is usually based on the surgeon's experience and personal conviction, rather than on scientifically valid

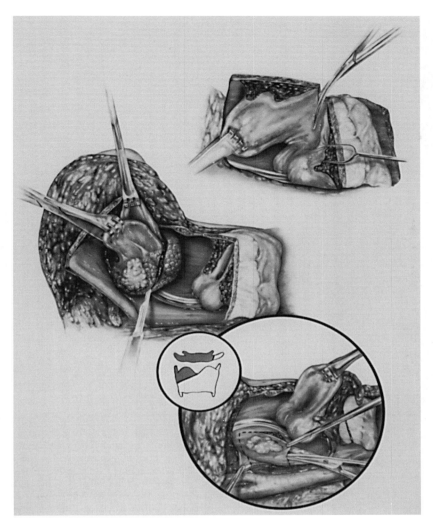

Fig. 32–29. Schematic representation of an extended subtotal supraglottic laryngectomy procedure. Top, epiglottic tumor and base-of-tongue lesion. Bottom, superior hypopharyngeal tumor.

knowledge. Two factors must be taken into consideration: (1) the incidence of occult metastasis, which ranges from 3% to 60% depending on primary laryngeal tumor location; and (2) the incidence of misdiagnosed palpable nodes, which is perhaps as high as 25%.[153]

Opponents of elective neck dissection point mainly to the amount of unnecessary neck surgery that would be done.[154] They note that even if in a given lesion the chance for occult metastasis were 40%, 6 of every 10 operations would have been done needlessly. These surgeons prefer to rely on a close follow-up postoperatively and perform therapeutic neck dissection if clinically positive nodes appear. Their belief is that therapeutic neck dissection, when done as a delayed secondary procedure, still provides survival rates comparable with those of a combined procedure in which neck dissection was elected.

As a general rule, it would seem proper to perform elective neck dissection in any patient with head and neck cancer in whom the expected occult metastasis rate is 25% or greater. The first surgical attack on malignancy is the most opportune time for cure. All lymphatic channels are removed in an en bloc resection in continuity with a primary lesion. The same channels will be cut, with the possibility of tumor dissemination, if only the primary tumor is removed. Neck dissection adds minimal morbidity to the surgery, particularly if modified to allow the sternocleidomastoid muscle and eleventh nerve to remain. It has certainly shown its value in the increased survival rates of certain aggressive lesions, such as carcinoma of the supraglottic larynx and laryngopharynx.

Elective neck dissections can often be modified to achieve a good functional and cosmetic result. These less-radical and less-mutilating procedures were initially reported by Suarez in 1963.[155] Later, they were popularized by Bocca.[156] Their major aim is to preserve the sternomastoid muscle, jugular vein, and spinal accessory nerve, although some surgeons advocate removal of the sternomastoid muscle to facilitate the operation.[157] A carefully executed functional neck dissection can produce survival rates similar to those seen with radical neck dissection.[158] These techniques

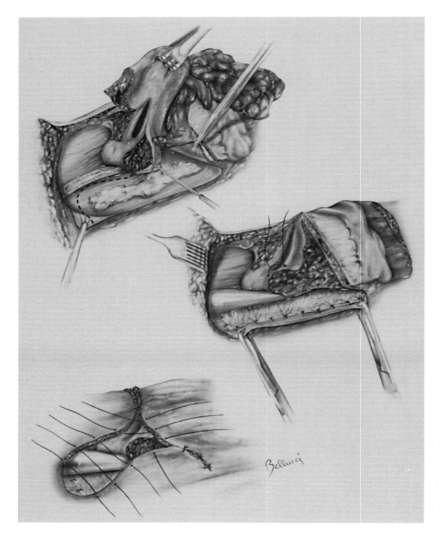

Fig. 32–30. Schematic representation of a partial laryngopharyngectomy. Top, tumor in hypopharynx and pyriform sinus. Middle, exposure of the pyriform, fixation of the arytenoid by a reverse King maneuver, and the use of split-thickness skin graft (today, major defects are corrected with myocutaneous flaps). Bottom, perichondrial and strap muscle closure.

are effective in elective neck, secondary neck, and contralateral neck dissections.

The extension of the neck dissection down to the paratracheal lymphatic bed is advocated for the control of occult metastases from unilateral carcinomas of the larynx and hypopharynx.[159] Bilateral paratracheal lymph node dissection should be considered for subglottic disease or contralateral tumor extension. Care needs to be taken to avoid injury to the thoracic duct on the left and the accessory thoracic duct on the right as well as to preserve a viable biopsy-proved parathyroid gland by reimplantation in the neck or forearm.

BILATERAL NECK DISSECTION. Bilateral neck dissection is performed if disease is found or suspected in the lymph nodes of both sides of the neck and the primary lesion can be controlled. Lesions of the midline, the base of the tongue, the epiglottis, and the subglottis have a propensity for bilateral metastasis.

Once bilateral neck dissection is decided on, the only other decision is whether it should be done as a one-stage or a two-stage operation. Although the former would seem to approach the ideal in cancer surgery, that is, removal of a primary carcinoma en bloc with all its lymphatic drainage above the clavicles, the morbidity caused by bilateral *radical* neck dissections has prevented its unquestioned acceptance. Severe facial and intraoral edema demands that a tracheotomy be performed concomitantly. The real damage, however, lies in the cerebral edema that occurs as the sequel of ligation of both internal jugular veins and the isolated cases of blindness secondary to retinal venous stasis. Although the vertebral venous system should be adequate to handle the increased blood flow, it may require time to accommodate to the new hemodynamic state. Insertion of a spinal catheter to relieve the increased intracranial pressure may be considered. A planned two-stage procedure seems to be a safer choice. Performance of modified or conservative neck dissections that allow the internal jugular veins to remain intact is an alternative. The use of conservative

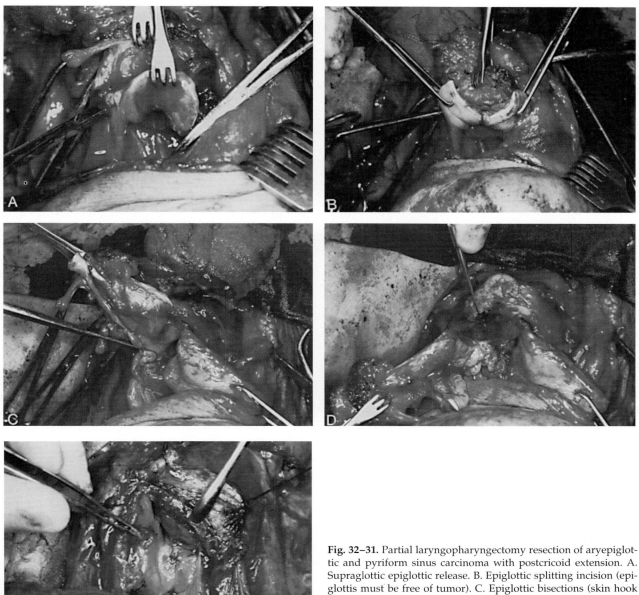

Fig. 32–31. Partial laryngopharyngectomy resection of aryepiglottic and pyriform sinus carcinoma with postcricoid extension. A. Supraglottic epiglottic release. B. Epiglottic splitting incision (epiglottis must be free of tumor). C. Epiglottic bisections (skin hook on posterior tumor extent). D. Tumor resection includes hemiepiglottis, arytenoid and aryepiglottic folds, pyriform sinus, and cricoid rostrum (with neck dissection). E. Reconstruction of the posterior defect with residual hemiepiglottis.

neck dissections, partial node dissections, and radio-sterilization of neck disease is covered in another section of this chapter.

RECURRENT CANCER OF THE LARYNX. Patients with therapeutic failures can be successfully salvaged by irradiation or by radical or conservative surgery. Cervical recurrence after neck dissection is treated by full-course radiation therapy. Tumors persisting after full-course irradiation are resected if feasible. Resection of the recurrent tumor is radical; sacrifice of the carotid artery is indicated if necessary. Postradiation neck recurrences, not amenable to surgery, can be treated by cryotherapy, chemotherapy, and photoradiation.

LARYNGEAL CARCINOMA WITH DISTANT METASTASIS. Occasionally, patients with laryngeal carcinoma have suspected pulmonary metastasis. If the chest lesion is deemed resectable, laryngeal surgery is performed, followed by thoracotomy. If the pulmonary lesion is not resectable, palliative irradiation to the primary site and metastatic foci is the treatment of choice unless palliation can be better achieved with surgery at the primary site.

Reports on distant metastasis with laryngeal carcinoma vary greatly. A large proportion of such metastases remain undetected during the lifetime of the patient. Approximately 75% of patients who die of the disease have undetected distant metastasis. Generally, 7 to 12% of patients with laryngeal carcinomas at presentation have distant metastasis, and 35 to 90% of autopsies on patients who die of laryngeal carcinomas show distant metastases. The latter are usually small (3 mm or less), and 75% are unnoticed during the life of the patient.[160–163] The greatest incidence is usually reported with supraglottic carcinomas. Little correlation with the degree of tumor differentiation exists, however. Distant metastases are rare in the absence of regional metastases. The primary site of distant metastasis is usually the lung; 50 to 80% of all distant metastases occur there. Once distant spread has been diagnosed, the expected survival is approximately 1 year. Interestingly, 10% of autopsy specimens also show the presence of a second primary tumor.[164] Lung metastases from the hypopharynx usually manifest themselves in 18 months, and those from the endolarynx usually appear in about 30 months. Endolaryngeal metastasis is generally to the mediastinal nodes or pleura (associated with pleural effusions). Large metastases to the lung parenchyma and pulmonary atelectasis are rare. In such situations, secondary tumors must be excluded. Metastases to the mediastinum and para-aortic lymph nodes, lung hilum, and bone are associated with pulmonary metastases in 60 to 80% of patients. Noteworthy is that lung metastases are usually osteolytic and account for 10 to 35% of all distant metastases. These are preterminal and are associated with a life expectancy of less than 4 months. The most common sites are the lower thoracic and lumbar vertebrae and the ribs. Other sites include the femur, ethmoid, tibia, fingers, and temporal bone. Liver metastases occur in 80% of all patients with distant disease spread. These lesions are small and usually multiple. Surprisingly, cardiac metastases are found in 10% of all cases. They are usually to the myocardium and can grow into the atrium and ventricle.[165] Lymphocytic and hematogenous skin metastases occur relatively frequently in the cervical and peristomal skin areas. These are usually associated with persistent tumors in the tracheostomal area. They occur early after treatment and rarely later than 3 years after therapy. Reports indicate that stomal recurrences occur in 3 to 15% of patients who have undergone total laryngectomy and are associated with greater than 2 cm subglottic tumor extension.[166]

SURGICAL COMPLICATIONS. The earlier complications are diagnosed and treated, the less the morbidity and mortality. In many instances, astute clinical observations before and during initiation of therapy and meticulous surgical technique alleviate future problems. Operative mortality is usually less than 0.1%.

The overall incidence of complications in conservation surgery is approximately 18%. In general, the greater the surgical resection and the higher the radiation dose, the more and greater are the complications encountered. For example, the complication rate in hemilaryngectomy is less than 2%, but in partial hemilaryngectomy with high-dose preoperative radiation or total laryngectomy following full-course radiation, it may approximate 50%. In essence, all laryngeal surgery is contaminated because the secretions from the oropharynx, hypopharynx, and esophagus are continuous with the open neck wound.

HEMATOMA AND EMPYEMA. Hematomas can be prevented by meticulous surgical technique and drainage. Drainage should be achieved with continuous vacuum suction and large "Hemovac"-style catheters. The neck is examined and palpated twice daily. Most hematomas occur in the first 24 postoperative hours. They should be evacuated, and bleeding should be controlled in the operating room under sterile conditions. Purulent drainage or subcutaneous accumulations are drained with adequate dependent incisions, and the wound is packed open. The earlier drainage is performed, the less devitalization of tissue and skin flap necrosis will occur.

In hemilaryngectomy, the most common site of hemorrhage is the cut edges of the thyroid gland or branches of the superior laryngeal artery and vein in the superior aspect of the resection. With SSL procedures, the bleeding is usually from the superior anastomotic site or the cut edges of the base of the tongue. In total laryngectomy, bleeding can occur from vessels that were cut during surgery (superior laryngeal) or dehiscence of the anastomotic repair of the pharyngoesophagus.

FISTULA. The overall incidence of fistula formation after resection of head and neck cancer is about 10%. Early recognition and control are important to prevent tissue sloughing. The fistula should be converted to a direct tract by the shortest route to the skin to prevent undermining skin flaps. In addition, fistulas should be rerouted in such a manner as to facilitate future reconstruction. Most fistulas close in time, but with larger defects, the use of pedicled skin flaps or myocutaneous flaps decreases the morbidity and the hospital stay. Generally, meticulous mucosal closure and lower preoperative radiation doses (or better fractionation dosage pattern) decrease the rate of fistula formation.

In hemilaryngectomy, the fistula rate is less than 0.1%. The most common cause is improper closure of the anterior defect with improper mucosal or muscle flap alignment or improperly placed through-and-through sutures. In SSL procedures, pharyngeal fistulas are relatively unusual and result from improper or tight closure in postradiated tumors. The fistulas tend to be lateral at the junction of the trifurcation of the base of the tongue, the pharynx, and the residual larynx.

Fistulas are the most common complication of total laryngectomy. The frequency varies from 6 to 66%, with an average of 15 to 30%.[167] Fistulas are more common following radiotherapy. Other factors that influence fistula formation are nutritional status, anemia, alcohol abuse, diabetes, preoperative sepsis, preoperative tracheotomy, hemorrhage, wound infection, and meticulousness of the closure (straight line closures are less likely to result in a fistula). Joseph and associates noted that fistula rates are as high as 75% in patients who undergo salvage surgery for radiation failures, compared with 23% with planned preoperative radiation and 8% for primary surgery.[168] Of course, fistulas predispose to tissue necrosis, skin loss, and carotid artery rupture. Today, rapid debridement, removal of necrotic tissue, diversion of the fistula tract, and closure with myocutaneous flaps are the methods of choice for control (Fig. 32–32).

SKIN LOSS. Skin loss is a result of poor vascularity of the neck flaps caused by previous radiation, incorrectly placed incisions, and other complications (most commonly fistulas and infections). Once the wound is clean and granulation is present, split-thickness skin or pedicled skin flaps may be used to resurface the wound. If the carotid artery is exposed, it must be covered as soon as possible.

CAROTID ARTERY EXPOSURE. Carotid artery exposure, if not corrected, can lead to vessel necrosis and rupture, central nervous system complications, and often death because of exsanguination. In all procedures in which a radical neck dissection is performed en bloc with resection of the primary tumor, the carotid artery is covered with dermal grafts, well-vascularized skin, or skin of myocutaneous flaps. This affords protection if the vessel is uncovered. A dermal graft, when exposed to air, grows skin to cover the carotid artery and to increase the vessel wall vascularity because of proliferating vasa vasorum.

If a fistula is adjacent to the carotid artery, a nondelayed chest flap sutured to the lateral aspect of the fistula will prevent secretions from bathing the vessel. A secondary reconstruction can be then used to close the fistula.

If a carotid artery is ruptured, pressure is applied to control bleeding, blood is given to correct the hypovolemia, and ligation proximal and distal to the rupture is performed.

STRICTURES. Tracheal stomal strictures can often be avoided by accurate approximation of the skin to the tracheal mucosa (cartilage must not be exposed) and by prevention of trauma and infection. Delayed flaps and Z-plasty reconstruction are successful in correcting tracheostomal stenosis.

In conservation surgery, hypopharyngeal and supraglottic stenoses are rare. Most are associated with extensive primary resections and can be corrected by frequent dilations and bougienage. Resection of the structure and reconstruction with split-thickness skin, pedicled or free skin flaps, or myocutaneous pedicled or free flaps correct stenoses that do not respond to dilatation (Fig. 32–33).

Strictures are not unusual in hemilaryngectomies and variations of these methods. These are usually small and are located in the anterior commissure area. They can be resected with a carbon dioxide laser under microscopic control. In supraglottic surgery, laryngeal stenosis secondary to chronic edema (especially when the false vocal folds are not completely removed), scar contracture, and arytenoid ankylosis occur in 10% of patients.

CHYLE LEAKS. Chyle leaks are manifested early

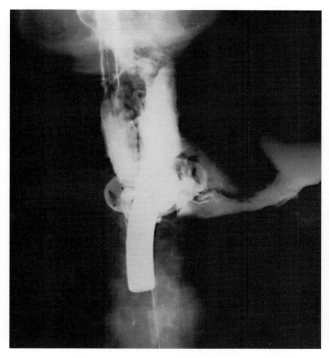

Fig. 32–32. Fistula demonstrated by barium swallow following partial pharyngolaryngectomy for a radiation failure of a pyriform sinus tumor.

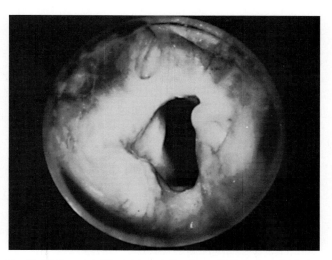

Fig. 32–33. Supraglottic stricture following subtotal supraglottic laryngectomy.

through suction drainage catheters. Initially, the drainage is clear, but when the patient starts oral or tube feeding, the fluid becomes cloudy, pale, or whitish.

The treatment depends on the amount of drainage occurring and the status of the skin flaps. In general, pressure dressing should be used only if the viability of the flaps is unquestioned. Diets low in fat should be adhered to until drainage decreases. Large leaks require opening the wound, locating and ligating the thoracic duct, and suturing a free muscle graft over the area.

PULMONARY COMPLICATIONS. Bronchopneumonia and atelectasis in the early postoperative period (first 3 to 4 days) are infrequent, and, if they do occur, they are caused by aspiration. Systemic antibiotic administration, humidification, and tracheal hygiene rapidly clear the infection.

Pneumothorax occurs in the first 36 hours postoperatively. Frequent auscultation and chest radiographs delineate the problem and facilitate correction. Pulmonary embolism is extremely rare and usually is not massive.

The incidence of pulmonary complications after surgery for head and neck cancer averages about 6%.

CARDIAC COMPLICATIONS. Myocardial infarction and congestive heart failure, in the older population, occur in about 4 to 5% of the patients within 2 years of therapy. In the immediate postoperative period, the mortality among patients with myocardial infarction is 4 to 5%.

WOUND INFECTION. The incidence of wound sepsis is small, even though the surgical procedures are contaminated from pharyngeal secretions. If high doses of radiation have been used preoperatively, or if the tumor is septic, laryngeal cartilage perichondritis can develop. This is treated with systemic antibiotics and occasionally by debridement and reconstruction.

Clinicians debate whether to use preoperative and postoperative antibiotics. The microorganisms are usually coliform or staphylococcal (nosocomial). We use pre-, intra-, and postoperative antibiotic coverage.

EDEMA. Severe facial swelling and cerebral edema may occur with simultaneous or staged radical neck dissections. For this reason, preservation of the internal jugular vein may be considered if the clinical situation permits. A tracheotomy is indicated with simultaneous staged or late contralateral neck dissections to avoid airway obstruction from laryngeal edema. The incidence of airway obstruction is 0.8%.

POSTSURGICAL REHABILITATION. Regardless of the method chosen for the patient for voice restoration following laryngectomy, the only appropriate approach is that of a multispecialty team. This care must be orchestrated by the head and neck surgeon and delivered by specialists including surgical nurses trained in head and neck postoperative care, nutritionists trained in the special dietary needs of patients who have had

aerodigestive tract reconstruction, and speech-language pathologists trained in voice and swallowing rehabilitation. After the earliest stages of recovery, communication skills need to be addressed, to mitigate the depression that is typical following the loss of the larynx. The patient should already have met with and be familiar with the speech-language pathologist trained in voice restoration and rehabilitation. Thus, after the operation, the initial contact will serve to reinforce what has been explained to the patient and what to expect. Apart from needing the technical skills to care for the head and neck wounds, the nurses involved in the patient's care need to exercise special attention to the patient's inability to communicate verbally. Call buttons and intercom systems need to be adapted to identify patients who may be able to signal a need but have no means to describe that need to the nursing personnel. A note pad, an electronic communication board, or a computer can make this transition much easier and safer.

RESTORATION OF PHONATION FOLLOWING TOTAL LARYNGECTOMY. The use of tracheoesophageal or pharyngeal shunts is successful in 60 to 88% of cases. These shunts may be prosthetic or created from the patient's tissues. Singer and Blum, as well as others, have introduced tubes to shunt air from the trachea to the hypopharynx. A permanent tracheotomy is required. The procedure, although conceptionally not new, is easier to perform and has a variable success rate, as discussed later in this chapter. Shunting operations essentially communicate the trachea with the esophagus or hypopharynx, producing esophageal speech. In the past, multiple procedures have been developed, but frequently these were associated with a high degree of failure and complications, and the success rate was low. Newer techniques have been developed by Singer and Blum[169–172] and by others. The procedures consist of making a puncture hole in the back wall of the trachea communicating with the front wall of the esophagus. The techniques may be done while the patient is under general or local anesthesia. After creation of a puncture, the Singer-Blum or other prosthesis is inserted and is taped into position using the flanges on the prosthesis. There is a one-way valve on the distal tip of the prosthesis, which is inserted into the esophagus. This allows air to pass from the trachea through the prosthesis and into the esophagus. The one-way valve prevents aspiration from the esophagus into the trachea. If the patient wishes to speak, he or she inhales deeply and covers the tracheal stoma, and as the patient exhales, air is shunted into the esophagus, producing esophageal speech.

The Panje prosthesis is a similar device, except it has inner and outer flanges similar to those of an ear ventilation tube, so the prosthesis does not have to be taped in place. It is held in position by the flanges. The perforation between the esophagus and trachea may be performed using the same techniques. A small metal inserter is used to insert the prosthesis. All patients are counseled extensively by speech-language pathologists preoperatively, and speech therapy continues postoperatively until the patient develops adequate speech.

The success rate for puncture procedures has been variable, but it is usually stated to be high. Singer and Blum reported a success rate of 88% in 129 patients; Panje reported an 80% success rate in 40 patients. Thawley noted a 76% success rate in 22 patients. Some patients may develop good speech results, but over a longer period, patients may not want the burden of having to clean and insert the prosthesis daily; some patients may discontinue wearing the prosthesis. The long-term success rate seems to be about 60 to 70%.

Patient selection is critical because the ability to care for the fistula and the prosthesis is important. Manual dexterity is important for the patient to be able to manipulate and place the prosthesis daily and also to be able to occlude the airway consistently for voice production on exhalation. Reasonably good pulmonary function is necessary to force air from the trachea through the prosthesis into the esophagus. Some patients lack motivation or are not physically able to care for the prosthesis and fistula consistently. Complications include cervical adenitis, subcutaneous emphysema, narrowing of the tracheal lumen, improper placement of the fistula, displacement of the prosthesis with subsequent stenosis of the fistula, enlargement of the fistula producing aspiration, leakage around the prosthesis, tissue breakdown of the anterior esophagus (in heavily irradiated patients), and neoglottal stenosis. In some patients, failure to produce speech may be caused by spasm of the neopharynx and/or esophageal inlet. Even though the prosthesis is in correct position, spasm prevents passage of air through the esophagus. These patients should usually be evaluated preoperatively by passing a small catheter into the esophagus. Air is then inflated into the esophageal area, and the patient is asked to speak. If the patient is having significant spasm, this will be apparent on the test, and these patients usually are poor candidates for the procedure. This problem can be corrected by cricopharyngeal and inferior constrictor myotomy or by pharyngeal plexus neurectomy.[172a]

About 60% of patients develop a useful buccoesophageal voice after total laryngectomy. In general, men are more adept at this. Training in this technique is instituted before surgery in all patients by a consulting speech and language pathologist.

Lessons in esophageal speech are instituted by the third to sixth week postoperatively. Because circumstances differ for every patient, numerous methods of instruction must be used. Patients near a large city have access to classes conducted by a trained speech-language pathologist. In another situation, the patient may join a "Nu Voice" or "Lost Chord" club. With group teaching, the patient has the incentive to learn by comparing methods of talking with others who have had a similar operation. Other patients may be taught by a teacher in the local chapter of the American Cancer Society. Finally, in smaller communities, former patients are available to help others in the neighborhood who have had similar operations.

No underlying anatomic or physiologic factor has been found to account for the lack of voice in many patients who do not develop it. Patients with extensive surgical removal, including a major part of the pharynx and portions of the tongue as well as the larynx, can often talk expertly. The one anatomic factor of significance in the production of a voice after a laryngectomy appears to be the integrity of the musculature of the tongue and floor of the mouth. Unimpeded motion of these structures is necessary both to initiate the act of swallowing and to phonate distinctly. Other factors include hypopharyngeal resonance, muscular coordination, accessory muscle function, physical status of the individual, and motivation.

Important factors in failure of esophageal speech are incoordination and spasm of the cricopharyngeal muscle, severe loss of hypopharyngeal or esophageal mucosa, narrowness of the neoglottic lumen, and reduced pharyngoesophageal transit time. Age is significant because this technique is more difficult for the older patients to learn; similarly, the voice, when present, is not as well understood in older patients. Reasonably high esophageal air pressures are required. The technique of taking in air to produce voice can be learned by anyone who takes the necessary time and effort to master the method. Patients who are unmotivated or who do not persevere in learning to talk by this method should be supplied with an artificial larynx. A small minority of patients cannot develop a voice after extensive effort, and use of an artificial larynx in this group is adequate.

A period of mental depression commonly follows laryngectomy but diminishes when the patient learns to compensate for the lost vocal function in one way or another. Most patients can be rehabilitated satisfactorily, but severe mental depression may lead to death by suicide in rare instances.

The physical capacity for work may be reduced from general causes such as protracted illness with weakness attributable to age. Special causes, such as loss of glottic closure, rendering fixation of the muscle of the shoulder girdle difficult, or sacrifice of the spinal accessory nerve with cervical node dissection, which interferes with the function of the shoulder muscles, may lessen the ability to perform heavy work. Physical therapy is used in all cases.

Laryngectomized patients are particularly sensitive to dust and smoke in the air, and the improper humidification of overheated buildings in the winter leads to dryness and crusting in the trachea (tracheitis sicca) with subsequent bleeding. Although bronchitis occurs frequently, pneumonia is only rarely observed.

Patients who fail to develop esophageal speech and who do not desire to use an electronic vibrator are candidates for a variety of reconstructive procedures.

Surgical reconstructive methods using direct anastomosis of the trachea to hypopharynx (neoglottic reconstruction) are generally dangerous because of aspiration.[173] In 1960, Asai presented a three-stage laryngoplasty procedure. In the first stage, a high pharyngostoma is created, and in the second, a tracheostoma is made in the anterior tracheal wall below the cut edge of the trachea.[174] Finally, the tracheostoma and pharyngostoma are connected by a tube fashioned out of skin. A tracheostomy cannula is required permanently. Montgomery described two types of modifications of this concept.[175] One was the creation of an esophageal tube, which is brought out through the anterior neck flap as an esophagostoma and later covered by a skin-lined tube to communicate it with the tracheostoma. Another was the creation of a valve pharyngostoma.

RESTORATION OF PHONATION FOLLOWING CONSERVATION SURGERY. Phonation problems are not major with conservation surgery. Reconstructive techniques and postoperative care assume more prominence in reconstituting deglutition and respiration, however.

RESTORATION OF DEGLUTITION FOLLOWING TOTAL LARYNGECTOMY. In many patients, direct esophageal reconstruction is possible after total laryngeal extirpation. When a tumor involves extralaryngeal areas, however, composite resections involving the hypopharynx or esophagus may be indicated. The reconstruction of a large pharyngostoma or cervical esophagus has been a problem to which much attention was addressed in the past. Several techniques are available for reconstruction: (1) creation of a neoesophagus from split-thickness skin graft stented over a mold; (2) mobilization of regional full-thickness skin flaps from the cervical or pectoral region; (3) utilization of a portion of the larynx; (4) intestinal transplantation, replantation, or anastomosis; and (5) utilization of myocutaneous flaps, either pedicled or free.

Techniques in reconstruction of surgical defects after partial or total laryngectomy have included primary closure, random flaps, and myocutaneous flaps. Each of these techniques has been successful to some degree. The functional results regarding deglutition, however, are less than satisfactory as a result of aspiration. Frequently, simultaneous or delayed total laryngectomy is performed to deal with the pulmonary complications. Various types of laryngoplasty do not uniformly correct the problems of aspiration and deglutition associated with subtotal glossectomy. One experience included eight patients who had advanced squamous cell carcinoma of the tongue base, vallecula,

and supraglottic larynx. All patients underwent partial or subtotal glossectomy and laryngectomy. The mucosal defect was reconstructed with a pectoralis myocutaneous flap. To reestablish voice, a primary tracheopharyngeal shunt was created with the use of a portion of cricoid and upper trachea. The majority of these patients had successful rehabilitation of deglutition, mastication, and speech.[176]

RESTORATION OF DEGLUTITION FOLLOWING CONSERVATION SURGERY. Generally, by the tenth or fourteenth day after operation, all skin sutures have been removed. The clinician must determine the adequacy of the laryngeal airway, which may be accomplished by obstructing the tracheostomy tube. The patient's voice may be husky with the tracheostomy occluded. The patient is first allowed to swallow thickened gruel, such as cereal thinned with water. The tracheostoma should be closed. In most instances, the patient first coughs the material out of the tracheostomy tube in spite of repeated efforts to keep the tube clean.

Effective deglutition is impaired early in the postoperative course because these patients display only weak efforts at swallowing because of pain and discomfort in the neck. The most effective part of swallowing is at the terminal phase of the voluntary act, when the tongue pushes the bolus into the hypopharynx. Patients do not attempt this until they consciously overcome the pain to bolt the food into the hypopharynx effectively. The use of analgesic drugs helps to overcome this discomfort.

The *supraglottic swallow* is the mainstay of the rehabilitation strategy in patients who have undergone conservation laryngeal surgery. Depending on the extent and nature of the resection performed and the cooperation of the patient, the technique can be mastered by most patients. The maneuver can be summarized briefly as follows: the primary element involves the starting of every swallowing effort with a breath-holding Valsalva maneuver. This is followed by a rapid ingestion and swallowing effort. The material that is inevitably deposited on the closed larynx and therefore is at risk to be aspirated is expelled out with two brisk coughing gestures with the air inhaled at the start of the cycle. This is followed by a second swallow that serves to clear the channel.

The ability to swallow different foods varies from patient to patient. Some patients handle liquids, especially carbonated liquids, better than solids; others do better with semisolids such as Cream of Wheat. A trial-and-error approach is necessary. The patient needs supplemental intravenous or nasogastric feedings for 3 or 4 days.

Foods that are handled with the greatest difficulty are milk and water. These two substances are the last to be swallowed with ease. It takes 3 to 7 days from the time the patient first relearns deglutition before an estimated 50% of semisolids are swallowed.

The patient is told to close off the tracheostomy opening with the finger each time he or she swallows to prevent escape of air. Usually, rapid adaptation of swallowing without aspiration develops in 2 to 3 days. The tracheostomy tube is removed, and the tracheal fistula is occluded at the same time. If aspiration persists and indirect laryngoscopy shows good glottic closure, the Levine or Dobhoff tube is reinserted and the patient is sent home for 3 weeks. A percutaneous feeding gastrostomy is a good alternative and removes any impediment to rehabilitation of swallowing that the nasogastric tube might present. Initiating and performing the act of deglutition requires strenuous activity. Certain patients need these extra 3 weeks to gain weight and strength before deglutition is successful.

Occasionally, aspiration and poor glottic closure persist. In such cases, surgical reconstruction may be indicated. This can be done by a variety of surgical techniques.

After vertical partial laryngectomy, aspiration is not common unless the patient has glottic insufficiency or arytenoid defects that were not corrected at the time of the initial procedure. Secondary repairs are possible with muscle or cartilage implantation. The injection of Teflon paste has also been used. Aspiration is relatively more common after supraglottic surgery, especially when coupled with irradiation. Several studies showed an aspiration rate of 25 to 75% after SSL.[177,178] Many patients have recurrent aspiration pneumonia and pulmonary scarring.[179] Mortality from pulmonary complications has been reported to be as high as 25 to 40%.[180,181] Some clinicians advocate complete laryngectomy if intolerable aspiration occurs. In three-quarter laryngectomy, most patients learn to swallow eventually without intolerable aspiration. In PLP procedures, however, both fistula formation (18%) and chronic aspiration are relatively common. The aspiration rate is similar to that of SSL procedures.

Radiotherapy

The development of new knowledge in the field of radiation biology was accelerated in 1956 with the development of in vitro tissue culture techniques to measure cellular reproduction after treatment by radiation. Since that time, much information has been provided that helps to explain the effects of radiation on tumors and normal tissue (Fig. 32–34). For instance, it was previously assumed that tumor cells were more sensitive to radiation than normal cells and that this was the reason radiation was able to cure some tumors and yet not irreversibly damage adjacent normal structures. Provided cells are irradiated during a sensitive portion of the cell cycle, most mammalian cells, tumor cells included, have similar radiosensitivity. Various tissues containing dividing cells differ markedly in their apparent response to irradiation because these tissues contain differing proportions of sensitive proliferating

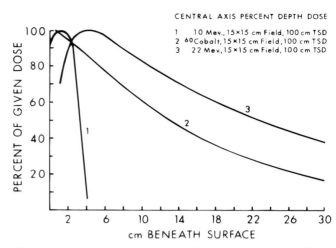

Fig. 32–34. Graphic representation of linear energy transfer (LET), that is, the physical determination of energy deposited per unit path length or tissue penetrability by different voltages of radiation.

cells. For example, brain and liver are less sensitive to the effects of radiation than tissues with rapid turnover of cells such as gut, bone marrow, testis, ovaries, and oral mucosa. Similarly, tumors with a large portion of proliferating cells (a high growth fraction) are more sensitive to the effects of radiation. By fractionating radiation or by delivering small increments of dose on a daily basis over long periods of time, normal cells in the irradiated volume that are not in the most sensitive portions of the cell cycle are given sufficient time to repair radiation injury. This ability to repair radiation injury prevents total destruction of the population of normal cells and preserves the integrity of normal tissues during the course of radiation. Once radiation treatment is completed, cells that are still viable within the irradiated volume and cells that migrate from adjacent unirradiated tissues actively divide and repopulate the irradiated tissue.

Tumor cells are also capable of repairing radiation injury during the course of fractionated radiation; this can result in regrowth of the tumor into a clinically detectable recurrence. Radiation therapists have learned that tumors can be controlled and normal tissues preserved by using fractionated courses of radiation, that is, 200 centiGrays (cGy) per day to total doses of 6000 to 7000 cGy. Despite this knowledge, significant numbers of patients still have tumor recurrence and radiation injury. Four points must therefore be remembered:

1. Tumor cells are not more sensitive to radiation than normal cells of the parent tissue; that is, all mammalian cells have roughly the same sensitivity to ionizing radiation. In radiobiologic terms, death or failure to reproduce (mitosis) is the end point of therapy. Therefore, the difference in the radiation-induced death of osteoclasts in the

mandible and of the mucosal cells of small bowel is not greater than a factor of 2; that is, both are of about equal sensitivity to radiation.

2. Radiation not only slows the growth of tumor cells, it also directly destroys some of them.
3. Tumor cells do not necessarily divide more rapidly than normal cells, but they tend to accumulate and lose their surface markers.
4. Tumor cells can be preferentially destroyed because of the therapeutic ratio developed by fractionation.

Experience shows that radiotherapy and surgery should be considered partners in management of laryngeal cancer. Nevertheless, because of the many irradiation techniques and surgical procedures, no standardized approach has been adopted. Few controlled studies in head and neck cancer have been conducted to prove the value of adjuvant radiation, preoperative or postoperative, and little proof exists that adjuvant radiation improves local control or survival for any number of tumors in the head and neck, including those of the oral cavity, oropharynx, larynx, and pyriform sinus. The claims of improved benefit from adding radiation to surgery have been based on comparing a group of patients sequentially treated by preoperative radiation and surgery with a historical control group treated by surgery alone. The major advantages of preoperative radiation are that it reduces tumor bulk and allows the surgeon more easily to gain margins and to perform more conservation surgery. The other proved advantage is that radiation is capable of controlling presumed microscopic nodal metastases in patients with clinically and radiographically N0 necks.

A correlation exists among dose, fractionation, tumor site, and operative complications. Complications are greater when higher doses of preoperative radiation are used, and the incidence of serious complications such as fistula and carotid artery rupture is higher in tumors of the laryngopharynx than in tumors of the oral cavity. This is because suture lines in the laryngopharynx are in close proximity to the carotid artery axis, and suture lines in the oral cavity are distant. A literature review is extremely confusing because of the paucity of controlled studies defining the value of adjuvant radiation in the treatment of head and neck tumors. The studies that exist provide little useful information because of differing end-point measurements.

Radiation therapy has been used basically for three different purposes: (1) primary cure (with surgery for failures); (2) radiotherapy and surgery in planned combinations; (3) radiotherapy for definitive treatment in selective cases; and (4) radiotherapy alone as palliation. Radiotherapy has also been used in combination with induction chemotherapy for the protocol treatment of advanced head and neck cancers (see the section of this chapter on organ preservation).

Combined therapy has included an initial resection followed by planned full-course postoperative radiation therapy. An attempt is made to begin the postoperative radiation within 3 to 6 weeks of the surgical excision.

Postoperative radiation for laryngeal and hypopharyngeal tumors is designed to prevent recurrence in the laryngeal remnant, pharynx, neck, tracheostoma, and superior mediastinum. Fields, therefore, encompass all these areas and are directed in an anteroposterior direction to irradiate the primary tumor, lymphatics, and tracheostoma in a single field. In the absence of electrons, it is simplest to use anteroposterior photon fields with compensating filters to ensure dose homogeneity and a posterior spinal block to reduce dose to the spinal cord. With electrons, one can effectively irradiate the pharynx, neck, and tracheostoma and spare the spinal cord by delivering 4000 cGy anteroposteriorly with photons and an additional 2000 cGy to the anterior field with 10 MeV electrons. Postoperative doses range from 5000 to 6000 cGy in 5 to 6 weeks and should probably approach the higher dose because hypopharyngeal tumors are aggressive, with relatively high rates of primary and regional recurrence. The concept behind this combined therapeutic approach is to allow maximal resection followed by full-course radiotherapy to minimize complications and to maximize the cure rate.

Megavoltage radiation such as cobalt 60 (1.25 MeV gamma rays) and 2 to 25 MeV x rays produced by Van de Graaff generators, linear accelerators, and betatrons are superior to kilovoltage x rays produced by lower-energy equipment. Megavoltage radiation has four advantages compared with kilovoltage radiation: (1) skin sparing; (2) increased penetrability; (3) relative elimination of preferential absorption in bone reducing bone shielding; and (4) less scattering of radiation outside the treatment volume. In head and neck tumors, skin sparing is important because it allows delivery of high doses of radiation without interruption because of moist desquamation of skin. Increased penetrability of high-energy x rays (20 to 25 MeV) is particularly advantageous for treatment of midline tumors such as those of the nasopharynx because the dose can be concentrated centrally, sparing superficial structures such as parotid glands, temporomandibular joints, and mandible. Megavoltage radiation is important in treatment of tumors of the oral cavity and oropharynx because the beam is not preferentially absorbed by the mandible, which shields tumors in these locations. Well-collimated megavoltage beams without much side scatter are important when it is necessary to deliver high doses of radiation for tumors in close proximity to the central nervous system, such as those of the nasopharynx and pharyngeal wall.

Some megavoltage machines produce electrons that are attenuated differently than electromagnetic radiation such as gamma rays and x rays. If one graphs percentage dose versus depth in tissue, the dose contributed by electrons falls precipitously beyond a certain point in tissue, depending on the energy of the beam and the attenuating material. This precipitous falloff in dose beyond a certain depth in tissue allows one to protect structures such as the parotid gland. The electron beam, therefore, is helpful in treatment of parotid gland tumors or temporal bone lesions in which one wishes to confine the dose to the side of the lesion, thereby sparing normal structures such as the parotid gland on the opposite side. All megavoltage radiations, that is, cobalt 60 gamma rays, high-energy x rays, and electrons, have a similar linear energy transfer (LET), which is energy deposited per unit of path length. Interest has increased in high LET radiation or particulate radiation such as neutrons, pi mesons, and other heavy particles in the treatment of head and neck cancers because these radiation techniques are effective in the destruction of hypoxic portions of tumors. The major failing of current ionizing megavoltage radiation is believed to be its inability to destroy the central hypoxic portions of a tumor. The technology for production of neutron beams and other particulate radiation beams is currently evolving and will undoubtedly improve in the future (see Fig. 32–34).

Radiation therapy should be considered the primary modality for the following lesions: (1) small, superficial cancers of one or both membranous true vocal folds that do not involve the anterior commissure or vocal process, extend subglottically, or fix the vocal fold; (2) lesions of the free border of the epiglottis that are smaller than 1 cm; and (3) lesions in patients who are poor surgical risks.

Our present method includes postoperative radiotherapy of 5000 to 6500 cGy when indicated; the dose is given over a 6-week period. This is used in the following situations: (1) T2 to T3 supraglottic carcinomas; (2) T2 to T3 glottic carcinomas; (3) all carcinomas that extend more than 1 cm subglottically; (4) T2 to T3 marginal (aryepiglottic fold) carcinomas; (5) all pyriform carcinomas; and (6) carcinomas that extend beyond the confines of the larynx.

Ipsilateral neck nodes are irradiated in all patients with tumors that have a high incidence of metastasis (greater than 25%) when neck dissection is not performed. Thus, in supraglottic, aryepiglottic fold, pyriform fossa, or subglottic carcinomas, the homolateral neck nodes are irradiated after surgery, even if none are palpable. All patients whose necks have palpable lymph nodes that have metastases are considered for irradiation and surgery.

Chemotherapy

Chemotherapy for laryngeal cancer (see Chap. 34) has generally been relegated to palliative efforts for the patient with advanced disease. Methotrexate and 5-fluorouracil are capable of producing significant, although short-lasting, tumor regression in an advanced setting. Agents such as hydroxyurea have been used in combination with radiotherapy for advanced lesions. Bleomycin, 15 mg/m^2 body surface area, given over a 6-week period, has also been used. The overall response rate for laryngeal carcinomas is about 30 to 50% for bleomycin given intravenously. This drug can be combined with vincristine for greater effectiveness because vincristine increases the number of mitoses. The major complication of bleomycin has been progressive pulmonary fibrosis. Another agent that has been introduced is doxorubicin, but experience is limited.[182] Daunorubicin, cyclophosphamide, aclarubicin, sodium diethyldithiocarbamate,[183] esorubicin,[184] VP16–213,[185] and cisplatin have also been used in the treatment of head and neck squamous carcinoma, frequently with relatively good initial, but poor final, success rates.[186]

Since the majority of the foregoing reports were published, interest in attempting to establish the benefit of chemotherapy in the treatment of advanced head and neck carcinoma has returned. The emphasis has been on attempts to preserve the larynx in patients with tumors warranting total laryngectomy as standard treatment (see the section of this chapter on organ preservation). The outcomes are at best minimally changed, and the treatment regimens are complicated with a variety of agent mixtures followed by radiotherapy or even delivered concomitantly. No one has yet to report significantly improved survival in patients with newly treated disease in any of the reports when compared with ablative or conservative surgery followed by radiotherapy. Vokes and associates reported on a series of patients treated with a combination of cisplatin, fluorouracil, and leucovorin for the treatment of recurrent head and neck carcinoma; the regimen significantly reduced distant spread of disease and increased the probability of survival.[187] Hamasaki and Vokes published two comprehensive reviews of the current state of chemotherapy and combined modality therapy in the treatment of advanced head and neck carcinoma[188,189] (see Chap. 34).

The duration of life for patients in whom primary surgical or radiotherapy procedures fail may be relatively long. During this period, the pain from bone involvement caused by local extension and progressive respiratory distress caused by tumor in the thoracic inlet may be considerable. In this setting, even moderate palliation may be extremely gratifying.

Advances in the identification of cell lines that are more or less susceptible to various chemotherapeutic agents in vitro may lead to individualized treatment of squamous cell carcinoma in vivo, with less toxicity and more effective tumor kill.[186]

Other drugs have been used in recent experimental

trials, including those that modify differentiation. The most important of these include the retinoic acid analogues, notably *cis*-retinoic acid and its derivatives. Results from the use of these drugs are preliminary, but they do show great promise for arresting the progression of disease.[190] Antihormonal therapy for laryngeal cancers that demonstrate surface receptors for steroid hormones has been proposed.[191] Mattox and colleagues and Urba and associates investigated the role of androgen and estrogen blockade on the growth of recurrent laryngeal carcinoma, respectively.[192,193] Neither group found marked responses, although both types of hormone receptors have been found in laryngeal tumor tissues.

Hyperthermia

Advances have been made in the treatment of surface tumors with hyperthermia[194] or a combination of hyperthermia and radiotherapy. For this method of treatment, tumors are exposed to heat at their surfaces, or in their interiors by means of implanted probes, to 102 to 105°F for varying lengths of time. Although this method of treatment is still experimental in that few controlled trials have been accomplished, it appears to have promise as an adjuvant to chemotherapeutic and radiotherapeutic approaches and may be synergistic with these other methods of treatment.[195]

Photoradiative Therapy

Techniques that involve administration of a drug producing a photosensitizing effect in tumors have begun to be applied to the treatment of head and neck carcinoma in various sites. After administration of the substance, light is applied to the tumor, and tumor necrosis is produced. Currently, this treatment is in the clinical trial stage, but it will probably prove useful in the therapy of advanced and recurrent disease and may be useful in the treatment of early invasive carcinoma or carcinoma in situ. Superficial tumors and intraluminal cancers causing obstruction have been reported to respond,[196] providing at least symptomatic benefit.

Immune Modulation

Generally, when metastases occur to the lymph nodes, the initial region of involvement is in the subcapsular or marginal sinus areas. This implies that capsular rupture need not be related to the degree of lymphocyte replacement by tumor. Another observation is that tumor emboli often travel the afferent lymphatic vessels in a tangential course within the capsule before they enter the marginal sinus. Thus, the capsule may be involved initially. Generally, metastases of greater than 2 cm in size show capsular rupture.

Changes are often seen in regional lymph nodes draining a carcinomatous region. These may precede metastasis to the lymph node. These changes include sinus histiocytosis, germinal center hyperplasia, paracapsular vascular engorgement, and cellular infiltration with plasma and mast cells. Some lymph nodes show loss of lymphocytes and fibrosis.[197] Some researchers consider cellular infiltration of lymph nodes as a crude "malignancy index." Increased cellular infiltration is considered favorable, and depletion and fibrosis are considered signs of cellular immune deficiency and poor prognosis. Others believe that no such specific relationships exist.[198–204]

Studies have targeted possible immune deficiencies as promoting causes of head and neck cancer formation and progression. For instance, a study indicated that the peripheral blood lymphocyte natural killer (NK) activity of cancer patients was significantly less than that of the controls, and that a spectrum of NK suppression exists in draining lymph nodes of patients with head and neck squamous cell carcinoma, the level of activity depending on the degree of nodal tumor involvement.[205]

Other changes in cellular immunity have been extensively documented in patients with laryngeal carcinoma. Increases in T lymphocytes have been found in venous blood-draining cancerous regions.[206] Attempts have been made at evaluating delayed hypersensitivity using the dinitrochlorobenzene reaction, with a reduction in T-lymphocytes manifested by a reduced delayed hypersensitivity to dinitrochlorobenzene.[207] One often notes reduction of blast cell transformation, immunoglobulin levels, total lymphocyte numbers, lymphokines, interferon activity, and cellular migration. Cellular immune deficits are reported to be related to multiple carcinomas in the head and neck,[208] and changes in cellular immunity appear to occur after radiation therapy.[209–211]

Changes in the function of the hormonal immunity system also occur in laryngeal cancer. For example, changes in IgE levels may be related to tumor persistence.[212] Prostaglandin levels often change in patients with laryngeal cancer.[213]

These types of studies have led to theories of possible immunomodulatory treatment of head and neck carcinoma in the future,[214,215] although attempts to treat laryngeal carcinomas with immunotherapy have not yet been successful.[216]

Palliative Management of Terminal Disease

Palliative procedures and measures are defined as those that are used to prolong life in a socially more acceptable and physically comfortable way. In general, this includes the terminal care of the patient with incurable carcinoma. The setting for this care can include the hospital, intermediary care facilities, and the patient's home. Personnel administering such care include physicians, clinic and floor nurses, social workers, pharmacists, and patients and their families. The patients needs control of local disease, proper nutrition, alleviation of pain, maintenance of proper hygiene, and support.

Patients with advanced laryngeal carcinoma are prone to nutritional deficits, particularly from carcinomatous obstruction of the esophageal introitus or a past history of alcoholism or odynophagia. If patients can maintain a reasonable dietary intake, they may be capable of being more ambulatory, happier, and more self-sufficient. If oral intake is not possible, feeding by means of a transnasal polyvinyl catheter with individualized formulas is indicated. Occasionally, a cervical esophagostomy, gastrostomy, or jejunostomy for feeding purposes is indicated.

General wound care and hygiene are important for the physical and mental well-being of the patient. Ulcerated, odoriferous, and septic wounds can be cleaned by topical solutions of hydrogen peroxide, neomycin, saline, and povidone-iodine solutions. Local debridement by wet or dry dressings and cryosurgery is effective. Oral hygiene is maintained by a dentist and oral hygienist, oral irrigations, and mucolytic agents. The tracheal protection of humidification is critical, especially in the winter or in a dry climate.

Pain is often a dehumanizing and agonizing experience. Its control is paramount in palliation. After analysis of the sites of pain production, drug therapy is used, beginning with the mildest analgesic agents and resorting to narcotics in rotation when needed. In the terminally ill patient, concerns about drug dependence are irrelevant.

Severe pain in the head and neck region resulting from cancer can, in many instances, be relieved by interrupting the innervation of the painful area. Sensory (cranial and spinal) rhizotomy and gasserian ganglionectomy by a neurosurgeon may be indicated.

Cancer care is clostly, and all resources, medical and social, must be woven into the scheme to aid the victim. The patient's own emotional and physical strengths and those of the family must be marshaled in palliation. Assistance can also be obtained from major tax-supported agencies (Social Security, Veterans Administration, state departments of public welfare, state departments of health, and state rehabilitation commissions, etc.), and from voluntary health agencies (American Cancer Society, Lost Chord Club, American Red Cross, Chamber of Commerce, and various church and service organizations such as Kiwanis, Lions, Optimist, Rotary, Salvation Army, United Fund, and Community Chest).

Prognosis

The natural history and biologic behavior of laryngeal and laryngopharyngeal cancers differ. The prognosis of patients with laryngeal cancers is more favorable because the tumors are well differentiated and localized, and they infrequently metastasize at early stages.

Laryngopharyngeal cancers are characterized by less cellular differentiation, greater submucosal extension, a higher incidence of cervical metastasis, and a poorer survival rate. The most important factors that influence survival are (1) location of primary lesion, (2) lesion size, (3) cervical metastasis, and, possibly, (4) cellular differentiation.

Location and Lesion Size

GLOTTIC. The location of the tumor determines its biologic behavior. Tumors that are confined to the glottis and true vocal folds are usually well differentiated, slow-growing lesions that extend in predictable ways (see Figs. 32–5 and 32–8). Some evidence indicates that they extend locally along blood vessel planes. They can extend anteroposteriorly to both the anterior commissure and the opposite vocal fold (see Fig. 32–9). They can infiltrate the vocal ligament and vocalis muscle and extend to the ventricle and the supraglottis or subglottic area (see Figs. 32–8 and 32–9). Cartilage invasion is late and usually occurs at the anterior commissure area (see Fig. 32–15). Extralaryngeal spread occurs late in the course of the disease, generally under the inferior thyroid cornu and cricothyroid membrane. Ossification of thyroid cartilage appears to increase incidence of cartilage invasion. When glottic tumors invade the base of the epiglottis and anterior commissure, the incidence of inner perichondrium or thyroid cartilage destruction and extension outside the cartilaginous larynx is approximately 75%. The main limitations of direct tumor extension are Broyles' ligament anteriorly and the conus elasticus laterally.

SUPRAGLOTTIC. Supraglottic tumors are large and bulky, with central areas of necrosis and heaped-up margins (see Fig. 32–7). They invade locally and have a tendency to travel cephalad. A barrier appears temporarily to prohibit their extension directly to the glottis (see Fig. 32–14). These tumors can invade the epiglottis, false vocal fold, and aryepiglottic fold. Tumors can follow the mucosal surface and climb up the epiglottis. They extend extralaryngeally through the vallecula to involve the base of the tongue, traveling by way of the aryepiglottic fold. They can invade the pyriform sinus and endolarynx. Invasion through the foramina of the epiglottic cartilage is not uncommon. This can lead to vallecular and base-of-tongue invasion submucosally. The epiglottis is usually divided into two portions in relation to the hyoid bone. The lower the lesion on the epiglottis (infrahyoid), the worse the prognosis. Invasion of the preepiglottic space allows tumors to enter the deeper laryngeal structures on both sides of the larynx and to invade the paraglottic space posteriorly.

SUBGLOTTIC. Subglottic tumors are broader, less fleshy, and have a lesser propensity to ulcerate. These lesions have a higher tendency for submucosal and circumferential growth and extension. Primary subglottic tumors are rare (about 2%), but glottic lesions with subglottic extension are more common (about 25%). They extend extralaryngeally by way of the cricothyroid membrane and tend to involve the hypopharynx, trachea, and thyroid gland by direct extension.

SUPERIOR HYPOPHARYNX. Cancers of the superior hypopharynx involve the vallecular surface of the epiglottis, vallecula, and base of the tongue (posterior to the circumvallate papillae). These tumors tend to invade locally the intrinsic and extrinsic lingual muscles, the epiglottis, aryepiglottic folds, and preepiglottic space.

INFERIOR HYPOPHARYNX AND PYRIFORM SINUS. Inferior hypopharynx and pyriform sinus tumors are large and bulky, with extensive local and submucosal invasion. They can extend to the base of the tongue, aryepiglottic fold, false vocal folds, and supraglottis. They extend extralaryngeally by destroying cartilage, invading the cricothyroid membrane, extending posterior to the free margin of the thyroid ala, breaking through the pyriform apex, or invading the glossoepiglottic and aryepiglottic folds (see Fig. 32–12).

Cervical Metastasis

Important factors in determining final survival rates are the presence of tumor in cervical lymph nodes and whether this metastatic disease has become extranodal at the time of discovery.[217] In general, survival decreases by more than one third when clinically positive lymph nodes are present. The incidence of metastasis is determined by the location, size, and possibly cellular differentiation of the primary tumor; that is, laryngopharyngeal tumors metastasize more readily, and tumors larger than 2 cm are more likely to have metastasis. The highest correlation with metastasis is the location of the tumor. Nevertheless, there is a 25% error in positive metastatic lymph node diagnosis on palpation. Moreover, that survival rate can be increased by administering postoperative adjuvant radiotherapy in patients with clinically positive neck lymph nodes, even after neck dissection.[217]

Patterns of lymph node response may be indicative of future prognosis; in one study,[218] the lymph nodes of 32 patients operated on for carcinomas of the larynx and pharynx were evaluated for the pattern of lymph node response. Pattern 1 (predominantly lymphocytes) and pattern 2 (predominantly germinal centers) showed fewer nodal metastases than pattern 3 (nonstimulated nodes). Well-differentiated carcinomas predominated in patterns 1 and 2, whereas moderately and poorly differentiated tumors predominated in pattern 3. Patterns 1 and 2 predominated in clinical stages I through III, and pattern 3 predominated in stage IV. Survival decreased progressively from pattern 1 to pattern 3.

GLOTTIC TUMORS. The incidence of tumor metastases from carcinoma in situ is extremely low. The incidence

of cervical node metastasis with T1 glottic lesions is low (0.5 to 3%). Generally, the larger and more deeply infiltrative the lesion, the higher the incidence of local metastases. For tumors 2 cm or less in size, metastases are about 15%, and for tumors larger than 2 cm, this rate rises to 40%. Transglottic carcinoma has a local metastatic rate of up to 50%.[202] Glottic tumors with extension to arytenoid have a low metastasis rate also, but it is higher than that of tumors that do not extend to the arytenoid (about 4%). Anterior commissure tumors have a metastatic rate of around 8%. Ventricular carcinomas and transglottic tumors have similar metastatic rates of approximately 50%. Subglottic tumor extensions of more than 2 cm have an incidence of metastases of 30 to 40%. These tumors, however, are hard to evaluate because they metastasize to the paratracheal nodes, Delphian node (precricothyroid membrane), superior deep chain along the internal jugular vein, and the low neck contralaterally. In our series of over 600 cases, 13% had positive nodes. Tumors that fix a vocal fold have metastatic rates of 14 to 30%.[219] The one exception to this finding is a positive midline deep lymph node (Delphian node) that occurs in about 5% of T3 glottic lesions, especially those with cordal fixation and subglottic extension. In these cases, the cricothyroid membrane, thyroid gland, and upper tracheoesophageal nodes are usually involved (40%) and must be resected with the primary tumor. If the patient is staged as N > 0 with a laryngeal cancer and has a lesion that extends to the midline or beyond, Patel and Snow recommend the elective treatment of the contralateral neck.[220]

SUPRAGLOTTIC TUMORS. Supraglottic carcinoma metastatic rate at the time of initial diagnosis is 35 to 45%.[202,221] In T2 supraglottic carcinomas, the metastatic rate is 43%.[222] Contralateral metastases are manifested in 40 to 50% of patients within 2 years of the presence of the disease in the ipsilateral lymph node.[219]

Marginal aryepiglottic fold carcinomas behave like hypopharyngeal tumors. The frequency of metastases is about 60%, usually to the jugular chain and paratracheal region.

SUBGLOTTIC TUMORS. The incidence of cervical metastasis in primary subglottic tumors or glottic tumors with more than 5 mm subglottic extension is about 25%. Some reports, however, indicate a higher incidence of paratracheal node metastasis (60%). In an analysis of lesions, 5 of 8 patients with primary subglottic tumors and 10 of 17 with glottic tumors with subglottic extension had positive lymph nodes. In our series, 2 of 5 patients with subglottic tumors and 5 of 132 with glottic tumors with subglottic extension of less than 10 mm had clinically positive nodes on initial examination. One fourth of patients, however, developed metastatic recurrence after therapy (20% in the neck and 4% distant metastasis).

TRANSGLOTTIC TUMORS. The incidence of cervical

metastasis is 30 to 50%, with about 20% being nonpalpable nodes. McGavran and associates reported 31% and Bauer and colleagues 38% metastasis in series of transglottic tumors.[202,223] If the lesion involves only the true and false vocal folds, the incidence of metastasis is about 10%. If the tumor involves the epiglottis, true vocal folds, and false vocal folds, the incidence of metastasis is 50%, 25% being occult positive nodes.

HYPOPHARYNGEAL TUMORS. The incidence of cervical metastasis in the hypopharynx is high, being around 66% (more than two thirds are not palpable).

Pyriform sinus carcinomas have the highest metastatic rates of all laryngeal cancers; at the time of diagnosis, neck metastases can be found in 70 to 85% of these patients. These metastases are usually to the middle deep jugular chain. Contralateral metastases are found in 10% of patients at presentation. Even small (T1 to T2) lesions metastasize early.[224] These metastases tend to be large and fixed and therefore are palpable in 60 to 70% of cases. Posterior pharyngeal wall, hypopharyngeal, and postcricoid carcinomas have an estimated metastatic rate of 80%. These figures, however, are not firm,[219,225] especially in the latter case, because lesions of the upper mediastinum are rarely diagnosed pretherapeutically.

BILATERAL OR LATE CONTRALATERAL CERVICAL NODE METASTASIS. Patients with bilateral palpable cervical adenopathy present most frequently with supraglottic and base-of-the-tongue cancers. The incidence of bilateral palpable cervical nodes in 138 patients with supraglottic lesions was 5%. The incidence of bilateral palpable lymph nodes with vallecula and base-of-the-tongue lesions is about 10%. A significant number of patients with supraglottic and superior hypopharyngeal cancers develop late contralateral nodes. The incidence of late contralateral metastasis, if ipsilateral lymph nodes are histologically positive, is 30 to 35%.

Peristomal Recurrence

Paratracheal node disease is considered to be a significant risk factor for peristomal recurrence of cancer. Based on a report by Weber and associates,[159] the presence of histologically positive metastases to this lymphatic bed was associated with a 0% survival beyond 42 months in 645 patients. These investigators advocate the elective unilateral dissection of this area (zone 6) in cancers of the larynx, hypopharynx, and cervical esophagus and advocate the bilateral dissection of this area in bilateral disease and for subglottic tumors. Esteban and colleagues reported the occurrence of peristomal recurrences in relation to tumor size, bulk, and subglottic extension.[226] They failed to find a relationship between the incidence of peristomal recurrence and the presence of positive lymph nodes in the neck dissections. They explained this finding by reporting that dissection of the paratracheal lymph nodes is not routinely done by their group. This finding seems to

further support the indication for elective dissection of these lymph nodes in patients with the previously listed tumors. Contrary to the opinions of the foregoing, Brennan and associates presented their data on 227 laryngectomies and found an 8% incidence of thyroid gland metastases.[227] These occurred exclusively in T3 and T4 tumors. Based on their finding, these investigators stated that elective thyroidectomy was only indicated in tumors of this T stage or with subglottic extension. In other laryngeal disease, they found the resection to have too low a yield.

Cellular Factors

Other cellular factors may play a role in determining prognosis by influencing metastatic potential. In one study,[228] a total of 246 previously untreated patients with head and neck carcinoma expressed deficient NK activity. Some 164 consecutive patients underwent definitive therapy subsequent to NK cell assessment and were followed-up for a minimum of 12 months (median = 16 months); 23 developed recurrent disease in distant sites. The risk of subsequently (1) developing distant metastases, (2) developing regional metastases, and (3) dying of progressive cancer was inversely related to pretreatment NK values. NK cell function within the peripheral blood of the patient with head and neck cancer could be related to the percentage of some NK cell subsets. On the basis of these data, the authors concluded that in vitro measured NK cell function identifies a population at increased risk for developing distant metastases, and thus NK function can influence final outcome.

Another study found alterations in T-lymphocyte subpopulations in patients with head and neck cancer;[229] the mean helper-to-suppressor cell ratio (T4:T8) increased progressively with increasing tumor stage and was significantly elevated among patients with cancer as a group and in patients with advanced (stage III or IV) disease, compared with 40 normal subjects. Decreased disease-free survival was significantly associated with elevated T4:T8 ratios and low-percentage T8 and T11 cell levels. The prognostic significance of the percentage of T8 (cytotoxic-suppressor) cell levels persisted even after adjusting for known prognostic factors of tumor stage, T class, N class, and tumor site. These correlations provide new insight into immune alterations in squamous cell carcinoma of the head and neck that may prove useful in identifying patients with early clinical disease who have a poor prognosis.[229]

Results of Treatment

The choice of radiotherapy or surgery as the primary treatment for small laryngeal carcinomas is the subject of much debate. The cure rates are similar, with the differences obviated by the combination of salvage surgery for the T2 tumors treated with radiotherapy.[230-233] Clinicians need to appreciate the many relevant concerns apart from those of cure percentages in the choice of treatment for these lesions.[234] The reliability of the patient is an important concern when choosing radiotherapy. A noncompliant patient is unlikely to cooperate with a treatment regimen that lasts 4 to 6 weeks. Conversely, a patient who depends largely on the voice for livelihood should be considered for radiotherapy. Patients with lesions that are difficult to survey should be considered for primary surgical treatment. General physical health, pulmonary reserve, literacy, access to transportation for daily treatment, and need for primary surgical treatment of neck disease are all concerns that should enter into the decision process. The surgeon's comfort with laser or conservation laryngeal resection, the patient's access to rehabilitation services, and the experience of the radiotherapist all should be considered. The clinician should also have an appropriate level of concern for the treatment costs. Comparison of the laser treatment of small carcinoma in situ to full-course radiotherapy is skewed to the side of surgical treatment, with radiation reserved for incomplete resection, recurrence, or another primary tumor.[235,236] Anterior commissure and arytenoid tumor extensions tend to decrease the curative potential of radiotherapy and are more appropriately treated by conservative surgery.[237] On the other hand, the extension of the lesion to the interarytenoid mucosa or the postcricoid mucosa virtually demands a total laryngectomy for surgical treatment. Attempting to cure these lesions with radiotherapy is therefore sensible, with laryngectomy reserved for salvage. The surveillance of postcricoid lesions is difficult and should include endoscopy under anesthesia for early posttreatment follow-up to avoid the undetected progression of the cancer into the cervical esophagus.

Glottic Carcinoma

HEMILARYNGECTOMY. Overall results from cordectomy by means of endoscopic or laryngofissure approaches has been good, in the range of 85 to 98%. One example is the result of Neel and colleagues, who reported only a 2% death rate from carcinoma.[238] The cure rates from frontoanterior and frontolateral partial laryngectomy procedures are difficult to compare because of a wide difference in indications, but they approach 85% overall. The results for frontolateral resections are slightly worse, in the range of 58 to 68%.[239]

Cure rates after classic hemilaryngectomy are in the range of 95% for T1 and 70 to 80% for T2 lesions.[240] This includes extended hemilaryngectomies requiring arytenoid removal, although patients with bilateral disease and T3 lesions do more poorly (58 to 60% 5-year survival).[241] After radiation failure, hemilaryngectomy produces cure rates from 60 to 80%.[242]

In our experience, 281 patients underwent hemilaryngectomy for true vocal fold carcinoma. In 278, no

TABLE 32–2. Glottic Carcinoma: Overall Survival Rates at 3 Years

Treatment	No. of NEDs	No. of Patients Treated	3-Year NED (%)
Hemilaryngectomy	241	281	86
Salvaged	14	19	74
Total	255	281	91
Total laryngectomy	128	182	70
Salvaged	18	35	51
Total	146	182	80
Overall survival	401	463	87

NED, No evident disease.

clinically palpable lymph nodes were noted before surgery, and 3 patients had positive clinical nodes. The therapeutic success rate, expressed as 3-year determinate survival rate, for the former group is as follows: T1N0, 87%; T2N0, 82%; T3N0, 94%; T2N1, 100%; and T1N2, 0%. The overall cure rate for the hemilaryngectomy group was 86% or 241 of 281 patients. At 3 years, no evidence of disease (NED) was seen (Table 32–2). The 3-year NED survival by stage was as follows: stage I, 87%; stage II, 82%; and stage III, 90%. Fourteen of 19 patients were salvaged by total laryngectomy and irradiation, for a 74% salvage rate. The 3-year NED overall survival for this group was 91% (Table 32–3).

These results have been improved on in recent series of 111 consecutive patients with glottic carcinomas treated by hemilaryngectomy. Primary cure rate for hemilaryngectomy was 90%. In this series, 11 patients had recurrences. Five of 6 patients with local recurrences and 2 of 5 with neck recurrences were salvaged by combined radiotherapy and surgery, for a salvage rate of 64% and an overall cure rate of 96%.

ANTERIOR COMMISSURE EXTENSION. Of 586 patients treated for glottic carcinoma, 5 (1%) had pure anterior commissure lesions, 78 (13%) had unilateral vocal fold tumors extending across the anterior commissure, and 97 (17%) had bilateral vocal fold cancers involving the anterior commissure. Fifty-four (31%) had greater than 5 mm subglottic extension. Eleven (8%) patients presented with clinically positive cervical lymph nodes. Surgical treatment resulted in overall absolute 3-year

TABLE 32–3. Glottic Carcinoma: Survival by Stage (3-Year NED)

Stage	Hemilaryngectomy No. of Patients	Percentage (%)	Total Laryngectomy No. of Patients	Percentage (%)
I	177 of 205	87	19 of 20	95
II	45 of 55	82	32 of 47	69
III	19 of 21	90	77 of 114	68
IV	—	—	0 of 1	0

NED, No evident disease.

TABLE 32–4. Anterior Commissure (AC) Tumors: Absolute 3-Year NED Survival by Site and Procedure

Primary Site	Hemilaryngectomy		Total Laryngectomy	
	No. of Patients	Percentage (%)	No. of Patients	Percentage (%)
AC only	1 of 2	50	0 of 2	0
TVC (unilateral) with AC	31 of 42	74	16 of 22	73
TVC (bilateral) with AC	13 of 17	76	35 of 58	60
Total	45 of 61	74	51 of 82	62

NED, No evident disease; TVC, tumor of the vocal fold.

NED survival rates of 74% (45 of 61) for hemilaryngectomy and 61% (19 of 31) for therapeutic irradiation. The survival rates decreased progressively with each increasing stage of disease. The best survival, 24 of 29 patients (83%), occurred in patients with stage I unilateral vocal fold lesions with anterior commissure involvement (Table 32–4).

Patients with stage II lesions have an approximate 75% 3-year NED survival. Patients with stage III and IV lesions were treated with total laryngectomy, and the survival was 51 of 82 patients or 62%.

Frequent recurrence was noted after therapeutic irradiation (6 to 30%) or total laryngectomy (16 to 58%) for bilateral true vocal fold lesions involving the anterior commissure. Local recurrence appeared to correlate with the primary site and size of the lesion. Neck recurrence (34%) was highest in patients with bilateral vocal fold-anterior commissure lesions. Only three patients had local recurrence after hemilaryngectomy. Most of the patients who developed recurrent tumors did so within 1 year (80%), and 96% of the recurrences occurred with 3 years of primary therapy.

ARYTENOID EXTENSION. In glottic carcinoma with extension to the arytenoid cartilage, a hemilaryngectomy with removal of a greater part or all of the arytenoid was performed in 79 patients. Good functional results and an overall cure rate of 90% (3-year NED) were reported. The survival (cure rate + salvage rate) for patients with these lesions was 94%.

TOTAL LARYNGECTOMY. Local recurrences after total laryngectomy for glottic or vocal fold carcinoma are rare, but the recurrences are commonly caused by supraglottic extension to the base of tongue, transthyroid cartilage extensions, invasion of the marginal areas and hypopharynx, or greater than 2 cm subglottic extension (recurrences on the tracheal stump). The overall local recurrence rate after total laryngectomy for all types of carcinomas is 5 to 10%. Thus, the overall cure rate is determined by the control of local metastasis.

In our experience, 182 patients with glottic carcinoma were treated by total laryngectomy with or without neck dissection. One hundred forty-nine had no clinically palpable lymph nodes, and 33 had positive nodes. The therapeutic success rates, expressed as 3-year NED determinate survival for the former group, was as follows: T1N0, 95%; T2N0, 69%; T3N0, 68%; and T4N0, 45%. The 3-year determinate NED survival classified by stage was as follows: stage I, 95%; stage II, 69%; stage III, 68%; and stage IV, 0% (only 1 case). The overall cure rate for the total laryngectomy group was 77% (3-year NED). Eighteen of 35 patients were salvaged by secondary surgical resections or postoperative radiation, for a 51% salvage rate. The overall survival for this group was 80% (3-year NED).

The overall cure rate after total laryngectomy for all types of vocal fold cancers is in the range of 55 to 80%.[243] Subglottic extension of 2 cm or more reduces the cure rate to 40 to 50%.[143,152,244] Treatment of supraglottic extension by total laryngectomy procedures produces an overall cure rate of 65 to 73%.[245,246] Reviews indicate an overall 50 to 70% 5-year tumor-free survival for all glottic carcinomas treated by total laryngectomy, but these data are not pertinent today because most lesions requiring total laryngectomy are treated by combined-modality therapy (usually including pre- or postoperative radiotherapy). The salvage of patients with radiotherapy failures by total laryngectomy produces variable 5-year survival results of 30 to 65%, depending on the location of the primary tumor and the speed of diagnosis of the local recurrence. Nevertheless, most patients die of metastasis rather than local recurrence.[247]

RADIOTHERAPY. In a series of 100 consecutive early carcinomas of the larynx, a 5-year determinate survival of 82% in T1 lesions and 77% in T2 lesions was reported. The conclusion was that irradiation was not as effective in T2 as in T1 lesions. The overall cure rate was 78%, and the salvage rate was 62%. Horiot and colleagues,[248] in an analysis of 366 patients with early glottic carcinoma, reported a 90.5% cure rate for T1 and 86% for T2 carcinomas. Geopfert and associates noted an overall cure rate for invasive carcinoma of 88% for T1 and 74% for T2 lesions.[249] Wang and O'Donnell reported a 90% survival in T1 glottic tumors.[249a] In lesions of the membranous vocal fold there was 92% survival, in those of the anterior commissure 81%, and in the posterior third of the vocal fold 76%, with an overall survival of 88%. With fixation of the vocal fold, however, the cure rate dropped to 63%. Stewart reported a survival of 95% for T1, 72% for T2, 50% for T3, and 25% for T4 glottic cancers treated by irradiation with an overall survival of 85%.[250] Hibbs and colleagues reported a cumulative survival of 76% (35 patients),[251] and Boles and Komorn noted a cure rate of 74% (12 patients) with radiation therapy for T2 glottic lesions.[252] Lederman and Dalley,[253] in a larger series (137 patients), obtained a 65% cumulative survival for T2 lesions.

In other series of radiation therapy for glottic carcinoma, equally good results seem the rule. A composite result of 38 reported series for T1 vocal fold cancer yields an overall cure rate of 83.7%. Further evaluation of 12 separate reports of radiation therapy for T1 glottic tumor treated in the 1980s gives a cure rate range of 80 to 91%.[254–257] Bilateral vocal fold involvement reduces the cure rate by 5 to 8%. An amalgamation of 15 reports indicates that between 5 and 33% of patients with T1 glottic carcinomas have local recurrence after irradiation. Women have a slightly better prognosis than men.[258]

A compilation of 25 reported series for irradiation of T2 glottic carcinoma showed a 64% overall cure rate. This figure has not changed since the early 1970s.[259] Results from the 1980s, however, varied widely, with cure rates ranging from 31 to 87%. Thus, overall cure rates for T2 glottic carcinomas seem about 20% worse than do those for T1 lesions. This may indicate a wide diversity in tumors treated; for example, superficial lesions have a 70 to 90% cure rate, and deeper lesions with hypomobility of vocal folds have a cure rate of 50 to 65%.[260] The percentage of patients with tumor persistence following irradiation ranges from 14 to 60%, with an average of 275 in 13 studies.

Anterior commissure invasion denotes a poorer prognosis. The results of 8 studies show cure rates reported from 64 to 96%. The recurrence rates vary from 24 to 80%. The treatment by radiation may depend on the accuracy of the radiotherapist, as well as on the extent of invasion of the tumor into the anterior commissure.[237] The techniques of anterior partial laryngectomy allow the safe and oncologically sound resection of anterior commissure carcinomas Zohar and associates reported a series of 67 patients with T1 and T2 lesions and found a 91% and 89% surgical cure rate, respectively, and a 76 and 56% cure rate, respectively, for primary radiotherapy.[261] They also reported that in 54% of patients failing primary radiotherapy, a total laryngectomy had to be performed for local control.

Patients with T3 glottic carcinomas treated by irradiation alone have a cure rate of 20 to 55%, with an average of 40%. Local recurrence rate is 45 to 65%.[262]

Patients with T4 glottic carcinomas treated by irradiation are cured from 10 to 20% of the time, based on five separate studies.[263]

The problems of comparing the results of treating different patient populations with different therapeutic modalities are obvious. No final answer can be given without a universally accepted staging and classification system, as well as standardized end-result reporting. Although hemilaryngectomy may be only slightly more advantageous than irradiation in treating T1 glottic lesions, it definitely appears superior for the cure of T2 and selective T3 lesions. A slightly better salvage rate (74%) after hemilaryngectomy also increases the patients' chances for eventual cure.

Finally, to demonstrate the difficulty in interpretation of retrospective studies, we cite the example of a prospective randomized trial,[264] performed in patients with advanced squamous cell carcinomas of the oral cavity, larynx, and pharynx, to examine the effect of adjuvant postoperative radiation therapy on local-regional recurrence and survival following "curative" resection. Fifty-one patients with stage III or IV squamous cell carcinoma treated from 1981 through 1984 were randomized to receive either surgery alone (n = 27) or surgery with postoperative radiation (n = 24). Five patients were excluded from the study after randomization because of ineligibility or protocol violations. Overall recurrence rates of 55.6% and 36.8% were noted in the surgery and surgery with adjuvant radiotherapy arms, respectively (p = NS). No significant differences in overall survival were noted between the two treatment arms, however. Therefore, the effects of surgery and/or irradiation, in combination, on recurrence and long-term survival of patients with laryngeal cancer are still unclear.

CONSERVATION SURGERY AFTER RADIATION THERAPY. Several studies support the possibility that conservation laryngeal surgery can be performed after radiation failure, provided such a resection was possible before treatment. Davidson and colleagues reported a series of 88 patients who underwent surgical attempted curative resection following failure of primary radiotherapy (61%) and combined-modality treatment (39%).[265] These patients were followed for a median time of 4.4 years, and the reported 5-year survival rate was 35%. Forty-one percent retained a functional larynx, with a 48% postsurgical complication rate. Survival probability correlated with the tumor found before salvage surgery and not with the original T stage. The authors maintained that the residual or recurrent tumor needed to be restaged and the decision should be based on this assessment.

In a retrospective study, Lavey and Calcaterra reported the results of a series of 25 patients demonstrating an 80% 5-year survival rate with vertical partial laryngectomy following primary radiotherapy failure.[266] They did not, however, find an increase of postsurgical complications. Their review of the literature found the range of conservation laryngectomy after radiotherapy to have a 75 to 100% (82% cumulative) initial control rate and a 86% minimum control rate (96% cumulative) in the reports of 14 separate series.

Another group studied the likelihood that surgical complications would result in radiation failures that required total laryngectomy. Natvig and colleagues reported a four- to sixfold increase in the proportion of patients having postoperative fistulas after radiotherapy.[267]

TABLE 32–5. Supraglottic Carcinoma: 3-Year Determinate Survival after Subtotal Supraglottic Laryngectomy

	Lesion		Nodes		
Stage	No. of Patients	No. (%)	No. of Patients	N1–3 (%)	
T1	64 of 78	82	8 of 14	58	
T2	23 of 34	79	8 of 12	61	
T3	7 of 10	70	2 of 3	66	
T4	9 of 12	75	8 of 13	73	
No of Patients	136			41	

Supraglottic Carcinoma

SUBTOTAL SUPRAGLOTTIC LARYNGECTOMY. If indications are respected carefully and surgery is performed properly, the cure rates from SSL procedures equal that of total laryngectomy. Based on numerous studies, the overall cure rate is 60 to 80% (90% for T1) to about 46 to 60% for T3 lesions that extend to the marginal zone (aryepiglottis).[268,269] Local recurrence rates are about 10%, and patients are salvageable by total laryngectomy.[270] The overall recurrence-free survival rate today from three-quarter laryngectomy is about 65 to 75%.[271–273]

Of the 177 patients with supraglottic squamous cell carcinomas treated with and without preoperative radiation and SSL and neck dissection, 136 had no clinically palpable lymph nodes and 41 had positive nodes. The 3-year determinate survival rate based on the T classification of all lesions is as follows: T1, 83%; T2, 79%; T3, 70%; and T4, 75% (Table 32–5).

The 3-year determinate cure rate for the four stages was as follows: stage I, 82%; stage II, 79%; stage III, 69%; and stage IV, 50%. The overall 3-year determinate survival was 76% (Table 32–6).

T1N0M0 lesions treated successfully with SSL in 64 of 78 patients had a 3-year determinate cure rate of 82%. Of 34 patients with T2N0M0 lesions, the 3-year cure rate was 79%. For those with T3N0M0 lesions, the cure rate was 70% (7 of 10 patients), and for those with T4N0M0 lesions, 9 of 12 (75% 3-year determinate cure rate) were successfully treated. The overall cure rate was 76%. The salvage rate from secondary modalities

TABLE 32–6. Supraglottic Carcinoma Treated by Subtotal Supraglottic Laryngectomy: 3-Year Determinate Survival by Stage

Stage	No. of Patients	Percentage (%)
I	64 of 78	82
II	28 of 36	78
III	39 of 57	68
IV	3 of 6	50
Overall		76

of treatment is 47%. The overall survival (3-year NED) is 82%.

T3 lesions of the supraglottis, those with vocal fold fixation, were treated by preoperative radiation, total laryngectomy, and radical neck dissection. In 22 of 35 patients, resection of the lesion was successful, and the 3-year determinate survival was 66%.

Of the 22 patients treated by radiation alone, the 3-year determinate survival rate was 7 of 22 or 33%.

In the literature, the 5-year survival rate after total laryngectomy ranges from 45 to 60%, and after full-course radiation therapy from 7 to 56%, with an average of 20%. Improvement in survival rates has been reported for radiation therapy and combined high-dose preoperative radiation and total laryngectomy.

On the basis of available data, we believe that conservation therapy is the treatment of choice in supraglottic carcinoma. Our results compare favorably with those of patients given irradiation alone[249,274] for small T1 and T2 lesions and are superior for T3 and T4 lesions. These results are in accord with those of total laryngectomy.[274] If a comparison is made on the basis of physiologic restitution of phonation and deglutition, conservation surgery is superior to irradiation and total laryngectomy as a combined modality of treatment.

ARYTENOID EXTENSION. One study found 63 patients to have supraglottic cancer with extension to the arytenoid. Twenty patients had positive lymph nodes confirmed by pathologic study. Seven (18%) of these patients had occult positive lymph nodes. Forty-three of 59 patients (73%) had no recurrence of their cancer more than 3 years after therapy. Twelve patients developed recurrent cancer after primary treatment. A strong correlation existed between tumor recurrences and patient survival with the presence of positive or fixed lymph nodes. All recurred within 3 years. Six of the 12 (50%) patients with recurrences were salvaged with a combination of surgery and irradiation. A further study of 31 similar patients has been reported, with similar results.[275]

Our observations support the hypothesis that patients with clinically positive neck lymph nodes have a better prognosis for resection without recurrence if preoperative radiation is given (50% as compared with 64.5%).

RADIOTHERAPY. The records of patients with stage I and II epidermoid carcinoma of the supraglottic larynx treated at the Memorial Sloan-Kettering Cancer Center (MSKCC), New York, and at the Rotterdam Radio-Therapeutic Institute (RRTI), The Netherlands, between 1965 and 1979, were reviewed.[276] At the MSKCC, the treatment modality of choice for the primary tumor as well as for the neck was surgery; in the 79 patients treated by surgery, an elective neck dissection was performed on 31. At the RRTI, however, the initial treatment for the primary tumor and the neck was radiation therapy. One hundred and one patients were treated, of whom 79% (80 of 101) had radiation therapy to the primary tumor as well as to both sides of the neck. Twenty-nine percent of the patients from MSKCC (23 of 79) had relapses in the neck. The relapse rate was identical between the patients who did not have an elective radical neck dissection and those who did. Among the patients who had relapses in the neck, 65% (15 of 23) later died of the cancer, whereas among those who did not, none have died of supraglottic larynx cancer. Twenty-three percent (23 of 101) of the patients of the RRTI had relapses in the neck. Those who received radiation therapy to the primary tumor only had relapses regionally in 38% (8 of 21); treatment of both sides of the neck reduced the incidence of nodal recurrence to 19% (15 of 80). The majority of patients who had relapses in the neck eventually died of the cancer, that is, 57% (13 of 23). The conclusion was reached that, so far, elective radiation to both sides of the neck is the preferable treatment.

A recent study of patients with advanced operable squamous cell carcinoma of the supraglottic larynx or hypopharynx, randomly allocated to receive either preoperative radiation therapy (5000 cGy) or postoperative radiation therapy (6000 cGy), showed that local-regional control was significantly better for patients assigned to receive postoperative radiation therapy (65%) than for those assigned to receive preoperative radiation therapy (48%, P = 0.04). This was because of a higher rate of both persistent and recurrent local and regional disease in the preoperative group. Survival was also better in the postoperative group (38%) compared with the preoperative group (33%, P = 0.10). Because of these results, the authors suggested that the use of definitive radiation therapy with surgical rescue as an ethically justified alternative treatment for these tumors remains a question for further research.[277]

Composite averages for irradiation cure rates of supraglottic carcinomas indicate a wide variation of results by individual radiotherapists. Generally, the larger the lesion, the lower the cure rate. The overall cure rate, based on six studies, for patients with T1 supraglottic carcinoma ranges from 80 to 93%.[249,278] For those with T2 supraglottic carcinomas, the cure rate ranges between 50 and 77%, with those with suprahyoid tumors having a better prognosis.[279] Thus, patients with T1 and T2 tumors have a combined cure rate range of 50 to 89% (based on six studies). The cure

rate for patients with T3 tumors ranges from 20 to 67%. The cure rate for those with T4 tumors ranges from 15 to 55%. The overall cure rate for all patients with supraglottic carcinomas treated by irradiation alone ranges from 38 to 48%.

Subglottic and Glottic-Subglottic Carcinoma

In a study of 591 patients, 5 (1%) had primary subglottic tumors, and 132 (22%) had glottic tumors with subglottic extension. Seventy-five percent of the patients with glottic primary tumors with subglottic extension were stage II, and 25% were stage III. Two of 5 patients with primary subglottic carcinoma had neck metastases on initial examination. Two of 3 patients treated surgically were alive 5 years after treatment with no evidence of disease, and 1 died of uncontrolled primary disease. Two patients treated by irradiation died with uncontrolled primary disease.

One of 5 patients with primary glottic tumors (22%) had extension greater than 5 mm subglottically. Of 132 patients with subglottic extension, 52 (39%) had 5- to 9-mm subglottic extension, and 26 (20%) had greater than 20-mm subglottic extension. Fifty-five percent of these lesions arose from 1 vocal fold, and 41% involved 1 or both true cords, and the anterior commissure. Seventy-five percent of patients were stage II, and 25% were stage III. Five patients had nodal metastasis.

The 3-year survival for hemilaryngectomy in these patients was 52 of 63 (83%), for total laryngectomy 29 of 46 patients (63%), and for therapeutic irradiation 10 of 16 patients (63%). Survival of patients with stage II lesions, with less than 10 mm subglottic extension, was 43 of 47 (92%). Patients with stage II and III lesions with subglottic extension greater than 10 mm had significantly decreased survival rates of 69% and 50%, respectively. Patients with unilateral vocal fold lesions (even with anterior commissure involvement), with less than 10-mm subglottic extension, had the best prognosis (90% survival).

Tumor recurrences occurred in 25 of 132 patients (19%). Tumors with greater than 20-mm subglottic extension showed a more frequent rate (10 of 26 patients) of recurrence (Table 32–7).

Aryepiglottic Zone Carcinoma

A subpopulation of supraglottic cancer cases was reported in a recent compilation in 1994 by Spector.[33] Although it includes many of the patients reported on previously, the study focused on a specific subtype of

TABLE 32–7. Overall Survival by Stage: Subglottic Extension

Stage	5–9 mm	10–14 mm	15–19 mm	>20 mm	Total
II	43 of 47 (92%)	15 of 26 (58%)	8 of 13 (62%)	9 of 13 (69%)	75 of 99 (76%)
III	3 of 5 (60%)	8 of 11 (73%)	2 of 4 (50%)	7 of 13 (54%)	20 of 33 (61%)
Total	46 of 52 (88%)	23 of 37 (62%)	10 of 17 (59%)	16 of 26 (62%)	95 of 132 (72%)

supraglottic tumors that had their epicenter on the aryepiglottic folds, the so-called "marginal tumors." This set is made up of 315 patients all meeting the same selection criteria described previously and followed-up for a minimum of 4.8 years. They were all treated surgically or with radiotherapy or both at Barnes Hospital (St. Louis, MO) between January 1961 and December 1991. Their mean age was 62.4 years, with a male-to-female ratio of approximately 5:1. Each had a mean presenting symptom duration of approximately 4.8 months, with 80% having T3 or T4 lesions and 56% having neck metastases. The most important finding of this retrospective compilation came from the delineation of a subpopulation of aryepiglottic fold tumors that appear to have a different tumor biology characterized by a less aggressive course. Grossly, these tumors were found to present as an exophytic and infiltrating mass on endoscopy. Fifty-seven patients had this type of lesion, making up 18% of the total. These were compared with 258 patients who were found to have tumors with a different gross morphology, that is, of a superficially spreading minimally ulcerating form.

The cumulative local-regional control rate was 77% for the entire retrospective period. The cumulative disease free survival was 66%, 57%, 55%, and 55% at 5, 10, 15, and 20 years, respectively. Patients with infiltrating exophytic tumors had an overall 10% greater disease-free survival rate than those with superficially spreading tumors (Fig. 32–35). The 5-year survival rates were predictable according to T stage: T1, 87%; T2, 80%; T3, 78%; and T4, 41% (Fig. 32–36). Node status predicted a significant effect on survival such as a marked difference between N0 and N > 0 with a 25% greater 5-year disease-free survival and N1 > N2 to N3 with an 18% difference in the 5-year survival rate. On a selected basis, patients with small T1 and T2 tumors could be equally treated by radiation or surgery. Overall, surgery out performed radiation therapy alone, with 5-year survival rates of 61 and 34%, respectively (Fig. 32–37). Predictably, combined surgery and radiation (pre- or postoperatively) gave the highest cure rates, with an overall 5-year survival rate of 67.2%. The combined local-regional control rate was 77%.

These findings confirm our previous observations that aryepiglottic fold lesions behave more as hypopharyngeal tumors than supraglottic tumors and must be considered separately.[249] The less common bulky and infiltrative tumors appear to be the exception, however, and behave more like endolaryngeal cancers. Smaller T1 and T2 lesions are treated with PLP and radical neck dissection. For large T3 and T4 lesions, total laryngectomy and neck dissection with postoperative radiation therapy are the treatment of choice.

Pyriform Sinus Carcinoma

Between 1964 and 1991, 408 patients with pyriform squamous cell carcinoma were treated either with sur-

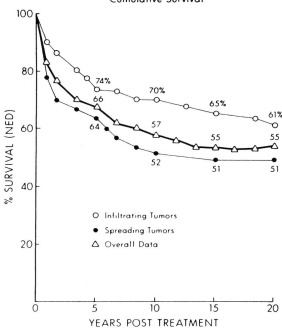

ARYEPIGLOTTIC FOLD CARCINOMA
Cumulative Survival

○ Infiltrating Tumors
● Spreading Tumors
△ Overall Data

YEARS POST TREATMENT

Fig. 32–35. Aryepiglottic fold carcinomas demonstrate a difference in their overall survival at 3 to 20 years. Infiltrative lesions have a better prognosis (10 to 15%) than spreading tumors over the entire follow-up period ($X^2 = 28.50$; $p = 0.01$). The overall data are dominated by the spreading tumor group, which was the largest group (82% of the cases).

gery, surgery with radiation, or radiation alone. Their mean age was 60.3 years (range 29 to 83 years), and the male-to-female ratio was 5:1. There was an average duration of symptoms of 3.9 months (range 1 to 32 months), and 89% had an alcohol and/or smoking history; 87% were stage III or IV at presentation, with 67% having T3 or T4 lesions and 69% having neck metastases.

Before 1978, preoperative radiotherapy was used. Since then, postoperative radiotherapy has been used. Conservation surgery was used whenever the tumor configuration was amenable to such methods (N = 207). This mostly consisted of PLP. Otherwise, total laryngectomy and partial or total pharyngectomy was the treatment (N = 157). Radiotherapy was used as a single modality in 33 cases. Since 1982, PLP defects have been closed with pectoralis major myocutaneous flaps that have more recently included microvascular free transfer of tissue. Postoperatively, 6000 cGy were given to the primary site and both sides of the neck if the margins were negative. This was boosted to 6500 to 7000 cGy in when negative margins were not attainable.

The breakdown of tumor size and configuration was divided into categories by the number of walls of the pyriform sinus that were invaded. The patient distribu-

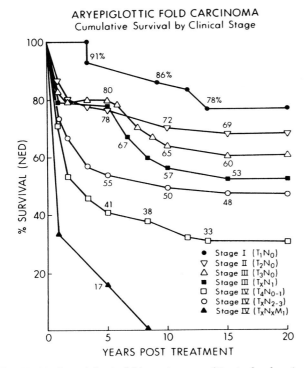

ARYEPIGLOTTIC FOLD CARCINOMA
Cumulative Survival by Clinical Stage

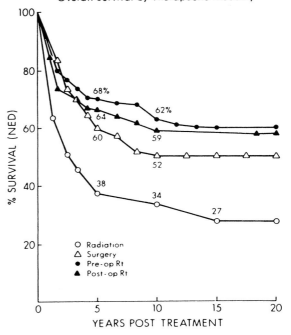

ARYEPIGLOTTIC FOLD CARCINOMA: ALL STAGES
Overall Survival by Therapeutic Modality

Fig. 32–36. Aryepiglottic fold carcinomas ultimate local-regional control ($X^2 = 15.00$, p < 0.001), T stage ($X^2 = 32.56$; p < 0.001), and neck metastases ($X^2 = 11.86$, p < 0.001) determine long-term survival. The lesions delineate themselves well by their clinical stage, except for some stage II and III lesions, which do not define themselves well in terms of 5-year disease-free survival ($X^2 = 5.278$, p = 0.15). Over the long-term survival period (> 20 years), however, they tend to demonstrate specific survival stratification.

Fig. 32–37. Aryepiglottic fold carcinomas treated by various therapeutic modalities demonstrate overall differences in survival. Single-modality therapies have a poorer outcome than combined-therapy groups ($X^2 = 7.48$; p = 0.01). Among the single modality-therapy groups, radical radiation had poorer results than the surgical groups ($X^2 = 5.48$; p = 0.07). In the combined-therapy groups, both conservation surgery ($X^2 = 0.01$; p = 0.91) and total laryngectomy ($X^2 = 0.46$, p = 0.50) had similar results with preoperative and postoperative adjuvant radiation. The surgical groups had similar results to the combined therapy groups for the first 3 years of follow-up; thereafter, the combined therapy groups demonstrated their advantage.

tion with the cancer confined to a single pyriform sinus wall (N = 48), centering on the medial wall adjacent to the larynx (N = 267), or extending to two or three walls, the postcricoid larynx, or the pyriform apex inferiorly (N = 93) was generated for analysis in this retrospective study. The overall local-regional control rate was 71%. The cumulative survival rate over all treatment modalities and stages was 54%, 34%, 24%, and 20% for the 5-, 10-, 15-, and 20-year follow-up, respectively (Fig. 32–38). The survival analysis was based on the product-limit method of the Kaplan-Meier algorithm. The survival curves by treatment demonstrated a consistent benefit to surgery followed by radiotherapy (see Fig. 32–38). Cure rates were significantly related to both T stage and nodal status, with T-1 + T-2 > T-3 + T-4 (28% difference) and N1 having a 26% lower cure rate. N > 1 had a 12% lower cure rate.

Other factors contributing to the already poor prognosis of these patients included a high second primary malignancy rate (6.2%), intercurrent disease fatalities (9.5%), and distant metastases (17.7%). The therapeutic complication rate was 19% overall, with 3.6% leading to death. The use of postoperative radiotherapy and flap reconstruction techniques have decreased the overall complication rate markedly.

Patients with hypopharyngeal tumors requiring total laryngectomy have a grave prognosis. Approximately 20 to 30% develop secondary primary tumors, and 30% have incurable disease at presentation. Small hypopharyngeal tumors have a cure rate of 47 to 66% when no lymph nodes are palpable in the neck.[280,281] Treatment is usually by combined radiation and surgery. The overall cure rate for all lesions is 25 to 35%.[282] The overall 5-year survival ranges from 15 to 25%. Distant metastases occur in 15 to 20% of patients at presentation and are mostly to the lung and liver. Patients who require a total laryngopharyngectomy with reconstruction have an even worse prognosis. Harrison achieved a 3-year NED survival of 29%, and Lam reported a 9% survival.[283–285]

Few randomized trials of hypopharyngeal carcinomas treated by irradiation alone have been conducted. Only 10% of the tumors at presentation are T1 and T2. In these patients, the irradiation cure rate is 20 to 40%. The overall cure rate for all hypopharyngeal carcinomas treated by irradiation alone ranges from 0 to 20%, and for T3 and T4 tumors, it ranges from 0 to 4%.

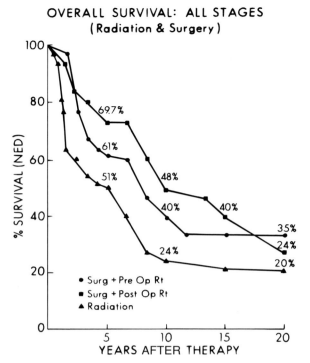

OVERALL SURVIVAL: ALL STAGES
(Radiation & Surgery)

69.7%

61%

51%

48%

40%   40%

24%

35%

24%

20%

• Surg + Pre Op Rt
■ Surg + Post Op Rt
▲ Radiation

% SURVIVAL (NED)

YEARS AFTER THERAPY

Fig. 32–38. Cumulative disease-free long-term survival for all the patients with pyriform fossa carcinomas in this study. The data are presented as disease-specific survival (Kaplan-Meier analysis).

More specifically, the 5-year cure rate for patients with pyriform carcinomas treated by irradiation alone is 13 to 20%. For those with postcricoid carcinoma, the cure rate for irradiation alone is 7 to 12%. Patients with posterior hypopharyngeal wall carcinoma have a radiation cure rate of 10 to 20%. Combined therapy is recommended for all hypopharyngeal tumors.

Neck Dissection

The results of neck dissection depend on many variables. Among these are stage of disease, selection of the case, quality of surgery, and type of metastasis (e.g., extracapsular spread, fixed nodes, degree of differentiation, location of metastatic nodes). Generally, the prognosis is worse for multiple metastases, miliary metastases, capsular rupture, soft tissue extension, invasion of vascular and neural structures, metastasis larger than 3 to 5 cm in diameter, low and posterior neck metastasis, and metastasis to high lymph nodes in the base of the skull.[286–288]

The prognosis for patients needing secondary neck dissections after radiation failures is also worse, with a recurrence rate of 45%.[289] In patients with radiation failures, capsular rupture of lymph nodes is present in 22% of lymph nodes less than 1 cm in diameter, 52% of nodes from 2 to 3 cm, and 74% of nodes larger than 3 cm in diameter. Snyderman and colleagues determined that 3-year NED survival following radical neck dissection is 71% without capsular rupture and 45%

with a ruptured lymph node capsule.[290] Preoperative planned radiotherapy produces variable results. Some have claimed improved results from neck dissection.[291] Others have found persistent metastases in 50% of the radiated specimens,[292] or no changes in metastatic recurrence.[293] Some investigators claim that pre- and postoperative radiation treatments are equally effective in reducing recurrence rates.[294] Some studies favor postoperative over preoperative radiation.

Local recurrences after radical neck dissection for N1 disease are 14%, for N2, 26%, and for N3, 34%. In patients who have surgery combined with irradiation, the recurrence rate drops to 2 to 25%.[295,296] DeSanto and associates noted the following recurrence rates after combined therapy: N0, 7%; N1, 20%; N2, 30%.[297]

Patients with bilateral neck metastases have a poor prognosis. The 5-year survival rates range from 25 to 50% in the most favorable circumstances.[298] Others report 5-year NED cure rates of 5 to 16%.[299]

A modification of the neck dissection occasionally needed in recurrent disease is the "superior mediastinal dissection." First introduced by Watson in 1962, it requires resection of a portion of the sternum.[300] Kleitsch, Minor, and Wardell, and Cannon introduced the sternal tracheotomy and transsternal mediastinal dissection; Sisson and associates reintroduced and modified these methods for extensive tumors at the thoracic inlet.[301] If these methods are performed electively, the prognosis is considerably better and the complications are fewer than when they are performed for necrotic, recurrent disease. Harrison reported that 14 of 22 patients survived 3 years or more.[302] Sisson had a 48% survival of patients from stomal recurrences for 1 year, 29% for 3 years, and 17% for 5 years (3 of 18 cases). The perioperative mortality is high because of hemorrhage from the brachiocephalic vessels, mediastinitis, and osteomyelitis. Total thyroid and parathyroid gland removal is required in most cases, and this results in hormonal and calcium deficiencies that need to be corrected.[303]

Organ Preservation

A resurgent interest has been noted in the use of radiotherapy combined with induction chemotherapy for the treatment of advanced squamous cell carcinoma of the head and neck.[187–189,304–310]

No study to date has demonstrated any improvement in survival when compared with the standard of care, that is, surgery combined with radiotherapy. Laryngeal cancer treatment has been given particular attention in this area based on the importance of avoiding the ablative surgical treatment of total laryngectomy, hence the concept of "organ preservation." The highest profile of these studies is the 1991 publication by the Department of Veterans Affairs (VA) Laryngeal Cancer Study Group.[310] This preliminary report presented the results of 332 patients treated with 2 to 3 cycles of dual-agent chemotherapy followed by definitive radiotherapy versus primary surgical treatment and postoperative radiotherapy. The median follow-up period for this report was 33 months, ranging from 11 to 66 months. The most important claim made the VA report is the preservation of the larynx in 66% of the patients in the nonsurgical arm of the study. Although 66% of the patients randomized to the experimental arm of the study had laryngeal preservation, only 39% had what was described as a "functional organ." The criteria for this designation were not described anywhere in the report, although all patients had a pretreatment assessment of their speech and voice according to the description in their methods section. The attendant morbidity of a patient with a larynx that produces no voice, fails to protect the airway, or results in chronic pain related to swallowing or speaking efforts is high, and this morbidity is often the basis for proceeding with laryngectomy. The nonfunctional organs that were *preserved* likely were designated as such based on one or more of these conditions. The quality-of-life issues that become apparent in patients left after therapy with this type of nonfunctional organ were not addressed, nor was the incidence of laryngectomies that were performed to treat this nonfunctional status.

The most common criticism cited about the VA study is the absence of a pure radiotherapy arm. No rationale was given for this lack in the preliminary paper. In a follow-up report (delivered in the form of the Rosenthal Foundation Award Lecture, 1993),[304] however, the project heads of the VA study acknowledged the criticism and stated that such a design would have been unethical because such treatment was already known to be less efficacious than the standard therapy of surgery followed by radiation. Although this is easy to understand, we still have no way to distinguish the effect of the chemotherapy on the curative potential of the radiotherapy from the results of this paradigm. Because the protocol isolates the subjects responding to the chemotherapy treatment, the population subjected to the radiotherapy is clearly biased. Unfortunately, this would be true even if a radiotherapy arm was used. The issue is one of tumor biology. Chemotherapy can be seen as a bioassay of tumor susceptibility to radiotherapy instead of contributing to the treatment of the cancer itself. Apart from rebutting the design critiques, the authors also reported some of the data from the original study, now with a 60-month median follow-up. They described a further 15% drop in the survival curve for the chemotherapy-radiotherapy group, as well as a 10% drop in the proportion of subjects left with "functional larynges."

The second point of published criticism is based on the finding that 31 subjects (10%) had primary tumors that were T1 and T2 in size.[230] These lesions are well known to be able to be highly curable by either surgery or radiotherapy. Although these patients may have had stage III disease by virtue of nodal disease, they were by definition not candidates for the study in so far as their treatment would not have necessitated total laryngectomy, as described in the materials and methods section. This injection of heterogeneity would skew the results of the primary tumor response data as well as the data on local recurrences. Although the number of patients represent a small proportion of the total N, the likelihood that these patients make up a large proportion of the survivors is high because their cure rates by standard surgery or radiation therapy followed by surgical salvage are well above 80%.

Other authors have published laryngeal preservation data that compare multiagent induction chemotherapy followed by radiotherapy or surgery. Karp and associates reported in 1991 that of 35 patients entered into their study, only 2 had salvage laryngectomy, claiming a 94% laryngeal preservation and a 2-year local control of 52%.[311] Twelve of the 35 patients had T1 or T2 primary tumors. Nineteen subjects had N0 or N1 disease. Eight of the 35 subjects were alive at the time of the report. Six of them were considered to be free of disease, with a follow-up range of 13 to 48 months (13 to 109 months for all surviving subjects). Of those surviving considered NED, 4 had T1 or T2 disease, 1 had a T3 of the larynx (N0), and 1 had a T4 of the hypopharynx (N3). Ten patients had local treatment failures, although all but 2 refused surgery or were considered inoperable. Three of those with local treatment failures also had distant disease, along with 4 others with treatment failures because of metastases.

Kraus and colleagues presented the MSKCC experience with laryngeal preservation in patients with hypopharyngeal cancers.[312] They reported the treatment of 25 patients, 8 of whom were considered to have had organ preservation or 32%. Of these 8, 4 were dead at the time of the report, 2 had died of other causes (NED), and 2 had died of uncontrolled regional or distant disease. Of the 17 patients not considered to have curative responses to chemotherapy and radiation, 10 underwent laryngectomy. Only 1 of these was successfully treated and died NED of other causes. One died of uncontrolled distant disease, and 8 had local treatment failures after failed salvage attempts. The other 7 patients with treatment failures were considered inoperable after being diagnosed with persistent disease after chemotherapy and radiation.

We believe that the development of successful organ preservation protocols is important. The benefits to the patient with advanced head and neck carcinoma from this pursuit, however, have thus far been limited and have not generated any appreciable survival increase. The hazard is that nonuniversity medical centers are using these alternative treatment reports as *standard* methods without the multispecialty support to treat the failures. These experimental treatments are *research protocols* and are not intended to be considered the standard of care. Surgically resectable advanced head and neck carcinoma should be resected and treated postoperatively with radiotherapy. This is the standard of care.

Chemotherapy

In 1988, a pilot study for resectable stage III and stage IV squamous cell carcinoma of the head and neck was performed, using a cytoreduction phase of preoperative radiation with cisplatin, followed by an eradicative treatment phase with radical surgery (group 1) versus radical dose radiation and cisplatin (group 2), followed by adjuvant chemotherapy with 5-fluorouracil infusion and cisplatin delivered at 4-week intervals for 6 cycles following initial radiation therapy to the primary site. A total of 43 patients were treated; 14 were classified with stage III carcinoma, 28 with stage IV, and 1 patient was not staged. Of 43 patients, 2 did not complete therapy. Forty-one patients completed the eradicative phase of treatment. Complete tumor clearance at the end of the eradicative treatment phase was 88% (36 of 41 patients). Actuarial recurrence-free survival was 61% at 3 years. Among 36 patients with complete tumor clearance after the eradicative treatment phase, no statistically significant difference for overall and recurrence-free survival was seen between group 1 and group 2.[313] Other studies show no benefit from the use of *cis*-diaminedichloroplatinum (CDDP).[314]

Another study compared a sequential program of induction chemotherapy followed by definitive treatment, arm A, with an alternation of chemotherapy and radiotherapy (three courses of 20 Gy in 10 daily fractions), arm B.[315] The same chemotherapy was used in both arms: vinblastine, bleomycin, methotrexate, and leucovorin. One hundred sixteen patients entered the study; 55 received chemotherapy in arm A and 61 in arm B. The patients all had previously untreated squamous cell carcinoma of the head and neck. Forty-five patients had stage III and 71 had stage IV disease. The two arms of the study were fully comparable. After 3 years, 116 patients were evaluable for survival, whereas 112 were evaluable for toxicity and 105 for response. There were 14 complete responses (CR) and 11 partial responses (PR), for an overall response rate (ORR) of 52% in arm A, and 30 CRs and seven PRs, for an ORR of 64.9% in arm B. The difference in terms of CR between the two arms was statistically significant (P less than 0.03). Progression-free survival (PFS) was also statistically different, with an advantage for arm B (P less than .05), but without differences in overall survival.

Other studies have also shown the efficacy of induction chemotherapy[316] in patients with advanced carcinoma, both as a treatment modality and as a predictor of future performance after completion of all treatment. Simply changing the scheduling of chemotherapeutic agents currently used[317] may provide some future control of disease proliferation as well.

Chemoprevention

Chemoprevention can be defined as the medical strategies to prevent second primary cancers from developing in *at risk* patients. Second primary tumors form at a rate of 3 to 7% per year.[304] Based on the presumption that cancers develop from premalignant lesions such as leukoplakia, the role of the retinoids in reversing leukoplakia has been eagerly studied. Unfortunately the toxicity of this class of drugs is substantial, causing compliance problems with a constellation of side effects including cheilitis, dermatitis, conjunctivitis, and hypertriglyceridemia. Moreover, the majority of the responding lesions recurred or progressed within 3 months of the cessation of the therapy.[318] In 1993, Lippman and associates reported the results of a National Cancer Institute study prospectively comparing the effect of 13-*cis*-retinoic acid to β-carotene on 70 subjects.[319] Although the 13-*cis*-retinoic acid group responded well, decreasing the degree of dysplasia in 43%, and halting progression in 92%, the β-carotene group had a 55% progression rate.

Other vitamin A analogues are active in vitro and in vivo against squamous cell carcinoma in animals and against certain epithelial precancers and cancers in humans. A prospective, multi-institutional, randomized phase II trial of isotretinoin in advanced head and neck squamous cell carcinoma, using 40 patients randomly assigned to receive isotretinoin or methotrexate, was performed. Overall, the study patients had extremely poor prognoses, that is, low performance statuses and recurring disease after surgery and/or irradiation. Three objective responses (16%), including 1 complete response, occurred in the 19 evaluable isotretinoin-treated patients. Only one minor response (5%) occurred in the methotrexate-treated group. Toxicity occurred with both drugs, but it was manageable and never life-threatening in the retinoid group. High-dose isoretinoin has also be investigated as an adjuvant chemotherapeutic agent after surgery and radiotherapy. Although no significant reductions of the primary disease were found, the incidence of second primary tumors was significantly reduced.[320] These results and the established activity of retinoids in oral leukoplakia and in the prevention of second primary tumors (a precursor of head and neck cancer) indicate the need for further study of this class of drugs in head and neck cancer.[190]

Another class of chemopreventive drugs receiving attention is that of the antioxidant and neucleophile *N*-acetyl-*l*-cysteine (NAC). This drug has been used for many years as a mucolytic agent in the treatment of acute and chronic bronchitis. It is currently being investigated as a chemopreventive agent because of the presumed role that oxidants have in carcinogenesis. It is thought to act at the earliest stages of carcinogenesis, perhaps before and just after genetic injury to the cell, whereas the retinoids are thought to act much later in the process.[321] NAC has been found effective in several animal models of cancer including dimethylbenz-anthracene (DMBA)-induced mouse skin papillomas model, the Swiss albino mouse urethane-induced disease, and other gastrointestinal malignancy models. The Euroscan project is using NAC and retinyl palmitate in the largest chemoprevention study using patients who have undergone curative treatment for head and neck cancer and those with oral leukoplakia. This drug appears to be safe and have few side effects.[322]

Radiotherapy

In vitro survival parameters of 14 human head and neck squamous cell carcinoma tumor cell lines cultured from patients who suffered local treatment failure after a curative course of radiotherapy were determined. The radiobiologic parameters determined included D, DO, n, and surviving fractions at 100, 200, and 300 cGy. When compared with in vitro radiobiologic parameters of tumor cells cultured from head and neck cancer patients before radiotherapy, human sarcoma cell lines derived from patients not receiving therapeutic radiation, normal human diploid fibroblasts, or other human tumor cell lines reported in the literature, the human tumor cells derived from radiotherapy failures are radioresistant. This may explain some radiation failures that occur occasionally in patients treated primarily with this modality.[323]

Hyperfractionation therapy may reduce radiation failures. In one study,[324] 144 patients with 148 moderately advanced to advanced primary squamous cell carcinomas of the head and neck received treatment with curative intent (7000 to 8000 cGy) with twice-a-day irradiation. The 5-year actuarial rates of neck control were 100% for N0 (45 patients), 90% for N1 (25 patients), 77% for N2 (23 patients), 50% for N3A (9 patients), and 70% for N3B (42 patients). The 5-year actuarial rates of continuous disease control above the clavicles were 73% for stage III, 64% for stage IVA, and 32% for stage IVB. The actuarial 4-year rate of continuous disease control above the clavicles was 78% for stage II. For patients whose disease was controlled above the clavicles, distant metastases developed in 4% of patients with stage II and III disease and in 18 of patients with stage IV disease. Radiation complications after irradiation alone to the primary site correlated with total dose. The actuarial 5-year survival rates, according to modified AJCC stage, were 59% for stage III, 37% for stage IVA, and 23% for stage IVB. The actuarial 4-year survival rate for stage II was 69%. Compared with historical control groups treated with once-a-day, continuous course irradiation, twice a-day treat-

ment produced local control results that were higher by 10 to 15 percentage points.

Most authors believe that it is not appropriate to try to extirpate advanced squamous cell carcinoma by operation alone. Evidence indicates that postoperative radiation therapy is more effective in local-regional control, at least in certain sites, than preoperative radiation therapy, and patient acceptance of the treatment plan in which the radiation therapy is administered after the operation is better.[325]

Hyperthermia

Hyperthermia shows promise as an adjuvant treatment. In one study,[194] 41 patients with superficial malignant tumors not previously treated with radiotherapy were treated with hyperthermia and definitive radiotherapy. After protocol radiotherapy, protocol hyperthermia, delivered twice weekly, was to start within 15 minutes after irradiation. It consisted of 60 minutes of heat to a tumor temperature of 43°C. Skin or subcutaneous necrosis occurred within 6 months in 2% of the patients; 12% experienced thermal blisters. Fourteen patients were followed-up for 6 months or more (after treatment); none of these experienced late toxicities more severe than telangiectasias. Complete responses were observed in 51% of these patients. Local disease control was maintained at nearly this level for at least 2 years. Logistic regression analyses showed site and histology, greatest tumor diameter, and average tumor temperature to be significantly related to the response. Based on these promising findings, the Radiation Therapy Oncology Group has instituted a randomized phase III study evaluating radiation therapy with or without hyperthermia in this patient population.

OTHER MALIGNANT TUMORS

Verrucous Carcinoma

Verrucous cancer of the larynx is a lesion that appears histologically benign but has a clinically malignant course. Verrucous carcinoma clinically appears sessile, with multiple heavy, broad filiform projections. It has heaped-up accumulations of dirty brown debris and is cauliflower-like in appearance. Hyperkeratosis with deep, swollen rete pegs is present histologically. Invasion and destruction of cartilage may be present. Verrucous cancer represents a lesion that does not have a histologic diagnosis of invasive cancer but that must be treated as such. The biologic behavior is that of slow but persistent growth with symptoms present for many years. Regional or distant metastases are not known to occur. The lesion is usually amenable to conservative surgery, although total laryngectomy may be required in advanced cases. Irradiation therapy is inef-

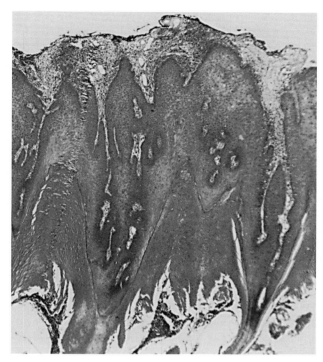

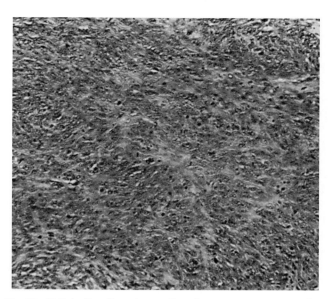

Fig. 32–40. Spindle cell carcinoma. Pseudosarcomatous perineoplastic stroma intermixed with squamous cell carcinoma. ×175, hematoxylin and eosin stain.

Fig. 32–39. Verrucous carcinoma of the larynx. ×45, hematoxylin and eosin stain. Note heaped-up keratin and deep rete pegs (Courtesy Dr. W. Bauer).

fective and may be contraindicated, because of reports of "malignant degeneration" of these tumors when irradiated. Elective neck dissection is usually not indicated, and the prognosis is excellent (Fig. 32–39).

Spindle Cell Carcinoma

"Spindle cell carcinoma" or "pseudosarcomatous carcinoma" refers to a squamous cell carcinoma accompanied by a highly reactive stroma. The underlying stroma may, in fact, appear to be sarcomatous, but the lesion should be treated like any squamous cell carcinoma. Pseudosarcomatous carcinoma appears as a dirty, ragged, fleshy lesion of large bulk and may have small areas of ulceration and necrosis (Fig. 32–40).

Carcinoid

Goldman and associates first demonstrated a carcinoid tumor in the larynx in 1969.[326] Over 200 cases have since been described.[327–329] These lesions mainly affect men between the ages of 50 and 70 years. Most tumors develop in the aryepiglottic folds, the false vocal folds, the pharyngoepiglottic folds, and the endoluminal surface of the epiglottis.[330,331] On more rare occasions, the first finding is a metastatic neck node.[332] The carcinoid syndrome, which is secondary to secretion of biogenic amines, has not been described with laryngeal tumors. The majority of these 200 cases were of a subtype called

atypical carcinoid that is thought to be much more aggressive than the rare typical form and has approximately a 50% 5-year survival rate.

Laryngoscopic examination shows a small, red nodule in the supraglottis that is covered by intact mucosa. Microscopic, histochemical, and ultrastructural studies give results indistinguishable from those of carcinoids elsewhere in the body. Treatment is surgical, with an emphasis on laryngeal conservation; modified neck dissections are performed when lymph node involvement is present. Long-term survival, even with distant metastasis, is the rule. The lesions appear to be radioresistant.

Adenocarcinoma

Adenocarcinomas may occur in any area of the larynx. They may be sessile or polypoid mucosal covered masses that do not have areas of ulceration. Most lesions occur in the supraglottic region and less often in the subglottic region. They are characterized by late, distant metastasis despite adequate surgical control of the primary tumor. Nine of 888 patients with primary laryngeal malignancies (1955 to 1971) had primary adenocarcinomas of the larynx (0.1%). Seven were supraglottic, and 2 were subglottic tumors. Six patients had large lesions (T3 and T4), 5 had clinical evidence of cervical metastasis, and 2 had pulmonary metastases. Four patients were alive without disease (6 months to more than 10 years). One patient was salvaged by secondary radical resection. Two died of pulmonary metastasis and one of delayed diffuse metastases. Average survival time was 3.6 years. Whicker and associates,[333] in a review, stated that in 27 patients, adenocarcinoma was more common (appearing in 12 patients) than adenoid cystic adenocarcinoma (9 patients) or mucoepidermoid carcinoma (6 patients). Twenty patients either died or remained alive with persistent disease. Adenocarcinoma of the larynx is a lethal disease that can recur many years after primary therapy with diffuse metastasis (Fig. 32–41).

Minor Salivary Gland Tumors

Pleomorphic Adenoma

The most common salivary gland tumor in the larynx is pleomorphic adenoma, first described by Lynch in 1929.[334] Since then, approximately a dozen such lesions have been described.[335,336] These usually arise in the aryepiglottic folds or epiglottis in the third to seventh decade of life. They rarely cause symptoms until they are large (3 to 4 cm in diameter). The main presenting symptoms are dysphagia and fluctuant dysphonia. These tumors are spheroid and have an intact overlying mucosa. They can be removed endoscopically (when small) or by lateral pharyngotomy (when large).

Mucoepidermoid Tumor

Masson and Berger first described this lesion in 1924.[337] Later, it was fully described by De and Tribedi.[338] Mucoepidermoid tumors arise from the ductal system of the minor salivary glands and have a mixture of epidermoid and mucous secretory cells. Myoepithelial cells are absent. These can be benign or malignant, depending on the degree of dedifferentiation. Since the first description of the lesion in the larynx in 1968, about 30 cases have been reported.

Mucoepidermoid tumors are rounded and mucosally covered and can occur anywhere in the larynx. The supraglottic area predominates as the most common site. The treatment of choice is surgical, using con-servation techniques. Malignant variants often demonstrate early metastasis to cervical lymph nodes. Clear cell carcinoma is considered a variant of this tumor; the "clear" cells contain large quantities of glycogen or mucus.[339–343]

The prognosis of the low-grade variety is excellent, whereas the high-grade mucoepidermoid, otherwise know as adenosquamous, is extremely aggressive and has a low survival percentage. Conservation laryngeal resections are reserved only for small, low-grade tumors. Total laryngectomy with or without radical neck dissection is indicated for the high-grade variety. Radiotherapy has not been found to be of any value in treating this tumor.[344]

Adenoid Cystic Carcinoma

This tumor comprises 0.25 to 1% of all laryngeal cancers. First described by Broeckart in 1912, adenoid cystic carcinomas, or cylindromas, have been reported over 80 times in the literature.[345,346] No age or sex predisposition is seen in patients with these tumors. Most such tumors arise in the subglottic region, near the tracheal junction. The lesion is usually rounded and submucosal, with mucosal hyperemia. Lymph node and distant hematogenous spread occurs early in the course of the disease and is more prevalent with supraglottic tumors than with subglottic lesions, which are more common.

In the subglottic region, adenoid cystic carcinomas usually arise from the posterior laryngeal wall, and they tend to invade the trachea, thyroid gland, esophagus, and larynx directly. This causes a circumferential reduction of the lumen of the trachea, with extensive growth before respiratory compromise. The resultant dyspnea, which is aggravated by exertion or lying down, may be the presenting symptom. Other symptoms include dysphagia, choking, referred otalgia,

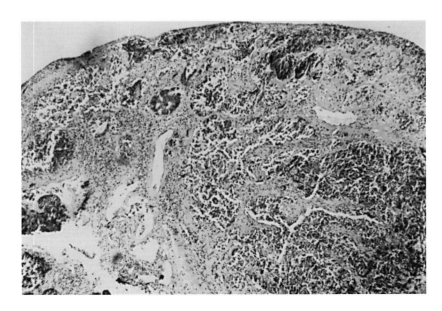

Fig. 32–41. Poorly differentiated adenocarcinoma of the subglottic larynx. ×90, hematoxylin and eosin stain.

wheezing, coughing, and hemoptysis. Paralysis of the recurrent laryngeal nerves is common in the latter course of this process, with hoarseness a late finding. As with adenoid cystic carcinomas at other locations, there is associated perineural and perivascular tumor spread and spread along other tissue planes (i.e., tracheoesophageal party wall, perithyroidal). These lesions are best delineated by CT scan with contrast.

The cure rate is poor, with the average survival ranging from 1 to 3 years. In patients who survive longer than 10 to 15 years, late distant metastases (lungs, bones, and brain) are not uncommon because hematogenous spread is common in both the early and late course of the disease. Prophylactic neck dissection is not advocated, and the use of radiotherapy is controversial. Some studies indicated a prolonged survival after radiation treatment, albeit with tumor persistence.[347–350]

Vascular Tumors: Kaposi's Sarcoma

Kaposi's sarcomas may be present as isolated lesions or associated with acquired immunodeficiency syndrome (AIDS). Approximately two dozen laryngeal cases have been reported. Most are associated with cutaneous or oral mucosal lesions, and in all instances laryngeal involvement occurs in the late stages of the disease. Almost all patients have cervical lymphadenopathy. An aggressive form of the disease has recently been described in Central Africa.[351–353]

Myogenic Tumors

Rhabdomyosarcoma

These most frequent sarcomas of infants and adolescents are common in the orbit, nasopharynx, temporal bone, and pharynx. Only 3% occur in the larynx. Approximately 30 cases have been reported in the literature.[30] Sutow and colleagues reported 1 laryngeal case in 57 patients from the Intergroup Rhabdomyosarcoma Study.[354] A slight male predilection (2:1) is reported. Rhabdomyosarcomas occur in the vocal folds, subglottis, and interarytenoid space. Rarely, they have been described in the pyriform fossa and aryepiglottic folds. Laryngeal tumors are usually of the embryonal botyroid type. Some tumors are pedicled, and pieces may be coughed up after choking episodes. Clinically, these lesions appear exophytic, but histologically they are invasive. Early hematogenous and lymphatic metastases are common to the cervical lymph nodes, lung, brain, and viscera. Treatment consists of chemotherapy, irradiation, and limited surgery. Late recurrences are not unusual.[355,356]

One study presented the long-term follow-up of five pediatric patients with laryngeal rhabdomyosarcoma; all patients were alive after a median time of 14.5 years. All but one received multimodality therapy including

conservative resection, often leaving positive margins, followed by chemotherapy and radiation. These investigators strongly advocate this conservative approach and do not believe there to be an indication for radical surgery.[357]

Leiomyosarcoma

About a dozen leiomyosarcomas have been reported in the larynx. Mainly found in older men, these lesions are mostly in the supraglottis. Vascular metastases can occur late in the course of the disease.[358]

Sarcomas

Clinical Appearance

Sarcomas may be sessile or pedunculated and are generally covered with mucosa. They show no area of ulceration and frequently occur in subglottic regions.

Synovial Sarcoma

These are rare laryngeal tumors; approximately 50 have been reported in the hypopharynx and larynx.[359] They can occur at any age, but most commonly in the 20- to 30-year age group. Most such tumors arise in the prevertebral fascia and extend to the hypopharynx in the pyriform fossae or posterior hypopharyngeal wall. Origins have also been reported in the hyoid and preepiglottic space. Other locations include the aryepiglottic fold, false vocal folds, medial pyriform wall, and interarytenoid space. These tumors have initially vague symptoms until they enlarge enough to cause obstruction, dysphagia, dysphonia, and dyspnea. They can be nodular or pedicled and are covered by shiny, smooth mucosa. The prognosis is better than that for lesions of the extremities. Early metastases to the lung are common, and late recurrences have been reported. Aggressive surgery is the treatment of choice.[360–362]

Fibrosarcoma

This is the most common sarcoma of the larynx. Citelli first described this lesion in 1912. Over 70 cases of laryngeal sarcoma are reported in the literature.[363] These tumors are found most commonly in men (4:1 ratio) in the fifth to seventh decades of life. They often arise in the anterior vocal fold region. They grow large and become exophytic, and occasionally they are pedunculated. They are gray or red and are covered with mucosa. Symptoms are nonspecific, but hoarseness and positional dyspnea are common. Metastases, when they occur, are hematogenous. Most lesions are well differentiated and relatively slow growing. The overall cure rate is approximately 70%.[364]

Fibrous Histiocytoma

These tumors have been described in the larynx. They usually arise deeply within the larynx, that is, in fascia or muscles. They usually present as exophytic poly-

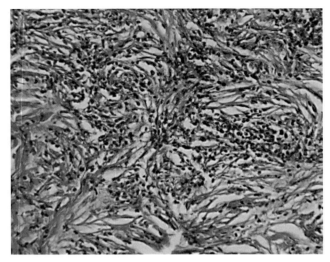

Fig. 32–42. Malignant fibrous histiocytoma. ×350, hematoxylin and eosin stain.

poid, mucosally covered tumors. Metastases occur frequently. The tumors metastasize by both lymphatic and hematogenous routes. The main symptoms are obstructive and are determined by the tumor location. The main therapeutic approach is surgical. Little experience is reported with radiation and chemotherapy (Figs. 32–41 and 32–42).[365–367]

Liposarcoma

These tumors occur exclusively in men and originate in the supraglottis or pyriform fossa. They may be exophytic or infiltrative. Their behavior is determined by the differentiation of the tumor. Recurrence rates are high, and these tumors may recur even 15 years after therapy. If metastases occur, it is early in the course of the disease, and they are hematogenous to the liver and lungs. Multicentric tumors have been reported. Primary therapy is surgical.[368–371]

Chondrosarcoma

Approximately 300 chondrosarcomas or chondromas have been reported in the larynx. In 1 series, 2 chondromas and 31 chondrosarcomas arising in the larynx were reported.[372] These are low-grade malignant tumors, about 80% of which arise in men in the rostrum of the cricoid cartilage, whereas 15% arise from the thyroid cartilage. The remainder arise from the arytenoid cartilage and epiglottis.[372,373] These tumors are round and firm and are covered by a violaceous mucosa. The most common symptoms are slowly increasing dyspnea and dysphagia. Hoarseness occurs late in the disease. Frequently, these tumors are diagnosed radiologically by a stippled appearance with dystrophic calcification. Approximately 15% of patients have distant metastases, although local recurrences are much more common. Partial resection conservation

surgery is often attempted first because of the low-grade malignancy of these lesions and the desire to preserve the patient's voice as long as possible.[374–376] Radiation and chemotherapy have not proved effective. With surgery, cure rates have been reported to approach 90%.[377]

Oat Cell Carcinoma

The small cell undifferentiated carcinomas are rare in the larynx, even though they comprise approximately 10 to 15% of lung tumors. Approximately 90 cases have been described in the literature.[378] The male-to-female ratio is 3:1, and the tumor is found more commonly in smokers. The most common location is in the subglottis.[379,380] The main symptoms are cough, hemoptysis, increasing dyspnea, and hoarseness. Vocal fold paralysis is present almost universally at the time of diagnosis. At the time of diagnosis, 66% of patients have neck metastases and 30% have distant metastases (liver, lung, bones, and brain).

These cells have been shown by electron microscopy to contain neurosecretory granules and are associated with paraneoplastic syndromes (presumably on a hormonal basis). One of the major paraneoplastic syndromes is hypercalcemia; others that can occur include Eaton-Lambert syndrome (pseuodomyasthenia) and Schwartz-Bartter syndrome (elevated antidiuretic hormone levels).

Extralaryngeal tumor spread is common, especially to the thyroid gland. In three reported cases, the tumor occurred after radiation therapy or ^{131}I therapy for thyroid disease.[381] The best approach today is triple therapy, that is, induction chemotherapy, surgery (usually total laryngectomy and bilateral neck dissection), and postoperative irradiation.[382,383] The overall cure rate is less than 10%.

Hematologic Malignant Disease

Approximately 1 to 3% of all thyroid carcinomas invade the larynx or upper trachea.[384–386] Lymphoreticular tumors often arise in the head and neck region. Approximately 30% present as primary tumors of the head and neck, but they are rare in the larynx. About 60 cases of non-Hodgkins lymphoma in the larynx have been described. Mostly, they manifest as infiltration of the false vocal folds and aryepiglottic folds, with submucous infiltration or nodule formation,[387,388] and with symptoms of dyspnea and stridor.[389,390] The origin of these tumors is said to be the lymphoid follicles in the vestibular fold.

Leukemic infiltrates usually invade the spaces of the thyroid cartilage or laryngeal skeleton, with rare submucosal infiltration.

Biot, in 1907, first described extramedullary plasmacytoma of the larynx. About 70 cases have been reported. Most arise in the supraglottis of men in the fourth to seventh decades of life.[391,392] They may be infiltrative or pedunculated and are yellowish, with a mucosal covering. Biopsy is usually followed by brisk bleeding. About 20% of patients with solitary extramedullary plasmacytoma have cervical lymph node extensions or metastases,[393] and about the same percentage eventually develop generalized multiple myeloma, with a latency period as long as 10 to 20 years. Treatment is generally by irradiation for solitary disease, combined with chemotherapy for generalized disease.

Metastases to the Larynx

Metastases to the larynx are rare. Ehrlich noted at autopsy that 8% of patients with malignant disease had laryngeal metastasis, although only 50 cases of metastasis to the larynx have been reported. The most frequent are clear cell renal carcinoma and melanoma. Less common metastases arise from the breast and bronchi; slightly less common are prostatic and gastrointestinal adenocarcinomas. Most metastases are hematogenous, by way of the prevertebral venous plexus to the marrow spaces of the larynx or soft tissue of the supraglottis. Melanomas tend to metastasize to soft tissues, usually early in the disseminated course of the disease. Hypernephromas usually metastasize to the supraglottis (i.e., epiglottis, aryepiglottic folds, and false vocal folds). They are extremely vascular and may produce hemoptysis. Bronchogenic carcinomas and breast carcinomas metastasize mainly to the marrow spaces of ossified cartilage.[394]

SUGGESTED READINGS

1. Pearse AGE: The APUD cell concept and its implications in pathology. Pathol Annu 9:27, 1974.
2. Pesce C, et al: APUD cells of the larynx. Acta Otolaryngol Suppl 98:118, 1984.
3. Moisa II: Neuroendocrine tumors of the larynx. Head Neck Surg 13:498, 1991.
4. Van Vroonhoven J, et al: Presurgical devascularization of a laryngeal paraganglioma. Arch Otolaryngol Head Neck Surg 108:600, 1982.
5. Andrews AH: Glomus tumors of the larynx: case report. Ann Otol Rhinol Laryngol 66:1034, 1955.
6. Blanchard CL and Saunders WH: Chemodectoma of the larynx: case report. Arch Otolaryngol Head Neck Surg 61:472, 1955.
7. Marks PV and Brookes GB: Malignant paragangliomas of the larynx. J Laryngol Otol 97:1183, 1983.
8. Ali S, et al: Pain-inducing laryngeal paragangliomas. J Laryngol Otol 97:181, 1983.
9. Suchanek E: Neurinoma des Kehlkopfeinganges. Mischr Ohreheilk 59:613, 1925.
10. Cummings C, Montgomery WW, and Bologh K: Neurogenic tumors of the larynx. Ann Otol Rhinol Laryngol 78:76, 1969.
11. Delozier HG: Intrinsic malignant schwannoma of the larynx: a case report. Ann Otol Rhinol Laryngol 91:336, 1982.
12. Colledge L: Two tumours of the peripheral nerves. J Laryngol Otol 45:409, 1930.
13. Maisel R and Ogura JH: Neurofibromatosis with laryngeal involvement. Laryngoscope 89:132, 1974.
14. Jafek BW and Stein FH: Neurofibroma of the larynx occurring with von Recklinghausen's disease. Arch Otolaryngol Head Neck Surg 98:77, 1973.
15. Abrikosoff AJ: Uber Myome Ausgeheit von der quergenstreeften willkurtichen Juskulatur. Virchows Arch (A) 260:215, 1926.
16. Garancis JC, et al: Granular cell myoblastoma. Cancer 25:342, 1970.
17. Sobel JH, et al: Granular cell myoblastoma: an EM and cytochemical study illustrating the genesis and aging of myoblastoma cells. Am J Pathol 65:59, 1971.
18. Ivatury R, et al: Granular cell tumor of the larynx and bronchus. Ann Thorac Surg 33:69, 1982.
19. Weisman RA, et al: Granular cell myoblastoma involving the recurrent laryngeal nerve. Arch Otolaryngol Head Neck Surg 106:294, 1980.
20. Garud O, et al: Granular cell tumor of the larynx in a 5 year old child. Arch Otolaryngol Head Neck Surg 94:45, 1984.
21. Phillips JH and Ruh HO: Angioma of the larynx, especially its relationship to chronic laryngitis. Am J Dis Child 5:123, 1913.
22. Sweetser TH: Hemangioma of the larynx. Laryngoscope 31:797, 1921.
23. Mizono G and Dedo H: Subglottic hemangioma in infants: treatment with CO_2 laser. Laryngoscope 94:638, 1989.
24. Hawkins DB, et al: Corticosteroid management of airway hemangiomas: long-term followup. Laryngoscope 94:633, 1984.
25. Jokinen K, et al: Cryocauterization in the treatment of subglottic hemangioma in infants. Laryngoscope 91:78, 1984.
26. Jaffe BF: Unusual laryngeal problems in children. Ann Otol Rhinol Laryngol 82:637, 1973.
27. Myer CM and Breitcher GO: Laryngeal cystic hygroma. Head Neck Surg 6:706, 1983.
28. Ruben RI, et al: Cystic lymphangioma of the vallecula. J Otolaryngol 4:180, 1975.
29. Pesavento G and Ferlito A: Hemangiopericytoma of the larynx: a chemico-pathological study with review of the literature. Laryngoscope 96:1065, 1982.
30. Kleinsasser O and Glanz H: Myogenic tumors of the larynx. Arch Otolaryngol Head Neck Surg 225:207, 1979.
31. Nuutinen J, et al: Angioleiomyoma of the larynx: report of a case and review of the literature. Laryngoscope 93:961, 1983.
32. Shibater K, et al: Laryngeal angiomyoma (vascular leiomyoma): clinicopathologic findings. Laryngoscope 90:1880, 1980.
33. Spector JG, et al: Squamous cell carcinoma of the pyriform sinus: a nonrandomized comparison of therapeutic modalities and long term results. Laryngoscope (in press).
34. Brockmuehl F: Die Behandlung und Prognose des Kehlkopfkrebes in der DDR von 1956–1966 und epidemiologisch Gesichtspunken. Berlin, Habel, 1977.
35. Ringertz N: Cancer incidence in Finland, Norway, Iceland, and Sweden. Acta Pathol Microbiol Scand Suppl 224:1, 1971.
36. DeRienzo DP, et al: Carcinoma of the larynx. Arch Otolaryngol Head Neck Surg 117:681, 1991.
37. Wynder EL, et al: Environmental factors in cancer of the larynx: a second look. Cancer 38:1591, 1976.
38. Tuyns AJ: Aetiology of head and neck cancer: tobacco, alcohol and diet. Bearing of basic research on clinical otolaryngology. Adv Otorhinolaryngol 46:98, 1991.
39. Jackson CE and Jackson CL: Cancer of the larynx: its increasing incidence. Arch Otolaryngol Head Neck Surg 67:45, 1941.
40. Kenneway EL and Kenneway WM: Further study of the incidence of cancer of the lung and larynx. Br J Cancer 1:260, 1947.
41. Terracini B, et al: Descriptive epidemiology of cancer of the larynx in the province of Torino, Italy. Tumori 64:448, 1978.
42. Barclay THC and Rao NN: The incidence and mortality rates

for laryngeal cancer from total cancer registries. Laryngoscope *85*:254, 1975.

43. Martensson B: Epidemiological aspects of laryngeal carcinoma in Scandinavia. Laryngoscope *85*:1185, 1975.

44. Destefani E, et al: Laryngeal cancer in Uruguay 1958–1981: an epidemiologic study. Cancer *55*:214, 1988.

45. Cutler SJ and Young JL: Demographic patterns of cancer: incidence in the U.S. In: Persons at High Risk For Cancer. Edited by Franmerri JE. New York, Academic Press, 1975.

46. Krajina Z, et al: Epidemiology of laryngeal cancer. Laryngoscope *85*:1155, 1975.

47. Mancuso TF, et al: Relation of place of birth and migration in cancer mortality in the U.S.: a study of Ohio residents 1959–1967. J Chronic Dis *27*:459, 1954.

48. Staszewski J: Cancer of the upper alimentary tract and larynx in Poland and Polish-born Americans. Br J Cancer *29*:389, 1974.

49. Atkinson L: Some features of the epidemiology of cancer of the larynx in Australia and Papua New Guinea. Laryngoscope *85*:1173, 1975.

50. Iwamoto H: An epidemiologic study of laryngeal cancer in Japan. Laryngoscope *85*:1162, 1975.

51. VICC Cancer Incidence in Five Continents: A Technical Report. Berlin, Springer, 1966.

52. Doll R: The epidemiology of cancer. Cancer *5*:2475, 1980.

53. Simarak S, et al: Cancer of the oral cavity, pharynx/larynx, and lung in North Thailand: a case control study and analysis of agar smoke. Br J Cancer *36*:130, 1977.

54. Martin G: Multiple maligne tumoren bei patienten mit Larynxkarzinomen. Laryng Rhinol Otol *58*:756, 1979.

55. Wagenfeld DJ, et al: Second primary respiratory tract malignancies in glottic carcinoma. Cancer *46*:1883, 1980.

56. Wagenfeld DJ: Second primary respiratory tract malignant neoplasms in supraglottic carcinoma. Arch Otolaryngol Head Neck Surg *107*:135, 1981.

57. Boysen M and Loven JO: Second malignant neoplasms in patients with head and neck squamous cell carcinomas. Acta Oncol *32*:238, 1993.

58. Vratec DP: Multiple primary malignancies associated with index cancers of the oral, pharyngeal, and laryngeal areas. Trans PA Acad Ophthalmol Otolaryngol *32*:177, 1979.

59. Moore C: Cigarette smoking and cancer of the mouth, pharynx, and larynx: a continuing study. JAMA *218*:553, 1971.

60. Savary M, et al: Multiple primary malignancies: bearing of basic research on clinical otolaryngology. Adv Otorhinolaryngol *46*:165, 1991.

61. Engelen AM, et al: Yearly chest radiography in the early detection of lung cancer following laryngeal cancer. Eur Arch Otorhinolaryngol *249*:364, 1992.

62. US Dept Health, Education, and Welfare: Smoking and Health. Washington, DC, 1964.

63. Smoking and health now. R Soc Health J *90*:40, 1970.

64. World Health Organization (WHO): Smoking and Its Effects on Health. WHO technical report, series no. 568. WHO, Geneva, 1975.

65. Breslow NE and Eustrom JE: Geographic correlations between cancer mortality rates and alcohol-tobacco consumption in the US. J Natl Cancer Inst *53*:631, 1974.

66. Wynder EL and Stillman SD: Comparative epidemiology of tobacco related cancers. Cancer Res *37*:4608, 1977.

67. Wynder EL and Stillman SD: Impact of long term filter cigarette usage on lung and larynx cancer risk: a case control study. J Natl Cancer Inst *62*:471, 1979.

68. Kalin HA: The Dorn Study of Smoking and Mortality among U.S. Veterans. National Oral Cancer Institute Monographs 19, 1966.

69. Boyle P, et al: Recent advances in epidemiology of head and neck cancer. Curr Opin Oncol *4*:471, 1992.

70. Wynder EL, et al: Environmental factors in cancer of the larynx: a second look. Cancer *38*:1591, 1976.

71. Blot, WJ: Alcohol and cancer. Cancer Res *52(suppl)*:2119s, 1992.

72. Stevens J: Synergistic effect of alcohol on epidermoid carcinogenesis in the larynx. Otolaryngol Head Neck Surg *87*:751, 1979.

73. Rothman KJ: The proportion of cancer attributable to alcohol consumption. Prev Med *9*:174, 1980.

74. Auerbach O, et al: Histologic changes in the larynx in relation to smoking habits. Cancer *25*:92, 1970.

75. Hamburger F, et al: Carcinoma of the larynx in hamsters exposed to cigarette smoke. Animal model: susceptible inbred line of Syrian hamsters. Am J Pathol *95*:845, 1979.

76. Trell E, et al: Aryl hydrocarbon hydroxylase inducibility and laryngeal cancer. Lancet *2*:140, 1976.

77. Loury MC, Johns ME, and Danes BS: In vitro hyperdiploidy in head and neck cancer: a genetic predisposition? Arch Otolaryngol Head Neck Surg *113*:1230, 1987.

78. Loning T, et al: HPV DNA detection in tumours of the head and neck: a comparative light microscopy and DNA hybridization study. ORL J Otorhinolaryngol Relat Spec *49*:259, 1987.

79. Kashima H, et al: Demonstration of human papilloma virus capsid antigen in carcinoma *in situ* of the larynx. Ann Otol Rhinol Laryngol *95*:603, 1986.

80. Brandwein MS, et al: Analysis of prevalence of human papilloma virus in laryngeal carcinomas. Ann Otol Rhinol Laryngol *102*:309, 1993.

81. Schantz SP: Carcinogenesis, markers, staging, and prognosis of head and neck cancer. Curr Opin Oncol *5*:483, 1993.

82. Carter RL: Pathology of squamous carcinomas of the head and neck. Curr Opin Oncol *5*:491, 1993.

83. Marschick H: Sekundare Laryngocoele bei carcinoma laryngis. Abl Has Nas U Ohrenheilk *10*:104, 1927.

84. Micheau C, et al: The relationship between laryngocoeles and laryngeal carcinomas. Laryngoscope *88*:680, 1978.

85. Pietrantoni L, et al: Laryngocoele and laryngeal cancer. Ann Otol Rhinol Laryngol *68*:100, 1959.

86. Dolcetti R, et al: p53 over-expression is an early event in the development of human squamous-cell carcinoma of the larynx: genetic and prognostic implications. Int J Cancer *52*:178, 1992.

87. Truelson JM, et al: DNA content and histologic growth pattern correlate with prognosis in patients with advanced squamous cell carcinoma of the larynx. Cancer *70*:56, 1992.

88. Gandour-Edwards RF, et al: DNA content of head and neck squamous carcinoma by flow and image cytometry. Arch Otolaryngol Head Neck Surg *120*:294, 1994.

89. Celin SE, et al: The association of laryngoceles with squamous cell carcinoma of the larynx. Laryngoscope *101*:529, 1991.

90. Nakayama M, et al: Sulcus vocalis in laryngeal cancer: a histopathologic study. Laryngoscope *104*:16, 1994.

91. von Eicken C and Soerusen: Larynxcarcinomen nach alter Rontgenschadigung. Abl Has Nas U Ohrenheilk *21*:71, 1934.

92. Peller S: Lung cancer among mine workers in Joachimsthal. Hum Biol *11*:130, 1939.

93. King ER, et al: Carcinoma of larynx occurring in a patient receiving therapeutic doses of I[131]. Arch Otolaryngol Head Neck Surg *59*:333, 1954.

94. Aaronsen JP and Olofsson J: Irradiation-induced tumours of the head and neck. Acta Otolaryngol Suppl (Stockh) *360*:178, 1979.

95. Lawson S and Som M: Second primary cancer after irradiation of laryngeal cancer. Ann Otol Rhinol Laryngol *84*:771, 1975.

96. Richards SH, et al: Postcricoid carcinoma and the Patterson-Kelly syndrome. J Laryngol Otol *85*:141, 1971.

97. Larsson LG, et al: Relationship of Plummer-Vinson disease to cancer of the upper alimentary tract in Sweden. Cancer Res *35*:3308, 1975.

98. Wynder EL, et al: Environmental factors in cancer of the upper alimentary tract: a Swedish study with special reference to

Plummer-Vinson (Patterson-Kelly) syndrome. Cancer *10:*470, 1957.

99. Chisholm M: The association between webs, iron and post cricoid carcinoma. Postgrad Med *50:*215, 1974.

100. Flanders WD and Rothman KJ: Occupational risk for laryngeal cancer. Am J Public Health *72:*369, 1982.

101. Klayman MB: Exposure to insecticides. Arch Otolaryngol Head Neck Surg *88:*116, 1968.

102. Manning KP, et al: Cancer of the larynx and other occupational hazards of mustard gas workers. Clin Otolaryngol *6:*165, 1981.

103. Moss E: Oral and pharyngeal cancer in textile workers. Ann NY Acad Sci *271:*301, 1976.

104. Stall PM and McGill T: Exposure to asbestos and laryngeal carcinoma. J Laryngol Otol *89:*513, 1971.

105. Liddell FDK: Laryngeal cancer and asbestos. Br J Ind Med *47:*289, 1990.

106. Parnes SM: Asbestos and cancer of the larynx: is there a relationship? Laryngoscope *100:*254, 1990.

107. Roels H: Histopathology of laryngeal tumours. Acta Otorhinolaryngol Belg *46:*127, 1992.

108. Lubsen H and Olde Kalter PHMT: Premalignant laryngeal lesions. Acta Otorhinolaryngol Belg *46:*117, 1992.

109. Schwarz R, et al: Fine needle cytology in the evaluation of head and neck masses. Am J Surg *159:*482, 1990.

110. Abram AC, et al: Fine needle aspiration (FNA) in diagnosing recurrent squamous cell carcinoma of the head and neck: truth or consequences? Laryngoscope *103:*1073, 1993.

111. Bremerich A and Stool W: Die Rehabilitation nach Laryngectomme ans der Sicht der Betroffenen. HNO *33:*220, 1985.

112. Higginson J: Patient delay in reference to stage of cancer. Cancer *15:*50, 1962.

113. Parker JT and Hill JH: Panendoscopy in screening for synchronous primary malignancies. Laryngoscope *98:*147, 1988.

114. Shaha A, et al: Is routine triple endoscopy cost-effective in head and neck cancer? Am J Surg *155:*750, 1988.

115. el-Gazzar AH, et al: Experience with thallium-201 imaging in head and neck cancer. Clin Nucl Med *13:*286, 1988.

116. Watkinson JC, et al: An evaluation of the uptake of technetium-99m (v) dimercaptosuccinic acid in patients with squamous carcinoma of the head and neck. Clin Otolaryngol *12:*405, 1987.

117. Soo KC, et al: Radioimmunoscintigraphy of squamous carcinomas of the head and neck. Head Neck Surg *9:*349, 1987.

118. Westhofen M: Ultrasound B-scans in the follow-up of head and neck tumors. Head Neck Surg *9:*272, 1987.

119. van den Brekel MWM, et al: Lymph node staging in patients with clinically negative neck examinations by ultrasound and ultrasound-guided aspiration cytology. Am J Surg *162:*362, 1991.

120. Vinzenz K, et al: Diagnosis of head and neck carcinomas by means of immunological tumour markers (Beta-2-microglobulin, immunoglobulin E, ferritin, N-acetyl-neuraminic acid, phosphohexose isomerase). J Craniomaxillofac Surg *15:*270, 1987.

121. Piccirillo JF, et al: New clinical severity staging system for cancer of the larynx. Ann Otol Rhinol Laryngol *103:*83, 1994.

122. Rajah V, et al: Histoplasmosis of the oral cavity, oropharynx, and larynx. J Laryngol Otol *107:*58, 1993.

123. Ramadan H, et al: Laryngeal tuberculosis: presentation of 16 cases and a review of the literature. Otolaryngology *22:*39, 1993.

124. Hautant A: Ma technique de l'hemilaryngectomie, ses resultats. Otorhinolaryngol Int *5:*217, 1930.

125. Neel HB, et al: Laryngofissure and cordectomy for early cordal carcinoma: outcome in 182 patients. Otolaryngol Head Neck Surg *88:*79, 1980.

126. Alonso JM: Conservative surgery of cancer of the larynx. Trans Am Acad Ophthalmol Otolaryngol *51:*633, 1947.

127. Dedo HH: Supraglottic laryngectomy: indications and techniques. Laryngoscope *78:*1183, 1968.

128. Tsuji H, et al: Head and neck reconstruction with microvascular tissue transfer and its surgical indication: our experience. Acta Otolaryngol Suppl *500:*131, 1993.

129. Shindo ML and Sulivan MJ: Soft-tissue microvascular free flaps. Otolaryngol Clin North Am *27:*173, 1994.

130. Lyndiatt WM, et al: Microvascular reconstruction of the head and neck cancer patient. Nebraska Med J *78:*375, 1993.

131. Haughey BH, et al: Vibratory segment function after free flap reconstruction of the pharyngoesophagus. Laryngoscope *105:*487, 1995.

132. Mladick RA, et al: Cricopharyngeal myotomy: application and technique in major oropharyngeal resection. Arch Surg *102:*1, 1971.

133. Wilkins SA: Indications for section of the cricopharyngeus muscle. Am J Surg *108:*533, 1964.

134. Berlin BP, et al: Manometric studies of the upper esophageal sphincter. Ann Otol Rhinol Laryngol *86:*598, 1977.

135. Lauerman S, et al: Cricopharyngeal myotomy in SSL: an experimental study. Laryngoscope *82:*447, 1972.

136. Litton WB and Leonard JR: Aspiration after partial laryngectomy: a cineradiographic study. Laryngoscope *79:*887, 1969.

137. Patterson N: A plea for the window resection instead in dealing with certain laryngeal carcinomas. J Laryngol *47:*81, 1932.

138. Norris CM: Technique of extended frontolateral partial laryngectomy. Laryngoscope *68:*1240, 1958.

139. Moser F: Horizontal resection of the larynx in limited indication of Oeser stage II. Arch Ohrenheilk *178:*275, 1961.

140. Pleet L, et al: Partial laryngectomy with imbrication and reconstruction. Trans Am Acad Ophthalmol Otolaryngol *84:*882, 1977.

141. Calearo CV and Teatini GP: Horizontal glottectomy. Laryngoscope *88:*1529, 1978.

142. Majer EH and Reeder W: Modification of laryngectomy and preservation of the air passage. Arch Ohrenheilk *173:*442, 1958.

143. Labayle J: Laryngectomy with reconstitution of the larynx: methods and results. Probl Actuels Otorhinolaryngol 185, 1973.

144. Hofmann Saquez R: A new technique for subtotal laryngectomy and reconstruction. J Fr Otorhinolaryngol *57:*666, 1950.

145. Foderl O: Zur Technik der Larynxextirpation. Arch Klinik Chir *58:*803, 1899.

146. Serafin I: Restoration of laryngeal function after laryngectomy. Adv Otorhinolaryngol *16:*95, 1969.

146a. Staffieri A and Valearo C: Peristomal recurrences. Acta Otorhinolaryngol Ital *10(suppl 30P):*95, 1990.

147. Sisson G, et al: Total laryngectomy and reconstruction of a pseudoglottis:problem and complication. Laryngoscope *88:*639, 1987.

148. Mozolewski ES, et al: Arytenoid vocal shunt in laryngectomized patients. Laryngoscope *85:*853, 1975.

149. Weisberger EC and Lingeman RE: Modified supraglottic laryngectomy and resection of lesions of the base of the tongue. Laryngoscope *93:*20 1983.

150. Pearson BW: Subtotal laryngectomy. Laryngoscope *91:*1904, 1981.

151. Meyer EH and Reeder W: Concerning the modification of laryngectomy and management of the airway. Arch Ohrenheilk *173:*442, 1958.

152. Piquet JJ, et al: Reconstruction surgery of the larynx. Fr Otorhinolaryngol *31:*589, 1982.

153. Reed G and Raluzzi DD: Neck dissection. Otolaryngol Clin North Am *2:*547, 1969.

154. Staley CJ and Herzon FS: Elective neck dissection in carcinoma of the larynx. Otolaryngol Clin North Am *3:*543, 1970.

155. Suarez O: El problema de las metastasis linfaticas y alejadas del cáncer de larynge e hypofaringe. Rev Otorhinolaryngol Santiago *23:*83, 1963.

156. Bocca E and Pignataro O: A conservation technique in radical neck dissection. Ann Otol Rhinol Laryngol *76:*975, 1967.

157. Deutsch EG, et al: The conservation neck dissection. Laryngoscope 95:561, 1985.

158. Moliari B, et al: Retrospective comparison of conservative and radical neck dissection in laryngeal cancer. Ann Otol Rhinol Laryngol 89:578, 1980.

159. Weber RS, et al: Paratracheal lymph node dissection for carcinoma of the larynx, hypopharynx, and cervical esophagus. Otolaryngol Head Neck 108:11, 1993.

160. Papae RJ: Distant metastases from head and neck cancer. Cancer 53:342, 1984.

161. Alonso JM: Metastasis of laryngeal and hypopharyngeal carcinoma. Acta Otolaryngol (Stockh) 64:353, 1967.

162. Abramson A, et al: Distant metastasis from carcinoma of the larynx. Laryngoscope 81:1503, 1971.

163. Mummer CS and Chusid CA: Distant metastases from primary malignancies of the endolarynx. Laryngoscope 71:524, 1961.

164. O'Brien P, et al: Distant metastases in epidermoid carcinoma of the head and neck. Cancer 27:304, 1971.

165. Barton RP, et al: Cardiac metastases from primary carcinoma of the larynx. J Laryngol Otol 93:833, 1979.

166. Bonneau RA and Lehman RH: Stomal recurrences following laryngectomy. Arch Otolaryngol Head Neck Surg 101:408, 1975.

167. Lundgren J and Olofsson J: Pharyngocutaneous fistulae following total laryngectomy. Clin Otolaryngol 4:12, 1979.

168. Joseph D and Shumrick D: Risk of head and neck surgery in previously irradiated patients. Arch Otolaryngol Head Neck Surg 97:381, 1973.

169. Singer MI: Tracheoesophageal speech: vocal rehabilitation after total laryngectomy. Laryngoscope 93:1454, 1983.

170. Singer MI and Blum ED: Tracheoesophageal puncture: a surgical prosthetic method for postlaryngectomy speech restoration. In: Third International Symposium on Plastic and Reconstructive Surgery of the Head and Neck. New Orleans, 1979.

171. Singer MI and Blum ED: An endoscopic technique for restoration of voice after laryngectomy. Ann Otol Rhinol Laryngol 89:529, 1980.

172. Singer MI and Blum ED: A selective myotomy for voice restoration after total laryngectomy. Arch Otolaryngol Head Neck Surg 107:670, 1981.

172a. Singer MI, Blom ED, and Haymaker RC: Pharyngeal plexus neurectomy for alaryngeal speech rehabilitation. Laryngoscope 96:50, 1986.

173. Alajmo E: Conservation surgery of cancer of the larynx in the elderly. Laryngoscope 95:203, 1985.

174. Asai R: Laryngoplasty after total laryngectomy. Arch Otolaryngol Head Neck Surg 95:114, 1972.

175. Montgomery WW: Postlaryngectomy vocal rehabilitation after laryngectomy. Arch Otolaryngol Head Neck Surg 95:76, 1972.

176. Mitrani M and Krespi YP: Functional restoration after subtotal glossectomy and laryngectomy. Otolaryngol Head Neck Surg 98:5, 1988.

177. Field JK and Spandidos DA: Expression of oncogenes in human tumours with special reference to the head and neck region. J Oral Pathol Med 16:97, 1989.

178. Staple HH and Ogura J: Cineradiology of the swallowing mechanism following subtotal laryngectomy. Radiology 87:226, 1966.

179. Murray GM: Pulmonary complications following SSL. Clin Otolaryngol 1:241, 1976.

180. Leonard JR and Litton WB: Selection of patients for conservation surgery of the larynx. Laryngoscope 81:232, 1971.

181. Sirrale U, et al: The problem of advanced supraglottic carcinoma. Laryngoscope 85:1633, 1975.

182. Gottlieb JA, et al: Recent developments in chemotherapy for head and neck cancer. In: Neoplasia of Head and Neck. Chicago, Year Book, 1974.

183. Paredes J, et al: Prospective randomized trial of high-dose cisplatin and fluorouracil infusion with or without sodium di-ethyldithiocarbamate in recurrent and/or metastatic squamous cell carcinoma of the head and neck. J Clin Oncol 6:955, 1988.

184. Frustaci S, et al: Phase II study of esorubicin (4′-deoxydoxorubicin) in locally advanced or metastatic head and neck carcinoma. Invest New Drugs 5:307, 1987.

185. Clerico M, et al: Phase II trial of VP16-213 in squamous cell carcinoma of the head and neck. Eur J Cancer Clin Oncol 23:577, 1987.

186. Wustrow TP, et al: Multiparametric flow cytometry of human squamous cell carcinoma lines from the head and neck. Otolaryngol Head Neck Surg 98:552, 1988.

187. Vokes EE, et al: Favorable long-term survival following induction chemotherapy with cisplatin, fluorouracil and leucovorin and concomitant chemoradiotherapy for locally advanced head and neck cancer. J Natl Cancer Inst 84:877, 1992.

188. Hamasaki VK and Vokes EE: Chemotherapy in head and neck cancer. Curr Opin Oncol 4:504, 1992.

189. Hamasaki VK and Vokes EE: Chemotherapy and combined modality therapy in head and neck cancer. Curr Opin Oncol 5:508, 1993.

190. Lippman SM, et al: Treatment of advanced squamous cell carcinoma of the head and neck with isotretinoin: a phase II randomized trial. Invest New Drugs 6:51, 1988.

191. Somers KD, et al: Growth of head and neck squamous cell carcinoma in nude mice: potentiation of laryngeal carcinoma by 17 beta estradiol. J Natl Cancer Inst 80:688, 1988.

192. Mattox DE, et al: Androgen receptors and antiandrogen therapy for laryngeal carcinoma. Arch Otolaryngol, 110:721, 1984.

193. Urba SG, et al: Tamoxifen therapy in patients with recurrent laryngeal squamous carcinoma. Laryngoscope 100:76, 1990.

194. Scott R, et al: Hyperthermia in combination with definitive radiation therapy: results of a phase I/II RTOG Study. Int J Radiat Oncol Biol Phys 15:711, 1988.

195. Herman TS, et al: Effect of hyperthermia on cis-diamminedichloroplatinum (II) (rhodamine 123)2[tetrachloroplatinum(II)] in a human squamous cell carcinoma line and a cis-diamminedichloroplatinum (II) resistant subline. Cancer Res 48:5101, 1988.

196. Keller GS, et al: Photodynamic therapy in otolaryngology—head and neck surgery. Arch Otolaryngol 111:758, 1985.

197. Mady MA, et al: Concerning cellular defense in carcinoma of the larynx. Arch Immunol Ther Exp (Warsz) 24:69, 1976.

198. Bennet SH, et al: Prognostic significance of host response on cancer of the larynx or hypopharynx. Cancer 28:1255, 1971.

199. Zoller M, et al: Guidelines for prognosis in head and neck cancer with nodal metastases. Laryngoscope 88:135, 1978.

200. Santoris A, et al: Natural killer mediated cytotoxicity in patients with laryngeal carcinoma. Ann Otol Rhinol Laryngol 93:109, 1984.

201. Brunetti F, et al: Prospects and limitations of systematic monitoring in patient with laryngeal cancer. Acta Otolaryngol (Stockh) 87:393, 1979.

202. McGavran M, et al: The incidence of cervical lymph node metastasis from epidermoid carcinoma of the larynx. Cancer 14:55, 1961.

203. Gilmore BR, et al: Carcinoma of the larynx: lymph node reaction patterns. Laryngoscope 88:1333, 1978.

204. Berlinger NT, et al: Prognostic significance of lymph node histology in patients with squamous cell carcinoma of the larynx. Laryngoscope 86:792, 1976.

205. Mickel RA, et al: Natural killer cell cytotoxicity in the peripheral blood, cervical lymph nodes, and tumor of head and neck cancer patients. Cancer Res 48:5017, 1988.

206. Katz AE: Immunologic staging of patients with carcinoma of the head and neck. Laryngoscope 93:445, 1983.

207. Makimoto KA, et al: Observations on immunologic parameters in laryngeal cancer patients. Arch Otolaryngol Head Neck Surg 238:241, 1983.

208. Tewfik H, et al: DiGeorge syndrome associated with multiple squamous cell carcinoma. Arch Otolaryngol Head Neck Surg *103*:105, 1977.

209. Jacobson P and Wahren JS: Elevated plasma CEA during radiotherapy for glottic carcinomas of the larynx. Can J Otol *4*:46, 1975.

210. Turpley J, et al: Prolonged depression of cellular immunity in cured laryngopharyngeal cancer patients treated with irradiation therapy. Cancer *35*:638, 1975.

211. Rafta S, et al: Changes in cell-mediated immunity in patients undergoing radiotherapy. Cancer *41*:1076, 1978.

212. Veltri RW, et al: Immune monitoring protocol for patients with carcinoma of the head and neck: preliminary results. Ann Otol Rhinol Laryngol *87*:692, 1978.

213. Berlinger JT: Deficient immunity in head and neck cancer due to excessive monocyte production of prostaglandins. Laryngoscope *94*:1407, 1984.

214. Boscia R, et al: Evaluation of therapeutic potential of interleukin 2 expanded tumor-infiltrating lymphocytes in squamous cell carcinoma of the head and neck. Ann Otol Rhinol Laryngol *97*: 414, 1988.

215. Schantz SP, et al: The relationship of circulating IgA to cellular immunity in head and neck cancer patients. Laryngoscope *98*: 671, 1988.

216. Hirsch R, et al: Immunostimulation of patients with head and neck cancer: in vitro and preliminary clinical results. Arch Otolaryngol Head Neck Surg *109*:298, 1983.

217. Carr BI: Cancer in Bangladesh: a model for some problems and proposed solutions in the Third World. Cancer Detect Prev *9*: 195, 1986.

218. Soto Ortega I, et al: Lymph node response and its relationship to prognosis in carcinomas of the head and neck. Clin Otolaryngol *12*:241, 1987.

219. Biller HF, et al: Delayed contralateral cervical metastases with laryngeal and laryngopharyngeal cancer. Laryngoscope *81*: 1499, 1971.

220. Patel P and Snow GB: Metastases of carcinoma of the larynx. Acta Otorhinolaryngol Belg *46*:141, 1992.

221. Breiting E, et al: Spread and mode of metastases of supraglottic laryngeal carcinoma. ORL J Otolaryngol Relat Spec *41*:288, 1979.

222. Cummings CW: Incidence of nodal metastases in T2 supraglottic carcinoma. Arch Otolaryngol Head Neck Surg *99*:268, 1974.

223. Bauer WC, Edwards DL, and McGavran MH: A critical analysis of laryngectomy in the treatment of epidermoid carcinoma of the larynx. Cancer *15*:263, 1962.

224. Kirshner J: Pyriform sinus cancer: a clinical and laboratory study. Ann Otolaryngol Rhinol Laryngol *184*:793, 1975.

225. Harrison DFN: Pathology of hypopharyngeal cancer in relation to surgical management. J Laryngol Otol *89*:367, 1970.

226. Esteban F, et al: Risk factors involved in stomal recurrence following laryngectomy. J Laryngol Otol *107*:527, 1993.

227. Brennan JA, et al: The intraoperative management of the thyroid gland during laryngectomy. Laryngoscope *101*:929, 1991.

228. Schantz SP, et al: Evidence for the role of natural immunity in the control of metastatic spread of head and neck cancer. Cancer Immunol Immunother *25*:141, 1987.

229. Wolf GT, et al: Alterations in T-lymphocyte subpopulations in patients with head and neck cancer: correlations with prognosis. Arch Otolaryngol Head Neck Surg *113*:1200, 1987.

230. Myssiorek D: The role of surgery in early stage glottic carcinoma. Cancer Invest *10*:391, 1992.

231. Ton-Van J, et al: Comparison of surgery and radiotherapy in T1 and T2 glottic carcinomas. Am J Surg *162*:337, 1991.

232. Murty GE, et al: Carcinoma in situ of the glottis: radiotherapy or excision biopsy? Ann Otol Rhinol Laryngol *102*:592, 1993.

233. Mendenhall WM, et al: T1-T2 vocal fold carcinoma: a basis for comparing the results of radiotherapy and surgery. Otolaryngol Head Neck Surg *10*:373, 1988.

234. Thomas JV, et al: Early glottic carcinoma treated with open laryngeal procedures. Arch Otolaryngol Head Neck Surg *120*: 264, 1994.

235. Sung DI, et al: Primary radiotherapy for carcinoma in situ and early invasive carcinoma of the glottic larynx. Int J Radiat Oncol Biol Phys *5*:467, 1979.

236. Fein DA, et al: Carcinoma in situ of the glottic larynx: the role of radiotherapy. Int J Radiat Oncol Biol Phys *27*:379, 1993.

237. Rucci L, et al: Glottic cancer involving anterior commissure: surgery vs. radiotherapy. Head Neck *13*:403, 1991.

238. Neel HB, et al: Laryngofissure and cordectomy for early cordal carcinoma: outcome in 182 patients. Otolaryngol Head Neck Surg *88*:79, 1980.

239. Kirchner JA and Som ML: The anterior commissure technique of partial laryngectomy: clinical and laboratory observations. Laryngoscope *85*:1308, 1975.

240. Ogura JH, et al: Glottic cancer with extension to the arytenoid. Laryngoscope *85*:1825, 1975.

241. Usinski S, et al: Hemilaryngectomy for T3 (fixed cord) epidermoid carcinoma of the larynx. Laryngoscope *86*:1563, 1976.

242. Biller HF, et al: Hemilaryngectomy following radiation failure for carcinoma of the vocal folds. Laryngoscope *80*:249, 1970.

243. Iwamoto H: An epidemiological study of laryngeal cancer in Japan (1960–1969). Laryngoscope *85*:1162, 1975.

244. Sessions D, et al: Carcinoma of the subglottic area. Laryngoscope *85*:814, 1976.

245. Coates HL, et al: Carcinoma of the supraglottic larynx: a review of 221 cases. Arch Otolaryngol Head Neck Surg *102*:686, 1976.

246. Rowley JH, et al: Supraglottic carcinoma: a 10 year review at the University Hospital. Laryngoscope *82*:1264, 1972.

247. Poncet P: Total laryngectomy for salvage in cancers of the glottic region. Laryngoscope *81*:1430, 1975.

248. Horiot JC, et al: Analysis of failures in early vocal fold cancer. Radiology *103*:663, 1972.

249. Goepfert H, et al: Optimal treatment for the technically resectable squamous cell carcinoma of the supraglottic larynx. Laryngoscope *85*:14, 1975.

249a. Wang CC and O'Donnell AR: Cancer of the larynx: five year results with emphasis on radiotherapy. N Engl J Med *252*:743, 1955.

250. Stewart JG: The steepness of the dose response curve both for tumor cure and normal tissue injury. Laryngoscope *85*:1107, 1975.

251. Hibbs GG, Ying D, and Hendrickson FR: Radiotherapy for early stages of vocal fold cancer. Ann Otol Rhinol Laryngol *78*:319, 1969.

252. Boles R and Komorn R: Carcinoma of the laryngeal glottis, A five-year review at a university hospital. Laryngoscope *79*:909, 1969.

253. Lederman J and Dalley VM: The treatment of glottic cancer: the importance of radiotherapy to the patient. J Laryngol Otol *79*:767, 1965.

254. Chacko DC, et al: Definitive irradiation of T1-T4N0 larynx cancer. Cancer *51*:994, 1983.

255. Dickens WJ, et al: Treatment of early vocal fold carcinoma. Laryngoscope *93*:216, 1985.

256. Kondo M: Radiation therapy of early glottic carcinoma: a Japanese experience. Acta Radiol *21*:381, 1982.

257. Mittal B, et al: Role of radiation in the management of early vocal fold carcinoma. Int J Radiat Oncol Biol Phys *9*:997, 1983.

258. Jorgensen K, et al: Laryngeal carcinoma. I. Treatment results. Acta Med Scand Suppl *18*:282, 1979.

259. Vermund H: Role of radiotherapy in cancer of the larynx as related to TNM systems of staging. Annu Rev Cancer *25*:485, 1970.

260. Olofsson J: Vocal fold fixation in laryngeal carcinoma. Acta Otolaryngol (Stockh) *75*:496, 1973.

261. Zohar Y, et al: The controversial treatment of anterior commissure carcinoma of the larynx. Laryngoscope 102:69, 1992.

262. Harwood A, et al: Management of T3 glottic cancer. Arch Otolaryngol Head Neck Surg 106:637, 1980.

263. Kazem J and van den Broek P: Planned preoperative radiotherapy vs. definitive radiotherapy for advanced carcinoma. Laryngoscope 94:1355, 1984.

264. Kokal WA, et al: Postoperative radiation as adjuvant treatment for carcinoma of the oral cavity, larynx, and pharynx: preliminary report of a prospective randomized trial. J Surg Oncol 38: 71, 1988.

265. Davidson J, et al: The role of surgery following radiotherapy failure for advanced laryngopharyngeal cancer. Arch Otolaryngol Head Neck Surg 120:269, 1994.

266. Lavey RS and Calcaterra TC: Partial laryngectomy for glottic cancer after high-dose radiotherapy. Am J Surg 162:341, 1991.

267. Natvig K, et al: Fistulae following laryngectomy in patients treated with irradiation. J Laryngol Otol 107:1136, 1993.

268. Ogura JH, et al: Results of conservation surgery for cancers of the supraglottis and pyriform sinus. Laryngoscope 90:591, 1980.

269. Laccourrege H, et al: Carcinoma of the laryngeal margin. Head Neck Surg 5:500, 1983.

270. Bocca E, et al: Supraglottic laryngectomy: 30 years experience. Ann Otol Rhinol Laryngol 92:14, 1983.

271. Zigner J: Vertical subtotal laryngectomy. Laryngoscope 87:101, 1972.

272. Sessions D: Extended partial laryngectomy. Ann Otol Rhinol Laryngol 89:556, 1980.

273. Sekula J: The subtotal operation in the treatment of cancer of the larynx. Laryngoscope 77:1966, 1967.

274. Wang CC, Schulz MD, and Miller D: Combined radiation therapy for carcinoma of the supraglottis and pyriform sinus. Laryngoscope 82:1883, 1972.

275. Zhu SC: The results of 31 patients of supraglottic-vertical hemilaryngectomy. Aust NZ J Surg 58:213, 1988.

276. Levendag P and Vikram B: The problem of neck relapse in early stage supraglottic cancer: results of different treatment modalities for the clinically negative neck. Int J Radiat Oncol Biol Phys 13:1621, 1987.

277. Kramer S, et al: Combined radiation therapy and surgery in the management of advanced head and neck cancer: final report of study 73–03 of the Radiation Therapy Oncology Group. Head Neck Surg 10:19, 1987.

278. Mendenhall WM, et al: Squamous cell carcinoma of the supraglottic larynx treated with radical irradiation. J Radiol Oncol Biol Phys 10:2223, 1984.

279. Wang CC: Megavoltage radiation therapy for supraglottic carcinoma: results of treatment. Radiology 109:183, 1973.

280. Briant TD, et al: Carcinoma of the hypopharynx: a 5-year followup. J Otolaryngol 6:353, 1977.

281. Carpenter RJ, et al: Cancer of the hypopharynx: analysis of treatment and results in 162 patients. Arch Otolaryngol Head Neck Surg 102:717, 1976.

282. Razak MS, et al: Carcinoma of the hypopharynx: success and failure. Am J Surg 134:489, 1977.

283. Harrison DFN: Surgical management of hypopharyngeal cancer. Arch Otolaryngol Head Neck Surg 105:149, 1979.

284. Lam KH, et al: Surgical treatment of hypopharyngeal carcinoma: cervical esophagus. Ann Acad Med Singapore 9:317, 1980.

285. Stell PM: Esophageal replacement by transposed stomach. Arch Otolaryngol Head Neck Surg 91:166, 1970.

286. Johnson JT, et al: The extra-capsular spread of tumours in cervical node metastasis. Arch Otolaryngol Head Neck Surg 107: 725, 1981.

287. Snow GB, et al: Prognostic factors in neck node metastasis. Clin Otolaryngol 7:185, 1982.

288. Vikrach B, et al: Failure in the neck following multi-modality

289. Moliari R: Indicazioni limiti e resultati degli svuotamenti laterocervicali tradizional. Tumori 60:573, 1974.

290. Snyderman NL, et al: Extracapsular spread of carcinoma of the cervical lymph nodes. Cancer 56:1597, 1985.

291. Strong E: Preoperative radiation and radical neck dissection. Surg Clin North Am 49:271, 1989.

292. Goldman JL, et al: Serial microscopic studies of radical neck dissection: Studies in a combined radiation and surgery programme for advanced cancer of the larynx and laryngopharynx. Arch Otolaryngol Head Neck Surg 89:620, 1969.

293. Ogura J and Biller H: Elective neck dissection for pharyngeal and laryngeal cancers. Ann Otol Rhinol Laryngol 80:646, 1971.

294. Lindborg R and Jesse RH: Treatment of cervical lymph node metastasis from primary lesions of the oropharynx, supraglottic larynx, and hypopharynx. Am J Roentgenol 102:132, 1968.

295. Goffinet D, et al: Combined surgery and post-operative irradiation in the treatment of cervical lymph nodes. Arch Otolaryngol Head Neck Surg 110:736, 1984.

296. Jesse RA and Fletcher GH: Treatment of the neck in patients with squamous cell carcinoma of the head and neck. Cancer 39:868, 1977.

297. DeSanto L, et al: Neck dissection and combined therapy: study of effectiveness. Arch Otolaryngol Head Neck Surg 111:659, 1975.

298. Nichols RT: Bilateral neck dissection. Am J Surg 117:377, 1969.

299. Krajina Z, et al: The problem of unilateral and bilateral neck dissection. Acta Otolaryngol (Stockh) 80:317, 1975.

300. Watson WL: Cancer of the trachea 15 years after treatment for cancer of the larynx. J Thorac Surg 12:142, 1942.

301. Sisson GA, et al: Mediastinal dissection: indications and newer techniques. Laryngoscope 87:759, 1977.

302. Harrison DFN: Resection of the manubrium. Br J Surg 64:374, 1977.

303. Sisson GA, et al: Transsternal radical neck dissection for control of stomal recurrences: end results. Laryngoscope 85:1504, 1975.

304. Hong WK, et al: Recent advances in head and neck cancer: larynx preservation and cancer chemoprevention: the seventeenth annual Richard and Hinda Rosenthal Foundation award lecture. Cancer Res 53:5113, 1993.

305. Vokes EE, et al: Cisplatin and fluorouracil chemotherapy does not yield long-term benefit in locally advanced head and neck cancer: results from a single institution. J Clin Oncol 9:1376, 1991.

306. Vokes EE, et al: Cisplatin, fluorouracil, and leucovorin augmented by Interferon Alfa-2b in head and neck cancer: a clinical and pharmacologic analysis. J Clin Oncol 11:360, 1993.

307. Forastiere AA, et al: Randomized comparison of cisplatin plus fluorouracil and carboplatin plus fluorouracil versus methotrexate in advanced squamous-cell carcinoma of the head and neck: a Southwest Oncology Group study. J Clin Oncol 10:1245, 1992.

308. Jacobs C, et al: A phase III randomized study comparing cisplatin and fluorouracil as single agents in combination for advanced squamous cell carcinoma of the head and neck. J Clin Oncol 10:257, 1992.

309. Vakaet L and van Eijkeren M: The role of chemotherapy in the management of advanced laryngeal cancer. Acta Otorhinolaryngol Belg 46:213, 1992.

310. Wolf GT, et al: Induction chemotherapy plus radiation compared with surgery plus radiation in patients with advanced laryngeal cancer. N Engl J Med 324:1685, 1991.

311. Karp DD, et al: Larynx preservation using induction chemotherapy plus radiation therapy as an alternative to laryngectomy in advanced head and neck cancer. Am J Clin Oncol 14: 273, 1991.

312. Kraus DH, et al: Larynx preservation with combined chemo-

therapy and radiation therapy in advanced hypopharynx cancer. Otolaryngology Head Neck Surg *111*:31, 1994.

313. Chang H, et al: Advanced head and neck cancer: response to and toxicity of multimodality therapy. Radiology *168*:863, 1988.

314. Keldsen N: Cisplatin as second line chemotherapy in advanced or recurrent squamous cell carcinoma of head and neck region. Acta Oncol *26*:357, 1987.

315. Merlano M, et al: Sequential versus alternating chemotherapy and radiotherapy in stage III-IV squamous cell carcinoma of the head and neck: a phase III study. J Clin Oncol *6*:627, 1988.

316. Clark JR, Fallon BG, and Frei E 3d: Induction chemotherapy as initial treatment for advanced head and neck cancer: a model for the multidisciplinary treatment of solid tumors. Important Adv Oncol 175, 1987.

317. Browman GP, et al: Methotrexate/fluorouracil scheduling influences normal tissue toxicity but not antitumor effects in patients with squamous cell head and neck cancer: results from a randomized trial. J Clin Oncol *6*:963, 1988.

318. Vokes EE, et al: Head and neck cancer. N Engl J Med *328*:184, 1993.

319. Lippman SM, et al: Comparison of low-dose isotretinoin with *β*-carotene to prevent oral carcinogenesis. N Engl J Med *328:* 15, 1993.

320. Hong WK, et al: Prevention of second primary tumors with isotretinoin in squamous-cell carcinoma of the head and neck. N Engl J Med *323*:795, 1990.

321. De Vries N and De Flora S: *N-Acetyl-l-cysteine.* J Cell Biochem Suppl *17F*:270, 1993.

322. De Vries N: Second primary tumors in laryngeal cancer. Acta Otorhinolaryngol Belg *46*:153, 1992.

323. Weichselbaum RR, et al: Radioresistant tumor cells are present in head and neck carcinomas that recur after radiotherapy. Int J Radiat Oncol Biol Phys *15*:575, 1988.

324. Parsons JT, et al: Hyperfractionation for head and neck cancer. Int J Radiat Oncol Biol Phys *14*:649, 1988.

325. Snow JB Jr: Surgical management of head and neck cancer. Semin Oncol *15*:20, 1988.

326. Goldman NC, et al: Carcinoid of the larynx. Arch Otolaryngol Head Neck Surg *90*:64, 1969.

327. Tawai S, et al: Laryngeal carcinoid tumor: light and EM studies. Cancer *48*:2256, 1981.

328. Nonomura A, et al: Primary carcinoid tumor of the larynx and review of the literature. Acta Pathol Jpn *33*:1041, 1983.

329. Govaerts PJ: Clinical oncology: case presentations from oncology centres: 2. Carcinoid of the larynx. Eur J Cancer *28A*:1755, 1992.

330. Mills SE and Foders ME: Atypical carcinoid tumor of the larynx: a light microscopic and ultrastructural study. Arch Otolaryngol Head Neck Surg *110*:58, 1984.

331. Capper JW: A malignant carcinoid tumor of the supraglottic larynx. J Larnyngol Otol *95*:963, 1981.

332. Blok DH, et al: Carcinoid of the larynx: a report of 3 cases and a review of the literature. Laryngoscope *95*:715, 1985.

333. Whicker JH, et al: Adenocarcinoma of the larynx. Presented at the American Laryngological Association, Palm Beach, FL, April 27, 1974.

334. Lynch RC: Report of a case of mixed tumor of the parotid type growing from the posterior aspect of the thyroid cartilage. Ann Otol Rhinol Laryngol *38*:706, 1929.

335. Yoshida T, et al: Benign neoplasms of the larynx: a 10 year review of 38 patients. Auris Nasus Larynx *10(suppl)*:61, 1983.

336. Aakznik MS: Pleomorphic adenoma of the larynx. J Laryngol Otol *99*:611, 1985.

337. Masson P and Berger L: Epitheliomas à double metaplasie de la parotide. Bull Assoc Fr Cancer *13*:366, 1924.

338. De MN and Tribedi BP: A mixed epidermoid and mucous secretory carcinoma of the parotid gland. J Pathol Bacteriol *49*:432, 1939.

339. Arcidiacono DG and Lomeo DG: Tumori mucoepidermoidale salivare. Ann Otol Rhinol Laryngol *15*:95, 1963.

340. Bahodur S, et al: Mucoepidermoid carcinoma of the larynx. J Otolaryngol S Aust *5*:236, 1985.

341. Bruder WJ, et al: Mucoepidermoid carcinoma of the larynx: a case report and review of the literature. Ann Otol Rhinol Laryngol *89*:103, 1980.

342. Gatti WM, et al: Mucoepidermoid carcinoma of the larynx. Arch Otolaryngol Head Neck Surg *106*:52, 1980.

343. Spiro RH, et al: Mucous gland tumor of the larynx and laryngopharynx. Ann Otol Rhinol Laryngol *85*:496, 1987.

344. Snow RT and Fox AR: Mucoepidermoid carcinoma of the larynx. J Am Osteopath Assoc *91*:182, 1991.

345. Broeckart J: Hyalogenes cylindrom des larynx. Z Laryng Rhinol *5*:51, 1912.

346. Ferlito A, et al: Biological behavior of laryngeal adenoid cystic carcinoma. ORL J Otorhinolaryngol Relat Spec *45*:245, 1983.

347. Tewfik TL, et al: Adenoid cystic carcinoma of the larynx. J Otolaryngol *12*:151, 1983.

348. Putney FJ, et al: Salivary gland tumors of the head and neck. Laryngoscope *64*:285, 1954.

349. Olofsson JA, et al: Adenoid cystic carcinoma of the larynx: a report of 4 cases and review of the literature. Cancer *40*:1307, 1977.

350. Donovan DJ and Carley J: Adenoid cystic carcinoma of the subglottic region. Ann Otol Rhinol Laryngol *92*:491, 1983.

351. Abemayor E and Calcaterra T: Kaposi's sarcoma and community acquired immune deficiency syndromes: an update with emphasis on its head neck manifestations. Arch Otolaryngol Head Neck Surg *109*:536, 1983.

352. Marcusen DC and Svoy DC: Otolaryngologic and head and neck manifestations of acquired immunodeficiency syndrome (AIDS). Laryngoscope *95*:401, 1985.

353. Coyas A, et al: Kaposi's sarcoma of the larynx. J Laryngol Otol *97*:647, 1983.

354. Sutow WW, et al: Three year relapse-free survival rates in childhood rhabdomyosarcoma of the head and neck. Cancer *49*:2217, 1982.

355. Kodar A, et al: Rhabdomyosarcoma of the larynx treated by laser surgery, combined with radiotherapy and chemotherapy. Med Pediatr Oncol *11*:279, 1983.

356. Liebner EJ: Embryonal rhabdomyosarcoma of the head and neck in children: correlation of stage, radiation dose, local control and survival. Cancer *37*:2777, 1976.

357. Mara ADP, et al: Rhabdomyosarcoma of the larynx in children: a series of five patients treated in the Institut Gustave Roussy (Villejuif, France). Med Pediatr Oncol *19*:110, 1991.

358. Frank DL: Leiomyosarcoma of the larynx. Arch Otolaryngol Head Neck Surg *34*:493, 1941.

359. Roth TA, et al: Synovial sarcoma of the neck: a followup study of 24 cases. Cancer *35*:1248, 1975.

360. Applebaum E, et al: Synovial sarcoma of the hypopharynx. Otolaryngol Head Neck Surg *91*:452, 1983.

361. Quinn HJ: Synovial sarcoma of the larynx treated by partial laryngectomy. Laryngoscope *94*:1158, 1984.

362. Jennstrom P: Synovial sarcoma of the pharynx: report of a case. Am J Clin Pathol *29*:957, 1984.

363. Swain R, et al: Fibrosarcoma of the head and neck: a clinical analysis of 40 cases. Ann Otol Rhinol Laryngol *83*:439, 1974.

364. Van den Branden J, et al: Le sarcome vrai de larynx. Rev Laryngol Otol Rhinol (Bord) *82*:876, 1961.

365. Rolander T, et al: Fibrous xanthoma of the larynx. Arch Otolaryngol Head Neck Surg *96*:168, 1972.

366. Ogura JH, et al: Malignant fibrous histiocytoma of the head and neck. Laryngoscope *90*:1429, 1980.

367. Canalis RF, et al: Malignant fibrous xanthoma of the larynx. Arch Otolaryngol Head Neck Surg *101*:135, 1975.

368. Olte T and Kleinsasser O: Liposarcoma of the head and neck. Arch Otolaryngol Head Neck Surg 323:285, 1981.

369. Ferlito A: Primary pleomorphic liposarcoma of the larynx. J Otolaryngol 7:161, 1978.

370. Tobey DN, et al: EM in the diagnosis of liposarcoma and fibrosarcoma of the larynx. Ann Otol Rhinol Laryngol 88:867, 1979.

371. Krausen T, et al: Liposarcoma of the larynx: a multicentric or a metastatic malignancy? Laryngoscope 87:1116, 1977.

372. Neel HB and Unn HK: Cartilaginous tumours of the larynx: a series of 35 patients. Otolaryngol Head Neck Surg 90:201, 1982.

373. Hyams VJ and Rabuzzi DO: Cartilaginous tumours of the larynx. Laryngoscope 80:755, 1970.

374. Cantrell RW, et al: Conservative surgical treatment of chondrosarcoma of the larynx. Ann Otol Rhinol Laryngol 89:567, 1980.

375. Dauirani KK and Tucker H: Chondroma of the larynx: surgical technique. Arch Otolaryngol Head Neck Surg 107:399, 1981.

376. Swerdlow RS, et al: Cartilaginous tumours of the larynx. Arch Otolaryngol Head Neck Surg 100:269, 1974.

377. Hoffer ME, et al: Laryngeal chondrosarcoma: diagnosis and management. Ear Nose Throat J 71:659, 1992.

378. Olofsson J and Van Nostrand AW: Anaplastic small cell carcinoma of the larynx: case report. Ann Otol Rhinol Laryngol 81:284, 1972.

379. Medina JE, et al: Oat cell carcinomas of the larynx and Eaton-Lambert syndrome. Arch Otolaryngol Head Neck Surg 110:123, 1984.

380. Ibrahim NBN, et al: Extrapulmonary oat cell carcinoma. Cancer 54:1645, 1984.

381. Coakley JF: Primary oat cell carcinoma of the larynx. J Laryngol Otol 99:301, 1985.

382. Gnepp DR, et al: Primary anaplastic small cell (oat cell) carcinoma of the larynx: review of literature and case presentation. Cancer 51:1731, 1983.

383. Posner MR, et al: Small cell carcinomas of the larynx: results of combined modality treatments. Laryngoscope 93:946, 1983.

384. Friedman M, et al: Laryngotracheal invasion by thyroid carcinoma. Ann Otol Rhinol Laryngol 91:363, 1982.

385. Lawson V: The management of airway involvement in thyroid tumors. Arch Otolaryngol Head Neck Surg 109:86, 1983.

386. Segal K, et al: Carcinoma of the thyroid gland invading larynx and trachea. Clin Otolaryngol 9:21, 1984.

387. Ehrlich A: Tumors involving thyroid cartilage. Arch Otolaryngol Head Neck Surg 59:177, 1954.

388. Schirling B, et al: Leukemic involvement of larynx. Arch Otolaryngol Head Neck Surg 85:658, 1967.

389. Swerdlow JB, et al: Non-Hodgkins lymphoma limited to the larynx. Cancer 53:2546, 1984.

390. Bouttens F and Curvelier C: Non-Hodgkins lymphoma presenting as a solitary laryngeal tumor. J Belg Radiol 64:357, 1981.

391. Barat M and Sciubba J: Extramedullary plasmacytoma. Arch Otolaryngol Head Neck Surg 110:820, 1984.

392. Maniglia AJ and Xe JW: Plasmacytoma of the larynx. Laryngoscope 93:741, 1984.

393. Fishkin B, et al: Cervical lymph node metastasis as the first manifestation of localized extremedullary plasmacytoma. Cancer 38:1641, 1976.

394. Abermayor F, et al: Metastatic cancer to the larynx: diagnosis and treatment. Cancer 52:1944, 1983.

33 Nutrition of the Head and Neck Patient

William D. DeWys

Nutritional care of patients with cancer or trauma of the head and neck requires a knowledge of nutritional requirements, alterations in these requirements by effects of disease and treatment, and technical aspects related to route of administration of nutrients. Weight may be lost because of decreased caloric intake, increased caloric requirement, or both.[1,2] Trauma patients often are unable to eat adequately and moderately may have increased caloric requirements related to stress and the healing process. In patients with cancer, decreased eating is often the major determinant of negative caloric balance, which is accompanied in some patients by a modest overall increase in caloric requirement. Specific metabolic needs, such as the need for amino acids, may be increased with trauma or cancer, and these needs may be met by breakdown of normal tissue such as muscle if nutrient intake is inadequate.

Caloric intake may be decreased because of 1) local effects, 2) systemic effects, or 3) treatment effects. In patients with head and neck cancer, local disease effects are often the predominant cause of deficient caloric intake. Systemic effects such as fever or pain may decrease appetite. With multimodality therapy of cancer, treatment effects such as mucous membrane damage and nausea may further reduce caloric intake.

RATIONALE FOR NUTRITIONAL INTERVENTION

Nutritional support may improve the patient's sense of well-being; may reduce complications related to trauma, cancer, or treatment; and may improve the overall outcome of treatment. Malnourished patients have an increased risk of postoperative morbidity and mortality.[3] Controlled clinical trials of nutritional sup-

port for trauma and cancer patients have shown reduced morbidity in patients who receive enteral or parenteral alimentation compared with patients who received conventional nutritional care. In a controlled trial of jejunostomy feeding versus no supplemental feeding in patients with major trauma, nitrogen balance improved in the enterally fed group, and septic morbidity decreased from 29% to 9%.[4] Patients who have cancer and receive parenteral nutrition had fewer wound and anastomatic complications (10% vs. 23%)[5], fewer postoperative complications and a reduced mortality,[6] a significant reduction in the incidence of postoperative wound infections,[7] and reduced problems with wound healing, reduced incidence and severity of pneumonia, and reduced postoperative mortality.[8] A review article estimated that parenteral nutrition could reduce the odds of major postoperative complications to between $\frac{1}{2}$ and $\frac{2}{3}$ of that in the control group and could reduce postoperative mortality to $\frac{1}{2}$ of that in the control group.[9] Advantages for preoperative nutritional therapy were seen in those patients who had a low baseline serum albumin (<3.5 g/dl) or weight loss suggesting that nutrition should begin preoperatively for undernourished patients but nutritional support may be started at the time of surgery for adequately nourished patients.

Patients who cannot eat adequately because of tumor obstruction, surgical resection, or other complications should receive enteral or parenteral nutrition until these problems are resolved. If a cachectic patient is judged to be unable to tolerate aggressive radiation therapy or chemotherapy without nutritional support, enteral or parenteral feeding should be considered as part of an overall treatment plan.[10] In patients who receive radiation therapy, nutritional support may reduce the need to suspend radiation therapy because of mucosal reaction or poor performance status.[11]

ROUTES OF ADMINISTRATION OF NUTRIENTS—ORAL VS. ENTERAL VS. PARENTERAL

The choice of route of feeding is based on consideration of the advantages and disadvantages of each route and the results of comparative studies.[12,13] Oral feeding has advantages of simplicity and patient enjoyment but may be limited by the patient's appetite or ability to swallow. Enteral feeding has advantages compared with oral feeding in that the volume administered is more controlled. Enteral feeding has advantages compared with parenteral feeding in that the tube and solutions need not be sterile, the solutions are inexpensive, feeding requires limited supervision, the intestinal mucosa is stimulated (advantageous for subsequent return to normal eating), and insulin production is stimulated so that exogenous insulin is rarely needed. Disadvantages of enteral feeding include nasopharyngeal irritation (with nasogastric route), abdominal cramps and diarrhea, and risk of pulmonary aspiration.

Advantages of parenteral feeding include use when the gastrointestinal tract is not functional or cannot accept a large volume, use when any risk of pulmonary aspiration is unacceptable (severe chronic lung disease), and use when the patient does not tolerate a nasogastric tube and cannot or does not accept a gastrostomy or jejunostomy tube. Disadvantages of parenteral feeding include the need for insertion of a central venous line with the attendant risks of pneumothorax, hemothorax, and venous thrombosis; the requirement for sterile handling of all tubes and solutions; greater supervision than enteral feeding; and complications of fluid overload, mineral imbalances, and sepsis. Overall the enteral route is often preferable to the parenteral route.

Comparative studies of feeding by different routes tend to report either equal effectiveness or slightly greater effectiveness for parenteral feeding than for enteral feeding. In a randomized study of jejunal feeding versus parenteral feeding in trauma patients, average daily caloric intakes, nitrogen balance, and complication rates were comparable.[14] In a study of protein metabolism in patients with esophageal cancer, both jejunal feeding and parenteral feeding tended to stabilize nutritional status and whole-body protein economics. Parenteral nutrition appeared to be slightly more efficacious.[15] In a study of patients with head and neck cancer, patients who received parenteral feeding on average maintained their weights whereas enterally fed patients lost an average of 5% body weight. No differences existed in surgical complications, and the survival analysis favored the enteral group.[16] In a study of patients with esophageal cancer, a group receiving parenteral feeding gained weight more rapidly, achieved positive nitrogen balance more quickly,

and had a tendency toward lower incidence of wound complications but the later difference was not statistically significant.[17]

TECHNICAL CONSIDERATIONS IN PROVIDING NUTRITIONAL SUPPORT FOR THE HEAD AND NECK PATIENT

Enteral feeding requires the insertion of a nasogastric tube, a gastrostomy tube or a jejunostomy tube (via laparotomy or via an endoscopically directed percutaneous technique).[18,19] The patient receiving nasogastric or gastrostomy feeding should have the head of the bed elevated to minimize pulmonary aspiration. Enteral feeding may be given as a continuous infusion or by periodic infusion of a bolus. Continuous infusion may be better tolerated by the patient with a prior poor caloric intake, but bolus feeding is more convenient for ambulatory patients. The tube should be aspirated periodically to check for retention.

Parenteral administration of nutrition requires the insertion of a large catheter into a central vein to minimize phlebitis and hemolysis related to the administration of hypertonic solutions. The catheter can be inserted into the subclavian vein and maintained as described by Grant.[20] In the patient with head and neck cancer or trauma, the presence of a tracheostomy, fistula formation, or drooling of oral secretions, a sterile polyurethane adhesive sheet may be applied to cover the catheter site and to separate it from the tracheostomy or fistula.[21]

ESTIMATING NUTRITIONAL NEEDS

Estimating the nutritional needs of a patient must take into account the baseline nutritional status and the ongoing nutritional requirements. Assessment of baseline nutritional status can be based on a weight loss history,[5,22] and measurement of serum albumen[23] and total iron-binding capacity. Weight loss may be considered significant if it is greater than 1% per week or greater than 10% total. Correction of weight loss or of protein deficits must be considered in the nutrition plan.

Nutritional requirements that must be considered include calories, protein, lipid, minerals, and vitamins. Calorie requirements are approximately 30 to 35 kcal/kg body weight for the average adult without complications.[24] To this baseline requirement, one may add for regain of lost weight, the stress of surgery, and the stress of a severe infection. Protein requirements are approximately 1 g/kg for the patient without complications but may be higher with stress, with protein loss such as through a fistula, or with a need for correction

ORDER 1   **PLEASE SELECT BASE SOLUTION, A, B, OR C BY PROVIDING REQUESTED INFORMATION**

A ☐ **Standard Central**	**B** ☐ **Standard Peripheral**	**C** ☐ **Non-Standard**
5% Amino Acids 17.5% Dextrose 3% Fat (Approximately 1.1 KCal/ml)	3.5% Amino Acids 5% Dextrose 4% Fat (Approximately 0.7 KCal/ml)	☐ Central ☐ Peripheral _____ Amino Acids (Gm/day) (A) _____ Dextrose (KCal/day) (D) _____ Fat (KCal/day) (F) ***(ml/day) = (Minimum volume = $\dfrac{(D + F)}{2}$ + 10A)

ORDER 2   **CONTINUOUS TPN VOLUME AND FLOW RATE**   **OR   CYCLIC TPN SCHEDULE**

☐ 1000 ml (42ml/hr)   ☐ 2400 ml (100ml/hr)
☐ 1500 ml (62ml/hr)   ☐ 3000 ml (125ml/hr)
☐ 2000 ml (83ml/hr)   ☐ _____ ml/hr
***The order vol. of non-standard sol. must be ≥ min. vol. calc. in box C above

Total _____ ml over _____ hours

Infuse _____ ml/hr × _____ hours

then _____ ml/hr × _____ hours

then _____ ml/hr × _____ hours

ORDER 3   **PLEASE DETERMINE ELECTROLYTE COMPONENT OF TPN**

Additive	☐ **Standard** Standard Electrolytes Per Day	☐ **Non-Standard** Non-Standard Electrolytes Per Day	Recommended Adult Requirements
Sodium	70 mEq		60–100 mEq/d
Potassium	60 mEq		60–100 mEq/d
Calcium	10 mEq		10–15 mEq/d
Magnesium	15 mEq		10–20 mEq/d
Chloride	52 mEq	Electrolytes will be balanced with chloride	
Phosphate	20 mmole		20–45 mmole/d
Acetate	50 mEq		Alkalosis and NG suctioning may require avoiding acetate
Multivitamins	10 ml		10 ml meets AMA guidelines
Trace Element	5 ml		5 ml meets AMA guidelines
Vitamin K	1 mg		1 mg/d
Regular Insulin	_____ units		
H_2 Receptor Antagonist	_____ _____ drug mg/day		Pepcid (famotidine) 40 mg/day or Tagamet (cimetidine) 900 mg/day or Zantac (ranitidine) 150 mg/day

TPN ORDERS SHOULD BE IN THE PHARMACY BY 1300. FOR ANY NEW ORDER RECEIVED AFTER 1300, THE STANDARD FORMULA WITHOUT FAT WILL BE PROVIDED UPON CONFIRMATION. FOR ANY QUESTIONS PLEASE CALL THE IV PHARMACIST AT EXT. 3124.

SPECIAL INSTRUCTIONS: ☐ Activate Total Parenteral Nutrition Monitoring Orders
☐ Nutrition Consult

_____

_____

Date: _____ Time: _____ Dr. Signature: _____ Page: _____

PATIENT IDENTIFICATION

Fig. 33–1. Order form for parenteral nutrition.

of undernutrition as judged by a low serum albumen or iron-binding capacity. Postoperative requirements for maintaining positive nitrogen balance in surgical patients have been 40 to 45 kcal/kg body weight and 1.2 to 1.5 g protein/kg body weight.[25]

Lipid requirements to prevent fatty acid deficiency are low and can be met by infusion of 500 ml of a lipid suspension 1 to 2×/week. However, approximately 30% of nonprotein calories should be provided as fat, based on the upper limit of carbohydrate that can be metabolized,[26] body tissues such as liver and muscle can use fat directly for energy, fat in the prescription minimizes the risk of developing fatty liver (because of excess carbohydrate), and reduces the glucose load, which reduces the need for exogenous insulin.

PARENTERAL NUTRITION—PRESCRIBING AND MONITORING

For parenteral nutrition, the prescription of calories, protein, and additives should be tailored to each patient and is facilitated by use of a total parental nutrition (TPN) order form (Figure 33–1). For most patients a standard TPN solution that contains 30% of nonprotein calories as fat can be used, and the amount is based on the calculated caloric requirements (Figure 33–1). To the base solution, one adds either standard or tailored amounts of major minerals (sodium, potassium, calcium, magnesium, chloride, acetate or bicarbonate, and phosphate), trace elements (zinc, manganese, copper, and chromium [available as trace metal additives]), and standard amount of a multivitamin preparation as shown in Figure 33–1. If imbalances or deficiencies of any of these components exist, nonstandard amounts are added aimed at correcting imbalances. Insulin may be added depending on the results of blood glucose monitoring. The orders should be rewritten periodically based on the results of patient clinical progress and nutritional monitoring. In addition, patients receiving long-term parenteral nutrition should receive vitamin K (1 mg/day IV or 10 mg/week IM) and IM injections of folate 1 mg per week and vitamin B12 1 mg per month.

During nutritional support, monitoring is necessary to minimize complications and maximize the nutritional benefits. The patient should be weighed daily. A weight gain of more than 0.2 kg/day suggests fluid accumulation and the possible need for diuretics. Blood sugar should be monitored every 6 hours for 72 hours and then every 24 hours when starting parenteral feeding because the high glucose load may overwhelm the patient's insulin production and require exogenous insulin. Other monitoring guidelines are

TABLE 33–1. Monitoring during Nutritional Therapy

All parameters listed below should be measured before starting nutritional therapy.

Parameters should be monitored according to the following schedules:
  Weight and intake and output—daily
  Blood glucose—every 6 hours for 72 hours, then daily until glucose is <150 mg/dl for several days
  Chem 6—Daily for 1 week
  Chem 24-Prothrombin time, Total iron-binding capacity, Magnesium—weekly

presented in Table 33–1. The site of catheter insertion should be inspected on alternate days, and the temperature should be measured periodically to monitor potential infectious complications.

PRESCRIBING THE FORMULA FOR ORAL OR ENTERAL FEEDING

Advice on oral nutrition can be provided by a registered dietician. The dietician can estimate the patient's current intake and requirements, educate the patient about the importance of good nutrition, guide the patient in the use of nutritional supplements, and monitor the patient's progress.[27] Use of oral nutritional supplements is enhanced by offering the patient the option

TABLE 33–2. Representative Products for Oral or Enteral Feeding

Category	Description	Example
Standard isotonic	Ready to use, suitable for most tube-fed patients, requires digestion, provides complete balanced nutrition, within a reasonable volume, isotonic, lactose free.	Osmolite
High nitrogen	Provides more protein and electrolytes to meet the needs of the anabolic patient.	Osmolite-HN
Hypertonic, calorically dense	Higher caloric density for hypermetabolic and fluid-restricted patients. May cause dehydration due to decreased free water.	Magnacal
Chemically defined	Requires minimal digestion, for patients with impaired-GI function. (poor taste so use enterally only)	Criticare
Modular Protein Carbohydrate Fat	Individual nutrients can be added to foods or nutritional formulas to provide desired level of protein, carbohydrate, and/or fat.	Promod Karo Syrup Microlipid

of tasting several preparations (commercially available supplements and Carnation Instant Breakfast) and selecting based on taste preference.[28]

For oral supplementation or for enteral nutrition, a number of products are available, but the physician needs to know only a limited number to meet the needs of most patients. An isotonic, lactose-free formula is preferred for most patients (Table 33–2). This type of formula contains 1 kcal/ml so the estimated caloric requirement per day equals the volume per day. These formulas are nutritionally complete including minerals and vitamins so no additives are needed. Other products provide higher amounts of nitrogen, higher caloric density, more easily digestible formulas or modular formulas to meet specific patient requirements (Table 33–2). When beginning enteral feeding, a half-strength solution should be used for the first few days to minimize abdominal discomfort and diarrhea.

TRANSITIONS

After prolonged parenteral feeding, atrophic changes may occur in the gastrointestinal system (mucosa and muscle), and the patient may not be able to resume intake by mouth immediately. A transition period may be required during which the parenteral feeding is gradually reduced while the patient gradually increases his/her ability to use the digestive system. An interim period of enteral feeding may facilitate the transition to oral feeding. This transition must be individualized and may extend over a week or more.

CONCLUSIONS

Attention to good nutrition is an important part of good medical care. The goal of nutritional support is to maintain or replete the patient's nutritional status, to maximize recovery and healing, and to minimize complications. In the trauma patient, aggressive nutritional support may reduce wound and respiratory complications. In the patient with cancer, aggressive nutritional support may be a worthwhile adjunct to aggressive surgery, radiation therapy, and chemotherapy, especially when these anticancer therapies are used in combinations.

SUGGESTED READINGS

1. DeWys WD: Pathophysiology of cancer cachexia: current understanding and areas for future research. Cancer Res 42:721s, 1982.
2. DeWys WD, Kisner D: Principles of nutritional care of the cancer patient. In Principles of Cancer Treatment. Edited by SK Carter, E Glatstein, and RB Livingston. New York, McGraw-Hill Book Co., 1982.
3. Buzby GP, et al: Prognostic nutritional index in gastrointestinal surgery. Am J Surg 139:160, 1980
4. Moore EE, Jones TN: Benefits of immediate jejunostomy feeding after major abdominal trauma—a prospective, randomized study. J Trauma 26:874, 1986.
5. Daly JM, et al: Parenteral nutrition in esophageal cancer patients. Ann Surg 196:203, 1982.
6. Holter AR, Fischer JE: The effects of perioperative hyperalimentation on complications in patients with carcinoma and weight loss. J Surg Res 23:31, 1977.
7. Heatley RV, Williams RH, Lewis MH: Preoperative intravenous feeding—A controlled trial. Postgrad Med J 55:541, 1979.
8. Mueller JM, Brenne U, Dienst J: Preoperative parenteral feeding in patients with gastrointestinal cancer. Lancet 1:68, 1982.
9. Klein S: Clinical efficacy of nutritional support in patients with cancer. Oncology 7(Supplement):87–92, 1993.
10. Nixon DW: The value of parenteral nutrition support: chemotherapy and radiation treatment. Cancer 58:1902, 1986.
11. Nayel H, el-Ghoneiny E, el-Haddad S: Impact of nutritional supplementation on treatment delay and morbidity in patients with head and neck tumors treated with irradiation. Nutrition 8:13–18, 1992.
12. DeWys WD: Nutritional care of the cancer patient. JAMA 244:374, 1980.
13. DeWys WD, Kubota TT: Enteral and parenteral nutrition in the care of the cancer patient. JAMA 246:1725, 1981.
14. Adams S, et al: Enteral versus parenteral nutrition support following laparotomy for trauma: a randomized prospective trial. J Trauma 26:882, 1986.
15. Burt ME, Stein TP, Brennan MF: A controlled, randomized trial evaluating the effects of enteral and parenteral nutrition on protein metabolism in cancer-bearing man. J Surg Res 34:303, 1983.
16. Sako K, et al: Parenteral hyperalimentation in surgical patients with head and neck cancer: A randomized study. J Surg Oncol 16:391, 1981.
17. Lim STK, et al: Total parenteral nutrition versus gastrostomy in the preoperative preparation of patients with cancer of the oesophagus. Br J Surg 68:69, 1981.
18. Gauderer MWL, Ponsky JL: A simplified technique for constructing a tube feeding gastrostomy. Surg Gynecol Obstet 152:83, 1981.
19. Sriram K, Gray DS: Home enteral hyperalimentation catheter: Surgical technique and problem-solving. Nutr Support Serv 4:32, 1984.
20. Grant JP: Handbook of Total Parenteral Nutrition Philadelphia, WB Saunders Co., 1980.
21. Vazquez RM: Tracheostomy and subclavian catheterizations. Surg Gynecol Obstet 152:342, 1981.
22. Studley HO: Percentage of weight loss: a basic indicator of surgical risk in patients with chronic peptic ulcer. JAMA 106:458, 1936
23. Rhoads JE, Alexander CE: Nutritional problems of surgical patients. Ann NY Acad Sci 63:268, 1955.
24. National Academy of Sciences: Recommended Dietary Allowances. Washington, D.C., U.S. Government Printing Office, 1974.
25. Moghissi K, Teasdale PR: Parenteral feeding in patients with carcinoma of the esophagus treated by surgery: energy and nitrogen requirements. J Parenter Enteral Nutr 4:371, 1980.
26. Wolfe RR, et al: Investigation of factors determining the optimal glucose infusion rate in total parenteral nutrition. Metabolism 29:892, 1980.
27. Kelly K: An overview of how to nourish the cancer patient by mouth. Cancer 58:1897, 1986.
28. DeWys WD, Herbst SH: Oral feeding in the nutritional management of the cancer patient. Cancer Res 37:2429, 1977.

34 Chemotherapy of Head and Neck Cancer

Janardan D. Khandekar

The ultimate objective of chemotherapy is to cure the patient of malignant disease. This is currently possible in at least 10 types of disseminated cancer, occurring predominantly in children, adolescents, and young adults. In most disseminated solid tumors, cure is not yet possible, although significant palliation and lengthening of survival can be achieved.

In the United States, head and neck cancer accounts for only 5% (or 40,000 patients) of patients in whom malignancy develops, but the associated pronounced cosmetic and functional deformities and malnutrition heighten its importance. These tumors challenge the expertise of head and neck surgeons, radiation and medical oncologists, prosthodontists, pathologists, dieticians, physiatrists, nurses, and social workers.

Traditionally, chemotherapy had been used only after failure of irradiation and/or surgery to control head and neck tumors. The local therapeutic modalities, however, do not cure a sizeable percentage of patients. Although patients with limited disease (T_{1-2}, N_0, M_0) can be treated effectively with local modalities such as surgery and radiation, with 60% or more 2-year disease-free survival, more than 70% of patients with extensive disease (T_{3-4}, N_0, M_0) have recurrence at 2 years after these treatments. Drug therapy for cancer began approximately 45 years ago, but until lately it has had little impact on the cure rate of head and neck tumors. In the last few years, multiple studies have emerged involving a variety of combinations of drugs used not only for recurrent and advanced disease, but also as primary treatment for head and neck tumors. Chemotherapy is emerging as an important adjunct to surgery and/or radiation.

THE CELL CYCLE

Malignant tissues are made up primarily of dividing cells, which synthesize DNA at some point in their life cycles, and nondividing cells. The dividing cells pass through four different phases (Fig. 34–1). Mitosis (M) occupies a discrete phase of the cell cycle. After the division, the cell enters the G1 phase. This phase is then followed by DNA synthesis, which is termed the S phase. After completion of the DNA synthesis, the cell then enters a phase of apparent rest (G2) before the initiation of the next mitosis.

In most dividing cells, the period for S, G2, and M phases are of relative constant duration. Variation of the length of the cell cycle occurs in the G1 phase. When the proliferating cells stop dividing, they do so in the G1 phase. This phase seems to hold the key to the proliferative activity of the tissue. When the cell cycle time (time taken for a proliferative cell to move from one mitosis to another) is short, and thus the proliferative activity is high, the G1 is of brief duration. When proliferative activity is slow, the G1 phase is long.

It is not clear how a mammalian eukaryotic cell decides to leave the G1 phase and to start DNA synthesis. Based on the differences in RNA content, two distinct subcompartments, G1A and G1B, have been recognized. It is postulated that after the mitosis, cells reside in the low RNA—G1A compartment and an increase in RNA above this critical level is required for G1 cells to be able to initiate DNA replication. The G1 cells with high RNA values are in G1B. During the S phase, biosynthesis of enzymes essential for pyrimidine and nucleic acids is accentuated, and the DNA content of the cell doubles. The phase of DNA synthesis is then complete and the cell enters G2 phase. None of the phases is quiescent, and RNA and protein synthesis occurs throughout each of them.

The molecular mechanisms that control cell cycle are being elucidated rapidly. Cell cycle control is based on two key families of proteins. The first is the family

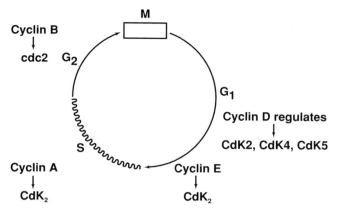

Fig. 34–1. The cell cycle phases: M, mitosis; G_1, preceding DNA synthesis; S, DNA synthesis; G_2, premitotic resting.

of cyclin-dependent protein kinases (CdK), which phosphorylates selected proteins. The second is a family of specialized activating proteins called cyclins that bind to the CdK molecules and control their ability to phosphorylate appropriate target proteins. Thus, two checkpoints that exist in the cell cycle are at G1/S and G2/M phases in the cycle.

In addition to differences in the biochemical mechanism of action, discussed later, antineoplastic agents also differ in the point in the cell cycle at which they act. The drugs can be grouped as follows on the basis of their effects of phases of the cell cycle:

1. *S phase specific:* These are the agents that inhibit the DNA synthesis that occurs in the S phase of the cell cycle. Drugs such as methotrexate (MTX) inhibit not only DNA, but also RNA and protein synthesis, and are called S phase specific.
2. *Non S specific:* Alkylating agents and antitumor antibiotics exert a direct effect on DNA, and thus their activities are not dependent on the phase of the cell cycle.
3. *Antimitotics:* Plant alkaloids such as vincristine arrest mitosis during metaphase.

Studies of the cell kinetics indicate that the often-held belief that all malignant tumors are rapidly proliferating is not necessarily true. The mean doubling time of human tumors (time taken by a tumor to double its volume) can be as short as 1 week in Burkitt's tumor, or as long as several years in some adenocarcinomas.

Malignant tumor formation occurs when any of the following three events occur together or separately: (1) The growth fraction, defined as proportion of tumor cells in mitotic cycle at a given time, becomes large; (2) the cell cycle time becomes shorter; on average, the cell cycle time of tumors is 2 days, which is not faster than normal cells; (3) normally, renewal of normal cells is accompanied by cell loss, an active process known as "programmed" cell death or apoptosis. When this cell

loss is reduced, tumor formation can occur. This seems to be the major factor in the production of most tumors.

Epidermoid neoplasms have approximately 35% growth fraction (dividing cells) as contrasted to 3 to 5% in breast cancer, and virtually 100% in embryonal tumors. Because most of the chemotherapeutic agents act on these dividing cells, epidermoid cancers would be intermediate in their response to drugs. A recent work suggests that, at the metastatic site, a tumor may still be proliferating rapidly, whereas the parent neoplasm has a low growth fraction. Chemotherapy given to these patients may still be useful. Methods for measurement of cell kinetic parameters in patients are cumbersome, however. The results of therapy based on these considerations are also at present not much different from those with conventional therapy. Nevertheless, newer advances in this field may considerably alter the present practice of chemotherapy.

MODE OF ACTION OF ANTINEOPLASTIC AGENTS

The DNA synthesized during the S phase of the cell cycle acts as a selective template for the production of specific forms of messenger, ribosomal, or transfer RNA. The specific sequences of the messenger RNA determine which enzymes will be synthesized in the cell. The enzymes, in turn, are responsible for the structure, function, metabolism, and proliferative rate of the cells.

Most of the clinically useful antineoplastic drugs appear to work by inhibition of synthesis of either enzymes or substrates essential for the nucleic acid synthesis and/or function. Based on the mechanism of drug action, agents that are useful in head and neck tumors can be classified as follows:

1. Antimetabolites. These drugs inhibit purine or pyrimidine biosynthesis. MTX, for example, inhibits formation of reduced folates, which are essential for thymidine synthesis.
2. Drugs that interfere with the structure or function of the DNA molecule. Alkylating agents such as cyclophosphamide (CTX) change the structure of DNA, thereby arresting cell replication. On the other hand, antibiotics such as dactinomycin and doxorubicin bind and intercalate with nucleotide sequences of the DNA molecule and thereby block messenger RNA production.
3. Mitotic inhibitors. Vinca alkaloids, such as vincristine and vinblastine, arrest cell division by disrupting the microfilaments of the mitotic spindle.

Chemotherapy drugs with little or no activity in head and neck cancer are not being considered here.

TABLE 34–1. Systemic Single-Agent Chemotherapy

Drugs*	Response Rate (%)
Carboplatin	25
Ifosfamide	25
Paclitaxel	36
Methotrexate	47
Cisplatin	29
Bleomycin	15
Cyclophosphamide	36
Chlorambucil	15
5-Fluorouracil	15
6-Mercaptopurine	12
Vinblastine	29
Doxorubicin	16
Semustine	15
Hexamethylmelamine	12
Dibromodulcitol	22
Hydroxyurea	38
Nitrogen Mustard	8
CCNU	5
DTIC	5
Mitoxantrone	15
Mitomycin-C	15

* *MTX emerges as the most effective single agent, although bleomycin, cisplatin, cyclophosphamide, hydroxyurea, vinblastine, 5-fluorouracil, ifosfamide, and paclitaxel also have considerable activity. By conservative estimate, at least one third of the patients with advanced carcinoma experience more than 50% regression of their tumor masses.*

The activity of various drugs in head and neck cancer is shown in Table 34–1.

GENERAL TOXICITY OF ANTINEOPLASTIC AGENTS

Most of these agents act on the proliferative fraction of cells. Therefore, an undesirable consequence of this drug action is the damage that is inflicted on the normal cells undergoing rapid cell division. These tissues are the cells of the hair follicles, skin, the gastrointestinal mucosa, and the normal bone marrow elements. Clinically, damage to these tissues is manifested by alopecia, stomatitis, nausea, vomiting, anemia, leukopenia, and thrombocytopenia. In addition to these effects, special problems can occur with each drug, and these are discussed briefly. The chemotherapeutic agents are immunosuppressive, less so when the drug is given intermittently rather than on a continuous schedule.

ADJUVANT AND NEOADJUVANT CHEMOTHERAPY

Much emphasis has been placed on the use of single-agent or combination chemotherapy before surgery or radiation in advanced stage III head and neck tumors. Such a strategy is based on the following factors: un-treated tumors with intact vascular supply have better drug delivery, as compared with tumors given prior radiation and that develop scar tissue; regression of primary and nodal tumors can permit subsequent local therapies such as surgery and radiation to have enhanced efficacy; reducing the bulk of initially unresectable lesions can allow better eventual surgical removal; eradication of subclinical micrometastasis at the earliest possible time can thereby reduce risk of systemic relapse; tolerance of intensive combination chemotherapy is better in patients with better performance and nutritional status; a subpopulation of patients can be identified who might further benefit from additional adjuvant chemotherapy after local treatments; and lastly, the extent of surgical resections can perhaps be reduced. Results of induction chemotherapy are presented later in the chapter.

Adjuvant chemotherapy can be defined as the administration of drugs in conjunction with surgery and/or radiation. This type of therapy has been effective in several cancers, including breast cancer. Adjuvant chemotherapy has also been used in patients with head and neck cancer, and the results are summarized later in this section. It is unlikely that a treatment program such as MTX, which produces only partial response (reduction of measurable disease by greater than 50%) in a minority of patients with overt metastatic disease, will prove effective in the eradication of micrometastasis.

Pulmonary metastasis up to 0.3 cm in diameter is barely detectable radiologically, but contains up to 10^8 neoplastic cells. Induction of complete remission (defined as complete disappearance of the measurable tumor) would result in 90 to 99% destruction of tumor cells. Large numbers of viable tumor cells still remain to allow definitive treatment. In contrast, micrometastatic disease is easier to eradicate for several reasons. Large growth fraction of smaller tumors decreases as the tumor enlarges. In the experimental tumor system, when the tumor is disturbed, the noncycling cells reenter the cell cycle. Because most antitumor agents, including methotrexate, have a greater killing effect on proliferating cells, treatment is far more effective in the presence of large growth fraction (microscopic tumor). The second reason for the apparent success of adjuvant chemotherapy is related to the so-called log kill hypothesis. Chemotherapeutic agents kill cells by first-order cell kinetics, i.e., they destroy a certain percentage and not a number of tumor cells. This hypothesis also explains the necessity for repeated prolonged chemotherapy, because the number of tumor cells destroyed decreases as the tumor becomes smaller. This is in contrast to immunotherapy, which kills by zero-order kinetics, i.e., a known number of cells is destroyed. A major limitation of immunotherapy, however, is its ineffectiveness in the presence of large, bulky tumors. Thus, these two modalities may complement each other.

The blood supply of tumors may also be an important factor in the effectiveness of therapy against microscopic disease. The small tumor foci have a greater blood supply than the large, bulky tumors. This can be explained by the fact of geometry that, in a spheroidal tumor, the cell population grows in proportion to the cube of the radius, whereas the surface increases only as the square of the radius. Thus, in small tumors, delivery of antineoplastic agents is more efficient. Surgery or radiation usually compromises the blood supply of tumors, and this may explain the high responsiveness of the totally untreated neoplasms. Finally, chronic debilitation caused by advanced disease may interfere with the effectiveness of the drug and increase the toxicity of chemotherapeutic agents.

COMBINATION CHEMOTHERAPY

A combination of drugs gives better results than single-agent therapy. These results may be explained on the basis of a number of theoretical and practical considerations. Multiple-action agents may prevent the emergence of resistant tumor clones because these drugs may have dissimilar modes of action. With computer-simulated models, it has been proposed that sequential, non–cross-resistant chemotherapy regimens may be superior in eradicating the resistant clones of tumor cells. Similarly, by acting on different phases of the cell cycle, the drugs may have additive or synergistic effects. Finally, with the combination of drugs with different spectrums of clinical toxicity, administration of full or nearly full doses of each of the active agents is possible. As discussed later in this chapter, some of these principles are being applied in the treatment of head and neck cancer.

MULTIPLE DRUG RESISTANCE

Resistance to natural product drugs, either inherent or acquired, remains a major problem in cancer chemotherapy. This kind of resistance, known as multidrug resistance, has been acquired by the tumor cells to drugs that are structurally and functionally unrelated. Initially, this type of drug resistance was due to the presence of a p-glycoprotein encoded by human multiple-drug resistance gene. Subsequently, p-glycoprotein is inserted in the plasma membrane and acts as an ATP-driven drug efflux pump. Other proteins, such as multidrug resistance associated protein, have also been implicated in this drug resistance. Many other mechanisms, such as altered blood delivery of drugs, activation of target enzymes as well as modulation of DNA, may also confer drug resistance.

PROGNOSTIC FACTORS

To appreciate the results of chemotherapy, knowledge of the natural history and prognosis of head and neck cancer is essential.

These neoplasms originate from the laryngeal, nasopharyngeal, and oropharyngeal tissues, from the paranasal sinuses, and from the salivary glands. Most tumors in these areas are squamous cell carcinomas. Squamous cell tumors of the head and neck, however, are a heterogeneous group of lesions, and response to chemotherapy depends on the site of origin, histologic differentiation, and stage of the tumor. MacComb and Fletcher have reviewed the data on 3- and 5-year survival according to the site of the primary lesion in patients treated with radiation and/or surgery. Similarly, the response rates to MTX vary from 18% in tumors that arise from the hypopharynx, to 67% in cancer that occurs in the palate. The degree of tumor differentiation may be another important prognostic factor. For example, bleomycin (BLM) is more effective against well-differentiated cancers. Patients with better performance status (ambulatory) and adequate nutrition seem to have a higher response rate and survival. Flow cytometry, which measures the percentage of the cells in S-phase of the cell cycle, as well as ploidy, is being used increasingly to assess prognosis in cancer patients. Data on flow cytometry in head and neck cancer is scant. More recently, abnormalities in expression of gene products such as p53 have been associated with poor prognosis. Finally, previous treatment may alter the response to the chemotherapy. Thus, in evaluating a chemotherapy regimen, one must carefully consider prognostic factors.

A history of heavy drinking and smoking is often associated with the development of squamous cell cancers. In parts of the Orient and Africa, nasopharyngeal cancer is the prevalent lesion and is often associated with high titers of antibodies to Epstein-Barr (EB) virus. Epstein-Barr virus may have etiologic significance in these tumors. In addition to squamous cell cancers, other types of cancers also occur in the head and neck region. These include lymphoepithelioma, lymphoma, adenocarcinoma, sarcoma, plasmacytoma, and salivary gland tumors. Therapy of these types of cancer is not discussed in this section.

INDICATIONS FOR CHEMOTHERAPY FOR HEAD AND NECK CANCER

Chemotherapy is indicated in recurrent or inoperable head and neck cancers. The impact of this treatment in advanced or recurrent head and neck cancers is modest. Chemotherapy is also used in the neoadjuvant setting preceding either radiation or surgery. A randomized clinical trial using cisplatin and 5-FU followed by radiation was equal to that of total laryngectomy. This trial has revived the issue of organ preservation and the use of optimum preoperative or preradiation chemotherapy.

SPECIFIC CHEMOTHERAPEUTIC AGENTS

A number of systematic studies have been performed on the response of head and neck cancer to chemotherapeutic agents. There is not enough uniformity to date to allow evaluation of responses in terms of pretreatment performance status, specific primary sites, or previous therapy. This limitation is further compounded by poor pretherapy nutritional status of these patients. Malnutrition caused by local tumor, surgical extirpation, radiation, fibrosis, fistulas, and adversion to protein, owing to change in taste, is aggravated by systemic toxicity of the antineoplastic agents. Because of the site of the disease or areas of induration or ulceration, accurate measurement of the two perpendicular diameters of the lesions essential for measuring response is often difficult. These considerations, along with heterogeneity of the head and neck tumors as discussed previously, make precise analysis of the response rates of the particular tumor sites impossible. Only complete responders live significantly longer.

Methotrexate (MTX)

Methotrexate was the first active chemotherapeutic agent for patients with head and neck cancer. It is still regarded as a standard therapy to which new agents or combinations should be compared. It has been given by multiple schedules, including intermittent, weekly, or biweekly IV dosage. The intermittent schedule of administration is, perhaps, superior (50% response) to daily low dosages or daily dosages for 5 consecutive days once a month (29% response). Complete remissions, however, are unusual and short-lived. Responding patients experience exacerbation of disease within $3\frac{1}{2}$ to 4 months.

The biochemical effects of MTX have been studied extensively. As shown in Figure 34–2, MTX acts primarily by inhibiting the activity of the enzyme dihydrofolate reductase, which converts dihydrofolate to tetrahydrofolate. The reduced folates are required for the formation of thymidylate, which then becomes incorporated into DNA. Other evidence suggests that the drug also inhibits purine biosynthesis. More recently, MTX forms polyglutamates within the cell. Polyglutamates inhibit DNA synthesis. Leucovorin, which is N5,N10 formyltetrahydrofolate, supplies the product of the inhibited reaction. Leucovorin thus prevents the three major effects of MTX inhibition: DNA, RNA, and protein synthesis. Thymidine also prevents the anti-

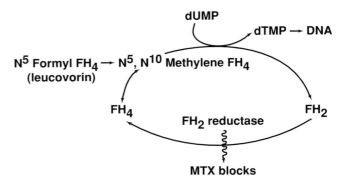

Fig. 34–2. Biochemical effects of MTX and leucovorin. FH_2, dihydrofolate; FH_4, tetrahydrofolate; dUMP, deoxyuridylate; dTMP, thymidylate.

thymidine effects of MTX without interfering with the antitumor effects of the drug. The rationale for clinical investigations of these regimens is derived from experimental findings in L1210 murine leukemia. A carrier-mediated cell membrane transport mechanism is shared by folates and MTX. Tumor cells may lack this transport mechanism. When concentrations of 10^{-3} to 10^{-4} of MTX are achieved, however, (this is possible only when the drug is given in large amounts), the drug enters the cell by a passive transport. Leucovorin and its metabolite, N5,N10 methylene tetrahydrofolate, share a common transport mechanism with MTX. Leucovorin thus can rescue normal host cells because they contain the carrier transport sites. On the other hand, leucovorin does not enter and rescue epidermoid cancers of the head and neck because these tumors lack transport sites.

Response durations to MTX are comparatively short-lived because of development resistance to the drug. Mechanisms of resistance to MTX include decreased transport of the drug across cell membranes; amplification of the gene for dihydrofolate reductase (gene amplification results in more copies of the gene and thus the enzyme, and increased enzyme level results in decreased inhibition by MTX); and decreased formulation of polyglutamates, which results in decreased inhibition of DNA synthesis. A better understanding of the mechanisms of drug resistance will perhaps lead to better therapy. Trimetrexate is a lipid-soluble quinazoline analog of MTX. It was synthesized with a view to circumvent resistance because of defective transport of MTX. However, in a phase III study in head and neck cancers, it was not superior to MTX in efficacy.

The main side effects of MTX, when given weekly or biweekly, include bone marrow suppression, stomatitis, mucositis, and sometimes nausea, vomiting, and diarrhea. Sometimes unexpected and apparently sudden severe toxicity from the drug can occur, and the factors underlying this unusual host response are not known. Low serum and red blood folate in some patients may be responsible for these reactions. Because MTX is excreted by the kidneys, dehydration and impaired creatinine clearance may potentiate drug toxicity. MTX, when given orally, is absorbed slowly and erratically.

Pharmacology and Toxicity of High-Dose MTX (HDMTX)

Although the combination of MTX and leucovorin has been used clinically for more than a decade, factors such as the optimal time of MTX infusion and the timing and dose of leucovorin required to prevent MTX toxicity have been defined poorly. Because fatal gastrointestinal toxicity develops in mice exposed to inhibitive concentrations of MTX for longer than 48 hours, leucovorin should be given within 42 hours from the onset of infusion.

Nephrotoxicity remains the principal limiting factor of HDMTX therapy. Administration of this therapy often causes an increase in serum creatinine and a decrease in creatine clearance. High-dose MTX is not myelosuppressive, a feature that permits its combination with other bone marrow suppressive agents. Bone marrow suppression and nephrotoxicity sometimes occur, however. Other side effects of this therapy include nausea, occasional violent vomiting, diarrhea, and, on rare occasions, cutaneous vasculitis and pneumonitis. Therefore, HDMTX should be given in an institution where appropriate supportive measures are available.

The overall response rate to moderate- to high-dose MTX is higher than that for conventional doses of MTX (approximately 50% versus 30% respectively). The numbers of complete responders and response durations are not greatly improved, however. Four prospective randomized studies comparing conventional-dose with moderate- and HDMTX show no statistically significant differences in response rates.

Thus, there is no evidence that HDMTX improves survival over that of standard-dose MTX. Therefore, the use of HDMTX, because of its potential high morbidity and cost, should probably be relegated to a clinical trial setting.

5-Fluorouracil (5-FU)

5-FU and its deoxynucleoside, 5-fluoro-2'deoxyuridine (5-FUdR), are both prodrugs that require intracellular metabolism for cytotoxicity. Three different targets are affected by these fluoropyrimidines. The metabolite of 5-FU, 5-FdUMP, forms a stable complex with thymidylate synthetase, inhibiting de novo thymidylate synthesis and thus causing cell death by thymidine starvation. Further, 5-FU may induce DNA damage by two distinct mechanisms: fraudulently being incorporated into DNA, causing DNA fragmentation and cell death, and inhibiting DNA repair. The degree of inhibition of thymidylate synthetase can be augmented by exogenous folates. This forms the basis for using leucovorin with 5-FU. Metabolites of 5-FU can also be incorporated into RNA to affect its maturation or function. The combination of 5-FU and cisplatin is being used increasingly in induction therapy of head and neck cancers.

Cisplatin, and Other Platinum Analogs

The antitumor properties of cisplatin (P) were identified by Rosenberg and his colleagues, stirring new enthusiasm in the treatment of advanced head and neck cancer. A major attraction of cisplatin is its lack of hematologic toxicity. Earlier, however, its use resulted in significant nephrotoxicity. Patients should not receive cisplatin unless their kidney functions are adequate. Adequate saline hydration with mannitol infusion prevents cisplatin-induced nephrotoxicity. An overall response rate of approximately 30% with a small number of complete remissions has been reported in most of the studies with cisplatin. The duration of remissions is approximately 4 months for partial remitters, and 6 to 8 months for complete responders. A randomized trial using high-dose (120 mg/M^2) or a low-dose (60 mg/M^2) of cisplatin showed that response rates were 16.1% and 17.7%, respectively. Thus 80 to 120 mg/M^2 of cisplatin given IV with mannitol diuresis and appropriate antiemetics is an acceptable regimen. Its major side effects include nausea and vomiting (partially ameliorated by newer antiemetics such as ondansetron, metochlorpromide) nephro- and ototoxicity, mild myelosuppression, or peripheral neuropathy and, in chronic dosage, hypomagnesemia. Other platinum derivatives have also received considerable attention. Carboplatin appears to be active, with 25% response rate, whereas iproplatin has no activity.

Bleomycin (BLM)

As a single agent, this drug appears less effective than MTX, but probably differences in trial design preclude meaningful comparisons in nonrandomized studies. The response rates to BLM vary (6 to 45%). Predominant side effects of this agent include mucositis and dose-dependent interstitial pulmonary fibrosis. It is recommended that BLM should not be given over an accumulated dose of 200 mg/M^2. An attractive feature of this drug is its lack of myelosuppression, making it suitable for combination chemotherapy.

Taxol (Paclitaxel)

This agent represents the first of a new class of antineoplastics that has activity in head and neck cancer. It is obtained from the bark of the Pacific Yew taxus brevifolia, and has a unique mechanism of action on the microtubules. Taxol binds preferentially to microtubules. The initial scarcity of the drug has been eliminated by newer techniques such as semisynthesis of the compound and harvesting of needles of the tree.

This drug, which is active in breast, ovarian, and lung cancers, achieves responses in 40% of the patients with advanced head and neck cancer. It is usually administered over a period of 24 hours by continuous infusion to avoid hypersensitivity reactions such as bradycardia and hypotension. The latter usually is eliminated by pretreatment with corticosteriods, H2 blockers, and benadryl. The other toxicities include alopecia, myelosuppression, and peripheral neuropathy. At higher dosages, support with growth factors such as growth–colony-stimulating factor (G-CSF) is necessary. A related drug known as taxotere is active in this disease. Currently, randomized trials are evaluating the role of paclitaxel when added to cisplatin in the treatment of advanced head and neck cancers.

Other Chemotherapeutic Agents

As shown in Table 34–1, although the data are limited, cyclophosphamide (CTX), vinblastine, and hydroxyurea also have some activity in these tumors. Cyclophosphamide is an alkylating agent that acts on nonreplicating and replicating cells. The drug has no antineoplastic action in vitro. Activation of CTX occurs primarily in the liver. The drug can be given intravenously or orally. The common toxic effects of the drug include nausea, alopecia, bone marrow suppression, and hemorrhagic cystitis. This drug has considerable activity in the head and neck tumors, and trials should be undertaken to assess its value in combination chemotherapy.

Vinblastine, derived from vinca alkaloids, acts on the mitotic phase of the replicating cells. The drug probably combines with tubulin, a protein required for metaphasic spindle formation. Unlike its congener vincristine, vinblastine is myelosuppressive, but less neurotoxic. Hydroxyurea is a radiomimetic agent, and its use is discussed later. Doxorubicin, a broad-based antitumor agent, gave only a 16% response rate in all but one study. This drug causes bone marrow suppression and has dose-limiting cardiotoxicity. 13-cis-retinoic acid has modest activity (15% response rate) and is being evaluated singly or in combination with α-interferon in the treatment and prevention of head and neck tumors.

COMBINATION CHEMOTHERAPY

Combinations Without Cisplatin

Combination chemotherapy has been successful in treating hematologic, testicular, and ovarian cancers. In head and neck cancers, combination chemotherapy is being used with some success. An extensive review of this literature suggests that only combinations that contain MTX and BLM, with or without cisplatin, have any relevance in this disease.

Several two-drug combinations using both BLM and MTX have been reported, but the superiority of any of these treatments over the two agents given alone has not been demonstrated clearly. Similarly, a number of other chemotherapeutic agents added to the BLM and MTX therapy have been reported to produce a response rate from 13 to 100% with median remission durations of 2 to 6 months. Table 34–2 summarizes the results of some of these studies.

Combinations have been designed on the principles of biochemical pharmacology and tumor cell kinetics. In these studies, the complete response rate and the duration of response were not significantly improved by any of these combinations.

TABLE 34–2. Combination Chemotherapy Regimens That Achieved at Least a 50% Remission Rate

Author	Drugs	No. of Responses/ No. of Patients	% Response
Amer	BLM + VCR + CTX	8/14	57
Cortes	BLM + CTX + MTX + 5-FU	22/40	55
Holoye	BLM + VCR + CTX + MTX + 5-FU	11/20	50
Holoye	BLM + CTX + MTX + 5-FU	13/22	59
Auersberg	BLM + VCR + MTX	19/38	50
Price	BLM + VCR + MTX	43/68	63
Reg. A	LV + 5-FU + Steroids		
Price	BLM + 5-FU + MTX + LV	14/17	82
Reg. B	Doxo + 5-FU + Steroids		
Rowland KM	DDP, 5-FU	18/34	53
Forastiere AA	Carboplatin + 5-FU	14/28	50
Vogl SV	MTX, 5-FU, Bleo, DDP	23/46	50

Combinations That Contain Cisplatin in Advanced Disease

Bleomycin and cisplatin have been combined in a variety of schedules. In patients with prior exposure to chemotherapy, the response rate is low. The two nephrotoxic agents, cisplatin and MTX, have also been combined in a schedule to preclude nephrotoxicity. In this regimen, MTX was given on days 1 and 15, BLM on days 1, 8, and 15, with cisplatin on day 4 of every 3-week cycle. Workers at Wayne State University have shown a high response rate with 5-FU infusion concurrent with allopurinol followed by high-dose cisplatin. In two nonrandomized pilot studies, bolus injection of 5-FU inferior results compared with those of continuous-infusion therapy. The studies also indicate that altering the combination of cisplatin and 5-FU by substituting carboplatin for cisplatin did not affect activity, whereas substituting doxorubicin, mitoguazone, or etoposide for 5-FU reduced response rates.

Attempts have also been made to increase the effectiveness of chemotherapy by altering combination chemotherapy to prevent emergence of drug resistance. In one study, courses one, three, and five were given with 5-FU and cisplatin, and courses two and four consisted of weekly doses of HDMTX followed by 5-FU + leucovorin. Twenty-one of 46 entered patients (46%) achieved complete remission. Unfortunately, considerable myelosuppression, mucositis, and skin toxicity developed, and 15 patients dropped out of the study.

Several investigators have compared single versus combination chemotherapy. Some of these studies are shown in Table 34–3. Combination chemotherapy with cisplatin produced higher response rates and significantly more complete remissions. In two studies, combination chemotherapy with 5-FU and cisplatin as compared with MTX resulted in significantly higher response rates. The combined therapy with 5-FU and cisplatin was also superior in producing response rates when compared with cisplatin or infusional 5-FU given

alone. However, overall, no difference existed in the median survival, although 40% of patients treated with combination were alive at 9 months of follow-up, as compared with 24% of patients given cisplatin and 27% patients given 5-FU.

From the variety of clinical studies summarized in the preceding text, head and neck cancer is responsive to multiple agents that differ in their biochemical actions and toxicity. Combination chemotherapy may produce a higher remission rate, although its effect on survival in advanced head and neck cancer has not been established. Such combination therapy, however, may have a major role in combined modality approach, which is discussed later.

INTRA-ARTERIAL CHEMOTHERAPY (IA)

It was postulated that administration of anticancer agents by the IA route, resulting in high local concentration and/or long exposure of the tumor to the drug, would improve the rate as well as the duration of response. Furthermore, by systemic administration of metabolic products of chemotherapeutically inhibited reaction, the drug toxicity could be minimized. Use of IA MTX with systemic leucovorin is based on these considerations. Although these methods have improved the response rates somewhat (overall 53% with MTX), the responses were not long-lasting. Four centers have reported IA cisplatin as a single drug with high overall response rate with complete remission rates in approximately 30% of the patients.

In the past, faulty placement of catheters, major problems of bleeding, and embolization have plagued IA therapy. Improved techniques of transfemoral catheterization and a 2-hour infusion may reduce potential vascular catastrophes. One must be cautious in this approach, however, because in the past, improved results with IA MTX were related possibly to selection of low-risk patients.

TABLE 34–3. Selected Randomized Trials with Cisplatin-Based Combination Chemotherapy

Author	Agents	Response Rate %	Complete Response %
Abele	MTX, BLM, hydroxyurea	27	3
	vs MTX, BLM, hydroxyurea + P	66	17
Cabel	ABO	28	5
	vs PABO	50	16
Vogl	MTX	35	8
	vs MTX, BLM + P	48	16
Liverpool	P vs MTX	14 vs 6 vs	
	vs P + 5-FU, vs P + MTX	12 vs 11	
Forastiere	P + 5-FU	32 vs	6 vs
	vs C + 5-FU vs MTX	21 vs 10	2 vs 2

ABO = methotrexate, bleomycin, vincristine; PABO = cisplatin, methotrexate, bleomycin, vincristine; P = cisplatin; C = carboplatin.

In conclusion, at present, IA chemotherapy should be given only by an experienced team, preferably as part of a controlled trial. Its general use does not seem indicated.

MULTIDISCIPLINARY APPROACH

Patients should be seen by an oral assessment team to evaluate the status of their oral mucosa and teeth. Patients who receive combination chemotherapy often develop significant mucositis; appropriate management by this team, with dental extractions if necessary, and use of oral antibiotics and antifungal agents, may prevent some oral complications of therapy.

Chemotherapy Combined with Surgery

Combined chemotherapy and surgery can be combined in two different ways. Chemotherapy may be used before surgery. The second approach is to use post-therapy adjuvant therapy to eradicate micrometastasis.

Sufficient theoretical reasons exist to combine chemotherapy with surgery. Preoperative chemotherapy reduces tumor size and facilitates subsequent operation. This may improve overall survival. Another advantage could be to minimize the extent of surgery. Postoperative therapy may destroy malignant cells that exist beyond resection margins or that have already metastasized to distant sites. Some potential disadvantages of a combined modality approach exist. Use of chemotherapy may delay definitive surgery or radiation. Should a tumor prove resistant to the drug, further tumor growth may occur. The antineoplastic therapy may cause leukopenia, resulting in postoperative wound infections or a delay in healing. Before beginning chemotherapy, the patient must be seen by the head and neck surgeon and/or radiation therapist and the extent of the tumor appropriately marked on the skin or otherwise documented. Otherwise, the surgeon may have difficulty finding the original margins of the tumor, resulting in less than optimal resection.

The group at the National Cancer Institute treated 30 consecutive patients with head and neck tumors preoperatively with 36-hour infusion of HDMTX. Twenty-three of these patients responded, and their disease-free survival rate was superior to that of similar patients treated at the same institution without preoperative chemotherapy. Others have used IM MTX with systemic leucovorin along with operative treatment. Hong and associates used a similar regimen and described a 76% response rate, with 20% complete remissions. In 14 patients who initially had inoperable disease, the tumor became operable after chemotherapy. Ibeus and associates pretreated 22 patients with cisplatin followed by BLM infusion and MTX. These and other studies indicate that advanced squamous cell carcinoma of the head and neck can be debulked effectively with appropriate pretreatment chemotherapy. Patients who exhibit complete response to chemotherapy have a better prognosis than patients who do not respond. This observation, though, does not establish that chemotherapy is responsible for better results because patients who are responsive to chemotherapy may have an intrinsically favorable course. All of these are pilot studies and controlled trials will be necessary to determine the ultimate effect on the survival (Table 34–4).

The result of six controlled trials of neoadjuvant (induction) chemotherapy have been published in full-length papers and abstracts. In a large randomized trial, 462 patients with resectable stage III and IV cancers were assigned randomly to induction chemotherapy with a single course of cisplatin and BLM, followed by either standard treatment or standard treatment followed by maintenance chemotherapy with six cycles of monthly cisplatin, or standard treatment only. At median follow-up of 61 months, overall survival and disease-free survival were no different among the three groups. Distant relapse rates were reduced for patients randomized to maintenance chemotherapy. This needs to be evaluated further, but the response rates in this

TABLE 34–4. Selected Induction Chemotherapy Regimens for Advanced Head and Neck Cancers (Neoadjuvant Therapy)

Author	Drugs	No. of Patients	Response Rate (%)
Al-Sarraf	DLM, cisplatin, VCR	77	79
Cognetti	MTX, cisplatin, BLM, VCR	123	63.4
Elias	Cisplatin + VBLM + MTX + LV	22	73
Ervin	BLM + cisplatin + MTX + LV	114	78
Glick	Cisplatin + BLM	29	48
Hong	Cisplatin + BLM	58	72
Kirkwood	MTX + LV	21	52
Kish	5-FU + cisplatin	26	87.5
Randolph	BLM + cisplatin	21	71
Tarpley	MTX + LV	33	77

study were low, at 37%. Whether a minimum of three cycles of induction chemotherapy should have been given, as others have done, also needs to be studied. Critical analyses of other neoadjuvant trials indicate major deficiencies because treatments were given with either one or two cycles of a noncisplatin-containing regimen, or else the definitive therapy with radiation or follow-up was inadequate.

To summarize, to date, no trial has demonstrated improved survival as a result of induction or adjuvant chemotherapy. Such a therapy reduces distant metastasis, but local or regional failure rates are not changed. Newer, more aggressive induction regimens have been introduced, but their impact on survival is unknown.

Combined Radiation and Chemotherapy

Some of the reasons for combining chemotherapy with radiation are similar to those for integrating surgery and drugs. These include the following: 1) reduction in the tumor cell mass, thereby facilitating more effective radiation therapy. (The center of the tumor contains hypoxic cells, and conventional radiotherapy is ineffective in the absence of oxygen. Reduction in tumor cell mass would result in a smaller number of hypoxic cells.); 2) control of distant metastasis; and 3) modification of the DNA molecule by drugs, resulting in sensitization of the cell to subsequent radiation.

Many drugs can increase radiation-induced damage, but often such effects are accomplished at the expense of greater damage to normal tissues. Besides chemotherapeutic drugs, other agents, such as nitroimidazoles, also increase the sensitivity of the tissues to radiation. Ideally, these radiosensitizers distribute themselves in a greater concentration in the tumor cells than in the surrounding normal tissues. This would provide the best ground work for increased selective tumor destruction. Nitroimidazoles produce neurotoxicity and, so far, results combining radiation with these agents have not been encouraging. A large number of chemotherapeutic agents have been used in conjunction with radiation, but a detailed analysis of these studies is beyond the scope of this text. A brief overview of the results, however, will be considered.

Several agents such as hydroxyurea, 5-FU, and MTX singly have been used with radiation. Although initial studies showed beneficial effects in combining hydroxyurea with radiation, randomized studies did not confirm this advantage. Similarly, studies of the Radiation Therapy Oncology Group in 712 patients showed improved local control and disease-free survival, but no prolongation of survival in patients given MTX with radiation and those given radiation only. Further, this combination produced increased mucositis. In an earlier randomized study, however, 5-FU IV, in conjunction with radiation, produced improved survival in patients with oral cavity and oropharyngeal lesions.

In a randomized study, Fu et al. used BLM (5 U IV twice weekly) during radiation therapy, followed by BLM, 15 U IV, and MTX weekly for 16 weeks after completion of radiation therapy. The complete response (CR) rate was 67% in the combined modality group, but the survival curves were not different. In another study, patients were randomized to radiation or radiation + mitomycin-C, 15 m/M^2 on day 5. At 60 months, disease-free survival was significantly better (75%) in patients who received combination therapy than in those who received radiation alone (55%).

Concomitant administration of cisplatin and radiotherapy in patients with locally advanced and inoperable tumors of the head and neck led to a 69% CR rate. A similar approach with a different schedule resulted in 98% local and regional control, with persistence of the control in 87% of the patients at a minimum follow-up of 24 months. Several investigators have used cisplatin and 5-FU with radiation in various schedules and dosages.

Toxicity is increased because of the combined treatments, and radiation may have to be interrupted. Such interruptions in radiation delivery produce decreased response rates. Three published trials have randomized patients into either concomitant radiation and combination chemotherapy or induction chemotherapy (using the same drugs) followed by radiation. The group receiving concomitant therapy had a better disease-free and overall survival. Merlano and colleagues from Italy reported a study with stage III and IV disease in which patients were randomized to either radiation of three, 2-week courses with chemotherapy or radiation alone. The complete response rate in combined group was 42%, as compared with 22% in those with radiation alone. Median survival increased by 5 months in the combined group.

In summary, randomized clinical trials have shown modest survival benefits by combining chemotherapy such as 5-FU used singly or in combination with cisplatin and radiation. However, local failure rates remain high, and more research is needed to improve local and regional control of tumor.

ORGAN PRESERVATION

A major goal of combined chemotherapy and radiation is to decrease morbidity. The organs in the head and neck area are of paramount importance for normal daily function, and therefore organ preservation has assumed an important role. An emerging concept not only in the chemotherapy of cancer, but also in all of cancer treatment is the impact that the disease and/or treatment may have on the quality of life. The case in point is that of laryngeal preservation by substituting combined radiation and chemotherapy for laryngectomy. In a large randomized trial, laryngeal preservation was feasible in 64% of the patients who received induction chemotherapy with 5-FU and cisplatin followed by radiation therapy. Because radiation alone was not used as one of the treatment arms, the trial is being repeated at this time. This and other organ preservation studies at other sites of head and neck cancer are currently under investigation.[1]

TREATMENT OF OTHER RARE TUMORS OF THE HEAD AND NECK

Salivary Gland Tumors

These tumors are treated with surgery and radiation. The most active agents used in the treatment of salivary gland tumors are MTX, 5-FU, doxorubicin, cyclophosphamide, and cisplatin. A combination of these drugs produces palliative results. Adenoid cystic carcinomas are rare, but respond to doxorubicin or mitoxantrone.

Nasopharyngeal and Paranasal Sinus Carcinoma

Surgery of these tumors is usually difficult. Traditionally, these tumors are treated with radiation, but systemic relapses are common. Induction chemotherapy with a combination of cisplatin, BLM, 5-FU, and MTX with leucovorin, in patients with stage III and IV disease, produced a 75% response rate. With radiation, a 2-year failure-free survival of 57% was achieved. Paranasal sinus tumors show a response to cisplatin with 5-FU infusion.

Prevention

Head and neck cancers are caused primarily by smoking and chewing tobacco. Primary prevention, therefore, continues to be of paramount importance. Patients with head and neck cancer who continue to smoke during radiation therapy have a lower response rate and survival than those patients who quit, even at that stage. Second primary cancer develops at an annual rate of 3 to 7% in patients with head and neck cancers that are treated successfully with surgery or radiation. Strategies have been devised to prevent the second primary cancers by administration of chemicals that suppress carcinogenesis, and thus prevent invasive cancer. This strategy, known as chemoprevention, has assumed great importance in recent years.

Leukoplakia is the usual premalignant lesion of the head and neck cancer. Several studies have examined the ability of synthetic (such as 13-cis-retinoic acid) and natural retinoids in reversing leukoplakia. Initial studies indicated a high response rate, but also a rapid relapse when therapy is stopped. Multiple trials are un-

derway with either reduced dosages of 13-cis-retinoic acid or with longer duration of therapy to prevent invasive cancer in patients with leukoplakia.

High-dose 13-cis-retinoic acid reduces the development of second cancer after treatment of primary head and neck tumors. A large randomized study is underway to evaluate the role of retinoids in secondary prevention in this disease.

CHEMOTHERAPY COMBINED WITH IMMUNOTHERAPY AND HYPERTHERMIA

Cancer immunobiology is discussed in Chapter 35. The tumor-related host immunosuppression is further accentuated by chemotherapeutic drugs. Because patients with head and neck tumors often have a defect in their cell-mediated immunity, several biologic response modifiers, such as levamisole, thymosine and its subfractions, autologous tumor cell vaccines, interferon, and interleukin are being evaluated with or without chemotherapy. To date, with the exception of interferon, none of these agents have shown significant antitumor effects. Interferon alone or in combination with 13-cis-retinoic acid or 5-FU is being evaluated.

Hypoxic cells, often present in head and neck tumors, are particularly resistant to cell killing by radiation. Hyperthermia is effective against hypoxic cells. Hyperthermia induced by focused ultrasound, radiofrequency or microwave has been evaluated in patients with head and neck tumors. Experimental evidence indicates that chemotherapeutic agents such as cisplatin or BLM may be synergistic with hyperthermia. In a randomized study, Arcangeli et al. showed that a combination of radiation and hyperthermia gave a 79% complete response rate, versus 42% for the lesions treated with radiotherapy alone. However, more studies are needed.

SUMMARY AND CONCLUDING REMARKS

In summary, induction chemotherapy may play a major role in the management of advanced head and neck cancers. The role of chemotherapy in recurrent head and neck cancer is modest. The side effects of the chemotherapeutic agent, particularly nausea and vomiting, can be ameliorated to a great extent by the use of antiemetics such as lorazepam, serotonin antagonists, corticosteroids, phenothiazines, and synthetic cannabinoids. Neutropenia can be reversed by colony stimulating factors such as G-CSF. Chemical modulation, such as use of 5-FU + leucovorin, may play an increasing role in improving therapeutic response of these tumors. Understanding of drug resistance, e.g., de novo or acquired, has improved in recent years.

Defective transport of drugs, gene amplification of target enzymes, defective metabolism of prodrug to active metabolites, increased drug inactivation, altered DNA repair, altered targets, and expression of multidrug resistant gene complex are some of the mechanisms important in chemotherapy.

In patients with stage IV carcinoma of the head and neck, significant palliation can be achieved by chemotherapy; however, a cure for patients with advanced recurrent head and neck tumors is still not possible. A better understanding of the mechanisms of drug resistance is forthcoming, and may improve our ability to treat these patients. The role of chemotherapy may be in combination with surgery and radiation. Tumors of certain specific sites (oral cavity) may benefit from adjuvant chemotherapy. Chemotherapy administered before radiation and/or surgery may significantly improve the response rate. Whether this improvement translates into longer survival remains to be seen. Trimodality treatments with cisplatin, radiation, and hyperthermia may further improve local control rate, but if improved local control can be obtained, systemic disease will continue to be an ever-increasing challenge.

In patients with head and neck tumors, malnutrition is a significant factor in the outcome of therapy. Chemotherapy may further aggravate this problem. Poor nutrition leads to immunosuppression, which may lead to tumor enhancement. Chapter 33 discusses at length the role of nutrition in the head and neck patient.

Cancer is a genetic disease and its genesis is controlled by dysregulation of oncogenes and tumor suppressor genes. Cytogenetic and molecular analysis of the head and neck cancers have shown chromosomal changes in regions of 1p22 and 11q13 and amplifications or mutations in *Ras, c-myc,* and p53 genes. This line of inquiry opens up the possibility of developing specific genetically directed therapies in head and neck cancers.

SUGGESTED READINGS

Bowman GP, Wong G, Hodson I, et al: Influence of cigarette smoking on the efficacy of radiation therapy in head and neck cancer. N Engl J Med *328*:159–63, 1993.

Decker J, Goldstein JC: Risk factors in head and neck cancer. N Engl J Med *306*:1151, 1982.

Field JK: Oncogenes and tumour-suppressor genes in squamous cell carcinoma of the head and neck. Oral Oncol, Eur J Cancer *28B*(1):67–76, 1992.

Khandekar JD, Lawrence GA: Fundamentals in Cancer Management. Niles, IL, Mel Publishers, Inc., 1982.

Lippman SM, Batsakis JG, Toth BB, et al: Comparison of low-dose isotretinoin with beta carotene to prevent oral carcinogenesis. N Engl J Med *328*:15–20, 1993.

MacComb W, Fletcher G: Cancer of the Head and Neck. Baltimore, Williams & Wilkins, 1967.

Rosenberg B, Van Camp L, Krigas T: Inhibition of cell division in

Escherichia Coli by electrolysis products from a platinum electrode. Nature *205*:698–699, 1965.

Schantz SP, Harrison LB, Hong WK: Cancer: Principles and Practice of Oncology, 4th Ed. Edited by DeVita VT, Hellman S, and Rosenberg SA. Philadelphia, JB Lippincott Co., 1994, pp. 574–654.

Schuller DE: Do otolaryngologist head and neck surgeons and/or chemotherapy have a role in the treatment of head and neck cancer. Arch Otolaryngol Head Neck Surg *117*:498–50, 1991.

Tepperman BS, Fitzpatrick PJ: Second respiratory and upper digestive tract cancers after oral cancer. Lancet *2*:547, 1981.

Vokes EE: Head and neck cancer. Semin Oncol *21*:No.3, 1994.

Vokes EE, Weichselbaum RR, Lippman SM, Hong WK. Head and neck cancer. N Engl J Med *328*:184–94, 1993.

Mechanism of Action and Toxicity of Antineoplastic Agents

Chabner B, Collins JM: Cancer Chemotherapy, Principles and Practice. Philadelphia, JB Lippincott Co., 1990.

DeVita VT: Principles of chemotherapy. Cancer: Principles and Practice of Oncology, 4th Ed. Edited by DeVita VT, et al. Philadelphia, JB Lippincott Co., 1994, pp. 276–292.

Khandekar JD, Lawrence GA: Fundamentals in Cancer Management. Niles, IL, Mel Publishers, Inc., 1982, pp. 75–99.

Adjuvant Chemotherapy

Fazekas JT, Sommer C, Kramer S: Adjuvant intravenous methotrexate or definitive radiotherapy alone for advanced squamous cancers of the oral cavity, oropharynx, supraglottic larynx, or hypopharynx. Int J Radiat Oncol Biol Phys *6*:533, 1980.

Frei E, Canellos GP: Dose: a critical factor in cancer chemotherapy. Am J Med *69*:585, 1980.

Glick JH, Taylor SG: Integration of chemotherapy into a combined modality treatment plan for head and neck cancers: A review. J Radiat Oncol Biol Phys *7*:229, 1980.

Schebel FM: Rationale for adjuvant chemotherapy. Cancer *3*:2875, 1977.

Combination Chemotherapy

Abele R, Honegger HP, Grossebacher R, et al: A randomized study of methotrexate, bleomycin, hydroxyurea with versus without cisplatin in patients with previously untreated and recurrent squamous cell carcinoma of the head and neck. Eur J Clin Oncol *23*:47, 1987.

Amrein P: Current chemotherapy of head and neck cancer. J Oral Maxillofac Surg *49*:864–70, 1991.

Clavel M, Cognetti F, Dodion P, et al: Combination chemotherapy with methotrexate, bleomycin, and vincristine with or without cisplatin in advanced squamous cell carcinoma of the head and neck. Cancer *60*:1173, 1987.

Golde JH, Coldman AJ, Gudauskas JA: Rationale for use of alternative non-cross resistant chemotherapy. Cancer Treat Rep *626*:439, 1982.

Kish J, Ensley J, Jacobs, et al: A randomized trial of cisplatin (CACP) + 5-fluorouracil (5-FU) infusion and CACP + 5-FU bolus for recurrent and advanced squamous cell carcinoma of the head and neck. Cancer *56*:227, 1985.

Stell PM, et al: The Liverpool Head and Neck Oncology Group: A phase III randomized trial of cisplatinum, methotrexate, cisplatinum + methotrexate, and cisplatin + 5-FU in end stage squamous carcinoma of the head and neck. Br J Cancer *61*:311–315, 1990.

Biology of Head and Neck Cancer

Decker J, Goldstein JC: Risk factors in head and neck cancer. N Engl J Med *306*:1151, 1982.

Millar D: The etiology of nasopharyngeal cancer and its management. Otolaryngol Clin North Am 13:467, 1982.

VanRensburg SJ: Epidemiologic and dietary evidence on specific nutritional disposition of esophageal cancer. Natl Cancer Inst Monogr 67:243, 1981.

Chemotherapy for Head and Neck Cancer

Clark JR: Induction chemotherapy for advanced head and neck cancer. Important Adv Oncol 3:23, 1987.

Khandekar JD, DeWys WD: Chemoimmunotherapy of head and neck cancer. Am J Surg 135:688, 1978.

Kirkwood JM, Canellos GP, Ervin TJ, et al: Increased therapeutic index using moderate dose MTX and leucovorin twice weekly vs. weekly high-dose MTX-leucovorin in patients with advanced squamous carcinoma of the head and neck: A safe new effective regimen. Cancer 47(10):2414, 1981.

Muggia FM, Rozencweig M, Louis AE: Role of chemotherapy in head and neck cancer: Systemic use of single agents and combinations in advanced disease. Head Neck Surg 2:196, 1980.

Veronesi A, Zagonel V, Tirelli U, et al: High-dose versus low-dose cisplatin in head and neck carcinoma: A randomized study. J Clin Oncol 3:1105, 1985.

Woods RL, Rox RM, Tattersall MHN: Methotrexate treatment of squamous cell head and neck cancers: Dose response evaluation. Br Med J 282:600, 1981.

Intra-Arterial Chemotherapy

Baker SR, Forastiere A, Wheeler R, et al: Intra-arterial chemotherapy for head and neck cancer—An update on the totally implantable infusion pump. Arch Otolaryngol Head Neck Surg 113:1183, 1987.

Collins JM: Pharmacologic rationale for regional drug delivery. J Clin Oncol 2:498, 1984.

Mortimer JE, Taylor ME, Schulman S, et al: Feasibility and efficacy of inter-arterial cisplatin in locally advanced (stage III and IV) head and neck cancers. J Clin Oncol 6:969, 1988.

Schuller DE, Wilson HE, Smith RE, et al: Preoperative reductive chemotherapy for locally advanced carcinoma of the oral cavity, oropharynx, and hypopharynx. Cancer 51:15, 1983.

Combination Chemotherapy, Radiation, and/or Surgery

Al-Sarraf M, Pajak TF, Marcial VA, et al: Concurrent radiotherapy and chemotherapy with cisplatin in inoperable squamous cell carcinoma of the head and neck. An RTOG study. Cancer 59:259, 1987.

Clark JR, Fallon BG, Chaffey JT, et al: Nasopharyngeal carcinoma: The Dana-Farber Cancer Institute experience with 24 patients treated with induction chemotherapy and radiotherapy. Ann Otol Rhinol Laryngol 96:608, 1987.

Fu KK, Phillips TL, Silverberg IJ, et al: Combined radiotherapy and chemotherapy with bleomycin and methotrexate for advanced inoperable head and neck cancer. An update of a Northern California Oncology Group randomized trial. J Clin Oncol 5:1410, 1987.

Merlano M, Vitale V, Rosso R, et al: Treatment of advanced squamous-cell carcinoma of the head and neck with alternating chemotherapy and radiotherapy. N Engl J Med 327:1115–21, 1992.

Murthy AK, Taylor SG, Showel J, et al: Treatment of advanced head and neck cancer with concomitant radiation and chemotherapy. Int J. Radiat Oncol Biol Phys 13:1807, 1987.

Peppard SB, Al-Sarraf M, Powers WE, et al: Combination of cisplatinum (cisplatin) vincristine (oncovin) and bleomycin (COB) prior to surgery and/or radiotherapy in advanced untreated epidermoid cancer of the head and neck. Laryngoscope 90:1273, 1980.

Richards GJ, Chambers RG: Hydroxyurea in the treatment of neoplasms of the head and neck: A resurvey. Am J Surg 126:513, 1973.

Sartorelli AC: Therapeutic attack on hypoxic cells of solid tumors: Presidential address. Cancer Res 48:775, 1988.

Vogl SE, Lerner H, Kaplan BH, et al: Failure of effective initial chemotherapy to modify the course of stage IV (MO) squamous cancer of the head and neck. Cancer 50:840, 1982.

Vogler WR, et al: Methotrexate therapy with or without citrovorum factor in carcinoma of the head and neck, breast, and colon. Cancer Clin Trials 2:227, 1979.

Wolf GT, Howly WK, Fisher SG: The Department of Veterans Affairs Laryngeal Cancer Study Group: Induction chemotherapy plus radiation compared with surgery plus radiation in patients with advanced laryngeal cancer. N Engl J Med 324:1685–90, 1991.

Chemoimmunotherapy, Hyperthermia, and Radiation Sensitizers

Arcangeli G, Benassi M, Cividalli A, et al: Radiotherapy and hyperthermia: Analysis of clinical results and identification of prognostic variables. Cancer 60:950, 1987.

Coleman CN, Bump EF, Kramer RA: Chemical modifiers of cancer treatment. J Clin Oncol 6:6709, 1988.

Herman TS, Teicher BA, Jochelson M, et al: Rationale for use of local hyperthermia with radiation therapy and selected anticancer drugs. Int J Hyperthermia 4:143, 1988.

35 Cancer Immunology

Ray O. Gustafson and H. Bryan Neel, III

At the beginning of the twentieth century, microbiologists established the foundation for the science of immunology and descriptions of the development of host resistance to infectious disease. As a logical extension, the field of tumor immunology grew out of speculation that immune mechanisms might be involved in host defense against malignant disease.

In the laboratory, when biologists harvested tumor tissue from one animal and attempted to propagate it in a second animal, the tumor transplant was rejected quickly. This phenomenon stimulated intense interest and investigation, but the nascent field of tumor immunology was arrested in the 1930s with the demonstration that rejection of transplanted tumors was simply a manifestation of the general phenomenon of rejection of foreign tissues. Although this observation led to the study of major histocompatibility complexes, formed the basis for organ transplantation, and resulted in the discovery of cell-mediated cytotoxicity, it dampened the search for an immunologic basis for tumor resistance for many years.

Renewed interest in the field of tumor immunology arose in the 1940s and 1950s from the work of Gross,[1] Foley,[2] Prehn and Main,[3] and Klein et al[4] after the development of highly inbred (syngeneic) strains of mice. In experiments using the chemical carcinogen methylcholanthrene (MCA) to induce murine sarcomas, these investigators conclusively demonstrated the ability of tumors to elicit a tumor-specific immune response.

As outlined in a review by Ritts and Neel,[5] resistance to subsequent transplantation of grafts of the same tumor could be induced by tumor excision or amputation, use of subtake tumor dose or cells that had been damaged irreversibly in their reproductive capacity by irradiation or chemicals, or necrosis in situ by ligation release,[6,7] cryosurgery,[8-11] or electrocoagulation. In a series of classic experiments, mice from which tumors had been excised showed a reduced rate of growth at the challenge site compared with that of controls, indicating existence of immunity after excision. Mice from which tumors had been eradicated in situ by cryosurgery, ligation release, or electrocoagulation showed a reduced rate of tumor take and growth at the challenge site compared with controls and with mice subjected to tumor excision, indicating even greater immunity after necrosis of tumor in situ. The pattern of differential immunity is consistently seen after challenge with graded doses of tumor cells and in other tumor-host systems.[12]

All of these experiments strongly suggested that tumor cells must express unique surface determinants that can be recognized by the immune system as nonself, and these determinants were termed "tumor-specific antigens (TSA)." Tumor immunologists subsequently have been concerned with the identification and characterization of tumor-associated antigens, processing and presentation of tumor-associated antigens, subsequent humoral and cellular immune responses, and manipulation of the immune system in the diagnosis and therapy of malignant disease. A thorough understanding of the basic science of immunology is a prerequisite for the study of cancer immunology, and the reader is referred to Chapter 4.

SIGNIFICANCE OF THE IMMUNE RESPONSE

Although tumor immunology is a young field, it has stimulated a great deal of research, and yet the actual clinical significance of the immune response to malignant disease remains unclear. In 1959, Thomas[13] suggested that the host possessed a normal homeostatic cellular mechanism that was active in preventing establishment of "nonself," and Burnet[14] later termed this homeostatic mechanism immunosurveillance.

Among the more impressive indirect data establishing the phenomenon of surveillance in cancer are the observations that the frequency of neoplasia ranges from 10 to 15% in patients who have cellular immunodeficiency diseases—10,000 times that of an actuarially matched population[15]—and is 0.7% in patients who have received selective immunosuppresive therapy, primarily at the cellular level, for kidney transplantation. The neoplasia observed to occur in children with T-cell deficiency syndromes is most often (more than 60%) of the reticuloendothelial system. Spontaneous, complete regression of established tumors is uncommon, but cases are well documented; on the other hand, every physician has observed apparently "cured" patients for many years only to discover metastases as long as 20 years after ablation of the primary neoplasm. Lymphocytic infiltration of solid tumors, including squamous cell carcinoma of the head and neck, is associated with a better prognosis.[16] Surgeons, particularly those working with diseases of the head and neck, know that identification of viable tumor cells in wound washings or in circulation does not reliably predict local recurrence or survival.[17] Finally, immunologic mechanisms are weak at the extremes of age, early childhood and late adulthood, and these are the times when the incidence of malignancy is greatest.

According to the theory of immunosurveillance, response against malignancy in the host has been attributed primarily to mature, specifically immune T cells. Accordingly, it was anticipated that T-cell–deficient laboratory animals, such as the congenitally athymic nude mouse, would lack resistance against malignancy and would be subject to a significantly higher incidence and more rapid progression of malignancy than its immunocompetent counterpart. Several reports have taken the failure to demonstrate such a significantly higher incidence of malignant change in the nude mouse as convincing evidence against the theory of immunosurveillance.[18–21] Studies of cell-mediated immunity (CMI), however, have provided additional information that diminishes the controversy surrounding immunosurveillance.

First, the nude mouse possesses high natural killer (NK) reactivity, which offers a potential explanation for its low incidence of spontaneous malignancy and its resistance to growth of malignant tissue transplants.[22] Additionally, Talmadge and associates[23] have shown that malignant cells that are highly susceptible to natural killing in vitro grow poorly in normal mice but disseminate rapidly in the NK-deficient beige mouse. In humans, depressed to absent NK reactivity has been found in patients with Chédiak-Higashi disease and a hereditary form of malignant melanoma.[24] Furthermore, Takasugi et al[25] and Pross and Baines[26] compared in vitro NK reactivity of a large number of cancer patients with various controls and demonstrated a correlation between increased tumor burden and depressed NK reactivity. Thus, there are several lines of evidence to associate the role of immunosur-

veillance with the NK phenomenon. Although NK activity may not be a critical factor in host defense against established tumors, evidence is accumulating to support the role of the NK cell in the control of metastatic disease.[27]

Escape of a tumor from immunosurveillance and the outcome of tumor growth are thought to be related to the heterogeneity of the tumor cell population, the type of host immune response, and the presence of specific suppressor cell mechanisms at the tumor site.[28] Tumor heterogeneity is characterized by differences in antigenicity, surface receptors, growth rate, and metastatic capability among cells within the same tumor.[29] Such heterogeneity has been demonstrated in preliminary studies of cell lines of primary and metastatic head and neck squamous cell carcinomas,[30] and it may contribute to tumor escape from cytotoxic T lymphocyte responses.

Lymphocytic blastogenic transformation induced by phytohemagglutinin (PHA) and by specific antigens, as an in vitro correlate of delayed cutaneous hypersensitivity, is impaired in some patients with cancer. Because the end point of such studies is unrelated to the inflammatory response, it is concluded that there is a cellular immune defect or diminution in CMI. At least on an operational level, the failure to manifest cellular immunity in cancer is caused by a deficit or a malfunction, or both, of T lymphocytes.

Immunologic testing, performed at the time of diagnosis and clinical staging and before treatment has been instituted, can provide information that will predict, or assist in predicting, patients in whom cancer is most likely to recur. Testing could also serve as a basis on which adjuvant forms of therapy can be instituted. In a prospective study of squamous cell carcinomas of the head and neck,[31] patients were categorized into two groups: those who remained tumor-free and those who had cancer recurrence. The study revealed that pretreatment phytohemagglutinin- and concanavalin A-induced blastogenesis were more often depressed in patients in whom clinically apparent recurrence eventually developed than in patients without recurrence. This finding is consistent with the hypothesis that cellular immune function, as measured in the laboratory by nonspecific blastogenesis, can identify, within the staging system, subpopulations of patients who are less likely to survive after conventional therapy (Table 35–1). In this study, T-lymphocyte and B-lymphocyte enumerations were not of any predictive value. However, other studies have demonstrated consistently reduced T-cell numbers and activity in patients with advanced head and neck cancers.[32–33]

Other studies[34–36] reported increased levels of suppressor T cells in the peripheral blood and regional lymph nodes of head and neck cancer patients, whereas another study[37] reported increased ratios of helper T cells to suppressor T cells in patients with head and neck cancer. These findings suggest that

TABLE 35–1. Pretreatment Test Results (Mean) by Stage of Disease in Patients Who Remained Tumor-Free and in Patients Whom Cancer Recurred*

Parameter	Tumor-Free			Recurrence		
	Stage I	Stage II	Stage III	Stage I	Stage II	Stage III
T cells						
No.	2,213	1,537	2,342	2,876	1,881	1,824
%	79	75	74	65	77	71
B cells						
No.	458	413	537	720	448	592
%	18	20	20	16	17	25
Blastogenesis (cpm)						
Phytohemagglutinin	44,000	34,200	51,250	27,500	22,500	10,400†
Concanavalin A	38,666	36,500	28,500	14,000†	24,500	15,000†
Pokeweed mitogen	12,000	22,300	25,500	24,000	13,250	14,200

* From Ryan RE Jr, Neel HB III, and Ritts RE Jr: Correlation and preoperative immunologic test results with recurrence in patients with head and neck cancer. Otolaryngol Head Neck Surg 88:58, 1980. By permission of the American Academy of Otolaryngology—Head and Neck Surgery, Inc.

† Significantly different from respective tumor-free stage value (P < 0.05).

complex changes in cellular immune regulation may be more important than total T-cell number in explaining the failure of immunosurveillance and that ineffective cytotoxic responses may be caused by inappropriate stimulation of suppressor cell activities. In a detailed series of experiments, Wolf et al[38] have shown that (1) T lymphocytes comprise the major lymphocyte component infiltrating head and neck carcinomas, (2) suppressor T cells are the dominant cell type in tumor parenchyma but that both helper and suppressor T cells are equally represented in tumor stroma, and (3) a direct correlation exists between the extent of helper cell parenchymal infiltration and clinical outcome in head and neck cancer patients. In a subsequent flow cytometry study of T-cell subsets in patients with previously untreated head and neck cancers, this group of investigators provided firm evidence that decreased proportions of cytotoxic/suppressor cells are associated frequently with advanced head and neck cancers and portend a poor prognosis.[39]

The humoral immune system may interfere with the host response to tumor, contributing to a failure of immunosurveillance. Elevated titers of immunoglobulin A (IgA) have been demonstrated in the sera of head and neck cancer patients,[40,41] and it has been proposed that the IgA functions as a blocking factor of lymphocyte-mediated cytotoxicity, at least in unique forms of nasopharyngeal carcinoma.[42,43] Furthermore, Seder et al,[44] reported successful palliative treatment of advanced head and neck cancers in patients with plasmapheresis and hypothesized mediation of the beneficial response by a reduction of circulating immunosuppressive factors.

CLINICAL APPLICATIONS OF TUMOR IMMUNOLOGY

The orchestrated activity of the immune system is capable of providing a natural defense against malignant disease, and a significant aspect of tumor immunology is concerned with manipulation of the immune system in the diagnosis and treatment of cancers that evade surveillance. Current emphasis is on tumor markers, monoclonal antibodies, and biologic response modifiers.

Tumor Markers

Oncogenesis is associated frequently with detectable changes in the serum content of various substances, which are referred to as tumor markers.[45] Many different types of tumor markers have been described. One scheme[46] groups them as (1) markers indicating a predisposition to malignant changes, (2) markers indicating inflammation of tumor necrosis, (3) markers relevant to tumor metabolism, (4) hormone receptors,[47] and (5) oncogenic virus antigens. The three basic categories of use for tumor markers include screening of high-risk populations, distinguishing between malignant tumors or between benign and malignant processes, and following the course of a tumor over time.[48]

Although there is growing evidence for the existence of tumor-specific antigens in squamous carcinomas of the head and neck,[18] two of the most widely used markers in the practice of head and neck oncology are calcitonin and Epstein-Barr (EB) virus-associated antigens. Jackson et al[49] demonstrated the value of serum calcitonin levels as a screening test for family members of patients with medullary carcinoma of the thyroid and for post-treatment surveillance for recurrent disease.

A wealth of biologic, biochemical, and immunologic evidence supports an association between the EB virus and nasopharyngeal carcinoma (NPC). Immunologic studies have identified antibodies against certain EB virus-associated antigens and support the concept that these markers are of value in the diagnosis and management of patients with NPC[50–53] The most specific tests are those that measure the IgA antibody response to EB virus-induced viral capsid antigen (VCA) and the immunoglobin G (IgG) antibody response to early antigen (EA); the VCA (IgA) is the more specific of the two tests.[52] The VCA (IgA) and EA tests complement the process of diagnosis of NPC and are of special value in directing attention to the nasopharynx in patients with occult or small NPCs.[53–55]

The antibody-dependent cellular cytotoxicity (ADCC) assay titrates sera for antibody to the EB virus-induced membrane antigen complex and predicts the clinical course and prognosis of patients with World Health Organization (WHO) types 2 and 3 NPC.[56] High ADCC titers at diagnosis signify a better prognosis. It is a significant risk factor and has been incorporated into a new staging (scoring) system for NPC.[57]

A striking relationship exists between the antibody titers and the histopathologic type of NPC. In a prospective collaborative study of NPC in North American patients,[52,53,58] antibody titers were consistently elevated in cases of WHO types 2 and 3, averaging 85% positive. In cases of WHO type 1, however, the incidence of positive tests was similar to that for control groups.[52] Further refinement of these tests may lead to their use in screening programs in areas of the world with a high incidence of NPC.

The cellular adhesion molecules, a group of all-surface antigens, mediate affinity of binding and play key roles in a variety of immune functions. Intercellular adhesion molecule 1 (ICAM-1) has been expressed on all lines of head and neck squamous cell cancer, with amplified expression after interferon treatment.[59] Further studies are in progress to assess the contribution of ICAM-1 to the generation of an immune response against squamous cell carcinoma of the head and neck.

Monoclonal Antibodies

Antigen-specific monoclonal antibodies are products of hybridomas, which typically result from the fusion of immune-stimulated murine spleen cells with an appropriate B-cell tumor. Although this technology was first reported as recently as 1975,[60] it has generated an explosion of research on the diagnostic and therapeutic applications of monoclonal antibodies.[61]

In the diagnosis of malignant disease, monoclonal antibodies have been "tagged" with a radionuclide, injected into the patient's blood stream, and then visualized with a radiation scanner radioimmunodetection or RAID. The potential clinical applications for RAID in malignant disease include presurgical extent of disease staging, postsurgical evaluation of residual disease, confirmation of viable tumor identified by other methods, identification of disease recurrence in patients with rising serum tumor-marker titers, and confirmation of tumor targeting of antibody for immuno-

therapy. The best current indications for RAID are the detection of occult tumors and the confirmation of tumor sites revealed by other radiologic methods. Most studies of RAID have used ovarian and colorectal cancers, and with several thousand patients studied, between 60 and 90% of known lesions have been identified correctly. With the use of pancarcinoma antibodies and monoclonal agents with greater specificity, the tumor indications for RAID are expanding.

Several strategies have been followed in the therapeutic application of monoclonal antibodies. One strategy has involved administration of unconjugated, naked monoclonal antibody to produce complement-dependent or antibody-dependent all-mediated cytotoxicity, to directly interfere with the growth or differentiation of tumor cells by binding to them, and to enhance the activities of other agents such as interferon and interleukin-2.

Another monoclonal antibody therapeutic strategy has involved the coupling of conventional cytotoxic agents to tumor-seeking monoclonal antibody, with the expectations of decreased host toxicity and increased antitumor efficacy. Similarly, the conjugation of biological toxins with carrier antibodies to produce potentially therapeutic immunotoxin has been explored. Despite their theoretic appeal, both of these approaches have been hampered by problems of conjugating agent to monoclonal antibody and the production of human antibodies against the murine monoclonal antibody and agent. Finally, with advances in the chemistry of antibody radiolabeling, a variety of radionuclides are being investigated for radioimmunotherapy, with the prospect of sparing normal tissues from intensive radiation. Despite its theoretic appeal, radioimmunotherapy presents formidable obstacles, including bone narrow toxicity, a low dose of radiation delivered to tumor, and limited use of multiple treatment courses because of mouse monoclonal antibody antigenicity. Monoclonal antibodies are not yet "magic bullets," but they do hold exciting prospects for enhanced oncologic selectivity and efficacy. In head and neck oncology, monoclonal antibodies have been used primarily in the laboratory for characterization of tumor-associated antigens and study of lymphocyte subpopulations.[18,38]

Biologic Response Modifiers

Biologic response modifiers (BRMs) are agents that modify the host's response to tumor, and the two broad classes of BRMs include those agents that enhance intact immune systems and those that reconstitute impaired immune mechanisms. The attenuated live mycobacterium bacillus Calmette-Guérin (BCG), a member of the first class, was the first BRM to enter a large-scale clinical trial. Although intralesional BCG therapy for early-stage malignant melanoma has resulted in tumor regression,[62] the systemic efficacy of BCG has not been confirmed.

The interferons, members of the second class of BRMs, are a group of glycoproteins that possess potent antiviral and antitumor activities related to their abilities to enhance NK activity, inhibit cell proliferation, and regulate immune responsiveness. The three types of interferon (IFN) include leukocyte-derived IFN-α, fibroblast-derived IFN-β, and T-lymphocyte-derived IFN-y. Genetic engineering has resulted in the availability of each type of IFN in cloned recombinant form, and IFN-α has been approved for the treatment of hairy cell leukemias; clinical trials of recombinant IFN-β and IFN-y are still in the preliminary stage. Because IFN-y possesses such potent immunomodulatory effects, its phase I trial results have been awaited with interest. Richtsmeier[63] reported an oncolytic effect of IFN-y on squamous cell carcinoma tissue cultures and speculated that the lack of success in published phase I trials may be caused by a suboptimal treatment protocol. Questions, concerning the optimal IFN dose and schedule, the mechanisms of IFN antitumor actions, the type of IFN for a particular tumor, and the incorporation of IFN into existing chemotherapy protocols, must be answered before the precise role of IFN can be defined.[64]

Another member of the second class of BRMs is the lymphokine interleukin-2 (IL-2), which plays a key role in the modulation of humoral and T-cell cytotoxicity reactions by helper T cells. The activity of helper T cells is often reduced in cancer patients, as a result either of the disease or therapy, and treatment of these patients with exogenous IL-2 may enhance helper T-cell activity.[65] Interleukin-2 also has been used to stimulate lymphocytes with antitumor reactivity in vitro, producing ''lymphokine-activated killer'' (LAK) cells. In a technique referred to as adoptive immunotherapy, the LAK cells are infused back into the lymphocyte donor cancer patient for tumor-specific cytotoxicity.[66] This technique has been extended to amplify effector lymphocyte oncolytic activity.[67] Specifically, tumor-infiltrating lymphocytes, harvested from melanomas, have been expanded in culture with IL-2 and reinfused resulting in impressive disease regression. Although these techniques are cumbersome and toxic, they are novel approaches to immunotherapy that are capable of achieving partial regressions in selected patients with advanced disease unresponsive to other treatment. Both the in vitro and in vivo applicability of these techniques in treatment of squamous cell carcinoma of the head and neck have been demonstrated,[68,69] and current related research is focused on the immunomodulation of the LAK cell phenomenon.[70] Advances such as these support the concept that a more rational approach to immunotherapy will evolve as the gap between the basic laboratory and the bedside further is narrowed.

The threads that bind the fabric of cancer immunology is immune recognition and elimination of malignant cells.[71] Numerous animal models provide support for an effective host response to cancer, but why then, in many instances, do tumors escape the immune system? The same defenses that maintain tolerance to self presumably act to impair the immune response to cancer. Tumor lysis requires the orchestration of a complex scheme of cells and factors, and the science of cancer immunology has proven to be an intricate, challenging field of investigation. The prospect for the future of tumor immunology and of patients with cancer remains bright. Although the observations we have described give apparent insight into oncogenesis and may be useful clinically, they require substantial validation, particularly in long-term clinical correlation, cell type of cancer, and staging. Without such information, the exact significance for perturbations of the immune mechanism is difficult to perceive, much less to consider a logical basis for rational immunotherapy. Some patients with cancer die with functioning, intact immune systems. We know little about the significance of these findings. Is cancer a manifestation of an immune deficiency or are the immune perturbations secondary to the process—further evidence of systemic nature of this disease?

SUGGESTED READINGS

1. Gross L: Intradermal immunization of C3H mice against a sarcoma that originated in an animal of the same line. Cancer Res 3:326, 1943.
2. Foley EJ: Antigenic properties of methylcholanthrene-induced tumors in mice of the strain of origin. Cancer Res 13:835, 1953.
3. Prehn RT, Main JM: Immunity to methylcholanthrene-induced sarcomas. J Natl Cancer Inst 18:769, 1957.
4. Klein G, Sjögren HO, Klein E, et al: Demonstration of resistance against methylcholanthrene-induced sarcomas in the primary autochthonous host. Cancer Res 20:1561, 1960.
5. Ritts RE Jr, Neel HB III: An overview of cancer immunology. Mayo Clin Proc 49:118, 1974.
6. Lewis MR, Aptekman PM: Atrophy of tumors caused by strangulation and accompanied by development of tumor immunity in rats. Cancer 5:411, 1952.
7. Takeda K, Aizawa M, Kikuchi Y, et al: Tumor autoimmunity against methylcholanthrene-induced sarcomas of the rat. Gann 57:221, 1966.
8. Neel HB III, Ketcham AS, Hammond WG: Requisites for successful cryogenic surgery of cancer. Arch Surg 102:45, 1971.
9. Neel HB III, Ketcham AS, Hammond WG: Experimental evaluation of in situ oncocide for primary tumor therapy: Comparison of tumor-specific immunity after complete excision, cryonecrosis and ligation. Laryngoscope 83:376, 1973.
10. Neel HB III, Ritts RE Jr: Tumor-specific immunity and the otolaryngologist. Ann Otol Rhinol Laryngol 82:323, 1973.
11. Neel HB III, Ritts RE Jr: Transfer of tumor-specific immunity with syngeneic spleen cells and serum from mice that have large tumors and metastases. Cancer 40:1643, 1977.
12. Neel HB III, Ritts RE Jr: Immunotherapeutic effect of tumor necrosis after cryosurgery, electrocoagulation, and ligation. J Surg Oncol 11:45, 1979.

13. Thomas L: Discussion. In: Cellular and Humoral Aspects of the Hypersensitive States. Edited by Lawrence HS. New York, P.B. Hoeber, 1959, pp 529–532.

14. Burnet FM: The concept of immunological surveillance. Prog Exp Tumor Res 13:1, 1970.

15. Gatti RA, Good RA: Occurrence of malignancy in immunodeficiency diseases: A literature review. Cancer 28:89, 1971.

16. Catalona WJ, Sample WF, Chretein PB: Lymphocyte reactivity in cancer patients: Correlation with tumor histology and clinical stage. Cancer 31:65, 1973.

17. Arons MS, Smith RR: Distant metastases and local recurrence in head and neck cancer. Ann Surg 154:235, 1961.

18. Möller GH, Möller E: Considerations of some current concepts in cancer research (Editorial). J Natl Cancer Inst 55:755, 1975.

19. Outzen HC, Custer RP, Eaton GJ, et al: Spontaneous and induced tumor incidence in germfree "nude" mice. J Reticuloendothel Soc 17:1, 1975.

20. Rygaard J, Povlsen CO: The nude mouse vs. the hypothesis of immunological surveillance. Transplant Rev 28:43, 1976.

21. Schwartz RS: Another look at immunologic surveillance. N Engl J Med 293:181, 1975.

22. Herberman RB, Holden HT: Natural cell-mediated immunity. Adv Cancer Res 27:305, 1978.

23. Talmadge JE, Meyers KM, Prieur DJ, et al: Role of NK cells in tumour growth and metastasis in *beige* mice. Nature 284:622, 1980.

24. Marx JL: Natural killer cells help defend the body. Science 210:624, 1980.

25. Takasurgi M, Ramseyer A, Takasugi J: Decline of natural nonselective cell-mediated cytotoxicity in patients with tumor progression. Cancer Res 37:413, 1977.

26. Pross HF, Baines MG: Spontaneous human lymphocyte-mediated cytotoxicity against tumour target cells. I. The effect of malignant disease. Int J Cancer 18:593, 1976.

27. Schantz SP, Goepfert H: Multimodality therapy and distant metastases. The impact of natural-killer cell activity. Arch Otolaryngol Head Neck Surg 113:1207, 1987.

28. Wolf GT: Tumor immunology, immune surveillance and immunotherapy of head and neck squamous carcinoma. In: Head and Neck Oncology. Edited by Wolf GT. Boston, Martinus Nijhoff, 1984, pp 375–410.

29. Fidler IJ, Kripke ML: Tumor cell antigenicity, host immunity, and cancer metastasis (Editorial). Cancer Immunol Immunother 7:201, 1980.

30. Carey TE, Kimmel KA, Schwartz DR, et al: Antibodies to human squamous cell carcinoma. Otolaryngol Head Neck Surg 91:482, 1983.

31. Ryan RE Jr, Neel HB III, Ritts RE Jr: Correlation and preoperative immunologic test results with recurrence in patients with head and neck cancer. Otolaryngol Head Neck Surg 88:58, 1980.

32. Olkowski ZL, Wilkins SA Jr: T-Lymphocyte levels in the peripheral blood of patients with cancer of the head and neck. Am J Surg 130:440, 1975.

33. Wanebo HJ, Jun MY, Strong EW, et al: T-cell deficiency in patients with squamous cell cancer of the head and neck. Am J Surg 130:445, 1975.

34. Balaram P, Vasudevan DM: Quantitation of Fc receptor-bearing T-lymphocytes (T_G and T_M) in oral cancer. Cancer 52:1837, 1983.

35. Saxon A, Portis J: Lymphoid subpopulation changes in regional lymph nodes in squamous head and neck cancer. Cancer Res 37:1154, 1977.

36. Yata J, Shimbo T, Sawaki S: Changes in T-cell subsets and their clinical significance in cancer patients. In: Nasopharyngeal Carcinoma: Etiology and Control. Edited by DeThe G, Ito Y. Lyon, IARC Scientific Publication No. 20, 1978, pp 511–521.

37. Wolf GT, Lovett EJ III, Peterson KA, et al: Lymphokine production and lymphocyte subpopulations in patients with head and neck squamous carcinoma. Arch Otolaryngol 110:731, 1984.

38. Wolf GT, Hudson JL, Peterson KA, et al: Lymphocyte subpopulations infiltrating squamous carcinomas of the head and neck: Correlations with extent of tumor and prognosis. Otolaryngol Head Neck Surg 95:142, 1986.

39. Wolf GT, Schmaltz S, Hudson J, et al: Alterations in lymphocyte-T subpopulations in patients with head and neck cancer; Correlations with prognosis. Arch Otolaryngol Head Neck Surg 113:1200, 1987.

40. Katz AE, Yoo TJ Harker LA: Serum immunoglobulin A (IgA) levels in carcinoma of the head and neck. Trans Am Acad Ophthalmol Otolaryngol 82:131, 1976.

41. Wara WM, Wara DW, Phillips TL, et al: Elevated IgA in carcinoma of the nasopharynx. Cancer 35:1313, 1975.

42. Mathew GD, Qualtiere LF, Neel HB III, et al: IgA antibody, antibody-dependent cellular cytotoxicity and prognosis in patients with nasopharyngeal carcinoma. Int J Cancer 27:175, 1981.

43. Sundar SK, Ablashi DV, Kamaraju LS, et al: Sera from patients with undifferentiated nasopharyngeal carcinoma contain a factor which abrogates specific Epstein-Barr virus antigen-induced lymphocyte response. Int J Cancer 29:407, 1982.

44. Seder RH, Vaughan CW, Oh S-K, et al: Tumor regression and temporary restoration of immune response after plasmapheresis in a patient with recurrent oral cancer. Cancer 60:318, 1987.

45. Veltri RW, Maxim PE: Tumor immunity and tumor markers in head and neck cancer. In: Head and Neck Oncology. Edited by Wolf GT. Boston, Martinus Nijhoff, 1984, pp 411–430.

46. Pruet CW, Ghosh BC: Antigens and markers in head and neck cancer. In: Tumor Markers and Tumor-Associated Antigens. Edited by Ghosh BC and Ghosh L. New York, McGraw-Hill, 1987, pp 313–317.

47. Berg NJ, Neel HB III, Weiland LH, et al: A new assay to assess steroid-hormone responsiveness in head and neck cancer. Laryngoscope 97:286, 1987.

48. Longo DL: Tumor markers: Current status of the quest—Introductory overview. Semin Oncol 14:85, 1987.

49. Jackson CE, Tashjian AH Jr, Block MA: Detection of medullary thyroid cancer by calcitonin assay in families. Ann Intern Med 78:845, 1973.

50. Henle G, Henle W: Epstein-Barr virus-specific IgA serum antibodies as an outstanding feature of nasopharyngeal carcinoma. Int J Cancer 17:1, 1976.

51. Klein G: The Epstein-Barr virus. In: The Herpesviruses. Edited by Kaplan AS, New York, Academic Press, 1973, pp 521–555.

52. Neel HB III, Pearson GR, Taylor WF: Antibodies to Epstein-Barr virus in patients with nasopharyngeal carcinoma and in comparison groups. Ann Otol Rhinol Laryngol 93:477, 1984.

53. Neel HB III, Pearson GR, Weiland LH, et al: Application of Epstein-Barr virus serology to the diagnosis and staging of North American patients with nasopharyngeal carcinoma. Otolaryngol Head Neck Surg 91:255, 1983.

54. Neel HB III: A prospective evaluation of patients with nasopharyngeal carcinoma: An overview. J Otolaryngol 15:137, 1986.

55. Neel HB III, Pearson GR, Weiland LH, et al: Immunologic detection of occult primary cancer of the head and neck. Otolaryngol Head Neck Surg 89:230, 1981.

56. Neel HB III, Pearson GR, Taylor WF: Antibody-dependent cellular cytotoxicity: Relation to stage and disease course in North American patients with nasopharyngeal carcinoma. Arch Otolaryngol 110:742, 1984.

57. Neel HB III, Taylor WF, Pearson GR: Prognostic determinants and a new view of staging for patients with nasopharyngeal carcinoma. Ann Otol Rhinol Laryngol 94:529, 1985.

58. Neel HB III, Pearson GR, Weiland LH, et al: Anti-EBV serologic tests for nasopharyngeal carcinoma. Laryngoscope 90:1981, 1980.

59. Scher RL, Koch WM, Richtsmeier WJ: Induction of the intercellular adhesion molecule (ICA M-1) on squamous cell carcinoma by interferon gamma. Arch Otolaryngol Head Neck Surg 119:432, 1993.

60. Köhler G, Milstein C: Continuous cultures of fused cells secreting antibody of predefined specificity. Nature 256:495, 1975.

61. Goldenberg DM: New developments in monoclonal antibodies for cancer detection and therapy. CA Cancer J Clinic 44:43, 1994.

62. Morton DL, Eilber FR, Holmes EC, et al: Present status of BCG immunotherapy of malignant melanoma. Cancer Immunol Immunother 1:93, 1976.

63. Richtsmeier WJ: Interferon gamma induced oncolysis: An effect on head and neck squamous carcinoma cultures. Arch Otolaryngol Head Neck Surg 114:432, 1988.

64. Krown SE: Interferons and interferon inducers in cancer treatment. Semin Oncol 13:207, 1986.

65. Gillis S, Conlon PJ, Cosmon D, et al: Lymphokines: From conjecture to the clinic. Semin Oncol 13:218, 1986.

66. Rosenberg SA: The adoptive immunotherapy of cancer using the transfer of activated lymphoid cells and interleukin-2. Semin Oncol 13:200, 1986.

67. Rosenberg SA, Packard BS: Aebersold PM, et al: Use of tumor-infiltrating lymphocytes and interleukin-2 in the immunotherapy of patients with metastatic melanoma. N Engl J Med 319:1676–1680, 1988.

68. Leess FR, Bredenkamp JK, Lichtenstein A, Mickel RA: Lymphokine-activated killing of autologous and allogeneic short-term cultured head and neck squamous carcinomas. Laryngoscope 99:1255, 1989.

69. Melioli G, Margarino G, Scala M, et al: Perilymphatic injections of recombinant interleukin-2 (rIL-2) partially correct the immunologic defects in patients with advanced head and neck squamous cell carcinoma. Laryngoscope 102:572, 1992.

70. Clayman GL, Taylor DL, Liu FJ, et al: Serum and acute phase protein modulation of the effector phase of lymphokine-activated killer cells. Laryngoscope 103:299, 1993.

71. Lynch SA, Houghton AN: Cancer immunology. Curr Opin Oncol 5:145, 1993.

36 Laser Surgery in the Head and Neck

Robert H. Ossoff, Jack A. Coleman, Jr., James A. Duncavage, and Lou Reinisch

The use of lasers in otolaryngology has seen the addition of new surgical procedures and the refinement of conventional surgical procedures. The carbon dioxide (CO_2) laser is still the most commonly used laser for surgery of the upper aerodigestive tract. In fact, in a recent review of laser use at Vanderbilt University Medical Center, the use of lasers by the Department of Otolaryngology had increased by 16% from 1989 to 1992.[1] In addition, the use of the CO_2 laser increased at a rate of 20% in this same period. The use of the CO_2 laser for treating lesions of the oral cavity, pharynx, larynx, and tracheobronchial tree has been facilitated by previous experience with the techniques of endolaryngeal microsurgery.[2] The introduction of the microspot for CO_2 laser microsurgery has further refined the use of the CO_2 laser for endoscopic surgery.[3,4] The super pulsed CO_2 laser and the argon and the KTP/532 lasers are being used for stapedotomy with increasing frequency.

The neodymium:yttrium aluminum garnet (Nd:YAG) laser, with and without contact probes, continues to be used for obstructing lesions of the tracheobronchial tree,[5,6] and for cavernous hemangiomas of the head and neck.[7] The use of the Nd:YAG contact probes for head and neck surgery is still being explored. The KTP/532 laser has been used by many otolaryngologists for pharyngeal tonsillectomy, although there appear to be no major benefits of using the laser over conventional techniques in routine tonsillectomies.[8–10] The continuous and flash-pumped yellow dye lasers are used to treat port wine stains with excellent results.[11–13] The concept of photodynamic therapy to treat malignancies of the upper aerodigestive tract is still under active investigation.[14–24]

One of the newest tools for laser surgery is the free-electron laser (FEL).[25] The FEL differs from conventional lasers in that the lasing medium is a beam of electrons traveling near the speed of light. The laser output can be tuned continuously from 10 μm to 2 μm and produces short pulses of light with a high peak intensity (on the order of 10 MW). Current tissue ablation studies with the FEL have identified the amide absorption bands near 6.0 μm to have remarkable ablation properties.[26] In this wavelength range, a portion of the laser intensity is absorbed directly by the protein structure of the tissue and a portion is absorbed by the water. The laser energy, therefore, compromises the structural integrity of the tissue as the water is ablated. Although it is not envisioned that every hospital will have a free-electron laser, newer lasers emitting light in the region of 6.0 μm will probably be the next major revolution in laser surgery.

LASER BIOPHYSICS

LASER is an acronym for light amplification by the stimulated emission of radiation. A laser is an optical device containing a lasing medium, an excitation source and a resonant cavity.[27,28] The atoms of the lasing medium have discrete energy states. Transitions between these energy states normally involve the absorption or emission of electromagnetic radiation. The absorption of radiation promotes the system to a higher-energy state. The emission of radiation accompanies the transition to a lower-energy state. The quantized light from one atom or molecule making a single energy transition is termed a photon of light. A photon can, therefore, be thought of as a single minimum quantity of light.

In a stable system, an atom can interact with a photon and rise to a higher-energy state; this process is called absorption. Similarly, this same atom in the high-energy state can emit a photon and decay to a more stable atomic state; this is called spontaneous emission. If a photon interacts with an atom that is

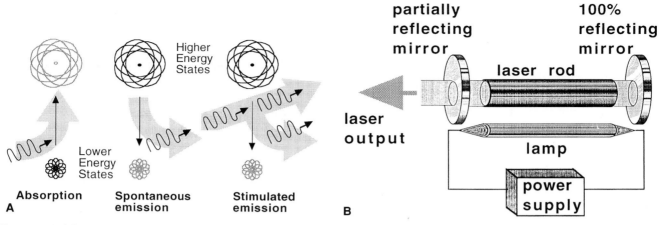

Fig. 36–1. A. Schematic illustration of absorption, spontaneous emission and the stimulated emission of light. B. Typical arrangement of an optical resonating chamber with the lasing medium; excitation from a lamp and two mirrors providing optical feed back.

already in a high-energy state and decay of that atomic system occurs, then two photons are released: the original photon and the second photon emitted by the decay of the high-energy system. These two photons are of equal wavelength and are coordinated in time and space (coherent). This process is called stimulated emission and is the underlying principle of laser physics (Fig. 36–1A).[29]

Typically, surgical lasers have an optical resonating chamber (cavity) with two end mirrors; the space between these mirrors is filled with a lasing medium such as argon, Nd:YAG or CO_2.[30] In the first laser made, the lasing medium was a ruby crystal.[31] An external energy source such as an electric current excites the lasing medium within the optical cavity. This excitation causes many atoms of the lasing medium to be raised to a higher-energy state. When more than half the atoms in the resonating chamber have reached a particular excited state, a population inversion has occurred. Spontaneous emission is taking place in all directions; light (photons) emitted in the direction of the long axis of the laser is retained within the optical cavity by multiple reflections between the precisely aligned end mirrors. One mirror is completely reflective and the other partially transmissive (Fig. 36–1B). Stimulated emission occurs when a photon interacts with an excited atom in the optical cavity, yielding pairs of identical photons that are of equal wavelength, frequency, and energy and are in phase with each other. This process takes place at an increasing rate with each passage of the photons through the lasing medium; the mirrors serve as a positive-feedback mechanism for the stimulated emission of radiation by reflecting the photons back and forth. The partially transmissive mirror emits some of the radiant energy as laser light. The radiation leaving the optical cavity through the partially transmissive mirror quickly reaches an equilibrium with the pumping mechanism's rate of replenishing the population of high-energy state atoms.*

The radiant energy thus emitted is extremely intense and unidirectional or collimated.[32] Finally, the light is coherent both temporally and spatially. Temporal coherence means that the photons alternate sinusoidally in phase with one another, whereas spatial coherence means that the photons are equal and parallel across the wave front. These properties of monochromaticity, intensity, collimation, and coherence distinguish the organized radiant energy of a laser from the disorganized radiant energy of a light bulb.

After emission of the radiant energy through the partially reflective mirror, the laser beam can be passed through a fiber. The fiber allows transmission of the laser energy to occur at the distal end of the fiber. The total internal reflection of the optical fiber causes the collimation of the laser beam to be lost. The result is a divergent beam at the fiber tip.

The laser beam can also be passed through a lens that focuses the radiant energy to a small beam waist, or spot size, ranging from approximately 0.1 to 2.0 mm. The focusing lens usually is treated with special optical coatings to allow the helium-neon aiming beam and the invisible CO_2 beam to be focused coplanar. This lens is characterized by a specific focal length that determines the distance from the lens to the target tissue for focused use.

Surgical lasers typically permit end-user control of three variables: 1) focal length spot size (mm); 2) power

---

* We have used the term atom in the preceding discussion when referring to the lasing material. In reality, the lasing material is often molecules, ions, atoms, semiconductors or even free electrons in a particle accelerator. In these other systems it does not have to be the bound electron that is excited. It can be many different excitations, including molecular vibrations or the kinetic energy of the accelerated free electron.

(watts); and 3) exposure time (seconds). Power, measured in watts, is perhaps the least useful parameter in medicine and may be kept constant with varying effects, depending on the spot size and duration of exposure. For example, if the time of exposure is kept constant, the relationship between power and depth of tissue injury becomes logarithmic as the spot size is varied.

Power density, on the other hand, is the most useful way of monitoring the surgical effects of the laser. It is a measure of the power output of the laser in watts over the cross-sectional area of the laser beam in square centimeters:

POWER DENSITY $= $ POWER (watts)$/\pi \times r^2$ (cm^2)

Furthermore, power density (irradiance) is a measure of the concentration of radiant energy of the laser beam. Here, if the time of exposure is kept constant, the relationship between power density and depth of injury is linear as the spot size is varied. Therefore, surgeons should calculate the appropriate power density for various procedures; such calculations allow the surgeon to control tissue effects predictably when changing from one focal length to another or when using different surgical lasers.

Radiant exposure (RE) expressed as joules/cm^2 is equal to the power density (watts/cm^2) multiplied by the time of exposure in seconds.

$$RE = \text{Power Density} \times \text{time}$$

This is a measure of the total amount of laser energy per unit area of exposed target tissue. Although radiant exposure documentation is used in the international laser literature, power density (irradiance) is the most

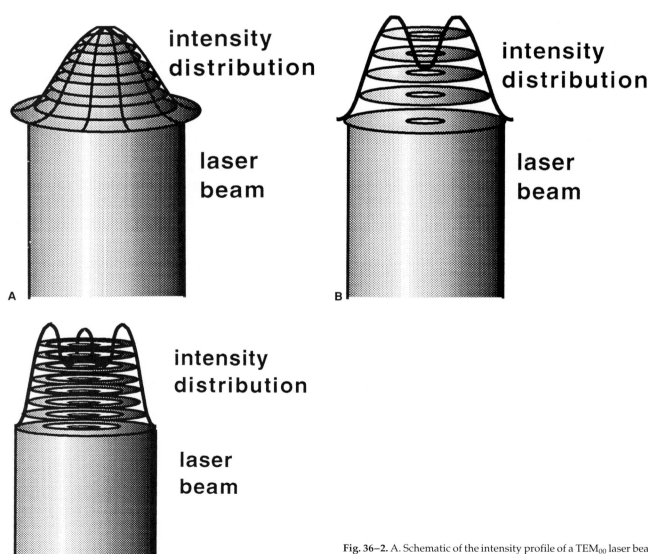

Fig. 36–2. A. Schematic of the intensity profile of a TEM$_{00}$ laser beam. B. Schematic of the intensity profile of a TEM$_{01*}$ laser beam. This beam has a doughnut shape. C. Schematic of the intensity profile of a TEM$_{11*}$ laser beam. This beam has a target shape.

meaningful measurement to the surgeon during the procedure.

Carbon dioxide lasers can emit radiant energy with different beam configurations that ultimately determine the depth of tissue damage and vaporization across the spot size. Transverse electromagnetic mode (TEM) refers to the intensity distribution over the spot area and determines the shape of the focused laser spot. The most fundamental TEM is TEM_{00}. In this mode, if the laser beam is cut in cross section, it appears circular, with the power density of the beam following a Gaussian distribution (Fig. 36–2A). In other words, the power density is greatest at the center of the beam and diminishes progressively toward the periphery. Thus, the center of the beam can be used for vaporization and the periphery for coagulation.

TEM_{01*} (Fig. 36–2B) and TEM_{11*} (Fig. 36–2C) modes have a more complex distribution of energy and cause characteristic variations in tissue ablation depth. In fact, there are cold spots in the center of their beams. Additionally, they cannot be focused to as small a spot size as TEM_{00} mode lasers. Most carbon dioxide surgical lasers manufactured in the last 5 years produce a TEM_{00} beam profile.

Although simple ray diagrams normally show parallel light to be focused to a point, the actual situation is more complicated. A lens will focus a gaussian beam to a beam waist or a finite size. This beam waist is the minimum spot diameter, d, and can be written as

$$d \sim \frac{2f\lambda}{D}$$

where f is the focal length of the lens, λ is the wavelength of light and D is the diameter of the laser beam incident on the lens (Fig. 36–3). The beam waist occurs not at one distance from the lens, but over a range of distances. This range is termed the depth of focus and can be written as

$$\text{depth of focus} \sim \frac{\pi d^2}{2\lambda}$$

We realize the depth of focus every time we focus a camera. With a camera, a range of objects is in focus, and we can set the focus without carefully measuring the distance between the object and the lens. Notice from the equations that a long focal length lens (a large f) leads to a large beam waist. A large beam waist also translates as a large depth of focus.

The size of the laser beam on the tissue (spot size) can therefore be varied in two ways. Because the minimum beam diameter of the focal spot increases directly with increasing the focal length of the laser focusing lens, the surgeon can change the focal length of the lens to obtain a particular beam diameter. As the focal length becomes smaller, there is a corresponding decrease in the size of the focal spot; also, the smaller the spot size is for any given power output, the greater the corresponding power density. The second way the surgeon can vary the spot size is by working either in or out of focus. The minimum beam diameter and highest power concentration occur at the focal plane, where much of the precise cutting and vaporization is carried out (Fig. 36–4A). As the distance from the focal plane increases, the laser beam diverges or becomes defocused (Fig. 36–4B). Here, the cross sectional area of the spot grows larger and thus lowers the power density for a given output. As one can readily see, the size of the focal spot depends on both the focal length of the laser lens and whether the surgeon is working in or out of focus.

Figure 36–5 demonstrates these concepts using arbitrary ratios accurate for a current model TEM_{00} CO_2 laser. The laser lens setting (focal length) and working distance (focus/defocus) combinations shown determine the spot size of the laser beam. The height of the various cylinders represents the relative fluence of the light incident on the tissue.

The equations for power density and radiant exposure demonstrate that the surgeon can vary the amount of energy delivered to the target tissue by varying the power output, cross section area of the beam, and time of exposure. The power output of the CO_2 laser can be varied between 1 and 100 watts. Tissues with less water content require a greater power output to achieve the desired effect. The cross-sectional area of the laser beam for lasers with a lens (spot size) can be varied in two ways. First, as the focal length becomes smaller, there is a corresponding decrease in the size of the spot. The smaller the spot size for any given power output, the greater the corresponding power density becomes. Second, the surgeon can vary the cross-sectional area of the beam by working either in focus or out of focus.

The use of a fiber to deliver the laser energy to tissue causes the laser beam to lose its collimation (unidirectional). The result is that the closer the fiber tip is to the tissue, the smaller is the spot size or area of laser energy distribution. As the fiber is moved away from the tissue, the spot size will increase, causing a dilution of the laser energy over the larger area.

The third means by which the surgeon can vary the amount of energy delivered to the target tissue is by

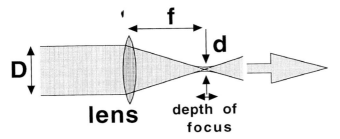

Fig. 36–3. Schematic of the diffraction limited spot size or beam waist of a parallel beam of light focused by a lens.

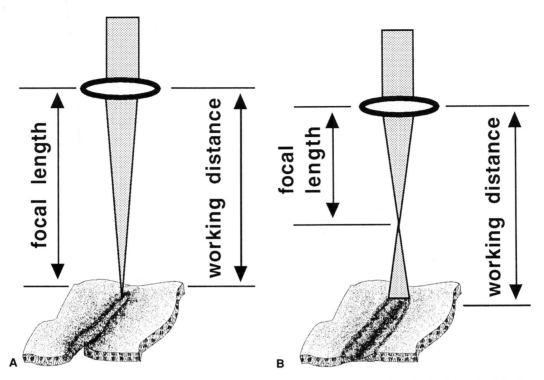

Fig. 36–4. A. Schematic illustration of the laser incising tissue with the working distance equal to the focal length of the lens. B. Schematic illustration of the laser excising tissue with the working distance not equal to the focal length of the lens.

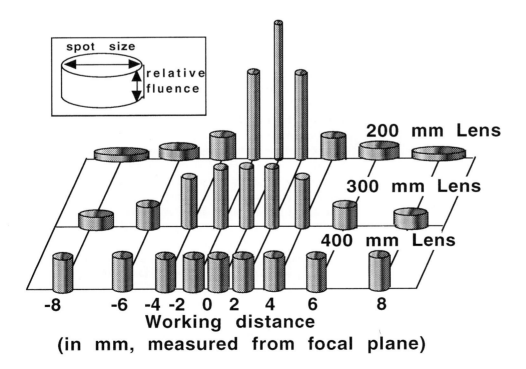

Fig. 36–5. Graph of the fluence and spot size for three different focal length lenses, working at and near the focal length of the lens. The cylinder diameter is proportional to the spot diameter for a current model carbon dioxide laser. The height of the cylinder is proportional to the fluence of the laser. We arbitrarily set the lowest fluence equal to one.

TABLE 36–1. Time Scales

1 second (s)					
1 millisecond (ms)	10^{-3} s				
1 microsecond (μs)	10^{-3} ms	10^{-6} s			
1 nanosecond (ns)	10^{-3} μs	10^{-6} ms	10^{-9} s		
1 picosecond (ps)	10^{-3} ns	10^{-6} μs	10^{-9} ms	10^{-12} s	
1 femtosecond (fs)	10^{-3} ps	10^{-6} ns	10^{-9} μs	10^{-12} ms	10^{-15} s

varying the exposure time. The longer the tissue is exposed to the laser beam, the greater the amount of radiant exposure (joules/cm^2) that is delivered to the target tissue. The time can be varied by working in either the continuous or the pulsed mode, with the pulse duration ranging from 0.05 to 0.5 second.

Laser energy can also be delivered over a short time, from milliseconds to femtosecond ranges. A continuous wave laser can be pulsed in the millisecond range. A noncontinuous or pulsed laser can deliver pulses of laser energy in a duration as short as several femtoseconds (10^{-15} seconds) (Table 36–1). The pulsed laser delivers energy with high-peak powers. One needs to visualize a train of pulses with high peaks but short time durations (Fig. 36–6). The high peaks are the peak intensities in watts that can be obtained by pulsed lasers. The average power delivered to tissue is expressed by the pulses/second times peak power times the pulse width. On a continuous wave laser, the meter reads in watts. On a pulsed laser, however, the meter reads in joules (watts times seconds). Pulsed lasers and super pulsing of a continuous wave laser permit the laser to produce a high-peak power. A pulsed Nd:YAG ophthalmologic laser can produce 6.7×10^6 watts per pulse. The pulse duration can be as short as 30×10^{-12} seconds. If we remember that power density or irradiance is the amount of watts divided by the area, we can see that the pulsing of the laser permits high wattage with resultant high-power densities. These high-power densities can cause nonthermal tissue interactions. The flash-pumped yellow dye laser is an example of a pulsed laser used to treat port wine stains. Some CO_2 lasers and the KTP/532 laser deliver laser energy in a quasicontinuous wave or pulsed mode.

In summary, by varying the power output of the laser unit, the spot size or cross-sectional area of the beam or the time of exposure, the surgeon can adjust the laser to incise, coagulate, or vaporize the target tissue.

TISSUE EFFECTS

The actual tissue effects produced by the radiant energy of a laser vary with the specific wavelength of the laser used. The interaction of laser energy with living tissue can produce three distinct reactions. First, the laser energy can be absorbed by chromophores within the tissue. The resulting effect can be the production of heat. This is the thermal effect seen in most conventional laser systems in use today.

Second, the radiant energy of a laser can stimulate or react with specific molecules within a cell. This reaction can cause a chemical change to occur within the cell. This effect is termed photochemical. An example is the reaction that occurs with injection of a photosensitizing drug into tissue and the biochemical effect that is produced when the drug is activated by the stimulating effect of radiant laser energy.

Third, the use of short pulses of high wattage laser energy can disrupt cellular architecture because of the production of sound waves or photoacoustic shock waves.[33] This mechanical disruption of tissue is an example of a nonthermal tissue effect.

The radiant energy of a laser can interact with tissue in four ways. With each laser, one effect normally predominates over the other three effects. The radiant laser energy can be transmitted through the tissue with little of the energy absorbed by the surrounding tissue. The first interaction is transmission. The transmission of laser energy can be understood by remembering the effect of argon laser energy on water. The energy of the argon laser passes through or is transmitted through clear liquids without being absorbed signifi-

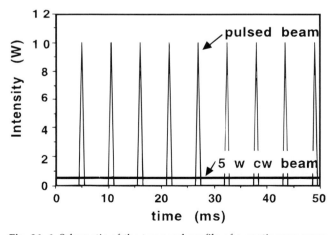

Fig. 36–6. Schematic of the temporal profile of a continuous wave laser and a pulsed laser. The continuous wave laser produces a constant 5 W laser output. The pulsed laser produces pulses of light, each 100 W in peak intensity and on for 5 ms with a repetition rate of approximately 18 Hz.

cantly. The second interaction is absorption. The absorption of laser energy by tissue is a complex process depending on the laser wavelength and the color of the tissue. The laser wavelength and the amount of color have an effect on energy absorption. The CO_2 laser is essentially colorblind. The visible lasers, however, are color-dependent on energy absorption. The third interaction is scattering. Laser energy is also scattered forward into tissue and backward away from tissue. The scattering coefficient depends on the wavelength. The shorter the wavelength, the more strongly scattered is the laser energy. Therefore the laser energy of visible lasers is more strongly scattered than for lasers in the infrared region of the electromagnetic spectrum. The last laser tissue effect is reflection of laser energy from the tissue surface in addition to limiting the penetration of the laser into the tissue.

The radiant energy of a laser produces a thermal effect when it is absorbed by the tissue and converted to heat.[34-36] When the target absorbs a specific amount of radiant energy to raise its temperature to approximately 60° to 65° C, protein denaturation starts to occur. Blanching of the tissue surface is visible and the deep structural integrity of the tissue is disturbed. When the absorbed laser light heats the tissue to approximately 100° C vaporization of intracellular water occurs. This causes vacuole formation, cratering, and tissue shrinkage (Fig. 36–7). Carbonization, disintegration and smoke and gas generation with destruction of the laser-radiated tissue occurs at several hundred degrees centigrade.

If the radiant energy is absorbed poorly by the target tissue, excess thermal damage to adjacent tissues occurs.[37,38] Reflection of the energy at the tissue surface or transmission of poorly absorbed energy through the target tissue makes it necessary to prolong the time of exposure of the target tissue to the laser energy to achieve the desired ablation. This prolonged exposure of the target tissue causes an increased thermal effect with resultant damage to the surrounding nontarget tissue.

In the center of the wound is a volume of tissue vaporization; just a few flakes of carbon debris are noted. Immediately adjacent to this volume is a zone of thermal necrosis measuring approximately 100 μm wide. Next is a volume of thermal conductivity and repair, usually 300 to 500 μm wide. Small vessels, nerves, and lymphatics are sealed in the zone of thermal necrosis; the minimal operative trauma combined with the vascular seal probably account for the notable absence of postoperative edema characteristic of laser wounds.

Studies that compare the histologic properties of healing and the tensile strength of the healing wound after laser and scalpel-produced incisions on experimental animals have been performed. In 1971, Hall demonstrated that the tensile strength in a CO_2 laser-induced incision was less up to the twentieth day of healing and became the same by the fortieth day.[39] In 1981, Norris studied the healing properties of CO_2 laser incisions on the hog histologically.[40] He showed that scalpel-induced incisions exhibited better tissue reconstruction than laser-induced incisions up to the thirtieth day, after which time both incisions exhibited similar results.

In 1982, Finsterbush et al. measured the tensile strength of CO_2 laser incisions in rabbits and compared them to scalpel wounds.[41] They gently removed the charring and debris on the wound edges before closure. The laser beam-induced wounds were significantly stronger than those done by scalpel for the first 19 days. In 1983, Buell and Schuller created CO_2, laser incisions in pigs and compared them to scalpel incisions.[42] They found the laser wound to be weaker in tensile strength than the scalpel wounds for the first 3 weeks. Research on wound healing from lasers has

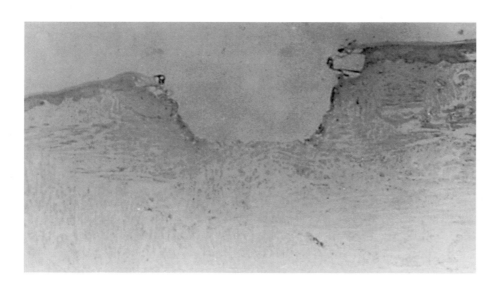

Fig. 36–7. Laser crater on the ventral rsurface of the canine tongue. Note the center area of tissue ablation, surrounded by an area of protein denaturation and tissue edema (H&E × 10).

confirmed the delay in the healing of laser incisions.[43,44] Analysis of the healing process and the effect of the laser on components of the healing process are beginning to provide details about the laser wound healing delay.[45,46]

LASER TYPES AND APPLICATIONS

Six types of lasers are in use in otolaryngology/head and neck surgery, and many more are in various states of development. The characteristic potential for the clinical application of a particular surgical laser is determined by its light emission paradigm, i.e., pulse character and wavelength, and by its absorptive characteristics in tissue. The surgeon should therefore consider the properties of each wavelength at the time that he or she chooses to use a particular laser. This facilitates the accomplishment of the surgical goal with minimal morbidity and maximal efficiency.

Argon Lasers

Argon lasers produce a visible blue-green light with discrete wavelengths of 488 and 514 nm. The radiant energy from an argon laser is transmitted readily through clear aqueous tissues such as those of the cornea, lens, and vitreous humor because it has a low water-absorption coefficient. Certain tissue pigments, such as melanin and hemoglobin, effectively absorb the argon laser light. When low levels of this blue-green laser light interact with highly pigmented tissues, a localized coagulation within these tissues takes place. The clinician uses this selective absorption of the argon laser by pigmented tissue to photocoagulate pigmented lesions such as port wine hemangiomas and telangiectasias.[47-51] Used in this application, the radiant energy from the argon laser passes through the overlying skin with some absorption by melanin and β-carotene and reaches the pigmented target tissue, causing protein coagulation. A second-degree burn occurs in the overlying epidermis. Gradual blanching of the laser-photocoagulated area occurs over several months.

Focusing the argon beam to a small spot size causes its power density to increase sufficiently to result in vaporization of the target tissue. Otologists have used this laser to perform stapedotomy procedures because of its ability to be focused into a very small beam. This procedure was popularized by Perkins.[52] Because bone reflects most visible light, including the blue-green radiant energy of argon laser, a small drop of blood should be placed on the stapes to initiate absorption. Other middle-ear applications of the argon laser include lysis of middle-ear adhesions, ossicle sculpturing, and spot welding of grafts in tympanoplasty.[53-59]

Advances in fiberoptic technology have allowed development of a series of hand-held argon laser microprobes, which have been call Endo-Otoprobes.[60-62] The optical fiber-transmitting laser energy is contained within the Endo-Otoprobe, which is hand-held like a surgical instrument in the operative field. Because Endo-Otoprobes are hand-held and available in a variety of angles, use of these probes allows the surgeon to use the laser in a direction different from the visual field of the microscope, facilitating aiming the laser beam around a corner without having to use an expensive and delicate micromirror.

Because the blue-green light from the argon laser readily penetrates the eye to the retina, special amber colored safety glasses are required for all personnel in the operating room.

Nd:YAG Laser

Neodymium:yttrium aluminum garnet (Nd:YAG) lasers produce light that has a wavelength of 1064 nm and is therefore invisible. Because the water-absorption coefficient of this laser is low, its radiant energy can be transmitted through clear liquids, which facilitates its use in the eye or other water-filled cavities, such as the urinary bladder or synovial capsule. The absorption of its energy by tissue depends on pigment; therefore, most of the energy is scattered both forward and backward through the tissue. The zone of damage produced by impact with the Nd:YAG laser is not limited as with the CO_2 laser. A homogeneous zone of thermal coagulation and necrosis may extend 4 mm from the impact site, and precise control is not possible.

These characteristics make the Nd:YAG laser an excellent surgical tool for tissue coagulation. Vaporization and incision can be performed with this wavelength, but precision is lacking and tissue damage is difficult to control. Attachment of synthetic sapphire contact tips to the end of the quartz fiberoptic delivery system allows the Nd:YAG laser to be used for incision and vaporization with increased precision and diminished tissue damage.[7,63,64]

The Nd:YAG laser beam can be transmitted through flexible fiberoptic endoscopes. A separate fiber passed down the biopsy channel of the endoscope transmits the laser beam. Extruded quartz or sapphire tips in many shapes have been introduced.[63,65,66] These are sometimes called sculpted tips and are used once and discarded. They appear to be reasonably effective in delivering the laser light to a small volume and providing some limitation to the lateral thermal damage. The major applications for Nd:YAG lasers to date are treatment of acute gastrointestinal hemorrhage[67] and palliation of obstructing bronchial carcinomas[68,69] and esophageal carcinomas.[70-73] Other applications include photocoagulation of hemangiomas[74,75] of the head and neck and photocoagulation of intranasal hereditary hemorrhagic telangiectasia.[76,77]

Nd:YAG lasers are typically available in 15- to 110-watt units. Because the invisible light from the Nd:YAG laser can cause retinal damage easily, specially colored safety glasses are required for all personnel in the operating room.

Pulsed Yellow Dye Laser

The pulsed yellow dye laser operates at a visible wavelength of 585 nm. The laser beam is pulsed to deliver energy for only 360 microseconds. This laser was specifically developed for use in treating port wine stains.[11–13,42,78] Oxyhemoglobin has an absorption peak near 577 nm. Although this absorption peak is less than at 418 nm, it does permit deeper laser penetration into tissue. Tan showed at 585 nm; there is maximal hemoglobin absorption with a minimum of scattering and minimal absorption by melanin and other pigments.[79] When the duration of the laser pulse is shorter than the time for the heat energy to be conducted away to adjacent tissues, the thermal relaxation time, excessive tissue heating can result. For cutaneous microvessels, 20-μsec pulses from a pulsed dye laser causes vessel wall fragmentation and hemorrhage. Garden et al. found that longer pulse widths caused no significant hemorrhage.[11] The pulse width of 360 μsec caused thermal denaturation of the vessel, producing a more desirable clinical outcome. The epidermis showed no evidence of damage when the laser was used at recommended threshold exposures.

The yellow dye laser has special electrical and plumbing requirements. Special safety eye wear is required.

Argon Tunable Dye Laser

The argon tunable dye laser system works on the principle of the argon laser making a high-intensity beam that is focused on dye that is circulating continuously in a second laser optically coupled to the argon laser. The argon laser beam energizes the dye, causing it to emit laser energy at a longer wavelength than the pump beam. By varying the type of dye and using a tuning system, different wavelengths can be obtained. The laser energy from this dye laser can then be transmitted through flexible fiberoptics and delivered through endoscopic systems or inserted directly into tumors. The major clinical use of this laser is with selective photodynamic therapy (PDT) of malignant tumors after the intravenous injection of a photosensitizer, typically, a hematoporphyrin derivative.[16,20,22,80–82] The argon tunable dye laser is tuned to emit laser light at 630 nm when using hematoporphyin derivatives.

After the intravenous injection, the photosensitizer disseminates to all the cells of the body, rapidly moving out of normal tissue, but remaining longer in neoplastic tissue. After a few days a differential in concentration exists between the tumor cells and the normal cells. When the tumor is exposed to red light (630 nm), the photosensitizer absorbs the light; the absorption of this red light causes a photochemical reaction to occur. Toxic oxygen radicals such as singlet oxygen are produced within the exposed cells causing selective tissue destruction and cellular death. Because there is less photosensitizer in the normal tissues, a much less severe or no reaction occurs. The main technical problem is getting enough light to the target area. The argon tunable dye laser system has helped to solve this problem. Additional research to increase the laser intensity and simplify the sometimes cumbersome setup is being conducted with gold vapor lasers.[82,23]

The premise of treating selected neoplasms with a photosensitizer followed by activation with light is valid. The overall potential and exact place of maximum value of this form of treatment remain to be established. Areas that are promising include carcinoma of the urinary bladder,[84] endobronchial lesions of the lung,[85] selected carcinomas of the upper aerodigestive tract,[86] skin cancers,[87] and metastatic dermal breast cancers.[88] Trials are being conducted in certain specialties on intraoperative PDT in conjunction with conventional surgery.[85]

Manyak et al reported in 1988 that patients who underwent PDT for recurrence of a primary head and neck neoplasm generally did not have improved survival despite successful local tumor eradication.[89] Photodynamic therapy may be indicated for either curative or palliative treatment of endobronchial malignancies. Prospective studies are underway to examine the efficacy of PDT for endobronchial neoplasms.

The argon dye laser requires special electrical and plumbing installation. Special eye wear is required. In addition, prolonged photosensitivity is the most common side effect encountered by the patients.

KTP/532 Laser

The KTP/532 laser is an optically pumped, solid-state laser that produces a visible 0.532 μm (532 μm) beam with an emerald green color. This laser is a frequency-doubled Nd:YAG laser that produces all of its output at 532 μm. The Nd:YAG laser rod is pumped continuously with a krypton arc lamp and Q-switched. The Nd:YAG laser wavelength is frequency-doubled by placing a KTP (potassium titanyl phosphate) crystal in the beam path, which halves the wavelength, producing the characteristic 532 μm output. Like the argon laser, the radiant energy from the KTP laser is transmitted through clear aqueous tissues because it has a low absorption coefficient. Certain tissue pigments, such as melanin and hemoglobin, absorb the KTP laser light effectively. When low levels of green laser light interact with highly pigmented tissues, a localized coagulation takes place within these tissues. The KTP/532 laser can be selected for procedures requiring precise surgical excision with minimal damage to surrounding tissue, vaporization, or photocoagulation. The power density chosen for a given application determines the tissue interaction achieved at the operative site.

The KTP/532 laser is transmitted through a flexible fiberoptic delivery system that can be used in association with a micromanipulator attached to an operating microscope or free-hand in association with various hand-held delivery probes having several different tip angles. These hand-held probes facilitate use of the KTP/532 laser for benign and malignant oral cavity applications,[90,91] functional endoscopic sinus surgery and other intranasal applications,[92,93] and otologic applications.[59,94–97] Examples of hand-held KTP/532 laser applications include tonsillectomy, turbinectomy, stapedotomy, excision of acoustic neurinoma, and excision of benign and malignant laryngeal lesions. Use of the micromanipulator facilitates middle-ear and microlaryngeal laser surgery because it is performed more conventionally using a carbon dioxide laser.

The KTP/532 laser is typically available as a unit that delivers between 0.5 and 20 watts with fiber diameters of 200, 400, and 600 μm. These units have special electrical and plumbing requirements that require advanced planning.

Because the visible green light from the KTP/532 laser can penetrate into the eye and cause retinal damage, special wavelength specific safety glasses must be worn by the surgeon and all personnel in the operating room.

Other Lasers

To have a more controlled laser effect with less damage to adjacent tissue, several lasers in the near to mid-infrared region are being investigated. These include the erbium:YAG (Er:YAG) and the holmium:YAG (Ho:YAG). The Er:YAG lases at the infrared peak of water absorption at 2.94 μm. The extinction length in water is less than 2 μm. The laser produces clean incisions with a minimal amount of thermal damage to the adjacent tissue.[98] The Er:YAG laser has been successful in ablating bone and cartilage in laboratory investigations.[99,100] There are some concerns about the negative consequences of the photoacoustic signal that accompanies the ablation.[101] Two negative aspects to this laser exist. The wavelength is too long to be transmitted through normal optical fibers. This gives a distinct advantage to lasers that produce light that can be transmitted through fibers. More importantly, the thermal propagation is so short there is practically no tissue coagulation and no hemostasis. This laser is therefore unsuitable for use in highly vascular tissue.

The Ho:YAG laser operates at 2.1 μm. This wavelength can be transmitted effectively through fibers. The extinction length in water is approximately 0.4 mm, which suggests that this laser light should interact with tissue similar to the CO_2 laser. The Ho:YAG has been combined with a fiberoptic endoscope for sinus surgery.[102,103] The hemostasis is good and the soft-bone ablation is controlled.[104–106] Adjacent thermal damage zones vary from 130 to 220 μm.

There is also work with other materials that lase in the near infrared region of the spectrum, such as the cobalt:magnesium fluoride laser (tunable from 1.8 to 2.14 μm).[107] Alexandrite lasers (750 μm)[108] and titanium sapphire lasers (tunable from 0.6 to 1.0 μm) have also been considered.[109] Ultimately, many parameters such as cost, reliability and size, in addition to the tissue response, will influence the choice of lasers in medicine.

Carbon Dioxide Laser

Carbon dioxide (CO_2) lasers produce light with wavelength of 10.6 μm in the mid-infrared, and therefore invisible, range of the spectrum. The site where the invisible CO_2 laser beam will impact the target tissue is indicated by a built-in coaxial helium-neon laser beam that is red. To increase the visibility of the aiming beam, some newer lasers have a green aiming beam. It acts as an aiming guide for delivery of the invisible carbon dioxide laser beam. The CO_2 laser has a high water-absorption coefficient, is independent of tissue color, and is well absorbed by all soft tissues that are high in water content; the thermal effects of adjacent nontarget tissue are minimal. The extinction length of this wavelength is approximately 0.03 mm in water and in soft tissue; reflection and scattering are negligible. These properties make the CO_2 laser versatile for use in otolaryngology/head and neck surgery.

With current technology, the radiant energy from a CO_2 laser cannot be transmitted readily through existing fiberoptic endoscopes. Research and development of a suitable flexible fiber for transmission of the CO_2 wavelength are being carried out on an international level.[110] At present, the invisible radiant energy emitted from the optical resonating chamber of a CO_2 laser must be mechanically conveyed by means of a series of mirrors through an articulating arm to the target tissue.[111] Transmission through rigid nonfiber optic endoscopes facilitates use of the CO_2 laser for bronchoscopy, laparoscopy, and arthroscopy. Hollow and flexible waveguides are available for clinical use, but there is considerable loss of energy and limitations on maximum incident energy.

Carbon dioxide surgical lasers can operate in both continuous and pulsed modes. They can be used free-hand for macroscopic surgery, adapted to the operating microscope for microlaryngoscopy, or adapted to a bronchoscopic coupler for rigid bronchoscopy.[112–115]

Carbon dioxide lasers are typically available in 25- to 100-watt units. They are self-contained and have no special electrical or plumbing requirements.

Although the beam cannot penetrate the eye to the retina, it can cause corneal or scleral burns.[116,117] Therefore, protective glasses are required; ordinary glass or plastic correctional lenses have been satisfactory. Clear plastic safety glasses have also provided adequate protection. Hard contact lenses stop the beam, but all the uncovered portions of the eye are unprotected from any misdirected laser radiation.

MACROSCOPIC APPLICATIONS. Macroscopic applications of the CO_2 laser are numerous. In the oral cavity, benign tumors can be excised or ablated with the laser.[118-123] A one-stage tongue release can be performed effectively; we have found this procedure helpful in rehabilitating patients after composite resection with tongue-flap reconstruction.[124] Speech and deglutition can be improved in selected cases. Multiple areas of leukoplakia can be excised precisely and ablated;[86,118,125,126] in most instances, a graft is not necessary to resurface the operative field. Selected superficial carcinomas can be excised with the use of the laser, and large recurrent or inoperable tumors can be debulked for palliation.[72,123,127]

Within the nasal cavities and paranasal sinuses, the CO_2 laser is used to treat choanal atresia, hypertrophic inferior turbinates, squamous papilloma, recurrent inverted papilloma, and hereditary hemorrhagic telangiectasia.[128-133] For this last condition, we believe the Nd:YAG laser to be a more efficacious instrument.

Lingual tonsillectomy, excision of tonsillar neoplasms, serial excision of the palatine tonsils, and excisions of neoplasms of the posterior pharyngeal wall can be performed with the help of this laser.[119,134,135] Peritubal adenoid tissue and recurrent papilloma in the nasopharynx can be ablated by reflecting the radiant energy of the CO_2 laser off a front surface or stainless steel mirror.

Facial plastic surgical applications include excision of rhinophyma,[136-139] excision of benign and malignant skin tumors,[140] and ablation or dermabrasion of nevi and tattoos.[141-144]

Procedures have been introduced to the United States from Europe that allow a serial ablation of the uvula and soft palate to treat patients with snoring problems successfully.[145] Preliminary European studies have shown that the procedure may have application in the treatment of sleep apnea. Performed in an ambulatory setting under local anesthesia, this procedure is associated with much less pain and perioperative morbidity for the patient than with conventional surgery. Additionally, there is no risk of airway obstruction, no hospitalization, and no lost time from work. For these reasons, it has become popular.

MICROSCOPIC APPLICATIONS. **Benign Laryngeal Disease.** The carbon dioxide laser has been used more in microlaryngeal surgery than in any other area of interest to the otolaryngologist/head and neck surgeon. This laser has universal applications in microscopic

surgery of benign laryngeal disease.[114] Its advantages of increased precision and decreased postoperative edema must be weighed against the disadvantages of risks of laser-associated complications and increased operating time. With experience, the drawbacks become limited and the advantages open new horizons. Although knowledge of its use permits the otolaryngologist to apply the CO_2 laser in practically all microlaryngeal procedures for benign laryngeal disease in a safe and effective manner, it is not the only surgical tool to be used for any given operative procedure.

Surgery for recurrent respiratory papillomatosis has advanced with the use of the laser.[130,131,146] Initial disappointment in its inability to cure the disease has been tempered by its effectiveness in preserving normal laryngeal structures and maintaining the translaryngeal airway with an efficiency previously unattained.[146,148] Surgery in children for webs, subglottic stenoses, capillary hemangiomas, and other lesions is also significantly enhanced by the precision, preservation of normal tissue, and predictable minimal postoperative edema associated with judicious use of the carbon dioxide laser.[150-154]

Surgery in adults for polyps, nodules, leukoplakia, papilloma, cysts, and other benign laryngeal conditions also finds advantage with this laser.[155,156] In fact, the laser has created an era of conservation surgery for benign disease. Classically, laryngeal surgery has consisted of vocal cord stripping with healing by remucosalization. Now, more normal tissue can be preserved and more limited spot ablations performed; even flaps of mucosa may be mobilized and advanced in the larynx with endoscopic laser techniques.[114] The laser has lowered the risks to the integrity of the anterior commissure of the larynx during one-stage operations on both cords by its ability to ablate areas and to leave adjacent tissue 0.1 mm away undisturbed by mechanical or other effects.

Biopsy may be performed with the laser, even with a small spot size machine, although there is some tissue vaporization. Scissors and cup forceps still have a role for small lesion biopsy. Surgical judgment is obviously important. In extensive areas of suspicious disease, the laser (with a small spot size) is used appropriately for excisional biopsy.

Webs and subglottic stenoses are incised effectively with the laser.[157-160] Fewer than 50% of anterior commissure webs recur after laser resection. Yet some lasers have such large spot sizes that their use is inappropriate for the procedure. Stenosis can also be treated as long as treatment requires simple tissue ablation with minimal associated edema. If skeletal support is needed, the laser does not provide this, and other techniques should be used.

Endoscopic arytenoidectomy has been performed for many years.[161-164] The addition of the laser allows the surgeon to vaporize the mucosa and underlying arytenoid cartilage layer by layer precisely in a dry field. The precision associated with its use facilitates performance of this operation even by surgeons who had difficulty in mastering the conventional techniques of endoscopic arytenoidectomy. Other microscopic applications of the CO_2 laser include excision of internal laryngoceles and excision of hypopharyngeal diverticula.[165–168] In the latter application, a specially designed endoscope facilitates performance of the operation.

The introduction of the adult subglottiscope has extended the microscopic control and delivery of the CO_2 laser radiation to the subglottis and upper trachea.[169] Selected stenosis in this area have been treated successfully using microtrapdoor flaps.[170,171]

Malignant Laryngeal Disease. Endoscopic management of malignant laryngeal disease is not a new concept. In 1920, Lynch reported 39 patients with early glottic cancers that he successfully treated with transoral excision.[172] New and Dorton in 1941 reported a 90% cure rate with transoral excision and diathermy.[173] Lillie and DeSanto in 1973 reported 98 patients with early glottic carcinoma who were treated with transoral excision; all were cured, although 5 of these patients required further treatment.[174] Hemostasis was provided by electromicrocautery.

The transoral treatment of squamous cell carcinoma of the larynx using the CO_2 laser is therefore an obvious extension of the application of this surgical instrument.[175–177] The advantages of precision, hemostasis, and decreased postoperative edema allow the laryngologist to perform exquisitely accurate and bloodless endoscopic surgery of the larynx. The laser has facilitated a renaissance in the endoscopic management of early vocal cord carcinomas.[178,179]

Three distinct advantages exist with this modality of treatment. First, with the laser, bulky tumors of the anterior commissure area or vocal fold can be removed to obtain an accurate assessment of its extent for purposes of staging and treatment. Additionally, previously biopsied tumors of the vocal cord may represent a diagnostic problem with respect to their extent. The laser may be used to excise the area surrounding the biopsy site.

Inexact staging after direct laryngoscopy is common. By definition, a T_1 carcinoma of the true vocal cords requires cord mobility as defined by the indirect examination. This implies that the tumor is confined to the surface epithelium and has not deeply invaded the vocalis muscle. Our experience agrees with that of previous investigators that vocal cord mobility by itself is a poor indicator of tumor invasion of the underlying muscle.[180] Deep invasion of the vocalis muscle by the cancer has been found after excisional biopsy in many patients who were staged T_1 by the indirect examination. Cancer in these patients should realistically be reclassified as T_3 squamous cell carcinoma.

Airway re-establishment is a second advantage of the CO_2 laser in treating patients with laryngeal carcinoma. The laser can be used to reduce the amount of tumor obstructing the airway, thereby avoiding the need for a preoperative tracheotomy.

The third advantage of using the CO_2 laser in the treatment of laryngeal cancers is that endoscopic excision of laryngeal carcinoma using the CO_2 laser may be curative. The experience of Strong et al,[123] Ossoff et al,[180] Blakeslee et al,[181] and Hirano et al,[182] appears to support the previous work of Lillie and DeSanto,[174] New and Dorton,[173] and Lynch.[172]

Our current treatment plan for the endoscopic management of T_1 vocal cord carcinoma includes an excisional biopsy with the CO_2 laser.[180] Supravital staining with toluidine blue can be performed as a diagnostic aid before biopsy. The surgical specimen is labeled and sent for frozen section examination. Any questionable margins are controlled by frozen section. If the tumor is histologically T_3 or T_4, the patient is treated later by conventional surgical techniques (partial or total laryngectomy).

Otosclerosis. The CO_2 laser possesses ideal tissue interaction characteristics for surgery in the oval window for the performance of primary stapedotomy and revision stapedectomy.[183] A small spot size microscopic coupler should be used in these cases.

Bronchoscopic Applications. Successfully coupling the CO_2 laser to a ventilating bronchoscope represented a logical extension of the clinical application of the CO_2 laser.[127,184] Specifically, use of the CO_2 laser coupled to a ventilating bronchoscope allows the surgeon to perform hands-off endoscopic surgery through the long and narrow operative field of a ventilating bronchoscope. The advantages of precision, hemostasis, decreased postoperative edema, and decreased scarring facilitate visualization and control over the final result of the operation.

Current indications for bronchoscopic CO_2 laser surgery include management of recurrent respiratory papillomatosis[130,131,146,148] or granulation tissue involving the trachea,[185] and resection of selected areas of tracheal stenosis.[158–160,186,187] Tracheal and proximal endobronchial adenomas and webs can also be resected using the CO_2 laser.[188] Finally, patients with selected obstructing tracheal and proximal endobronchial cancers can have their airways re-established as a means of palliation using the laser bronchoscope.[189] The major contraindication to this procedure is extraluminal compression of the trachea by an extrinsic tumor. The Nd:YAG laser is preferred over the CO_2 laser for this latter application.[190,191]

Anesthetic Techniques for CO_2 Laser Surgery

Optimal anesthetic management of patients for laser surgery of the larynx must include attention to the safety of the patient, the requirements of the surgeon, and the hazards of the equipment.[192,193]

Because of the time required to accurately align and manipulate the laser, most patients require general anesthesia for this type of operation. Any nonflammable general anesthetic is suitable, and both halothane and enflurane are in this category. Because of the fire hazard, the inspired concentration of oxygen is important. Mixtures of helium, nitrogen, or air plus oxygen are used to maintain the FIO_2 below 40%, but also to ensure adequate oxygenation. Intravenous supplementation of inhalation anesthesia with small doses of narcotic and/or tranquilizers are used to shorten the emergence period after anesthesia. Total intravenous anesthesia with reversible short-acting narcotics and tranquilizers plus jet ventilation is another acceptable anesthetic technique for microlaryngeal laser surgery. The use of the adult subglottiscope requires the use of jet ventilation and total paralysis.

Advantages of CO₂ Laser Surgery

The greatest advantage of the CO_2 laser is precision, which allows the surgeon to make accurate lesions. When the CO_2 laser is coupled to the operating microscope with a micromanipulator, surgical accuracy can be achieved within 0.1 mm. The smallest spot sizes are in the range of 0.01 mm (200 mm objective) to 0.3 mm (400 mm objective) with current technology. This control, provided by the micromanipulator, is significantly more than is available with hand-held microlaryngeal cupped forceps. The second major advantage of the CO_2 laser is hemostasis. Characteristically, the laser coagulates vessels up to 0.5 mm in diameter, but has the ability to coagulate larger vessels up to 2 mm in diameter under certain circumstances. Vessels larger than 2 mm must be clamped and ligated. The third advantage of the CO_2 laser is decreased postoperative edema. A fourth advantage is decreased postoperative pain. Pain has been reported to be reduced or absent after use of the CO_2 laser. This probably results from the thermal sealing of nerve endings in the operative wound. Other advantages that have been attributed to the CO_2 laser include decreased postoperative scarring and uncomplicated wound healing.

Precautions for CO₂ Laser Surgery

Certain precautions are necessary when using the CO_2 laser. First, to reduce the risk of ocular damage, the patient's eyes should be protected by a double layer of moistened eye pads, and all operating room personnel should wear protective glasses. Additionally, a sign should be placed outside the operating room door warning all persons entering the room to wear protective glasses because the laser is in use. Corneal damage can occur from direct or reflected laser beam irradiation to the eyes. Second, all exposed skin and mucous membranes of the patient outside of the surgical field should be protected by a double layer of moistened surgical towels.

Protection of the endotracheal tube from either direct or reflected laser beam irradiation is of primary importance.[194-198] Should the laser beam strike an unprotected endotracheal tube carrying oxygen, ignition of the tube could cause a catastrophic, intraluminal, blowtorch-type airway fire. Red rubber endotracheal tubes wrapped circumferentially with reflective tape have been used successfully in the past to reduce the risk of intraluminal fire. New metallic endotracheal tubes and silicone endotracheal tubes specially designed for use in microlaryngeal laser surgery also reduce the risk of intraluminal fire.[199-206] The cuff of the endotracheal tube should be inflated with methylene blue saline to act as a heat-sink. The placement of water-saturated neurosurgical cottonoids below the vocal cords to protect the cuff of the endotracheal tube further reduces this risk. These cottonoids should be moistened frequently during the procedure. The development of the operating platform placed in the subglottic larynx can minimize the possibility of an airway fire even further. Should the cuff become deflated by an errant hit of the laser beam, the tube should be removed and replaced with a new one. The cottonoids must be counted like surgical sponges at the completion of the procedure. Perhaps the single most important safety precaution related to reducing the risk of an intraluminal endotracheal tube fire is using mixtures of oxygen (FIO_2 40% or less) and helium for ventilating the patient during microlaryngeal laser surgery.

Additional precautions must be taken to provide for adequate smoke evacuation from the laryngoscope, bronchoscope, or oral cavity to allow for safety as well as visualization of the operative field.[206-209]

Complications of CO₂ Laser Surgery

Many of the possible complications of CO_2 laser surgery have been mentioned in the general discussion of precautions for laser surgery. These include corneal burns, skin burns, misdirected burns from direct or reflected energy, and endotracheal tube ignition.[210-212]

Other complications associated with the use of the CO_2 laser include trauma to the vocal cords during intubation with the aluminum foil-wrapped endotracheal tube, intraoperative airway obstruction secondary to a foreign body (aluminum foil tape or cottonoids), tracheal perforation, acquired glottic web, subglottic stenosis, vocal cord fibrosis, arytenoid perichondritis, delayed bleeding, and delayed postoperative airway obstruction.[213-218]

Great care must be exercised when wrapping the red rubber endotracheal tube circumferentially with the reflective metal tape. We recommend using one quarter-inch tape because it wraps better than larger sizes with fewer subsequent folds, kinks, or rough spots. As previously mentioned, the cottonoids must be counted at the end of the procedure. Additionally, the endotracheal tube should be inspected for areas of possible dislodged aluminum tape.

Tracheal perforation is a distinct possibility when performing laser bronchoscopy. Using the laser in the single or repeat pulse mode should allow the surgeon to differentiate among mucosa, perichondrium, and tracheal cartilage. Using the laser in the continuous mode often makes that necessary distinction difficult.

Acquired glottic web can occur if laser surgery is performed bilaterally at the anterior commissure.[219,220] Subglottic stenosis can result from accidental laser irradiation to the subglottic larynx while working at the anterior or posterior commissure.[221] We recommend using the operating platform to protect the mucosal tissues of the subglottis. Vocal cord fibrosis results from vaporizing vocalis muscle during the process of laser surgery to the true vocal cords.[220,222] This complication can be avoided by proper control of the power density while working on the true vocal cords. Close observation also prevents this complication; a small amount of tissue retraction occurs within the laser impact point when the vocalis muscle is penetrated by the laser beam. Arytenoid perichondritis can occur after deliberate or accidental cartilage exposure during endoscopic laser surgery. Parenteral antibiotics help to minimize this complication.

Delayed postoperative bleeding often occurs if vessels larger than 1 mm are treated by laser coagulation. In dealing with bleeding vessels, those that would ordinarily need to be clamped and ligated if the laser were not being used should still be clamped and ligated. Only vessels less than 1 mm should be coagulated with the CO_2 laser. Although delayed postoperative airway obstruction associated with using the CO_2 laser is rare, it can occur within 18 hours of the operative procedure. The most frequent time for airway edema to occur has been between 1 hour and 6 hours postoperatively. We do not recommend performing outpatient endoscopic microlaryngeal laser procedures. When performing laser surgery in the oral cavity under local anesthesia, patients should remain in the day surgery suite for up to 6 hours postoperatively to observe them for edema or possible airway obstruction before discharge.

SUGGESTED READINGS

1. Duncavage JA, Smith SL: Patterns of laser use at Vanderbilt University Medical Center. Lasers Surg Med Suppl 5:38, 1993.
2. Andrews AH, Polanyi TG(eds.): Microscopic and endoscopic surgery with the CO_2 laser. Littleton, MA, John Wright-PSG, Inc., 1982.
3. Ossoff RH, Werkhaven JA, Raif J, et al: Advanced microspot microslad for the CO_2 laser. Otolaryngol Head Neck Surg 105: 411–414, 1991.
4. Shapshay SM, Wallace RA, Kveton JF, et al: New microspot mi-
5. Ossoff RH: Bronchoscopic laser surgery: which laser when and why. Otolaryngol Head Neck Surg 94:378, 1986.
6. Unger M: Neodymium:YAG laser therapy for malignant and benign endobronchial obstructions. Clin Chest Med 6:277, 1985.
7. Apfelberg DB, Maser MR, White DN, et al: Combination treatment for massive cavernous hemangioma of the face: YAG laser photocoagulation plus direct steroid injection followed by YAG laser resection with sapphire scalpel tips, aided by superselective embolization. Lasers Surg Med 10:217–223, 1990.
8. Joseph M, Reardon E, Goodman M: Lingual tonsillectomy: A treatment for inflammatory lesions of the lingual tonsil. Laryngoscope 94:179–184, 1984.
9. Krespi YP, Har-El G, Levine TM, et al: Laser laryngeal tonsillectomy. Laryngoscope 99:131–135, 1989.
10. Kuhn F: The KTP/532 laser in tonsillectomy. KTP/532 clinical update. Laserscope, San Jose, Calif., No. 06, April, 1988.
11. Garden JM, Polla LL, Tan OT: The treatment of port-wine stains by the pulsed dye laser. Analysis of pulse duration and long-term therapy. Arch Dermatol 124:889–896, 1988.
12. Tan OT, Kershmann R, Parrish JA: The effect of epidermal pigmentation on selective vascular effects of pulsed laser. Lasers Surg Med 4:365, 1984.
13. Tan OT, Stafford TJ, Murray S, et al: Histologic comparison of the pulsed dye laser and copper vapor laser effects on pig skin. Lasers Surg Med 10:551, 1990.
14. Schweitzer VG, Visscher D: Photodynamic therapy for treatment of AIDS-related oral Kaposi's sarcoma. Otolaryngol Head Neck Surg 102:639–649, 1990.
15. Cortese DA, Kinsey JH: Hematoporphyrin-derivative phototherapy for local treatment of cancer of the tracheobronchial tree. Ann Otol Rhinol Laryngol 91:652, 1982.
16. Dougherty TJ, Grindey GB, Fiel R, et al: Photoradiation therapy II. cure of animal tumors with hematoporphyrin and light. J Natl Cancer Inst 55:115–121, 1975.
17. Dougherty TJ, Kaufman JE, Goldfarb A, et al: Photoradiation therapy for the treatment of malignant tumors. Cancer Res 38: 2628–2635, 1978.
18. Dougherty TJ: Photodynamic therapy. Photochem Photobiol. 58: 895–900, 1993.
19. Davis RK: Photodynamic therapy in otolaryngology-head and neck surgery. Otolaryngol Clin North Am 23:107–119, 1990.
20. Gluckman JL: Hematoporphyrin photodynamic therapy: is there truly a future in head and neck oncology? Reflections on a 5-year experience. Laryngoscope 101:36–42, 1991.
21. Manyak MJ, Russo A, Smith PD, et al: Photodynamic therapy. J Clin Oncol 6:380, 1988.
22. Gluckman JL, Zitsch RP: Photodynamic therapy in the management of head and neck cancer. Cancer Treat Res 52:95–113, 1990.
23. Petrucco OM, Sathananden M, Petrucco MF, et al: Ablation of endometriotic implants in rabbits by hematoporphyrin derivative photoradiation therapy using the gold vapor laser. Lasers Surg Med 10:344, 1990.
24. Wenig BL, Kurtzman DM, Grossweiner LI, et al: Photodynamic therapy in the treatment of squamous cell carcinoma of the head and neck. Arch Otolaryngol Head Neck Surg 116:1267–1270, 1990.
25. Brau CA: Free-electron lasers. Science 239:1115–1121, 1988.
26. Edwards G, Logan R, Copeland M, et al: Tissue ablation by a free-electron laser tuned to the amide II band. Nature 371: 416–419, 1994.
27. Polanyi TG: Laser physics. Otolaryngol Clin North Am 16: 753–774, 1983.
28. Schawlow AL, Townes CH: Infrared and optical masers. Phys Rev 112:1940, 1958.

29. Einstein A: Zur Quanten Theorie der Strahlung. Phys Zeit *18*: 121, 1917.

30. Fuller TA: The physics of surgical lasers. Lasers Surg Med *1*: 5–14, 1980.

31. Maiman TH: Stimulated optical radiation in ruby. Nature *187*: 493, 1960.

32. Fuller TA: The characteristics of operation of surgical lasers. Surg Clin North Am *64*:843–849, 1984.

33. Doukas AG, McAuliffe DJ, Flotte TJ: Biological effects of laser-induced shock waves: structural and functional cell damage in vitro. Ultrasound Med Biol *19*:137–146, 1993.

34. LeCarpentier GL, Motamedi M, McMath LP, et al: Continuous wave laser ablation of tissue: analysis of thermal and mechanical events. IEEE Trans Biomed Eng *40*:188–200, 1993.

35. Verdaasdonk RM, Borst C, van Gemert MJ: Explosive onset of continuous wave laser tissue ablation. Phys Med Biol *35*:1129–44, 1990.

36. Reinisch L: Laser induced heating and thermal propagation: a model of tissue interaction with light. Proc Conf Lasers Elect Optics *11*:TuR4, 1989.

37. McKenzie AL: How far does thermal damage extend beneath the surface of CO_2 laser incisions? Phys Med Biol *28*:905–912, 1983.

38. Walsh JT Jr, Flotte TJ, Anderson RR, et al: Pulsed CO_2 laser tissue ablation: effect of tissue type and pulse duration on thermal damage. Lasers Surg Med *8*:108–118, 1988.

39. Hall RR: The healing of tissues incised by carbon dioxide laser. Br J Surg *58*:222–225, 1971.

40. Norris CW, Mullarry MB: Experimental skin incision made with the carbon dioxide laser. Laryngoscope *92*:416–419, 1982.

41. Finsterbush A, Rousso M, Ashur H: Healing and tensile strength of CO_2 laser incisions and scalpel wounds in rabbits. Plast Reconstr Surg *70*:360–362, 1982.

42. Buell BR, Schuller DE: Comparison of tensile strength in CO_2 laser and scalpel skin incisions. Arch Otolaryngol *109*:465–467, 1983.

43. Middleton WG, Tees DA, Ostrowski M: Comparative gross and histological effects of the CO2 laser, Nd-YAG laser, scalpel, Shaw scalpel and cutting cautery on skin in rats. Otolaryngol *22*: 167–170, 1993.

44. Kyzer MD, Aly AS, Davidson JM, Reinisch L, Ossoff RH: Sub ablation effects of the KTP laser on wound healing. Lasers Surg Med *13*:62–71, 1993.

45. Pogrel MA, Pham HD, Guntenhoner M, et al: Profile of hyaluronidase activity distinguishes carbon dioxide laser from scalpel wound healing. Ann Surg *217*:196–200, 1993.

46. Luomanen M, Virtanen I: Fibronectins in healing incision, excision and laser wounds. Oral Path Med *20*:133–138, 1991.

47. Apfelberg DB, Maser MR, Lash H, et al: The argon laser for cutaneous lesions. JAMA *245*:2073–2075, 1981.

48. Cosman B: Experience in the argon laser therapy for port-wine stains. Plast Reconstr Surg *65*:119–129, 1980.

49. Tan OT, Carney JM, Margolis R, et al: Histologic responses of port-wine stains treated by argon, carbon dioxide, and tunable dye lasers. A preliminary report. Arch Dermatol *122*:1016–1022, 1986.

50. Parkin JL, Dixon JA: Argon laser treatment of head and neck vascular lesions. Otolaryngol Head Neck Surg *93*:211–216, 1981.

51. Kluger PB, Shapshay SM, Hybels RL, et al: Neodymium-YAG laser intranasal photocoagulation in hereditary hemorrhagic telangiectasia: an update report. Laryngoscope *97*:1397–1401, 1987.

52. Perkins RC: Laser stapedotomy for otosclerosis. Laryngoscope *90*:228–240, 1980.

53. Hodgson RS, Wilson DF: Argon laser stapedotomy. Laryngoscope *101*:230–3, 1991.

54. Vollrath M, Schreiner C: Influence of argon laser stapedotomy on inner ear function and temperature. Otolaryngol Head Neck Surg *91*:521–526, 1983.

55. McGee TM: The argon laser in surgery for chronic ear disease and otosclerosis. Laryngoscope *93*:1177–1182, 1983.

56. DiBartolomeo JR, Ellis M: The argon laser in otology. Laryngoscope *90*:1786–1796, 1980.

57. Escudero LH, Castro AO, Drumond M, et al: Argon laser in human tympanoplasty. Arch Otolaryngol *105*:252–253, 1979.

58. Hanna E, Eliachar I, Cothren R, et al: Laser welding of fascial grafts and its potential application in tympanoplasty: an animal model. Otolaryngol Head Neck Surg *108*:356–366, 1993.

59. Wanamaker HH, Silverstein H: Compatibility of the argon and KTP lasers with middle ear implants. Laryngoscope *103*:609–613, 1993.

60. Horn KL, Cherini S: Otologic argon laser surgery using an endolaryngealotoprobe system. Abstracts of Second International Laser Surgery Congress, Nashville, Tennessee, June 22–26, 1986.

61. Horn KL, Gherini S, Griffin GM Jr: Argon laser stapedectomy using an endootoprobe system. Otolaryngol Head Neck Surg *102*:193–198, 1990.

62. Rauch SD, Bartley ML: Argon laser stapedectomy: comparison to traditional fenestration techniques. Am Otol *13*:556–560, 1992.

63. Apfelberg DB, Lane B, Marx MP: Combined (team) approach to hemangioma management: arteriography with superselective embolization plus YAG laser/sapphire-tip resection. Plastic Reconstr Surg *88*:71–82, 1991.

64. Mehta AC, Livingston DR, Golish JA: Artificial sapphire contact endoprobe with Nd-YAG laser in the treatment of subglottic stenosis. Chest *91*:473–4, 1987.

65. Hukki J, Krogerus L, Costren M, et al: Effects of different contact laser scalpels on skin and subcutaneous fat. Lasers Surg Med *8*: 276–282, 1988.

66. Iwasaki M, Sasako M, Konishi T, et al: Nd-YAG laser for general surgery. Lasers Surg Med *5*:429–438, 1985.

67. Matthewson K, Swain CP, Bland M, et al: Randomized comparison of Nd YAG laser, heater probe, and no endoscopic therapy for bleeding peptic ulcers. Gastroenterol *98*:1239–1244, 1990.

68. Castro DJ, Saxton RE, Ward PH, et al: Flexible Nd:YAG laser palliation of obstructive tracheal metastatic malignancies. Laryngoscope *100*:1208–1214, 1990.

69. Dumon JF, Reboud E, Garbe L, et al: Treatment of tracheobronchial lesions by laser photoresection. Chest *81*:278–284, 1982.

70. Eckhauser ML: The neodymium-YAG laser and gastrointestinal malignancy. Arch Surg *125*:1152–1154, 1990.

71. Eckhauser ML: Palliative therapy of upper gastrointestinal malignancies using the Nd-YAG laser. Am Surg *56*:158–162, 1990.

72. Rontal E, Rontal M, Jacob HJ, et al: Laser palliation for esophageal carcinoma. Laryngoscope *96*:846–850, 1986.

73. Dumon JF, Shapshay S, Bourcereau J, et al: Principles for safety in application of Neodymium-YAG laser in bronchology. Chest *86*:163–168, 1984.

74. Shapshay SM, David LM, Zeitels S: Neodymium:YAG laser photocoagulation of hemangiomas of the head and neck. Laryngoscope *97*:323–330, 1987.

75. Apfelberg DB, Maser MR, White DN, et al: Benefits of contact and noncontact YAG laser for periorbital hemangiomas. Ann Plastic Surg *24*:397–408, 1990.

76. Illum P, Bjerring P: Hereditary hemorrhagic telangiectasia treated by laser surgery. Rhinology *26*:19–24, 1988.

77. Kluger PB, Shapshay SM, Hybels RL, et al: Neodymium-YAG laser intranasal photocoagulation in hereditary hemorrhagic telangiectasia: an update report. Laryngoscope *97*:1397–1401, 1987.

78. Garden JM, Bakus AD: Clinical efficacy of the pulsed dye laser in the treatment of vascular lesions. Dermatol Surg Oncol *19*: 321–326, 1993.

79. Tan OT, Morrison P, Kurban AK: 585 nm for the treatment of port-wine stains. Plast Reconstr Surg *88*:547–548, 1991.

80. Rausch PC, Rolfs F, Winkler MR, et al: Pulsed versus continuous wave excitation mechanisms in photodynamic therapy of dif-

ferently graded squamous cell carcinomas in tumor-implanted nude mice. Euro Arch Oto-Rhino-Laryngol 250:82–87, 1993.

81. Okunaka T, Kato H, Conaka C, et al: Photodynamic therapy of esophageal carcinoma. Surg Endoscopy 4:150–153, 1990.

82. Shikowitz MJ: Comparison of pulsed and continuous wave light in photodynamic therapy of papillomas: an experimental study. Laryngoscope 102:300–310, 1992.

83. Petrucco OM, Sathananden M, Petrucco MF, et al: Ablation of endometriotic implants in rabbits by hematoporphyrin derivative photoradiation therapy using the gold vapor laser. Lasers Surg Med 10:344–348, 1990.

84. Dougherty TJ, Marcus SL: Photodynamic therapy. Euro Cancer 28A:1734–1742, 1992.

85. Pass HI: Photodynamic therapy in oncology: mechanisms and clinical use. Natl Cancer Inst 85:443–456, 1993.

86. Grant WE, Hopper C, Speight PM, et al: Photodynamic therapy of malignant and premalignant lesions in patients with 'field cancerization' of the oral cavity. Laryngol Otol 107:1140–1145, 1993.

87. Lui H, Anderson RR: Photodynamic therapy in dermatology: recent developments. Dermatol Clinics 11:1–13, 1993.

88. Khan SA, Dougherty TJ, Mang TS: An evaluation of photodynamic therapy in the management of cutaneous metastases of breast cancer. Euro Cancer 29A:1686–1690, 1993.

89. Manyak MJ, Russo A, Smith PD, et al: Photodynamic therapy. Clin Oncol 6:380–391, 1988.

90. Ikeda M, Takahashi H, Karaho T, et al: Amelanotic melanoma metastatic to the epiglottis. Laryngol Otol 105:776–779, 1991.

91. Oas RE Jr, Bartels JP: KTP-532 laser tonsillectomy: a comparison with standard technique. Laryngoscope 100:385–388, 1990.

92. Kass EG, Massaro BM, Komorowski RA, et al: Wound healing of KTP and argon laser lesions in the canine nasal cavity. Otolaryngol Head Neck Surg 108:283–292, 1993.

93. Levine HL: Endoscopy and the KTP/532 laser for nasal sinus disease. Ann Otol Rhinol Laryngol 98:46, 1989.

94. Bartels LJ: KTP laser stapedotomy: is it safe?. Otolaryngol Head Neck Surg 103:685, 1990.

95. Thedinger BS: Applications of the KTP laser in chronic ear surgery. Am Otol 11:79–84, 1990.

96. Lesinski SG, Palmer A: Lasers for otosclerosis: CO2 vs. Argon and KTP-532. Laryngoscope 99:1–8, 1989.

97. Pillsbury HC: Comparison of small fenestra stapedotomies with and without KTP 532 laser. Arch Otolaryngol Head Neck Surg 115:1027, 1989.

98. Herdman RC, Charlton A, Hinton AE, et al: An in vitro comparison of the Erbium: YAG laser and the carbon dioxide laser in laryngeal surgery. Laryngol Otol 107:908–911, 1993.

99. Nelson JS, Orenstein A, Liaw LH, et al: Mid-infrared erbium: YAG laser ablation of bone: the effect of laser osteotomy on bone healing. Lasers Surg Med 9:362–374, 1989.

100. Gonzalez C, van de Merwe WP, Smith M, et al: Comparison of the erbium-yttrium aluminum garnet and carbon dioxide lasers for in vitro bone and cartilage ablation. Laryngoscope 100:14–17, 1990.

101. Li ZZ, Reinisch L, Van de Merwe WP: Bone ablation with Er: YAG and CO2 laser: study of thermal and acoustic effects. Lasers Surg Med 12:79–85, 1992.

102. Shapshay SM, Rebeiz EE, Bohigian RK, et al: Holmium: yttrium aluminum garnet laser-assisted endoscopic sinus surgery: laboratory experience. Laryngoscope 101:142–149, 1991.

103. Shapshay SM, Rebeiz EE, Pankratov MM: Holmium:yttrium aluminum garnet laser-assisted endoscopic sinus surgery: clinical experience. Laryngoscope 102:1177–1180, 1992.

104. Kautzky M, Trodhan A, Susani M, et al: Infrared laser stapedotomy. Eur Arch Oto Rhino Laryngol 248:449–451, 1991.

105. Treat MR, Trokel SL, Reynolds RD, et al: Preliminary evaluation of a pulsed 2.15-micron laser system for fiberoptic endoscopic surgery. Lasers Surg Med 8:322–326, 1988.

106. April MM, Rebeiz EE, Aretz HT, et al: Endoscopic holmium laser laryngotracheoplasty in animal models. Ann Otol, Rhinol Laryngol 100:503–507, 1991.

107. Schomacker KT, Domankevitz Y, Flotte TJ, et al: Co:MgF2 laser ablation of tissue: effect of wavelength on ablation threshold and thermal damage. Lasers Surg Med 11:141–51, 1991.

108. Schlenk E, Profeta G, Nelson JS, et al: Laser assisted fixation of ear prostheses after stapedectomy. Lasers Surg Med 10:444–447, 1990.

109. Frederickson KS, White WE, Wheeland RG, et al: Precise ablation of skin with reduced collateral damage using the femtosecond-pulsed, terawatt titanium-sapphire laser. Arch Dermatol 129:989–993, 1993.

110. Merberg GN: Current status of infrared fiber optics for medical laser power delivery. Lasers Surg Med 13:572–576, 1993.

111. Ossoff RH, Karlan MS: Instrumentation for CO2 laser surgery of the larynx and tracheobronchial tree. Surg Clin North Am 64:973–980, 1984.

112. Ossoff RH, Karlan MS: Instrumentation for microlaryngeal laser surgery. Otolaryngol Head Neck Surg 91:456–460, 1983.

113. Ossoff RH, Karlan MS: A set of bronchoscopes for carbon dioxide laser surgery. Otolarynol Head Neck Surg 91:336–337, 1983.

114. Karlan MS, Ossoff, RH: Laser surgery for benign laryngeal disease. Conservation and ergonomics. Surg Clin North Am 64:981–994, 1984.

115. Ossoff RH, Karlan MS: Universal endoscopic coupler for carbon dioxide laser surgery. Ann Otol Rhino Laryngol 91:608–609, 1982.

116. Leibowitz HM, Peacock GR: Corneal injury produced by carbon dioxide laser radiation. Arch Ophthalmol 87:713, 1969.

117. Fine BS, Fine S, Peacock GR, et al: Preliminary observations on ocular effects of high-power, continuous CO2 laser irradiation. Am J Ophthalmol 64:209–222, 1967.

118. Chu FWK, Silverman S Jr, Dedo HH: CO2 laser treatment of oral leukoplakia. Laryngoscope 98:125–130, 1988.

119. Duncavage JA, Ossoff RH: Use of the CO2, laser for malignant disease of the oral cavity. Lasers Surg Med 6:442–444, 1986.

120. Guerry TL, Silverman S Jr, Dedo HH: Carbon dioxide laser resection of superficial oral carcinoma: Indications, technique, and results. Ann Otol Rhinol Laryngol 95:547–555, 1986.

121. McDonald GA, Simpson GT: Transoral resection of lesions of the oral cavity with the carbon dioxide laser. Otolaryngol Clin North Am 16:839–847, 1983.

122. Nagorsky MJ, Sessions DG: Laser resection for early oral cavity cancer: Results and complications. Ann Otol Rhinol Laryngol 96:556–560, 1987.

123. Strong MS, Vaughan CW, Jako GJ, Polanyi T: Transoral resection of cancer of the oral cavity: the role of the CO2 laser. Otolaryngol Clin North Am 12:207–218, 1979.

124. Liston SL, Giordano A Jr: Tongue release using the CO2 laser. Laryngoscope 91:1010–1011, 1981.

125. Roodenburg JL, Panders AK, Vermey A: Carbon dioxide laser surgery of oral leukoplakia. Oral Surg Oral Med Oral Path 71:670–674, 1991.

126. Chiesa F, Tradati N, Sala L, et al: Follow-up of oral leukoplakia after carbon dioxide laser surgery. Arch Otolaryngol Head Neck Surg 116:177–180, 1990.

127. Shapshay SM, Davis RK, Vaughan CW, et al: Palliation of airway obstruction from tracheobronchial malignancy: Use of the CO2 laser bronchoscope. Otolaryngol Head Neck Surg 91:615–619, 1983.

128. Healy GB, McGill T, Jako GJ, et al: Management of choanal atresia with the carbon dioxide laser. Ann Otol Rhinol Laryngol 87:658–662, 1978.

129. Mittelman H: CO2 laser turbinectomies for chronic obstructive rhinitis. Lasers Surg Med 2:29–36, 1982.

130. Simpson GT, Strong MS: Recurrent respiratory papillomatosis;

the role of the carbon dioxide laser. Otolaryngol Clin North Am 16:887–894, 1983.

131. Strong MS, Vaughan CW, Cooperband SR, et al: Recurrent respiratory papillomatosis: Management with the CO2 laser. Ann Otol Rhinol Laryngol 85:508–516, 1976.

132. Siegel MB, Keane WM, Atkins JF Jr, et al: Control of epistaxis in patients with hereditary hemorrhagic telangiectasia. Otolaryngol Head Neck Surg 105:675–679, 1991.

133. McCombe AW, Cook J, Jones AS: A comparison of laser cautery and submucosal diathermy for rhinitis. Clin Otolaryngol 17:297–299, 1992.

134. Wouters B, van Overbeek JJ, Buiter CT, et al: Laser surgery in lingual tonsil hyperplasia. Clin Otolaryngol 14:291–296, 1989.

135. Puar RK, Puar HS: Lingual tonsillitis. South Med J 79:1126–1128, 1986.

136. Shapshay SM, Strong MS, Anastasi GW, et al: Removal of rhinophyma with the carbon dioxide laser. Arch Otolaryngol 106:257–259, 1980.

137. Gjuric M, Rettinger G: Comparison of carbon dioxide laser and electrosurgery in the treatment of rhinophyma. Rhinology 31:37–39, 1993.

138. Har-El G, Shapshay SM, Bohigian RK, et al: The treatment of rhinophyma. 'Cold' vs laser techniques. Arch Otolaryngol Head Neck Surg 119:628–631, 1993.

139. Haas A, Wheeland RG: Treatment of massive rhinophyma with the carbon dioxide laser. J Dermatol Surg Oncol 16:645–649, 1990.

140. Kirschner RA: Cutaneous plastic surgery with the CO2 laser. Surg Clin North Am 64:871–883, 1984.

141. Levine H, Bailin P: Carbon dioxide laser treatment of cutaneous hemangiomas and tattoos. Arch Otolaryngol 108:236–238, 1982.

142. Fairhurst MV, Roenigk RK, Brodland DG: Carbon dioxide laser surgery for skin disease. Mayo Clin Proc 67:49–58, 1992.

143. Dinehart SM, Gross DJ, Davis CM, et al: Granuloma faciale. Comparison of different treatment modalities. Arch Otolaryngol Head Neck Surg 116:849–851, 1990.

144. Sunde D, Apfelberg DB, Sergott T: Traumatic tattoo removal: comparison of four treatment methods in an animal model with correlation to clinical experience. Lasers Surg Med 10:158–164, 1990.

145. Kamami YV: Laser CO2 for snoring. Preliminary results. Acta Oto-Rhino-Laryngol Belgica 44:451–456, 1990.

146. Kattner MN, Clark GD: Recurrent respiratory papillomatosis. Nurse Anesth 4:28–35, 1993.

148. Ossoff RH, Werkhaven JA, Dere H: Soft-tissue complications of laser surgery for recurrent respiratory papillomatosis. Laryngoscope 101:1162–1166, 1991.

149. Shapshay SM, Rebeiz EE, Bohigian RK, et al: Benign lesions of the larynx: should the laser be used?. Laryngoscope 100:953–957, 1990.

150. Kay GA, Lobe TE, Custer MD, et al: Endoscopic laser ablation of obstructing congenital duodenal webs in the newborn: a case report of limited success with criteria for patient. J Pediatr Surg 27:279–281, 1992.

151. Werkhaven JA, Weed DT, Ossoff RH: Carbon dioxide laser serial microtrapdoor flap excision of subglottic stenosis. Arch Otolaryngol Head Neck Surg 119:676–679, 1993.

152. Ossoff RH, Tucker JA, Werkhaven JA: Neonatal and pediatric microsubglottiscope set. Ann Otol Rhinol Laryngol 100:325–326, 1991.

153. Bagwell CE: CO2 laser excision of pediatric airway lesions. J Pediatr Surg 25:1152–1156, 1990.

154. McGill TJI, Friedman EM, Healy GB: Laser surgery in the pediatric airway. Otolaryngol Clin North Am 16:865–870, 1983.

155. Vaughan CW: Transoral laryngeal surgery using the CO2 laser: Laboratory experiments and clinical experience. Laryngoscope 88:1399–1420, 1978.

156. Vaughan CW: Use of the carbon dioxide laser in the endoscopic management of organic laryngeal disease. Otolaryngol Clin North Am 16:849–864, 1983.

157. Dedo HH, Sooy CD: Endoscopic laser repair of posterior glottic, subglottic and tracheal stenosis by division or micro-trapdoor flap. Laryngoscope 94:445–450, 1984.

158. Holinger LD: Treatment of severe subglottic stenosis without tracheotomy: a preliminary report. Ann Otol Rhinol Laryngol 91:407–412, 1982.

159. Lebovics RS, Hoffman GS, Leavitt RY, et al: The management of subglottic stenosis in patients with Wegener's granulomatosis. Laryngoscope 102:1341–1345, 1992.

160. Whitehead E, Salam MA: Use of the carbon dioxide laser with the Montgomery T-tube in the management of extensive subglottic stenosis. Laryngol Otol 106:829–831, 1992.

161. Ossoff RH, Karlan MS, Sisson GA: Endoscopic laser arytenoidectomy. Lasers Surg Med 2:293–299, 1983.

162. Ossoff RH, Sisson GA, Duncavage JA, et al: Endoscopic laser arytenoidectomy for the treatment of bilateral vocal cord paralysis. Laryngoscope 94:1293–1297, 1984.

163. Ossoff RH, Duncavage JA, Shapshay SM, et al: Endoscopic laser arytenoidectomy revisited. Ann Otol Rhinol Laryngol 99:764–771, 1990.

164. Netterville JL, Aly A, Ossoff RH: Evaluation and treatment of complications of thyroid and parathyroid surgery. Otolaryngol Clin North Am 23:529–552, 1990.

165. Komisar A: Laser laryngoscopic management of internal laryngocele. Laryngoscope 97:368–369, 1987.

166. Van Overbeek JJM, Hoeksema PE, Edens ET: Microendoscopic surgery of the hypopharyngeal diverticulum using electrocoagulation or carbon dioxide laser. Ann Otol Rhinol Laryngol 93:34–36, 1984.

167. Benjamin B, Gallagher R: Microendoscopic laser diverticulotomy for hypopharyngeal diverticulum. Ann Otol Rhinol Laryngol 102:675–679, 1993.

168. van Overbeek JJ: Meditation on the pathogenesis of hypopharyngeal (Zenker's) diverticulum and a report of endoscopic treatment in 545 patients. Ann Otol Rhinol Laryngol 103:178–185, 1994.

169. Ossoff RH, Duncavage JA, Dere H: Microsubglottoscopy: an expansion of operative microlaryngoscopy. Otolaryngol Head Neck Surg 104:842–848, 1991.

170. Duncavage JA, Piazza LS, Ossoff RH, et al: The microtrapdoor technique for the management of laryngeal stenosis. Laryngoscope 97:825–828, 1987.

171. Beste DJ, Toohill RJ: Microtrapdoor flap repair of laryngeal and tracheal stenosis. Ann Otol Rhinol Laryngol 100:420–423, 1991.

172. Lynch RC: Intrinsic carcinoma of the larynx with a second report of the cases operated on by suspension and dissection. Trans Am Laryngol Assoc 42:119, 1920.

173. New GB, Dorton HE: Suspension laryngoscopy and the treatment of malignant disease of the hypopharynx and larynx. Mayo Clin Proc 16:411, 1941.

174. Lillie JC, DeSanto LW: Transoral surgery of early cordal carcinoma. Trans Am Acad Ophthalmol Otolaryngol 77:192, 1973.

175. Koufman JA: The endoscopic management of early squamous carcinoma of the vocal cord with the carbon dioxide surgical laser: clinical experience and a proposed subclassification. Otolaryngol Head Neck Surg 95:531–537, 1986.

176. Wetmore SJ, Key JM, Suen JY: Laser therapy for T1 glottic carcinoma of the larynx. Arch Otolaryngol Head Neck Surg 112:853–855, 1986.

177. Rothfield RE, Myers EN, Johnson JT: Carcinoma in situ and microinvasive squamous cell carcinoma of the vocal cords. Ann Otol Rhinol Laryngol 100:793–796, 1991.

178. Rice DH, Wetmore SJ, Singer M: Recurrent squamous cell carcinoma of the true vocal cord. Head Neck 13:549–552, 1991.

179. Myers EN, Wagner RL, Johnson JT: Microlaryngoscopic sur-

gery for T1 glottic lesions: a cost-effective option. Ann Otol Rhinol Laryngol *103*:28–30, 1994.

180. Ossoff RH, Sisson GA, Shapshay SM: Endoscopic management of selected early vocal cord carcinoma. Ann Otol Rhinol Laryngol *94*:560–564, 1985.

181. Blakeslee D, Vaughan CW, Shapshay SM, et al: Excisional biopsy in the selective management of T_1 glottic cancer: a three-year follow-up study. Laryngoscope *94*:488–494, 1984.

182. Hirano M, Hirade Y, Kawasaki H: Vocal function following carbon dioxide laser surgery for glottic carcinoma. Ann Otol Rhinol Laryngol *94*:232–235, 1985.

183. Lesinski SG, Newrock R: Carbon dioxide lasers for otosclerosis. Otolaryngol Clin North Am *26*:417–441, 1993.

184. Andrews AH Jr, Horowitz SL: Bronchoscopic CO_2 laser surgery. Lasers Surg Med *1*:35–45, 1980.

185. Katlic MR, Burick AJ, Lucchino DB: Experiences with laser bronchoscopy. Penn Med *94*:247, 1991.

186. Simpson GT, Strong MS, Healy GB, et al: Predictive factors of success or failure in the endoscopic management of laryngeal and tracheal stenosis. Ann Otol Rhinol Laryngol *91*:384–388, 1982.

187. Duncavage JA, Ossoff RH, Toohill RJ: Carbon dioxide laser management of laryngeal stenosis. Ann Otol Rhinol Laryngol *94*:565–569, 1985.

188. Stanley PR, Anderson T, Pagliero KM: Laser photoresection in the preoperative assessment of a bronchial adenoma. Thorax *43*:741–742, 1988.

189. Shapshay SM, Strong MS: Tracheobronchial obstruction from metastatic distant malignancies. Ann Otol Rhinol Laryngol *91*:648–651, 1982.

190. Sutedja G, Koppenol W, Stam J: Nd-YAG laser under local anaesthesia in obstructive endobronchial tumours. Respiration *58*:238–240, 1991.

191. Edell ES, Cortese DA, McDougall JC: Ancillary therapies in the management of lung cancer: photodynamic therapy, laser therapy, and endobronchial prosthetic devices. Mayo Clin Proc *68*:685–690, 1993.

192. Keon TP: Anesthetic management during laser surgery. International Anesthesiology Clin *30*:99–107, 1992.

193. Spiess BD, Ivankovich AD: Anesthetic management of laser airway surgery. Semin Surg Oncol *6*:189–193, 1990.

194. Burgess GE, LeJeune FE: Endotracheal tube ignition during laser surgery of the larynx. Arch Otolaryngol *105*:561–562, 1979.

195. Cozine K, Rosenbaum LM, Askanazi J, et al: Laser-induced endotracheal tube fire. Anesthesiology *55*:583–585, 1981.

196. Hirshman CA, Smith J: Indirect ignition of the endotracheal tube during carbon dioxide laser surgery. Arch Otolaryngol Head Neck Surg *106*:639–641, 1980.

197. Ossoff RH, Duncavage JA, Eisenman TS, et al: Comparison of tracheal damage from laser-ignited endotracheal tube fires. Ann Otol Rhinol Laryngol *92*:333–336, 1983.

198. Treyve E, Yarington CT, Thompson GE: Incendiary characteristics of endotracheal tubes with the carbon dioxide laser. Ann Otol Rhinol Laryngol *90*:328–330, 1981.

199. Hawkins DB, Joseph MM: Avoiding a wrapped endotracheal tube in laser laryngeal surgery: experiences with apneic anesthesia and metal laser-flex endotracheal tubes. Laryngoscope *100*:1283–1287, 1990.

200. Fried MP, Mallampati SR, Liu FC, et al: Laser resistant stainless steel endotracheal tube: experimental and clinical evaluation. Lasers Surg Med *11*:301–306, 1991.

201. Sosis MB, Dillon F: Prevention of CO2 laser-induced endotracheal tube fires with the laser-guard protective coating. J Clin Anesthesiol *4*:25–27, 1992.

202. Sosis MB: Which is the safest endotracheal tube for use with the CO2 laser? A comparative study. J Clin Anesthesiol *4*:217–219, 1992.

203. Sosis MB, Dillon FX: A comparison of CO2 laser ignition of the Xomed, plastic, and rubber endotracheal tubes. Anesth Analgesia *76*:391–393, 1993.

204. Hayes DM, Gaba DM, Goode RL: Incendiary characteristics of a new laser-resistant endotracheal tube. Otolaryngol Head Neck Surg *95*:37–40, 1986.

205. Fontenot R Jr, Bailey BJ, Stiernberg CM, et al: Endotracheal tube safety during laser surgery. Laryngoscope *97*:919–921, 1987.

206. Tomita Y, Mihashi S, Nagata K, et al: Mutagenicity of smoke condensates induced by CO_2 laser irradiation and electrocauterization. Mutat Res *89*:145–149, 1981.

207. Wenig BL, Stenson KM, Wenig BM, et al: Effects of plume produced by the Nd:YAG laser and electrocautery on the respiratory system. Lasers Surg Med *13*:242–245, 1993.

208. Baggish MS, Poiesz BJ, Joret D, et al: Presence of human immunodeficiency virus DNA in laser smoke. Lasers Surg Med *11*:197–203, 1991.

209. Abramson AL, DiLorenzo TP, Steinberg BM: Is papillomavirus detectable in the plume of laser-treated laryngeal papilloma? Arch Otolaryngol Head Neck Surg *116*:604–607, 1990.

210. Ossoff RH: Laser Safety in Otolaryngology-Head and Neck Surgery: Anesthetic and educational considerations for laryngeal surgery. Laryngoscope *99*:1–26, 1989.

211. Ossoff RH, Karlan MS: Safe instrumentation in laser surgery. Otolaryngol Head Neck Surg *92*:664, 1984.

212. Ossoff RH, Hotaling A, Karlan MS, et al: The CO_2 laser in otolaryngology--head and neck surgery: a retrospective analysis of complications. Laryngoscope *93*:1287, 1983.

213. Alberti PW: The complications of CO_2 laser surgery in otolaryngology. Acta Otolaryngol *91*:375–381, 1981.

214. Fried MP: A survey of the complications of laser laryngoscopy. Arch Otolaryngol *110*:31–34, 1984.

215. Healy GB, Strong MS, Shapshay S, et al: Complications of CO_2 laser surgery of the aerodigestive tract: experience of 4416 cases. Otolaryngol Head Neck Surg *92*:13–18, 1984.

216. Meyers A: Complications of CO_2 laser surgery of the larynx. Ann Otol Rhinol Laryngol *90*:132–134, 1981.

217. Mohr RM, McDonnell BC, Unger M, et al: Safety considerations and safety protocol for laser surgery. Surg Clin North Am *64*:851–859, 1984.

218. Spilman LS: Nursing precautions for CO_2 laser surgery. Symposium Proceedings, The Laser Institute of America *37*:63, 1983.

219. Crockett DM, McCabe BF, Shive CJ: Complications of laser surgery for recurrent respiratory papillomatosis. Ann Otol Rhinol Laryngol *96*:639–644, 1987.

220. Wetmore SJ, Key JM, Suen JY: Complications of laser surgery for laryngeal papillomatosis. Laryngoscope *95*:798–801, 1985.

221. Cotton RT, Tewfik TL: Laryngeal stenosis following carbon dioxide laser in subglottic hemangioma: Report of three cases. Ann Otol Rhinol Laryngol *94*:494–497, 1985.

222. Durkin GE, Duncavage JA, Toohill RJ, et al: Wound healing of true vocal cord squamous epithelium after CO2 laser ablation and cup forceps stripping. Otolaryngol Head Neck Surg *95*:273–277, 1986.

IV IMAGING OF THE HEAD AND NECK

Galdino E. Valvassori and Mahmood A. Mafee

37 Computed Tomography, Magnetic Resonance

Mahmood F. Mafee

The development of computerized tomography (CT) and magnetic resonance imaging (MRI) has been regarded as the most important contribution to diagnostic medical imaging techniques since Roentgen discovered the x-ray in 1895. Computers were first used in nuclear medicine in the 1960s, but it was the introduction of CT in 1971, an invention of Godfrey N. Hounsfield who won the Nobel prize for his pioneering research, that accelerated interest in the application of computers to the broader aspects of radiology. Like CT, MRI has proven to be a major breakthrough in diagnostic medical imaging. Based on pioneering work of Paul Lauterbur[1] in the early 1970s, MRI with its continued refinement is considered to be the most important medical imaging advance of the century.

The technique of CT employs a narrow highly collimated scanning radiographic beam and a scintillation-crystal photomultiplier, or xenon-ionization detectors with high detection efficiency, to monitor the radiographic absorption throughout the part of the body being studied.[2] The data collected are processed by a computer, which, by solving thousands of equations instantaneously, produces a true tomographic section.[2-4] The reconstruction of the subject cross-section resides in the computer as a series of digital numbers, usually referred to as "CT numbers."[2] These numbers are related to the linear radiograph attenuation of the material in the volume element (Voxel) at the location of interest.[2]

Zero is arbitrarily chosen to represent water. The numbering system −500 to +500 used on the original EMI scanner is referred to as Old Hounsfield Units (OHU).[2] The numbering system, −1000 or less to +1000 or more, is referred to now as Hounsfield Units (HU). In this system, air is black (dense air, −1000 HU) and bone is white (dense bone, +1000). Fat absorbs the radiograph less than water and more than air,

therefore, its CT numbers will be negative, usually between −50 to −140 HU. The CT number of circulating blood is (+40 to +50), congealed blood (+50 to +80), calcium (+80 to +500), muscle (+30 to +40), cerebral spinal fluid (+5 to +12), bone (+100 to +1000), and air (−100 to −1000).[5]

The viewing devices (console) provided with CT scanners usually have a set number of gray scales (e.g. 50, 100, 150, 300, 1000 or more). The range of CT numbers covered by these gray scales (the contrast) is adjustable (e.g., window-width control)(Fig. 37–1).[2] The location of the center of the gray scale also is adjustable (window-level control) (Fig. 37–1). This manipulation of window-width (image contrast) and window-level (mean level, Fig. 37–1) by the CT radiologist at the console gives the most effective diagnostic information, ensuring that the diagnostic sensitivity is limited by the recorded image and not the observer's eye.[4] A window width of 80 units with the level of 35 examines values ranging from +75 to −5. With the window level = L = +35, and window width = W = +80 setting, values higher than +75 will be white, those lower than −5 will be black, and those values between +75 and −5 will be shades of gray (Fig. 37–1).

Nuclear Magnetic Resonance (NMR) Phenomenon and Magnetic Resonance Imaging

Magnetic resonance imaging[6] is a fascinating field and has introduced an entirely new and important parameter in the evaluation of abnormalities of the head and neck and neurologic disorders.[7-11]

Historical Background

In 1936, D. J. Gorter[12] using calorimetric techniques, described his unsuccessful attempt to observe the Li

(Lithium) nuclear magnetic resonance in LiCl (Lithium Chloride). In 1938, I. Rabi and coworkers[13] described the first successful molecular beam nuclear magnetic resonance. Subsequent to successful molecular beam nuclear magnetic experiments, Gorter and Broer, in 1942,[14] again attempted to observe nuclear magnetic resonance in powders of LiCl and KF (potassium flouride), but no resonance was observed. Despite Gorter's failure, two independent groups, Felix Bloch and coworkers[15] and Edward Purcell and coworkers[16] in 1946, were successful in demonstrating NMR in condensed matter, work for which they shared the Nobel prize in physics in 1952.

Historically, the impetus of the development of MRI is attributable to Lauterbur,[1] who in 1973, by using the interaction of magnetic fields, generated the first two-dimensional MRI. This depicted the proton-density and the spin lattice relaxation time (T1) distribution (see section of MR phenomena) in two 1-mm tubes of water.[1] Subsequently, numerous NMR techniques have been developed generating data from a point, line, plane or multiple planes, within a volume as well as from the entire volume.[17]

THE MAGNETIC RESONANCE PHENOMENON

Elementary Physics

In discussing radiographs and their effects on atoms, we are concerned with their extranuclear structure, that is the arrangement of planetary (orbital) electrons outside the nucleus. In the MR phenomenon, we are concerned with nuclear structures of atoms, that is, the nucleons ("nucleon" is the generic term for a proton or neutron). The existence of nuclear spin and nuclear angular momentum, the entity essential to MR phenomenon, was first suggested by the Austrian physicist Wolfgang Pauli in 1924[7] when he observed the behavior of light in a magnetic field. Since then, it has been verified that atomic nuclei have an angular momentum arising from their inherent property of rotation, or spin. Pairs of protons or neutrons, however, align in such a way that their spins cancel out, and a net spin (net rotation) will therefore exist for a nucleus only when it contains an odd (unpaired) proton, an odd neutron, or both.[18] Since protons carry a positive charge, the nuclei have an associated electric charge distribution, and therefore the spin generates a current flowing about the spin axis, which in turn generates a small magnetic field. Each nucleon of non-zero spin has an inherent magnetic field (magnetic dipoles) and a magnetic moment (a magnetic moment is a vector quantity represented by an arrow which describes the magnetic field's strength and direction), or dipole, associated with it that can be thought of as behaving like

a tiny spinning bar magnet with north and south poles (Fig. 37–2). Therefore these tiny spinning magnets can interact with the electromagnetic field.[17–19] In a sample of materials, the nuclear magnets (magnetic moments or dipoles) will be pointing in random directions,[17–19] and the result of many nuclei in a random arrangement is that there is no net magnetization (one cancels the other) in any direction (Fig. 37–2A). However, if the nuclei are placed in an external static magnetic field, the randomly oriented magnetic dipoles respond to the force of the field by trying to line up in the direction of the field (Fig. 37–2B). In the magnetic field, therefore, there is a net (sum) magnetization produced parallel to, and in the same direction as the applied field (Fig. 37–2B). The magnetic behavior of the entire population of nuclei can be defined as a macroscopic, or bulk magnetization vector or moment (M), (Fig. 37–2B) that represents the net effect of all the magnetic moments of the nuclei of a given nuclear species in the sample.

In the absence of an external magnetic field, the net magnetization is, of course, zero due to random orientation of nuclei. When the external magnetic field BO (Fig. 37–2) is imposed on the sample, however, the nuclear dipoles become oriented parallel to the applied field, and the net magnetization (spin vector, M) (Fig. 37–2B) yields a finite equilibrium that will point in a direction parallel to the external magnetic field BO (Fig. 37–2). This direction conventionally defines the longitudinal (Z) axis (Fig. 37–2C). By convention, the spin system is presented in a cartesian coordinate system (X,Y,Z), with the axis Z parallel with the direction of the external magnetic field BO (Fig. 37–2).

Precession Motion

Let us focus particular attention on the nuclei of the hydrogen atoms, protons, which, from the standpoint of the MR phenomenon, are particularly favorable nuclei. From now on, the hydrogen atom is referred to as proton. Each proton can be regarded as a small freely suspended bar magnet spinning rapidly about its magnetic axis. If a group of protons are placed in a static magnetic field of particular strength (BO), the magnetic moment of each proton experiences a couple (from the north and south pole), a force or torque tending to turn its magnetic moment (M) parallel to the static magnetic field (Fig. 37–2). Because it spins, the proton responds to this couple by rotation about the line of force (like a gyroscope precessing about the gravitational force), and therefore its axis is tilted and begins to precess (rotate) about the direction of the magnetic field in a movement known as "precession" (Fig. 37–2C). The precessional motion traces a cone in a manner analogous to the wobbling of a toy top as it spins and tries to orient itself in the earth's gravitational field. The frequency of the precessional motion given by the famous theorem of Larmor and the Larmor equation, w (omega) = 8 (gamma) × B_O, states that the frequency of the precessional motion (W) is proportional to the couple and therefore to the strength of the applied static external magnetic field (B_O), and the constant of proportionality gamma, the so-called gyromagnetic properties (or ratio) of the specific nucleus.[8] The equation shows that as the magnetic field changes, so does the nuclear precessional rate of motion (angular frequency W or Larmor frequency). This is an important point in MRI because it enables us to locate the origin of the MR signal and to pinpoint spatially the source of each frequency (W).

Nuclear Magnetic Resonance

Resonance is a physical phenomenon that permits the transfer of energy from an object, particle, or system vibrating mechanically or electronically, to another similar object, particle, or system, causing the latter to vibrate at the same frequency. When a substance containing nuclei of non-zero spin is placed in a magnetic field, a resonance condition is produced, which means there will be a strong interaction, or resonant effect.[20] The nuclei then can absorb energy at a sharply defined frequency from electomagnetic radiation and re-emit the energy as electromagnetic radiation of the same frequency after the incident beam has been turned off.[7,18,19] Either the absorption or the re-emission can be measured. To secure this resonant effect, the applied electromagnetic radiation (pulse) from the RF (radiofrequency) generator (Fig. 37–2D) must have just the same frequency as the Larmor precession frequency (natural resonant frequency) of the sample (that is, it has to be resonant). Hence, the name ''nuclear magnetic resonance'' (NMR) has been designated for the phenomenon. In short, the precession is a resonance effect and if a system has a natural resonance (frequency resonance, frequency of oscillation) energy needs can most efficiently be imparted to the resonance frequency. For example, at the field strength of 1.5 Tesla (1 Tesla = 10,000 Gauss), a pulse at 63.87 MHz (megahertz) will excite hydrogens (protons), whereas a pulse at 25.86 MHz will excite phosphorus nuclei.[21]

Relaxation Phenomenon and Times

As mentioned earlier, in the presence of a static magnetic field, BO nuclei with non-zero spin orient themselves with the magnetic field lines that point in the ''Z'' direction at a state of equilibrium ''rest'' (Fig. 37–2). At equilibrium, the nuclei possess their lower energy level. When an electromagnetic radiation (radio frequency) or RF pulse (wave) is used at a sharply designated frequency (Larmor frequency) because of resonant condition, some of the nuclei can absorb energy from the RF pulse, become excited (attain higher energy level) and change the direction of their magnetic moments. When the RF pulse is turned off, the excited nuclei relax and return to their original orientation (equilibrium, lower energy level) losing the excess energy by emitting electromagnetic radiation (the source of the MR signal) of the same frequency as the applied RF pulse by transferring energy to surrounding (lattice) molecules. This process is called ''relaxation'' and is characterized by two sample-related relaxation time constants: the longitudinal (spin-lattice) relaxation time (T1) and the transverse (spin-spin) relaxation time (T2). When the RF pulse of specific frequency (Larmor frequency) is applied, it affects the NMR-sensitive nuclei in two ways: 1) the RF pulse excites the nuclei and makes them move into a higher energy level, and 2) the net magnetization vector (M) (Fig. 37–2) will precess along the direction of the main field (Z axis) with an ever-increasing angle depending on the intensity and duration of the RF pulses (Fig. 37–3A). The magnetization vector (M) will consequently spiral down toward the x-y plane (90 degree pulse) and then continue to rotate in the x-y plane (Fig. 37–3A). The magnetization vector M can be considered as having a component, Mz (longitudinal magnetization), along the Z axis (Figs. 37–2, 37–3) and a component, Mxy (transverse magnetization), in the x-y plane perpendicular to the field axis (Z) (Fig. 37–3A). At equilibrium, the ''longitudinal magnetization'' Mz is equal to the net magnetization M and the ''transverse magnetization'' Mxy is zero (Fig. 37–3). After RF excitation, the precessional angle (Figs. 37–2, 37–3) continues to increase as long as the RF pulse is applied (Fig. 37–3). The precessional frequency (cycles per second), however, remains constant, being fixed by the inherent properties of the nuclei and the strength of the static magnetic field, BO. After the excitation of the RF pulse, Mz decreases and Mxy increases (Figs. 37–2, 37–3). The RF needed to tip the vector (M) through an angle of 15 degrees is described as a 15-degree pulse. Pulses of 90 and 180 degrees cause corresponding increases in the precessional angle.[18] After a 90 degree pulse, the vector (M) will be in the x-y plane and when the nuclei are flipped through 180 degrees the net magnetization vector (M) will be in the opposite direction of the main field BO. The ''transverse magnetization'' Mxy is time-dependent and has a rotational or ''precessional property'' in the x-y plane. Such a rotating magnetic current acts as a radiator of RF energy and therefore, according to Faraday's law of induction, can induce a current (voltage) in a receiver coil (inductance antenna) in the x-y plane (Fig. 37–2). Immediately after the application of a specific pulse through the transmitting coil (Fig. 37–2), the transverse magnetization Mxy continues to rotate freely in the x-y plane, generating an induced current (signal) that can be detected either by the same coil (acting as transmitting and receiving coil) that transmitted the pulse or by a specific receiver coil. The emitted signal is called the free induction signal or the free induction decay (FID). The magnitude and length of the FID (NMR signal) is determined by the relaxation times.[20]

T1 Relaxation Time

The T1 (T one) relaxation time represents the time constant required for the net magnetization vector (M) to return to its equilibrium after it has been perturbed by the RF pulse. In other words, T1 is the time that characterizes the recovery of the net magnetization (M) after it is perturbed to its equilibrium state in the field direction (Figs. 37–2, 37–3A). The alignment of nuclei is not instantaneous, but rather grows exponentially, increasing to approximately 63% of its final value within a period equal to the time constant (T1). It will reach 95% of the final value at a time equal to three times the constant. Therefore, in reality, T1 is the time that characterizes the recovery (return of excited spin to equilibrium) of 63% of nuclear magnetization. T1 is called "spin-lattice relaxation" because the thermal equilibrium state, hot state (excited spin) to cold state (spin at rest or equilibrium) is reached through an exchange of energy with its molecular environment or lattice. The alternative term, "longitudinal relaxation time," is used to reflect the fact that T1 characterizes the behavior of the Mz component of the magnetic vector (M) (Fig. 37–3A) when magnetization reverts to its equilibrium orientation in the direction of the applied field (Z) (Fig. 37–3A). Basically, T1 is a measure of how fast energy can be transferred from the spinning nuclei to the lattice by random collision between molecules or the rate at which thermal equilibrium is restored after being disturbed.

T2 Relaxation Time

As mentioned, the nuclear magnetic resonance signal picked up after an RF pulse is known as FID (free induction delay). The signal is proportional to the magnetization in the sample and would be produced continuously if the individual nuclear spins were able to maintain their coherence (synchronization) with no shifting of their relative phases.[19] The FID signal, however, decays because of spin–spin ("dipole–dipole") interaction (magnetic interaction of neighboring nuclei) and the inhomogeneity of the static magnetic field BO, both causing fluctuation in local magnetization with resultant fluctuation (any error) in precessional frequency (around Larmor frequency) of the individual proton. This causes the resonance of protons within the sample to lose synchronization and their vectors to develop a phase difference (Figs. 37–2, 37–3). The signal decays exponentially in time, with a time constant characterized by the T2 (Fig. 37–3). Basically, T2 is the time taken for the transverse magnetization, Mxy

to decrease by 63% of its original value. In a period three times as long as this, the transverse magnetization will have almost disappeared. In short, T2 relaxation time is the time taken for the decay of FID or MR signal to decrease by 63% of its original intensity value.

For water, T1 and T2 are several seconds, the precise value depending on the purity of water. For cellular water, T1 and T2 are shorter. T1 is shorter in liquids (seconds) than in solids (minutes). In solids and/or in a sample of materials at low temperatures, where the atoms and molecules move about very little, transfer of thermal energy is slow, and therefore, T1 can last for hours.[18] T1 is short in liquids because of the mobility of the atoms and molecules and the consequent rapid transfer of thermal energy.

For protons in pure water, T1 and T2 are approximately equal.[18] T2 is short in solids (microseconds) and long in fluids. In pure fluids, because of rapid motion of the atoms and molecules (random process), the magnetic field contribution from neighboring nuclei average zero, and only the main magnetic field determines the resonant frequency. T2 in this case is very long. If the nuclei find themselves in impure liquids where water molecules attach to proteins and have low translational and rotational speeds, this averaging random process of the magnetic field contribution from neighboring nuclei is more effective and the resonant frequency is therefore different (rapid phase difference and loss of coherence) for each nucleus; this makes T2 short. Solids, on the other hand, have fixed atoms and molecules that maintain local field variations (spin–spin, or dipole–dipole interaction), which result in a rapid loss of coherence and a very short T2. Relaxation rates are affected by viscosity, temperature, and the presence of dissolved ions and molecules.[19]

NMR Spectroscopy and Chemical Shift

Nuclear magnetic resonance spectroscopy is a plot of signal intensity versus resonance frequency. The appearance of NMR spectra depends on the density and molecular environment surrounding a nucleus. The presence of neighboring atoms and the "shielding currents" that are associated with the distribution of electrons around adjacent atoms slightly modifies the strength of local magnetic fields at particular nuclei and hence modifies the resonance frequency,[17–19,21] so that the details of molecular structure change the NMR frequency of a nucleus in that molecule. The extent of this field change depends on the electronic environment of the observed nucleus and consequently identical nuclides have slightly different resonance frequencies (lines) if they are residing in different chemical structures (environments). For example, the resonant frequency of a hydrogen proton within a water molecule differs slightly from that of a hydrogen proton within a fat molecule, and the resonant frequency of a

31P nucleus bound in an ATP molecule varies slightly from that of a 31P nucleus within a phosphocreatine molecule. These small but specific displacements or shifts in frequency produce separate absorption peaks in a spectrum (chemical shift) which are "fingerprints" of the molecular conformations and directly aid in the determination of chemical structure.[18,21] The chemical shift is measured and listed in ppm (parts per million) with respect to the signal from a reference such as signal of tetramethylsilane (TMSi). The chemical shift is of paramount importance in analytical chemistry, since it allows the assignment of different signal (lines) in an NMR spectrum to corresponding substances or molecular groups. For example, the proton spectrum of acetic acid CH3-COOH provides two lines. One line represents the three protons of the methyl group and another line for carboxyl proton. The three protons of the methyl group have an identical electronic environment surrounding so their signal appears as a single resonance line. In 31P spectra of muscle tissue, the signal of phosphocreatine is used as reference signal. The 31P spectrum of a muscle typically shows five signals that are related to inorganic phosphate, phosphocreatine, and the three phosphorus atoms of ATP (alpha, beta and gamma).

Currently, NMR spectroscopy is one of the most powerful tools used in chemical analysis.[18] The combined MRI, in-vivo spectroscopy, has become a routine procedure to provide morphologic as well as noninvasive biochemical "noninvasive biopsy" information of internal structures of human tissues.[22–25]

High Resolution In-Vivo Proton (1H) Magnetic Resonance Spectroscopy of Human Tissues

For more than 45 years, NMR has been used in chemical analysis and in the study of molecular behavior.[18,19] A simple method used in early NMR spectroscopy was to place a small sample in an extremely homogeneous magnetic field and subject it to an RF pulse of progressively increasing frequency from a coil wrapped around the sample. As the frequency passed through a resonance, the absorption of RF energy from the generator increased (Fig. 37–2).[19] A pen recorder graphing absorption against frequency would demonstrate a peak wherever there was a resonance. The size of the peak would be proportional to the abundance of the nuclei concerned. With the advent of wide-bore superconducting magnets, metabolism can be monitored in excised perfused organs[26] and more recently, in organs in vivo.[22,23,27] Most of the spectroscopic work done thus far has used the phosphorus 31P nucleus.[26] An alternative is 1H NMR, which is more sensitive than 31P-NMR.[23,26] MR spectra of live human tissues have been performed by several authors[22,23] in which the major resonances were due to water and fat pro-

tons.[22,27] Luyten and den Hollander[22] recorded resonances from N-acetylasparate and phosphocreatine-creatine in the human brain. Barany et al[23] recorded several resonances from known metabolites that were assigned tentatively to metabolites N-acetylaspartate, glutamate, phosphocreatine and creatine, choline derivatives and taurine.[34] They reported the presence of urea, various amino acids, and nucleotides in some cancerous tissues.[23] They concluded that the presence of a large nucleotide pool is a characteristic of tumor tissue involved in rapid nucleic acid synthesis.[23] Proton is the most sensitive biological nucleus and is a constituent of virtually all the organic molecules that are metabolized in the body. Therefore, protein spectroscopy has the potential for tissue-specific markers and metabolic indicators. In medicine, this technique is used to obtain biochemical information and understand and differentiate biochemical processes in pathologic entities.

Magnetic Resonance Imaging

The basic concept of imaging is simple. The fundamental Larmor equation states that the resonance frequency (W) of a particular nucleus with constant gyromagnetic ratio[8] is proportional to the field strength (B_O). Magnetic resonance scanners apply a strong time-dependent linear magnetic field gradient (super-imposed for a short period on the main field) to the sample. This introduces spatial dependence into the corresponding NMR signal[28] so the resonance frequency depends on the location of the nuclei relative to the gradient.[1,20,28,29] The frequency directly gives the locations of the nuclei along an axis in that direction. If the FID of a sample of protons is observed in a gradient after an RF pulse, each volume element in the sample can be labeled (coded) by having a different resonant frequency for the protons contained within it. Once the frequency information (location) has been collected by the receiver coil, computerized equipment can decode and change the spatial information into digital data and plot it as an image.[28,29]

Clinical Use of T1-Weighted, Proton-Weighted, and T2-Weighted MRI

Magnetic resonance scanners produce images that represent one or more of NMR parameters. These are 1) hydrogen (proton) density (also called spin-density); 2) the state of motion of hydrogen; 3) the tissue relaxation times T1 and T2; and 4) chemical shift. All forms of unprocessed MR signals depends on nuclear spin density.

The ability to rotate net magnetization (M) (Figs. 37–2, 37–3) from the direction of the static magnetic field (BO) into some other orientation by applying a RF pulse is fundamental to MR spectroscopy and imaging techniques because it provides a flexible method for investigating relaxation processes and other phenomena.[19] By choosing an appropriate pulse sequence, the intensity of an MR image can be made to reflect one or more of several NMR parameters inherent to the tissue being examined.[18] Although the proton density, chemical makeup, T1 and T2, and motion represent intrinsic tissue properties, the transition of these parameters onto the MR image is also dependent on the particulars of the imaging technique used to form that image. This subject has been described by many authors in several articles.[30,31]

The 90-degree and 180-degree pulses are used for NMR techniques.[19] In forming an MR image, the RF pulse must be applied repeatedly. After each 90-degree pulse, the magnetization of the sample is reduced to zero, as this rotates the longitudinal magnetization vector (M) into the transverse (x-y) plane to become transverse magnetization Mxy (Figs. 37–2, 37–3A). Therefore, the longitudinal component of magnetization Mz is zero. The longitudinal magnetization will recover exponentially with a time constant of T1. Rapid repetition of pulses (irradiation of sample) would not allow much recovery of magnetization and little signal would be detected after each successive 90-degree exciting pulse. Thus, a certain time (repetition time = TR) is introduced between successive RF pulses. As the TR increases, the signal and imaging time increase. After RF pulse, the FID signal decays exponentially in time with a time constant T2. The interval between application of RF pulse and reception of a signal or spin echo is called echo time or time of echo (TE). As TE increases, signal decreases (Fig. 37–3A), and contrast between tissues of different values of T2 changes. If the signal is obtained immediately after RF excitation, it will not undergo any T2 decay, and therefore, although it is a strong signal, it has no T2 dependence. If instead, the signal is obtained sometime after RF excitation, the available signal, although weaker, has an exponential dependence on T2. Strong signals (proton-weighted and T1-weighted images) yield better signal-to-noise levels or ratio and therefore better spatial resolution. With better optical resolution, anatomy is better appreciated. However, in the image the differences due to T2 relaxation time (T2-weighted image) contribute to contrast resolution with better pathologic details to the extent that T2 often contribute to tissue characterization.

Saturation Recovery (SR) Sequence

Various pulse patterns that emphasize different aspects of the evoked NMR signal can be exploited to alter the contrast of NMR images.[18] In a "saturation-recovery" (SR) pulse sequence which is not very commonly used, in forming an MR image, the RF pulses must be applied repetitively for signal averaging purposes.

A series of 90 degree pulses is applied with an interpulse spacing, time of repetition, (TR) longer than the decay time T2 and roughly the same length as T1 time.[18] This sequence is also known as the Repeated FID Technique. If the sequence is repeated with TR long enough for the magnetization vector (M) (Figs. 37–2 and 37–3A) to be realigned completely from the xy plane to the Z-direction (full recovery of magnetization), the detected FID signal has an initial amplitude which has no significant T1 and T2 dependence. In this situation the signal is mostly dependent on the proton density (proton or density weighted image) of the sample. In SR sequence, to avoid T1 dependence, a TR much greater than T1 (at least three times greater) must be applied. If in a SR pulse sequence, TR is much shorter than the T2 of the sample, the signal will not decay to zero between successive pulses, creating a condition known as steady-state free precession. In this situation there occurs only partial recovery of magnetization along the z-direction. As a result, the following 90-degree pulse rotates a reduced magnetization vector (Mz) through 90 degrees, which results in a smaller transverse magnetization (Mxy). The precession of this reduced Mxy in the x-y plane induces a signal of smaller amplitude in the receiving coil (Figs. 37–2, 37–3A). In this situation, tissues with short T1 produce a stronger signal than tissues with long T1. This is because the magnetization of the nuclei with shorter T1 will recover more than that of nuclei with longer T1. Therefore, after successive 90-degree pulse, the nuclei with more recovery of their magnetization Mz (Figs. 37–2, 37–3A) produce a stronger signal. The signal strength of each FID in this repeated FID or SR sequence is given by the formula $I = P(1 - e - TR/T1)$, where I is the intensity, P is the spin (proton) density, TR is the repetition time and T1 is the longitudinal relaxation time. In SR method, when the TR is long, the contrast is dependent on the proton density, and when the TR is shorter, the image intensity is dependent on the tissue proton density and T1 relaxation time as seen from this equation.

Inversion Recovery (IR) Pulse Sequence)

Another pulse sequence that is more commonly used than SR sequence is inversion recovery (IR) pulse sequence, which uses a 180-degree (inverting) pulse, followed by a 90-degree (read) pulse.[17] The signal amplitude is given by the formula $I = P(1 - 2e - TR/T1)$. Because of application of 180-degree pulse and the fact that magnetization must be allowed to recover after 180-degree inverting pulse, the IR sequence is slower than SR in data collection. Both SR and IR are used to obtain T1-weighted images. In IR, the dynamic range of the signal response is increased two times over the

SR sequence and therefore more T1-dependent (heavily T1-weighted) images with greater contrast enhancement can be obtained using IR sequence. However, the price paid is an increased time for the IR sequence. In general, greater contrast enhancement of an image is acquired by using an IR pulse sequence and greater spatial resolution of an image is acquired by using a SR pulse sequence of equal time.[17]

On SR and IR pulse sequence, regions with long T1 will have less signal than regions of short T1 and hence will appear dark on an image. However, as seen from these equations, long TR, SR, or IR images show contrast only by differences in spin density, i.e., the concentration of proton (P) in the sample.[17] Water has a long T1, and fat has a short T1. Therefore, on both SR and IR, (proton and T1 weighted images), the water appears dark, and fat appears bright.

Spin-Echo (SE) Pulse Sequence

In the spin-echo pulse sequence, which is the most used technique, a 90-degree pulse is first applied so that a coherent arrangement of the spins in the sample is obtained, and the net magnetization is directed at right angles to the field, which induces a signal that decays as the spins dephase.[19] After an interval, a 180-degree pulse is applied which has the effect of rephasing or refocusing (collecting together the spins) the dephasing spins. T2 data are acquired by using the principle of the SE pulse sequence.[17]

T1 weighted (T1W) MR images can be obtained using the SE pulse sequence with a short TR (repetition time or time of repetition) of 400 to 800 msec and a short TE (echo time) of 20 to 25 msec. The multiple-echo pulse sequence of long TR, (1500 to 3000 or more msec) and short TE (20 to 25 msec) provides proton density (proton-weighted = PW) MR images. Long TR (1500 to 3000 or more msec) and long TE (40 to 120 or more msec) provide the T2-weighted (T2W) MR images.

The viewing devices (console) provided with MR scanners, like CT scanners, have a set number of gray scales that can be used to adjust the contrast. The MR parameters (TR, TE) and pulse sequences (SR, IR, SE), the strength of the magnet (e.g., 1.5 Tesla) and the time and number of images in each series of pulse sequences are recorded on the screen and reflected on each frame of hard-copy MR films. Therefore, a simple method for beginners is to look for TR and TE to recognize the T1W, PW, and T2W images. A short TR (less than 800 msec) and short TE (20 to 25 msec) is a T1W image (see Fig. 37–68A). A long TR (more than 800 msec) and short TE (20 to 30 msec) is a PW image (Figs. 37–18B, 37–26) and a long TR and TE (more than 40 msec) is a T2W image (Figs. 37–51B and 37–67B). T1W images and PW images provide better anatomic details (Figs.

37–18, 37–67, and 37–68), and T2W images are best for pathologic details (Figs. 37–67, 37–68).

Magnetic Resonance Angiography (MRA) and Venography (MRV)

Magnetic resonance angiography (MRA) and venography (MRV) are noninvasive techniques used to depict blood vessels in a projective format similar to conventional invasive angiography, without the use of ionizing radiation or iodinated contrast materials (Fig. 37–3B,C). On standard SE pulse sequences, rapidly moving blood will usually yield a signal void regardless of the orientation of the plane of the image. Therefore, MRA must employ certain radiofrequency (RF) pulse sequences to produce signal from flowing blood. In MRA, the appearance of flowing blood depends on two main flow related effects: time-of-flight (TOF) and phase contrast (PC).

Time-of-flight MRA refers to motion of blood into and out of the plane of section. Stationary tissues remain in the plane of section and are frequently affected by selective RF pulses. If the TR is short relative to the T1 relaxation time, the tissue will become saturated by the RF pulses and produce no signal and subsequently appear dark. "Saturation" refers to a process whereby RF irradiation is used to excite protons so there is no net longitudinal magnetization. The same process is used in chemical shift fat suppression technique to produce fat-suppressed T1W MR images. Blood from outside the section is unaffected by the section-selective RF pulse and therefore the protons are fully magnetized. When the magnetized protons of the flowing blood enter the saturated plane, an intense signal is produced. This is called flow-related enhancement or paradoxical enhancement.

In phase contrast (PC) MR angiography, two images are acquired, each with a field gradient pulse applied of equal magnitude, but opposite polarity. This produces phase shifts from the stationary tissues within the plane of sections which are also of equal but opposite magnitude. For blood flowing at a constant velocity, the moving protons are not at the same location for both gradient pulses and a net non-zero phase shift is produced. Images are subtracted by the computer producing a pure flow image.[32]

Technical advances, such as the development of the two-dimensional (2D) and three-dimensional (3D) gradient-echo (GRE) pulse sequences (Fig. 37–15), led to more widespread use of MRA and MRV. These noninvasive techniques of studying blood flow not only permit the evaluation of the vascular anatomy of the head and neck but also provide information on flow direction, velocity and blood vessel patency. Both TOF and PC MR angiography can be obtained as a series of 2D images or as a 3D data set. This leads to the logical terminology of 2D TOF, 3D TOF, 2D PC and 3D PC for the two fundamental approaches to vascular MRI techniques. In our experience, MRA has been most valuable for vascular lesions such as aneurysm, dissecting carotid artery, detailed evaluation of dural venous sinuses (Fig. 37–3B,C), thrombosis of the jugular vein arteritis, glomus complex tumors, and for providing a vascular map in tumors of the head and neck.

Clinical application best suited for 2D TOF MRA include mapping dural venous sinus, evaluating the vascular structures of the neck for evidence of thrombosis or invasion by tumor (Figs. 37–37D, 37–38C, and 37–61H), evaluating for carotid or vertebral dissection, and assessing the draining veins of arterial venous malformations. 2D TOF MRV can be used to evaluate suspected intracranial venous thrombosis; however, thrombus may appear bright (as a result of the short T1 of methemoglobin) and can be confused for a patent venous sinus resulting in a false negative examination.[32]

Clinical applications best suited for 3D TOF MRA in the head and neck include evaluation of intracranial aneurysm and assessment of vascular malformations. PC MRA scan times are longer compared with TOF. Clinical applications best suited for 3D PC MRA include evaluating pathology, which has slow blood flow or when better background suppression is needed; demonstrating venous thrombosis; evaluating large volume (whole head); and assessing AVM (arteriovenous malformations).[32]

Standard Film Radiography Versus CT and MRI

The modern diagnostic radiology department is equipped with a variety of medical imaging systems. Each has advantages and limitations. Plain film radiography is simple, fast, inexpensive, and produces sharp images of high-contrast structures (air, fluid, bone) (Figs. 37–4 to 37–11); however, high-contrast objects can obscure low-contrast objects, and the presence of overlying objects can sometimes be misleading.

Tomography

Standard-linear or complex-motion tomography such as polytomography is aimed at improving visualization of localized areas of the body. A radiologic image derived from standard tomographic methods has at least two limitations as far as diagnostic specificity is concerned: 1) the presence of a background blur of structures above and below the focal plane, and 2) a large proportion of the detected radiation is that which has been scattered from the patient.[2] These two properties limit the ability of this type of system to image adequately the subtle differences in subject contrast (i.e., the linear radiograph attenuation coefficient) ob-

served in soft tissues of the human body.[2] Even if the two limitations discussed previously could be reduced to "acceptable" levels, the conventional radiographic films and screens are inherently nonuniform (less sensitive than the computer) and would limit subject-contrast discrimination (resolution) to possibly 3 to 5%, which is greater than the range for some soft tissue. Because of these limitations, standard tomography such as polytomography is no longer used if a CT unit is available.

Computed tomography and MRI allow the reconstruction of tissue contrast in true cross sections (i.e., without being influenced by nearby or distant tissues in the section), with excellent tissue-contrast discrimination (resolution).[2] Both modalities, and in particular MRI, provide the best anatomic cross-sectional imaging technology available to date. The chief advantages of CT in diagnostic radiology are as follows: 1) blurred background and superimposed overlying structures, as in standard tomography, are removed[2,4]; 2) a true tomographic section is obtained that is almost an exact representation of a tissue attenuation coefficient, which may be used to identify and quantitate particular tissues; 3) the CT image is stored and displayed digitally so that the image contrast can be manipulated during viewing, giving the most effective diagnostic information.[2,4] The majority of present CT scanners cannot take direct sagittal (lateral) sections. This has been available with the use of a special head holder developed by Mafee et al. at the University of Illinois at Chicago Medical Center (Fig. 37–12). By using an intravenous iodinated-contrast medium during CT scanning, the vascular structures will be better differentiated from the adjacent areas. The new generation high-resolution scanner, with a smaller pixel (picture element), the combination of thin section (1 to 1.5 mm) and extended bone range possibility (expansion of the Hounsfield unit scale up to 4000 units, i.e., +3000 to −1000), provides clear definition and differentiation of soft-tissue structures, while also providing superior bone detail to complex motion tomography (Figs. 37–13, 37–17).

Dynamic CT

One limitation of conventional CT scanning is that it is a static imaging technique giving essentially an anatomic and morphologic image. The routine iodinated contrast-enhanced CT also provides a static picture of the distribution of the iodinated-contrast material within the various tissues. With the development of the high-resolution scanner, with both short-scan time and interscan delay, rapid-sequence CT imaging (dynamic CT) could be performed following the time course of the passage of the bolus of iodinated contrast material through an organ.[33–35] A CT dynamic study consists of a rapid sequence of short-duration scans of the same section taken during and after a peripheral bolus injection (10 to 15 sec) of iodinated contrast material. The scanning sequence is initiated with the start of the injection so that the first scan is completed before the contrast reaches the selected section and a baseline reference scan is available (Figs. 37–44, 37–46). The passage of contrast material through a cross section creates a dynamic image field exhibiting local density changes during the scan interval.[33] The reconstructed images from a dynamic study can be used to derive a set of CT numbers versus time curves (Figs. 37–30B, 37–44B, 37–45B). In these computer-generated curves, density is plotted on the y-axis and time on the x-axis. Rapid-sequence CT imaging allows for sequential imaging throughout the arterial, capillary and venous phases, provides information about vascular anatomy (CT angiography), locates major vessels, and eliminates the possibility of vascular lesions in the differential diagnosis of a head and neck tumor (Figs. 37–44 to 37–46).[33,34] Another application of dynamic CT for visualization of vascular structures is rapid-sequential dynamic CT with automatic table incrementation: "dynamic incrementation scanning."[33,34] The rapid-sequence CT scanner has the capability of quickly acquiring adjacent axial or coronal images while integrating table motion (incrementally between scans) so that several adjacent (contiguous) sections may be obtained through an area of interest during a short period and immediately after the intravenous injection of a bolus of contrast material. This technique allows sequential images throughout the arterial and venous phases, which improves delineation of vascular structures and thus resolves a common clinical problem encountered with regular contrast infusion CT scanning, i.e., whether a rounded image represents a vascular structure, a neoplasm or both (Figs. 37–46A and 37–44 to 37–47).[33,34] In glomus complex tumors or vascular lesions, dynamic CT scanning allows visualization of the sequential enhancement of the carotid arteries and jugular veins. The tumor becomes densely opacified for a short time as the intravenously injected bolus of iodinated contrast material traverses the vascular bed of a particular tissue section (Figs. 37–44 to 37–47).[33–35]

Magnetic Resonance Imaging (MRI)

One of the advantages of MRI is the ability to obtain transverse (axial) and direct coronal, sagittal, and oblique images without needing to change the position of the patient. The contrast relationships of different tissues on MRI are much different than on CT scanning (Fig. 37–13). The technical factors of various pulse sequences to obtain MR image, in addition to physical and biochemical composition of the sample, play a significant role in tissue contrast in MR images. Water such as in vitreous (see Fig. 37–13B) has long T1 and T2 relaxation times and would appear as a hypointense (dark) in T1-weighted (T1W) and proton-weighted

(PW) (proton-density) (Fig. 37–13B) images, and as a hyperintense (bright) in T2-weighted (T2W) MR scans. The lens has an intermediate signal intensity (gray) in T1W and PW scans (Fig. 37–13B) and appears as a hypointense image in T2W scans.

Fat has short T1 and intermediate T2 relaxation times and would therefore appear as a hyperintense image in T1W and PW (Fig. 37–13B) scans and as a hypointense image in T2W scans. Tissues of intermediate structure (muscles) have an intermediate signal on T1W and PW scans and a low signal on T2W MR scans (Fig. 37–13B). Solid structures such as cortical bone, enamel, dentin and fibrous tissues (sclera, tendons, fascias) are hypointense (dark) on T1W, PW, and T2W scans because of their sparsity of mobile hydrogen atoms. The cortical bone would appear black, whereas the medullary cavity will be bright because of signals from fat content. Air in paranasal sinuses, because of the lack of hydrogen atoms, appears dark in all MR scans. In most pulse sequences, vascular structures such as carotid arteries and internal jugular veins are identified readily as low-signal intensity (dark) structures. With normal rapid blood flow, excited spins are carried away from the selected imaging section before a signal (echo) is formed (signal void phenomenon), creating a dark image with signal intensity similar to that of air, cortical bone, enamel and dentin.

Dynamic MRI

Fast-scan or narrow flip angle MRI (dynamic MRI) is performed using the gradient echo (GRE) pulse sequence such as "GRASS" technique. The GRASS, which stands for gradient recalled acquisition in the steady state, is a new imaging technique. Its prime characteristics is the ability to provide T1, T2 and PW images in a short time. A striking feature of GRASS images is the high-intensity appearance of vascular structures, "MR angiography," especially when vessels transect the image slice (Fig. 37–15). All MR scans, except where mentioned, were performed with a superconductive magnet of 1.5 Tesla (Tesla = 10,000 gauss). GRASS images are obtained with TR = 25 to 30 msec, TE = 12 to 15 msec, and a variable flip angle (10 to 30 degrees).

Tissue Characterization of T1W and T2W Images

Damadian and coworkers[36] showed that malignant tissues, except melanotic tumors, have a long T1 and T2 relaxation time. Nonmelanotic tumors, therefore, are hypointense on T1W scans and would appear as hyperintense images on T2W scans. Melanotic lesions on T1W and PW MR scans would appear hyperintense and become hypointense on T2W MR scans.[37,38]

Normal CT and MRI of the Face and Neck

A complete description of the anatomy of the face and neck is discussed in this volume. Emphasis here is placed on the structures that are most pertinent to understanding CT and MRI scans in the broad field of otolaryngology.

Orbits, Ethmoid and Sphenoid Sinuses

Because fat, fluid, and bone are natural contrast material, the orbit is the ideal structure for a highly detailed CT and MRI scan. A scan taken through the orbits shows the relationship of the ethmoid sinuses, sphenoid sinuses, pituitary fossa, cavernous sinuses, and temporal lobes with the orbit (Fig. 37–13). The cortical bones, which appear as hyperdensity on CT images (Fig. 37–13A), are seen on MR as hypointense images because of little MR signal from them (Fig. 37–13B). The bone marrow appears on MRI as hyperintense image due to the presence of fat. The air is seen as a dark image on both CT (low electron density) and MR (low proton density) images (Fig. 37–13).

The ethmoid sinuses are positioned between the orbits and comprise approximatley 10 to 12 cells within the labyrinth of the ethmoid bone. The fine-bone septa of the ethmoid labyrinth, the lamina papyracea, olfactory groove, cribriform plate, and maxillofacial bony structures will be best imaged by extended-bone window high-resolution CT (Fig. 37–14).[39,40] The anatomic landmarks of the ethmoid bone and ostiomeatal unit, such as uncinate process, infundibulum, middle meatus-ethmoid complex, ethmoid bullae, middle turbinate, cribriform plate (as well as the opening of the maxillary sinuses) are best evaluated on coronal and sagittal CT images (Fig. 37–16).[41–43] The sphenoid sinuses are paired cavities within the sphenoid bone. They are rarely symmetrical, and the intersphenoid septum is variable. The internal carotid canal may protrude into the sphenoid sinus, and the intersphenoid septum may extend toward the bulging internal carotid canal. A bony septum separates the sphenoid sinuses from the ethmoid sinuses anteriorly (Figs. 37–13A, 37–14, 37–16A). The optic nerves within the orbit can be visualized with both CT and MRI. The intracanalicular portion of the optic nerve is best seen on MRI (Fig. 37–13B). The lateral orbital wall separates the orbit from the middle cranial and temporal fossae (Figs. 37–13, 37–14). Two of the "lateral 3 lines" or "triple line shadows" (orbital wall and middle cranial-fossa line), seen in plain film submentovertical (base view) projection (Fig. 37–6) are imaged in this section (Figs. 37–13A and 37–14). The temporal (innominate) line is also visualized (Fig. 37–14).

Base of the Skull

The unique ability of CT to image both bone and soft tissue structures with excellent tissue contrast discrimination (resolution) makes it ideal to study the base of the skull and temporal bones. Both CT and MRI provide an accurate assessment of the total extent of disease and precise identification of intraorbital or intracranial extension of the tumor or inflammatory process. Computed tomography is superior to MR for a detailed bony process (Fig. 37–17), and MR is superior to CT for a detailed soft tissue process (Fig. 37–18). In many instances they are complementary to each other. Use of the extended bone CT range (scale) high-resolution scan is a major imaging advantage and provides the best diagnostic bone detail available to date (Fig. 37–17).

Maxillary Sinus, Nasal Cavity, and Nasopharynx

The maxillary sinuses, nasal cavities, nasal septum, conchae, and turbinates are seen on axial (horizontal) and coronal (frontal) CT and MR images (Figs. 37–16 to 37–19). The nasolacrimal ducts are visualized in axial and coronal sections. The ethmoid-maxillary plate, separating the ethmoid and maxillary sinuses on each side, is best seen in coronal sections.

Computed tomography and MR examinations of the nasopharynx delineate the air-containing cavity of the nasopharynx, the mucosal surfaces, and the deep fascial planes (Fig. 37–19). The cartilaginous end of the eustachian tube bulges into the airway, producing the mucosal prominence known as the torus tubarius.

The pharyngeal recesses or fossae of Rosenmuller extend posteriorly and superiorly to the tori (Fig. 37–19B). The pharyngeal openings of the eustachian tubes are visualized on the anterior and inferior surfaces of the tori (Fig. 37–19). Scans taken using a modified Valsalva's maneuver show distension of both the eustachian tubes and lateral recesses. On axial and coronal CT and MR images obtained during respiration, air is rarely seen more than 3 to 5 mm within the eustachian tube opening. The tympanic end of the eustachian tube can easily be seen in thin (1 to 1.5 mm) axial sections. The intrapharyngeal muscles (levator and tensor veli palati and salpingopharyngeus) lie between the pharyngobasilar fascia and the mucosa. The pharyngobasilar fascia is not seen as a separate discrete structure on CT images. The levator veli palatini is the major contributor to intrapharyngeal muscle density seen on CT.[44] The muscle belly produces a characteristic oval image just deep to the mucosa posterior to the torus (Fig. 37–19). The tensor veli palatini opens the eustachian tube and can be imaged on MR as a distinct muscle bundle (Fig. 37–18B). The prevertebral musculature (mainly the longus capitis muscles) is identifiable readily on CT and MRI scans and is seen as symmetrical in Figures 37–18 and 37–19. The parapharyngeal space (PPS), filled with loose fibrofatty tissues, lies between the pharyngeal muscles and the lateral and medial pterygoid muscles. This space is subdivided by a consistent layer of fascia into prestyloid and poststyloid compartments. The relationship between the medial pterygoid fascia, representing the medial wall of the masticator space, and the fascia of the tensor veli palatini, representing the medial wall of the prestyloid parapharyngeal space, allows better preoperative differentiation and perhaps more accurate diagnosis. Specifically, tumors that arise in the prestyloid parapharyngeal space are most often of salivary gland origin.[45] We have seen neurogenic tumors and hemangiopericytoma in the prestyloid PPS. Tumors that arise in the masticator space are unlikely to be of salivary gland origin. Tumors that arise in the poststyloid PPS are most often of neurogenic or chemoreceptor (paraganglion) origin. The fat content of the parapharyngeal space allows one to identify it as hypointense (dark) on CT scan (Fig. 37–19) and hyperintense (bright) on T1W and PW MR images (Fig. 37–18B).

Infratemporal Fossa

The boundaries and content of the infratemporal fossa or zygomatic fossa were once difficult to image using radiographic techniques before the advent of CT scanning. It can be evaluated in detail by CT and MRI, in axial, coronal, and sagittal sections. The infratemporal fossa is an irregularly shaped cavity medial and deep to the zygomatic arch. It is bound anteriorly by the infratemporal surface (posterior wall) of the maxilla and ridge from its zygomatic process (Figs. 37–18 and 37–19). It lies lateral to the parapharyngeal space[5,45,46] and is bound medially by a line from the styloid process to the lateral pterygoid plate[44] and laterally by the zygomatic arch and the articular tubercle of the temporal bone.[46] Above the level of the zygomatic arch, the infratemporal fossa is continuous with the temporal fossa. Inferiorly, the infratemporal fossa has no floor but is continuous with the space external to the buccinator muscle and buccal space (Fig. 37–20).[44] This space contains most of the mandible, the pterygoid, masseter, and part of the temporalis muscles, the deep lobe of the parotid gland, the internal, maxillary vessels, the mandibular and maxillary nerves, and the pterygoid plexus of veins.[5,44,46] The foramen ovale, foramen spinosum, and alveolar canal open into it.[46]

Pterygomaxillary Fissure

Along the superior and medial parts of the infratemporal fossa are two fissures that meet at right angles. The horizontal limb is the inferior orbital fissure, which is shown best in coronal and axial CT sections (Fig. 37–17), and the vertical limb is the pterygomaxillary fissure, which is formed by the divergence of the maxilla from the pterygoid process of the sphenoid and shown best in sagittal (Fig. 37–12B) and horizontal

(axial) CT images. The pterygomaxillary fissure connects the infratemporal fossa with the pterygopalatine fossa and transmits the terminal part of the internal maxillary artery and veins.[46] The pterygopalatine or sphenomaxillary or sphenopalatine fossa is a small, pyramidal space at the angle of junction of the inferior orbital fissure and pterygomaxillary fissure at the apex of the orbit (Fig. 37–12B). It is bound by the infratemporal (posterior) surface of the maxilla, the vertical plate of the palatine bone and the base of the pterygoid process (Fig. 37–12). It communicates with the nasal cavity by the sphenopalatine foramen; with the infratemporal fossa by the pterygomaxillary fissure; and with the orbit by the inferior orbital fissure. Five foramina open into it, including the foramen rotundum, the pterygoid, vidian canal, pharyngeal canal, and sphenopalatine foramen, which in turn lead to the pterygopalatine canal. The fifth foramen is placed inferiorly at the junction of the anterior and posterior walls and leads into the greater palatine canal. The fossa contains the maxillary nerve, pterygopalatine ganglion, and the terminal part of the internal maxillary artery.[39,46] Many of the superficial and deep muscles of the face are imaged on CT and MRI scans at the level of the nasopharynx. The lateral pterygoid muscle is a short, thick muscle, somewhat conical in shape, which extends almost horizontally between the infratemporal fossa and the condyle of the mandible (Fig. 37–18). It has its origins in the lateral surface of the lateral pterygoid plate and lateral surface of the greater wing of the sphenoid bone and inserts into the articular disc of the temporomandibular joint and the condyle of the mandible (Figs. 37–18A and 37–19).[5,39,46] The main mass of the medial pterygoid muscle lies deep and inferior to the lateral pterygoid muscle (Figs. 37–18 and 37–19) and arises from the medial surface of the lateral pterygoid plate, palatine bone, and maxilla and inserts into the angle and ramus of the mandible (Fig. 37–20).[39,46] In axial CT section taken at the level of the low-nasopharynx and soft palate, the medial pterygoid muscle occupies a position on the inside of the ramus of the mandible, similar to that of the masseter on the outside (Fig. 37–20). Both pterygoid muscles can be visualized in a coronal section taken at the level of the infratemporal fossa (Fig. 37–19B). The masseter is a thick, somewhat quadrilateral muscle that arises from the zygomatic process of the maxilla and the zygomatic arch and inserts into the angle and lateral surface of the ramus and the lateral surface of the coronoid process of the mandible.[39,46] In axial and coronal sections, the masseter is seen as a thick, somewhat quadrilateral muscle, anterior and inferior to the parotid gland, occupying a position on the outside of the ramus of the mandible (Figs. 37–18 to 37–20). The temporalis is a broad, radiating muscle, arising from the whole of the temporal fossa.[5,39,46] It passes inferiorly deep to the zygomatic arch and inserts into the medial surface, apex and anterior border of the coronoid process and anterior aspect of the ramus of the mandible (Figs. 37–18 and 37–19A).[5,39,46] The temporalis muscle is seen anterolateral to the lateral pterygoid muscle and pterygoid process as it inserts on the coronoid process (Figs. 37–18 and 37–19A). Symmetrical low-density fascial-fatty planes are seen on CT scans between the lateral pterygoid and infratemporal muscles. They are continuous with the symmetrical fat pad just anterior to the infratemporal muscles and posterior to the posterior wall of the maxillary sinus. Obliteration of these fascial-fat planes is usually indicative of extension of a neoplastic or inflammatory process into them.

Carotid Sheath

The carotid sheath, forming a tubular investment for the carotid artery, internal jugular vein, and vagus nerve, is within the retrostyloid parapharyngeal space,[5,39,46] abutting but separated from the infratemporal fossa by the "styloid diaphragm," an aponeurotic sheet of the pharyngobasilar fascia passing from the pharyngeal wall to the styloid process and its muscles.[5] Intravenous iodine-contrast material is given to define the internal carotid artery and internal jugular vein from the density of cranial nerves 9 to 12, the sympathetic trunk, normal lymph nodes, and the density of three muscles arising on the styloid process (i.e., stylohyoideus, stylopharyngeus and styloglossus) (Fig. 37–19A).

SALIVARY GLANDS

Parotid Gland

The parotid gland, which lies immediately inferior and anterior to the external ear, is divided into a deep lobe that curves around the posterior margin of the ramus of the mandible and extends deeply inward toward the lateral parapharyngeal wall (Figs. 37–18 and 37–20).[46,47] The main portion of the gland is superficial and is connected to the deep lobe by an isthmus. On a CT scan, the parotid gland is seen as a low-density (lucent) image with its superficial lobe somewhat flattened and quadrilateral in form in children and young adults. Its density is low but may be the same as the submandibular gland. It is placed between the ramus of the mandible, the mastoid process, and sternocleidomastoideus (Figs. 37–18 to 37–20). Not uncommonly, a prominent indentation by the sternocleidomastoid muscle is seen on CT or MRI scans over the posterior aspect of the gland, which should not be mistaken for a mass. The superficial lobe is broad and can reach nearly to the zygomatic arch. Stensen's duct crosses the masseter muscle, pierces the buccinator muscle and

mucous membrane of the mouth, and opens in the cheek opposite the second upper molar tooth. The gland and duct can be visualized with CT contrast sialography. The parotoid glands demonstrate an intermediate signal intensity on T1W and PW MR scans that enables the clinician to define the gland-muscle interface (Fig. 37–18).

Submandibular Gland

The submandibular gland is situated in the submandibular triangle, reaching anteriorly to the anterior belly of the digastric muscle and posteriorly to the stylomandibular ligament, which intervenes between it and the parotid gland.[46] It extends superiorly deep to the inferior border of the mandible, in the submandibular fossa to the medial side of the body of the mandible, opposite the second and third molar teeth (Figs. 37–21 to 37–25).[46,47] The mylohyoid muscle indents the anterior surface of the gland (Figs. 37–21, 37–24, 37–25). The lower part of the gland is covered by the skin, superficial cervical fascia, platysma, and deep cervical fascia (Figs. 37–23, 37–25). The submandibular duct (Wharton's duct) runs anteriorly between the mylohyoid, hyoglossus, and genioglossus muscles and the sublingual gland to open in the caruncula sublingualis. The entire gland and duct can be visualized with CT sialography (Fig. 37–22). Both submandibular and sublingual glands are visualized distinctly after intravenous infusion of iodine contrast (Fig. 37–23).

The sublingual gland is situated beneath the mucous membrane of the floor of the mouth, at the site of the frenulum of the tongue, in contact with the sublingual depression on the inner surface of the mandible close to the symphysis.[46] Its excretory ducts are multiple. The larger one (Bartholin's duct) opens into the submandibular duct.[46] Sometimes the sublingual gland can be visualized during sialography of the submandibular gland (Fig. 37–24). Because of marked enhancement, both the submandibular and sublingual glands are visualized by CT incremental dynamic study (Fig. 37–25). The parotid, submandibular, and sublingual glands are seen on MR images with exquisite anatomic details (Fig. 37–26).

Oropharynx, Oral Cavity, and Upper Neck

The detailed anatomy of the oropharynynx, oral cavity and neck can be found in another section of this volume. For the purpose of this section of the book, the cross-sectional anatomy visible in MR and CT images should be reviewed and defined. Several CT and MR images of the normal oropharynx and upper neck are shown in Figures 37–20 to 37–26. Magnetic resonance images are all spin density or proton weighted for uniformity. In the axial CT section taken at the level of the alveolar process of the maxilla, the soft palate is shown blending with the upper portion of the oropharynx (Fig. 37–20). The hard palate is limited laterally by the alveolar process of the maxilla (Fig. 37–20). The medial pterygoid muscle is seen as a distinct quadrilateral image occupying a position on the inside of the ramus of the mandible. Medial to the medial pterygoid muscles, the symmetrical low-density (lucent) parapharyngeal spaces are shown. Also visualized are the masseter muscle, retromandibular vessels, parotid gland, styloid process, and retrostyloid neurovascular structures (Fig. 37–20). In an axial CT section or MR taken at the level of the tongue (Figs. 37–21 to 37–26), the oropharynx, palatine tonsils, submandibular glands, extrinsic and intrinsic muscles of the tongue, external and internal carotid arteries, internal jugular veins, and part of the mandible are among the many structures that are visualized clearly (Fig. 37–26). The differential enhancement of the vascular structures of the neck versus other structures is best demonstrated with the incremental CT dynamic technique (Fig. 37–23). On MR scans, the vascular structures are demonstrated as hypointense images (void signal) without need for contrast injection (Fig. 37–26).

Larynx and Hypopharynx

Computed tomography of the neck represents a major advance in laryngology.[48–58] The ability of CT to show accurately mucosa, deep laryngeal tissues and laryngeal cartilages makes it an ideal radiologic imaging method for evaluation of the larynx. The characteristic configurations of the hyoid bone and the thyroid, cricoid, and arytenoid cartilages greatly facilitate the orientation of CT scanning.[48,49,52,56] A section taken at the level of the hyoid bone (Fig. 37–27) demonstrates the free portion of the epiglottis, valleculae, glossoepiglottic folds, pharyngoepiglottic folds, and superior portion of the piriform sinuses. In scans taken caudally, the preepiglottic space, the epiglottis, the aryepiglottic folds, the piriform sinuses, thyroid cartilage (Fig. 37–28), false cords, corniculate cartilages, true vocal cords, arytenoid cartilages, cricoid cartilage, cricothyroid articulation, conus elasticus, trachea, thyroid gland, and vascular structures will be visualized (Figs. 37–28 to 37–36).

On CT scans, the preepiglottic space (Fig. 37–28) is seen anterior to the epiglottis as a low-density (lucent) image because of its high-fat content.[48] On MR scans, this space is seen as a hyperintense image. The epiglottis is rarely calcified (Fig. 37–36B). Therefore, in an axial section it is imaged as a sharply delineated anteriorly convex curved image, separating the preepiglottic space from the laryngeal vestibule (Fig. 37–36C). The aryepiglottic folds make the posterolateral limit of the laryngeal vestibule[48] and separate the laryngeal vestibule from the posteriorly and laterally located piriform sinuses lying between the aryepiglottic folds and thyroid cartilage[48] (Figs. 37–28, 37–30D). The ventricular folds (false vocal cords) are two thick folds of mucous membrane that contain both fat and minor salivary gland structures.[46,57] At the level of the false vocal cords, the airway is pear-shaped (Fig. 37–29). The soft tissues of the false cords are less dense on CT scans than the true vocal cords. The level of this examination will always be apparent because of the shape of the airway and the fact that the corniculate and arytenoid cartilages (in their upper portions) are usually imaged with the false cords. At this level, the upper portion of the thyroid gland is imaged overlying the thyroid cartilage (Fig. 37–29). The remainder of the gland is seen on CT scans as a triangular, dense image (due to iodine content) in the lower sections taken down to the upper tracheal rings (Figs. 37–31, 37–36). The junction of the false and true vocal cords (laryngeal ventricle) reveals a diamond-shaped contour if contiguous thin sections are obtained[54] (Fig. 37–30C).

True Vocal Cords and the Rima Glottidis

When the transition is made to the glottis, the airway assumes a triangular appearance (Fig. 37–30A, B). The rima glottidis is a fissure between the vocal cords and includes the vocal process of the arytenoid cartilages. It is limited dorsally by the mucous membrane, passing between the arytenoid cartilages at the level of the true vocal cord (Fig. 37–30).[46,54] The true vocal cords can be seen arising from the vocal process of the arytenoids and extending to the midpoint of the thyroid cartilage as they attach to the anterior commissure region of the larynx immediately subjacent to the point of fusion of the paired thyroid alae (Fig. 37–30A, B).[48,49,54,57] The true vocal cords have a dense vocal ligament along their free margin (Fig. 37–30B, C).[48,49,54,57] At its widest, the true vocal cord measures 5 mm in thickness,[49] and tapers to a thickness of one to two mm anteriorly where it meets with the contralateral true vocal cord to form the anterior commissure (Fig. 37–30B). Minor soft-tissue thickening in this area usually suggests the presence of anterior commissure extension by the tumor.[57] If the neck is not positioned properly, slight asymmetry of the true vocal cords will be present (Fig. 37–30B).

The anatomy of the rima glottidis and its function can be evaluated by obtaining CT scans during quiet breathing, forced inspiration, phonation, and Valsalva and modified Valsalva maneuvers.[54] The rima glottidis has two parts: intermembranous, the ventral 3/5th between the cords (glottis vocalis), and the intercartilaginous, dorsal 2/5th between the arytenoid cartilages (glottis respiratoria). It is the narrowest part of the larynx, but its width and shape vary with the movements of the vocal cords and arytenoid cartilages during respiration and phonation. In a state of rest (e.g., in quiet respiration), the intermembranous part of the rima is triangular (Fig. 37–30A, B), its apex is ventrally located at the anterior commissure and its base is represented by a line between the arytenoids (Fig. 37–30A, B).[54] The intercartilaginous part is somewhat semicircular in shape (Fig. 37–30A, B) and should be smooth and symmetric on a CT scan.[54] During closure of the rima glottidis, (e.g., when Valsalva's or modified Valsalva's maneuver is employed) both the true vocal cords and the arytenoid cartilages are adducted (Fig. 37–30C). During forced inspiration, the vocal cords undergo extreme abduction; the arytenoid cartilages are rotated laterally and their vocal processes move widely apart. During phonation, the intermembranous and intercartilaginous space of the glottis is reduced, owing to adduction of the vocal cords and adduction and medial rotation of the arytenoid cartilages (Fig. 37–30C).[54]

Subglottis and Cricoid Cartilage

The subglottis is well imaged by CT and MRI. The undersurface of the true vocal cords forms the superior limits of the subglottis (Fig. 37–31). The cricoid cartilage and the membrane and ligaments that attach to it make up the remaining boundaries of the subglottic space.[46,54] It must be remembered that the cricoid cartilage, which has a signet-ring shape, slopes inferiorly as it is followed anteriorly. The cricothyroid distance approximates 1.5 cm anteriorly,[57] although the cricoid rises to the level of the vocal cords at the cricoarytenoid articulations posteriorly (Fig. 37–30A, B).[57] This is a critical transition point as anterior soft-tissue extension in the subglottis does not produce cartilage involvement until it has made the full inferior infiltration to the level of the cricoid cartilage. However, posterior extension of glottic cancer provides easy access to the high-rising cricoid signal. When the transition is made to the subglottis, the airway first assumes an ovoid (Figs. 37–31, 37–32) and then a circular appearance (Figs. 37–31, 37–34). The mucosa in the subglottic region is thin and should be smooth and symmetric in all sections. Minor soft-tissue thickening in this area always suggests the presence of some abnormality.

Measurements of the transverse and anteroposterior diameters of the subglottis and the postcricoid-prevertebral soft-tissue thickness in 20 individuals (26 to 73 years) who were scanned for possible herniated disc or cervical cord lesion have been made. At the level of the undersurface of the true vocal cord (Figs. 37–31, 37–32), and at the widest area (at the level of the posterior undersurface of the cords), the transverse diameter measured 1.38 to 1.58 cm, with an average of 1.47 cm. The anteroposterior diameter measured 2.20 to 2.40 cm, with an average of 2.24 cm. The prevertebral soft-tissue (from the anterior margin of the vertebra to the posterior margin of the cricoid lamina) measured 0.82 to 0.96 cm, with an average of 0.87 cm. The transverse and anteroposterior diameters of the subglottic region, measured in a section obtained at the cricothyroid ar-

ticulation (Figs. 37–33, 37–34) were as follows: the transverse diameter, at the widest area (midportion), measured 1.60 to 1.76 cm with an average of 1.64 cm, and the anteroposterior diameter measured 2.08 to 2.36 cm with an average of 2.12 cm. The prevertebral soft tissue measured 0.70 to 0.98 cm with an average of 0.85 cm. When the transition is made to the trachea, the airway shows a posterior indentation because of the esophagus, which appears as a round soft-tissue image posterior to the trachea (Fig. 37–36).

The calcification and ossification of the thyroid cartilage may be occasionally uniform, and therefore, on CT its boundaries are delineated clearly (Fig. 37–30). Frequently, however, its calcification and ossification are irregular and asymmetric. Therefore, care must be taken in evaluating thyroid cartilage involvement by CT.[47,52,54–57] The paralaryngeal fat planes marginate the internal cortices of the thyroid cartilage (Fig. 37–32) and are seen as low-density fatty regions that are actually an inferior and lateral extension of the preepiglottic space (Fig. 37–32).[48,49,57] Obliteration of the paralaryngeal fatty planes usually indicates tumor infiltration.[57] The cricoid cartilage (Fig. 37–33), however, is frequently well calcified and its boundaries clearly delineated (Figs. 37–32, 37–34). Characteristically, it has a dense cortex and a lucent medullary portion (Figs. 37–32, 37–34). The arytenoid cartilages are frequently calcified and often appear symmetric (Fig. 37–30). Asymmetric calcification of the arytenoid cartilages should not be mistaken for tumor involvement.[56]

Magnetic resonance imaging, because of its superior spatial resolution and three-dimensional capability, is superior to CT for delineating the anatomy and pathology of the larynx (Fig. 37–36B–E). MRI provides maximum information on the extent of the tumor. Disadvantages of MRI are as follows: 1) MRI frequently requires 45 to 60 minutes scanning time, during which time any patient motion, including heavy breathing, swallowing, and coughing, can degrade the image; 2) MRI is contraindicated in patients with cardiac pacemakers, cochlear implants, and those with ferromagnetic objects in the body; 3) MRI is, unfortunately, the most expensive of all diagnostic imaging modalities.

APPLICATIONS OF MRI AND CT IN PATHOLOGIC CONDITIONS OF THE HEAD AND NECK

Base of the Skull and Neck

With MRI and CT, the diagnosis and management of patients with disease involving the skull base, nasopharynx, and head and neck lesions have been advanced significantly. Primary and secondary tumors of the base of the skull cause expansion, destruction, or sclerotic reaction of the bones of the skull base.[5,59]

Benign lesions such as primary cholesteatoma (Fig. 37–37) and cholesterol granuloma (Fig. 37–38) involving the base of the skull demonstrate characteristic bone expansion with CT showing a low-density image (because of desquamated debris and cholesterol content) and no enhancement after intravenous injection of iodinated-contrast medium (Fig. 37–37).[58–61] Although cholesteatomas may not be differentiated from cholesterol granulomas on CT scans, they often can be easily differentiated by MRI. On T1W images epidermoid cysts and cholesteatomas are seen as a hypointense or isointense image relative to brain and appear hyperintense to brain on T2W MR images (Fig. 37–37B, C).[60] Cholesterol granulomas, however, appear as a hyperintense image on both T1W and T2W MR scans (Fig. 37–38A, B). Cholesterol granulomas may be homogeneous or heterogeneous. The heterogeneity of signal is usually due to hemosiderin debris.[60] Unlike cholesteatomas and cholesterol granulomas, lesions such as jugular fossa schwannoma and glomus jugulare tumors demonstrate bone destruction and usually appear as increased density in noncontrast CT and show moderate to marked enhancement after intravenous infusion of contrast medium (Fig. 37–39).[58] On T1W MR scans, schwannomas are seen as a hypointense image to brain and become hyperintense on T2W MR scans. Glomus tumors also have similar MR appearance; however, they usually show signal void (dark) areas because of their increased vascularity. The intracranial extension of a base of the skull lesion is best demonstrated on postcontrast enhanced CT or MRI. Destruction of the jugular fossa and hypoglossal canal is demonstrated in Figure 37–40 in a patient with liposarcoma of the base of the skull who presented with 12th nerve palsy. The same appearance may be present on CT of a patient with metastatic carcinoma or lymphoma, including multiple myeloma. As far as the glomus complex tumors are concerned, CT reveals the bone destruction and total extent of the disease and gives accurate assessment of middle-ear (Fig. 37–41), intracranial (Fig. 37–42), extracranial (Fig. 37–43), and nasopharyngeal extension (Fig. 37–44).[33,58,59] Dynamic CT has been valuable in the diagnosis and differentiation of glomus complex tumors (Figs. 37–44B, 37–45B, and 37–46) from other pathologic entities such as meningioma (Fig. 37–47) and metastatic and recurrent neck tumors.[33,58,59] The MRI features of glomus jugulare tumors and their pre- and postembolization angiographic characteristics are illustrated in Figure 37–47.

Nasopharynx

Magnetic resonance imaging and CT scans of the nasopharynx are indispensible in patients with clinically diagnosed nasopharyngeal disease in whom information concerning the extent of disease is necessary (Figs. 37–48 to 37–52) and in those patients in whom a search is being made for an unknown primary tumor of the head and neck (Fig. 37–53). Hypertrophied and normal lymphoid tissue is seen commonly within the nasopharynx (Fig. 37–54).[44] Adenoidal tissue is usually symmetric and has a lobulated pattern (Fig. 37–54). Benign lymphoid tumor of the nasopharynx is limited to the mucosa and is smooth in outline (Fig. 37–55). Any extension into the deeper plane with obliteration of the facial planes should be considered evidence of a more aggressive lesion (Figs. 37–50, 37–53, and 37–56).[44,49] Extension of the nasopharyngeal carcinoma into the nasal cavity (Fig. 37–48), infratemporal fossa, orbit, and cranial cavity is best demonstrated by contrast enhanced CT examination (Fig. 37–49) or MRI. Dynamic CT study or dynamic MR study should be used to differentiate lesions such as juvenile angiofibroma (Fig. 37–57) and for any nasopharyngeal hypervascular lesion such as extension of the glomus tumor along the eustachian tube into the nasopharynx (Figs. 37–44 and 37–52).

Benign lesions of the nasopharynx such as inflammatory processes (Fig. 37–58), Tornwaldt's bursa, parapharyngeal cyst, polyps, papillomas, juvenile angiofibromas, neuromas, fibromas, and lipomas are all well suited for MRI and CT.[5,48,62]

Infratemporal Fossa and Parapharyngeal Space

Infection (Figs. 37–59, 37–60), and both benign (Fig. 37–61A, B) and malignant (Fig. 37–61C) tumors of the infratemporal fossa and parapharyngeal space, are manifested by obliteration of the normal soft-tissue planes and/or by a mass effect.[5,59,63] Tumors and inflammatory processes in these areas are difficult to assess clinically.[5] However, they are identified readily by MRI and CT (Fig. 37–61). Tumors of the PPS are rare, accounting for only 0.5% of head and neck neoplasms.[59] Neuromas of the vagus, trigeminal, sympathetic chain (Fig. 37–61E) and hypoglossal nerves and neurofibromas that arise within the parapharyngeal space present as rounded masses bulging into the nasopharynx.[48,59] The benign nature of the tumor is often predicted by an evaluation of CT and MRI scans, which show mass effect but not obliteration or invasion of the fascial planes (Fig. 37–61A, B). Tumors of the mandible usually are confined to the bone; however, extension deep into the adjacent infratemporal fossa may occur (Fig. 37–62). Extension of the nasal, maxillary, and ethmoid sphenoidal lesions into the infratemporal fossa and the pterygopalatine fossa can be delineated clearly by MRI and CT scans.

Parotid Glands

Acute infection of the parotid gland manifests itself as diffuse swelling of the gland. An abscess is seen on a CT scan as a discrete low-density (lucent) image (Fig.

37–63). The inflammatory processes of adjacent structures, such as an abscess of the masseter and sternocleidomastoid muscles, can be diagnosed and differentiated from a parotid abscess (Fig. 37–64). The diagnosis of chronic parotitis, which results from ductal obstruction because of stone and recurrent parotitis and chronic punctate sialadenitis (benign lymphoepithelial disease, Mikulicz's syndrome, Sjögren's syndrome) of the parotid or submandibular gland can be accomplished more readily with conventional sialography.[47] Computed tomography of the parotid gland performed with or without contrast infusion (Fig. 37–65) and CT contrast sialography (Fig. 37–66) can locate parotid masses. Magnetic resonance imaging, similar to CT, is extremely useful and has replaced CT in the evaluation of salivary gland masses (Figs. 37–67, 37–68). The differentiation of extrinsic mass versus intrinsic parotid tumor is a simple matter if MRI or CT is used,[50,63] whereas this problem can be extremely difficult to resolve by conventional sialography (Fig. 37–69).[47]

Tumors that are 1 cm in diameter or less are exceedingly difficult to demonstrate by conventional sialography, especially if they are peripherally located.[47] On CT scans, small-mass lesions can be seen because they have a different CT appearance in noncontrast and contrast infusion CT as compared with normal parts of the gland.[47] On CT sialography, they appear as a filling defect (Fig. 37–66). Magnetic resonance imaging, because of its superior contrast resolution, is more sensitive than CT scan and sialography for the evaluation of salivary gland tumors. Conventional sialography is the study of choice for the evaluation of chronic sialopathy, including Sjögrens syndrome.

Oropharynx, Hypopharynx, and Neck

Infection, trauma, and benign and malignant tumors in this area are evaluated adequately by clinical examination, plain films, barium swallow, and cine esophogram. The ability of MRI and CT to provide superficial and deep information and soft-tissue identification (fat, air, fluid, calcium, blood) makes them the most complete technique for the diagnosis of pathologic conditions in these regions.[5] Branchial cleft cysts (Fig. 37–70), ranula (Fig. 37–71), cystic hygroma (Figs. 37–72, 37–73), thyroglossal duct cysts (Fig. 37–74), cellulitis and abscesses are all well suited for MRI and CT. Deep soft-tissue edema and hematoma can be readily recognized in trauma patients (Fig. 37–75). The total extent of deep-seated malignant tumors, associated lymphatic-chain involvement and vascular encasement can be better determined with a contrast-enhanced CT examination (Figs. 37–76, 37–77).[5,33] The carotid body and glomus vagale tumors, although uncommon, are considered frequently in the differential diagnosis of cervical masses.[34,35] With infusion CT, the differential enhancement of these lesions from adjacent muscles and vascular structures may not be sufficiently diagnostic to distinguish them from a vascular tumor (Fig. 37–78), lymph node, or other abnormal solid lesion (Fig. 37–79).[34] Dynamic CT clearly visualizes the sequential enhancement of the carotid arteries and internal jugular veins, and the tumor becomes densely opacified for a short time as the intravenously injected bolus of contrast material traverses the vascular bed of the tumor (Figs. 37–45A, 37–46A–B, 37–78, 37–79). With MR, glomus vagale and carotid body tumors (Figs. 37–69, 37–80) can be distinguished from other lesions such as neurofibromas (Fig. 37–81). Glomus-complex tumors are highly vascular (Fig. 37–82), and, therefore, on dynamic CT or dynamic MR (GRASS), this increased vascularity can be demonstrated, allowing differentiation of them from other lesions (Figs. 37–69, 37–80, and 37–81).

Benign and malignant lesions of the pharynx and oral cavity can be visualized by MRI scanning. Figure 37–83 shows a lymphangiohemangioma of the tonsillar region, and Figure 37–84 shows a carcinoma of the tonsil and soft palate with bilateral nodal metastases. With MR, a primary tumor and metastatic nodal involvement can be identified readily (Figs. 37–84, 37–85). Figure 37–86 demonstrates the value of MRI, including dynamic MR, in the evaluation of a recurrent tonsillar cancer and thrombosis of the internal jugular vein. Tumors of the tongue and floor of the mouth (Fig. 37–87), posterior pharyngeal wall (Fig. 37–88), and hypopharynx (Fig. 37–89) are readily evaluated by MRI.

Larynx

Computed tomography has made a major contribution to the radiologic evaluation of the larynx.[48–51,54,55,57] Computed tomography is the procedure of choice in the investigation of laryngeal trauma, especially in the acute phase, because it provides evidence of mucosal disruption, hematoma formation, fracture and cartilage displacement, and an axial display of the airway (Figs. 37–90, 37–91).[53,57] Benign lesions of the larynx are generally diagnosed by clinical examination rather than radiologic techniques. Laryngeal cysts and laryngoceles are well suited for CT. Computed tomography is able to define the extent of the laryngocele more precisely than either clinical examination or conventional radiographic techniques. Using CT, a laryngocele appears as a well-circumscribed air-filled enlargement that represents extension and elongation of the normal appendice of the laryngeal ventricle (saccule) (Fig. 37–92).[48] When the laryngocele is filled with fluid (complicated laryngocele), it appears on CT as a low-density, smoothly marginated mass along the lateral wall of the larynx and may be difficult to differentiate from an aryepiglottic-fold cyst.

Malignant Tumors of the Larynx

The ability of CT and MRI to demonstrate accurately mucosal, deep laryngeal tissue, and associated lymphatic-chain involvement makes either of them an ideal imaging method for evaluation of laryngeal tumors[44,48,50,54,57] (Fig. 37–93). Computed tomography has its major value in the pretreatment TNM staging of laryngeal cancer.[57] Tumor involvement of the anterior and posterior commissure (Fig. 37–93), subglottic region (Fig. 37–94), and trachea (Fig. 37–95) is best evaluated by CT.[57] Cartilage involvement (Fig. 37–96) and extension of the tumor in the paralaryngeal and paraglottic space (Figs. 37–97, 37–98) can be demonstrated in a manner not available before the introduction of CT. Computerized tomography will permit the consistent detection of lymph nodes greater than 1.5 cm in diameter (Fig. 37–96),[57] and they are almost always tumor-bearing. Lymph nodes between 1 to 1.5 cm, may represent tumor or reactive hyperplasia.[57]

Computed tomography is very helpful in the evaluation of tumor extension, specifically in the axial dimension.[48,49,54,55,57] Its primary application is in the evaluation of T3 and T4 laryngeal cancer.[57] Magnetic resonance imaging of the larynx can provide valuable information (Fig. 37–98B–I). With MRI, however, motion artifact related to respiration and blood flow can cause significant distortion of the images. For lesions such as chondrosarcoma of the larynx, maximum information is obtained by combination of CT and MRI (Fig. 37–98G–I).

Paranasal Sinuses and Nasal Cavity

The traditional approach to the radiologic evaluation of lesions of the paranasal sinuses and face have been standard plain-film radiography followed by polytomography.[39] Because these techniques are not capable of imaging soft-tissue structures, extension of lesions into the orbit, cranial cavity, pterygopalatine fossa, infratemporal fossa, and parts of the neck can only be inferred from adjacent bone involvement.[39] The inherently superior contrast resolution of CT and a precise three-dimensional effect of the combined axial and coronal sections have established CT as the method of choice in the staging of maxillofacial neoplasms and the evaluation of chronic and complicated inflammatory processes of the paranasal sinuses and face.[5,39] Magnetic resonance imaging has been used to demonstrate maxillofacial anatomy and certain pathology. Familiarity with CT dictates that the MR evaluation complement and not be a substitute for the CT evaluation. Magnetic resonance imaging is superior to CT for the evaluation of the extent of soft tissue involvement and intracranial invasion of sinonasal tumors. A detailed discussion of the various diseased entities of the paranasal sinuses and nasal cavity is limited by the scope of this chapter; although certain conditions will be described to illustrate the role of CT and MRI in the evaluation of patients with paranasal sinus and nasal diseases.

Conventional plain films still provide the best screening studies in various pathologic conditions of the sinuses and in maxillofacial trauma and give orientation and direction to further examinations using CT.[43,64] Developmental anomalies, such as a palato-maxillary cleft, are more clearly seen using CT (Fig. 37–99). The appearance of lesions of the paranasal sinuses and face on a CT scan usually does not provide sufficient evidence for a specific histologic diagnosis; however, cystic (Fig. 37–100), cartilaginous, and osseous tumors are an exception (Fig. 37–114A). Fibrous dysplasia also frequently shows characteristic islands of bone formation within a dense, rather uniform, stroma on a CT scan.

Infection

Conventional radiography is adequate for the diagnosis of acute sinusitis. Even though antibiotics have cut down on the incidence of complicated sinusitis with orbital involvement, it still occurs and may even be the first sign of sinus infection in children.[65] Infection can spread from sinuses to orbit by direct extension. It can also spread by way of numerous valveless communicating veins between the sinuses and the orbit.[65] In complicated sinusitis, CT is the best method to demonstrate the nature and the source of the problem. The orbital extension of sinusitis include: orbital periostitis, subperiosteal induration (phlegmon) (Fig. 37–101), subperiosteal abscess (Fig. 37–102), orbital cellulitis, orbital abscess and ophthalmic veins thrombophlebitis (Fig. 37–103).[65] Should the infection spread from the sinuses into the cranial cavity, one or more of the following complications may ensue: cavernous sinus thrombosis, meningitis, or epidural (Fig. 37–103), subdural, or brain abscess.[65]

Periostitis and osteomyelitis of the frontal bone can complicate frontal sinusitis (Fig. 37–103C, D).[65] An infection of the frontal sinus severe enough to involve the orbit may also extend through the posterior plate of the frontal sinus to involve the anterior cranial fossa (Fig. 37–103C, D).[65] Orbital complications that result from sphenoid sinusitis can best be evaluated with CT and MRI scans (Fig. 37–104).

Chronic inflammatory disease is often associated with sclerosis of the walls of the sinuses and ethmoidal trabeculae (Figs. 37–105, 37–106).[5] Fungi, particularly aspergillus, may be considered possible causative agents.

Polyposis of the paranasal sinuses and nasal cavity (Fig. 37–107 and mucocele of the maxillary (Fig. 37–108), frontoethmoid (Fig. 37–109), and sphenoid sinuses (Fig. 37–110A) are best evaluated by CT and MRI scans.[5,39,43,66] Mucoceles and benign tumors tend to expand the area of origin by virtue of their slow growth.[5,39,66] The gradual pressure, atrophy, and erosion of the bone by the enlarging soft-tissue mass of the mucocele and the expansile low-density appearance on CT (Figs. 37–108 to 37–110), with no enhancement after contrast infusion (except around the inflamed capsule and peripheral calcifications), make the CT diagnosis of mucocele almost certain. Mucoceles may extend into the orbit or intracranially from the frontal ethmoid, and sphenoid sinuses (Fig. 37–110). Computed tomography is the diagnostic method of choice for the diagnosis and management of the mucocele. Magnetic resonance can provide valuable information regarding intracranial extension of a mucocele. Mucoceles are most often hyperintense on both T1W and T2W MR images (Fig. 37–110B, C). Calcifications and inspissated mucus can be easily missed by MRI. At times, a sinus filled with inspissated mucus can appear as a perfectly aerated and normal sinus. Magnetic resonance imaging should be used as a complementary study to evaluate mucoceles.

Tumors of the Paranasal Sinuses

Computed tomography has made significant contributions to the radiographic evaluation of tumors of the paranasal sinuses and other head and neck tumors.[66–68] Computed tomography and MRI have also been valuable in the management of malignant tumors, particularly in the planning of portals for radiation therapy.[69,70,71]

Conventional radiography is adequate for the diagnosis of paranasal osteoma. Computed tomography, however, is indicated when there is orbital extension or other complications (Fig. 37–111). Malignant tumors of the nasal cavity and paranasal sinuses account for only 0.2 to 0.8% of all malignant neoplasms and only 3% of all tumors occurring in the head and neck.[70,71] Approximately 50 to 65% of malignant sinonasal tumors arise within the maxillary sinuses, 10 to 25% in the ethmoid sinuses, 0.1 to 4% in the frontal and sphenoid sinuses, and 15 to 30% in the nasal cavity.[70] Malignant tumors of the nasal cavity (Fig. 37–112) and paranasal sinuses (Fig. 37–113) destroy bone and invade the adjacent soft-tissue structures (Figs. 37–112 and 37–113). Extension into the orbit, pterygopalatine fossa, infratemporal fossa (Fig. 37–113A, B), and cranial cavity can best be demonstrated by contrast-enhanced CT or MRI (Fig. 37–113C–F). Osteogenic or chondrogenic sarcomas of the paranasal sinuses show on CT scans as irregular islands of tumor, bone formation, and marked bone destruction (Fig. 37–114A).[70] On the other hand, osteoclastoma or giant cell tumor produces bone destruction as well as bone expansion (Fig. 37–114B). Early subperiosteal extension of a neoplastic condition is best evaluated by CT scans. CT

remains the study of choice for osseous and chondrogenic lesions such as osteoma, osteoid osteoma, osteoblastoma, ossifying fibroma, osteogenic and chondrogenic sarcomas and developmental conditions such as fibrous dysplasis.[43,70] Although CT is more specific in the diagnosis of osteogenic and chondrogenic sarcomas, MRI is more sensitive for the determination of the extent of their soft tissue components as well as the presence of subtle or obvious intracranial spread.[43] Magnetic resonance imaging is superior to CT in differentiating inflammatory conditions from neoplastic processes.[70,71] Most inflammatory lesions are hyperintense on T2W MR images as opposed to most malignant tumors, lymphoreticular proliferative, myeloproliferative and chronic granulomatous disorders.[43,70] Most tumors of the sinonasal cavities are not as hyperintense as the surrounding inflammation and retained secretions, and therefore, MRI plays an important role in the mapping and staging of these tumors. The intraorbital and intracranial complications of sinus surgery for tumors or inflammatory conditions are often best demonstrated by MRI.

Trauma

Conventional plain-film examination and selective complex-motion tomography can be used for radiologic diagnosis of the isolated maxillofacial fracture.[40] These modalities are clinically accessible, cost effective, and diagnostic. In complex maxillofacial trauma, CT provides the most effective imaging modality.[40] Current generation scanners with extended bone range on scale imaging possibilities provide superior bone detail to polytomography.[40] The orbit is superbly suited to CT scanning. Orbital findings in trauma are well documented.[5,40,73,74] The fracture fragments and foreign bodies projecting into the orbit and fat and muscle herniation projecting into the ethmoid or maxillary sinuses are readily identified together with any hematoma and/or pneumo-orbit (Fig. 37–115). CT is the procedure of choice for evaluation of the position of the Silastic implant for the repair of orbital floor fracture (Fig. 37–116). The fracture of the lamina papyracea, which is difficult to image conventionally, can be imaged with axial and coronal sections (Figs. 37–115C, 37–117C).

The intracranial and intraorbital extension of complex maxillofacial fractures, shattering craniofacial fractures, and medial and lateral orbital wall and orbital apex fractures can be imaged in a manner not previously possible.[40] The axial dimension of posterior maxillary, alveolar, and pterygoid plate fractures and the posterior extensions of the LeFort group of fractures are particularly suited to axial CT imaging (Fig. 37–117).[40] Displacement and rotation of the malar bone and bone fragments in tripod fractures can best be demonstrated with axial CT (Fig. 37–118A). Sphenoid sinus fractures can be evaluated by axial and particularly by direct coronal section (with extended bone range technique) and sagittal reformatted images. The coronal CT sections should be taken only in the injured patient who is facially stable and is without cervical spine injury. In a sphenoid sinus fracture, opacification of the sinus with blood or CSF can be readily recognized with CT scan.

Three dimensional (3-D) reconstruction of CT images is a well-established imaging modality which has been investigated in various clinical settings. Perhaps one of its most useful applications is in trauma. Rotational abnormalities may be better appreciated on 3-D images (Fig. 37–118B).

CSF Leak and Pneumocephalus

In trauma patients, the recognition of free air within the cranial cavity and cisternal and ventricular system is the result of a dural and subarachnoid tear. This can occur at any number of sites: the posterior wall of the frontal sinus, the roof of the ethmoid labyrinth, the cribriform plate, the walls of the sphenoid sinus, the middle cranial fossa, and beyond.[40] Localization of the fracture site and bone fragments in axial and, if possible, direct coronal display, utilizing the extended bone range technique and thin sections (1 to 1.5 mm) in critical areas is mandatory. Contrast examination with intrathecal, water soluble, iodinated contrast material is not indicated at this stage since most acute CSF leaks will close spontaneously or with operative fracture reduction alone.[40] In persistent CSF leaks, all such fistulae should undergo CT cisterography (Fig. 37–119).[40,75–77] The examination must be carried out during a period of active CSF rhinorrhea or otorrhea for effective imaging results.[75–77] Other examinations, such as a radionuclide CSF scan, are not needed.[40] When the leak is large, MRI may be sufficient to make the correct diagnosis.

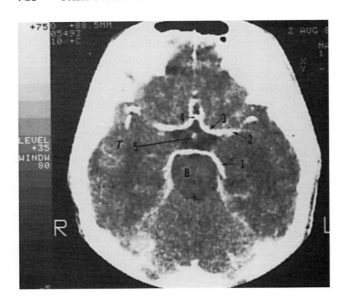

Fig. 37–1. Normal circle of Willis. Postcontrast axial CT scan of the lower head at the level of the suprasellar cistern demonstrates the enhanced pituitary stalk (5) in the center of the low-density starshaped suprasellar cistern. The posterior cerebral (1), middle cerebral (2), anterior cerebral (3), anterior communicating (4) arteries are well seen as high-density images because of their higher iodine contrast content. This image was obtained with a window width of +80 (+75, −5) and window level of +35. With this setting, values higher than +75 will be white (bones), and those lower than −5 will be black (air in the frontal sinus). Note the differential enhancement of the white and gray matter in the brain stem (B) and temporal lobe (T). The gray matter by virtue of its richer vascularity shows more enhancement than white matter. The CSF fluid (suprasellar cistern, cerebral aqueduct) appears as a low-density image in CT.

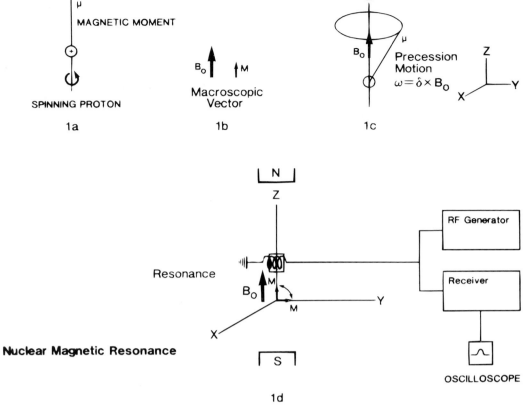

Nuclear Magnetic Resonance

Fig. 37–2. Nuclei of odd number of neutrons or protons or both such as hydrogen (proton) have a net spin or "nuclear angular momentum." Each spinning nucleus generates a magnetic field and hence a magnetic moment which is a vectoral quantity with both direction and magnitude (1a). Nuclear magnets of the nuclei with spin will be pointing in random directions. Therefore, there is no net magnetization in any direction. If the nuclei are placed in an external static magnetic field B_o, (1b), the randomly oriented magnetic moments line up in the direction of field at a state of equilibrium. The magnetic behavior of the entire population of nuclei is defined as a macroscopic or bulk magnetization vector M (1b). When a proton is placed in a magnetic field B_o, (1c), it experiences a couple (from the north and south poles) tending to turn its magnetic moment parallel to the field. Because it spins, the proton responds to this force like a gyroscope and its axis of the magnetic moment vector M wobbles or precesses about the direction of the magnetic field B_o (1c). The frequency (W) of this precessional motion is unique for each nuclear magnetic sensitive element and is given by the famous theorem of Larmor (w = $8 \times B_o$). By convention, the spin system is presented in a cartesian coordinate system (x,y,z) with the Z axis parallel with the external magnet field B_o. When the spin system (M) is placed in an external magnetic field (B_o), besides the creation of precession, another phenomenon, a resonance condition is produced in which the nuclei can absorb energy at sharply defined frequency (Larmor frequency) from an electromagnetic pulse (wave) and re-emit the energy as electromagnetic radiation of the same frequency after the incident beam has been turned off. Let us wind a coil around a nuclear magnetic sensitive specimen and place it inside a magnet (with north, N, and south, S, poles) as shown in (1d) and supply it with radiofrequency (RF) current at Larmor frequency. A short pulse of such resonant RF current can be arranged to tip the net magnetization vector (M) through 90 degrees into the xy plane (1d) which is perpendicular to B_o. This is called 90 degree pulse. The magnetization M now continues to rotate in the x-y plane at the same frequency and induces a voltage (current) in a receiver coil (antenna) in the x-y plane. If the pulse is then turned off, the excited spin system (the nuclei) return to their state of equilibrium and lose the excess energy. The vector (M) continues to rotate freely in the x-y plane, causing the induced current (signal) in the antenna to fade. This decaying signal is called the "free induction decay" (FID), which can be amplified, detected and displayed on an oscilloscope or fed into a computer to provide pictorial information. The return of excited spin system to the state of equilibrium, the so-called relaxation, is characterized by two sample related time constants. T1 (spin-lattice relaxation time) is the time constant required for the net magnetization (M) to return from x-y plane to its equilibrium along Z axis. T2 (spin-spin relaxation time or transverse relaxation time) is the time constant of the decay of FID.

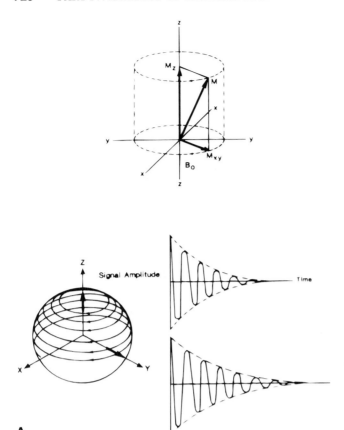

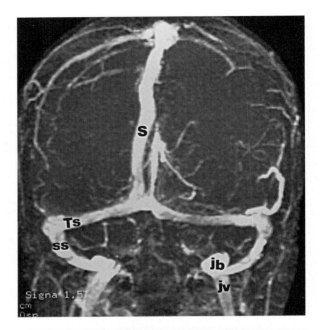

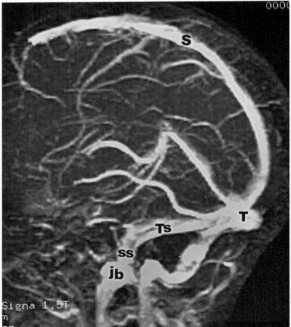

A

Fig. 37–3. A. The precessing net magnetization vector (M) can be considered as having a component, Mz, along the axis of the main field (BO) and a component, Mxy, in a plane perpendicular to the field axis such as xy plane (top image). At equilibrium the net magnetization is aligned with main field so Mz has its maximum (Mz = M0 and Mxy has its minimum (zero) magnitude. After a 90 degree pulse the Mxy has its maximum and Mz its minimum (zero) magnitude. Following application of an RF pulse, the net magnetization vector M, will precess at an ever increasing angle to the main field direction (bottom image), with the precession occurring at the inherent or natural Larmor frequency. If the RF pulse is long enough or strong enough, the net magnetization vector (M) spirals down toward the xy plane (bottom image). When the RF pulse is turned off, the spin system would relax and the excess energy is released as decaying signal (FID) with a time constant of T2. The T2 relaxation time for most tumors (T) is longer than normal tissue (N). In other words, the NMR signal of the tumor (lower decaying pulse) decays longer than the normal tissue (upper decaying pulse). B. MR venogram: TdTOF coronal venography shows normal venous structures. S, Superior sagittal sinus; Ts, transverse sinus; ss, sigmoid sinus; Jb, jugular bulb; Jv, internal jugular vein. C. Sagittal MR venogram shows normal venous structures. S, Superior sagittal sinus; T, torcula herophili; Ts, transverse sinus; ss, sigmoid sinus; Jb, jugular bulb.

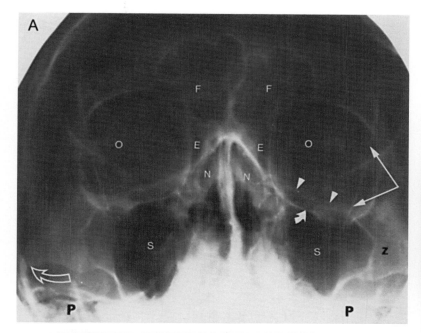

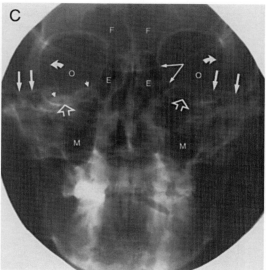

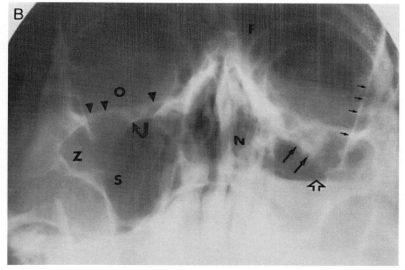

Fig. 37–4. A. Waters view showing maxillary sinuses (S), frontal sinuses (F), nasal cavity (N), body of zygoma (Z), orbit (O), inferior orbital rim (arrowheads), floor of orbit (curved arrow), temporal line (crossed arrows), zygomatic arch and petrous pyramid (P). B. Waters view shows blow-out fracture (depressed floor) of the left orbit (arrows) with associated air-fluid level (hollow arrowheads). Note soft tissue swelling of eyelid and cheek. F, Frontal sinus; N, nasal cavity; O, orbit; S, maxillary sinus; Z, zygoma. Arrowheads point to inferior orbital rim and curved arrow points to normal floor of the right orbit, and short arrows refer to innominate line. C. Caldwell view showing the maxillary (M), ethmoid (E), and frontal (F) sinuses. Notice orbits (C), inferior orbital rim (short arrows), orbital floor (hollow arrow), lamina papyracea (crossed arrows) and innominate lines (curved arrow).

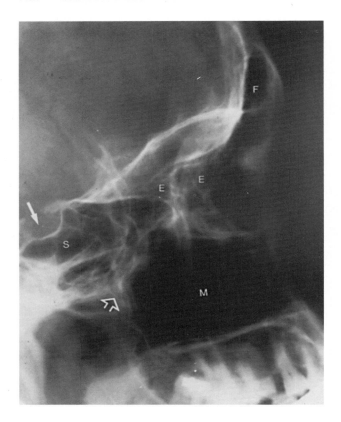

Fig. 37–5. Lateral view showing the sphenoid sinus (S), sella turcica (arrow) and pterygoid plates (hollow arrows), maxillary sinus (M), ethmoid air cell (E), and frontal sinus (F).

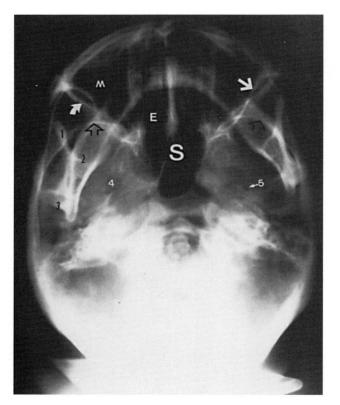

Fig. 37–6. Basal view showing the sphenoid (S), ethmoid (E) sinuses. Notice the "3 lines." Sinus line (arrow), orbital line (curved line), middle cranial fossa line (hollow arrow). Note maxillary sinuses (M), coronoid process (1), mandible (2), mandibular condyle (3), foramen ovale (4) and foramen spinosum (5).

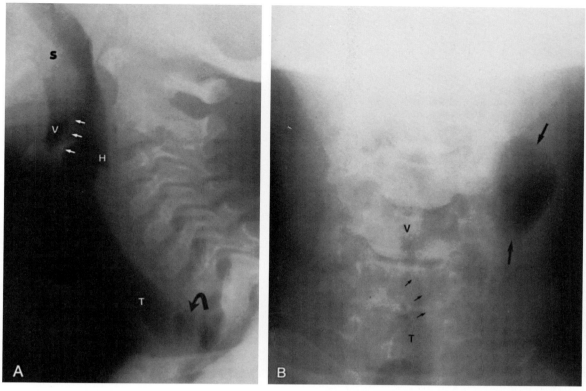

Fig. 37–7. A. Normal lateral view of neck, showing the soft palate (S) valleculae (v) epiglottis (arrows), hypopharynx (H), trachea (T) and apex of the lungs (curved arrow). B. Frontal view of neck showing the trachea (T), subglottic space (small arrows), air in the laryngeal vestibule (V) and a large laryngocele (large arrows).

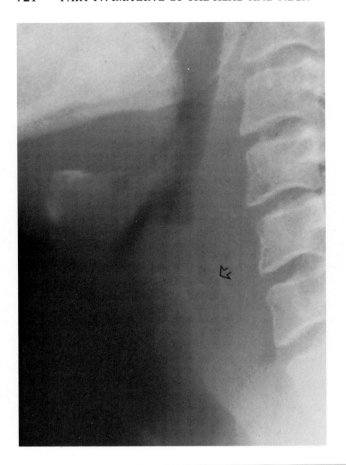

Fig. 37–8. Fish bone and edema of the retropharyngeal space. Lateral neck showing marked increased thickness of the prevertebral space (compare with normal Fig. 37–7A). Note the fish bone (arrow). Anterior to fish bone are partially calcified cricoid and thyroid cartilages.

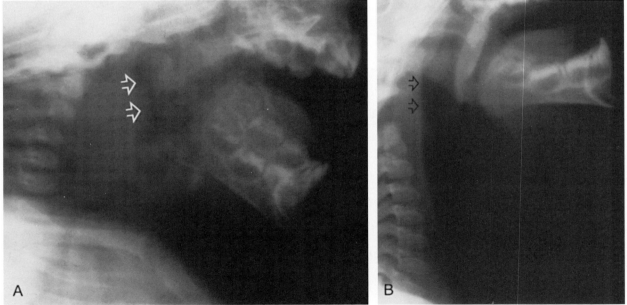

Fig. 37–9. Normal neck of an infant. Lateral neck taken with flexion during expiration (A) and with head in extension (same patient), during inspiration (B). In A, there is bulging of the retropharyngeal soft tissue (arrows), mimicking a retropharyngeal abscess or cellulitis. In B, the thickness of retropharyngeal soft tissue is normal (arrows).

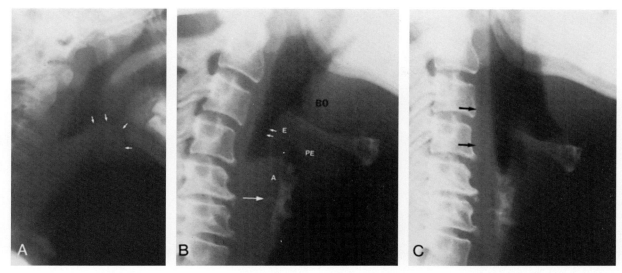

Fig. 37–10. Epiglottitis and angioneurotic edema. A. Lateral neck film showing marked enlargement of the epiglottis (arrows). Notice marked thickening of aryepiglottic folds. B. Lateral neck in another patient with angioneurotic edema showing thickening of epiglottis (E), aryepiglottic folds (small arrows), arytenoid region (A), pre-epiglottic space (PE), and base of tongue (BO). The large arrow points to cricoid cartilage. C. Lateral neck of same patient as in B, showing marked resolution of edema. There is now slight retropharyngeal soft tissue thickening (edema) (arrows).

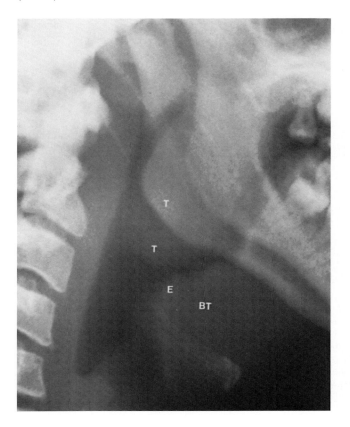

Fig. 37–11. Tonsillitis and retropharyngeal abscess. Lateral neck shows large tonsils (T) with edema of epiglottis (E) and base of tongue (BT). The prevertebral soft tissue is thickened as a result of early cellulitis.

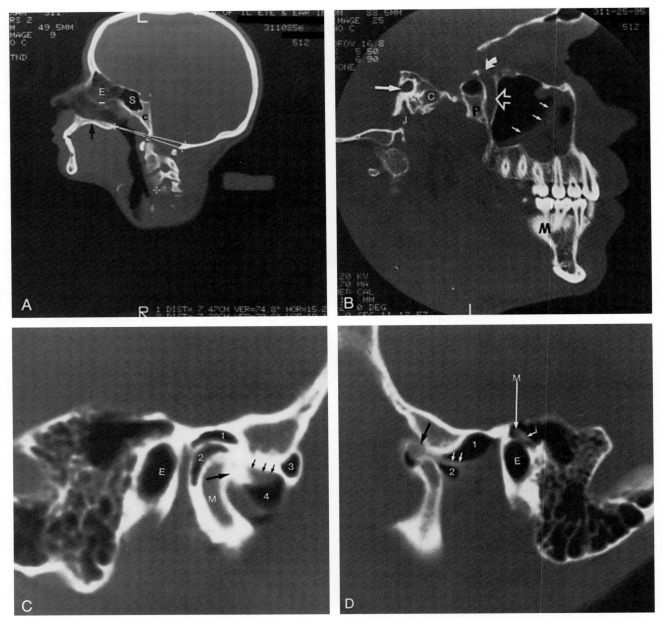

Fig. 37–12. A. Direct sagittal CT of the midline head showing the hard palate (arrow), sphenoid sinus (S), clivus (C), ethmoid air cells (E), and craniocervical junction. B. Sagittal CT showing mucosal thickening of the maxillary sinus (short arrows), pterygomaxillary fissure (hollow arrow), pterygoid plate (P), pterygopalatine fossa and inferior orbital fissure (curved arrow), carotid canal (C), jugular fossa (J), internal auditory canal (long arrow), and mandible (M). C. Sagittal CT air-iodinated contrast arthrogram of left temporomandibular joint (TMJ) showing dislocation of the disc (short arrow). Notice air in the superior (1) and inferior (2) joint spaces as well as in the anterior recess of the superior (3) and inferior (4) joint spaces. Notice iodinated contrast in the inferior joint space (large arrowhead). E, External auditory canal; M, mandible. D. Sagittal CT air-iodinated contrast arthrogram of right TMJ during open mouth position showing dislocated disk (arrow). Air is seen in the superior (1) and inferior (2) joint spaces. Note stretching of retrodiscal zone (arrows). E, External auditory canal; I, incus; M, malleus.

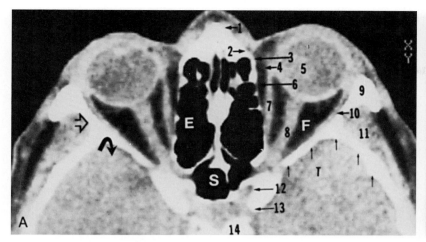
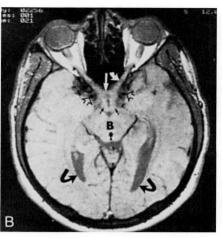

Fig. 37–13. A. Normal ethmoid: Axial CT scan through the plane of optic nerves showing the nasal bone (1), nasal process of maxilla (2), lacrimal bone (3), periorbital fat (4), globe (5), lamina papyracea (6), medial rectus (7), optic nerve (8), zygomatic process of frontal bone (9), lateral rectus muscle (10), temporal fossa (11), temporal line (curved arrow), cranial opening of optic canal (12), anterior clinoid (13), posterior clinoid process (14). Note ethmoid (E) and sphenoid (S) sinuses and retroglobar fat (F). Two of the "triple lines" seen in the submentovertical projection (Fig. 37–6E), the orbital line (posterior wall of the orbit) (open arrow) and middle cranial fossa line (arrows) are seen. B. Proton-weighted axial MR scan showing optic nerves, optic chiasm (long white arrow), hypothalamus (short black arrows), brain stem (B) and cerebral aqueduct (arrowhead). Note visualization of intracanalicular segment of the optic nerve (curved white arrow) which is hardly seen in CT scan. Notice that in this PW image the water in vitreous cavity and cerebrospinal fluid in lateral ventricles (curved black arrows) are hypointense and fat in the retrobulbar space as well as in the subcutaneous space is hyperintense. The blood vessels are hypointense (hollow arrows).

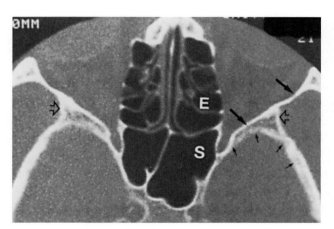

Fig. 37–14. Normal ethmoid and sphenoid sinuses. High-resolution axial CT scan at the level of the middle orbit, using the extended bone CT range technique showing: the ethmoid labyrinth (E) with their intact and sharply delineated septa, and sphenoid sinuses (S). Note the spheno-ethmoidal plate, intersphenoid septum, and sharply delineated orbital (long arrows) and anterior middle cranial fossa (short arrows) lines. Part of the innominate lines are also well visualized (hollow arrows). The innominate line (see Fig. 37–6) is related to the outer cortex of the greater wing of the sphenoid bone.

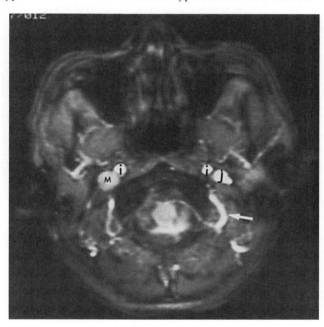

Fig. 37–15. Schwannoma of acoustic nerve extending into the jugular fossa. GRASS (gradient recalled acquisition in the steady state) image shows the hyperintense internal carotid artery (i), internal jugular vein (j), vertebral artery (arrow), and hyperintense mass (M) within the right jugular vein.

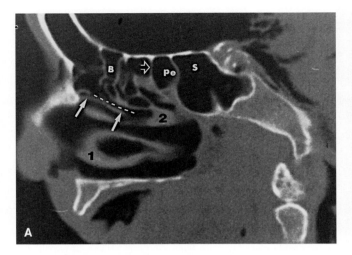

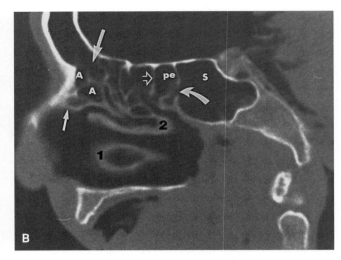

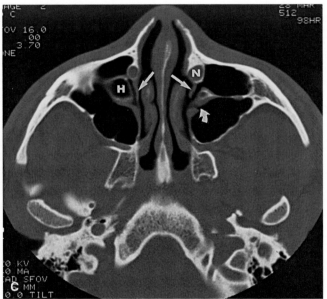

Fig. 37–16. A. Sagittal CT scan shows uncinate process of the ethmoid (arrows), infundibulum (broken line), bulla (B), basal lamella (hollow arrow) posterior ethmoid sinus (Pe), sphenoid sinus (S), and middle (2) and inferior (1) turbinates. B. Sagittal CT scan shows inferior turbinate (1), middle turbinate (2), uncinate process (small straight arrow), agger nasi cell (A), frontal recess (large straight arrow), basal lamella (hollow arrow), posterior ethmoid sinus (pe), sphenoid sinus (s), and sphenoid sinus ostium (curved arrow). C. Axial CT scan shows nasolacrimal canal (N), ostium of maxillary sinus (curved arrow), and Haller cells (H). *(continued)*

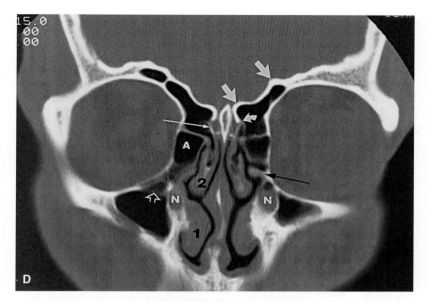

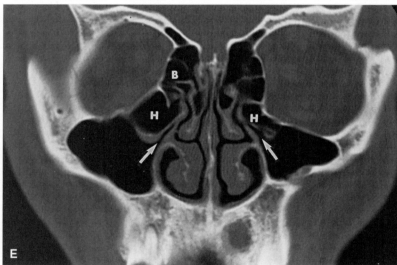

Fig. 37–16. *(continued)* D. Coronal CT scan, same patient as in C, shows inferior turbinate (1), middle turbinate (2), nasolacrimal duct (N), uncinate process (long black arrow), Haller cell (hollow arrow), agger nasi cell (A), lateral lamella (long white arrow), fovea ethmoidalis (double white arrows), and canal for ethmoidal artery (curved arrow). E. Coronal CT scan, same patient as in C and D, shows bulla (B), Haller cells (H), and maxillary ostia (arrows), opening into the infundibulum.

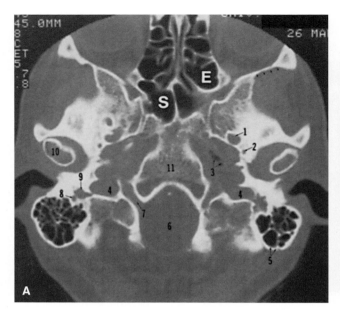
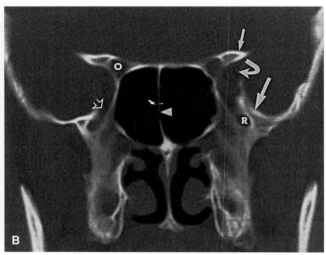

Fig. 37–17. Normal base of the skull. A. High-resolution axial CT scan at the level of the clivus (11), using the extended bone CT range technique showing: the ethmoidal labyrinth (E), sphenoid sinuses (S), posterior wall of the orbit (arrowheads), foramen ovale (1), foramen spinosum (2), air in the eustachian tube (3), jugular fossa (4), mastoid air cells (5), foramen magnum (6), hypoglossal canal (7), vertical portion of the facial nerve canal (8), lateral extension of the right jugular fossa (9), mandibular condyle (10). B. Coronal CT scan shows anterior clinoid (small straight arrow), superior orbital fissure (curved arrow), greater wing of sphenoid (large arrow), foramen rotundum (R), intersphenoid septum (arrowhead), inferior orbital fissure (hollow arrow), and optic canal (o).

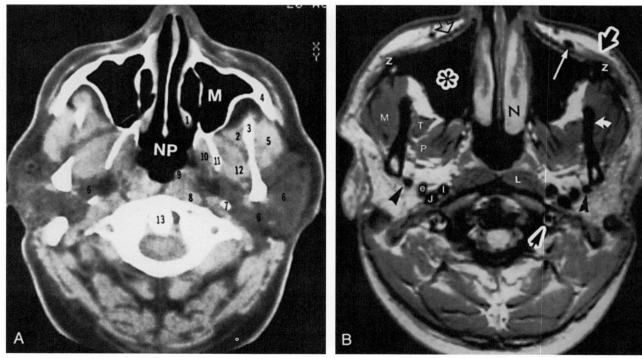

Fig. 37–18. Normal nasopharynx, maxillary sinus and infratemporal fossa. A. Axial CT scan through the midportion of the maxillary sinuses (M) and upper odontoid process (13) showing: nasal septum, inferior turbinate (1), nasopharynx (NP), temporalis muscle (2), coronoid process (3) zygoma (4), masseter muscle (5), parotid gland (6), styloid process (7), longus capitis muscle (8), torus tubarius (9), tensor veli palati muscle (10), lateral pterygoid plate (11), lateral pterygoid muscle (12). The density seen behind the torus is mainly caused by levator veli palati muscle. The tensor veli palati is rarely seen as a distinct muscle bundle. Part of the density seen medial to the lateral pterygoid plate is caused by tensor veli palati muscle (10). Medial to the deep lobe of parotid (6), the symmetric low-density parapharyngeal spaces are seen. Posterior to the styloid process, are seen the densities of the petrostyloid neurovascular structures. B. Axial proton-weighted MR scan showing, quadratus labii superioris (open arrow), orbicularis oculi and zygomaticus muscles (white and black arrow), angular vein (white arrow), zygomatic bone (Z), maxillary antrum (*), nasal turbinate (N) masseter muscle (M), pterygoid muscles (P), mandible (curved arrow), retromandibular vein (arrowhead), vertebral artery (white and black arrowhead), longus colli muscle (L), external (E) and internal (I) carotid arteries, internal jugular vein (J), and temporalis muscle (T).

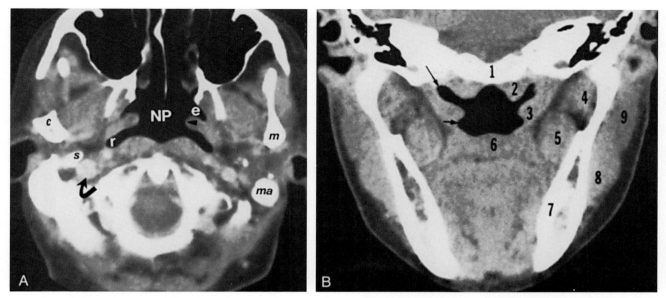

Fig. 37–19. A. Normal nasopharynx. Axial CT through the mid-nasopharynx (NP) with the patient instructed to blow against closed mouth. Note torus tubarius (arrowheads) and extension of air into the eustachian tube (e) (anterior to tori) and Rosenmuller fossae (r) (posterior to tori). Note enhancement of the retrostyloid vascular structures (internal jugular) (curved arrow) after intravenous iodine contrast infusion. The upper part of the parotid gland is seen posterior to the mandible (m) and anterior to the mastoid process (ma). s, Styloid process; c, mandibular condyle. B. Semicoronal CT section of the nasopharynx showing the: clivus (1), longus capitis muscle (2), torus tubarius (3), lateral (4), and medial (5) pterygoid muscles, soft palate (6), mandible (7), masseter muscle (8), and parotid gland (9). Note eustachian tube opening (lower arrow) just inferior to the tori (3), and superior extension of Rosenmuller fossae (upper arrow).

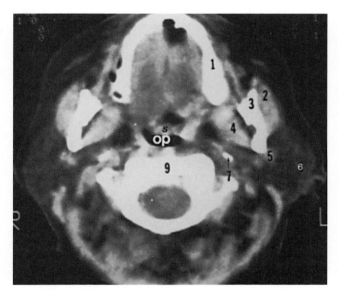

Fig. 37–20. Axial CT section of the oropharynx showing the alveolar ridge (1), masseter muscle (2), mandible (3), medial pterygoid muscle (4), retromandibular vein (5), parotid gland (6), styloid process (7), odontoid process (9), oropharynx (op), and soft palate (s). Note symmetrical parapharyngeal fat densities just medial to the medial pterygoid muscles.

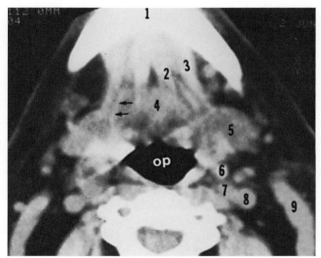

Fig. 37–21. Axial CT section of the oropharynx (op) at the level of the tongue showing the mandible (1), geniohyoid muscle (2), myelohyoid muscle (3), intrinsic muscles of the tongue (4), submandibular gland (5), external (6) and internal (7) carotid arteries, internal jugular vein (8), and sternocleidomastoid muscle (9). The hyoglossus and styloglossus muscles are along the lateral border of the tongue (arrows).

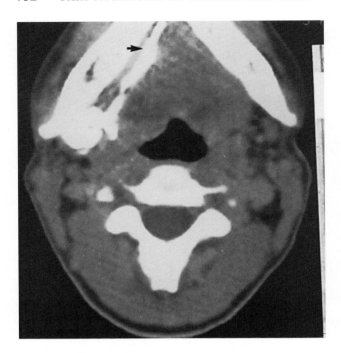

Fig. 37–22. CT sialogram showing the right submandibular gland and the Wharton's duct (arrowhead). Note atrophic submandibular gland on the left side.

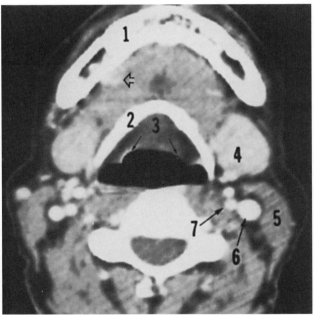

Fig. 37–23. Axial CT scan of the oropharynx showing the mandible (1), hyoid bone (2), base of the tongue (3), epiglottis (arrows), submandibular gland (4), sternocleidomastoid muscle (5), internal jugular vein (6), internal carotid artery (7), and anterior to that the external carotid artery. The submandibular (4) and sublingual glands (open arrowhead) are intensely enhanced during rapid infusion of iodine-contrast material.

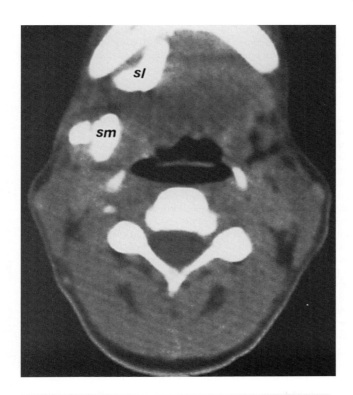

Fig. 37–24. Normal axial CT sialogram of the submandibular (sm) and sublingual (sl) glands.

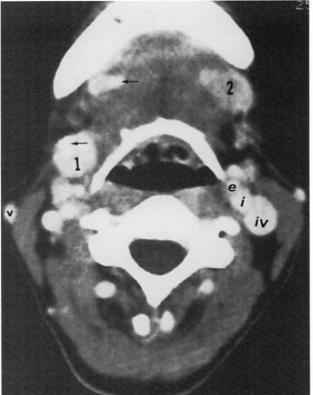

Fig. 37–25. Axial CT scan of the oropharynx showing marked enhancement of the submandibular (1) and sublingual (2) glands. Arrows point the residual pantopaque in the glands from previous CT pantopaque sialography (see Fig. 37–24). Note atrophic left submandibular gland (compare with Fig. 37–23) and intense enhancement of the internal (i), external (e) carotid arteries, and internal (iv) and external (v) jugular veins.

Fig. 37–26. All MR (A through M) are proton density 2000/20 of the same, normal subject. A. This section passes through the lower margin of the mandible (black and white arrow) and through the body of the third cervical vertebra. The section passes through the lower part of the tongue and through the oral portion of the pharynx (P), just above the epiglottis (small white arrows). The submandibular glands (curved arrows) are cut through their middle portion. The platysma (open arrow) and external jugular vein (black arrow) are seen. The hyoglossus muscle (white arrow), and the stylohyoid muscle (arrowhead) and the tendinous portion of digastric (lateral to styloid) muscle are seen medial to the submandibular gland. (1) Mylohyoid muscle; (2) intrinsic muscle of the tongue with associated intermuscular fat; (3) median raphe; e, external carotid artery; GH, geniohyoid muscle; I, internal carotid artery; J, internal jugular vein; L, longus colli muscle; S, sternocleidomastoid muscle. B. This section passes through the body of the mandible, just above the mental foramen, through the lower margin of the axis. It cuts the tongue just above the level of the foramen cecum (small white arrow) and the inferior margin of the palatine tonsil (T). Little of the parotid gland (6) is seen in this section. The maximal anteroposterior extension of the sublingual gland is seen (1), and the submandibular gland (2) is also demonstrated. Note the intrinsic muscle of the tongue (5), the genioglossus (g), the pharynx (P), masseter (M), mylohyoid (white and black arrowhead), stylohyoid and digastric muscles (3), a possible lymph node as well as digastric muscle (4), sternocleidomastoid muscle (S), spinal accessory nerve (small black arrow), auricular nerve (long black curved arrow), internal carotid artery (i), external carotid artery (e), internal jugular vein (J), retromandibular vein (black arrow), anterior facial vein (short black curved arrow), styloglossus muscle posterior to hyoglossus muscle (white arrowheads), and constrictor pharyngeal muscles (open arrow). C. This section passes through the mandible, near the junction of the ramus and the body; section passes through the tongue at the level of the upper portion of the sublingual gland (white arrowheads). The high-density image medial to the mandible is caused by to sublingual gland and fat in the fascial planes. Section passes through the pharynx (P) at the level of the middle portions of the tonsils (3). The tongue shows the following muscles: genioglossus (g), hyoglossus (white arrow), styloglossus (black arrowheads), and mylohyoid (black and white arrowhead). Note internal black arrows), platysma (black arrow), parotid gland (6), digastric muscle (5), stylohyoid muscle (4), external jugular vein (curved arrow), and sternocleidomastoid muscle (s). D. This section is 3 mm superior to C and shows various structures: genioglossus muscle (gg), septum linguae (white arrow), stylohyoid muscle (black arrowhead), stylopharyngeus muscle (white arrowhead), tonsils (T), oropharynx (P), longitudinal (6) and transverse (7) muscle fibers of the tongue, hyoglossus (1), mylohyoid (2), internal pterygoid (3) and masseter (4) muscles, parotid gland (5), posterior belly of digastric muscle (black arrow), sternocleidomastoid muscle (s), retromandibular vein (open arrow), external jugular vein, (black and white arrow), external carotid (e) and internal carotid (i) arteries, and internal jugular vein (j). *(continued)*

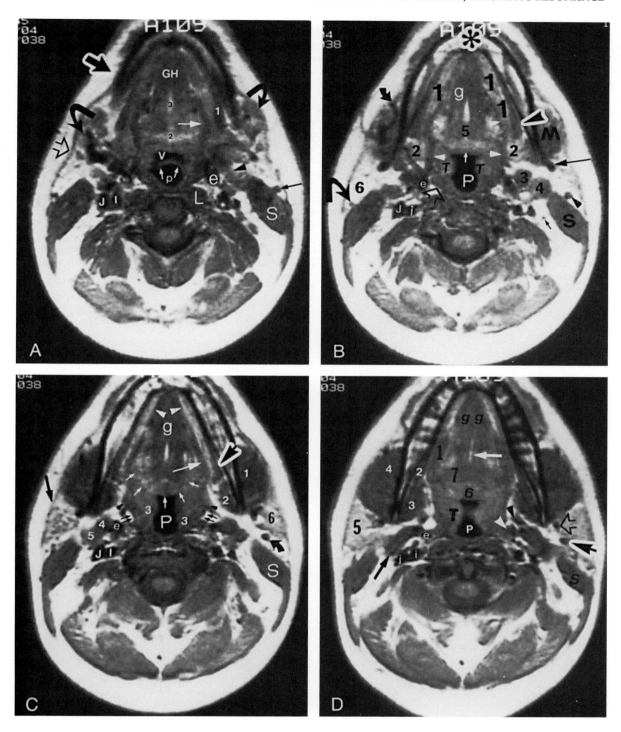

Fig. 37–26. *(continued)* E. This section is 3 mm superior to D and passes through the upper portion of the tongue and shows the uvula (U), palatine tonsil (T), oropharynx (P) and posterior belly of digastric (black arrow), stylohyoid (open arrow), and stylopharyngeus (black arrowheads) muscles. The styloglossus and stylopharyngeus muscles are seen medial to stylohyoid muscle and lateral to internal carotid artery (I). Note glossopalatine muscle (white arrow), parotid gland (PG), spinal accessory nerve (white arrowhead), superior longitudinal muscle fibers of the tongue (1), transverse muscle fibers (2), buccinator muscle (3), masseter muscle (4), internal pterygoid muscle (5), constrictor pharyngeal muscle (small black and small white arrows), retromandibular vein (small black and white arrows), retromandibular vein (black and white arrow), and internal jugular vein (J). F. This section is 3 mm superior to E and shows superior longitudinal muscle fibers of the tongue (1), transverse muscle fibers (2), buccinator muscle (3), orbicularis oris muscle (4), masseter muscle (5), internal pterygoid muscle (6), parotid gland (7), posterior belly of digastric (8), sternocleidomastoid (9), splenius capitis (10) and superior constrictor pharyngeal muscles (small white and small black arrows), uvula (u), pharynx (P), parapharyngeal fat space (PS), internal carotid (i), external carotid (e), arteries internal jugular vein (j), anterior facial vein (black arrow), intraparotid facial nerve (curved arrow), retromandibular vein (black arrowhead), stylopharyngeus (s), and stylohyoid (open arrow) muscles. G. This section is 3 mm superior to F and passes through the lower alveolar process of maxilla and just below the palatine process of the maxilla. The section passes through the upper part of the ramus of the mandible (R). Following structures are seen; quadratus labii superioris (1), buccinator (2), masseter (3) and internal pterygoid (4) muscles parotid gland (5), sternocleidomastoid (6), splenius capitis (sc) digastric (7), lateral rectus capitis (8), anterior rectus capitis (9), longus capitis (10) and pharyngopalatinus (11) muscles, superior constrictor pharyngeal muscle (small white and small black arrows), styloid muscle group (joined arrows), platysma muscle (white and black arrow), anterior facial vein (long black arrow), retromandibular vein (black arrowhead), external carotid artery (e), internal carotid artery (i), internal jugular vein (J), the mucous membrane of the hard palate, which shows the medial raphe (curved arrow), and numerous mucous glands, which are represented by small white areas. H. This is the T2-weighted MR scan of G. Note hypointensity of all muscles and hyperintensity of mucosal linings.

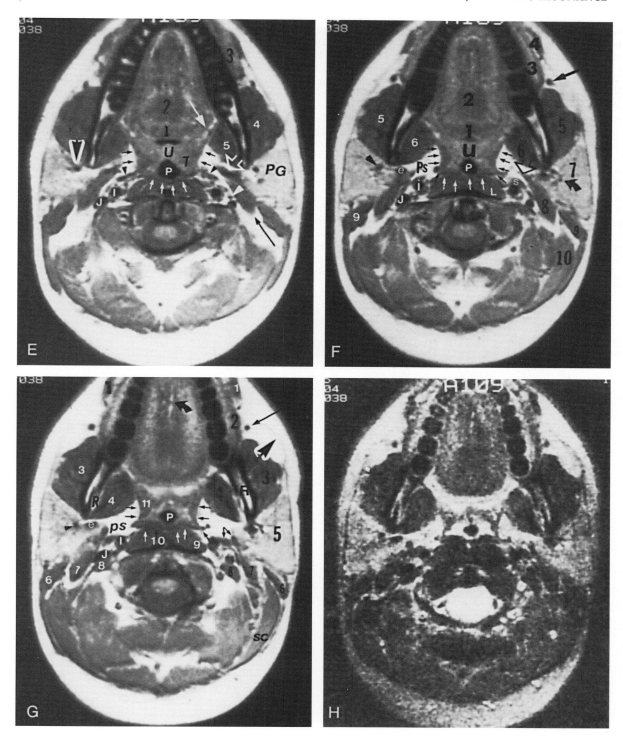

Fig. 37–26. *(continued)* I. This section is 3 mm superior to G and passes through the lower alveolar process of the maxilla and upper part of the ramus of the mandible (white arrow) and shows the following structures; quadratus labii superioris (1), buccinator (2), masseter (3) and internal pterygoid muscles (4), parotid gland (5), anterior rectus capitis (6), longus capitis (7), lateral rectus capitis (8), digastric (9), splenius capitis (sc) and superior constrictor muscles (small white and small black arrows), pharynx (P), soft palate (s), parapharyngeal space (ps), pharyngeal vein (black arrowhead), retromandibular vein (black arrowheads), external carotid (e), internal carotid (i) arteries, internal jugular vein (J), pharyngopalatinus muscle (large white arrows), hard palate (H) and platysma muscle (white and black arrowhead): note part of the levator veli palatini muscle (curved white arrows). J. This section is 3 mm superior to I and passes through the mid-alveolar process of the maxilla and upper end of the coronoid process of the mandible and mastoid portion of the temporal bone (8). The following structures are seen: quadratus labii superioris (1), buccinator (2) and masseter muscles (3), parotid gland (4), medial pterygoid (5), lateral pterygoid (6) and temporalis muscles (7), mastoid process (8), anterior rectus capitis (9), longus capitis (L), splenis capitis (sc), levator veli palatini (white arrows) and pharyngopalatinus muscles (small black arrows), nasopharynx (P), buccopharyngeal space (white arrow), buccal fat (BF), and platysma muscle (black arrows). K. This section is 3 mm superior to J and passes through the upper alveolar process of the maxilla and upper part of the mandibular ramus. The following structures are seen: buccal fat (1), soft palate (2), parapharyngeal fat (3), parotid gland (4), medial pterygoid (5), lateral pterygoid (6), temporalis (7) and masseter muscles (8), mandible (9), eustachian tube (e), nasopharynx (P), longus capitis muscle (L), and, immediately posterior to that, anterior rectus capitis muscle. Notice buccinator (B) and quadratus labii superioris (Q) muscles hard palate (H), anterior facial vein (black arrowhead), levator veli palatini (long black arrow) and tensor veli palatini (short black arrow) muscles, mandibular nerve (short white arrow), and pharyngeal vein (long white arrow). L. This section is 3 mm superior to K and passes through the upper alveolar process of the maxilla. The following structures are seen: hard palate (H), nasopharynx (P), adenoidal pad (1), mandible (lower condyle) (2), lateral pterygoid muscle (3), parotid gland (4), temporalis muscle (5), masseter muscle (6), buccal fat (7), zygomaticus muscle (curved black arrow), levator veli palatini muscle (white arrow), tensor veli palatini muscle (black arrow), and anterior facial vein (arrowhead). *(continued)*

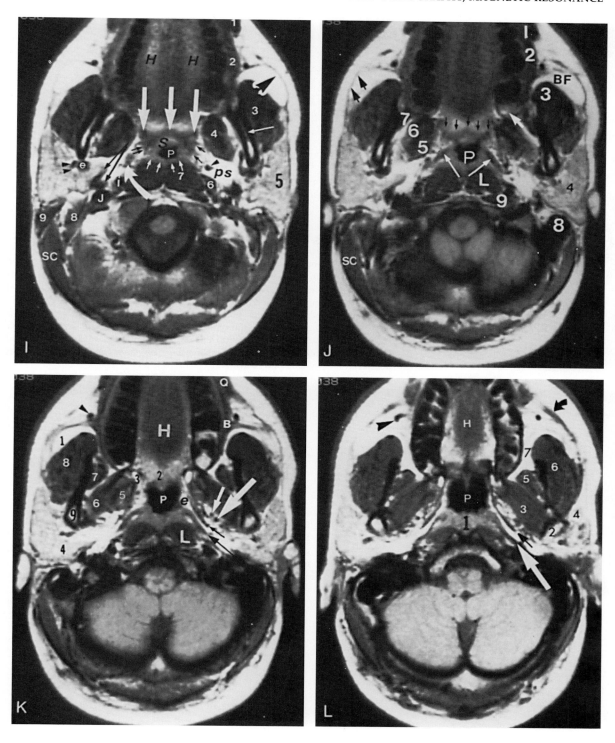

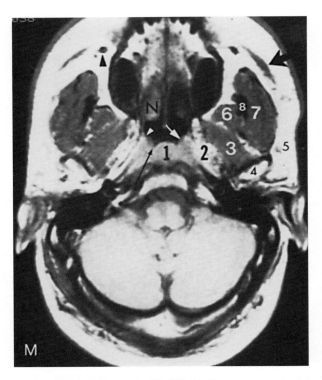

Fig. 37–26. *(continued)* M. This section is 3 mm superior to L and passes through the maxilla and lower part of the nasal cavity. Note the pharyngeal openings of the eustachian tube (white arrowhead), the cartilaginous portion of the eustachian tube (torus tubarius) (white arrow), the pharyngeal recess or Rosenmuller fossa (long black arrow), adenoidal pad (1), parapharyngeal space (2), lateral pterygoid muscle (3), mandible (condyle)(4), parotid gland (5), temporalis muscle (6), masseter muscle (7), coronoid process (8), zygomaticus muscle (short black arrow), anterior facial vein (black arrowhead), and nasal turbinate (N). (From Mafee MF, et al: Head and neck: High magnetic field resonance imaging versus computed tomography. Otolaryngol Clin North Am 21:513–546, 1988.)

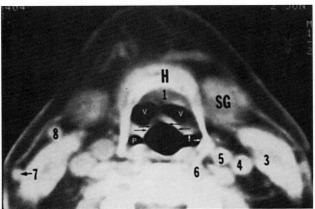

Fig. 37–27. Axial CT scan of the oropharynx showing the hyoid bone (H), base of the tongue (1), and posterior to that the valleculae (V). Note the epiglottis (black arrows), pharyngoepiglottic folds (white arrows), upper part of the piriform sinuses (p), submandibular gland (SG), sternocleidomastoid muscles (3), internal jugular vein (4), common carotid artery (5), longus colli muscle (6), external jugular vein (7). The platyma muscle is overlying the lateral facial vein (8).

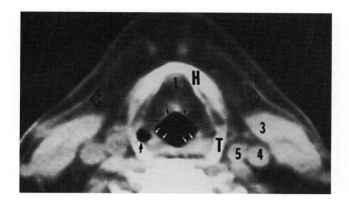

Fig. 37–28. Axial CT scan of the larynx and hypopharynx at the level of the superior cornua of the thyroid cartilage (T) showing the inferior part of the hyoid bone (H), preepiglottic space (1), epiglottis (black arrows) and aryepiglottic folds (white arrows), platysma muscle (open arrowheads), sternocleidomastoid muscle (3), internal jugular vein (4), common carotid artery (5). Air is seen in the right piriform sinus (arrow).

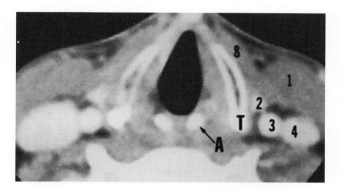

Fig. 37–29. Axial CT scan of the larynx at the level of the false vocal cords showing the superior portion of the arytenoid cartilage (A), thyroid cartilage (T), thyroid gland (2), common carotid artery (3), internal jugular vein (4), sternocleidomastoid muscle (1), and infrahyoid strap muscle (8). Note asymmetry of the internal jugular veins, with the right being larger than the left.

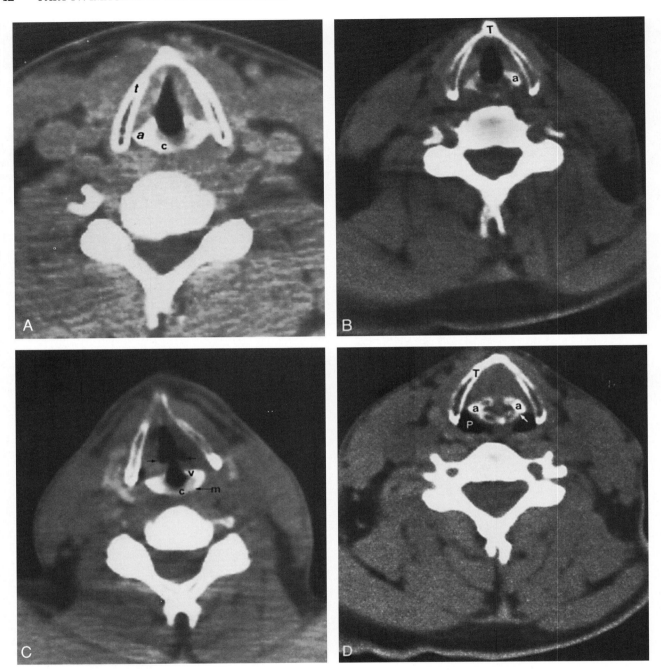

Fig. 37–30. A. Rima glottidis in quiet respiration. Note the symmetry and smooth appearance of the true vocal cords and arytenoid cartilages (a). Notice that the widest part of the glottic aperture is opposite the vocal processes of the arytenoid cartilages. The intermembranous part of the rima glottidis is triangular, and the intercartilaginous part is semicircular in shape. Notice the symmetry in the distance between the thyroid (t) and arytenoid (a) cartilages. B. Normal true vocal cord. Axial CT scan obtained during quiet breathing showing the thyroid cartilage (t), arytenoid cartilages (a) and their vocal processes, and the upper part of the cricoid cartilage (c). Notice the slight asymmetry of the true vocal cords, which is caused by asymmetric position of the cords in the section. C. Normal true vocal cords. CT scan of the larynx during expiratory phonation showing the cricoid lamina (c), the vocal (v) and the muscular (m) processes of the arytenoid cartilages. The adducted true vocal cords and partially volumed laryngeal ventricles (arrows) are shown. D. Closure of the rima glottidis. This is the same patient and the same CT scan level as in A; however, during scanning the patient was requested to hold his breath. Notice closure of the glottic aperture caused by approximation of the true vocal cords. The true vocal cords and the arytenoid cartilages (a) are adducted. Notice rotation of the arytenoid cartilages as compared with A. The cricoarytenoid articulation (arrows) is demonstrated in this breath-holding scan. P, Piriform sinus; T, thyroid cartilage. (From Mafee MF, et al: Radiology, *147*:123, 1983.)

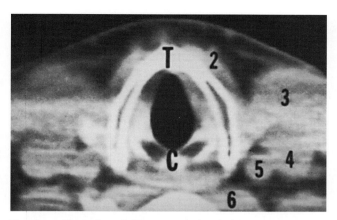

Fig. 37–31. Normal axial CT scan at the level of the undersurface of the true vocal cords showing the thyroid cartilage (T), infrahyoid strap muscle (2), sternocleidomastoid muscle (3), internal jugular vein (4), common carotid artery (5), longus colli muscle (6), and the cricoid lamina (C).

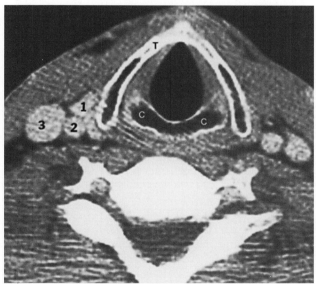

Fig. 37–32. Normal axial CT scan at the level of the undersurface of the true vocal cords using extended bone CT range technique. Notice the sharply delineated thyroid (T) and cricoid (c) cartilages. The cortices and medullary portion of the both cartilages are well outlined. The cricoid cartilage frequently shows this dense cortical and low-density medullary appearance. There is a paraglottic low-density sharply delineated line abutting the medial cortex of the thyroid cartilage on each side. Obliteration of this line and loss of cortical outline of the thyroid cartilage usually indicate thyroid cartilage involvment by tumor. Notice thyroid gland (1), common carotid artery (2) and internal jugular vein (3).

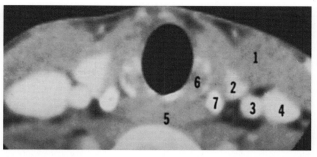

Fig. 37–33. Normal axial CT scan at the level of the upper subglottic region. The cricoid cartilage is partially calcified (6). Notice the sternocleidomastoid muscle (1), thyroid gland (2), common carotid artery (3), internal jugular vein (4), postcricoid region (5), and inferior cornua of the thyroid cartilage (7).

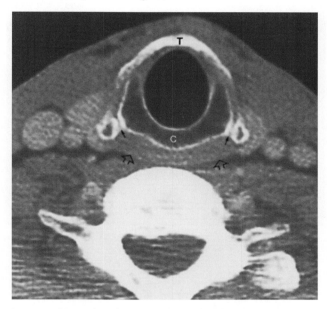

Fig. 37–34. Normal axial CT scan obtained at the cricothyroid articulation (arrows) using the extended bone range CT technique. Notice the symmetric, sharply outlined subglottic space. Note cricoid (C) and thyroid (T) cartilages and the inferior constrictor pharyngeal muscle (hollow arrows) just posterior to the cricoid cartilage.

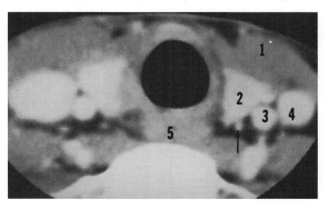

Fig. 37–35. Normal axial CT scan at the lower subglottic region showing the sternocleidomastoid muscle (1), thyroid gland (2), common carotid artery (3), internal jugular vein (4), postcricoid pharyngeal musculature (5), and inferior thyroid artery (arrow).

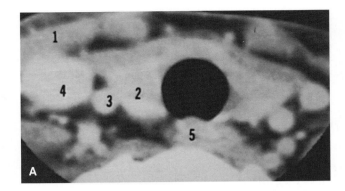

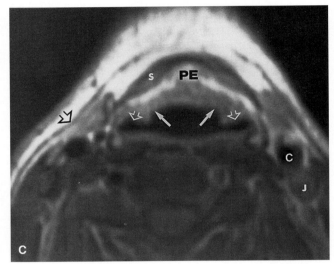

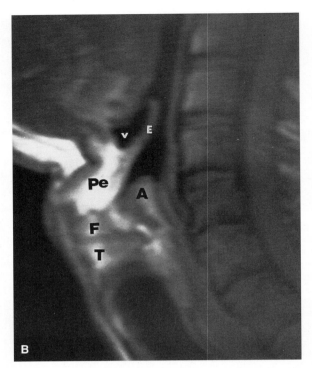

Fig. 37–36. A. Normal axial CT scan at the level of the first tracheal ring showing the sternocleidomastoid muscle (1), thyroid gland (2), common carotid artery (3), internal jugular vein (4), and esophagus (5). B. T1W sagittal MR scan shows epiglottis (E), Vallecula (v), pre-epiglottic space (pe), arytenoid region (A), false vocal cord (F) and true vocal cord (T). C. PW axial MR scan shows strap muscle (S), preepiglottic space (PE), epiglottis (solid arrows), pharyngoepiglottic folds (hollow white arrows), common carotid artery (C), internal jugular vein (J) and platysma muscle (hollow black arrow). *(continued)*

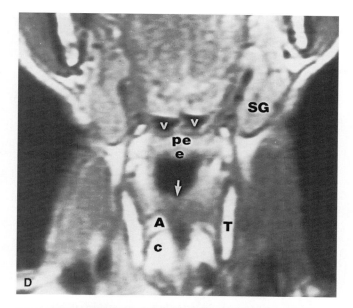

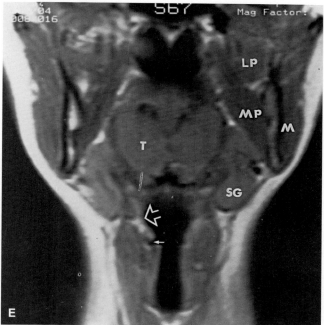

Fig. 37–36. *(continued)* D. T1W curved coronal MR scan shows submandibular glands (SG), valleculae (V), preepiglottic space (pe), epiglottis (e), interarytenoid region (arrow), arytenoid cartilage (A), cricoid cartilage (c) and thyroid cartilage (T). E. T1W curved coronal MR scan shows lateral pterygoid muscle (LP), medial pterygoid muscle (MP), masseter muscle (M), tongue (T), submandibular gland (SG), aryepiglottic fold (hollow arrow) and laryngeal ventricle (small arrow).

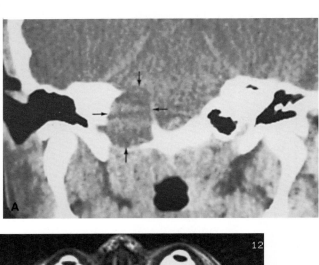

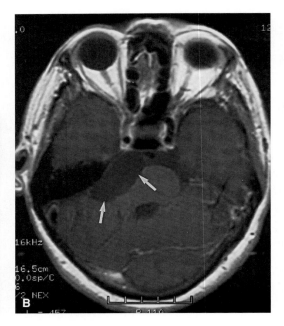

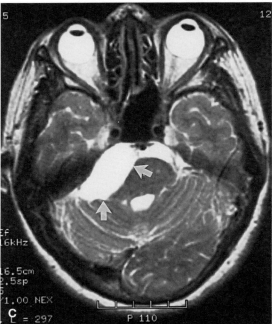

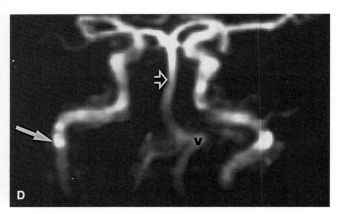

Fig. 37–37. Primary cholesteatoma (epidermoid cyst). A. Contrast-enhanced coronal CT scan showing a nonenhanced low-density image in the region of the right petrous apex (arrows). Note moderate enhancement only in the peripheral portion (capsule) of the lesion. Lack of enhancement, relatively low density, its expansile nature, and smooth border of the destroyed bone are almost characteristic of an epidermoid cyst. (From Mafee MF, Valvassori GE, Dobben GD: Role of Radiology in surgery of the ear and skull base. In: Symposium on complications in surgery of the ear and skull base. Edited by Wiet RJ. Otolaryngol Clin North Am *15*:723–754, 1982.). B. Cerebellopontine angle (CPA) epidermoid. After injection of Gd-DTPA, T1W MR scan shows an unenhanced hypointense mass (arrows). C. T2W MR scan. The epidermoid is seen as a hyperintense image (arrows). D. Three-dimensional TOF MR angiogram shows normal right (solid arrow) and left internal carotid arteries, vertebral (v) and basilar (hollow arrow) arteries. MRA clearly shows that the epidermoid cyst has not affected the right internal carotid artery.

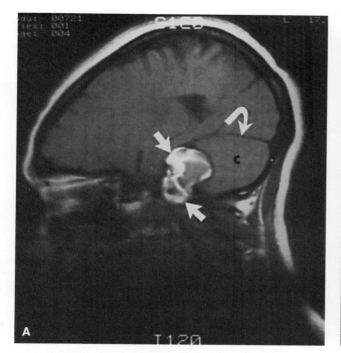

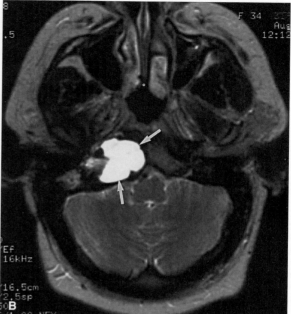

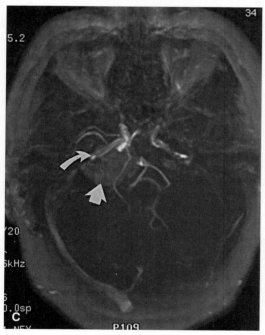

Fig. 37–38. Cholesterol granuloma. A. Sagittal T1W MR scan showing a large lesion (arrows) involving the base of the skull and extending into the posterior fossa. Notice the tentorium cerebelli (curved arrow) and cerebellum (c). B. Cholesterol granuloma. T2S axial MR scan shows a hyperintense mass (arrows). C. Three-dimensional TOF MR angiogram shows the cholesterol granuloma (straight arrow) and petrous portion of right internal carotid artery (curved arrow). Note that the artery is not involved.

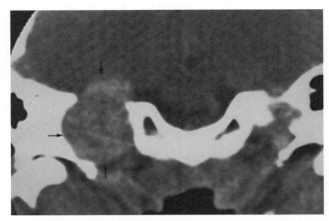

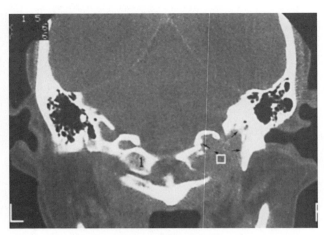

Fig. 37–39. Schwannoma of the jugular fossa. Contrast-enhanced coronal CT scan showing a moderately enhanced soft tissue mass in the region of the right enlarged and eroded jugular fossa (arrows). The extra- and intracranial components of the tumor are clearly visualized. Note the smooth border of the destroyed bone similar to that in Figure 37–37, which is indicative of the slow-growing nature of the lesion, as opposed to irregular bone destruction seen with the malignant process in Figure 37–40. (From Mafee MF, Valvassori GE, and Dobben GD: The role of radiology in surgery of the ear and skull base. Otolaryngol Clin North Am 15:723, 1982.)

Fig. 37–40. Liposarcoma of the base of the skull. Contrast-enhanced coronal CT scan showing extensive bone destruction of the right jugular fossa and occipital condyle (arrows). Note erosion of the right occipital condyle as compared with the left one (1).

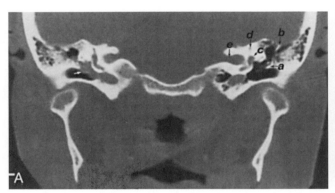

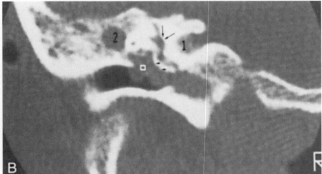

Fig. 37–41. A. Glomus jugulare. Coronal CT scan showing extension of a glomus jugular tumor into the left middle ear (white arrow). The left jugular fossa was enlarged and eroded in more posterior sections. Note lateral wall of attic (a), tegmen (b), vestibule (c), superior semicircular canal (d), and internal auditory canal (e). B. Glomus jugulare. Contrast-enhanced coronal CT scan through the left temporal bone. This is the same patient as in A one year after radiation therapy. The size of the tumor in the middle ear is more or less the same. Note opacification of the mastoid antrum (2) and mastoid air cells with thickening of the trabeculae. The cursor measurement of 115 indicates marked enhancement, and hence, the hypervascular nature of the middle ear lesion. Note the basal turn of the cochlea (arrowheads), internal auditory canal (1), and the vestibula (arrows). (From Mafee MF, et al: High resolution and dynamic sequential computed tomography (CT). CT use in the evaluation of glomus complex tumors. Arch Otolaryngol Head Neck Surg 109:691–696, 1983.)

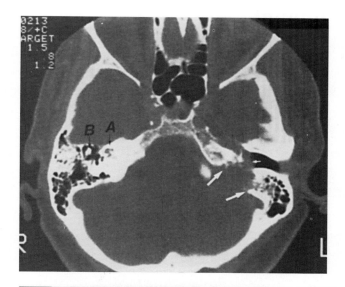

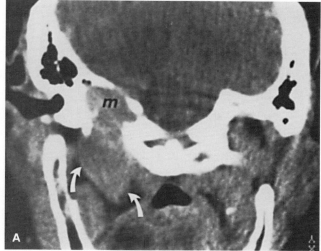

Fig. 37–42. Glomus jugulare. Contrast-enhanced axial CT scan using extended bone range CT technique showing marked destruction of the left petrous bone in a patient with glomus jugulare tumor. Note extension into the middle ear (white arrow) and posterior cranial fossa (black arrows). Right cochlea (A), malleus (B), and posterior to that, the incus. (From Mafee MF, et al: High resolution and dynamic sequential computed tomography: use in the evaluation of glomus complex tumors. Arch Otolaryngol Head Neck Surg *109*:691–696, 1983.)

Fig. 37–43. A. Coronal CT scan showing soft tissue mass (m) in region of right enlarged and eroded jugular fossa. Note extension of tumor along carotid sheath down to level of soft palate. B. Coronal T₁W MR scan shows a large mass in the left jugular fossa (arrows).

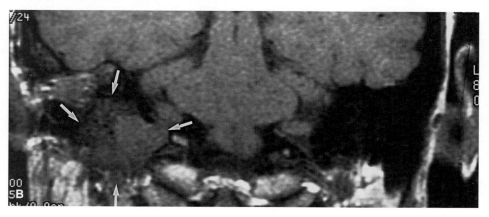

Fig. 37–43. *(continued)*

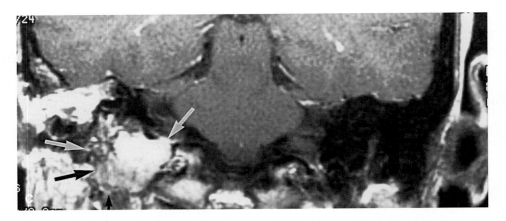

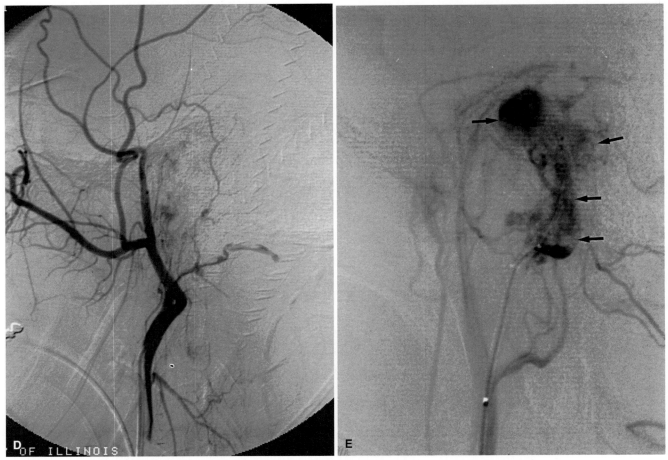

Fig. 37–43. *(continued)* C. Coronal post-Gd-DTPA T$_1$W MR scan shows marked enhancement of the lesions (arrows). D. Standard angiogram shows marked vascularity of the tumor (arrows). E. Post embolization angiogram shows marked decrease in tumor vascularity. At surgery tumor was completely resected and patient recovered with no neurological deficit. (Case Courtesy of Arvind Kumar, MD, University of Illinois at Chicago Medical Center.)

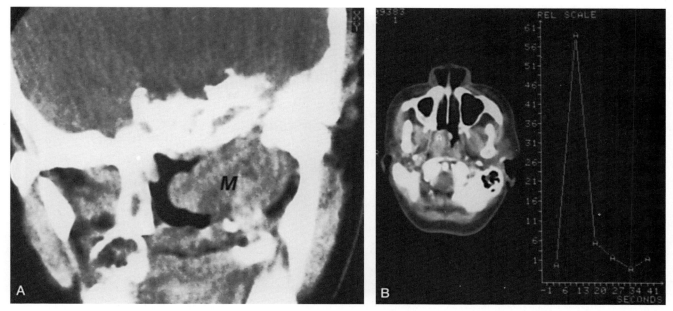

Fig. 37–44. A. Extension of glomus jugulare tumor into the nasopharynx. Contrast-enhanced coronal CT scan showing the large right paranasopharyngeal mass (M) protruding into the nasopharynx. B. Computer-generated density-time curve obtained from a dynamic CT scanning demonstrates nasopharyngeal mass (A) and a high peak in this region indicative of hypervascularity of the lesion. Note rapid wash-out (downslope) of the curve. This pattern of the curve is characteristic of glomus complex tumors and arteriovenous malformation and aneurysm. (From Mafee MF: Dynamic CT and its application to otolaryngology: head and neck surgery. J Otolaryngol *11*:307–318, 1982.)

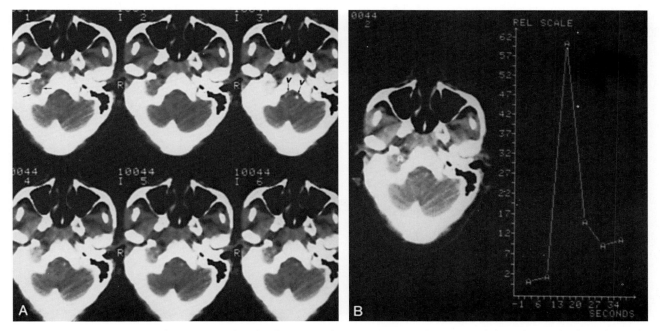

Fig. 37–45. A. Dynamic CT scan of a patient with right glomus jugulare tumor. Note enlargement of the right jugular fossa (arrows) and intense enhancement of the tumor in the third section (arterial phase) (v, vertebral artery) and rapid wash-out of contrast. B. Glomus jugulare tumor. Computed generated density-time curve demonstrates a high peak with rapid wash-in (up-slope) and rapid wash-out (down-slope) phases characteristic of glomus tumors. (From Mafee MF: High resolution and dynamic sequential computed tomography (CT): CT use in the evaluation of glomus complex tumors. Arch Otolaryngol Head Neck Surg *109*:691–696, 1983.)

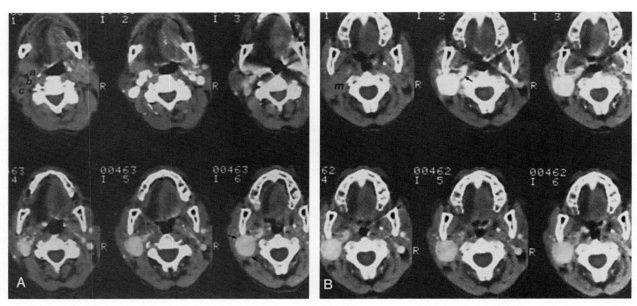

Fig. 37–46. A. Glomus vagale tumor. Incremental dynamic CT scan with the first section obtained at the level of the tongue and extending superiorly (with automatic table incrementation) to the level of the superior alveolar ridge in this patient with a large right neck mass. Notice sequential enhancement of the external (a) and internal (b) carotid arteries and the internal jugular vein (c). A rounded enhancing mass is recognized in section Nos. 5 and 6 (arrows), which show a prominent feeding vessel (see B). B. Glomus vagale tumor. Dynamic CT scan performed at the level of right neck mass in the same patient in A. Note intense enhancement of paravertebral mass (m) in the second section and rapid wash-out of contrast in the remainder of the sections. The glomus tumors often behave like an AV malformation in CT dynamic study. Note the large artery (most likely ascending pharyngeal artery) (arrows) feeding this tumor. Note also the marked atrophy of the right side of the tongue in this patient with twelfth nerve palsy caused by superior extension of the tumor into the posterior cranial fossa and with associated destruction of the hypoglossal canal. (From Mafee MF, et al: High resolution and dynamic sequential computed tomography (CT): CT use in the evaluation of glomus complex tumors. Arch Otolaryngol Head Neck Surg *109*:691–696, 1983.)

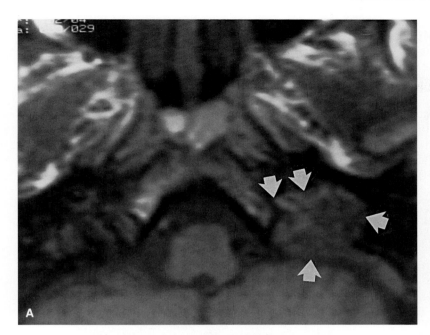

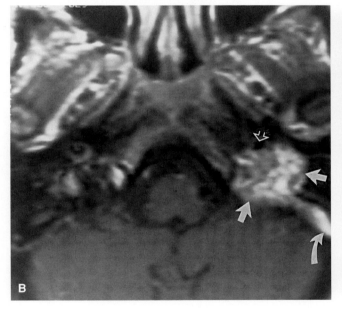

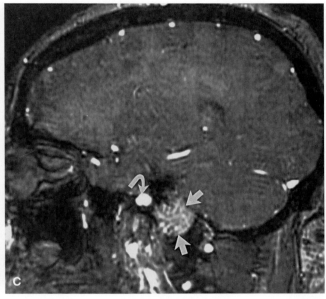

Fig. 37–47. Glomus jugulare tumor. A. T1W axial precontrast MR scan shows a large mass (arrows) in the left jugular fossa. B. T1W axial postcontrast MR scan shows marked enhancement of the glomus tumor (straight arrows). Notice normal internal carotid artery (hollow arrow) and sigmoid sinus (curved arrow). C. GRASS (gradient recalled acquisition in the steady state) image shows tumor vascularity (straight arrows) and normal internal carotid artery (curved arrow). *(continued)*

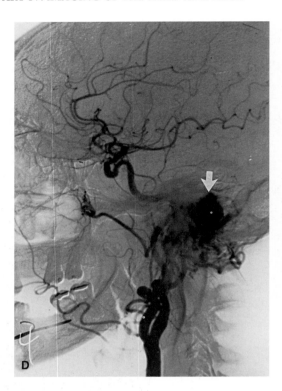

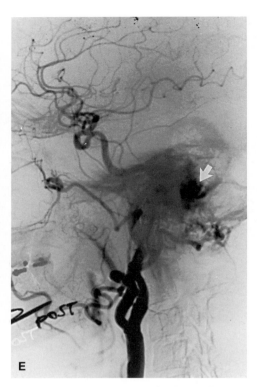

Fig. 37–47. *(continued)* D. Standard angiogram shows marked vascularity (arrow) of another patient with a glomus jugulare tumor. E. Postembolization angiogram of some patient in D shows decreased vascularity of the tumor bed.

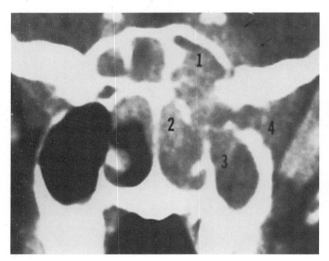

Fig. 37–48. Nasopharyngeal carcinoma. Postcontrast semicoronal CT scan of the nasopharynx showing large nasopharyngeal tumor (2) with extension into the sphenoid sinus (1), maxillary sinus (3), and infratemporal fossa (4). There was also tumor extension into the apex of the orbit and along the cavernous sinus (arrows). Note extensive irregular bone destruction of the floor of the sphenoid sinus.

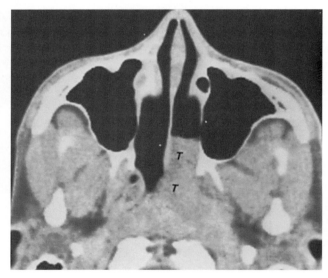

Fig. 37–49. Nasopharyngeal carcinoma. Axial CT scan of the nasopharynx showing large soft tissue tumor (T), occupying the left side of the nasopharynx and extending into the left nasal cavity.

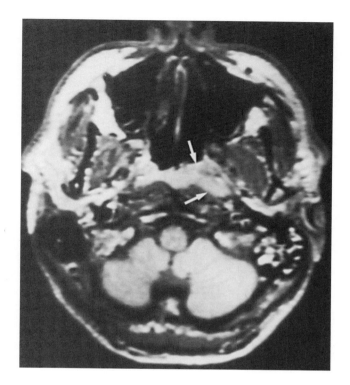

Fig. 37–50. Nasopharyngeal carcinoma. PW MR scan showing an infiltrative process involving the left Rosenmuller fossa (arrows).

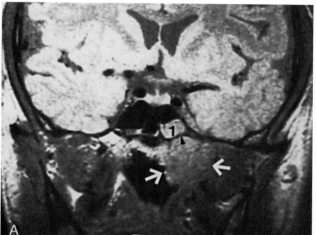

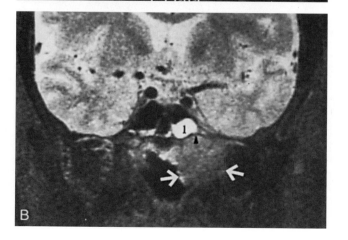

Fig. 37–51. Squamous cell carcinoma of the nasopharynx. Proton weighted (A) and T2 weighted (B) MR scans show the tumor (arrows) and a retention cyst (1) in the left sphenoid sinus. Note the difference between the signal of tumor and cyst in T2-weighted (B) MR scan. The bone of the base of the skull adjacent to the tumor is not involved (arrowhead).

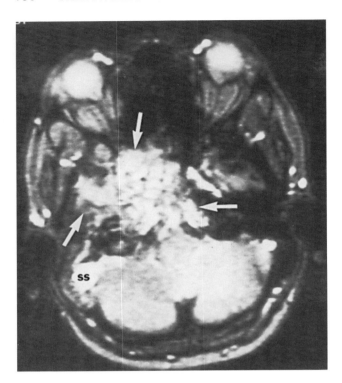

Fig. 37–52. Diffuse glomus tumor extension in the nasopharynx. Dynamic MR shows extensive mass (arrows) in the base of the skull with extension into the nasopharynx. With this MR dynamic GRASS (gradient recalled acquisition in the steady state) technique vascular tumors appear bright. Notice hyperintensity of vasculatures. ss, Sigmoid sinus.

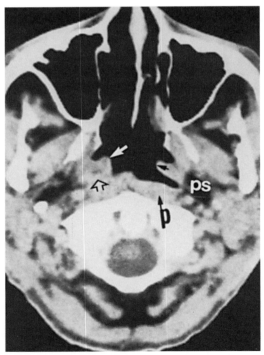

Fig. 37–53. Clinically unrecognized nasopharyngeal tumor. Notice normal torus tubarius on the left (arrowhead), and anterior to that the normal eustachian tube opening, and posterior to that the normal Rosenmuller fossa and parapharyngeal space (ps). Notice enlargement of the right torus tubarius (white arrow) and early infiltration in the adjacent portion of the parapharyngeal space by a soft tissue mass (hollow arrow). Biopsy of this lesion revealed carcinoma. P, Left paravertebral muscle, longus capitis muscle.

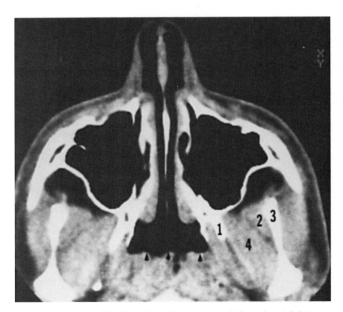

Fig. 37–54. Adenoid. There is enlargement of the adenoidal tissue with a lobulated pattern and a wavy but smooth mucosal (arrowheads) appearance. (1) Lateral pterygoid plate, (2) temporalis muscle, (3) coronoid process, (4) lateral pterygoid muscle.

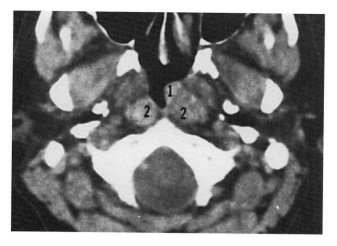

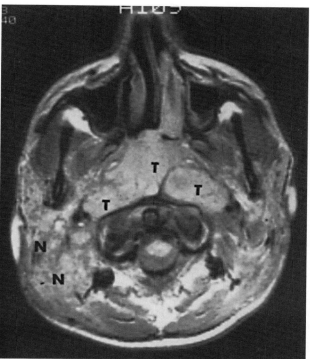

Fig. 37–55. Lymphoid hyperplasia. CT scan showing a superficial soft tissue bulge (1) over the nasopharyngeal mucosa on the left side. The low-density deep fascial planes are intact. A lucent zone is seen between the mass and prevertebral muscle density (2).

Fig. 37–56. Poorly differentiated carcinoma with lymphoid stroma in a 16-year-old male with 4-month history of nasal stuffiness, fever, and neck masses. Proton-weighted MR scan shows massive nasopharyngeal tumor (T) with large neck nodes (N).

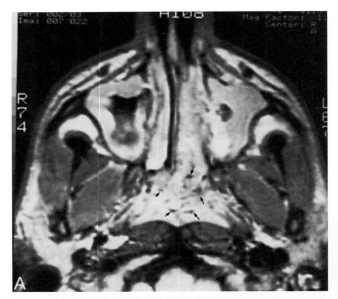

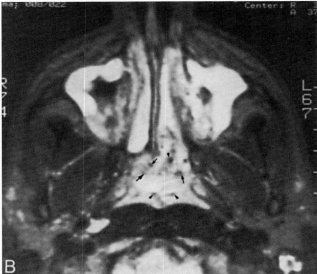

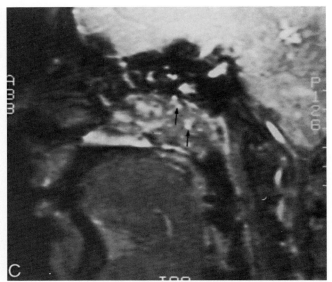

Fig. 37–57. Angiofibroma. Proton-weighted (A) and T2-weighted (B) axial scans. The tumor is poorly outlined with areas of low signal, representing blood vessels (arrows). C. GRASS (gradient recalled acquisition in the steady state) sagittal image shows areas of hyper-intesity (arrows), indicative of highly vascular mass. Notice inflammatory changes in the maxillary sinuses.

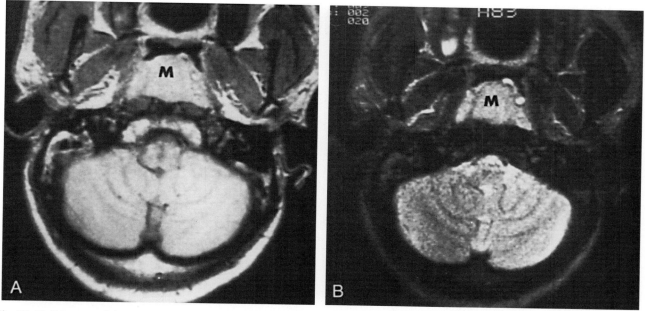

Fig. 37–58. Scleroma of the nasopharynx. Proton-density (A) and T2-weighted (B) axial MR scans show a mass (M) in the nasopharynx.

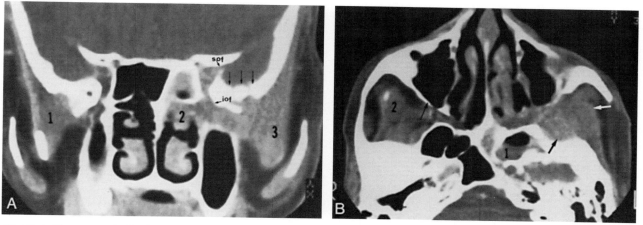

Fig. 37–59. A. Mucormycosis. Semicoronal CT scan showing a soft tissue density in the left nasal cavity (2) and left sphenoid sinus, with bone destruction along the superior aspect of the medial wall of the left nasal cavity and soft tissue infiltration along the inferior orbital fissure (iof) and into the apex of the left orbit along the superior orbital fissure (sof) (compare with the density of the right inferior and superior orbital fissures). There is also involvement of the left infratemporal fossa (3) with an irregularity of the bone of the left middle cranial fossa (arrows) caused by osteomyelitis. B. Mucormycosis. Postcontrast axial CT scan of the same patient in A showing soft tissue density in the left sphenoid sinus (1) and left nasal cavity, with extension into the left infratemporal fossa causing obliteration of the deep fascial plane (arrows). Compare with normal right infratemporal fossa (2). Note also involvement of the posterior portion of the left maxillary sinus as compared to the right side (arrow).

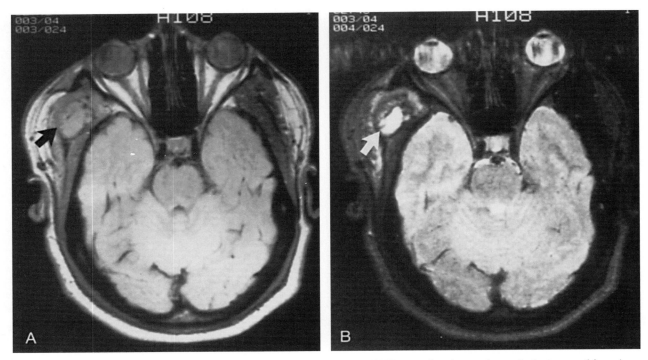

Fig. 37–60. Temporal fossa abscess. Proton weighted (A) and T2-weighted (B) axial MR scans showing an abscess in the temporal fossa (arrows). This abscess developed after a dental procedure.

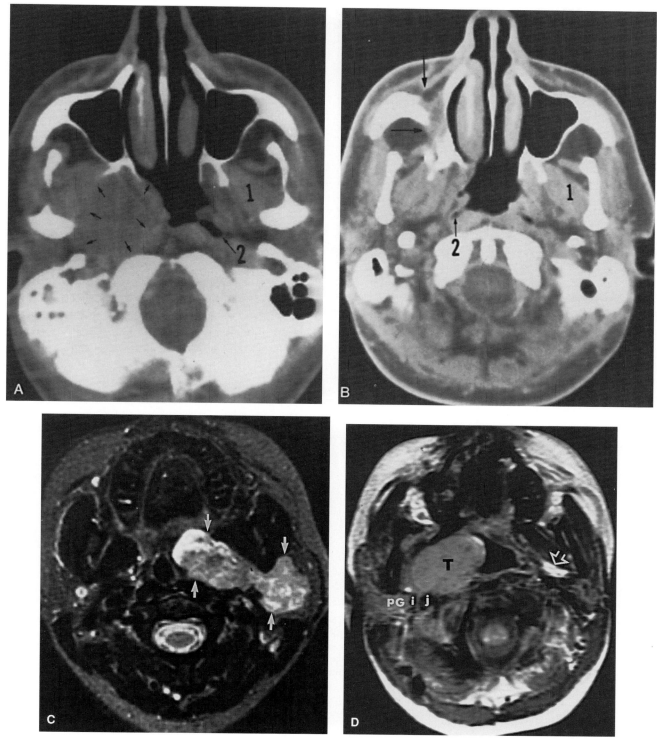

Fig. 37–61. A. Paranasopharyngeal neurofibroma. Axial CT scan in a patient with a 12-year history of a recurrent right serous otitis media showing a large, smoothly marginated mass (arrows) in the right parapharyngeal region that is protruding into the nasopharynx. Note normal Rosenmuller fossa on the left (2) and its obliteration on the right. Note also expansion of the pterygoid fossa without bone destruction as well as distortion of the right pterygoid muscle, all of which indicate the benign and slow-growing nature of the lesion. (1) Left lateral pterygoid muscle. B. Parapharyngeal neurofibroma. Axial CT scan of the same patient in A following extended-transantral removal of the right parapharyngeal tumor. The superficial landmarks of the right nasopharynx (effaced in A) are symmetrically and normally seen in this CT scan. Notice extension of air in the right Rosenmuller fossa (2) and right eustachian tube, and the symmetrical appearance of lateral pterygoid muscles (1) and parapharyngeal spaces. Note postsurgical changes of the right maxillary sinus (arrows). C. Malignant tumor of the parotid. T2W axial MR scan shows a large mass involving the deep lobe of the left parotid, extending into the parapharyngeal space (arrows). This was reported as being compatible with liposarcoma. D. Parapharyngeal adenocarcinoma. PW axial MR scan shows a large tumor (T) involving the right parapharyngeal space. Notice normal left parapharyngeal space (arrow). i, Internal carotid artery; j, internal jugular vein; PG, parotid gland. *(continued)*

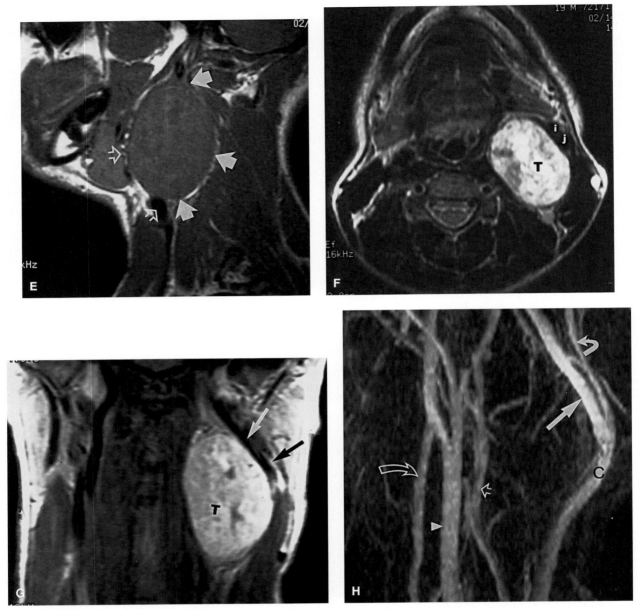

Fig. 37–61. *(continued)* E. Parapharyngeal schwannoma. T1W sagittal MR scan shows a large mass (large arrows), resulting in anterior displacement of the internal carotid artery (hollow arrows). F. T2W axial MR scan same case as E shows marked hyperintensity of the tumor (T). i, Internal carotid artery; j, internal jugular vein. G. Coronal MR scan, same patient as in F shows the tumor (T) and laterally displaced carotid artery (arrows). H. 2D TOF MR angiogram showing laterally displaced common (c), internal (straight arrow), and external (curved arrow) carotid arteries. Note left vertebral artery (hollow arrow), right common carotid artery (arrowhead and right vertebral artery (curved hollow arrow).

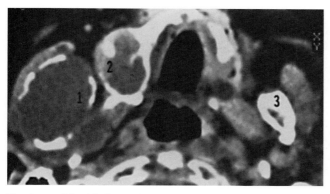

Fig. 37–62. Mandibular and maxillary cysts. CT scan showing an expansile low-density cyst of the right mandible and a right superior alveolar ridge cyst (2) in a patient with basal cell nevus syndrome. The left mandible appears normal (3). Notice the low-density of the right medial pterygoid muscle caused by extension of the right mandibular cyst (1) into the right infratemporal fossa.

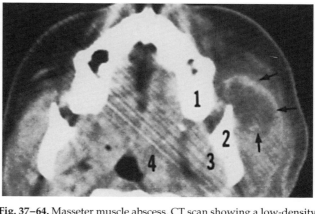

Fig. 37–64. Masseter muscle abscess. CT scan showing a low-density image along the anterior aspect of the left masseter muscle (arrows) caused by an abscess. (1) Superior alveolar ridge, (2) mandible, (3) medial pterygoid muscle, (4) and upper aspect of the left tonsil.

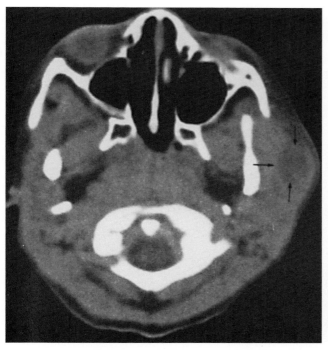

Fig. 37–63. Parotid gland abscess. CT scan of the parotid glands showing a round low-density image (arrows) caused by an abscess.

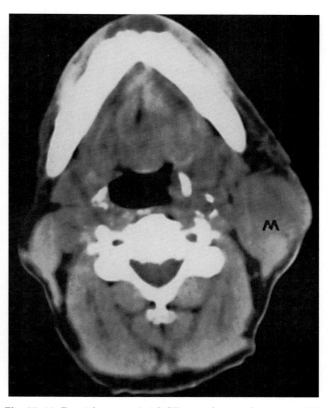

Fig. 37–65. Parotid tumor. Axial CT scan shows a large mass (M) involving the left parotid gland.

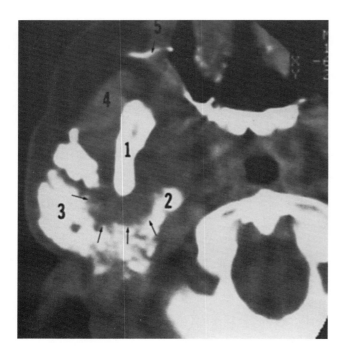

Fig. 37–66. Axial CT sialogram of a parotid tumor. A large tumor (arrows) is seen involving the superficial and deep lobe of the right parotid gland. The lesion is sharply delineated from the surrounding gland tissue which is filled with contrast. (1) Mandible; (2) deep lobe of parotid; (3) superficial lobe of parotid; (4) masseter muscle; (5) contrast in the Stensen duct.

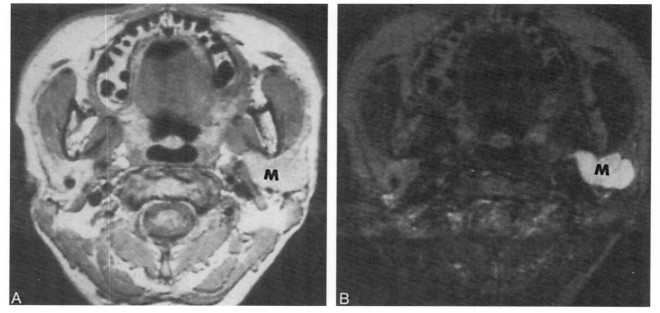

Fig. 37–67. Pleomorphic adenoma. Proton-weighted (A) and T2-weighted (B) axial MR scans show a well-defined mass (M) involving the left parotid gland.

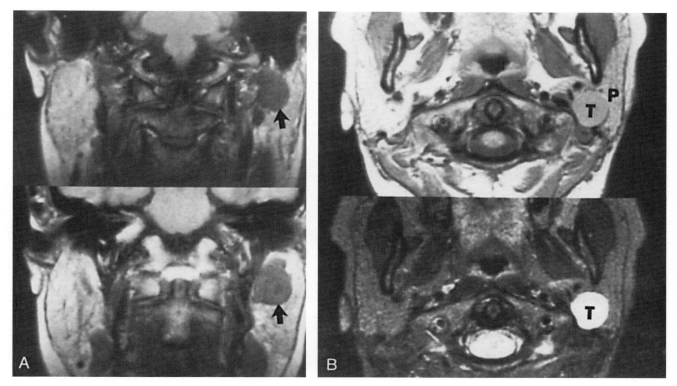

Fig. 37–68. Facial neuroma arising within the parotid gland. A. T1-weighted MR scan showing a hypointense mass (arrows). B. Proton-weighted (top) and T2-weighted (bottom) axial MR scans showing the tumor (T) within the parotid gland (P). Notice hyperintensity of the tumor in T2W image.

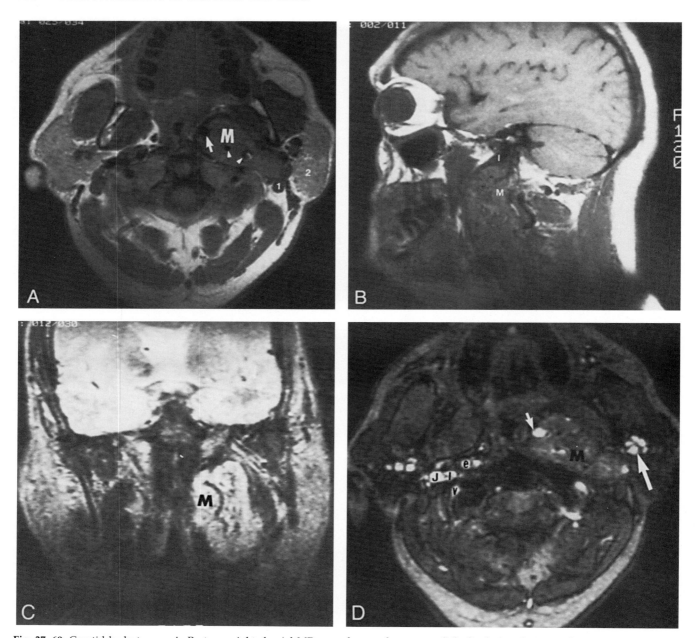

Fig. 37–69. Carotid body tumor. A. Proton-weighted axial MR scan shows a large mass (M), displacing the internal carotid artery (arrow) toward the parapharyngeal space. Note prominent vessels within the mass (arrowheads). (1), Posterior belly of digastric; (2), parotid gland. B. Sagittal T1W MR scan showing the carotid body tumor mass (M). Note marked anterior displacement of the internal carotid artery (I) and serpiginous low-density vascular structures within the mass. C. T2W coronal MR scan, showing hyperintense mass (M), with several tortuous low-density images representing prominent vessels within the mass. The location of the mass as seen in sagittal and coronal MR scan is high, raising the possibility of glomus vagale, rather than carotid body tumor. D. Dynamic GRASS (gradient recalled acquisition in the steady state) axial MR image showing the tumor (m). Note hyperintensity of arteries and veins in this section. e, External carotid artery; I, internal carotid artery; J, internal jugular vein; v, vertebral artery. Note retromandibular veins (large arrow) and displaced left internal carotid artery (small arrow). (From Mafee MF, et al: Head and neck high field magnetic resonance imaging versus computed tomography. Otolaryngol Clin North Am 21:513–540, 1988.)

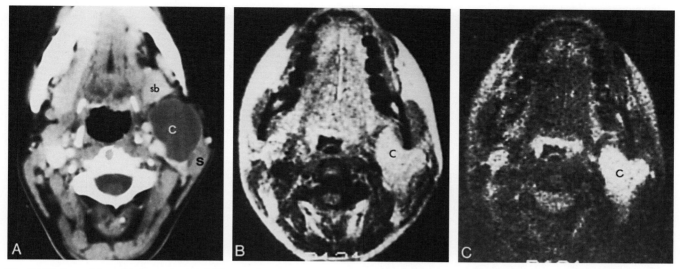

Fig. 37–70. Second branchial cyst. A. Axial CT scan showing the bronchial cyst (c), sternocleidomastoid muscle (S), and submandibular gland (sb). B. Proton-weighted axial MR scan showing the cyst (c). C. T2-weighted axial MR scan showing the cyst (c) as a hyperintense image.

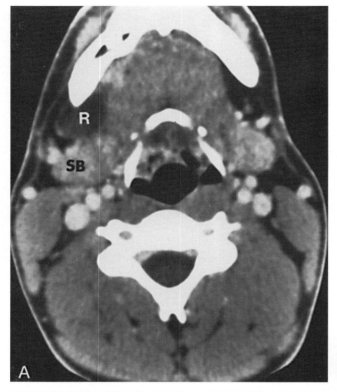

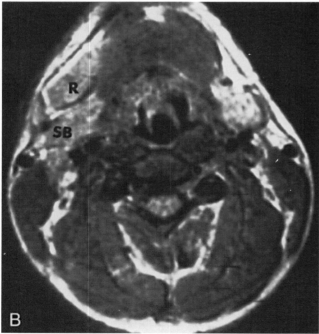

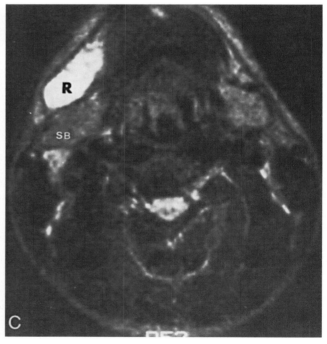

Fig. 37–71. Ranula. A. Axial CT scan showing the ranula (R) and submandibular gland (SB). B. Proton-weighted axial MR scan. Note ranula (R) and submandibular gland (SB). C. T2-weighted axial MR scan shows the ranula (R) and submandibular gland (SB).

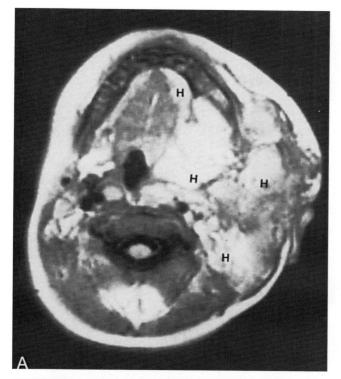

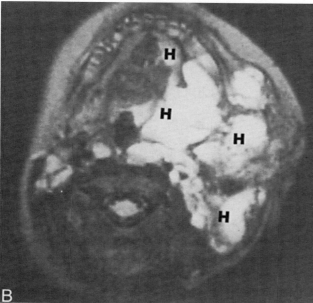

Fig. 37–72.

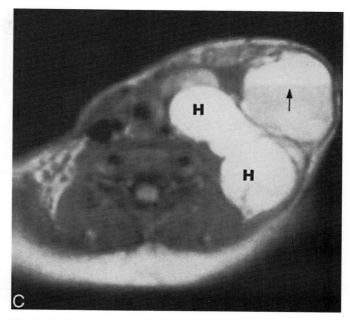

Fig. 37–72. Cystic hygroma. Axial proton-weighted (A), T2-weighted (B), and proton-weighted (C) MR scans showing extensive posterior and anterior cystic hygroma (H). The lesion appears predominantly hyperintense, which is believed to be the result of proteinaceous fluid. Note fluid-fluid level in C (arrow) related to hemorrhage.

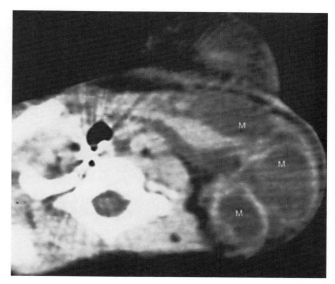

Fig. 37–73. Cystic hygroma. CT scan showing multiloculated low-density masses (M). Cystic hygromas are characteristically seen on CT as hypodense images.

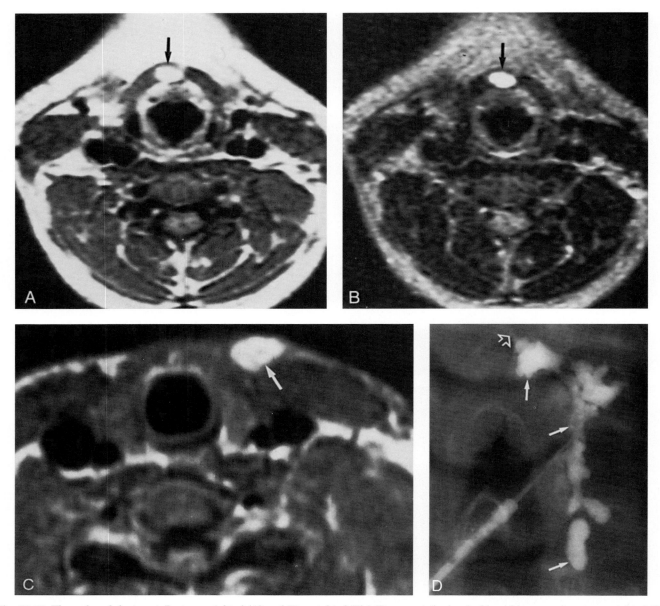

Fig. 37–74. Thyroglossal duct cyst. Proton-weighted (A) and T2-weighted (B) MR scans at the level of hyoid bone, and proton-weighted (C) MR scan at the level of midcricoid showing a hyperintense cyst (arrows). D, Fistulogram of the same patient as in A to C following injection of iodinated contrast in the fistula demonstrating branched thyroglossal duct cyst (arrows), which extends from the base of the tongue (hollow arrow) down to the laryngotracheal level.

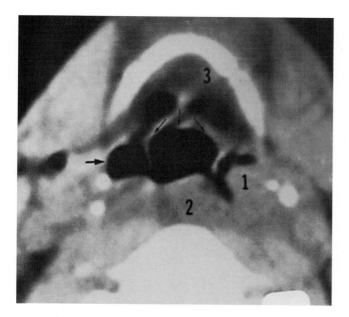

Fig. 37–75. Posttraumatic hematoma of the hypopharynx. CT scan showing high-density bulge along the posterior aspect of the superior portion of the left piriform sinus (1) protruding into the lumen of the left piriform sinus as compared with normal right side (arrow). Note soft tissue thickening of the posterior pharynx wall (2) caused by edema and hematoma. The epiglottis (arrows), valleculae, and partially volumed base of the tongue (3) are also shown.

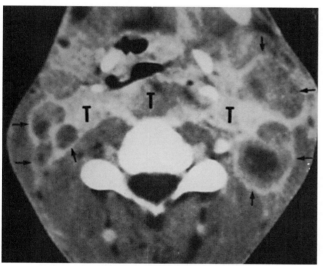

Fig. 37–76. Pharyngeal carcinoma. Postinfusion contrast-enhanced CT scan showing a large enhanced, partially necrotic (low-density areas) tumor (T) involving the posterior pharyngeal wall, left tonsillar fossa, left side of the epiglottis, and left side of the base of the tongue, extending beyond the midline, involving the right side of the upper part of the hypopharynx. Note multiple, well circumscribed ring-like enhancing lesions caused by necrotic lymph nodes (arrows). The carotid sheath vessels are engulfed by the metastatic lymph nodes at this level.

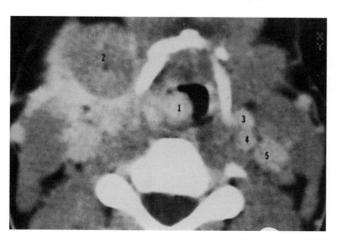

Fig. 37–77. Lymphoma. Postcontrast CT scan showing an enhancing soft tissue mass in the right tonsillar region (1), and a large neck mass (2) with thick peripheral enhancement. The external (3) and internal (4) carotid arteries and the internal jugular vein (5) are visualized. The right external and internal carotid arteries are displaced but not engulfed by the process.

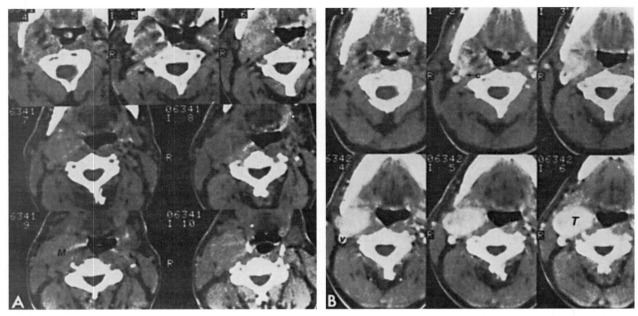

Fig. 37–78. A. Carotid body tumor. Contiguous CT sections obtained following contrast infusion technique. A mass (M) is seen behind the mandible in the third section and can be followed down to the last section obtained at the level of the hyoid bone. B. Contiguous axial CT sections obtained with dynamic technique. Note identification of internal carotid artery (c) and internal jugular vein (v) and intense enhancement of carotid body tumor (T). (From Mafee MF, et al: High resolution and dynamic sequential computed tomography CT. CT use in the evaluation of glomus complex tumors. Arch Otolaryngol Head Neck Surg *109*:691–696, 1983.)

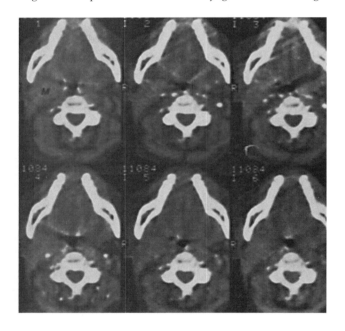

Fig. 37–79. Metastatic lymph nodes. Dynamic CT scan of a patient with right neck metastatic lymph node. Note differential enhancement of the vascular structures as compared with the enhancement of the tumor (M). (From Mafee MF, et al: High resolution and dynamic sequential computed tomography (CT): CT use in the evaluation of glomus complex tumors. Arch Otolaryngol Head Neck Surg *109*:691–696, 1983.)

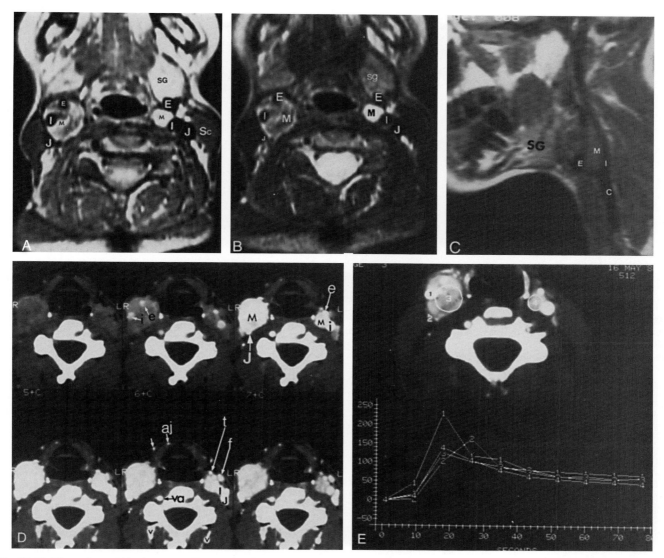

Fig. 37–80. Bilateral carotid body tumors. Proton-weighted (A) and T2-weighted (B) axial MR scans showing bilateral masses (M), submandibular gland (SG), carotid (E and I) arteries and internal jugular vein (J). C. T1-weighted sagittal MR scan showing the right carotid body mass (M), common (C), internal (i) and external, sternocleidomastoid muscle (SC), (E) arteries and submandibular gland (SG). D. Dynamic CT scan showing the sequential enhancement of external (e) and internal (i) carotid arteries and internal jugular vein (J). Notice intense enhancement of carotid body tumors (M). Note vertebral artery (Va), deep paravertebral venous plexus (v), facial vein (f), superior thyroid artery (t), anterior jugular vein (aj), and anterior facial vein (white arrow). E. Density-time curve shows characteristic arterial peak of carotid body tumors (3,4). (1) Carotid artery; (2) internal jugular vein. (From Mafee MF, et al: Head and neck high field magnetic resonance imaging versus computed tomography. Otolaryngol Clin North Am 21:513–546, 1988.)

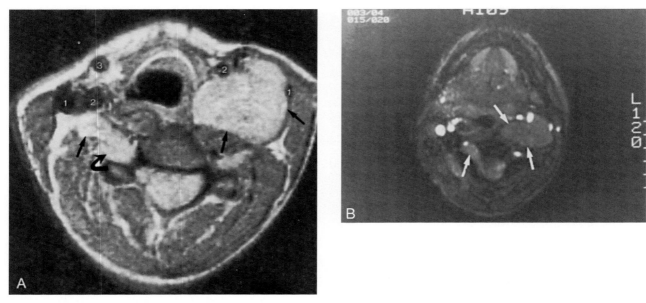

Fig. 37–81. Neurofibroma. A. PW, axial MR scan shows bilateral masses (arrows), in this patient with neurofibromatosis. On the left side the tumor has widened the neuroforamen (curved arrow). (1) internal jugular vein; (2) internal carotid artery; (3) anterior jugular vein. B. Dynamic GRASS (gradient recalled acquisition in the steady state) axial MR scan shows the neurofibromas (arrows). Notice hyperintensity of the vascular structures.

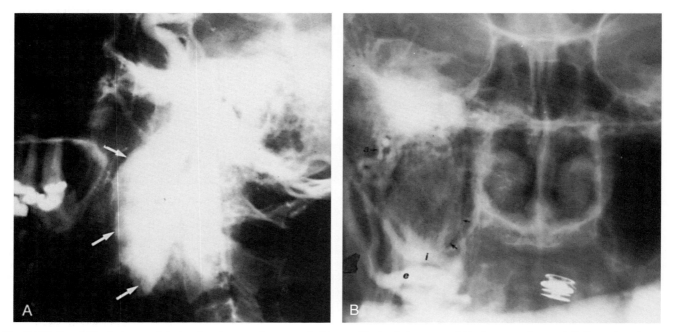

Fig. 37–82. Carotid body tumor. A. Lateral angiogram shows marked tumor blush of a large carotid body tumor (arrows). B. Frontal angiogram of another patient with large glomus jugulare tumor showing the tumor blush (large arrows) and involvement of the internal jugular vein (small arrows). Notice the displaced internal (i) and external (e) carotid arteries. Notice also a large ascending pharyngeal artery (a).

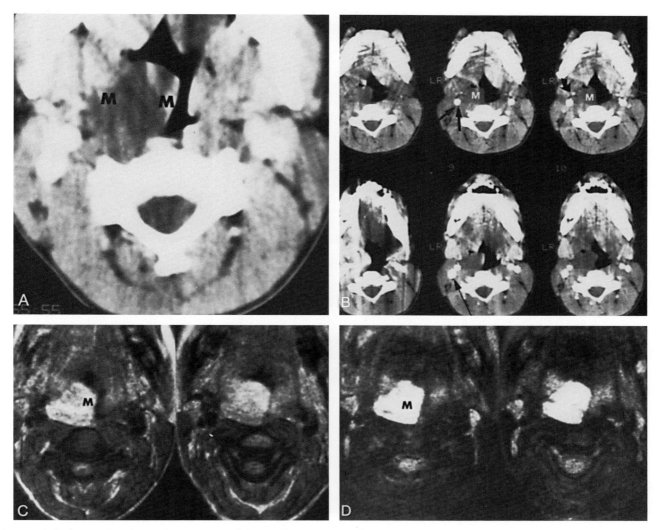

Fig. 37–83. Cavernous lymphangiohemangioma of the oropharynx. A. Axial contrast CT scan shows a low-density mass (M) involving the right tonsil and posterolateral wall of the oropharynx. B. Serial dynamic CT scan shows sequential enhancement of external carotid (curved arrow) and internal carotid (arrows) arteries and internal jugular vein (long arrow). Note that the mass (M) is not enhanced. Artifacts are seen in the fourth section. C. Proton-weighted MR scans showing the cavernous lymphangiohemangioma (M). D. T2-weighted MR scans showing the lymphangiohemangioma (M). (From Mafee MF, et al: Head and neck: high field MRI versus computed tomography. Otolarngol Clin North Am *21*:513–546, 1988.)

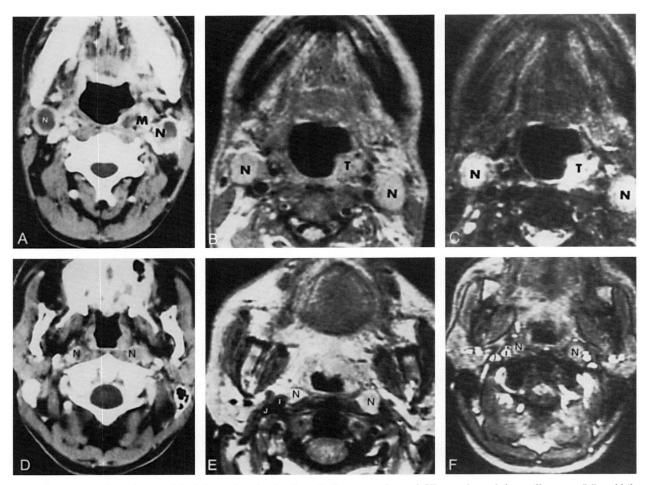

Fig. 37–84. Squamous cell carcinoma of the left tonsil and soft palate. A. Contrast-enhanced CT scan shows left tonsillar mass (M) and bilateral necrotic lymph nodes (N). PW (B) and T2W (C) MR scans show tumor (T) and enlarged lymph nodes (N). Necrotic nature of the lymph nodes is better appreciated on CT scan (A). Notice that tumor and nodal metastases have identical signal characteristics in this patient. D. Axial CT scan obtained superior to A, showing bilateral retropharyngeal lymph nodes (N). E. PW MR scan shows bilateral retropharyngeal lymph nodes (N). Note hyperintensity of all vascular structures. e, External carotid artery; I, internal carotid artery; J, internal jugular vein. (From Mafee MF, et al: Head and neck: high field MRI versus computed tomography. Otolaryngol Clin North Am 21:513–546, 1988.)

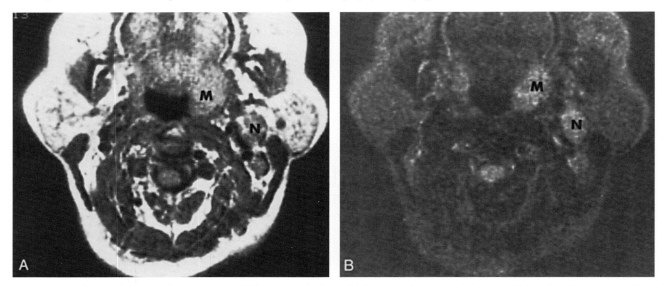

Fig. 37–85. Lymphoma of the tonsillar region. PW (A) and T2W (B) axial MR scans show a tonsillar mass (M) and a deep enlarged lymph node (N). (From Mafee MF, et al: Head and neck: high field MRI versus computed tomography. Otolaryngol Clin North Am 21:513–546, 1988.)

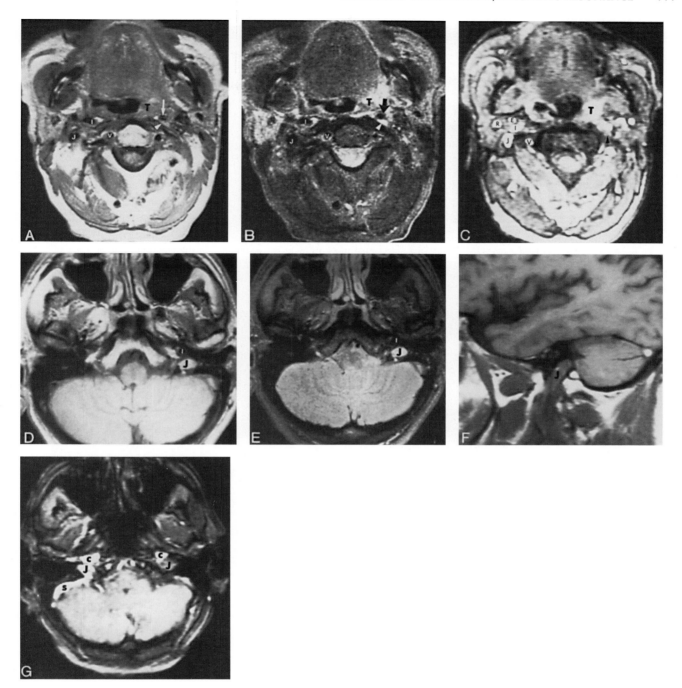

Fig. 37–86. Recurrent squamous cell carcinoma of the soft palate and tonsil with involvement of internal jugular vein. PW (A) and T2W (B) MR scans show tumor (T) in the left tonsillar and glossopalatine arch. The left internal carotid (arrow) is seen as a hypointense (arrowhead), compared to the normal side. I, Internal carotid artery; J, internal jugular vein; v, vertebral artery. C. Dynamic GRASS (gradient recalled acquisition in the steady state) MR image shows hyperintensity of tumor (T) and all vasculature including the thrombosed left internal jugular vein (arrowhead). R, Retromandibular vein. D and E. PW (D) and T2W (E) MR scans showing increased signal of left internal jugular vein (J) and hypointense left internal carotid artery (I). F. Sagittal, T1W MR scan showing the thrombosed left internal jugular vein (J). G. Dynamic (GRASS) image shows hyperintensity of all vasculature. Note assymetry of signal of internal jugular vein (J). c, Internal carotid artery; s, sigmoid sinus. (From Mafee MF, et al: Head and neck: high field magnetic resonance versus computed tomography. Otolaryngol Clin North Am 21:513–546, 1988.)

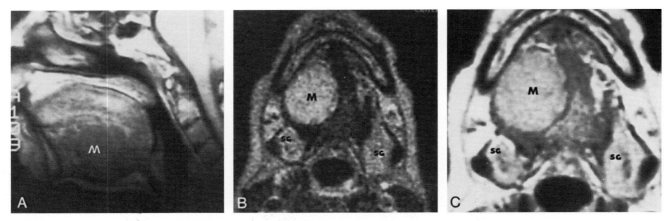

Fig. 37–87. Pleomorphic adenoma of right submandibular region. A. T1W sagittal MR scan shows a hypointense mass (M) in the submandibular region. B. PW MR scan showing a mass (M) of intermediate signal intensity, which is isointense to submandibular gland (SG). C. T2W MR scan showing the mass (M), which is slightly hyperintense to normal submandibular gland (SG). This tumor was thought to arise from minor salivary gland of the floor of the mouth. (From Mafee MF, et al: Head and neck: high field MRI versus computed tomography. Otolaryngol Clin North Am 21:513–546, 1988.)

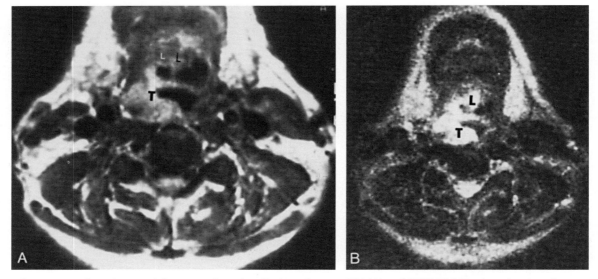

Fig. 37–88. Squamous cell carcinoma of the posterolateral wall of oropharynx. PW (A) and T2W (B) MR scans showing the tumor (T) and lymphoid tissues (lingual tonsil) at the base of the tongue (L). As seen the tumor in this patient cannot be distinguished from the lymphoid tissue on T2W MR image (B). (From Mafee MF, et al: Head and neck: high field MRI versus computed tomography. Otolaryngol Clin North Am 21:513–546, 1988.)

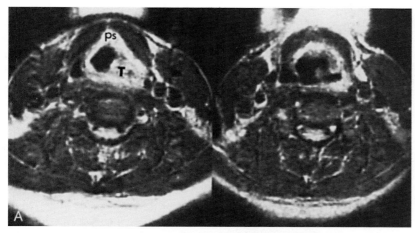

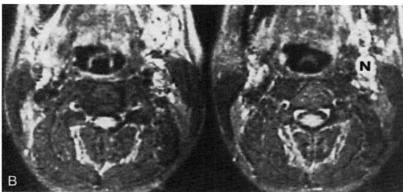

Fig. 37–89. Squamous cell carcinoma of the piriform sinus. A. PW MR scans showing the tumor (T) and the fatty-areolar tissue in the preepiglottic space (PS). As seen, the tumor boundaries cannot be distinguished from normal fatty tissues in these PW MR scans. T2W MR scan is needed for the distinction. B. PW MR scans, obtained superior to A, showing enlarged lymph node (N).

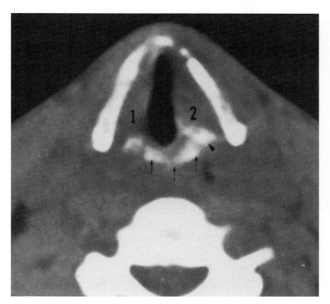

Fig. 37–90. CT scan showing enlargement (hematoma) of the left true vocal cord (2). The left arytenoid cartilage (arrowhead) is rotated medially. The signet portion of the cricoid cartilage (arrows) and right vocal cord (1) appear normal.

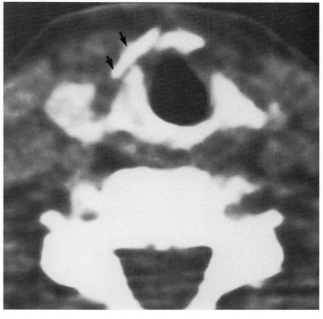

Fig. 37–91. CT scan at the level of the inferior margin of the true vocal cords showing a displaced fragment of fractured thyroid cartilage (arrows). Compare with Figure 37–32.

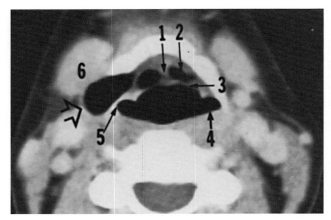

Fig. 37–92. Laryngocele. The laryngocele bulges outside the larynx laterally (open arrow). (1) Median glossoepiglottic fold; (2) vallecula; (3) tip of the epiglottis; (4) upper portion of pyriform sinus; (5) pharyngoepiglottic fold; and (6) submandibular gland.

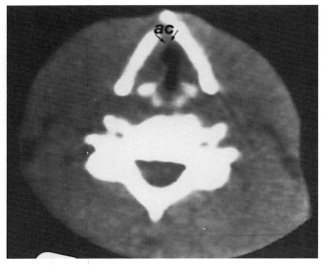

Fig. 37–93. Carcinoma of the true vocal cords. CT scan obtained at the level of the true vocal cords during quiet breathing. The right true vocal cord is enlarged by tumor. The bulk of it is seen along its posterior phonating edge and in the region of the right arytenoid cartilage. Note enlargment of the most anterior portion of the right true vocal cord, involving the anterior commissure (ac) and extending beyond the midline. Note also increased soft tissue and asymmetrical appearance of interarytenoid region, which is indicative of posterior commissure involvement. Compare this figure with Figure 37–30A. (From Mafee MF, et al: Computed tomography of the larynx. *Radiology 147*:123, 1983.)

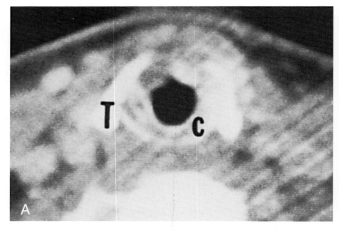

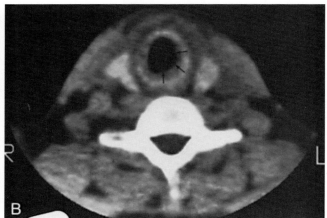

Fig. 37–94. A. CT scan showing narrowing caused by tumor involvement along the anterior portion of the subglottic space. C, Cricoid cartilage; T, thyroid cartilage. B. CT scan obtained at the lowest portion of the cricoid cartilage showing tumor involvement on the left side (arrows). (From Mafee MF, et al: Computed tomography of the larynx. *Radiology 147*:123, 1983.)

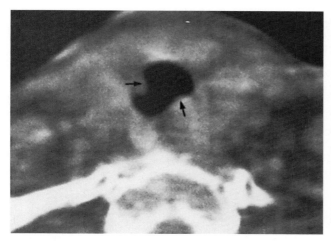

Fig. 37–95. CT scan showing tumor involvement (arrows) involving the thyroid gland and trachea.

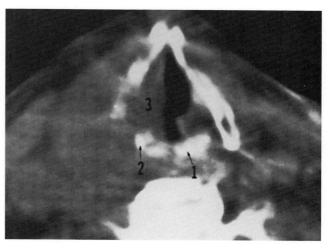

Fig. 37–96. CT scan showing a large tumor involving the right true vocal cord which is fixed in paramedial position (3). Note extension of tumor between partially destroyed thyroid cartilage and partially destroyed right arytenoid cartilage (2). Note tumor extension outside of the larynx into the neck. (1) Left arytenoid cartilage.

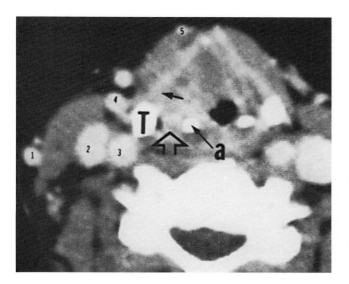

Fig. 37–97. Postcontrast CT scan showing a large tumor involving the right false vocal cord, epiglottis, and extending beyond the midline involving the left false vocal cord. The thyroid cartilage (T) is partially calcified and the thyroid alae, seen as a faint increased density with the tumor involving the right ala (arrow) and extending into the paraglottic space (open arrowhead) between the thyroid cartilage and right arytenoid cartilage (a) which is displaced medially. (1) External jugular vein; (2) internal jugular vein; (3) common carotid artery; (4) posterior facial vein; (5) and anterior jugular vein.

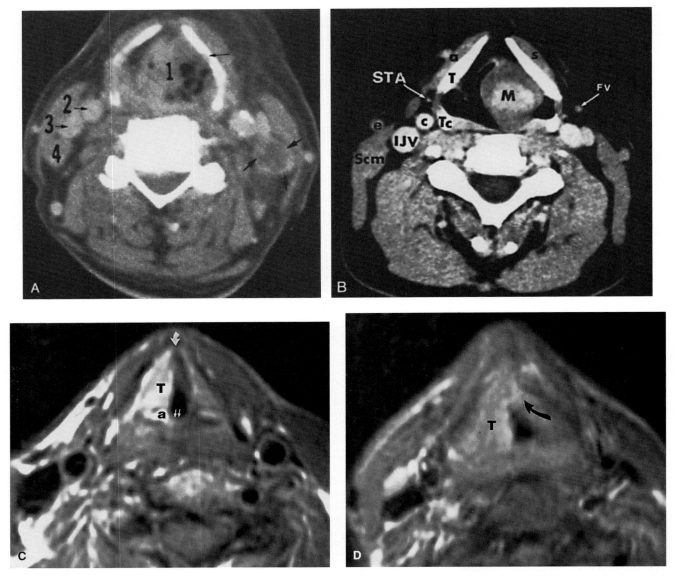

Fig. 37–98. A. CT scan showing a large necrotic exophytic tumor arising from the left aryepiglottic fold (1). Note tumor involvement of the left thyroid ala (arrow), epiglottis, and extension beyond the midline with involvement of the right aryepiglottic fold and destruction of the posterior aspect of the right thyroid ala. Note large left necrotic lymph node (arrows) and right large lymph node (4). Common carotid artery (2), and internal jugular vein (3). B. Leiomyoma of larynx (M) for comparison with squamous cell carcinoma (A). a, Anterior jugular vein; c, common carotid artery; e, external jugular vein; FV, facial vein; IJV, internal jugular vein; s, strap muscles; SCM, sternocleidomastoid; STA, superior thyroid artery. C. Glottic carcinoma. PW axial MR scan shows tumor (T) involving the entire right true vocal cord. Note normal anterior (curved arrow) and posterior (arrows) commissures. The arytenoid cartilage (a) is normal. D. Supraglottic carcinoma. PW axial MR shows tumor (T) involving the right false vocal cord and extending beyond the midline to involve the left false vocal cord (curved arrow). *(continued)*

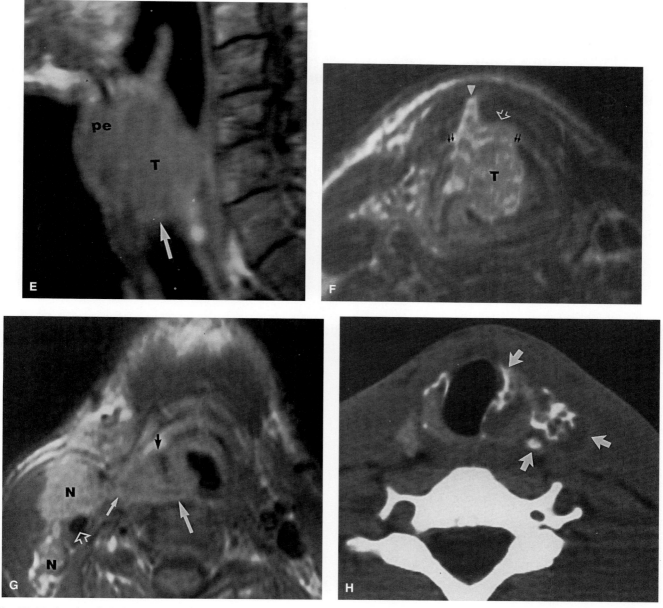

Fig. 37–98. *(continued)* E. Supraglottic carcinoma. T1W sagittal MR scan, same patient as in C, shows large supraglottic tumor (T) with involvement of the preepiglottic space (pe) and with extension into the immediate subglottic space (arrow). F. Supraglottic carcinoma. T2W axial MR scan shows large tumor (T) with involvement of thyroid cartilage (small arrows), extending into the preepiglottic space (hollow arrow) and strap muscles (arrowhead). G. Carcinoma of right pyriform sinus. PW axial MR scan shows a large mass (arrows) involving the right side of the hypopharynx. Note multiple metastatic lymph nodes (N). The common carotid artery (hollow arrow) is intact. H. Chondrosarcoma of the cricoid cartilage. Axial CT scan shows a large mass (arrows) with foci of calcification, involving the cricoid cartilage. Note expansion and partial erosion of the cricoid cartilage. *(continued)*

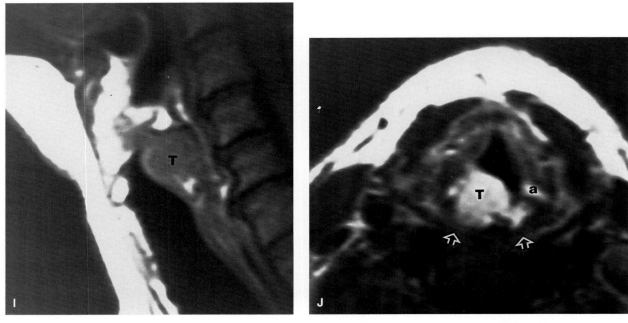

Fig. 37–98. *(continued)* I. Chondrosarcoma of the cricoid cartilage. T1W sagittal MR scan shows large tumor (T) involving the posterior portion of the larynx. J. T2W axial MR scan, same patient as in H, shows hyperintense tumor (T) involving the right side of the cricoid cartilage as well as right arytenoid cartilage. Note normal left arytenoid cartilage (a) and tumor extension into the hypopharynx (arrows).

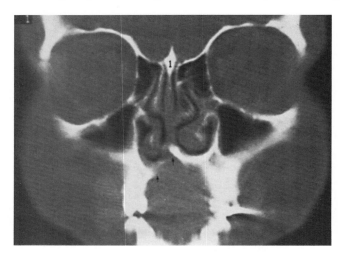

Fig. 37–99. Coronal CT showing a right palatomaxillary cleft (arrows). Note crista galli (1), cribriform plate, roof of the ethmoid sinuses (olfactory plates), lamina papyracea, and middle and inferior turbinates.

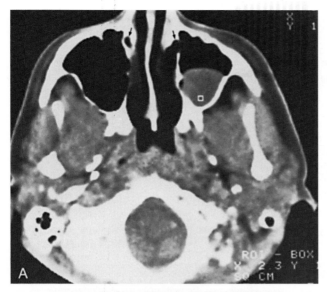

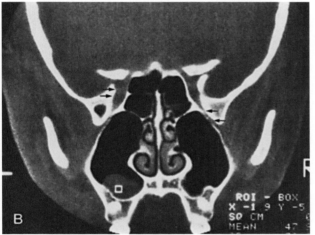

Fig. 37–100. A. CT scan showing a smoothly marginated soft tissue image with cursor measurement of water density (mean = 5) in the left maxillary sinus. This is characteristic of a retention cyst. Notice the nasolacrimal canals (arrows). B. Coronal CT scan showing a mucous cyst with cursor measurement of 47.9 on the floor of the left maxillary sinus. The mucous cysts usually show a high CT number compared with retention cysts. Note excellent bone details and visualization of the nasal turbinates, maxilloethmoid plate, and superior and inferior orbital fissures (upper and lower arrows).

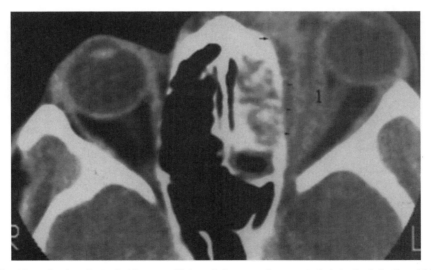

Fig. 37–101. Ethmoid periostitis and subperiosteal phlegmon. Note soft tissue replacement of air in the left ethmoid labyrinth with thickening of the trabeculae. The left lamina papyracea is thickened and in some areas dehiscent. These findings are indicative of periostitis. Note soft tissue swelling (not leading yet to necrosis and abscess formation) in the left periorbita (arrowheads), resulting in displacement of the left medial rectus muscle (1). Notice proptosis of the left eye and marked periorbital edema and inflammation anterior to the orbital septum (arrow).

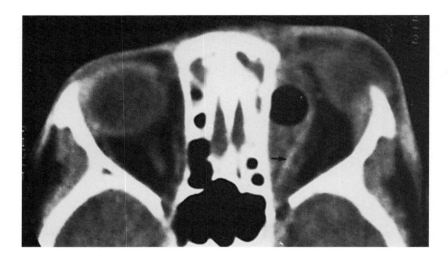

Fig. 37–102. CT scan showing proptosis of the left eye and a subperiosteal abscess. A large gas pocket is seen (dark round area) within the abscess. Note displaced left medial rectus muscle (arrow).

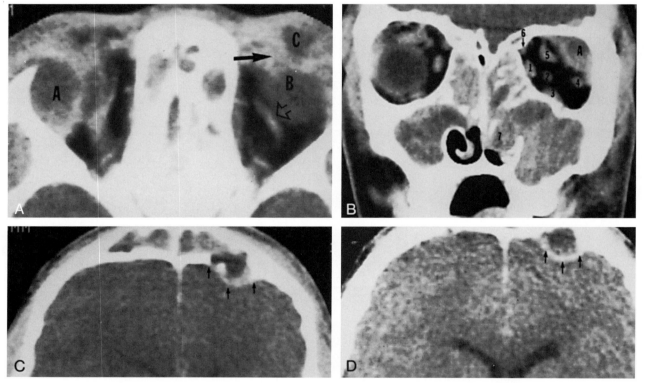

Fig. 37–103. A. CT scan showing increased density of the ethmoid labyrinth, and bilateral retro-orbital soft tissue inflammation (cellulitis) (A and B). Note also a low-density image involving the left upper eyelid (C). The eyelid lesion (C) was drained and 3 ml of pus was removed. Hollow arrowhead points to superior ophthalmic vein, and the arrow points to the retroseptal granulation tissue. B. Postcontrast semicoronal CT scan of the same patient in A showing enhancing soft tissue densities (polyps and hyperplastic mucosa) involving the maxillary and ethmoid sinuses. Notice polyp in the right nasal cavity (7) and periorbital cellulitis involving the right orbit (A). (1) Medial rectus muscle; (2) optic nerve; (3) inferior rectus muscle; (4) lateral rectus muscle; (5) superior rectus muscle; (6) and superior oblique muscle. C. CT scan of same patient in A and B showing increased density of the frontal sinuses with erosion of the posterior table of the left frontal sinus (arrows). D. Postcontrast CT scan obtained 5 mm superior to C, showing enhancement along the exposed and displaced dura (arrows).

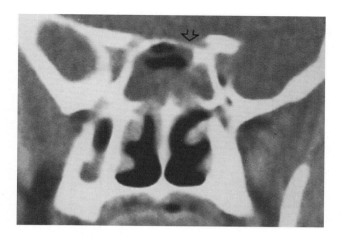

Fig. 37–104. Acute sphenoid sinusitis. Coronal CT scan showing opacification of sphenoid sinuses with demineralization of the roof of the right sphenoid sinus (arrow) close to the optic canal.

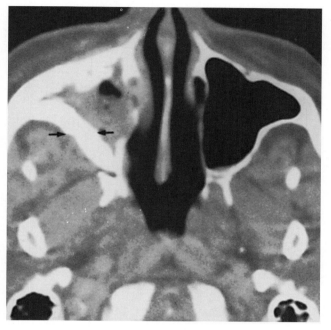

Fig. 37–105. CT scan showing marked hyperplastic mucosa with periosteal thickening (arrows) (osteoblastic sinusitis).

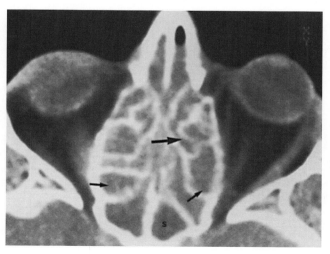

Fig. 37–106. Chronic hypertrophic polypoid sinusitis. Postcontrast axial CT scan showing enhanced soft tissues in the ethmoid labyrinth (arrows), sphenoid sinuses (s), and nasal cavity in this patient with nasal and paranasal polyposis.

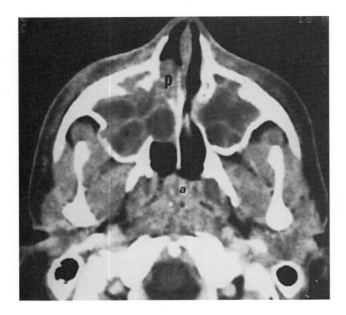

Fig. 37–107. Nasal and paranasal polyps. Postcontrast axial CT showing polyp in the right nasal cavity (p) and enhancing soft tissue in the maxillary sinuses. Note large adenoid (a).

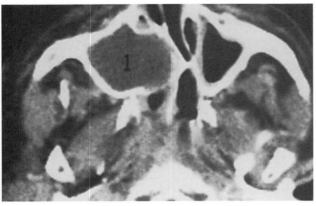

Fig. 37–108. CT scan showing expansion and replacement of the right maxillary sinus (1) by a soft tissue of low density, which is characteristic of a mucocele.

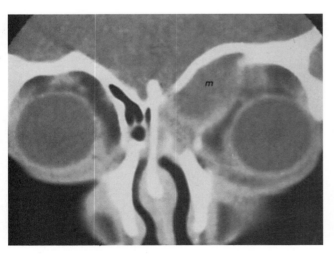

Fig. 37–109. Mucocele of the ethmoid sinus. Postcontrast coronal CT scan showing expansion and replacement of the supraorbital recess of the left ethmoid sinus by a soft tissue of relatively low density (m). There is erosion and lateral displacement of the lamina papyracea and the superiomedial rim of the left orbit.

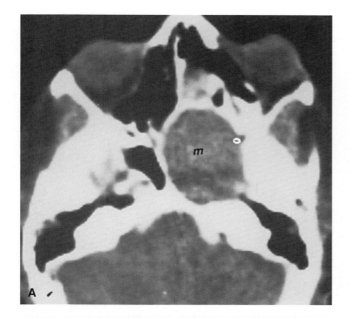

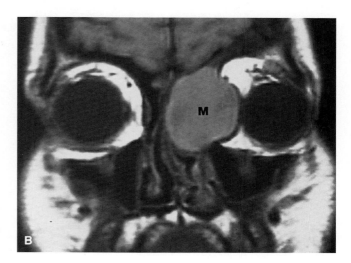

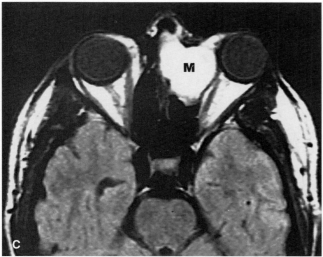

Fig. 37–110. A. CT scan showing expansion and replacement of the left sphenoid sinus by soft tissue of low density, which is characteristic of a mucocele (m). B. Mucocele of the left ethmoid sinus. T1W coronal MR scan shows expansile rather hyperintense mass (M), involving left ethmoid sinus. C. PW axial MR scan, same patient as in B, shows that the mass (M) is markedly hyperintense.

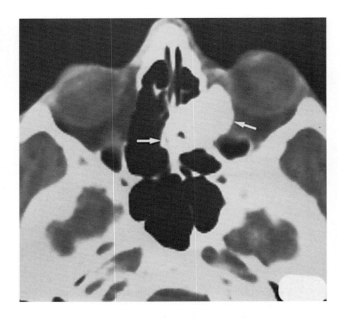

Fig. 37–111. CT scan showing a left ethmoid sinus osteoma extending into the left orbit (arrows).

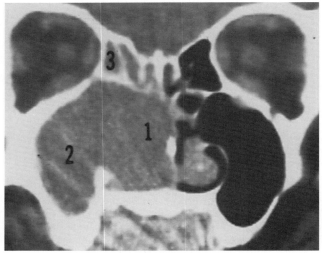

Fig. 37–112. Carcinoma of the nasal cavity. Postcontrast coronal CT scan showing a large tumor in the left nasal cavity (1), extending into the left maxillary sinus (2) and left ethmoid sinus (3). Note destruction of the medial wall of the left maxillary sinus and partial destruction of the maxilloethmoidal plate.

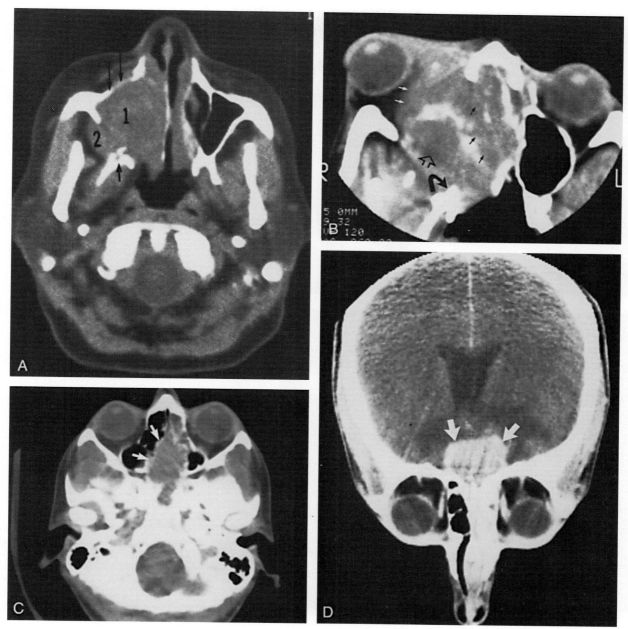

Fig. 37–113. A. Carcinoma of the right maxillary sinus. Postcontrast axial CT scan showing a large mass involving the right maxillary sinus (1) and extending into the right nasal cavity. There is erosion of the anterior wall of the maxillary antrum (arrows). Note destruction of the posterior wall of the right maxillary sinus and extension of tumor into the right infratemporal fossa (2). Note tumor in the right pterygopalatine fossa with partial erosion in the pterygoid portion of the right sphenoid bone (arrow). B. Rhabdomyosarcoma; axial CT scan shows large mass in the right ethmoid sinus (black arrows) with extension into the right orbit (white arrows). Note extension of tumor in the superior portion of the right maxillary sinus (hollow arrow) with tumor seen in the pterygopalatine fossa (curved arrow). C. Esthesioneuroblastoma; axial CT scan shows a mass in the left ethmoid sinus (arrows) with opacity of the sphenoid sinuses. D. Coronal CT scan of same patient as in C, showing markedly enhanced mass (arrows) in the anterior cranial fossa caused by extension of tumor along the cribriform plate into the cranium. *(continued)*

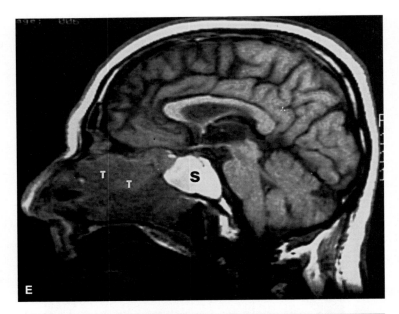

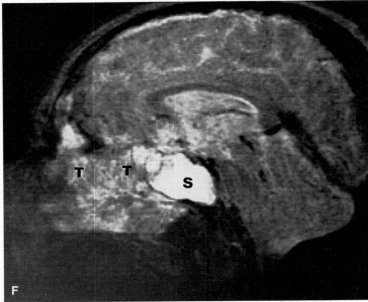

Fig. 37–113. *(continued)* E. Adenocarcinoma of the nasal cavity and ethmoid sinus. T1W sagittal MR scan shows large tumor (T) within the nasal cavity and ethmoid cells. Note hyperintensity of retained secretion in the sphenoid sinus (S). F. T2W sagittal MR scan, same patient as in E. The tumor (T) appears hyperintense. The retained fluid remains hyperintense within the sphenoid sinus (S).

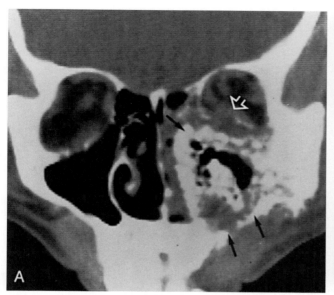

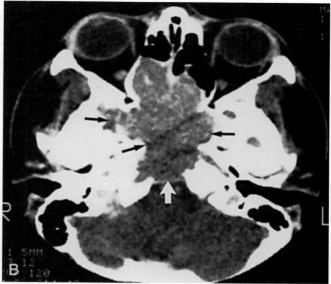

Fig. 37–114. A. Osteogenic sarcoma, CT scan showing a large maxillary tumor with irregular islands of bone formation (arrows) and with marked bone destruction. Notice invasion of the floor of the orbit (hollow arrow). B. Giant cell tumor of the sphenoid bone; axial CT shows destructive tumor of the sphenoid bone (black arrows) with extension into the posterior ethmoid cells. Notice destruction of the clivus (white arrow) and exposed dura.

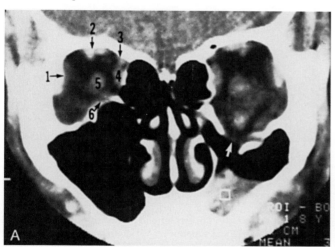

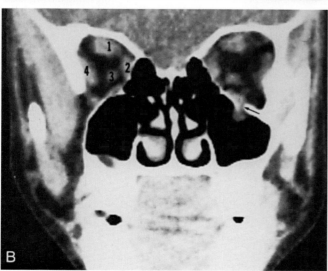

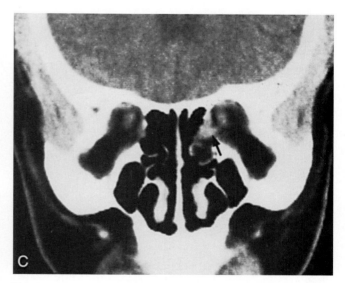

Fig. 37–115. A. Coronal CT scan showing "blow-out fracture" of the right orbital floor with displacement of the periorbital fat and fractured fragments into the right maxillary sinus (arrow). Notice fluid in the right maxillary sinus with cursor measurement of 36, which is indicative of hemorrhage. (1) Lateral rectus muscle; (2) superior rectus muscle; (3) superior oblique muscle; (4) medial rectus muscle; (5) optic nerve; (6) and inferior rectus muscle. B. Coronal CT scan showing fracture of the floor of the right orbit (arrow) and with the inferior rectus partially hooked over the fracture site. (1) Superior rectus muscle; (2) medial rectus muscle; (3) optic nerve; and (4) lateral rectus muscle. C. Coronal CT scan showing fracture of the right medial orbital wall with entrapment of the medial rectus muscle (arrow).

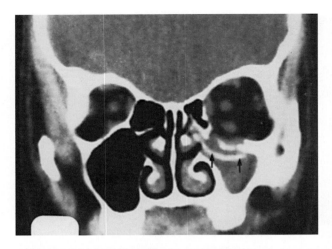

Fig. 37–116. Coronal CT scan showing displacement of the silastic implant into the left maxillary sinus (arrows). Notice associated maxillary sinusitis and scar formation on the floor of the left orbit.

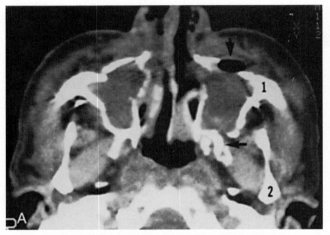

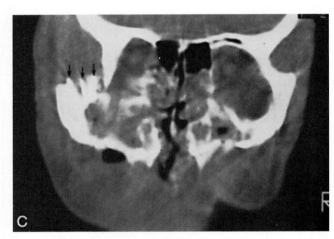

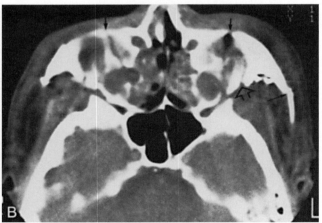

Fig. 37–117. A. Complex maxillofacial fracture. Axial CT scan showing fractures of the anterior and medial wall of both maxillary sinuses. Note marked soft tissue swelling of the face, air in the subcutaneous tissue (arrow), opacification of the maxillary sinuses caused by hematoma, fracture of the left zygoma (1), fracture of the left pterygoid plates (posterior arrow), and normal mandible (2). B. Axial CT scan obtained 1 cm superior to A. Note bilateral fractures of the inferior orbital rim (anterior arrows), extending along the zygomaticomaxillary suture on the left, and involving the posterior wall of the left maxillary sinus (open arrowhead). Note fractures of the left zygomatic arch (arrow), the floor of the right orbit, and the posterior wall of the right maxillary sinus. C. Coronal CT scan of the same patient in A and B. Note separation of the left frontozygomatic suture (arrows) and lateral displacement of the left fractured malar bone. Note fractures of the anterior wall of both maxillary antra, shattered fractures of the ethmoid and floor sinuses of both orbits.

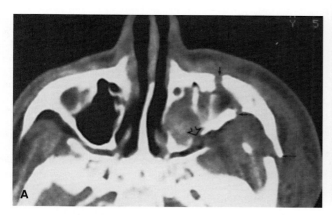

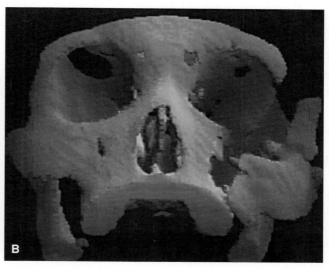

Fig. 37–118. A. Malar fracture. Axial CT scan showing fractures involving the inferior orbital rim and left malar bone, which extend along the left zygomaticomaxillary suture (small arrows). Notice fracture of the left zygomatic arch, fracture of the posterior wall of the left maxillary sinus (open arrowhead), and bone fragments within the left maxillary antrum with associated left antral submucosal hematoma. B. Malar fracture. Three-dimensional image reformation from regular CT scans showing the fractures and displacement of the malar bone.

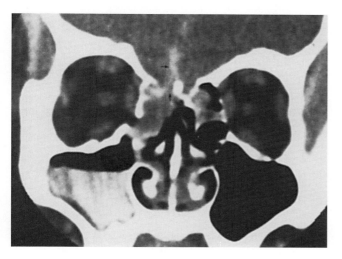

Fig. 37–119. CSF rhinorrhea. Coronal CT scan after intrathecal injection of metrizamide showing contrast-enhanced subarachnoid space of the anterior cranial fossa (upper arrow) just above the crista galli. Note fracture of the left cribriform plate (lower arrow) and presence of metrizamide (high density) within the ethmoid labyrinth and air metrizamide fluid level in the left maxillary sinus.

SUGGESTED READINGS

1. Lauterbur PC: Image formation by induced local interactions: examples employing nuclear magnetic resonance. Nature 242: (Mar. 16) 190–191, 1973.
2. McCullough EC: Basic physics of x-ray computed tomography. In: Computed Tomography. Edited by Korobkin M, Newton TH. St. Louis, C. V. Mosby Co., 1977.
3. Hounsfield GN: Picture quality of computed tomography. Am J Roentgenol 127:3–9, 1976.
4. Boyd DP: Physics II computed tomography. In: Computed Tomography. Edited by Norman D, Korobkin M, Newton TH. St. Louis, C. V. Mosby Co., 1977.
5. Carter BL: Computed tomography part III. In: Radiology of the Ear, Nose and Throat. Edited by Valvassori GE, et al. Stuttgart, Georg Thieme, 1982.
6. Basosi R, Niccolai N, Tiezzi E, et al: Nuclear and electron spin relaxation techniques for delineation of bioinorganic and biological activities. Bull Magnet Res 7:119–139, 1985.
7. Mafee MF, Rasouli F, Spigos DG, et al: Magnetic resonance imaging in the diagnosis of nonsquamous tumors of the head and neck. Otolaryngol Clin North Am 19:523–536, 1986.
8. Mafee MF, Compos M, Raju S, et al: Head and neck, high field magnetic resonance imaging versus computed tomography. Otolaryngol Clin North Am 21:513–546, 1988.
9. Mafee MF, Valvassori GE, Kumar A, et al.: Tumors and tumor-like conditions of the middle ear and mastoid: Role of CT and MRI: An analysis of 100 cases. Otolaryngol Clin North Am 21: 349–375, 1988.
10. Mafee MF, Heffez L, Campos M, et al.: Temporomandibular joint: Role of direct sagittal CT air-contrast arthrogram and MRI. Otolaryngol Clin North Am 21:575–588, 1988.
11. Mafee MF: Acoustic neuroma and other acoustic nerve disorders: Role of MRI and CT: An analysis of 238 cases. Semin Ultrasound CT MRI 8:256–283, Sept. 1987.
12. Gorter CJ: Paramagnetic relaxation. Physica 3:503, 1936.
13. Rabi II, et al: A new method of measuring paramagnetic moment. Phys Rev 53:318, 1938.
14. Gorter CJ, Broer LJF: Negative results of an attempt to observe nuclear magnetic resonance in solids. Physica 9:591, 1942.
15. Bloch F, et al: Nuclear induction. Phys Rev 69:127, 1946.
16. Purcell EM, Torrey HG, Pound RV.: Resonance absorption by nuclear magnetic moments in a solid. Phys Rev 69:37, 1946.
17. Rosen BR, Brady TS: Principles of nuclear magnetic resonance for medical application. Semin Nucl Med 13:308–318, 1983.
18. Pykett IL, Newhouse JH, Buonanno FS, et al: Principles of nuclear magnetic resonance imaging. Radiology 143:157–168, 1982.
19. Gore JC, Emery EW, Orr JS, et al: Special articles. Medical nuclear magnetic resonance imaging. I. Physical principles. Invest Radiol 16:269–274, 1981.
20. Hawkes RC, Holland GN, Moore WS, et al.: Nuclear magnetic resonance imaging: An overview. Radiography 551:253–255, 1980.
21. Principles of MR Imaging. Philips Medical Systems. Printed in the Netherlands, 1984.
22. Luyten PR, den Hollander, JA, et al: Observation of metabolites in the human brain by MR spectroscopy. Radiology 161: 795–798, 1986.
23. Barany M, Langer BG, Glick PP, et al: In-vivo H-1 spectroscopy in humans at 1.5T. Radiology 167:839–844, 1988.
24. Mafee MF: Magnetic resonance imaging and its simplifications for ophthalmology in Ophthalmology Annual. Edited by Reinecke RD. New York, Raven Press, pp. 193–264, 1989.
25. Mafee MF: MRI and in-vivo proton H-1 spectroscopy of the lesions of the globe. Semin Ultrasound CT MRI 9:1988.
26. Fan TWM, Higashi RM, Lane AN, et al.: Combined use of 1-H-NMR and GC-MS for metabolic monitoring and in-vivo 1-H-NMR assignments. Biochim Biophys Acta 882:154, 1986.
27. Bottomley PA, Edelstein WA, Foster TH.: In-vivo solvent-suppressed localized hydrogen nuclear magnetic resonance spectroscopy: a window to metabolism? Proc Natl Acad Sci 82: 2148–52, 1985.
28. Bottomley PA: NMR imaging techiques and applications: A review. Rev Sci Instrum 53:1319–1337, 1982.
29. Smith SL: Nuclear magnetic resonance imaging. Anal Chem 57: 597–608, 1985.
30. Wehrli FW, Macfall JR, Newton TH: Parameters determining the appearance of NMR images. In: Modern Neuroradiology. Vol II. Edited by Newton TH, Potts DV. San Anselmo, CA, Clavadel Press, 1983.
31. Wehrli FW, Macfall JR, Shutts D, et al: Mechanisms of contrast in NMR imaging. J Comput Assist Tomogr 8:369–380, 1984.
32. Pisaneschi MJ, Mafee MF, Samii M: Applications of magnetic resonance angiography in head and neck pathology. Otolaryngol Clin North Am 1994 (In press).
33. Mafee MF: Dynamic CT and its application to otolaryngology and head and neck surgery. J Otolaryngol 11:5, 1982.
34. Shugar MA, Mafee MF: Diagnosis of carotid body tumors by dynamic computerized tomography. Head Neck Surg 4:518–21, 1982.
35. Mafee MF, Valvassori GE, Shugar MA, et al. High resolution and dynamic sequential computed tomography (CT). CT use in the evaluation of glomus complex tumors. Arch Otolaryngol Head Neck Surg 109:691–696, 1983.
36. Damadian R, et al. Human tumors by NMR. Physiol Chem Phys 5:381, 1973.
37. Mafee MF, et al.: Malignant uveal melanoma and simulating lesions: MR imaging evaluation. Radiology 160:773, 1986.
38. Mafee MF, Peyman GA, Peace JH, et al.: Magnetic resonance imaging in the evaluation and differentiation of uveal melanoma. Ophthalmology 94:341–8, 1987.
39. Hesselink JR, et al.: Computerized tomography of the paranasal sinuses and face—part I and II. J Comp Asst Tomogr 2:559, 1978.
40. Noyek AM, Kassel EE, Gruss JS, et al.: Sophisticated CT and complex maxillo facial trauma. Laryngoscope 92:1–17, 1982.
41. Mafee MF, Chow JM, Meyers R: Functional endoscopic sinus surgery: anatomy, CT screening, indications, and complications. Am J Radiol 160:735–744, 1993.
42. Chow JM, Mafee MF: Radiologic assessment pre-operative to endoscopic sinus surgery. Otolaryngol Clin North Am 22: 691–701, 1989.
43. Mafee MF: Modern imaging of paranasal sinuses and the role of limited sinus computerized tomography; consideration of time, cost and radiation. ENT J 8:532–546, 1994.
44. Mancuso AA, Bohman L, Hanafee WN, et al: Computed tomography of the nasopharynx: normal and variation of normal. Radiology 137:113, 1980.
45. Curtin HD: Separation of the masticator space from the parapharyngeal space. Radiology 163:195, 1987.
46. Clemente CD: Gray's Anatomy, 30th American Ed., Philadelphia, Lea & Febiger, 1984.
47. Hanafee WN.: Sialography—Part V. In: Radiology of the Ear, Nose and Throat. Edited by Valvassori GE, et al. Stuttgart, Georg Thieme, 1982.
48. Hanafee WN: Radiology of the pharynx and larynx—Part IV. In: Radiology of the Ear, Nose and Throat. Edited by Valvassori GE, et al. Stuttgart, Georg Thieme, 1982.
49. Mancuso AA, et al.: The role of computed tomography in the management of cancer of larynx. Radiology 124:243, 1977.
50. Mafee MF: Normal CT anatomy of the larynx. Radiol Clin North Am 22:251, 1984.
51. Ward PH, Hanafee W, Mancuso A, et al.: Evaluation of the computerized tomography, cinelaryngology and laryngology

in determining the extent of laryngeal disease. Ann Otol Rhinol Laryngol *88*:454–456, 1979.

52. Pullen FW: The use of computerized tomography in otolaryngology. Trans Am Acad Ophthalmol Otolaryngol *84*:622–627, 1977.

53. Mancuso AA, Hanafee WN: Computerized tomography of the injured larynx. Radiology *133*:139, 1979.

54. Mafee MF, Schild JA, Valvassori GE, Capek V: Computed tomography of the larynx: correlated anatomy and pathologic macrosection studies. Radiology *147*:123–128, 1983.

55. Schild JA, Mafee MF, Valvassori GE, et al: Laryngeal malignancies and computerized tomography—a correlation of tomographic and histopathologic findings. Ann Otolaryngol Rhinol Laryngol *91*:571–575, 1982.

56. Archer CR, Yeager BL: Evaluation of laryngeal cartilages by computed tomography. J Comput Assist Tomogr *3*:604, 1979.

57. Noyek AM, Shulman HS, Steinhardt M: Contemporary laryngeal radiology a clinical perspective. J Otolaryngol *11*:178–85, 1982.

58. Mafee MF, Valvassori GE, Dobben GD: Role of Radiology in surgery of the ear and skull base. In: Symposium on complications in surgery of the ear and skull base. Edited by Wiet RJ. Otolaryngol Clin North Am *15*:723–754, 1982.

59. Mafee MF, Carter BL, (eds). Valvassori—Imaging of the head and neck. Georg Thieme Verlag, Stuttgart, 1994.

60. Mafee MF, Kumar A, Heffner DK: Epidermoid cyst (cholesteatoma) and cholesterol granuloma of the temporal bone and epidermoid cysts affecting the brain. Neuroimag Clin North Am *3*:561–578, 1994.

61. Mafee MF, Aimi K, Valvassori GE. Computed tomography in the diagnosis of primary tumors of the temporal bone. Laryngoscope *94*:1423–1430, 1984.

62. Bohman L, et al: CT approach to benign nasopharyngeal masses. AJNR *1*:513, 1980.

63. Som PM, Braun IF, Shapiro MD, et al. Tumors of the parapharyngeal space and upper neck: MR imaging characteristics. Radiology *104*:823–829, 1987.

64. Mafee MF. Imaging methods for sinusitis. JAMA *20*:2808, 1993.

65. Hawkins DB, Clark RW: Orbital involvement in acute sinusitis. Clin Pediatr *16*(5):464, 1977.

66. Som PM, Shugar JMA: The classification of ethmoid mucoceles. J Comput Assist Tomogr *4*:199, 1980.

67. Gould LV, Cummings CW, Raguzzi DD, et al.: Use of computerized axial tomography of the head and neck region. Laryngoscope *87*:1270–6, 1977.

68. Zimmerman RA, Bilaniuk LT: Computed tomography of sphenoid sinus tumors. Comput Axial Tomogr *1*:25, 1977.

69. Chernak ES, et al: The use of computed tomography for radiation therapy treatment planning. Radiology *117*:613, 1975.

70. Mafee MF: Nonepithelial tumors of the paranasal sinuses and nasal cavity. Role of CT and MR Imaging. Radiol Clin North Am *31*:75–90, 1993.

71. Chow JM, Leonetti JP, Mafee MF: Epithelial tumors of the paranasal sinuses and nasal cavity. Radiol Clin North Am *31*:61–75, 1993.

72. Grove AS, Fr.: Orbital trauma evaluation for computed tomography. Comput Tomogr *3*:264, 1981.

73. Zilka A: Computed tomography of bow-out fracture of the medial orbital wall. AJNR *2*:427, 1981.

74. Drayer BP, et al: Cerebrospinal fluid rhinnorhea demonstrated by metrizamide cisternography. Am J Roentgenol *129*:149, 1977.

75. Nabawi P, Mafee MF, Phillips J, et al: The success rate of metrizamide CT cisternography in the evaluation of cerebrospinal fluid (CSF) rhinnorhea. Comput Radiol (In press).

76. Manelfe C, et al: Cerebrospinal fluid rhinnorhea—evaluation with metrizamide. Am J Neuroradiol *3*:25, 1982.

38 Imaging of the Temporal Bone

Galdino E. Valvassori

The temporal bone is unique in the human body because it contains, in the small volume of a cubic inch, a concentration of vital osseous and membranous structures surrounded by a more or less extensive system of pneumatic cells. Because of the different densities of its bony components and of the air- and fluid-filled spaces around and within them, the temporal bone lends itself to accurate visualization and assessment by various imaging procedures.

Conventional radiography, computed tomography, magnetic resonance, and arteriography are the techniques currently used to study the temporal bone and auditory-vestibular pathways. The otolaryngologist should know how to select the proper procedure for the anatomic area and the clinical problem under investigation.

CONVENTIONAL RADIOGRAPHY

Today, the use of conventional radiography is limited to evaluation of the mastoid pneumatization and assessment of the position and integrity of cochlear implant electrodes. The latter cannot be established by tomographic techniques because the wires often are visualized in several contiguous sections, and therefore, their continuity cannot be demonstrated. Only three projections are of practical interest: the lateral or Schuller's, the frontal or transorbital, and the oblique or Stenvers'. The other special projections have historic significance but no useful clinical application.

Schuller's or Rungstrom's Projection

The Schuller's projection is a lateral view of the mastoid obtained with a cephalocaudad angulation of the x-ray beam of 25 to 30 degrees. The patient's head is turned so that the sagittal plane of the skull becomes parallel to the table top and the side under examination is closer to the film. Proper centering is obtained by placing the external auditory meatus of the side to be examined 1 cm above the center of the film or of the table top.

The extent of the pneumatization of the mastoid, distribution of the air cells, degree of aeration, and status of the trabecular pattern are the main features of this projection (Fig. 38–1). The anterior plate of the vertical portion of the sigmoid sinus groove (corresponding to the most lateral part of the posterior aspect of the petrous pyramid) casts an almost vertical line, slightly concave posteriorly in its upper portion, superimposed on the air cells. At its upper extremity, this line joins another line that slopes gently forward and downward to form the sinodural angle of Citelli. The latter line is produced by the superior aspect of the lateral portion of the petrous pyramid. The more medial portion of the superior petrous ridge, from the arcuate eminence to the apex, has been displaced downward by the angulation of the x-ray beam and casts a line that extends forward and downward, crossing the epitympanic area, and more anteriorly, the neck of the mandibular condyle. Above this line, the upper portion of the attic with the head of the malleus is usually visible. Finally, the temporomandibular joint is outlined.

Transorbital Projection

This view can be obtained with either the patient's face to or away from the film. The patient's head is flexed on the chin until the orbitomeatal line is perpendicular to the table top. For better details, each side should be obtained separately, and the central x-ray beam should be directed at the center of the orbit of the side under examination and perpendicular to the film.

The petrous apex is outlined clearly but foreshortened because of its obliquity to the plane of the film. The internal auditory canal is visualized in its full

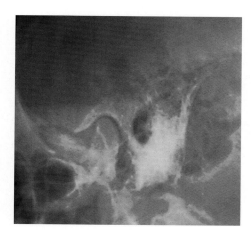

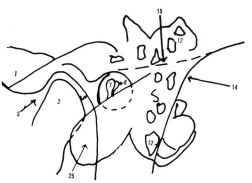

Fig. 38–1. Schuller's projection: (1) root of the zygoma; (2) condyle of the mandible; (3) temporomandibular joint; (7) malleus; (8) incus; (12) air cells; (14) anterior plate of the sigmoid sinus; (15) dural plate; (25) petrous apex.

length as a horizontal band of radiolucency extending through the petrous pyramid (Fig. 38–2). At the medial end of the canal, the free margin of the posterior wall casts a well-defined and smooth margin, concave medially. Often, the radiolucent band of the internal auditory canal seems to extend medially to the lip of the posterior wall into the petrous apex. This band is not caused by the internal auditory canal but is produced by the medial extension of the upper and lower lips of the porus (opening) of the canal and by the interposed groove. Lateral to the internal auditory canal, the radiolucency of the vestibule and of the superior and horizontal semicircular canals are usually detectable. The apical and middle coils of the cochlea are superimposed on the lateral portion of the internal auditory canal, whereas the basilar turn is visible underneath it and the vestibule.

Stenvers' Projection

The patient is positioned facing the film, with the head slightly flexed and rotated 45 degrees toward the side opposite the one under examination. The lateral rim of the orbit of the side under investigation should lie in close contact with the table top. The x-ray beam is angulated 14 degrees caudad.

The entire petrous apex is visualized in its full length lateral to the orbital rim (Fig. 38–3). The porus of the internal auditory canal seen on the face appears as an oval-shaped radiolucency open medially and limited laterally by the free margin of the posterior canal wall. Lateral to the porus, the internal auditory canal appears foreshortened. The vestibule and semicircular canals, especially the posterior, which lies in this projection in a plane parallel to the film, are usually recognizable. On the outside, the entire mastoid is outlined, with the mastoid process free from superimpositions.

COMPUTED TOMOGRAPHY

Computed tomography (CT) has replaced multidirectional tomography as the study of choice for the diagnosis and assessment of intratemporal pathology.

Computed tomography is a radiographic technique that allows measurement of small absorption coefficients and differentials not recognizable by previously available recording or displaying systems.

The scan is initiated at a chosen level and the x-ray tube, collimated to a thin or pencil beam, rotates

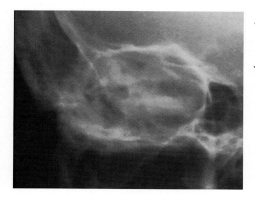

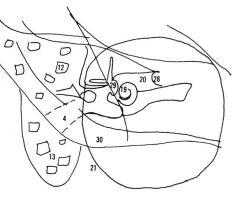

Fig. 38–2. Transorbital projection: (4) external auditory canal; (12) air cells; (13) mastoid process; (19) cochlea; (20) internal auditory canal; (21) orbital rim; (28) medial lip of the posterior wall of the internal auditory canal; (29) vestibule; (30) base of the skull.

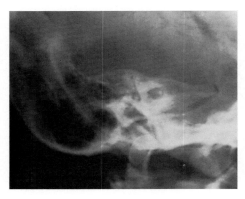 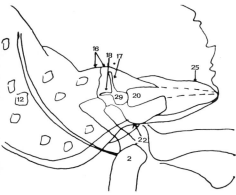

Fig. 38–3. Stenvers' projection: (2) condyle of the mandible; (12) air cells; (16) arcuate eminence; (17) superior semicircular canal; (18) horizontal semicircular canal; (20) internal auditory canal; (22) basilar turn of the cochlea; (25) petrous apex; (29) vestibule.

around the patient. The transmitted x-rays are picked up by detectors arrayed along the circumference of the tube trajectory, converted into electronic current and amplified and transmitted to the computer for storing and processing. The computer analyzes this data and develops an image on a 320/320 picture element (pixel) matrix, where the brightness of each point is proportional to the attenuation coefficient.

Spatial resolution of CT is measured by the volume of tissue represented by the displayed pixel. In the later generation of CT scanners, spatial resolution has been reduced to 0.1 cubic millimeter by a special software reconstruction technique of the area of interest. Narrowing the collimator of the x-ray beam and the aperture of each detector has reduced the slice thickness to 1.5 mm.

The study is often performed after intravenous injection of iodinated contrast agents that produce an increase in density value or enhancement of several anatomical structures and pathologic tissues.

Enhancement of the lesion after intravenous administration of contrast material allows the recognition of vascular lesions such as a glomus tumor and vascular structures such as the jugular bulb and the internal carotid artery. Further differentiation of the type of vascular lesions can be obtained by prefixed dynamic scanning, in which six or more consecutive scans of a single preselected section demonstrating the mass are obtained in 30 seconds. The exposure starts simultaneously with the bolus injection of 30 to 45 ml of contrast material. A curve, characteristic of the type of lesion, is obtained by plotting amount of enhancement expressed in CT numbers versus time.

CT Projections of the Temporal Bone

Horizontal or Axial Projection
This is the basic projection of the CT study. It is comfortable for the patient, who lies supine on the table, and is easy to obtain and reproduce. It allows a good demonstration of the external, middle, and inner ear

(Fig. 38–4), except for the structures parallel to the plane of section, such as the tegmen.

Coronal or Frontal Projection
The patient lies on the table, either prone or supine, with the head overextended. The gantry of the scanner is often tilted to compensate for an incomplete extension of the head. This projection is indispensable to complement the axial sections (Fig. 38–5), but often difficult to obtain, particularly in young children and older people.

Twenty Degrees Coronal Oblique Projection
This projection is a modification of the coronal for the study of the medial wall of the tympanic cavity. The medial or labyrinthine wall of the middle ear forms an angle, open posteriorly, of 15 to 25 degrees with the midsagittal plane of the skull. The patient is first positioned as for the coronal projection, and the head is then rotated 20 degrees toward the side under examination so that the medial wall becomes perpendicular to the plane of section. For this projection, we position the patient prone with the head overextended and the chin resting on a special head holder devised by Dr. Zonneveld in Holland. This projection is particularly useful for the study of the oval window, promontory, and tympanic segment of the facial canal (Fig. 38–6). It should be used in all patients with otosclerosis.

Sagittal or Lateral Projection
It is impossible or extremely difficult to obtain direct sagittal sections. However, computer-reconstructed sagittal images can be obtained from the raw data collected for the horizontal sections. This is particularly true if fast or spiral CT is used, and thin sections at 1-mm increments are obtained. Although these images are not as satisfactory as the direct sections, they are usually sufficient for the demonstration of the mastoid segment of the facial canal and of the vestibular aqueduct.

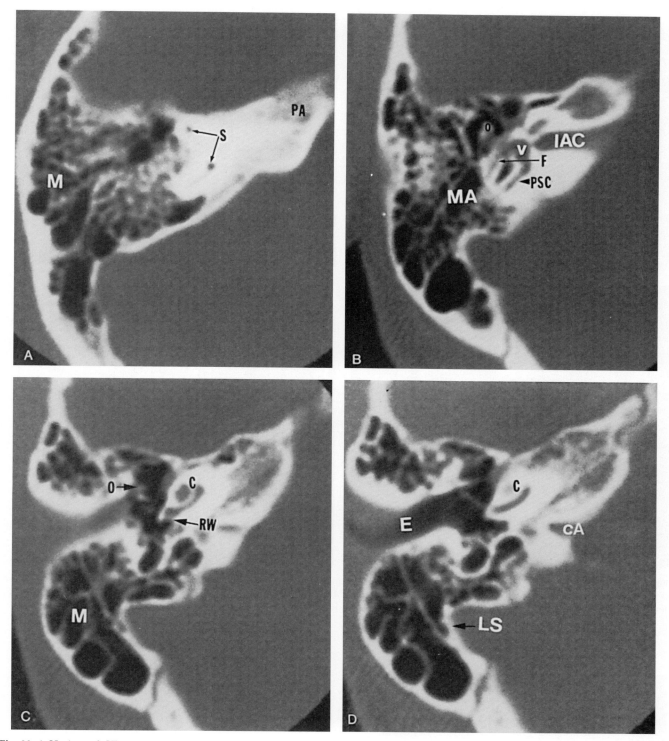

Fig. 38–4. Horizontal CT sections of a normal right temporal bone, in sequence from top to bottom: A. M, Mastoid; S, superior semicircular canal; PA, petrous apex. B. MA, Mastoid antrum; O, ossicles; V, vestibule; F, facial nerve canal; IAC, internal auditory canal; PSC, posterior semicircular canal. C. C, Cochlea; RW, round window. D. E, External auditory canal; CA, cochlear aqueduct; LS, lateral sinus plate.

MAGNETIC RESONANCE IMAGING

Magnetic resonance imaging (MRI) is an imaging modality capable of producing cross sections of the human body in any plane without exposing the patient to ionizing radiation. Magnetic resonance images are obtained by the interaction of hydrogen nuclei or protons of the human body, high magnetic fields, and radio frequency pulses. The strength of the MR signal to be converted into imaging data depends on the con-

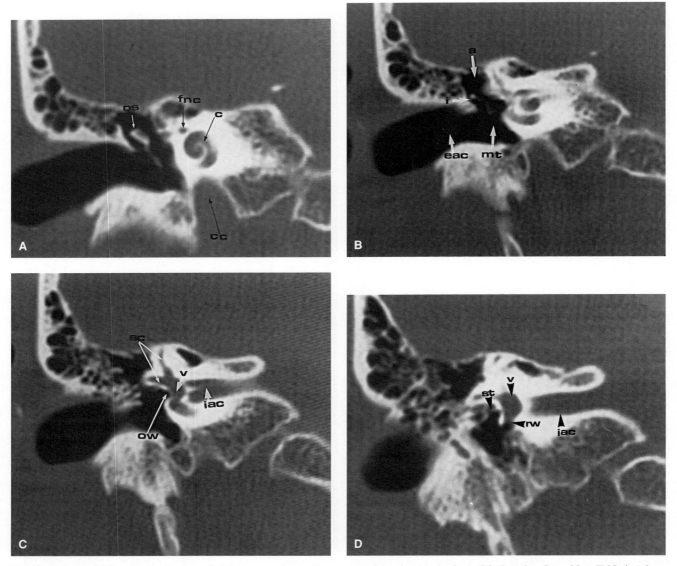

Fig. 38–5. Coronal CT sections of a normal right temporal bone in sequence from front to back. A. OS, Ossicles; C, cochlea; FNC, facial nerve canal; CC, carotid canal. B. EAC, External auditory canal; A, attic; MT, mesotympanum; I, incus. C. OW, Oval window; V, vestibule; SC, semicircular canals; IAC, internal auditory canal. D. RW, Round window; ST, sinus tympani.

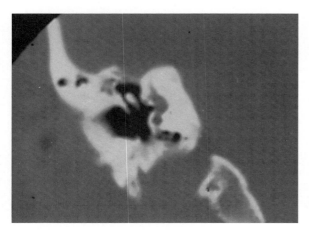

Fig. 38–6. Twenty-degree coronal oblique section of a normal right temporal bone. The oval window forms a well-defined opening in the lateral wall of the vestibule underneath the horizontal semicircular canal and above the promontory.

centration of the free hydrogen nuclei or protons and on two magnetic relaxation times, T1 and T2, which are tissue-specific. One of the characteristics of MR is the possibility of changing appearance and therefore information of the images by changing the contribution of the T1 and T2 relaxation times. This is accomplished by varying the time between successive pulses (TR or repetition time) and the time that the emitted signal or echo is measured after the pulse (TE or echo time).

Examination is performed with the patient supine and the plane extending from the tragus to the inferior orbital rim perpendicular to the table top.

Different projections are obtained by changing the orientation of the magnetic field gradients without moving the patient's head. Axial, coronal, and sagittal projections are usually obtained.

T1 images obtained by a short TR and TE offer the best anatomical delineation. T2 images obtained with long TR and TE better differentiate normal from pathologic tissues.

Air, cortical bone, and calcifications contain few free protons and therefore appear in the images as dark areas of no signal. Fat and body fluid are rich in free protons and produce signals of high intensity, fat in

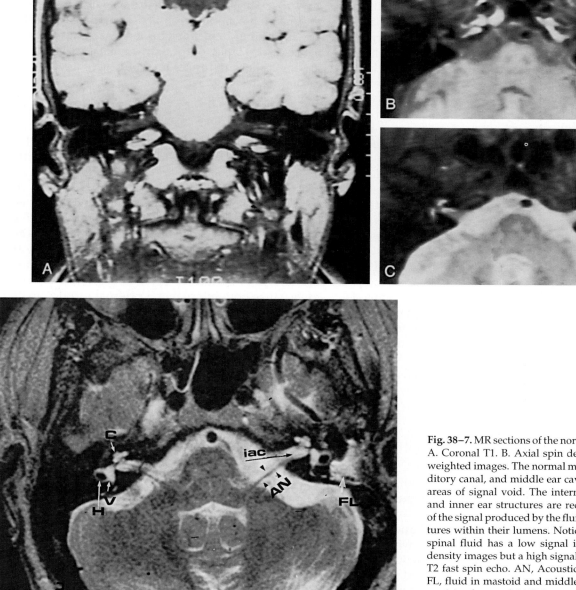

Fig. 38–7. MR sections of the normal temporal bone. A. Coronal T1. B. Axial spin density. C. Axial T2-weighted images. The normal mastoid, external auditory canal, and middle ear cavity appear as dark areas of signal void. The internal auditory canals and inner ear structures are recognizable because of the signal produced by the fluid and neural structures within their lumens. Notice that the cerebrospinal fluid has a low signal in the T1 and spin density images but a high signal in the T2. D. Axial T2 fast spin echo. AN, Acoustic nerve; C, cochlea; FL, fluid in mastoid and middle ear; H, horizontal semicircular canal; IAC, internal auditory canal; V, vestibule.

the T1, and fluid in the T2 weighted images. Blood vessels usually appear as areas of signal void because the stimulated protons of the circulating blood have moved out of the section before their emitted signals can be detected. Because cortical or nondiploic bone and air emit no signal, the normal mastoid, external auditory canal, and middle ear appear in the MR images as dark areas without pattern or structures within them. The petrous pyramid is equally dark except for a gray or white cast of the inner ear structures and internal auditory canal produced by the fluid within their lumens (Fig. 38–7).

Pathologic processes are demonstrated by MRI whenever the hydrogen density and relaxation times of the pathological tissues are different from the normal. The intravenous injection of ferromagnetic contrast agents (gadolinium DPTA and gadolinium chelate) has improved the recognition and differentiation of pathological processes. Because the contrast material does not penetrate the intact blood barrier, normal brain does not enhance except for structures such as the pituitary gland and several cranial nerves that lack a complete blood-brain barrier. Enhancement of brain lesions occurs whenever the blood-brain barrier is disrupted, provided there is sufficient blood flow to the lesions. Extra-axial lesions such as meningiomas and neuromas lack a blood-brain barrier and therefore undergo a strong enhancement.

Fluid, blood, and soft tissue masses within the temporal bone are identified readily by MRI as areas of abnormally high-signal intensity. The exact location, extent, and involvement of bony structures such as the ossicles, scutum, and labyrinthine capsule cannot be detected, however. For this reason, CT remains the study of choice for the assessment of intratemporal pathology with the exception of the petrous apex.

The images shown in this chapter were obtained with a super-conducting magnet and a magnetic field of 15,000 gauss or 1.5 tesla. The higher the magnetic field, the higher the signal-to-noise ratio and therefore the thinner the sections that can be obtained. A further improvement in details has been accomplished for structures close to the surface of the body by the use of surface receiver coils.

ANGIOGRAPHY

Gradient-echo techniques and flow-encoding gradients have enabled the development of magnetic resonance angiography (MRA).

Time of flight (TOF) angiography is a gradient-echo technique in which the stationary tissues within the imaging plane are saturated with the magnetic field so that they will not produce a signal. Blood flowing within the same plane is unsaturated and will be the only tissue to produce a signal.

Phase-contrast (PC) angiography is acquired differently. Instead of saturating the stationary tissues with radio frequency pulses, a bipolar gradient of magnetization is applied to the entire slice, first with a positive value and then with a negative value. In the stationary tissues, the two opposite gradients cancel each other out. In the flowing blood, however, the two opposite gradients cannot cancel each other out because the blood will have moved to a different plane in the region before the inverse gradient is applied.

The obtained slices are reconstructed into projection images, which can be rotated in different planes to separate vessels and eliminate superimposition. Magnetic resonance angiography of the intracranial vasculature has been particularly useful in the demonstration of aneurysms in the region of the circle of Willis (Fig. 38–8), arteriovenous malformation (AVM) (particularly a small dural AVM that may not be visible on routine spin-echo images), and vasoocclusive pathology including dural sinus thrombosis. Magnetic resonance angiography of the extracranial circulation provides excellent information about the patency of the carotid and vertebral arteries. These vessels may be compressed or displaced by neck masses and their lumens stenosed or obstructed by thrombosis or atheromatous plaques.

Conventional angiography is seldom required for the diagnosis of vascular tumors or anomalies within or adjacent to the temporal bone. Arteriography is, however, mandatory for identifying the feeding vessels of lesions, usually glomus tumors, whenever embolization or surgical ligation is contemplated. Subtraction is necessary to delineate the vascular mass and feeding vessels, which are otherwise obscured by the density of the surrounding temporal bone. The injection should be performed in the common carotid artery to visualize both internal and external carotid circulation. A vertebral arteriogram may also be performed.

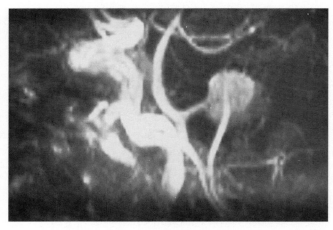

Fig. 38–8. MRA demonstrating an aneurysm of the left vertebral artery. The aneurysm compresses the acoustic nerve and mimics an acoustic neurinoma.

Retrograde jugular venography is rarely used for the diagnosis of a high jugular bulb or glomus tumor. The study is done by percutaneous puncture of the vein with a Seldinger needle.

PATHOLOGIC CONDITIONS

The pathologic conditions of the ear and temporal bone will be reviewed by anatomic location. Seven sites of involvement are considered: mastoid, external auditory canal, middle ear, inner ear, petrous pyramid, facial nerve canal, and cerebellopontine angle.

Mastoid

Conventional views and CT are used for the study of this region.

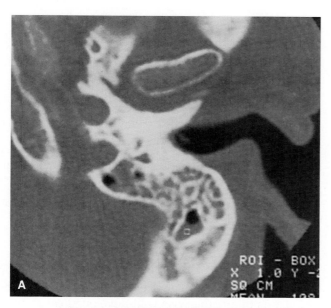

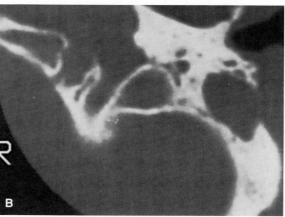

Fig. 38–9. A. Acute mastoiditis. This axial CT section of the left mastoid shows clouding and air-fluid levels within the air cells. The trabecular pattern is intact. B. Coalescent mastoiditis, axial CT section of the left mastoid. A large coalescent cavity is noticed in the mastoid with erosion of the outer cortex and formation of a subperiosteal abscess.

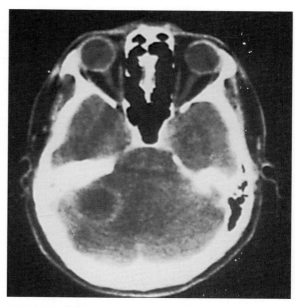

Fig. 38–10. Cerebellar abscess, axial CT section of the posterior cranial fossa obtained after infusion of contrast material. The abscess appears as an area of low density surrounded by a ring of enhancement.

Acute Mastoiditis
The early findings of acute mastoiditis are diffuse and homogeneous clouding of the middle ear cavity and mastoid air cells, and often air-fluid levels within the air cells (Fig. 38–9A). With the progression of the process, the mastoid trabeculae become first demineralized and then destroyed, with formation of coalescent areas of suppuration (Fig. 38–9B). Involvement of the posterior sinus plate often leads to thrombophlebitis of the lateral sinus and to posterior fossa abscesses (Fig. 38–10), whereas erosion of the tegmen may lead to extension of the infection into the middle cranial fossa.

Chronic Mastoiditis
The mastoid is often poorly pneumatized, and the mastoid antrum and mastoid air cells appear nonhomogeneously cloudy. Reactive new bony formation produces thickening of the trabeculae (Fig. 38–11), which may lead to complete obliteration of the air cells (sclerotic mastoiditis).

Eosinophilic Granuloma
Lytic lesions of variable size are observed in the mastoid and temporal squama. In the involved areas, the trabecular pattern is completely erased and the mastoid cortex may be thinned out, destroyed, or expanded (Fig. 38–12).

External Auditory Canal

Computed tomography is the study of choice, but MRI may add useful information whenever the lesion ex-

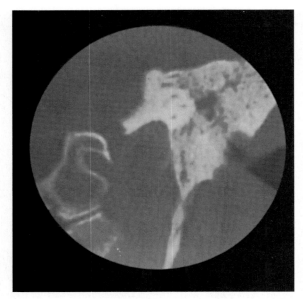

Fig. 38–11. Chronic mastoiditis, coronal CT section. The trabeculae are thickened and the air cells cloudy and partially obliterated.

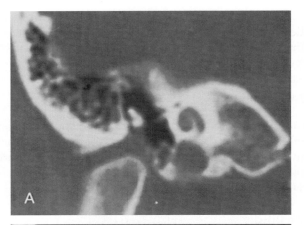

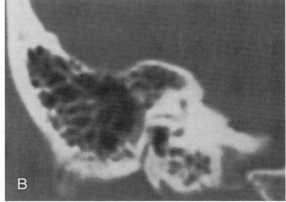

Fig. 38–13. Agenesis of the right external auditory canal, coronal CT sections. A. The external auditory canal is absent and the mandibular condyle is displaced posteriorly and lies lateral to the atretic plate. The middle ear cavity is aerated and normal in size, but the head of the malleus and body of the incus appear malformed and fused. B. The mastoid is well pneumatized and clear. The vertical segment of the facial canal is rotated slightly outward.

tends outside the confines of the canal into the adjacent structures.

Congenital

Microtia of varying degrees is often associated with dysplasia of the external auditory canal, although no direct correlation exists between the two anomalies. The degree of malformation of the external auditory canal varies from complete agenesis of the tympanic

bone (Fig. 38–13) and canal to stenosis of its lumen and atresia of an otherwise well-developed canal by a bony plate, usually lateral. The small tissue tag and pit often observed in patients with atresia of the canal often have no topographic relationship to the underlying mastoid and middle ear.

Trauma

Fractures of the external auditory canal are the result of a longitudinal fracture of the temporal bone, direct trauma to the anterior wall after a blow to the mandible, or projectile missiles such as bullets or metallic fragments from industrial accidents. Longitudinal fractures usually pass from the temporal squama into the superior canal wall. The fracture often extends to the anterior canal wall and temporomandibular joint.

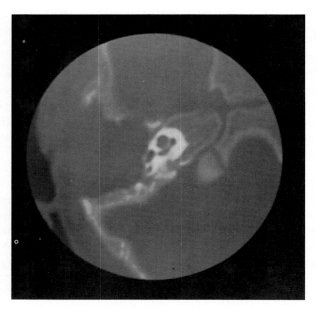

Fig. 38–12. Eosinophilic granuloma, axial CT section of the right ear. A large lytic lesion involves the right mastoid, external auditory canal and middle ear. A soft tissue mass fills the cavity.

Necrotizing External Otitis

This condition, also known as malignant external otitis, is an acute osteomyelitis of the temporal bone that occurs in debilitated, diabetic and immunosuppressed patients and is usually caused by the Pseudomonas bacterium. The infection starts in the external canal and spreads rapidly to the other portions of the temporal bone and adjacent areas. Computed tomography reveals erosion of the external canal, particularly of its floor, and stenosis of the lumen of the canal caused by soft tissue swelling. The infection may then spread inferiorly along the undersurface of the temporal bone to the facial nerve at the stylomastoid foramen, anteriorly to the temporomandibular fossa, posteriorly to the mastoid, and medially into the middle ear and petrous pyramid (Fig. 38–14).

External Auditory Canal Cholesteatoma

This lesion is caused either by blockage of the canal, with consequent accumulation of epithelial debris (keratosis obliterans), or by dyskeratosis with localized accumulation of debris on the floor of the canal (invasive keratitis). In the first type, a soft tissue mass fills and expands the canal medial to the site of stenosis or obstruction (Fig. 38–15). In the second type, the lumen of the canal is patent, but areas of bony erosion are demonstrated in the involved portion of the canal.

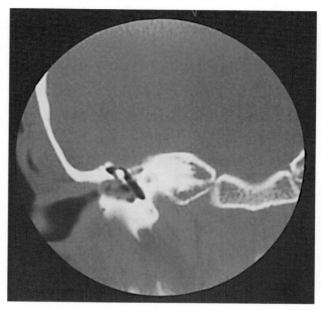

Fig. 38–15. External auditory canal cholesteatoma, coronal section of the right ear. The cholesteatoma fills and obstructs the bony external auditory canal. The cholesteatoma erodes the inferior margin of the lateral wall of the attic and extends into the attic lateral to the ossicles.

When the cholesteatoma is large and erodes the anulus, it may extend into the middle ear cavity.

Carcinoma

Carcinoma of the temporal bone usually arises in the external auditory canal. The CT findings vary with the extent of the lesion. In an early lesion, portions of the bony wall of the external auditory canal are eroded (Fig. 38–16). When further destruction occurs, the tumor may spread anteriorly into the temporomandibular fossa; posteriorly into the mastoid, where it often reaches the facial canal; and medially into the middle ear, jugular fossa, petrous pyramid, and labyrinth. Extension into the mastoid and petrous pyramid causes a typical moth-eaten appearance because of infiltration of the bone.

Middle Ear and Ossicular Chain

Computed tomography is the study of choice for pathologic processes that arise in the middle ear and involve the ossicular chain.

Because granulation tissue enhances after the injection of paramagnetic agents, MRI with contrast is useful in some cases to differentiate granulation tissue from fluid and cholesteatoma, which have a similar density in the CT sections.

Congenital

Malformations of the middle ear space vary from minor hypoplasia to complete agenesis. In the majority

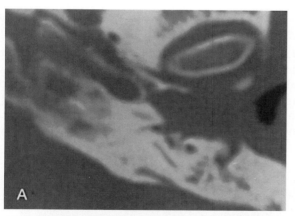

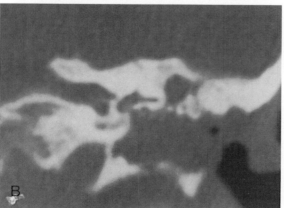

Fig. 38–14. Necrotizing external otitis. Axial (A) and coronal (B) CT sections of the left ear. There is erosion of all walls of the external auditory canal with stenosis of the lumen of the canal caused by soft tissue swelling. The infection has eroded the lateral wall of the attic and spread into the middle ear.

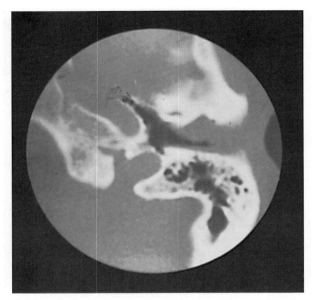

Fig. 38–16. Carcinoma of the left external auditory canal, axial CT section. The anterior wall of the external auditory canal is eroded by an adjacent soft tissue mass. The lesion does not extend into the middle ear cavity.

of the cases with an atretic external auditory canal, the middle ear cavity is normal in size and aerated. The head of the malleus and body of the incus are often fused (Fig. 38–13A) and fixed to the atretic plate at the level of the malleus neck. If the middle ear cavity is grossly hypoplastic, the malleus and incus form a rudimentary amalgam that is often in an ectopic position (Fig. 38–17). A congenital anomaly may be confined to the ossicular chain, which may be malformed or fixed.

Malformations of the stapes superstructures and fixation of the stapes footplate are not uncommon, isolated defects. Computed tomography sections in 20-degree coronal oblique projection are indispensable for the study of the stapes and oval window. The jugular bulb sometimes projects into the hypo- or mesotympanum. The bulb may be covered by a thin bony shell or may be exposed in the middle ear, often in contact with the medial surface of the tympanic membrane, and thus mimicking a glomus tumor. Whenever the diagnosis is in doubt, we perform a dynamic CT study at the level of the middle-ear mass. A high jugular bulb is characterized by a high venous peak at 20 to 25 seconds. A jugular venogram is seldom necessary. The intratemporal segment of the carotid artery may take an ectopic course through the middle ear. In these cases, the CT examination shows a soft tissue mass extending throughout the entire length of the middle ear cavity to regain its normal position in the petrous apex (Fig. 38–18). The proximal portion of the carotid artery, rather than being located underneath the cochlea, enters the temporal bone through a canal or defect in the floor of the posterior hypotympanum. A dynamic CT study produces a graph with a high arterial peak at 10 to 15 seconds. A carotid arteriogram may be used to confirm the anomalous course of the artery.

Trauma

The middle ear cavity is usually involved in longitudinal fractures of the temporal bone. Computed tomography permits precise evaluation of the course of the fracture and status of the ossicular chain. A fracture line may disappear at a certain level only to reappear

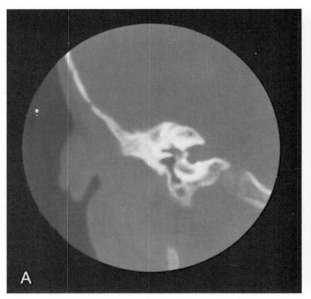
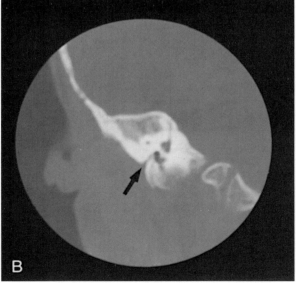

Fig. 38–17. Congenital malformation of the right external and middle ear, coronal CT sections. A. Agenesis of the external auditory canal with hypoplasia of the attic and rudimentary ossicular mass. B. Notice the lack of development of the mastoid pneumatization and the outward rotation of the vertical segment of the facial canal (arrow).

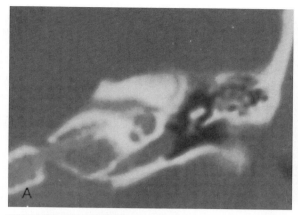

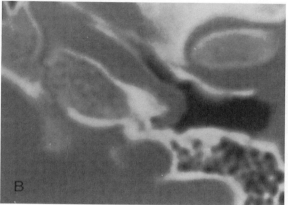

Fig. 38–18. Ectopic left internal carotid artery. Coronal (A) and axial (B) CT sections. The ectopic carotid artery courses throughout the entire length of the middle ear cavity. Notice the absence of the proximal portion of the carotid canal normally seen underneath the cochlea and of the bony wall dividing the anterior mesotympanum from the horizontal segment of the carotid canal.

a few millimeters distant. This apparent gap is not caused by interruption of the fracture line but rather by a change in its course so that the fracture becomes invisible in some of the sections. The tegmen is usually involved, and cerebrospinal fluid otorrhea or rhinorrhea occurs whenever the dura is torn. Anterior extension of the fracture may reach the eustachian tube, which becomes obstructed. Conductive hearing loss is usually secondary to disruption of the ossicular chain (Fig. 38–19). The body of the incus is usually rotated and displaced superiorly, posteriorly, and laterally. Interruption at the incudostapedial area results from a fracture of the lenticular process of the incus or the stapes superstructure and from a dislocation of the incudostapedial joint.

Meningocele and Meningoencephalocele

A soft issue mass contiguous to a defect in the tegmen of the mastoid suggests the possibility of a meningocele or meningoencephalocele. If the brain and meninges herniate into the small space of the antrum or epitympanum, the constant pulsation of the cerebrospinal

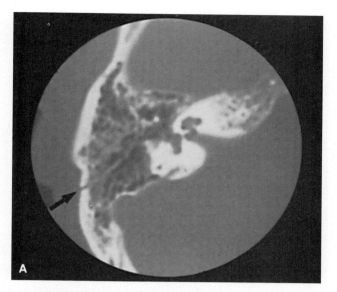

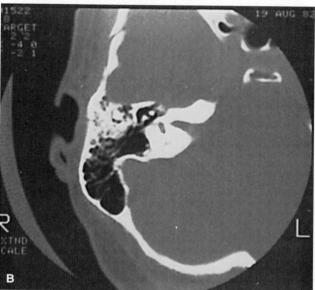

Fig. 38–19. A. Longitudinal fracture of the right temporal bone, axial CT section. The longitudinal fracture extends from the cortex of the posterior portion of the mastoid to the posterosuperior canal wall (arrow). The fracture reaches the attic and disrupts the ossicular chain. The body of the incus is displaced lateralward and posteriorly. B. Longitudinal fracture of the right temporal bone. This horizontal CT section demonstrates fractures of the temporal squama and mastoid with bleeding into the adjacent air cells as well as interruption of the ossicular chain at the incudomalleolar joint.

fluid is transmitted through the walls of the meningocele to cause a gradual resorption of the surrounding bony walls. Computed tomography demonstrates the bony defect in the tegmen and a soft tissue mass filling the mastoid cavity (Fig. 38–20A). This soft tissue lesion cannot be reliably differentiated from a recurrent cholesteatoma, since the absorption coefficients of both lesions are similar. A more definite diagnosis of meningoencephalocele is reached by injecting, by means of

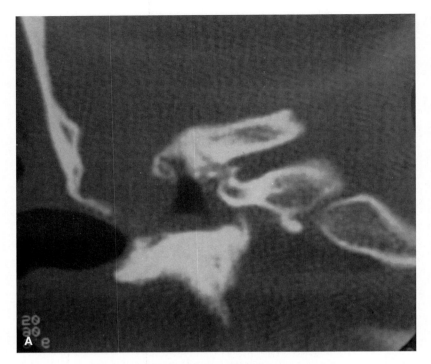

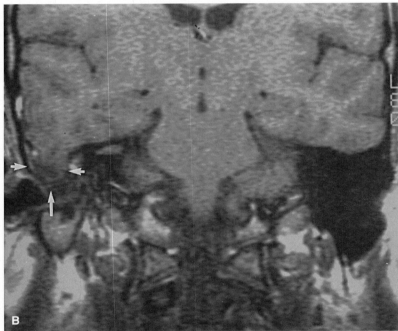

Fig. 38–20. Meningoencephalocele, post modified radical mastoidectomy. A. coronal CT section showing a large defect in the tegmen of the cavity with a soft tissue mass underneath it. B. T1 coronal MR image clearly identifying the soft tissue mass as a brain herniation.

lumbar puncture, a small amount of metrizamide that will diffuse in the subarachnoid space and produce an enhancement of the herniated mass. The differentiation between a meningocele and a cholesteatoma can best be made by MR. On MR, cholesteatoma appears as a lesion of medium signal in the T1 and high signal intensity in T2 images. A meningocele will have the same characteristics as cerebrospinal fluid: low signal intensity in T1 and high intensity in the T2 images. On MR, meningoencephaloceles have the same character-

istics of the adjacent brain, which are quite different from a cholesteatoma (Fig. 38–20B).

Acute Otitis Media
The CT sections demonstrate a nonspecific and diffuse clouding of the middle ear cavity. The tympanic membrane is often swollen and bulges externally.

Chronic Otitis Media
There are two types of chronic otitis media. In chronic suppurative otitis media, a partial, nonhomogeneous

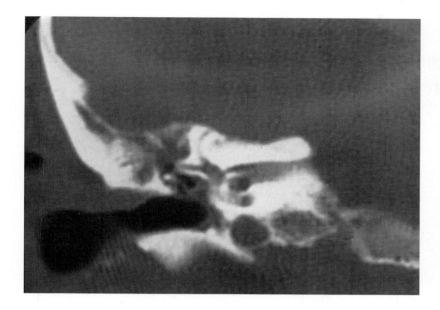

Fig. 38–21. Right chronic otitis media, coronal CT section. The tympanic membrane is thickened and retracted. The mesotympanum is markedly contracted, and the mastoid air cells appear cloudy. Lateral wall of the attic and incudo-stapedial junction are intact.

clouding of the middle ear cavity is caused by granulation tissue, polyps, and fluid or pus. Because the tympanic membrane is perforated, some aeration of the middle ear space is present. Erosion of the long process of the incus is a common finding, whereas erosion of the body of the incus and head of the malleus is rare unless a cholesteatoma is present. In chronic adhesive otitis media, the middle ear space is contracted because of retraction of the tympanic membrane on the promontory (Fig. 38–21). The handle of the malleus is foreshortened, and the long process of the incus is often thinned out or eroded. In these cases, the retracted tympanic membrane may be attached to the head of the stapes with formation of a natural myringostapediopexy. Tympanosclerotic deposits are recognizable by CT whenever they are sufficiently large and calcified. The deposits appear as punctate or linear densities within the tympanic membrane or the mucosa covering the promontory. Large deposits of tympanosclerosis in the attic may surround and fix the ossicles.

Cholesteatoma

Congenital cholesteatomas appear as well-defined soft tissue masses often producing an outward bulge of the intact tympanic membrane (Fig. 38–22). If there is an accompanying serous otitis media, the fluid may obscure the mass as the entire tympanic cavity becomes cloudy. If the lesion extends into the attic, the medial aspect of the lateral wall of the attic is eroded from within.

Acquired cholesteatomas produce a soft tissue mass in the middle ear and typical erosion of the lateral attic wall, posterosuperior canal wall, and ossicles. If the middle-ear cavity is aerated, the soft tissue mass is well outlined. When fluid or inflammatory tissue surrounds the cholesteatoma, the margin of the mass is obscured

because the x-ray densities of cholesteatoma, inflammatory tissue, and fluid are similar. Magnetic resonance imaging with contrast may be useful in these cases to differentiate the enhancing granulation tissue from fluid and cholesteatoma. Different patterns of x-ray findings are observed. Cholesteatomas that arise from the pars flaccida of the tympanic membrane produce erosion of the anterior portion of the lateral wall of the attic and of the anterior tympanic spine (Fig. 38–23). The lesion extends into the attic lateral to the ossicles, which may become medially displaced. Cholesteatomas arising from the pars tensa, usually

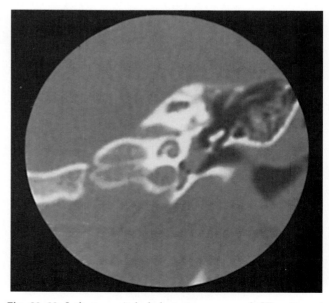

Fig. 38–22. Left congenital cholesteatoma, coronal CT section. A well-defined soft tissue mass lies in the mesotympanum and extends from the intact tympanic membrane to the promontory. The remainder of the middle ear cavity and the mastoid are well aerated.

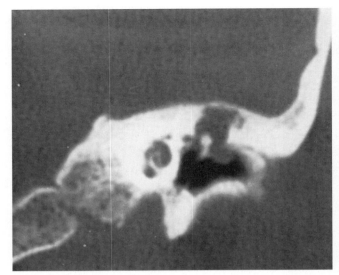

Fig. 38–23. Left attic cholesteatoma, coronal CT section. The lateral wall of the attic is eroded by a soft tissue mass extending into the attic lateral to the ossicles. A polyp protrudes into the external auditory canal through the perforation of the pars flaccida of the tympanic membrane.

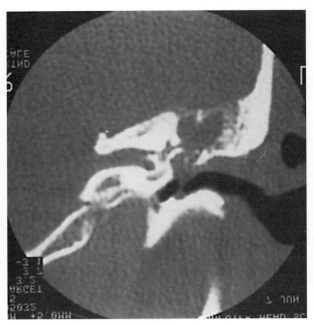

Fig. 38–25. Left cholesteatoma with fistula of the horizontal semicircular canal, coronal CT section. A soft tissue mass fills the upper portion of the mesotympanum and attic. Notice the flattening of the medial wall of the attic and the erosion of the capsule covering the lateral end of the horizontal semicircular canal.

from the posterosuperior margin of the membrane, appear as a soft tissue mass in the middle ear eroding the long process of the incus and extending into the attic medial to the ossicles which may be displaced laterally (Fig. 38–24). The lateral wall of the attic is usually intact, but the posterosuperior canal wall is often eroded. Sometimes a cholesteatoma may involve both the pars flaccida and tensa, producing a mixed x-ray pattern. In advanced cholesteatomas of all types, extensive bony destruction occurs, and no distinct pattern remains. The ossicles in the attic, particularly the body of the incus, are eroded; the aditus is widened; and the mastoid antrum becomes enlarged, cloudy, and smooth in outline because of erosion of the air cells lining the walls of the antrum. Further extension into

the mastoid causes destruction of the trabeculae with formation of large cavities. Erosion of the tegmen may lead to meningeal and intracranial complications. Labyrinthine fistulas occur most commonly in the lateral portion of the horizontal semicircular canal. The CT sections show flattening of the normal convex contour of the horizontal semicircular canal and erosion of the bony capsule covering the lumen of the canal (Fig. 38–25). Further complications of cholesteatoma are extension into the petrous pyramid, which usually occurs in well pneumatized bones, and erosion of the facial canal, which may lead to facial paralysis.

Tumors

Osteomas are frequent in the external auditory canal, but also occur in the middle ear, where they may cause conductive hearing loss by impinging on the ossicular chain. Glomus tumors, also called chemodectomas or nonchromaffin paragangliomas, arise in the middle ear or jugular fossa from minute glomus bodies. Glomus tympanicum tumors arise from glomus bodies along Jacobson nerve on the promontory. The CT sections reveal a soft tissue mass of variable size, usually in the lower portion of the middle ear cavity (Fig. 38–26A). As the lesion enlarges, it may cause a lateral bulge of the tympanic membrane, smooth erosion of the promontory, and involvement of the mastoid and hypotympanic air cells. If the lesion erodes into the jugular fossa, it becomes indistinguishable from a glomus jugulare. A dynamic CT study of a preselected section

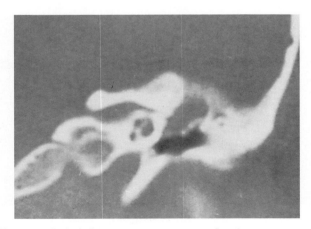

Fig. 38–24. Left cholesteatoma, pars tensa perforation type, coronal CT section. The cholesteatoma extends into the attic medial to the ossicles and displaces the ossicles laterally.

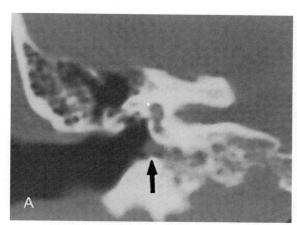

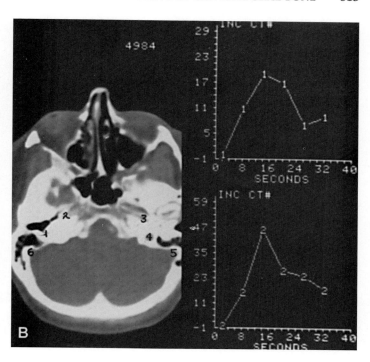

Fig. 38–26. Right glomus tympanicum. A. Coronal CT section showing a small soft tissue mass in the lower portion of the middle ear cavity (arrow). B. Dynamic CT study of the preselected section showing the mass. Graphic display of the circulation in the tumor (1) and internal carotid artery (2). Notice the high peak of the curve at the tumor site at quasiarterial time.

showing the tumor mass generates a curve with a high quasiarterial peak (Fig. 38–26B) rather than the high but delayed venous peak of a high jugular bulb. Selective arteriography with subtraction is indicated to identify feeding vessels before embolization. Carcinomas extend into the middle ear from the external auditory canal. Adenocarcinoma is rare and produces a nonspecific soft tissue mass, often eroding the walls of the middle ear.

Otosclerosis

Otosclerosis that involves the oval window causes fixation of the stapes and consequent conductive hearing loss. A 20-degree coronal oblique is far superior to the other projections for the study of the oval window. In active otosclerosis or otospongiosis, the margin of the oval window becomes decalcified so that the window seems larger than normal. In mature otosclerosis, the oval window becomes narrowed (Fig. 38–27) or closed, and in severe cases the entire oval window niche is obliterated by calcified otosclerotic foci. The x-ray assessment is useful before surgery to confirm the clinical diagnosis, and in some bilateral cases for selection of the ear to be operated on. More important is the study of the post-stapedectomy ear in determining the cause for recurrent or persistent hearing loss and of immediate or delayed vertigo. Computed tomography can demonstrate protrusion of the prosthesis into the vestibule, reobliteration of the oval window with fixation of the strut, dislocation of the medial end of the prosthesis from the oval window, and separation of the lateral end of the strut from the incus or necrosis of the long process of the incus.

Inner Ear

Both CT and MRI are used for the study of the inner ear structures. Computed tomography is best for the study of the labyrinthine capsule; MRI is best for the assessment of the membranous labyrinth.

Congenital

Most cases of congenital sensorineural hearing loss have abnormalities limited to the membranous laby-

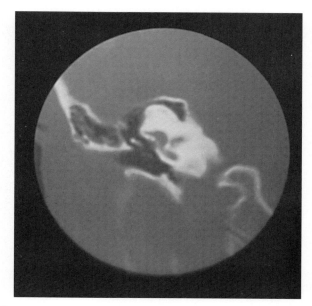

Fig. 38–27. Right stapedial otosclerosis, 20-degree coronal oblique CT section. The oval window appears partially closed by a thickened footplate. The cochlear capsule is normal.

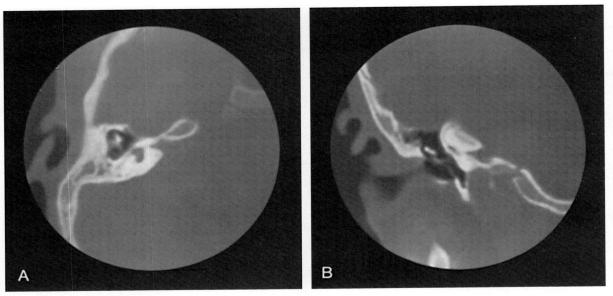

Fig. 38–28. Michel malformation of the right inner ear structures. Axial (A) and coronal (B) CT sections. The middle ear cavity is normal, but the petrous pyramid is hypoplastic. The cochlea is absent or markedly hypoplastic. Notice the cavity in the region of the vestibule with rudimentary semicircular canals.

rinth and therefore not demonstrable by present imaging studies. Defects in the otic capsule are visible by CT. Anomalies may involve a single structure or the entire capsule. The most severe anomaly is the Michel type, which is characterized by hypoplasia of the petrous pyramid and almost complete lack of development of the inner ear structures (Fig. 38–28). A less severe but more common malformation is the Mondini defect, which is characterized by hypoplasia or absence of the bony partitions between the cochlear coils, a

short but wide vestibular aqueduct and dilation of the vestibule, and ampullated ends of the semicircular canals (Fig. 38–29). Enlargement of the vestibular aqueduct, hypoplasia of the cochlea, and internal auditory canal, and deformity of the vestibule and semicircular canals may occur as isolated anomalies. Dilation of the cochlear aqueducts may be responsible for cerebrospinal fluid gush, which sometimes occurs during a stapedectomy for congenital footplate fixation or otosclerosis.

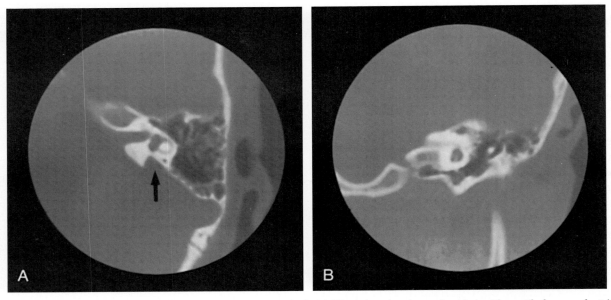

Fig. 38–29. Mondini malformation of the left inner ear structures. A. Axial CT section showing a short but wide vestibular aqueduct (arrow) and a moderate dilatation of the vestibule. B. Coronal CT section. The cochlea appears normal in size, but the absence of the bony partition between the cochlear coils causes the appearance of an empty cochlea.

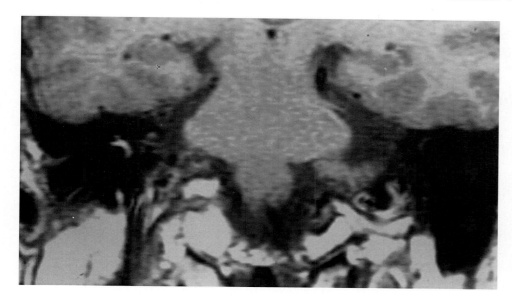

Fig. 38–30. Labyrinthine concussion with bleeding. This T1 coronal MR section shows an area of high signal intensity within the right vestibule and adjacent portion of the semicircular canals.

Trauma

Bleeding within the lumen of the inner ear structures may occur after trauma. If bleeding occurs by concussion without actual fracture, MR may be indicated to confirm the diagnosis. The study should be performed at least 2 days after the injury to allow the transformation of deoxyhemoglobin into methemoglobin, which has a bright signal in both T1 and T2 images (Fig. 38–30).

The inner ear structures are seldom crossed by longitudinal fractures of the temporal bone but are usually involved in transverse fractures. These fractures typically cross the petrous pyramid at a right angle to the longitudinal axis of the pyramid and extend from the dome of the jugular fossa to the superior petrous ridge (Fig. 38–31). Laterally placed fractures involve the promontory, vestibule, horizontal and posterior semicircular canals, and occasionally the tympanic segment of the facial nerve. Medially situated fractures involve the vestibule, cochlea, fundus of the internal auditory canal, and common crus.

Labyrinthitis

Enhancement within the lumen of the bony labyrinth is often observed in MRI obtained after injection of contrast material in patients with acute bacterial and viral labyrinthitis and sudden deafness (Fig. 38–32).

Chronic labyrinthitis varies from a localized reac-

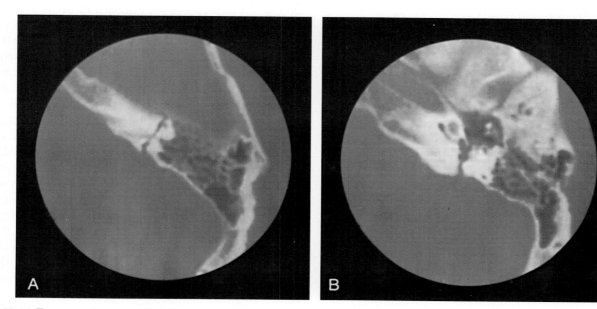

Fig. 38–31. Transverse fracture of the left petrous pyramid. A and B. Axial CT sections. The fracture extends from the superior petrous ridge to the undersurface of the temporal bone crossing the superior semicircular canal, vestibule, and promontory of the cochlea.

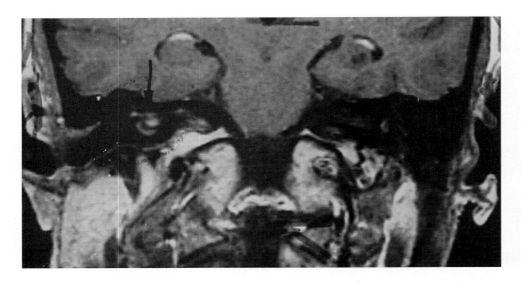

Fig. 38–32. Acute labyrinthitis, presumably viral. This T1 coronal MR image obtained after injection of gadolinium DPTA reveals enhancement within the lumen of the right cochlea (arrow).

tion caused by a fistula of the bony labyrinth to a diffuse process. The lumen of inner ear is partially or totally filled with granulation and fibrous tissues. Osteitis of the bony labyrinth occurs, which may lead to a partial or complete bony obliteration of the lumen (Fig. 38–33). Whereas bony obliteration of the inner ear is readily identified by CT, fibrous obliteration is only recognizable by MRI. In the T2 images, the high signal seen within the normal inner ear structures is absent, therefore making involved structures no longer recognizable.

Labyrinthine Schwannomas

In the past, small schwannomas have been found within the vestibule and cochlea during postmortem dissection of the temporal bones. These lesions are usu-

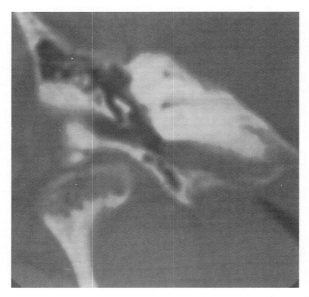

Fig. 38–33. Obliterative labyrinthitis, coronal CT section of the right ear. Notice the complete bony obliteration of the cochlear lumen.

ally not recognizable by CT but are well demonstrated as small enhanced masses in MR examinations performed after injection of contrast material (Fig. 38–34).

Otosclerosis

Otosclerosis involving the cochlear capsule is often responsible for sensorineural hearing loss by an unknown mechanism. Cochlear otosclerosis is caused by progressive enlargement of the perifenestral foci or by single or multiple foci in other locations in the cochlear capsule. The CT findings vary with the stage of maturation of the process. In the active or spongiotic phase, small areas of demineralization are first observed in the normally sharp contour of the capsule. These foci may enlarge and become confluent, producing large areas of demineralization and finally complete dissolution of the capsule. A typical sign of active cochlear otosclerosis is the "double ring" caused by confluent spongiotic foci within the thickness of the capsule (Fig. 38–35A, B). In the mature or sclerotic stage, localized or diffuse areas of thickening of the capsule are present. A precise and quantitative assessment of the involvement of the cochlear capsule is accomplished by CT densitometric readings. The contour of the cochlear capsule is scanned with the smallest cursor (0.25 × 0.25 mm) and 31 densitometric readings obtained. A profile of the density of the capsule is obtained by plotting densitometric values versus the 31 points where the readings were made. The obtained curve is then compared with the densitometric profile of the normal capsule, which was previously determined (Fig. 38–36). Variations in density exceeding the standard deviation of 10 to 15% are considered significant (Fig. 38–37). With comparison of the original densitometric profile with follow-ups, the evolution of the otosclerotic process and whether surgical or medical treatment was performed can both be established to determine

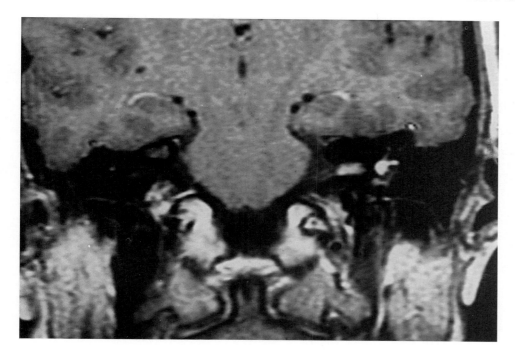

Fig. 38–34. Left labyrinthine schwannoma, T1 coronal MR image after injection of contrast material. An enhancing soft tissue mass fills the vestibule and extends into the horizontal semicircular canal. A second, seemingly not connected, mass is seen within the left internal auditory canal.

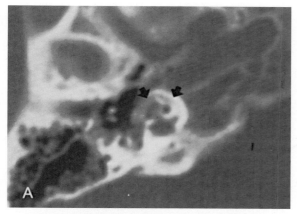

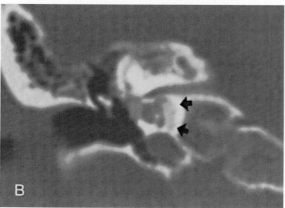

Fig. 38–35. Cochlear otosclerosis. Axial (A) and coronal (B) CT sections. Multiple spongiotic foci are noticed in the cochlear capsule with formation of a double ring (arrows).

if any change has occurred in the maturation and extent of the disease.

Petrous Pyramid

Glomus Jugulare Tumors

These tumors arise from minute glomus bodies found in the jugular fossa. The typical CT findings include erosion of the cortical outline and enlargement of the jugular fossa, erosion of the septum dividing the jugular fossa from the outer opening of the carotid canal, and erosion of the hypotympanic floor with extension of the tumor in the middle ear cavity (Fig. 38–38). As the lesion enlarges, the posteroinferior aspect of the entire petrous pyramid becomes eroded, as well as the adjacent aspect of the occipital bone including the hypoglossal canal. Large tumors protrude extradurally in the posterior cranial fossa and inferiorly below the base of the skull along the jugular vein. These extensions are better demonstrated by MRI in which the tumor appears in both T1 and T2 weighted images as a mass of medium signal intensity containing several small areas of signal void produced by blood vessels (Fig. 38–39). After the injection of contrast material, the tumor undergoes a moderate enhancement. The signal intensity of the glomus tumor is differentiated easily from the surrounding intra- and extracranial structures. In addition, MRI allows determination of displacement, encroachment, narrowing, or obstruction of the jugular vein and internal carotid artery because these large vessels are well visualized with no need for invasive vascular procedures. Jugular venography and carotid arteriography are seldom needed, and ca-

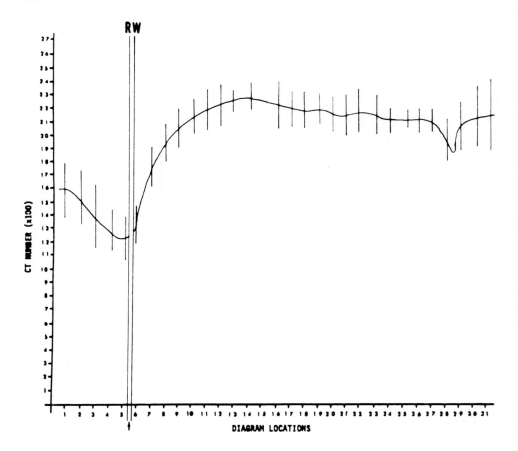

Fig. 38–36. Densitometric profile of the normal cochlear capsule with standard deviations.

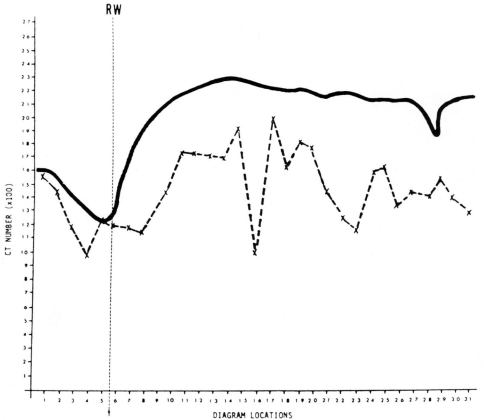

Fig. 38–37. Densitometric profile of the patient shown in Figure 38–35 (interrupted line). Comparison with the densitometric profile of the normal capsule (solid line) shows a diffuse demineralization of the cochlear capsule more severe in the region of the middle and apical coils.

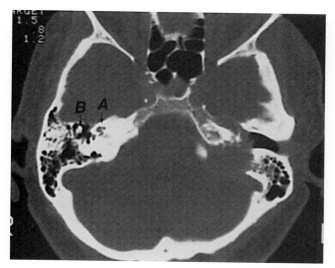

Fig. 38–38. Left glomus jugulare tumor, axial CT section. The posterior aspect of the left temporal bone in the region of the jugular fossa is eroded. A soft tissue mass extends into the middle ear cavity through a large defect in its posterior wall. A. Cochlea. B. ossicles on right side.

rotid arteriography is limited to pre-embolization studies.

Congenital Cholesteatomas and Cholesterol Granulomas

Congenital cholesteatomas may arise in the petrous pyramid. In the CT images, the involved area of the pyramid appears expanded by a cyst-like low-density lesion (Fig. 38–40), which often reaches and erodes the internal auditory canal and labyrinth. A CT study with

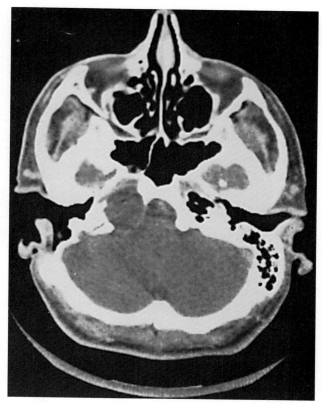

Fig. 38–40. Congenital cholesteatoma of the right petrous pyramid, axial CT section. There is destruction of the right petrous apex by an expansile cystic lesion of low density.

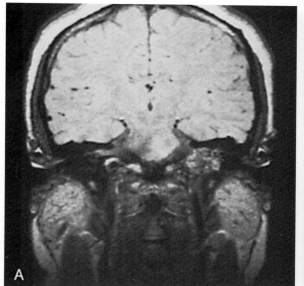
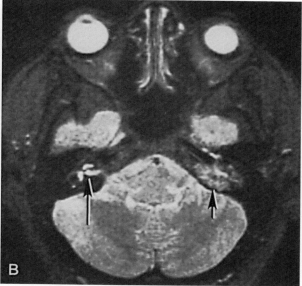

Fig. 38–39. Left glomus jugulare tumor. Coronal T1 (A) and axial T2 (B) MR images. A nonhomogeneous soft tissue mass of medium signal intensity is noticed in the region of the left jugular fossa (short arrow). The mass erodes the floor of the internal auditory canal and extends within the canal lumen. Compare with the normal right side (long arrow).

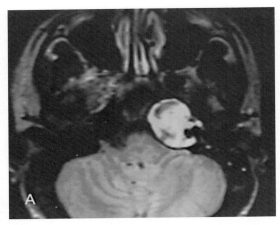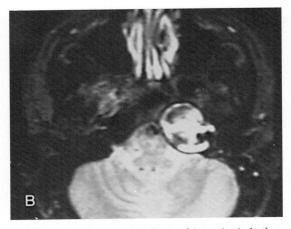

Fig. 38–41. Cholesterol granuloma. Axial spin density (A) and axial T2 (B) MR images. A mass of high signal intensity in both sequences is demonstrated in the left petrous apex. The areas of signal void within the mass are produced by deposits of hemosiderin.

infusion shows no enhancement of the mass except for its capsule. By CT, a congenital cholesteatoma of the petrous apex is difficult to differentiate from a cholesterol granuloma cyst that occurs in extensively pneumatized petrous pyramids. The two lesions can be differentiated by MR because congenital cholesteatomas produce a signal of medium intensity in the T1 images and high intensity in T2, whereas cholesterol granulomas have a similar high signal in both T1 and T2 sequences (Fig. 38–41). In addition, areas of signal void are observed in cholesterol granulomas produced by deposits of hemosiderin.

Meningiomas

These tumors arise from the meningeal covering of the temporal bone and from the meningeal extension into the internal auditory canal. The latter mimics, both clinically and in imaging, the appearance of an acoustic schwannoma. Meningiomas that arise from the petrous ridge are usually recognizable in the CT images as highly enhancing masses producing hyperostotic or lytic changes in the adjacent petrous pyramid. In meningiomas en plaque, only the bony changes are recognizable. MRI obtained after injection of paramagnetic contrast demonstrate a strong and usually homogeneous enhancement of the tumor. Enplaque lesions are recognizable as areas of enhancing meningeal thickening (Fig. 38–42).

Paget's Disease

This often affects the calvarium and the base of the skull including the petrous pyramids. The disease usu-

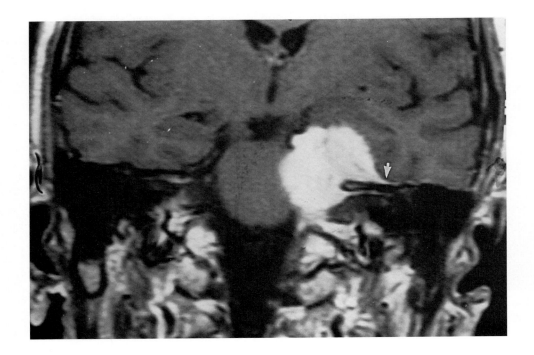

Fig. 38–42. Meningioma, coronal T1 MR section after injection of contrast material. A large enhanced mass extends above and below the left side of the tentorial notch. The tumor spares the internal auditory canal. Notice the lateral enplaque extension (tail sign) of the lesion (arrow).

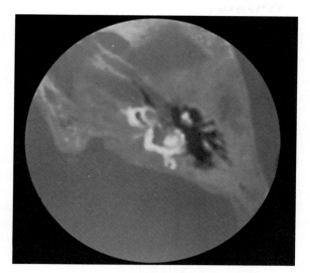

Fig. 38–43. Paget's disease, axial CT section of the left temporal bone. Notice the severe demineralization of the petrous pyramid and mastoid with thinning of the otic capsule, particularly of the cochlea.

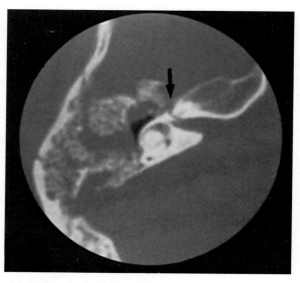

Fig. 38–44. Longitudinal fracture of the right temporal bone, axial CT section. The fracture passes from the mastoid through the attic into the petrous pyramid anterior to the labyrinth. The fracture reaches and involves the facial canal at its anterior genu (arrow).

ally spreads from the petrous apex laterally and produces a typical washed-out appearance of the involved pyramid caused by extensive demineralization (Fig. 38–43). The internal auditory canal is usually involved first, followed by the otic capsule, which becomes first thinned out and then completely erased. In the late stage of the disease, deposition of irregularly mineralized bone occurs and results in thickening of the petrosa, narrowing of the internal auditory canal, and fixation of the footplate of the stapes.

Facial Nerve

Computed tomography is the study of choice of the facial canal. The examination should be performed in two or three planes to visualize the various segments of the canal. MR visualizes the facial nerve itself, particularly when the nerve is thickened.

Congenital Anomalies

Congenital anomalies involve the size and course of the facial canal. The canal may be partially or completely absent, hypoplastic, or unusually narrow. Minor variations of the course of the facial nerve are common and of no clinical significance. More severe anomalies should be identified to avoid serious damage of the nerve during surgery. The horizontal segment may be displaced inferiorly to cover the oval window or lie exposed on the promontory. In congenital atresia of the external auditory canal, the mastoid segment of the facial canal is rotated laterally. The rotation varies from minimal obliquity to a true horizontal course (Figs. 38–13B, 38–17B).

Trauma

Traumatic lesions of the intratemporal portion of the facial nerve occur in approximately 20% of longitudinal fractures of the temporal bone and 50% of transverse fractures. The most common site of involvement in longitudinal fractures is the anterior genu (Figs. 38–44, 38–45), and in transverse fractures the labyrinthine or intracanalicular segments. The facial nerve may be transected by the fracture, compressed, or

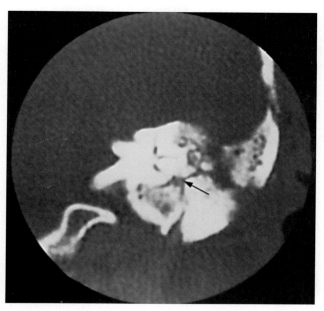

Fig. 38–45. Comminuted fracture of the left mastoid, coronal CT section. Multiple fractures are noticed in the mastoid. One of the fractures passes underneath the posterior semicircular canal and transects the vertical segment of the facial canal (arrow).

sheared by a depressed fragment of the canal wall, or simply contused by the violent shock.

Facial Neuritis

Moderate bilateral enhancement of the normal facial nerve, particularly in the region of its anterior genu, is often observed in MRI obtained after injection of contrast material.

Asymmetric enhancement of the facial nerve more prominent on the paralyzed side is common in patients with Bell's palsy and Ramsey Hunt syndrome. In Bell's palsy, the involvement is segmental and usually confined to the anterior genu and adjacent labyrinthine and tympanic segments. In Ramsey Hunt syndrome,

the involvement by the herpes zoster virus is more consistent and often extends to the nerve within the internal auditory canal (Fig. 38–46).

In viral neuritis, the nerve is usually not thickened. In sarcoidosis, the involvement is similar to Bell's palsy, but the nerve is moderately thickened.

Tumors

Primary tumors of the facial nerve are rare. Facial neurinomas cause thickening of the nerve and expansion of the canal (Fig. 38–47A). Further enlargement of the lesion results in erosion of the bony canal, extension into the middle-ear space, and involvement of the mastoid and petrous pyramid. Magnetic resonance imag-

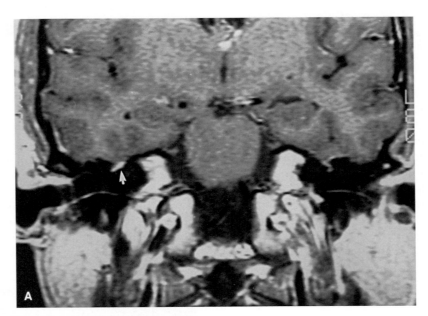

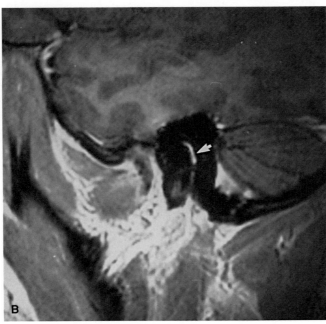

Fig. 38–46. Facial neuritis. Coronal (A) and sagittal (B) T1 MR images after injection of contrast material. There is enhancement of the right facial nerve in the regions of the anterior genu and proximal portion of the mastoid segment (arrows).

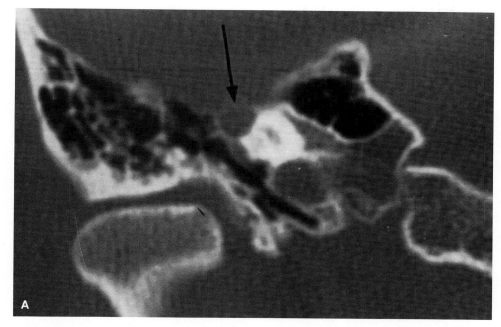

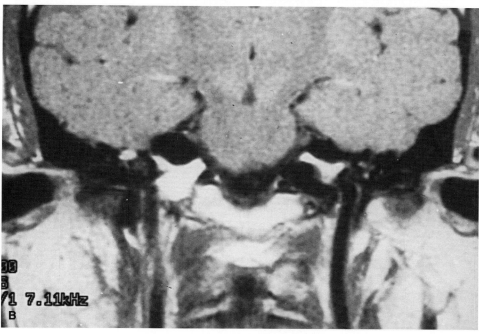

Fig. 38–47. Facial neurinoma. A. Coronal CT section revealing expansion of the right facial canal at the anterior genu (arrow). B. The coronal T1 MR section obtained after injection of gadolinium DPTA shows the actual enhancing tumor mass.

ing is useful to differentiate large facial nerve neurinomas from other lesions. The mass has a nonspecific low signal in T1 and high signal in T2-weighted images, but changes to bright in T1 images obtained after injection of gadolinium DPTA (Fig. 38–47B). The facial canal, particularly its vertical segment, is often involved by carcinoma arising in the external auditory canal and malignancies arising in the parotid gland and extending into the temporal bone.

Cerebellopontine Angle Tumors
Acoustic Schwannomas. Acoustic schwannomas account for 90% of the tumors of the cerebellopontine

angle. These tumors usually arise within the internal auditory canal, which becomes enlarged. Expansion of the internal auditory canal, shortening of its posterior wall and erosion of the crista falciformis are well visualized in high-definition CT images targeted for bone. Both sides should always be examined to compare significant differences. Acoustic schwannomas are not visualized in plain CT scans because the tumor is isodense to the surrounding brain and is not surrounded by edema. After infusion of iodinated contrast material, the mass enhances and becomes visible (Fig. 38–48). Intracanalicular lesions and cisternal masses smaller than 0.8 cm usually are not visualized by the

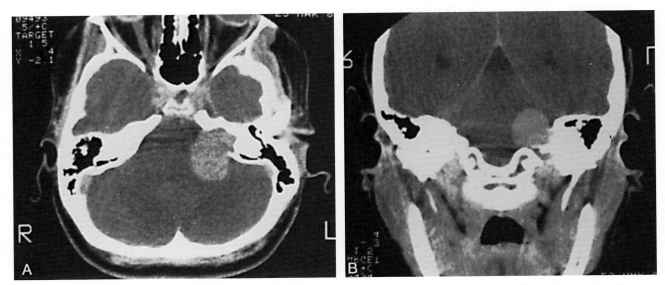

Fig. 38–48. Left acoustic schwannoma, postinfusion study. A. Horizontal CT section. B. Coronal CT section. The left internal auditory canal appears grossly expanded and eroded. A large tumor mass fills the canal and the cerebellopontine cistern. Notice the displacement to the right of the brain stem and fourth ventricle.

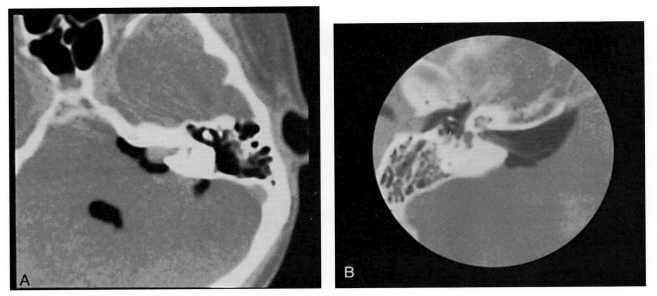

Fig. 38–49. Left acoustic schwannoma. A. The CT pneumocisternogram demonstrates a tumor mass filling the left internal auditory canal and slightly protruding into the cerebellopontine cistern. Notice the uninvolved portion of the eighth cranial nerve extending from the medial aspect of the tumor to the brain stem. B. The right cerebellopontine cistern and internal auditory canal are well filled by air. The eighth cranial nerve courses from the brain stem through the cistern to the internal auditory canal.

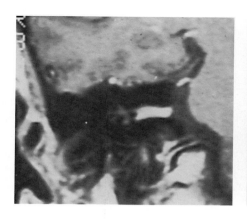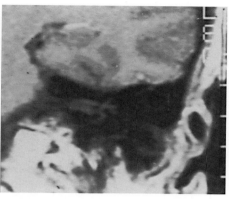

Fig. 38–50. Right acoustic schwannoma. T1 coronal MR section obtained after injection of Magnevist. An enhanced soft tissue mass fills but does not expand the right internal auditory canal. The left acoustic nerve is normal.

infusion technique, and a CT pneumocisternogram is indicated. This examination requires a spinal puncture for the injection in the subarachnoid space of air, CO_2, or O_2. With proper positioning, the gas is moved into the cerebellopontine angle under investigation, and several thin sections are obtained. In normal cases, the gas fills the cerebellopontine cistern and the internal auditory canal outlining the seventh and eighth cranial nerves. If a small tumor is present, the gas outlines the localized swelling of the nerve; if the tumor is large, it outlines the convex medial aspect of the mass obstructing the canal (Fig. 38–49).

Magnetic resonance imaging is the study of choice for diagnosis of acoustic schwannomas without exposing the patient to ionizing radiation and without the necessity for spinal puncture. In the plain study, the tumor appears in the T1 images brighter than cerebrospinal fluid and isointense to gray matter. In the T2 sections, neurinomas are brighter than brain but isointense to cerebrospinal fluid. Large tumors easily are identified in both sequences, but small lesions can be detected only in the T1 images because in the T2 they are obscured by the isointense cerebrospinal fluid. A final diagnosis of small tumors is achieved by injecting intravenously paramagnetic agents. Gadolinium DPTA (Magnevist) concentrates in the tumor and produces a shortening of the T1 relaxation time with consequent marked increase of the MR signal in the T1 images (Figs. 38–50 to 38–52). Tumors as small as 1 mm can be diagnosed by this technique.

Meningioma. Meningiomas account for approximately 3 to 4% of the cerebellopontine angle tumors. The lesion has a signal intensity less than the brain in the T1 sequences. In the T2 images, the lesion has variable characteristics, either a pathognomonic further decrease in signal intensity or a nonspecific increase in brightness. After intravenous injection of Magnevist, meningiomas show in the T1 images a marked increase in signal intensity similar to that seen in acoustic schwannomas. Unlike the latter tumor, meningiomas

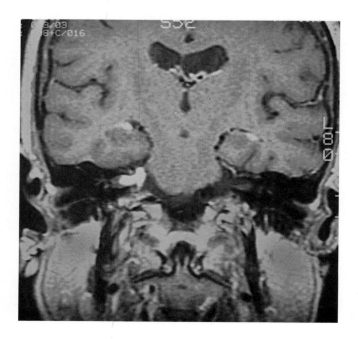

Fig. 38–51. Acoustic schwannoma. This coronal T1 MR image obtained after injection of contrast material shows an enhancing soft tissue mass filling the medial two thirds of the right internal auditory canal. The mass extends into the cerebellopontine cistern but does not reach the brain stem.

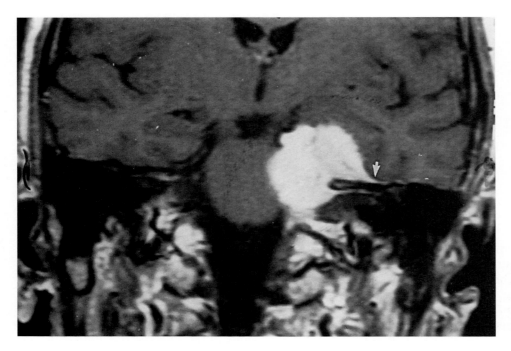

Fig. 38–52. Acoustic schwannoma, coronal T1 MR section after injection of contrast material. A large enhancing tumor expands the left internal auditory canal and fills the cerebellopontine cistern. The mass indents the brain stem.

usually arise in the cerebellopontine cistern and spare the fundus or the entire internal auditory canal.

SUGGESTED READINGS

1. Valvassori GE, Buckingham RA: Tomography and cross sections of the ear. Philadelphia, WB Saunders Co.; Stuttgart, Georg Thieme Verlag, 1975.
2. Curtin HD: Congenital malformations of the ear. Otolaryngol Clin North Am 21:317–336, 1988.
3. Phelps PD, Lloyd GAS: Traumatic lesions of the temporal bone. Radiology of the Ear. Oxford, Blackwell Scientific Publications, pp. 68–75, 1983.
4. Mafee MF, Singleton EL, Valvassori GE, et al: Acute otomastoiditis and its complications: Role of CT. Radiology 54:391–397, 1985.
5. Valvassori GE, Dobben GD: CT Densitometry of the cochlear capsule in otosclerosis. AJNR 6:661–667, 1985.
6. Mafee MF, Valvassori GE, Kumar A, et al: Tumors and tumor-like conditions of the middle ear and mastoid: role of CT and MRI. Otolaryngol Clin North Am 21:349–375, 1988.
7. Seltzer S, Mark AS: Contrast enhancement of the labyrinth on MR scans in patients with sudden hearing loss and vertigo: evidence of labyrinthine disease. AJNR 12:13–16, 1991.
8. Gerbarski SS, Telian SA, Niparko JK: Enhancement along the normal facial nerve in the facial canal: MR imaging and anatomic correlation. Radiology 183:391–394, 1992.
9. Rodgers GK, Applegate L, De La Cruz A, et al: Magnetic resonance angiography: analysis of vascular lesions of the temporal bone and skull base. Am J Otol 14:56–62, 1993.
10. Casselman JW, Kuhweide R, Ampe W, et al: Pathology of the membranous labyrinth: comparison of T1- and T2-weighted and gadolinium-enhanced spin-echo and 3DFT-CISS imaging. AJNR 14:59–69, 1993.
11. Casselman JW, Kuhweide R, Deimling M, et al: Constructive interference in steady state-3DFT MR imaging of the inner ear and cerebellopontine angle. AJNR 14:47–57, 1993.
12. Valvassori GE, Carter BL, Mafee MF: Imaging of the head and neck. Stuttgart, Georg Thieme Verlag, 1995.

V THE EAR

James B. Snow, Jr.

39 Development of the Human Ear

Ronan O'Rahilly and Fabiola Müller

Prenatal life is divided into embryonic and fetal periods. The embryonic period, which comprises the first 8 weeks, is subdivided into 23 developmental stages, the details of which have been described elsewhere.[1] A summary of the developing ear in relation to embryonic stages has been published by O'Rahilly.[2]

EXTERNAL EAR

The auricle is usually considered to develop from a series of auricular hillocks[3] around pharyngeal cleft 1. These elevations are noticeable in pharyngeal arches 1 and 2 at 5 weeks (stage 15) and are basically six in number, three on each arch, by 6 weeks (stage 17) (Fig. 39–1). The external acoustic meatus, representing pharyngeal cleft 1, appears as a "keyhole" between the hillocks. The hillocks, however, soon lose their identity (stage 19), so that the details of their contribution to the formation of the auricle are disputed. Perhaps the mandibular hillocks (1 to 3 in Fig. 39–1) contribute to the tragus and the crus of the helix, and the hyoid hillocks (4 to 6) to the helix and the antitragus. Nevertheless, the hillocks are transitory features and may be incidental rather than fundamental to the development of the auricle.[4]

The auricles are situated ventrolaterally at first but, by the end of the embryonic period, an apparent shift has occurred, whereby they adopt a dorsolateral position.[5]

During the embryonic period, ectodermal cells fill the meatus. This meatal plug becomes resorbed during the fetal period, and its medial end becomes the external layer of the tympanic membrane.[6] Pharyngeal cleft 1 corresponds to the cartilaginous part of the external acoustic meatus, and the temporary epithelial core to the osseous portion. The auricle increases in length throughout life.[7] Atresia or hypoplasia of the external acoustic meatus may arise from defects of various elements of the temporal bone: the tympanic part, styloid process, and tegmen tympani.[8]

MIDDLE EAR

The possible developmental interrelationships between the internal ear and the middle and the external ear are still uncertain. Moreover, the early development of the middle ear needs much further investigation. "Our ignorance of the morphogenesis of the middle and external ear far exceeds our knowledge."[9]

The tympanic cavity develops from the tubotympanic recess (Fig. 39–2A), which frequently is described as a diverticulum of pharyngeal pouch 1,[10] or of pouches 1 and 2. It may, however, arise independently of the pharyngeal pouches because pharyngeal pouch 1 disappears at "exactly the period when" the recess develops.[11,12]

The auditory ossicles become distinguishable at 6 to 7 weeks (stages 16 to 19) (Fig. 39–3). Their derivation, however, is not entirely clear. The malleus and incus arise from the cartilage of pharyngeal arch 1, and the stapes from that of 2 (Fig. 39–4A). However, the head of the malleus and the body and short crus of the incus may arise from arch 1, whereas the handle of the malleus, possibly the long crus of the incus, and the head and crura of the stapes come from arch 2 (Fig. 39–4B).[13] All components of the ossicles may be of neural crest origin. The base of the stapes seems to develop in the lateral wall of the otic capsule; it occupies the fenestra vestibuli (oval window).

A small vessel, the stapedial artery, traverses the stapedial condensation.[14] It is derived from aortic arches 2 and 1, and then appears as a branch of the internal carotid. It is well developed at 6 to 7 weeks (stages 18 and 19), when it divides into a superior (supraorbital) and an inferior (maxillomandibular) division (Fig. 39–5A). Later connections with the external

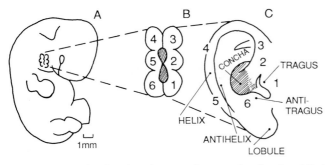

Fig. 39–1. A. and B. Six elevations on pharyngeal arches 1 and 2 at 6 weeks (stage 17). C. One interpretation of the relationship between the auricular hillocks and the adult auricle.

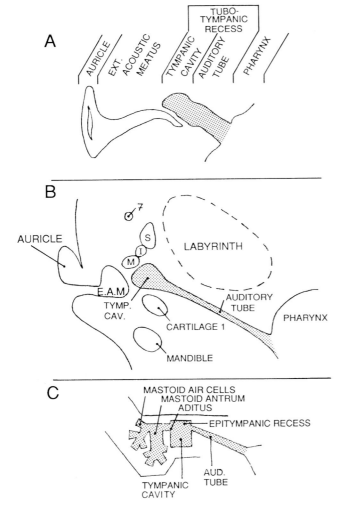

Fig. 39–2. General development of the external and middle ear. A. Drawing shows that the pharyngotympanic (so-called auditory) tube and the tympanic cavity are derived from the tubotympanic recess (stippled). B. Plan shows the close relationship between the external acoustic meatus (E.A.M.) and the tympanic cavity (separated by the future tympanic membrane). Close by are the facial nerve (7), the auditory ossicles (S,I,M = stapes, incus, malleus), the cartilage of pharyngeal arch 1, and the beginning mandible. C. Drawing emphasizing the developmental continuity of the auditory tube, tympanic cavity, epitympanic recess, aditus ad antrum, mastoid antrum, and mastoid air cells.

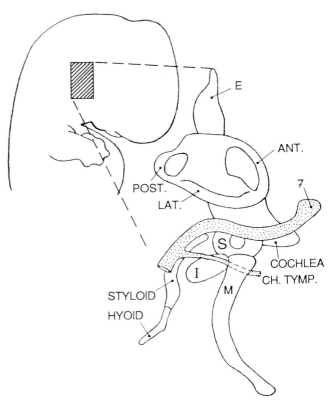

Fig. 39–3. Components of the ear at 6 weeks (stage 18). All three semicircular ducts are separated off in the vestibular part of the otic primordium, and the cochlear duct is becoming elongated in the cochlear portion. The skeletal primordia are laid down in mesenchyme and cartilage, and the chorda tympani passes between the incus and the malleus (proximal part of cartilage of pharyngeal arch 1). ANT., Anterior semicircular duct; CH. TYMP., chorda tympani; E, endolymphatic appendage; I, incus; LAT, lateral semicircular duct; M, malleus (which at this stage is part of Meckel's cartilage); POST., posterior semicircular duct; S, stapes.

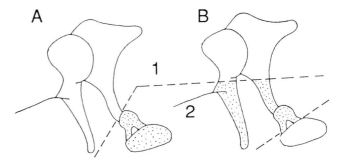

Fig. 39–4. Derivation of auditory ossicles. A. Traditional view, in which most of the ossicles are thought to arise from pharyngeal cartilage 1 and the stapes from cartilage 2. B. Anson's interpretation, in which the malleus and incus are each derived from cartilages 1 and 2, the head and crura of the stapes from cartilage 2, and its footplate from the otic capsule.

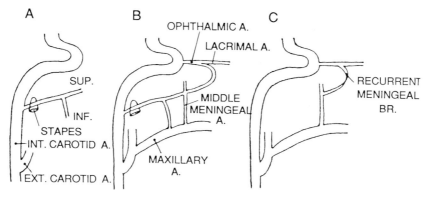

Fig. 39–5. The stapedial artery. A. At 6 weeks (stage 18), the stapedial artery is surrounded by the mesenchymal primordium of the stapes and gives off a superior and an inferior branch, the superior going to the orbit and the inferior to pharyngeal arch 1. B. Anastomoses between the inferior branch and the maxillary artery result in the formation of the definitive vessels to the maxillary and mandibular regions. The connection between the superior branch and the maxillary artery forms the middle meningeal. The superior branch also connects with the ophthalmic artery. By this connection, the lacrimal artery, formerly a tributary of the superior branch, becomes connected to the ophthalmic artery. C. The ophthalmic connection is largely being interrupted. A remnant forms the recurrent meningeal branch of the lacrimal artery, which still joins the middle meningeal. In about 2% of people, the connection persists to such a degree that the ophthalmic artery arises from the middle meningeal.

carotid (Fig. 39–5B and C) alter its disposition, so that by 9 weeks (40 mm) only small rests of the stapedial system remain. In rare instances, the stapedial artery may persist.

The tensor tympani and the stapedius, which develop during the embryonic period (stages 18 to 20), arise from pharyngeal arches 1 and 2, respectively, and hence are supplied, largely, by the mandibular and facial nerves, respectively.

The gelatinous tissue in the tympanic cavity becomes absorbed during the fetal period, when various pouches and mucosal folds are formed.[15,16] The epithelium of the tympanic cavity progressively envelops the auditory ossicles and the chorda tympani and closes the fenestra cochleae (round window). It also forms the internal layer of the tympanic membrane. A portion of the tympanic cavity, the epitympanic recess (Fig. 39–2C), or "attic," is situated above the level of the tympanic membrane, and it contains the head of the malleus and the body and short crus of the incus. Details of the developing hypotympanum are available.[17] Later expansions of the tympanic cavity become the mastoid antrum and, postnatally, the mastoid air cells (Fig. 39–2C). The middle ear reaches its adult size during the second half of prenatal life. Several views of the ear and of the temporal bone in infancy have been provided by Bosma.[18]

THE TEMPORAL BONE

The temporal bone consists of four main elements: petromastoid, styloid, squamous, and tympanic.[19]

1. The future petromastoid part is derived from the otic capsule (Fig. 39–6A), which appears first as a mesenchymal condensation around the otocyst (4½ weeks: stage 14), then becomes chondrified (6 weeks: stage 17), and later (13 to 14 weeks: 94 to 116 mm) begins to ossify from many centers. A wing from the petrous part (Fig. 39–6B) grows over the tympanic cavity, for which it acts as a roof termed the tegmen tympani. The tegmen becomes more and more covered by the squamous part (Fig. 39–6C and D). After birth, the mastoid component grows anteroinferiorly to form the mastoid process (Fig. 39–6E), which becomes a definite projection at approximately 1 to 2 years. Pneumatization begins at about the time of birth.

2. The styloid part (Fig. 39–6) develops from the cartilage of pharyngeal arch 2, which appears at 6 weeks, first in mesenchyme (stage 17) and then as cartilage (stage 18). The proximal portion of the styloid process ossifies before birth, and the distal part after birth. The styloid process fuses with the petromastoid part during the first postnatal year.

3. The squamous part begins to ossify intramembranously on the side of the calvaria at 8 to 8½ weeks (Fig. 39–7A) (29 to 35 mm). It includes the zygomatic process and the mandibular fossa (Fig. 39–6D). The squamous fuses with the petromastoid part during the first postnatal year.

4. The tympanic part develops first as an incomplete ring (Fig. 39–6C) that begins to ossify intramembranously at 8½ to 9 weeks (35 to 40 mm). The squamous and tympanic parts meet at the squamo-tympanic fissure, which, when traced medially, displays the lower margin of the teg-

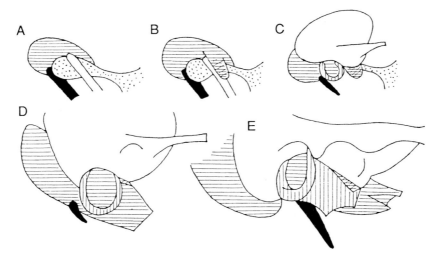

Fig. 39–6. Frazer's developmental analysis of the temporal bone. Right lateral views. A. At about 6 weeks, the petrous part (horizontal lines) is related to the tubotympanic recess (stippled) and pharyngeal cartilages 1 (white) and 2 (black). B. A (cross-hatched) "wing" (the tegmen tympani) is thrown laterally from the petrous part over the tympanum. C. At the end of the embryonic period, the squamous part (white) has begun to appear, and early in the fetal period, the tympanic ring (vertical lines) develops. Cartilage 2 is forming the styloid process (black). D. The squamous covers more and more of the tegmen. E. The tympanic plate (vertical lines) has developed. A sliver of tegmen (which is a portion of the petrous) is still visible between the mandibular fossa of the squamous part and the tympanic plate. The squamotympanic fissure is seen to divide into petrosquamous and petrotympanic fissures, as in adult. The mastoid part is a derivative of the petrous temporal, and hence the temporal bone consists of four main elements: petrous (petromastoid), styloid, squamous, and tympanic.

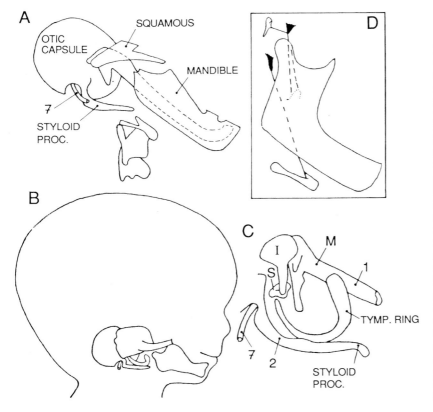

Fig. 39–7. Development of the temporal bone, auditory ossicles, and mandible. Right lateral views. At about 9 weeks, showing the otic capsule (which represents the petrous temporal), squamous temporal, styloid process, and facial nerve (7). The cartilage of pharyngeal arch 1 is giving rise proximally to portions of the malleus and incus; distally it is covered by the developing mandible. The hyoid, thyroid, and cricoid cartilages are also shown. (Based on Macklin CC: The skull of a human fetus of 43 millimeters greatest length. Contrib Embryol Carnegie Inst *10:* 57–103, 1921.) B. At about 12 weeks, showing the squamous temporal, below which the tympanic ring and styloid process are visible (M,I,S = malleus, incus, stapes), and the cartilages of pharyngeal arches 1 and 2, the tympanic ring, and the styloid process and facial nerve (7). The tympanic membrane is omitted. (B and C are based on Hertwig's model as shown by Kollmann J: Handatlas der Entwicklungsgeschichte des Menschen. Vol. 1, Jena, Fischer, 1907.) D. The adult mandible and hyoid bone. The spine of the sphenoid (black) is connected with both the malleus and the mandible, so that a malleosphenomandibular ligament (representing the course of pharyngeal cartilage 1) can be described.[21] The styloid process (black) is connected to the hyoid bone by the stylohyoid ligament (representing the course of pharyngeal cartilage 2).

men tympani, thereby giving rise to petrosquamous and petrotympanic fissures (Fig. 39–6E). The tympanic ring unites with the squamous part shortly before birth. After birth, the tympanic ring grows laterally and inferiorly to form the tympanic plate (Fig. 39–6E). In its growth, it may form a small, temporary foramen in the floor of the meatus. The tympanic plate forms the sheath of the styloid process.

The development of the auditory ossicles is associated with that of the temporal bone (Fig. 39–7). They begin as mesenchymal condensations at 6 weeks (stages 16 and 17) and, as pharyngeal bars 1 and 2 begin to chondrify (stage 18), the malleus, incus, and stapes become more clearly identifiable (stage 19), although the stapes may not be cartilaginous until 8 weeks. The anterior process of the malleus shows a special ossific center at 8½ to 9 weeks (34 to 40 mm). The incus and malleus begin to ossify after 13 weeks (108 to 120 mm), and the stapes a few weeks later (139 to 148 mm).[20]

The anterior ligament of the malleus (which is prolonged through the petrotympanic fissure to reach the spine of the sphenoid) and the sphenomandibular ligament (Fig. 39–7D) are remains of the fibrous sheath of the first pharyngeal cartilage. These bands consist of a single formation, the "malleo-spino-mandibular ligament," which extends not only to the lingula of the mandible but also as far as the mental region.[21]

INTERNAL EAR

The first indication of the internal ear is the otic disc, which appears at 20 days (stage 9) in the surface ecto-derm opposite the rhombencephalic neural fold[22] (Fig. 39–8). Epithelio-mesenchymal interactions between the disc and the adjacent mesenchyme are necessary, and the proximity of the hindbrain is also crucial. The many experimental studies (e.g., organ culture) of the otocyst of the chick and mouse are outside the scope of this chapter.

The disc becomes invaginated; the otic pit is thereby formed (stage 11); the connection with the surface becomes narrowed to a pore (stage 12); and the resulting otic vesicle, or otocyst, finally becomes completely closed from the surface (stage 13) (Fig. 39–8). Programmed cell (apoptosis) death occurs in the epithelium.[23] Otic (neural) crest cells emerge from the wall of the vesicle[22,24] and contribute, at least in part, to the vestibular and possibly the cochlear (spiral) ganglion.[25,26] The association between hypopigmentation and abnormalities of the cochlea and the saccule in certain syndromes has been attributed to the common origin of melanocytes and a part of the vestibulocochlear ganglion from neural crest.[27]

The dorsomedial portion of the otic vesicle gives rise to the endolymphatic appendage (stage 14), whereas the ventral portion develops into the cochlear duct. As a result of an inductive effect of the otic vesicle, the mesoderm around the otocyst becomes condensed to form the otic capsule (stages 14 and 15).

At 5½ weeks, three elevations that resemble plates appear in the main portion of the otic vesicle (stage 16). They represent the future anterior, posterior, and lateral semicircular ducts. The central parts of these hollow plates become thinner, and the adjacent epithelial layers fuse and disappear, so that a "hole" is formed in each of the semicircular ducts (stage 18) (Fig. 39–9). The ducts open into the future utricle, which

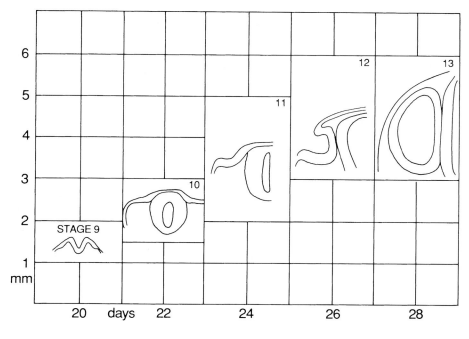

Fig. 39–8. Graph shows timing of the development of the otic vesicle (otocyst). The primordium is laid down as a thickening in the surface ectoderm at about 20 days (stage 9). A seeming rotation of the otic disc takes place at 22 days (stage 10). The otic pit forms within a few days (stages 11 and 12), and the vesicle is evident at 4 weeks (stage 13). Note that the relationship with the neural tube becomes more and more intimate. The numerals within the rectangles indicate Carnegie stages.

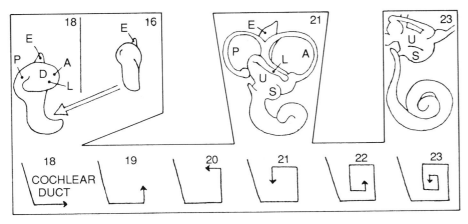

Fig. 39-9. Development of the membranous labyrinth from 6 to 8 weeks. The upper row of drawings shows the labyrinth at 37 (stage 16), 44 (stage 18), 52 (stage 21), and 57 (stage 23) days. The lower row is a series of schemes to show the progressive coiling of the cochlear duct (stages 18 to 23). At 6 weeks it is L-shaped, and by 8 weeks it has acquired almost 2 1/2 turns. A, Anterior semicircular duct; E, endolymphatic appendage; L, lateral semicircular duct; P, posterior semicircular duct; S, saccule; U, utricle.

becomes separated from the cochlear duct by the saccule. Each duct develops an ampulla at one end (see stage 21 in Fig. 39–9 and stage 23 in Fig. 39–10).

The L-shaped cochlear duct soon begins to curl (stage 19) and attains almost 2½ turns by 8 weeks (stage 23) (Fig. 39–9).

As a result of inductive action by the otocyst, the

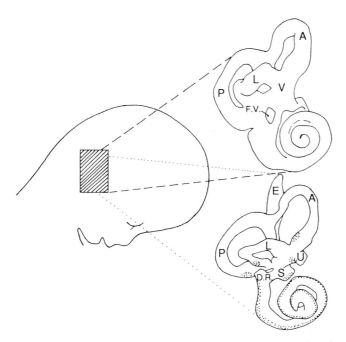

Fig. 39-10. The cartilaginous (future osseous) (upper drawing) and membranous (lower drawing) labyrinths at 8 weeks (29 mm, probably stage 23). The advanced form of the membranous labyrinth is evident, and the condensation (otic capsule) around it has followed it closely as the cartilaginous labyrinth. (Based on Martin J and Anson BJ: Otic capsule and membranous labyrinth of the 29 mm. (crown-rump) human embryo. Arch Otolaryngol 27:279–303, 1938.) In the membranous labyrinth, the six neuroepithelial areas (three ampullary crests, two maculae, and one spiral organ) are indicated by stippling. A, Anterior semicircular duct; E, endolymphatic appendage; D.R., ductus reuniens; F.V., fenestra vestibuli (oval window); L, lateral semicircular duct; P, posterior semicircular duct; S, saccule; U, utricle; V, vestibule.

otic capsule begins to chondrify (stage 19) and then unites with the base of the skull. It is separated from the semicircular ducts by reticular tissue.

Unexpectedly, the first nerve fibers to reach the otic vesicle are efferent fibers of the vestibular nerve.[28] Thickenings in the epithelial wall of the otic vesicle become related to the ingrowth of nerve fibers from the vestibular and cochlear (spiral) ganglia. Six specialized neuroepithelial areas become established: three ampullary crests in the semicircular ducts (one in each ampulla), two maculae (one in the utricle and the other in the saccule), and one spiral organ along the length of the cochlear duct (Fig. 39–10).

Early in the fetal period, the epithelial floor of the cochlear duct becomes thickened (Fig. 39–11), and the tectorial membrane appears. The thickening rests on the basilar membrane and forms the spiral organ, in which hair cells develop. By the middle of prenatal life, the fetus can hear and respond to sounds. Moreover, because the fetus is almost weightless as it floats in a subgravity state, it may orient itself by labyrinthine-activated kicking and hence actively influence its position in utero.[29]

The first indication of a periotic space occurs early (30 to 40 mm) in the fetal period.[30] Coalescence of spaces within the periotic reticulum results in a vestibular cistern. The scala tympani also appears early (43 mm), and the scala vestibuli arises (50 mm) as an extension of the cistern. The scalae then communicate with each other at the helicotrema (130 mm) (Fig. 39–11). The margins of the cavities within the cartilaginous otic capsule are advancing constantly or receding, so that "a suitable suite of chambers is always provided for the enlarging membranous labyrinth."[30] Although excavation is usually attributed to dedifferentiation resulting in the removal of cartilage previously laid down, histochemical studies do not support this concept and indicate rather that histiocytes with an ability to chondrolyse are responsible for cavitation.[31]

Approximately 14 ossific centers develop in the cartilaginous otic capsule in a variable order (Fig.

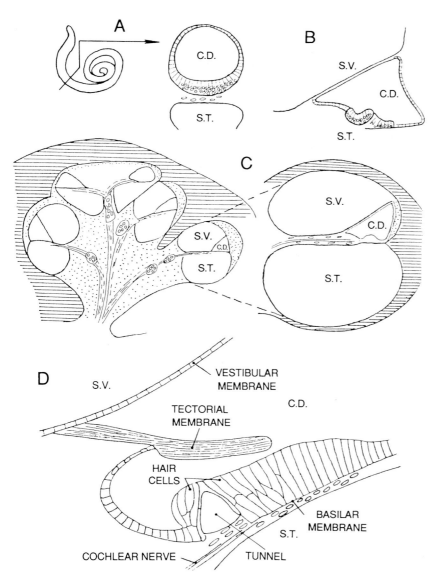

Fig. 39–11. Development of the cochlea. A. The cochlear duct at 10 weeks, with a section showing the cochlear duct in relation to the scala tympani, which is the first of the perilymphatic spaces to appear. B. At 14 weeks, showing the cochlear duct between the two scalae. The spiral organ is differentiating. C. At about 16 weeks, showing various turns of the cochlea. Cochlear nerve fibers and groups of neurons that constitute the spiral (cochlear) ganglion are indicated. The cartilaginous otic capsule is represented by horizontal lines. D. At 25 weeks, including further details of the spiral organ. C.D., Cochlear duct; S.T., scala tympani; S.V., scala vestibuli.

39–12).[31] Ossification begins at approximately 15 weeks (126 mm; Noback and Robertson give 94 to 116 mm).[20] The cartilaginous otic capsule is almost completely converted into bone by the middle of prenatal life (202 mm).

The later development of the aqueduct of the cochlea and the periotic duct have received special attention.[33] The periotic duct is regarded as an extension of the subarachnoid space rather than an appendage of the internal ear. Details of the development of the blood vessels to the internal ear (7.5 to 9.4 mm) are also available.[34]

Pigment derived from neural crest is found in the internal ear, chiefly in the stria vascularis, where melanocytes are considered to be essential for the endocochlear potential of the endolymph. One type of congenital sensorineural deafness (Waardenburg syndrome) is caused by a defective gene in chromosome 2. The neural crest is affected and melanocytes of the stria are deficient.

THE POSTNATAL EAR

Although the rest of the labyrinth attains its adult size by the middle of prenatal life, the aqueduct of the vestibule and the endolymphatic sac continue to grow postnatally.[35]

In infancy, the external acoustic meatus is short, straight, and fibrocartilaginous. The tympanic membrane faces more caudally than laterally. The tympanic ring and membrane, tympanic cavity, and auditory ossicles are all of adult size. The mastoid process develops gradually during childhood; hence the facial nerve

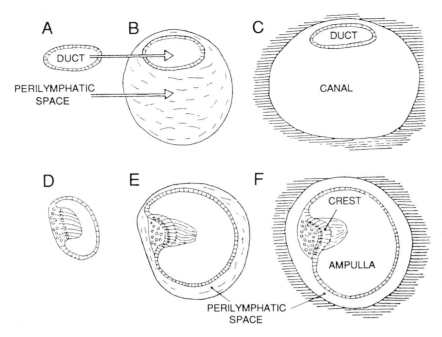

Fig. 39–12. Development of a semicircular duct. The semicircular duct in A (8 weeks) becomes surrounded by the perilymphatic space in B (12 weeks). In C (22 weeks) the semicircular canal is delineated by the cartilaginous otic capsule (horizontal lines). The development of the ampullary crest within an ampulla is shown in D through F (8, 10, and 13 weeks, respectively). (Based largely on Bast TH and Anson BJ: The Temporal Bone and the Ear. Springfield, IL, Charles C Thomas, 1949.)

is exposed during infancy. The auditory tube, which is more horizontal, is 17 to 21 mm in length in the newborn (approximately 35 mm in the adult).

SUGGESTED READINGS

1. O'Rahilly R, Müller F: Developmental Stages in Human Embryos, Including a Revision of Streeter's "Horizons" and a Survey of the Carnegie Collection. Washington, DC, Carnegie Institution of Washington, 1987.
2. O'Rahilly R: The timing and sequence of events in the development of the human eye and ear during the embryonic period proper. Anat Embryol 168:87–99, 1983.
3. Aghemo GF, Fortunato G: Observations on the development of the auricle in man. Panminerva Med 11:10–12, 1969.
4. Streeter GL: Development of the auricle in the human embryo. Contrib Embryol Carnegie Inst 14:111–138, 1922.
5. Gerhardt HJ, Otto HD: The intratemporal course of the facial nerve and its influence on the development of the ossicular chain. Acta Otolaryngol 91:567–573, 1981.
6. Nishimura Y, Kumoi T: The embryonic development of the human external auditory meatus. Acta Otolaryngol 112: 496–503, 1992.
7. Pellnitz D: Über das Wachstum der menschlichen Ohrmusckel. Arch Ohr-Nas-Kehlk-Heilk 171:334–340, 1958.
8. Politzer G, Mayer EG: Über angeborenen Verschluss und Verengerung des äusseren Gehörgangs und ihre formale Genese. Virchows Arch (A) 258:206–231, 1925.
9. Van de Water TR, Maderson PFA, Jaskoll TF: The morphogenesis of the middle and external ear. Birth Defects 16:147–180, 1980.
10. Kanagasuntheram R: A note on the development of the tubotympanic recess in the human embryo. J Anat 101:731–741, 1967.
11. Goedbloed JF: De vroege ontwikkeling van het middenoor. Leiden, p 116, 1960.
12. Goedbloed JF: The early development of the middle ear and the mouth-cavity. A study of the interaction of processes in the epithelium and the mesenchyme. Arch Biol Liège 75:207–243, 1964.
13. Hanson JR, Anson BJ, Strickland EM: Branchial sources of the auditory ossicles in man. Arch Otolaryngol Head Neck Surg 76:100–122, 200–215, 1962.
14. Lazorthes G, Gouazé A, Salamon G: Vascularisation et circulation de l'encéphale. Vol. 1, Paris, Masson, 1976.
15. Schurig, H: Die Individualität der Entwicklung sowie der Ausreifung der Bindesubstanzen in der fetalen Paukenhöhle und die Variabilität der Schleimhaut. Arch Ohr Nas Kehlk Heilk 177:404–416, 1961.
16. Proctor B: Surgical anatomy and embryology of the middle ear. Trans Am Acad Ophthalmol Otolaryngol 67:801–814, 1963.
17. Spector GJ, Ge X-X: Development of the hypotympanum in the human fetus and neonate. Ann Otol Rhinol Laryngol 90(Suppl 88):1–20, 1981.
18. Bosma JF: Anatomy of the Infant Head. Baltimore, Johns Hopkins University Press, 1986.
19. Frazer JE: Anatomy of the Human Skeleton (revised by A.S. Breathnach). 6th ed. London, Churchill, 1965.
20. Noback CR, Robertson GG: Sequences of appearance of ossification centers in the human skeleton during the first five prenatal months. Am J Anat 89:1–28, 1951.
21. Bossy J, Gaillard L: Les vestiges ligamentaires du cartilage de Meckel. Acta Anat (Basel) 52:282–290, 1963.
22. O'Rahilly R: The early development of the otic vesicle in staged human embryos. J Embryol Exp Morphol 11:741–755, 1963.
23. Represa JJ, Moro JA, Gato A et al.: Patterns of epithelial cell death during early development of the human inner ear. Ann Otol Rhinol Laryngol 99:482–488, 1990.
24. Politzer G: Die Entstehung des Ganglion acusticum beim Menschen. Acta Anat (Basel) 26:1–13, 1956.
25. Müller F, O'Rahilly R: The development of the human brain, the closure of the caudal neuropore, and the beginning of secondary neurulation at stage 12. Anat Embryol 176:413–430, 1987.
26. Müller F, O'Rahilly R: The development of the human brain from a closed neural tube at stage 13. Anat Embryol 176: 413–430, 1988.

27. Deol MS: The relationship between abnormalities of pigmentation and the inner ear. Proc R Soc Lond (A) *175*:201–217, 1970.

28. Müller F, O'Rahilly R: The first appearance of the future cerebral hemispheres in the human embryo at stage 14. Anat Embryol *176*:495–511, 1988.

29. Editorial: Fetal ear function and fetal position. Can Med Assoc J *91*:348–349, 1964.

30. Streeter GL: The histogenesis and growth of the otic capsule and its contained periotic tissue-spaces in the human embryo. Contrib Embryol Carnegie Inst *7*:5–54, 1918.

31. Andersen H, Matthiessen ME, Jørgensen MB: The growth of the otic cavities in the human foetus. Acta Otolaryngol (Stockh) *68*:243–249, 1969.

32. Bast TH, Anson BJ: The Temporal Bone and the Ear. Springfield, IL, Charles C Thomas, 1949.

33. Spector GJ, Lee D, Carr C, et al: Later stages of development of the periotic duct and its adjacent area in the human fetus. Laryngoscope Suppl *90*:1–31, 1980.

34. Kellner G, Richter OB: Über die Entwicklung der Gefässe des Innenohres beim Menschen. Monatsschr Ohr-heilk Laryngorhinol *96*:187–209, 1962.

35. Kodama A, Sando I: Postnatal development of the vestibular aqueduct and endolymphatic sac. Ann Otol Rhinol Laryngol *91* (Suppl) *96*:3–20, 1982.

36. Macklin CC: The skull of a human fetus of 43 millimeters greatest length. Contrib Embryol Carnegie Inst *10*:57–103, 1921.

37. Kollmann J: Handatlas der Entwicklungsgeschichte des Menschen. Vol. 1, Jena, Fischer, 1907.

38. Martin J, Anson BJ: Otic capsule and membranous labyrinth of the 29 mm. (crown-rump) human embryo. Arch Otolaryngol *27*:279–303, 1938.

40 Anatomy of the Ear

David F. Austin

THE TEMPORAL BONE

The temporal bone not only contains the sense organs of hearing and balance, together with the sound conduction apparatus, but also contributes to the cranial vault and zygoma. The temporal bones 1 and 2 are situated at the sides and base of the skull and consist of five parts: the squama, mastoid, petrous, tympanic, and styloid process (Figs. 40–1 to 40–3).

The *squamous portion* of the temporal bone is largely thin and convex outward. Its external surface affords attachment to the temporalis muscle, which is bounded inferiorly by the temporal line, an important surgical landmark. The suprameatal triangle, another landmark, is a fossa situated just superior and posterior to the external meatus. The triangle is bounded at the meatus by the suprameatal spine (spine of Henle). This triangle approximates, on the external surface of the temporal bone, the position of the mastoid antrum. The zygomatic process projects forward from the lower part of the squama, and with the squama and tympanic bone serves to bound the mandibular fossa. A suture line runs through the fossa, the petrotympanic fissure (glaserian fissure), which leads to the middle ear and transmits the tympanic branch of the internal maxillary artery. A canal separated slightly from the fissure, the canal of Huguier, transmits the chorda tympani nerve.

The *tympanic portion* is an incomplete cylinder that, together with the squama superiorly, forms the bony external auditory meatus, a canal roughly 2 cm in length by 1 cm in diameter. Anteriorly, it also serves to bound the mandibular fossa. The medial end of the tympanic bone contains a sulcus that holds the fibrous anulus of the tympanic membrane. A thin plate that extends posteriorly contains a socket in which the styloid process is held. The posterior margin of the tympanic bone articulates with the mastoid portion to form the tympanomastoid fissure, which transmits the auricular branch of the vagus nerve.

The greatest volume of the temporal bone is formed by the *mastoid portion* posteriorly and inferiorly. Because it is extensively pneumatized, however, it has no greater mass than the other portions. The mastoid process projects inferiorly behind the external meatus. This serves as the attachment for the sternocleidomastoid, splenius capitis, and longissimus capitis muscles. From the inferior aspect, there is a deep groove, the mastoid notch (digastric fossa), which holds the digastric muscle. In the interior of the mastoid process, when a mastoidectomy is being performed, this groove presents as the digastric ridge and is an important landmark because the stylomastoid foramen, which transmits the facial nerve, is located at the anterior extremity of this ridge. The superior surface of the mastoid is a thin plate of bone overlying the tympanic antrum, known as the tegmen mastoideum. Posteriorly, together with the posterior surface of the petrous portion, it forms the anterior border of the posterior cranial fossa. It has a deep groove that is formed by the lateral or sigmoid sinus. Two smaller channels that are directed medially contain the superior and inferior petrosal sinuses.

The *petrous portion* is usually called the petrous pyramid and contains the otic labyrinth. Superiorly, it forms the inferior surface of the middle cranial fossa. Posteriorly, bounded by the attachment of the tentorium cerebelli, it helps to form, together with the mastoid portion, the anterior face of the posterior cranial fossa. The superior face of the petrous is marked by the arcuate eminence, which is the protrusion formed by the superior semicircular canal. Anterior to this is the fossa that contains the geniculate ganglion, occasionally covered by a thin plate of bone, and a groove extending forward from this fossa, which contains the greater superficial petrosal nerve and a branch of the middle meningeal artery. Medially, there is a depression in which lies the semilunar ganglion. The posterior face of the bone presents

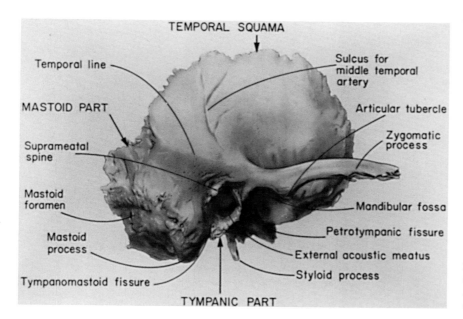

Fig. 40–1. Right temporal bone, lateral view. (From Anson BJ and Donaldson JA: Surgical Anatomy of the Temporal Bone and Ear. Philadelphia, WB Saunders, 1981.)

several landmarks, the most obvious being the porus acusticus, or mouth of the internal auditory canal, which transmits the seventh and eighth cranial nerves as well as the internal auditory artery. The lateral end of the internal auditory meatus is divided horizontally by the crista falciformis. The superior compartment contains the facial nerve anteriorly and the superior branch of the vestibular nerve posteriorly. The inferior compartment transmits the cochlear division anteriorly and the inferior branch of the vestibular nerve posteriorly. A shallow depression in the middle of the posterior face ends in a duct running posteriorly under a thin ledge of bone and marks the external position of the endolymphatic sac. The

cochlear aqueduct opens just below the internal auditory canal at the base of the petrous bone. The lateral aspect of the petrous bone constitutes the medial wall of the middle ear and will be described under that section. At the petrous apex, a hiatus is present between the tentorium and the petrous, which forms a canal for the passage of the fifth cranial nerve (Meckel's cave). The sixth cranial nerve runs through a notch just below the posterior clinoid process (the medial attachment of the tentorium) and above the articulation of the petrous and sphenoid (Dorello's canal). Disease in the petrous apex will produce irritation and dysfunction of the fifth and sixth cranial nerves—Gradenigo's syndrome.

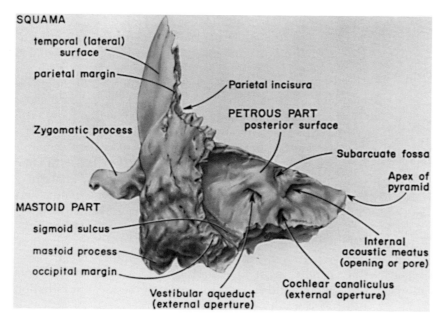

Fig. 40–2. Left temporal bone, posterolateral view. (From Anson BJ and Donaldson JA: Surgical Anatomy of the Temporal Bone and Ear. Philadelphia, WB Saunders, 1981.)

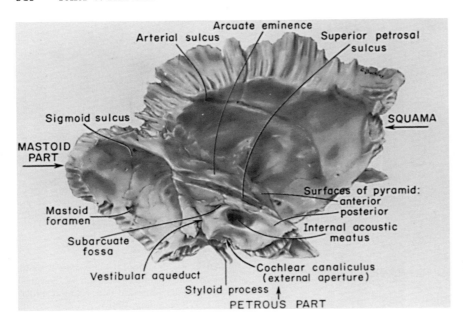

Fig. 40–3. Left temporal bone, medial view. (From Anson BJ and Donaldson JA: Surgical Anatomy of the Temporal Bone and Ear. Philadelphia, WB Saunders, 1981.)

THE EAR

Both anatomically and functionally, the ear is divided into three parts: the external ear, the middle ear, and the inner ear (Fig. 40–4).

The External Ear

The external ear is the portion of the ear external to the tympanic membrane. It consists of the auricle and the passage leading to the tympanic membrane, the external auditory canal.

The auricle is a convoluted plate of elastic cartilage covered with skin and fixed in position by both muscles and ligaments. The major convolutions of the auricle are the helix and antihelix, the tragus and antitragus, and the concha, which is a funnel-like depression leading to the meatus (Fig. 40–5). The lobule is the only portion of the auricle that does not contain cartilage. The cartilage of the auricle is continuous with that of the external meatus.

The external auditory canal is formed in its outer third by an extension of the cartilage of the auricle and in its inner two thirds by the tympanic and squamous portion of the temporal bone. It is bounded medially by the tympanic membrane. The cartilaginous portion of the canal differs markedly in structure from the bony portion. The cartilage is firmly attached to the temporal bone but maintains some mobility because of fibrous channels in the cartilage, the fissures of Santorini, which may also transmit infection or tumor between the canal and the parotid gland. The skin covering the cartilaginous portion of the canal is loosely applied and contains numerous hair follicles and ceruminous and sebaceous glands.

The bony external canal is curved anteriorly and inferiorly and narrows in its midportion to form an isthmus. It constitutes two thirds of the total length of the meatus, which averages 3½ cm. The diameter of the canal varies but averages 7 by 9 mm, the vertical dimension being the greater. The skin of the bony canal is applied closely to bone, the subcutaneous layers condensing to form the periosteum. Fibrous tissue enters the two suture lines in the canal, making elevation of the canal skin particularly difficult over these sutures. As the tympanic membrane is approached, the skin gradually thins, forming a layer five to seven cells thick over the meatal surface of the tympanic membrane. The drum and bony canal skin have a self-cleaning property because of migration of the keratin layer of epithelium from the drum outward to the cartilaginous portion. This migration is rather rapid near the attachment of the malleus handle, decelerates circumferentially from the umbo and becomes slow as the canal is reached.

The tympanic membrane is composed of three layers, the squamous cell epithelial layer bounding the external ear medially, the mucosal layer bounding the middle ear laterally, and the fibrous layer lying between. The fibrous layer is composed of both circumferential and radial fibers and gives the tympanic membrane its shape and consistency. The radial fibers insert into the periostium of the malleus handle and into the fibrous anulus, creating the functionally significant conical shape. The circumferential fibers give strength without interfering with free vibration, whereas some tangential fibers reinforce the architecture. These architectural characteristics of the tympanic membrane allow it to approach the ideal in radiation of vibratory energy.

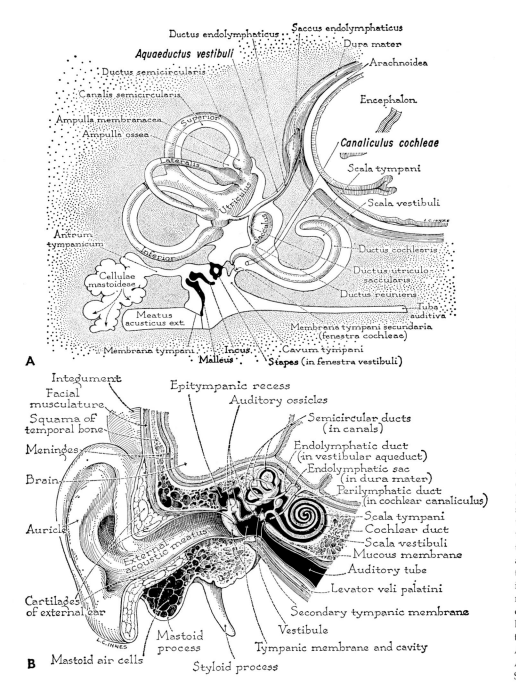

Fig. 40–4. A. Parts of the ear (diagrammatic): the membranous duct system for the endolymph; the surrounding osseous labyrinth containing the perilymph; the tympanic cavity; the auditory tube and pneumatic spaces (with which the cavity is continuous); and the contained auditory ossicles. The tympanic cavity (of the middle ear) is separated from the external acoustic meatus (of the outer ear) by the tympanic membrane and from the vestibule (of the inner ear) by the base, or footplate, of the stapes, anchored in the vestibular (oval) window by the annular ligament. The labyrinths are not wholly sequestered systems. The perilymphatic spaces of the osseous labyrinth communicate with those of the cranial arachnoid through the cochlear canaliculus (or aqueduct); the endolymphatic sac of the membranous labyrinthine system is lodged in the dura mater, which it reaches through the vestibular aqueduct. (Courtesy of Dr. Barry J. Anson). B. General relationships of parts of the ear (semidiagrammatic). (From Anson BJ and McVay CB: Surgical Anatomy. 5th ed. Philadelphia, WB Saunders, 1981.)

The most prominent landmark in the tympanic membrane is the manubrium (handle) of the malleus whose superior limit is marked by the lateral or short process, a short thumblike projection directed laterally. The manubrium is flat and rounded inferiorly, ending at the apex or umbo of the tympanic membrane. Because of the conical shape of the drumhead, a light reflex projects anteroinferiorly from the umbo. At the periphery of the tympanic membrane, the fibrous layer thickens and coalesces to form the tympanic anulus, which is inserted into the sulcus of the tympanic bone.

Superiorly, the tympanic ring is incomplete so that the fibrous layer is bounded by the anterior and posterior mallear folds. The superior arch of the margin of the tympanic membrane formed by the squamous portion of the temporal bone is termed the incisura tympanica or notch of Rivinus. The segment of tympanic membrane superior to the mallear folds and bounded by the rivinian notch is completely lacking a fibrous layer and is thus called the pars flaccida (Shrapnell's membrane). The larger, inferior portion is called the pars tensa of the tympanic membrane.

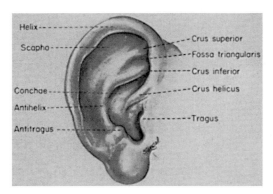

Fig. 40–5. The anatomy of the auricle.

The Middle Ear

The middle ear consists of the space between the tympanic membrane and the capsule of the inner ear, the ossicular and muscular contents of this space, and the appendages; the auditory (eustachian) tube; and the mastoid air cell system (Fig. 40–6). The superior and inferior limits of the tympanic membrane divide the tympanic cavity into the epitympanum or attic, the mesotympanum, and the hypotympanum.

The *hypotympanum* is a shallow space that lies inferior to the tympanic membrane. Its bony surface presents a scalloped appearance because of the presence of cuplike air cells. This wall covers the jugular bulb. Occasionally a dehiscence permits the jugular to present in the lower tympanic cavity.

The *mesotympanum* is bounded medially by the otic capsule, inferior to the level of the tympanic portion of the facial nerve. The curved eminence that covers the basal turn of the cochlea lies immediately medial to the drumhead and is termed the promontory. Several shallow channels in the promontory contain the nerves that make up the tympanic plexus. Posterior to the promontory, located superiorly and inferiorly, respectively, are the oval (vestibular) and round (cochlear) windows, each placed at the bottom of a niche. These two depressions communicate at the posterior limit of the mesotympanum by a deep curved fossa, the tympanic sinus. The oval window contains the stapedial footplate, which is placed in the sagittal plane. The round window is protected from view because it is placed in a mostly transverse plane anterior to a lip that extends from the promontory. The round window is closed by a thin membrane, the secondary tympanic membrane. The posterior wall of the mesotympanum is formed by the bone covering the descending portion of the facial nerve. This bone is usually pneumatized with the cells, often communicating with the mastoid air cell system. Superiorly on this wall, a conical projection, the pyramidal eminence, encloses the stapedius muscle and transmits its tendon. A branch of the seventh nerve runs to the muscle. Lateral to the pyramidal eminence is the foramen for the chorda tympani nerve, which runs inferiorly through a curved canal to join the facial canal near or at the stylomastoid foramen.

A clinically important space, the posterior sinus or facial recess, occurs immediately lateral to the facial canal and pyramidal process, being bounded laterally by the posterosuperior tympanic anulus and superiorly by the short process of the incus inserting into the incudal fossa (Fig. 40–7). The space leads from the posterosuperior middle ear cavity to the aditus ad antrum and frequently hides disease. Approaching this space from the mastoid antrum allows exposure of the structures of the posterior tympanum and the facial nerve.

The anterior extremity of the tympanic portion of the facial canal is marked by a hooklike projection of

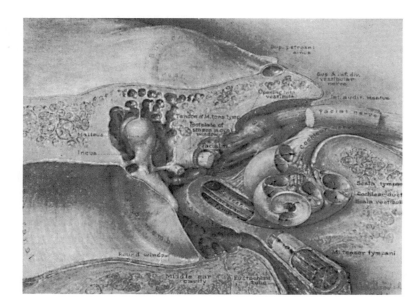

Fig. 40–6. Section through the middle ear and labyrinth. (From three unpublished drawings of the human ear. Max Brodel, WB Saunders, 1946.)

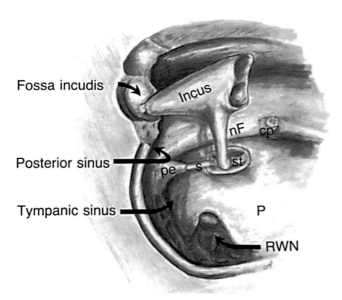

Fossa incudis

Posterior sinus

Tympanic sinus

Fig. 40–7. Recesses of the posterior tympanum. RWN, Round window niche; P, promontory; pe, pyramidal eminence; s, stapedius tendon; st, stapes; nF, facial nerve; cp, cochleariform process.

the posterior end of the canal of the tensor tympani muscle, the cochleariform process, which turns the tendon of the tensor laterally into the middle ear. The canal of the tensor tympani runs forward into the superior surface of the eustachian tube and marks the anterosuperior limit of the mesotympanum.

The anterior wall of the mesotympanum contains the tympanic orifice of the eustachian tube superiorly and forms the bony covering of the ascending carotid canal inferiorly. This wall is usually well pneumatized and may have bony dehiscences.

The *epitympanum* contains the bulk of the incus and malleus. Superiorly, it is bounded by a thin projection of the petrous, the tegmen tympani, which is continuous with the posterior tegmen mastoideum. The otic capsule forms the medial attic wall, which is marked by the bulge of the lateral semicircular canal. Anteriorly, the ampullary region of the superior canal may be approached, and anteriorly yet is the region of the geniculate ganglion, marking the anterior extremity of the attic space. The anterior wall is separated by a narrow space from the malleus head and may contain entrances of some of the air cells pneumatizing the root of the zygoma. The lateral attic wall is formed by the squamous, which continues laterally as the superior bony external canal wall. Posteriorly, the attic narrows into the entrance to the mastoid antrum, the aditus ad antrum.

Auditory Ossicles

The auditory ossicles form a system of bony levers and columns that transmits vibratory mechanical energy to the periotic fluid. The system is composed of the malleus (hammer), the incus (anvil), and the stapes (stir-

rup) (Fig. 40–8). The malleus and incus operate largely as a unit, rotating in response to movements of the drumhead through an axis, which may be approximated by a line drawn between the anterior mallear ligament and the ligament of the incus at the tip of the short process. These movements are maintained in unison by the interlocking form of the incudomalleal joint. This rotational motion is transferred into the piston-like action of the stapes at the incudostapedial joint.

The malleus consists of the handle (manubrium), neck, head, and two processes, lateral or short process and anterior process. The head is contained within the attic space, whereas the neck lies behind the pars flaccida of the tympanic membrane. The handle is contained within the drum membrane, serving as the attachment for the fibers of the tunica propria. Viewed from the lateral aspect, the axis of the malleus is straight, but in the sagittal plane, the head forms an angle of approximately 45 degrees with the inwardly slanting manubrium. The tensor tympani tendon inserts on the medial surface of the upper end of the manubrium. The articular surface on the head is notched to clasp firmly a similar surface on the incus. This joint has a narrow space and thin articular ligament. The malleus is suspended by the anterior mallear ligament, a superior ligament attached to the tegmen, and a lateral ligament between the base of the short process and the margin of the notch of Rivinus.

The incus has a body that narrows to form the short process, which is attached by the incudal ligament in the fossa incudis, and an inferiorly directed long process. The long process arises near the articular surface, descends parallel to the malleus handle, and ends with a short accessory process, the lenticular process, which arises at a right angle to articulate with the stapes. This joint is shaped in a mild ball and cup fashion, with a joint space and articular ligament.

Except for the cartilaginous articular surfaces and the cartilaginous malleus handle, the incus and malleus are formed of replacement bone, with a heavy periosteal layer and a small true marrow cavity. The adult stapes has been excavated completely, however, consisting of a thin shell of periosteal bone that forms the framework, with cartilage remaining on the articular surface of the head and the vestibular surface of the base.

The *stapes* is shaped like a stirrup, consisting of a head, neck, anterior and posterior crura, and a base or footplate. The head supports the shallow cup-shaped articular surface, then constricts slightly to form the short neck. The crura are bowed, the posterior more than the anterior, and terminate by fusing with the flat reniform base. The obturator aspect of the neck and crura is extensively excavated, leaving a hollow shell of periosteal bone. The stapedius tendon inserts on a

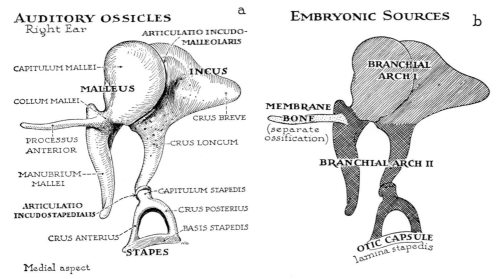

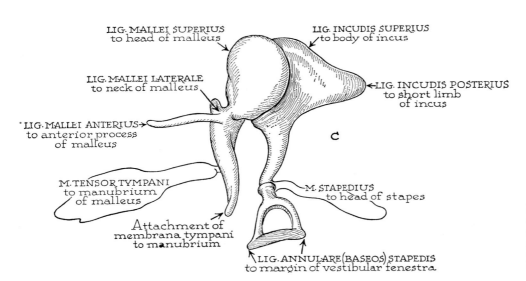

Fig. 40–8. Auditory ossicles: their adult form, embryologic derivation, and muscles and ligaments. (From Anson BJ [Ed]: Morris' Human Anatomy. 12th ed. New York, McGraw-Hill, 1966.)

small prominence on the posterior surface of the neck of the stapes.

Tympanic Muscles

Two muscles are contained within the middle ear: the tensor tympani and the stapedius (Fig. 40–8).

The tensor tympani muscle arises from the walls of the semicanal of the tensor tympani. This canal lies just superior to the bony auditory canal and is open toward the auditory canal, thus the term "semicanal." The muscle fibers collect and become tendinous at the tympanic end of the semicanal, which is marked by the cochleariform process. This process serves to turn the tendon lateralward into the middle ear. The tendon inserts on the upper portion of the manubrium of the malleus. The tensor tympani is innervated by a branch of the fifth cranial nerve. Its action causes the drumhead to be pulled inward, thus tensing it and raising

the resonant frequency of the sound conduction system as well as attenuating low-frequency sound.

The stapedius muscle arises within its canal in the pyramidal eminence, the fibers being attached to the periosteum of this canal. The fibers collect and form the stapedius tendon, which inserts on the posterior aspect of the neck of the stapes. The stapedius is innervated by a branch of the seventh cranial nerve given off as it passes the stapedius during its second turn. The action of the stapedius pulls the stapes posteriorly around a pivot at the posterior lip of the stapes base. This stiffens the stapes, attenuating sound transmission and raising the resonant frequency of the ossicular chain.

These actions can be controlled voluntarily by some individuals but are usually a part of the reflex activity of the ear. Although the purpose of this activity was thought to be to protect the inner ear from the trauma of loud sounds, animal investigation has indicated the possibility of vegetative and species survival function.

Auditory (Eustachian) Tube

The auditory tube extends from the anterior superior wall of the mesotympanum to the nasopharynx. The anatomy of the tube varies considerably, ranging from its pharyngeal cartilaginous portion to the tympanic bony portion. The pharyngeal orifice is surrounded by a hook-shaped cartilage within the torus tubarius. Contraction of the anteriorly attached tensor veli palatini muscle causes the cartilaginous tube to assume a more cylindric shape and become patent. The mucosal lining of the cartilaginous portion is similar to that of the pharynx, having many mucous glands. The submucosa contains numerous lymphoid aggregates. The cartilaginous portion runs posteriorly and superiorly for two thirds of the total length of the auditory tube (4 cm), where it joins the bony or tympanic portion of the tube. The point of union is the narrowest part of the tube, the isthmus, and there is a gradual widening to the largest diameter at the tympanic orifice. During this course, the mucosa gradually thins to become similar to the cuboidal or low columnar tympanic mucosa. A few mucous glands continue through the tympanic portion. The inferior wall of the bony auditory tube overlies the carotid canal. The superior wall contains the semicanal of the tensor tympani muscle.

Nerve Supply of External and Middle Ear

The auricle and external meatus receive sensory branches from the auriculotemporal branch of the fifth nerve anteriorly, from the greater and lesser auricular nerve posteriorly, and by branches arising from the glossopharyngeal and vagus nerves. The branch from the vagus is known as Arnold's nerve, the stimulation of which may cause a cough reflex when the external ear is being cleaned. The posterior superior portion of the bony canal may be supplied by sensory branches of the facial nerve (Fig. 40–9).

The promontory of the middle ear contains the tympanic plexus (Jacobson's plexus). This receives Jacobson's nerve, a branch of the glossopharyngeal arising from the petrosal ganglion below the ear. After entering the tympanic plexus, the fibers run forward, leaving the middle ear with a branch of the facial, the lesser superficial petrosal nerve. After a short course through the cranial cavity on the anterior aspect of the temporal bone, the fibers terminate in the otic ganglion to innervate primarily the parotid gland. The tympanic plexus receives sympathetic fibers from the carotid plexus by superior and inferior caroticotympanic branches.

The chorda tympani enters the middle ear just below the posterosuperior lip of the tympanic sulcus and runs forward lateral to the long process of the incus, then under the neck of the malleus just above the attachment of the tensor tympani tendon. It exits through the petrotympanic fissure after running medial to the anterior mallear ligament.

Mastoid Anatomy

PNEUMATIC. The pneumatic air cell system arises in conjunction with the enlarging temporal bone as an outgrowth of the middle ear and antrum. Air cell groups may be classified by the point of developmental origin. The cells developing from the antrum are the largest group, forming in the enlarging mastoid process. *Mastoid cells* are external to a commonly occurring plate of bone marking the fusion of the antral process of the petrous and the tympanic process of the squama (petrosquamous suture), known as Körner's septum. Internal to the septum are the *antral cells,* which are extensions medially from the original antrum into the petrous. These may invade the petrous deeply to outline the semicircular canals and internal auditory canal. The sigmoid sinus may be surrounded with a *sinus group,* and the squama may be invaded. An anterior and lateral extension of these cells may invade the zygoma (*zygomal cells*) and communicate with the attic. The *mastoid tip cells* occasionally form a large coalescent area in the extremity of the mastoid process.

The middle ear tympanic cells form several divergent groups, which pneumatize the petrous. The largest of these is made up of the *carotid air cells,* which surround the carotid canal and merge with the *subtubal group* of air cells that arise from the auditory tube. The *apical cells* of the petrous arise mainly from this group, as do the *precochlear cells.* Also differentiated are *precarotid, postcarotid,* and *supracarotid* groups of air cells. A *supracochlear* group of air cells may arise from the medial attic wall and extend above the cochlea and around the geniculate ganglion, sometimes merging with antral cells around the superior semicircular canal. Cells that arise from the posterior middle ear may communicate anterior to the facial nerve with the mastoid cells or even serve as a point of origin for the mastoid cells. The *retrofacial cells* arise from the tympanic sinus and pneumatize the petrous medial to the facial nerve. Eradication of disease from these last two groups of air cells presents a surgical risk to the facial nerve.

The extent of pneumatization of the temporal bone varies among individuals. This is determined by both hereditary and environmental factors. Otitis in infancy and childhood can inhibit further pneumatization and cause sclerosis. On the other hand, limited pneumatization of the temporal bone may predispose the ear to infection.

SURGICAL. The surgical anatomy of the mastoid deserves special study because it involves picturing the internal margins of the mastoid after removal of the air cell system. This anatomic configuration is thus created surgically and consists of exposing, but not injuring, the important structures bordering the *mastoid cavity.*

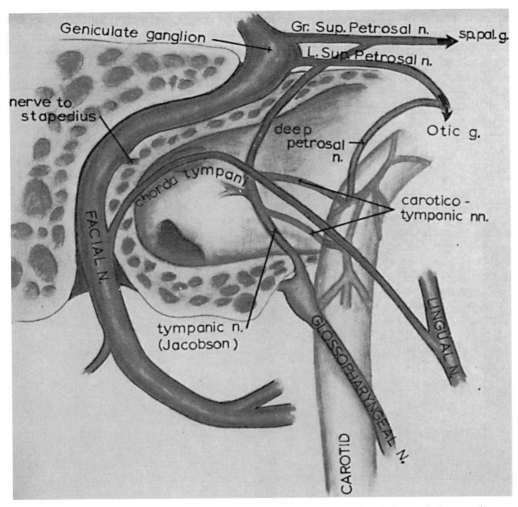

Fig. 40–9. The facial nerve and its relationships (diagrammatic). sp.pal.g., Sphenopalatine ganglion.

The posterior limit of the mastoid cavity is formed by the bone that overlies the posterior dura. The major landmark is the large convex channel running from the superolateral corner to the posteromedial corner formed by the lateral sinus. The superior limit of this wall forms an acute angle with the mastoid tegmen, the sinodural angle. The tegmen forms the upper wall of the cavity. Inferiorly, the mastoid tip forms the wall superficially, with the digastric ridge projecting into the space medial to the tip. The cavity is limited anteriorly by the posterior wall of the external auditory canal and the vertical segment of the facial nerve lying at the base of this wall (Fig. 40–10). This portion of the facial nerve extends roughly from the fossa incudis to the anterior end of the digastric ridge.

The medial wall of the mastoid cavity presents several landmarks. The lateral and posterior semicircular canals occupy the major portion of this wall. The triangle between the external prominence of these canals and the posterosuperior corner of the mastoid is known as Trautmann's triangle, from which a group of antral cells invades the petrous deeply to the region of the internal auditory canal. Visualization of the medial wall may be confused by the presence of Körner's septum, which divides the cells into superficial and deep regions. The antrum is not reached until this septum is removed and the previously mentioned landmarks identified.

The Inner Ear

Contained within the petrous portion of the temporal bone is the otic capsule, in turn containing the periotic labyrinth, which surrounds the essential structure of the inner ear, the membranous labyrinth (Fig. 40–11). The membranous labyrinth is the continuous series of epithelial lined tubes and spaces of the inner ear that contains the membranous endolymph. The membranous labyrinth is divided into three interconnected parts with separate functions: the pars superior or vestibular labyrinth, the pars inferior or cochlea, and the endolymphatic duct and sac.

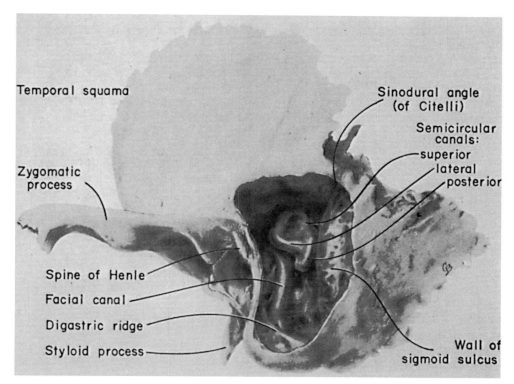

Fig. 40–10. Mastoid cavity in a left temporal bone. Complete exenteration of the air cells, demonstrating the relation of the facial (fallopian) canal to the semicircular canals and to the sulcus for the sigmoid part of the transverse (venous) sinus of the dura mater. The facial canal, in passing lateralward and downward, lies close to the mastoid wall of the tympanic cavity. Surgically, the tip cells are removed with the facial canal as the anterior limiting boundary and the wall of the sigmoid sulcus serving as the posterior boundary. The sulcus, on the medial wall of the mastoid part of the temporal bone, curves from above and behind in a direction downward and forward. The floor of the space is elevated by the so-called digastric ridge. On the external surface of the mastoid process a corresponding depression occurs; this is the mastoid incisure (or digastric fossa of the older terminology). The sigmoid sulcus meets the "roof" of the cavity at an acute angle; externally the angle thus formed is represented by the junction of the middle with the posterior cranial fossa. The roof is the bone of the anterior surface of the petrous pyramid; it is covered by the meningeal layers of the cerebrum. (From Anson BJ and Donaldson JA: Surgical Anatomy of the Temporal Bone and Ear. Philadelphia, WB Saunders, 1981.)

The *vestibular labyrinth* consists of the saccule, utricle, and semicircular ducts. The semicircular ducts arise and end at the utricle, each being directed in a plane perpendicular to the other in the axis of the petrous pyramid. These are the superior, posterior, and lateral or external or horizontal ducts. The posterior limb of the superior duct joins into a common crus with the superior limb of the posterior duct to enter the utricle, while each of the remaining limbs is separate. Near the origin of each semicircular duct is a cystic dilation termed the ampulla, which contains the end-organ of balance, the crista.

The sensory organs within the inner ear are constructed of essentially the same elements, but each is organized in a specialized manner to respond to a particular type of mechanical stimulus. These elements include supporting cells; sensory cells that contain nonmotile cilia on their free surface, the hair cells; and a gelatinous, cushionlike structure lying on the hair cells, principally composed of mucopolysaccharides secreted by the supporting cells.

The crista ampullaris forms a ridge across the ampulla perpendicular to the direction of fluid motion. This ridge is capped by a layer of hair cells supported between flask-shaped cells. A semilunar cap of gelatinous material, the cupula, extends from the hair cells to the opposite wall of the ampulla to form a valve which is deflected by the smallest fluid motion in either direction (Fig. 40–12). Two types of cuboidal cells, light and dark, run along the base of the ridge, then up on the walls of the ampulla at each end of the crista to form the planum semilunatum, which seems to have both a secretory and an absorptive function. The cupula has a definite structure, with channels running through it that contain for at least part of their length the cilia of the hair cells. There is a thin, clear zone between the hair cells and the cupula.

The semicircular ducts are located eccentrically within the surrounding periotic space (semicircular canals), being attached along their greater curvature to the endosteum of the otic capsule. The remaining space within the semicircular canals is crossed with sparsely distributed arachnoid-like trabeculae through which circulates the periotic fluid (perilymph). The periotic

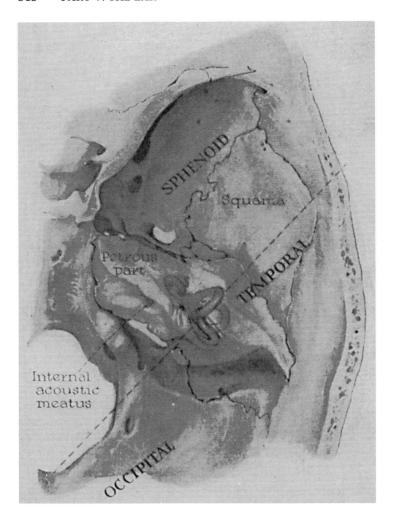

Fig. 40–11. Position of the right osseous (perilymphatic) labyrinth in the skull. (From Anson BJ [Ed]: Morris' Human Anatomy. 12th ed. New York, McGraw-Hill, 1966.)

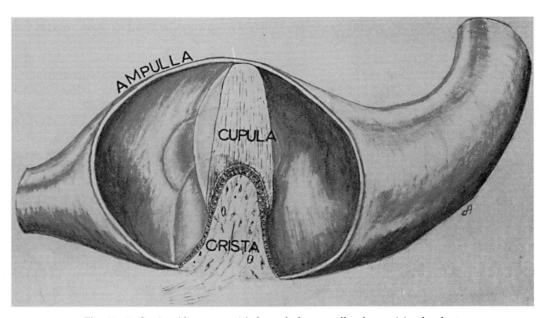

Fig. 40–12. Section (diagrammatic) through the ampulla of a semicircular duct.

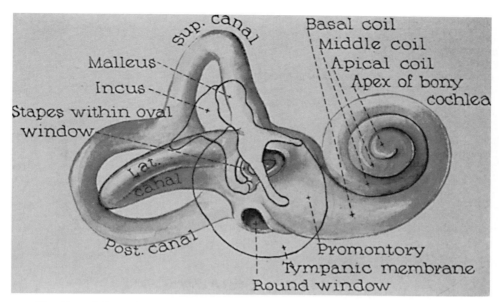

Fig. 40–13. Relationship of the tympanic membrane and ossicles with the bony labyrinth.

spaces join anteriorly into a single large cistern, the vestibule, containing the utricle and saccule. The lateral wall of this space contains the oval window, closed by the stapes footplate (Fig. 40–13).

In addition to serving as a reservoir for the semicircular duct fluid flow, the utricle has an otolithic endorgan or macula lying on its floor in the horizontal

plane and occasionally extending slightly up the anterior wall. The maculae are flat structures composed of hair cells between supporting cells (Fig. 40–14). The gelatinous cushion (otolithic membrane) overlying the hair cells is flat and firmly attached to the cilia. There is a free space between the undersurface of the otolithic membrane and the free surface of the hair cells through

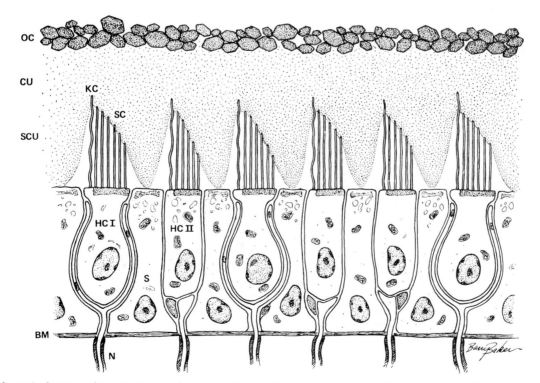

Fig. 40–14. Schematic drawing of a cross section of a macula. The gelatinous substance is divided into cupular (CU) and subcupular (SCU) layers. There are two types of hairs: kinocilia, labeled KC (one per hair cell), and stereocilia, labeled SC (many per hair cell). OC, Otoconia; HC I, type I hair cell; HC II, type II hair cell; N, nerve fiber; BM, basement membrane; S, supporting cell.

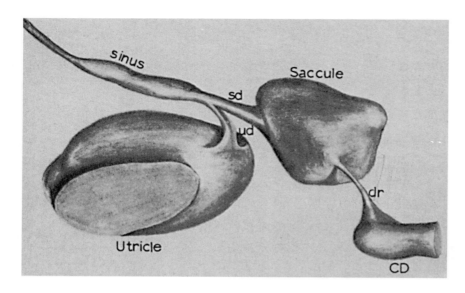

Fig. 40–15. Detail of the endolymphatic duct system (after Anson). sd, Saccular duct; ud, utricular duct; dr, ductus reuniens; CD, cochlear duct.

which the cilia project. Embedded on the surface of the otolithic membrane are numerous small calcareous deposits adding additional mass.

The utricular duct leaves the anterior face of the utricle and curves posteriorly around the anterior wall, creating a deep, valvelike fold over the orifice of the duct first described by Bast and termed the utriculoendolymphatic valve. The valve is structured to permit inflow of endolymph but not outflow. An actual valvular function has yet to be demonstrated. The utricular duct joins with a similar channel from the saccule, the saccular duct, to form the endolymphatic duct (Figs. 40–15 to 40–17). After an initial dilation, the sinus of the endolymphatic duct, it narrows to enter a bony channel through the otic capsule, the vestibular aqueduct. The aqueduct parallels the common crus of the posterior and superior semicircular canals, then swings in a lateral and posterior direction to emerge on the posterior face of the petrous bone, usually just medial to the lateral extremity of the posterior semicir-

cular canal. The vestibular aqueduct gradually enlarges and contains abundant vascular connective tissue around the endolymphatic duct. Within the terminal portion of the aqueduct, the duct enlarges and the lining membrane becomes rugose to form the proximal portion of the endolymphatic sac, which is contained within the bony aqueduct. The distal external portion gradually becomes smooth and is contained within the dural covering of the posterior face of the petrous pyramid. The end of the sac terminates in close relationship to the sigmoid sinus. Numerous active granular cells similar to others with secretory activity are found in the lining membrane of the endolymphatic sac.

The saccule is much smaller than the utricle but similar in structure. The saccule supports a macular structure on its medial wall in the vertical plane extending slightly onto the anterior wall. Both the utricle and saccule are entirely surrounded by perilymph except where the nerves enter at the macular region. A small

Fig. 40–16. Membranous labyrinth. Adult anatomy, demonstrated by a reconstruction (6-month-old infant) and by a semidiagram. a. The utricle communicates broadly with the common arm of the superior and posterior semicircular ducts; together they assume the form of an open V. The tube-shaped utricle, lying in the elliptical recess of the vestibule, is continuous with the three semicircular ducts. The utricle opens widely into its canalicular ducts. On its anterolateral surface is situated the acoustic macula. The saccule has the form of an elongated oval. It occupies the spherical recess. The saccule is connected with the utricle indirectly, through the saccular and the utricular (or utriculoendolymphatic) ducts; in the opposite direction (toward the cochlea) the connections are the reuniting duct (*ductus reuniens*) and the vestibular cecum, a cul-de-sac of the cochlear duct proper. These enter and leave the saccule on the latter's inferior surface; as a result, the saccule is set off from its dependent communications. The acoustic macula is situated on the anteromedial surface. b. The endolymphatic duct, far from being a quill-like tube with a mushroom-shaped terminal expansion, is regionally modified in a constant fashion. The opening into the utricle, for example, is slitlike in form, the orifice being bounded by a folding of the apposed walls of the utricle and the endolymphatic duct. The proximal part of the latter duct is expanded into a sinuslike enlargement that occupies the internal aperture of the vestibular aqueduct. Continuing toward the external aperture, the duct narrows into an isthmus. While still intraosseous, the duct becomes a flattened cecal dilatation, the endolymphatic sac. The *saccus* is prolonged beyond the aperture, to rest in a shallow impression on the posterior surface of the petrous pyramid. The cochlear part of the membranous labyrinth is formed by the cochlear duct. It begins in a recess of the vestibule and extends within the osseous spiral canal, through basal, middle, and apical coils, where it ends blindly in the cupular cecum. The cochlear duct is in large part triangular in cross section. Its outer wall is held by periosteal connective tissue to the osseous cochlea. It contains the spiral organ (Corti), a highly differentiated structure that contains the termination of the cochlear nerve. (From Anson BJ and Donaldson JA: Surgical Anatomy of the Temporal Bone and Ear. Philadelphia, WB Saunders, 1981.)

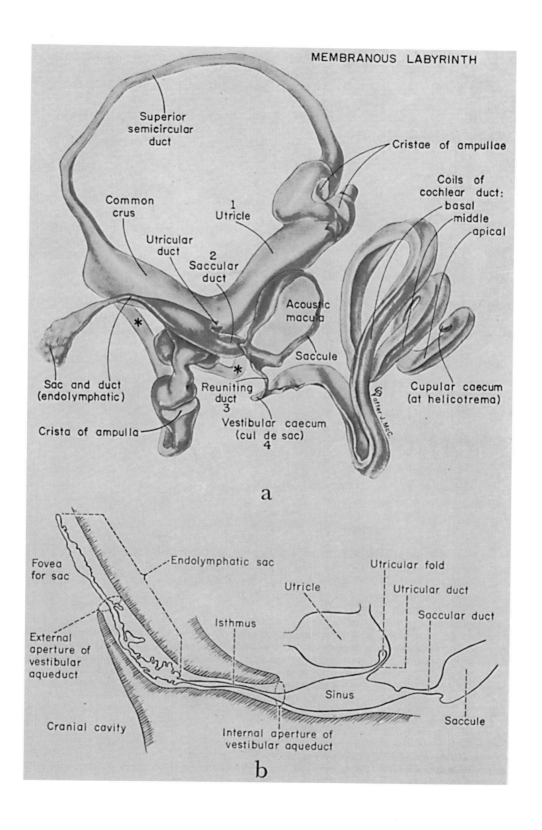

MEMBRANOUS LABYRINTH

Superior semicircular duct

Cristae of ampullae

Coils of cochlear duct:
basal
middle
apical

Common crus

1
Utricle

Utricular duct

2
Saccular duct

Acoustic macula

Saccule

*

Cupular caecum (at helicotrema)

Sac and duct (endolymphatic)

Reuniting duct
3

Crista of ampulla

Vestibular caecum (cul de sac)
4

a

Fovea for sac

Endolymphatic sac

Utricular fold

Utricle

Utricular duct

Saccular duct

External aperture of vestibular aqueduct

Isthmus

Cranial cavity

Sinus

Saccule

Internal aperture of vestibular aqueduct

b

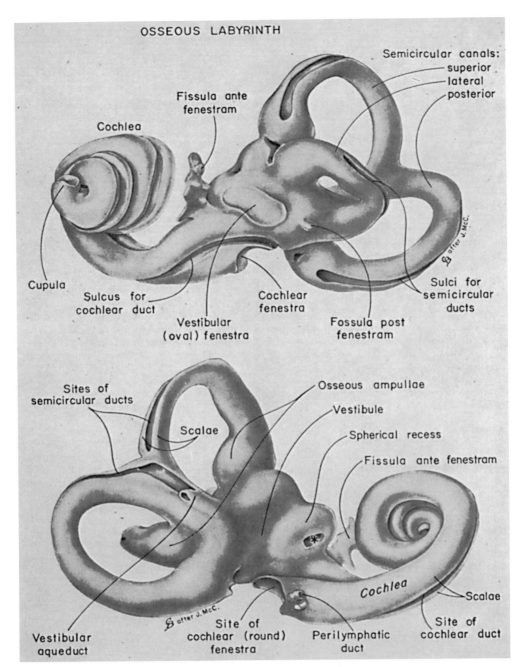

OSSEOUS LABYRINTH

Semicircular canals:
— superior
— lateral
— posterior

Fissula ante fenestram

Cochlea

Cupula

Sulcus for cochlear duct

Vestibular (oval) fenestra

Cochlear fenestra

Fossula post fenestram

Sulci for semicircular ducts

Sites of semicircular ducts

Scalae

Osseous ampullae

Vestibule

Spherical recess

Fissula ante fenestram

Cochlea

Scalae

Vestibular aqueduct

Site of cochlear (round) fenestra

Perilymphatic duct

Site of cochlear duct

Fig. 40–17. Osseous labyrinth, shown by a reconstruction of the contained perilymphatic system of spaces. Lateral and medial aspects. The bony labyrinth, here represented as the contained perilymphatic space, consists of three parts: a middle, the vestibule; the cochlea, situated anteromedially; the three semicircular canals, placed posterolaterally in the petrous part of the temporal bone. The vestibule is roughly oval-shaped. The medial wall (see lower figure) forms part of the fundus of the internal meatus. Two deepened areas of unequal size are present on this wall; the posterior one, the elliptical recess, serves for reception of the utriculus; the anterior small rounded area, the spherical recess, receives the saccule. In the latter, the perforated area (medial cribrose macula, at *) transmits the saccular branch of the vestibular nerve. The bony semicircular canals are three curved tubes, each of which is continuous at two points with the space of the vestibule. The lateral, or "horizontal," canal produces the *prominentia* in the wall of the epitympanic recess. Its plane is not exactly horizontal. The other two canals run in approximately vertical planes. The superior canal stands at a right angle to the axis of the petrous pyramid; it gives rise to the *eminentia arcuata* on the anterior surface of the pyramid. The posterior canal lies almost parallel to the posterior surface of the pyramid. One of the two ends of each semicircular canal presents a flask-shaped enlargement, the osseous ampulla (entrance for an ampullary nerve). The nonampullated ends of the superior and posterior canals unite to form a *crus commune*. The corresponding semicircular duct occupies the periphery of the canal (represented here by sulci between scalae). The cochlea, or "snail," is cone-shaped with the axis placed horizontally. The base, with the modiolus, is directed toward the fundus of the internal acoustic meatus. It curls upon itself into about two and three-quarter turns. The basal turn projects into the tympanic cavity as the *promontorium*. The cochlear duct, like each of the semicircular ducts, occupies the outer aspect of a coil (here shown as a continuous sulcus). In the macerated bone (that is, in a skeletal preparation) the perilymphatic space is carried into three offsets, which cross the bone to the opposite surface of the pyramid. These appendages are the following: vestibular aqueduct, cochlear canaliculus (or aqueduct), fissula ante fenestram (and, inconstantly, a fossula post fenestram). The so-called perilymphatic "duct" is the network of interstices among the fibrils of periotic connective tissue in the canaliculus. (From Anson BJ and Donaldson JA: Surgical Anatomy of the Temporal Bone and Ear. Philadelphia, WB Saunders, 1981.)

duct leaves the wall of the saccule to run along the floor of the vestibule and enter the cochlear duct. This is termed the ductus reuniens and is the sole endolymphatic communication of the cochlea with the remainder of the labyrinth.

Cochlea

The pars inferior of the labyrinth is formed in a spiral of 2½ to 2¾ turns, with a total length of approximately 35 cm. Both the cochlear duct and the periotic space are complex structures that form a system of three tubular chambers, the scala vestibuli, the scala media or cochlear duct, and the scala tympani (Fig. 40–18).

The cochlea is supported by the modiolus, a central spiral of membrane bone anchored to the otic capsule by septa, which serve to separate and delineate the turns of the cochlea. The fibers of the auditory portion of the eighth nerve ascend within the modiolus, reaching their termination at the hair cells through small channels in the osseous spiral lamina, a projection outward from the modiolus that anchors the cochlear duct centrally. The cell bodies of these neurons are grouped along the modiolus at the base of the spiral lamina to form the spiral ganglion.

The cochlear duct (scala media) is triangular, expanding from a narrow attachment at the bony spiral lamina to a broad attachment external to the otic capsule by means of a band of fibrous tissue, the spiral ligament. The boundary adjacent to the scala tympani forms the principal attachment, a strong, radially fibrous extension of the bony spiral lamina called the basilar membrane, which supports the end-organ of hearing, the organ of Corti, on its surface. The border between the scala vestibuli and the cochlear duct is formed by a delicate two-cell layer membrane, Reissner's membrane. Externally, a vascular strip extends along the cochlear duct, containing a surface of granular secretory type cells, the stria vascularis.

The periotic spaces, scala vestibuli and scala tympani, around the cochlear duct are joined only at the termination of the cochlear spiral. Here the bony spiral lamina ends in a hooklike projection, the hamulus, which forms a round opening with the top of the modiolus, the helicotrema. Through the helicotrema the two periotic scalae communicate. The scala tympani ends

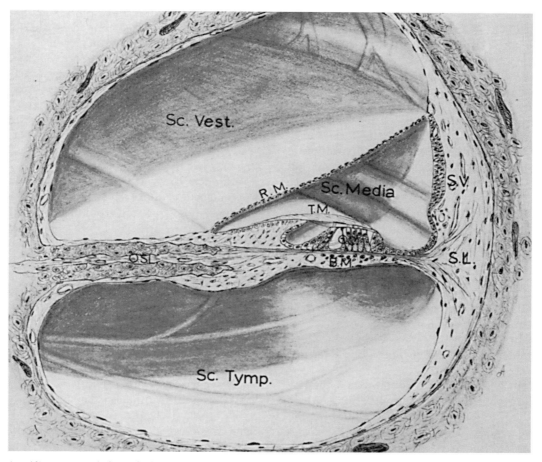

Fig. 40–18. Section (diagrammatic) through the cochlea. Sc. Vest., scala vestibuli; R.M., Reissner's membrane; Sc. Media, scala media; T.M., tectorial membrane; O.C., organ of Corti; B.M., basilar membrane; S.V., stria vascularis; S.L., spiral ligament; O.S.L., osseous spiral lamina; Sc. Tymp., scala tympani.

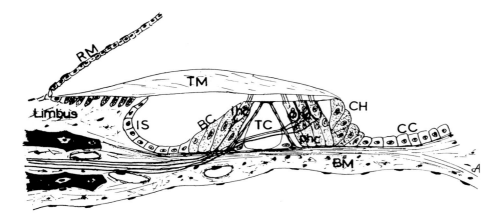

Fig. 40–19. Detail of organ of Corti. RM, Reissner's membrane; TM, tectorial membrane; IS, inner sulcus; BC, border cells; ihc, inner hair cells; TC, tunnel of Corti; ohc, outer hair cells; phc, phalangeal cells; CH, cells of Hansen; CC, cells of Claudius; BM, basilar membrane.

proximally in a blind pouch into which the fenestra rotunda (round window) opens. The scala vestibuli opens directly into the vestibule. A bony passage communicates between the termination of the scala tympani and the subarachnoid space, the cochlear aqueduct. This contains a trabecular network of connective tissue, the so-called periotic duct, which may allow exchange of spinal fluid and perilymph. Paralleling the cochlear aqueduct is a separate channel that contains the cochlear vein.

The *organ of Corti* is a complex structure that consists of three basic parts: supporting cells, hair cells, and a gelatinous-contacting membrane, the tectorial membrane (Fig. 40–19). Together with its supporting structure, the basilar membrane, it varies continuously throughout its length. At the basal end, the basilar membrane is narrow and stiff, becoming broad and more flaccid in the apical portion. The tectorial membrane and organ of Corti follow a similar variation in structural characteristics along their length, resulting in a "tuning" of the cochlear duct. As a result of these characteristics, high-frequency sound energy is concentrated at the basal end of the cochlea, while lower frequencies spread progressively along the length of the organ of Corti.

The hair cells are arranged in a single row of inner hair cells and three to five rows of outer hair cells. These are separated by an inverted V formed by the tonofibrils of the inner and outer pillar cells, resulting in a strong central supporting structure. The space between the pillars is called the tunnel of Corti, which seems to contain a fluid other than endolymph, termed "cortilymph."

The hair cells are supported by elongated phalangeal cells. The free ends bear nonmotile cilia, which rest against the inferior surface of the tectorial membrane. The remainder of the supporting cells have a changing shape, tall near the hair cells and becoming shorter away from them to give the organ of Corti a sloping shape. These cells are named the cells of Hansen, cells of Claudius, and border cells. The tectorial

membrane is supported centrally by the limbus, a thick plate of cells resting on the bony spiral lamina. The limbus also serves as the attachment for Reissner's membrane. The tectorial membrane is attached firmly at its free edge to the cells of Hansen, creating a space between the hair cells and the tectorial membrane containing the cilia of the hair cells. This space is continuous with a rather large space medially between the tectorial membrane and the medial edge of the basilar membrane, the internal spiral sulcus. The medial boundary of this space is lined by a distinct group of cuboidal cells, the inner sulcus cells.

The basilar membrane averages 32 cm in length. The width varies about sixfold, averaging 0.08 mm at the base to 0.498 mm at the apex. There are about 24,000 transverse fibers along the length of the membrane.

The organ of Corti contains approximately 15,500 hair cells. These are grouped in an inner row of 3500 and three to five outer rows containing 12,000. Near the base are three rows of outer hair cells. Another row is added in the middle turns and occasionally a fifth row near the apex. The cross-sectional area varies about 4½-fold, ranging from 0.0053 mm 2 at the base to 0.0223 at the apex.

The spiral ligament and tectorial membrane also vary in a similar manner and degree along their lengths.

Approximately 26,000 ganglion cells exist in the spiral ganglion of an adult with good hearing. A greater concentration of cells are present near the basal portion than in the upper turns.

The hair cells receive the termination of several neurons, which form a basket around the base. Two types of nerve endings are found, one being efferent, the other afferent in function. The afferent system principally is related to the inner hair cells while the outer hair cells receive the main efferent innervation. Single afferent dendrites and the efferent split to end on several hair cells. The axons run through the canaliculi of the bony spiral lamina to the dendrites the cells of the spiral ganglion in the canal of Rosenthal at the base of the lamina. The axons then run through channels in the core of the modiolus, coiling to form the auditory portion of the eighth nerve. These fibers enter the pons in the region of the two cochlear nuclei, dorsal and ventral.

The nerve fibers of the vestibular labyrinth are slightly more complexly arranged, separated into superior and inferior divisions. The superior division is made of fibers from the cristae of the lateral and superior semicircular canals and the macula of the utricle. The inferior division receives fibers from the crista of the posterior canal and the macula of the saccule. The ganglia containing the cell bodies of these fibers, Scarpa's ganglia, are contained within the internal acoustic meatus. The nerve trunk then runs medially to enter the pons near the auditory portion of the acoustic nerve, where the fibers are divided intricately among several vestibular nuclei (Chapter 43).

Fluids of the Inner Ear

It was formerly thought that there were two fluid systems of the inner ear, the endolymph and the perilymph (otic fluid and periotic fluid). The perilymph was thought to be derived from spinal fluid, entering through the periotic duct. The endolymph was thought to be formed by secretory cells of the stria vascularis and absorbed by the endolymphatic sac. Recent observations have thrown great doubt on these traditional concepts; not only have the sites of fluid formation and absorption been doubted, but also the possibility of two or three separate types of fluid being contained within the otic labyrinth has been added.

Perilymph

Much evidence has accumulated in recent years to indicate that little, if any, perilymph originates from cerebrospinal fluid. Anatomically, the cochlear aqueduct is a narrow channel filled with loose areolar tissue without true ductal tissue. Fluid ingress through this channel should be slow at best. Clinically, this is verified at stapes surgery, when only a slow renewal of perilymph is usually seen. Abnormally patent cochlear aqueducts have been seen in temporal bone specimens that are correlated with a massive flow of perilymph when the oval window is open. These patients usually demonstrate diminished cochlear function before surgery.

Chemically, the fluid resembles extracellular fluid, high in sodium content and low in potassium (140 mEq/L versus 5.5 to 6.25 mEq/L). The protein content averages 200 mg per 100 ml, which is considerably greater than that of the CSF. Other chemical differences outlined in Table 40–1 indicate the probability that perilymph is largely formed as an ultrafiltrate of plasma from the vessels in the walls of the periotic spaces. Perilymphatic fluid balance would thus be largely under the control of the balance of hydrostatic and os-

motic pressure, as is most extracellular fluid. An important but yet unmeasured factor in this balance is the amount and state of polymerization of mucopolysaccharides present in this fluid.

Endolymph

Although it has been believed that the stria vascularis is responsible for the formation of endolymph, many other areas play a role. Certain spaces within the otic ducts contain substances dissimilar to endolymph.

Endolymph (Table 40–1) is high in potassium content (140 to 160 mEq/L) and low in sodium (12 to 16 mEq/L), as is intracellular fluid. The protein content is slightly lower than that of perilymph. Radioactive labeling experiments have shown the basilar membrane to be impermeable to these ions, whereas Reissner's membrane is engaged actively in transporting K^+ into the scala media against this concentration gradient. The transport activity is shown by rapid appearance of the labeled K^+ from the scala media into the capillaries of the stria vascularis. Cells of the stria are actively engaged in both absorption and secretion of endolymph. In a similar manner, cells of the planum semilunatum of the ampullae and on the slopes of the cristae are also active in the formation and absorption of endolymph.

There is a longitudinal flow of endolymph to the endolymphatic sac. Small particulate matter and radioactive sulfur gravitate to this structure. Fluid found in the sac is dissimilar to endolymph elsewhere in that it has a high concentration of protein (5 g/100 ml), with a concentration of sodium and potassium similar to that of serum. These findings indicate a high absorption of fluid in this region. Absorptive-type cells contained in the rugose walls of the sac give an anatomic basis for this assumption.

Fluid within the tunnel of Corti ("cortilymph") is different from endolymph, and one investigator has suggested that it is formed from CSF passing along the fibers of the auditory nerve through the canaliculi of the bony spiral lamina. Neurophysiologic knowledge supports this view because neural transmission should be impossible in the high potassium concentration of endolymph and the fibers terminating on the outer hair cells pass through the tunnel of Corti.

The space between the hair cells and the overlying membranes (cupula, otolithic, and tectorial) contains a substance different from endolymph. Little is known of this material, but it has a high viscosity, is structureless, and resembles in other characteristics a concentrated mucopolysaccharide. This is apparently secreted by the supporting cells of the sensory organs.

Fluid Pressure Dynamics

Another function of the intracranial extension of both the otic and periotic spaces is the maintenance of equilibrium between perilymphatic and endolymphatic

TABLE 40–1. Chemical Composition of Inner Ear Fluids

Mean Value	Perilymph	Endolymph	Cap. Serum	CSF
Na$^+$ (mEq/L)	143	12–16	141	141
K$^+$ (mEq/L)	5.5–6.25	143.3 (140–160)	5.9	2.9
Protein (mg%)	200 (89–326)	150?	7170	30
Glucose (mg%)	104		104	67
Free cholesterol (mg%)	1.5			0.035
Total cholesterol (mg%)	12		28	
MDH (IU)	95.6–136		63.5	18.3
LDH (IU)	127–155		151	1.9
PO$_3^-$ (mM/L)	0.72		0.95	0.36
Ca^{++} (mM/L)	1.16	1.07	2.44	1.12
Lactate (mM/L)	6.78		4.63	3.94

MDH = Malate dehydrogenase
LDH = Lactate dehydrogenase

fluid pressure. Normal vestibular and cochlear function depends on stability of fluid pressures. Not only are variations in hydrostatic pressure constantly present, as with change in body position, coughing, or straining, but also the inner ear is exposed to changes in the atmospheric pressure in the middle ear through the round and oval windows. The endolymphatic sac can compensate for changes in perilymphatic pressure, because similar CSF pressure changes will be transmitted to both fluid systems simultaneously, maintaining equilibrium. Air pressure variations directed into the perilymphatic space may be compensated for by a reservoir action of the endolymphatic sac and slight release of perilymph through the cochlear aqueduct.

Although the details of this mechanism remain largely conjectural, it is obviously effective, as demonstrated by the ability of man to function both in the depths of the sea and in the reaches of outer space.

BLOOD SUPPLY TO THE EAR

The blood supply to the ear is formed in two completely independent circulations—one that supplies the external and middle ear, and one that supplies the inner ear—with a complete lack of anastomosis between the two.

The external ear is supplied mainly by the auriculotemporal branch of the superficial temporal artery anteriorly and by branches of the posterior auricular division of the external carotid artery posteriorly.

The middle ear and mastoid are supplied by an abundant anastomosing arterial circulation. The anterior tympanic branch of the facial artery enters through the petrotympanic fissure. The anterior wall of the mesotympanum also transmits small branches from the carotid artery to the tympanum, the caroticotympanic arteries. Superiorly, the middle meningeal gives off the superior tympanic branch, which enters the middle ear through the petrosquamous fissure. The middle meningeal also gives off the superficial petrosal artery, which runs with the greater superficial petrosal nerve to enter the facial canal at the hiatus containing the geniculate ganglion. This vessel anastomoses with a branch of the posterior auricular artery, the stylomastoid artery, which enters the facial canal inferiorly through the stylomastoid foramen. A branch of this last artery, the posterior tympanic artery, runs through the canaliculus of the chorda tympani to enter the middle ear with this nerve. An important artery enters from the inferior aspect of the middle ear, the inferior tympanic branch of the ascending pharyngeal artery. This is the major supplier of glomus jugulare tumors of the middle ear.

The ossicles receive an anastomosing blood supply from the anterior tympanic artery, the posterior tympanic artery, a vessel running with the stapedius tendon, and branches from the plexus of vessels on the promontory. The vessels run in the mucosal covering of the ossicles, sending nutrient vessels into the bone. The long process of the incus seems to have the most tenuous blood supply, commonly suffering necrosis when there is inflammatory or mechanical interference with its circulation.

The inner ear receives its blood supply from the internal auditory artery, usually arising from the anterior inferior cerebellar artery but occasionally arising directly from the basilar artery. This is an end artery receiving no known anastomosing vessels.

Soon after entering the internal auditory meatus, the artery divides into three branches. One branch accompanies the vestibular nerve and supplies that nerve, semicircular ducts, utricle, and saccule. The second branch, the vestibulocochlear artery, supplies the saccule, utricle, posterior semicircular canal, and basilar turn of the cochlea. The terminal branch is the cochlear artery. This enters the modiolus, where it gives rise to the spiral vessels running through the base of the bony spiral lamina. Branches leaving the spiral arteries run through the canaliculi to the base of the organ of Corti.

Other branches leaving the spiral arteries supply the walls of the scala vestibuli and scala tympani, both terminating at the stria vascularis.

Two other vessels enter the inner ear without anastomosis. One enters at the subarcuate eminence to supply the intercanalicular bone; the other supplies the endolymphatic sac and duct.

The venous drainage of the external and middle ear is accomplished by vessels accompanying the arterial supply. A mastoid emissary vein communicates between the external mastoid cortex and the lateral sinus.

The venous drainage of the inner ear is accomplished by three routes. The cochlear return is by the internal auditory vein draining the middle and apical turns. The cochlear vein drains the basilar turn of the cochlea and the anterior vestibule, leaving through a channel paralleling the cochlear aqueduct to empty into the inferior petrosal sinus. A third venous channel follows the endolymphatic duct to drain into the sigmoid sinus. This plexus drains the posterior labyrinth.

FACIAL NERVE

The facial nerve (Fig. 40–9) leaves the pons in two functional divisions, the motor division and the nervus intermedius, the latter containing the special sensory fibers of taste and parasympathetic fibers. The nerve enters the temporal bone through the internal acoustic meatus, running along the anterosuperior portion. The nerve then enters a bony channel, the facial canal (fallopian canal), which runs through the temporal bone from the anterosuperior fundus of the internal auditory canal to the stylomastoid foramen. Initially, the nerve runs a lateral and superior course between the cochlea and superior semicircular canal to approach the junction of the petrous with the middle ear. Here in a shallow fossa just under the dura covering the superior face of the petrous is the geniculate ganglion. A branch, the greater superficial petrosal nerve, runs forward through a channel in the petrous to innervate the lacrimal gland. A smaller branch runs into the middle ear, the lesser superficial petrosal nerve, to join the tympanic plexus.

The trunk of the facial nerves makes a right angle turn to enter the middle ear just above the cochleariform process and runs posteriorly just inferior to the lateral semicircular canal. During this course, it forms a portion of the superior wall of the oval window niche. This part of the facial canal is often dehiscent, allowing the nerve trunk to bulge into the oval window niche, partially occluding it.

In the region above the pyramidal eminence and medial to the fossa incudis, the facial makes a second turn downward to begin its vertical portion. At this turn, the nerve gives off a branch to the stapedial muscle. As the facial canal nears its inferior limit, a tributary channel, the canaliculus of the chorda tympani, is given off at an acute angle to return to the posterosuperior middle ear. This canaliculus contains the fibers of the chorda tympani nerve. The facial nerve then leaves the temporal bone through the stylomastoid foramen, after which the main trunk turns forward to run between the superficial and deep lobes of the parotid gland to be distributed to the muscles of the facial expression (Chapter 59).

SUGGESTED READINGS

Anson BJ (Ed): Morris' Human Anatomy. 12th ed. New York, McGraw-Hill Book Co, 1966, Chapter X, Part II.

Anson BJ, Bast TH: In: The Ear and Temporal Bone in Otolaryngology. Edited by Schenck HP. Vol I. Hagerstown, Prior, 1955, Chapter I.

Anson BJ, Donaldson JA: Surgical Anatomy of the Temporal Bone and Ear. Philadelphia, WB Saunders Co, 1981.

Bast TH, Anson BJ: The Temporal Bone and the Ear. Springfield, Ill, Charles C Thomas, Publisher, 1949.

Clemente CD: Gray's Anatomy, 30th Ed. Philadelphia, Lea & Febiger, 1985.

English GM: Otolaryngology. Philadelphia, JB Lippincott Co., 1994.

Rauch S: Membrane problems of the inner ear and their significance. J Laryngol Otol 80:1144, 1966.

Simmons FB: Perceptual theories of middle ear muscle function. Ann Otol Rhinol Laryngol 73:724, 1964.

Spondelin H: The innervation of the outer hair cell system. Am J Otol 3:274, 1982.

Thalmann R, et al: Amino acid profile in inner ear fluids and cerebrospinal fluid. Laryngoscope 92:321, 1982.

41 Molecular Biology of the Ear

David J. Lim and Allen F. Ryan

Molecular biology is a branch of modern biology in which biological phenomena and processes are studied using physical, biochemical, cellular and genetic principles at the molecular level. This emerging science has contributed to major advances in our understanding of cellular function in health as well as in disease. It also has resulted in a deeper understanding of the molecular pathogenesis of many diseases and the revolutionary development of new approaches in diagnosis, prevention, and treatment of diseases, including gene therapy. This chapter will review the rapidly developing important molecular methodologies which have made contributions to advance our understanding of the cellular functions and dysfunctions of the ear in molecular terms.

MOLECULAR METHODOLOGY

The rapid expansion of molecular research has been the result of the introduction of several powerful methodologies for isolating gene sequences and characterizing their expression. At the center of these methodologies are gene cloning techniques, which rely upon the replication of DNA sequences in bacteriophages and plasmids, generating large amounts of DNA which can be screened, characterized and sequenced.[1] Another crucial method is reverse transcription of messenger RNA (mRNA), in which viral enzymes capable of copying RNA into DNA are used to generate complementary DNA (cDNA) copies of mRNAs isolated from tissue. Reverse transcription and cloning have allowed the rapid discovery of new genes, usually based upon homology with known DNA sequences, or upon assay of functional characteristics when cDNAs are cloned in expression vectors. This has lead to the isolation of many families, some quite extensive, of genes encoding related proteins. Other widely used methods in molecular biology include the polymerase chain reaction (PCR) for amplification of DNA sequences present in low copy numbers,[2] and in situ mRNA hybridization for the localization of gene expression to individual cells.[3] (Terms which are frequently used in molecular biology are listed in Table 41–1, and a number of important concepts and methods are illustrated in Figs. 41–1–41–5).

Gene Expression Systems

The expression of cloned genes in biological systems ranging from bacteria and *Xenopus* oocytes[4] (Fig. 41–6), to eukaryotic cell lines and intact mammals has become a major tool in biological research. The expression of functional proteins in cells has added to our knowledge of numerous molecules such as neuronal receptors, ion channels, and transcription factors. Targeted mutations in the translated sequences of genes have made fundamental contributions to the molecular determinants of protein function, as in studies which identify the functional domains of potassium channels and provide evidence to support a "ball-and-chain" model of their action[5,6] and amino acid sequences governing interaction between subunits of ion transport ATPases.[7] The use of different promoter elements and mutations within promoters has dramatically increased our understanding of the control of gene expression.[8]

Transgenic Animals

The influence of genes in the organism has been studied by placing the gene sequences of interest under control of tissue-specific promotor sequences which target expression to given tissue, and inserting these transgenes into the DNA of mice to create a transgenic animal (Fig. 41–7). The resultant transgenic animals then display the effects of transgene expression, and can be used to document the effects of genes and/or

TABLE 41–1. Terms Used in Molecular Methods

Alternative splicing	Different ways of assembling exons to produce different mature mRNAs.
Base pair (bp)	A combination of A with T or G with C formed by hydrogen bonding between two antipararell strands of a DNA double helix.
cDNA clone	A vector containing a cDNA molecule from another organism.
cDNA	A single strand of DNA complementary to a mRNA, and synthesized from it by reverse transcription.
DNA library	A set of cloned genomic DNA fragments from an organism or cDNAs from a cell type or tissue.
Exon	Any segment of an interrupted gene that is represented in a mature mRNA. Segments of DNA separating exons are called introns.
Gene family	A group of genes related by sequence similarity.
Genomic clone	A selected host cell with a vector containing a fragment of genomic DNA from a different organism.
Genomic DNA	All DNA sequences of an organism.
Host Cell	A cell (usually a bacterium) in which a vector can be propagated.
Hybridization	Localization of mRNA or DNA in a cell or tissue section by hydrogen bonding of complementary sequences found in a probe which can be detected.
Library	A complete set of genomic clones from an organism or of cDNA clones from one cell type.
Linkage analysis	A means of identifying the chromosomal location of genes based on the frequency of recombination between the gene of interest and known loci.
Oligonucleotide	A short DNA sequence, usually less than 100 base pairs.
PCR	The Polymerase Chain Reaction. Exponential amplification of a DNA sequence using paired oligonucleotide primers, DNA polymerase to extend the primers by synthesizing new DNA strands and thermal cycling to denature the duplex DNA and allow a new round of primer binding.
Phage	Bacteriophage, a bacterial virus, often engineered to carry inserted DNA, as in DNA libraries.
Plasmid	A small, circular, extrachromosomal DNA molecule capable of replicating independently in a host cell.
Polymorphism	Two or more alleles of the same gene (i.e. Rh+ or Rh− individuals) in a breeding population.
Promoter	A region of DNA involved in binding RNA polymerase to initiate transcription.
Recombination	A reciprocal exchange of DNA between sister chromatid during meiosis.
Restriction enzyme	A bacterial enzyme that recognizes and cleaves a particular short DNA sequence. Often used to cut and join two DNA sequences, as in cloning.
Reverse transcription	DNA synthesis from an RNA template, mediated by a retroviral enzyme called reverse transcriptase.
RNA splicing	Removal of introns from an RNA sequence to produce a mature mRNA.
Transfection	A method for introducing exogenous DNA into eukaryotic cells.
Transgene	An artificial gene constructed from a promoter active in the tissue or cell to be studied, a coding sequence of interest, and a termination sequence.
Transgenic	Animal (or plant) that has stably incorporated one or more genes from another cell or organism.
Transcript	The RNA product produced by template-dependent RNA synthesis from a DNA sequence.
Transcription	RNA synthesis on a DNA template, mediated by an enzyme called RNA polymerase.
Transcription	Loosely applied term to any protein required to initiate or regulate transcription factor in eukaryotic or prokaryotic cells.
Translation	Synthesis of protein on an mRNA template.
Transposon	DNA elements that can transpose themselves (move) from one position in a DNA molecule to another.

promoters.[9] A serendipitous byproduct of this technique has been insertional mutations. In a few percent of transgenic animals, insertion of the transgene disrupts an endogenous gene and produces a morphological or behavioral change completely unrelated to the transgene. In these animals, the mutation site is marked by the inserted DNA sequence,[10,11] simplifying the process of localizing the mutated gene and its normal counterpart. Insertional mutagenesis has lead to the identification of several new genes, including genes controlling limb development[12] and motor control.[13] However, transgenic insertions are frequently extremely complex often involving deletion of hundreds of kilobases at or near the site of transgene insertion. For this reason, the identification of genes mutated by insertion in transgenic animals has sometimes proven to be difficult, if not impossible.

Several insertional mutations in transgenic animals which affect the inner ear have been identified. For example, Crenshaw[15] found that one out of 14 lines of mice with a v-src transgene showed behavior consistent with an inner ear defect. The inner ear of these animals showed collapse and degeneration of the pars superior of the inner ear at about one month of age. This was preceded by a period of severe endolymphatic hydrops, suggesting that the gene disrupted in

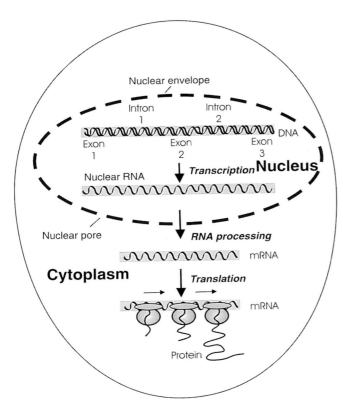

Fig. 41–1. Summary of steps by which proteins are synthesized by DNA in eukaryotic cell. A nuclear envelope with pores segregates the DNA from cytoplasm. (Adapted from Gilbert, 1994).

the mutation affects inner ear fluid balance. The gene has been localized to a 6 cM region on chromosome 1, near the interleukin 1 receptor.[16]

Gene Knockouts (Gene Targeting)

A method by which a gene knockout can be created is illustrated in Fig. 41–8. Single gene knockouts can be lethal or have extensive effects on development and adult function. For example, knockouts of single POU-domain genes, transcription factors which contribute to cell differentiation, are typically lethal shortly after birth, and deletion of the genes encoding the neurotro-

phins or their receptors can produce serious deficits in sensory neurons. Alternatively, knockouts can have little influence, since the process of development appears to have a high degree of redundancy. An example is the regulation of differentiation in muscle, in which several factors act to drive a cell toward the muscle phenotype.[22]

Molecular Diversity (Gene Families)

Gene cloning has revealed the existence of many families of genes which mediate important aspects of cell function, including the genes that encode neuronal receptors such as acetylcholine receptors.[23–24] The first of these receptor genes were identified by injecting RNA molecules transcribed in vitro from cDNA clones isolated from brain cDNA libraries into *Xenopus* oocytes. When exposed to the appropriate transmitter, the oocytes showed intracellular potential changes consistent with the presence of specific receptors on their surfaces. Subsequent low-stringency screening of cDNA libraries for related sequences yielded families of receptor genes.[25–34]

Other gene families that have been isolated recently include voltage-gated potassium channels,[35] Ca-ATPases,[36] G-proteins and numerous growth factors and their receptors.[37] Several gene families consist of subunits which can be assembled in a variety of combinations, leading to increased diversity of functional expression from a limited set of genes. For example, the nicotinic acetylcholine receptor consists of α and β subunits. The existence of genes encoding several different α and β subunits allows a multitude of different combinations, each with different functional properties.[23] The non-NMDA (*N*-methyl-*D*-aspartate) glutamate receptors have been hypothesized to amalgamate as hetero-pentamers of subunits, with each subunit isoform capable of complexing with several other isoforms.[38,39] This provides the potential for a very large number of structurally and functionally different glutamate receptors, explaining in part the high level of pharmacological diversity observed at synapses utilizing the same neurotransmitter. In addition, mRNA transcribed from a single gene can often

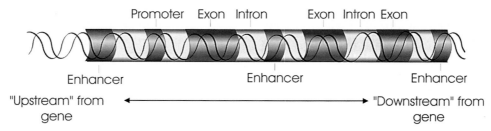

Fig. 41–2. Basic structure of a developmentally regulated gene is illustrated. The promoters of most genes encoding proteins are found at the 5′ (upstream) end of the gene. Enhancers are often even farther upstream, but they can also occur within an intron of the gene or at the 3′ end. Proteins that bind to promoters and enhancers interact to regulate transcription of the gene. (Adapted from Gilbert, 1994).

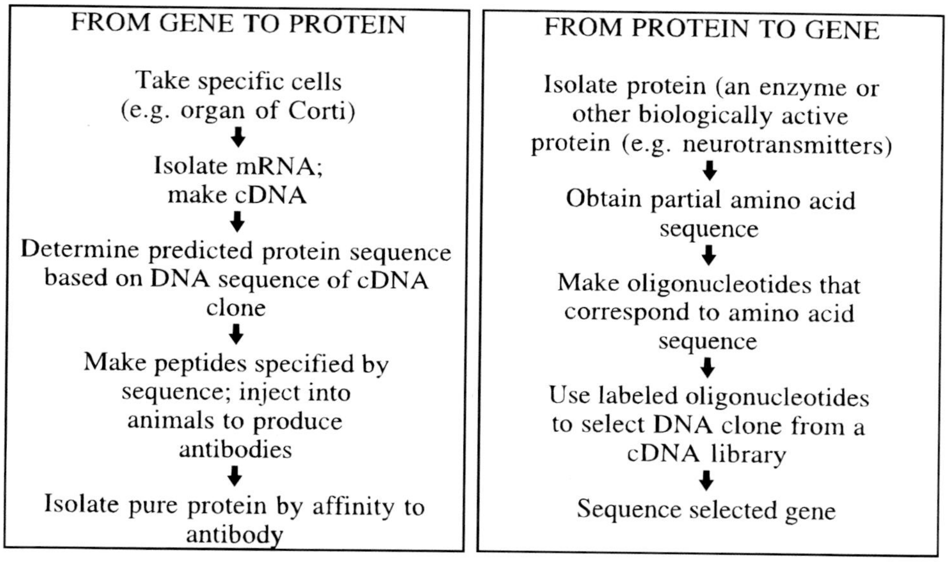

FROM GENE TO PROTEIN

Take specific cells
(e.g. organ of Corti)

↓

Isolate mRNA;
make cDNA

↓

Determine predicted protein sequence
based on DNA sequence of cDNA
clone

↓

Make peptides specified by
sequence; inject into
animals to produce
antibodies

↓

Isolate pure protein by affinity to
antibody

FROM PROTEIN TO GENE

Isolate protein (an enzyme or
other biologically active
protein (e.g. neurotransmitters)

↓

Obtain partial amino acid
sequence

↓

Make oligonucleotides that
correspond to amino acid
sequence

↓

Use labeled oligonucleotides
to select DNA clone from a
cDNA library

↓

Sequence selected gene

Fig. 41–3. It is now possible to identify an mRNA of interest (such as obtained from the inner ear or even the organ of Corti) and to use it to isolate the protein it encodes without knowing the function of that protein. Conversely, it is also possible to sequence part of a protein that has a specific function and then to synthesize an oligonucleotide that can be used to identify and isolate the gene that encodes the complete protein. Adapted from Gilbert, 1994.

be assembled into mRNAs encoding functionally different forms of the protein product from different combinations of exons by the process of alternative splicing, leading to even greater variation.[36] Increased understanding of the molecular basis for functional diversity of proteins may be one of the most significant contributions of molecular biology.

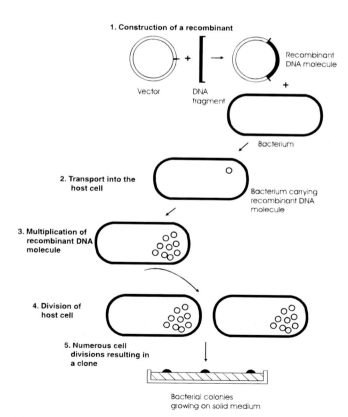

Fig. 41–4. The basic steps in gene cloning are schematically illustrated. Adapted from Brown, 1990.

Molecular Genetic Methods

Molecular methods have also transformed the field of genetics. Gene localization by kindred analysis classically depended upon the linkage of a phenotypic trait associated with a genetic disorder to a relatively small number of phenotypic traits controlled by genes whose locations were already known. Recently, several developments have lead to a dramatic increase in our ability to localize genes. The number of genetic markers at known locations in the genome increased exponentially after the introduction of molecular methodology, from a few dozen in the early 1980s, to nearly 10,000 in 1991,[40] and the number continues to increase. This increase was the result of several critical technical developments. The isolation of large numbers of restriction enzymes to cut DNA at specific locations has lead to the discovery of many restriction fragments at defined chromosomal locations whose length differs between individuals (a phenomenon called polymorphism; the more polymorphic a marker, the more useful it is for gene localization). These differences can readily be identified by Southern blotting (Fig. 41–9). Another family of markers has been developed by exploiting the tendency of DNA to form repeating sequences called minisatellites. Repeats of short DNA sequences, or of C-A or G-T pairs, are ubiquitous in the genome, often highly polymorphic, and can be identified by PCR. In animals, interspecies crosses between the laboratory mouse, *Mus musculus,* and closely related mouse species such as *Mus spretus,* have been used to generate markers at many loci.

Taken together, these developments have greatly increased both the ease of linkage analysis and the number of defined chromosomal loci against which to test a given phenotype for linkage. This has allowed more precise localization of the genes determining traits of

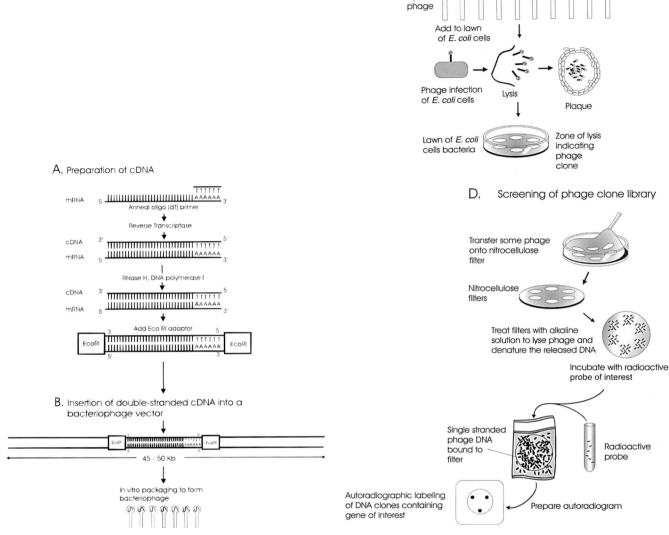

Fig. 41–5. Schematic illustration of protocol to make cDNA libraries. (Step A) Messenger RNA (mRNA) is isolated from a tissue of interest and reverse transcribed into cDNA. This cDNA represents all of the genes being expressed in the tissue. It is made double-stranded in a nick translation reaction, where RNAse H nicks the mRNA strand creating a primer for second strand DNA synthesis by DNA polymerase I. Sequences (adapters) that allow ligation into a cloning vector are added to double stranded cDNA. (Step B) The cDNA can then be inserted into specially modified vectors, in this case bacteriophages. (Step C) Phages containing the recombinant DNA will infect E. Coli and reproduce, making many copies and eventually lysing the bacteria forming plaques. (Step D) The plaques are transferred to nitrocellulose paper and treated with alkali to lyse the phages and denature the DNA in place. These filters are then incubated in a radioactive probes. This can be a short DNA sequence (oligonucleotide), a cDNA or other DNA fragment. In the case of differential cDNA library screening, the same phage library is screened with radioactive cDNA probes reverse transcribed from mRNA isolated from two different tissues. This allows the identification of a relatively abundant mRNA that would be found in one type of tissue but not in the other. Adapted from Gilbert, 1994.

interest, increasing the chance that the genes can be identified at the molecular level by fine mapping, chromosome walking, testing of candidate genes within a region, and/or exon trapping. The proliferation of gene markers has contributed to the location, and in many cases, identification of genes involved in diseases such as retinoblastoma,[41] and Duchenne muscular dystrophy.[42]

MOLECULAR BIOLOGY OF THE INNER EAR

Molecular biological studies of the organs of hearing and balance of the inner ear have increased rapidly in recent years leading to the identification of many genes involved in inner ear function. In order to isolate genes that are important for development, maintenance, and

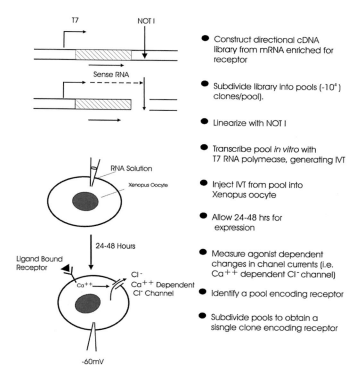

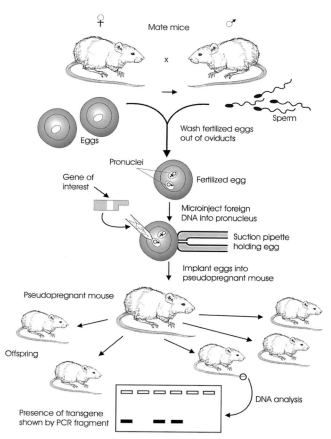

Fig. 41–6. Expression cloning using *Xenopus* oocytes. The steps required to generate *in vitro* transcripts from pools of directional cDNA library clones are shown. Included are *in vitro* transcription, injection into *Xenopus* oocytes and voltage clamp assay for a ligand-evoked opening of the calcium-dependent chloride channel. Shaded boxes indicate the receptor-coding region. (Adapted from Battey et al., 1993).

Fig. 41–7. Schematic illustration of production of transgenic mice using the microinjection technique. A transgene is constructed from promoter that directs expression in the tissue of interest, the gene to be studied and a termination sequence. Fertilized eggs are collected from mated females, and the transgene is injected into one of the two pronuclei. The injected eggs are transferred to foster mothers, which are female mice made pseudopregnant by mating with vasectomized males. Three weeks after birth, the offspring are checked for the presence of the transgene by Southern blot analysis of DNA extracted from a small piece of the tail. Screening can be performed rapidly using the polymerase chain reaction if suitable primers are available. Three of the offspring carry the transgene in the example given. Adapted from Watson et al., 1993.

normal functioning of the inner ear, it is necessary to construct an CDNA library based on the mRNAs from the inner ear including sensory organs. Several of such cDNA libraries are now available: guinea pig organ of Corti;[43] human fetal cochlea;[44] mouse inner ear;[45] and rat outer hair cells.[46] These libraries are increasingly used for screening gene products of interest in the inner ear.

Another area in which substantial progress has been made is in the identification of genes where mutation leads to inherited loss of hearing, or deafness genes.

Deafness Genes

Several genes involved in inherited auditory disorders have recently been linked to specific chromosomal locations. Usher syndrome type I (US-I) has been linked to at least three loci,[47–49] suggesting considerable genetic heterogeneity in this disease. Usher II (US-II) also appears to be linked to at least two loci.[50–52] Branchio-oto-renal syndrome has been localized to chromosome 8q,[53] and X-linked deafness with perilymph gusher has been localized to a small segment of Xq.1.[54–56] While the localization of genes causing nonsyndromic hereditary hearing impairment is considerably more prob-

lematic, progress has also been made. Leon et al.[57] localized the gene for a dominant form of nonsyndromic hereditary hearing impairment to chromosome 5q31 in a large Costa Rican kindred and recently Coucke et al.[58] localized the gene for an autosomal dominant form of nonsyndromic hereditary hearing impairment to chromosome 1p32. Guilford a[59], b[60] have localized one form (NSRD1) of recessive, nonsyndromic hereditary hearing impairment to chromosomes 13q12 and other form (NSRD2) to 11q13.5. Recently additional genes responsible for nonsyndromic recessive deafness (NARD1) mapped to the pericentimeric region of chromosome 17.[61] A nonsyndromic form of X-linked deafness has also been localized to Xp11.[62] Efforts to identify these and other genes associated with heredi-

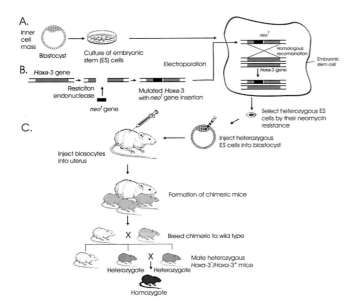

Fig. 41–8. Schematic illustration of technique for gene targeting using *Hoxa*-3 gene as an example. A. Embryonic stem (ES) cells are cultured from inner cell mass. B. The cloned *Hoxa*-3 gene are cut with a restriction enzyme, and the neomycin resistance gene is inserted into the region that encodes the DNA-binding site of the protein. The mutant *Hoxa*-3 gene are introduced into ES cells, where homologous recombination exchanges a wild-type gene for the mutant copy. These cells are selected with neomycin, heterozygous ES cells are inserted into the inner cell mass of a wild-type embryo, and the blastocyst is returned to the uterus. The resulting mouse is a chimera composed of heterozygous *Hoxa*-3 tissues and wild-type *Hoxa*-3 tissues. Mating the chimeric mice to wild-type mice produces heterozygous Hoxa-3 offspring if the ES cells contributed to the germ line in the chimeras. These heterozygous mice can be bred together, and some of their progeny should be homozygous mutants of *Hoxa*-3 gene. Adapted from Gilbert 1994.

tary hearing impairment and deafness by fine mapping and cloning are ongoing.

Several genes involved in hereditary hearing impairment and deafness have already been identified, and mutations characterized. Alport syndrome has been associated with a mutation in the gene encoding the basement membrane collagen (COL4A5).[63,64] Waardenburg syndrome type I (WS-I) was linked to 2q37,[65] after a *de novo* cytogenetically visible inversion[66] defined a candidate region. Since this locus is homologous to a gene which causes a similar mutation in *splotch* mice,[67,68] it has been quickly confirmed that the same gene, *PAX3*, was mutated in several WS-I families.[69,70] The NIDCD Waardenburg Syndrome Consortium reported the remarkable finding that all 41 WS-I kindreds analyzed were linked to the *PAX3* gene locus.[71] WS-III may also be caused by *PAX3* mutations,[72] however WS-II does not appear to involve this gene.[71] The gene defect in the *shaker*-1 mouse, proposed as a model for Usher syndrome, was localized near a gene encoding myosin VII. When tested as a candidate gene, it proved to have a mutation.[73] This in turn lead

to the screening of Usher syndrome families, and the resultant identification of myosin VII as the gene responsible for Usher syndrome IB.[74] Similarly, testing of candidate genes near the linkage site for X-linked deafness with stapes fixation (DFN3) lead to the identification of the mutated gene as *Brain*-4 which encodes a transcription factor with a POU domain (POU3F4).[75] This transcription factor is one member of a gene family that is expressed in the cochlea during development.[76] A defect in mitochondrial DNA which increases susceptibility to aminoglycoside ototoxicity, and which, in combination with an autosomal mutation, leads to maternally inherited nonsyndromic deafness, has been recently characterized.[77–79]

The mouse microphthalmia (*mi*) gene encodes a basic-helix-loop-helix-zipper protein and mutation of this gene resulted in loss of pigmentation in eye, inner ear and skin, microphthalmia, and early onset deafness.[80] A line of transgenic mice, VGA-9, containing mouse vasopressin-β-galactosidase fusion constructs exhibited a complete loss of skin pigmentation, microphthalmia, and cochlear abnormalities.[81] In the homozygous transgenic mice, cochlea abnormalities included an abnormal stria, deficient melanocytes (intermediate cells) and presumed secondary degeneration of the outer hair cells. An interesting aspect of this transgenic mice is the phenotypic similarity to mice with mutations at the *mi* gene locus.[81] Breeding experiments confirmed that VGA-9 transgenic insertion was allelic with the *mi* gene. Using human melanocyte cell lines and unrelated human donors, Tachibana et al.[82] obtained cDNA and genomic clones of the human homolog of mouse *mi*, and mapped this gene to a human chromosome 3p12.3-p14.1. Hughes et al.[83] mapped a gene for Waardenburg syndrome type II (WSII) close to human homolog of the *mi* gene at chromosome 3p12-p14.1.

Linkage of neurofibromatosis-2 to chromosome 22q[84,85] leads to fine-scale mapping[86] and then to identification of a mutated gene, which encodes a new member of the family of 4.1 cytoskeletal associated proteins known as merlin.[87,88] NF2 is an autosomal dominant inherited disease characterized by bilateral vestibular schwannomas and other central nervous system tumors, and is often associated with hearing impairment caused by cochlear nerve compression.

Linkage and identification of mutations causing deafness and vestibular disorders has immediate clinical significance, since it allows genetic testing and counselling and may eventually provide a basis for gene therapy. It is also proving to be an important means of identifying genes whose expression is important for normal cochlear development and function.

Inner Ear Pathology

It has been known that melanin granule-bearing cells such as intermediate cells in the stria vascularis of the

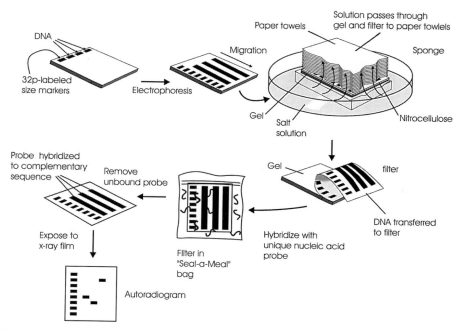

Fig. 41–9. Schematic illustration of Southern blotting. DNA digested with restriction enzymes is loaded onto a gel and electrophoretically separated by molecular size. After the fragments of DNA are separated, the DNA is denatured into single strands. The gel is then placed on a support on top of filter paper saturated with buffer. A nitrocellulose or nylon filter is placed on top of the gel, and absorbent towels are placed on top of the filter. The transfer buffer makes its way through the gel, nitrocellulose paper, and towels by capillary action, taking the DNA with it. The single-stranded DNA sticks to the filter. The filter is then removed, the DNA immobilized on to the filer, and the filter is hybridized with a radioactively labeled probe. The position of the DNA fragment complementary to the probe appears as a band on X-ray film, which reflects the position of the DNA fragment in the gel. Adapted from Watson et al., 1993.

cochlea and dark cell-associated melanocytes in the vestibular organs are derived from melanoblasts (melanocyte precursor) of the neural crest in early development. Failure of neural crest melanoblast to migrate to the target inner ear tissue in steel/dickie *(Sld)* mutant mice led to poor strial development, resulting in failure to generate a positive endocochlear potential needed for sensory transduction, which causes deafness.[89] It is believed that the steel locus encodes a mast cell growth factor (MGF) and the *Sld* mutation results in a protein lacking both transmembrane and cytoplasmic domains of the membrane-bound growth factor.[90] It is not yet established, however, whether the *Sld* mutation affects melanoblast migration, proliferation, differentiation or survival of melanoblasts.[89] Recently, a transgenic mice, created by insertion of SV40/tyrosinase promoter expression vector, developed intermediate cell-derived strial tumors and melanocyte-derived vestibular tumors.[91]

Inner Ear Development

Because of the highly ordered structure of the inner ear sensory organs (e.g., tonotopic organization of the cochlea, central (striolar) vs peripheral part of sensory epithelium of the vestibule), the development, particularly in respect to pattern formation, of the inner ear

is an important area in which molecular methods can make a significant contribution. To develop such intricate inner ear sensory organs, highly complex spatiotemporal enactment of developmental events must be orchestrated via selected pattern of transcriptional regulation.[92] Many genes involved in development of the inner ear have been identified using molecular techniques. For example, both gene expression studies and insertional mutagenesis have demonstrated that several transcription factors and growth factors make significant contributions to the induction, early embryonic development, and terminal differentiation of the cochlea.

Thyroid hormone[93] and retinoids[94,95] affect the ear development. Spatial and temporal pattern of expression of thyroid hormone receptors (TRs) was investigated using in situ hybridization in the rat embryo.[96] They found that as early as embryonic day 12.5, both TRβ1 and TRβ2 mRNAs are restricted only to the part of inner ear which gives rise to the cochlea. In contrast, the TRα1 and TRα2 transcripts are localized in the part of otic vesicle which gives rise to the vestibular organs.[97]

Bone morphogenetic proteins (BMPs) are members of transforming growth factor-ß (TGFß) superfamily. Recently, Oh and Wu[98] investigated BMP (BMP-4, 5, 7) expression during the ear development in chick otocyst. In situ hybridization analysis showed that BMP-4 mRNA was present in the future ampullae of the three semicircular canals in embryonic day 2.5–3. BMP-5 mRNA, however, was only found transiently in the future ampulla of the posterior semicircular canal. BMP-7 mRNA, on the other hand, was initially expressed in most part of the otocyst and became restricted to specific regions by embryonic day 3. These investigators suggested that BMPs may play an important role in the differentiation of inner ear sensory organs.

Exposure of chick otic vesicle to retinoic acid (RA) in culture induced precocious differentiation of sensory epithelium.[99] Exposure of developing mouse cochlea from embryonic day 13 to 16 in culture to RA induced supernumerary hair cells presumably through alteration of the cell fate of existing (supporting) cells.[100] The action of RA is believed to be mediated through RA receptors (RAR and RXR), which are members of the intracellular receptor superfamily (or steroid/thyroid hormone receptor superfamily). Interestingly, *in situ* hybridization analysis of mRNAs encoding the protein RARß showed that it is strongly expressed both in mesenchyme and in the sensory epithelium of the developing mouse inner ear.[101] On the other hand, the cytoplasmic retinoic acid binding protein II (CRABP II), which is believed to be involved in controlling the intracellular concentration of free retinoids, is expressed within the cochlear epithelium.[102] Recently, Sanne and Wu[103] investigated the expression of mRNA encoding CRABP I in developing chick inner ear. CRABP I expression was localized mostly in the dorsal and anterior region of the otic pit, but later in development the expression was localized in entire otocyst, except in the most ventral portion. It has been also known for many years that close proximity of hindbrain tissue is necessary for the induction of the otocyst during inner ear embryogenesis.[104] During the period of this induction, it was noted that Int-2, a member of the fibroblast growth factor (FGF) family also known as FGF-3, is expressed at high levels in hindbrain and later on in the developing inner ear.[105,99] Whether FGF-3 might be the inductive factor was tested by Represa et al.[106] by inhibiting FGF-3 expression using antisense oligonucleotides in an in vitro model of otocyst development. They found that the otocyst failed to form when FGF-3 expression was inhibited. Abnormal inner ear development was also noted in a mouse with a targeted mutation in FGF-3,[107] although the defect was much more modest, perhaps due to compensatory increases in the expression of other FGFs.[106] FGF-1 mRNA is expressed in postnatal cochlear hair cells, and in auditory and vestibular neurons from around birth until adulthood.[108] FGF receptors are expressed on neonatal cochlear hair cells,[109] and FGF-2 protects neonatal hair cells from neomycin ototoxicity in vitro.[110]

Nerve growth factors (NGFs) in concert with basic fibroblast growth factor (bFGF) and transforming growth factor β (TGFβ1), and neurotrophins, such as neurotrophin 3 (NT-3), brain derived neurotrophic factor (BDNF), are necessary for survival and neurite extension in auditory and vestibular neurons during both early and late stages in ear development.[111–115] mRNAs encoding both BDNF and NT-3 are expressed in the inner ear during development.[116,117] Cochlear and vestibular neurons both respond to NGFs and BDNF and NT-3 in vitro.[18] Inhibition of BDNF and NT-3 expression using antisense oligonucleotides prevents neurite extension in vitro.[118] Finally, using mutant mice with knockout of BDNF gene or TN-3 gene or both genes, Ernfors et al.[18,115] demonstrated that BNDF is critical for survival of vestibular ganglion and maintenance of both afferent and efferent innervation. These data are consistent with observations in mice lacking a functional NT-3 gene reported by Farinas et al.[19] In the cochlea, BNDF-gene-deleted mice showed loss of presumptive type II ganglion cells and afferent innervation to outer hair cells, while NT-3 gene deleted mice showed loss of presumptive type I ganglion cells and majority of afferent innervation. The double mutants lose all vestibular and cochlear ganglion cells.[18]

Neurotransmitters

Afferent and efferent (medial and lateral) systems and the innervation patterns of the auditory organ are relatively well established. Although remarkable progress has been made in recent years, our knowledge concerning the inner ear neurochemistry is yet to be completed.[119–123] Afferent neurotransmission between the cochlear hair cells and spiral ganglion neurons is mediated by an as-yet unidentified neurotransmitter. Based on pharmacologic evidence, the strongest candidate for this transmitter is glutamate or a related amino acid.[1,125] Recently, the expression of mRNAs encoding glutamate receptors has been detected in spiral ganglion neurons. These include members of the AMPA,[76] NMDA,[1] and kainate[1,127] glutamate receptor families. These observations strongly support the hypothesis that an excitatory amino acid like glutamate is one of the cochlear afferent neurotransmitters. The primary efferent neurotransmitter between the brainstem and cochlea is thought to be acetylcholine, with other transmitters, including GABA, opioid and other peptides, and possibly ATP, also being involved. Members of several neuronal receptor gene families have been shown to be expressed in the cochlea. Expression of genes encoding nicotinic,[1,130] muscarinic[131] and metabotropic[132] acetylcholine receptors, GABA receptors[133] and ATP receptors[134] has been documented in the cochlea, while preproenkephalin mRNA has been found in cochlear and vestibular efferent cell bodies in the brainstem.[135] In particular, the α9 member of the nicotinic acetylcholine receptor has been shown to be strongly expressed in cochlear hair cells, and to match exactly the pharmacology of the outer hair cell response to this transmitter.[1] In general, the diversity of receptor and transmitter expression associated with the efferent system matches the complex pharmacology of the inner ear.

Inner Ear Fluid Regulation

Differences in the ionic composition between endolymph and perilymph have been shown to play a critical role in the inner ear function. It is therefore not surprising that the expression of genes encoding a number of ion transport enzymes[135,136] and ion channels[137] has been found in the inner ear. Of particular interest are the Na, K-ATPase genes, since this enzyme appears to be the most important determinant of the composition of perilymph and endolymph. In the stria vascularis, the α1 and β2 isoforms are the only ones expressed.[135] This combination is not found in isolation in any other tissue in the body. However, the β2 subunit is associated with transporting sodium against a high electrochemical gradient. In order for the stria transport sodium against the highest gradient in the body, perhaps this unique composition of the enzyme is required.

Hair Cell Transduction

The major function of the sensory hair cells in the inner ear is to transduce mechanical energy into neural information. The sensory cells of both the cochlea and the vestibular sensory organs are mechanoreceptors equipped with geometrically arranged sensory stereociliary bundle on each sensory cell surface. Deflection of the ciliary bundle by mechanical force toward the kinocilium (or basal body in the case of the cochlea) are excitatory, and toward the opposite direction is inhibitory for neural discharges. Deflection of the stereociliary bundle toward the excitatory direction is now known to open transduction channels located on the upper part of the stereocilia.[138–140] The opening of the transduction channels is believed to be mediated by a filamentous structure connecting the tip of the lower stereocilium to the neighboring taller stereociliary surface and known as the tip-links.[141,142]

Most of the molecules responsible for the hair cell transduction process have yet to be identified. However, some progress has been made in the transduction channel,[143,137] and the adaptation motor in vestibular sensory hairs.[144] The precise location of the transduction channels is not yet established. It is believed to be associated with tip-links, because the calcium chelator BAPTA eliminates both transduction current as well as tip-links.[142] Hackney et al.[143] used an antibody to amiloride sensitive sodium channel to label the side of the stereocilia just below the tip-link attachment site.[143]

To retain sustained sensitivity during transient displacement, the vestibular sensory cell must adapt to sustained stimuli. Adaptation of vestibular sensory cell is thought to be mediated by a "slipping" of tip-link attachment and by an active "tensioning".[145] Readjusting tension of the tip-link is necessary for the adaptation of the vestibular sensory cells.[144,146] This tensioning is suggested to be mediated by 120 kDa myosin motors which are presumably located in the insertional plaque and runs on the surface of the stereociliary actin filaments as guides.[144,146,147]

The discoveries of the acoustic emission[148] and the electromotor activity of the dissociated outer hair cells (OHCs) in mammals[149,150] led to the concept of active hearing. According to this concept, amplification of auditory sensitivity and sharp tuning of the basilar membrane frequency response is the result of motor activity by the outer hair cell. There is strong evidence that this motor activity is driven by multiple molecular motors which are an integral part of the cell membrane.[151,152]

Based on homology with known proteins and on physiology, some progress has been made in identifying genes underlying important aspects of hair cell transduction, with candidates being identified for the outer hair cell motor protein.[153,154] For example, voltage-gated ion channels show a voltage-dependent alteration in molecular shape that appears rapid enough to be compatible with OHC electromotility.[153] According to these investigators, one model for ion channel pore opening involves shape changes in the S4 segment of voltage-dependent ion channels, which appears to consist of nested alpha-helices that slide relative to one another with changes in transmembrane voltage. They suggested that the OHC motor might be evolutionarily related to an ion channel and used PCR to clone S4-related sequences from organ of Corti cDNAs.

Although, definitive evidence is still lacking, several lines of evidence suggest that these intramembranous particles may include anionic channel proteins.[154] Recent data obtained from a cDNA clone isolated from a guinea pig organ of Corti library suggests that a new isoform of the anion exchanger 2 (AE2) protein may be involved.[155]

Inner Ear Proteins

Genes important for inner ear function have often been highlighted by mutational analysis. An additional paradigm for identifying functionally important proteins is to look for genes whose pattern of expression is limited to the inner ear, and test if these genes are important for inner ear function creating animal models with non-functional mutant versions of these genes. To date, very few genes showing a pattern of expression limited to the inner ear have been reported.

The organ of Corti-specific proteins OCP I and OCP II have been identified,[156] and recently OCP II has been cloned.[157] Tectorial membrane proteins (tectorins) with little homology to known proteins have been also cloned.[158]

An inner ear-specific novel structural protein in sun fish saccule has been cloned and characterized.[159] A cDNA, obtained by differential screening of a saccular cDNA library, that encodes an inner ear-specific collagen molecule was identified. The predicted amino acid sequence of this protein showed 40% identity and 56% over all homology with collagen types VIII and X.[159] In situ hybridization with an antisense saccular collagen cRNA showed that transcripts encoding this protein are localized only to the edge of the saccular epithelium indicating that these specialized epithelial (supporting) cells may secrete this protein which is believed to be a component of the otolithic membrane.[159]

Much of the molecular data generated to date has involved identification of novel gene sequences for structural proteins, and has not been well integrated into the functions of the inner ear. Future studies will be needed to test the importance of these genes and others for normal inner ear function.

GENE THERAPY IN ANIMAL MODELS

The use of gene therapy for disorders of the ear remains a prospect for the future. However, research on this topic gives promise to the idea that at least some inner ear conditions might be treated using molecular biological methodologies. For example, mutations that delete a critical gene can, in some instances, be corrected by supplementing the missing gene product. Yoo et al.[160] studied the *shiverer* mouse, which has a neurological disorder caused by a mutation in the gene encoding myelin basic protein and characterized by defects in the myelination of nerve tracts. These mice show deficits in both the amplitude and latency of auditory brainstem responses (ABRs) due to abnormal conduction in auditory nerve fibers. When a transgene encoding normal myelin basic protein was integrated into the genome of *shiverer* mice, the ABR deficits were partially corrected. A similar approach, combined with in vitro fertilization, might someday be used to treat certain devastating genetic disorders in humans.

A more practical form of therapy is one that can be used in the adult organism. For example, there is a great interest in developing methods to preserve spiral ganglion cells after the loss of sensory cells in the organ of Corti due to various causes. Acidic fibroblast growth factor (aFGF) is believed to be involved in such a function.[108] Therefore, sustained availability of such factor(s) near the ganglion cells will support their survival and maintenance. It is generally accepted that subjects with surviving ganglion cells will have a better chance

of successful cochlear implant. Ryan and Luo[161] explored the molecular biological methods to deliver such a factor in the inner ear. They injected into the adult mouse inner ear of fibroblasts which had been genetically engineered to secrete high levels of acidic FGF into the inner ear of adult mice. In order to suppress proliferation, the fibroblasts were irradiation, and they found that the irradiated cells were well tolerated in the cochlea, with few side effects, and continued to produce the growth factor for several weeks. Because the ganglion cells are bathed with fluid freely communicating with perilymph, growth factors secreted by the fibroblast in the spiral ligament will be available to the ganglion cells. Staecker et al.[162] also found that inner ear injections of fibroblasts engineered to produce brain derived neurotrophic factor (BDNF) promoted survival of spiral ganglion neurons after hair cell destruction in guinea pigs. However, the use of non-irradiated cells in this study lead to destructive over-proliferation. While preliminary, these studies demonstrate theoretical possibilities of molecular genetic-based therapy for diseases in the human inner ear.

MOLECULAR PATHOGENESIS OF OTITIS MEDIA

Purification and sequencing of gene products are important in understanding for the pathogenesis of OM. Cloning bacterial genes has allowed investigators to produce a number of mutant or genetically engineered bacteria, in which a gene is either deleted or altered.[163] These mutants or genetically engineered bacteria can be used to probe the molecular mechanisms of bacteria-host interaction, virulence factors, and immunogenicity. The genetically engineered bacteria can also be used to mass produce recombinant outer membrane proteins for vaccine candidates. Although not yet fully explored, transgenic and gene knockout animals are being developed for the study of host defense mechanisms against infection.

Bacterial Adherence

To be a successful pathogen on a mucous membrane, bacteria must be able to colonize, evade host defense, and express toxins that damage host cells and tissues. To accomplish these goals, the bacteria must be able to adapt to the new environment by altering their phenotypic expression through transcriptional regulation. Although the exact mechanisms by which bacteria attach to the mucosal surface are poorly understood, it is generally believed that receptor-ligand mediated bacterial binding plays a major role, even though non-receptor ligand binding may also play a role in the adherence. The host receptor for *streptococcus pneumoniae* is now known to be GlcNacβ1–3Gal,[164] whereas the host receptor for nontypeable *H. influenzae* is not yet fully characterized. However, several of the bacterial ligands of the nontypeable *H. influenzae* (NTHi) have been described. The suggested ligands include 22 kDa pilin,[165] 27.5 kDa LKP pilin,[166] 36.4 kDa fimbrin[167,168] and 120 kDa high molecular weight outer membrane proteins (HMW1, HMW2),[169–173] which may mediate bacterial binding to the host epithelial cell surface. Pilin is a subunit of the rigid, tubular surface appendage pilus and mediates hemagglutination. Fimbrin is a subunit of the surface appendage fimbria, which is a nontubular filament, thinner than pili and nonhemagglutinating.[166,168]

The gene encoding LKP1 pilus (27.5 kDa) from an NTHi strain obtained from a middle ear effusion has been cloned and expressed in *E. coli*, and the recombinant pili were capable of mediating both the binding of bacteria to the buccal mucosa and hemagglutination.[166] Coleman et al.[165] cloned and sequenced the gene encoding the 22 kDa hemagglutinating pilin from another strain of NTHi, and found the DNA sequence to be 77% identical to that of the *H. influenzae* type b pilin gene, and showed 68% homologous via the derived amino acid sequence. Because only less than 5% of middle ear isolates and 35% nasopharyngeal isolates expressed pili,[174] the precise role of the pili in the pathogenesis of otitis media is unclear.

While it has not yet been established that fimbrial expression is mandatory for the establishment of infection, there is good evidence which indicates that 100% of nontypeable *H. influenzae* isolates from the middle ear of patients with chronic otitis media with effusion are fimbriated.[175] Sirakova et al.[168] sequenced and cloned a 36.4 kDa fimbrial protein from another strain of NTHi recovered from middle ear effusion. The translated amino acid sequence of fimbrin was found to be homologous with various members of OmpA family of proteins of other gram-negative bacteria,[176] and with type b *Haemophilus influenzae* outer membrane protein P5, which showed 92% identity. Disruption of fimbrin gene resulted in a mutant lacking fimbrial expression and loss of immunoreactivity to the antisera directed against isolated fimbrial proteins.[168] Importantly, this isogenic mutant showed reduced adherence to the human oropharyngeal cells in vitro and significantly reduced induction of otitis media through intranasal inoculation of NTHi in the chinchilla animal model. Thus, fimbrin is not only an adhesin mediating bacterial adherence but is also a virulence factor for NTHi.[168]

Although the exact mechanism or role of the fimbria in the pathogenesis of otitis media is not clear, one possibility is that when fimbrin is expressed, it may help to establish an intimate association between the bacteria and host cell.[175] It is possible that through such an interaction, bacterial toxins can be delivered to the host cell causing cell injury and mediating inflammatory cell responses.

Virulence Factors

Endotoxin plays an important role in the pathogenesis of otitis media.[177] Recent evidence indicates that phase variation of the endotoxin lipooligosaccharide (LOS) is a virulence factor in type b *H. influenzae*.[178] Phase variation is a reversible switch between two stable genotypes. Phase variation provides bacteria with an advantage in evading host immune response, and becoming a successful pathogen. The genes responsible for phase variation have been identified and three *lic* genes (*lic1*, *lic2*, and *lic3*) are known to be responsible for variable translation of the *lic* loci, which enables a number of different LOS structures to be produced from a limited set of genes.[178–181] Although the loss of phase variation did not affect bacterial colonization, it has affected the ability to invade the blood stream from the respiratory epithelium when the genes are inactivated.[180] It is possible that similar phase variation of LOS may also exist in *NTHi* as well.

Pneumococcal proteins pneumolysin and autolysin, contribute significantly to the virulence of pneumococci.[182] *S. pneumoniae* type 3 mutants deficient in production of either pneumolysin or autolysin were constructed by transformation of DNA from derivatives of a rough strain, in which the respective genes had been interrupted by insertion-duplication mutagenesis using internal fragments of the cloned genes in the vector.[182] Both the pneumolysin-negative and the autolysin-negative strains had significantly reduced virulence in mice, as judged by survival time after intraperitoneal challenge. When pneumolysin and autolysin productions are restored by back-transformation of the mutants with an intact copy of the respective cloned gene, the mean survival time was indistinguishable from that of mice challenged with wild-type strain. Thus, the pneumolysin and autolysin are important virulence factors in type 3 pneumococci.[182] Mice challenged with a genetically-modified mutant strain of pneumococcus were unable to express active pneumolysin. Pre-immunization of such mice with autolysin failed to provide any significant protection against the challenge.[183] These authors suggested that the most important contribution made by autolysin to the virulence of *S. Pneumoniae* may be its role in mediating the release of pneumolysin from the pneumococcal cytoplasm during infection.

MOLECULAR BIOLOGICAL APPROACHES IN THE DEVELOPMENT OF VACCINES

The intention of this section is not meant to be a review on current otitis media vaccines, but rather it is intended to focus on the molecular biological aspects of the vaccine development. Excellent reviews on the otitis media vaccine development are available.[184,162,185]

Nontypeable *Haemophilus Influenzae* Vaccines

Several lines of evidence suggest that a number of outer membrane proteins *(OMPs)* of nontypeable *Haemophilus influenzae* are potential candidates for vaccine against this organism. The genes encoding several of these outer membrane proteins have been cloned, sequenced, and expressed.[186–190] This nucleotide sequence information together with mapping of bactericidal epitopes molecules of OMPS which enabled investigators to define the structure and function of these outer membrane proteins and identify domains that are conserved across the strains.[191,192] Such information is critical in selecting antigens as vaccine candidates. Among those identified as potential vaccine candidates, NTHi outer membrane protein P6 (peptidoglycan-associated lipoprotein), which is common to both nontypeable and type b *Haemophilus* is the most promising because P6 is a target of bactericidal antibodies in convalescent sera. A truncated P6 gene without the signal peptide has been constructed by Green and his associates,[193] and the recombinant protein encoded by this construct is capable of eliciting bactericidal antibody in vitro. Using a monoclonal antibody, Murphy and Kirkham[190] identified a region of P6 encoding an epitope recognized by bactericidal antibody.

Another *Haemophilus* outer membrane protein known as P6 cross-reactive protein (PCP) is also considered to be an excellent vaccine candidate, because polyclonal antisera against PCP is bactericidal. The PCP is antigenically conserved and present in both type b and NTHi. Deich et al.[194] recently cloned and sequenced this protein.

Other *Haemophilus* outer membrane proteins are believed to mediate bacterial adherence which are also considered as potential vaccine candidates include pilin and fimbrin. Antibody response to such proteins by immunization can block the bacterial adherence mediated by these proteins, thus reducing colonization and infection.[174,168] Another vaccine candidate is a group of high-molecular-weight surface-exposed proteins of NTHi which are related to the filamentous hemagglutinin protein of *Bordetella pertussis*.[172] The high-molecular-weight proteins are known to be critical adhesion molecules,[171] but also are major targets of human serum antibody.[195] To further characterize these proteins, Barenkamp and Leninger[196] cloned and sequenced genes encoding two related high-molecular-weight proteins (120-Kda and 125-Kda).

Streptococcus pneumoniae Vaccines

Many new vaccines including multivalent polysaccharide vaccines and polyvalent pneumococcal conjugate vaccines are under development and being field-tested,[162,184,185] and they will not be covered here.

Pneumococcal proteins autolysin and pneumolysin contribute significantly to the virulence of this organism. Autolysin and a defined toxoid derivative of pneumolysin were tested for efficacy in a mouse model as antigens protecting against challenge with virulent, wild-type *S. pneumoniae,* and the result showed that each antigen alone provided significant protection.[183] When mice were challenged with a genetically-modified mutant strain of pneumococcus unable to express active pneumolysin, pre-immunization of mice with autolysin failed to provide any significant protection against the challenge.[183] When mice were immunized with a genetically engineered toxoid version of pneumolysin derived from serotype 2 pneumococcus, and challenged with twelve strains of pneumococci (capsular types 1–6, 7F, 8, 18c), pneumolysin toxoid conferred protection against nine pneumococcal serotypes.[197] Thus, these investigators suggested that pneumolysin toxoids warrant consideration for inclusion in pneumococcal vaccines.

DNA Vaccines Against Respiratory Viruses

Acute otitis media is frequently preceded by a viral upper respiratory infection. Recent data using PCR demonstrated that a high number of middle ear effusions contained evidence of upper respiratory viruses,[198] and upper respiratory viral infection is causally related to the bacterial otitis media. It has been shown that attenuated influenza viral vaccine conferred protection against pneumococcal otitis media in chinchilla.[199] Thus, preventing upper respiratory viral infection will reduce the incidence of acute otitis media. In recent years, clinical trials have been initiated with live attenuated vaccines for respiratory syncytial virus (RSV), influenza, and parainfluenza viruses and adenovirus.[184] Such trials can provide an excellent opportunity to test the above hypothesis. In a clinical trial in Finland, attenuated influenza virus was administered to children under 4 years old. During a 6-week epidemic, 83% of the children were protected from confirmed influenza A-associated acute otitis media, and 36% from acute otitis media in general.[200] However, efficacies of viral vaccines against disease in susceptible populations are modest at best owing to rapid changes of viral surface antigens and heterogeneity of surface antigens among different strains, as well as incomplete knowledge of the characteristics of protective immunity of different upper respiratory viruses.[184]

Most of the current viral and bacterial vaccines are largely using surface antigens. However, such an approach poses a serious problem, because a microbe's surface structures frequently change at a rapid rate rendering vaccines useless. For example, evolution of the genes for surface proteins of influenza virus occurs so fast that a new vaccine must be made every year to be effective. However, proteins in the interior of viruses are more highly conserved (stable) than those of the surface. A recent discovery that plain DNA from a virus injected into the body could function as a vaccine may provide a new opportunity to develop an effective viral vaccine.[201] In a recent report, investigators described the results of experiments on mice using DNA from influenza virus.[202] The opponents to the viral DNA vaccines caution a theoretical possibility of activation of an oncogene, which may induce cancer in the host.

MOLECULAR MECHANISMS OF ANTIBIOTIC RESISTANCE AMONG OTITIS MEDIA PATHOGENS

Antibiotic Resistance to *Haemophilus Influenzae*

The genetic basis of ampicillin and chloramphenicol resistance in *H. influenzae* has been well characterized, and the principal mechanism of the resistance is largely enzymatic.[203] The gene that encodes the beta-lactamase enzyme is located within a large gene segment, transposon A.[204] Mendelman et al.[205] reported a small number of strains which demonstrate ampicillin resistance in the absence of beta-lactamase production, which is believed to be mediated by alterations in one or more of penicillin-binding proteins (PBPs). The PBPs 3a and 3b showed decrease in affinity for beta-lactams in antibiotic resistant strains.[206] The gene for the altered PBPs was recently cloned.[207] The genetic basis for resistance of *H. influenzae* type b to chloramphenicol has been elucidated and it is believed to be caused largely by the enzyme, acetyltransferase. The genetic sequence that codes for this enzyme is also located within a transposon.[208] Molecular cloning and mechanisms of trimethoprim resistance in *H. influenzae* were elucidated by cloning the gene for trimethoprim resistance into a cosmid vector and transducing recombinant plasmids into E. coli.[209] The results indicated that the acquisition of trimethoprim resistance involved a chromosomally mediated rearrangement or change of nucleotide sequences. The mechanism of trimethoprim resistance is overproduction of dihydrofolate reductase.[209]

Antibiotic Resistance to *S. pneumoniae*

Penicillin resistance to *Streptococcus pneumoniae* is believed to be mediated by changes in the production of altered PBPs.[210] The PBPs 1a, 2b, and 2x have been cloned and sequenced.[210–212] No beta-lactamase-mediated penicillin resistance was reported in pneumococci. Dowson and his associates[211] investigated a pen-

icillin binding protein PBP2b from several sensitive and resistant pneumococci and demonstrated a major change in the carboxyl-terminal sequence. It is postulated that this change is responsible for the development of penicillin resistance.

MOLECULAR EPIDEMIOLOGY AND DIAGNOSIS

Molecular biological techniques have been used to diagnose bacterial and viral diseases and fingerprint specific organisms in epidemiologic surveys.[213] Using a sensitive total genomic DNA restriction fingerprinting method, different isolates of *H. influenzae* has been identified.[214–218] Restriction endonuclease analysis of bacterial chromosomal DNA was used to compare NTHi obtained from middle ear effusions with that of the nasopharynx of patients with otitis media. The restriction digest profiles of strains isolated simultaneously from the middle ear effusion and nasopharynx of an individual child were identical, whereas the restriction profiles of strains isolated from different children were different from one another.[215] In this study, the isolates from recurring episodes of NTHi in six children were different from those which cause the initial episode.

Like in the NTHi, another gram-negative bacteria *Branhamella catarrhalis* was subject to restriction fragment mapping for epidemiological study for this newly emerging pathogen for otitis media. Dickson et al.[219] was able to finger print and compare *B. catarrhalis* isolates obtained from middle ear effusions and those from nasopharynges of the same patients using restriction fragment mapping following digestion of genomic DNA with restriction endonuclease such as *Pst*I and *Cla*I. This micro-organism was considered as a normal flora of the nasopharynx of healthy children as well as adult. However, it became increasingly associated with acute purulent otitis media and otitis media with effusion in recent years. Therefore, it is important to learn about strains that are pathogens versus non-pathogens, and restriction fragment mapping technique allows investigation of the epidemiology of this micro-organism reliably.

Polymerase chain reaction (PCR) assay based on the amplification of pneumolysin gene fragments in sera was developed to diagnose acute pneumococcal pneumonia.[220] Analysis of DNA restriction patterns of genomic DNA provided a sensitive measure of genetic similarity between strains and provided a convenient method for use in epidemiologic studies.

FUTURE DIRECTION

The explosive pace of development of molecular techniques does not allow us in this chapter to do justice to all aspects of molecular biology that are relevant to otology. We have just begun to scratch the surface of many important areas of biology of the ear with these new tools. Availability of such powerful techniques is already beginning to impact on our understanding of cellular functions and malfunctions on a molecular level. Identification of genes important for the formation of the ear, maintenance and normal function of the sensory and nonsensory cells of the inner ear are now possible, and discovery of many new genes of importance will be accelerated. Many more transgenic animals and gene knockout animals of interest will be made available and these animals will propel our knowledge concerning specific gene functions important for the ear.

Although only limited attempts have been made, many innovations for the gene- or gene-based therapy will allow scientists to develop new approaches (e.g. antisense oligonucleotide therapy) to prevent or cure human diseases, which currently cannot be ameliorated.

For otitis media, molecular biological techniques already have made a major impact on our understanding of bacterial pathogenesis at the molecular level. We are beginning to understand the molecular mechanisms involved in bacteria-host interaction. A number of otitis media-causing bacterial surface antigens important for the protective host immune response have now been identified, and their genes are cloned. Molecular methods will allow us to incorporate this new knowledge in developing strategies to prevent and treat otitis media. Although the molecular biology of host responses including immune response, cytokine regulation, inflammatory cell mobilization, B and T cell activation and mucin regulation were not covered in this chapter, there is a large body of knowledge that is relevant for understanding of the pathogenesis and progression of otitis media. Rapid progress is being made in these areas including identification of genes regulating various aspect of host responses, which will impact on the way we manage otitis media in the future.

In summary, molecular biologic techniques are no longer an esoteric scientific curiosity, but are beginning to be used in diagnosis, new vaccine development, and even gene therapy. Many more molecular-based innovative approaches will become available in the future which will ultimately change our understanding and treatment of these diseases.

SUGGESTED READINGS

1. Sambrook J, Fritsch ER, Maniatis T: Molecular cloning: a laboratory manual; (2nd ed.) Cold Spring Harbor Lab Press, Cold Spring Harbor, NY, 1989.
2. Saiki RK, Gelfand DH, Stoffel S, Scharf SJ, Higuchi R, Horn GT, Mullis KB, Erlich HA: Primer-directed enzymatic amplification of DNA with a thermostable DNA polymerase. Science 239: 487–491, 1988.
3. Simmons DM, Arriza JL, Swanson LW: A complete protocol for in situ hybridization of messenger RNAs in brain and other tissues with radiolabeled single-stranded RNA probes. J Histotechnol 12:169–181, 1989.
4. Battey JF, Fathi S, Wada E, Hellmich MR, Way J M: Molecular genetic approaches to the analysis of neuropeptide receptors; Cell Physiol and Biochem 3:3–230, 1993.
5. Hoshi T, Zagotta WN, Aldrich RW: Biophysical and molecular mechanisms of Shaker potassium channel inactivation; Science 250:533–538, 1990.
6. Zagotta WN, Hoshi T, Aldrich RW: Restoration of inactivation of mutants of Shaker potassium channels by a peptide derived from ShB; Science 250:568–571, 1990.
7. Fambrough DM, Lemas MV, Hamrick M, Emerick M, Renaud KJ, Inman EM, Hwang B, Takoyasu K: Analysis of subunit assembly of Na, K-ATPase; Amer J Physiol 6:579–589, 1994.
8. Siddique MAQ, Goswami SK, Qasba P, Shen R, Zhou MD: Regulation of muscle tissue specific transcription: analysis of chicken cardiac myosin light chain 2 gene promoter; Proc 1st World Cong Cell Molec Biol: p345, 1991.
9. Rosenfeld MG, Crenshaw EB, Lira SA, Swanson L: Transgenic mice: applications to the study of the nervous system; Ann Rev Neurosci 11:353–72, 1988.
10. Gridley T, Soriano P, Jaenish R: Insertional mutagenesis in mice; Trends Genet 3:162–166, 1987.
11. Naori H, Kumura M, Otami H, Yokoyama M, Koizumi T, Katusuki M, Tanaka O: Transgenic mouse model of hemifacial microsomia: cloning and characterization of insertional mutation region on chromosome 10; Genomics 23:515–519, 1994.
12. Xiang X, Benson KF, Chada K: Minimouse: disruption of the pygmy locus in a transgenic insertional mutant; Science 7: 967–969, 1990.
13. Gordon JW, Uehlinger J, Dayani N, Talansky BE, Gordon M, Rudomen GS, Newmann PE: Analysis of the hotfoot (ho) locus by creation of an insertional mutation in a transgenic mouse; Devel Biol 137:349–358, 1990.
14. Meisler MH: Insertional mutation of "classical" and novel genes in transgenic mice; Trends Genet 8:341–344, 1992.
15. Crenshaw EB III, Ryan AF, Dillon SR, Kalla K, Rosenfeld MG: Wocko, a neurological mutant generated by insertional mutagenesis in a transgenic mouse pedigree; J Neurosci 11:15–1530, 1991.
16. Friedman TB, Liang Y, Weber JL, Hinnant JT, Barbetr TD, Winata S, Arhya IN, Asher JH Jr: A gene responsible for profound congenital nonsyndromal recessive deafness maps to the pericentromeric region of chromosome 17; Am J Hum Genetic 55:Supplement #68, 1995.
17. He X, Treacy MN, Simmons DM, Ingraham HA, Swanson LW, Rosenfeld MG: Expression of a large family of POU-domain regulatory genes in mammalian brain development; Nature 340:35–42, 1989.
18. Ernfors P, Lee K-F, Jaenisch R: Mice lacking brain-derived neurotrophic factor develop with sensory deficits; Nature 368: 147–150, 1994.
19. Farinas I, Jones KR, Backus C, Wang XY, Reichardt LF: Severe sensory and sympathetic deficits in mice lacking neurotrophin-3; Nature 369:658–661, 1994.
20. Klein R, Smeyne RJ, Wurst W, Long LK, Anerbach BA, Joyner AL, Barbacid M: Targeted disruption of the trkB neurotrophin receptor gene results in nervous system lesions and neonatal death; Cell 75:113–122, 1993.
21. Smeyne RJ, Klein R, Schnapp A, Long LK, Bryant S, Lewin A, et al: Severe sensory and sympathetic neuropathies in mice carrying a disrupted Trk/NGF receptor gene; Nature 368:6–9, 1994.
22. Gu W, Schneider JW, Condorelli G, Kaushai S, Mahdavi V,

Nadal-Ginard B: Interaction of myogenic factors and the retinoblastoma protein mediates muscle cell commitment and differentiation; Cell 72:309–3, 1993.

23. Boulter J, Connoly J, Deneris E, Goldman D, Heinemann S, Patrick J: Functional expression of two neural nicotinic acetylcholine receptors from cDNA clones identifies a gene family; PNAS 84:7763–7767, 1987.

24. Wada K, Ballivet M, Boulter J, Connolly J, Wada E, Deneris ES, et al: Functional expression of a new pharmacological subtype of brain nicotinic acetylcholine receptor; Science 7:330–334, 1988.

25. Bettler B, Boulter J, Hermans-Borgmeyer I, O'Shea-Greenfield A, Heneris ES, Moll C, et al: Cloning of a novel glutamate receptor subunit, GluR5: expression in the nervous system during development; Neuron 5:588–95, 1990.

26. Boulter J, Hollmann M, O'Shea-Greenfield A, Hartley M, Deneris E, Maron C, Heinemann S: Molecular cloning and functional expression of glutamate receptor subunit genes; Science 9:1033–1037, 1990.

27. Hollmann M, O'Shea-Greenfield A, Rogers SW, Heinemann S: Cloning by functional expression of a member of the glutamate receptor family; Nature 342:643–648, 1989.

28. Keinanen K, Wisden W, Sommer B, Werner P, Herb A, Verdoorn TA, Sakmann B, Seeburg PH: A family of AMPA-selective glutamate receptors; Science 9:556–560, 1990.

29. Drewe J, et al: Cloning of rat brain potassium channels a new member of the RCK family and representatives of two novel families; Neurosci Abstr 20:671, 1990.

30. Tempel BL, Jan YN, Jan LY: Cloning of a probable potassium channel gene from mouse brain; Nature 332:837–839, 1988.

31. Hererra V, Emanuel JR, Ruiz-Opazo N, Levenson R, Nadal-Ginard B: Three differentially expressed Na,K-ATPase a subunit isoforms: structural and functional implications; J Cell Biol 105:1855–1865, 1987.

32. Vassallo PM, Dackowski W, Emmanuel JR, Levenson R: Identification of a putative isoform of the Na,K-ATPase β subunit: Primary structure and tissue-specific expression; J Biol Chem 4:4613–4618, 1989.

33. Mercer RW, Schneider JW, Savitz A, Emmanuel J, Benz EJ, Levenson R: Rat-brain Na,K-ATPase β-chain gene: primary structure, tissue specific expression, and amplification in ouabain resistant HeLa C+ cells; Mol Cell Biol 6:3884–3890, 1986.

34. Shull GE, Greeb J, Lingrel JB: Molecular cloning of three distinct forms of the (Na + K +)ATPase a subunit from rat brain; Biochemistry 25:8125–8132, 1986.

35. Young RM, Shull GE, Lingrel JB: Multiple mRNAs from rat kidney and brain encode a single Na+,K+ATPase β subunit protein; J Biol Chem 2:4905–4910, 1987.

36. Hammes A, Oberdorf S, Strehler EE, Stauffer T, Carafoli E, Vetter H, Neyses L: Differentiation-specific isoform MRNA expression of the calmodulin-dependent plasma membrane Ca-ATPase; FASEB J 8:4–435, 1994.

37. Johnson DE, Williams LT: Structural and functional diversity in the FGF receptor multigene family; Adv Cance Res 60:1–41, 1993.

38. Heinemann S, Bettler B, Boulter J, Deneris E, Gasic G, Hartley M, et al: The glutamate receptor gene family: evidence that the GluR1, GluR2, GluR3 subunits form multiple glutamate receptors; Sidia Research Foundation Transmitter Amino Acid Receptors: Structures, Transduction and Models for Drug Development, Royal Society, London, Oct, 1990.

39. Wenthold RJ. Structure and distribution of glutamate receptors: Subunit-specific antibody studies; Neurosci Facts 3:2–3, 1992.

40. Farrer LA: Gene localization by linkage analysis; In Molecular Biology and Genectics, (Grundfast, K, ed.) Otolaryngol Clin N Amer 25:907–922, 1992.

41. Lee WH, Bookstein R, Hong F, Young LJ, Shew JY, Lee EY: Human retinoblastoma gene: cloning, identification and sequencing; Science 235:1394–1399, 1987.

42. Koenig M, Hoffman EP, Bertelson CJ, Monaco AP, et al: Complete cloning of the Duchenne muscular dystrophy (DMD) cDNA and preliminary genomic organization of the DMD gene in normal and affected individuals; Cell 50:509–517, 1987.

43. Wilcox ER and Fex J: Construction of a guinea pig organ of Corti cDNA library; Hear Res, 1992.

44. Robertson NG, Khetarpal U, Gutierrez-Espeleta GA, Bieber FR, Morton CC: Isolation of known and known genes from a human fetal cochlear cDNA library using subtractive hybridization and differential screening; Genomics 23:42–50, 1994.

45. Ryan AF, Batcher S, Brunm D, O'Driscell K, Harris JP: Cloning genes from an inner ear cDNA library; Arch Otolaryngol 119:17–1220, 1993.

46. Beisel KW, Kennedy JE, Morley BJ: Construction and assessment of a rat outer hair cell unidirectional cDNA library; Abst Assoc Res Otolaryn #323, p81, 1995.

47. Kaplan J, Gerber S, Bonneau D, Rozert JM, et al: A gene for Usher syndrome type I (USH1A) maps to chromosome 14q; Genomics 14:979–987, 1992.

48. Smith RJH, Lee EC, Kimberling WJ, Daiger SP, Pelias MZ, Kents BJB, et al: Localization of two genes for Usher syndrome type I to chromosome 11; Genomics 14:995–1002, 1992a.

49. Kimberling WJ, Moller CG, Davenport S, Priluck IA, Beighton PH, Greenberg J, et al: Linkage of Usher syndrome type I gene (USH1B) to the long arm of chromosome 11; Genomics 14:988–994, 1992.

50. Kimberling WJ, Weston MD, Moller C, Davenport SLH, Shugart YY, Priluck IA, et al: Localization of Usher syndrome type II to chromosome 1q; Genomics 7:5–9, 1990.

51. Lewis RA, Ottenid B, Stauffer D, Lalouel JM, Leppert M, et al: Mapping recessive ophthalmic diseases: Linkage of the locus for Usher syndrome type II to a DNA marker on chromosome 1q; Genomics 7:250–256, 1990.

52. Dahl SP, Weston MD, Kimberling WJ, Gorin MB, Shugart YY, Kenyon JB: Possible genetic heterogeneity of Usher syndrome type 2: A family unlinked to chromosome 1q markers; Abst 8th International Congress of Human Genetics; (Washington) #1077, 1991.

53. Smith RJH, Coppage KB, Ankerstjerne JKB, Capper DT, Kumar S, Kenyon J, et al: Localization of the gene for branchiootorenal syndrome to chromosome 8q; Genomics 14:841–844, 1992b.

54. Cremers FPM, Van de Pol TJR, Diergaarde PJ, Wieringa B, Nussbaum RL, Schwartz M, Ropers HH: Physical fine mapping of the choroideremia locus using Xq deletions associated with complex syndromes; Genomics 4:41–46, 1989.

55. Merry DE, Lesko JG, Susnoski DM, Lewis RA, Lubinsky M, Trask B, et al: Choroideremia and deafness with stapes fixation: A contiguous gene deletion syndrome in Xq; Amer J Hum Genet 45:530–540, 1989.

56. Bach I, Brunner HG, Beighton P, Ruvalcaba RHA, Reardon W, Pembrey ME, et al: Microdeletions in patients with gufsher-associated, X-linked mixed deafness (DFN3); Amer J Hum Genet 50:38–44, 1992.

57. Leon PE, Raventos H, Lynchm E, Morrow J, King M-C: The gene for an inherited form of deafness maps to chromosome 5q31; PNAS 89:5181–5184, 1992.

58. Coucke P, Van Camp G, Djoyodiharjo B, Smith SD, Frants RR, Padberg GW, Darby JK, Huizing EH, Cremers CWRJ, Kimberling WJ, Oostra BA, Van De Heyning PH, Willems PJ: Linkage of autosomal dominant hearing loss to the short arm of chromosome 1 in two families; New England J of Med 331:425–431, 1994.

59. Guilford P, Ben Arab S, Blanchard S, Levilliers J, Weissenbach J, Belkahia A, Petit C: A nonsyndromic form of neurosensory, recessive deafness maps to the pericentromeric region of chromosome 13q; Nature Genet 6:–, 1994a.

60. Guilford P, Ayadi H, Blanchard S, Chaib H, Le Paslier D, Weissenbachi Drira M, Petiti C, et al: A human gene responsible for neurosensory nonsyndromic recessive deafness is a candidate homologue of the mouse sh-1 gene; Hum Molec Genet 3: 989–993, 1994b.

61. Friedman R: Wocko: a transgenic insertional inner ear mutation; (Ph.D. Thesis) Dept. of Molecular Pathology, UCSD, Dec, 1994.

62. Lalwani AK, Brister JR, Fex J, Grundfast KM, Pikus AT, Ploplis B, et al: A new non-syndromic X-linked sensorineural hearing loss linked to the DMD locus; Amer J Human Gen 55:685–94, 1994.

63. Barker DF, Hostikka SL, Zhou J, Chow LT, Oliphant AR, Gerken SC, et al: Identification of mutations in the COL4A5 collagen gene in Alport syndrome; Science 8:12–1227, 1990.

64. Tryggvason K, Zhou J, Hostikka SL, Snows TB: Molecular genetics of Alport syndrome; Kidney Intnatl 43:38–44, 1993.

65. Foy C, Newton V, Wellesley D, Harris R, Read AP: Assignment of the locus for Waardenburg syndrome type I to human chromosome 2q37 and possibly homology to the Splotch mouse; Amer J Human Gen 46:1017–1023, 1990.

66. Ishikiriyama S, Tonoki H, Shilbuya Y, Chin S, Harada N, Abe K, Niikawa NS: Waardenburg syndrome type I in a child with de novo inversion (2) (q35-q37.3); Amer J Med Genet 33: 505–507, 1989.

67. Epstein DJ, Vekemans M, Gros P: Splotch (SP²H), a mutation affecting development of the mouse neural tube, shows a deletion within the paired homeodomain of Pax-3; Cell 67:767–774, 1991.

68. Tassabehji M, Newton VE, Leverton K, Turnbull R, Seemanova E, Kunze J, et al: PAX3 gene structure and mutations: close analogies between Waardenburg syndrome and the Splotch mouse; Hum Mol Genet 3:(7):1069–74, 1994.

69. Tassabehji M, Read AP, Newton VE, Harris R, Balling R, Gruss P: Waardenburg's syndrome patients have mutations in the human homologue of the Pax-3 paired box gene; Nature 355: 635–636, 1992.

70. Baldwin CT, Hoth CF, Amos JA, da-Silva EO, Milunsky A: An exonic mutation in the HuP2 paired domain gene causes Waardenburg's syndrome; Nature 355:637–638, 1992.

71. Farrer LA, Arnos KS, Asher JH Jr, Baldwin CT, Diehl SR, Friedman TB, et al: Locus heterogeneity for Waardenburg Syndrome is predictive of clinical subtypes; Am J Human Gen 55:7–737, 1994.

72. Hoth CF, Milunsky A, Lipsky A, Sheffer R, Clarren SK, Baldwin CT: Mutations in the paired domain of the human PAX3 gene cause Klein-Waardenburg syndrome (WS-III) as well as Waardenburg syndrome type I (WS-I); Amer J Hum Genet 52: 455–562, 1993.

73. Gibson F, Walsh J, P Mburu, Varela A, Brown KA, Antonio M, et al: A type VII myosin encoded by the mouse deafness gene shaker-1; Nature 374:62–64, 1995.

74. Weil D, Blanchard S, Kaplan J, Gullford P, Gibson F, Walsh J, et al: Defective myosin VIIA gene responsible for Usher syndrome type 1B; Nature 374:60–61, 1995.

75. de Kok YJM, Vander Maarel SM, Bitner-Glindzicz M, Huber I, Monaco AP, Malcolm S, et al: Association between X-linked mixed deafness and mutations in the POU domain gene POU3F4; Science 7:3:685–688, 1995.

76. Ryan AF, Brumm D, Kraft M: Occurrence and distribution of non-NMDA glutamate receptor mRNAs in the cochlea; Neuro Rep 2:543–646, 1991.

77. Jaber L, Shohat M, Bu X, Fischel-Ghodsian N, Yang H, Wan SJ, Rotter JI: Sensorineural deafness inherited as a tissue specific mitochondrial disorder; Med Genet :86–90, 1992.

78. Prezant TR, Shohat M, Jaber L, Pressman S, Fischel-Ghodsian N: Biochemical characterization of a pedigree with mitochondrially inherited deafness; Amer J Med Genet 44:465–472, 1992.

79. Fischel-Ghodsian N, Prezant TR, Bu X, Oztas S: Mitochondrial ribosomal RNA gene mutation in a patient with sporadic aminoglycoside ototoxicity; Am J Otolaryngol 14:(6):399–403, 1993.

80. Hodgkinson CA, Moore KJ, Hakayama A, Steingrimsson E, et al: Mutations at the mouse microphthalmia locus are associated with defects in a gene encoding a novel basic-helix-loop-helix-zipper protein; Cell 30:74:395–404, 1993.

81. Tachibana M, Hara Y, Jyas D, Hodgkinson C, Fex J, Grundfast K, Arnheiter H: Cochlear disorder associated with melanocyte anomaly in mice with a transgenic insertional mutation; Mol Cell Neuro 3:433–445, 1992.

82. Tachibana M, Perez-Jurado LA, Nakayama A, Hodgkinson CA, Li X, Schneider M, et al: Cloning of MITF, the human homolog of the mouse microphthalmia gene and assignment to chromosome 3p14.1-p12.3; Hum Mol Genetic 3:4:553–557, 1994.

83. Hughes AE, Newton VE, Liu XZ, Read AP: A gene for Waardenburg syndrome type 2 maps close to the human homonolgue of the microphthalmia gene at chromosome 3p12-p14.1; Nat Genet 7:(4):509–12, 1994.

84. Seizinager BR, Martuza RL, Gusella JF: Loss of genes on chromosome 22 in tumorigenesis of human acoustic neuroma; Nature 322:644–647, 1986.

85. Rouleau GA, Wertelecki W, Haines JA, Hobbs WJ, Trofatter J, Seizinager BR, et al: Genetic linkage of bilateral acoustic neurofibromatosis to a DNA marker on chromosome 22; Nature 3: 6–8, 1987.

86. Frazer KA, Boehnke M, Budarf ML, Wolff RK, Emanuel BS, Myers RM, and Cox DR: A radiation hybrid map of the region on human chromosome 22 containing the neurofibromatosis type 2 location; Genomics 14:574–584, 1992.

87. Trofatter JA, MacCollin MM, Rutter JL, Murrell JR, Duyao MP, Parry DM, et al: A novel moesin-, radixin-like gene is a candidate for the neurofibromatosis 2 tumor suppressor; Cell 72: 791–800, 1993.

88. McCollin M, Ramesh V, Jacoby LB, Louis DN, et al: Mutational analysis of patients with neurofibromatosis 2; Am J Hum Genet 55:(2):314–20, 1994.

89. Steel KP, Davidson D, Jackson I: Melanoblast migration in embryonic steel-dickie mice mutants which later show deafness associated with white spotting; Assoc Res Otlaryng, MidWinter Meeting Abst #131, p46, 1992.

90. Brannan CI, Lyman SD, Williams DE, Eisenman J, Anderson DM, Cosman D, Bedell M, Jenkins N, Copeland N: Steel-Dickie mutation encodes a c-kit ligand lacking transmembrane and cytoplasmic domains; PNAS 1:88(11):4671–4, 1991.

91. Wright CG, et al: Abnormalities of the stria vascularis and dark cell epithelium in transgenic mice with ocular melanoma; Assoc Res Res Otolaryng, MidWinter Meeting Abst 535:134, 1994.

92. Corey DP and Breakefield XO: Transcription factors in inner ear development; PNAS 91:433–436, 1994.

93. Uziel A: Periods of sensitivity to thyroid hormone during the development of the organ of Corti; Acta Otolaryng Suppl4: 23–27, 1986.

94. Granstrom G: Retinoid-induced ear malformations; Otolaryn Head Neck Surg 103:702–709, 1990.

95. Jarvis BL, Johnston MC, Sulik KK: Congenital malformations of the external, middle, and inner ear produced by isotretinoin exposure in mouse embryos; Otolaryn Head Neck Surg 102: 391–401, 1990.

96. Bradley DJ, Towle HC, Young WS: Spatial and temporal expression of alpha-and beta-thyroid hormone receptor mRNAs, including the beta 2-subtype, in the developing mammalian nervous system; J Neurosci 12:(6):28–302, 1992.

97. Bradley DJ, Towle HC, Young WS III: Alpha and beta thyroid hormone receptor (TR) gene expression during auditory neurogenesis: evidence for TR isoform-specific transcriptional regulation in vivo; PNAS 18:91(2):439–43, 1994.

98. Oh SH and Wu D: Expression of bone morphogenetic protein 4,

5 and 7 in the developing chick inner ear; Assoc Res Otolaryng, MidWinter Meeting Abst #422, p106, 1995.

99. Represa J, Leon Y, Miner C, Goraldez F: The *int-2* proto-oncogene is responsible for induction of the inner ear; Nature *353:* 561–563, 1991.

100. Kelley MW, Xu X-M, Wagner MA, Warchol ME, Corwin JT: The developing organ of Corti contains retinoic acid and forms supernumerary hair cells in response to exogenous retinoic acid in culture; Develop *119:*1041–1055, 1993.

101. Dolle P, Ruberte E, Leroy P, Morris-Kay G, Chambon P: Retinoic acid receptors and cellular retinoid binding proteins. I. A systematic study of their differential pattern of transcription during mouse organogenesis; Develop *110:*1133–1151. 1990.

102. Ruberte E, Friedrich V, Morriss-Kay G, Chambon P: Retinoic acid receptors and cellular retinoid binding proteins. III. Their differential transcript distribution during mouse nervous system development; Develop*115:*973–989, 1992.

103. Sanne J-L, and Wu D: Expression of retionoic acid binding protein I in the Developing Chick otocyst; Am Soc Cell Biol Abst, 1995.

104. Van De Water TR: Development mechanisms of mammalian inner ear formation;[1,2,3] Hearing Sci 2:50–107, 1984.

105. Wilkinson DG, Bhatt S, McMahon AP: Expression pattern of the FGF-related proto-oncogene int-2 suggests multiple roles in fetal development; Devel *105:*131–136, 1989.

106. Represa J: NGF gene-related neurotrophins differentially regulated development of embryonic auditory and vestibular neurons; Inner Ear Neuropharmacology Int Sympo; Montpellier, France #23, 1994.

107. Mansour SL, Goddard JM, Capecchi MR: Mice homozygous for a targeted disruption of the proto-oncogene *int-2* have developmental defects in the tail and ear; Devel *117:*13–, 1993.

108. Luo L, Koutnouyan H, Baird A, Ryan AF: Acidic and basic FGF NRNA expression in the adult and developing rat cochlea; Hear Res *69:*182–93, 1993.

109. Datzert S, Baird A, Ryan AF: Selective ablation of neonatal cochlear outer hair cells by FGF-2-saporin: evidence for high-affinity FGF receptors; In preperation.

110. Low W, Baird A, Ryan AF: Protection of cochlear hair cells form aminoglycoside injury by basic fibroblast growth factor; Assoc Res Otolaryng, MidWinter Meeting Abst #18, p200, 1995.

111. Lefebvre PP, Staecker H, Weber T, Van De Water TR, Rogister B, Moonen G: TGF*B*₁ modulates bFGF receptor message expression in cultured adult auditory neurons; Neuro Report 2: 305–308, 1991a.

112. Lefebvre PP, Van De Water TR, Represa J, Liu W, Bernd P, Modlin S, Moonen G, Mayer MB: Temporal pattern of nerve growth factor (NGF) binding in vivo and the in vitro effects of NGF on cultures of developing auditory and vestibular neurons; Acta Otolaryngol *111:*304–311, 1991b.

113. Lefebvre PP, Van De Water TR, Weber T, Rogister B, Moonen G: Growth factor interactions in cultures of dissociated adult acoustic ganglia: neuronotrophic effects; Brain Res *567:*306–312, 1991c.

114. Lafebvre PP, Van De Water TR, Staecker H, Weber T, Galinovic-Schwartz V, Moonen G, Ruben RJ: Nerve growth factor stimulates neurite regeneration but not survival of adult auditory nerve in vitro; Acta Otolaryngol *112:*8–3, 1992.

115. Ernfors P, Loring J, Jaenisch, Van De Water TR: Function of the neurotrophins in the auditory and vestibular systems: Analysis of BDNF and NT-3 gene knockout mice; Assoc Res Otolaryngol MidWinter Meeting Abst #759, p190, 1995.

116. Pirvola U, Ylikoski J, Palgi J, Lehtonen E, Arumae U, Saarma M: Brain-derived neurotrophic factor and neurotrophin 3 mRNAs in the peripheral target fields of developing inner ear ganglia; PNAS *89:*9915–9919, 1992.

117. Ylikoski J, Privola U, Moshnyakow M, Palgi J, et al: Expression patterns of neurotrophin and their receptor mRNAs in the rat inner ear; Hear Res *65:*1–2:69–78, 1993.

118. Staecker H, Lefebvre P, Liu W, Ruttner B, Moonen G, Van De Water TR: Brain dirived neurotrophic factor and its influence otocyst; Abst Assoc Res Otolaryngol MidWinter Meeting #104, p, 1993.

119. Kim DO: Functional roles of the inner-and outer-hair-cell subsystems in the cochlea and brainstem; Hearing Sci 7:2–2, 1984.

120. Schwartz AM: Auditory nerve and spiral ganglion cells: morphology and organization; Neurobiol Hear *15:*271–2, 1986.

121. Warr WB, Buinan JJ Jr., White JS: Organization of the efferent fibers: The lateral and medial olivocochlear systems; In Neurobiol Hear: The Cochlea: edited by Altshuler RA, Hoffman DW, and Bobbin, RP (eds); Raven Press pp333–348, 1986.

122. Altshuler RA and Fex J: Efferent Neurotransmitters; Neurobiol Hear: The Cochlea; Altshuler RA, Hoffman DW, and Bobbin RP (eds); Raven Press pp383–396, 1986.

123. Hunter C, Doi K, Wenthold RJ: Neurotransmission in the auditory system; In Molecular Biology and Genetics (Grundfast, K. ed.) Otolaryngol Clin N Am 25:(5):1027–52, 1992.

124. Wenthold RJ and Martin MR: Neurotransmitters of the auditory nerve and central auditory system; Hearing Sci 10:342–369, 1984.

125. Hunter C, Petralia RS, Vu T, Wenthold RJ: Expression AMPA-selective glutamate receptor subunits in morphologically defined neurons of the mammalian cochlear nucleus; J Neurosci *13:*1932–1946, 1993.

126. Kuriyama H, Albin RL, Altschuler RA: Expression of NMDA-receptor MRNA in the rat cochlea; Hear Res *69:*1–2:5–20, 1993.

127. Wenthold RJ, Niedzielski AS, Hunter C, Petralia RS, Wang Y-X, Mathura J: Expression of glutamate receptors in spiral ganglion neurons. Inner Ear Neuropharrmacology Symposium, Montpellier, France, Sept. 1994.

128. Niedzielski AS and Wenthold RJ: Expression of AMPA, kainate, and NMDA receptor subunits in cochlear and vestibular ganglia; J Neurosci *15:*2338–2353, 1995.

129. Elgoyhen AB, Johnson DS, Boulter J, Vetter DE, Heinemann S: Alpha 9: acetylcholine receptor with novel pharmacological properties expressed in rat cochlear hair cells: Cell *18:*705–15, 1994.

130. Housley GD, Batcher S, Kraft M, Ryan AF: Nicotinic acetylcholine receptor subunits expressed in rat cochlea detected by polymerase chain reaction; Hearing Res *75:*47–53, 1994.

131. Drescher DG, Upadhyay S, Wilcox, Fex J: Analysis of muscarinic receptor subtypes in the mouse cochlea by means of PCR; J Neurochem *59:*765–767, 1992.

132. Eybalin M and Safieddine S: Neurotransmitters and neuromodulators in the cochlea; Inner Ear Neuropharmacology Symp, Montpellier, France, Sept. 1994.

133. Drescher DG, Green GE, Khan KM, Kajela K, Beisel KW, Morley BJ, Gupta AK: Analysis of GABA-A receptor subunits in the mouse cochlea by means of PCR: J Neurochem *61:*1167–1170, 1993.

134. Housley GD, Raybould NP, Taylor L: Variation in conductances activated in response to extracellular ATP and tonotopic-dependent expression of P2 purinoceptors in the sensory hair cells of the inner ear; Inner Ear Neuropharmacology Symp, Montpellier, France, 1994.

135. Ryan AF and Watts AG: Expression of genes coding for a and *β*isoforms of Na/K-ATPase in the cochlea of the rat; Cell Molec Neurosci *2:*179–187, 1991.

136. Fina M and Ryan AF: Expression of mRNAs encoding subunit isoforms of the Na, K-ATPase in the vestibular labyrinth of the rat; Cell Molec Neurosci *5:*604–613, 1994.

137. Killick R and Richardson G: Isolation of clones for the a-subunit of the epithelial Na channel from chick cochlear cDNA library; Inner Ear Neuropharmacology Symp, Montpellier, France, Sept. 1994.

138. Corey DP and Hudspeth AJ: Ionic basis of the receptor potential in a vertebrate hair cell: Nature *1:*675–677, 1979.

139. Corey DP and Hudspeth AJ: Kinetics of the receptor current in bullfrog saccular hair cells; J Neurosci *3:*962–976, 1983.

140. Hudspeth AJ: Extracellular current flow and the site of transduction by vertebrate hair cells: J Neurosci 2:(1):1–10, 1982.

141. Pickles JO, Comis SD, Osborne MP: Cross-links between stereocilia in the guinea pig organ of Corti, and their possible relation to sensory transduction; Hear Res 15:103–112, 1984.

142. Assad JA, Shepherd GMG, Corey DP: Tip-link integrity and mechanical transduction vertebrate hair cells; Neuron 7: 985–994, 1991.

143. Hackney CM, Furness DN, Benos DJ, Woodley JF, Barratt J: Putative immunolocalization of the mechanoelectrical transduction channels in mammalian cochlear hair cells; Proc Roy Soc B 8:5–2, 1992.

144. Gillespie PG, Wagner MC, Hudspeth AJ: Identification of a 120 kd hair-bundle myosin located near stereociliary tips; Neuron 11:581–594, 1993.

145. Howard J and Hudspeth AJ: Mechanical relation of the hair bundle mediated adaptation in mechanoelectrical transduction by the bullfrog's saccular hair; PNAS 84:3064–3068, 1987a.

146. Solc CK, Derfler BH, Duyks GM, Corey DP: Molecular cloning of myosins from the bullfrog saccular macula: a candidate for the hair cell adaptation motor; Auditory Neuro 1:63–75, 1994.

147. Hudspeth AJ and Gillespie PG: Pulling springs to tune transduction: adaption by hair cells; Neuron 12:109, 1994.

148. Kemp DT: Stimulated acoustic emissions from within the human auditory system; J Acoust Soc Am 64:1386–1391, 1978.

149. Brownell WE, Bader CR, Bertrand D, and de Ribaupierre Y: Evoked mechanical responses isolated cochlear outer hair cells; Science 227:194–196, 1985.

150. Kachar B, Brownell WE, Altschuler R, Fex J: Electrokinetic shape changes of cochlear outer hair cells; Nature 322:365–367, 1986.

151. Dallos P, Evans BN, Hallworth R: Nature of the motor element in electrokinetic shape changes of cochlear outer hair cells; Nature 350:155–157, 1991.

152. Kalinec F, Holley MC, Iwasa K, Lim DJ, and Kachar B: A membrane-based force generation mechanism in auditory sensory cells; PNAS 89:8671–8675, 1992.

153. Ryan AF and Housley GD: Molecular cloning of sequences containing s4-like regions from the rat organ of Corti; Abst Conf Mole Biol Hearing & Deafness, p 74, 1992.

154. Kalinec R and Kachar B: Inhibition of outer hair cell electromotility by sulfhydryl specific reagents; Neurosci Lett 157:134–231, 1993.

155. Negrini C, Rivolta M, Kalinec F, Kachar B: Cloning of an organ of Corti AE2 isoform with a truncated C-terminal domain; Abstr Inner Ear Biol 31: 61, 1994.

156. Thalmann I, Suzuki H, McCourt DW, Comegys TH, Thalmann R: Partial amino acid sequences of organ of Corti proteins OCP1 and OCP2: A progress report; Hear Res 64:191–198, 1993.

157. Chen HJ, Thalmann I, Adams JC, Avraham KB, Copeland NG, Jenkins NA, Beier DR, Corey DP, Thalmann R, Duyk GM: Cloning, molecular analysis and tissue distribution of Ocp2, gene encoding a putative transcription-associated factor predominantly expressed in the auditory organs. Cell, in press.

158. Legan K, Killick R, Goodyear R, Richardson G: Expression of the 41 Kda chick tectorin MRNA is restricted to the striolar region within the lagenar macula; Abstr Inner Ear Biol 31:48, 1994.

159. Davis JG, Oberholtzer JC, Burns FR, Greene MI: Molecular cloning and characterization of an inner ear-specific structural protein; Science 7:1031–134, 1995.

160. Yoo TJ, Fujiyoshi T, Readhead C, Hood L: Restoration of auditory evoked potential by myelin basic protein (MBP) gene therapy in shiverer mice; Assoc Res Otolaryng MidWinter Meeting Abstr #586, p147, 1993.

161. Ryan AF and Luo L: Delivery of a recombinant growth factor into the mouse inner ear by implantation of transfected cell line; Assoc Res Otolaryng MidWinter Meeting Abstr #18, p47, 1995.

162. Staecker H, Kopke R, Lefebvre P, Malgrange B, Liu W, Moonen G, and Van De Water TR: The effects of neurotrophins on adult auditory neurons in vitro and in vivo; Assoc Res Otolaryn MidWinter Meeting Abstr #18, p177, 1995.

163. Ryan AF, Bakaletz LO, Barenkamp SJ, Forney LJ, Samuelson AG: New Technology: Molecular Biology; In Recent Advances in Otitis Media; Report of the Fifth Research Conference; Ann Otol Rhinol Laryng Suppl 164:103:2:46–52, 1994.

164. Andersson B and Svanborg-Eden C: Attachment of Streptococcus pneumoniae to Human Pharyngeal Epithelial Cells; Respiration 55:(suppl):49:49–52, 1989.

165. Coleman T, Grass S, Munson R Jr: Molecular cloning, expression, and sequence of the pilin gene from nontypeable Haemophilus influenzae M37; Infect Immun 59:1716–22, 1991.

166. Kar S, To C-MS, and Brinton CC Jr: Cloning and expression in escherichia coli of LKP pilus genes from a nontypeable Haemophilus influenzae Strain; Infect Immun 58:4:903–908, 1990.

167. Bakaletz LO, Ahmed MA, Forney LJ, Kolattukudy PE, and Lim DJ: Cloning and sequence analysis of a pilin-like gene from an otitis media isolate of nontypeable Haemophilus influenzae (strain #11); J Infectious Dis 165:S201, 1992.

168. Sirakova T, Kollatukudy PE, Murwin D, Billy J, Leake E, Lim DJ, et al: Role of fimbriae expressed by nontypeable Haemophilus influenzae (NTHi) in the pathogenesis of and protection against otitis media and the relatedness of the fimbrin subunit to outer membrane protein A.; Infect Immun 62:2002–2020, 1994.

169. Barenkamp SJ and Leininger E: Cloning, expression, and DNA sequence analysis of genes encoding nontypeable Haemophilus influenzae high-molecular-weight surface-exposed proteins related to filamentous hemagglutinin of bordetella pertussis; Infect Immun 60:1302–1313, 1992.

170. Barenkamp SJ and St. Geme III JW: Genes encoding high-molecular-weight adhesion proteins of nontypeable Haemophilus influenzae are part of gene clusters; Infect Immun 62:8:3320–33, 1994.

171. St. Geme III JW, Falkow S, and Barenkamp SJ: High-molecular-weight proteins of nontypeable Haemophilus influenzae mediate attachment to human epithelial cells; PNAS 90:75–79, 1993.

172. Barenkamp SJ: Cloning, expression, and DNA sequence analysis of genes for nontypeable Haemophilus influenzae high molecular weight outer membrane proteins which are targets of bactericidal antibody; In: Lim DJ, Bluestone CD, Klein JO, Nelson JD, Ogra PL eds. Recent Advances in Otitis Media. Proceedings of the Fifth International Symposium. Hamilton, Canada: Decker Periodicals; 379–80, 1993.

173. Bakaletz LO and Barenkamp SJ: Localization of high-molecular-weight adhesion proteins of nontypeable Haemophilus influenzae by immunoelectron microscopy; Infect Immun 62: 4460–4468, 1994.

174. Brinton CC Jr, Carter MJ, Derber DB, Kar S, Kramarik JA, To ACC, et al. Design and development of pilus vaccines for Haemophilus influenzae diseases; Pediatric Infect Dis J 8: S54–S61, 1989.

175. Bakaletz LO, Tallan BM, Hoepf TM, DeMaria TF, et al: Frequency of fimbriation of nontypeable Haemophilus influenzae and its ability to adhere to chinchilla and human respiratory epithelium; Infect Immun 56:(2):331–5, 1988.

176. Spinola SM, Griffiths GE, Shanks, Blake MS: The major outer membrane protein of Haemophilus ducreyi is a member of the Ompa family of proteins; Infect Immun 61:1346–1351.

177. DeMaria TF, Yamaguchi T, Lim DJ: Quantitative cytologic and histologic changes in the middle ear after the injection of nontypeable Haemophilus influenzae endotoxin; Am J Otolaryngol 10:(4):2361–6, 1989.

178. Weiser JN, Lindberg AA, Manning EJ, Hansen EJ, Moxon ER: Identification of chromosomal locus for expression of lipopoly-

saccharide epitopes in Haemophilus influenzae; Infect Immun 57:3045–52, 1989a.

179. Weiser JN, Love JM, Moxon ERL: The molecular mechanism of phase variation of H influenzae lipopolysaccharide; Cell 17: 657–665, 1989b.

180. Weiser JN, Maskell DJ, Butler PD, Lindberg AA, Moxon ER: Characterization of repetitive sequences controlling phase variation of Haemophilus influenzae lipopolysaccharide; J Bacteriol 172:3304–9, 1990a.

181. Weiser JN, Williams A, Moxon ER: Phase-variable lipopolysaccharide structures enhance the invasive capacity of Haemophilus influenzae; Infect Immun 58:3455–7, 1990b.

182. Berry AM, Paton JC, Hansman D: Effect of insertional inactivation of the genes encoding pneumolysin and autolysin on the virulence of Streptococcus pneumolysin pneumoniae type 3; Microb Pathog 12:(12):87–93, 1992.

183. Lock RA, Hansman D, Paton JC: Comparative efficacy of autolysin and pneumolysin as immunogens protecting mice against infection by Streptococcus pneumoniae; Microb Pathog 12:(2): 137–43, 1992.

184. Ogra PL, Barenkamp SJ, Mogi G, Pelton SI, Juhn SK, Karama P, et al: Microbiology, immunology, biochemistry and vaccination; Recent Advance in Otitis Media. Report of the fifth Research Conference Ann Otol Rhino Laryng Suppl 164 103:8: 27–43, 1994.

185. Karma PH, Bakaletz LO, Giebink GS, Mogi G, Rynnel-Dagoo B: Present views on possibilities of immunoprophylaxis of acute otitis media in infants and children; In Immunological Aspects of Otitis Media Int J Ped Otolaryn, In Press.

186. Nelson MB, Murphy TF, van Keulen H, Rekosh D, Apicella MA: Studies on P6, and important outer-membrane protein antigen of Haemophilus influenzae; Rev Infect Dis 10:Suppl 2: S331–6, 1988.

187. Nelson MB, Munson RS, Apicella MA, Sikkema DJ, et al: Molecular conservation of the P6 outer membrane protein among strains of Haemophilus influenzae: analysis of antigenic determinants, gene sequences, and restriction fragment length polymorphisms; Infect Immun 59:(8):58–63, 1991.

188. Deich RA, et al: Cloning of genes encoding a 15,000-dalton peptidoglycan-associated outer membrane lipoprotein and an antigenically-related 15,000-dalton protein from Haemophilus influenzae; J Bacteriol 170:489–498, 1988.

189. Sikkema DJ and Murphy TF: Molecular analysis of the P2 porin protein of nontypeable Haemophilus influenzae; Infect Immun 60: (12):5204–11, 1992.

190. Murphy TF and Kirkham C: Amino acid sequence of a surface-exposed epitope of the P6 outer membrane protein of nontypable Haemophilus influenzae; In: Lim DJ, eds. Abstracts of the Fifth International Symposium on Recent Advances in Otitis Media, Ft. Lauderdale, Florida:120–1, 1993.

191. Martin D, Munson R Jr, Grass S, et al: Mapping of B-cell epitopes on the outer membrane P2 porin protein Haemophilus influenzae by using recombinant proteins and synthetic peptides; Infect Immun 59:1457–64, 1991.

192. Haasse EM, Yi K, Morse GD, Murphy TF: Mapping of bactericidal epitopes on the P2 porin protein of nontypeable Haemophilus influenzae; Infect Immun 62:(9):3712–22, 1994.

193. Green BA, Metcalf BJ, Quinn-Dey T, Kirkley DH, Quataert SA, Deich RA: A recombinant non-fatty acylated form of the Hi-PAL (P6) protein of Haemophilus influenzae elicits biologically active antibody against both nontypeable and type b H influenzae: Infect Immun 58:3272–8, 1990.

194. Deich RA, Anilionis A, Fulginiti J, et al: Antigenic conservation of the 15,000-dalton outer membrane lipoprotein PCP of Haemophilus influenzae and biologic activity of anti-PCP antisera; Infect Immun 58:3388–93, 1990.

195. Barenkamp SJ and Bodor FF: Development of serum bactericidal activity following nontypeable Haemophilus influenzae acute otitis media; Pediatr Infect Dis J 9:333–339, 1990.

196. Barenkamp SJ and Leininger E: Cloning, expression, and DNA sequence analysis of genes encoding nontypeable Haemophilus infleunzae high-molecular-weight surface-exposed proteins related to filamentous hemagglutinin of Bordetella pertussis; Infec Immun 60:4:1302–1313, 1992.

197. Alexander JE, Lock RA, Peeters CC, Poolman JT, et al: Immunization of mice with pneumolysin toxoid confers a significant degree of protection against at least nine serotypes of Streptococcus pneumoniae; Infect Immun 62:(12)5683–8, 1994.

198. Okamoto Y, Kudo K, Ishikawa K, et al: Presence of respiratory syncytial virus genomic sequences in middle ear fluid and its relationship to expression of cytokines and cell adhesion molecules; J Infect Dis 168:(5):1277–81, 1993.

199. Giebink GS: Studies of Streptococcus pneumoniae and influenzae virus vaccines in the chinchilla otitis media model; Pediatr Infect Dis J 8:(Suppl):S42–S44, 1989.

200. Heikkinen T, Ruuskanenn O, Waris M, Eigler T, Arola M, Halonen P: Influenza vaccination in the prevention of acute otitis media in children; Am J Dis Child 145:445–8, 1991.

201. Robinson HL, Hunt LA, Webster RG: Protection against a letal influenza virus challenge by immunization with hemoagglutinin-expressing plasmid DNA; Vaccine 11:(9):957–60, 1993.

202. Montgomery DL, Shiver JW, Leander KR, Perry HC, et al: Heterologous and monological protection against infleunzae A by DNA vaccination: optimization of DNA vectors; DNA Cell Biol 12(9):777–83, 1993.

203. Needham CA: Haemophilus influenzae: antibiotic susceptibility; Clin Microbiol Rev 1:8–227, 1988.

204. DeGraff J, Elwell OP, Falkow S: Molecular nature of two beta-lactamase-specifying plasmids isolated from Haemophilus influenzae type b; J Bacteriol 1:439–46, 1976.

205. Mendelman PM, Chaffin DO, Stull TL, et al: Characterization of non-beta-lactamase-mediated ampicillin resistance in Haemophilus influenzae; Antimcrob Agents Chemother :235–44, 1984.

206. Clarioux N, Picard M, Brochu A, Rousseau N, et al: Molecular basis of the non-beta-lactamase-mediated resistance to beta-lactam antibiotics in strains of Haemophilus influenzae isolated in Canada; Antimicrob Agents Chemother 36:7:1504–13, 1992.

207. Matouin R and Bryan LE: DNA probe technology for detection of Haemophilus influenzae; Mol Cell Probes 1(3):2–32, 1987.

208. Roberts MC, Swenson CD, Owens LM, Smith AL: Characterization of chloramphenicol-resistant Haemophilus influenzae; Antimicrob Agents Chemother 18:610–5, 1980.

209. de Groot R, Campos J, Moseley SL, Smith AL: Molecular cloning and mechanism of tripethoprim resistance in Haemophilus influenzae; Amtibicrob Agents Chemother 332(4):477–84, 1988.

210. Klugman KP: Pneumococcal resistance to antibiotics; Clin Microbiol Rev 3:171–96, 1990.

211. Dowson CG, Hutchinson A, Spratt BG: Extensive remodeling of the transpeptidase domain of penicillin-binding protein 2B of a penicillin-resistant South African isolate of Streptococcus pneumoniae; Molec Microbiol 3:95–102, 1989.

212. Klugman KP, Coffey TJ, Smith A, Wasas A, et al: Cluster of an erythromycin-resistant variant of the Spanish multiply resistant 23F clone of Streptococcus pneumoniae in South Africa; Eur J Clin Microbiol 13:(2):171–4, 1994.

213. Soares S, Kristinsson KG, Musser JM, Tomasz A: Evidence for the introduction of a multiresistant clone of serotype 6B Streptococcus pneumoniae from Spain to Iceland in the late 1980's; J Infect Dis 168:1:158–63, 1993.

214. Owen RJ: Chromosomal DNA fingerprinting—a new method of species and strain identification applicable to microbial pathogens; J Med Microbiol 30:89–99, 1989.

215. Loos BG, Bernstein JM, Dryja DM, Murphy TF, Dickinson DP: Determination of the epidemiology and transmission of nontypeable Haemophilus influenzae in children with otitis media

by comparison of total genomic DNA restriction fingerprints; Infect Immun 57:2751–7, 1989.

216. Bernstein JM, Dryja DM, Loos BG, Dickinson D: Restriction fragment mapping nontypeable *Haemophilus influenzae:* a new tool to study this middle ear pathogen; Otolarylngol Head Neck Surg 100:200–6, 1989.

217. Ueyama T, Kuron U, Shirabe K, Takeshita M, Mogi G: Detection of Haemophilus influenzae in the nasopharynx and middle ear effusions by polymerase chain reaction; In Proc Recent Advance in Otitis Media; (Lim, D. J. et al, ed.), Decker Periodicals, pp595–599, 1993.

218. Hotomi M, Fujihara K, Kunimoto M, Yamanaka N: Detection of Haemophilus influenzae in middle ear effusions by the polymerase chain reaction; In Proc Recent Advances in Otitis Media; (Lim, D. J., et al, ed.), Decker Periodicals, pp601–605, 1993.

219. Dickinson DP, Loos GB, Loos GB, Dryja DM, Bernstein JM: Restrictions fragment mapping of *Branhamella catarrhalis:* A new tool for studying the epidemiology of this middle ear pathogen; J of Infect Dis 158:205–208, 1988.

220. Salo P, Ortqvist A, Leinonen M: Diagnosis of bacteremic pneumococcal pneumonia by amplification of pneumolysin gene fragment in serum; J Infect Dis 171:(2):479–82, 1995.

FURTHER SUGGESTED READINGS

Gilbert SF: Genes and development: Introduction and techniques; Development Biology (4th ed) Sinauer Associates, Inc., pp34–76, 1994.

Bockaert J: G proteins and G-protein coupled receptors: structure, function and interactions; Curr Opin Neurobiol 1:32–42, 1991.

Battey J, Davis L, Kuehl M: Basic Methods in Molecular Biology; (2nd ed.), Appleton & Lang, 1994.

Battey J, Fathi S, Wada E, Hellmich MR, Way JM: Molecular genetic approaches to the analysis of neuropeptide receptors; Cell Physiol & Biochem 3:3–230, 1993.

Watson JD, Gilman M, Witkowski J, Zoller M: Recombinant DNA; (2nd ed.), Scientific American Books, 1992.

Darnell J, Lodish H, Baltimore D: Molecular Cell Biology; (2nd ed.), Scientific American Books, 1990.

Glick RB and Pasternak JJ: Molecular Biotechnology: Principles & Applications of Recombinant DNA, ASM Press, 1994.

Brown TA: Gene Cloning: An Introduction; (2nd ed.), Chapman & Hall, 1990.

42 Physiology of the Auditory and Vestibular Systems

Brenda L. Lonsbury-Martin, Glen K. Martin, and Anne E. Luebke

INTRODUCTION TO THE AUDITORY SYSTEM

General Principles

Over the past 15 years, there have been major advances in our knowledge about how the ear achieves its high sensitivity, sharp frequency tuning, impressive dynamic range, and excellent temporal resolution. This new wisdom has led to a new understanding about the distinct functions of the inner and outer hair cells of the cochlea. Traditionally, the transfer of acoustic information from the environment to the higher centers of analysis in the central auditory nervous system was considered to be a passive process. According to this notion, the salient features of sound, including frequency, magnitude, and timing attributes, were principally encoded by peripheral processes, and then simply passed relatively unaltered along the ascending system, from one structure to another, in a forward traveling manner. With the discovery that the healthy ear can generate sounds in the form of otoacoustic emissions and that outer hair cells mechanically vibrate in response to depolarizing stimuli, the role of the cochlea in analyzing acoustic signals is considered to represent an active process. Given the assumption that the vibromechanical aspects of outer hair cell function underlie the production of otoacoustic emissions, and the awareness that the major portion of the cochlear-efferent system innervates this class of auditory sensory cell, central auditory-system structures may also modify peripherally generated responses in an active manner. Thus, rather than conceptualizing the role of the auditory system as a passive analyzer of environmental sounds, the modern view is to consider it as an active participant in controlling acoustic information so that the most meaningful features are registered.

AUDITORY APPARATUS

A traditional approach toward understanding the primary sensitivity, frequency-tuning, and timing functions of the peripheral part of the auditory system is to divide the periphery into three discrete parts. In this manner, the unique contributions that the external, middle, and inner ear (i.e., cochlea) make to the overall analysis of sound can be best appreciated.

External Ear

The external ear or pinna of the mammal is regarded as a simple funnel that collects and crudely filters sound. Given the immobility of the human external ear, it is assumed that these classical frequency-tuning functions are performed passively. However, evidence from experimental studies suggest that the human pinna serves two functions: (1) it aids in sound localization, especially front-to-back and high-to-low differentiations, where interaural time differences between ears provide no clues; and (2) it, along with the external ear canal, increases acoustic pressure at the tympanic membrane in the 1.5- to 5-kHz range, which is the frequency range important for speech perception. Evidence for the sound-localizing function of the human external ear includes the demonstration of accurate sound localization in patients with monaural hearing, and the loss of this localization ability when the pinna of the hearing ear is strapped to the head. In addition, abnormally poor sound localization around an "imperfectly" remodeled pinna has been reported.[1]

In summarizing available data on the role that the external ear plays in boosting sound pressure at the tympanic membrane, Shaw[2] described the contributions of the different parts of the head and neck and external ear by successively adding their distinct com-

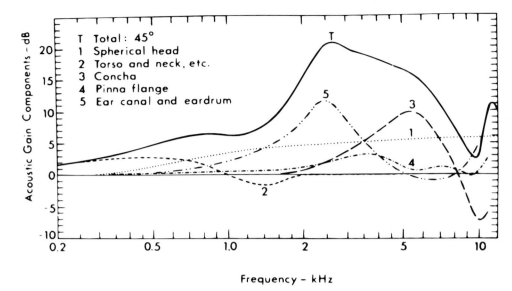

Fig. 42–1. Pressure gain contributed by the individual components of the outer ear in man. The total (T) curve plots the overall gain based upon the addition of the various components in the order listed with the sound source positioned 45° from straight ahead. Reprinted with permission from Shaw EAG: The external ear. In: Handbook of Sensory Physiology, Vol. V/1: Auditory System, Anatomy Physiology (Ear). Edited by W.D. Keidel, and W.D. Neff. New York: Springer-Verlag, 1974.[2]

ponents in a model. According to this analysis (Figure 42–1), most of the individual components of the external ear provide complementary gains resulting in a significant increase in sound pressure from approximately 2 to 7 kHz. When the overall additive effect is appreciated (''T'' in Figure 42–1), at certain frequencies, this gain is substantial, resulting in sound-pressure increases on the order of 20 dB.[2]

Studies of models of the human external ear suggest that the pinna extracts information about sound location by altering the transmission properties of different frequencies according to the location of the sound source relative to the pinna. For example, when the sound source is behind the ear, interference of directly transmitted sound with sound waves scattered off the pinna flange alters the response in the 3- to 6-kHz range. Thus, the external ear modifies the spectrum of the incoming sound allowing an individual to make judgments about the location of unknown sound sources. This localization ability suggests that the central part of the auditory system can use very subtle spectral cues in the analysis of environmental sounds.[2,3]

Middle Ear

Figure 42–2 outlines the anatomy of the middle and inner ears. The middle-ear ossicles form a transmission pathway that conducts sound energy from the tympanic membrane, at the interface of the external and middle ear, to the oval window of the cochlea. The discussion of middle-ear function is separated into two categories: 1) ''impedance matching'' between the air of the external environment and the fluids (perilymph and endolymph) of the cochlea, and 2) the acoustic reflex of the middle-ear muscle system.

The widespread use of surgical modification of mid-

dle-ear structures to improve hearing and the usefulness of immittance audiometry make the concept of acoustic impedance and its relationship to middle-ear function important. Accordingly, the discussion of the middle ear begins with some basic principles of acoustic impedance.

Transmission of Acoustic Energy through the Middle Ear

Figure 42–3A diagrams the route for the conduction of sound energy through the middle ear into the cochlear portion of the inner ear. The ossicular chain consisting of the malleus, incus, and stapes can be thought of as a lever system. The tympanic membrane moves the manubrium or handle of the malleus. The long process of the incus and manubrium move together, because the malleoincudal joint is essentially fixed. In contrast, the joint between the incus and the stapes is flexible. Therefore, because the stapes is fixed at its postero-inferior border, movement of the tympanic membrane causes it to rock in and out of the oval window. The changes in acoustic pressure caused by the stapes moving in and out of the oval window are transmitted instantaneously by the perilymph through the cochlear partition, then out the round window. Pressure transmission through the cochlear partition causes it to move either upward or downward, depending on the direction of the pressure change. This pressure change initiates a mechanical traveling wave, shown in Figure 42–3B, that reaches a maximum at some point on the basilar membrane depending on the frequency of the stimulating sound. The traveling wave moves from the base to the apex of the cochlea largely due to reduced stiffness in the apical direction. As discussed below, this traveling-wave disturbance causes the hair cells in the organ of Corti to stimulate the cochlear-nerve

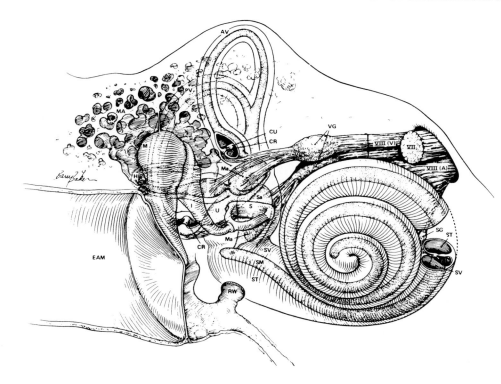

Fig. 42–2. Schematic drawing of the inner ear (labyrinth), which consists of a series of tunnels within the petrous portion of the temporal bone. The osseous labyrinth (outer tunnel) is clear, and the membranous labyrinth (inner tunnel) is stippled. SV = scala vestibuli, ST = scala tympani, SM = scala media, SG = spiral ganglion, containing the cell bodies of the cochlear nerve, VG = vestibular ganglia, containing the cell bodies of the vestibular nerve, VIII (A) = cochlear part of the eighth cranial nerve, VIII (V) = vestibular part of the eighth cranial nerve, VII = facial nerve, Ma = macula, CU = cupula, CR = crista, Sa = sacculus, U = utriculus. Semicircular canals are labeled AV (anterior vertical), PV (posterior vertical), and H (horizontal). EAM = external auditory meatus, RW = round window, M = malleus, I = incus, S = stapes, MA = mastoid air cells in temporal bone.

endings, thus, signaling to the central part of the auditory system that a sound stimulus has occurred.

At high sound levels (−100 to 110 dB SPL), the mode of vibration of the ossicular chain changes. Thus, instead of rotating about its short axis, as shown in Figure 42–3A, the stapes footplate turns about its long axis.[4] Because this change results in less efficient sound transmission through the middle ear, it may serve a protective function. Interestingly, the change in vibration mode occurs at the threshold of feeling, thus, suggesting that the somatic sensation caused by excessive sounds may be due to the detection of the altered ossicular vibration by middle-ear bone and tendon receptors.

IMPEDANCE MATCHING BY THE MIDDLE EAR. Hearing by terrestrial animals requires transmission of sound from an air to fluid environment. A useful way to appreciate the problem in conducting sound effectively between two distinct media is to recall how difficult it is to listen to sounds produced even a few inches above the surface while swimming underwater. Thus, direct transmission of sound across an air/water boundary is extremely inefficient. The inefficiency occurs because the specific acoustic impedances of air and water differ greatly, and whenever energy is transmitted between media with different specific impedances, much of the energy is reflected back from the boundary between the two media. To help solve this problem, the middle ear matches reasonably well the impedances of the air and cochlea, and thereby greatly increases the efficiency of transmitting acoustic energy from the environment into the cochlea.

The term impedance describes the opposition of a system to movement. Thus, the more force required to move a mechanical system at a given speed, the greater its impedance. Figure 42–4 illustrates the principles of mechanical impedance. If the force applied to a system and the speed that it moves in response are known, the impedance of the system may be calculated as follows:

Mechanical impedance

$$= \frac{\text{force}}{\text{velocity}} = \sqrt{R^2 + \left(2\pi\, fM - \frac{S}{2\pi\, f}\right)^2}$$

(equation 1)

The impedance of a mechanical system involves a complex relationship between the three physical parameters illustrated in Figure 42–4. Together, mass (M), stiffness (S), and frictional resistance (R) (i.e., friction) determine the mechanical impedance of the middle-ear system. Friction, the *resistive* component of impedance, consumes energy and is independent of the driving frequency (f). Stiffness and mass store energy and thus they comprise the *reactive* component of impedance. For example, once the "fluid" filled cylinder in Figure 42–4 is set in motion, it tends to continue because of inertia, and if the spring representing stiffness is compressed, it tends to push backward. As shown by equation 1, stiffness reactance (S) decreases with frequency (f), and mass reactance (M) increases with frequency. The equation also reveals that stiffness and mass reactance are of opposite sign (− and +, respectively), thus, indicating that there is a particular

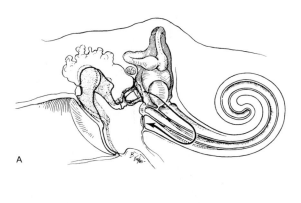

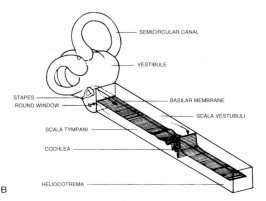

SEMICIRCULAR CANAL

VESTIBULE

STAPES
ROUND WINDOW

BASILAR MEMBRANE

SCALA VESTUBULI

SCALA TYMPANI

COCHLEA

HELIOCOTREMA

Fig. 42–3. A. Transmission of tympanic-membrane movement into the cochlea via the ossicles. The system at rest is unstippled. The stippled ossicles and dashed cochlear partition illustrate the system when the tympanic membrane is pushed inward by a sound wave. B. Inward pressure (arrows) initiates a traveling wave that migrates toward the apex of the cochlea. This propagation depends largely on fluid coupling and the fact that the basilar membrane changes in stiffness with the traveling wave moving from a region of highest stiffness (base) to a point of lower stiffness (apex). Reprinted with permission from Zweig G, Lipes R, Pierce JR: The cochlear compromise. J Acoust Soc Am 59:975, 1976.[269]

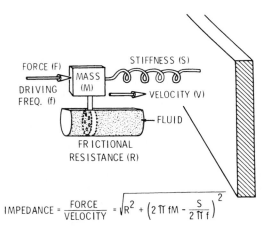

FORCE (F)

DRIVING
FREQ. (f)

MASS
(M)

STIFFNESS (S)

VELOCITY (V)

FLUID

FRICTIONAL
RESISTANCE (R)

$$\text{IMPEDANCE} = \frac{\text{FORCE}}{\text{VELOCITY}} = \sqrt{R^2 + \left(2\pi fM - \frac{S}{2\pi f}\right)^2}$$

Fig. 42–4. Principles of mechanical impedance. Frictional resistance is represented by a "dashpot"—a perforated piston operating inside a fluid-filled cylinder. The diagram could be converted to a representation of acoustic impedance by interposing a cylinder, or diaphragm, between the driving force and the driven mass and expressing the displacing input as pressure (force per unit area).

resonant frequency where stiffness reactance equals mass reactance and, hence, the total reactance is zero. At the resonant frequency, impedance is minimal.

Acoustic impedance represents a special type of mechanical impedance in which force is replaced by pressure (force per unit area) and the system is driven by sound. Thus, Figure 42–4 could be converted into a sketch of an acoustic system by interposing a piston, or membrane, between the force and the mass.

When air conducts sound, the stiffness component of its acoustic impedance is determined by the elastic coupling between air molecules, the mass component is determined by the mass of the air molecules, and the frictional component is determined by frictional resistance between the molecules. Because water is much denser and less compressible than air, it might seem at first that mass and stiffness create the principal difference between the acoustic impedance of the cochlea and that of air. However, Figure 42–4 demonstrates that transmission of energy into the cochlea does not involve compression of the cochlear fluid itself. In addition, the elastic restorative forces of the cochlear partition and round window tend to cancel out the effect of the fluid's mass. Thus, the effective acoustic impedance of the cochlea is primarily resistive.[5]

As noted earlier, a primary function of the middle ear is to provide a means of "matching" the low impedance of air with the high cochlear impedance resulting from fluid flow and the distensibility of the cochlear membranes that separate the endolymph from the perilymph. Impedance matching by the middle ear is achieved by three factors that include: (1) the area of the tympanic membrane relative to the oval window, (2) the lever action of the middle-ear ossicles, and (3) the shape of the tympanic membrane. The principles behind these factors are depicted in the three diagrams of Figure 42–5. By focusing the incident sound pressure from the large area of the tympanic membrane onto the small area of the oval window (Figure 42–5A), the effectiveness of energy transfer between the air of the external-ear canal and the fluids of the cochlea is increased greatly. In the human, the area ratio of the tympanic membrane and the oval window is about 20:1. However, the tympanic membrane does not vibrate as a whole.[4,6] Thus, the effective area ratio is only about 14:1. The ossicular chain also contributes to the transformer action of the middle ear by a levering action that increases the vibration amplitude (Figure 42–5B). The ossicular-chain lever ratio is around 1.3:1. A final factor influencing the efficiency of energy transfer depends on the conical shape of the tympanic membrane that allows a buckling action to occur. The buckling motion of the tympanic membrane results in an increased force and decreased velocity to produce approximately a four-fold increase in the effectiveness of energy transfer.[7] Together, these ac-

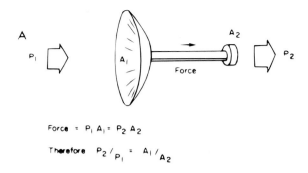

$$\text{Force} = P_1 A_1 = P_2 A_2$$

$$\text{Therefore } P_2/P_1 = A_1/A_2$$

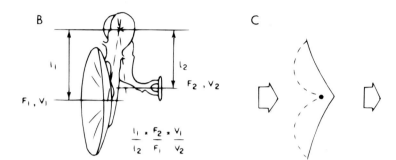

$$\frac{l_1}{l_2} = \frac{F_2}{F_1} = \frac{V_1}{V_2}$$

Fig. 42–5. Illustration of the three principles of impedance matching performed by the middle ear. A. The primary factor is the ratio of the area of the tympanic membrane to that of the oval window. B. The lever action acts to increase the force and decrease the velocity. C. Buckling motion of the tympanic membrane also increases the force while reducing the velocity. Reprinted with permission from Pickles JO: An Introduction to the Physiology of Hearing. New York: Academic Press, 1982.[3]

tions of the middle-ear system result in an estimated overall transformer ratio of 73:1.

MIDDLE-EAR MUSCLES. In primates, the stapedius muscle contracts reflexively in response to intense sound stimuli, but the tensor tympani muscle probably does not.[8,9] In laboratory animals such as the cat, rabbit, and guinea pig, both muscles contact in response to loud sound. However, the threshold of the tensor tympani is often higher than that of the stapedius muscle. A four-neuron reflex arc consisting of the cochlear afferent nerve fibers, neurons of the ventral cochlear nucleus, neurons of the medial superior olive, and facial motor neurons comprises the stapedius-reflex pathway illustrated in Figure 42–6 for the rabbit. The reflex arc for the tensor tympani muscle is slightly different in that neurons of the ventral nucleus of the lateral lemniscus are also involved.[9] From the neural pathway depicted in Figure 42–6, clinical abnormalities of the acoustic reflex implicate pathology at the level of the lower brainstem.

In Figure 42–7, the sensitivity of the stapedius reflex in human is plotted as a function of sound frequency. The reflex-threshold curve evoked by pure tones parallels the audibility threshold curve, but is about 80 dB above it.[10] Not surprisingly, because of their greater overall energy levels, broadband stimuli (e.g., white noise) elicit the reflex more effectively than do pure tones.[10,11] Experimental evidence indicates that the stapedius-reflex threshold decreases with increasing stimulus duration with a time constant of about 200 ms.[12] This value approximates the time constant of temporal summation for the percepts of loudness and sensitivity. These findings, along with the clinical observation that the stapedius reflex exhibits "recruitment" in patients with cochlear hearing loss,[13] suggest that the acoustic-reflex threshold correlates more with subjective loudness than with absolute stimulus intensity.

Contraction of the middle-ear muscles can also be caused by nonauditory factors including: (1) spontaneous contractions, (2) body movements,[8] (3) vocaliza-

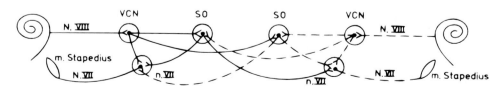

Fig. 42–6. Neural pathway for the acoustic middle-ear reflex in the rabbit. Reflex is mainly a chain of four neurons with a small ipsilateral three-neuron link. N. VIII = auditory nerve; N. VII = facial nerve; VCN = ventral cochlear nucleus; SO = superior olive; n. VII = facial nerve motoneuron. Reprinted with permission from Moller AR: Auditory Physiology. New York: Academic Press, 1983.[270]

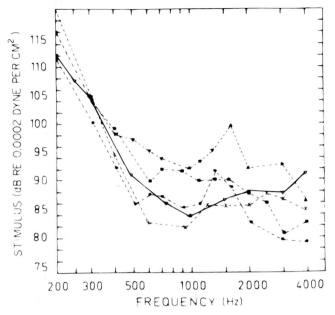

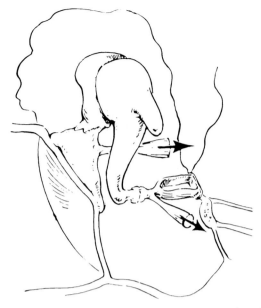

Fig. 42–7. Sensitivity of the human acoustic reflex. Dashed lines from four subjects plot intensities required to elicit an acoustic reflex with 10% of the maximum obtainable amplitude (measured with an immittance technique). The solid line is the threshold of audibility raised 80 dB. Reprinted with permission from Moller AR: The sensitivity of contraction of the tympanic muscles in man. Ann Otol Rhinol Laryngol 71:89, 1962.[10]

Fig. 42–8. Action of the middle-ear muscles. The view is from behind the head. The muscles are not drawn to scale. The tensor tympani muscle (above) attaches to the handle of the malleus and pulls it backward, tensing the tympanic membrane. The stapedius muscle (below) attaches to the neck of the stapes and pulls the posterior-inferior border of the stapes down and into the oval window.

tion[8] (i.e., contractions begin prior to vocalization), (4) movement of facial muscles[8] involving only the tensor tympani, (5) stimulation of the external ear canal,[14] and (6) voluntary contractions.[15]

As diagrammed in Figure 42–8, the stapedius muscle moves the stapes footplate backward and into the oval window, whereas the tensor tympani muscle pulls the manubrium inward. The effects of these contractions on the transmission of pure tones through the middle ear are illustrated in Figure 42–9.[15,16] In summary, the transmission of low-frequency sounds is attenuated by contraction of either muscle,[11] but the stapedius is probably a somewhat better attenuator than the tensor tympani.

The function of the human acoustic reflex has been studied by recording: (1) gross muscle potentials via the electromyogram,[8] (2) pressure changes in the external canal,[17] and (3) acoustic-immittance changes[11,13] (the clinical application of acoustic-impedance measurements has come to be known as immittance audiometry—the terms of 'impedance' and 'immittance' are used interchangeably). In Figure 42–10, the time course is shown for the human stapedius reflex as recorded by the immittance-change method. The latency or time to the first detectable change generally varies from 10–30 ms, whereas the reflex decays over about 500 ms after the onset of the stimulus. The initial reduction in impedance is frequency-dependent.

One major function of the middle-ear muscles is to

support and stiffen the ossicular chain.[11] In addition, because loud sounds are attenuated by the actions of the acoustic reflex, it seems reasonable to propose that another function of the muscles is to protect the inner ear against the damage that can be caused by over-

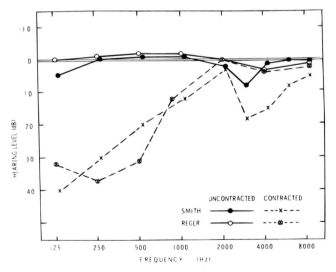

Fig. 42–9. Effect of middle-ear muscle contractions on pure-tone thresholds. The curves were obtained from normal subjects with the ability to voluntarily contract their middle-ear muscles.[15,16] Although the effect of voluntary contraction may differ from the effect of normal involuntary contraction, the general observation that middle-ear muscle contractions preferentially attenuate low frequencies is probably valid.

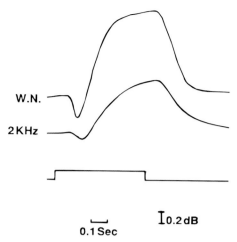

Fig. 42–10. Time course of human stapedius contractions in response to white noise (W.N.) and 2-kHz pure-tone stimuli. Bottom trace shows stimulus time course. The stimuli were 90 dB above normal threshold and were delivered to the right ear. The muscle contractions were recorded from the left ear by the acoustic immittance-change method. Records courtesy of Dr. James Jerger.

exposure to excessive sounds. This notion is supported by the results of a study in which the amount of temporary threshold shift was assessed in patients suffering from acute Bell's palsy in which the stapedius muscle was completely paralyzed.[18] These patients showed a greater threshold shift in the affected ear after exposures to low-frequency noise than in the opposite ear with a normal stapedius reflex. However, whether this protective effect is a "true" function of the stapedius reflex has been criticized on the basis that the continuous loud sounds against which the reflex is supposed to protect do not exist in nature.[19]

An alternative middle-ear muscle function could be to attenuate low-frequency masking sounds which might otherwise interfere with auditory function. Contractions during chewing and other facial and body movements would attenuate the resultant internal body sounds (which are largely low frequency), while preserving sensitivity to high-frequency external sounds. The low-frequency attenuation produced by contractions prior to vocalization may also be functionally important. Observations that support a middle-ear muscle role in vocalization and in speech discrimination are: (1) patients with otosclerosis show significant deficits when administered the delayed feedback test for malingering,[20] (2) stutterers have a deficit in the prevocalization middle-ear muscle contraction,[21] and (3) absence of the stapedius reflex results in decreased speech discrimination when the level of speech is raised above 90 dB.[21]

COCHLEA

The cochlea performs two basic functions as a: (1) transducer that translates sound energy into a form

suitable for stimulating the cochlear-nerve endings, and (2) encoder that programs the features of an acoustic stimulus so that the brain can process the information contained in the stimulating sound. Each of these functions is considered below.

Transducer Function

Anatomy

As shown in Figure 42–11A, the cochlea is divided into three tubes or scalae. The middle tube or scala media is the cochlear extension of the membranous labyrinth and is filled with a potassium-rich, sodium-poor electrolyte fluid called endolymph. The outer two tubes, scala vestibuli and scala tympani, constitute the osseous labyrinth, which is divided by the scala media and filled with perilymph, a sodium-rich, potassium-poor electrolyte fluid. When the cochlea is activated by sound, the scala media and its contents, bounded superiorly by Reissner's membrane and inferiorly by the basilar membrane, tend to move as a unit. This space is referred to as the "cochlear partition."[4]

The contents of scala media are illustrated in Figure 42–11B. The cochlear-nerve fibers synapse at the bases of the hair cells in the organ of Corti. The dendrites of the cochlear nerve enter scala media through the habenula perforata, where they lose their myelin sheaths. The reticular lamina and the tectorial membrane are two membranes in the organ of Corti that are particularly critical in stimulus transduction. The reticular lamina, supported by the rods of Corti, resembles a stiff net with its webbing enmeshing the apical surfaces of the hair cells. Together, the rods of Corti and the reticular lamina provide the skeletal support of the organ of Corti.

The boundary separating the high-potassium and high-sodium electrolytes is formed by the reticular lamina. As diagrammed in Figure 42–12, tight junctions—generally thought to present a barrier against ionic diffusion—are observed by scanning-electron microscopy (SEM) between all cells that face the endolymphatic space. Figure 42–12 also indicates that the junctions between nonsensory epithelium (e.g., cells of Hensen and Claudius, cells lining the spaces of Nuel, and the cells of Reissner's membrane) are not as "tight" (dotted line) as the junctions between the sensory cells and the basal cells (solid line) of the stria vascularis.[22] The fluid within the organ of Corti (i.e., between the basilar membrane and the reticular lamina) has been termed cortilymph.[23] However, the fluid in this space is in free communication with the perilymph of scala tympani via relatively large channels through the basilar membrane.[24] Thus, cortilymph is probably identical to perilymph with respect to its electrolyte content.

The tectorial membrane resembles a rather stiff, oval, gelatinous tube. It is attached to the limbus by a

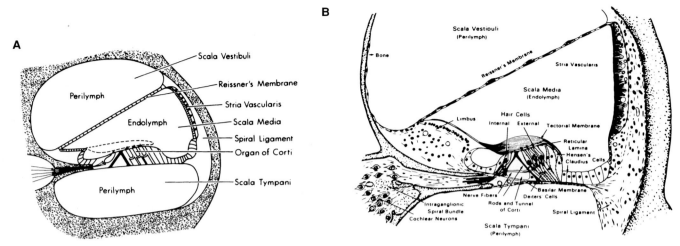

Fig. 42–11. A. Simplified drawing depicting a cross-section through one turn of the cochlea showing the three compartments (scalae). The middle compartment (scala media) is filled with potassium-rich endolymph. The other two partitions (scala tympani and scala vestibuli) make up the osseous labyrinth. This compartment is filled with sodium-rich perilymph. **B.** Semi-diagrammatic representation of a cross section of the guinea pig cochlear duct. A: Reprinted with permission from Salt AN, Konishi T: The cochlear fluids: Perilymph and endolymph. In: Neurobiology of Hearing: The Cochlea. Edited by R.A. Altschuler, D.W. Hoffman, and R.P. Bobbin. New York: Raven Press, 1986.[271]; B: Reprinted with permission from Davis H: Advances in the neurophysiology and neuroanatomy of the cochlea. J Acoust Soc Am 34:1377, 1962.[272]

flexible membranous band that allows it to move up and down like the cover of a book.[25]

Mammals have three rows of outer hair cells (OHCs). A fourth row of OHCs is seen in an occasional cross section, especially in primates, but there is no

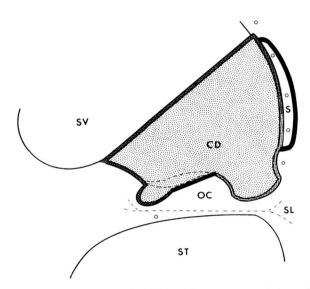

Fig. 42–12. The perilymph/endolymph barriers around the scala media and stria vascularis. The dotted line represents "intermediate-to-tight" tight junctions, whereas the solid line represents "very tight" tight junctions. The circles represent blood vessels, which all have tight junctions that separate them from the intracochlear spaces. SV = scala vestibuli, ST = scala tympani, CD = cochlear duct, OC = organ of Corti, S = stria vascularis, SL = spiral ligament. (Reprinted with permission from Jahnke K: The fine structure of freeze-fractured intercellular junctions in the guinea pig inner ear. Acta Otolaryngol Suppl 336:1, 1975.[22]

well-defined fourth row.[26] There is only one row of inner hair cells (IHCs). The finger-like projections present on the apical surface of the hair cells are called stereocilia. The detailed arrangement of the stereocilia on the hair-cell apices are unique to each class of receptor, and are illustrated in the SEM photomicrograph of Figure 42–13. The IHC stereocilia form a longitudinally oriented, relatively shallow curve, whereas the OHC cilia make a radially oriented "V", with a notch at the apex marking the site of the missing kinocilium that degenerates embryonically during development of cochlear hair cells. The OHC stereocilia vary systematically in length in that they are longest at the apex of the "V" and shorten progressively from the apex to the distal limbs. Whereas the longest OHC stereocilia attach to the undersurface of the tectorial membrane, it is probable that the shorter cilia do not.[27,28] However, an interconnecting network of fine fibrils links the entire bundle of stereocilia, both laterally and from tip-to-tip, so that it moves as a unit.[29]

Until recently, little was known about stereocilia bundles. However, their importance in the transduction process has stimulated considerable research directed toward understanding the morphological and physiological properties of hair-cell bundles and their separate stereocilia. The detailed structure and arrangement of individual hair-cell bundles varies across species, and even as a function of position along the organ of Corti. However, a number of general features of stereocilia bundles and individual cilia has been described: (1) each bundle consists of 30 to 150 stereocilia arranged in several rows of decreasing length; (2) individual cilia range from 0.2 to .08 μm in diameter and

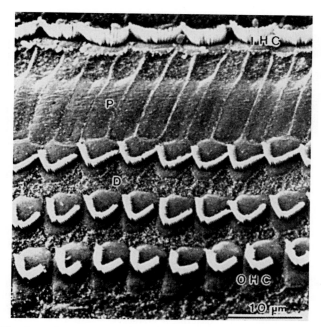

Fig. 42–13. Scanning-electron micrograph of the surface of the organ of Corti after removal of the tectorial membrane. A single row of inner hair cells (IHC) has cilia arranged in a linear (or shallow "U") pattern, whereas the three rows of outer hair cells (OHC) have stereocilia arranged in a "V" pattern. D = Deiter's cells, P = pillar cells. Reprinted with permission from Harrison RV, Hunter-Duvar IM: An anatomical tour of the cochlea. In Physiology of the Ear. Edited by Jahn, A.F., and Santos-Sacchi, J. New York: Raven Press, 1988.[273]

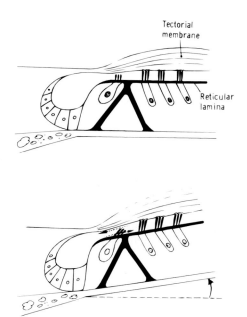

Fig. 42–14. Translation of basilar membrane displacement (as shown in Fig. 42–3) into bending of the hair-cell cilia. Shearing action between the tectorial membrane and the reticular lamina bends the OHC cilia, which are attached to both structures. Streaming movement, imparted to the fluid between the reticular lamina and the tectorial membrane, may bend the IHC cilia, which are not attached to the tectorial membrane. IHC-cilia deflection may be longitudinal (i.e., perpendicular to the page) rather than radial, as depicted.

increase in length from cochlear base to apex; and (3) each stereocilium is covered with a charged-cell coat material that has been postulated to keep individual stereocilia from fusing together.[30]

Using various techniques Flock and coworkers[31,32] demonstrated that stereocilia contained the proteins actin and fimbrin. Whether or not stereocilia are associated with motile responses due to their muscle-like composition is still not fully resolved. However, the unidirectional orientation of the actin filaments[33] suggests these proteins serve a structural rather than a contractile role.

Functional studies of the mechanical properties of stereocilia[34] showed that the cilia are stiff and pivot at their bases. When too much force is applied, the stereocilia break as if they were brittle. Noise-exposure studies have also demonstrated the vulnerability of stereocilia to damage.[30] The tallest stereocilia are affected first by becoming floppy due to alterations to their membrane and cytoskeleton. With continued noise exposure, the stereocilia fuse and then are destroyed resulting in permanent hearing loss. The earliest measurable hearing changes resulting from noise exposure probably involve changes in the stereocilia of the cochlea's hair cells.[30]

Mechanical Transduction
The final mechanical event in the cochlear-transduction process is the bending of the stereocilia as illustrated in Figure 42–14. Basilar-membrane deformation causes a shearing action between the reticular and tectorial membranes. Because the long OHC cilia are attached to both membranes, they are bent. In contrast, the IHC cilia, and possibly also the shorter OHC cilia, which are not attached to the tectorial membrane, bend in response to some mechanism other than displacement shear. One proposition is that this process may involve fluid streaming between the sliding parallel plates formed by the two membranes.[35,36] Fluid streaming would result from differences between the relative velocities of the two membranes rather than by their relative displacements. Thus, the IHCs may be velocity sensors and the OHCs displacement sensors.[37,38] (See, however, other propositions.[39])

Von Bekesy noted that the shearing action between the reticular and tectorial membranes could reduce the displacement amplitude of the stimulating energy while increasing its force.[4,40] Thus, the shearing action may serve to match the impedances of fluid- and solid-transmission media as the middle ear matches air and fluid impedances.

Cochlear Electrical Potentials
Using gross microelectrode methods, three cochlear bioelectric events have been extensively studied: (1) the endocochlear potential (EP), (2) the cochlear microphonic (CM), and (3) the summating potential (SP).

Whereas the EP is present at rest; the CM and SP appear only when sound stimulates the ear.

Endocochlear Potential

The EP is a constant (dc), +80-mV potential, which can be recorded with an electrode in scala media.[41] The majority of evidence indicates that the stria vascularis generates the EP.[42] Because it is extremely sensitive to anoxia and chemical agents interfering with oxidative metabolism,[43] its existence likely depends on the active metabolic-ion pumping processes of the stria vascularis. The anatomical distribution of the EP closely approximates the limits of the endolymphatic compartment formed by the tight-junction boundaries shown in Figure 42–12. The augmentation of the voltage drop cross the apical ends of the hair cells that the EP provides is thought to be critically important in cochlear transduction.[44]

Cochlear Microphonics and Summating Potentials

When the appropriate stimulus is applied, most sensory end organs generate bioelectric events called receptor potentials. These potentials differ from action potentials in that they are graded rather than all-or-none, they have no latency, they are not propagated, and they have no apparent post-response refractoriness.[45] The SPs and CMs are the receptor potentials of the cochlea, and they can be recorded indirectly from gross electrodes on the round window or directly from the fluid spaces within the organ of Corti.

The CM reproduces the alternating (ac) waveform of the stimulating sound (hence the name "microphonic").[46] The SP, illustrated in the lowest inset at the top left of Figure 42–15, represents the dc shift that follows the "envelope" of the stimulating sound.[47] As depicted in Figure 42–15, both the CM and SP are generated across the hair-bearing end of the hair cells.[41,48] Based on experimental findings,[49] it is assumed that the generator site for the receptor potentials is at the apical tips of the stereocilia.

Results of intracellular recordings from IHCs and OHCs suggest that IHCs generate the SP and the OHCs generate the CM.[39] Generation of the SP requires some form of rectification of the acoustic waveform (i.e., alteration from a waveform that oscillates above and below the baseline to a waveform that is entirely above or below the baseline). It is quite straightforward to model the mechanical coupling of the free-floating IHC cilia in such a way as to produce the mechanical rectification. Thus, the concept that the IHCs generate the SP fits well with what is known about the morphology of this class of hair cell. Other evidence, however, derived from recording in the fluid spaces of the cochlea with OHCs selectively damaged by kanamycin,[50] suggests that both the IHCs and OHCs contribute to the volume-recorded SP and CM, with the OHCs dominating the production of both potentials.

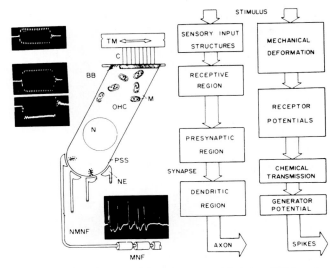

Fig. 42–15. Generator sites of cochlear potentials (upper left from top to bottom: sound stimulus, cochlear microphonic, and summating potential) and functional diagram of the cochlear transducer mechanism (at right). TM = tectorial membrane, C = cilia, OHC = outer hair cell body, N = cell nucleus, M = mitochondria, PSS = presynaptic structures, NE = afferent nerve endings, NMNF = nonmyelinated segment of nerve fiber, MNF = myelinated segment of nerve fiber, BB = basal body. Reprinted with permission from Dallos P: The Auditory Periphery. New York: Academic Press, 1973.[35]

Generation of the CM can be understood by examination of the resistance-battery model of Davis[51] depicted in Figure 42–16. In this conceptualization, the EP serves as the "battery" that provides the driving force to move current through the high resistance of

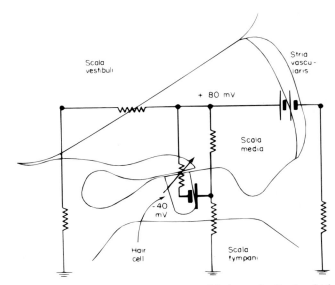

Fig. 42–16. Diagram of Davis' battery model of transduction in which the positive endocochlear potential and negative intracellular potential provide the force to drive current through the variable resistances at the top of the hair cells. Reprinted with permission from Pickles, J.O.: An Introduction to the Physiology of Hearing. New York: Academic Press, 1982.[3]

the reticular lamina in which the apical ends of the hair cells are embedded. The traveling wave displaces the basilar membrane resulting in the deflection of the stereocilia and changes in hair-cell resistance. Thus, hair cells acting as variable resistors modulate current flow across the reticular lamina to produce a time-varying potential, the CM, that follows the waveform of the input stimulus.[3]

Role of the Cochlear Potentials in Stimulus Transduction

Wever and Bray's discovery of the CM[52] led to the hypothesis that cochlear nerve-fiber endings are stimulated electrically.[53] However, with the electron microscope, the morphology of the interface between the afferent-nerve endings and the hair-cell bases was unmistakably that of a chemical synapse. The chemical-synapse-like structures found there include a synaptic cleft (i.e., a uniform space between the hair-cell and nerve-fiber membranes), synaptic vesicles, and a synaptic bar in the form of an electron-dense disc surrounded by vesicles that resemble the synaptic ribbon of the retina.[54]

The presence of subcellular organelles consistent with a chemical synapse at the hair cell/cochlear-nerve junction supports the current view that a chemical transmitter released by the hair cell stimulates the cochlear-nerve endings.[54] Thus, cochlear-receptor potentials are probably either directly involved in the cause-and-effect chain leading to chemical stimulation of the cochlear nerve, or they are intimately related to a process that is directly involved, but does not stimulate the cochlear-nerve fibers electrically.[35,51]

Current thinking about cochlear transduction, which originates primarily from the studies of Hudspeth and coworkers[55] is illustrated in Figure 42–17. In this formulation, displacement of the hair-cell bundle opens the transduction channels located at the tips of the stereocilia to allow potassium (K^+) to flow into the cell. This influx of K^+ depolarizes the cell causing calcium (Ca^{++}) channels at the base of the hair cell to open, thus, admitting Ca^{++} into the cell. The Ca^{++} ions stimulate the transmitter vesicles to fuse with the hair-cell membrane and release transmitter into the synaptic cleft. Transmitter substance then diffuses across the synaptic space to initiate action potentials in the adjacent cochlear-nerve fibers.

Cochlear Transmitters

One area of intense research interest in the study of cochlear transduction leading to intercellular communication has been the identification of the afferent-transmitter substance that is released onto the primary-afferent neurons at the bases of the IHCs and OHCs. In combination with these studies, other efforts have attempted to characterize the efferent neurotransmitter released on the OHCs, and on afferent endings terminating on the OHCs, by efferent neurons originating in the brainstem. Recent evidence indicates that the afferent neurotransmitter is probably a single excitatory amino acid, or a structurally related compound, which is responsible for initiating cochlear-nerve action potentials. Besides this chemical transmitter substance, other chemicals called modulators, that influence the action of the transmitter, are also believed to be released into the synaptic cleft.[56,57]

In the search for neurotransmitters, several criteria have been established which are requisite for the identification of transmitter substances.[58] These criteria require that: (1) the transmitter must produce the same response when applied to the synapse as the natural stimulation of presynaptic elements; (2) extraneous substances that alter natural synaptic transmission such as blocking agents should produce the same effect on the transmitter candidate; (3) stimulation of presynaptic elements should release the transmitter substance; (4) the transmitter substance must be shown to

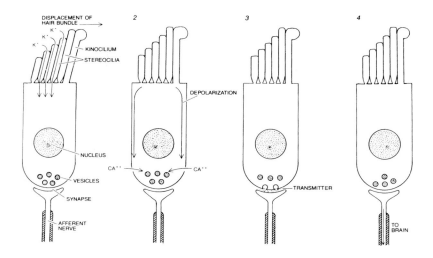

Fig. 42–17. Schematic representation of the major steps involved in transduction in hair cells. Deflection of the hair bundle (1) opens the transduction channels to allow potassium to flow into the hair cell. This results in a reduction of potential difference (depolarization). Depolarization spreads instantly to the lower part of the cell (2) causing calcium channels to open. Calcium ions (3) cause transmitter vesicles to fuse with the basal part of the cell membrane. Fusing vesicles release transmitter substance into the synaptic cleft. Transmitter (4) diffuses across the synaptic cleft to initiate an action potential in the cochlear-nerve fiber. Reprinted with permission from Hudspeth, A.J.: The hair cells of the inner ear. Sci Am *248*:54, 1983.[55]

exist presynaptically; (5) enzymes responsible for the synthesis of the transmitter candidate must be present; and (6) a mechanism must be demonstrated that can deactivate the transmitter once it has been released into the synaptic cleft. To date, concrete evidence for the auditory transmitter in the mammalian cochlea is scanty when compared to the findings of other studies of the central nervous system. That is to say, all of the criteria have yet to be met for any candidate afferent-transmitter substance. However, based upon our present ability to satisfy the above criteria, one of the most likely afferent transmitter substances is believed to be the excitatory amino acid glutamate.[59,60]

Documentation regarding the efferent transmitter in the mammalian cochlea is considerably stronger with the most persuasive evidence favoring acetylcholine. The strongest support for acetylcholine comes from a set of experiments demonstrating that anticholinergic compounds block the effects of efferent stimulation, but do not influence afferent cochlear activity.[61] From other histochemical and immunostaining studies of the mammalian cochlea, there is considerable evidence for a GABA-ergic (τ-aminobutyric acid) efferent innervation of the OHCs as well as the IHC afferents including: (1) measurements of the uptake of tritiated GABA;[62] (2) immunostaining for GAD (glutamic acid decarboxylase);[63] and (3) immunostaining for GABA.[63] Interestingly, evidence that isolated OHCs stain for GABA,[64] and that GABA application to isolated OHCs induces membrane hyperpolarization and membrane elongation[65] infers that the functional consequences of this candidate transmitter substance is inhibition of the electromechanical transduction process. For more in depth treatment of recent studies of cochlear transmitters, readers are encouraged to consult an excellent review.[66]

Coding in the Cochlea

The cochlea must encode acoustic features into properties of neural activity. The principal acoustic parameters to be encoded are frequency, intensity, and temporal pattern, whereas the basic biologic variables available for neural encoding are place (i.e., the location of the activated cell), amount of neural firing, and temporal pattern of firing. The cochlear encoding of frequency and intensity is addressed below.

Frequency Coding
In the late nineteenth century, two opposing theories of frequency coding in the auditory periphery were proposed. These classic theories have influenced subsequent thinking about cochlear frequency coding. The place theory of Helmholtz held that the basilar membrane acts as if it were a series of tuned resonators, analogous to a set of piano strings. Each tuned resonator vibrates sympathetically to a different frequency

and thus selectively stimulates a particular nerve fiber. Rutherford's frequency theory, later termed telephone theory, proposed that all frequencies activate the entire length of the basilar membrane, which transmits, essentially unchanged, the temporal pattern of the auditory stimulus. According to the telephone theory, it remains for more central neural structures to "decode" these temporal patterns in order to educe the features of the acoustic stimulus.

Evidence for Place Coding: Mechanical and Neural Tuning Curves
Von Bekesy used optical methods to make the first direct observations of the mechanical-place analysis of stimulus frequency in the cochlea.[4] Subsequent observations with more sensitive techniques (Mossbauer, capacitive probe, laser interferometric methods) confirmed the general nature of von Bekesy's results but, as will be discussed, have modified his conclusions in several important details.[67]

The principal features of the mechanical responses that von Bekesy observed are illustrated in Figure 42–18. Each pure-tone cycle elicits a traveling wave that moves along the cochlear partition from base to apex.[4] As it travels, the wave's amplitude increases slowly, passes through a maximum, then declines rapidly (Fig. 42–18A). As the frequency of the stimulating tone is increased, the maximum of the traveling wave moves basally toward the oval window.

The inset at the bottom of Figure 42–18B illustrates the tuned behavior of the vibration of a specific locus on the cochlear partition that results from the traveling-wave patterns generated by stimuli of different frequencies (top four plots). The bottom plot of Figure 42–18B, called a cochlear mechanical-tuning curve, was obtained by plotting the vibration amplitude of a single cochlear partition point against the exciting frequency. The frequency that generates the maximum vibration of a specific place on the cochlear partition is that point's characteristic frequency (CF). Thus, the plot at the bottom of Figure 42–18B illustrates the mechanical-tuning curve for a place on the cochlear partition with a CF of 150 Hz. Mechanical-tuning curves at all cochlear-partition locations have the same general shape, i.e., a rapid fall off for frequencies above the CF (>150 Hz), and a gradual drop off for frequencies below the CF (<150 Hz).

Microelectrode recordings from single hair cells and cochlear-nerve fibers yield an analog of the cochlear mechanical-tuning curve. Figures 42–19 and 42–20, respectively, show examples of neural tuning curves obtained from primary cochlear-nerve fibers with traditional glass micropipets,[68] and mechanical tuning curves for the 9-kHz point on the basilar membrane made by a laser-Doppler vibrometer for a number of vibration criteria.[69] Essentially, neural tuning curves are plots of response threshold against frequency (Fig.

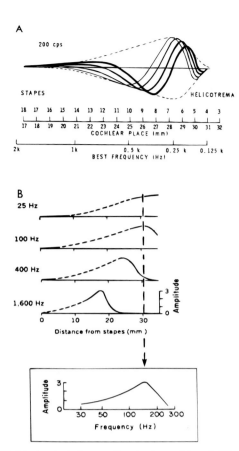

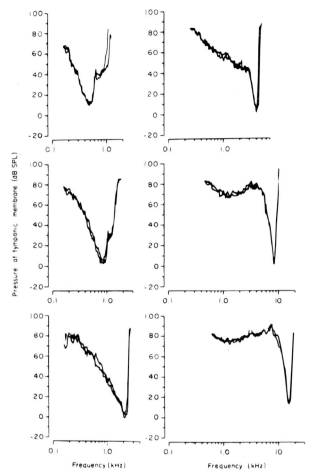

Fig. 42–18. Mechanical place coding in the cochlea. A. The cochlear partition is "uncoiled" showing the traveling-wave response to a pure-tone stimulus. Vertical distance represents the amount of cochlear partition displacement. The four progressively darker lines show cochlear partition positions at three successive instants during one cycle of a 200-Hz stimulation tone. Darker lines represent later points in time. The fine dashed line shows the "envelope" of cochlear-partition displacement. Scale at bottom shows linear distance along the cochlear partition measured from helicotrema (upper scale), from stapes (middle scale), and also in terms of one commonly used cochlear-partition "frequency map"[274] (bottom scale). Note the expected peak in displacement-pattern envelope at about the 0.2-kHz point on the frequency map. B. The top four curves are envelopes of traveling-wave responses to pure-tone stimuli of varying frequencies. Each envelope depicts a point on the partition approximately 30 mm from the stapes (indicated by the vertical dashed line). Only the upper half of the envelope traced in A is shown. At bottom, the response of a single cochlear point is plotted against frequency. This is the mechanical tuning curve of this point. Reprinted with permission from von Bekesy G: Experiments in Hearing. Translated and edited by E.G. Wever. New York: McGraw-Hill, 1960.[4]

Fig. 42–19. Representative tuning curves (frequency-threshold curves) of cat single cochlear nerve fibers are shown for six distinct frequency regions. In each panel, two fibers from the same animal, of similar CF and threshold are shown, indicating the constancy of tuning under such circumstances. Reprinted with permission from Liberman MC, Kiang NYS: Acoustic trauma in cats. Acta Otolaryngol Suppl *358*:1, 1978.[68]

42–19), and similar tuning curves can be recorded from single neurons throughout the auditory neural pathway. Note the relatively similar tuning capabilities of the nerve fiber with the 9-kHz CF (middle panel at right of Fig. 42–19), and the most sensitive membrane-velocity response (thick solid line of Fig. 42–20) with respect to frequency selectivity (−2-kHz bandwidth at 10 dB above threshold) and the tip-to-tail distance of about 80 dB.

The tuning curves of primary auditory-nerve fibers have the same basic shape (steep high-frequency slope, shallow low-frequency slope) as the mechanical tuning curves. Thus, the mechanical-place code of the cochlea is clearly imprinted upon the cochlear nerve's neural response pattern. However, when neural tuning curves first began to be investigated systematically, it appeared that they were more sharply tuned than mechanical tuning curves.[70] In addition, it was observed (Fig. 42–19) that the neural tuning curves could be divided into a sharply tuned "tip" region, with the peak of the tip at CF, and a less sharply tuned (though still more sharply tuned than the mechanical tuning curve) low-frequency "tail" region.[71]

The apparent large difference between neural and mechanical tuning led to the postulate of a "sharpening" mechanism, i.e., a "second filter, occurring within the cochlea subsequent to the displacement pattern of

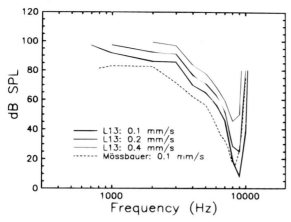

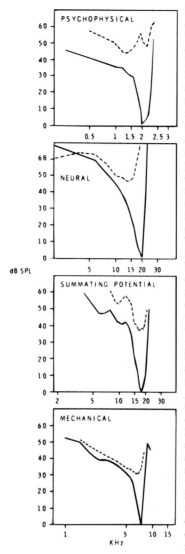

Fig. 42–20. Isoresponse contours (tuning curves) for basilar-membrane velocity responses to tone pips recorded from the chinchilla with the laser-vibrometer (solid lines). The ordinate indicates the sound pressure level required at any particular frequency to elicit a given velocity amplitude (0.1, 0.2, or 0.4 mm/s, indicated as the parameter). For the laser-vibrometry responses, sound pressure levels were interpolated logarithmically using a series of isointensity contours for basilar-membrane responses to tone pips. For comparison, a 0.1-mm/s tuning curve is shown which is representative of results obtained using the Mossbauer technique (dashed line) at approximately equivalent basilar-membrane sites in normal chinchillas. Reprinted with permission from Ruggero MA, Rich NC: Application of a commercially manufactured Doppler-shift laser velocimeter to the measurement of basilar-membrane vibration. Hear Res 51:215, 1991.[69]

Fig. 42–21. Collection of tuning curves from several authors illustrating "de-tuning" with damage. The tuning curves illustrated were obtained from humans ("psychophysical") and from animals at the primary-auditory neuron ("neural"), cochlear-receptor potential ("summating potential"), and basilar membrane ("mechanical") levels. The psychophysical tuning curves were obtained by a tone-on-tone masking procedure.[275] The dashed curve is from a hearing-impaired listener; the solid curve is from a normal listener. The "notch" in the detuned hearing-impaired curve may be a technique-related artifact created by detection of combination tones or beats made by combining masker and test tones. The neural tuning curves were obtained from guinea pigs before (solid curve) and 20 min after (dashed curve) acoustic trauma.[76] The summating-potential curves are 10 μV-isoamplitude curves obtained from intracellular hair-cell recordings. The dashed line is an example of an "insensitive" cell (presumably damaged in the course of exposure); the solid line is from a "sensitive" cell.[39] The mechanical tuning curves illustrate the range of results obtained from different animals in the course of Rhode's Mossbauer-technique measurements.[276]

the basilar membrane.[70] The search for the cochlear second filter was the subject of intensive research for a number of years until it became apparent that the second filter as a separate component of the organ of Corti did not exist. However, the results of this research altered several basic concepts of how the cochlea works and, in addition, led to important new insights into the physiological vulnerability of the cochlea.

Cochlear Tuning

Two characteristics of cochlear tuning are critical to the determination of its location and mechanism. First, the process by which filtering takes place is too rapid to permit a neural delay; thus, there is no possibility that tuning is sharpened by some sort of neural "lateral inhibition" analogous to that occurring at higher levels in the auditory pathway.[72] The second important characteristic of cochlear filtering is that it is physiologically vulnerable. Almost all damaging agents—including hypoxia,[73] ototoxic drugs,[74] local mechanical damage,[75] and acoustic trauma[76]—detune the neural tuning curves so that they closely approximate the broader mechanical tuning curves. As Figure 42–21 shows, the detuning by damaging agents occurs not only for neural tuning curves, but also for mechanical tuning curves, SP tuning curves measured with electrodes placed intracellularly in IHCs, and psychophys-

ical tuning curves from humans with cochlear deficits. Until recently, the vulnerability of mechanical tuning curves was a controversial point. The first published "modern" mechanical tuning curves measured using Mossbauer and capacitive-probe techniques were tuned about as sharply as von Bekesy's.[77] However, even at this early stage, the sharpness obtained by different laboratories differed.[78]

The sharpness of cochlear mechanical tuning is extremely vulnerable and, even when great care is taken, the surgical and other manipulations necessary to obtain mechanical-tuning curves unavoidably cause broadening of the mechanical frequency response.[67] Cochlear mechanical tuning curves obtained under conditions in which extreme precautions were taken to minimize cochlear damage have demonstrated tuning that is as sharp as that of neural tuning curves.[69] In addition, the existence of nonlinear behavior in the normal cochlear-mechanical response has been con-

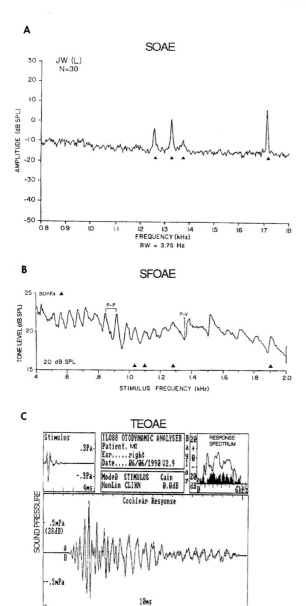

Fig. 42–22. Examples of three types of OAEs. A. Spectrum of the sound pressure level in the ear canal of a 26-yr old female showing four spontaneous OAEs within the 0.8- to 1.8-kHz frequency range. Spectral average was based on 30 samples. Arrowheads = frequencies of spontaneous OAEs. B. Ear-canal record for a 23-yr old male evoked by a continuous 20-dB SPL pure tone swept slowly (150 s) from 0.4 to 2 kHz. Peaks (P) and valleys (V) in the trace indicate regions of stimulus-frequency OAE activity in which the elicited returning emitted response moves in and out of phase with the sweeping tone. Arrowheads = frequencies of coexisting spontaneous OAEs. C. An example of the ILO88 record displayed on screen and in hard-copy forms, which includes visual representations of the temporal course of two averages of the poststimulus response acquired by separate buffers (below), the form of the eliciting stimulus (above left), in this case a click based on an 80-μs rectangular pulse with a peak level of about 82 dB SPL, and a spectrum (top right) of the response showing both the emission (unshaded) and background noise (shaded) components. Basic information concerning the patient and stimulus mode is noted above (center). Reprinted with permission from Lonsbury-Martin BL, Martin GK,

firmed. Thus, the search for the second filter ended with the conclusion that there is no second filter, and that the sharpness of tuning observed at the primary-neuron level is already accomplished at the level of the mechanical-traveling wave.

The question remains, however, of how the physiological vulnerable sharpening of mechanical tuning is accomplished. One critical consideration in answering this question is the calculation by Kim and coworkers that mechanically tuning a location on the basilar membrane requires the local addition of mechanical energy.[79] The discovery that otoacoustic emissions (OAEs) are produced by the healthy cochlea[80] and can be recorded simply from human and animal ear canals, provided indirect evidence for the presence of such a mechanical-energy generator within the cochlea. The results of further studies on OAEs in vertebrates and more recent investigations of the biophysical properties of isolated OHCs have implicated micromechanical processes at the level of the OHCs as being responsible for the normal frequency selectivity of the cochlea.

The OAEs, which can be classified into two general categories, those which are elicited with acoustic stimuli (evoked OAEs) and those which occur in the absence of stimulation (spontaneous OAEs), can be recorded using averaging techniques by a sensitive subminiature-microphone assembly inserted snugly into the outer-ear canal. Over the past 15 years, all four types of emissions, illustrated in Figures 42–22 and 42–23, including the transient-evoked (Fig. 42–22A), stimulus-frequency [continuous pure tone (Fig. 42–22B)], spontaneous [no stimulus (Fig. 42–22C)], and distortion-product [two simultaneous pure tones (Fig. 42–23)], have been studied extensively. The following facts support the notion that OAEs come from the cochlea and are related to the active frequency-filtering process: 1) the frequency of the click-evoked OAE varies considerably from subject to subject, and across subjects there is a systematic relationship between the emission's delay (i.e., latency) and its frequency.[81] This suggests that the origin of OAEs is the cochlear bandpass-filtering mechanism; 2) stimulation of the crossed-olivocochlear bundle, which preferentially provides efferent innervation to the OHCs, modulates the magnitude of OAEs;[82,83] and 3) the emission is extremely sensitive to the detrimental effects of cochlear pathology, acoustic trauma, and ototoxic drugs.[84,85] The most parsimonious interpretation of the existence of the various OAE types, their duration, bandwidth, and delayed-onset characteristics, and their relationship to the activity of the cochlear-efferent

Balkany T: Clinical applications of otoacoustic emissions. *In* Highlights of the Instructional Courses—1994. Edited by F.E. Lucente. Alexandria VA: Am Acad Otolaryngol Head Neck Surg 1994.[188]

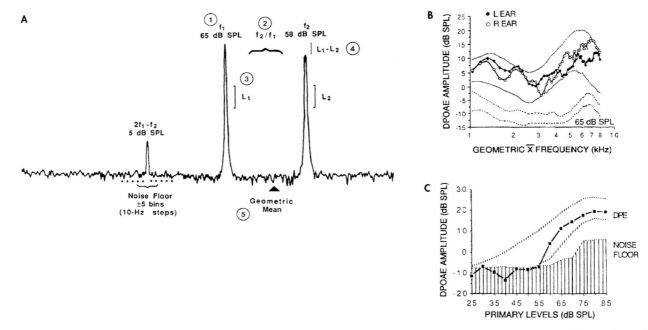

Fig. 42–23. Distortion-product OAEs. A. Distortion-product OAE at $2f_1-f_2$ is shown in the spectrum of the ear-canal sound. Note the position of the geometric-mean frequency (5) with respect to the primary tones (f_1,f_2) and the frequency range over which the noise floor is measured relative to that of the emission (dotted region surrounding the distortion-product OAE frequency). B. Typical distortion-product OAE frequency/level function or "audiogram" elicited by 75-dB SPL primaries is shown for the right (open circles) and left (solid circles) ears of a normal-hearing person. The pairs of long (above) and short (below) dotted lines represent the ranges of average activity and their related noise-floor levels, respectively, associated with normal function. C. Typical response/growth or input/output (I/O) curve depicts the growth of the distortion-product OAE with progressive increases in the levels of the primary tones. The pair of dotted lines above depicts the normal range of emission levels, whereas the striped lines below represent the average noise floor. Reprinted with permission from Lonsbury-Martin BL, Whitehead ML, Martin GK: Clinical applications of otoacoustic emissions. J Sp Hear Res 34:964, 1991).[180]

system is that they originate in the OHCs which possess a mechanical energy that generates the frequency-selective output of the cochlea.

Brownell and Zenner and their colleagues[86–88] were first to show in *in vitro* preparations of mammalian hair cells that OHCs display electromotility. Using mechanical trituration to dissociate single OHCs from other organ of Corti tissues and video-enhanced imaging to directly visualize the isolated OHC, these investigators used both intracellular and transcellular electrical stimulation[87] or pharmacological (K^+, cholinergic chemicals) agents[86–88] to elongate and shorten OHCs along their resting lengths. Because it has been demonstrated that hair cells possess both actin and myosin,[89] it was originally presumed that some aspect of the active motile mechanism is mediated, as in muscle, by interactions between these molecules. However, as more details developed about OHC electromotility, including the knowledge that they mechanically vibrate at frequencies up to 30 kHz, it became clear that a fast-acting motor molecule,[90] or some instantaneous physical phenomenon induced by an electrokinetic process,[91] formed the basis of the ability of the OHC to vibrate in response to changes in the receptor potential.

Inner Versus Outer Hair-Cell Function
Figure 42–24 illustrates salient characteristics of IHC and OHC anatomy, and Figures 42–25 and 42–26 illus-

trate respectively their afferent and efferent innervation. There are many differences between IHCs and OHCs in terms of their morphology, biochemistry, physiology, and afferent- and efferent-innervation patterns. Phylogenetically, OHCs are much younger than IHCs, being present only in the mammalian cochlea. In keeping with their relative phylogenetic youth, OHCs develop later embryologically,[92] are more easily compromised by various damaging agents, and have many unique characteristics that distinguish them from hair cells in other mechano-receptor systems.

The OHCs and IHCs are functionally different, but our concept of the nature of this difference is changing. The classic view that the relatively insensitive IHC system carries the frequency-place code, whereas the OHCs comprise a sensitive low-level detector system that has poor place-coding ability has been abandoned in favor of more recent notions based on the active biomechanical functioning of the organ of Corti. That the OHCs possess effector abilities supports the proposal of Kim[93] that these receptors are bidirectional transducers that are capable of converting acoustic energy into neural energy (mechano-electrical transduction) and electrical into mechanical energy (electro-mechanical transduction). Kim[93] elaborated on this notion by postulating the existence of two distinct but parallel cochlear subsystems that use OHCs as the modulators

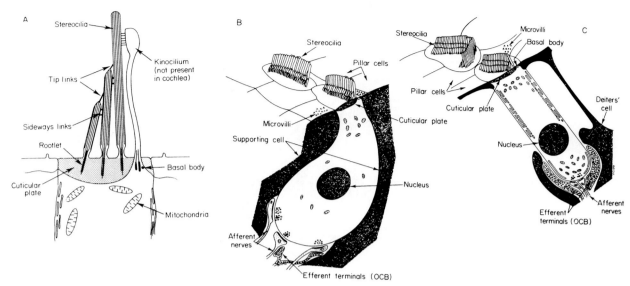

Fig. 42–24. Schematic drawing of cochlear hair cells. A. The common structures on the apical portion of acousticolateral hair cells include rows of stereocilia which are graded in height and joined by cross-links. The tip links may be involved in transduction, opening the transducer channels. The kinocilium is not present in the mature cochlea, although it is present in vestibular cells. B and C. Inner hair cells are shaped like a flask (B), and OHCs are shaped like a cylinder (C). OCB = olivocochlear bundle. Reprinted with permission from Pickles JO: An Introduction to the Physiology of Hearing, 2nd Edition. New York: Academic Press, 1988.[277]

and IHCs as the carriers of auditory information. Table 42–1 presents a summary of a comparison of the two subsystems.

The vulnerable filter sharpening described previously involves some kind of interaction between the IHC and OHCs including: (1) selective damage to OHCs causes detuning of neural-tuning curves (Fig. 42–27),[94] which presumably are from IHC fibers; (2) crossed olivocochlear-bundle stimulation, which presumably affects only OHCs (see below), strongly depresses the compound auditory-nerve click-evoked ac-

tion potential, which apparently originates entirely from IHC fibers; (3) crossed olivocochlear-bundle stimulation also reduces the amplitude of the receptor potential recorded intracellularly from IHCs;[95] (4) crossed olivocochlear-bundle stimulation as well reduces the firing rate and synchronization index,[96] and shifts the dynamic range of cochlear-nerve fibers;[97] and (5) a trapezoid acoustic stimulus elicits from a cochlear-nerve fiber a spike train with a complex time course suggesting combined IHC and OHC influences, whereas selective damage to OHCs by kanamycin

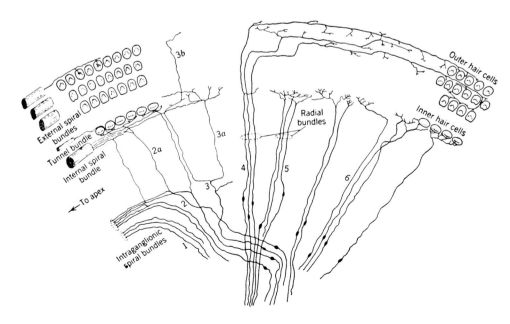

Fig. 42–25. Diagram of the cochlea's afferent-innervation pattern. The view is through Reissner's membrane, looking "down" on the organ of Corti. Principal fiber bundles are 1 and 2, intraganglionic-spiral bundles (fibers labeled "1" are efferent-olivocochlear fibers); 2a and 3a = internal-spiral fibers, 4 = external spiral fibers, traveling in radial bundle to innervate OHCs, 5 and 6 = radial fibers, innervating IHCs. The "V" shape of cilia pattern on the OHCs and the shallower "U" pattern on the IHCs are shown in the upper corners of the diagram. Reprinted with permission from Wever EG: Theory of Hearing. New York: John Wiley & Sons, 1949.[112]

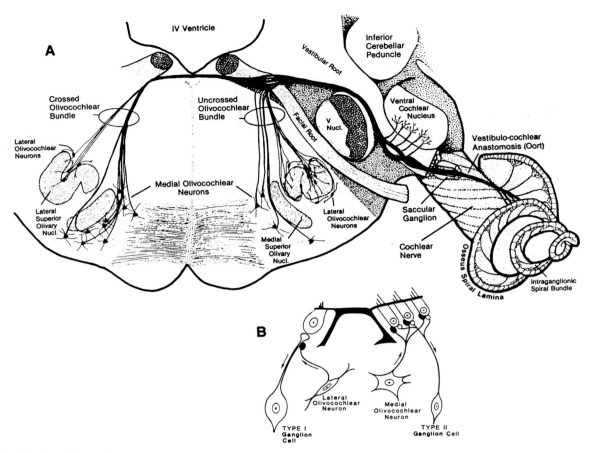

Fig. 47–26. The descending auditory system. A: Origination in the brainstem, distribution, and termination within the cochlea of the olivocochlear-bundle efferent fibers of the cat. B. Organization of the lateral and medial olivocochlear (OC) systems. Lateral OC neurons project to the region beneath the IHCs where they form axo-dendritic contacts on the dendrites of Type I spiral ganglion cells. Medial OC neurons project to the region beneath the OHCs and synapse directly with them. A: Reprinted with permission from Warr WB, Guinan JJ, Jr, White JS: Organization of the efferent fibers: The lateral and medial olivocochlear systems. In Neurobiology of Hearing: The Cochlea. Edited by R.A. Altschuler, D.W. Hoffman, and R.P. Bobbin. New York: Raven Press, 1986.[120] B: Reprinted with permission from Spangler KM, Warr WB: The descending auditory system. In Neurobiology of Hearing: The Central Auditory System. Edited by R.A. Altschuler, R.P. Bobbin, B.M. Clopton, and D.W. Hoffman. New York: Raven Press, 1991.[141])

treatment simplifies the trapezoidal-response pattern in a way compatible with isolated IHC influence.[38]

The precise mechanism by which OHCs influence the response of IHCs is unknown at this time. However, because the physiologically vulnerable cochlear filter-sharpening process appears to involve basilar-membrane vibrations, the mechanism requires that the OHCs directly influence the mechanical vibration of the basilar membrane. A corollary to this conclusion is that the OAEs recorded from the human ear canal reflect OHC function. Indeed, one intensely studied subfield of OAE research is focused on using emitted responses to evaluate the normality of central-auditory processing based on the influence of the descending efferent system on OHC-generated activity.[98,99]

Clinical Consequences

The existence of a vulnerable cochlear-filtering process and a related cochlear emission that can be recorded noninvasively have some important implications for our understanding of pathophysiologic processes in the cochlea. First, although it is unlikely that the majority of cases exhibiting severe tinnitus are related to spontaneous OAEs,[100,101] emissions may elucidate the mechanism of at least some kinds of tinnitus.[102] Moreover, by separating the sensory from the neural aspects of ear dysfunction, OAEs may reveal the critical underlying causes of some common diseases like Meniere's disease,[103] and sudden idiopathic sensorineural hearing loss.[104] Second, as shown by Figure 42–28, detuning of the neural response in cochlear pathologic conditions may also explain recruitment.[105] As previously described, detuning caused by cochlear pathology eliminates the low-threshold, sharply tuned tip region of the tuning curve, but preserves the high-threshold tail region. Elimination of the tip region raises threshold, but preservation of the tail region preserves neural responsiveness at high intensities. Thus, the loudness

TABLE 42–1. Differences Between Inner and Outer Hair Cells

	Inner Hair Cells	Outer Hair Cells
Anatomy (Fig. 43–24)		
Cell shape	Flask (35 μm × 10 μm)	Cylinder [25 μm (base) to 45 μm (apex) × 7 μm]
Relation to supporting cells	Closely approximated to inner phalangeal cell processes	Contact Deiters supporting cells only at apical and basal ends and are surrounded by large perilymph-filled spaces of Nuel
Cilia	Longitudinally oriented shallow curve	Radially oriented "V"-shaped curve
	Not obviously attached to tectorial membrane	Attached to tectorial membrane
Location of cell nucleus	Central	Basal
Organelles	Resemble hair cells in other systems	Several unique features including submembrane cisternae, numerous mitochondria parallel to cell membrane, Hensen bodies
Afferent Innervation (Fig. 43–25)		
	Convergent via radial fibers	Divergent via spiral fibers
	95% of fibers in auditory nerve come from IHCs	95% of fibers in auditory nerve come from OHCs
	All published nerve-fiber studies are probably from IHCs	No convincing neurophysiologic demonstration of population of nerve fibers from OHCs
	Nerve endings plentiful and show typical chemical synapse morphology	Nerve endings relatively sparse; morphology differs from chemical synapse
Efferent Innervation (Fig. 43–26)		
	Small neurons near LSO	Large neurons near MSO
	Primarily ipsilateral via uncrossed-olivocochlear bundle	Primarily contralateral via crossed-olivocochlear bundle
	Small endings primarily on afferent nerve terminals	Large endings on OHCs
	Acetylcholinesterase activity poorly visualized	Acetylcholinesterase activity easily visualized
	Enkephalin-like immunoreactivity	Aspartate aminotransferase immunoreactivity
	Distributed evenly along cochlear length	Distributed preferentially in middle and basal cochlea
Physiology		
Resting membrane potential	−35 to 45 mV	−70 mV
Basal cells		
ac receptor potential	0.6 mV	3 mV
dc receptor potential	12 mV	Immeasurable
Apical cells		
ac receptor potential	10 mV	5 mV
dc receptor potential	5 mV	3 mV
Biochemistry		
Intracellular glycogen	Scarce	Plentiful

function (bottom right plot) is made abnormally steep, because threshold is elevated. However, at high intensities, loudness is normal, because a normal number of neurons are responding.

Evidence for Telephone Coding

The aforementioned evidence for place coding has not invalidated Rutherford's telephone theory because there is also considerable evidence for a telephone code at low frequencies. For example, cochlear tuning becomes progressively poorer as frequency is lowered, and below about 100 Hz, there are no cochlear partition amplitude maxima and no tuned auditory units.[70] Thus, the physiologically observed frequency-place code becomes progressively worse as frequency is lowered.

A neural telephone code has been demonstrated which, in contrast to the place code, becomes progressively better as frequency is lowered. Analyzing the spike discharges of single cochlear-nerve fibers to low-frequency stimulation has demonstrated "phase-locking" to the individual cycles of the eliciting tone that preserves the temporal-firing pattern.[106] Compiling large numbers of single-unit spikes into spike-discharge histograms has shown an impressive ability of single auditory-unit discharges to reproduce the waveform of the stimulating sound. The upper limit of this phenomenon is generally estimated at about 4 kHz, but critical inspection of quantitative single-unit data suggests that phase-locking becomes poor at around 2.5 kHz.[107] Analogous waveform-reproducing whole-nerve responses have also been recorded.[108]

Another line of evidence supporting the importance of the encoding of phase or timing information comes

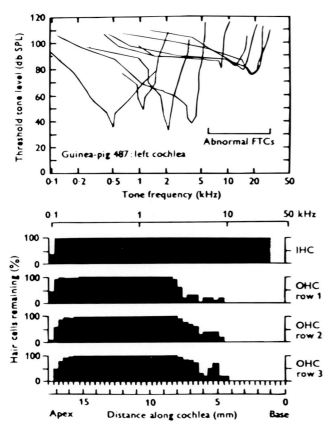

Fig. 42–27. Correlation between detuning of neural tuning curves and OHC damage. Results are shown from a kanamycin-treated guinea pig in which the IHCs were intact throughout the cochlea. In the high-frequency region, however, OHCs were damaged and tuning curves, presumably from fibers coming from this region, were detuned. This result suggests that the OHCs participate in the process by which cochlear tuning curves are sharpened. Reprinted with permission from Evans EF, Harrison RV: Correlation between cochlear outer hair cell damage and deterioration of cochlear nerve tuning properties in the guinea pig. J Physiol 256:43, 1976.[94]

from the outcome of studies of the responses of cochlear-nerve fibers to speech sounds. The work of Kiang[109] addressed the limitations of fiber discharge rate-place encoding in neurally representing the frequency components in speech signals, especially those of moderate to high intensities. More recently, the single-unit population studies of Sachs and Young and co-workers on the representation of speech sounds in hundreds of cochlear-nerve fibers have demonstrated that the temporal pattern of fiber discharges in the form of phase locking provides considerable information about the frequency content of the stimulus at all levels of stimulation.[110,111] These population measures of temporal synchrony were based on Fourier transforms of period histograms from fibers with CFs near each frequency component of the sound. Such measures were combined to provide discharge-rate profiles for groups of active nerve fibers. Because information concerning rate, timing, and place is represented

in these measures, these spectra provide details concerning temporal fine structure from a localized cochlear region and thus represent a type of temporal-place code.

Telephone-Place Theory of Frequency Coding

One short-coming of the telephone theory became apparent when neural refractoriness was discovered. This process imposed a physical limitation on nerve-fiber firing at the very short time intervals associated with high-frequency stimuli. Thus, to reconcile in part the effects of neural refractoriness on the telephone theory, Wever[112] published an auditory-frequency coding theory, which he termed the volley theory, but which has since become known as the telephone-place or frequency-place theory. Wever advanced an interesting evolutionary argument in support of the telephone-place code theory. Primitive ears (as found in fish, amphibians, and lower reptiles) are telephone coders that cannot analyze high audio frequencies, because of the inherent limitation of the rate at which nerve fibers can respond. Therefore, as evolution progressed, place coding had to be added to allow analysis of high frequencies, which are important in sound localization and directionality.

Our own use of sounds in communication is greatly aided by our keen sensitivity to the frequency region between 1–4 kHz, and though our sensitivity falls off beyond 4 kHz, we still depend on the higher frequencies for many of our discriminations of consonants and sharp transients. The appearance and elaboration of the place principle for frequency representation therefore was a major event in the evolution of the ear.[112]

Intensity Coding

"Loudness" is the approximate subjective correlate of the physical dimension of sound intensity. It is generally assumed that the neural correlate of loudness is the "amount" of nervous activity—amount meaning the total number of action potentials delivered by a population of nerve fibers over a given time period. Thus, loudness is encoded as a combination of the number of fibers firing and the rate at which they are firing.

Figure 42–29 compares plots of stimulus level versus single cochlear-nerve fiber firing rates (left), and stimulus level versus subjective loudness (right). The agreement in the general shapes of the curves supports the view that the amount of cochlear-nerve firing encodes loudness. On closer scrutiny, however, it is apparent that firing rate changes only over a 20-dB sound-intensity range, whereas loudness varies over a 100-dB range. This limited dynamic range is a general property of all primary cochlear neurons.[113]

The obvious way to solve this loudness-encoding problem is to assume that additional nerve fibers are "recruited" as stimulus level is increased. This process

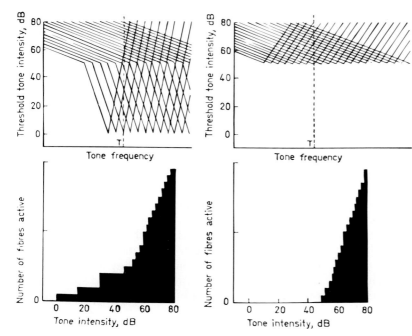

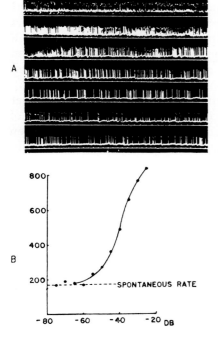

Fig. 42–28. Possible explanation of recruitment (elevated threshold and abnormal growth of loudness) based on detuning with pathology. Solid diagrams at bottom depict increase in number of active cochlear fibers as tone intensity is increased in normal (left) and abnormal (right) ears. The tone's frequency is indicated by the dashed line in the upper diagram. Because the effect of disease is to remove the sharply tuned "tips" but leave the broadly tuned "tails" relatively unaffected, the threshold of the "pathological" cochlea is increased, but as tone intensity is increased into the normal tail regions, the number of active fibers responding becomes normal; hence, loudness grows abnormally rapidly from the elevated threshold. Reprinted with permission from Evans EF: The sharpening of cochlear frequency selectivity in the normal and abnormal cochlea. Audiology *14*:419, 1975.[105]

would increase the total "number of discharges per unit time" by increasing the number of fibers firing rather than the firing rate for an individual fiber. However, most studies of cochlear-nerve single units agree that the thresholds of the nerve-fiber population fall within a relatively restricted stimulus range, i.e., within 20 to 30 dB of behavioral threshold.[114] Thus, there is no possibility of recruiting additional fibers as sound level is increased more than 60 dB above thresh-

old. The "fiber-recruitment" hypothesis also creates problems for frequency-place coding, because adding new responding fibers as stimulus level is increased would quickly require the spread of activity to fibers of adjacent CFs. This tradeoff between the ability to recruit new fibers and the ability to place-code is especially bothersome for explaining the perception of complex sounds where multiple frequencies must be distinguished simultaneously. Thus, the dynamic-

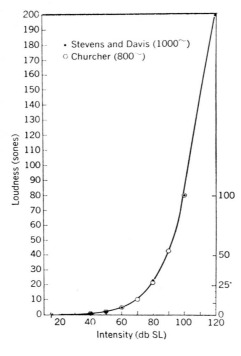

Fig. 42–29. Effects of sound intensity on subjective loudness[275] (right) and cochlear-nerve fiber firing rate (left). The shapes of the curves are similar, but the dynamic range of the single cochlear-nerve fiber is much narrower than that of the auditory system as a whole. Above the cochlear-nerve firing-rate curve are shown single-fiber responses[278] to sounds of progressively increasing intensity. Subjective loudness curve from Gulick WL: Hearing, Physiology and Psychophysics. New York: Oxford University Press, 1971.[275] Cochlear-nerve curve reprinted with permission from Katsuki Y, Sumi T, Uchiyama H, Watanabe T: Electric responses of auditory neurons in cat to sound stimulation. J Neurophysiol *21*:569, 1958.[278])

range problem becomes apparent.[115] The dynamic range of cochlear-nerve fibers, i.e., the range over which the spike rate changes as stimulus level is altered, is too narrow to account for (at least, in simple terms) the extent over which the human ear discriminates sound levels.

Several subsequent observations shed light on the dynamic-range problem. Evans and Palmer[116] discovered that approximately two-thirds of the cells in the dorsal cochlear nucleus had dynamic ranges that extend to well over 100 dB, and thus could easily "code" loudness over the necessary sound-intensity range. However, the problem of the input pathway to these dorsal cochlear nucleus cells remains to be resolved. In addition, some cochlear-nerve units have been found which do, after all, have wide dynamic ranges, but these are only a minority of the total cochlear-nerve fiber population.[117] Studies have also demonstrated that relative degrees of phase-locking[111] of different frequency components in complex sounds could code the relative intensity levels of the frequency components. However, because phase-locking does not occur above 3 to 4 kHz, this mechanism could not account for the loudness coding of high frequencies.

Another approach to the dynamic-range problem is the concept of an "automatic-gain control" operating at the input of the auditory system.[115] Such a control mechanism would feed back a decreased gain-command signal to the input to maintain the cochlear output within an acceptable operating range. Possibilities for such a control system include the middle-ear reflex and the olivocochlear efferent system.

Viemeister[118] concluded from his review of the psychophysical and physiological literature relevant to intensity encoding in cochlear-nerve fibers that a localized rate code "seems theoretically possible and, at present, appears to be the best candidate for a general intensity code." The conclusion that rate information from a frequency-specific population of active nerve fibers provides the neural basis for a code of stimulus intensity is consistent with the findings discussed above concerning the encoding of high-level speech sounds by a population of cochlear-nerve fibers.

Efferent Auditory System

Anatomy

Rasmussen[119] established the existence of a chain of descending auditory neurons that links auditory cortex to hair cells, and that parallels the classic afferent projection pathway (discussed below). The olivocochlear bundle, the final link in the descending chain, originates in the superior olivary complex.

Figure 42–26A summarizes schematically the origins, course and distribution of the olivocochlear bundle to one cochlea, whereas Figure 42–26B analyzes the principal relationships between the two afferent and the two efferent innervations of the organ of Corti.[120] The olivocochlear bundle is divided into crossed and uncrossed components. The crossed component is composed primarily of relatively large myelinated fibers which originate in large "globular" neurons surrounding the medial region of the superior olivary complex.[121] Most of the uncrossed component is composed of small fibers,[122] a large percentage of which may be unmyelinated, and which originate in the small fusiform neurons in the lateral region of the superior olivary complex.[121] The majority of the large crossed fibers innervate OHCs, whereas most of the small uncrossed fibers predominately innervate IHCs.[121]

The crossed olivocochlear fibers decussate just beneath the floor of the fourth ventricle, then enter the vestibular nerve. At this point they are joined by the uncrossed fibers. The combined crossed and uncrossed fibers travel in the vestibular nerve until, at the saccular portion, they cross into the cochlear nerve via the vestibulocochlear anastomosis. Within the cochlea, efferent fibers have been identified among the external spiral fibers (3b in Fig. 42–25), the tunnel spiral fibers, and the internal spiral fibers.[123,124]

Physiology

In cases in which olivocochlear axons have been labeled histochemically and traced following single nerve-fiber recordings, the labeled fibers terminate beneath OHCs in cochlear regions with best frequencies corresponding to the CFs of the fiber.[125,126] Such direct recordings from efferent axons within the periphery have demonstrated that these units possess thresholds and tuning-curve properties that are essentially identical to those of primary afferents with similar CFs.[125] Although the proportion of olivocochlear neurons that can be excited by ipsilateral and contralateral stimuli is consistent with the predominant efferent innervation to a given cochlea, many units are binaurally responsive.[127]

The effects of stimulating the crossed-olivocochlear bundle are almost certainly mediated by the release of a cholinergic mediator at the OHCs.[128] It has long been known that stimulating the crossed-olivocochlear bundle in the floor of the fourth ventricle causes depression of the cochlear nerve's response to sound stimulation and a simultaneous increase in the amplitude of the cochlear microphonic.[129]

Much less is known about the uncrossed-olivocochlear bundle. Stimulation of the uncrossed bundle decreases the click-evoked action potential amplitude, but the effect is much less than for the uncrossed bundle.[96] In addition, unlike the crossed bundle, the terminations of the uncrossed bundle do not show high concentrations of acetylcholinesterase[130] and curare does not block the effect of stimulating the uncrossed bundle (although strychnine does).[128] Thus, the uncrossed system may not be cholinergic.

Functional Significance

The function of the olivocochlear-efferent system is at present unknown. Several attempts to demonstrate functional deficits after sectioning the crossed-olivocochlear bundle have failed.[131] A series of more recent studies has systematically examined the effects of electrically stimulating the crossed-olivocochlear bundle on cochlear nerve-fiber dynamic ranges that have been compressed by broadband-noise stimulation.[97] The restoration of dynamic range in the presence of background noise supports the notion that the cochlear-efferent system may function to improve the discriminability of complex signals i.e., the signal-to-noise ratio. However, the hypothesis that the olivocochlear system primarily provides some sort of input-gating mechanism may not be completely correct.

The most recent and unexpected of the effects of stimulating the crossed-olivocochlear bundle is a decrease in the amplitudes of OAEs that are generated mechanically by the cochlea and recorded in the ear canal. Mountain[82] was first to report that electrical stimulation of the olivocochlear-efferent system directly affected the active nonlinearities in OHC mechanics inferred from decreases in distortion-product OAEs. A number of other studies evaluating the influence of contralateral acoustic stimulation with wideband noise on OAEs recorded ipsilaterally reported small reductions in click-evoked OAEs[98] and in $2f_1$-f_2 distortion-product OAEs.[132] The influence of contralateral stimulation on OAEs also supports the notion that the cochlear-efferent system is involved in the modulation of OHC micromechanics. These effects, along with the reductions in neural-discharge rate and tuning, suggest that the function of the crossed-olivocochlear bundle is to allow the central auditory system to govern the mechanical properties of the basilar membrane by controlling the vulnerable cochlear-tuning mechanism previously discussed. Because detuning a frequency-bandpass system increases damping, the detuning effect of the crossed-olivocochlear bundle could be useful as a method of improving auditory time resolution (e.g., to improve speech perception). The consensus view[91] at present is that the active transduction process[133] is regulated in some way through efferent innervation of the OHCs. Also, the olivocochlear-efferent system could relate to extending the dynamic range of the auditory system.[134]

In addition, other experimental results[135] suggest that the olivocochlear system may help protect against acoustic trauma. In this work, it was discovered that the amount of threshold shift induced by overstimulation of one ear could be reduced by the presentation of a simultaneous tone to the contralateral ear thus inferring that activating the efferent system reduced

the effects of over-exposure. One intriguing line of current research on the traumatic effects of noise exposure is the notion of "training" the cochlea to become less susceptible to damaging sounds.[136,137] Although the underlying mechanism(s) responsible for the protective effect is, at present, unknown, the most likely site is the crossed cochlear-efferent system. Indeed, Le-Page[138] demonstrated that loud sound induces a mechanical baseline shift in the position of the cochlear partition. It is highly probable that such a gain-control system is effected by cochlear efferents.

CENTRAL AUDITORY PATHWAY

Each of the five primary senses sends information into the brain via two separate pathways: (1) a direct or specific pathway, and (2) a nonspecific pathway. The nonspecific pathway involves structures in the core of the neuraxis, collectively known as the reticular system. In the reticular system, all sensory modalities share the same gross neural structures (hence the name "nonspecific"). Ascent via the nonspecific structures is multisynaptic and hence is characterized by long delay times.

The direct pathways for each sensory modality are separate and involve long axonal processes, with a minimal number of synapses; consequently, compared to the indirect pathway, transmission along the direct pathways involves minimal delay times. The synapses of the direct pathways tend to congregate in well-defined neural structures called nuclei.

Clinically, lesions of the central auditory system are localized according to their level in the direct-projection pathway. Therefore, the following discussion emphasizes this pathway.

Anatomy

Figure 42–30 diagrams the direct auditory-projection pathway. The numbers in each nucleus indicate neuronal "order" (determined by the number of synapses). The auditory-projection pathway is more complex than the pathways of other sensory systems, possibly because it developed relatively late on the phylogenetic scale, and had to incorporate pieces of other already developed neuronal systems. Although the basic "wiring diagram" depicted in Figure 42–30 has remained relatively unchanged for many years, it should be emphasized that within the last 15 years tremendous advances have been made in the development of methods for describing neuronal connectivity.[139] These breakthroughs have relied upon the discovery that when certain amino acids, conjugated enzymes (e.g., horseradish peroxidase conjugated lectin from soy bean), sugars, or immunocytochemicals (e.g., polyclonal or monoclonal antibodies) are injected

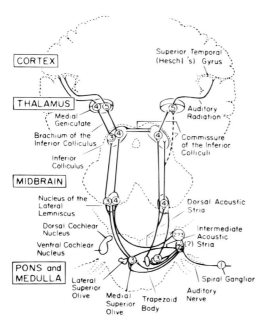

Fig. 42–30. Diagram of the direct auditory-projection pathway. Numbers indicate approximate neuron "order" as determined by the number of synapses traversed. Dashed lines labeled with question marks indicate two areas of uncertainty: (1) whether the dorsal cochlear nucleus primarily contains second- or third-order neurons; and (2) whether any nerve fibers bypass the inferior colliculus.

into a neuronal or fluid (e.g., cochlear duct) region of interest they will be taken up by the cells or nerve-fiber endings in this region and transported by the normal cellular process of axonal transport in both retrograde and anterograde directions. Other techniques make use of such labels as lipophitic dyes (e.g., DiI), which can be retrogradely transported in fixed tissue by diffusion. Visualization of the location of cellular projections or the cellular/subcellular location of labeled substances at the light and electron-microscope levels is achieved either by autoradiography, in the case of radioactive compounds, or by catalyzation of histochemical reactions, which are typically viewed under epifluorescence or darkfield. With recent refinement of these tract-tracing and cell-component labeling techniques using immunohistochemical markers, virtually all projection pathways and cell types of the auditory system have been described. Lagging far behind our description of the connections of the neural pathway for hearing is our understanding of how this network of interconnections interacts to produce our complex auditory sensations. Presented below, is a brief description of the major projections of the auditory pathway sufficient to understand the transfer of information within the auditory system, without consideration of the many lesser connections revealed by modern immunocytochemical-staining techniques. The reader is referred to several comprehensive reviews that provide more details of the intricate interconnections of the central part of the auditory system.[140,141]

Cochlear Nucleus

Central processing of the information carried in the cochlear nerve begins in the cochlear nucleus (CN), the first obligatory synapse for all nerve fibers. Upon entering the CN, the cochlear portion of the eighth nerve bifurcates into two branches, one which sends fibers to synapse in the anteroventral cochlear nucleus (AVCN), and the other which synapses in the posteroventral cochlear nucleus (PVCN) and dorsal cochlear nucleus (DCN). The distribution of fibers within the CN is not random, but follows an orderly pattern of tonotopic projection throughout the nucleus with low-frequency fibers projecting ventrally and high-frequency fibers distributed dorsally. Thus, both neurophysiologic and anatomic observations show that cochlear place is represented in an orderly manner throughout the projection pathways of the central part of the auditory system.[142] The security of tonotopic organization is also apparent in the "multiple representation" of the stimulus-frequency domain. For example, typically, along any one penetration of a microelectrode trajectory within a principal nucleus, there are two or more breaks in the orderly progression of best frequencies. Thus, as in the direct-projection pathways of all sensory systems, multiple representation of the receptor surface occurs. It is likely that nerve-fiber branching in the various nuclei, as described for the CN, is the anatomic basis of this multiple-frequency representation.[143]

All cochlear-nerve fibers display relatively uniform response characteristics to pure-tone stimuli compared to the activity of CN cells when categorized by the use of a poststimulus time (PST) histogram.[113] The PST plots the number of nerve discharges that occur in small time bins within the period that begins slightly before and extends throughout the duration of the stimulus. Poststimulus-time histograms are shown for a cochlear-nerve fiber and various CN cells in Figure 42–31. The CN consists of at least nine different cell types described for their anatomical characteristics revealed by various staining techniques.[144] It can be seen from the unit-activity patterns of Figure 42–31 that the uniform response characteristics of cochlear-nerve fibers are soon elaborated upon by the various cells of the CN to produce a variety of response types named after the patterns seen in the PST.[145] When examined in the frequency-intensity domain, some CN cells exhibit complex response patterns that describe regions of excitation and inhibition produced by a pure-tone stimulus. An example of such complex response patterns shown by cells in the CN is shown in Figure 42–32.[145]

Three fiber pathways project information from the CN to higher brainstem centers. These fiber tracts include: 1) the ventral-(trapezoid body), 2) intermediate-, and 3) dorsal-acoustic striae. The ventral-acoustic stria, originating from AVCN and PVCN regions, projects ventrally and medially to send fibers ipsilaterally to

CELLS IN THE COCHLEAR NUCLEUS

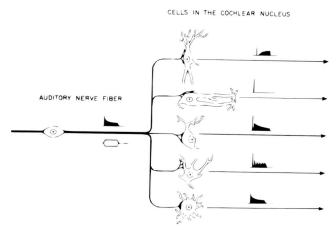

AUDITORY NERVE FIBER

Fig. 42–31. Diagram showing the diverse single-unit response types obtained from cells in the cochlear nucleus compared to the uniform response pattern found for fibers of the cochlear nerve. The PST histograms were obtained by presenting short 25- to 50-msec tone bursts at the unit's CF. Response types from top to bottom are: pauser; on$_1$; primary-like with notch; chopper; primary-like. Cell types presumably associated with these response patterns from top to bottom are: pyramidal, octopus, globular, multipolar, and spherical. Reprinted with permission from Kiang NYS: Stimulus representation in the discharge patterns of auditory neurons. In The Nervous System, Vol 3: Human Communication and Its Disorders. Edited by D.B. Tower. New York: Raven Press, 1975.[279]

the lateral (LSO) and medial superior olives (MSO), and then to the medial nucleus of the trapezoid body (MTB). The fibers then cross the midline to terminate on the contralateral MSO and MTB, but do not innervate the LSO on the opposite side. Thus, for any one

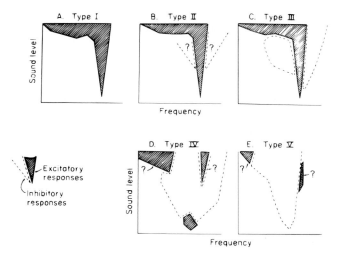

Fig. 42–32. Tuning curves of excitation and inhibition in the cat cochlear nucleus are shown in order of increasing amounts of inhibition (A–E). Purely excitatory responses as in A are predominant in the AVCN. Greater amounts of inhibition are found towards the DCN (D and E). Question marks show variable or uncertain features. Reprinted with permission from Young ED: Response characteristics of neurons of the cochlear nuclei. In Hearing Science: Recent Advances. Edited by C.I. Berlin. San Diego: College-Hill Press, 1984.[145]

ear, connections are bilateral only to the MSO and MTB.[146]

The intermediate-acoustic stria, the primary output of the PVCN, sends some fibers ipsilaterally to a group of cells around the superior olivary complex (SOC) called the periolivary nucleus (PON), whereas other fibers ascend in the lateral lemniscus (LL). This pathway also crosses the midline to innervate the same structures on the contralateral side. Fibers of the intermediate-acoustic stria which enter the LL synapse within the nucleus. The dorsal-acoustic stria, the principal output of the DCN, bypasses the SOC to synapse in the contralateral dorsal nucleus of the LL and the inferior colliculus (IC).[146]

Superior Olivary Complex

The SOC is composed of the LSO, MSO, MTB, and PON. The SOC receives fibers from both cochlear nuclei and consequently receives information from both ears. This feature allows this group of nuclei to monitor the arrival time and level of sounds to both ears and provides the cues for the localization of sound in space based upon the stimulus arrival time and intensity to both ears.[146] In fact, localization of sound in the horizontal plane provides the most straightforward relationships that have been observed between central auditory single-unit behavior and psychophysical function. As sound to one ear is made progressively louder, or earlier, than sound to the opposite ear, some SOC units change abruptly from inhibitory to facilitatory response patterns. By assuming a facilitatory contralateral input and an inhibitory ipsilateral input (or *vice versa*), the neurophysiologic behavior of these units can be explained. Thus, slight binaural differences in level and/or arrival time provide the auditory cues for localization of sound in the horizontal plane (sound lateralization). The acoustic image is located on the side of the louder or earlier sound. As a whole, the SOC represents the lowest level in the auditory system at which binaural processing takes place. However, at all levels in the auditory projection pathway above the trapezoid body, there are units that are sensitive to binaural time and level differences.[147,148]

Lateral Lemniscus

The LL is the major ascending projection from the CN and SOC to the IC, and contains both contralateral and ipsilateral fibers from lower auditory-brainstem structures. Although there are three distinct nuclei within the LL, historical emphasis has been simply on its function as a connection between the SOC and IC. Recently, these nuclei have received more attention in attempts to define their role in auditory processing.

Inferior Colliculus

The IC receives synapses from the majority if not all of the fibers projecting from the lower auditory nuclei.

The three neuronal areas that make up the IC are the central, external and pericentral nuclei. The predominate termination zone for the ascending-auditory projections is in the ventrolateral region of the central nucleus. This region receives inputs from the SOC and a heavy contralateral input from the DCN. Other major projections come ipsilaterally from the MSO and bilaterally from the LSO. The function of the IC is far from completely understood with many neurons exhibiting complex excitatory/inhibitory interactions. A simple view is that the IC integrates the frequency-analysis features of the DCN with the localization abilities of the SOC.[146]

Medial Geniculate

The medial geniculate (MG) is the thalamic-relay nucleus for auditory information. All auditory projections from the IC to the auditory cortex pass through the MG. This nucleus is also composed of three divisions, the ventral, dorsal, and medial nuclei.[148] The ventral nucleus receives heavy ipsilateral projections from the ventrolateral portion of the central nucleus of the IC. This portion of the MG projects to the AI, AII and Ep regions of auditory cortex (see below). Again a wide variety of single-unit response types have been recorded in the MG. In attempting to understand the MG's role in auditory processing, special efforts have been made to examine MG single-unit responses to complex sounds. Thus, David[150] and associates and Keidel[151] demonstrated that MG neurons in the unanesthetized cat were responsive only to specific parameters of complex speech sounds. In general, it has been extremely difficult to attribute specific feature-extraction capabilities to neurons in the higher auditory nuclei which cannot be explained by complex responses already present at the level of the CN.

Auditory Cortex

The auditory cortex has been most extensively studied in the cat and can be divided into three areas based upon similarity of Nissl-stained cytoarchitectural details.[152] These include a primary area AI, a secondary area AII, and a remote projection region Ep. In humans and nonhuman primates, the primary auditory-projection area is located on the temporal lobe, but hidden by the Sylvian fissure. The ventral division of the MG projects almost entirely to AI,[153] which can be considered the primary auditory core. Surrounding auditory areas receive projections from all divisions of the MG. Like the auditory-relay nuclei, the auditory cortex is also tonotopically organized. As might be expected by the many intricate interconnections of the auditory system prior to input arriving at the cortex, the understanding of cortical processing has been a complex and difficult task. One approach to solving the problem of cortical function has been the use of ablation studies in which the auditory cortex is removed after training

an animal to perform a specific auditory task. These studies have demonstrated that cortical ablation does not result in a complete loss of function as does similar lesions in the visual system. In fact, for many simple tasks, no long-term deficits can be detected.[146] Based upon these results it is reasonable to assume that auditory cortex is involved in numerous details of more complex auditory processing. Consequently, it is unlikely that one simple unifying concept will be uncovered that describes the functional role of the auditory cortex.

Although there have been many studies of single-unit activity in the auditory nuclei over the past 50 years, they have thus far yielded few unifying principles about the data-processing mechanisms of the auditory nervous system. However, a number of recent studies suggest that in many instances the brain makes use of patterns of activity distributed over many cells to extract relevant information.[154] Consequently, if future studies focus on describing the responses of individual cells without viewing their participation, as a whole, in some functional unit, they may be doomed to result in failure as a means of understanding central-auditory processing.

AUDITORY-EVOKED ELECTROPHYSIOLOGIC RESPONSES

Modern averaging techniques have made it possible to record from humans, with surface electrodes, electrical responses reflecting the entire auditory pathway, from cochlea to cortex.[155,156] Clinical applications of this technique have expanded rapidly. In this section some basic physiologic principles are discussed upon which clinical application of auditory-evoked potentials are based.

Two major classes of human auditory-evoked potentials generated by acoustic transients (clicks) are used clinically. One class is recorded with an electrode located as close to the cochlea as possible (either "extra-tympanic" located on the external ear-canal skin, or "trans-tympanic," penetrating the eardrum to rest on the medial wall of the middle ear). Tests based on this class of auditory-evoked potentials have been termed electrocochleography (ECoG). The second class of auditory-evoked potentials is recorded between one electrode located on the vertex and another near the external ear (either on the mastoid or ear-lobe). This latter class of evoked potentials has been subdivided conventionally according to onset-latency range into early, middle, and late responses.

Electrocochleographic Responses: Auditory-Nerve Action Potential, Cochlear Microphonic, Summating Potential

Description of the Responses

Figure 42–33 shows a typical example of cochlear and cochlear-nerve click-evoked potentials recorded from

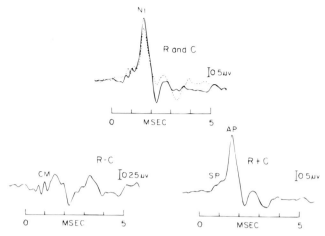

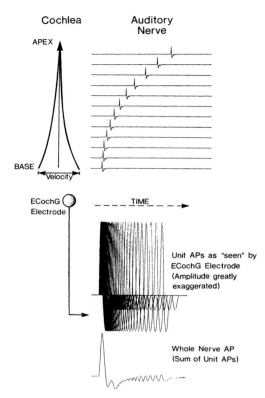

Fig. 42–33. Examples of cochlear and cochlear-nerve electrical responses to clicks recorded from the human outer-ear canal. The cochlear potentials are the cochlear microphonic (CM) and summating potential (SP). The neural action potential (AP) typically has a large negative peak, labeled N_1 in the upper record. At top, labeled R and C, are shown separate condensation (dashed line) and rarefaction (solid line) rectangular-pulse click responses recorded from external auditory meatus (EAM) with nasion "reference." At bottom left, labeled R − C, is the waveform produced by subtracting C from R responses. At bottom right, labeled R + C, is the waveform produced by adding C and R responses. Upward deflections represent negativity at EAM, and time-scale zeroes are set at the leading edge of the rectangular pulse driving the earspeaker. Click rate was 8/sec; click intensity was 115 dB peak equivalent SPL. Each C and R response is the average of 1,000 single sweeps.

Fig. 42–34. Summation of the single-unit spikes (amplitude exaggerated) picked up by a distant ECoG electrode to form the whole-nerve AP. Note that the highly synchronized spikes from the basal end of the cochlea sum more effectively than the poorly synchronized spikes from the apical end of the cochlea. The records of unit APs and whole-nerve AP at bottom are from a simplified computer experiment. Reprinted with permission from Elberling C: Simulation of cochlear action potentials recorded from the ear canal in man. In Electrocochleography. Edited by R.J. Ruben, C. Elberling, and G. Salomon. Baltimore: University Park Press, 1976.[157])

the ear canal. Evoked responses to clicks of opposite polarity are shown at top center. The auditory-nerve action potential (AP) has two or more ear-canal negative peaks designated N, N_1, N_2, N_3, and so forth. Each peak lasts about 1 msec and, in normal ears, N_1 is always the larger peak. The CM appears as a series of sinusoidal oscillations, typically about 3 kHz, on the leading edge of the N_1 peak. The SP appears as an ear-canal negative hump on the leading edge of the N_1 peak, with the CM oscillations superimposed.

The auditory-nerve AP (Fig. 42–33) is the sum of the waveforms of single-fiber auditory-nerve spikes as seen by the distant recording electrode as illustrated in Figure 42–34.[157] The single-unit spikes are triggered by the passage of the cochlear-traveling wave. Thus, spikes from basal (high-frequency) fibers appear at the recording electrode earlier than spikes from apical (low-frequency) fibers. Because the degree to which single neural-unit responses contribute to the evoked potential is determined largely by their synchrony, high-frequency (basal) fibers contribute more effectively to the whole-nerve AP and also to the brainstem auditory-evoked response (ABR) than do low-frequency fibers.

This principle leads to several important conclusions for clinical applications: (1) broadband-click APs preferentially reflect high-frequency fiber activity[158]

and, as a corollary, high-frequency clicks are more effective generators of auditory-evoked potentials than low-frequency clicks;[159] (2) high-frequency hearing loss due to selective removal of basal units tends to bias the broadband click-evoked AP and ABR toward more apical units. Therefore, high-frequency cochlear deficits prolong N_1 peak latencies;[158] and, (3) a low-frequency deficit does not cause a corresponding basalward shift, because of the already existing heavy bias toward basal units in the normal response. Therefore, low-frequency cochlear deficits have no apparent effect on AP and ABR latencies. Because the CM response follows the waveform of basilar-membrane vibration, it reverses polarity when click polarity is reversed, whereas the "envelope-following" SP does not. The neural response also maintains the same polarity. Thus, adding together responses to opposite-polarity clicks cancels out the polarity-reversing CM and allows a better view of the SP (bottom right of Fig. 42–33). In contrast, subtracting the condensation and rarefaction responses preserves the CM, while canceling the SP and most of the AP (bottom left of Fig. 42–33).

The cochlear-receptor potentials (CM, SP) can also be separated from the AP because receptor potentials are nonrefractory and do not adapt, whereas neural responses do. Thus, masking and increasing click rate are often used in clinical testing to selectively depress the neural response while preserving the CM and SP.

Reliable methods for separation of the SP from the other cochlear potentials have made this response useful in the diagnosis of Meniere's disease.[160] A number of studies have demonstrated that the SP is enlarged in a certain percentage of Meniere's patients.[161] Evidence supporting the notion that SP enlargement is specifically related to endolymphatic hydrops is provided by observations that manipulations expected to reduce fluid accumulation within the endolymphatic space (e.g., glycerol administration) often shrink abnormally enlarged SPs.[162]

Vertex-Recorded Auditory-Evoked Potentials

Description of the Responses

Figure 42–35 shows examples of early (top traces), middle (middle traces), and late (bottom traces) vertex-recorded auditory-evoked potentials generated by broadband clicks. Commonly used peak designations are also shown. In all traces, upward deflection represents negative voltage at the vertex ("referred" to an electrode on the mastoid). Note the differences in the time and voltage scales. The early response, commonly termed the ABR, is the smallest and also is the most recently discovered.

Auditory Brainstem Response (ABR)

An example of an ABR is shown in the top section of Figure 42–35 in which the peaks of this response are labeled with Roman numerals I–VII. It can be seen that the ABR occurs approximately between 1 and 8 msec after stimulus onset. Wave V is typically the largest and most robust of the potentials and waves beyond V are seldom used clinically. Studies in humans[163] and animals[164] suggest wave V is generated at the lateral lemniscus. Thus, the ABR is probably not useful in detecting abnormalities at or above the level of the inferior colliculus.[165] However, for the lower brainstem, the ABR is one of the best audiologic tests for detecting dysfunction.

The ABR is one of the most frequently-used auditory evoked-potential procedures because the variables which affect this response have been well-described and it provides a good measure of cochlear sensitivity and retrocochlear status. Clinically the response can be interpreted by quantitative measures of peak latencies, interpeak intervals, and interpeak-latency differences. In addition, the presence or absence of the various waves are noted as well as waveform morphology.[166]

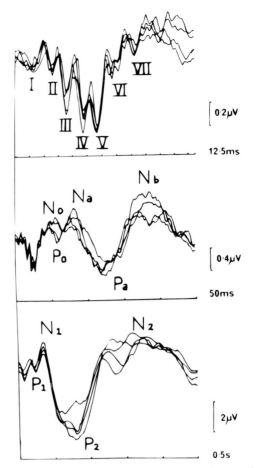

Fig. 42–35. Averaged human click-evoked potentials, recorded with vertex-mastoid electrodes. Upward deflection represents negativity at the vertex. From top to bottom, the time base is slowed to demonstrate progressively later responses. At top is the ABR (polarity is opposite the response recorded with a nasopharyngeal electrode); in the center is the MLR; and at bottom is the late "vertex" (LAER) response. Each tracing represents the average of 1,024 single responses. Several tracings are superimposed in each record to give an idea of variability. Roman numerals and letters identify individual peaks of the various responses according to accepted convention. Reprinted with permission from Picton TW, et al.: Human auditory evoked potentials. I. Evaluation of components. Electroencephalogr Clin Neurophysiol 36:179, 1974.[156]

Middle-Latency Response (MLR)

The MLR, labeled N_0, P_0, Na, Pa, and so forth (middle panel of Fig. 42–35), occurs between 8 and 40 msec after the auditory stimulus.[167] In animals, Wave Pa appears to be generated in primary auditory cortex by cortical elements on the side contralateral to stimulation.[168] However, in humans Pa seems to be generated in both hemispheres, even with monaural stimulation. Human cortical mapping localizes this potential to the region of the Sylvian fissure,[169] whereas studies based on clinical correlations indicate involvement of thalamocortical projections to the primary-auditory area located along Heschel's gyrus in the genesis of this response. Site-of-lesion studies suggest that Wave Na originates in the midbrain including such structures as the medial geniculate and thalamocortical projections.[169]

Although the MLR is not used nearly as frequently as ABR, useful clinical information can be obtained from this response particularly in conjunction with ABR testing. The MLR is robust at all frequencies including low-frequencies below 1000 Hz and, consequently offers a complementary index of high- and low-frequency hearing.[170] The MLR can also be useful in assessment of central auditory-system disorders, neurological evaluation, and most recently, as a tool for cochlear implant assessment.[171] The most significant disadvantage of MLR is that subject variables such as sleep state or sedation can severely reduce the amplitude of this potential. Thus, behavioral state must be controlled for, to obtain meaningful results.

Late Auditory-Evoked Response (LAER)

The relatively high-amplitude LAER, labeled P_1, N_1, and so forth (also called the vertex potential), occurs between 50 and 250 msec after the stimulus (bottom panel of Fig. 42–35). It is a cortical response, but its long latency suggests that the LAER is not generated within the primary-auditory cortex, but rather that it originates in "associative" cortex.[156] These potentials are often very dependent on the subject's state of alertness and consequently have received little use in clinical situations.

Auditory-Brain Mapping

One technique that is receiving considerable attention as a new and potentially powerful diagnostic tool is the use of auditory-brain mapping. Methods for this procedure are highly similar to those used to obtain the traditional evoked responses already described. The primary difference is that brain mapping simultaneously records the electrical activity from an array of scalp electrodes. Although this mass of data could be viewed as many evoked potentials, the human observer cannot readily interpret such a massive amount of data. Therefore, brain mapping was developed using computer-processing techniques to provide a visual display of the potential fields between all of the electrodes simultaneously. This method reduces the data into a multicolored or shaded plot in which intense activity is usually given the most brilliant color or the darkest shading. An example of the typical electrode placements and the derivation of a simple brain map are shown in Figure 42–36. With this type of visual output, patterns of activity in normal patients can be established and abnormalities easily visualized in pathological cases. Computer techniques also allow the clinician to view the patterns of activity throughout the duration of the stimulus to produce a "motion picture" of the evoked-electrical activity that occurred

over time. This method allows for the visualization of the spatiotemporal patterns of brain activity. Because the data are stored in the computer, a number of advanced mathematical-processing methods, that permit further refinement of the data, can be applied to aid in the detection of subtle abnormalities. For more information on this topic, the reader is referred to several comprehensive reviews.[172,173]

Magnetoencephalography

Magnetoencephalography involves the completely noninvasive recording of weak cerebral magnetic fields, which represent about one part in 10^9 of the earth's geomagnetic field, outside the head.[174] The neuromagnetic technique was made possible by the invention of SQUID (superconducting quantum interference device) magnetometers. Using a whole-head neuromagnetometer, magnetic brain signals are averaged by time-locking them to the onset of acoustic stimulation. It is assumed that the probable sources of cerebral magnetic fields are the electric currents in the synapses of synchronously activated cortical pyramidal neurons, and the sinks or volume currents, to complete the electrical circuit, are generated in the surrounding tissue. The development of multichannel systems increased the speed and convenience of neuromagnetic recording and made it feasible to apply magnetoencephalography (MEG) for clinical purposes.

Based on the accurate spatio-temporal resolution of whole-head Magnetoencephalography, Hari and colleagues have been instrumental in applying MEG to investigate the activity of the auditory projection areas, particularly with respect to language-related sites.[174] A schematic illustration of a typical experimental setup for auditory measurements is illustrated in Figure 42–37, and shows the relationship of the SQUID to the patient's head. The inset above indicates the isocontours across the scalp for the component of the magnetic field which is generated by the active region of the auditory cortex. An example of the averaged magnetic responses from measurement sites anterior (above) and posterior (below) to the Sylvian fissure of the right hemisphere (i.e., along the superior surface of the temporal lobe) are shown for one subject for a spoken word (solid line) and noise bursts (dashed lines) on the left side of Figure 42–38. The right side of Figure 42–38 illustrates the effects of increasing the duration of the onset of the word in another subject. It is clear that sound evokes a complex magnetic waveform, which lasts several hundred milliseconds after stimulus onset. Interesting and clinically useful data have been obtained about the perception of speech of deaf patients with cochlear prostheses by examining the activity of their auditory cortices with MEG.[175] Information of this 'real-time' sort implies that neuromagnetic recording may be used to assess functional

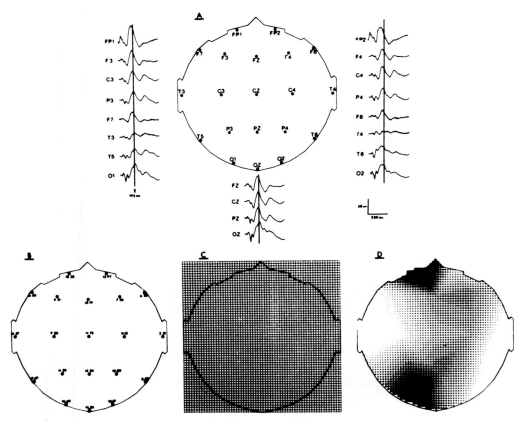

Fig. 42–36. Example of the construction of topographic images from evoked-potential data. A. Individual evoked potentials are shown at the electrode locations indicated in the diagram. B. Mean voltages are shown for the time interval 192 msec after the stimulus. The head region is then divided into a 64 × 64 matrix (C) to produce 4,096 spatial domains. Each spatial domain is assigned a voltage derived by linear interpolation from the three nearest recording locations. The visual image is then constructed (D) by fitting a discrete-level, equal-interval intensity scale to the points. Although a visual-evoked potential was used to create this topographic map, the same procedure is used for mapping auditory data. Reprinted with permission from Duffy FH: Auditory brain mapping. In Physiology of the Ear. Edited by A.F. Jahn, and J. Santos-Sacchi. New York: Raven Press, 1988.[173]

disorders in more detail than what is possible by other clinical evidence, and thus it is likely to become an important diagnostic tool of the future.

Evoked Otoacoustic Emissions

One of the principal benefits of OAEs with respect to clinical testing is that they provide an objective and noninvasive measure of cochlear activity which is completely independent of retrocochlear activity. In particular, OAEs measure the functional responses of OHCs which are uniquely sensitive to agents that damage hearing. Kemp,[80] the pioneer investigator into the basic features of OAEs, has also been instrumental in establishing one class of evoked emissions, the click-based transient-evoked OAE (Fig. 42–22C), as a potentially useful indicator of the various causes of ear disease including Meniere's disease and acoustic neurinoma.[103] In addition, Kemp and coworkers have also established the use of the click-evoked OAE as a method of screening for hearing dysfunction in newborns.[176,177,178]

Because of the frequency specificity of the eliciting pure tones, distortion-product OAEs (Fig. 42–23) also hold great promise for having a beneficial clinical applicability. This frequency specificity permits distortion-product OAEs to be measured after averaging the responses to only a few stimuli. Thus, under computer control, the fine resolution of these emissions in both the stimulus frequency and level domains permits the precise determination of the boundary between normal and abnormal hearing. Data from our laboratory[179,180] illustrate this feature of distortion-product OAEs in Figure 42–39A, which show the development of ototoxicity during a course of anti-neoplasm therapy with cis-platinum. Comparing the OAE findings with behavioral hearing (top), note the abrupt change in hearing and emission activity between 2 and 3 kHz (open circles), which accurately followed the 40-dB loss in hearing sensitivity produced by the ototoxic agent.

Based on their ability to distinguish between the relative contribution that sensory and neural components of the cochlea make to a hearing loss, OAEs promise to facilitate identification of the anatomic sub-

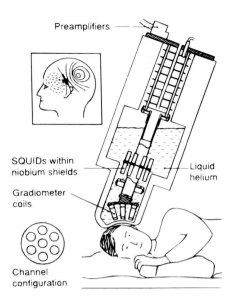

Fig. 42–37. Schematic illustration of a typical experimental set-up for auditory measurements. The most important parts of the seven-channel dc SQUID instrument used are shown, with the mid-points of the different channels separated by 36.5 mm. The inset above depicts isocontours across the scalp for the radial component of the magnetic field, generated by an active area in the auditory cortex; the arrow illustrates the location of the equivalent current dipole. Reprinted with permission from Hari R, Lounasmaa OV: Recording and interpretation of cerebral magnetic fields. Science *244*:432, 1989.[174]

strate of complex ear diseases. For example, the records shown in Figure 42–39B represent a typical pattern of audiometric loss in early Meniere's disease, which is accompanied by thresholds that are >40 dB HL and, not unexpectedly, no transient OAEs (bottom left) and abnormally low-level distortion-product OAEs (solid circles). Together, these results imply that the OHC system is involved in this patient's disease. However,

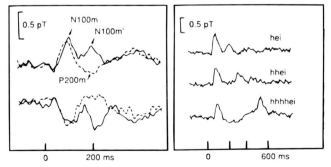

Fig. 42–38. Averaged magnetic responses from the auditory cortex. Left. Averaged magnetic response (n = 120) to 'hei' words (solid lines) and noise bursts (dashed lines) from the right hemisphere in one subject; the upper curves are from an anterior and the lower ones from a posterior measurement location near the ends of the Sylvian fissure. The passband was 0.05 to 70 Hz. Right. Effect of increasing the duration of 'h' in another subject. Reprinted with permission from Hari R, Lounasmaa OV: Recording and interpretation of cerebral magnetic fields. Science *244*:432, 1989.[174]

other patients with Meniere's disease, who show a similar hearing loss, can demonstrate rather robust distortion-product OAEs, even for test frequencies where behavioral thresholds are >50 dB HL.[181] Such differential findings for patients with Meniere's disease suggest that OAEs can distinguish between disease states that involve either OHCs (Fig. 42–39B) or other cochlear processes which are probably neural in origin. A comparable example of this feature of OAE testing to contribute toward differentiating between cochlear versus non-cochlear involvement in hearing disease is illustrated in Figure 42–40 for two patients diagnosed with acoustic neurinomas. The patient in Figure 42–40A displays the expected outcome for OAE testing in the presence of a retrocochlear disease; i.e., in the presence of a moderate hearing loss on the tumor side (solid circles), both transient and distortion-product OAEs are measurable. However, it is clear for the patient in Figure 42–40B diagnosed with a right-sided (open circles) acoustic neurinoma that the tumor has modified cochlear function in a manner that mimics the frequency configuration of the hearing loss. Thus, in certain retrocochlear disorders such as tumors of the cerebellopontine angle, cochlear function can be adversely affected, probably due to compromise of the vascular supply to the inner ear.

One benefit of OAE testing illustrated in Figure 42–39B is its sensitivity to changes in hearing status, which are mediated by the OHC system. In this instance, at the time the patient returned for follow-up testing (open circles), her hearing had improved, particularly over the low-frequency test range. The 20 to 30 dB improvement in low frequency hearing was mirrored by a similar increase in distortion-product OAEs, and by the ability to now measure transient OAEs.

In addition to the clinical applications noted above for OAEs, a number of studies have also demonstrated the utility of using emitted responses to understand the fundamental basis of a number of cochlear pathologies including the effects of noise-induced[182] or hereditary hearing loss,[183] congenital hearing disorders,[181] ototoxicity,[184] bacterial meningitis,[185] and presbyacusis[186] on both transient-evoked and distortion-product OAEs. The interested reader is encouraged to refer to several comprehensive reviews concerning the strengths and limitations of the clinical application of OAEs.[187,188]

INTRODUCTION TO THE VESTIBULAR SYSTEM

General Principles

The nonauditory part of the inner ear consists of two functional subdivisions: (1) the semicircular canals (two vertical and one horizontal), and (2) the otolith organs (the saccule and the utricle). The semicircular canals sense head rotation (angular or vectoral acceler-

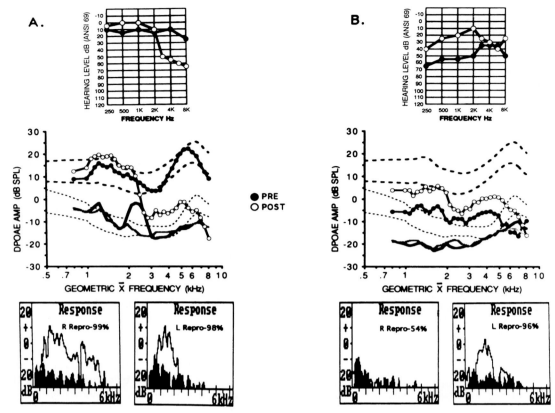

Fig. 42–39. Conventional audiograms (top), distortion-product OAE frequency/level (middle) functions ("audiograms") relating emission magnitude to stimulus frequency (in 0.1 octave steps from 0.8 to 8 kHz) for primary-tone levels of 75 dB SPL, and click-evoked OAEs (bottom) elicited by the 'default' mode of the ILO88 Otodynamic Analyzer. **A.** Behavioral hearing and evoked OAE findings for the right ear of an 8-yr-old female comparing pre- (solid circles) versus post-treatment (open circles) responses following a course of anti-neoplasm therapy with cis-platinum. Immittance and speech-testing results were normal for the baseline session, and were not tested during the post-treatment examination. **B.** Audiometric and OAE results for the left ear of a 49-yr-old female for two test sessions separated by about 2 weeks. The patient complained of a fluctuating hearing loss, tinnitus, aural fullness, and episodic dizziness of several months duration. Immittance findings were normal, whereas the speech-discrimination score (SDS) and speech-reception threshold (SRT) improved from 72 to 96% and 55 to 25 dB HL, respectively, at the last evaluation period. Reprinted with permission from Balkany T, Telischi FF, McCoy MJ, Lonsbury-Martin BL, Martin GK: Otoacoustic emissions in otologic practice. Am J Otol Suppl 15:29, 1994.[179]

ation), whereas the otolith organs are stimulated by the effects of gravity and linear acceleration of the head. The primary function of the utricle is to signal head position relative to gravity. Ablation of the saccule produces a less significant deficit than ablation of the utricle; hence, the function of the saccule is less well-defined than that of the utricle. In fact, it has been proposed that the saccule is a low-frequency auditory receptor.[189] However, a series of systematic studies using single-unit recordings have revealed that saccular-nerve fibers respond only to linear acceleration.[190–192] These findings suggest that the saccular system provides the high-level vertical acceleration signals required to elicit the motor response necessary to land optimally from a fall.[193]

The vestibular system is one of three sensory systems that function to maintain body balance and equilibrium. The other two are the somatosensory (chiefly proprioceptive) and visual systems. Loss of propri-

oception (e.g., as in tabes dorsalis) or vision causes significant balance and equilibrium difficulty. With bilateral vestibular function loss, difficulties occur only when one of the other systems is disrupted (e.g., when walking in the dark or on a soft surface), or when balance must be maintained under particularly difficult conditions (e.g., walking on a narrow beam).[194] The most significant functional deficits occur when the vestibular system suffers acute, asymmetrical damage and generates "false" head position or head-rotation signals.

In addition, the vestibular system maintains the field of gaze during head and body motion and provides control of the head, neck, trunk and limbs during locomotion and all other volitional acts.

Anatomy

The top portion of Figure 42–2 illustrates the general anatomic plan of the vestibular apparatus. There are

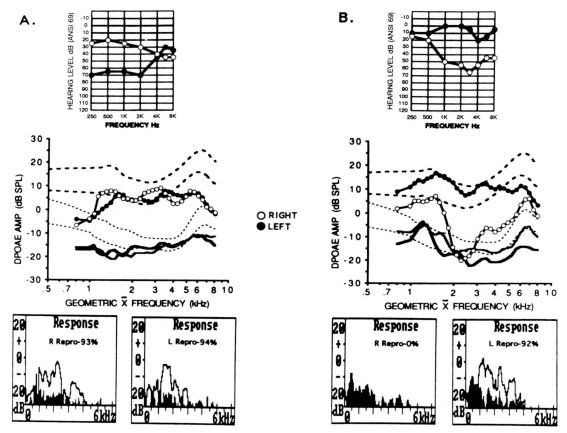

Fig. 42–40. Audiometric and OAE findings for two patients with acoustic neurinomas confirmed by magnetic-resonance imaging. **A.** A 39-yr-old male with an acoustic tumor on the left side who had normal tympanograms, but absent reflexes bilaterally. Although speech testing was normal for the right ear (open circles), the SDS and SRT were 0% and 70 dB HL, respectively, for the involved left ear (solid circles). **B.** A 47-yr-old female with a right-sided acoustic neurinoma. Whereas her tympanograms were normal, the only measurable acoustic-reflex threshold was for ipsilateral stimuli at 1 kHz. Speech testing was normal for the left ear, whereas the right ear was associated with a SDS of 60% and a SRT of 35 dB HL. Reprinted with permission from Balkany T, Telischi FF, McCoy MJ, Lonsbury-Martin BL, Martin GK: Otoacoustic emissions in otologic practice. Am J Otol Suppl 15:29, 1994.[179]

many similarities with cochlear anatomy. For example, both end organs are located in a tunnel that is hollowed out of the petrous portion of the temporal bone (embryologically, both organs come from the same tunnel). The tunnel is divided into an outer perilymph-filled bony labyrinth and an inner endolymph-filled membranous labyrinth. In addition, as in the cochlea, the receptor cells of the vestibular apparatus are ciliated and the cilia extend into a gelatinous matrix.

The three semicircular canals are oriented orthogonally or at right angles to each other. They can be thought of as lying in a bottom corner of a box. The horizontal (or lateral or external) canal is in the plane of the bottom of the box, and the anterior-vertical (or superior) and posterior-vertical (or posterior) canals are in the planes of the two sides of the box. In man, the entire canal complex is tilted upward about 30 degrees (30°). In the physiologic position, the head is bent forward about 30° from earth horizontal plane; therefore, the 30°-upward tilt puts the horizontal canal in the horizontal position under everyday conditions.[195] The su-

perior and posterior canals are oriented in vertical planes that form an angle of approximately 45° with the saggital head planes. Each semicircular canal lies parallel to one of the canals in the opposite vestibular labyrinth. Thus, the right horizontal canal is coplanar with the left horizontal canal, while the right superior and posterior canals are coplanar with the left posterior and superior canals, respectively.

The sensory epithelia (cristae) of the semicircular canals are located in enlarged areas (ampullae) at one end of each canal. The nonampullated ends of the vertically oriented superior and posterior canals connect to form the common crus. The bony vestibular aqueduct originates in the vestibule (entrance to the inner ear) and connects to the cerebrospinal-fluid space medially. Within the vestibular aqueduct is the fibrous endolymphatic duct that establishes a route between the membranous vestibule and the cranial meninges where the duct ends in the endolymphatic sac. The utriculosaccular duct, connecting the utricle and saccule, permits communication between the saccule and endolym-

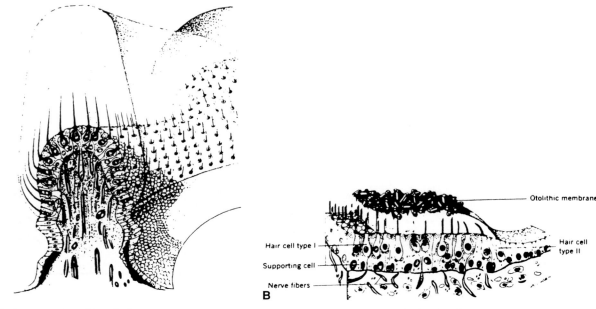

Fig. 42–41. Sensory receptors of vestibular system. **A.** Schematic drawing of the crista ampullaris illustrating the sensory cells, their hair bundles (cilia) that protrude into the cupula, and their innervating nerve fibers. **B.** Schematic drawing of a macula, showing how the cilia of the hair cells are embedded in a gelatinous membrane to which are attached calcium carbonate crystals (i.e., otoconia). A: Reprinted with permission from Wersall J: Studies on the structure and innervation of the sensory epithelium of the cristae ampullaris in the guinea pig. Acta Otolaryngol Suppl *126*:1, 1956.[280] B: Reprinted with permission from Iurato S: Submicroscopic Structure of the Inner Ear. Oxford: Pergamon Press, 1967.[281]

phatic duct. Although there is no agreement concerning the site of endolymph absorption, it is likely that the potassium-rich fluid is absorbed in the endolymphatic sac.[196] The ductus reuniens connects the saccule with the cochlear duct.

Figure 42–41A shows the anatomy of the crista. It is a saddle-shaped mound of tissue, attached to the ampullar wall at right angles to the long axis of the ampulla. The hair cells are on the surface of the crista. The ampullar nerve fibers travel through the center of the crista to synapse at the hair cell bases. The hair-cell cilia protrude from the surface of the crista into the fan-shaped cupula, a gelatinous structure consisting of mucopolysaccharides within a keratin framework.[197] The cupula partitions the semicircular canal by covering the top of the crista and extending to the opposite bony ampullar wall.

The sacculus and utriculus are two sacs in the membranous labyrinth, located in the vestibule. Their receptor organs, called maculae, can be seen in Figure 42–41B as patches of epithelia on the membranous labyrinth walls. The utricular macula lies on the floor of the utricle approximately in the plane of the horizontal semicircular canal. The saccular macula lies on the anteromedial wall of the saccule and is oriented principally in the vertical plane.

Figure 42–42 shows the structure of the macula. It consists of hair cells which are surrounded by supporting cells. The hair-cell cilia are attached to a gelatinous otolithic membrane. On the top of the gelatinous membrane is a layer of calcium carbonate crystals called statoconia (otoliths). The otoliths are denser than the surrounding endolymph[198]—hence their differential response to gravity and other inertial forces.

Figure 42–43 summarizes electron-microscopic observations of vestibular hair-cell morphology. First, as shown by Figure 42–43A, there are two types of hair cells in both the macula and the crista.[199] Type I hair cells are flask-shaped and have "chalice"-type afferent nerve endings that surround all but the hair-bearing end. Efferent nerve terminals synapse with the afferent calyx near its base. Type II hair cells have a cylindrical or test-tube shape and have several small bouton-type nerve endings that represent both afferent and efferent innervation only at the cell's base. Type I hair cells are concentrated in the central apex of the crista and the central part of the macula; type II hair cells are more numerous toward the peripheral region of the end organ.[200] Although significant amounts of filamentous actin occur at the apical surfaces of both the sensory cells and the supporting cells in the hair-cell containing regions of the vestibular organs,[201] motile properties such as the fast rates of lengthening and shortening which have been observed for cochlear OHCs have not been shown for vestibular hair cells. However, there is preliminary evidence that slow motility is exhibited by type II hair cells.[202]

The electron microscope has also demonstrated two types of cilia: (1) stereocilia, and (2) kinocilia[203] (Fig.

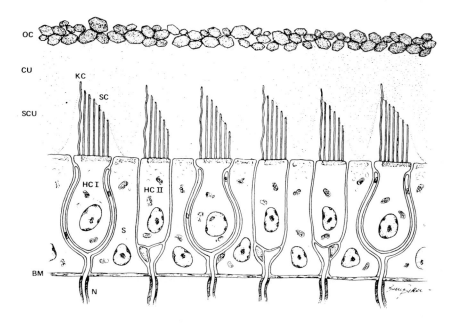

Fig. 42–42. Schematic drawing of a cross section of a macula. The gelatinous substance is divided into cupular (CU) and subcupular (SCU) layers. There are two types of cilia: kinocilia, labeled KC (one per hair cell), and stereocilia, labeled SC (many per hair cell). OC = otoconia, HC I = type I hair cell, HC II = type II hair cell, N = nerve fiber, BM = basement membrane, S = supporting cell.

42–43B). Each hair cell has only one motile kinocilium and a bundle of 60 to 100 stereocilia.

Stereocilia are relatively rigid, club-like rods, varying systematically in length in a "pipe-organ" fashion,

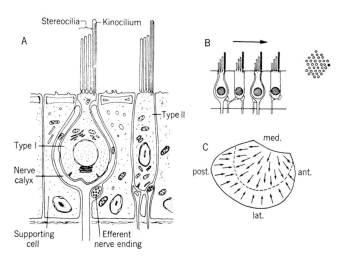

Fig. 42–43. Microanatomy of the vestibular hair cells. **A.** Schematic drawing of two hair cell types. **B.** Diagram showing morphologic polarization of the hair cells. Arrow shows direction of cilia bending that produces excitation. At right is a cross section through the hair-bearing end of the hair cell showing many stereocilia (open circles) and one kinocilium (filled circle). **C.** A diagrammatic surface view of the human utricular macula. Arrows indicate direction of polarization. Dashed line is the linea alba. A: Reprinted with permission from Brodal A: Neurological Anatomy in Relation to Clinical Medicine. New York: Oxford University Press, 1969.[216] B and C: Reprinted with permission from Lindeman HH, et al.: The sensory hairs and the tectorial membrane in the development of the cat's organ of Corti. Acta Otolaryngol 72:229, 1971,[281] and Wersall J, et al: Ultrastructure of the vestibular end organs. In Myotatic, Kinesthetic and Vestibular Mechanisms. Edited by A.V.S. de Reuck, and J. Knight. Boston: Little, Brown, 1968.[199]

that extend, at the apical end of the hair cell, from a dense cuticular plate that consists of actin and myosin.[124] They are not homogeneous as was originally thought. Rather, they contain longitudinally oriented microfilaments[204] composed of actin.[31] The membrane enveloping the stereocilia is a thickened continuation of the hair-cell cuticular membrane.[205] The stereocilia are constricted at their base and, when deflected, move like stiff rods pivoting around the basal-constricted area.[34] Recent work has demonstrated interconnections between stereocilia via fibrils or tip links.[206]

Kinocilia end in a basal body, located just beneath the hair-cell membrane. Within each kinocilium, there are nine peripherally arranged double-tubular filaments, positioned regularly around two centrally located tubular filaments. This 9-plus-2 tubule pattern is found in many motile cilia (e.g., respiration epithelia, oviduct epithelium, unicellular flagellates).[207] Stereocilia are coupled to the kinocilium as well as to each other so that during deflection, all cilia are stimulated as one bundle.[49]

On each hair cell, the single kinocilium is located to one side of the bundle of stereocilia. In both maculae and cristae, hair cells in the same area tend to have kinocilia on the same side of the stereocilia bundle. Thus, the vestibular sensory epithelium has a morphologic "directional polarization"[203] that is determined by the direction of the cilia alignment. Figure 42–43C illustrates the directional polarization of the utricular macula. The kinocilia all tend to point toward a line of demarcation called the striola (or linea alba) running across the approximate center of the macula. In the saccule, the kinocilia point away from the striola. In the horizontal canal crista, kinocilia point toward the

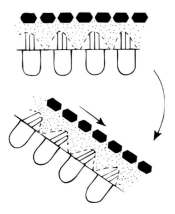

Fig. 42–44. Diagrammatic representation of the conversion of a head tilt to bending of the hair-cell cilia by the macula.

utricle, whereas in the pair of vertical cristae, they point away from the utricle. Thus, vertical and horizontal cristae are morphologically polarized in opposite directions.[200]

Transduction and Coding

Mechanical Events

As in the cochlea, the final mechanical event in vestibular transduction is the bending of the hair-cell cilia. Figure 42–44 illustrates transduction by the macula. When the macular surface is tilted, the heavy otoliths tend to slide downward, carrying the gelatinous membrane and attached cilia with them.

Figure 42–45 shows a simplified diagram of a semicircular canal. It consists of a circular, narrow-bore tube in the temporal bone filled with endolymph. The tube originates from, and returns to, a reservoir (the utricle), but each canal may be treated, for practical purposes, like a fluid ring. In this diagram "H" is the angular rotation of the head in the plane of a canal. When the head under goes an angular acceleration [H (d^2H/dt^2)], the fluid is left behind because of its inertia.

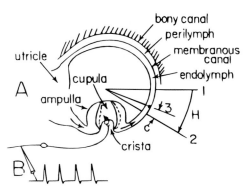

Fig. 42–45. Transduction of head velocity by the semicircular canals. **A.** Axis 1 represents an axis fixed in space. Axis 2 moves with the head as it is displaced through angle H. Axis 3 moves with the endolymph as it is displaced relative to the canal by the angle c which is proportional to cupula deflection indicated by the dashed lines. **B.** Deflection of the cupula alters the rate of impulses carried by primary vestibular afferent fibers. (Courtesy of D.A. Robinson.)

This causes the endolymph to flow relative to the canal and to push on a gelatinous mass called the cupula, which lies across the canal blocking it. The cupula is attached to the ampulla wall around its entire periphery and billows, like a sail (Fig. 42–45 dashed lines) under endolymph pressure.[208,209] Normal deflections are tiny, in the range of 0.01 to 3 mm.[210] The subsequent strain on the hair cells, by the bending of their cilia embedded in the cupula, creates a generator potential that modulates the discharge rate (R_{v1}) of primary vestibular-afferent fibers.

The overall behavior of the cupula and canal was described by Steinhausen.[211] If "c" is some measure of cupula (and thus endolymph) displacement, the force balance equation for the canal is:

$$mc + rc + kc = mH$$

where "m" represents the net, equivalent moment of inertia of the endolymph, "r" is the lumped effect of viscous drag on fluid flow (c), and "k" represents the stiffness of the gelatinous cupula. The term $m[H(d^2H/dt^2)]$ is the driving force on the endolymph due to head acceleration. During most natural head movements the inertial reactance $m[c(d^2c/dt^2)]$ and cupula restoring force kc are very small compared to the viscous term $r[c(dc/dt)]$, because the narrowness of the tube creates a high resistance to flow. Consequently, the above equation can be reduced to $r[c(dc/dt)] = m[H(d^2H/dt^2)]$ or, integrating both sides, $c = m/r[H(dH/dt)]$.

Thus, the discharge rate (R_{v1}) which is proportional to cupula deflection (Fig. 42–46), carries a signal into the central nervous system proportional to head velocity, not acceleration. In other words, a constant head acceleration applies a constant force on the endolymph, causing it to flow at a constant velocity. Consequently, cupula *position*, the integral of flow, must be proportional to head *velocity*, the integral of head acceleration.

In the squirrel monkey the typical resting discharge rate is 90 spikes/s.[212] The discharge rate, R_{v1}, increases for deflection of the cupula in one direction and decreases in the other. On the abscissa of Fig. 42–46, B(dH/dt) may be substituted for c, in which case the slope of the line, S_v, for the average fiber, is 0.4 (spikes/s)/(deg/s). Thus, the signal sent from the canal to the brainstem on the average fiber for most normal head movements is $R_{v1} = 90 + 0.4$ H(dH/dt)].

Response of Primary-Vestibular Neurons

Microelectrode studies in higher mammals have demonstrated the following characteristics of primary vestibular neuron activity: most of the primary-vestibular neurons called regular units have a high (-100/s) and remarkably uniform spontaneous discharge.[213] When one listens to their spikes on a loudspeaker, the neurons make a characteristic "motorboat" sound. There is also a small population of irregular neurons with a

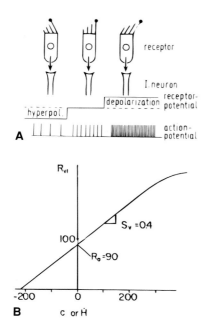

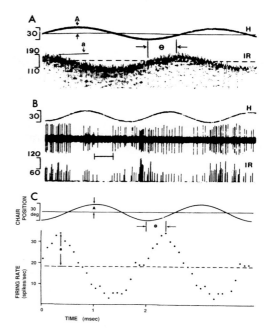

Fig. 42–46. Motion transduction by vestibular hair cells. **A.** At rest there is a resting rate of action potential discharge in the primary vestibular afferents (center). Shearing forces on the hair cells cause either depolarization (right) or hyperpolarization (left) depending on whether the stereocilia are deflected toward or away from the kinocilium (indicated by longest cilium, with beaded end), respectively. This modulates the discharge rate in the vestibular nerve. **B.** Vestibular-nerve discharge rate, R_{v1}, is 90 spikes/s at rest (R_o) in the squirrel monkey and changes approximately linearly with cupula deflection. When the latter is expressed in equivalent head velocity, the slope of the line, S_v, is about 0.4 (spikes/s)/(deg/s) for the average vestibular-afferent fiber. A: Reprinted with permission from Baloh R, Honrubia V: Clinical Neurophysiology of the Vestibular System, 2nd Edition. Philadelphia: F.A. Davis, 1990.[283] B: Reprinted with permission from Zee DS, Leigh RJ: The Neurology of Eye Movements, 2nd Edition. Philadelphia: F.A. Davis, 1991.[284]

Fig. 42–47. Peripheral vestibular neuron responses to sinusoidal rotation stimulation in the alert monkey. **A.** A regular (high-rate) neuron. **B.** An irregular neuron. Sinusoidal curve (H) plots head position. The records immediately below the sinusoidal traces show intervals between neuronal spikes. The height of vertical bars on these records is proportional to the interval between spikes. Because one of these bars occurs for every spike, their frequency reflects the frequency of the recorded spikes. **C.** Response of unit in B averaged over 10 cycles; 0 is the phase lag of firing rate (i.e., the shortest interval between spikes) which occurs at about the 0 crossing of the head-position signal. Thus, firing rate at the output of the semicircular canal is related most closely to head velocity.

lower rate and less regular spontaneous discharge. The high-rate regular units have small-diameter, slowly conducting axons that predominantly innervate the periphery of the end organ (type II hair-cell region of the crista), whereas the low-rate irregular neurons come from the center of the crista where most type I hair cells are located.[190] The high, regular spontaneous firing rate of the primary neurons permits the bidirectional sensitivity of the vestibular hair-cell receptors.

When the head rotates causing cupula displacement and a stimulatory deflection of hair-cell cilia, the semicircular-canal afferents change their discharge rate above, in response to hair-cell depolarization, and below, in response to hair-cell hyperpolarization, the resting rate depending on the direction of rotation.[214] When the head rotates sinusoidally at velocities encountered during normal function, ampullar-nerve discharge rate varies sinusoidally (Fig. 42–47). The phase relationship between head position and head velocity (phase lag of about 90°) is such that the maximum discharge rate occurs at the head's zero crossing;

i.e., at the head's maximum velocity. Thus, the ampullar-afferent discharge rate codes head-angular velocity. The adequate stimulus is actually angular acceleration, but the hydrodynamics of the semicircular-canal system are such that the head's acceleration is integrated to give a velocity output.[215]

Similarly, with the macular afferents, accurate coding by discharge rate of the head's position relative to gravitational vertical can be demonstrated in all species. The more complex orientation of the macular hair cells makes directional correlates more difficult to establish than for semicircular-canal afferents. However, Fernandez and Goldberg[190] studied large populations of saccular and utricular neurons and were able to demonstrate neural "sensitivity vectors" among the neuronal populations that corresponded to the relative orientations of the saccular and utricular maculae.

CENTRAL VESTIBULAR PATHWAY

Anatomy

Primary-Afferent Connections

The vestibular system functions primarily as an afferent-reflex input to the motor system. In general, vestibular pathway-mediated reflexes involve three muscular systems: extrinsic oculomotor, cervical, and antigravity.

As might be expected, the semicircular canals (rotation sensors) connect primarily with the extrinsic oculomotor and cervical muscles (i.e., the muscles that compensate for head rotation), whereas the otolith organs (position sensors) connect primarily with the antigravity muscles. Figure 42–48 outlines these major central vestibular connections.[216]

Scarpa's (vestibular) ganglia, in the internal auditory canal within the vestibular portion of the eighth nerve, contain the bipolar ganglion cells of the first-order vestibular neurons. The vestibular nerve can be divided into superior and inferior divisions that innervate the sensory epithelia of the canal and otolithic end organs. The superior portion innervates the cristae of the superior and horizontal semicircular canals, the utricular macula, and a small region of the saccular macula. The inferior division of the vestibular nerve innervates the crista of the posterior semicircular canal and the remaining part of the saccular macula. Centrally, all first-order vestibular neurons synapse in the vestibular nucleus complex, which occupies a considerable area beneath the floor of the fourth ventricle

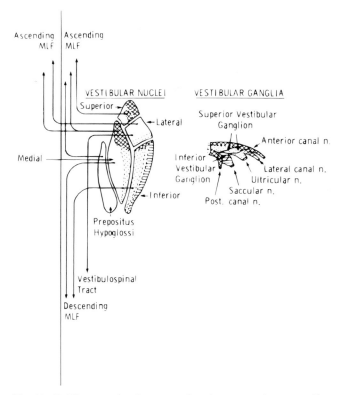

Fig. 42–48. Diagram of major connections between primary-vestibular neurons in the vestibular ganglia and the vestibular nucleus. Also shown are major outflows from the vestibular nucleus. Vestibulocerebellar connections are excluded. The primary-afferent connections are modified from Carpenter MG: Human Neuroanatomy, 7th Edition. Baltimore: Williams & Wilkins, 1976.[285]

and lies across the pontomedullary boundary. Upon entering the brainstem, the vestibular axons bifurcate into the ascending rostral and descending caudal divisions.

The vestibular nucleus complex consists of four distinct subnuclei (Fig. 42–48): (1) the superior (Bechterew's or angular), (2) lateral (Deiters'), (3) medial (Schwalbe's or principal or triangular), and (4) inferior (spinal or descending) nuclei. There is recent anatomic evidence that the nucleus prepositus hypoglossi (classically thought to relate to taste) has strong efferent and afferent vestibulo-oculomotor [via the medial longitudinal fasciculus (MLF)] and cerebellar projections. In addition, microelectrode recordings from awake monkeys have demonstrated that prepositus neurons fire in relation to both vestibular- and visual-induced eye movements.[217] Studies on the activity of ocular motor neurons in alert monkeys have shown that the neural commands for all conjugate eye movements (vestibular, optokinetic, saccadic, and pursuit) have both velocity and position commands.[218,219]

The vestibular input to prepositus is di-synaptic and reciprocally organized (ipsilateral input excitatory/ contralateral input inhibitory). In addition, if cells in the monkey's nucleus prepositus hypoglossi are lesioned by kainic acid, the monkey's eye movements only reflect the velocity command.[220] A great amount of neurophysiologic evidence indicates that the position command is obtained from the velocity command by the mathematical process of integration. That is, a neural network located in the nucleus prepositus hypoglossi integrates, in the mathematical sense, velocity-coded signals; thus, the prepositus is included in the diagram of the vestibular-nuclear complex in Figure 42–48.

As indicated in Figure 42–49, each subnucleus has a unique set of connections with the periphery and with specific regions of the central nervous system including the spinal cord, cerebellum, and brainstem oculomotor nuclei (III, IV, VI). Most of the semicircular-canal afferents terminate in the superior nucleus and rostral portion of the medial-vestibular nucleus. Both of these nuclei in turn project to the oculomotor nuclei of the extraocular muscles via the ascending MLF. The superior nucleus projects only to the ipsilateral MLF, whereas the medial nucleus projects bilaterally. The medial nucleus, via the medial vestibulospinal tracts in the descending MLF, also sends bilateral descending projections to spinal anterior-horn cells that control the cervical musculature.[221] Thus, the input and output of the superior and medial vestibular nuclei provide a possible anatomic basis for the nystagmus and head-turning-reflex responses to semicircular-canal stimulation (see below).

The otolith organs (particularly the utriculus) project primarily to the inferior nucleus and caudal part of the lateral nucleus. Outputs from these nuclei

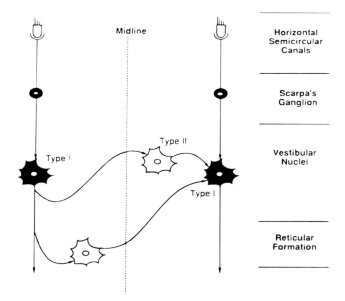

	Horizontal Semicircular Canals
	Scarpa's Ganglion
	Vestibular Nuclei
	Reticular Formation

Fig. 42–49. Interrelation of type I and type II secondary vestibular neurons. Dark neurons are excitatory and light neurons inhibitory. Reprinted with permission from Baloh R, Honrubia V: Clinical Neurophysiology of the Vestibular System, 2nd Edition. Philadelphia: F.A. Davis, 1990.[283]

in turn project downward to the ventral-horn region throughout the length of the spinal cord via the lateral vestibulospinal tract. Thus, the afferent and efferent connections of the lateral vestibular nucleus provide the anatomic basis for antigravity-muscle responses in the limbs (extensors of the legs and flexors of the arms) to postural change. The otolith organs have relatively sparse connections to the extraocular muscles. These may be the connections that produce the ocular counter-rolling response to head tilt.[222]

Vestibulocerebellar Connections

Primary Vestibular Fibers
Primary-vestibular neurons project not only to the vestibular nuclei, but also to the cerebellum. Most of these fibers are distributed to the ipsilateral flocculus and nodulus and the medially located uvula[223] Because of this innervation by primary-vestibular fibers, these three cerebellar areas have been termed collectively the vestibulocerebellum. As will be discussed, the primary-vestibular input to the vestibulocerebellum appears to be important in controlling the vestibulo-oculomotor reflex (VOR). As will be discussed, the primary-vestibular input to the vestibulocerebellum and the climbing fiber input from the inferior olive, appear to be important in controlling the VOR.

Secondary Vestibular Fibers
The vestibulocerebellum receives secondary fibers primarily from the medial and inferior vestibular nuclei,

but also from the other divisions. In addition, the fastigial nucleus and the cortex of the vermis receive a strong, somatotopically organized projection from the lateral vestibular nucleus. Since this nucleus is the primary origin of the vestibulospinal tract, connections to it from the cerebellum are probably important in regulating antigravity reflexes that help to maintain an upright body posture.[224]

Projections to Cerebral Cortex

Whether or not the vestibular system has a direct cortical projection has long been a controversial question. The functional corollary to this question is whether or not we can consciously appreciate a sensation due to vestibular stimulation. This question also has generated debate, because most of the subjective sensations produced by vestibular stimulation (e.g., vertigo) are secondary to motor reflex or to autonomic responses, and it is difficult or impossible to separate a primary vestibular sensation from the secondary sensations.[193]

Experiments employing electrical stimulation of the vestibular nerve have demonstrated relatively short-latency localized cortical responses in both the cat and the monkey.[225,226] The cat's vestibular area is adjacent to both auditory and somatosensory fields, but in the monkey (and therefore probably also in the human), it is located near the face area of the somatosensory field on the postcentral gyrus. Deecke et al.[227] demonstrated that the ventroposteroinferior (VPI) nucleus is the thalamic relay for the vestibulocortical projection. The VPI nucleus lies adjacent to the thalamosomatosensory representation of the face. Prior to this study, the function of the VPI nucleus was unknown.

Physiology of Vestibular Nuclei

General Characteristics of Neuronal Responses
Microelectrode studies of responses of vestibular nucleus neurons to electrical stimulation of individual ampullary nerves and to "natural" stimuli (rotation and tilt) have established the following general characteristics: (1) neurons can be classified as tilt responders (otolith units) or rotation responders (canal units); (2) the locations of these two types correspond with that expected from the anatomic projections of otolith and semicircular canal afferents on the vestibular-nuclear complex. Thus, the tilt responders are found primarily in the areas innervated by the sacculus and utriculus (inferior nucleus and caudal part of lateral nucleus), and the rotation responders are found mainly in the areas innervated by the semicircular canals (superior nucleus and rostral part of medial nucleus); and (3) among the rotation responders, pathways from individual canals seem to be preserved. Thus, for example, a neuron that responds to vertical rotation or to electrical stimulation of a vertical-ampullary nerve does not

TABLE 42–2. Characteristics of Canal-Responding Units in Vestibular Nucleus

	Input Side	Response Directionality	Response Time Course	Latency	Gain	Spontaneous Activity
Type I (67%)	Ipsilabyrinth	Same as 1°	—	—	—	—
Kinetic (56%)	Ipsilabyrinth	Same as 1°	Fast decay	Long (multisynaptic)	High	None
Tonic (11%)	Ipsilabyrinth	Same as 1°	Slow decay	Short (monosynaptic)	Low	High level
Type II (29%)	Contralabyrinth	Opposite 1°				
Type III (3%)	?	Facilitated both directions				
Type IV (<1%)	?	Inhibited both directions				

respond to horizontal rotation or to stimulation of a horizontal ampullary nerve and *vice versa.*

Classification of Neuronal-Response Types

Both canal and otolith vestibular nucleus units preserve the basic properties of the primary-afferent input, but some respond in the same direction (e.g., ipsilateral horizontal rotation increases firing rate); others respond in the opposite direction. A few of the vestibular nucleus neurons respond with either inhibition or facilitation in both directions. Table 42–2 outlines the characteristics of the canal units. The type I (response same as primary) units are innervated by the ipsilateral labyrinth, whereas the type II (response opposite that of primary) units are innervated by the contralateral labyrinth.

The analogous classification for otolith responders subdivides all types into: (1) "a" units (increases on ipsilateral tilt), (2) "b" units (decrease on ipsilateral tilt), (3) "y" units (increase by tilt in both direction), and (4) "o" units (decrease by tilt in both directions). Analogous to the canal units, the relative populations of these units are a > b > y > o.[228,229]

Commissural Inhibition

Many of the contralateral (type II) semicircular-canal responses listed in Table 42–2 are abolished when a midline dorsal-brainstem incision is made which interrupts vestibular-crossing fibers. Thus, the "opposite-primary" type II responses are probably elicited by inhibitory input from type I neurons from the opposite labyrinth. Figure 42–49 summarizes the simplest of the probable neuronal interconnections responsible for this contralateral inhibition.

The commissural-inhibitory system is also important in the mechanism of compensation following labyrinthectomy. Immediately after labyrinthectomy, the type I units on the labyrinthectomized side have no spontaneous activity and do not respond to rotation. However, within a few days, the deafferented type I units regain their spontaneous activity and, via inhibition from the contralateral pathway, also regain their normal response to rotation. The mechanisms by which this recovery process occurs are unknown, but a contributing factor is lowered threshold of the deaf-ferented type I neuron for contralateral input.[230] Fetter and Zee[231] showed that visual experience was not necessary for the acquisition, or for the maintenance of this recovery process.

Vestibulo-Ocular Reflex (VOR)

Although there are neural connections between the maculae and the extraocular muscles, they are less important in humans, both functionally and clinically than are the semicircular-canal connections. This discussion will therefore focus on the reflex connection between the semicircular canals and the extraocular muscles.

An important function of the semicircular canals is to provide afferent input to a VOR which generates eye movements that compensate for head movements by maintaining a stabilized visual image on the retina during rotation (compensatory eye movements). Figure 42–50 diagrams the neural connections that stabilize gaze during head movement.

The following simple experiment demonstrates this "compensatory eye-movement" function of the semicircular canals. First, with head motionless, fixate on a finger while the finger is being moved back and forth in front of the eyes. Then hold the finger motionless and rotate the head back and forth at the same rate, while still maintaining fixation on the finger. In the "canal-assisted" (head rotating, finger motionless) situation, it can be readily appreciated that visual fixation is more easily maintained on the finger than in the first situation where only visual information on target movement is available.

Anatomic Connections

The VOR is subserved by a simple three-neuron pathway: motions detected by the end organ are transduced into neural impulses that are sent via the vestibular nerve to the vestibular nuclei and rostrally through the ascending MLF to the oculomotor nuclei of the extraocular muscles. Secondary vestibulo-ocular connections via the reticular formation have been described, but functionally these are less important than the "direct" three-neuron MLF vestibulo-ocular pathway.

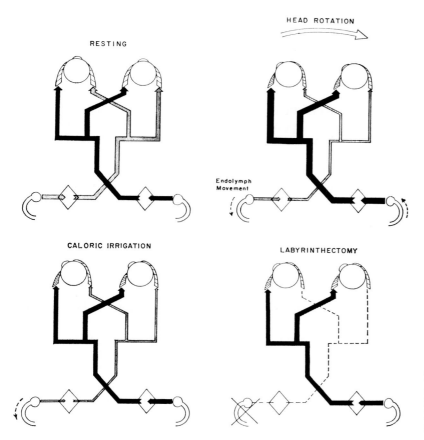

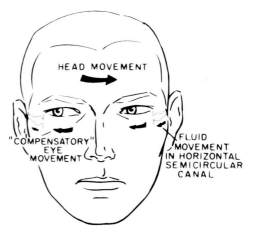

Fig. 42–50. Generation of the vestibular (slow) phase of different kinds of nystagmus. The thickness of the lines connecting the semicircular canal to the extraocular muscles is proportional to the intensity of neural discharge along the nerve pathways.

Inhibitory-crossed connections at the levels of both vestibular (already described) and oculomotor nuclei probably also participate in the VOR. The crossed-inhibitory oculomotor connections subserve antagonistic extraocular muscles.[232] These inhibitory interconnections are important in the formation of conjugate-eye movements.

Functional Connections

Investigations have uncovered many details of facilitatory and inhibitory interactions between neurons of the vestibular-nuclear complex and motor neurons of the extraocular muscles. For a review, the reader is referred to Wilson and Melvill-Jones.[229] However, in older experiments, the effect of mass stimulation of individual ampullar nerves on eye movements provides the clinician with the most useful integrative concepts of the functional organization of the VOR. Results of all these ampullar nerve-stimulating experiments agree on the principle (illustrated by Fig. 42–50): *Stimulation of an ampullar nerve generates conjugate-eye movements away from the side stimulated and in the plane of the canal stimulated.*

This principle allows a straightforward description of the events leading from endolymph movement in the horizontal canal to the compensatory-eye move-

ment depicted in Figure 42–51: (1) head movement to the left generates endolymph movement to the right in the left canal. This is toward the ampulla and therefore increases ampullar-nerve discharge rate; (2) the increased ampullar-nerve output (by the aforementioned rule) causes conjugate-eye deviation away from the

Fig. 42–51. A compensatory-eye movement, initiated by the horizontal semicircular canals. The eyes move in the direction of endolymph movement. If rotation of the head is continued at an ever-increasing speed, the compensatory eye movement becomes the slow phase of a rotational nystagmus.

side stimulated (i.e., to the right, which is opposite to the direction of head movement); (3) similarly, head movement to the left generates ampulofugal movement in the right canal, which decreases neural output; and (4) decreased neural output inhibits the extraocular muscles, causing the eyes to deviate conjugately to the left, thus, providing an output that is synergistic to the conjugate right-eye deviation generated by the output of the opposite canal. Figure 42–50, upper right, depicts this sequence of events.

Functionally, the VOR provides more than a simple 1–1 transfer of information from the semicircular canal to the extraocular muscles. It will be recalled that the response of the ampullary nerves reflects head velocity, yet the ocular rotation at the vestibular reflex output reflects head position. Therefore, at some point in the transfer from vestibular input to ocular output, some form of neural integration must occur that converts the velocity signal at the input into the displacement signal at the output. The location of this integrator, as noted above, is the nucleus prepositus hypoglossi.[220]

Control of the Gain of the VOR

In studies of the VOR, the concept of gain is important. Gain of the VOR is simply the amplitude of eye rotation divided by amplitude of the head rotation. Generally, amplitudes of eye and head rotation are expressed as angles.

Because eye rotation is supposed to be equal and opposite to head rotation (in order to fully compensate and leave gaze steady), it might seem at first that the ideal VOR gain would be −1. However, there are many real-life situations where the ideal VOR gain is not "−1." Functionally, such situations can be divided into long-term (slow) and short-term (fast) adjustments. The short-term, or fast, vestibulo-ocular gain adjustments occur in the course of visual-tracking tasks where both the head and the eyes follow the fixation target at varying relative velocities. For example, in a tracking task where the head and eyes must move in the same direction, the VOR must be completely suppressed. In the clinical-test situation, this visual suppression of the VOR is observed as suppression of caloric or rotational nystagmus during visual fixation.

An example of functionally beneficial long-term vestibulo-ocular gain control is the situation where a prescription for new glasses has been received. The change in magnification of the visual image changes the speed with which the visual image moves across the retina (e.g., increasing magnification would increase the speed of movement of retinal images). Therefore, to maintain a stable retinal image after new glasses have been obtained, the VOR gain must be adjusted for the new magnification levels. Such adjustments have been demonstrated experimentally in humans by testing the VOR-rotational response in the

dark after long-term periods of wearing highly-corrective lenses.[233]

An extreme example of the plasticity of the VOR gain is provided by reversing prisms. Reversing-prism glasses causes a normal visual image to be reversed right-to-left; hence, movement of the visual image when the head or eyes are rotated horizontally is exactly opposite of normal. Even in this extreme example, humans and other animals[234,235] have been shown to function normally after a few days of wearing the prisms—even in situations requiring visually-controlled movements during head movements (e.g., mountain climbing).[236] Testing the VOR in humans after a few days of wearing reversing prisms has demonstrated actual reversal (i.e., conversion of negative to a positive gain) of the VOR.[237]

There is strong evidence that the vestibulocerebellum plays an important role in both short-[238] and long-term[239] control of the VOR gain. The strong primary-vestibular afferent projection to the vestibulocerebellum and equally strong projection from the vestibulocerebellum to the oculomotor portion of the vestibular-nuclear complex have already been described. There is also a strong input to the vestibulocerebellum from the retina by way of the inferior olivary climbing fibers. Most of these visual units detected in the vestibulocerebellum are "movement detectors."[240] They are thus ideally suited to provide information on "retinal slip" of the visual image, which is needed to modify vestibulo-ocular gain control. The visual and vestibular inputs to the cerebellum converge upon Purkinje cells of the flocculus cortex. Furthermore, experiments on alert monkeys, in which rotation of the animal's visual environment and its head were controlled independently, showed that visual and vestibular inputs modulate Purkinje cell output in ways exactly appropriate for the functionally useful control of the VOR gain.

Ablation experiments further support the role of the flocculonodular lobes in control of VOR gain. It has been demonstrated, for example, that removal of the vestibulocerebellum eliminates suppression of caloric nystagmus by visual fixation.[241] An analogous "failure of fixation suppression" (FFS) of nystagmus is also observed in humans with cerebellar lesions.[242] However, clinical data suggest that FFS can be produced by lesions in the brainstem and (less frequently) cerebral hemispheres as well as the cerebellum.[242]

Robinson[235,239] has reported a striking ablation experiment that demonstrates the role of the flocculus in causing long-term (plastic) changes in VOR gain. Cats wore reversing prisms for several days and VOR gain was measured each day by rotating the cats in the dark. After several days, as expected, VOR gain dropped from 0.9 to 0.1. When the vestibulocerebellum was removed, the vestibulo-ocular gain promptly increased to about 1.2. Furthermore, it proved impossible to reinstate the VOR gain decrease by continued prism-wearing after removal of the vestibulocerebellum. In addition, Miles et al.[243] uncovered results in the monkey that implicated synaptic changes at other sites, especially in the brainstem. More recently, Lisberger[244] provided further evidence that the modifiable synapses were located between vestibular primary afferents and those second-order and/or possibly third-order, vestibular neurons that also received synapses from Purkinje cells. Finally, Luebke and Robinson[245] reversibly silenced the flocculus of alert cats adapted to either high-gain or to low-gain VOR. This reversible floccular shutdown did not alter the adapted VOR gain, yet the animals were subsequently unable to modify their VOR gain while the flocculus was silenced.

Clinical Considerations of Vestibular Reflexes

General Pattern

The vestibular system functions primarily as an afferent input for motor reflexes and, at rest, most primary-vestibular neurons have high and remarkably regular spontaneous discharge rates. For purposes of the following clinically oriented discussion, the spontaneous vestibular neuronal activity will be referred to as the resting discharge.

Normally, with the head at rest in the neutral position, the resting discharges in the two vestibular nerves are equal. Vestibulo-motor reflexes are elicited when inputs from the two vestibular end organs or their central projections are made unequal (unbalanced). They can be unbalanced by an abnormality involving one side to a greater degree than the other. In this case, we term the resultant vestibular reflex spontaneous. Vestibular input from the two sides can also be unbalanced by stimulating one or both of the vestibular end organs. In this case, the resultant vestibular reflex is termed "induced."

When a vestibular input imbalance is unusually large or prolonged, a constellation of stereotyped motor responses occurs.[246] These responses are head-turning, falling (or swaying), past-pointing, vertigo (a sensation of rotation), and nystagmus (a rhythmic back-and-forth eye movement with alternate slow phases in one direction and fast phases in the opposite direction). These slow and fast eye movements are termed the slow and fast phases of vestibular nystagmus. The head-turning, falling, past-pointing, and nystagmus slow phase are all in the same direction, i.e., away from the ear with the greater output. In this discussion, the reference is to the nystagmus slow (vestibular) phase. The clinical convention is to designate nystagmus direction by fast (central) phase, presumably because these movements can be easily observed. Thus, the indicated reflex directions may be the opposite of those to which the reader is accustomed. Fast-phase nystagmus is in the direction of the angular ac-

celeration. The rotation sensation (vertigo) may be referred either to the subject's body (subjective vertigo) or to the environment (objective vertigo). If the body rotates, the apparent rotation of the environment is in the same direction as the nystagmus slow phase; if the environment rotates, the rotation sensation is in the opposite direction.

Methods of Eliciting

Vestibular responses can be generated by rotational, caloric, and galvanic stimulation of the vestibular periphery. The caloric and rotational responses are discussed in the following section. The galvanic vestibular response occurs when an electrical current is applied to the head in the vicinity of the ear.[247] Electrical current applied in this manner elicits the entire constellation of vestibular responses, except vertigo (although subjects may report a slight sense of disorientation). If the current is positive, the nystagmus slow phase, past-pointing, and body-sway responses are toward the stimulated ear; if the current is negative, these responses are away from the stimulated ear.

Because the galvanic stimulus probably acts at a retrolabyrinthine location (either vestibular nerve, Scarpa's ganglia, or more central location), it has been suggested as a means of differentiating vestibular end organ from vestibular-nerve lesions. However, this procedure has not found widespread clinical acceptance, possibly because of uncertainty over the exact locus of action. For example, patients with their vestibular nerves sectioned intracranially still have a recognizable body-sway galvanic response,[247] suggesting that at least part of the action of the galvanic stimulus is central to the vestibular nerve (brainstem or possibly cerebellum).

Vestibular Nystagmus

Vestibular nystagmus occurs when the semicircular-canal system is overstimulated. For example, if the head is continuously rotated in one direction at an ever-increasing speed, the semicircular-canal initiated compensatory-eye movement becomes repeatedly interrupted by rapid, snap-back movements and hence becomes a rotational nystagmus. Because the relatively slow compensatory eye-movement phase of the nystagmus comes from the semicircular-canal system, it is called the vestibular or slow phase of the nystagmus. Conversely, because the fast, snap-back eye movement comes from the brain, it is called the central or fast phase of the nystagmus.

Caloric nystagmus is produced by a temperature change in the region of the vestibular apparatus. In the clinical laboratory, this temperature change is usually produced by running cold or warm water into the external auditory canal. The temperature change is conducted through bone to the semicircular canals. Since the horizontal semicircular canal is closest to the irri-

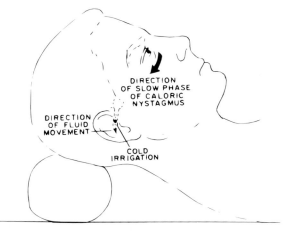

Fig. 42–52. The mechanism of cold-caloric nystagmus. The density of the cooled portion of the endolymph (darkened) is increased, causing it to fall, thereby producing endolymph movement. The slow phase of the caloric nystagmus is in the direction of endolymph movement.

gating water, it is the most affected; hence, caloric nystagmus is almost entirely in the horizontal plane.

Figure 42–52 illustrates the generation of caloric nystagmus. The subject is in the supine position, with his head elevated 30° to bring the horizontal canal into the vertical position. The cold-caloric irrigation cools the endolymph in part of the horizontal canal. This cooled endolymph becomes slightly denser than the surrounding endolymph and thus falls, causing the eyes to rotate toward the irrigated ear. This vestibular eye movement is repeatedly interrupted by a rapid central eye movement in the opposite direction. A cold caloric nystagmus is thus created, with its slow phase toward, and its fast phase away from, the irrigated ear.

Although the slow phase is the vestibular phase of vestibular nystagmus, it is the clinical convention to designate the direction of the vestibular nystagmus by the direction of the fast phase. This convention originated because the fast phase is easier to observe than the slow phase.

Neural Mechanisms of Nystagmus
Figure 42–50 diagrams the neural mechanisms of different kinds of vestibular nystagmus. This figure shows the physiologic rather than the anatomic form of the horizontal VOR system. It is drawn to reflect the fact that increased neural activity from a horizontal semicircular canal rotates the eyes horizontally away from the canal.[248]

At rest, both canals generate equal neural activity (the resting discharge, described previously). Unbalancing the vestibular inputs from the two ears generates vestibular nystagmus (if the imbalance is prolonged). Caloric and rotational stimuli unbalance the vestibular input via the normal transducer action of the semicircular canals. Lesioning one labyrinth by op-

eration or disease causes a pathologic imbalance by eliminating or reducing the resting discharge on the involved side.

THE FUTURE

Regeneration of Hair Cells

A great amount of study has focused over the past 10 years on the ability of vertebrate hair cells to regenerate. One popular model has been the bird in which it has been shown that the sound-damaged sensory epithelium, the basilar papilla, is capable of undergoing significant structural repair.[249,250,251] Detailed morphologic examination of damaged cochleas showed that immediately after over-exposure, there is a substantial loss of hair cells, an expansion of the surrounding supporting-cell surface area,[252] and a degeneration of the tectorial membrane overlying the region of the lost hair cells.[253] In the days following the overstimulation, the regenerative processes repair many of the damaged structures so that the hair cells are almost completely replaced by regenerated hair cells,[254] cochlear ganglion cells appear to form new synapses with the regenerated hair cells,[255] and a new tectorial membrane is partially regenerated over the lesioned area.[253] In parallel to the structural repair is a considerable recovery of auditory function as measured with physiological techniques.[256] Other investigators have documented the capacity of the avian cochlea and vestibular sensory epithelium to repair itself following aminoglycoside toxicity.[257] Using cell proliferation-marker procedures (i.e., triticated-thymidine autoradiography, proliferating cell nuclear-antigen immunochemistry), it has been well-documented that the supporting cells are the precursors or progenitors of the regenerated cochlear[258] and vestibular[259] hair cells.

The knowledge that noise- or drug-damaged hair cells of birds, and possibly guinea pigs, can regenerate has motivated researchers to learn how to stimulate the regrowth of the sensory cells of the human inner ear. It is quite likely that, in the future, individuals with hearing impairment will regain certain of their abilities to hear by growing new hair cells.

Molecular Basis of Hearing and Balance

A current view is that many of the acquired hearing disorders have a genetic basis. Thus, differential susceptibility to the adverse effects of ototoxins or exposure to loud sounds likely involves as yet undiscovered heritable factors. Although the field of molecular biology has made significant advances toward interpreting the human genome through genetic mapping, many of the essential proteins involved in either auditory or vestibular function have yet to be identified. The basic recombinant-dioxyribonucleic acid (DNA) technology used to identify gene sequences which encode proteins consists of isolating and reversely transcribing the template for translating a gene, i.e., the messenger ribonucleic acid (mRNA). By applying techniques such as the polymerase chain reaction (PCR) to amplify the identified DNA sequences, or by cloning DNA fragments into bacterial vectors, quantities large enough to permit sequence analysis can be produced.

One step in identifying the genes expressed in a tissue such as the cochlea is to create a gene library containing independent recombinants. To this end, mRNA is isolated from the cochlea using techniques that preserve the mRNA from undergoing natural degradation by RNases. The isolated mRNA is transcribed into complementary DNA (cDNA) copies using reverse transcriptase. A devised bacteriophage-expression vector is used to ligate the cDNA copies, which are amplified by replicating the phage in bacteria to obtain large quantities of DNA. The library is typically screened using a subtractive strategy to identify gene sequences expressed in the tissue from which the library was constructed. Related studies isolate individual cDNA clones so that inserts can be identified and used for *in situ* hybridization to determine the cochlear tissue in which the message for a particular replication factor is expressed. In this manner, cloned molecules are hybridized against frozen sections of the inner ear and exposed to x-ray film to produce autoradiographs. Following a specified exposure period, the sections are developed and counterstained with a fluorescent agent and evaluated under dark-field and fluorescence microscopy.

Complementary DNA (cDNA) libraries have been constructed for the cochleas of several laboratory animals including the chicken[260] and rat.[261] Wilcox and Fex[262] have created an even more specific tissue cDNA library for the organ of Corti of the guinea pig, as well as for the semicircular canal cristae ampullaris.[263] In addition, Metcalf et al.[264] have cloned a type of myosin that may be involved in the motor responsible for vestibular adaptation. Molecular cloning of more specific components of cochlear cells has also been demonstrated for a G protein α-subunit,[265] a DNA-replication factor,[260] a mineralcorticoid type I receptor,[266] and a nicotinic subtype of an acetylcholine receptor.[267] In contrast to the few studies on molecular cloning in the auditory and vestibular systems, many studies have been described in the literature that report using *in situ* hybridization to inner ear tissues of previously cloned molecules to assess the cellular distribution of the mRNA of a particular gene using immunohistochemical methods.[268] From the great number of molecular studies being conducted in the auditory and vestibular fields, it is clear that the application of these powerful tools will dramatically expand our knowledge of the fundamental basis of hearing and balance mechanisms in the near future.

SUGGESTED READINGS

1. Shaw EAG, Teranishi R: Sound pressure generated in an external-ear replica and real human ears by a nearby point source. J Acoust Soc Am 44:240, 1968.
2. Shaw EAG: The external ear. *In* Handbook of Sensory Physiology, Vol. V/1: Auditory System, Anatomy Physiology (Ear). Edited by W.D. Keidel, and W.D. Neff. New York, Springer-Verlag, 1974.
3. Pickles JO: An Introduction to the Physiology of Hearing. New York, Academic Press, 1982.
4. Bekesy G, von: Experiments in Hearing. Translated and edited by EG Wever. New York, McGraw-Hill, 1960.
5. Moller AR: An experimental study of the acoustic impedance of the middle ear and its transmission properties. Acta Otolaryngol 60:129, 1965.
6. Tonndorf J, and Khanna SM: The role of the tympanic membrane in middle ear transmission. Ann Otol Rhinol Laryngol 79:743, 1970.
7. Khanna SM, and Tonndorf J: Tympanic membrane vibration in cats studied by time-averaged holography. J Acoust Soc Am 51:1904, 1972.
8. Salomon G, and Starr A: Electromyography of middle ear muscles in man during motor activities. Acta Neurol Scand Suppl 39:161, 1963.
9. Borg E: On the neuronal organization of the acoustic middle ear reflex, a physiological and anatomical study. Brain Res 49:101, 1973.
10. Moller AR: The sensitivity of contraction of the tympanic muscles in man. Ann Otol Rhinol Laryngol 71:89, 1962.
11. Moller A: Acoustic reflex in man. J Acoust Soc Am 34:1524, 1962.
12. Djupesland G, and Zwislocki JJ: Effect of temporal summation on the human stapedius reflex. Acta Otolaryngol 71:262, 1971.
13. Jerger J: Clinical experience with impedance audiometry. Arch Otolaryngol 92:311, 1970.
14. Klockhoff IH: Middle ear muscle reflexes in man. Acta Otolaryngol Suppl 164:1, 1961.
15. Reger SN: Effect of middle ear muscle action on certain psychophysical measurements. Ann Otol Rhinol Laryngol 69:1179, 1960.
16. Smith HD: Audiometric effects of voluntary contraction of the tensor tympani muscles. Arch Otolaryngol 38:369, 1943.
17. Holst HE, et al: Ear drum movements following stimulation of the middle ear muscles. Acta Otolaryngol Suppl 182:73, 1963.
18. Zakrisson JE, et al.: Auditory fatigue in patients with stapedius muscle paralysis. Acta Otolaryngol 79:228, 1975.
19. Simmons FB: Perceptual theories of middle ear muscle function. Ann Otol Rhinol Laryngol 73:724, 1964.
20. Harford ER, and Jerger JF: Effect of loudness recruitment on delayed speech feedback. J Speech Hear Res 2:361, 1959.
21. Borg E, and Zakrisson JE: The activity of the stapedius muscle in man during vocalization. Acta Otolaryngolog 79:325, 1973.
22. Jahnke K: The fine structure of freeze-fractured intercellular junctions in the guinea pig inner ear. Acta Otolaryngol Suppl 336:1, 1975.
23. Engstrom H: The cortilymph, the third lymph of the inner ear. Acta Morphol Neer Scand 3:195, 1960.
24. Nadol JB Jr: Intercellular fluid pathways in the organ of Corti of cat and man. Ann Otol Rhinol Laryngol 88:2, 1979.
25. Steele KP: Tectorial membrane. In Neurobiology of Hearing: The Cochlea. Edited by R.A. Altschuler, D.W. Hoffman, and R.P. Bobbin. New York, Raven Press, 1986.

26. Smith CA: Structure of the cochlear duct. *In* Evoked Electrical Activity in the Auditory Nervous System. Edited by R. Naunton, and C. Fernandez. New York, Academic Press, 1978.

27. Engstrom H, and Ades HW: The ultrastructure of the organ of Corti. *In* The Ultrastructure of Sensory Organs. Edited by I. Friedman. Amsterdam, North Holland, 1973.

28. Lim D: Morphological relationship between the tectorial membrane and the organ of Corti—scanning and transmission electron microscopy. J Acoust Soc Am *50*:92, 1971.

29. Flock A: Physiological properties of sensory hairs in the ear. *In* Psychophysics and Physiology of Hearing. Edited by E.F. Evans, and J.P. Wilson. New York, Academic Press, 1977.

30. Nielsen DW, and Slepecky N: Stereocilia. *In* Neurobiology of Hearing: The Cochlea. Edited by RA Altschuler, DW Hoffman, and RP Bobbin, New York, Raven Press, 1986.

31. Flock A, and Cheung HC: Actin filaments in sensory hairs of inner ear receptor cells. J Cell Biol *75*:339, 1977.

32. Flock A, Bretscher A, and Weber K: Immunohistochemical localization of several cytoskeletal proteins in inner ear sensory and supporting cells. Hear Res *6*:75, 1982.

33. Slepecky N, and Chamberlain SC: Distribution and polarity of actin in the sensory hair cells of the chinchilla cochlea. Cell Tissue Res *224*:15, 1982.

34. Flock A, Flock B, and Murray E: Studies on the sensory hairs of receptor cells in the inner ear. Acta Otolaryngol *83*:85, 1977.

35. Dallos P: The Auditory Periphery. New York, Academic Press, 1973.

36. Steele CR: A possibility for sub-tectorial membrane fluid motion. *In* Basic Mechanisms in Hearing. Edited by A.R. Moller. New York, Academic Press, 1973.

37. Dallos P, et al.: Cochlear inner and outer hair cells: Functional differences. Science *177*:356, 1972.

38. Zwislocki JJ: Phase opposition between inner and outer hair cells and auditory sound analysis. Audiol *14*:443, 1975.

39. Russell IJ, and Sellick PM: The responses of hair cells to low frequency tones and their relationship to the extracellular receptor potentials and sound pressure level in the guinea pig cochlea. *In* Neuronal Mechanisms of Hearing. Edited by J. Syka, and L. Aitkin. New York, Plenum, 1981.

40. Bekesy G von: Shearing microphonics produced by vibrations near the inner and outer hair cells. J Acoust Soc Am *25*:786, 1953.

41. Tasaki I, Davis H, and Eldredge DH: Exploration of cochlear potentials in guinea pig with a microelectrode. J Acoust Soc Am *26*:765, 1954.

42. Tasaki I, and Spyropoulos CS: Stria vascularis as source of endocochlear potential. J Neurophysiol *22*:149, 1959.

43. Konishi T, and Kelsey E: Effect of cyanide on cochlear potentials. Acta Otolaryngol *65*:381, 1968.

44. Tasaki I, and Fernandez C: Modification of cochlear microphonics and action potentials by KCl solution and by direct currents. J Neurophysiol *15*:497, 1952.

45. Davis H, Derbyshire AJ, Lurie JH, and Saul LJ: The electric response of the cochlea. Am J Physiol *107*:311, 1934.

46. Tasaki I, Davis H, and Legouix JP: The space-time pattern of the cochlear microphonic (guinea pig) as recorded by differential electrodes. J Acoust Soc Am *24*:502, 1952.

47. Davis H, Deatheridge BH, Eldredge DH, and Smith CA: Summating potentials of the cochlea. Am J Physiol *195*:251, 1958.

48. Konishi T, and Yasuno T: Summating potential of the cochlea in the guinea pig. J Acoust Soc Am *35*:1448, 1963.

49. Hudspeth AJ: Extracellular current flow and the site of transduction by vertebrate hair cells. J Neurosci *2*:1, 1982.

50. Dallos P, and Cheatham MA: Production of cochlear potentials by inner and outer hair cells. J Acoust Soc Am *60*:510, 1976.

51. Davis H: A model for transducer action in the cochlea. Cold Spring Harbor Symp Quant Biol *30*:181, 1965.

52. Wever EG, and Bray CW: Action currents in the auditory nerve in response to acoustical stimulation. Proc Natl Acad Sci *16*: 344, 1930.

53. Davis H, Tasaki I, and Goldstein R: The peripheral origin of activity with reference to the ear. Cold Spring Harbor Symp Quant Biol *17*:143, 1952.

54. Brownell WE: Cochlear transduction: An integrative model and review. Hear Res *6*:335, 1982.

55. Hudspeth AJ: The hair cells of the inner ear. Sci Am *248*:54, 1983.

56. Bobbin RP, Bledsoe SC Jr, Winbery SL, and Jenison GL: Actions of putative neurotransmitters and other relevant compounds on Xenopus laevis lateral line. *In* Auditory Biochemistry. Edited by D.G. Drescher. Springfield, IL: Charles C. Thomas, 1985.

57. Bledsoe SC Jr: Pharmacology and neurotransmission of sensory transduction in the inner ear. Sem Hear *7*:117, 1986.

58. Werman R: A review: Criteria for identification of a central nervous system transmitter. Comp Biochem Physiol *18*:745, 1966.

59. Bledsoe SC Jr, Bobbin RP, and Puel J-L: Neurotransmission in the inner ear. *In* Physiology of the Ear. Edited by A.F. Jahn, and J. Santos-Sacchi. New York: Raven Press, 1988.

60. Kuriyama H, Jenkins O, and Altschuler RA: Immunocytochemical localization of AMPA selective glutamate receptor subunits in the rat cochlea. Hear Res *80*:233, 1994.

61. Bobbin RP, Bledsoe SC Jr, and Jenison GL: Neurotransmitters of the cochlea and lateral line organ. *In* Hearing Science: Recent Advances. Edited by C.I. Berlin. San Diego: College-Hill Press, 1984.

62. Schwartz IR, and Ryan AF: Uptake of amino acids in the gerbil cochlea. *In* Neurobiology of Hearing: The Cochlea. Edited by R.A. Altschuler, D.W. Hoffman, and R.P. Bobbin. New York, Raven Press, 1986.

63. Fex J, and Altschuler RA: Neurotransmitter-related immunocytochemistry of the organ of Corti. Hear Res *22*:249, 1986.

64. Plinkert PK, Mohler H, and Zenner HP: A subpopulation of outer hair cells possessing GABA receptors with tonotopic organization. Arch Otorhinolaryngol *246*:417, 1989.

65. Gitter AH, and Zenner HP: τ-aminobutyric acid receptor activation of outer hair cells in the guinea pig cochlea. Eur Arch Otorhinolaryngol *249*:62, 1992.

66. Eybalin M: Neurotransmitters and neuromodulators of the mammalian cochlea. Physiol Rev *73*:309, 1993.

67. LePage EL, and Johnstone BM: Nonlinear mechanical behaviour of the basilar membrane in the basal turn of the guinea pig cochlea. Hear Res *2*:183, 1980.

68. Liberman MC, and Kiang NYS: Acoustic trauma in cats. Acta Otolaryngol Suppl *358*:1, 1978.

69. Ruggero MA, and Rich NC: Application of a commercially manufactured Doppler-shift laser velocimeter to the measurement of basilar-membrane vibration. Hear Res *51*:215, 1991.

70. Evans EF: The frequency response and other properties of single fibers in the guinea-pig cochlear nerve. J Physiol *226*:263, 1972.

71. Kiang NYS, and Moxon EC: Tails of tuning curves of auditory-nerve fibers. J Acoust Soc Am *55*:620, 1974.

72. Moller AR: Studies of the damped oscillatory response of the auditory frequency analyzer. Acta Physiol Scand *78*:299, 1970.

73. Evans EF: Auditory frequency selectivity and the cochlear nerve. *In* Facts and Models in Hearing. Edited by E. Zwicker and E. Terbardt. New York, Springer-Verlag, 1974.

74. Kiang NYS, Moxon EC, and Levine RA: Auditory nerve activity in cats with normal and abnormal cochleas. *In* Ciba Symposium on Sensorineural Hearing Loss. Edited by G.E.W. Wolstenhome, and J. Knight. London, Churchill Press, 1970.

75. Robertson D: Cochlear neurons: Frequency selectivity altered by perilymph removal. Science *186*:153, 1974.

76. Cody AR, and Johnstone BM: Single auditory neuron response during acute acoustic trauma. Hear Res *3*:3, 1980.

77. Johnstone BM, and Boyle AJ: Basilar membrane vibration examined with the Mossbauer technique. Science 158:389, 1967.

78. Rhode WS: Measurement of vibration of the basilar membrane in the squirrel.monkey. Ann Otol Rhinol Laryngol 83:619, 1974.

79. Kim DO, Neely ST, Molnar CE, and Matthews JW: An active cochlear model with negative damping in the partition: Comparison with Rhode's ante- and post-mortem observations. In Psychophysical, Physiological, and Behavioral Studies in Hearing. Edited by G. van den Brink, and F.A. Bilsen. Delft, Delft University Press, 1980.

80. Kemp DT: Stimulated acoustic emissions from within the human auditory system. J Acoust Soc Am 64:1386, 1978.

81. Wit HP, and Ritsma RJ: Evoked acoustical responses from the human ear: Some experimental results. Hear Res 2:253, 1980.

82. Mountain DC: Changes in endolymphatic potential and crossed olivocochlear bundle stimulation alter cochlear mechanics. Science 210:71, 1980.

83. Siegel JH, and Kim DO: Efferent neural control of cochlear mechanics? Olivocochlear bundle stimulation affects cochlear biomechanical nonlinearity. Hear Res 6:171, 1982.

84. Anderson SD: Some ECMR properties in relation to other signals from the auditory periphery. Hear Res 2:273, 1980.

85. Kemp DT, and Chum R: Properties of the generator of stimulated acoustic emissions. Hear Res 2:213, 1980.

86. Brownell WE: Microscopic observation of cochlear hair cell motility. Scan Elect Microsc III:1401, 1984.

87. Brownell WE, Bader CR, Bertrand D, and de Ribaupierre Y: Evoked mechanical responses of isolated cochlear outer hair cells. Science 227:194, 1985.

88. Zenner HP, Zimmermann U, and Schmitt U: Reversible contraction of isolated mammalian cochlear hair cells. Hear Res 18:127, 1985.

89. Flock A: Hair cells, receptors with a motor capacity? In Hearing, Physiological Bases and Psychophysics. Edited by R. Klinke, and R. Hartman. New York, Springer-Verlag, 1983.

90. Dallos P, Evans BN, and Hallworth R: Nature of the motor element in electrokinetic shape changes of cochlear outer hair cells. Nature 350:155, 1991.

91. Brownell WE: Outer hair cell electromotility and otoacoustic emissions. Ear Hear 11:82, 1990.

92. Rubel EW: Ontogeny of structures and function in the vertebrate auditory system. In Handbook of Sensory Physiology. Vol. IX: Development of Sensory Systems. Edited by M. Jacobson. New York, Springer-Verlag, 1978.

93. Kim DO: Functional roles of the inner- and outer-hair-cell subsystems in the cochlea and brainstem. In Hearing Science: Recent Advances. Edited by C.I. Berlin. San Diego, College-Hill Press, 1984.

94. Evans EF, and Harrison RV: Correlation between cochlear outer hair cell damage and deterioration of cochlear nerve tuning properties in the guinea pig. J Physiol 256:43, 1976.

95. Brown MC, Nuttal AL, and Masta RI: Intracellular recordings from cochlear inner hair cells: Effects of stimulation of the crossed olivocochlear efferents. Science 222:69, 1983.

96. Gifford ML, and Guinan JJ Jr: Effects of crossed-olivocochlear-bundle stimulation on cat auditory nerve fiber responses to tones. J Acoust Soc Am 74:115, 1983.

97. Winslow RL, and Sachs MB: Effect of electrical stimulation of the crossed olivocochlear bundle on auditory nerve response to tones in noise. J Neurophysiol 57:1002, 1987.

98. Collet L: Use of otoacoustic emissions to explore the medial olivocochlear system in humans. Br J Audiol 27:155, 1993.

99. Berlin CI, Hood LJ, Hurley A, and Wen H: Contralateral suppression of otoacoustic emissions: An index of the function of the medial olivocochlear system. Otolaryngol Head Neck Surg 110:3, 1994.

100. Penner MJ, and Burns EM: The dissociation of SOAEs and tinnitus. J. Sp. Hear. Res., 30:396, 1987.

101. Penner, M.J.: An estimate of the prevalence of tinnitus caused by spontaneous otoacoustic emissions. Arch Otolaryngol Head Neck Surg 116:418–423, 1990.

102. Wilson JP: Evidence for a cochlear origin for acoustic re-emissions, threshold fine-structure and tonal tinnitus. Hear Res 2:233, 1980.

103. Kemp DT, Bray P, Alexander L, and Brown AM: Acoustic emission cochleography—Practical aspects. Scand Audiol Suppl 25:71, 1986.

104. Sakashita T, Minowa Y, Hachikawa K, Kubo T, and Nakai Y: Evoked otoacoustic emissions from ears with idiopathic sudden deafness. Acta Otolaryngol Suppl 486:66–72, 1991.

105. Evans EF: The sharpening of cochlear frequency selectivity in the normal and abnormal cochlea. Audiol 14:419, 1975.

106. Brugge JF, Anderson DJ, Hind JE, and Rose JE: Time structure of discharges in single auditory nerve fibers of the squirrel monkey in response to complex periodic sounds. J Neurophysiol 32:386, 1969.

107. Rose JE, Brugge JF, Anderson DJ, and Hind JE: Phase-locked response to low-frequency tones in single auditory nerve fibers of the squirrel monkey. J Neurophysiol 30:769, 1967.

108. Boudreau JC: Neural volleying: Upper frequency limits detectable in the auditory system. Nature 208:1237, 1965.

109. Kiang NYS: Processing of speech by the auditory nervous system. J Acoust Soc Am 68:830, 1980.

111. Sachs MB, and Young ED: Encoding of steady state vowels in the auditory nerve: Representation in terms of discharge rate. J Acoust Soc Am 66:470, 1979.

111. Young ED, and Sachs MB: Representation of steady-state vowels in the temporal aspects of the discharge patterns of populations of auditory-nerve fibers. J Acoust Soc Am 66:1381, 1979.

112. Wever EG: Theory of Hearing. New York, John Wiley & Sons, 1949.

113. Kiang NYS, Watanabe T, Thomas EC, and Clark LF: Discharge Patterns of Single Fibers in the Cat's Auditory Nerve. M.I.T. Research Monograph No. 35. Cambridge, MA, Massachusetts Institute of Technology, 1965.

114. Kiang NYS: A survey of recent developments in the study of auditory physiology. Ann Otol Rhinol Laryngol 77:656, 1968.

115. Evans EF: The dynamic range problem: Place and time coding at the level of the cochlear nerve and nucleus. In Neuronal Mechanisms of Hearing. Edited by J. Syka, and L. Aitkin. New York, Plenum, 1981.

116. Evans EF, and Palmer AR: Responses of units in the cochlear nerve and nucleus of the cat to signals in the presence of band-stop noise. J Physiol 252:60P, 1975.

117. Palmer AR, and Evans EF: On the peripheral coding of the level of individual frequency components of complex sound levels. Exp Brain Res Suppl 2:19, 1979.

118. Viemeister NF: Intensity coding and the dynamic range problem. Hear Res 34:267, 1988.

119. Rasmussen GL: Anatomic relationships of the ascending and descending auditory systems. In Neurological Aspects of Auditory and Vestibular Disorders. Edited by W.S. Fields, and B.R. Alford. Springfield, Charles C. Thomas, 1964.

120. Warr WB, Guinan JJ Jr, and White JS: Organization of the efferent fibers: The lateral and medial olivocochlear systems. In Neurobiology of Hearing: The Cochlea. Edited by R.A. Altschuler, D.W. Hoffman, and R.P. Bobbin. New York, Raven Press, 1986.

121. Warr WB: The olivocochlear bundle: Its origins and terminations in the cat. In Evoked Electrical Activity in the Auditory Nervous System. Edited by R.F. Naunton, and C. Fernandez. New York, Academic Press, 1978.

122. Iurato S, et al.: Distribution of the crossed olivocochlear bundle in the chinchilla's cochlea. J Comp Neurol 182:57, 1978.

123. Spoendlin HH, and Gacek RR: Electronmicroscopic study of

the efferent and afferent innervation of the organ of Corti in the cat. Ann Otol Rhinol Laryngol 72:660, 1963.

124. Wright CG, and Preston RE: Degeneration and distribution of efferent fibers in the guinea pig organ of Corti. A light and scanning electron microscopic study. Brain Res 58:37, 1973.

125. Liberman MC, and Brown MC: Physiology and anatomy of single olivocochlear neurons in the cat. Hear Res 24:17, 1986.

126. Robertson D: Horseradish peroxidase injection of physiologically characterized afferent and efferent neurones in the guinea pig spiral ganglion. Hear Res 15:113, 1984.

127. Liberman MC: Response properties of cochlear efferent neurons: Monaural vs. binaural stimulation and the effects of noise. J Neurophysiol 60:1779, 1988.

128. Klinke R, and Galley N: Efferent innervation of vestibular and auditory receptors. Physiol Rev 54:316, 1974.

129. Desmedt JE: Physiological studies of the efferent recurrent auditory system. In Handbook of Sensory Physiology. Vol. V/2: Physiological (CNS), Behavioral Studies, Psychoacoustics. Edited by W.D. Keidel, and W.D. Neff. New York, Springer-Verlag, 1974.

130. Ishir D, and Balogh K Jr: Distribution of efferent nerve endings in the organ of Corti. Their graphic reconstruction in cochleae by localization of acetylcholinesterase activity. Acta Otolaryngol 66:282, 1968.

131. Igarashi M, Cranford JL, Nakai Y, and Alford BR: Behavioral auditory function after transection of crossed olivo-cochlear bundle in the cat. Acta Otolaryngol 87:79, 1979.

132. Moulin A, Collet L, and Duclaux R: Contralateral auditory stimulation alters acoustic distortion products in humans. Hear Res 65:193, 1993.

133. Davis H: An active process in cochlear mechanics. Hear Res 9:79–90, 1983.

134. Geisler CD: Hypothesis on the function of the crossed olivo-cochlear bundle. J Acoust Soc Am 56:1908, 1974.

135. Cody AR, and Johnstone BM: Temporary threshold shift modified by binaural acoustic stimulation. Hear Res 6:199, 1982.

136. Canlon B: The effect of acoustic trauma on the tectorial membrane, stereocilia, and hearing sensitivity: Possible mechanisms underlying damage, recovery, and protection. Scand Audiol Suppl 27:1, 1988.

137. Franklin DJ, Lonsbury-Martin BL, Stagner BB, and Martin GK: Altered susceptibility of $2f_1-f_2$ acoustic-distortion products to the effects of repeated noise exposure in rabbits. Hear Res 53:185, 1991.

138. LePage EL: Frequency-dependent self-induced bias of the basilar membrane and its potential for controlling sensitivity and tuning in the mammalian cochlea. J Acoust Soc Am 82:139, 1987.

139. Heimer L, and RoBards MJ: Neuroanatomical Tract-Tracing Methods. New York: Plenum, 1981.

140. Helfert RH, Snead CR, and Alschuler RA: The ascending auditory pathways. In Neurobiology of Hearing: The Central Auditory System. Edited by R.A. Altschuler, R.P. Bobbin, B.M. Clopton, and D.W. Hoffman. New York, Raven Press, 1991.

141. Spangler KM, and Warr WB: The descending auditory system. In Neurobiology of Hearing: The Central Auditory System. Edited by R.A. Altschuler, R.P. Bobbin, B.M. Clopton, and D.W. Hoffman. New York, Raven Press, 1991.

142. Moore JK: Cochlear nuclei: Relationship to the auditory nerve. In Neurobiology of Hearing: The Cochlea. Edited by R.A. Altschuler, D.W. Hoffman, and R.P. Bobbin. New York, Raven Press, 1986.

143. Lorente de No R: Anatomy of the eighth nerve: I. The central projection of the nerve endings of the internal ear. Laryngoscope 43:1, 1933.

144. Brawer JR, Morest DK, and Kane ES: The neuronal architecture of the cochlear nucleus of the cat. J Comp Neurol 155:251, 1974.

145. Young ED: Response characteristics of neurons of the cochlear nucleus of the cat. In Hearing Science: Recent Advances. Edited by C.I. Berlin. San Diego, College-Hill Press, 1984.

146. Thompson GC: Structure and function of the central auditory system. Sem Hear 4:81, 1983.

147. Brugge JF, Anderson DJ, and Aitkin LM: Responses of neurons in the dorsal nucleus of the lateral lemniscus of cat to binaural tonal stimulation. J Neurophysiol 33:441, 1970.

148. Goldberg JM, and Brown PB: Response of binaural neurons of dog superior olivary complex to dichotic tonal stimuli: Some physiological mechanisms of sound localization. J Neurophysiol 32:613, 1969.

149. Morest DK: The neuronal architecture of the medial geniculate body of the cat. J Anat 98:611, 1964.

150. David E et al.: Decoding processes in the auditory system and human speech analysis. In Psychophysics and Physiology of Hearing. Edited by E.F. Evans, and J.P. Wilson. New York: Academic, 1977.

151. Keidel WD: Information processing in the higher parts of the auditory pathway. In Facts and Models in Hearing. Edited by E. Zwicker, and E. Terhardt. New York, Springer-Verlag, 1974.

152. Rose JE: The cellular structure of the auditory region of the cat. J Comp Neurol 91:409, 1949.

153. Winer JA, Diamond IT, and Raczkowski D: Subdivisions of the auditory cortex of the cat: The retrograde transport of horseradish perioxidase to the medial geniculate and posterior thalamic nuclei. J Comp Neurol 176:387, 1977.

154. Phillips DP: Introduction to anatomy and physiology of the central auditory nervous system. In Physiology of the Ear. Edited by A.F. Jahn, and J. Santos-Sacchi. New York, Raven Press, 1988.

155. Coats AC: On electrocochleographic electrode design. J Acoust Soc Am 56:708, 1974.

156. Picton TW et al.: Human auditory evoked potentials. I. Evaluation of components. Electroencephalogr. Clin Neurophysiol 36:179, 1974.

157. Elberling C: Simulation of cochlear action potentials recorded from the ear canal in man. In Electrocochleography. Edited by R.J. Ruben, C. Elberling, and G. Salomon. Baltimore, University Park Press, 1976.

158. Coats AC: Human auditory nerve action potentials and brainstem evoked responses—Latency-intensity functions in detection of cochlear and retrocochlear abnormality. Arch Otolaryngol 104:709, 1978.

159. Coats AC: Electrocochleography: Recording techniques and clinical applications. Sem Hear 7:247, 1986.

160. Coats AC, Jenkins HA, and Monroe B: Auditory evoked potentials—The cochlear summating potential in detection of endolymphatic hydrops. Am J Otol 5:443, 1984.

161. Goin DW, Staller SJ, Asher DL, and Mischke RE: Summating potential in Meniere's disease. Laryngoscope 92:1383, 1982.

162. Moffat DA, et al.: Transtympanic electrocochleography during glycerol dehydration. Acta Otolaryngol 85:158, 1978.

163. Moller AR: Physiology of the ascending auditory pathway with special reference to the auditory brainstem response (ABR). In Assessment of Central Auditory Dysfunction: Foundations and Clinical Correlates. Edited by M.L. Pinheiro, and F.E. Musiek. Baltimore, Williams and Wilkins, 1985.

164. Wada S, and Starr A: Generation of auditory brainstem responses. III. Effects of lesions of the superior olive, lateral lemniscus, and inferior colliculus on the ABR in guinea pig. Electroencephalogr Clin Neurophysiol 56:352, 1983.

165. Musiek FE, Gollegly KM, Kibbe KS, and Verkest SB: Current concepts on the use of ABR and auditory psychophysical tests in the evaluation of brainstem lesions. Am J Otol Suppl 9:25, 1988.

166. Hosford-Dunn H: Auditory function tests. In Otolaryngology—Head and Neck Surgery. Edited by C.W. Cummings, et al. St. Louis, C.V. Mosby, 1986.

167. Kaga K, Hirik RF, Shimada Y, and Suzuki J: Evidence for a primary cortical origin of a middle latency auditory evoked potential in cats. Electroencephalogr Clin Neurophysiol 30:254, 1980.

168. McGee TJ, Ozdamar O, and Kraus N: Auditory middle latency responses in the guinea pig. Am J Otolaryngol 4:116, 1983.

169. Scherg M, and Von Cramer D: Topographical analysis of auditory evoked potentials: Derivation of components. In Evoked Potentials. II. Edited by R. Nodar, and C. Barber. Stoneham, MA, Butterworth, 1984.

170. Fifer RC, and Sierra-Irizzary B: Clinical applications of the auditory middle latency response. Am J Otol Suppl 9:47, 1988.

171. Kileny PR, and Kemink JL: Electrically evoked middle-latency auditory potentials in cochlear implant candidates. Arch Otolaryngol Head Neck Surg 113:1072, 1987.

172. Baran JA, Long RR, Musiek FE, and Ommaya A: Topographic mapping of brain electrical activity in the assessment of central auditory nervous system pathology. Am J Otol Suppl 9:72, 1988.

173. Duffy FH: Auditory brain mapping. In Physiology of the Ear. Edited by A.F. Jahn, and J. Santos-Sacchi. New York, Raven Press, 1988.

174. Hari R, and Lounasmaa OV: Recording and interpretation of cerebral magnetic fields. Science 244:432, 1989.

175. Hari R, Pelizzone M, Makela JP, Hallstrom Huttunen J, and Knuutila J: Neuromagnetic responses from a deaf subject to stimuli presented through a multi-channel cochlear prosthesis. Ear Hear 9:148, 1988.

176. Bray P, and Kemp DT: An advanced cochlear echo technique suitable for infant screening. Br J Audiol 21:191, 1987.

177. Kemp DT, and Ryan S: Otoacoustic emission tests in neonatal screening programmes. Acta Otolaryngol Suppl 482:73, 1991.

178. Kemp DT, and Ryan S: The use of transient evoked otoacoustic emissions in neonatal hearing screening programs. Sem Hear 14:30, 1993.

179. Balkany TJ, Telischi FF, Lonsbury-Martin BL, and Martin GK: Otoacoustic emissions in clinical practice. Am J Otol Suppl 15:29, 1994.

180. Lonsbury-Martin BL, Whitehead ML, and Martin GK: Clinical applications of otoacoustic emissions. J Sp Hear Res 34:964, 1991.

181. Martin GK, Ohlms LA, Franklin DJ, Harris FP, and Lonsbury-Martin BL: Distortion-product emissions in humans: III. Influence of sensorineural hearing loss. Ann Otol Rhinol Laryngol Suppl 147:29, 1990.

182. Hotz MA, Probst R, Harris FP, and Hauser R: Monitoring the effects of noise exposure using transiently evoked otoacoustic emissions. Acta Otolaryngol 113:478, 1993.

183. Fiore C, Cagini C, Menduno P, Toniassoni I, Desantis A, Pennacchi A, Ricci G, and Molini E: Evoked otoacoustic emissions behavior in retinitis pigmentosa. Documenta Ophthalmologica 87:167, 1994.

184. Zorowka PG, Schmitt HJ, and Gutjahr P: Evoked otoacoustic emissions and pure tone threshold audiometry in patients receiving cisplatinum therapy. Int J Ped Otorhinolaryngol 25:73, 1993.

185. Fortnum H, Farnsworth A, and Davis A: The feasibility of evoked otoacoustic emissions as an in-patient hearing check after meningitis. Br J Audiol 27:227, 1993.

186. Stover L, and Norton SJ: The effects of aging on otoacoustic emissions. J Acoust Soc Am 94:2670, 1993.

187. Hall JW, Baer JE, Chase PA, and Schwaber MK: Clinical application of otoacoustic emissions: What do we know about factors influencing measurement and analysis? Otolaryngol Head Neck Surg 110:22, 1994.

188. Lonsbury-Martin BL, Martin GK, and Balkany T: Clinical applications of otoacoustic emissions. In Highlights of the Instructional Courses—1994. Edited by F.E. Lucente. Alexandria, VA, Am Acad Otolaryngol Head Neck Surg, 1994.

189. Igarashi M, Miyata L, and Alford BR: Utricular ablation and dysequilibrium in squirrel monkeys. Acta Otolaryngol 74:66, 1972.

190. Fernandez C, and Goldberg JM: Physiology of peripheral neurons innervating otolith organs of the squirrel monkey. I. Response to static tilts and to long-duration centrifugal force. J Neurophysiol 39:970, 1976.

191. Fernandez C, and Goldberg JM: Physiology of peripheral neurons innervating otolith organs of the squirrel monkey. II. Directional selectivity and force-response relations. J Neurophysiol 39:985, 1976.

192. Fernandez C, and Goldberg JM: Physiology of peripheral neurons innervating otolith organs of the squirrel monkey. III. Response dynamics. J Neurophysiol 39:996, 1976.

193. Wendt GR: Vestibular functions. In Handbook of Experimental Psychology. Edited by S.S. Stevens. New York, John Wiley & Sons, 1951.

194. Cogan DG: Some objective and subjective observations on the vestibulo-ocular system. Am J Ophthalmol 45:74, 1958.

195. de Beer GR: Presidential address: How animals hold their heads. Proc Linn Soc Lond 159:125, 1947.

196. Juhn SK: Biochemistry of the labyrinth: A manual. Rochester, MN, Am Acad Ophthal Otolaryngol, 1973.

197. Dohlman GF: Critical review of the concept of cupula function. Acta Otolaryngol Suppl 376:1, 1980.

198. Carlstrom D, et al.: Electron microscopic and x-ray diffraction studies of statoconia. Laryngoscope 63:1052, 1953.

199. Wersall J, et al.: Ultrastructure of the vestibular end organs. In Myotatic, Kinesthetic and Vestibular Mechanisms. Edited by A.V.S. de Reuck, and J. Knight. Boston, Little, Brown, 1968.

200. Spoendlin H: Ultrastructure of the vestibular sense organ. In The Vestibular System and its Diseases. Edited by R.J. Wolfson. Philadelphia, University of Pennsylvania Press, 1966.

201. Anniko M, and Thornell LE: Cytoskeletal organization of the human inner ear. IV. Expression of actin in vestibular organs. Acta Otolaryngolog Suppl 437:65, 1987.

202. Zenner HP, and Zimmermann U: Motile responses of vestibular hair cells following caloric, electrical or chemical stimuli. Acta Otolaryngol 111:291, 1991.

203. Wersall J, et al.: Structural basis for directional sensitivity in cochlear and vestibular sensory receptors. Cold Spring Harbor Symp Quant Biol 30:115, 1965.

204. Engstrom H, Bergstrom B, and Ades HW: Macular utriculi and macular saculi in the squirrel monkey. Acta Otolaryngol Suppl 301:75, 1972.

205. Tilney LG, DeRosier DJ, and Mulroy MJ: The organization of actin filaments in the stereocilia of cochlear hair cells. J Cell Biol 86:244, 1980.

206. Assad JA, Shepherd GM, and Corey DP: Tip link integrity and mechanical transduction. Neuron 7:985, 1991.

207. Spoendlin H: Receptor ultrastructure. In Symposium on Hearing Mechanisms in Vertebrates. Edited by A.V. S. De Reuck, and J. Knight. Boston, Little Brown, 1968.

208. Hillman DE, and McLaren JW: Displacement configuration of semiciruclar canal cupulae. Neuroscience 4:1989, 1979.

209. McLaren JW, and Hillman DE: Displacement of semicircular canal cupula during sinusoidal rotation. Neuroscience 4:2001, 1979.

210. Oman CW and Young LR: Physiological range of pressure difference and cupula deflections in the human semicircular canal: theoretical considerations. Prog Brain Res 37:529, 1972.

211. Steinhausen W: The cupula. Z. Hals-, Nas. u. Ohrenheilk., 29:211, 1931.

212. Goldberg JM, and Ferenadez C: Physiology of peripheral neurons innervating semicircular canal of the squirrel monkey. J Neurophysiol 34:635, 1971.

213. Goldberg JM, and Fernandez C: Vestibular mechanisms. Ann Rev Physiol 37:129, 1975.

214. Keller EL: Behavior of horizontal semicircular canal afferents in alert monkey during vestibular and optokinetic stimulation. Exp Brain Res 24:459, 1976.

215. Fernandez C, and Goldberg JM: Physiology of peripheral neurons in innervating semicircular canals of the squirrel monkey. II. Response to sinusoidal stimulation and dynamics of peripheral vestibular system. J Neurophysiol 34:661, 1971.

216. Brodal A: Neurological Anatomy in Relation to Clinical Medicine. New York, Oxford University Press, 1969.

217. Baker R: The nucleus prepositus hypoglossi. In Eye Movements. Edited by B.A. Brooks, and F.J. Bajandos. New York, Plenum, 1977.

218. Robinson DA: Oculomotor unit behaviour in the monkey. J Neurophysiol 33:393, 1970.

219. Keller EL: The behavior of eye movement motoneurons in the alert monkey. Bibliotheca Ophthalmologica 82:7, 1972.

220. Cannon SC, and Robinson DA: Loss of the neural integrator of the oculomotor system from brainstem lesions in monkey. J Neurophysiol 57:1383, 1987.

221. Wilson VJ, et al.: Organization of the medial vestibular nucleus. J Neurophysiol 31:166, 1968.

222. Miller EF II, and Graybiel A: A comparison of ocular counter rolling movements between normal persons and deaf subjects with bilateral labyrinthine defects. Ann Otol Rhinol Laryngol 72:885, 1963.

223. Kotchabhakdi N, and Walberg F: Primary vestibular afferent projections to the cerebellum as demonstrated by retrograde axonal transport of horseradish peroxidase. Brain Res 142:142, 1978.

224. Kotchabhakdi N, and Walberg F: Cerebellar afferent projections from the vestibular nuclei in the cat: An experimental study with the method of retrograde axonal transport of horseradish peroxidase. Brain Res 31:591, 1978.

225. Andersson S, and Gernandt GE: Cortical projection of vestibular nerve in cat. Acta Otolaryngol Suppl 116:10, 1954.

226. Fredrickson JM, Frigge U, Scheid P, and Kornhuber HH: Vestibular nerve projection to the cerebral cortex of the rhesus monkey. Exp Brain Res 2:318, 1966.

227. Deecke L, et al.: The vestibular thalamus in the rhesus monkey. Adv Otorhinolaryngol 19:210, 1973.

228. Fujita Y, Rosenberg J, and Segundo JP: Activity of cells in the lateral vestibular nucleus as a function of head position. J Physiol 196:1, 1968.

229. Wilson VJ, and Melvill-Jones G: Mammalian Vestibular Physiology. New York, Plenum, 1979.

230. Precht W, Shimazu H, and Markham CH: A mechanism of central compensation of vestibular function following hemilabyrinthectomy. J Neurophysiol 29:996, 1966.

231. Fetter M, and Zee DS: Recovery from unilateral labyrinthectomy in rhesus monkey. J Neurophysiol 59:370, 1988.

232. Highstein SM: Abducens to medical rectus pathway in the MLF: A possible cellular basis for the syndrome of internuclear ophthalmoplegia. In Eye Movements. Edited by B.A. Brooks, and F.J. Bajandas. New York, Plenum, 1976.

233. Gauthier GM, and Robinson DA: Adaptation of the human vestibulo-ocular reflex to magnifying lenses. Brain Res 92:331, 1975.

234. Miles FA, and Fuller JH: Adaptive plasticity in the vestibulo-ocular responses of the rhesus monkey. Brain Res 80:512, 1974.

235. Robinson DA: Adaptive gain control of the vestibulo-ocular reflex by the cerebellum. J Neurophysiol 39:954, 1976.

236. Kohler I: Experiments with goggles. Sci Am 206:62, 1962.

237. Melvill-Jones G, et al.: Long-term effects of maintained vision reversal: Is vestibulo-ocular adaptation either necessary or sufficient? In Control of Gaze by Brainstem Neurons, Vol. 1: Developments in Neuroscience. Edited by R. Baker, and A. Berthoz. Amsterdam, Elsevier/North-Holland Biomedical, 1977.

238. Miles FA: The primate flocculus and eye-head coordination. In Eye Movements. Edited by B.A. Brooks, and F.J. Bajandas. New York, Plenum, 1977.

239. Robinson DA: Is the cerebellum too old to learn? In Eye Movements. Edited by B.A. Brooks, and F.J. Bajandas. New York, Plenum, 1977.

240. Simpson J, and Alley KE: Visual climbing fiber input to rabbit vestibulo-cerebellum: A source of direction-specific information. Brain Res 82:301, 1974.

241. Honrubia V, et al.: Effect of bilateral ablation of the vestibular cerebellum on visual-vestibular interaction. Exp Neurol 75:616, 1982.

242. Sato Y, et al.: Failure of fixation suppression of caloric nystagmus and ocular motor abnormalities. Arch Neurol 37:35, 1980.

243. Miles FA, Braitman DJ, Dow BM: Long-term adaptive changes in primate vestibulooocularreflex. IV. Electrophsyiological observations in flocculus of adapted monkeys. J Neurophysiol 43:1477, 1980.

244. Lisberger SG: The neural basis for learning of simple motor skills. Science 242:728–734, 1988.

245. Luebke AE, Robinson DA: Gain changes of the cat's vestibuo-ocular reflex after flocculus deactivation. Exp Brain Res 98:379, 1994.

246. McNally WJ, and Stuart WA: Physiology of the Labyrinth. Chicago, Am Acad Ophthalmol Otolaryngol, 1967.

247. Benson AJ, and Jobson PH: Body sway induced by a low frequency alternating current. Equilibrium Res 3:55, 1973.

248. Cohen B: Vestibulo-ocular relations. In The Control of Eye Movements. Edited by P. Bach-y-Rita, et al. New York, Academic Press, 1971.

249. Corwin JT, Jones JE, Katayama A, Kelly MW, and Warchol ME: Hair cell regeneration: The identities of progenitor cells, potential triggers, and instructive cues. In Regeneration of Vertebrate Sensory Receptor Cells (Ciba Foundation Symposium 160). Chichester, Wiley, 1991.

250. Rubel EW: Regeneration of hair cells in the avian inner ear. In Noise-induced Hearing Loss. Edited by A.L. Dancer, D. Henderson, R.J. Salvi, and R.P. Hamernik. St Louis, Mosby Yearbook, 1992.

251. Cotanche DA, Lee KH, Stone JS, and Picard DA: Hair cell regeneration in the bird cochlea following noise damage or ototoxic drug damage. Anat Embryol 189:1, 1994.

252. Cotanche DA: Regeneration of hair cell stereociliary bundles in the chick cochlea following severe acoustic trauma. Hear Res 30:181, 1987.

253. Cotanche DA: Video-enhanced DIC images of the noise-damaged and regenerated chick tectorial membrane. Exp Neurol 115:23, 1992.

254. Ryals BM, and Rubel EW: Hair cell regeneration after acoustic trauma in adult Coturnix quail. Science 240:1774, 1988.

255. Ryals BM, and Westbrook EW: TEM analysis of neural terminals on autoradiographically identified regenerated hair cells. Hear Res 72:81, 1994.

256. Cohen YE, and Saunders JC: The effects of sound overexposure on the spectral response patterns of nucleus magnocellularis in the neonatal chick. Exp Brain Res 95:202, 1993.

257. Weisleder P, and Rubel EW: Hair cell regeneration after streptomycin toxicity in the avian vestibular epithelium. J Comp Neurol 331:97, 1993.

258. Girod DA, Duckert LG, and Rubel EW: Possible precursors of regenerated hair cells in the avian cochlea following acoustic trauma. Hear Res 42:175, 1989.

259. Tsue TT, Watling DL, Weisleder P, Coltrera MD, and Rubel EW: Identification of hair cell progenitors and intermitotic migration of their nuclei in the normal and regenerating avian inner ear. J Neurosci 14:140, 1994.

260. Oberholtzer JC, Cohen EL, Davis JG: Molecular cloning of a chick cochlea cDNA encoding a subunit of DNA replication factor C/activator 1. DNA Cell Biol 13:87, 1994.

261. Ryan AF, Batcher S, Brumm D, O'Driscoll K, and Harris JP: Cloning genes from an inner ear cDNA library. Arch Otolaryngol Head Neck Surg *119:*1217, 1993.

262. Wilcox ER, and Fex J: Construction of a cDNA library from microdissected guinea pig organ of Corti. Hear Res *62:*124, 1992.

263. Wilcox ER, and Fex J: Construction of a cDNA library from microdissected guinea pig crista ampullaris. Hear Res *73:*65, 1994.

264. Metcalf AB, Chelliah, Y., and Hudspeth, A.J.: Molecular cloning of a myosin I beta isozyme that may mediate adaptation by hair cells of the bullfrog's internal ear. Proc Natl Acad Sci *91:* 118, 1994.

265. Tachibana M, Wilcox E, Yokotani N, Schneider M, and Fex J: G protein alpha subunits from cochlear tissues. Hear Res *62:* 82, 1992.

266. Furuta H, Mori N, Sato C, Hoshikawa H, Sakai S, Iwakura S, and Doi K: Mineralcorticoid type I receptor in the rat cochlea: mRNA identification by polymerase chain reaction (PCR) and in situ hybridization. Hear Res, *78:*175, 1994.

267. Elgoyhen AB, Johson DS, Boulter J, Vetter DE, and Heinemann S: α9: An acetylcholine receptor with novel pharmacological properties expressed in rat cochlear hair cells. Cell *79:*705, 1994.

268. Kuriyama H, Albin RL, and Altschuler RA: Expression of NMDA-receptor MRNA in the rat. Hear Res *69:*215, 1993.

269. Zweig G, Lipes R, and Pierce JR: The cochlear compromise. J Acoust Soc Am *59:*975, 1976.

270. Moller AR: Auditory Physiology. New York: Academic Press, 1983.

271. Salt AN, and Konishi T: The cochlear fluids: Perilymph and endolymph. *In* Neurobiology of Hearing: The Cochlea. Edited by R.A. Altschuler, D.W. Hoffman, and R.P. Bobbin. New York, Raven Press, 1986.

272. Davis H: Advances in the neurophysiology and neuroanatomy of the cochlea. J Acoust Soc Am *34:*1377, 1962.

273. Harrison RV, and Hunter-Duvar IM: An anatomical tour of the cochlea. *In* Physiology of the Ear. Edited by A.F. Jahn, and J. Santos-Sacchi. New York, Raven Press, 1988.

274. Greenwood DD: Critical bandwidth and the frequency coordinates of the basilar membrane. J Acoust Soc Am *33:*1344, 1961.

275. Gulick WL: Hearing, Physiology and Psychophysics. New York, Oxford University Press, 1971.

276. Rhode WS: Cochlear partition vibration—Recent views. J Acoust Soc Am *67:*1696, 1980.

277. Pickles JO: An Introduction to the Physiology of Hearing, 2nd Edition. London, Academic Press, 1988.

278. Katsuki Y, Sumi T, Uchiyama H, and Watanabe T: Electric responses of auditory neurons in cat to sound stimulation. J Neurophysiol *21:*569, 1958.

279. Kiang NYS: Stimulus representation in the discharge patterns of auditory neurons. *In* The Nervous System, Vol. 3: Human Communication and Its Disorders. Edited by D.B. Tower. New York, Raven Press, 1975.

280. Wersall J: Studies on the structure and innervation of the sensory epithelium of the cristae ampullaris in the guinea pig. Acta Otolaryngol Suppl *126:*1, 1956.

281. Iurato S: Submicroscopic Structure of the Inner Ear. Oxford, Pergamon Press, 1967.

282. Lindeman HH, et al.: The sensory hairs and the tectorial membrane in the development of the cat's organ of Corti. Acta Otolaryngol *72:*229, 1971.

283. Baloh R, and Honrubia V: Clinical Neurophysiology of the Vestibular System, 2nd Edition. Philadelphia, F.A. Davis, 1990.

284. Zee DS, and Leigh RJ: The Neurology of Eye Movements, 2nd Edition. Philadelphia, F.A. Davis, 1991.

285. Carpenter MB: Human Neuroanatomy, 7th Edition. Baltimore, Williams and Wilkins, 1976.

FURTHER SUGGESTED READINGS

Corwin JT, and Warchol ME: Auditory hair cells: Structure, function, development and regeneration. Ann Rev Neurosci *14:*301, 1992.

Counter SA: Electromagnetic stimulation of the auditory system: Effects and side-effects. Scand Audiol Suppl *37:*1, 1993.

Dallos P: The active cochlea. J Neurosci *12:*4575, 1992.

Dallos P, and Corey ME The role of outer hair cell motility in cochlear tuning. Cur Opin Neurobiol *1:*215, 1991.

Davis H: Mechanisms of the inner ear. Ann Otol Rhinol Laryngol *77:*644, 1968.

Dobie RA: Objective response detection. Ear Hear *14:*31, 1993.

Harrison JM, and Howe ME: Anatomy of the afferent auditory nervous system of mammals. *In* Handbook of Sensory Physiology, Vol. V/1: Auditory System, Anatomy Physiology (Ear). Edited by W.D. Keidel, and W.D. Neff. New York, Springer-Verlag, 1974.

Hudspeth AJ: Mechanoelectrical transduction by hair cells in the acousticolateralis sensory system. Ann Rev Neurosci *6:*187, 1983.

Margolis RH: Detection of hearing impairment with the acoustic stapedius reflex. Ear Hear *14:*3, 1993.

Osterhammel PA, Nielsen LH, and Rasmussen AN: Distortion product otoacoustic emissions. The influence of the middle ear transmission. Scand Audiol *22:*111, 1993.

Shallop JK: Objective electrophysiological measures from cochlear implant patients. Ear Hear *14:*58, 1993.

Stasche N, Foth HJ, Hormann K, Baker A, and Huthoff C: Middle ear transmission disorders—Tympanic membrane vibration analysis by laser-Doppler-vibrometry. Acta Otolaryngol *114:*59, 1994.

43 Evaluation of the Vestibular System

Alfred C. Coats

The four tests most commonly used in current clinical practice to evaluate patients with balance disorders are 1) the electronystagmography (ENG) test battery, 2) the low-frequency rotation test (rotary chair test), 3) the high-frequency rotation test (the vestibular autorotation test (VAT), and 4) computerized dynamic posturography (CDP). For each of these, the test and analysis techniques will be reviewed and the clinical significance of the results will be discussed. The discussion will, of necessity, be brief. For more detailed coverage of these and other, less frequently used balance tests, the reader is referred to current reviews.[1-4]

A significant advance in vestibulometry during the past decade has been the addition of computerized analysis. Therefore, computerized measurements will be featured in the discussion of test results and their clinical interpretation.

Use of training regimens to treat patients with balance disorders, a clinical paradigm known as "vestibular rehabilitation," has grown rapidly in recent years.[5-7] Vestibular rehabilitation has added a new dimension to the clinical application of vestibulometric results. Traditionally, vestibulometry has been used to localize deficits—usually to either the central nervous system or the peripheral vestibular system. However, when used to evaluate patients undergoing vestibular rehabilitation, some vestibulometric measurements have been found useful as a means of quantifying functional status without necessarily addressing the location of the abnormality causing the functional deficit. These functional status measurements are useful in designing, setting goals for, and monitoring the progress of, vestibular rehabilitation training programs. Therefore, the discussion of clinical significance will be divided into two categories: deficit localization and functional assessment.

In discussing localizing significance, abnormalities are classified as "central" (defined, according to the neurological convention used to classify cranial nerve deficits as central to the entrance of the vestibular nerve into the brainstem), "peripheral" (peripheral to the nerve-brainstem boundary) or "nonlocalizing" (abnormal, but by themselves, not providing localizing information).

ELECTRONYSTAGMOGRAPHY (ENG)

The ENG is essentially a battery of tests drawn from the otologic, neurotologic, and neurologic physical examinations. The tests are basically the same as those done in the office or at the bedside. The only substantial differences are 1) nystagmus is recorded by electro-oculography (EOG) rather than observed visually, and 2) techniques for inducing nystagmus are quantified with greater care.

Although there are no formal "standards" for clinical vestibulometry, there is a reasonable consensus concerning the tests to be included in the ENG examination and the basic techniques for performing them. Table 43-1 lists the tests that comprise the basic ENG examination, in the order in which they are typically performed.

Principle of Electro-oculography

The EOG is produced by a constant voltage generated within the retina (probably in the pigment epithelium), which is often called the "corneoretinal potential". Figure 43-1 illustrates the principle. The corneoretinal potential and the insulating properties of the sclera cause the eyeball to behave like an electrical dipole,[8,9] a common example of which is the flashlight battery. Rotation of the "battery" creates a voltage change that can be detected by electrodes placed on the surface of the head. This voltage change is amplified and either made to drive a recorder or sent to a computer. The EOG electrodes record only eye movements in the plane of

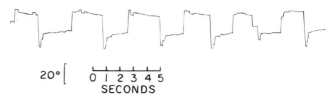

$20°$ [

0 1 2 3 4 5
SECONDS

Fig. 43–2. Example of ocular dysmetria manifested as "overshoots" when the patient looks back and forth between fixation points positioned 10° on either side of midline. In all records in this chapter, upward deflection represents eye movements to the right in horizontal eye movement and upward in vertical eye movement.

TABLE 43–1. Tests Comprising the ENG Examination

Calibration
Test for gaze nystagmus
Optokinetic test
Sinusoidal tracking test
Saccade velocity test
Dix-Hallpike test for paroxysmal nystagmus
Position test
Caloric test

the electrode pair. Consequently, two pairs of electrodes are required to record both horizontal and vertical eye movements.

Ocular Dysmetria Test

Ocular dysmetria is an overshoot or undershoot of the eye rotation that occurs when visual fixation is transferred from one place to another (a "refixation movement" or "saccade"). Overshoot dysmetria ("hypermetric" saccades) is thought to originate in the cerebellum,[10–12] but in practical clinical application it indicates either cerebellar or brainstem pathology. Undershoots of refixation saccades ("hypometric" saccades) are fairly common in clinically normal individu-

als,[13] hence are not as significant clinically as saccadic overshoot. However, undershoot dysmetria can be caused by visual deficits (e.g., hemianopsia and cataracts) and a variety of neurologic disorders, including cerebellar and brainstem disorders and Parkinson's disease.[14]

Because of the fleeting nature and small amplitude of the typical dysmetric eye movement, obtaining a graphic record of it has obvious advantages. Haring and Simmons[15] pointed out that ocular dysmetria may be recorded in the course of the routine ENG calibration ("calibration overshoot"). Thus, a valuable central sign may be detected during the ENG examination with virtually no investment in additional examination time. Figure 43–2 shows an example of overshoot ocular dysmetria recorded during a 20-degree eye-movement calibration of a patient with traumatic cerebellar injury.

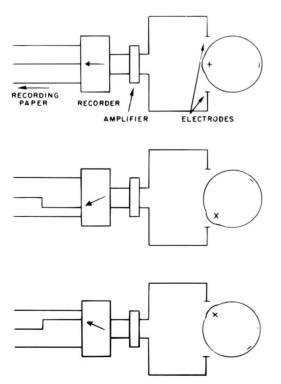

Fig. 43–1. The principle of electro-oculography. the corneoretinal potential is shown as a positive voltage (+) at the front of the eye and the negative voltage (−) at the back of the eye. Eye movement displaces the voltage difference between the front and back of the eye. This displacement is recorded by electrodes positioned in the plane of the eye movement.

Gaze Test

The gaze test examines for gaze nystagmus, defined as a nystagmus that is not present with the eyes centered but is present when the eyes are deviated away from center. The gaze test also examines for paresis of ocular rotation. Gaze nystagmus almost always demonstrates the following characteristics: 1) it is divided into slow and fast components, with the fast component in the direction of eye deviation; and 2) its amplitude and slow-component speed increase with increasing eye deviation.

Technique

When performing the gaze test in the ENG laboratory, the amount of eye deviation is quantified to rule out end-point nystagmus, which occurs in approximately 50% of normal individuals on extreme eye deviation (approximately 55 degrees from center) and probably in approximately 10% of normals with eyes deviated 40 degrees.[16,17] In the test for gaze nystagmus, the patient gazes steadily at fixation points 20 and 30 degrees to the right and left and above and below center. Gaze is maintained for 30 seconds in each of the eight eye positions.

Gaze nystagmus may be present but not recordable by EOG, either because its amplitude is too low or because it is rotary. In addition, paretic eye movements may be easier to observe visually than to record. Therefore, during the gaze test it is important to watch the patient's eyes while recording their movements.

Diagnostic Significance

Gaze nystagmus and gaze paresis usually indicate the presence of central nervous system pathology. Particularly if persistent for a month or more, these findings further suggest brainstem or cerebellar involvement.[18] Figure 43-3 illustrates a recording of gaze nystagmus in a patient with a brainstem glioma.

The major exceptions to the these statements of the localizing significance of gaze nystagmus are 1) intense spontaneous nystagmus (visible only behind closed eyelids), causing a unilateral horizontal-gaze nystagmus,[19-21] and 2) diphenylhydantoin (Dilantin, Parke Davis, Morris Plains, NJ) or barbiturates,[22-24] causing horizontal gaze nystagmus, which is usually bilateral, but may occasionally be unilateral.[25]

Sinusoidal-Tracking Test

Technique

The sinusoidal-tracking or ocular-smooth-pursuit test is most commonly performed by having the patient fix on a spot that is moving in a sinusoidal pattern.[26,27] Frequencies of 0.3 and 0.6 Hz are commonly used with the pattern subtending an angle of ±15 degrees from center gaze.[28] In this manner, eye tracking movements in both the vertical and horizontal directions are elicited.

Diagnostic Significance

An individual without neurologic or ocular abnormalities should be able to track the moving fixation point

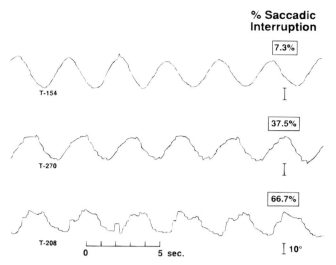

Fig. 43–4. Examples of horizontal sinusoidal tracking showing varying degrees of "saccadic interruption" or "breakup." Computer quantified measurements of saccadic interruption are shown to the right, and above each record.

smoothly (e.g., Figure 43–4, top) although brief fixations on other objects may occasionally interrupt the smooth sinusoidal pattern. In the abnormal tracking pattern, saccadic eye jerks in the direction of spot movement repeatedly "break up" the smooth sinusoidal pattern. This abnormality indicates the presence of central nervous system pathology.[29-32] However, it yields a high incidence of "false positive" results, defined as an isolated finding in a patient with no other objective abnormalities. Supporting this high false positive incidence are reports of abnormal ocular tracking tests in subjects taking mildly psychoactive drugs[33,34] and in healthy relatives of patients with schizophrenia.[35]

Figure 43–4 illustrates normal and abnormal sinusoidal tracking patterns and one method of computer quantifying them. The computer calculates "percent saccadic interruption" measurements,[28] shown at the right of the figure, by detecting interrupting saccades, measuring their amplitude, and dividing total interrupting saccade amplitude by total peak-to-peak tracking pattern amplitude. Many computerized ENG systems quantify saccadic interruption by calculating smooth pursuit "gain", which is the amplitude of the eye tracking pattern after saccade removal divided by the amplitude of the tracking stimulus. Although actual measurements may sometimes yield minor differences, percent saccadic interruption may, for practical clinical purposes, be converted to "gain" by subtracting it from 100%.

Sometimes another useful sinusoidal tracking abnormality may be seen—a tendency for gaze nystagmus to appear in an enhanced form at the extremes

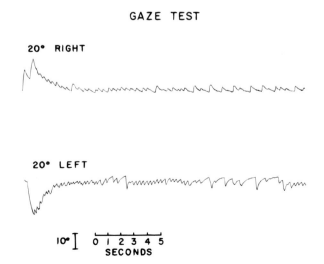

Fig. 43–3. Recording of bilateral, unequal horizontal gaze nystagmus from a patient with an intrinsic pontine glioma.

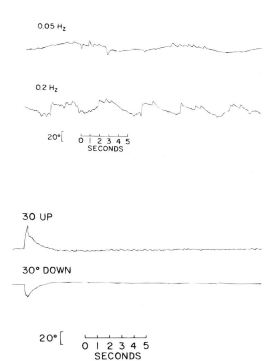

Fig. 43–5. Vertical sinusoidal tracking (top) and vertical gaze test (bottom) demonstrating nystagmus-like beats at the tracking pattern extreme corresponding to the direction of gaze producing the gaze nystagmus. The patient had a long history of multiple sclerosis.

of the sinusoidal pattern.[26] Figure 43–5 illustrates this pattern in a patient with an up-beating vertical gaze nystagmus. Often this tracking abnormality combines with gaze nystagmus and "breakup" patterns.

Saccadic Velocity Test

A saccade is a rapid (up to 800° second)[1,3,36,37] eye movement that typically occurs when eye position is shifted abruptly from one fixation point to another (e.g., between fixations during reading). Nystagmus fast components have many of the same characteristics as refixation saccades. Eye velocity during a saccade is difficult to measure manually but is easy to measure with digital processing techniques. When evaluating for an abnormality, saccade velocity is normalized against amplitude, because, in healthy subjects, saccade velocity increases with increasing saccadic amplitude.[28,37,38] Other saccade parameters that have been proposed for diagnostic use include saccade latency (time from refixation command to beginning of saccade), "saccade accuracy" (amplitude relative to the distance between refixation points), and saccade form (e.g., a single large refixation movement versus a response that is broken up into a series of small hypometric saccades).[39–41] Because it is sensitive to the subject's mental state,[42] saccade latency is regarded commonly as of less clinical utility than saccade velocity.

Technique

A typical saccade test is performed with the patient in front of a linear array of controlled fixation points (e.g., small lights or spots on a television screen).[28,36,41] Movements are recorded separately from each eye. The patient is asked to follow the fixation points while they illuminate and extinguish randomly. In this way saccades of varying amplitude, usually from 5° to 55, are recorded from each eye.

Diagnostic Significance

The basic principles used in interpreting saccade test results are:

1. Saccadic velocity is decreased when refixation is attempted in the direction of a paresis.[41,43] Thus, for example, a left lateral rectus paresis would cause a decrease in velocity of the abducting saccade in the left eye.[43]
2. Conjugate impairments of saccadic velocity are caused by central pathologic conditions, whereas uniocular impairments are caused by either peripheral oculomotor or medial longitudinal fasciculus deficits.[38,40,41,43–48] Table 43–2 summarizes the localizing significance of saccade abnormalities.
3. Anticonvulsants and benzeodiazapines can cause saccade slowing.[49–51]

Optokinetic Test

Optokinetic nystagmus (OKN) occurs when one looks at a moving repetitive pattern (black stripes on a white

TABLE 43–2. Localizing Significance of Saccade Abnormalities

Extraocular muscle paresis	Slowed velocity and normal amplitude in direction of paretic muscle—uniocular
Entrapment of extraocular muscle	Reduced amplitude and normal velocity in direction of entrapped muscle—uniocular
Medical longitudinal fasciculus syndrome	Adducting saccade of eye on side of lesion is slowed
	Abducting saccade of eye opposite lesion overshoots
Lesion of cerebellopontine angle	None
Lesions of pons and medulla	Slowed velocity in both directions—conjugate
Spinocerebellar degeneration	Slowed velocity in both directions—conjugate
Cerebellar lesions	Normal velocity
	Increased latency
	Tendency toward multiple low-amplitude saccades

background usually are used) that fills most or all of the visual field.[52,53] Optokinetic nystagmus has alternating slow (following) components in the direction of pattern movement and fast (refixation) components opposite the direction of pattern movement. It is involuntary if fixation on the moving pattern is maintained.

Technique

The optokinetic test consists, in essence, of eliciting oppositely directed OKN at equal stimulus speeds and examining the nystagmus for asymmetry and bilateral absence or deficiency. In most clinical ENG laboratories, the optokinetic test is performed with an optokinetic drum which can be either hand-operated or motor-driven (Fig. 43–6). In larger centers, the optokinetic test is performed by placing the patient inside a large, internally lighted cylinder which is usually included with the rotatory chair apparatus (Fig. 43–18).

When eliciting OKN with a hand-held drum, avoid eliciting a voluntary tracking pattern rather than the involuntary optokinetic reflex.[54] A "nystagmus" that has high amplitude and low frequency indicates that the patient is voluntarily tracking the optokinetic stimulus rather than generating an involuntary optokinetic reflex. This voluntary "look nystagmus" pattern is often seen when the patient is given too-detailed instructions (e.g., "Follow each stripe."). The high frequency, low amplitude "stare nystagmus" pattern, indicative of the involuntary optokinetic reflex, is best elicited by minimally instructing the patient (e.g., "Watch the stripes.") and encouraging when the appropriate pattern is seen on the record (Figure 43–7).

An important consideration is whether the hand-held optokinetic drum, which fills only approximately 30% of the patient's visual field, elicits "true" optokinetic nystagmus or whether it stimulates only the smooth pursuit system. Some authorities believe that only a full-field stimulus elicits "true" optokinetic nystagmus, presumably because circularvection (a sensa-

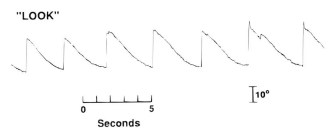

"STARE"

"LOOK"

Fig. 43–7. Recordings of "stare" (top) and "look" (bottom) optokinetic nystagmus. The "stare" optokinetic nystagmus (top) was obtained by instructing the subject to "watch the stripes go by". The "look" nystagmus was obtained by instructing the subject to "pick up one stripe as it comes around the edge of the drum and follow it to the opposite edge, then go back and pick up another stripe."

tion of self-rotation) is elicited by the full-field stimulus, but not by an optokinetic drum.[4,42,55]

However, "stare" OKN elicited with an optokinetic drum seems clearly different from a voluntary smooth pursuit response, because 1) normal smooth pursuit tests can be found in patients with optokinetic asymmetries demonstrated with a hand-held drum; 2) The high-frequency, low-amplitude "stare" OKN pattern is impossible to elicit voluntarily; 3) the incidence of saccadic interruption of the OKN fast components increases when drum speed is increased from 13°/sec to 26°/sec in contrast to voluntary pursuit, where incidence of saccadic interruption increases when tracking pattern speed is increased[28,56]; and 4) circularvection does not invariably accompany OKN. The presence or absence of circularvection is less dependent on the size of the stimulus than on whether or not the visual "background" moves or is stationary.[57,58]

In the clinical optokinetic test, vertical as well as horizontal OKN should be included, because if it is not, a significant number of abnormalities will be missed.[19,59] However, interpretation of the vertical optokinetic responses for asymmetry must take into account the fact that there is a tendency for upbeating OKN to predominate in clinically normal individuals.[28]

Quantification Methods

Two characteristics of OKN are analyzed: 1) absolute slow component speeds to test for bilateral diminution or reduced gain, and 2) right-left and up-down slow component speed differences to test for asymmetry. As discussed below, when testing with a hand-held drum the OKN asymmetry test is more useful clinically than the test for bilateral diminution.

Figure 43–8 shows examples of computer-quantified optokinetic responses. Two patterns of optokinetic asymmetry can be seen: 1) a "poorly formed" pattern

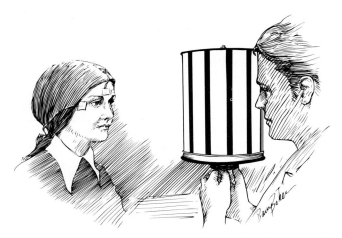

Fig. 43–6. Use of a hand-held drum, which can be either manually operated or motor driven, to elicit optokinetic nystagmus.

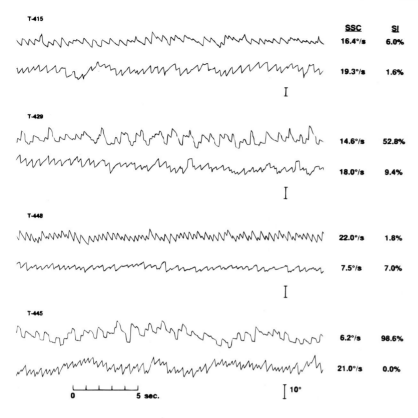

	SSC	SI
T-415	16.4°/s	6.0%
	19.3°/s	1.6%
T-429	14.6°/s	52.8%
	18.0°/s	9.4%
T-448	22.0°/s	1.8%
	7.5°/s	7.0%
T-445	6.2°/s	98.6%
	21.0°/s	0.0%

Fig. 43–8. Optokinetic tests illustrating varying degrees of asymmetry. All tests were obtained with a hand-held motor-driven drum. "SSC" = speed of slow component. SI = saccadic interruption.

where the OKN slow components are repeatedly interrupted by saccades in the direction of the slow components (a pattern reminiscent of smooth pursuit "breakup"), and 2) a slow component speed difference. The computer quantifies the responses by extracting and measuring the amplitude of interrupting saccades and measuring the average velocity of the remaining "pure" slow components. A "saccadic interruption" measurement is also calculated by expressing the total amplitude of the interrupting saccades as a percentage of the total slow component amplitude.

As shown in Figure 43–8, OKN asymmetry can appear as a predominantly saccadic interruption pattern (Record T-429), as a predominantly slow component speed difference (Record T-448), or as a combination of the two patterns (Record T-445). Optokinetic asymmetry can be quantified by expressing the difference between the oppositely directed optokinetic (OKN) slow component speeds as a percentage of their sum. When applying a 25 degree/second "equivalent stimulus speed" (the speed at which the eye would rotate if it followed the moving pattern exactly) stimulus with a motor-driven optokinetic drum, one study reported the limit of normal (95% confidence limits) for OKN asymmetry to be ±25% for the horizontal responses and +63% (up-beating predominant) and −31% (down-beating predominant) for the vertical responses.[28]

The saccadic interruption asymmetry measurement

can be obtained by subtracting the two percentages. Limit of normal for this measurement has been found to be ±10% for horizontal OKN and over ±100% for vertical OKN (indicating that the saccadic interruption measurement is not clinically useful with vertical OKN).[28]

Diagnostic Significance

OKN ASYMMETRY. An intense spontaneous nystagmus of peripheral vestibular origin, even if detectable only in the absence of visual fixation, can cause a predominance of the OKN beating in the direction of the spontaneous nystagmus.[60,61] If, however, intense spontaneous nystagmus in the direction of an OKN asymmetry is not present (easily determined by simply recording eye movements with the patient's eyes closed), and if peripheral ocular or oculomotor pathology can also be ruled out, OKN asymmetry indicates the presence of a central nervous system deficit.[19,52] If an OKN asymmetry is associated with a gaze nystagmus or gaze paresis, brainstem or cerebellar pathology, is probable.[19,27,62] If a normal gaze test accompanies an OKN asymmetry, a cerebral hemisphere is probably involved, and the fast component of the predominant OKN is commonly directed toward the involved side.[19,27] An isolated vertical OKN asymmetry suggests bilateral or midline lesions in the midbrain or upper pons.[27,59,63]

BILATERALLY DEFICIENT OKN. Although OKN is involuntary if fixation is maintained, in practice, OKN is under considerable voluntary control when elicited with an optokinetic drum because the patient can influence his OKN by varying his fixation on the drum.[27,52] Hence, lack of cooperation must always be suspected in cases of bilateral OKN diminution or absence—particularly if found when testing with an optokinetic drum. If, however, lack of cooperation can be ruled out, bilaterally absent or deficient OKN has essentially the same localizing significance as vertical OKN asymmetry, i.e., it suggests a high brainstem lesion, either bilateral or midline.[42]

Spontaneous Nystagmus

Spontaneous nystagmus may be defined as a nystagmus present with head upright and eyes centered. Although perhaps somewhat arbitrary, this definition has the virtue of being logical, because head upright with eyes centered is the best approximation of the "neutral" position in the human.

Technique

To record spontaneous nystagmus, vertical and horizontal eye-movement records are obtained with the patient's head upright and his eyes centered and open for 30 to 60 seconds then closed for an additional 30 to 60 seconds.

Diagnostic Significance

Pathologic spontaneous nystagmus may be classified according to its probable system of origin, i.e., vestibular, ocular, or central. This classification is analogous to Cogan's "otologic," "ocular," and "neurologic" divisions.[64] Others have proposed similar classifications.[65] The classification schema presented here includes a fourth category—"normal," which is required when considering nystagmus recorded in the absence of visual fixation.[66] Table 43–3 summarizes this clinical classification of spontaneous nystagmus.

TABLE 43–3. Classification of Spontaneous Nystagmus

Normal
  Vertical, behind closed eyelids
  Horizontal, behind closed eyelids <7.5°/sec (hand measured) or
    5°/sec (computer measured)
  Voluntary
Vestibular (Otologic)
  Fast and slow phases
  Horizontal
  Conjugate
  Suppressed by visual fixation
Ocular (Ophthalmologic)
  Congenital
  Occupational
Central (Neurologic)
  Diagnosis made by excluding other types

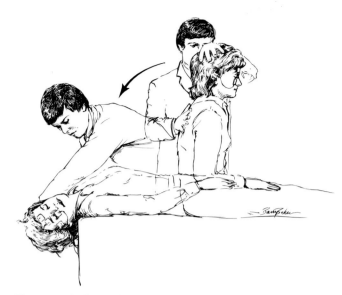

Fig. 43–9. The Dix-Hallpike maneuver for eliciting paroxysmal nystagmus.

Paroxysmal Nystagmus

Paroxysmal nystagmus is a burst of abnormal nystagmus elicited by the maneuver illustrated in Figure 43–9. Dix and Hallpike[67] first described this maneuver and the abnormal nystagmic response, which they termed "benign paroxysmal positional nystagmus." An important point of nomenclature is whether "positional" should be used when referring to the abnormal nystagmus elicited by the Dix-Hallpike maneuver. Independent observers have demonstrated that if the Dix-Hallpike maneuver and the position test both elicit nystagmus, the responses often are directed oppositely.[68,69] Figure 43–10 shows an example of this outcome. Therefore, "positional nystagmus of the benign paroxysmal type" depends not on the final head position but on the maneuver preceding it. Hence, use of the word "positional" in describing a positive response to the Dix-Hallpike maneuver may be invalid.

Technique

The Dix-Hallpike maneuver consists of bringing the patient rapidly from the sitting to the head-hanging-and-turned position. The maneuver is done once with the head turned in each direction (Figure 43–9). If either maneuver elicits paroxysmal nystagmus, it is repeated to see if the response "fatigues."

In the ENG-recorded paroxysmal nystagmus test, the eyes are closed and the nystagmic response is recorded rather than visually observed. Although paroxysmal nystagmus is usually primarily rotatory, it almost always has sufficient vertical or horizontal components to be recordable.[70–72] Because the vertical component is often predominant, however,[71,73] paroxysmal nystagmus frequently will be missed if vertical eye movements are not recorded.

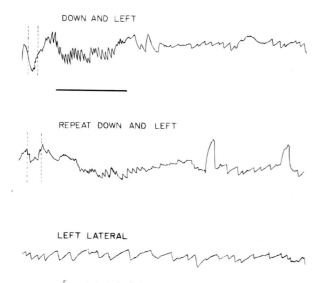

Fig. 43–10. Example of classic paroxysmal nystagmus coexisting with oppositely-directed positional nystagmus. The two top tracings show a right-beating paroxysmal nystagmus coexisting with a moderate left-beating positional nystagmus which is shown in the bottom trace taken from the position test. The black bar below the top records indicates approximate period of dizziness. The dashed lines indicate the period during which the Dix-Hallpike maneuver was in progress.

TABLE 43–4. Classification of Positional Nystagmus

Persistent—continues for at least 1 minute after assuming the test position

  Type I (direction changing)—beats in one direction in one (or more) positions

  Type II (direction fixed)—beats in the same direction whenever present

Transitory—goes away within 1 minute after assuming the test position; also called "type III positioning nystagmus"

response is considered "classic." A nonclassic paroxysmal nystagmus is a nonlocalizing sign.

Position Test

The position test looks for nystagmus in a series of standard head positions. Unlike the paroxysmal nystagmus test, movement into each position is as slow as possible to exclude the effect of head movement. Most authorities use Aschan and coworkers' modification of Nylen's classification as outlined in Table 43–4.[75-77] Figure 43–11 shows an example of type I (persistent, direction changing) positional nystagmus. Type III positional nystagmus includes all varieties of pathologic transient positional nystagmus. Because it

Diagnostic Significance

It is helpful to distinguish between "classic" and "nonclassic" paroxysmal nystagmus. Classic paroxysmal nystagmus is so named because it fits the definition of the response that Dix and Hallpike originally described.[67] Figure 43–10 shows an example of classic paroxysmal nystagmus. The essential criteria of classic paroxysmal nystagmus are: 1) dizziness, accompanying the nystagmus, 2) a latent period of 0.5 to 15 seconds between the arrival at the head-hanging-and-turned position and the beginning of the nystagmus, 3) transient nystagmus response, and 4) response to a repeat maneuver is less intense than the response to the original maneuver, i.e., the response "fatigues."

Classic paroxysmal nystagmus suggests peripheral vestibular pathology. Usually the involved ear is the ear that is down when the nystagmus is elicited. Patients with classic paroxysmal nystagmus tend to cluster into the following clinical types: 1) elderly patients (older than 65 years), 2) those with post-traumatic dizziness, 3) those with middle-ear pathology, and 4) those with prior surgical manipulation of the stapes or round window.[74]

Nonclassic paroxysmal nystagmus is a positive response to the Dix-Hallpike maneuver that does not meet one or more of the criteria of a classic response (e.g., it does not fatigue when the maneuver is repeated); except that, if a clear latent period is not present and the response meets the other three criteria, the

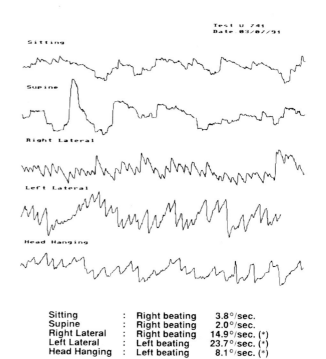

Sitting	: Right beating	3.8°/sec.
Supine	: Right beating	2.0°/sec.
Right Lateral	: Right beating	14.9°/sec. (*)
Left Lateral	: Left beating	23.7°/sec. (*)
Head Hanging	: Left beating	8.1°/sec. (*)

Fig. 43–11. Example of a low-intensity, right-beating spontaneous nystagmus (seen in the sitting position), with intense, direction-changing positional component (right-beating in the right lateral position and left-beating in the left lateral and head-hanging positions). Computer analysis results are shown at bottom. The (*) labels on the bottom three slow phase speed measurements indicate that the measurements are outside predetermined "normal" limits.

is, by definition, transient, type III ''positional'' nystagmus is often called ''positioning'' nystagmus. A transient positional nystagmus may be a partially-elicited paroxysmal nystagmus. However, some transient positional responses either do not have a typical ''paroxysmal'' time course or are accompanied by a negative Dix-Hallpike test.

Technique

Eyes-closed records of at least 30 seconds are obtained with the patient in the sitting, supine, right lateral, left lateral, and head-hanging positions. The records are interpreted for presence or absence of nystagmus, and, if nystagmus is present, its direction and slow-component speed are quantified. When the records are interpreted manually, a ''guesstimate'' of intensity usually is made (e.g., ''low'' = slow-component speed less than about 4.5°/sec; ''moderate'' = slow component speed between about 4.5 and 7.5°/sec, and ''intense'' = slow component speed greater than about 7.5°/sec).[78] With computer analysis a quantitative slow component speed measurement can be made conveniently. However, computer nystagmus slow component speed measurements tend to be about 25% less than manual measurements.[28,79]

Diagnostic Significance

LOW-INTENSITY POSITIONAL NYSTAGMUS. As with spontaneous nystagmus (Table 43–3), at least 80% of apparently healthy subjects have, in the absence of visual fixation, a positional nystagmus with a slow-component speed of less than 7.5°/second when hand measured or 5.5°/sec when computer measured.[66] Low-intensity positional nystagmus is therefore of doubtful pathologic significance.

MODERATE- AND HIGH-INTENSITY POSITIONAL NYSTAGMUS. Although some authors have reported a statistical tendency for direction-changing positional nystagmus to occur in central lesions and direction-fixed positional nystagmus to occur in peripheral lesions,[80,81] this tendency is not sufficiently strong to be useful clinically.[77,82–84] Therefore, positional nystagmus, either type I or type II, with a manually-measured or computer-measured slow component speed of more than 7.5°/second 5.5°/second respectively is a nonlocalizing abnormality.

Alcohol may cause positional nystagmus, usually direction changing, which may persist for as long as 48 hours after ingestion.[81,85,86] Therefore, when a direction-changing positional nystagmus is encountered as an isolated finding, the possibility of prior alcohol ingestion must be ruled out.

POSITIONING NYSTAGMUS. Because it is relatively uncommon, there has been little or no systematic study of the diagnostic significance of positioning nystagmus. Therefore, until better information is available, this finding must be considered nonlocalizing.

Bithermal-Caloric Test

Technique

In the bithermal-caloric test, cold and warm caloric responses are obtained from each ear, with the temperatures equally above and below body temperature.[87] Figure 43–12 illustrates a caloric irrigation. The patient is supine, with the head inclined 30° to bring the horizontal canal into the vertical position. Each ear is irrigated for 40 seconds, to produce a volume of approximately 250 mL, at temperatures of 31°C and 43°C. (Many laboratories use 30 second irrigations at 30°C and 44°C—the parameters originally proposed by Aschan, et al. However, the author believes that the longer duration and lower warm temperature gives a less variable thermal stimulus.) Just after the caloric response maximum has passed, the patient is asked to look at a target for about 20 seconds (e.g., the eyes

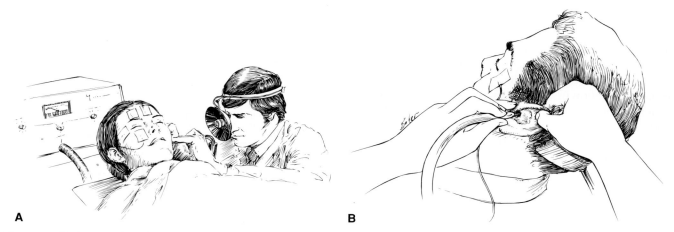

A   **B**

Fig. 43–12. Performing the caloric irrigation. A. A dual, constant termperature reservoir can be seen behind the patient. B. Tester's view of the irrigating tip inserted into the ear. A catch basin normally placed under the patient's ear, is not shown.

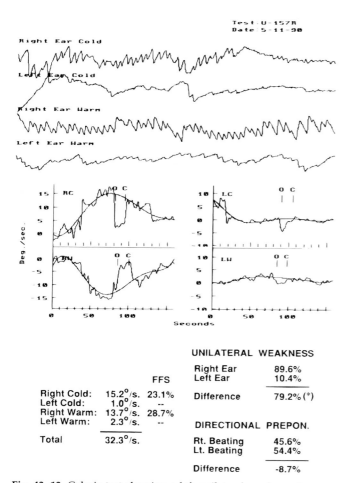

		FFS
Right Cold:	15.2°/s.	23.1%
Left Cold:	1.0°/s.	--
Right Warm:	13.7°/s.	28.7%
Left Warm:	2.3°/s.	--
Total	32.3°/s.	

UNILATERAL WEAKNESS

Right Ear	89.6%
Left Ear	10.4%
Difference	79.2% (*)

DIRECTIONAL PREPON.

Rt. Beating	45.6%
Lt. Beating	54.4%
Difference	-8.7%

Fig. 43–13. Caloric test showing a left unilateral weakness from a patient with a left acoustic neurilemmoma. The records at top show the raw nystagmus traces during the periods of maximum slow phase speed. Graphs in the center show the caloric response slow phase speed time courses. The more variable curves are 10 second moving averages of all slow phase speed data points. "O" = open; "C" = closed. The smooth curves are polynomials fitted to the 10 second moving average data, excluding data points during the eyes open periods. At bottom left are shown (1) the four maximum caloric nystagmus slow component speed measurements in degrees per second ("°/s") taken from the fitted polynomial peaks and (2) the failure of fixation suppression ("FFS") measurements. At bottom right are shown unilateral weakness and directional preponderance measurements. The "(*)" label indicates a result that is outside normal limits.

open-closed, "O-C", period in Figure 43–13 to test the ability of visual fixation to suppress caloric nystagmus.

A rest period of at least 5 minutes is allowed between the disappearance of one caloric response and the beginning of the next irrigation. Because large fluctuations in corneoretinal potential amplitude can occur,[88] the amplitude calibration should be repeated before each irrigation. To minimize central suppression of the caloric responses, the patient is instructed to perform aloud a "concentration task" (e.g., subtracting serial sevens) during each response.[89,90,91] The task's difficulty is adjusted to match the patient's ability.

Quantification Methods

MAXIMUM SLOW COMPONENT SPEED. Maximum slow component speed is used almost universally as the measure of caloric response intensity. The most direct way of manually measuring slow component speed is to measure the slow component's amplitude and duration and divide duration into amplitude. In terms of the record's appearance, this determines the slow component's steepness or slope. In manual measurements the effect of random slow-component speed fluctuations is minimized by averaging across several (at least 10) beats.

Computerized systems typically quantify a caloric response by first differentiating it to convert the eye position signal into an eye velocity signal, then removing saccades and other "artifacts" (e.g., eyeblinks) to obtain a "pure" slow component speed record. The pure slow component speed record is then subjected to a smoothing process, which varies from system to system, and the maximum slow component speed is determined from the maximum point of this smoothed curve.[28]

In the computer-quantified caloric test examples

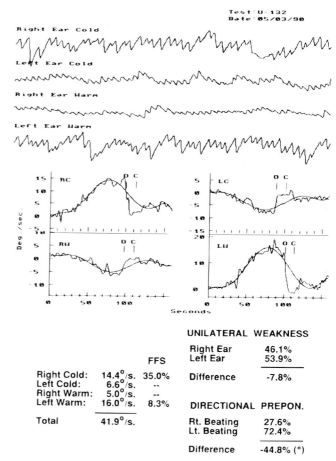

		FFS
Right Cold:	14.4°/s.	35.0%
Left Cold:	6.6°/s.	--
Right Warm:	5.0°/s.	--
Left Warm:	16.0°/s.	8.3%
Total	41.9°/s.	

UNILATERAL WEAKNESS

Right Ear	46.1%
Left Ear	53.9%
Difference	-7.8%

DIRECTIONAL PREPON.

Rt. Beating	27.6%
Lt. Beating	72.4%
Difference	-44.8% (*)

Fig. 43–14. Caloric test showing a directional preponderance to the left in a patient with probable left endolymphatic hydrops. Labeling conventions are as described in the Figure 43–13.

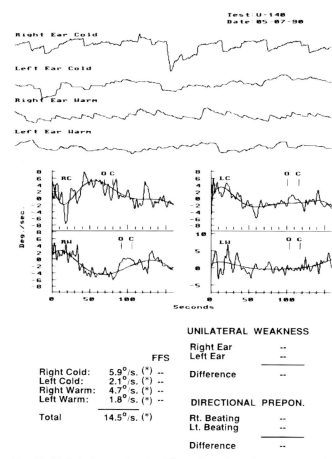

Test:U-140
Date:05-07-90

UNILATERAL WEAKNESS

	FFS	Right Ear	--
		Left Ear	--
Right Cold:	5.9°/s. (*) --		
Left Cold:	2.1°/s. (*) --	Difference	--
Right Warm:	4.7°/s. (*) --		
Left Warm:	1.8°/s. (*) --	DIRECTIONAL PREPON.	
Total	14.5°/s. (*)	Rt. Beating	--
		Lt. Beating	--
		Difference	--

Fig. 43–15. Caloric test showing bilateral weakness in a patient with probable gentamycin ototoxicity due to prophylactic administration during a hospital stay for cardiovascular surgery. The low caloric responses make intensities unilateral weakness, directional perponderance, and failure of fixation suppression measurements extremely variable, hence of doubtful diagnostic significance. The computer, therefore, does not calculate these measurements. All other labeling conventions are as described in the Figure 43–13.

shown herein (Figs. 43–14 to 43–17) two different methods of smoothing the slow-component speed time course plots are used. The more variable curves are obtained by taking 10 second moving averages of the data points, and the smoothest curves are obtained by fitting sixth order polynomials to the moving average data points. The fitted polynomials exclude data points during the eyes-open periods, hence represent approximations of what the caloric response time-courses would have been had the patient not opened his eyes.

UNILATERAL WEAKNESS AND DIRECTIONAL PREPONDERANCE. Caloric unilateral weakness (UW) is, essentially, a quantitative comparison of the responses from the right and the left ears. Directional preponderance (DP) is a comparison of right-beating with left-beating nystagmus. Absolute differences between caloric responses become more variable as the responses become more intense. Therefore, unilateral weakness and directional preponderance are expressed in relative

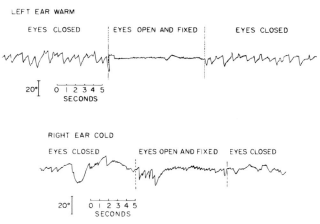

Fig. 43–16. Demonstration of "failure of fixation suppression" (FFS) of caloric nystagmus. The top record, obtained from a patient with a small right acoustic neurilemmoma, demonstrates normal suppression of caloric nystagmus by visual fixation. The bottom record demonstrates FFS. It was obtained from a patient with multiple sclerosis.

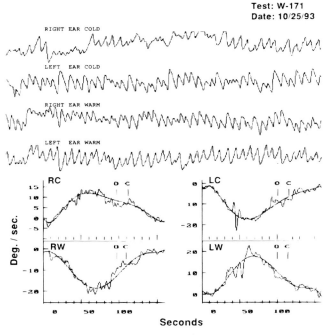

Test: W-171
Date: 10/25/93

UNILATERAL WEAKNESS

		FFS	Right Ear	46.1%
			Left Ear	53.9%
Right Cold:	12.4°/s. (*)	73.8% (*)		
Left Cold:	18.5°/s. (*)	87.1% (*)	Difference	-7.8%
Right Warm:	19.8°/s. (*)	71.3% (*)		
Left Warm:	19.0°/s. (*)	78.9% (*)	DIRECTIONAL PREPON.	
Total	69.7°/s.		Rt. Beating	55.0%
			Lt. Beating	45.0%
			Difference	10.0%

Fig. 43–17. Caloric test showing FFS obtained from a patient under evaluation for unsteadiness following severe head trauma. Labeling conventions are as described in the Figure 43–13.

terms, i.e., as a percentage of the total of all four responses intensities. Figure 43–13 illustrates a UW on the left, and Figure 43–14 illustrates DP to the left.

FAILURE OF FIXATION-SUPPRESSION. To test for "failure of fixation suppression" (FFS), the computer first obtains two slow component speed values from each eyes-open record segment: 1) an estimate of the eyes-closed slow component speed from the fitted polynomial, and 2) an actual eyes-open slow component speed from the moving average. The computer then calculates a "fixation index" by expressing the eyes-open speed as a percentage of the eyes-closed speed. Thus, the higher the percentage is, the less the fixation suppression. Many computerized ENG analysis systems calculate a more complex fixation index: (eyes closed slow component speed minus eyes open slow component speed divided by eyes closed slow component speed).[92] For these systems, the lower the percentage is the less the fixation suppression. Figure 43–16 contrasts FFS with the normal effect of visual suppression on caloric nystagmus, and Figure 43–17 shows a set of computer-quantified caloric responses that demonstrate failure of fixation suppression.

Diagnostic Significance

UNILATERAL WEAKNESS AND DIRECTIONAL PREPONDERANCE. The normal limit for UW is typically set at 20%, which is approximately twice the standard deviation obtained from most published normal bithermal caloric test series. Directional preponderance is more variable than UW, and there may be a "physiologic" DP in some normals. Typically, a DP of 20 to 30% is regarded as "questionably pathologic," whereas a DP greater than 30% is considered pathologic. A recent normative study of computer-quantified caloric tests yielded normal limits of ±21% for UW and ±24% for DP.[28]

A caloric UW can only be caused by a lesion of the vestibular end organ or the primary vestibular nerve fibers. It is therefore a peripheral finding.[27,82,93,94] Caloric DP can be caused by either peripheral or central pathology.[87,95] It is therefore a nonlocalizing abnormality.

BILATERAL WEAKNESS (BW). Caloric bilateral weakness is present when the average of the warm and cold caloric response maximum slow component speeds from each ear (e.g., (RC + RW)/2) is below a predetermined lower limit of normal. A recent normative study of the computer-quantified caloric tests yielded lower normal limit for maximum slow component speed of 8.6°/second.[28] Figure 43–15 shows a caloric test that demonstrates BW.

Caloric BW may be caused by either bilateral peripheral vestibular pathology, such as that produced by aminoglycoside toxicity, or central pathology that interferes with the vestibulo-ocular reflex. Most BWs, however, are caused by bilateral, peripheral vestibular

pathology. Furthermore, the occasional patient with BW caused by central pathology almost always has central oculomotor signs. In particular, the OKN test is often abnormal. Thus, BW is considered a peripheral sign with, however, the proviso that brainstem pathology has been ruled out.

In addition to its localizing significance, caloric BW provides useful information when planning a vestibular rehabilitation program. Since bilateral loss of vestibular function can never be restored, the patient with caloric BW cannot be expected to recover function in situations where maintenance of balance depends solely or primarily on vestibular input, e.g., walking on rough surfaces in the dark. Therefore, in setting the goals of a vestibular rehabilitation program for a patient with caloric BW, this inherent limitation of the program's expected benefits must be taken into account.[96–98]

FAILURE OF FIXATION SUPPRESSION. A recent study set upper limit of the computer-calculated fixation index at 58%.[28] In normal individuals, visual fixation either suppresses or abolishes caloric nystagmus. A number of reports suggest that failure to suppress caloric nystagmus with visual fixation indicates central nervous system pathology.[99,100] However, two benign causes must be ruled out: 1) sedation, particularly by barbiturates,[19] and 2) contact lenses, particularly if they are new or uncomfortable. In addition, as with all central ENG abnormalities, peripheral ocular or oculomotor pathology must be ruled out.

LOW-FREQUENCY ROTATION (ROTATING CHAIR) TEST

At the beginning of the twentieth century, Barany[101] pioneered the clinical use of rotational stimuli to assess function of the vestibular-controlled system which helps maintain eye stability during head movements (the vestibulo-ocular reflex, VOR). In current clinical practice, the Barany-style rotation test is done by seating the patient in a rotating chair and recording and analyzing the eye movements generated by the rotational stimulus. Because rotation is in the horizontal plane, this test evaluates only the function of the horizontal semicircular canal.

For technical reasons, it is difficult to obtain valid rotating chair test results at frequencies above approximately 1 Hz. As will be discussed, a clinically practicable method of applying high-frequency rotational stimuli (the Vestibular Autorotation Test) has been introduced. Therefore, to separate the traditional rotating chair test from this higher frequency rotational test, we refer to the rotating chair test as the "low-frequency rotation test."

In discussing clinical applications, the rotation test's advantages and disadvantages should be compared with those of the other classic vestibular test, the caloric test. The main advantages of the rotation test are 1) it requires less time and creates less patient discomfort, thus suiting it for repeat testing and for hard-to-test patients such as children; 2) the rotational stimulus can be quantified with greater precision than the caloric stimulus; 3) the rotation test covers a wider frequency range than the caloric test, which is basically an extremely low frequency stimulus—well below the normal frequency at which the VOR reflex operates in everyday life. The main disadvantages of the rotation test are 1) it stimulates both labyrinths simultaneously; hence, it cannot localize deficits involving individual labyrinths; and 2) the motor-driven rotating chair is expensive and occupies a large amount of laboratory space.

Technique

The patient is seated in a motor-driven rotating chair with his head fixed to the chair by either placing it in a headrest or attaching it to a headrest with a strap (Figure 43–18). The chair rotates in a sinusoidal pattern at a series of discrete frequencies—commonly 0.01–0.64 Hz in doubling steps. Several cycles at each frequency are averaged.

Eye movements generated in response to the rotational stimuli are recorded electro-oculographically and computer processed. The computer removes saccades and other non-VOR-mediated eye movements to extract a sinusoidal velocity signal as illustrated in

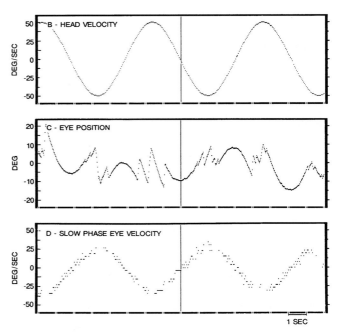

Fig. 43–19. Rotation test records from a clinically normal individual illustrating computer extraction of nystagmus fast components to leave only the slow component velocity trace (bottom trace). The middle ("eye position") trace is the horizontal EOG record. The top trace ("head velocity") plots velocity of the rotating chair. Upward deflection indicates rightward motion in all traces. Reprinted with permission from Stockwell C, Bojrab O: Background and technique of rotational testing. In Handbook of Balance Function Testing. Edited by Jacobson BP, Newman GW, Kartush JM. St. Louis: Mosby Year Book, 1993.

Figure 43–19. Eye velocity is compared with chair velocity to obtain *gain*, calculated as the ratio of eye velocity to head velocity, typically expressed as a decimal fraction. *component* is also computed. This is a measure of the time relationship between eye and head movement, expressed as a "component angle." Also, eye velocities in the opposite direction are compared to obtain a measurement of *asymmetry*, which may be expressed either as an absolute velocity difference or as a percentage of the total velocity.[102–104] Figure 43–19 shows an example of these measurements, as presented in the clinical report. Some laboratories also compare VOR gains with (patient rotated in the dark) and without (patient rotated while fixating a spot attached to the chair) visual fixation to obtain a quantitative "rotational FFS" measurement.[105,106]

Two major causes of inaccuracies in rotatory chair testing are 1) the effect of mental status on the response,[107] and 2) head movement relative to the chair. The latter contributes to the practical limitation of rotation chair test frequencies below 1 Hz because it is very difficult to prevent slippage of the head versus the chair at higher frequencies.[106] Also contributing to the practical upper-frequency limitation of rotation chair testing is the exponential increase in both bulk and cost

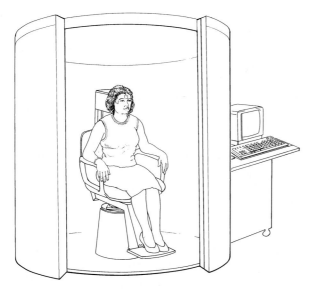

Fig. 43–18. Apparatus for administering the low-frequency rotational test. The patient, with EOG electrodes in place, is seated in a rotating chair inside a light-proof booth. The driving motor is inside the chair base. A computer, diagrammed at right, controls the pattern of chair rotation and analyzes the patient's eye movement signal.

of the torque motors required to rotate the human body accurately at higher frequencies.

Mental status must be carefully controlled during low-frequency rotation testing. If the subject imagines a visual scene moving in the opposite direction, VOR gain is approximately 0.9; if, in contrast, the patient imagines a visual scene moving in the same direction, VOR gain is only about 0.1. If the patient is distracted by mental arithmetic, gain is somewhere between 0.1 and 0.9. Most clinical laboratories use the intermediate situation—i.e., mental arithmetic with no visual scene imagined.[107]

Diagnostic Significance

Rotational component abnormalities and asymmetries are nonlocalizing. component abnormalities typically appear as increased low-frequency component leads.[102,108] This is the most common rotational abnormality. Occasionally it can be seen in patients with normal ENG examinations;[108] thus, the low-frequency rotation test can provide a useful objective sign of a VOR abnormality. Rotational asymmetry has the same diagnostic significance as caloric DP and, as with DP, often co-exists with spontaneous or positional nystagmus in the same direction as the predominant rotational response.[83]

Reduced rotational VOR gain has the same basic clinical significance as caloric BW—both in detecting bilateral peripheral vestibular deficits and in limiting the goals of a vestibular rehabilitation program. However, the caloric irrigation is a low-frequency stimulus, approximately one octave below the lowest rotational test frequency. Therefore, patients with caloric BW have reduced gains at low rotational frequencies but normal gains at higher frequencies.[103,109] Figure 43–20 shows a rotational test result from a patient with gentamycin ototoxicity and caloric BW illustrating this pattern. Both because it covers a wider frequency range and is more precisely quantified, reduced rotational gain is probably a more sensitive indicator of bilateral, peripheral vestibular pathology than caloric BW.[108]

Rotational FFS has the same clinical significance as caloric FFS—it indicates the presence of a central nervous system deficit. However, because it quantifies the VOR more precisely than the caloric test, rotational FFS is probably both a more sensitive and a more specific detector of central nervous system pathology than caloric FFS.

Because of the accuracy with which it quantifies the VOR and its minimal invasiveness, the rotation test is ideal for following the progress of a vestibulo-ocular reflex deficit—for example, to monitor vestibular compensation, as measured by amount of asymmetry, after an acute unilateral peripheral vestibular insult or to follow the progress of bilateral deficits in a patient receiving aminoglycoside antibiotic therapy.

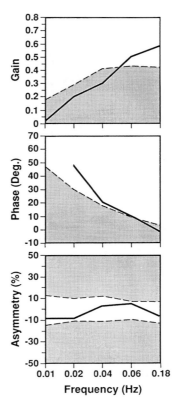

Fig. 43–20. Plots of gain, phase, and asymmetry versus rotation frequency from a rotation test demonstrating abnormally low gain and abnormally large phase leads over the low end of the frequency range tested. Abnormal areas (outside the 2 standard-deviation range of a clinically normal test population) are stippled. For clarity of representation, the eye velocity signal is inverted before measuring phase angle, so that an actual phase angle of 180° (i.e., head and eye moving in exactly opposite directions) would be expressed in the clinical report as a phase angle of 0°. The low gain at .01 Hz makes the phase angle measurement too variable to be useful; hence it is not plotted at this frequency.

HIGH-FREQUENCY ROTATION (VESTIBULAR AUTOROTATION) TEST

Fundamental functional differences exist (Table 43–5) between the low- and high-frequency VOR.[110–113] The low-frequency (below approximately 2 Hz) VOR supplements the smooth pursuit system to maintain visual fixation during voluntary head turning. In contrast, the high-frequency VOR (2 to 6 Hz) helps maintain eye stability during the rapid head movements that accompany running, jumping, and other locomotion-related activities.[114] Because of these functional differences, a test of the high-frequency VOR might be expected to

TABLE 43–5. Functional Differences Between the High- and Low-Frequency Vestibulo-Ocular Reflex

Stabilizes Eyes During	Low-Frequency VOR (Below 2 Hz) *Voluntary Head Rotation*	High-Frequency VOR (2–6 Hz) *Locomotion*
Modified by long-term visual input changes	Yes	No
Influenced by mental tasking	Yes	No
Interrupted by fast phases	Yes	No
Suppressed by visual fixation	Yes	No

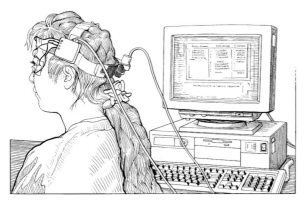

Fig. 43–21. Velocity sensor cylinder on the back of the head in position for vestibular autorotation testing. The EOG electrode connector terminal box, attached to the head strap, accepts the EOG electrode leads (R = right; L = left; U = up; D = down).

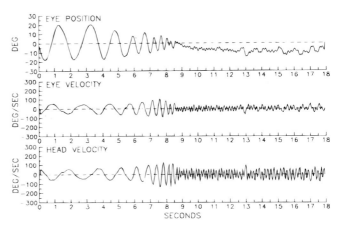

Fig. 43–22. Example of eye and head movement recordings from the vestibular autorotation test (VAT). The patient is asked to rotate his head back and forth at a progressively increasing frequency while fixating on a spot on the wall. The eye velocity record (center) is obtained by differentiating the eye position record (top trace). The head velocity record (bottom trace) is obtained from the velocity sensor (Fig. 43–21). This patient was diagnosed as having Meniere's disease and has decreased gains (eye velocities consistently less than head velocities).

demonstrate abnormalities not found by the low-frequency VOR test. However as noted, it is difficult-to-impossible to test the high frequency VOR with the rotating chair.

An alternative approach to testing the high-frequency VOR, pioneered by O'Leary and colleagues,[115] consists of strapping a velocity sensor to the head (Figure 43–21) so that head rotation is measured directly rather than quantified by controlling whole body rotation. The test based on this technique (termed by O'Leary the vestibular autorotation test, abbreviated VAT) has several unique advantages as a clinical tool: 1) it extends the upper frequency limit of VOR testing to approximately 6 Hz, thereby testing VOR functions not covered by the caloric or rotating chair test; 2) it is portable and inexpensive; 3) it is quick (the complete test takes less than a minute) and noninvasive; and 4) the vertical VOR, which is particularly important in maintaining eye stability during locomotion, can be tested conveniently.

Technique and Quantification Methods

With the velocity sensor in place, the patient is asked to rotate his head while fixating on a spot on the wall while eye movements are recorded by EOG. The velocity sensor can be rotated to record either vertical or horizontal head rotation. Two separate test runs are performed, one with vertical eye movements recorded during vertical head rotations, the other with horizontal eye movements recorded during horizontal head rotations. During each run a computer-generated warble tone guides the patient's head rotations, which begin at 0.5 Hz for 6 seconds (used for calibration), then increase progressively from 1 to 6 Hz for the remaining 12 seconds of the run. From the resultant

record (Fig. 43–22) the computer calculates, with Fourier analysis, vertical and horizontal VOR gain, component, and asymmetry at a series of discrete frequencies from 2 to 6 Hz. Figure 43–23 shows an example of a VAT showing reduced gain and abnormal component lead in a patient with gentamycin ototoxicity.

Although the patient is "fixating" on the visual target during the VAT test, the visual pursuit system is not effective at the velocities and frequencies used.[113] Therefore, the VOR is at least mostly, and probably entirely, responsible for the compensatory eye movements recorded in the VAT.

The following factors may contribute to inaccuracies

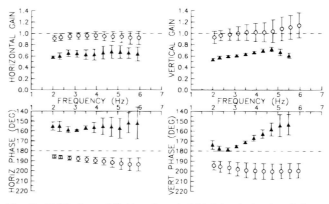

Fig. 43–23. Horizontal (left) and vertical (right) gain (top) and phase (bottom) plots of a VAT from a patient with gentamycin ototoxicity. Normal ranges are shown by the open circles with one standard deviation error bars. The data from the patient are shown by closed triangles with error bars showing one standard deviation ranges obtained from three trials.

in the VAT: 1) At the high frequencies and accelerations employed in the VAT, slippage of the head velocity sensor is inevitable. O'Leary has incorporated algorithms into his computer analysis program to compensate for this slippage. 2) The cervico-ocular reflex contributes to the compensatory eye movement response, and this contribution may be increased significantly in the presence of bilateral, peripheral vestibular pathology.[116]

Diagnostic Significance

Localization
The localizing significance of VAT abnormalities is the same as that of the low-frequency rotating chair test—i.e., reduced gain indicates bilateral, peripheral vestibular pathology, and abnormal component and asymmetry are nonlocalizing findings. However, because a higher, and functionally different frequency range is covered, and the vertical as well as the horizontal VOR is tested, the VAT often demonstrates abnormalities not detectable over the lower frequency range by either conventional ENG or the low-frequency rotation test. Published examples of cases in which only the VAT has detected abnormalities include decreased high frequency VOR gains in cisplatin ototoxicity[117] and increased high-frequency vertical VOR gains in Meniere's disease.[118]

Functional Assessment
The VAT can contribute greatly to assessing the patient's functional status. Because it covers the high-frequency VOR range, which stabilizes eyes during locomotion, its results tend to correlate more directly with symptoms of oscillopsia and unsteadiness on walking than do the results of the caloric and low-frequency rotation test. Also, VAT results can contribute to the design of vestibular rehabilitation programs. For example, vertical head shaking exercises would be much more likely than horizontal exercises to benefit a patient in which the VAT demonstrates only a vertical VOR abnormality.[119]

The short test duration, noninvasiveness, and portability of the VAT also make it ideal for repeat testing to chart the course of a functional deficit. It is thus well suited to provide objective measurements of vestibular training results or early warning of an impending vestibular deficit in a patient undergoing chemotherapy or aminoglycoside antibiotic therapy.

DYNAMIC POSTUROGRAPHY

The dynamic posturography examination, pioneered by Nashner and colleagues,[120] quantifies postural stability under varying conditions of sensory input and postural disturbance. It consists of two tests: 1) the sensory organization test (SOT), which quantifies body sway under conditions in which the sensory inputs providing information on body position (somatosensory, visual, vestibular) are either selectively removed, or "sway-referenced," and 2) the motor control test (MCT) in which postural responses to brief displacements of the support surface are recorded.

Dynamic posturography differs fundamentally in clinical significance from the ENG test battery and rotation tests in that 1) it assesses the descending vestibular pathways rather than the ascending vestibulo-ocular reflex pathways, and 2) it assesses the contribution of the somatosensory and visual systems to postural stability; whereas the ENG and rotation tests are limited to evaluation of VOR and oculomotor function.

Technique and Quantification Methods

General
Figure 43–24 diagrams the apparatus for performing dynamic posturography. The patient stands on movable force plates (one for each foot) that measure the force applied by the feet to the support surface during anterior–posterior body sway. The force plates also measure horizontal shear forces exerted by the feet against the support surface. Servomotors, controlled by signals from the force plates can tilt the force plates to coincide with the patient's body sway. In this way, the support surface can be "sway referenced" to eliminate ankle bending, hence eliminating most somatosensory information on body position. Also the plates

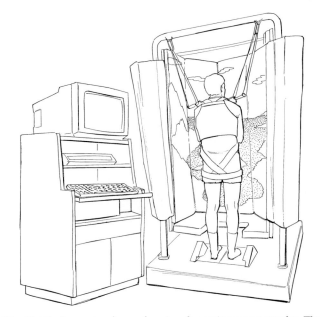

Fig. 43–24. Apparatus for performing dynamic posturography. The patient stands on movable force-measuring plates—one for each foot. The patient is supported by a harness to prevent falling. The visual field is filled by a semicircular screen with a scene painted on it.

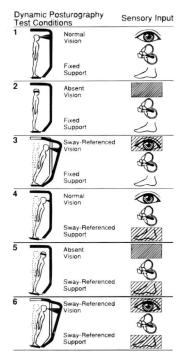

Dynamic Posturography Test Conditions — Sensory Input

1 — Normal Vision / Fixed Support

2 — Absent Vision / Fixed Support

3 — Sway-Referenced Vision / Fixed Support

4 — Normal Vision / Sway-Referenced Support

5 — Absent Vision / Sway-Referenced Support

6 — Sway-Referenced Vision / Sway-Referenced Support

Fig. 43–25. The six "sensory conditions" (numbers at left) of the sensory organization test (left column). In the right column are diagrammed the sensory inputs subserving body balance: vision, represented by an eye, vestibular, represented by a vestibular apparatus, and somatosensory, represented by a foot. Narrow crosshatching with no diagram indicates absent input (e.g., absent vision in condition 2). Wide crosshatching over the diagram indicates sway-referenced input (e.g., sway-referenced vision in condition 3). Adapted from Nashner LM: Computerized dynamic posturography. *In* Handbook of Balance Function Testing. Edited by Jacobson BP, Newman CW, Kartush JM. St. Louis: Mosby Year Book, 1993.

can be actively tilted or moved horizontally ("translated") to assess postural responses to balance disturbance. The test apparatus also includes a body-length shield painted with a scene which fills most of the patient's visual field. The shield can be tilted under force plate control to "sway reference" the visual surround.

Sensory Organization Test (SOT)

While the patient is standing on the force plates, sensory input can be controlled by either removing (by blindfolding) or sway referencing vision or sway referencing somatosensory input.[121] Figure 43–25 diagrams the six "sensory conditions" thereby achieved.

Figure 43–26 shows an example of a clinical report of a SOT. Body sway under each of the six sensory conditions is quantified as maximum peak-to-peak sway expressed as a percentage of a calculated maximum deflection achievable before falling (the "equilibrium scores," top, Fig. 43–26) and after falling (Fig. 43–27). From the equilibrium scores are calculated "sensory analysis scores" (bottom left, Fig. 43–26), which isolate the contributions of specific sensory systems to body stability. The sensory analysis score of each system (vestibular, visual, somatosensory) is cal-

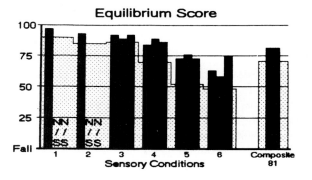

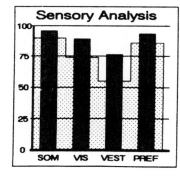
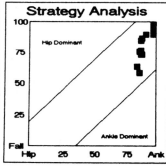
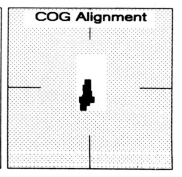

Fig. 43–26. Report of sensory organization test (SOT) results from a clinically normal subject. The upper plot shows equilibrium scores for the six sensory conditions. Each bar represents a trial, and there are up to three trials per condition. N/S means "not scored," indicating that the trial was not performed. At right, on the upper plot is the composite equilibrium score. At lower left are shown the four sensory analysis ratios. The lower center plot labelled "Strategy Analysis" quantifies the relative dominance of bending at the ankle (horizontal axis) and bending at the hip (vertical axis) while standing. The lower right plot shows average center of gravity ("COG") positions during all SOT trials. In all plots except Strategy Analysis, abnormal areas (two standard deviations from a population of scores from clinically normal subjects) are stippled. In the strategy analysis plot, the abnormal areas are labeled "Hip Dominant" and "Ankle Dominant." Reprinted with permission from Nashner LM: Computerized dynamic posturography. *In* Handbook of Balance Function Testing. Edited by Jacobson BP, Newman CW, Kartush JM. St. Louis: Mosby Year Book, 1993.

culated by expressing the equilibrium score yielded by the condition in which only the measured sense is active as a percent of the condition where all senses are operating normally. For example, in condition 4, vision is normal, but the platform is sway referenced; hence, somatosensory input is eliminated. Therefore, expressing the condition 4 equilibrium score as a percent of the condition 1 score isolates the ability of visual input to maintain balance. The set of sensory analysis scores also includes a "visual preference" score which is the sum of the two sway-referenced visual conditions (433 and 436) expressed as a percentage of the sum of the two vision-absent conditions (432 and 435). This score quantifies the extent to which sway-referencing the visual surround increases body sway.

Also calculated is a "strategy analysis" score (bottom center, Fig. 43–26), which quantifies the relative preponderance of bending at the ankles ("ankle strategy") versus bending at the hips ("hip strategy") while maintaining an upright position. The strategy analysis score is based on the premise that hip movement creates horizontal shear forces on the platform, while bending at the ankles does not. It is calculated by taking the ratio of the horizontal shear force's peak-to-peak amplitude to a theoretical peak-to-peak amplitude limit for a normal individual of similar weight. In normals, as body sway increases hip movements are increasingly used to maintain an upright position.

Therefore, the "normal range" of the hip strategy versus total sway plot forms a diagonal from the lower left to the upper right of the graph. Points falling in the lower right quadrant indicate abnormal dependence on ankle strategy; whereas points falling in the upper left quadrant indicate abnormal dependence on hip strategy.

The system also calculates alignment of the patient's center of gravity (COG) during the sensory organization test as the average COG position during each 20 second run (Fig. 43–26, bottom right).

Motor Control Test (MCT)

The motor control test records the strength and latency of the force exerted by the feet against the support surface to bring the body back into vertical alignment after the support surface is suddenly translated horizontally (Fig. 43–28). Response latency and asymmetry between the two feet are evaluated.

Diagnostic Significance

Deficit Localization

SENSORY ORGANIZATION TEST. The abnormal results of the sensory organization test are classified into six patterns.[122] Each pattern and its clinical significance are described below.

1. *Physiologically Inconsistent.* The easier 1, 2, and 3

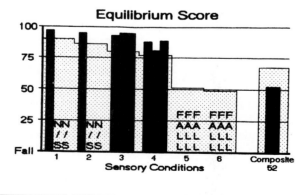

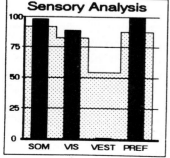
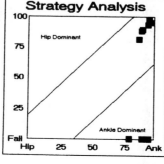
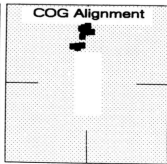

Fig. 43–27. Sensory organization test result from a patient with central vestibular system pathology. "FALL" = patient fell and was caught by the safety harness. The sensory analysis score for the vestibular system (lower left) is abnormally low. Conventions are the same as in Figure 43–26. From Nashner, L. M. Computerized dynamic posturography: Clinical Applications. *In* Handbook of Balance Function Testing. Edited by Jacobson, B. P., Newman, C. W., and Kartush, J. M. St. Louis, Mosby Year Book, 1993. (By permission)

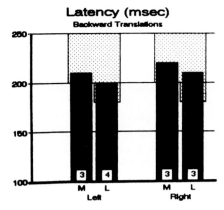
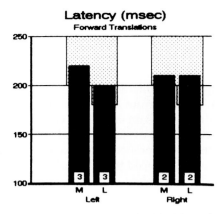

Fig. 43–28. Motor control test from a patient with sensory motor deficits following head trauma. The solid black bars show "latencies"—the delays, in milliseconds, from a sudden horizontal movement of the support plates to the patient's application of force at his feet to regain the upright position. M indicates a "medium" translation (1.25 cm in 250 ms); L indicates "large" translation (3.15 cm in 300 ms). The numbers in the clear boxes indicate the number of trials averaged to obtain the latencies. All latencies, both to backward (left graphs) and forward (right graphs) translations, are abnormally long. Reprinted with permission from Nashner LM: Computerized dynamic posturography: Clinical Applications. In Handbook of Balance Function Testing. Edited by Jacobson BP, Newman CW, Kartush JM. St. Louis: Mosby Year Book, 1993.

conditions yield more abnormal results than the harder 4, 5, and 6 conditions. If the better-performed 4, 5, and 6 conditions are still abnormal, the patient probably has a balance-and-equilibrium abnormality, but is exaggerating his symptoms. If the 4, 5, and 6 conditions are within the normal range, but the easier conditions are abnormal, the patient probably has normal balance and equilibrium function and, either deliberately or because of anxiety, is exaggerating his symptoms.[122,123] Also tending to support the presence of symptom exaggeration is a regular, sinusoidal sway pattern as opposed to the normal tendency for relatively long periods of stability to be interrupted by irregular, brief, but large sways.[123]

2. *Somatosensory Deficit.* Performance on condition 2 (standing on stable platform with eyes closed) is low relative to condition 1 (all inputs normal). This is the classic Romberg test[124] quantified. It indicates a somatosensory deficit that could be either a peripheral neuropathy or a deficit of the central somatosensory pathways.

3. *Visual Deficit.* Performance on condition 4 (somatosensory input eliminated but visual input normal) is low relative to condition 1. This abnormality indicates that either visual input is abnormal, or the ability of the central nervous system to process visual input is impaired.[122]

4. *Vestibular Deficit.* Performance on condition 5 (visual and somatosensory inputs both eliminated, leaving only vestibular input) is low relative to condition 1. This abnormality indicates the presence of either bilateral peripheral vestibular pathology,[125] uncompensated unilateral peripheral deficit,[126–128] or a deficit involving the central vestibular pathways.[120,129] Figure 43–27 shows an example of a SOT showing a vestibular deficit.

5. *Visual Preference.* Performance under conditions in which visual input is sway referenced (conditions 3 and 6) is poor relative to conditions in which visual input is simply eliminated (conditions 2 and 5). The cause of this disorder is unknown but occurs frequently in post-traumatic vertigo.[129]

6. *Multisensory Pattern.* Deficits are found in more than one sensory system. This abnormal pattern usually indicates the presence of central nervous system lesions, which extend beyond the central vestibular system.[130]

MOTOR CONTROL TEST. Abnormally long response latencies (Fig. 43–28) indicate the presence of either a peripheral sensory neuropathy[131] or a central nervous system deficit,[132–136] which could involve either the segmental spinal pathways that mediate lower motor responses to body displacement, or higher neural centers which have a descending influence on these segmental spinal pathways.

Functional Assessment

Dynamic posturography yields measurements that can help to 1) quantify the patient's functional balance-and-equilibrium deficit, 2) follow the course of a deficit, or 3) design and monitor the progress of a physical therapy program. As a functional assessment tool, dynamic posturography has the advantage of testing functions that often closely approximate the patient's actual complaints[137] (e.g., a problem with locomotion or standing). In designing a vestibular rehabilitation training program, the SOT has come to be regarded as essential in many laboratories[135,138,139] because it identifies the functional area upon which the training program should concentrate. For example, the program for a patient with normal vision whose SOT shows a visual deficit or abnormal visual preference pattern

TABLE 43–6. Localizing Significance of Vestibulometric Abnormalities

Test	Nonlocalizing	Peripheral	Central (R/O ocular for all abnormalities)
Calibration			Ocular dysmetria or "calibration overshoot" (R/O eyeblinks)
Gaze			Gaze NYS:
			Vertical
			Unilateral (R/O intense spontaneous NYS)
			Bilateral, equal (R/O sedation)
Optokinetic			Bilateral, unequal
			Asymmetry (R/O intense spontaneous NYS)
			Bilateral diminution (R/O lack of voluntary visual fixation and sedation)
Sinusoidal tracking			"Breakup" (R/O sedation)
Saccade velocity			Slowed velocities involving both eyes
Position	Vestibular spontaneous and positional NYS		Central spontaneous NYS
Paroxysmal NYS	Nonclassic	Classic	
Bithermal caloric	DP	UW	FFS (R/O sedation)
		BW (R/O central VOR interruption)	
Rotation (both Chair and VAT)	DP	Reduceed gain (R/O central VOR interruption)	FFS (R/O sedation)
Dynamic Posturography	Vestibular deficit SO pattern		Multisensory SO pattern (R/O peripheral) nonvestibular sensory abnormality
			Prolonged MCT latency (R/O peripheral neuropathy)

R/O = rule out, NYS = nystagmus, VOR = vestibulo-ocular reflex, DP = directional preponderance, UW = unilateral weakness, FFS = failure of fixation suppression, BW = bilateral weakness, MCT = motor control test, SOT = sensory organization test, VAT = vestibular autorotation test.

might concentrate on teaching the patient to make more effective use of vision.

The sensory organization test can also quantify an ineffective use of movement strategies (excessive hip movement at low sway amplitudes or excessive reliance on ankle strategy at high sway amplitudes). In such cases, a therapeutic program might emphasize training to use the appropriate strategy and repeat testing to track progress.[122]

A misaligned COG increases the risk of falling. If there are no musculoskeletal deficits that account for the abnormal COG alignment, biofeedback therapy using the dynamic posturography instrumentation can help teach patients to correct their abnormal alignment.[122,140]

SUMMARY OF CLINICAL SIGNIFICANCE OF VESTIBULOMETRIC TEST RESULTS

Tables 43–6 and 43–7 summarize the localizing and functional significance, respectively, of the vestibulometric test abnormalities discussed in this chapter.

TABLE 43–7. Functional Significance of Vestibulometric Abnormalities

Test	Abnormality	Significance
ENG	Caloric UW	Prognosis good for recovery of balance/equilibrium function.
	Caloric BW	If severe, cannot restore normal balance in situations where visual and somatosensory inputs are absent.
Rotating Chair	Reduced VOR gain	Same as Caloric BW
VAT	Vertical abnormality	Train high frequency vertical VOR.
	Horizontal abnormality	Train high frequency horizontal VOR.
Dynamic Posturography	Physiologically inconsistent	Balance-and-equilibrium system is normal if ENG And rotatory tests are abnormal.
	Sensory dysfunction	Train sensory modalities that remain functional.
	Visual preference	Train to suppress inappropriate visual input.
	Inappropriate hip or ankle strategy	Train to use appropriate strategy (R/O physiological inability to use appropriate strategy).
	COG misaligned	Train to maintain normal COG (R/O underlying musculoskeletal deficit).

ENG = Electronystagmography, VAT = Vestibular autorotation test, COG = center of gravity, UW = unilateral weakness, BW = bilateral weakness, VOR = vestibulo-ocular reflex, R/O = rule out.

REFERENCES

1. Baloh R, Honrubia V: Clinical Neurophysiology of the Vestibular System. Philadelphia, Davis, 1979.
2. Hart CW: Manual of Electronystagmography. Washington, D.C., Am Acad Otolaryngol Head Neck Surg 1987.
3. Jacobson BP, Newman CW, Kartoush JM: Handbook of Balance Function Testing, St. Louis, Mosby Year Book, 1993.
4. Leigh RJ, Zee DS: The Neurology of Eye Movements, Ed. 2. Philadelphia, F. A. Davis, 1993.
5. Herdman S: Vestibular Rehabilitation, Philadelphia, F. A. Davis, 1994.
6. Shepherd NT, Telian SA, Smith-Wheelock M: Habituation and balance retraining therapy. A retrospective review. Neurol Clin 8:459, 1990.
7. Shumway-Cock A, Horak FB: Rehabilitation strategies for patients vestibular deficits. Diagn Neurotol 440, 1990.
8. Carl JR: Principles and Techniques of Electro-oculography, Chapter 4, In Jacobson, B. P., Newman, C. W., Kartoush, J. M.: Handbook of Balance Function Testing, St. Louis, Mosby Year Book, 1993.
9. Kris C: Electro-oculography. In Medical Physics, Vol. 3 . Edited by Glasser, O., Chicago, Year Book Medical Publishers, 1960.
10. Ellenberger C, Jr, et al.: Ocular dyskinesia in cerebellar disease. Evidence for the similarity of opsoclonus, ocular dysmetria and flutter-like oscillations. Brain 95:683, 1972.
11. Higgins DC, Daroff RB: Overshoot and oscillation of ocular dysmetria. Arch Ophthalmol 75:742, 1966.
12. Ritchie L: Effects of cerebellar lesions on saccadic eye movements. J Neurosci 39:1246, 1976.
13. Troost BT, Weber RB, Daroff RB: Hypometric saccades. Am J Ophthalmol 78:1002, 1974.
14. Melville-Jones G, DeJong JD: Dynamic characteristics of saccadic eye movements in Parkinson's disease. Exp Neurol 31:17, 1971.
15. Haring RD, Simmons FB: Cerebellar defects are detectable by ENG calibration overshoots. Arch Otolaryngol 98:14, 1973.
16. Abel LA, Parker L, Daroff RD, et al: End point nystagmus. Invest Ophthalmol Vis Sci 17:539, 1977.
17. Shallo-Hoffman J, Schwarze H, Simonsz H, et al: A re-examination of end point and rebound nystagmus in normals. Invest Ophthalmol Vis Sci 31:388, 1990.
18. Daroff RB, Hoyt WF: Supranuclear disorders of ocular control systems in man. Clinical, anatomical and physiologic correlations—1969. In The Control of Eye Movements. Edited by Bach-y-Rita P, Collins CC, Hyde HE. New York: Academic Press, 1971.
19. Coats AC: Central electronystagmographic abnormalities. Arch Otolaryngol 92:43, 1970.
20. Hess K, Durstler MR, Reisine H: Analysis of slow phase eye velocity during the course of an acute vestibulopathy. Acta Otolaryngol (Stockh) Suppl 406:227, 1984.
21. Robinson DA, et al.: Alexander's law: Its behavior and origin in the human vestibulo-ocular reflex. Ann Neurol 16:714, 1984.
22. Kutt H, Winters W, Scherman R, et al: Diphenylhydantoin and phenobarbital toxicity. Arch Neurol 11:649, 1964.
23. Bergman PS, et al.: The effects of drugs on normal and abnormal ocular reflex. Neurology 16:714, 1984.
24. Rashbass C: Barbiturate nystagmus and mechanics of visual fixation. Nature 183:897, 1959.
25. Herishanu Y, Osimand A, Louzoun Z: Unidirectional gaze paretic nystgmus induced by phenytoin intoxication. Am J Ophthalmol 94:122, 1982.
26. Benitez JT: Eye-tracking and optokinetic tests. Diagnostic significance in peripheral and central vestibular disorders. Laryngoscope 80:834, 1970.
27. Jung R, Kornhuber HH: Results of electronystagmography in man. The value of optokinetic, vestibular and spontaneous nystagmus of neurologic diagnosis and research. In The Oculomotor System. Edited by Bender MB. New York: Harper & Row, 1964.
28. Coats AC: Normative data for the Janus ATAC computerized eye movement analysis. Houston: Life-Tech, 1992.
29. Baloh RW, Honorubia V, Sills A: Eye tracking and optokinetic nystagmus. Results of quantitative testing in patients with well-defined nervous system lesions. Ann Otol Rhinol Laryngol 86:108, 1977.
30. Coats AC: Electronystagmography. In Physiological Measures of the Audio-Vestibular System. Chapter 3. Edited by Bradford LF. New York: Academic Press. 1975.
31. Hartje W, et al: Diagnostic value of saccadic pursuit movement in screening for organic cerebral dysfunction. J Neurol 217:253, 1978.
32. Schalen L, Henriksson NG, Pyykko I: Quantification of tracking eye movements in patients with neurological disorders. Acta Otolaryngol (Stockh) 93:387, 1982.
33. Bittencourt PRM, Wade T, Smith HE, et al: Benzodiazepines impair smooth pursuit eye movements. Br J Clin Pharmacol 15:59, 1983.
34. Sibony PA, Evinger E, and Manning, K. A.: The effects of tobacco smoking on smooth pursuit eye movements. Neurol., 23:238, 1988.
35. Whicker L, Abel LA, Del O'Osso LF: Smooth pursuit eye movements in the parents of schizophrenics. Neurol Ophthalmol 5:1, 1985.
36. Baloh RW, et al.: Quantitative measurement of saccade amplitude, duration, and velocity. Neurology 25:1065, 1975.
37. Gavilan J, Gavilan C, Siera MJ: Saccadic movements. A computerized study of their velocity and latency. Acta Otolaryngol (Stockh) 96:429, 1983.
38. Baloh RW, et al.: The saccade velocity test. Neurology 25:1071, 1974.
39. Kimura Y, Kato I: Modification of saccade by various central nervous system dysfunctions. In Vestibular and Oculomotor Physiology. International Meeting of the Barany Society. Edited by Cohen B. New York: New York Academy of Sciences, 1981.
40. Troost BT, Weber RB, Daroff RB: Hypometric saccades. Am J Ophthalmol 78:1002, 1974.
41. Metz HS: Saccadic velocity measurements in internuclear ophthalmoplegia. Am J Ophthalmol 81:296, 1976.
42. Hain T: Interpretation and usefulness of ocular motility testing. Chapter 6, In Handbook of Balance Function Testing. Edited by Jacobson G, Newman C, Hunter L, Balber G. St. Louis: Mosby Year Book, 1992.
43. Metz HS, et al: Ocular saccades in lateral rectus palsy. Arch Ophthalmol 84:453, 1970.
44. Baloh RW, Yee RD, Honorubia V: Internuclear ophthalmoplegia. I. Saccades and dissociated nystagmus. Arch Neurol 35:484, 1978.
45. Aschoff JC, Cohen B: Changes in saccadic eye movements produced by cerebellar cortical lesions. Exp Neurol 32:1233, 1971.
46. Hanson MR, et al.: Selective saccadic palsy caused by pontine lesions: Clinical, physiological, and pathological correlates. Ann Neurol 20:209, 1986.
47. Mizutani T, Satoh J, Morimatsu Y: Neuropathologic background of oculomotor disturbances in olivopontocerebellar atrophy with special reference slow saccade. Clin Neuropathol 7:53, 1988.
48. Zee DS, et al.: Slow saccades in spinocerebellar degeneration. Arch Neurol 33:243, 1976.
49. Tedeshi G, et al.: Neuroocular side effects of carbanazepine and phenobarbital in epileptic patients as measured by saccadic eye movement analysis. Epilepsia 30:62, 1989.
50. Rothenberg SJ, Selkoe D: Specific oculomotor deficit after diazepam. I. Saccadic eye movements. Psychopharmacology 74:232, 1981.

51. Thurston SE, Leigh RJ, Abel LA, et al: Slow saccades and hypometria in anticonvulsant toxicity. Neurology 34:1593, 1984.

52. Smith JL: Optokinetic Nystagmus. Springfield: Charles C. Thomas, 1963.

53. Van Die G, Collewijn H: Optokinetic nystagmus in man. Role of central and peripheral retina and occurrence of asymmetries. Hum Neurobiol 1:111, 1982.

54. Honorubia V, Downey WL, Mitchell DM, et al: Experimental studies on optokinetic nystagmus. Acta Otolaryngol (Stockh) 65:441, 1968.

55. Zee DS, Yee RD, Robinson DA: Optokinetic responses in labyrinthine-defective human beings. Brain Res 113:423, 1976.

56. Coats AC: Unpublished observation. 1994.

57. Howard IP, Heckmann T: Circular vection as a function of the relative sizes, distances and positions of two competitive displays. Perception 18:657, 1989.

58. Howard IP: Personal communication, 1993.

59. Rosborg J, et al.: Vertical optokinetic nystagmus. Acta Neurol Scand 48:621, 1972.

60. Brandt T, Allum JHJ, Dichgans J: Computer analysis of optokinetic nystagmus in patients with spontaneous nystagmus of peripheral vestibular origin. Acta Otolaryngol (Stockh) 86:115, 1978.

61. Coats AC Central and peripheral optokinetic asymmetry. Ann Otol Rhinol Laryngol 77:938, 1968.

62. Davidoff RA, et al.: Optokinetic nystagmus and cerebral disease. Arch Neurol 14:73, 1966.

63. Smith JF: Vertical optokinetic nystagmus. Neurology 12:38, 1962.

64. Cogan DG: Neurology of the Ocular Muscles, 2nd Ed. Springfield: Charles C. Thomas, 1963.

65. Toglia JU, Moreno S: Labyrinthine versus central nystagmus: Electronystagmographic observation. Dis Nerv Syst 32:623, 1971.

66. Coats AC: Computer-quantified positional nystagmus in normals. Am J Otol 14:314, 1993.

67. Dix MR, Hallpike CS: Pathology, symptomatology and diagnosis of certain common disorders of the vestibular system. Proc R Soc Med 45:341, 1952.

68. Aschan G, Bergstedt M, Goldberg L, et al: Positional nystagmus in man during and after alcohol intoxication. Q J Stud Alcohol 17:381, 1956.

69. Stenger HH: Uber Lagerungsnystagmus unter besonderer berucksichtigung des gegenlaufigen transitorischen provokations-nystagmus bei lagewechsel in der saggitalebene. Arch F Ohren Nassen U Kehik 168:220, 1955.

70. Baloh RW, Honorubia V, Jacobson K: Benign positional vertigo: Clinical and oculographic features in 240 cases. Neurology 37:371, 1987.

71. Preber L, Silvershiold BP: Paroxysmal positional vertigo following head injury (studied by electronystagmography and skin resistance measurements). Acta Otolaryngol (Stockh) 48:255, 1957.

72. Stahle J, Terins J: Paroxysmal positional nystagmus—An electronystagmographic and clinical study. Ann Otol Rhinol Laryngol 74:69, 1965.

73. Cawthorne T: Positional nystagmus. Trans Am Otol Soc 42:265, 1956.

74. Schuknecht HF: Cupuloithiasis. Arch Otolaryngol 90:113, 1969.

75. Aschan G, et al: The effect of head movement on positional nystagmus—electronystagmography with an electric driven posture table. Laryngoscope 67:884, 1957.

76. Barber HO: Positional nystagmus: Testing and interpretation. Ann Otol Rhinol Laryngol 73:838, 1964.

77. Jongkees LBW: On positional nystagmus. Acta Otolaryngol (Stockh) Suppl 159:78, 1961.

78. Coats AC: The diagnostic significance of spontaneous nystagmus as observed in the electronystagmographic examination. Acta Otolaryngol (Stockh) 67:33, 1969.

79. O'Neill G, Oren WA: Computerized analysis of the caloric response. Arch Otolaryngol (Stockh) 104:400, 1987.

80. Henriksson NG, Pfaltz CD, Torok N, et al: A Synopsis of the Vestibular System. Basel: Gasser & Cie, 1972.

81. Nylen CO: Positional nystagmus (a review and future prospects). J Laryngol Otol 64:295, 1950.

82. Aschan G, Bergstedt M, Stahle J: Nystagmography. Recording of nystagmus in clinical neur-otological examinations. Acta Otolaryngol (Stockh) Suppl 129:1, 1956.

83. Baloh RW: Dizziness, Hearing Loss, and Tinnitus: The Essentials of Neurotology. Philadelphia: F. A. Davis, 1984.

84. Simmons FB, Gillam SF, Mattox DE: An Atlas of Electronystagmography. New York: Grune & Stratton, 1979.

85. Brandt, T.: Positional and positioning vertigo and nystagmus. J. Neurol. Sci. 95:3, 1990.

86. Hill R, et al: Influence of alcohol on positional nystagmus over 32-hour periods. Ann Otol Rhinol Laryngol 82:103, 1973.

87. Fitzgerald G, Hallpike CS: Studies in human vestibular function. I. Observations on the directional preponderance (nystagmusbereitschaft) of caloric nystagmus resulting from cerebral lesions. Brain 65:115, 1942.

88. Aantaa E: Light-induced and spontaneous variations in the amplitude of the electro-oculogram. Acta Otolaryngol (Stockh) Suppl 267:1, 1970.

89. Barber HO, Wright G: Release of nystagmus suppression in clinical electronystagmography. Laryngoscope 77:1016, 1967.

90. Coats AC: Directional preponderance and spontaneous nystagmus as observed in the electronystagmographic examination. Ann Otol Rhinol Laryngol 75:1135, 1966.

91. Kinley PE, McCabe PF, Ryu JH: Effects of attention-requiring tasks on vestibular nytagmus. Ann Otol Rhinol Laryngol 89:9, 1980.

92. Kato I, Nakamura TN, Koike Y, et al: Computer analysis of fixation-suppression of caloric nystagmus. ORL 44:277, 1982.

93. Jongkees LBW: Value of the caloric test of the labyrinth. Arch Otolaryngol Head Neck Surg 48:402, 1948.

94. Stahle J: Electro-nystagmography in the caloric and rotatory tests. Acta Otolaryngol (Stockh) Suppl 137:1, 1958.

95. Brookler KH: Directional preponderance in clinical electronystagmograph. Laryngoscope 80:747, 1970.

96. Herdman SJ: Management of balance disorders in vestibular deficiency. Rehab Manag 4:68, 1991.

97. Rycewicz C, Horak FD, Shumway-Cook A: Comparisons of Exercises and Medication for the Treatment of Peripheral Vestibular Dysfunction. In Posture and Gait: Control Mechanisms. Vol. II., Edited by Wollancott and Horak, Eugene. University of Oregon Books, 1992.

98. Nashner LW: Computerized Dynamic Posturography: Clinical Applications. In Handbook of Balance Function Testing. Edited by Jacobson BP, Newman CW, Kartush JM. St. Louis: Mosby Year Book, 1993.

99. Hart CW: Ocular fixation and the caloric test. Laryngoscope 77:2103, 1967.

100. Sato Y, et al.: Failure of fixation suppression of caloric nystagmus and ocular motor abnormalities. Arch Neurol 37:35, 1980.

101. Barany R: Physiologie und Pathologie Bongengangsapparates deim Menschn. Vienna: Deutiche, 1907.

102. Jenkins HJ: Rotatory testing. In Manual of Electronystagmography. Edited by Hart CW. Washington, DC. Am Acad Otolaryngol Head Neck Surg 1987.

103. Stockwell C, Bojrab D: Background and Technique of Rotational Testing. In Handbook of Balance Function Testing. Edited by Jacobson BP, Newman GW, Kartush JM. St. Louis: Mosby Year Book, 1993.

104. Wolfe JW, Engelken EJ, Kos CM: Low-frequency harmonic ac-

celeration as a test of labyrinthine function: Basic methods and illustrative cases. Otolaryngology *86*:130, 1978.

105. Baloh R, Honorubia V: Clinical Neurophysiology of the Vestibular System. Philadelphia: F. A. Davis, 1979.

106. Hyden D, Larsby B, Odkvist LM: Quantification of compensatory eye movements in light and darkness. Acta Otolaryngol (Stockh) Suppl *406*:2029, 1984.

107. Barr C, Schultheis L, Robinson D: Voluntary, nonvisual control of the human vestibulo-ocular reflex. Acta Otolaryngol (Stockh) *81*:365, 1976.

108. Stockwell CW: Vestibular function testing: Four-year update. *In* Otolaryngology, Head and Neck Surgery: Update II. Edited by Cummings. St. Louis: Mosby Year Book, 1989.

109. Furman J, Kamerer D: Rotational responses in patients with bilateral caloric reduction. Acta Otolaryngol (Stockh) *108*:355, 1989.

110. Jell R, Guedry F, Hixon W: The vestibuloocular reflex in man during voluntary head oscillation under three visual conditions. Aviat Space Environ Med *53*:541, 1982.

111. Jell R, Stockwell C, Turnispeed G, et al: The influence of active versus passive head oscillation and mental set on the human vestibulo-ocular reflex. Aviat Space Environ Med *59*:1061, 1988.

112. Melville-Jones F, Gonshor A: Oculomotor responses to rapid head oscillation (0.5–5.0 Hz) after prolonged adaptation to vision-reversal. Exp Brain Res *45*:45, 1982.

113. Meyer C, Lasker A, Robinson D: The upper limit of human smooth pursuit velocity. Vis Res *25*:561, 1985.

114. Grossman G, et al.: Performance of the human vestibulo-ocular reflex during locomotion. J Neurophysiol *62*:264, 1989.

115. O'Leary D, Davis NL: High-frequency autorotational testing of the vestibulo-ocular reflex. Neurol Clin *8*:297, 1990.

116. Kasai T, Zee D: Eye-head coordination in labyrinthine-defective human beings. Brain Res *144*:123, 1978.

117. Kitsiginis G-A, O'Leary D, Davis L: Vestibular autorotation testing of cisplatin chemotherapy patients. Adv Otorhinolaryn *42*: 250, 1988.

118. O'Leary D, Davis L: Vestibular autorotation in Meniere's disease. Otolaryngol Head Neck Surg *103*:66, 1990.

119. Davis L, O'Leary D, Lei S: Gentamycin vestibulo-toxicity: Detection, rehabilitation monitoring and modeling with active head movements. Abst Assn Res Otolaryngol, St. Petersburg Beach, Fl. 1993.

120. Nashner L, Black FO, Wall C: Adaptation to altered support and visual conditions during stance: Patients with vestibular deficits. J Neuro Sci *2*:536, 1982.

121. Nashner LM: Computerized dynamic posturography. *In* Handbook of Balance Function Testing. Edited by Jacobson BP, Newman CW, Kartush JM. St. Louis: Mosby Year Book, 1993.

122. Nashner LM: Dynamic Posturography: Clinical Applications. *In* Handbook of Balance Function Testing. Edited by Jacobson BP, Newman CW, Kartush JM. St. Louis: Mosby Year Book, 1993.

123. Sataloff R, Cevette M, Goebel J: Computerized dynamic posturography (CDP) in workers compensation cases. NeuroCom Breakfast Symposium. San Diego, CA, September 19, 1994. NeuroCom International, Portland, 1994.

124. Romberg MH: Manual of Nervous System Disease of Man. London: Sydenham Society, 1853.

125. Freyss G, Semont A, Vica E: Dynamic Body Stabilization: Equi-Tests System in Patients with Bilateral Vestibular Caloric Areflexia. *In* Posture and Gait: Control Mechanisms, Vol. I. Edited by Wallcott G, Horak F. Eugene: University of Oregon Books, 1992.

126. Black R, Shubert C, Peterka R: Effects of unilateral loss of vestibular function on the vestibulo-ocular reflex posture control. Ann Otol Rhinol Laryngol *98*:884, 1989.

127. Fetter M, Diener H, Dichgans J: Recovery of postural control after an acute unilateral vestibular lesion in humans. J Vestib Res *1*:373, 1991.

128. Goebel J, Paige G: Dynamic posturography and caloric test results in patients with and without vertigo. Otolaryngol Head Neck Surg *100*:553, 1989.

129. Black F, Nashner L: Postural control in four classes of vestibular abnormalities. *In* Vestibular and Visual Control of Posture and Locomotor Equilibrium. Edited by Igarashi M, Black F. Basel: S. Karger, 1985.

130. Voorhees R: Dynamic posturography findings in central nervous system disorders. Otolaryngol Head Neck Surg *103*:96, 1990.

131. Ledin T, Odkvist L, Vrethem M: Dynamic posturography assessment of polyneuropathic disease. J Vestib Res *1*:123, 1991.

132. Nashner L, Shumway-Cook and Marin O: Stance posture control in selected groups of children with cerebral palsy: Deficits in sensory organization and muscular coordination. Exp Brain Res *197*:393, 1983.

133. Nashner L, Friedman J, Wusteny D: Dynamic posturography assessment of patients with peripheral and central vestibular system deficits: Correlations with results from other clinical tests. Upsala, Sweden: Barany Society Abstracts, 1988.

134. Panzer V, Smith M, Marken R: Functional evaluation of clinical status in multiple sclerosis. Neurology *42*(S3):446, 1992.

135. Smith-Wheelock M, Shepard N, Telian S: Physical therapy program for vestibular rehabilitation. Am J Otol *12*:218, 1991.

136. Tian J-R, Herdman S, Zee D, et al: Postural instability in patients with Huntingdon's disease. Neurology *42*:1232, 1992.

137. Jacobson G, Newman C, Hunter L, et al: Balance function test correlates of the dizziness handicap inventory. J Am Acad Audiol *2*:253, 1991.

138. Herdman S: Management of balance disorders in vestibular deficiency. Rehab Manag *4*:68, 1991.

139. Shumway-Cook A, Horak F: Vestibular rehabilitation: An exercise approach to managing symptoms of vestibular dysfunction. Neurol Clin North Am *8*:444, 1990.

140. Shumway-Cook A, Anson D, Haller S: Postural sway feedback: Its effect on reestablishing stance stability in hemiplegic patients. Arch. Phys Med Rehabil *69*:395, 1988.

44 Diagnostic Audiology and Hearing Aids

James W. Hall III, Troy Hackett, and Mark Clymer

Within the past 20 years, dramatic advances in techniques and technology have occurred for hearing assessment and options for audiologic management of hearing-impaired children and adults. With auditory brainstem response (ABR) and otoacoustic emissions (OAE) techniques, newborn infants can be screened for hearing impairment within days after birth. These two electrophysiologic techniques, applied in a test battery with aural immittance measures (tympanometry and acoustic reflexes) and traditional behavioral audiometry permit accurate diagnostic hearing assessment of young and difficult-to-test children and contribute to prompt audiologic and otolaryngologic management of this patient population.

Techniques for the assessment and management of hearing disorders in adults have also undergone rapid development in recent years. Inexpensive, hand-held devices permit rapid, yet effective, hearing screening in the office. Computer-based instrumentation, and associated devices (e.g. compact disk players), contribute to more accurate and complete neurodiagnostic evaluation of peripheral and central auditory system function. The ABR, for example, is a noninvasive, sensitive, and inexpensive measure of cochlear and retrocochlear (eighth cranial nerve and auditory brainstem) auditory function that is available in most hospitals and other medical facilities. Most adults with sensory (inner ear) hearing loss do not require medical or surgical treatment. Fortunately, today these patients can often obtain benefit from hearing aid use. More than 80% of the hearing aids dispensed in the United States are small enough to fit within the ear canal, and the latest generation of hearing aids can be worn deep within the ear canal within millimeters of the tympanic membrane. Digital and programmable technology has been incorporated into hearing aids, resulting in successful hearing aid use by persons who, in the past, rejected conventional hearing aids. Electroacoustic documentation and adjustment of hearing aid performance within the ear canal permits more precise prescription of amplification for the individual patient.

The otolaryngologist is in a pivotal position to identify children and adults at risk for hearing loss, to work closely with audiologists in diagnostic hearing assessment, and to contribute to timely and appropriate intervention. In this chapter, we describe current techniques and strategies for hearing assessment of children and adults. We also summarize indications for hearing loss in infants and young children. The chapter inludes a review of hearing aid technology that is useful in the nonmedical management of hearing loss. This review is followed by a summary of the concerns held by the deaf community regarding hearing impairment management, which must be appreciated by the otolaryngologist. Finally, common audiologic terms and abbreviations are defined in a glossary.

BASIC AUDIOMETRY

Pure-tone Audiometry

Pure-tone audiometry, the most common hearing test, is a measure of hearing sensitivity for pure-tone stimuli (sinusoids). The normal hearing, young (younger than 20 years) ear responds to frequencies from as low as 20 Hz to as high as 20,000 Hz. With routine pure-tone audiometry, however, a more limited region of hearing sensitivity is assessed. Stimuli are pure tones that range in octave frequencies from 250 Hz up to 8000 Hz, and sometimes also including 3000 Hz and 6000 Hz. Hearing test results for these frequencies are graphed on an audiogram. Versions of audiogram forms differ. One rather comprehensive version is illustrated in Figure

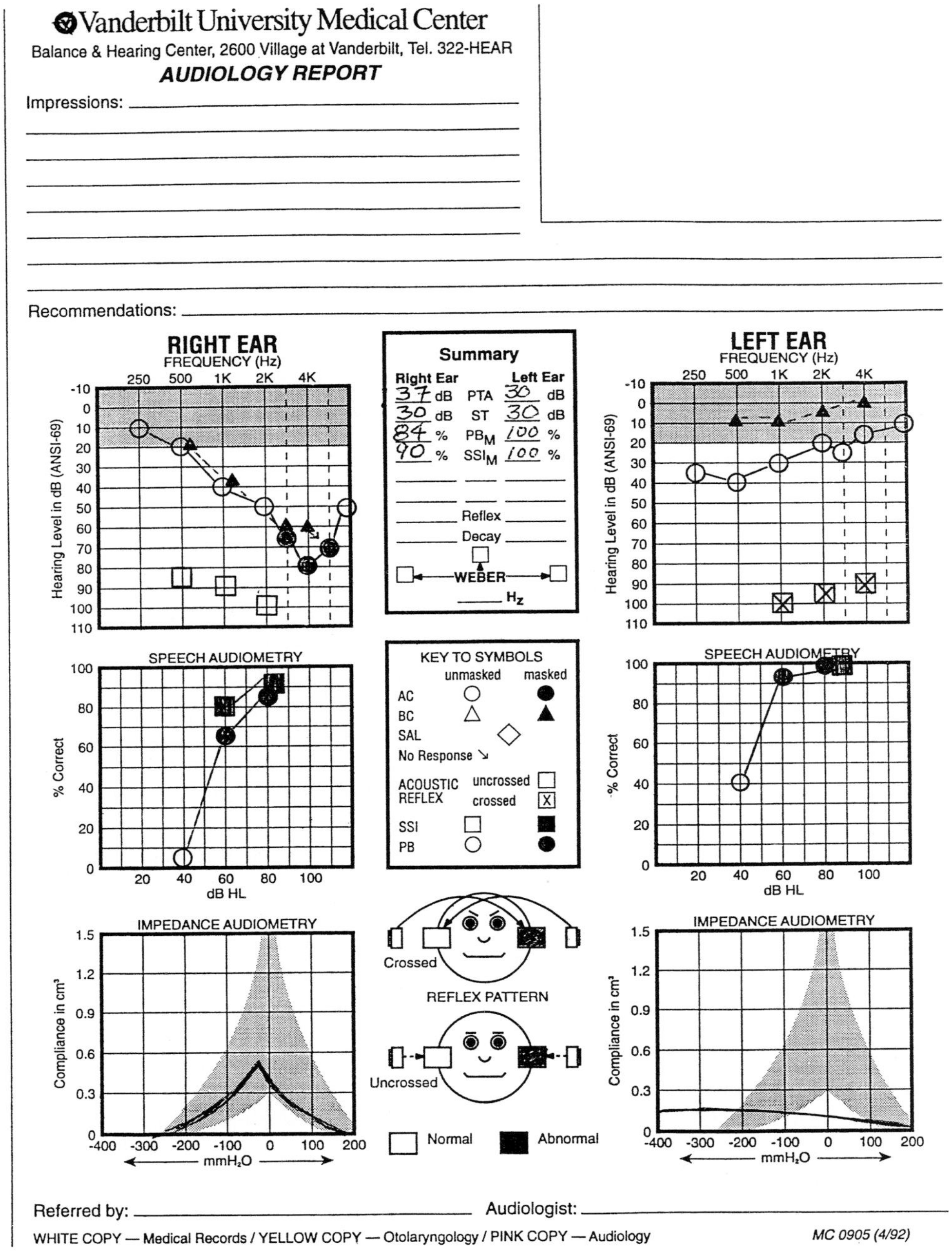

Vanderbilt University Medical Center

Balance & Hearing Center, 2600 Village at Vanderbilt, Tel. 322-HEAR

AUDIOLOGY REPORT

Impressions: _____

_____

_____

_____

_____

_____

_____

Recommendations: _____

RIGHT EAR — FREQUENCY (Hz) — Hearing Level in dB (ANSI-69)

LEFT EAR — FREQUENCY (Hz) — Hearing Level in dB (ANSI-69)

Summary		
Right Ear		Left Ear
37 dB	PTA	30 dB
30 dB	ST	30 dB
84 %	PB_M	100 %
90 %	SSI_M	100 %

Reflex _____
Decay _____
WEBER
_____ Hz

KEY TO SYMBOLS

	unmasked	masked
AC	○	●
BC	△	▲
SAL	◇	
No Response	↘	
ACOUSTIC REFLEX	uncrossed □	crossed ⊠
SSI	□	■
PB	○	●

SPEECH AUDIOMETRY — % Correct — dB HL

IMPEDANCE AUDIOMETRY — Compliance in cm³ — mmH₂O

Crossed

REFLEX PATTERN

Uncrossed

□ Normal   ■ Abnormal

Referred by: _____   Audiologist: _____

WHITE COPY — Medical Records / YELLOW COPY — Otolaryngology / PINK COPY — Audiology   *MC 0905 (4/92)*

Fig. 44–1. An example of an audiogram form including sections for reporting results for pure tone audiometry (top portion), speech audiometry (middle portion), and aural immittance measurement (bottom portion). Masking is indicated by filled symbols. Findings for the right ear represent a typical sensorineural audiometric pattern, whereas left ear findings typify a conductive hearing loss.

44–1. All audiograms include, at the least, a graph for plotting hearing threshold levels (HTLs) for pure-tone signals as a function of the frequency of pure-tone signals.

The unit of stimulus intensity is the decibel (dB), a logarithmic unit. The intensity of any sound is defined by a ratio of its sound pressure (or sound intensity) compared with a reference sound pressure (or sound intensity). This relationship for sound *intensity* is: dB {equi} 10 log 10 (sound intensity/reference intensity. For *sound pressure* the relationshiop is: dB {equi} 20 log 10 (sound pressure)/reference pressure. The reference sound pressure is the amount of pressure against the eardrum, caused by air molecules when a sound is present, that vibrates the eardrum and can just be detected by a normal human ear. The reference sound pressure, defined this way, is equivalent to several physical quantities (0.0002 dynes/cm2, 20 micropascals RMS or 2 × 10 (−5) Newtons/m2 RMS (root mean square). The intensity of sounds defined by this physical reference are described in dB sound pressure level (SPL). There is not a one-to-one relationship between the physical intensity of a sound and the dB. For example, a sound of 20 dB is not twice the intensity of 10 dB but, rather, 10 times as intense, and 30 dB is 100 times as intense as 10 dB.

Clinically, the intensity of sound is not usually described in dB SPL, with a physical reference level, but in *dB hearing level (HL)*, with a biologic reference level. On the audiogram (Figure 44–1) the dB scale has as its reference 0 dB, which is known as audiometric 0 (zero). This is the intensity level that corresponds to the average normal HTL, the faintest detectable intensity for each of the pure-tone test frequencies for a group of young normal hearers. The db HL scale is standardized. Currently, in the United States, the standard that is followed for this intensity scale was established by the American National Standards Institute (ANSI) in 1969. Audiometers are calibrated to this standard. Naturally, there is a well-defined and close relationship between dB HL and dB SPL. The third common unit for expressing sound intensity is *dB sensation level (SL)*. This describes the number of dB that a stimulus is above an individual person's hearing threshold. It is not standardized and has no meaning unless the type of stimulus is noted clearly (e.g. pure tone, click, speech) and the measure of hearing threshold also is described carefully (e.g., speech reception threshold, pure-tone average, behavioral click threshold).

Hearing thresholds are measured customarily, under earphones (air-conduction stimulation) for each ear. Recently developed insert earphones offer distinct advantages over the traditional supra-aural earphones, including comfort, reduced likelihood of ear canal collapse, greater interaural attenuation, and greater acceptance by young children. Whenever possible, ear-specific results are obtained also for children. With very young children who do not tolerate any type of earphones, hearing should be assessed with sounds delivered through loudspeakers. In these cases, information is only available for the better hearing ear, rather than for each ear separately. Pure-tone audiometry can also be conducted with stimuli presented by a bone conduction vibrator placed on the mastoid bone (just behind the ear).

During pure-tone audiometry, all equipment meets ANSI specifications, and testing is carried out according to clinical adaptations of psychoacoustic methods. The patient is instructed to listen carefully for the tones and to respond (usually by pushing a button that activates a response light on the audiometer or raising a hand) every time the patient thinks that a tone is heard. To eliminate interference by background (ambient) noise, hearing testing is carried in with the patient in a double-walled, sound-treated room that meets ANSI specifications for minimal noise. The goal of pure-tone audiometry is to determine the faintest intensity level that is just audible to the patient over the range of frequencies that are important for communication. A young, otologically normal person has hearing threshold levels of 0 dB HL across this frequency region. The clinically normal region on the audiogram, however, is from 0 to 20 dB HL. Thresholds in the 20 to 40 dB

HL region constitute a mild hearing loss, 40 to 60 dB HL thresholds define a moderate loss, and threshold levels greater than 60 dB HL are considered a severe hearing loss. As a reference, the intensity level of whispered speech close to the ear is less than 25 dB HL, conversational speech is in the 40 to 50 dB HL region, and a shouted voice within a foot of the ear is at about 80 dB HL. The most important frequencies for understanding speech are in the 500 through 2000 Hz region, although higher frequencies also contribute to discrimination between certain speech sounds. Often, hearing sensitivity within the "speech frequency" region is summarized with by calculating the *pure-tone average* or PTA (hearing thresholds for 500, 1000, and 2000 Hz divided by 3 and reported in dB). As a rule, hearing loss in the mild-to-moderate range will usually cause noticeable difficulty in communication for adults, and can have a very serious effect on speech and language acquisition in young children. Persons with severe hearing impairment can rarely understand or even hear speech to communicate effectively, without visual cues (e.g. speech reading) or amplification (the use of a hearing aid). With unaided profound hearing loss, communication must be largely nonauditory.

The validity of audiometric results depends on whether the patient's responses result from stimulation of the test ear. If a sound of greater than 40 dB HL is presented to one ear via standard earphones with supra-aural (resting on the outer ear) cushions, the acoustic energy may cross-over from one side of the head to the other, and stimulate the nontest ear. The mechanism for the cross-over is presumably bone-conduction stimulation caused by vibration of the earphone cushion against the skull at high stimulus intensity levels. The amount of sound intensity needed before the cross-over occurs is a reflection of *interaural attenuation,* that is, the sound insulation between the two ears provided by the head. Interaural attenuation is usually about 50 dB for lower test frequencies and 60 dB for higher test frequencies (such as those contributing to the ABR). With bone-conduction stimulation, interaural attenuation is very limited (about 10 dB) or may not be present at all. In other words, even a very faint sound presented to the mastoid bone of one ear by a bone-conduction vibrator may be transmitted through the skull to either or both inner ears.

Masking is the audiometric technique used to eliminate participation of the nontest ear when air- and bone-conduction stimulation exceeds interaural attenuation. A noise sound is presented to the nontest ear at the same time that the stimulus is presented to the test ear. If an adequate masking technique is used, stimulus sounds crossing over to the nontest ear are masked or "covered up" by the noise. Effective masking does not prevent cross-over from occurring but, rather, it prevents the nontest ear from responding to the test signal. Choosing the appropriate amount of masking for patient's with unilateral and, particularly, bilateral hearing impairment is sometimes difficult.

Comparison of the air- versus bone-conducted hearing thresholds is useful in determining whether a hearing loss is sensorineural (no air- vs. bone-conduction gap), conductive (normal bone conduction and a loss by air-conduction), or mixed (loss by bone conduction with a superimposed air- vs. bone-conduction gap). An example of a sensorineural pattern is shown under the right ear in Figure 44–1, whereas a conductive pattern is shown under the left ear. In performing pure-tone audiometry, stimuli presented to one ear should not cross over to activate the other (nontest) ear. A masking noise is generally used in the nontest ear to reduce this test problem. *Configuration* refers to hearing loss as a function of the test frequency. With the sloping configuration, hearing is better for low frequencies and then becomes poorer for higher frequencies. This high-frequency deficit pattern is common and often reflects a sensorineural hearing impairment. HTLs are comparable for air- vs. bone-conduction (i.e., there is no air-bone gap). A rising configuration is typified by poor hearing for lower frequency stimuli and better hearing for the high frequencies. The rising configuration can result from varied types of middle-ear pathology. Measurement of middle-ear function by immittance techniques, rather than pure-tone audiometry, is the approach of choice for differentiating among these types. One exception to the typical association of conductive hearing loss with rising configuration is Meniere's disease (Chapter 56). Meniere's disease is one cochlear lesion that produces a rising configuration. A flat audiometric configuration is often recorded from patients with mixed hearing impairment, and hearing thresholds do not vary systematically across the test-frequency range.

Speech Audiometry

Speech audiometry is a measure of how well a person hears speech signals, such as words or sentences. Speech audiometry procedures are used routinely to estimate hearing sensitivity for words or speech discrimination ability. Spondee reception threshold (SRT), also referred to as the speech threshold (ST), is the faintest intensity level at which a patient can repeat words correctly. Spondee words, two syllable words with equal stress on each syllable (e.g., baseball), are presented to the patient monaurally (one ear) via earphones. The intensity level of the spondee words is gradually decreased until the tester determines the dB level at which the patient can just repeat 50% of the words presented. The technique is comparable to the method for determining pure-tone thresholds described.

Because the PTA reflects hearing threshold levels in the speech frequency region and ST or SRT is measured with a speech signal, close agreement between PTA and ST is expected. These two values should be compared routinely. If the difference between PTA and ST exceeds + / − 7 dB, one or both of the measures may be invalid. An unusually good ST relative to PTA (e.g., ST of 10 dB and PTA of 50 dB) should alert immediately the tester to the possibility of malingering. This pattern of threshold findings is often an early sign that a patient is feigning or exaggerating a hearing loss. With young children (younger than 2 years) who sometimes cannot be evaluated completely with pure-tone audiometry, the ST may provide a useful indicator of the adequacy of hearing for speech/language acquisition.

Speech recognition for phonetically balanced (PB) words is the most common clinical procedure for estimating a person's ability to hear and understand speech. In this type of procedure, a list of 25 or 50 single-syllable words are presented to the patient via earphones at a fixed intensity level and the percentage of words correctly repeated by the patient is calculated by the tester. One ear is tested at a time, often at a "comfortable listening level" initially. Within the list of words, specific speech sounds (phonemes) occur approximately as often as they would in everyday English conversion. That is, sounds that are most common in conversational speech are most common in the word list and vice versa. Therefore, the word lists often are referred to as phonetically (or phonemically) balanced (PB).

At many test facilities, these words are spoken into a microphone by the tester, while the level is monitored with a VU meter, and then the words are routed to the patient through the audiometer so that the test ear and intensity level can be selected. However, this is a poor clinical practice as it is not standardized and introduces test variabilty and response inconsistency. Whenever possible, professionally produced (and commercially available) speech materials should be presented via tape recorder or compact disk player and through an audiometer, rather than spoken directly to the patient. A number of other, more sophisticated, speech audiometry test materials exist (e.g. dichotic word tests, sentences in the presence of a competing message) to assess central auditory processing abilities. One of the most useful special speech audiometry procedures clinically is synthetic sentence identification (SSI) with competing speech. The SSI was developed in 1968 because extensive clinical experience with the PB word recognition task revealed serious limitations. The SSI task requires the patient to listen for one of 10 sentences that are presented monaurally, usually via earphones. The term "synthetic" is used for the sentences because they lack syntax needed to be meaningful sentences. The patient is given a list of the 10 sentences, on a sheet and calls out the appropriate sentence number when one is heard. At the same time, the patient is listening for the sentences, the patient is hearing a ongoing story about Davy Crockett, in the same ear and at the same intensity level, but is instructed to pay no attention to the story. The tester calculates the percentage of sentences correctly identified per list (e.g., 80%). The SSI offers several unique clinical advantages over the word recognition test. It assesses a patient's ability to hear speech in the presence of competing speech, which is an everyday listening task, and eliminates the ambiguity of reliance on the patient's speech and the tester's hearing abilities in scoring results. In addition, SSI results are not unduly influenced by high-frequency hearing loss, since the sentences include more low-frequency speech information, mostly around 750 Hz (well within the speech-frequency region).

Immittance Measurement

Aural immittance (impedance) measures are electrophysiologic procedures that are an important part of the basic audiometry test battery. Immittance audiometry is an electrophysiologic measure of auditory function. Immittance is a term that combines two similar techniques for assessing middle-ear function (impedance and admittance). It was first described in patients with middle-ear lesions as early as 1946 but has only been routinely applied clinically since about 1970. Aural immittance measures are particularly valuable with young or uncooperative children because the tests do not require a behavioral response, that is, close attention and a conscious response to sounds.

A detailed discussion of the principles of immittance measurement is not within the scope of this chapter. Many recent and comprehensive texts, monographs, and journal articles exist on the topic. Briefly, the external-ear canal is sealed with a soft rubber probe tip. Connected to the probe tip is a machine that produces a tone that is delivered to the tympanic membrane and that can quantify middle-ear impedance or admittance (hence the generic term immittance) based on the intensity and other physical properties of the tone in the ear canal. Middle ears with low impedance more readily accept the acoustic energy of the tone whereas those with greater impedance (due, for example, to fluid within the middle-ear space) tend to reject energy flow. Thus, impedance (admittance) characteristics of the middle ear can be inferred, by the machine, from probe tone properties in the ear canal.

Tympanometry

Tympanometry, the continuous measurement of middle-ear impedance as air pressure is varied systematically in the ear canal, is a sensitive measure of tympanic-membrane integrity and middle-ear function (Figure 44–2). Compliance (the reciprocal of stiffness) of the middle ear is the dominant component of immittance and is usually described on the vertical dimension of a tympanogram. Tympanometry is popular clinically because it requires little technical skill and only several seconds of time, is an electrophysiologic (vs. behavioral) method that does not depend on cooperation of the patient, and yet provides valuable information on middle-ear function. Tympanometric patterns, in combination with audiogram patterns, permit differentiation among middle-ear disorders. The normal, or type A, tympanogram has a distinct peak in compliance within air pressures in the ear canal equivalent to 0 to ± 100 mm of water. This is in the normal range of middle-ear pressure. The height of the compliance peak must also be within a certain normal range, as indicated by the stippled area, for a tympanogram to be classified as normal. With the type B tympanogram, there is no peak in compliance but, rather, a flat pattern with little or even no apparent change in compliance as a function of pressure in the ear canal. This pattern is most often associated with fluid within the middle-ear space (e.g., otitis media), although other middle-ear lesions may give rise to a type B tympanogram as well. The type C tympanogram resembles the type A in that it has a distinct peak in compliance, but the peak is displaced to the negative pressure region on the horizontal dimension of the graph. By definition, a tympanogram is type C if the peak is at negative ear-canal pressure beyond-100 mm H_2O. This pattern is usually found in patients with eustachian tube dysfunction and inadequate ventilation of the middle-ear space. It often precedes the type B tympanogram in the development of otitis media.

A variation of the type A tympanogram is the type A_s. The "s" stands for shallow. Peak compliance is low, and outside of the stippled area. Put another way, middle-ear impedance is unusually high. The type A_s pattern is found in patients with fixation of the ossicular chain. Otosclerosis is a disease that often results in ossicular chain fixation, but a type A_s tympanogram does not invariably mean the patient has otosclerosis. An usually steep and high-compliance tympanogram is classified as type A_d (d for deep). The peak may actually exceed the upper compliance limits of the equipment. This type is found in patients with disruption of the ossicular chain, which leaves the middle ear extremely mobile and hypercompliant (i.e. little impedance). In the absence of serious hearing loss, however, this tympanogram pattern usually is associated with minor tympanic membrane abnormalities, such as scarring. Finally, if during the initial portion of tympanometry, the impedance machine records an abnormally large volume of air between the probe tip and presumably the tympanic membrane, the tester must suspect a perforation of the tympanic membrane. That is, the machine is measuring not just ear-canal volume but also volume of the middle-ear space. Average ear-canal volume as measured by impedance devices is about 1 ml in the adult, and slightly smaller in children. A volume equal to or greater than 2.5 ml, or a large

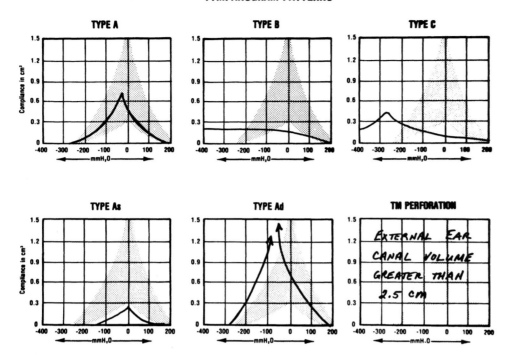

Fig. 44–2. Classification system for tympanograms. Adapted from Jerger JF: Clinical experience with impedance audiometry. Arch Otolaryngol *92*:11–24, 1970.

asymmetry in ear-canal volume between ears, is consistent with a hole in the tympanic membrane. This may be an actual perforation or an open middle ear ventilation tube.

Acoustic Stapedial Reflex Measurement

Measurement of acoustic reflex activity, contractions of the middle ear stapedial muscle to sound, is also clinically useful for estimating hearing sensitivity and differentiating among sites of auditory disorders (middle ear, inner ear, 8th cranial nerve, and auditory brainstem). The acoustic reflex is a contraction of the stapedius muscle in response to relatively high intensity sounds. The stapedius muscle, one of the smallest muscles in the body, is located in the middle ear. It is attached to the posterior part of the stapes, the innermost ossicle. When a high intensity stimulus (usually greater than 80 dB HL) is presented to either ear of a person with normal hearing or up to a moderate degree of cochlear loss, and normal middle ear function, the stapedius muscle reflexively contracts bilaterally. The afferent portion of the acoustic reflex arc is the eighth cranial nerve. Complex brainstem pathways lead from the cochlear nucleus on the stimulated side to the region of the motor nucleus of the seventh (facial) nerve on both sides (ipsilateral and contralateral to the stimulus) of the brainstem. The efferent portion of the arc is the seventh nerve that innervates the stapedius muscle. The muscle then contracts, causing increased stiffness (decreased compliance) of the middle ear. The small change in compliance that follows (within 10 msec)

stapedius muscle contraction is detected by the probe assembly of the impedance machine, just as compliance changes during tympanometry are detected.

Acoustic reflex measurement is a valuable diagnostic procedure because it can provide information, electrophysiologically, on the status of the auditory system from the middle ear to the brainstem. Distinctive acoustic reflex patterns for ipsilateral and contralateral stimulation and measurement arrangements characterize middle-ear, cochlear, eighth-nerve, brainstem and even facial-nerve dysfunction. Comparison of acoustic reflex threshold levels, ie. the lowest stimulus intensity level that activates the reflex, for tone versus noise stimuli permits estimation of the degree of cochlear hearing impairment. This technique is especially valuable in infants and difficult-to-test patients. Because impedance measures, including acoustic reflex, are electrophyisologic and not behavioral, they can be carried out with patients sedated, before or after ABR assessment. They can thus augment ABR information, especially on the status of the middle ear and cochlea.

Auditory-Evoked Responses

Auditory Brainstem Response

Auditory-evoked responses are electrophysiologic recordings of responses from within the auditory system that are activated by sounds. Auditory-evoked responses can be recorded clinically at all levels of the auditory system, from the cochlea to the cortex. Among these responses, the auditory brainstem response or

AUDITORY BRAINSTEM REPONSE (ABR)

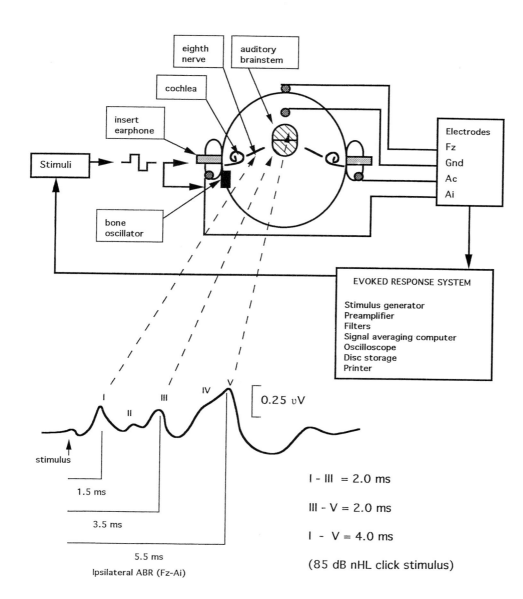

Fig. 44–3. Schematic of the instrumentation used for recording the auditory brainstem response (ABR) and major relations between auditory anatomy and waveform components. A simple strategy for analysis of ABR waveform in neurodiagnosis is also shown.

ABR (also referred to as the brainstem auditory-evoked response or BAER) is applied most often clinically. An ABR recording is shown schematically in Figure 44–3. The ABR is generated with transient acoustic stimuli (clicks or tone bursts) and recorded with surface electrodes placed on the forehead and the ears (mastoid, earlobe, or external-ear canal). By means of a fast computer, thousands of sound stimuli can be presented, and reliable ABR waveforms can be averaged in a matter of minutes. The ABR wave components arise from the 8th cranial nerve and auditory regions in the caudal and rostral brainstem (Figure 44–3).

Analysis of ABR waveforms evoked by high-intensity stimuli provides neurodiagnostic information on cochlear and retrocochlear auditory function. Early re-

ports on ABR in identification of retrocochlear disorders (e.g. acoustic neurinomas) described a success rate exceeding 95%. With the development of sophisticated neuroradiologic techniques, such as CT or MRI with enhancement, reports of normal ABR findings in patients with very small posterior fossa tumors have appeared in the literature. Nonetheless, ABR continues to be an excellent technique for initial diagnostic assessment of eighth nerve and auditory brainstem status in patients with signs and symptoms of retrocochlear disorders. ABR is also valuable in electrophysiologic monitoring of the eighth-nerve and auditory-brainstem function during certain neurotologic operations (e.g. vestibular-nerve section, posterior cranial fossa tumor removal).

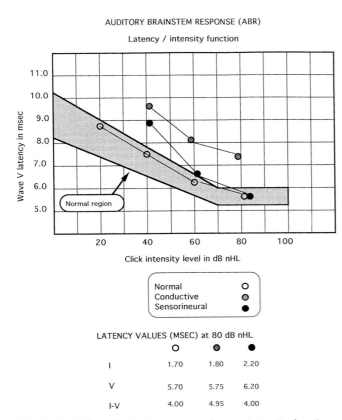

AUDITORY BRAINSTEM RESPONSE (ABR)

Latency / intensity function

Wave V latency in msec

Click intensity level in dB nHL

	Normal	○
	Conductive	◉
	Sensorineural	●

LATENCY VALUES (MSEC) at 80 dB nHL

	○	◉	●
I	1.70	1.80	2.20
V	5.70	5.75	6.20
I-V	4.00	4.95	4.00

Fig. 44–4. Auditory brainstem response latency-intensity functions associated with normal hearing, and conductive and sensory hearing loss (approximately 30 to 35 dB in the 1000 to 4000 Hz region). Latency for the ABR wave V component is plotted as a function of stimulus intensity level. Note the distinctly different patterns and latency values for these three clinical entities.

A major clinical advantage of ABR is that it can be reliably recorded from very young children, even newborn infants, and from children who are difficult-to-test by conventional audiometric techniques. ABR is not affected by patient state of arousal. In fact, because any patient movement produces muscle artifact that precludes valid recordings, children between the ages of 6 months and 5 years typically must be lightly sedated for ABR assessment. ABRs can also be recorded in the operating room under general anesthesia. By systematically reducing the intensity level of the stimuli and analyzing changes in the response (particularly the wave V latency), one can estimate a patient's hearing sensitivity level, at least for the high-frequency region, and can often determine the type of hearing loss, such as conductive versus sensorineural (Figure 44–4). The ABR can now be elicited also with abrupt, specially shaped tone-burst stimuli for estimation of hearing for specific audiometric frequency regions. In addition, bone-conduction stimulation of the ABR permits approximation of the degree of conductive-hearing component, even in young children who cannot be assessed adequately with behavioral audiometry.

The ABR is also used to determine brain-stem functional integrity in coma due to head trauma and other causes.

Electrocochleography

Electrocochleography (ECochG) has been applied in the assessment of peripheral auditory function for over 30 years. Currently, ECochG is performed most often for intraoperative monitoring of cochlear and eighth-nerve status and in the diagnosis of Meniere's disease. Optimal ECochG waveforms are recorded from a small needle electrode placed transtympanically onto the promontory, although ear canal or tympanic membrane electrode locations are also clinically useful. Three major components of the ECochG are the cochlear microphonic (CM), the summating potential (SP), and the action potential (AP). The CM and SP reflect cochlear bioelectric activity, whereas the AP is generated by synchronous firing of distal afferent eighth nerve fibers (Figure 44–5). In patients with Meniere's Disease, the characteristic ECochG finding is an abnormal enlargement of the relation between the SP and AP component amplitudes.

Otoacoustic Emissions

Otoacoustic emissions (OAE) are low-intensity sounds produced by the cochlea spontaneously and in re-

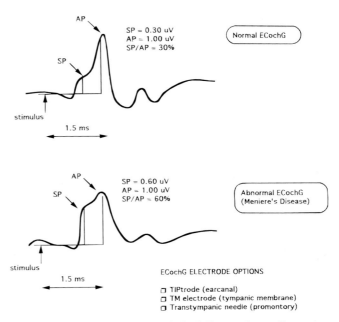

ELECTROCOCHLEOGRAPHY (ECochG)

AP

SP

SP = 0.30 uV
AP = 1.00 uV
SP/AP = 30%

Normal ECochG

stimulus

1.5 ms

AP

SP

SP = 0.60 uV
AP = 1.00 uV
SP/AP = 60%

Abnormal ECochG
(Meniere's Disease)

stimulus

1.5 ms

ECochG ELECTRODE OPTIONS

□ TIPtrode (earcanal)
□ TM electrode (tympanic membrane)
□ Transtympanic needle (promontory)

Fig. 44–5. Electrocochleography (ECochG) waveforms illustrating normal relation of summating potential (SP) and action potential (AP) in the top panel and abnormally enlarged SP/AP relation in a patient with Meniere's disease (bottom panel).

sponse to an acoustic stimulus. An acoustic stimulus, a click or a combination of tones, can activate outer hair cell movement or motility. This motility, in turn, generates mechanical energy within the cochlea, which is propagated outward, via the middle-ear system and the tympanic membrane, to the ear canal. Vibration of the tympanic membrane then produces an acoustic signal (the OAE), which can be measured by a sensitive microphone. When outer hair cells are damaged structurally or nonfunctional, otoacoustic emissions cannot be evoked by acoustic stimuli. The noninvasive nature of OAE recording, coupled with their accuracy and objectivity in assessing cochlear, in particular outer-hair cell, function suggests diverse potential clinical applications, ranging from auditory screening to sensorineural hearing impairment diagnosis. Considerable research is underway to document the effectiveness of otoacoustic emissions in hearing screening of infants, and in other clinical applications.

There are two broad classes of otoacoustic emissions: spontaneous and evoked. Spontaneous otoacoustic emissions (SOAE), present in only approximately 60% of persons with normal hearing, are measured in the ex-

ternal-ear canal when there is no external sound stimulation. A significant gender effect for SOAE has been confirmed with females demonstrating SOAE at twice the rate of males. *Evoked* oto acoustic emissions are elicited by low-to-moderate levels of acoustic stimulation in the external-ear canal and are classified according to characteristics of the stimuli used to elicit them or characteristics of the cochlear events that generate them. *Stimulus-frequency* otoacoustic emissions (SFOAE), which are technically difficult to record, are the least studied of the evoked otoacoustic emissions. *Distortion-product* otoacoustic emissions (DPOAE) are produced when two pure-tone stimuli at frequencies f_1 and f_2 are presented to the ear simultaneously. The most robust DPOAE occur at the frequency determined by the equation $2f_1-f_2$, whereas the actual cochlear frequency region that is assessed with DPOAE is between these two frequencies, and probably close to the f_2 stimulus (Figure 44–6). *Transiently evoked* otoacoustic emissions (TEOAE) are elicited by brief acoustic stimuli such as clicks or tonebursts (Figure 44–7). More than 250 literature citations describe investigations of DPOAE and TEOAE. Each of

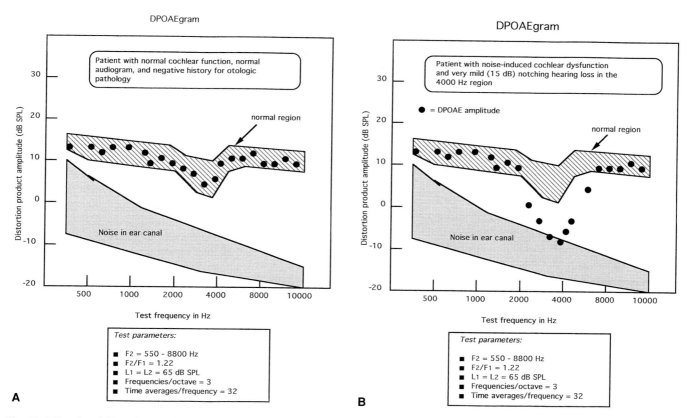

Fig. 44–6. Results of distortion product otoacoustic emission (DPOAE) measurement for a normal hearing subject (top panel) and for a patient with mild sensory hearing impairment (bottom panel) secondary to noise exposure. Replicated plots of DPOAE amplitude in dB SPL are shown as a function of the frequency of the stimuli (the geometric mean of the f_1 and f_2) in a "DP gram" (data collected with a Virtual Corportation 330 device).

KEY: normal ○ maybe abnormal ◔ abnormal ●	DIAGNOSTIC AUDIOLOGY TEST BATTERY PATTERNS					
	Site of Lesion					
TEST PROCEDURE	Middle ear	Cochlea	Eighth nerve	Brainstem Caudal	Brainstem Rostral	Cerebrum
Aural Immittance						
tympanometry	●	○	○	○	○	○
acoustic reflexes	●	◔	●	◔	○	○
Pure tone audiometry	◔	●	◔	○	○	○
Word recognition	○	◔	◔	○	○	○
Otoacoustic emissions	●	●	○	○	○	○
Diagnostic speech audiometry	○	○	●	●	●	●
Evoked Responses						
ECochG	◔	◔	○	○	○	○
ABR	●	◔	●	●	●	○
AMLR	○	○	○	○	○	●
P300/MMN	○	○	○	○	○	●

Fig. 44–7. Patterns of diagnostic audiometry test battery findings associated with different sites of lesions within the auditory system. For each site of lesions, audiometric results may vary depending on the specific type of pathophysiology and the extent of the pathology, and on whether the auditory stimulus is presented ipsilaterally or contralaterally to the lesion. Abbreviations are as follows: ABR {equi} auditory brainstem response; AMLR {equi} auditory middle latency response; P$_{300}$ {equi} endogenous cognitive response at about 300 msec; MMN {equi} mismatch negativity response.

these types of evoked OAE are likely to be incorporated into routine auditory assessment of children and adults.

Recently, interest in clinical application of OAE has increased considerably largely because of the outcome of a 1993 National Institutes of Health (NIH) Conference on the Early Identification of Hearing Impairment in Infants and Young Children. A Panel assembled by the NIH recommended that all infants be screened for hearing impairment within the first three months of life. The Panel specifically recommended a two-stage hearing screening approach that called for an initial screening with an OAE technique, and a secondary ABR screening of those infants failing the OAE screen. OAE will soon assume a central role in the early detection of hearing impairment in infants and young children. OAE are also likely to be valuable in neurotologic diagnosis. Evoked OAE are "preneural" and physiologically vulnerable to cochlear insults, whereas ABR is a time-tested clinical index of auditory system function at level of the 8th cranial nerve and auditory brainstem. ABR can also, of course, contribute to detection and quantification of conductive and sensory (cochlear) auditory disorders. Therein lies the power of using both OAE and ABR in conjunction with immittance, pure-tone and speech measurements, and even later-latency auditory-evoked responses, for systematic assessment of the auditory system from the tympanic membrane to the auditory cortex. Even though OAE will soon join the audiometric test battery for

everyday clinical assessment of cochlear status, ABR will continue to play a crucial role in auditory assessment.

Patterns of Auditory Findings

No single measure of auditory function is adequate for comprehensive hearing assessment. This is the assumption underlying the audiologic "crosscheck principle." For example, the pure-tone audiogram provides information on hearing sensitivity, at least for a handful of frequencies, but is not useful in distinguishing among middle-ear disorders, in differentiating sensory versus neural hearing loss, nor in identification of central auditory nervous system dysfunction. Immittance measurements are invaluable for analyzing middle-ear function, but are not measures of hearing. Normal tympanograms, for example, can be recorded in a patient with a nonfunctioning cochlea and, conversely, markedly abnormal tympanograms may be associated with only a mild hearing sensitivity deficit. Similarly, other auditory procedures (ABR, ECochG, OAE) also have their unique limitations for the complete assessment of hearing—assessment of the peripheral and central auditory nervous system.

Comprehensive and sensitive hearing assessment of children and adults is possible only with a battery of auditory procedures. By selecting the appropriate audiologic procedures, and properly analyzing the pattern of test findings, it is almost always possible to describe the site of disorder within the auditory system and the degree of auditory dysfunction. Information gained from careful interpretation of the pattern of auditory findings can contribute to the otologic diagnosis. Perhaps more importantly, this information is essential for prompt and effective medical, surgical, and audiologic management.

INDICATIONS FOR DIAGNOSTIC HEARING ASSESSMENT

Children

"Hearing loss, regardless of etiology, affects speech and language development of infants and young children. Communication deficits may initially occur within the first six months of life. Hearing loss in preschool- and school-age children interferes with educational development. Early identification of hearing loss, with prompt and appropriate intervention and managment, is essential if the child is to reach his or her communicative and educational potential . . . Monitoring a child's hearing at periodic and regular intervals during the first five years of life is the responsibility of *pediatricians* and *primary care physicians*" (Consensus Statement, 1992, pp. 508, 510). The 1994 Joint Committee on Infant Hearing developed specific sets of indicators for hearing impairment in neonates (birth to 28 days) and infants (29 days to 2 years). Joint Committee risk indicators for hearing impairment are summarized in Table 44–1. Parental concern about possible hearing loss is always an indication for audiologic assessment. Strategies for hearing screening and diagnostic hearing assessment vary depending on the age of the child. Otolaryngologists and audiologists must coordinate efforts in properly and promptly assessing and managing pediatric hearing impairment.

Adults

The first suspicion of hearing impairment in adult patients arises, in many cases, during the medical history. The patient may cite hearing loss as the chief complaint. Close questioning may reveal that the patient has difficulty hearing, especially difficulty understanding speech. Sometimes this problem is only apparent, or is most noticeable, under specific conditions, such as when the patient is speaking on the telephone or conversing in noisy environments, or conversing with certain persons (e.g. children or women whose voices tend to be fainter and higher pitched than men). The medical history may also produce other information which puts the patient at risk for hearing impairment, such as exposure to potentially damaging levels of recreational or work-related noise. A physical finding associated with auditory system involvement, of course, also indicates the need for audiologic assessment.

TABLE 44–1. Indicators Associated with Sensorineural and/or Conductive Hearing Loss in Children, as Recommended by the 1994 Joint Committee on Infant Hearing

Neonates: birth to 28 days when universal hearing screening is not available
   Family history of hereditary childhood sensorineural hearing loss

   In utero infections, such as cytomegalovirus, rubella, syphilis, herpes, and taxoplasmosis

   Craniofacial anomalies, including morphologic abnormalities of the pinna and ear canal

   Birthweight less than 1500 g (3.3 lb)

   Hyperbilirubinemia at a serum level requiring exchange transfusion

   Ototoxic medications including but not limited to the aminoglycosides used in multiple courses or in combination with loop diuretics

   Bacterial meningitis

   Apgar scores of 0–4 at 1 minutue or 0–6 at 5 minutes

   Mechanical ventilation lasting 5 days or more

   Stigmata or other findings associated with a syndrome known to include a sensorineural and/or a conductive hearing loss

Infants: 29 days to 2 years when health conditions develop that require rescreening
   Parent/caregiver concern regarding hearing, speech, language, and/or developmental delay

   Bacterial meningitis and other infections associated with sensorineural hearing loss

   Head trauma associated with loss of consciousness or skull fracture

   Stigmata or other findings associated with a syndrome known to include a sensorineural and/or a conductive hearing loss

   Ototoxic medications including but not limited to chemotherapeutic agents or aminoglycosides used in mulitple courses or in combination with loop diuretics

   Recurrent or persistent otitis media with effusion for at least 3 months

Infants: 29 days to 3 years who require periodic monitoring of hearing
   Indicators associated with delayed onset hearing loss include:
      Family history of hereditary childhood hearing loss
      In utero infections, such as cytomegalovirus, rubella, syphillis, herpes, or toxoplasmosis
      Neurofibromatosis type II and neurodegenerative disorders

   Indicators associated with conductive hearing loss include:
      Recurrent or persistent otitis media with effusion
      Anatomic deformities and other disorders that affect eustachian tube function
      Neurodengerative disorders

HEARING AIDS

A hearing aid is a prosthetic device that delivers an amplified acoustic signal into the ear canal. The use of some form of amplification to overcome the deleterious effects of a hearing impairment on communication has been used for centuries. The most simplistic "hearing aid" is made easily by cupping one's hand behind the ear. This technique is effective because a stronger acoustic signal is channeled into the ear canal. Another simple way to improve the reception of an acoustic signal is to move closer to its source. When the distance between the sound source and the listener is doubled, acoustic intensity is reduced by 6 decibels. Similarly, cutting the distance by one-half increases the intensity by 6 decibels. When the source of the acoustic signal is an electronic device, such as a television, reception can be easily enhanced by adjusting the volume control to deliver a more intense signal. All of these methods enhance the reception of a particular acoustic signal and demonstrate that amplification is often an effective means of improving one's ability to hear. Although there are a few exceptions, amplification can be used to improve hearing in virtually all forms of hearing impairment, as well.

Electronic hearing aids enhance signal strength by amplification of the acoustic signals that reach its microphone. The first hearing aids were large, undependable, and inefficient. Hearing aid design evolved rapidly with advances in electronics becoming smaller, reliable, and highly efficient. Today's hearing aids are technologically advanced electronic devices. The most sophisticated hearing aids fit completely within the ear canal and contain microprocessors that can be reprogrammed by remote control while being worn by the patient. Perhaps the most amazing aspect of hearing aid design is that most units are powered only by a single disposable button-type battery of less than 1.5 volts. Average battery life ranges between 10 and 14 16-hour days. The battery life of the most efficient units can exceed 21 days. Rechargable batteries are also available in some models.

Electronic hearing aids are comprised of three basic components: a microphone, amplifier, and receiver. The *microphone* is located externally and is activated by miniscule fluctuations in air pressure caused by the sound source. These vibrations are converted into an electrical impulse and delivered to the *amplifier*. At this stage the signal is amplified and filtered. The altered signal is delivered to the *receiver* which converts the electronic impulse into an acoustic signal. The amplified acoustic signal is then delivered into the ear canal. These components are housed in a plastic case designed to fit behind or in the ear. A user adjustable volume control is typically located conveniently on the surface of the hearing aid for easy manipulation by the patient. Many hearing aids are also available with a remote control device that can be used to adjust the volume or tone quality of the instrument.

Types of Hearing Aids

Currently, two basic categories of hearing aids exist, distinguished by the size and location of the instru-

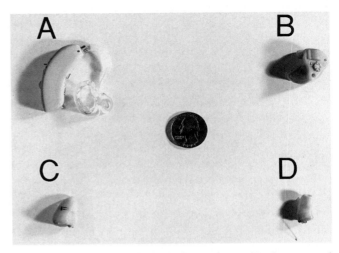

Fig. 44–8. Examples of major hearing aid designs. The four types of hearing aids are behind-the-ear (A), in-the-ear (B), and in-the-canal (C), and deep canal (peritympanic).

ment in relation to the outer ear: behind-the-ear (BTE) and in-the-ear (ITE). In-the-ear hearing aids are divided into three categories: custom in-the-ear (ITE), in-the-canal (ITC), and completely-in-the-canal (CIC). Each category can be further subdivided into programmable and nonprogrammable designs.

Behind-the-ear hearing aids are aptly named because the body of the instrument is designed to rest on the postero-superior aspect of the auricle (Figure 44–8). The receiver is coupled to the ear canal by a piece of acoustic tubing attached to a custom-made earmold. BTE hearing aids are extremely flexible because of their design and large size. Any degree of hearing loss (from mild to profound) can be managed with a BTE. A defective unit can be replaced by removing the tubing/earmold assembly and attaching it to a new unit. Changes in the size of the auricle in patients are inexpensively accomodated by making a new earmold. It is not necessary to modify the body of the hearing aid. For this reason BTE units have been a popular choice for children. In addition, the earmold can be made of materials with densities ranging from hard (lucite) to very soft (silicone rubber). The choice of earmold material can significantly add to the comfort and flexibility of the instrument. One disadvantage of BTE instruments is their vulnerability to perspiration. BTE hearing aids require frequent cleaning to maintain maximum performance. Another disadvantage is the location of the microphone. The ideal location of a microphone would be deep in the ear canal using the natural resonance of the auricle and ear canal. The microphones of BTE instruments are located above the auricle and are oriented anteriorly. The loss of natural cues must be compensated for by the hearing aid. BTEs account for less than 20% of annual hearing aid sales in the United States.

In-the-ear hearing aids are housed completely within a custom-made earmold designed to fit in the auricle and ear canal. The body of the hearing aid completely fills the concha and contains most of the electronic components, the battery, and a volume control. The antero-superior arm of the ITE hearing aid fits into the helix of the auricle inferior to the triangular fossa and functions primarily to keep the instrument in place. The microphone is sometimes located within this portion of the instrument. The medial portion fits partially into the ear canal and contains the receiver. ITE hearing aids are completely self-contained. There is no tubing or earmold assembly. The hearing aid is essentially built into the earmold. Properly fit ITE instruments are appropriate for mild-to-severe, and sometimes profound, losses of hearing. The location of the microphone close to the level of the ear canal is an advantage of the ITE style. However, the size of the instrument within the auricle minimizes the use of natural resonance. ITE instruments are highly reliable and less vulnerable to perspiration from the scalp. The custom-fit one-piece design is highly desirable, but creates a few problems. First, when an instrument must be repaired or replaced the patient is usually without it for several days. Sometimes a BTE loaner is provided, but this is not always an acceptable alternative. Second, ITE hearing aids can be difficult for some patients to insert and remove. Small children and adults with poor manual dexterity often need assistance inserting and removing their hearing aids, as well as adjusting the volume control. Almost 60% of hearing aid sales are ITE units.

In-the-canal instruments fit primarily into the ear canal. Only the face of the hearing aid is visible in the concha area. A wide range of hearing losses can be accomodated by a properly fitted ITC instrument, including severe sensorineural hearing loss. The location of the microphone is at the opening of the ear canal taking advantage of the acoustic properties of most of the auricle. Although the size of ITC instruments is a cosmetic advantage, there are a few disadvantages. First, there is less structure holding the hearing aid in place, thus they are more easily dislodged and frequently become lost. Second, their small size makes them more difficult to insert and remove. As with ITE units, children and adults with poor manual dexterity often need assistance. Third, the volume controls on ITC instruments are small. Manipulation of the volume control can be difficult for many patients, especially during the initial adjustment period. Aside from these potential problems, the ITC hearing aid is an extremely popular design accounting for over one-fourth of total instrument sales.

Completely-in-the-canal hearing aids are inserted deeply into the ear canal by the patient, and are essentially invisible to the casual observer. The medial aspect of the CIC hearing aid is located within 2 mm of the tympanic membrane (e.g., peritympanic). The instrument is retrieved by pulling on a nylon loop attached to its lateral surface. Aside from their obvious cosmetic appeal, CIC hearing aids take full advantage of the natural acoustic properties of the auricle and ear canal. Because of its proximity to the tympanic membrane, the acoustic signal is more efficiently transferred and requires less amplification. The volume of air between the medial surface of the hearing aid and the tympanic membrane in CIC fittings is approximately one-tenth of that found in a typical ITE or ITC fitting. The result is a gain of up to 15 decibels in sound pressure without additional amplification. The primary disadvantage is placement and removal of the hearing aid. Patients must be trained to place the instrument safely without damaging the tympanic membrane. The otolaryngologist may play an important role in evaluation of candidacy of patients for CIC hearing aids. Contraindications include perforated tympanic membrane, chronic or recurrent otitis media, chronic drainage, osteoma, petromastoidectomy, exostosis, cholesteatoma, and any other structural anomaly that would interfere with safe and effective use of the instrument. CIC instruments are relatively new to the market. At the time of this writing, no sales statistics are available for comparison.

Every major hearing aid manufacturer has incorporated at least one programmable unit into its line of hearing instruments. It is safe to speculate that sales of digitally programmable hearing aids will exceed analog hearing aids in the years to come. Programmable hearing aids differ in three primary ways: 1) number of channels; 2) number of memory settings; and 3) type of signal processing used. First, most of the instruments currently available operate with one channel. Additional channels allow for the simultaneous processing of different portions of the signal to maximize performance. Second, both single- and multiple-channel instruments can have multiple memories. Each memory, in turn, can be programmed to process the signal in a different way. This gives the patient a number of settings to choose from when the listening environment changes. Different memories can be accessed by using a remote control. Third, signal processing is used to enhance the reception of the signal (usually speech), particularly in unfavorable (noisy) listening conditions. A variety of algorithms are in use, but no single strategy is best for a given situation. Performance with respect to signal processing is situation- and patient-specific; therefore, it must be tailored to meet the needs of each patient on an individual basis. This requires a thorough knowledge of the listening needs of the patient and the characteristics of the hearing aid being used.

Signal Processing

The average listening environment is characterized by continual change. The relationship between the desired signal and background noise differs from moment to moment and from one location to the next. Normally hearing listeners are able to handle the changes quite well, even in very noisy environments. Fluctuations in the acoustic environment cause unique problems for the hearing-impaired listener, especially when the level of the background noise approaches or exceeds the level of the desired signal.

Signal-processing circuits are designed to enhance the reception of the signal actively in response to changes in the listening environment. The primary goal is to eliminate interference (noise) and clarify the signal (usually speech). This goal is accomplished by real-time alteration of the acoustic signal using sophisticated circuitry or digital processing. Traditional signal processing attempted to enhance the signal by reducing amplification at high levels (compressing limiting) and/or increasing amplification at lower levels (wide dynamic range compression). This approach is commonly referred to as *automatic gain control* (AGC). The balance between low and high frequencies is maintained in AGC circuitry. More recent approaches utilize compression to alter the balance between low and high frequencies. The combined approach is also known as *level dependent frequency response* (LDFR) after Killion et al. There are three types of LDFR processing. *Type 1* processing gradually reduces the amplification of low frequencies as the level of the acoustic signal increases. This strategy is designed to limit the amplification of low frequency noise found in many listening environments. Unfortunately, this approach is not effective in all listening environments and important speech cues are lost in the filtering process. *Type 2* processing gradually increases the amplification of high frequencies at low levels while reversing the process at higher levels. This method incorporates the amplification of important speech cues at low levels and reduces their volume at higher levels to avoid overamplification. *Type 3* processing utilizes multiple channel processing capabilities of programmable hearing aids to perform both Type 1 and Type 2 signal processing independently. This type is the most versatile, but is only available in multichannel programmable instruments.

Indications for Amplification

A hearing aid(s) is indicated whenever it can be demonstrated that the patient's ability to communicate will be significantly improved through the use of amplification. A hearing aid is not recommended under the following conditions: 1) when effective medical treatment can be implemented to restore normal hearing; 2) when the use of a hearing aid would interfere with or exacerbate pathology or its treatment; and 3) when a hearing aid fails to improve the ability of the patient to communicate significantly.

A common myth is that amplification is of no benefit in cases of sensorineural hearing loss. While there is no evidence correlating the use of a hearing aid with restoration, or treatment, of the impaired auditory system, hearing aids are routinely used to offset the *effects* of sensory hearing impairment. Sensory hearing loss accounts for over 90% of all types of hearing loss. In excess of 95% of all hearing aids are purchased by patients with sensorineural hearing loss. Amplification is an effective means of improving the communicative abilities of individuals with sensory hearing impairment, as attested by hundreds of research articles published throughout the last fifty years which directly or indirectly attest to the successful use of hearing aids in the audiologic habilitation of individuals with sensory hearing impairment.

Amplification is an extremely effective means of improving the hearing of patients with conductive hearing loss. A hearing aid is clearly not an acceptable alternative to effective medical treatment of the pathological condition, but it may be utilized after the course of treatment to offset residual hearing impairment. Residual conductive hearing loss is commonly present following placement of an ossicular prosthesis, for example. A hearing aid is often an effective means of further improving hearing sensitivity. In contrast, amplification is of little benefit to patients with retrocochlear (neural or central) auditory disorders. Amplification may actually exacerbate the effects of the disorder in some cases. The use of amplification must be carefully evaluated in all cases in which central impairment is suggested to determine efficacy. There are alternative strategies for audiologic management of patients with central auditory dysfunction. Perhaps the most common hearing instrument approach is recommendation of an assistive listening device for improvement of speech understanding by enhancement of the speech-to-noise relation.

Assessment of Hearing Aid Efficacy

There are several ways to assess the efficacy, or outcome, of amplification. Perhaps the most compelling evidence comes directly from the patient. After a brief period of hearing aid use, most patients are quite capable of determining whether the prescribed amplification has improved their ability to hear. This is understandable considering that the vast majority of individuals who purchase hearing aids cope with the hearing impairment for several years before deciding to try amplification. After very little experience wearing the new hearing aid, most patients are able to precisely describe the listening situations in which their hearing aid(s) are effective or ineffective. To quantify the valuable patient report, a number of *self-assessment inventories* have been developed for use by audiologists and hearing aid dispensers. These inventories are widely used to evaluate the initial fitting and assess the effectiveness of subsequent modifications.

In addition to the self-assessment inventories, there are numerous approaches for objectively assessing hearing aid efficacy in the clinic. These methods are collectively known as *functional tests* of hearing. Functional tests simply compare the results of audiologic tests with and without amplification. The *functional gain* test compares unaided and aided thresholds for pure tones and spondee words. These tests indicate whether the hearing aid has effectively improved thresholds for tones and/or speech. *Functional word-identification* tests compare unaided and aided scores on a variety of word-identification tasks. These tests indicate whether amplification improves the ability of the patient to identify isolated words, words in sentences, and words in the presence of various levels of background noise. Together, self-assessment inventories and functional tests can be used to index accurately the efficacy of the prescribed amplification. The information can also be used to recommend and evaluate subsequent modifications to the prescription.

Prescriptive Hearing Aid Fitting

It is a well-known phenomenon that two patients with identical audiograms will frequently require vastly different hearing aid configurations. Aside from the test battery conducted during a routine hearing aid evaluation, there are no standardized methods in use that can reliably objectify the process of hearing aid selection. The selection of appropriate amplification is a process of ongoing assessment and re-evaluation. It is rare when a hearing aid fitting is ideal on the first day. A period of adjustment and reconfiguration is usually required.

In recent years, attempts have been made to take some of the guesswork out of hearing aid selection. Procedures that are based on the results of routine audiometric tests have been adopted for prescribing a hearing aid. The prescription is not expected to be a panacea, but is intended to provide the dispenser with a valid approximation—a logical starting point. From there, the process of assessment and modification should be minimal. A number of prescriptive methods are in use, but no standard has been adopted. All hearing aid manufacturers use at least one prescriptive formula to aid in selection of an appropriate circuit or to program the instrument before it is shipped to the dispenser. Thereafter, the dispenser can adjust the instrument to accomodate the individual needs of the patient.

Early attempts at prescribing amplification were based on the assumption that the gain of the hearing aid must match the amount of the hearing loss. This frequently resulted in overamplification and rejection of the hearing aid. It was soon recognized that patients with sensory hearing loss required much less amplification than was originally assumed. Most of the prescriptive formulas in use today are based on the *half-gain rule*. According to this metric, a hearing loss of 50 decibels requires a gain of approximately 25 decibels to achieve the maximum benefit from amplification. Examination of the most widely used prescriptive formulas indicates rough approximation to the half-gain rule. Typically, slightly less gain is prescribed in the lower frequencies to minimize the amplification of background noise, while slightly more amplification is prescribed in the higher frequencies to enhance reception of speech cues.

Real-ear Verification of Hearing Aid Fit

Until recently, analysis of the acoustic properties of a hearing aid while in the ear of a patient was impossible. Yet, a valid method of measuring the performance of the hearing aid in vivo is especially important when trying to match a prescription or evaluate a problem fitting. Real-ear systems were developed to make this possible. Real-ear measurement systems use a specially designed probe microphone to measure the sound pressure in the ear canal at the eardrum. Silastic tubing attached to a sensitive microphone is inserted into the open ear canal. A broad band click or tonal series is presented via a loudspeaker approximately one meter away from the patient. The frequency response of the unoccluded ear is recorded and displayed graphically. Next, the hearing aid is inserted and adjusted to a comfortable level. The stimulus is presented again, recorded, and displayed. Subtraction of the unaided (open ear) response from the aided response yields a precise measure of the performance of the instrument in the ear of the patient. The hearing aid can then be adjusted to match the prescription. Rear-ear techniques are also extremely useful in troubleshooting problems with a fitting, as might be required when the hearing aid is not performing according to specifications. The reader is referred to a text by Mueller, Hawkins, and Northern for a comprehensive discussion real-ear technology, and a variety of clinical procedures based on the technique.

Monaural Versus Binaural Hearing Aid Fittings

A great deal of research has been devoted to the following question: when hearing loss is bilateral are two hearing aids better than one? The intuitive answer is, of course, that two hearing aids would best offset the effects of a hearing loss in both ears. The question persists, however, because many patients choose monaural fittings. This decision is usually made for cosmetic or financial reasons, although some patients claim to hear just as well with one hearing aid as with two, while others appear to hear better with a single instrument.

The benefits of binaural amplification have been well documented in the audiologic literature. The most commonly cited benefits are as follows:

1. Improved word-identification, particularly in noisy environments
2. Precise localization of the source of a sound;
3. A sense of "balanced hearing";
4. Less gain is required in binaural hearing aid fittings.

In addition to these advantages, a number of recent studies have appeared which document the effects of auditory deprivation in unaided ears. The research indicates that word-identification scores in the unaided ear decrease over time relative to scores in the aided ear in a monaural fitting. In contrast, this decrement is not observed in either ear after binaural amplification. Further, limited recovery in word-identification follows the subsequent provision of amplification to the deprived ear.

In consideration of the available evidence, binaural amplification is recommended unless specifically contraindicated. Valid contraindications to binaural amplification are as follows:

1. Unilateral hearing loss
2. Medical complication in one ear
3. One ear is unaidable due to insufficient residual hearing
4. Binaural amplification results in diminished word identification

Patient Accomodation to Amplification

Hearing-impaired listeners require a period of adjustment to become accustomed to wearing hearing aids. The average patient has developed a hearing loss over a period of many years before deciding to try a hearing aid. During this time considerable adaptation has occurred in the central auditory system. The sudden introduction of amplification initiates compensatory neurophysiologic changes that may take 5 to 6 weeks to develop. During this time adjustments to the hearing instruments are often needed to assist the patient in the process of accomodation. Patients are typically placed on a wearing schedule that gradually extends the length of time the hearing aids are worn each day. Some programs also restrict hearing aid use to quiet listening environments during the initial period of accommodation with systematic exposure to more demanding conditions as accommodation progresses.

A common problem arises when a patient is initially unhappy with the peformance of the hearing aid. According to federal law, a customer may return a hearing aid to the dispenser within 30 days without penalty. Unfortunately, 30 days is often an insufficient period to allow for complete accomodation and/or modification of the instrument. Therefore, prospective hearing-aid patients should receive counseling before, during, and after the initial fitting to avoid making a premature decision.

Current Trends in Prescriptive Amplification

New strategies for hearing aid selection and fitting are being developed to maximize the benefits of today's nonlinear hearing aids and, ultimately, to improve patient satisfaction with hearing aid use. The Independent Hearing Aid Fitting Forum (IHAFF), a group of dispensing audiologists, has developed an innovative, computer-based protocol. The IHAFF prescriptive hearing aid fitting protocol has four main goals: "1) soft speech and and environmental sounds, in as wide a bandwidth as possible, should be audible, 2) speech and environmental sounds that are comfortably loud for normal listeners should also be comfortably loud when amplified, 3) loud speech and environmental sounds should not be uncomfortable, and 4) circuit noise and distortion should be minimal at typically encountered input levels." With the IHAFF protocol, prefitting strategies are expanded, and essential. Essential components of these strategies are computer-assisted loudness-contour measurements with frequency-specific stimuli, using a loudness rating scale. Electroacoustic parameters of current sophisticated commercially available hearing aids, e.g. gain, output, and compresssion characteristics for various frequencies, are then adjusted to meet the objectives of the IHAFF protocol for an individual patient. Probe-microphone measurements, which are already applied in hearing aid fitting, are a critical part of these new strategies. Patient inventories of communicative handicap, such as the Abbreviated Profile of Hearing Aid Benefit, or APHAB are also an important feature of the hearing aid fitting and rehabilitative process and may contribute to both hearing aid selection and validation of effective amplification. IHAFF protocols are likely to have a positive impact on hearing aid selection and fitting.

ADVISING THE PARENTS OF YOUNG CHILDREN WITH HEARING IMPAIRMENT

Guidelines for the Otolaryngologist

Although the otolaryngologist is concerned directly with medical or surgical managment of aural diseases and disorders, an appreciation and understanding of the educational issues confronting the patients with hearing impairments, and their families, is important.

Otolaryngologists are involved in both recognition and diagnosis of hearing impairments and must be responsible for informing parents regarding the medical, surgical, and educational options available to their child. Otolaryngologists are asked by parents about options open to them. Otolaryngologists must, therefore, be aware of the scientific basis for intervention and education, so that hearing-impaired individuals and their parents understand and are aware of the options for hearing habilitation and language acquisition. This counselling should be based on as much scientific data as is available, and should include a rational and unbiased review of the communicative options available. Recognition of the controversial issues in this field as well as an understanding of their origins is essential if otolaryngologists are to fulfill their role in serving hearing-impaired individuals. Advances in medical technology have failed to resolve all of the problems confronting hearing-impaired individuals. Techniques such as cochlear implantation have raised questions about the best and most ethical approaches for educating the approximately 4000 deaf and severely hard-of-hearing individuals born each year in the United States.

Many of the controversial issues in education of the hearing impaired have been debated since the 1500s. Although valuable in understanding the current debates regarding management of severe hearing impairment, a historical overview of the education of deaf and profoundly hard of hearing individuals is beyond the scope of this chapter. Education of the hearing impaired in the United States was directly influenced by previous developments in Europe. After visiting with major figures in the education of the hearing impaired in Europe, Thomas H. Gallaudet established the American School for the Deaf, and later founded Gallaudet University in Washington D.C. which, along with the National Technical Institute for the Deaf in Rochester, NY, are the only American institutes of higher education dedicated exclusively to the needs of deaf individuals. He introduced a manual educational method that had been developed in France. Horace Mann (1796–1859) introduced an oral method to the United States, and this concept was advocated by Alexander Graham Bell and further developed by an otolaryngologist, Dr. Max A. Goldstein (1870–1942). Goldstein was Professor of Otology at the Beaumont Medical College, which later became St. Louis University. He founded the Central Institute for the Deaf in St. Louis, and stressed the development and use of residual hearing to assist in development of oral communication.

Historically, the development of techniques for educating hearing-impaired individuals, and the debate surrounding these techniques, led to two primary philosophies which are still in place today, and still generate considerable discussion. These are the Manual Visual Method, arising in France, and the Oral Auditory Method, arising in Germany. There are proponents of the strict use of signing and others who are proponents of the use of oral communication only. Recently, the majority practice is a combination of these methods. It is believed that the simultaneous method of using American Sign Language (ASL) signs in English word order achieves the best educational outcome for hearing-impaired individuals. Otolaryngologists must be aware of the four major educational methods in use today.

American Sign Language is a manual form of communication that evolved in the deaf community in America. Similar but different sign languages have evolved in other countries. It is a vast lexicon of hand shapes and motions, or signs, and has its own syntax and grammar. For this reason, it is a unique language that is different from English. Its status as a unique language leads to the notion that it is the native or natural language of deaf individuals, a concept which dates back to de I'Epee and the origins of the French Method. This concept is embraced by individuals in the deaf community. *Manual English* is another of the manual forms of communication. This is a variety of systems, which all use signs, finger spelling, and gestures to represent the English language manually. This differs from ASL in that it is a direct representation of the English language, conveyed manually. One element of Manual English is finger spelling, which allows an exact representation of written English. In the *Rochester method,* which is no longer in use, there are 26 handshapes which correspond to the 26 letters of the English language. Each word is spelled out using these symbols. *Cued Speech* also uses handshapes, but does so to supplement spoken language by cuing differences in sounds. In this sense, it may also be considered a form of combined communication. There are 8 handshapes which represent phonetic elements of speech which are not readily visible when utilizing speech reading. These handshapes are used as manual cues to supplement spoken language. Pidgin Sign English (PSE) is manual English which uses ASL signs in English word order. There are no inflectional signs, and the ASL signs are supplemented with finger spelling for proper names, etc. Signed English is a semantic representation of English, which also uses ASL signs in English word order, and adds additional signs for inflection. This is primarily used with children in the first 6 years of age.

In contrast to these manual methods, there are basically two forms of oral English. The *Acoupedic Method* proposed by Dr. Goldstein, places an emphasis on amplification and maximization of residual hearing, with minimizing speech reading. The more prevalent oral communication method used today is the *Oral Auditory Method.* This system employs speech and speech reading, with an emphasis on early and consistent use of high-quality amplification. An essential element in this educational method is early auditory training, which serves to maximize the beneficial effects of amplification and fully develop the child's residual hearing.

Manual Visual and Oral Auditory forms of communication when used together, are referred to as *Combined Methods. Total Communication* (also called simultaneous communication) uses sign language, finger spelling, and oral communication together. This is the most prevalent form of education of hearing-impaired individuals used today. In special schools, 97% of pupils are educated using Total Communication, and 70% of students in integrated schools are educated using this method. The goal of Total Communication is to use all forms of communication available to the child for language development. This may at first seem to be the most beneficial method, but it may lead to a reliance on signing and incomplete utilization of residual hearing if used too early in a child's education. Now that we have gained an increased understanding of the critical period of auditory development and the adverse effects of auditory deprivation, further research is needed to clarify the role of signing and Total Communication in a hearing-impaired child's education.

A variety of educational methods are available to the hearing-impaired individual. Considerations differ for hearing-impaired children of deaf parents who naturally teach their children ASL from birth and of hearing parents who account for more than 90% of the parents of deaf children, and who may or may not want to use ASL. The roles of the various methods in achieving English literacy are also important factors. How should parents of hearing-impaired children be counseled as they struggle to decide which method is best for their child? To make this decision, one would like to be able to answer some controversial questions. Are hearing-impaired children fundamentally different? Do they communicate differently from hearing children? Do they have a native language that is their natural form of communication? These questions, debated for four centuries, are even now not easily answered. To address these questions for our patients, an objective, rather than emotional approach should be taken. Professionals must ensure that parents of hearing-impaired infants and children know all of the options available to them and they should be supported in their decision making process. For those choosing the Oral Auditory approach, audiologists and otolaryngologists have a special responsibility to maximize the use of residual hearing through amplification and other signal processing strategies, such as vibrotactile devices and cochlear implantation.

The concept of a critical period of development during which the central nervous system exhibits maximal plasticity is central to any discussion regarding the education of hearing-impaired individuals. Should one maximize language development or use of residual hearing capability? Both language development or use of residual hearing share a critical period. Extensive experimental studies have shown that auditory system development includes a critical period of maximal neural plasticity. Experimental models using chicken, mice, owls, and cats have shown there is a detrimental effect of auditory deprivation, which is maximal if incurred during a critical developmental period in the animals' lives. Furthermore, these changes are irreversible if auditory deprivation is maintained beyond the critical period. Anatomic studies confirm a deprivation-related decrease in the size of auditory brainstem nuclei, in the cross-sectional area of cell bodies, and in cell size. Auditory deprivation also may result in physiologic alterations, such as increased latency and decreased duration of responses in inferior colliculus neurons in the rat, and absent or greatly decreased responses in inferior colliculus in the gerbil. Clinical investigations provide additional support for the concept of a critical period during the first 3 to 4 years of a child's life. Although precise studies of language development with ASL have not been accomplished, language development is subject to the same critical period.

In summary, each of the current educational methods available (oral auditory, manual visual, and total communication) have their proponents and opponents. Whenever appropriate, and with the support of parents and other caregivers, otolaryngologists should encourage and facilitate maximal use of residual hearing in an attempt to help hearing-impaired children to realize their full communicative potential. Debate regarding the optimal educational strategy, or strategies, for children with hearing impairment persists. Further research is needed on the early education of hearing-impaired children to refine optimal strategies for maximizing the development of their communication skills.

GLOSSARY

ABLB: Alternate binaural loudness balance. A traditional diagnostic auditory procedure for detecting "loudness recruitment" used in differentiating cochlear versus retrocochlear auditory dysfunction in unilateral hearing loss. The task is to balance the sensation of loudness for the better versus poorer hearing ear. Loudness recruitment is a cochlear auditory sign.

ABR (BAER): Auditory brainstem response. Electrical activity, evoked (stimulated) by very brief-duration sounds, that arises from the eighth cranial nerve and auditory portions of the brainstem. The ABR is usually recorded from the surface of the scalp and external ear with disc-type electrodes and processes with a fast signal averaging computer. ABR wave components are labeled with Roman numerals (e.g. I, III, V) and described by the latency after the stimulus (in msec) and the amplitude from one peak to the following trough (in microvolts).

AC: Air conduction. Audiometric signals presented via earphones to the ear canal.

AGC: Automatic gain control. A feature of some hearing aids which reduces over amplification at high input intensity levels.

air-bone gap: Difference in pure tone thresholds for air- versus bone-conducted signals. With calibrated audiometers, the normal ear and the sensorineurally-impaired ear show no air-bone gap, whereas conductive hearing losses are characterized by an air-bone gap.

audiologist: Hearing care professional who is educated and trained clinically to measure auditory system function and to manage non-medically persons with auditory and communcative impairments. Minimal educational requirements for audiologists are a Masters degree and certification and/or state licensure.

BC: Bone conduction. Audiometric signals presented via an oscillator to the skull (e.g. mastoid bone or forehead).

BCL: Bekesy comfortable level. A Bekesy audiometry procedure conducted at a comfortable loudness level versus threshold level.

Bekesy audiometry: Audiometric procedure performed with a Bekesy audiometer for differentiating cochlear versus retrocochlear auditory dysfunction. Bekesy audiometry is based on the comparison of responses to pulsed versus continuous tones varied across a wide frequency range. Four patterns of Bekesy responses were classified by Jerger.

BOA: Behavioral observation audiometry. A pediatric behavioral audiometry procedure in which motor responses to sounds (e.g. eye opening, head turning) are detected by a trained observer.

BTE: Behind-the-ear hearing aid design.

CIC: Completely-in-the-canal hearing aid design.

configuration: Shape or pattern of an audiogram, i.e. how hearing los varies as a function of the audiometric test frequency. There are three main configurations: rising (low frequency loss), sloping (high frequency loss) and flat.

CROS: Contralateral routing of signals. A hearing aid configuration in which a microphone is located on the severely or profoundly impaired ear and sounds are transduced and delivered electrically to the normal or mildly impaired ear.

crossover: Sound stimulus presented to one ear (the test ear) travels around the head (by air conduction) or across the head (by bone conduction) to stimulate the other (nontest) ear. See interaural attenuation.

dB HL: Decibel scale referenced to accepted standards for normal hearing (0 dB is average normal hearing for each audiometric test frequency).

dB nHL: Decibel scale used in auditory brainstem response measurement referenced to average behavioral threshold for the click stimulus of a small group of normal hearing subjects.

dB SL: Sound intensity is described in reference to an individual patient's behavioral threshold for an audiometric frequency or some other meaure of hearing threshold (e.g. the speech reception threshold).

dB SPL: Decibel scale referenced to a physical standard for intensity (e.g. 0.0002 dynes/cm^2).

dichotic: Simultaneous presentation of a different sound to each ear.

DPOAE: Distortion product otoacoustic emission

DPgram (DPOAEgram): Graph of distortion product otoacoustic emission amplitude in the ear canal (in dB SPL) as a function of the frequencies of the stimulus tones (in Hz).

ECochG: Electrocochleography. Evoked responses originating from the cochlea (the summating potential, or SP, and the cochlear microphonic, or CM) and the eighth cranial nerve (the action potential, or AP).

ENG: Electronystagmography. A test of vestibular function in which nystagmus is recorded with electrodes placed near the eyes during stimulation of the vestibular system.

ENoG: Electroneurography. Myogenic activity recorded from the facial muscles, usually in the nasiolabial fold, in response to electrical stimulation of the facial nerve as it exits the stylomastoid foramen.

gain: Increase in the amplitude or energy of an electrical signal with amplification.

Interaural attenuation: Insulation to the crossover of sound (acoustic or mechanical energy) from one ear to the other provided by the head. Interaural attenuation varies depending on whether the signal is presented by air-conduction (interaural attentuation >40 dB) or bone-conduction (interaural attenuation < 10 dB). Insert earphones offer maximum interaural attenuation.

ITC: In-the-canal hearing aid design.

ITE: In-the-ear hearing aid design.

malingering: Feigning ore exaggerating a hearing impairment. Also referred to as functional or nonorganic hearing loss.

masking (masker): Controlled background noise presented usually to the nontest ear in an audiometric procedure to prevent a response from the nontest ear (due to crossover when interaural attenuation is exceeded).

masking dilemma: Problem encountered in audiometric assessment of patient's with severe conductive hearing loss. The level of masking noise necessary to overcome the conductive component and adequately mask the nontest ear exceeds interaural attenuation levels. The masking noise may then crossover to the test ear, and mask the signal (e.g. pure tone or speech). In the masking dilemma, enough masking is too much masking. The masking dilemma can be reduced by the use of insert earphones. The SAL test is also helpful for measuring ear-specific bone conduction hearing thresholds in patients presenting the masking dilemma.

MCL: Most comfortable level. The intensity level of a sound that is perceived as comfortable.

MLD: Masking level difference. An audiometric procedure which compares a threshold response with masking noise presented in- versus out-of-phase with a pure tone or speech signal. Release from masking is a normal phenomenon reflecting auditory brainstem integrity.

MPO: Maximum power output. A measure of hearing aid performance. See SSPL.

OAE: Otoacoustic emissions. Sounds generated by energy produced by the outer hair cells in the cochlea and detected with a microphone placed within the external ear canal.

PB: Phonetically balanced. Word lists developed in the late 1940s which contain all the phonetic elements of general American english speech that occur with the approximate frequency of occurence in conversational speech.

PI: Performance-intensity. A measure of speech recognition or understanding as a function of the intensity level of the speech signal. See rollover.

PTA: Pure tone average. The arithmetic average of hearing threshold levels for 500, 1000, and 2000 Hz, or the speech frequency region of the audiogram. The PTA should agree within $+/- 7$ dB of the speech reception threshold (SRT).

REAR: Real ear aided response. A measure of hearing aid performance made with a probe microphone placed in the earcanal between the hearing aid and the tympanic membrane.

REUR: Real ear unaided response. A measure of sound made with a probe microphone placed in the earcanal.

rollover: Decrease in speech recognition performance (in percent correct) at high signal intensity levels versus lower levels. Rollover is an audiometric sign of retrocochlear auditory dysfunction.

SAL: Sensory acuity level. An audiometric procedure developed by Jerger for assessing bone conduction hearing in patients with serious conductive hearing loss. Air-conduction thresholds are determined without masking and then with masking presented by bone conduction to the forehead. The size of the masked shift in hearing thresholds corresponds to the degree of conductive hearing loss component.

SAT (SDT): Speech awareness threshold (speech detection threshold). The lowest intensity level at which a person can detect the presence of a speech signal. The SAT approximates the best hearing level in the 250 to 8000 Hz audiometric frequency region.

SSI: Synthetic sentence identification. A measure of central auditory function which involves identification of syntactically incomplete sentences (a closed set of 10 sentences) presented simultaneously with a competing message (an ongoing story about Davy Crockett).

SSPL: Saturation sound pressure level. A measure of the maximum power output (MPO) of a hearing aid.

SSW: Staggered spondaic word test. A measure of central auditory function developed by Katz which utilizes spondee words presented dichotically.

SISI: Short increment intensity index. A clinical procedure developed by Jerger for assessing the ability to detect a 1 dB increase in intensity. High SISI score is consistent with cochlear auditory dysfunction.

S/N: Signal-to-noise. The signal-to-noise ratio is the difference between the intensity level of a sound or electrical event and background acoustic or electrophysiologic energy.

SRT: Speech reception level. The lowest intensity level at which a person can accurately identify a speech signal (e.g. two syllable spondee words). See PTA.

tone decay test: Clinical measure of auditory adaption in which a tone is presented continuously to a hearing impaired ear until it becomes inaudible. There are numerous versions of tone decay tests. Excessive tone decay is a sign of retrocochlear auditory dysfunction.

TROCA: Tangible reinforcement operant conditioning audiometry. A pediatric behavioral audiometry technique which reinforces a response to auditory signals with food. TROCA is used mainly with mentally retarded or developmentally delayed children.

UCL/LDL: Uncomfortable level or loudness discomfort level. The intensity level of a sound that is perceived as too loud.

VRA: Visual reinforcement audiometry. A pediatric behavioral audiometry procedure which reinforces localization responses to acoustic signals with a visual event (e.g. an animal playing).

SUGGESTED READINGS

Burkey JM, Arkis PN: Word recognition changes after monaural, binaural amplification. Hearing Instruments 44(1):8–9, 1993.

Carhart R, Jerger JF: Preferred method for clinical determination of pure-tone thresholds. J Speech Hear Disord 24:330–345, 1959.

Cox RM, Alexander GC: The abbreviated profile of hearing aid benefit (APHAB). Presented at the annual meeting of the American Academy of Audiology, Richmond, VA, April 1994.

Cranmer-Briskey KS: 1992 hearing instruments dispenser survey results. Hearing Instruments 43(6):8–15, 1992.

Gatehouse S: The time course and magnitude of peripheral acclimatization to frequency responses: Evidence from monaural fitting of hearing aids. J Acoust Soc Am 92:1256–1268, 1992.

Gelfand S, Silman S, Ross L: Long-term effects of monaural, binaural, and no amplification in subjects with bilateral hearing losses. Scand Audiol 16:201–207, 1989.

Glasscock ME: Education of hearing-impaired children in the United States. Am J Otol 13:4–5, 1992.

Hall JW III (ed): Immittance Audiometry. Seminars in Hearing 8: 1987.

Hall JW, III. The acoustic reflex in central auditory dysfunction. In: Assessment of auditory dysfunction: foundations and clinical correlates. Edited by M Pinheiro, FE Musiek. Baltimore, Williams & Wilkins, pp. 103–130, 1985.

Hall JW III: Handbook of Auditory Evoked Responses. Needham MA: Allyn & Bacon, 1992.

Hall JW III (ed): Otoacoustic Emissions: Facts and Fantasies. Hearing J *45:* 1992.

Hall JW III: Otoacoustic emissions: the audiologic test procedure of the 1990s. Hearing J *45:7,* 1992.

Hall JW III, Bratt G, Schwaber MK, Baer JE: Dynamic Sensorineural Hearing Loss: Implications for Audiologists. J Am Acad Audiol *4:*399–411, 1993.

Hall JW III, Baer JE, Chase PA, et al: Clinical application of otoacoustic emissions: What do we know about factors influencing measurement and analysis? Otolaryngol Head Neck Surg *110:* 22–38, 1994.

Jahrsdoerfer RA, Hall JW III: Congenital malformation of the ear. Am J Otol *7:*267–269, 1986.

Jerger JF: Clinical experience with impedance audiometry. Arch Otolaryngol *92:*11–24, 1970.

Jerger J, Jerger S, Mauldin L: Studies in impedance audiometry. I. Normal and sensorineural ears. Arch Otolaryngol *96:*513–523, 1972.

Jerger J, Anthony L, Jerger S, et al: Studies in impedance audiometry. III. Middle ear disorders. Arch Otolaryngol *99:*165–171, 1974.

Jerger J, Hayes D: The cross-check principle in pediatric audiometry. Arch Otolaryngol Arch Otolaryngol *102:*614–620, 1976.

Jewett DL, Williston JS: Auditory evoked far fields averaged from the scalp of humans. Brain *4:*681–696, 1971.

Joint Committee on Infant Hearing: 1994 Position Statement. Audiol Today *5,* 1994.

Killion MC: The K-AMP hearing aid: An attempt to present high fidelity for persons with impaired hearing. Am J Audiol *2:* 52–74, 1993.

Killion MC, Staab WJ, Preves DA: Classifying automatic signal processors. Hearing Instruments *41* (8), 990.

Moore DR: Postnatal Development of the Mammalian Central Auditory System and the Neural Consequences of Auditory Deprivation. Acta Otolaryngol (Stockh) Suppl *421:*19–30, 1985.

Mueller HG, Hawkins DB, Northern JL: Probe Microphone Measurements: Hearing Aid Selection and Assessment. San Diego, Singular Publishing Group, Inc., 1992.

Mueller HG: Update on programmable hearing aids. Hearing J *47*(5): 13–20, 1994.

Mueller HG: Getting ready for the IHAFF protocol. Hearing J *47*(6): 10, 46–48.

National Institutes of Health Consensus Development Conference: Early identification of hearing impairment in infants and young children. 1993.

Northern JL, Downs M: Hearing Disorders in Children (4th ed). Baltimore: Williams & Wilkins, 1991.

Pillsbury HC, Grose JH, Hall JW: Otitis Media with Effusion in Children—Binaural Hearing Before and After Corrective Surgery. Arch Otolaryngol Head Neck Surg *117:*718–723, 1991.

Robertson D, Irvine DRF: Plasticity of frequency organization in auditory cortex of guinea pigs with partial unilateral deafness. J Comp Neurol *282:*456–471, 1989.

Schildroth A: Recent Changes in the Educational Placement of Dear Students. Am Ann Deaf *133:*61–67, 1988.

Selters WA, Brackmann D: Acoustic tumor detection with brain stem electric response audiometry. Arch Otolaryngol *103:*181–187, 1977.

Silman S, Gelfand S, Silverman C: Late-onset auditory deprivation: effects on manaural versus binaural hearing aids. J Acoust Soc Am *76:*1357–1362, 1984.

Silverman CA, Silman S: Apparent auditory deprivation from monaural amplification and recovery with binaural amplification: Two case studies. J Am Acad Audiol *1:*175–180, 1990.

Staab WJ: The peritympanic instrument: fitting rationale and test results. Hearing J *45*(10):21–26, 1992.

Updike C, Thornburg JD: Reading skills and auditory processing ability in children with chronic otitis media in early childhood. Ann Otol Rhinol Laryngol *101:*530–537, 1992.

Waldhauer F, Villchur E: Full dynamic range multiband compression in a hearing aid. Hearing J *9:*29–32, 1988.

Weir N: Otolaryngology—An Illustrated History. 1st ed. London, Butterworth & Co. Ltd., pp. 89–97, 1990.

Willot JF, Aitken LM, McFadden SL: Plasticity of auditory cortex associated with sensorineural hearing loss in adult mice. J Comp Neurol *329*(3):402–411, 1993.

45 Diseases of the External Ear

David F. Austin

AURICLE

The skin on the external surface of the auricle is attached firmly to the underlying cartilage with the connective tissue of the dermis condensing to form perichondrium. The skin on the undersurface of the auricle, by contrast, has a true subcutaneous layer. This feature of the auricular integument, combined with the exposed position of the auricle, is responsible for the majority of clinical problems that involve the auricle: trauma, exposure, and infection. Fluid accumulation consequent to these processes results in separation of perichondrium from the cartilage. Unless this process is promptly relieved, necrosis of cartilage will result because of interference with its nutritional perfusion from the vessels of the perichondrium.

Trauma

Trauma to the auricle occurs frequently and may cause contusion, laceration, or occasionally, loss of the entire auricle. In some instances, the auricle has been resutured successfully to the head with at least partial survival of the composite tissue. Repair of these injuries should follow ordinary principles of plastic surgery. Suturing of the anterior surface should be done with care and with complete control of hemorrhage because the thin skin is closely applied to the underlying cartilage. Extremely macerated areas may be removed by wedge excision with little resultant deformity compared to the severe scarring that might otherwise occur.

Hematoma of the auricle is not confined to fighters but is also common in children. Trauma is the most common cause, although small hemorrhages secondary to blood dyscrasias have been described. The external surface of the auricle is affected usually because of its exposed position (Fig. 45–1).

Blood collects rapidly after the injury, dissecting be-tween the perichondrium and cartilage. This creates a bluish swelling, usually involving the entire auricle although it may be confined to the upper half. If the lesion is not treated early, the blood organizes into a fibrous mass, causing necrosis of the cartilage because of interference with its nutrition. This mass of twisted scar, especially if formed from repeated trauma, creates the deformity known as "cauliflower ear."

Treatment is based on rapid evacuation of the collected blood. Because of the danger of perichondritis and its resultant severe scarring, aseptic surgical technique is required. Antibiotics whose spectrum includes *Pseudomonas aeruginosa (B. pyocyaneus)* should be used preoperatively and postoperatively.

The incision should be placed in the scapha, paralleling the helix. Sufficient exposure should be obtained to aspirate the entire hematoma. If delay has resulted in some "organization," sharp ring curettes may be used to remove the clot. Small rubber drains may be used to prevent reaccumulation of blood or serum and not left longer than 48 hours because of the risk of infection.

A tight pressure dressing (e.g., plaster gauze) that conforms to the shape of the auricle should be applied for a minimum of 48 hours. Small residual blebs may be aspirated with a syringe and needle, again with aseptic technique. The antibiotic should be continued for a 5-day period. Frequent observation is necessary to detect perichondritis quickly if it occurs. The treatment of this complication is discussed later.

Frostbite

Frostbite is prevalent in northern climates, and the auricle is frequently involved because of its exposed position and lack of subcutaneous or adipose tissue to insulate the blood vessels (Fig. 45–2). The factors of wind and humidity, as well as temperature, are important determinants of the severity of exposure.

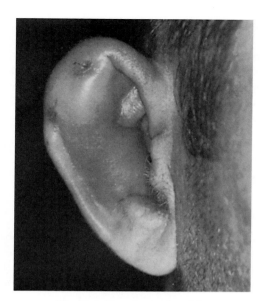

Fig. 45–1. Hematoma of auricle.

Initially there is vasoconstriction, leaving the ear, especially the edges of the helix, blanched and cold to the touch. Hyperemia and edema follow and are caused by a marked increase in capillary permeability. Ice crystallization of intracellular fluid may be primarily responsible for this, as well as cellular necrosis in the surrounding tissues. The ear becomes swollen, red, and tender, and blebs of tissue fluid may appear under the skin. The final stage of frostbite is caused by ischemia. The regional capillaries are filled with clumped red cells because of the slowed circulation through the distended capillaries and loss of serum through the capillary walls. If recovery of normal permeability does not occur within a few hours, intravascular clotting occurs, with permanent thrombosis and ischemic necrosis of the affected tissue.

Treatment of frostbite is based on the aforemen-

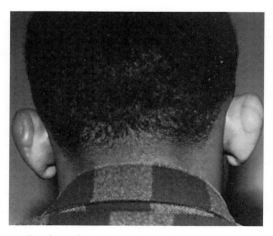

Fig. 45–2. Frostbite of auricle. Both auricles show massive vesiculation of the posterior surface.

tioned process and varies somewhat with its severity. The ear should be treated gently because of the risk of further damage to the already traumatized and devitalized tissue. Massaging with snow should thus be avoided, as should any other manipulation.

The ear is allowed to return slowly to body temperature. This may be done by placing the patient in a cool room or by directing a stream of cooled air over the affected area. With the onset of vasodilatation, burning and itching will be severe and should be controlled with analgesics. In children it may be necessary to restrain their hands. In severe or prolonged exposure, the use of heparin to prevent blood sludging and intravascular clotting is recommended. This should be continued until the extent of final injury can be determined. In every case the parenteral use of conjugated estrogen, bioflavonoids, and vitamin C can be used to reduce the abnormal capillary permeability. Antibiotics may be necessary to prevent infection of the devitalized tissue.

If necrosis of portions of the auricle takes place, this should be allowed to delineate completely before any surgical excision is done. Spontaneous separation of the necrotic tissue results in less loss of tissue and a better cosmetic result than if early surgery is undertaken. Infection of the gangrenous portion, however, indicates immediate surgical excision.

Perichondritis

Perichondritis of the auricle was once a complication of chronic otitis media or chronic external otitis. Spread of infection through an endaural incision can also result in perichondritis. Trauma with laceration and hematoma is an occasional cause. The usual infecting microorganism is *Pseudomonas aeruginosa* (*B. pyocyaneus*).

The onset of perichondritis is marked by a diffuse painful red swelling of the auricle (Fig. 45–3). The auricle feels hot and tender. The edema may spread to the postauricular region, causing the auricle to protrude. Elevation of temperature, regional adenopathy, and leukocytosis are common. Collections of serum in the subperichondral layer soon become purulent.

The treatment of perichondritis is difficult because of the antibiotic-resistant microorganism usually present. Prophylaxis, therefore, becomes paramount. Endaural incisions must avoid the auricular cartilage in any infected case. The most common errors involve making the meatal incision too far lateral, thus incising the concha or posterior cartilaginous wall of the canal, and making the superior incision too close to the helix, shaving its cartilage in so doing. An even more common error, and one more likely to cause perichondritis, is that of traumatizing the auricle with the shaft of the burr while drilling in the mastoid. This is often unnoticed because the operator's attention is directed to the point of the burr. Care must always be taken during

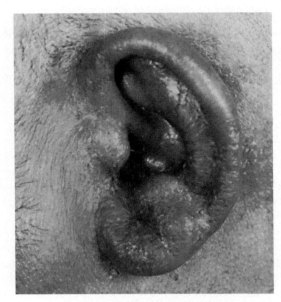

Fig. 45–3. Perichondritis of auricle.

mastoid surgery to avoid trauma to the auricle. Early diagnosis aids treatment greatly, and to this end it is felt that pressure dressings over the ear should not be left for more than 48 hours. If circumstances dictate the need for prolonged dressings, they should be changed daily with aseptic technique.

If perichondritis should develop, rapid institution of treatment is needed. Heat should be applied to the auricle. Hot, moist packs are the most effective, but dry heat is required if the infection follows surgery. Cultures should be taken and antibiotic treatment, which is directed toward a presumed infection with *Pseudomonas* should be started. If cultures reveal another microorganism to be causative, the antibiotic regimen may be changed at that time. Effective systemic antibiotics are tobramycin and ticarcillin administered together. Treatment is extended for 2 weeks, with regular checks on renal function and drug levels. Topical application is used in treating an otitis media or external otitis if present. The antibiotic should be continued for several days after apparent recovery because of the possibility of residual hidden areas of infection. The appearance of fluctuation indicates the need for incision and drainage. This should be done as described under hematoma of the auricle and drains left in place until the purulent discharge has ceased. Prognosis for a cosmetic result is poor because of the cartilage necrosis. Cosmetic reconstruction may be carried out, but this should be delayed for many months to ensure the complete elimination of residual infection.

TUMORS OF THE EXTERNAL EAR

Most tumors of the ear are similar to those occurring in other portions of the body. They derive from skin or its appendages, bone, neural tissue, or connective tissue. The major problem today, as in the past, is early diagnosis so that treatment may be carried out with a minimal loss of tissue, function, and life. Because the methods of removal of the neoplasms depend primarily on their location, the discussion will be subdivided by location and whether the tumor is benign or malignant.

BENIGN TUMORS OF THE AURICLE

Angiomas

Angiomas are congenital tumors and are the most common tumors of childhood. They may involve the auricle together with other areas of the face and neck. These tumors occur in various forms. *Capillary hemangioma* consists of masses of capillary-sized vessels and may be in the form of a large flat mass, the "port-wine stain," or spider nevus, which is a branching network of capillaries fed by a central larger vessel. The spider nevus is not a major problem, being small and fixed in size. Treatment, when necessary, usually consists of needle coagulation of the central vessel. The port-wine stain is much more of a problem, increasing in size gradually until adolescence, and is generally disfiguring.

Cavernous hemangioma is the most alarming of these lesions, consisting of raised masses of blood-filled endothelial spaces. Often termed a "strawberry tumor," it increases rapidly in size during the first year of life but usually regresses thereafter. Much less common is the *lymphangioma*. This has the appearance of multiple pale circumscribed lesions, like a cluster of fish or frog roe.

The major problem in these tumors is cosmetic. In general, the lesion should be allowed to regress maximally and the residual tumor treated. Various modalities have been recommended, including cryosurgery, surgical excision and skin grafting, radiation, electrolysis, and tattooing for port-wine stains. Most of these cases are handled by plastic surgeons, and consultation with those specializing in this field is recommended.

Cysts

Sebaceous cysts are common around the ear. They usually occur on the posterior surface of the lobule, in the skin over the mastoid process, and in the skin of the inferior or posterior cartilaginous canal (Fig. 45–4). These soft, nontender swellings may become infected and at these times may be confused with furuncle.

Treatment of sebaceous cyst is total excision. Incision and curettage, which has been recommended in the past, is followed by recurrence. Infection, if present, should be treated with heat and antibiotics before sur-

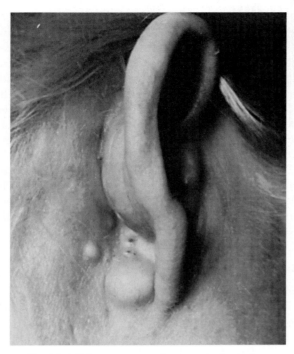

Fig. 45–4. Sebaceous cysts of retroauricular region.

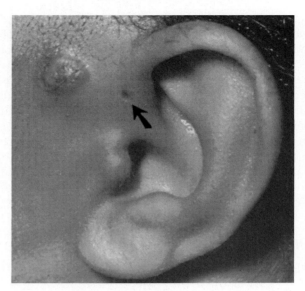

Fig. 45–5. Preauricular cyst and fistula. Arrow indicates the fistula opening. Anterior to this is an inflamed swelling caused by an infected preauricular cyst.

gery is attempted. The cyst is removed by sharp dissection, care being taken to keep the walls intact to ensure complete removal. The ductal tissue leading to the cyst as well as its external opening are removed by including this tissue with a small segment of the overlying skin.

Preauricular cyst and/or fistula is of congenital origin, arising because of disunion of the hillocks of the first and second branchial arches forming the auricle (Chapter 40). It presents as a small opening in the skin anterior to the insertion of the helix (Fig. 45–5). From this opening a long branched tract may run under the skin between the helix and tragus and anterior to the tragus. The tract, which is lined with squamous cell epithelium, is often cystic, and the patient is frequently seen initially because of infection of the cyst.

Treatment of a preauricular fistula should be avoided unless recurrent infection is present because of the difficulty of complete removal. Incomplete removal is associated with the formation of draining sinuses, requiring even more difficult and radical surgery for their elimination. The difficulty of the surgery is caused by the branching of the fistula, which makes it hard to define the complete extent of the tract. One suggestion to aid in removal is to inject the tract before surgery with methylene blue so that the stained tissue may be used as a rough guide to the extent of the fistula.

Fibroma

Fibromas occur only rarely about the external ear, most often in diffuse neurofibromatosis (von Reckling-

hausen's disease). They are firm, nontender, discrete swellings with slow growth. Surgical excision is indicated when they occlude the canal or create a cosmetic problem.

Keloid tumors represent a form of fibroma but more likely are pseudotumors caused by genetic susceptibility (Fig. 45–6). The formation of a keloid is stimulated

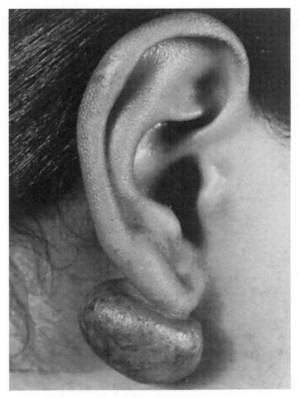

Fig. 45–6. Keloid of auricle that followed piercing of lobule.

by trauma to the skin and is made up of massive collections of collagen interspersed with active fibroblasts and normal thin collagenous strands. Keloid formation is seen most frequently in the dark-skinned races, particularly in blacks. Keloids around the ear are most frequently seen as pedunculated tumors on the lobule following ear lobe piercing. They may also occur in mastoidectomy and endaural scars, resulting in disfigurement or stenosis of the canal.

Treatment is excision. A frequently used treatment to prevent keloid reformation is the injection of a small amount of Kenalog (Bristol-Myers Squibb, New York, NY) into the surgical site.

Papilloma

Papillomas are seen in various forms both on the auricle and in the canal and arise in response to chronic irritation of the skin. The common wart is felt to have a viral cause. The basic lesion consists of hyperplasia of both the basal and prickle cell layers of the skin. Malignant changes are not rare in these lesions, but benign papillomas do not have the pleomorphism, mitotic activity, or disruption of the basement membrane seen with malignancy.

A *cutaneous horn* is formed when there is a heaping up of keratin in a circumscribed papilloma, creating a rough, hard, brownish horn-shaped tumor (Fig. 45–7). This is seen most frequently on the rim of the helix in elderly individuals with long exposure to the elements. The curious appearance leads the individual to seek medical attention, which consists of surgical excision.

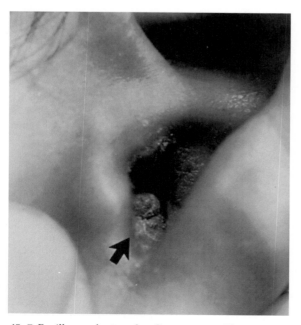

Fig. 45–7. Papilloma of external auditory meatus. This is a common wart (verruca vulgaris) that, because of the marked keratinization, may be called a cutaneous horn.

Keratoacanthoma is a rare lesion, important because of its similarity to carcinoma and its premalignant nature. It occurs usually after the fifth decade in men who work outdoors. The lesion consists of a peripheral heaping up of prickle cells with a central crater filled with a mass of keratin. The lesion tends to grow rapidly after its initial appearance and then slowly regresses, leaving a retracted scar. Although the disease is self-limited, excision biopsy is required to rule out the presence of a malignant tumor.

Senile keratoses are raised, flat-surfaced lesions on exposed surfaces of the skin of elderly individuals. The lesion has a color distinct from the surrounding normal skin, usually yellow, brown, or black. The lesion is discussed in Chapter 9.

Winkler's Disease

Painful nodular growth of the auricle is a rare tumor occurring on the top of the helix. It consists of tiny arteriovenous anastomoses with many nerve endings similar to a glomus body. It is seen mainly in men (90%) and is of unknown origin.

The main symptom causing the patient to seek medical attention is pain and tenderness. The lesion may be excised or injected with cortisone, which relieves the pain in most instances.

EXTERNAL AUDITORY CANAL

The external auditory canal, lined with squamous cell epithelium, is subject to all forms of dermatitis. Many of these problems are self-inflicted because of the common tendency to pick at our ears with fingers or other objects. Because of the gutter beyond the isthmus, water is difficult to remove. The skin then becomes macerated, creating a dank medium ideal for the growth of bacteria and fungus.

Cerumen

Ceruminous glands are contained in the superior canal wall and in the cartilaginous canal. Their secretion combines with the oily sebaceous secretion in the upper portion of the hair follicle to form a complex substance, cerumen. Cerumen forms a coating of the canal skin that mixes with the migrating keratin layer to give a protective surface which seems to have antibacterial action. The amount and speed of migration of cerumen varies; some individuals have a scanty amount and others tend to form obstructive masses.

Removal of cerumen may be done by irrigation or with instruments (Fig. 45–8). Irrigation is the most gentle means and should be used only if the tympanic membrane has been examined previously. A perforation allows the wash solution to enter the middle ear and

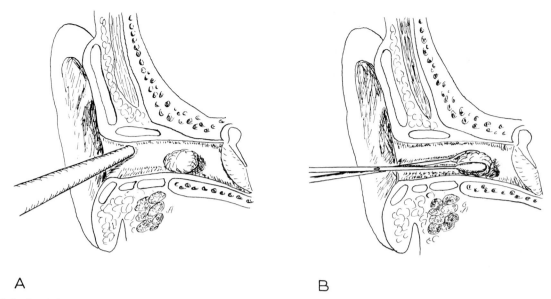

Fig. 45–8. Methods of cleaning the external ear canal. A. Irrigation: the stream of water is directed superiorly. B. Instrumentation: delicate Hartmann forceps is being used to grasp the object.

may cause otitis media and a too vigorous stream of water directed toward an atrophic drumhead may cause a perforation. The canal may be irrigated, either with a syringe or more easily with a pressure-driven irrigating bottle. The canal is straightened by pulling the auricle up and back. Under direct visualization, the water stream is directed along the superior canal wall so that the returning stream may push the cerumen from within. The outflow is caught in a basin held below the ear. Masses of impacted cerumen should be softened before removal to prevent trauma. A useful preparation for this is glycerite of peroxide used 2 or 3 days before cleaning. Cerumen-dissolving agents should be used cautiously because their action depends on enzymes or chemicals, which often irritate the canal and cause external otitis.

The most useful instruments for cleaning the canal are wire loops, dull ring curettes, and delicate Hartmann forceps. The cerumen and desquamated layer of epithelium are first gently separated from the canal skin. The posterior and superior canal walls are less sensitive and the separation is best done on these surfaces. The loosened cerumen is then grasped with the forceps and teased out. Inspection of the drumhead may show that further cleaning can be done with irrigation.

Foreign Bodies

The list of objects which have been recovered from the ear canal is impressive for its variety (Figs. 45–9 to 45–11). These objects may be animate or inanimate, vegetable, or mineral. Children are prone particularly to this affliction.

The major problem of foreign body removal is the isthmus of the canal. Attempts to remove the object occasionally result in pushing it beyond the isthmus. The foreign body, if smaller than the canal lumen, may be grasped with Hartmann forceps and removed. A larger object is removed by placing a hook or loop behind it and "pulling" it out. In some instances, a stream of water may be directed superiorly to push the object out as described for cerumen removal. Animate objects must be killed before removal. A cotton tampon mois-

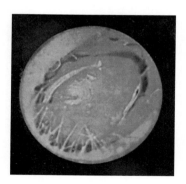

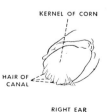

KERNEL OF CORN

HAIR OF
CANAL

RIGHT EAR

Fig. 45–9. Foreign body. A kernel of corn is tightly impacted in external canal.

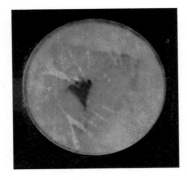

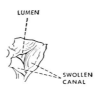

LUMEN

SWOLLEN CANAL

LEFT EAR

Fig. 45–10. Acute diffuse external otitis (swimmer's ear) with marked swelling of external canal.

tened with ether for 5 minutes is sufficient and then irrigation used to flush the insect out.

Unless children are calm during foreign body removal, it is best to use general anesthesia. Many instances of traumatic injury to the tympanic membrane or the ossicles have occurred because a child jumped

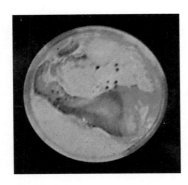

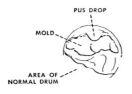

PUS DROP

MOLD

AREA OF NORMAL DRUM

LEFT EAR

Fig. 45–11. Chronic diffuse external otitis (otomycosis). The mold growth is confined chiefly to the upper half of the canal. A portion of normal membrane is seen inferiorly. A clog of purulent exudate is visible externally at the uppermost portion of the canal. From Buckingham RA: What's New. Abbott Laboratories, 1956, p. 196.

during an attempt to remove a foreign body. In all patients in whom the object is lodged beyond the isthmus, removal should be done with anesthesia.

External Otitis

All of the inflammatory processes that involve the skin of the external auditory canal are included in this term. Generalized skin disease may affect the ear together with other parts of the body. This discussion covers diseases peculiar to the ear.

For purposes of differentiation, these disorders may be classified as infectious, eczematoid, or seborrheic and may also be acute, recurrent, or chronic. Although at least 58 forms of external otitis have been cataloged, the foregoing simple classification includes more than 95% of patients with external otitis.

Symptoms

The symptoms of external otitis are common to the various forms, being dependent on the structure of the external canal rather than on the cause. The initial symptom is itching or pruritis within the canal due to beginning inflammation. This symptom is often confused with a deep-seated tickle referred to the ear from the mouth of the Eustachian tube and caused by mild inflammation in this region. It is usually accompanied by a scratching sensation in the throat at the base of the tonsil. Movement of the palatal muscles modifies this tickle, while movement of the auricle has no effect. The reverse is true of the itching due to external otitis. As the external otitis becomes more severe, the itching progresses to a painful sensation. Any movement of the auricle or cartilaginous canal, as in chewing, produces pain. Exudation and swelling now may cause hearing loss secondary to obstruction of the canal.

Aural discharge is initially watery but soon becomes purulent and thick when mixed with pus cells and desquamated epithelium. In chronic forms, the discharge is scanty or absent, with a coagulum forming in the canal. This is usually musty-or foul-smelling because of the action of saprophytic bacteria or fungi. Symptoms of toxicity with fever signify lymphatic spread. Adenopathy becomes evident in the upper anterior cervical triangle, in the parotid region, or in the postauricular groups with this spread of infection.

Diagnosis

INFLAMMATORY EXTERNAL OTITIS. Inflammatory external otitis may be divided into both localized and diffuse forms and acute and chronic forms.

1. *Acute localized external otitis* is an infection of a hair follicle, beginning as a folliculitis but usually extending to form a furuncle. The infecting microorganism is usually *Staphylococcus*. An occasional case, usually involving a furuncle, is caused by a blocked and infected sebaceous gland in the canal. Because heat and

humidity seem to lower the canal skin's resistance to infection, these cases occur with slightly increased frequency during the summer months.

If the patient is seen early, a diffuse red swelling can be visualized in one area of the cartilaginous canal, and may be sufficient to occlude the lumen. As localization takes place, a pustule is seen. Pain is severe in this condition, and examination is difficult. Discharge is not usually present until the abscess ruptures. Toxicity and adenopathy appear early.

2. *Acute diffuse external otitis (swimmer's ear)* is primarily a disease of the summer months and is the most common form of external otitis. Heat and humidity cause swelling of the stratum corneum of the skin, which blocks the follicular canals (Fig. 45–10). Introduction of extraneous moisture from swimming or bathing increases the maceration of the canal skin and creates a condition favorable to bacterial growth. These changes may also cause itching of the canal, which adds the possibility of trauma from scratching. This may follow the actual onset of infection, however. Except in tropical climates, where fungi are a significant infecting microorganism, *Pseudomonas aeruginosa* is the most common bacteria found.

As hyperemia and edema of the canal skin occur, intense itching occurs, which gradually becomes painful. The canal is diffusely inflamed and swollen, with tenderness on movement of the auricle. There is a copious serous discharge. As the disease progresses, the discharge becomes seropurulent and edema causes a partial or complete closure of the canal. Although the process usually is limited to the canal, involvement of the intertragic notch and lobule may occur. Small papules and vesicles are present on the surface of the canal skin, but usually are not noticed because of the difficulty of examination.

Systemic manifestations may occur, but not commonly. A special form of acute diffuse external otitis occurs in diabetics, "Malignant External Otitis," is discussed later in this chapter.

3. *Chronic diffuse external otitis,* caused by fungus infection, is relatively unusual in all but the southernmost regions of the United States. It has become a common practice to diagnose inappropriatly all chronic itching or tickling of the ear as caused by "fungus".

Fungi, usually *Aspergillus niger, Actinomyces,* or yeasts, create a chronic superficial redness of the bony canal wall. A musty-smelling exudate forms, with a gray, wrinkled appearance similar to that of wet newspaper. On the surface of this rather thick membrane will be seen the filaments of the fungus (Fig. 45–11). On the removal of the membrane, the skin has a smooth red shine. Itching is constant and intense but seldom progresses to pain. Systemic manifestations are rare unless superimposed bacterial infection takes place.

ECZEMATOID EXTERNAL OTITIS. This category includes all forms of hypersensitivity of the canal skin. The major causes of this type of external otitis are topical antibiotics or vehicles (dermatitis medicamentosa); allergy to various chemicals or metals used around the ear, such as hair sprays or earrings (contact dermatitis or dermatitis venenata); atopic reaction caused by ingested or inhaled antigen (atopic dermatitis); and infectious eczematoid dermatitis caused by contact of the skin with middle ear discharge. Neurodermatitis and psoriasis might be included in this group of problems, but since they have multiple manifestations, they are best managed by dermatologists and will not be discussed.

Each of these types represents a distinct form of allergy. In contact dermatitis, the local tissue contains the entire response, with no circulating antibodies present. Dermatitis medicamentosa is a particular variety of contact allergy. In atopy, circulating antibodies are present, as well as genetically determined defect of protein metabolism. In some instances, examples of both the Shwartzman and Arthus reactions may be present. Each of these forms of external otitis is characterized by histamine release in the tissues.

The entire ear canal, concha, intertragic notch, and lobule are usually involved (Fig. 45–12), although in some cases of contact dermatitis the process is limited to the lobule. The appearance is that of a confluent mass of weeping, crusted lesions of the hyperemic and edematous skin. This is similar to any lesion of the same type anywhere on the body, such as poison ivy.

SEBORRHEIC EXTERNAL OTITIS. This common form of

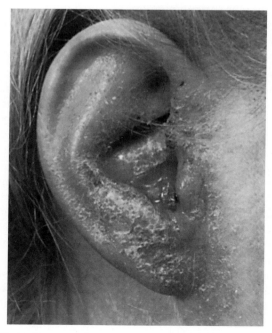

Fig. 45–12. Eczematoid external otitis. The external canal, concha, tragus, antitragus, and lobule are involved with confluent weeping, crusted lesions.

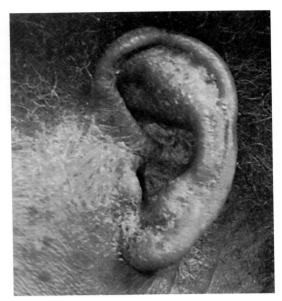

Fig. 45–13. Seborrheic external otitis. The typical greasy scaling is seen not only over the auricle, but also anterior to the ear and in the scalp.

external otitis is associated with seborrheic dermatitis of other regions, particularly the scalp (dandruff). This condition is of unknown cause but seems to have a hereditary factor.

The lesions are typified by a greasy scaling that has a yellowish appearance because of the abnormal sebum production (Fig. 45–13). Many patients are not aware of excess "oiliness," feeling that the scaling is caused by "dry skin." The external cartilaginous canal, concha, and postauricular regions are most often involved. The condition is usually recurrent rather than continuously present.

Treatment of External Otitis

Certain principles of management must be observed in every case of external otitis. These are frequent inspection and cleansing of the canal, control of pain, use of specific medication appropriate to the type and severity of disease, acidification of the canal, and control of predisposing causes.

Frequent inspection, with cleansing and drying of the ear canal, is undoubtedly the single most important factor in obtaining resolution of all forms of external otitis. During the summer months with their high humidity, special efforts are needed to maintain dryness within the canal.

The most efficient method of cleaning the ear canal varies with the state of inflammation. In patients with extremely edematous canals, cleaning must wait until the inflammation has subsided. If much soggy debris is present, irrigation with 3% saline solution or dilute alcohol (10 to 20%) should be performed. This is followed by gentle suction drying. Blotting with cotton-tipped metal applicators is sometimes necessary (some children do not tolerate the noise of suctioning), but this is usually time-consuming and induces more trauma. Burow's solution is often used in acute moist ears to obtain rapid resolution of edema and crusting but, when used, requires special cleaning because of the abundant desquamative debris. As soon as possible, these patients should be placed on a dilute alcoholic cleansing and drying solution (when its use will not cause burning). Seventy percent alcohol acidified to a pH of 5 is efficient for this purpose.

Relief of pain is urgent and usually requires narcotics. Oral codeine or hydrocodone is effective. The pain, caused by the edema and inflammation, is alleviated by the use of heat and hydroscopic solutions.

Acute localized external otitis should be treated the same as an abscess on any part of the body. If it is seen before suppuration has taken place, resolution may occur with the use of antibiotics only, used both topically and systemically. Because this infection is usually staphylococcic, appropriate antibiotics in therapeutic dosage are administered for 5 days. Polymyxin B and/or neomycin combined with corticosteroid in a liquid hydroscopic and acidified vehicle is commonly used. The use of opthalmic drops such as Tobradex (Alcon Labs., Fort Worth, TX) is effective since the antibiotic is more potent and the corticosteroid has a higher concentration. The patient should apply dry heat to the ear for at least 20 minutes 3 times a day. Bed rest is advisable in the more severe cases. The ear should be inspected at least every 2 days until localization or resolution has occurred. With localization, incision of an abscess is necessary.

Acute diffuse external otitis should be treated during the early stages in such a way as to relieve rapidly the edema that blocks the lumen of the canal. To accomplish this, it is usually necessary to insert moistened cotton into the canal to carry the medication to the affected skin. A small tampon is best for this because gauze wicks wad up and do not exert even pressure. The tampon is inserted gently with fine Hartmann forceps. The patient is instructed to apply the liquid medication to the cotton once or twice daily. Within 48 hours, the tampon should fall out of the canal because of an increase in the size of the lumen. After this time, the medication may be applied directly into the canal.

Topical medication is usually effective although adenopathy and toxicity indicate the need for systemic antibiotics (see perichondritis). Polymyxin B, tobramycin, or colistimethate are effective antibiotics against *Pseudomonas* and should be used in a hydroscopic vehicle, such as mildly acidified propylene glycol. Corticosteroids are a useful addition to these antibiotics. Chemical agents such as 2% aqueous gentian violet and 10% silver nitrate are bactericidal and may be applied directly to the canal skin.

As the inflammatory response lessens, 70% alcohol

may be added to keep the canal clean and dry. The antibiotic drops should not be used longer than 2 to 3 weeks because of the risk of contact dermatitis from the medication itself.

The patient should be warned of the possibility of future episodes, especially after swimming. To avoid this, the patient should keep the ear dry by the routine use of dilute alcohol three times weekly and by drying the ear with alcohol whenever it comes in contact with water. The patient should also be warned against scratching the ear or using cotton applicators in the ear.

Chronic diffuse external otitis is usually of fungal origin. This condition is most common in the fourth and fifth decades. It seems to regress as middle age is reached, although recurrence is common. During the age of activity, these patients should be seen periodically and urgently if there is any exacerbation.

When initially seen, the moist membrane is removed by gentle irrigation and suction. The underlying skin is hyperemic and bleeds easily. The skin should be painted with metacresol acetate. If superimposed bacterial infection is present, the ear should be powdered with a mixture of polymyxin B and chloramphenicol. For this, 250 mg of polymyxin B powder is mixed with 3 g of chloramphenicol powder and applied with a powder blower. When the hyperemia has begun to subside, dilute alcohol is added to the regimen and the powder and metacresol acetate gradually discontinued.

Although *seborrheic external dermatitis* may be linked to hormonal imbalance, treatment based on this etiology has been ineffectual. As will be pointed out in the discussion of eczematoid otitis, superimposed infection is often present in this condition and must be controlled before the basic seborrhea is treated.

Control of seborrheic dermatitis of the scalp is necessary to control the external otitis. The best agent for this is selenium sulfide in a shampoo (Selsun, Ross Labs., Columbus, OH) used once a week. At other times, a detergent-type shampoo should be used and oily rinses avoided. The canal and the concha are painted with 10% silver nitrate and dilute alcohol used daily to keep the canal clean and dry.

Eczematoid external otitis is perhaps the most difficult of all forms of external otitis to treat because the provocative agents usually remain undiagnosed. It may follow infectious external otitis or otitis media as a reaction either to the infecting microorganisms or to the medication used to treat them. It may seem psychosomatic at times, because it may follow emotional trauma. Atopic individuals may exhibit external otitis after being sensitized to milk, peanuts, or other foods. Once the canal skin has become a target tissue, allergens other than the original sensitizing agent may provoke an episode of external otitis, thus producing a chronic, recurrent disease.

The prime agents for producing a rapid response are the corticosteroids. Because infection often accompanies the acute episode, topical antibiotics are usually combined with the corticosteroid in the otic solution. Another agent that has been proven most efficient, particularly in the chronic forms of eczematoid otitis, is heparin. Heparin forms a chemical complex with histamine, preventing the local tissue reaction. In practice, heparin (1 mL containing 10,000 or 15,000 units) is added to a commercially prepared corticosteroid-antibiotic otic solution to produce more rapid of the clearing of the otitis.

Contact dermatitis may call for skin testing to find the offending chemical. The more common causes, such as hair spray or nail polish, can usually be detected by history. Any ear preparation used for more than 10 days may produce an eczematoid reaction. Polymyxin B and penicillin are both of significance in this regard. Atopy is detected by family history of allergy, asthma or hay fever. Skin manifestations in other areas of the body may be of great help in diagnosis.

The use of gentian violet is of help in drying and coating weeping areas. In chronic cases characterized by hypertrophy and fissuring of the skin, 10 and 25% silver nitrate painted on the canal is helpful. Dilute alcohol cleansing should be used between episodes to keep the canal clean and dry. Frequent inspection of the canal, even in quiescent periods, may help to treat subacute manifestations. In these cases, treatment may be individualized, and experience plus an open-minded acceptance of non-response to the first tried treatment so that another course may be adopted without undue delay is paramount to success.

Malignant External Otitis

This specific form of acute diffuse external otitis typically occurs in elderly patients with diabetes. Usually unilateral, it begins with the common symptom of itching, soon followed by painful discharge and swelling. Standard topical therapy is ineffectual and the disease progresses to involve the surrounding tympanic bone. The pain becomes intense, and profuse granulation develops, blocking the ear canal. The facial nerve may be involved, causing peripheral paresis or paralysis. Temporizing treatments are contraindicated as the disease will extend to the surrounding areas of the temporal bone: the mastoid: squamous, and petrous portions. Sequestration of the temporal bone and even death have occurred in a number of these patients.

The essential pathology is a progressive osteomyelitis with *Pseudomonas aeruginosa* as the infecting microorganism. The endothelial thickening accompanying advanced diabetes together with high blood sugar levels resulting from the active infection make adequate treatment difficult. Surgical debridement may be required but attempts at definitive surgical excision often result in even further extension of the process.

The standard treatment is hospitalization of the patient, treatment of the diabetes, if present, together with the use of high doses of antibiotics specific for *Pseudomonas* for an extended length of time. Aminoglycosides and synthetic penicillins are used together for a six week course. Tobramycin and Ticarcillin are the antibiotics currently used. Some cephalosporins have anti-*Pseudomonas* activity but are hampered by rapid emergence of resistance. Oral ciprofloxacin in high doses has recently been used to effect an earlier discharge from the hospital.

Special precautions must be taken during such a regimen because the aminoglycosides are nephrotoxic and ototoxic (Chapter 54). Blood levels must be obtained regularly to ensure adequate dosage. Creatinine levels should be obtained three times a week to measure renal function. Electrolyte disturbances such as hypokalemia may occur, and therefore regular determination of electrolytes should be performed. Periodic hearing tests should be obtained if possible, particularly of the uninvolved ear.

Chronic Stenosing External Otitis

This disease is an extreme form of hypertrophic reaction to uncontrolled external otitis. In these patients, there is a fibrous tissue proliferation in the subcutaneous layers combined with hyperkeratosis. Occasionally, a foreign body hidden deep within the canal, may be responsible for this reaction, and in rare instances neoplastic tissue has been found. These changes in the skin of the canal are irreversible and may also be responsible for the chronic infection caused by retention of moisture and debris in a narrow canal. Occasionally, fibrous hyperplasia of the pars media of the tympanic membrane occurs, resulting in a thick tympanic membrane.

The best treatment in most of these cases is surgery. The operation consists of complete removal of the involved skin, enlargement of the bony canal, if smaller than normal, and grafting with split-thickness skin. In many instances, the operation may be done with a meatal incision. In involving the cartilaginous canal, an endaural incision provides improved exposure. When an endaural incision is made, Lempert's technique of excising a semilunar segment of conchal cartilage is recommended. This enlargement of the canal orifice gives the advantage of improved access for postoperative care. The abnormal canal skin is removed entirely using sharp dissection. If the eardrum is involved, the fibrous tissue is removed until a layer of normal thickness remains. The denuded canal is enlarged, using burrs, to an optimum size, increasing gradually in diameter toward the exterior. A 10-mL slit-thickness graft is removed with a dermatome. This should be from an inconspicuous, hairless area such as the inguinal region ("bikini area") or the inner surface of the upper arm. The skin is placed in the canal to cover all exposed surfaces. If the tympanic membrane epithelium is removed, the skin is brought onto the drum. A firm, resilient packing is placed within a lining of plastic strips. Some overlapping of the graft is unavoidable but does not cause difficulty because the superfluous skin sloughs. In cases in which skin removal is limited to the bony canal, it is not necessary to place a graft because the epithelium regenerates without stenosis.

The canal is left alone for 2 or 3 weeks, after which it is cleaned and any granulating areas touched with 25% silver nitrate. Inspection and cleaning are carried out at biweekly intervals until healing is complete.

Keratosis Obliterans

Keratosis obliterans is a rare condition. Also referred to as destructive or invasive keratitis or canal cholesteatoma, it is characterized by the accumulation of large plugs of desquamated keratin in the bony portion of the external canal. Erosion of the bony canal occurs, usually of the inferior or posterior walls. These erosions may be so extensive as to undermine the tympanic annulus and expose the hypotympanum. Occasionally the descending portion of the facial nerve may be uncovered, calling for care in the removal of the keratin debris.

This condition is usually asymptomatic and discovered incidental to examination for conductive hearing loss. Removal of the keratin plug reveals the erosion of the canal. Occasionally the eroded area becomes a source of irritation and infection, producing pain and discharge from the canal.

The cause is unknown. It has been associated with chronic pulmonary disease and sinusitis. Bronchiectasis has been present in a high percentage of these patients, especially those with an onset before age 20.

The disease may be controlled in most cases by periodic cleaning as often as every 3 months. The use of dilute alcohol irrigations or glycerite of peroxide drops three times weekly is helpful. When erosion and infection are marked or uncontrollable, a free tissue graft placed under the skin in the affected region may be of benefit. A transmeatal skin flap is elevated to expose the eroded bone sometimes including the annulus. A free graft of temporalis fascia is removed through an incision above and behind the auricle. In cases with deep erosion, some muscle tissue may be left attached to the fascia to increase the thickness of the graft. The tissue is placed onto the erosion and the skin flap replaced over the graft. A light packing of absorbable gelatin holds the flap in place. Healing is usually rapid and the chronic infection is eliminated. Periodic cleaning may still be necessary.

BENIGN TUMORS OF THE EXTERNAL AUDITORY CANAL

Keloid, papilloma, sebaceous cyst, and melanoma may all involve the canal as well as the auricle.

Exostosis

Exostoses are the most common tumors of the external auditory canal. These benign outgrowths of bone are symptomless unless accompanied by the accumulation of debris against the tympanic membrane, resulting in infection or obstruction. Exostoses are usually seen as two or three smooth sessile protrusions on opposing surfaces of the bony canal near the annulus. In almost every case, a history may be obtained of frequent swimming, often in cold water. This fact possibly is of etiologic significance.

Osteoma occurs in the auditory canal as a single larger growth forming near the lateral end of the bony portion. These tumors are often pedunculated. All these growths are benign and may be ignored unless of sufficient size to obstruct the canal or cause repeated infection from retention of debris. Surgical removal involves elevating the skin from the surface of the bony growth and then removing the growth with motor-driven burrs. When the normal canal lumen has been restored, the skin is replaced over the bone of the canal and held in place with packing of absorbable gelatin sponge. In some instances, an exostosis interferes with tympanic surgery, in which case the described procedure becomes a part of the tympanoplasty, with the skin flap becoming a tympano-meatal flap.

Adenoma

Adenomas of various sorts occur in the canal. These are derived form sweat glands (epithelioma adenoides cysticum or ceruminoma), sebaceous glands, or aberrant salivary gland tissue. Differentiation of these tumors depends on microscopic examination because each appears as a smooth, skin-covered, polypoid mass arising from the canal wall. Symptoms are minimal unless the growth completely occludes the canal. Pain is a sign of malignancy.

The treatment is surgical excision. Some of these lesions occasionally become malignant, and pathologic examination is required in each case. Most of these adenomas may be removed through a transmeatal approach, although with larger growths an endaural incision may be needed.

Finally, any mass occurring within the external auditory canal, if persistent, should be removed for examination. Lesions thought to be polyps, granulomas, or other innocent forms have all on occasion proved to be malignant, usually squamous cell carcinoma. Because this disease is often associated with chronic discharge from the ear, patients with such discharge should be regarded particularly if the discharge does not respond to adequate treatment.

BENIGN TUMORS OF THE MIDDLE EAR

Because cholesteatoma and middle ear polyps will be discussed elsewhere in this book, chronic otitis media, the principal lesion in this group is the glomus jugulare tumor (nonchromaffin paraganglioma).

Glomus Jugulare Tumor

Although vascular tumors of the middle ear have been described since the onset of the twentieth century, it was not until 1941 that the basic tissue of origin, the glomus jugulare, was discovered and described by Stacey Guild. In 1945, Rosenwasser reported the removal of a tumor of the middle ear whose microscopic appearance resembled that of a glomus jugulare. Since that year, this tumor has proved to be the most common one arising in the middle ear.

The glomus jugulare is a tiny ($0.5 \times 0.5 \times 0.25$mm) glandular structure similar to the carotid body. It consists of nests of nonchromaffin staining cells clustered among thin-walled vascular channels. There are usually several of these in every temporal bone, being found on the top of the jugular bulb, along the course of Jacobson's nerve, the tympanic plexus, or Arnold's nerve. The function of these structures is unknown, the most probable being that they are chemoreceptors sensitive to CO_2 level of pH of the blood, as is the carotid body.

Histology

The glomus jugulare tumor is similar in cellular structure to the tissue of origin. It usually arises in the hypotympanum at the site of the entrance of Jacobson's nerve or in the adventitia of the jugular bulb. In many instances, these tumors have been seen to arise on the promontory. They occur five times more often in women than in men. The tumors are extremely vascular, consisting of vascular sinuses supplied by the ascending pharyngeal artery, which enters the tympanum along with Jacobson's nerve. Although the growth rate is variable, these tumors grow slowly as a rule, in some instances with 20 years elapsing between onset and diagnosis. These tumors only rarely metastasize, but they are destructive, growing by invasion into the surrounding structures. Instances of multicentric origin and association with carotid body tumors have been reported, indicating the need for a search for other similar tumors when a glomus tumor is found.

Symptoms

The earliest reported symptom is tinnitus, which is most often pulsatile. Hearing loss follows as the tumor enlarges; as it invades the tympanic membrane, bleeding and discharge occur because of secondary infection. Facial nerve paralysis is frequently present, and invasion along the course of the jugular results in multiple involvement of the ninth, tenth, eleventh, and twelfth cranial nerves. Invasion of the cochlea and petrous tip is a late occurrence, resulting in sensorineural hearing loss and rarely, paralysis of the fifth and sixth cranial nerves. Pain is not a common symptom.

Diagnosis

Examination in the early stages reveals a reddish swelling behind the tympanic membrane which, with magnification, may be seen to pulsate. If the drum is dull and the tumor is small, this appearance might be confused with the Schwartze sign in otosclerosis. As the tumor enlarges, it causes the inferior portion of the tympanic membrane to bulge (Fig. 45–14), and it finally breaks through to form a smooth dark red polypoid mass that bleeds easily (and often massively) on manipulation. Application of pressure with a Siegle otoscope causes the tumor to increase in pulsation as the pressure is raised until sudden blanching occurs after the systolic pressure is exceeded (Brown's test). Radiographic examination is of little value in early cases, but as the tumor advances, reveals the extent of bony destruction. In advanced tumors, external carotid angiography is helpful in delineating the extent of involvement. Diagnosis is confirmed by biopsy, which must be done carefully in the hospital operating room because of the severe bleeding that may occur. With an intact tympanic membrane, the biopsy is best done

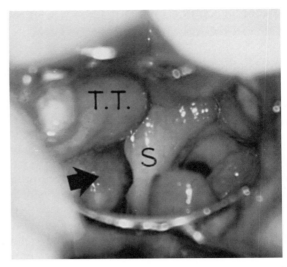

Fig. 45–15. Mirror view of nasopharynx showing extension of glomus jugulare down eustachian tube. At arrow, the tumor is protruding through the tumor orifice. T.T., Torus tubarius; S, posterior end of the nasal septum.

through a tympanotomy approach and combined with total excision.

Alford and Guilford introduced the concept of staging of glomus tumors, describing five clinical stages. The best treatment of the tumor varies with the stage of the disease.

STAGE 0. This stage is the earliest manifestation of a glomus tumor. The patient complains of hearing loss and/or pulsating tinnitus. There is normal hearing or a conductive hearing loss. The drumhead is intact but discolored. Radiographs will be normal.

STAGE I. Added to the above is aural discharge from involvement of the tympanic membrane by the tumor. Radiographs show clouding of the middle ear but no bone erosion. There is no nerve involvement.

STAGE II. Facial paralysis is now present, and there is sensorineural hearing loss. Radiographs show no bone erosion other than occasional enlargement of the jugular foramen.

STAGE III. Involvement of the jugular foramen adds paralysis of the cranial nerves IX, X, XI, and XII. There will be radiographic evidence of erosion of the petrous bone and enlargement of the jugular foramen.

STAGE IV. Intracranial extension has taken place (Fig. 45–15), and papilledema is present. Extensive involvement of the petrous bone has occurred, with paralysis of the third, fourth, fifth, and sixth cranial nerves.

Treatment

Treatment must be individualized because many early cases may be cured through surgical excision, but slow growth of the tumor usually dictates palliation in the far-advanced cases. Tumors (Stage I) involving only the middle ear may be completely excised through a tympanotomy. The exposure should be primarily of

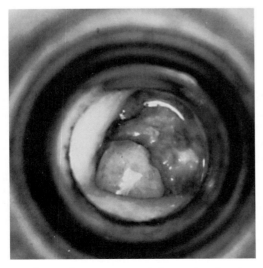

Fig. 45–14. Otoscopic appearance of glomus jugulare tumor. The tumor has eroded the tympanic membrane and is creating a serosanguineous otorrhea.

the hypotympanum. This is done by extending the meatal flap to include the inferior canal wall and removing the inferior tympanic sulcus with a diamond burr to expose the entire hypotympanic space. Extension into the attic or mastoid (Stage I or II) requires a radical mastoidectomy approach for adequate exposure. In extensive lesions, hemorrhage may be life-threatening, so that ligation of the ascending pharyngeal artery should be done if surgery contemplated. Cases involving the jugular foramen with cranial nerve paralysis (Stage III) have been operated on successfully, but this is such a formidable procedure, necessitating dissection and ligation of the lateral sinus and jugular vein in the neck, that in most instances partial removal combined with radiation is used. The easiest method of handling the tumor tissue is to expose the entire extent of the tumor and pack around it with small cotton or gauze packs while it is being removed to control the bleeding.

Radiation is often used in these cases, especially when complete removal is not possible. Although these tumors are somewhat radioresistant, x ray has a definite effect on their course, causing a slow regression in the size of the tumor. Tumor doses of 2400 to 6000 R given over a period of 2 to 4 weeks have been employed. Long-term periodic examination must follow any type of treatment.

MALIGNANT TUMORS OF THE EAR

Carcinoma

Eighty-five percent of cases of carcinoma of the ear present on the auricle, 10% on the external auditory canal, and 5% in the middle ear. Fortunately, in clinical practice these percentages represent a small incidence, 4 or 5 carcinomas per 20,000 patients. The onset is most often in the sixth or seventh decade of life, with approximately 80% of cases occurring in men. They may be of the squamous basal cell, carcinoma or adenocarcinoma. Squamous cell carcinoma of the middle ear is difficult to diagnose early in its course. Usually associated with chronic infection, pain, and bleeding, the tumor has a rough reddened surface that may be mistaken for granulation or polyp. Carcinomas of the skin of the face are discussed in Chapter 9. Adenocarcinoma arises from the skin appendages of the canal or the glandular elements of the middle ear.

Treatment

AURICLE. Early carcinoma of the auricle is usually treated with electrocautry and curettage with control rates of 98% to 99%. With cartilage invasion, excision is required with an associated cure rate of more than 90%.

EXTERNAL AUDITORY CANAL. The cure rate in carcinoma of the external auditory canal is less than 35%.

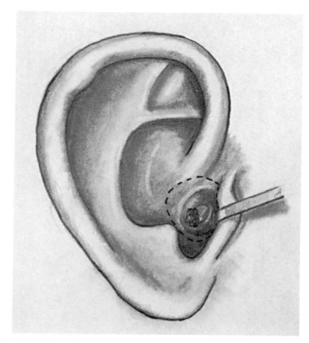

Fig. 45–16. Carcinoma of external auditory canal. The external meatus is isolated by the incision shown around the orifice of the canal (after Conley).

Wide excision of the lesion dictates complete removal of the cartilaginous and bony auditory canal by means of a mastoid approach which removes the canal en bloc without disturbance of the involved tissue. The surgery is usually supplemented with a postoperative tumoricidal dose of radiation.

The surgical approach initially isolates the external meatus from the auricle by incisions made widely around the canal orifice through the tragus and concha (Fig. 45–16). A postauricular incision then gives access to the mastoid cortex to allow an atticomastoidectomy to outline completely the superior and posterior bony canal walls (Fig. 45–17). The intramastoid portion of the facial nerve is dissected to permit transection of the bony external canal at the level of the facial canal. A perforating burr is used to make multiple holes through the facial canal into the posterior sinus and tympanic sinus of the middle ear to create a controlled fracture at this level. The same technique is used to separate the anterior canal wall from the anterior extremity of the lateral attic wall. These fractures are made with a thin osteotome. With further separation of the surrounding soft tissues, an en bloc specimen is removed containing the entire cartilaginous and bony canal with the tympanic membrane and malleus included. The resultant defect may be covered with a split-thickness skin graft.

Ceruminoma

This term indicates a rare tumor that arises from the apocrine (ceruminous) glands of the external auditory

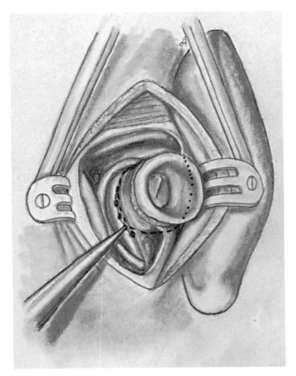

Fig. 45–17. Carcinoma of external auditory canal. The external auditory canal has been isolated by complete mastoidectomy and atticotomy. The facial nerve has been exposed and removed from the fallopian canal. A perforating bur is being used to outline a line that will be fractured through with chisel to free completely the entire auditory canal en bloc (after Conley).

canal, most often located within the meatus. Malignant types outnumber the benign by a 2:1 ratio and adenocystic carcinoma is most common. Males and females affected equally and the average age is about 48. Clinically a tumor mass obstructing the auditory canal to varying degrees is found. Roentgen evidence of bone erosion is usually absent. Surgical removal of the tumor is necessary.

Cystic Adenoid Carcinoma (Brooke's Tumor)

This tumor is a special form of carcinoma in which the cell type is thought to be derived from the germinal epithelium of the hair follicles and/or sweat glands. The lesion is exceedingly rare but may involve either the auricle or the external auditory canal. Clinically these tumors appear after puberty and are more common in females. They present as small painless, slowly enlarging nodules that do not ulcerate.

Histologically there are immature epidermoid cells arranged in cords, clumps, and alveoli plus concentric rings of cornifying epithelium around a core of homogenous material. These cells project from the basal layer of the skin or glandular ducts and commonly contain cystic areas filled with amorphous material. Metastasis is rare, but the prognosis is poor because of insidious progress and recurrence despite seemingly adequate treatment.

Malignant Melanoma

Melanoma may occur either on the auricle or in the external canal, more common in the former location. Diagnosis should be suspected with a pigmented lesion that begins to increase in size or change in color.

SUGGESTED READINGS

Alford BR, Guilford FR: Tumors of the glomus jugulare. Laryngoscope 72:763, 1962.

Brown JS: Glomus jugulare tumors revisited: a ten-year statistical follow-up of 231 cases. Laryngoscope 95:284, 1985.

Chandler JR: Malignant external otitis: Further considerations. Ann Otol Rhinol Laryngol 86:417, 1977.

Chen D, Johnson JT, Zini I, et al: Prosthetic auricular reconstruction. Otolaryngol Head Neck Surg 91:556, 1983.

Dayal VS, Lanfond G, Van Nostrand AW, et al: Lesions simulating glomus tumors of the middle ear. J Otolaryngol 12:175, 1983.

Derlacki EL: Repair of central perforations of the drum. Arch Otolaryngol 58:405, 1953.

Elsahy NI: Ear reconstruction with rotation-advancement composite flap. Plast Reconstr Surg 75:567, 1985.

Jones EH: External Otitis; Diagnosis and Treatment. Springfield, Charles C Thomas, 1965.

Konefal JB, Pilepich MV, Spector GJ, et al: Radiation therapy in the treatment of chemodectomas. Laryngoscope 97:1331, 1987.

Krespi YP, Ries WR, Shugar JM, et al: Auricular reconstruction with postauricular myocutaneous flap. Otolaryngol Head Neck Surg 91:193, 1983.

Lesser RW, Spector GJ, Deviveni VR: Malignant tumors of the middle ear and external auditory canal: A 20-year review. Otolaryngol Head Neck Surg 96:43, 1987.

Mclaurin JW: Persistent External Otitis. Laryngoscope 75:1699, 1965.

Mohs FE: Fixed-tissue micrographic surgery for melanoma of the ear. Arch Otolaryngol Head Neck Surg 114:625, 1988.

Paparella MM, Kurkjian JM: Surgical treatment for chronic stenosing external otitis. Laryngoscope 76:232, 1966.

Proud GO: Surgery for chronic, refractory otitis externa. Arch Otolaryngol 83:436, 1966.

Senturia BH: Disease of the External Ear. 3rd Ed., Springfield, Charles C Thomas, 1957.

Shockley WW, Stucker FJ Jr: Squamous cell carcinoma of the external ear: a review of 75 cases. Otolaryngol Head Neck Surg 97:308, 1987.

Sooy CD, Sooy FA: Transcanal management of benign middle ear lesions involving the anterior middle ear cleft. Laryngoscope 95:671, 1985.

Stell PM: Carcinoma of the external ear auditory meatus and middle ear. Clin Otolaryngol 9:281, 1984.

46 Reconstruction of the Outstanding Ear (Otoplasty)

Howard S. Kotler and M. Eugene Tardy, Jr.

ANATOMIC AND PATHOLOGIC FEATURES

The normal ear is a thin, shell-like structure having definite depressions and projections (Fig. 46–1). Many variations that may still be considered within normal limits are found. It is only when the ear protrudes abnormally (''outstanding'') or is absent that the defect is immediately noticeable. Large or small ears, which may be proportionately more deformed than an outstanding ear, may go unnoticed if they are placed in a normal relationship to the head. The normal *auricle, or pinna,* is described by Gray as ovoid, with its larger end directed upward. The prominent rim of the auricle is called the helix. Where the helix turns downward, a small projection, known as *Darwin's tubercle,* is frequently seen. This tubercle is evident at about the sixth month of fetal life, when the whole auricle has a slight resemblance to that of a macaque monkey. This fact has caused much speculation and controversy among anthropologists, but as yet the significance of this tubercle is not clear. Another prominence parallel with and anterior to the helix is called the anthelix; this divides above into the superior and the inferior crus between which is a shallow depression, the fossa triangularis. Some authors refer to these two crura as the posterior and anterior crura. The narrow, curved depression between the helix and the anthelix is called the *scaphoid fossa,* or ''boat-shaped ditch.'' The anthelix describes a curve around a deep cavity, the *concha,* which is divided into two parts by the crus helicis or the beginning of the helix; the upper part is termed the *cymba concha,* the lower part the *cavum concha.* Anterior to the concha and projecting back over the external auditory meatus is a small pointed eminence, the *tragus,* so called because it is generally covered on its undersurface by a tuft of hair, in the male resembling a

goat's beard. Opposite the tragus and separated from it by the *intertragic notch* is a small tubercle, the *antitragus.* Below this is the *lobule,* which is composed of areolar and adipose tissue with overlying epithelium. At the junction of the anthelix and the antitragus is a small space, which may be deep in some ears and is known as the *sulcus auriculae posterior.*

The auricle, with the exception of the lobules, is composed of a thin, flexible plate of yellow elastic fibrocartilage. The cartilage is 0.5 to 1 mm thick and covered on each surface by integument intimately applied and having a minimum of subcutaneous tissue. The skin is closely adherent to the surface of the cartilage except on its posterior surface and along the helix.

The cartilage of the auricle (Fig. 46–2) is a single piece that gives form to the ear and outlines the landmarks previously mentioned. It is absent from the lobule and is deficient between the tragus and the beginning of the helix. At the anterior part of the auricle, where the helix bends upward, is a small projection of cartilage called the *spina helicis.* At the lower part of the helix, the cartilage is prolonged downward as a tail-like process, the *cauda helicis,* which is separated from the anthelix by a fissure, the *fissura antitragohelicina.* The posterior aspect of the cartilage exhibits a transverse furrow, the *sulcus anthelicis transversus,* which corresponds to the inferior (anterior) crus of the anthelix and separates the *eminentia triangularis.* Another furrow exists at the central region of the concha, known as the *sulcus crusis helicis,* which corresponds to the continuation of the helical rim and separates the concha into two portions, the *cavum conchae* and the *cymba conchae.*

The ligaments of the auricle consist of two sets: 1) extrinsic, which connect the auricle with the side of the head; and 2) intrinsic, which connect various parts of its cartilage to each other and to the external auditory meatus.

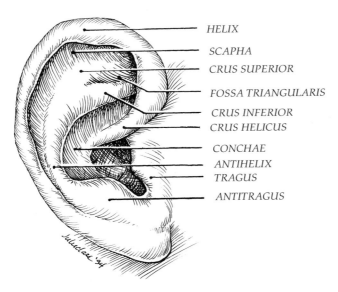

Fig. 46–1. The anatomy of the auricle.

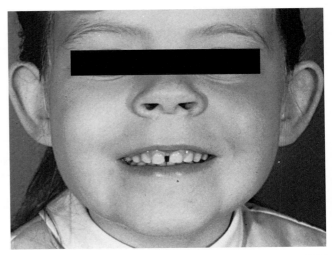

Fig. 46–3. Common auricular deformity with loss of anthelical fold and normal concha. Note normal lobule positioning and size.

The muscles of the auricle likewise consist of two sets: 1) extrinsic, which connect it with the skull and scalp and move the auricle as a whole; and 2) intrinsic, which extend from one part of the auricle to another. Because these muscles are rudimentary, they have no particular surgical importance save for the abundant blood supply coursing within the musculature. In the infraprimate mammals, these muscles are particularly well developed and are important in turning the auricle toward the source of a sound.

The motor innervation is by the temporal branch and the posterior auricular branch of the facial nerve. The sensory nerves are the great auricular nerve from the cervical plexus, the auricular branch of the vagus nerve, and the lesser occipital nerve from the cervical plexus.

The arteries of the ear are composed of the posterior auricular, from the external carotid artery; the anterior auricular, from the superficial temporal artery; and a branch from the occipital artery. The veins accompany the corresponding arteries. The lymphatics drain into the periauricular nodes.

CORRECTION OF PROTRUDING EARS CAUSATIVE FACTORS

Malformations of the auricle are not unusual and may range in severity from complete absence to macrotia. The protruding ear (failure of development of the anthelical fold) is by far the most common deformity (Fig. 46–3).

The embryonic origin of the external ear is still a controversial matter, but most observers agree that the six tubercles, or hillocks, of the first branchial groove, which appear about the fifth week of embryonic life, develop into the pinna. For convenience, these hillocks are numbered from 1 to 6; three hillocks develop on the mandibular arch and three on the hyoid arch of the first branchial groove. The tragus is derived from mandibular hillock 2, the helix from mandibular hillocks 2 and 3, the anthelix from hyoid hillocks 4 and 5, and the antitragus from hyoid hillock 6. The lobule represents the lower end of the auricular fold.

At the end of the third month of embryonic life, the hillocks are well defined and the ear begins to assume definite form. According to Evans, it is at this time that the greatest number of malformations occur. The ear

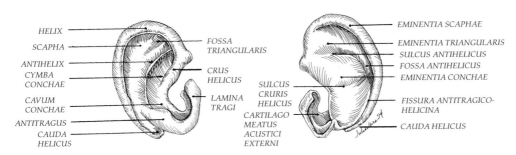

Fig. 46–2. The cartilage of the auricle from the lateral (left) and medial (right) surfaces.

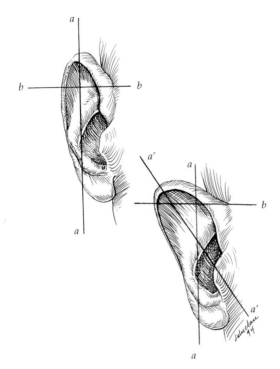

Fig. 46–4. The essential pathology of an outstanding ear. In the upper figure, the customary relation of the ear to the head is seen. The plane of the scapha, represented by a-a, makes a right angle with the plane of the concha, indicated by b-b. In the lower figure, a'-a' is seen to make a much broader angle with b-b.

mines the degree of protrusion of the ear, the outstanding ear deformity may be conceptualized as to the type and development of the anthelix—that is, the more obtuse the angle, the more the ear projects (Fig. 46–4).

Other pathologic factors are encountered less frequently. A heavy, concave concha protrudes the lower portion of the ear and is often accompanied by a thickened antitragus (Fig. 46–5).

Congenital deformities of the helical rim are usually

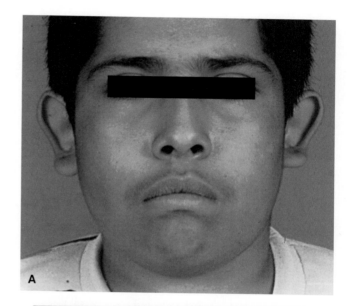

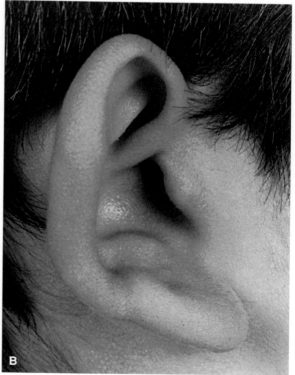

Fig. 46–5. Bilateral prominent ear deformity. Note overdeveloped concha with absent anthelix.

margin at this time is pointed, and because the crura of the anthelix are not formed, the ear protrudes from the head. Davis and Kitlowski stated that, at about the sixth fetal month, the margin curls, forming the helix; the anthelix becomes more definitely folded, and its crura appear. It is the folding of the anthelix and the development of the crura that are responsible for bring the ear closer to the head.

The protruding ear, therefore, is embryonically a congenital deformity, is inherited according to mendelian law, and may be a dominant or a recessive trait. Potter reported that a dominant gene may be transmitted through many generations.[1] She revealed the transmission through five generations of a malformation in which the ears were extremely cupped and protruding. A family tree embracing 92 members was obtained in the study. On the average, half of the members with this deformity had transmitted it to their children, whereas normal siblings married to normal persons had not transmitted the defect.

Therefore, the protruding ear in most instances is a congenital or hereditary deformity caused by maldevelopment of the anthelix. The angle between the concha and scapha is formed by the anthelix, and an absence or lack of development of the angle formed by the anthelix results in a protrusion of the auricle away from the head. Because the angle of the anthelix deter-

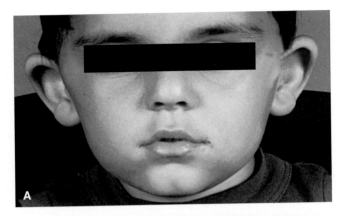

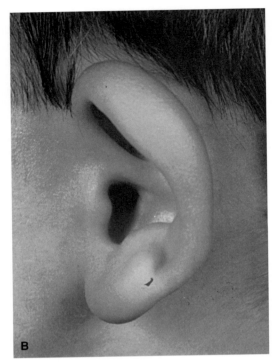

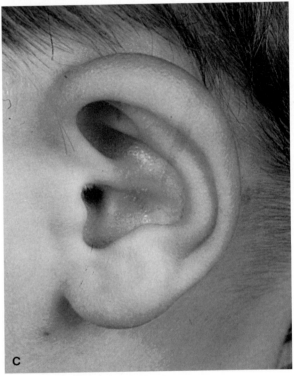

Fig. 46–6. Pre- and 6-month postoperative views of bilateral lop ear deformity. Anthelical fold is underdeveloped with prominent concha and minimally constricted superior helix.

associated with a thin, flat ear that may or may not be protruding but is frequently lopped forward at the upper pole (Fig. 46–6). If deformed, everted superior crus accompanies this deformity, it produces a vertical projection of the upper pole to form the satyr type of ear.

The protruding (microtic) ear differs from the usual protruding ear. The ear is folded on itself and smaller than normal. This is almost invariably caused by a short (usually thickened) helix and a deformed anthelix. The conchal cartilage in some instances is heavier than normal or may appear so because of a superimposition of the anthelix over the concha (Fig. 46–7).

The pinnae of humans and primates have poorly developed external musculature and mobility, that in comparison to lower animals serves little appreciable function in hearing. However immobile, the pinna does appear to assist high frequency localization of sounds originating in front and in back of the head. This occurs through the complementary intrinsic resonant frequency of the pinna (5 kHz) and external auditory canal (2.5 kHz). During normal hearing, a frequency dependent increase in a sound pressure level (SPL) of approximately 10 to 15 dB occurs in the frequency range from 1.5 kHz to 7 kHz. In lower animals, the auricle has function in determining direction of sound and protecting the internal auditory mechanism. Some animals, on stimulation of the tragus, close the auditory canal by an infolding of the auricle to serve as protection against water or insects. Henneberg and others observed that some mammals of the aquatic and semiaquatic group, such as the muskrat, seal, and beaver, can close the external ear when they are plunged into water. Rodents, moles, and other ground-

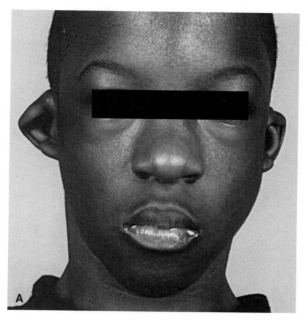
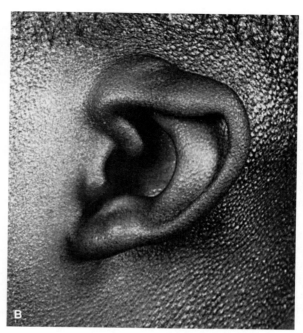

Fig. 46–7. Asymmetric, severe bilateral lop ear deformity. Note marked left helical fold constriction with contralateral complete effacement of superior helical fold.

burrowing animals are also capable of closing the external meatus.

The psychologic effects of protruding ears vary with the sensitivity of the individual. In pediatric patients, a feeling of insecurity is often evident. This is because unlike most visible malformations, the congenitally deformed ear produces reactions of mirth in other people. To be constantly reminded of, and ridiculed about a deformity, breaks all defense mechanisms of repression that a patient might have formed and subjects him or her to the development of any insecurity or inadequacy neurosis. Fortunately for these persons, this deformity can be corrected simply and satisfactorily, preferably at an early preschool age, before any real psychologic trauma can be inflicted. Many who appear unperturbed by their deformity may in fact be sensitive about it and suffer inwardly. Other patients who are not at all sensitive about their appearance or defects may desire a correction of the ears purely for economic or social reasons.

In examining the normal ear from behind, the concha forms a 90-degree angle with the head. The scapha likewise forms an angle of approximately 90 degrees with the concha, but this may vary as much as 10 to 15 degrees and still be within normal limits, according to Young. The rim of the helix turns slightly outward. The angle between the scapha and the concha is formed by the anthelix, and in its absence or underdevelopment, the angle may become obtuse, resulting in auricular protrusion away from the head. Since the angle of the anthelix more or less determines the degree of auricular protrusion, it follows that the more

obtuse the anthelical angle, the more the ear protrudes from the mastoid. The angle formed by the helix and the head is known as the auriculomastoid angle and is usually 30 degrees.

HISTORICAL SURVEY

The earliest reference to the correction of protruding ears was in 1845, by Dieffenbach, who advised removal of skin from the back of the ear followed by the suturing of the auricular cartilage to the periosteum of the mastoid bone.[2]

Ely in 1881, Keen in 1890, and Monks in 1891 all described similar operations but added the removal of a cartilaginous section from the posterior surface of the auricle. Monks classified protruding ears into firm and soft cartilaginous types, the former requiring cartilage and skin excision and the latter only skin excision. Haug in 1894, Joseph in 1896, and Morestin in 1903 described similar procedures; however, Morestin emphasized the complete sectioning of the cartilage from the superior to the inferior pole to prevent any recurrence of the protrusion.[3]

A variety of complicated operations were later described. Gersuny, in 1903, split the conchal cartilage into strips with removal of alternate sections. Payr, in 1906, used a cross-shaped, pedunculated strip of cartilage and perichondrium, which was passed under a loop of periosteum in the mastoid region. Ruttin, in 1910, and Luthi, in 1929, used fascia lata attached to the perichondrium at the inner edge of the helix and anchored it to periosteum over the mastoid. Alexander, in 1928, recommended a longitudinal incision through the conchal cartilage. The cartilage was then overlapped and held in position with catgut sutures between the cartilage and postauricular fascia.

In 1937, Eitner recommended an operation similar to the Joseph and Morestin procedures. The skin and perichondrium were incised horizontally and then undermined before the longitudinal removal of the cartilage.

None of the procedures described can possibly result in a normal-appearing ear. The scapha projects abnormally, while the ear appears flattened against the head. On a lateral view, the concha often appears deformed; sharp ridges and excess wrinkling of the skin are noted, along with absence of the anthelical fold.

The basic concept for the newer type of otoplasty was first described by Luckett, who in 1910 pointed out that the reason for protruding ears was the absence or underdevelopment of the anthelix.[4] If a new anthelix were made, the prominence of the ear could be overcome; furthermore, on a lateral view a more normal-appearing ear would result without the distortions of the concha and absence of the normal anthelical fold. Luckett's operation consisted of removing a crescent-shaped area of cartilage and skin from the posterior surface of the auricle over the line of the proposed anthelix and everting the edges of cartilage by the use of a Lembert suture, thereby forming a new anthelix.

Davis, in 1919 and again in 1937 with Kitlowski emphasized Luckett's basic concepts, which also served as the basis for Barsky's operation in 1938.[5,6] Davis and Kitlowski outlined the new anthelix along the inferior crus with brilliant green introduced by a needle through perforations in the skin from the anterior surface of the auricle. The skin on the posterior surface of the auricle, which had been removed from both the conchal and the mastoid regions, was discarded. The cartilage was split along the previously marked line and a section removed. The authors emphasized that the cartilage must be split through the entire length of the proposed anthelix to break its elasticity. Surgical gut sutures closed the perichondrium, and the edges were everted to form the new anthelix.

The objection to the Davis-Kitlowski procedure is that the normal postauricular sulcus is obliterated by the excessive removal of skin from the posterior surface of the auricle and from the mastoid region. Also, in the removal of cartilage only from the inferior crus, the superior crus may appear flat, and at times the ear appears to lop forward at its upper pole.

The Davis-Kitlowski procedure led to a modification in 1940 by New and Erich, who used mattress sutures externally to help hold the form of the new anthelix.[7] They also excised cartilage from the inferior crus but at times felt it necessary to remove a wedge of cartilage from the superior (posterior) crus to prevent the upper pole of the ear from falling forward. They cited Webster as stating that he had satisfactory results without incising the cartilage but by merely shaving the cartilage in the region of the anthelix. New and Erich, however, stated that the ear can be folded back with greater ease if a narrow strip of cartilage is excised.

Young in 1944 described a method similar to, but an improvement of, the Davis-Kitlowski procedures.[8] He stated that if the section of cartilage forming the new anthelix were removed correctly, the scapha could be slipped over the concha, and thus no external mattress or internal gut sutures would be needed to hold the new fold of the anthelix. The excision of cartilage was made in the region of the superior crus rather than in the inferior crus, although Young expressed the belief that an incision is sometimes necessary in the inferior crus. No skin, other than the excess, is sacrificed from the postauricular sulcus.

Young's procedure is a decided improvement over the Davis-Kitlowski method for two reasons: 1) the main excision of cartilage is from the superior crus, giving the ear a better appearance; 2) no skin is sacrificed from the postauricular sulcus; thus the ear is prevented from appearing too close to the head. The objection to Young's method is that a sharp ridge is produced in the region of the superior crus.

In 1947, McEvitt described a method similar to that used by Young. He advised the excision of cartilage at the anthelix and its crura and, in some cases, the placement of parallel incision to break the spring of the cartilage further. He emphasized the necessity in some cases of excising part of the antitragus and of crosscutting the remaining portion, a detail which most reports do not mention in correction of the extremely cupped type of ears. He stated that, in correcting some of the similar types of protruding ears, he has tended to removed less and less cartilage, and at times none.

Pierce, Klabunde, and Bergeron, in 1947, reported a procedure for correction of protruding ears that involved making eight to ten incisions almost through the cartilage. They stated the belief that the older operations leave a prominent ridge on the anterior surface of the auricle and that this new method gives an accurate representation of the normal fold. Five surgical gut sutures are used to hold back the anthelix fold and the ear. Excess skin is removed, and the remaining skin is sutured with Dermalon. This procedure represent an important advance because it is an attempt to prevent sharp ridges on the anterior surface of the ear.

LATER PROCEDURES

In 1949 and again in 1952, Becker described a method of correcting protruding ears based on the principle of incising the cartilage along natural lines, thereby allowing the ridges formed by those incisions to be hidden in the normal folds of the ear.[9,10] The only excision of cartilage was made in the anthelix region. This excision was supplemented in cases of marked cupping and protrusion by the removal of a section of cauda helicis. In other cases, a section of the upper border of the superior crus under the helical rim was also removed.

The cartilage excision from the anthelix was continued by an incision extending through and along the inferior crus. This incision (after 1953) was extended up from the inferior crus to meet the incision along the helical rim that outlined the superior crus and superior border of the triangular fossa. If the cartilage was unusually firm, the superior crus cartilage was crosscut incompletely, that is, by incisions that did not completely transect the cartilage. The cartilage was then undermined for a few millimeters from the anterior surface of the auricle to prevent any wrinkling of the anterior skin and to help mobilize or round the borders of the incised and excised cartilage. The excess skin, which is always present in varying amounts, was removed and the incision closed. External mattress sutures were placed in the region of the anthelix and in some cases through the superior crus region. A drain was inserted, and a fairly snug mastoid dressing applied.

The results of the foregoing procedure have been gratifying. Occasionally, however, the excision of cartilage from the anthelix left a slightly sharpened ridge. This was not objectionable to the patient but was disconcerting to the surgeon seeking perfection. Furthermore, to break the spring of the upper portion of the ear completely, the incision extending through the superior crus down through the fossa triangularis sometimes left a sharp ridge in the area near the juncture of inferior crus, triangular fossa, and new anthelix. To avoid this, the incision at the junction of anthelix, inferior crus, and triangular fossa was made incompletely through the cartilage. This was sometimes insufficient to break the spring of the firm, cartilaginous type of protruding ear, and to avoid cutting completely through in this area, Becker began depending on the incision along the upper pole of the superior crus. This maneuver allowed the incomplete transection of cartilage at the junction of the triangular fossa, inferior crus, and anthelix, thereby avoiding any sharpness in this area.

In 1956, Coverse and coworkers presented a method of minimal removal of cartilage from the anthelix region by a new concept of thinning the cartilage so that it may be tubed in its lower portion.[11] The incisions through the cartilage were the same as described, that is, along the natural folds, but instead a section of cartilage was thinned with a motor-driven brush and then rolled on itself with internal catgut fixation sutures. A

section of cartilage was removed from the conchal side of the anthelix when necessary. This method of tubing the cartilage created a smoother anthelix than the method of excising cartilage. The incision through the fossa triangularis, however, was retained by Converse.

Withers in 1955 presented a similar concept of using a burr to thin the cartilage of the superior crus but he retained the excision of anthelical cartilage.[12] Construction of a normal rounded anthelix and scaphoid fossa by cartilage resection was advocated by Farrior in 1959.[13] He advocated postauricular triangular excisions in parallel, folding the anthelix into normal position and maintaining it with mattress sutures. The anterior surface of the cartilage (and perichondrium) was not disturbed. In the early 1970's, however, interest grew in developing approaches for modification of the anterior surface of the ear. Experimental and clinical studies enlarged upon the concepts of directional cartilage curl away from the sides of the incision(s), with release of inherent interlocked stresses. Disruption of perichondrium appears to influence favorably the curling tendency toward the intact perichondrial side, possibly because of its unopposed contraction. However, this phenomenon is not observed with abrasion of the perichondrium and cartilage.

Stenstrom observed this phenomenon and aware of Gibson and Davis' studies on the bending tendency of rib cartilage, applied the principle to a technique for correcting outstanding ears.[14] His approach depends upon weakening the anterior cartilage surface and its inherent spring by variably strong "scratching" maneuvers. To accomplish sufficient weakening of ear cartilage, scratches are placed with a rasp over the entire anterior surface, but with special intensity over the anthelix, anterior and posterior crura, and posterior conchal wall. Especially resistant areas of cartilage are scratched more deeply, but scratches are not extended through cartilage because unnatural ridges may result. Consequent posterior curling accentuates the rounded anthelical fold. Precise segments of postauricular skin (the original incision for access to anterior surfaces) are measured and resected, stabilizing permanently the retropositioned ear. Kaye exploited the advantages of the Mustarde and the Stenstrom approaches.[15] Combining anterior striation with permanent mattress sutures placed through limited small anterior incisions, extensive undermining was thus avoided. Webster suggested correction of the deformity created by bulges on the cavum or cymba concha by serial excision of cartilaginous discs from the corresponding posterior eminentia, thus allowing the ear to settle anatomically against the mastoid. He likewise utilized precise postauricular skin excision to aid in the permanent positioning of the auricle.

Mattress Suture Otoplasty

During the mid-1960's, a corrective otoplasty procedure, developed primarily by Mustarde, gained ready acceptance and wide popularity. Vertically positioned nonabsorbable mattress sutures were inserted to recreate the natural shelving curve of the anthelical fold, blending gently into the scaphoid fossa. The principal advantages of this cartilage-sparing technique were as follows:

1. No through-and through cartilage incisions are necessary, thereby avoiding the potential sharp edges of other techniques.
2. Transperichondrial sutures may be positioned, test-tied, and then maintained (or replaced) as necessary to develop a natural anthelix. This eliminates the commitment of cutting through cartilage, a noncorrectable action.
3. The procedure is rapid and relatively easy to learn and teach, requiring less dissection of the ear and avoid surgical trauma.
4. The long range results are satisfactory.

Furnas augmented the Mustarde approach with variable addition of sutures from the concha to the mastoid periosteum, the scaphoid fossa to the temporalis fascia and the lobule to the sternocleidomastoid muscle surface.[16] The intent was to appose forcibly the protruding ear closer to the side of the head. Acceptable sequelae (when minimal) are listed as diminished depth of the postauricular sulcus, flattening of the conchal floor, and occasional ''post-like'' straightening of the normal curving line of the anthelical root.

Since the introduction of the mattress suture otoplasty technique, this procedure, with variations, has been performed on several hundred outstanding ears. Certain modifications have been introduced that have led to ease of operation and surgical safety. It must be emphasized that an operation is designed individually for each ear, depending on the existent deformity. Often a *combined* operation is accomplished, the basic mattress suture procedure being augmented by Becker's dissection technique to achieve surgical correction and natural appearance. Ears are commonly asymmetric, and therefore asymmetric operations are necessary.

Details descriptions of the *dissection technique* of Becker and the *mattress suture technique* modified by Tardy and Tenta follow. Mastery of the precise anatomy of the auricle (anterior and posterior), combined with a knowledge of the following two surgical procedures, allows the surgeon wide latitude in achieving natural correction of the many varieties of outstanding ear. No single technique suffices.

The Dissection Technique (Becker)

The hair is shaved for a distance of 2.5 cm from the ear and held away from the operative field with head drapes. The ears are washed with a detergent containing hexachlorophene followed by an antiseptic solution. With the patient lying on his or her back, the head is draped, and only one ear is exposed at a time. A comparison of the two ears is usually unnecessary during the operation because one can judge with fair accuracy when the ears are evenly placed to the head.

Either local or general anesthesia may be used. A complete encirclement of the ear is made with injections of the local anesthetic agent, and additional solution is infiltrated on the posterior surface and the anterior surface of the anthelix, the injections in the latter two regions being primarily to facilitate the dissection and for hemostasis.

Before the anesthetic solution is injected, an outline of the proposed incisions is made on the anterior surface of the ear and will subsequently be transferred to the posterior surface during the surgery. The ear is pressed back toward the mastoid region, and an excess section of skin will appear on the posterior surface. An outline of this excess of skin can then be made with methylene blue. It is well to outline this excess of skin before an anesthetic solution is injected, because the ballooning of the tissues interferes with the proper outline of the skin. The section of the skin is then removed (Fig. 46–8A).

The skin is dissected forward (toward the helical rim) just beyond the scaphoid eminence on the posterior surface of the auricle. Skin undermining should be kept to a minimum. Only the area necessary to expose the landmarks is undermined. The wide exposure shown on the illustrations is for diagrammatic purposes (Fig. 46–8B).

After dissection of the skin, the following landmarks should be exposed by further dissection. The cauda helicis and the fissura antitragohelicina are exposed. The sulcus anthelicis transversus (inferior crus) is exposed by blunt dissection to remove the small intrinsic muscle that covers the area. The eminentia triangularis is exposed. The eminentia scapha is exposed down to the inferior crus.

A series of needles is now inserted from the anterior surface of the ear through the scaphoid fossa along its entire length. The lightly shaded dots represent the markings made under the helical rim at the depth of the scaphoid fossa and follow this fossa around the entire ear to the inferior crus.

The needle that was used to pierce the anterior surface of the auricle in the scaphoid fossa (under the helical rim) is noted to follow the scaphoid eminence from the bisection of the cauda helicis around to the inferior crus. It then follows the anterior border of the proposed anthelix, which is noted on the anterior surface of the ear when the ear is folded back into normal position (Fig. 46–8C).

An incision through the cartilage is made along these markings. The cartilage should be cut completely through to the perichondrium on the anterior surface. It is then undermined with fine, flat scissor for about

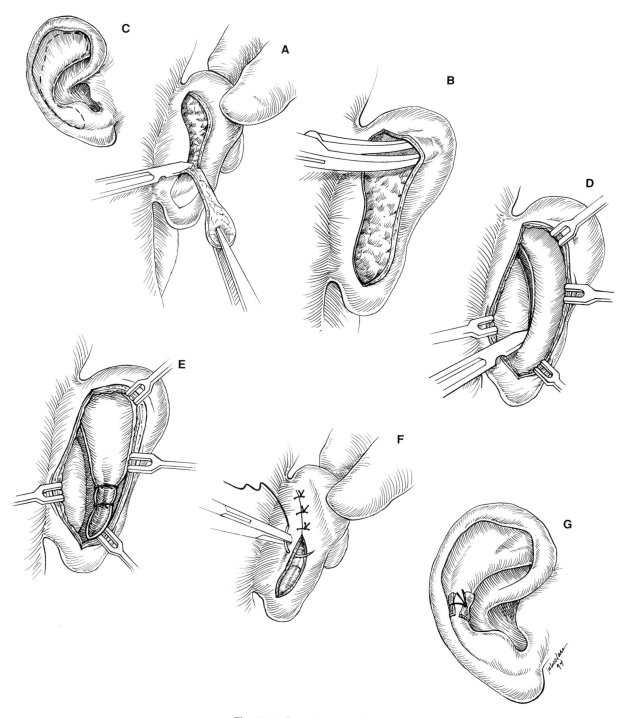

Fig. 46–8. Operative procedure.

4 or 5 mm, following completely around the incision. The lower pole, however, is completely dissected free from the anterior skin so that it is detached for a distance of about 0.75 to 1 cm (Fig. 46–8D). This allows the cartilage to curl on itself. The perichondrium over the center portion of the ear is completely removed by excision and scraping of the surface with a sharp scalpel (Fig. 46–8D). The removal of the perichondrium helps turn the borders of the ear cartilage inward. The perichondrium along the edges of the incision is left attached to aid in the healing and adherence of the outer edges united by sutures. The lower free end of the cartilage is then sutured together with 0000 chromic catgut (Fig. 46–8E).

An additional incision may be made through the eminentia triangularis if the upper pole of the ear seems to have any residual spring. The incision must not be completely through the cartilage at the lower end; otherwise, a sharp ridge will develop where the fossa triangularis meets the anthelix.

The skin incision is then sutured with continuous 5–0 mild chromic catgut. An external mattress suture may be placed through the borders of the newly formed anthelix to help maintain its position on the anterior surface of the auricle. The mattress suture is tied without tension over a small roll of Adaptic dressing rolled on itself (Fig. 46–8F, G). A narrow Penrose drain is usually inserted in the lower portion of the posterior incision and remains for 48 hours. Adaptic dressing is used to cover the ear and is followed by cotton packed into the convolutions. An external bandage is firmly applied.

In many patients, a section of antitragus is removed if the lower portion of the ear protrudes markedly. This area is just anterior to the lower pole, which has been sutured. In other patients with a large thick concha, it may be necessary to remove a section of conchal cartilage.

In patients in whom the anthelix appears too prominent after this method has been used, or if the spring of the cartilage appears inadequately broken, the catgut sutures are removed and a narrow section of cartilage is removed from the center of the anthelix almost up to the inferior crus. The cartilage is then sutured together with catgut.

The dressings are changed on the second day. The drain is removed and a new bandage applied. On the fifth day, the external mattress suture is removed and the ears are again firmly rebandaged. On the eighth or ninth day, the postauricular sutures are removed and a bandage is reapplied until the fourteenth day.

This method has been used in a large series of patients with excellent results. The methods first described by Becker in 1949 and again in 1952 resulted in a good correction.[9,10] The two objections to the first procedure were that 1) the anthelix fold was sometimes too sharp, and 2) the spring at the juncture of the fossa triangularis and inferior crus, if completely cut through, would leave a sharpened ridge that was often objectionable. In many patients with protruding ears in which the cartilage was soft, this latter incision was made only partially through the cartilage, and a better result was obtained.

The present method of following up through the inferior crus and then curving along the scaphoid sulcus at its upper end eliminates the complete transection of the cartilage at the junction of the triangular fossa, anthelix, and inferior crus.

The undermining of the cartilage, the complete freeing of the lower border, and the removal of the perichondrium from the center portion of the cartilage (i.e., the section of cartilage remaining between the two lateral cut edges) help the cartilage to roll on itself to duplicate the natural curve of the anthelix. This is further reinforced by the catgut sutures and an external mattress suture.

If this method does not adequately correct the ear or if the anthelix is too prominent, it is necessary to resect a section of cartilage from the new anthelix and/or from the conchal margin. In other cases, it may be necessary to extend an incision from the previous incision above the superior crus down through the eminentia triangularis.

As the surgeon concentrates on creation of an anthelical fold and superior pole position, the importance of the tail of the helix and lobule position are often overlooked. The lobule and cauda helicis are often times only minimally improved by these maneuvers. Therefore, achieving a balanced aesthetic result sometimes requires a more direct approach to lobule and cauda helicis repositioning.

The malpositioned helical tail is maintained by fibrous attachments between the cauda helicis and the cavum concha, bridging across the fissura antitragicohelicina. Simple posterior skin excision rarely produces adequate or permanent correction of the cartilaginous cauda helicis but may reduce the malpositioned lobule. Methods to improve this deformity advocated by Spira, include simple suturing of the lobule dermis to the scalp periosteum, while Furnas described suturing the fibrofatty tissue of the lobule to the insertion of the sternocleidomastoid muscle.[16,17] However, the techniques described by Webster, Elliot, Goulian and Conway involves direct suturing of the cauda helicis to the cavum concha.[18–20] These techniques achieve an aesthetic and permanent repositioning of the lower third of the malpositioned ear. Alternatively, an incision around the earlobe, freeing its anterior attachment from the skin of the face, may also be necessary if the lobe itself projects abnormally after adequate excision of the antitragus.

The postauricular sulcus is not obliterated, as occurs following the procedure in which a large skin excision from the mastoid and conchal regions is necessary to hold the ear back in position.

Mattress Suture Otoplasty (Tardy)

After use of hexachlorophene shampoo and a similar facial cleansing the evening before surgery, application of Betadine solution completes the periauricular skin preparation. General endotracheal anesthesia is used in children; adolescents and adults receive local infiltration anesthesia supplemented by continuously monitored intravenous analgesia. Apertured transparent plastic drapes allow frequent intraoperative auricular comparison to ensure symmetry of repair. Xylocaine, 1%, with 1:100,000 epinephrine (standard solution) infiltrates sparingly the postauricular subcu-

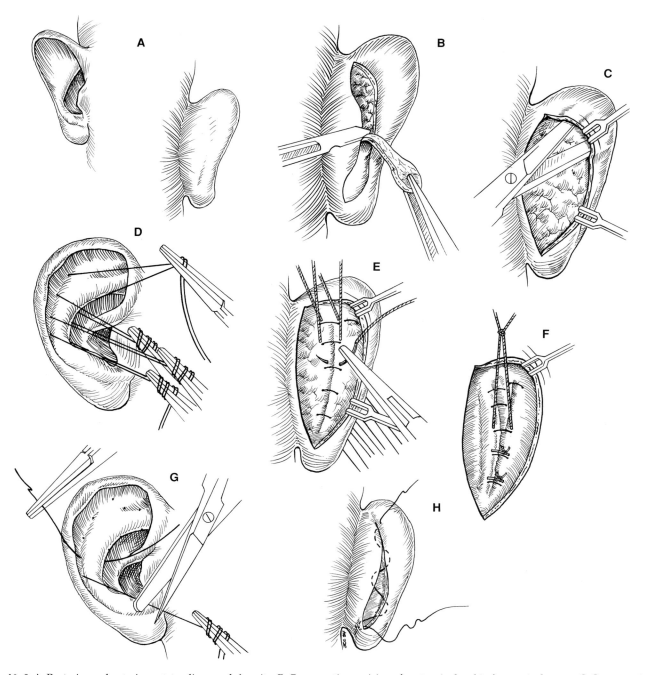

Fig. 46–9. A. Posterior and anterior outstanding ear deformity. B. Conservative excision of postauricular skin for surgical access. C. Conservative undermining of skin. D. Temporary silk sutures preplaced as guides to accurate placement of permanent buried transperichondrial mattress sutures. E. Preplaced temporary sutures indicate sites for mattress suture placement. F. Transperichondrial mattress sutures positioned and test-tightened to determine precise effect in creating new anthelical fold. G. Final positioning and ligation of transperichondrial mattress sutures. H. Preplaced temporary guide sutures removed. I. Postauricular incision closure is with running intradermal monofilament suture.

taneous tissues, aiding in dissection and promoting hemostasis (Fig. 46–9A).

An incision adequate to expose the posterior surface of the neoanthelical fold is created in fusiform fashion (Fig. 46–9B). It is necessary to remove a large portion of skin or to undermine extensively (Fig. 46–9C). Minimal dissection thereby diminishes surgical trauma and

promotes rapid healing, an advantage of mattress suture otoplasty. The posterior perichondrium is not stripped bare of subcutaneous tissue to facilitate postauricular scar formation in the posterior trough formed by the neoanthelical fold. This scar forms the eventual strength of the repair, relieving the buried mattress sutures of their original burden (revision operations reveal the presence of this important sheet of scar, retaining the retropositional attitude of the ear, even after removal of the mattress sutures). With the thumb and index finger, the neoanthelical fold is sited and created, blending naturally into the posterior crus. Temporary marking sutures of 4–0 black silk are next passed from anterior to posterior (Fig. 46–9D) to guide precisely the placement of the permanent mattress sutures. Black silk siting sutures eliminate the disadvantages of marking with ink or sharp needles.

Using the silk sutures as a guide, transperichondrial horizontal mattress sutures of white 4–0 braided nylon are positioned sequentially (Fig. 46–9E) from caudal to cephalic along the neoanthelical fold. It is essential that each suture encompass *both* the anterior and the posterior perichondrium in order to prevent ultimate tearing through of the suture. Seldom are less than four horizontal mattress sutures required, each sharing the retropositioning vector force until scar tissue cements the eventual position of the auricle. Each suture may be test-tightened to assess its effect (Fig. 46–9F); an unnatural-appearing fold is avoided by the removal and repositioning of the suture until exact sculpture of the auricle is achieved, a considerable advantage of the technique.

The auricle with a deep cavum conchae may require excision of a semilunar segment of cartilage within the cavum conchae at this point to construct the neoanthelix properly.

It is unnecessary to overcorrect the retropositioning of the auricle because sufficient properly positioned sutures maintain the correction precisely (Fig. 46–9G).

After meticulous hemostasis, a continuous running intradermal monofilament nylon suture completes the postauricular skin closure (Fig. 46–9H), thereby facilitating suture removal in 10 to 14 days. No drains are used. Frequent comparison of the two ears during surgery ensures symmetry and exacting repair. Mineral oil-soaked cotton, gauze fluffs, and Kerlex wraparound gauze comprise the support bandage, which is changed the morning after surgery and maintained thereafter for 36 to 72 hours. The use of nylon stocking caps during sleep is recommended to the patient to prevent inadvertent nocturnal trauma and displacement.

It is worthy of emphasis that the mattress suture procedure is frequently augmented by thinning, weakening, and even limited incision of cartilage to achieve natural and symmetric results. Knowledge of one technique only is obviously inadequate.

OTOPLASTY COMPLICATIONS

Although many of the complications encountered in otoplasty are common to any surgical procedure, some are specific to the operation itself. The auricle, by virtue of it's anatomic location and structure, is particularly predisposed to postoperative complications that would not otherwise present in head and neck procedures. Particularly important is the avascular cartilaginous framework and it's compromise if incisions are combined with unnecessary elevation of the thin skin-subcutaneous envelope. Undesirable anatomic sequelae or complications, both immediate and late may be avoided by completely understanding the preoperative deformity and how to manage all complications. While the following is not an exhaustive description of all potential complications, those mentioned are some of the most commonly encountered.

Pain/Tenderness

Postoperative pain in otoplasty should not be considered a normal course of events. While some patients may feel a periauricular "tightness", pain in the first few postoperative days may herald the presence of hematoma. Examination of the surgical site reveals a fluctuant mass under a tense, erythematous or dusky soft tissue envelope. Hematoma occurs frequently from inadequate hemostasis during the procedure, rebound vasodilation following injectable vasoconstrictors, occult coagulopathy or preoperative ingestion of salicylates. Similar to any of the facial plastic procedures performed in our center, we recommend a minimum interval of two weeks after aspirin ingestion. While not routine by other published methods, we also advocate the use of 2 postauricular rubber band drain that is removed on the first postoperative day.

An unsecured postoperative dressing generates shearing forces between the cartilaginous framework and the delicate, loosely adherent soft tissue envelope. Small collections of blood or serous fluid may coalesce and result in cartilaginous necrosis or in visible soft tissue irregularities. Following the management principles in traumatic auricular hematoma, the wound should be opened, drained and a pressure dressing applied. Needle aspiration is rarely successful as the organized clot is oftentimes loculated or too fibrous to permit removal through even the largest needle bore. Prophylactic antibiotics are essential to prevent additional infectious complications.

Postoperative pain may also be secondary to infection independent of hematoma. Infection may be either superficial in the skin or deep in the perichondrium or cartilage. Wound drainage with culture and sensitivity testing are imperative to determine resistant microorganisms and target antibiotic use better. Rarely, excision of devitalized or necrotic cartilage is necessary, with subsequent planned reconstruction.

Neural injury is indicated by hypesthesia or numbness in the absence of signs that classically indicate infection. Postoperative hypesthesia results from transected rami of the greater auricular nerve during postauricular dissection or suture traction injury. This discomfort usually subsides to a tolerable level or may disappear completely within four to six months postoperatively.

Postoperative Pinna Malpositioning

The best surgical efforts to create an aesthetically pleasing pinna may be defeated by any degree of postoperative trauma. Most patients comply with the recommended postoperative elastic headband use, but these are often displaced during sleep. Early postoperatively, poorly applied dressings may be displaced, resulting in hematoma with a newly created helix folded onto itself. Minor trauma to the pinna, uncomplicated by either hematoma, suture rupture or torn cartilage may be treated by headband repositioning or gentle taping of the ear. Careful inspection of the extent of malformation determines if re-operation is necessary.

Hypertrophic Scarring and Keloid Formation

Unlike most healing facial soft tissues above the mandible, the otoplasty patient is at risk for keloid formation and hypertrophic scarring. Rare in any anterolateral conchal incision, postauricular hypertrophic scarring and keloids are not uncommon. Conservative management includes intralesional triamcinolone injection with application of pressure. If the obliterated postauricular sulcus creates both an obvious aesthetic and functional deformity (as with poorly fitting eyeglasses), then surgical excision with subsequent triamcinolone injection may be required (Fig. 46–10).

Suture Complications

Relative to polyfilament suture, monofilament suture construction shows a lower incidence of long-term su-

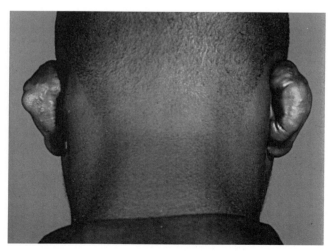

Fig. 46–10. Bilateral postauricular keloids 6 months following otoplasty. These were treated by conservative resection and sequential postoperative triamcinolone injection.

ture failure and rate of infection. This may justify its use despite the greater tendency for mechanical erosion through the thin postauricular skin envelope. Suture prominence or "bridging" beneath a thin posterior cover may be minimized by limiting the amount of skin excision and maintaining its full thickness.

Anatomic Deformity

Anatomic deformity following otoplasty represents either postoperative complication or an incomplete treatment of pre-existing deformity. These undesirable changes may not become evident until years after surgery, when the forces of scar contraction have produced their maximal effect. While some are only minimally visible to both patient and surgeon, others create functional deficits to the external auditory canal or postauricular sulcus. The following discussion is arranged by specific anatomic subunits and the common deformities produced in each.

Distortion of the External Auditory Canal
Conchal retropositioning requires suture fixation between the posterior concha and mastoid fascia. Sutures placed excessively posteriorward on the conchal cartilage or too far anteriorward on the mastoid fascia may narrow the external auditory meatus. Careful adjustment of these sutures under direct visualization, while insuring an adequate aesthetic result will prevent meatal stenosis.

Prominent Tragus
Repositioning a laterally displaced concha using concha-mastoid sutures may displace the tragus anteriorly. Resection of the postauricular muscle and fibrofatty tissue overlying the mastoid creates a deeper pocket for the concha, effectively avoiding this deformity.

Anthelical Overcorrection and Hidden Helix
Although not considered an anatomic deformity in the nonoperated auricle, a retropositioned helical rim relative to the anthelix is undesirable as a postoperative result. The most common cause is related to the overcorrection of the neoanthelix. Drawing Mustarde sutures too tight creates an overly acute anthelical angle, and consequently places the helical rim medial to the anthelix. This deformity is also seen as a result of excessive postauricular skin excision.

Telephone Deformity
Over-reducing the hypertrophic concha otherwise refractory to more conservative measures (i.e., concha-mastoid suture), results in a relative prominence of superior and inferior poles. Reminiscent of a hand-held receiver, this is known as a telephone deformity and is easily avoided by minimal conchal resection. If nec-

essary, adjunctive traction sutures placed superiorly and inferiorly will reform a more natural planar arrangement of the helix.

Sharp Cartilage Edges

Resection of the cartilaginous framework adjunctive to its repositioning may lead to visible anterior scars. Prominent creases indicate overlapping conchal margins, and a visible soft tissue cleft indicates the discontinuity of resection margins. Both are avoided by precise on-edge suture approximation.

Malposition of the Lobule

As attention is focused on creating an anthelical fold and position of the cavum concha, the lobule's final position is often neglected. The lobule and helix should lie approximately in the same plane and while this is common in the unoperated ear, it is also desirable as a postoperative result. The degree of lobule shift after cavum or helix manipulation determines in part the most appropriate surgical maneuver. Management options include simple excision of a soft tissue triangular segment from the posterior lobule surface, amputation of the cauda helicis or as proposed by Webster cauda repositioning relative to the concha.[18] Few patients require little more than soft tissue excision to realign the lobule with the helix. Amputation of the cauda helicis releases control of the lobule by the cauda helicis, and lobule protrusion tends to persist postoperatively. Moreover, this maneuver carries the additional complication when viewed anterolaterally of a visible contour irregularity at the cauda remnant. The repositioning of the cauda helicis, by dividing its fibrous attachments at the fissura antitragohelicina and then by suture fixation to the concha, is perhaps the most anatomic and stable method to correct gross deformity.

REFERENCES

1. Potter EI: A hereditary ear malformation transmitted through five generations. J Hered 28:255, 1937.
2. Dieffenbach JF: Die Operative Chirurgie. Leipzig, FA Bruckhaus, 1845.
3. Morestin PHM: De la reposition et du plissement cosmetiques due pavillon de l'oreille. Rev Orthop 4:289, 1903.
4. Luckett WH: A new operation for prominent ears based on the anatomy of the deformity. Surg Gynecol Obstet 10:635, 1910.
5. Davis JS, Kitlowski EA: Abnormal prominence of the ears: A method of readjustment. Surgery 2:835, 1937.
6. Barsky A: Principles and Practice of Plastic Surgery. Baltimore, Williams & Wilkins Co., 1950.
7. New GB, Erich JR: Protruding ears: A method of plastic correction. Am J Surg 48:385, 1940.
8. Young F: The correction of abnormally prominent ears. Surg Gynecol Obstet 78:541, 1944.
9. Becker OJ: Surgical correction of the abnormally protruding ear. Arch Otolaryngol Head Neck Surg 50:541, 1949.
10. Becker OJ: Correction of the protruding deformed ear. Br J Plast Surg 5:187, 1952.
11. Converse JM, et al: A technique for surgical correction of lop ears. Trans Am Acad Ophthalmol Otolaryngol 60:551, 1956.
12. Withers BT: Modern concept of surgical correction of protruding ears. Laryngoscope 65:1172–1193, 1955.
13. Farrior RT: A method of otoplasty: normal contour of the anthellix and scaphoid fossa. Arch Otolaryngol 69:400–408, 1959.
14. Stenstrom SL: The Stenstrom otoplasty. Clin Plast Surg 5:465–470, 1978.
15. Kaye BL: A simplified method correcting the prominent ear. Plast Reconstr Surg 40:44–48, 1967.
16. Furnas DF: Correction of prominent ears with multiple sutures. Clin Plast Surg 5:491–493, 1978.
17. Spira M, et al: Correction of the principal deformities causing protruding ears. Plast Reconstr Surg 44:150–154, 1969.
18. Webster GV: The tail of the helix as a key to otoplasty. Plast Reconstr Surg 44:455–461, 1969.
19. Elliot RA: Complications in the treatment of prominent ears. Clin Plast Surg 5:479–490, 1978.
20. Goulian D, Conway H: Prevention of persistent deformity of the tragus and lobule by modification of the Luckett technique. Plast Reconstr Surg 26:399–404, 1960.

47 Otitis Media and Middle Ear Effusions

Gerald B. Healy

Infections of the middle-ear space and their sequelae have plagued mankind from the beginning of time. First described by Hippocrates in 450 BC, this universally observed process continues to present one of the most perplexing medical problems of infancy and childhood, while being the leading cause of hearing loss in this age group. It is estimated that 70% of children will have had one or more episodes of otitis by their third birthday.[1] This disease process knows no age boundaries but occurs mainly in children from the newborn period through approximately age seven, when the incidence begins to decrease. It occurs equally in males and females. A racial prevalence exists, with a higher incidence occurring in specific groups such as Native Americans, Alaskan and Canadian Natives and Australian aboriginal children. African-American children appear to have less disease than do American white children, but this observation has yet to be adequately explained.

Important epidemiologic factors include, a higher incidence of otitis in children attending day care centers, a seasonal variation with more disease being present in the fall and winter vs. the spring and summer, and a genetic predisposition to middle-ear infection. Other epidemiologic factors include a lower incidence in breast fed children and a higher incidence in children with altered host defenses. These include anatomic changes such as cleft palate, as well as congenital and acquired immune deficiencies. One of the earliest signs of acquired immune deficiency syndrome (AIDS) in infants is recurring episodes of otitis media. This observation has been seen in more than 50% of neonates with AIDS.[2]

DEFINITION

Unfortunately, numerous terms have been used to describe the various inflammatory conditions of the middle ear-space (Table 47–1) This has resulted in both confusion and a lack of uniformity in reporting. An attempt to standardize nomenclature was undertaken in the early 1980s and will be used throughout this chapter when discussing this disease process.[3]

Otitis media represents an inflammatory condition of the middle-ear space, without reference to cause or pathogenesis.

Middle-ear effusion is the liquid resulting from otitis media. An effusion may be either serous (thin, watery); mucoid (viscid, thick); or purulent (pus). The process may be acute (0–3 weeks in duration); subacute (3–12 weeks in duration); or chronic (greater than 12 weeks in duration).

Otitis media may occur with or without effusion. In those cases without effusion, inflammation of the middle ear mucous membrane and tympanic membrane may be the only physical finding present. Occasionally, infection may involve only the tympanic membrane, (myringitis), without necessarily involving the mucosa of the middle-ear space.

This chapter will deal primarily with two disease processes:

1. Acute otitis media
2. Chronic otitis media with effusion

Acute otitis media represents the rapid onset of an inflammatory process of the middle-ear space associated with one or more local or systemic signs. This usually includes otalgia, fever, irritability, anorexia, vomiting, diarrhea, or otorrhea. Physical exam usually indicates a thickened, erythematous or bulging tympanic membrane with limited or no mobility to pneumatic otoscopy. Erythema of the tympanic membrane may be an inconsistent finding and may be absent in certain systemic illnesses such as immune deficiency, when the patient cannot mount a sufficient inflammatory response to present this more classical finding. The acute onset of fever, otalgia, and on occasion a

TABLE 47–1. Synonyms Used in the Past for Otitis Media

Acute Otitis Media	Otitis Media with Effusion
Suppurative	Serous
Purulent	Secretory
Bacterial	Mucoid
	Glue ear
	Middle ear effusion

purulent discharge is usually evidence of acute otitis media. Following such an episode, the patient may move into a subacute or even chronic phase where fluid is present in the middle-ear space although active infection may be absent.

Chronic otitis media with effusion indicates the presence of asymptomatic middle-ear fluid usually resulting in conductive hearing loss. The tympanic membrane may present numerous physical findings including thickening, opacification, and impaired mobility. An air-fluid level and/or bubbles may be observed through a translucent tympanic membrane. This entity is distinguished from acute otitis media in that the signs and symptoms of acute infection are lacking (e.g., otalgia, fever, otorrhea).

ETIOLOGY

Eustachian tube dysfunction is considered the major etiologic factor in the development of middle-ear disease. Politzer first proposed the *ex vacuo* theory of otitis in 1867.[4] The theory postulates that chronic negative pressure, secondary to eustachian-tube malfunction results in the development of a transudate into the middle-ear space. Numerous experiments have been carried out by many authors to substantiate this theory. It is traditionally maintained that the effusion is sterile and, therefore, therapy should be aimed chiefly at relieving eustachian-tube dysfunction. Most proponents of the theory have proposed that there are essentially two types of eustachian-tube obstruction resulting in middle-ear effusion: mechanical and functional. *Mechanical* obstruction may be either intrinsic or extrinsic. *Intrinsic mechanical obstruction* is usually caused by inflammation of the mucous membrane of eustachian tube or an allergic diathesis causing edema of the tubal mucosa. *Extrinsic mechanical obstruction* is caused by obstructing masses such as adenoid tissue or nasopharyngeal tumors.

Some observers believe that infants and younger children may suffer from *functional eustachian tube obstruction* as a result of either decreased tubal stiffness or an inefficient active opening mechanism. Proponents believe that either form of obstruction results in inadequate ventilation of the middle ear with resulting negative middle ear pressure. This theory supports the development of a rational medical or surgical approach to alleviate the obstruction, and thus overcome negative pressure.

The eustachian tube has three physiologic functions with respect to the middle ear:

1. *Ventilation* associated with equalization of air pressure in the middle ear with atmospheric pressure
2. *Protection* of the middle ear from sound and secretions
3. *Drainage* of middle-ear secretions into the nasopharynx with the assistance of the mucociliary system of the eustachian tube and middle-ear mucous membrane

The second etiologic theory was first suggested by Brieger in 1914 and proposes an inflammatory origin to otitis.[5] Since that time, several other authors have supported this theory. In 1958 Senturia reported a 41% incidence of positive bacterial cultures in 130 specimens taken from patients with a diagnosis of "serous otitis media".[5] Other series have supported this finding.[6] Sade's observation that the basic histopathologic mechanism in otitis media with effusion is an inflammatory hypertrophy of the middle-ear mucous membrane and hyperplasia of its mucous glands, also tends to support an inflammatory basis.[7]

Protein analysis of middle-ear effusions indicate a significantly higher concentration of total protein, lactate dehydrogenase, malate dehydrogenase, and acid phosphatase than in serum. This finding has led to the speculation that this material represents an exudate rather than a transudate giving further evidence that this is an inflammatory process. Some proponents of the inflammatory theory feel, however, that inflammation occurs secondary to eustachian-tube dysfunction and thus the inflammatory response is not the primary etiologic factor.

Numerous other factors may well contribute to the development of middle-ear disease. These include allergy, ciliary dysfunction, nasal and/or sinus disease, and immaturity of the immune system.

DIAGNOSIS

In most cases, a careful history and physical examination will lead to the diagnosis of otitis media.

A careful history should elicit classic symptoms of otitis. In the patient with the *acute* form of the disease, otalgia, fever, irritability, vomiting, and diarrhea may be present. Less frequently, otorrhea, vertigo, and facial paralysis may be associated with an acute infection of the middle-ear space. In those patients in whom infection has spread into the mastoid air cell system and beyond, swelling of the postauricular area may be present.

In *chronic otitis media with effusion,* hearing loss may be the only symptom. The most definitive part of the

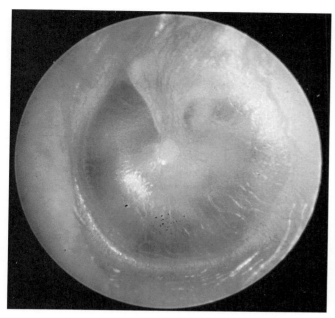

Fig. 47–1. Normal left tympanic membrane appearance at otoscopy.

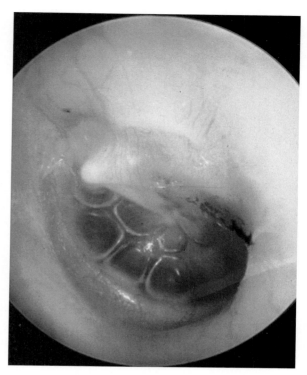

Fig. 47–2. Otitis media with effusion. Note air bubbles confirming the presence of fluid.

diagnosis is an appropriate physical examination to confirm the presence or absence of middle-ear pathology. A complete examination of the head and neck should be undertaken first, to identify the possibility of any predisposing condition such as craniofacial anomaly, nasal obstruction, palatal defect, or adenoid hypertrophy. In patients with unilateral otitis media, the nasopharynx should be visualized to rule out the possibility of tumor.

Otoscopy represents the most critical part of the examination to establish the diagnosis of otitis media (Fig. 47–1). Use of the pneumatic otoscope is essential. The existence of *chronic middle ear effusion* is most easily confirmed when there is a definite air fluid level or when bubbles are clearly visible within the middle ear space (Fig. 47–2). However, findings commonly associated with otitis media with effusion include a severely retracted tympanic membrane with apparent foreshortening of the handle of the malleus and a reduction in tympanic membrane mobility (Fig. 47–3). Occasionally, the tympanic membrane may be dull or thickened and has an amber hue (Fig. 47–4). In severe cases, middle-ear fluid may become purplish or blue indicating hemorrhage within the tympanic cavity.

The color of the tympanic membrane is important but is not conclusive in making a diagnosis. An erythematous tympanic membrane alone may not be indicative of a pathologic condition because the vasculature of the tympanic membrane may be engorged as a result of the patient's crying or the presence of fever.

Acute otitis media usually presents with a hyperemic tympanic membrane that is frequently bulging and has poor mobility (Fig. 47–5). Occasionally, perforation may be present, and purulent otorrhea is clearly visible.

The use of *tympanometry* has been popularized to confirm the findings of pneumatic otoscopy. This modality provides an objective assessment of the mobility of the tympanic membrane as well as the ossicular chain. By measuring tympanic membrane impedance, one can accurately predict conditions of the middle-ear space.

The ultimate diagnostic test to confirm the presence of otitis media involves aspiration of middle-ear con-

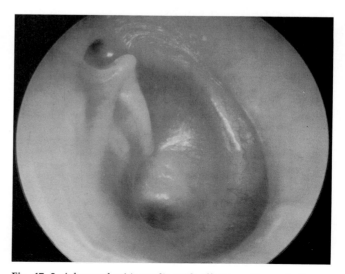

Fig. 47–3. Advanced otitis media with effusion with markedly retracted right tympanic membrane, with apparent foreshortened handle of the malleus and thick, mucoid effusion.

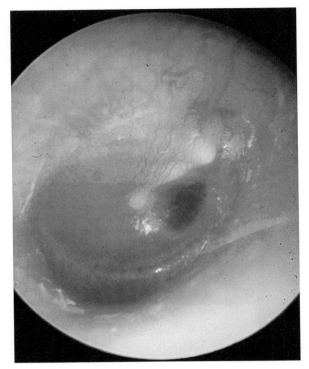

Fig. 47–4. Chronic otitis media with effusion, secondary to chronic effusion in the middle-ear space.

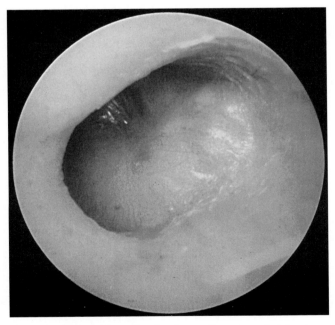

Fig. 47–5. Acute otitis media showing erythematous, bulging tympanic membrane.

tents. In acute situations, *myringotomy* or *tympanocentisis* may be undertaken to confirm the diagnosis, obtain material for culture, and relieve pus under pressure in an effort to avoid further complications. This may be necessary in patients who are unusually ill or

toxic secondary to otitis media or in patients with severe suppurative complications. It may also be necessary in those patients who are having an unsatisfactory response to antibiotic therapy, in toxic newborns, or in patients who are significantly immune deficient.

The *hearing loss* associated with otitis media should be documented whenever possible, especially in cases where chronic effusion is present. Although the presence of a conductive hearing loss does not confirm the diagnosis of chronic otitis media with effusion, its presence does contribute to the confirmation of middle-ear fluid. It is also important in documenting response to therapy.

MICROBIOLOGY

Numerous studies have documented the microbiology of otitis media.[8] Although the treatment of acute otitis media is directed toward the elimination of the bacteria from the middle-ear space, viruses may also play an important etiologic role in this disease process.[9] The most common bacterial pathogens responsible for acute infection include *Streptococcus pneumoniae,* and *Haemophilis influenzae.* These two microorganisms account for approximately 60% of the cases associated with bacterial infection. Group A *streptococcus, Branhamella catarrhallis, Staphylococcus aureus,* and gram-negative enteric bacteria are less frequent causes of otitis media (Fig. 47–6).

Because of the difficulty in obtaining viral cultures, less specific data are available regarding their occurrence in patients with otitis media. However, respiratory syncytial virus accounts for a majority of the viral infections of the middle-ear space.[9] Otitis media may accompany exanthematous viral infections such as infectious mononucleosis and measles.

Over the years, chronic effusions have been thought to be sterile. However, more recent studies have confirmed the presence of bacteria in middle-ear fluid, and studies show that the bacterial spectrum closely resembles that found in acute otitis media.[10] This information becomes increasingly important when consideration is

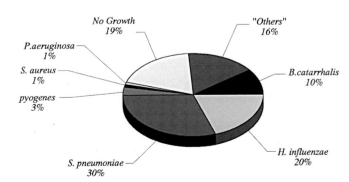

Fig. 47–6. Bacterial incidence in acute otitis media with effusion.

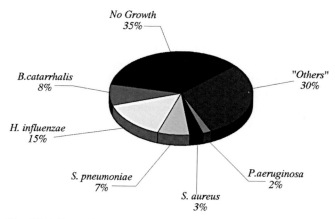

Fig. 47–7. Bacterial incidence in chronic otitis media with effusion.

TABLE 47–2. Daily Dosage for Common Antibiotic Agents in Acute Otitis Media

Agent	Dosage/24 hr
Amoxicillin	40 mg/kg in 3 doses
Ampicillin	50–100 mg/kg in 4 doses
Amoxicillin-clavulanate	40 mg/kg in 3 doses
Trimethoprim-sulfamethoxazole	8 mg (TMP) and 40 mg (SMZ) in 2 doses
Cephalexin	100 mg/kg in 4 doses
Cefixime	8 mg/kg in 1 dose
Cefprozil	15 mg/kg in 2 doses
Erythromycin-sulfisoxazole	40 mg/kg (E) and 120 mg/kg (S) in 4 doses

given to the treatment of patients with both of these disease processes (Fig. 47–7).

MANAGEMENT

Acute otitis media

Acute otitis media represents one point in a continuum of the disease process known as "otitis media." The current standard of care strongly indicates that patients diagnosed as having an acute middle ear process should receive antimicrobial therapy for at least 10 to 14 days. In light of the fact that culture material is usually not readily available, therapy is begun on an empiric basis with treatment being aimed at the more common microorganisms found in the acute process. Some have recommended withholding antimicrobial agents in certain cases.[11] However, in light of the fact that suppurative complications have markedly declined during the antibiotic era, antibiotic therapy is still strongly recommended in the acute process.[11]

The standard initial treatment for acute otitis media has been amoxicillin, 40 mg/kg/24 hr in three divided doses or oral ampicillin, 50–100 mg/kg/24 hr in four divided doses for 10 days. In children allergic to penicillin, a combination of erythromycin, 40 mg/kg/24 hr and sulfisoxazole, 120 mg/kg/24 hr in four divided doses may be substituted. If beta-lactamase producing H. influenzae or B. catarrhalis is suspected then either amoxicillin-clavulanate 40 mg/kg/24 hr in three divided doses, or trimethoprim-sulfamethoxazole, 8 mg of trimethoprim and 40 mg of sulfamethoxazole every 24 hours may be used in two divided doses. Cefixime (Suprax, Lederle Labs., Wayne, NJ) 8 mg/kg in one dose or cefprozil (Cefzil, Bristol-Myer-Squibb, Princeton, NJ) 15 mg/kg/24 hr in two divided doses may also be used effectively. A single intramuscular injection of ceftriaxone (Rocephin, Hoffman-Roche, Nutley, NJ) 50–100 mg/kg mixed with 1% xylocaine, not to exceed

1.5 cc, may be used in patients with vomiting (Table 47–2).

Most patients who are receiving antibiotic therapy for acute otitis media have significant improvement within 48 hours. If, in fact, the child has not improved or the condition has worsened, then tympanocentesis for culture and possibly myringotomy for drainage may be indicated. The patient may be reexamined some time during the course of therapy to ensure that the treatment has been efficacious.

Most children will have an effusion present at the completion of a 10- to 14-day course of antibiotic therapy. Such effusions may last up to 12 weeks before spontaneous clearance can be expected.[12]

Additional therapy such as analgesics, antipyretics, and oral decongestants (antihistamines and sympathomimetic amines) may be useful. Oral decongestants may relieve nasal congestion providing some aeration of the eustachian tube. Their efficacy has not been proven, however. The patient may remain in a subacute phase of the disease process for several weeks.

Repeated episodes of acute otitis media plague many children, especially during the first 3 to 4 years of life. Several issues should be considered and evaluated in the management of such patients. A search should be made for a concomitant source of infection in the upper respiratory tract such as chronic adenoiditis or chronic sinusitis. Mild immune immaturity, especially in the IGG subclass group may be responsible for this relentless process. Testing of immunoglobulins should be considered in relentless cases.

Such patients may be divided into two groups, the first being children who clear their effusion between episodes while the second is made up of patients who have a persistent effusion between episodes. In the latter group, chronic hearing loss becomes an additional major issue, especially as it impacts speech and language development.[1]

Several options are available for those patients who clear their effusion between episodes. The first option includes antibiotic therapy for each separate episode; a second option would be the use of antibiotic prophylaxis on a prolonged basis; while the third would include myringotomy and ventilation tube insertion. The administration of pneumococcal vaccine also may be useful if the patient is two years of age or older.

Amoxicillin, or a suitable substitute in penicillin allergic patients, may be given once daily at bedtime as prophylaxis. This form of therapy is usually administered during the months that otitis has its highest prevalence.

In children in whom the middle ear does not clear between acute episodes, ventilation tubes may be necessary to address the concomitant hearing loss associated with the process. Their use may also be necessary in those patients with antibiotic allergy or intolerance. Dosages of appropriate antimicrobial agents for use in acute otitis media are noted in Table 2.

Chronic Otitis Media with Effusion

Medical Therapy

Chronic otitis media with effusion may occur as a sequela to acute otitis media or in patients who have had no documented recent episodes of acute suppurative disease. Numerous associated factors must be considered and thus a careful history should be taken for the possibility of underlying allergy, sinus disease, or nasopharyngeal obstruction which may be secondary to hypertrophic adenoids or even neoplasm.

Numerous methods of management have been advocated over the years for the persistent form of the disease. Antihistamine-sympathomimetic amine preparations were used frequently to clear the effusion. However, controlled clinical trials have demonstrated a lack of efficacy.[13] The use of corticosteroids, either applied topically in the nose or given systematically, has been reported to be advantageous in clearing middle-ear fluid.[14] Unfortunately, there is a paucity of data to demonstrate efficacy and, therefore, their usage cannot be strongly recommended at this time.

The most effective medical therapy utilized to this point has been antibiotic administration. Numerous trials have concluded that some patients may respond to a 21- to 30-day course of full-dose antibiotic therapy.[15] The demonstration of viable bacteria in the middle-ear effusions of chronically diseased ears has lead to this recommendation. In light of the similarity of the bacteria spectrum, the same antibiotics recommended for acute otitis media may be used in this disease as well. This form of therapy is strongly recommended in any child who has not received antibiotic treatment before consideration is given to myringotomy and ventilation tube insertion, and/or adenoidectomy.

In children with concomitant disease of the upper respiratory tract such as chronic sinusitis or adenoiditis, consideration must be given to the simultaneous control of these diseases. In addition, systemic problems such as allergy or immunodeficiency must also be addressed if long term reversal of the middle-ear abnormality is to be achieved.

Surgery

The use of ventilation tubes with or without adenoidectomy has become the ultimate treatment of chronic otitis media with effusion. This surgical intervention immediately corrects the conductive hearing loss associated with the middle-ear process and diminishes the patient's tendency toward recurrent infection. It should be strongly considered in the following situations:

1. Recurrent acute otitis media
   a. Unresponsive antibiotic therapy
   b. Significant antibiotic allergy or intolerance
2. Negative middle ear pressure with impending cholesteatoma
3. Chronic effusion of the middle-ear space with a duration of greater than 3 months.
   a. Conductive hearing loss of greater than 15 db.
   b. Nasopharyngeal neoplasm for which chronic treatment such as radiation therapy may be necessary

Although some controversy exists over the use of ventilation tubes, they do provide a safe method for normalizing middle-ear pressure and in most cases, restoring hearing to normal. They are usually associated with minimal morbidity although tympanosclerosis or persistent perforation may be seen in a few instances. In most circumstances, it is difficult to determine whether these findings are a result of the underlying middle-ear pathology with middle-ear atelectasis or are secondary to the ventilation tube itself. Numerous types of tubes are available for ventilation of the middle-ear space, but basically they are all designed to provide equalization of pressure across the tympanic membrane (Fig. 47–8). Some designs favor a more

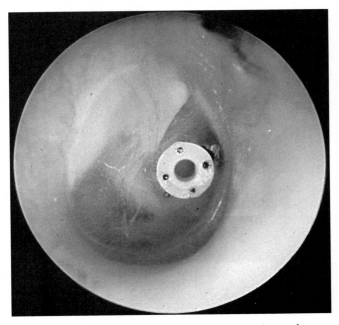

Fig. 47–8. Ventilation tube in place in right tympanic membrane.

lengthy intubation but also carry a slight risk of an increased incidence of persistent perforation upon extrusion.

Depending on the age of the patient, tube insertion may be carried out either under local or general anesthesia.

It is usually advisable to allow spontaneous extrusion of the tubes to occur. Most tympanostomy tubes remain in the tympanic membrane for approximately 6 to 12 months with some extruding earlier and some later.

The most common complication of tube insertion is otorrhea. This may be secondary to either reflux of nasopharyngeal secretions especially during an upper respiratory infection or as a result of pathogens entering the middle ear through the lumen of the ventilation tube. It is commonly believed that contaminated water that is allowed to enter the middle ear through the typanostomy tube may result in acute otitis media with otorrhea. In these instances, the external ear canal should be carefully cleaned, and a culture obtained from the middle ear by aspirating through the tympanostomy tube. After this has been accomplished, oral antibiotics should be initiated as well as topical antibiotic therapy. The usual treatment includes the use of antibiotic agents commonly prescribed for other forms of acute otitis media.

To avoid this possible complication, water protection of the ears is usually advised where contamination may be a possibility. This may be accomplished through the use of earplugs or cotton covered with petrolatum jelly, both of which can be inserted into the ear canal to provide adequate protection. In summary, tympanostomy tubes can provide a useful means of ventilating the middle-ear space, controlling hearing loss secondary to middle-ear effusion, and controlling recurrent infection.

Adenoidectomy may be useful as an adjunct to myringotomy in the treatment of middle-ear effusion.[16] Removal of adenoid tissue improves the ventilatory function of the eustachian tube thus allowing for appropriate equalization of pressure. Studies have also shown that the recurrence rate of acute otitis media may be reduced by adenoidectomy.[17] In addition, other confounding factors may warrant adenoidectomy such as evidence of chronic adenoiditis, nasal obstruction, or recurrent or chronic sinusitis, secondary to nasal obstruction.

CONCLUSION

The future solution to otitis media, acute or chronic, does not lie in current therapy regimens. Manipulation of the immune system to provide enhanced protection will probably result in a significant decrease of the incidence of this disease process.

Other factors such as the role of gastroesophageal reflux or the role of such substances as surfactant have yet to be determined.

Currently, otitis media represents a costly medical problem, worldwide. In some cultures, its morbidity with associated hearing loss, learning difficulties, and secondary central nervous system complications, are almost unmeasurable. This significant medical problem deserves more research attention that it receives so that significant costs and morbidity associated with it can be reduced.

REFERENCES

1. Teele DW, Klein JO, Rosner B. Otitis media with effusion during the first three years of life and the development of speech and language. Pediatrics 74:282–287, 1984.
2. Ammann AJ, Shannon K: Recognition of acquired immune deficiency syndrome (AIDS) in children. Pediatr Rev 7:101–107, 1985.
3. Senturia BH, Bluestone CD, Klein JO, et al: Report of the ad hoc committee on definition and classification of otitis media with effusion. Ann Otol Rhinol Laryngol 89(68):3–4, 1980.
4. Politzer A: Diagnose und theraphaie der ansammlung seroeser fluessigkeit in der thrommelhoehle. Wien Med Wochenschr 17:244–247, 1867.
5. Senturia BH: Studies concerned with tubo-tympanitis. Ann Otol Rhinol Laryngol 67:440–467, 1958.
6. Healy GB, Smith HG: Current concepts in the management of otitis media with effusion. Am J Otol 2:138–144, 1981.
7. Sade J: The biopathology of secretory otitis media. Ann Otol Rhinol and Laryngol 81:59–70, 1970.
8. Bluestone CD, Klein JO: Microbiology in otitis media in infants and children. Philadelphia, Pennsylvania: W.B. Saunders, 1988.
9. Klein JO, Teele DW: Isolation of viruses and mycoplasmas from middle ear effusions: A review. Ann Otol Rhinol Laryngol 85(Suppl.)25:140–144, 1976.
10. Healy GB, Teele DW: The microbiology of chronic middle ear effusions in young children. Laryngoscope 87:1472–1478, 1977.
11. VanBuchem FL, Peters MF, Van't Hof MA: Acute otitis media: A new treatment strategy. Par Med J (Clin) Res 290:1033–1037, 1985.
12. Teele DW, Klein JO, Rosner BA: Epidemiology of otitis media in children. Ann Otol Rhinol Laryngol 89(68):5–6, 1980.
13. Cantekin EI, Mendel EM, Bluestone CD, et al: Lack of efficacy of a decongestant-antihistamine combination for otitis media with effusion ("secretory" otitis media) in children. N Engl J Med 308:297–301, 1983.
14. Schwartz RH, Puglese J, Schwartz DM: Use of a short course of prednisone for treating middle ear effusion: A double-blind cross-over study. Ann Otol Rhinol Laryngol 89(Suppl. 68):296–300, 1980.
15. Healy GB: Antimicrobial therapy of chronic otitis media with effusion. Int J Pediatr Otorhinolaryngol 8:13–17, 1984.
16. Gates GA, Avery CS, Phihooa TJ, et al: Effectiveness of adenoidectomy and tympanostomy tubes in the treatment of chronic otitis media with effusion. N Engl J Med 317:1444–1488, 1987.
17. Paradise JL, Bluestone CD, Rogers KD: Efficacy of adenoidectomy for recurrent otitis media: Results from parallel random and non random trials. Pediatr Res 21:286–291, 1987.

48 Chronic Otitis Media

David F. Austin

DESCRIPTION

Chronic diseases of the middle ear classically have been divided into benign and dangerous forms. The danger of the bone-invading forms of chronic otitis media is caused by the presence of squamous epithelium within the middle ear cleft and is better considered under the proper term *cholesteatoma*.

The two benign forms of chronic otitis media are chronic suppurative otitis media and atelectatic ear disease. These benign forms can change, over time, their character with the development of secondary cholesteatoma, thus indicating the need for prompt surgery in all patients with these problems. In the usual otologic practice, each of these problems—cholesteatoma, chronic suppurative otitis, and atelectatic ear disease—share an equal incidence.

The onset of chronic ear disease is insidious, the patient usually presenting with fully developed symptomatic disease. Because the developmental stages of these diseases have not been observed or reported in the literature, the causes and pathogenesis remain totally conjectural.

The morbidity of chronic disease of the middle ear is twofold. The primary disability is caused by continuing or recurrent infection of the ear. The second area of disability is the attendant loss of function (hearing) caused by damage to the sound conduction mechanism and cochlear damage from toxicity or direct extension of the infectious process. Both these areas must be evaluated and treated in the patient with chronic otitis media to obtain complete resolution of the disease process.

Chronic Suppurative Otitis Media

Causes and Pathogenesis
Because patients present with fully developed disease, the developmental period remains enigmatic. A theory

as to pathogenesis appears in most modern texts and is accepted as fact. This hypothesis states that a necrotizing otitis media occurs, mostly in childhood, resulting in a large drum perforation. After the initial acute disease, the drumhead either remains perforate or heals with an atrophic membrane, which may then collapse into the middle ear, creating the picture of atelectatic otitis.

This hypothesis ignores several factors that throw strong doubts on its plausibility:

1. Almost all cases of acute otitis media resolve with complete healing of the tympanic membrane. Scarring, rarely present, is usually characterized by thickening rather than atrophy.
2. Necrotizing otitis media is rare because the use of antibiotics became established. I have seen fewer than a dozen instances in the past 25 years. The incidence of chronic otitis media, on the other hand, has not decreased over this period.
3. Patients with chronic otitis media do not give a history of such an acute episode of otitis as an initiating factor, but rather of a silent progress gradually increasing in disability until help is sought some years after the patient became aware of the problem. Children are not brought to medical care until a hearing disability is found by testing at school or chronic discharge becomes an annoyance.
4. Pediatricians observing children with acute otitis media, often recurrent, have not reported the development of chronic suppurative otitis, even with long term follow-up.

At this time, the pathogenesis of chronic suppurative otitis media remains unknown. It is most likely a primary process of the Eustachian tube-middle ear mastoid cell system. This process must have the characteristics of low-grade, insidious, and persistent activity, resulting in loss of portions of tympanic membrane and establishment of factors conductive to further chronicity.

The factors responsible for chronicity in suppurative middle ear disease are varied. Among them are the following:

1. Chronic Eustachian tube dysfunction caused by:
   a. Chronic or recurrent nose and throat infection
   b. Partial or complete anatomic obstruction of the Eustachian tube
2. Persistent perforation of the tympanic membrane
3. Involvement of the middle ear with squamous metaplasia or other irreversible pathology
4. Persistent obstruction to aeration of the middle ear or mastoid spaces (this may be caused by scarring, thickened mucosa, polyps, granulation tissue, or tympanosclerosis)
5. Areas of sequestration or persistent osteomyelitis in the mastoid
6. Constitutional factors such as allergy, debility, or altered defense mechanisms of the host

Pathology

Chronic suppurative otitis media is most often a recurrent rather than a constant disease. Chronicity is defined in time and stage rather than a uniform pathologic picture. Because the effects of tissue destruction, healing, and scarring are added to the overlying process of persistent or recurrent infection, the pathologic condition encountered is characterized by lack of uniformity. In general, the following patterns may be noted:

1. *The tympanic membrane* is perforated in its central portion. The size may vary from less than 20% of the drum area to the entire drum and portions of the anulus.

   Healing efforts may result in ingrowth of squamous epithelium into the middle ear. This ingrowth may extend only through the perforation or may line the entire middle ear space. Occasionally, extension of the media layer into the attic region results in pocketing and secondary acquired cholesteatoma (see Atelectatic Otitis Media). The formation of an atrophic two-layer membrane lacking in fibrous elements may be seen. This membrane is rapidly destroyed during active periods of infection.
2. *The mucosa* varies during stages of the disease. In quiescent periods, it appears normal unless the effects of infection have produced thickening or metaplasia into transitional epithelium. Squamous metaplasia has been described.

   During active infection, the mucosa becomes thickened and hyperemic, producing a mucoid or mucopurulent discharge. After treatment, the thickening and mucoid discharge may persist owing to chronic dysfunction of the Eustachian tube. Allergic factors or environmental may be responsible for this persistence of mucosal change.

   Mucosal thickening may completely seal the attic and mastoid spaces, filling these spaces with mucus. With time, cholesterin crystals are deposited in these mucous pockets, causing cholesterol granuloma. This process is irritative, producing granulation of the mucous membrane and giant cell infiltration of the mucus-cholesterin fluid and may also be seen in the middle ear in chronic secretory otitis media.

   During healing, the mucosa may exhibit the changes of tympanosclerosis. These consist of the formation of amorphous hyaline plaques in the submucosa, varying in size form thin layers to dense masses. In early stages, the mucosa assumes a thick, rubbery appearance. As healing progresses, the plaques become yellowish, with puttylike consistency. In time, calcium salts may be deposited, creating bony, hard masses. The sites of predilection for this process are in the annular region of the tympanic membrane, particularly antero-superiorly, and surrounding the ossicles. The process may result in further or complete fixation of the ossicular system, resulting in severe hearing loss.

   The mucosa may also show the formation of granulation tissue and/or polyps. This process is associated with long-standing persistent discharge or active infection. Polyp formation is commonly associated with the presence of squamous epithelium in the middle ear and may protrude through a small perforation, partially obstructing drainage and causing persistence of disease.
3. *The ossicles* may or may not be damaged. Commonly, the long process of the incus has undergone necrosis because of thrombotic disease of the mucosal vessels supplying the incus. Necrosis less commonly involves the malleus and stapes unless secondary squamous ingrowth has occurred, in which case the arch of the stapes and the handle of the malleus may be destroyed. This process is not caused by the osteomyelitis but is said to be caused by the formation of osteolytic enzymes or collagenase in the subepithelial connective tissue.
4. *Mastoid.* Chronic suppurative otitis media most often has its onset in childhood. Because *mastoid* pneumatization is most active between ages 5 and 10, this process of pneumatization is often halted or reversed by otitis media occurring at this age or earlier. As the chronic infection continues, the mastoid undergoes a process of sclerosis, reducing the size of the mastoid process. The antrum becomes smaller, and pneumatization is

limited to a few air cell tracts in the immediate vicinity of the antrum.

This concept is contrasted with the fact that the degree of pneumatization of the mastoid varies among individuals. Individuals with limited pneumatization (either from genetic cause or neonatal infection) are felt by some to have increased susceptibility to chronic otitis media. Radiographs show these changes in the cellularity of the mastoid so commonly that a radiological diagnosis of chronic mastoiditis is synonymous with the actual finding of a dense, small, sclerotic mastoid.

Severe forms of acute otitis media may also cause areas of osteitis or osteomyelitis of the walls or septa of the mastoid. This results, in time, in a continuous, foul, purulent discharge or sequestration of the bone.

Atelectatic Otitis Media

Many terms are presently applied to this common chronic disease pattern of the middle ear. "Adhesive otitis media," "middle ear cholesteatoma," and "marginal or posterior-superior perforation" are used interchangeably in describing the process referred to here as "atelectatic otitis." Because "secondary acquired cholesteatoma" is a complication of this disease process, it will be discussed in this section rather than the section on cholesteatoma.

Causes and Pathogenesis

In contrast to chronic suppurative otitis media, this type of chronic ear disorder develops over time. The typical patient has initially suffered from chronic secretory otitis, particularly in childhood but often extending into adulthood. Although many suffer from an unrelenting "blue drum" or "glue ear," recurrent acute secretory otitis may result in the same sequelae. Duration of the catarrhal process within the middle ear is probably a determining factor.

Over time, atrophy of the drumhead occurs, usually in the posterior-superior quadrant but also involving other portions, even including the entire tympanic membrane. Accompanying this atrophy is a collapse of the atrophic membrane into the middle ear—thus the term "atelectatic otitis." The degree of collapse depends entirely on the extent of atrophy of the tympanic membrane. Loss of elasticity of the drumhead prevents normal ventilation of the middle ear and thus creates chronicity entirely subsequent to the nature of the pathology, even if the Eustachian tube problem has cleared.

Progression of the retraction causes the atrophic membrane to drape over the incus and stapes, often resulting in necrosis of these structures. The aeration pathway to the attic is blocked, which, with time, re-

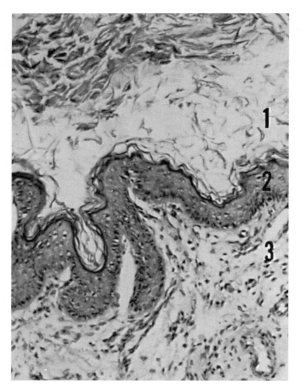

Fig. 48–1. Microscopic structure of cholesteatoma: (1) keratin debris; (2) epidermis (matrix); (3) subepithelium.

sults in the membrane retracting into these areas, causing secondary acquired cholesteatoma. This has the same characteristics of all cholesteatomas (Fig. 48–1): enlargement with keratin retention, bone destruction, and the onset of infection.

The above disease process seems clear-cut, yet the pathogenesis of the tympanic membrane atrophy is still unknown. Perforation with healing by a two-layered membrane is often cited, but the atrophy has been seen to occur without perforation. It is most likely the result of activation of collagenase by the underlying disease, which causes breakdown of the fibrous layers of the tympanic membrane, leaving only the squamous and mucosal layers intact.

Pathology

The major pathologic features of "atelectatic otitis" have been described in the previous section. The remaining pathologic feature is that of cholesterin granuloma. This process is the result of chronic blockage of the middle ear, attic, or mastoid ventilation pathways. These spaces fill with abnormal mucus ("glue"), and cholesterin crystals are deposited. The mucosa forms granulations, and breakdown of septa can occur. Apart from this sequela, infection of the middle ear is uncommon, occurring most often when contaminants are introduced through the canal, such as after swimming or showering. Extension of infection up the Eustachian tube causes breakdown of the atrophic membrane and

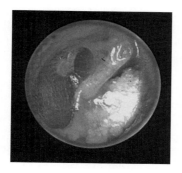

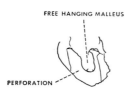

Fig. 48–2. Chronic otitis media. Massive central perforation. Recurrent discharge has been present for 30 years. (From Buckingham RA: What's New. Abbott Laboratories, 1956, p 196).

converts the pathologic pattern to that described with chronic suppurative otitis media (Figs. 48–2 and 48–3).

Cholesteatoma

Cholesteatoma (Figs. 48–4, 48–5) may be defined as the presence within the middle ear cleft of a squamous

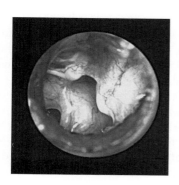

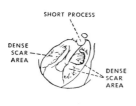

Fig. 48–3. Chronic otitis media. Healing of previous infections has resulted in dense tympanosclerotic plaque of the submucosa of the tympanic membrane. Fixation of the ossicular chain by tympanosclerosis caused a 40-dB conductive hearing loss. (From Buckingham RA: What's New. Abbott Laboratories, 1956, p 196).

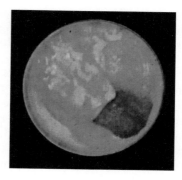

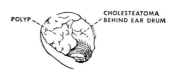

Fig. 48–4. Cholesteatoma. Polypoid granulation is forming at the mouth of an attic perforation. The posterosuperior tympanic membrane appears pearly white owing to downward growth of the cholesteatoma into this region of the middle ear. (From Buckingham RA: What's New. Abbott Laboratories, 1956, p 196.)

epithelial pocket or sac filled with keratin debris. Three types are recognized:

1. *Congenital cholesteatoma.* This is an epithelial cyst occurring within one of the bones of the skull (usually the temporal bone) without contact with

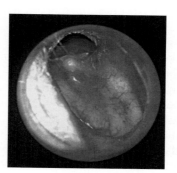

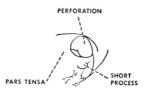

Fig. 48–5. Cholesteatoma. Large perforation of the pars flaccida leads into a cholesteatoma sac filled with hard black debris. (From Buckingham RA: What's New. Abbott Laboratories, 1956, p 196).

the external ear. It may occur deep in the temporal bone or in the squama. Increasing numbers are described as occurring in the mastoid or attic space.

2. *Primary acquired cholesteatoma.* This type of cholesteatoma develops in continuity with the perforation of the pars flaccida of the tympanic membrane. It first fills Prussak's space and then may enlarge to occupy the attic, mastoid antrum, and portions of the middle ear.

3. *Secondary acquired cholesteatoma.* This type of cholesteatoma has been described previously under Atelectatic Otitis Media.

Causes

The cause of primary acquired cholesteatoma has been the subject of debate since the latter half of the nineteenth century. Many theories have been proposed, but none as yet has been shown to be entirely causative in this disease. Among the postulates are:

1. Negative pressure in the attic, causing invagination of the pars flaccida and cyst formation.
2. Metaplasia of middle ear and attic mucosa caused by infection.
3. Invasive hyperplasia followed by cyst formation of the basal layers of the epidermis of the pars flaccida caused by the irritation of infection.
4. Congenital epidermal rests occurring in the attic region.
5. Invasive hyperkeratosis of the deep external meatal skin.

An important factor is the rapid proliferative ability of the drum epithelium, particularly in the pars flaccida and superior portion of the pars tensa.

Pathogenesis

Once a pocket or cyst of squamous epithelium has formed within the middle ear cleft, the progress of cholesteatoma is well-documented. Layers of desquamated epithelium interspersed with cholesterin crystals form and fill the sac. The surrounding epithelial matrix expands into the available spaces of attic, middle ear, and mastoid. Accompanying this process is the expansion is bony destruction of the attic walls, ossicles, and mastoid septa to accommodate the increasing size of the cholesteatoma.

It was thought that pressure caused the bone destruction occurring with the expanding cholesteatoma. The bone erosion is caused by the secretion of osteolytic enzymes or collagenase by the subepithelial connective tissue.

The osteolytic process is accompanied by osteogenesis within the mastoid as sclerosis takes place, thus limiting free space available for expansion of the cholesteatoma. The process of sclerosis is accelerated by the superimposition of infection. Cholesteatoma,

which develops free of infection, may allow normal pneumatization, creating the extremely difficult problem of widely pneumatized mastoid filled with cholesteatoma. This is particularly true of congenital cholesteatoma.

Infection of the cholesteatoma not only causes rapid sclerosis of the mastoid but also increases the osteolytic process and creates the danger of extension through the lateral semicircular canal, facial canal, attic, and mastoid tegmen, and lateral sinus plate and rapid dissolution of the ossicular system. This creates the need for prompt diagnosis and surgical intervention in these cases.

If the disease is allowed to run its course, any of the aforementioned complications may ensue, or complete destruction of the mastoid, middle ear, and posterior canal wall, resulting in "nature's radical mastoidectomy," may occur. Other cases reach a stage of apparent equilibrium, remaining quiescent unless further stimulated by infection.

Diagnosis

Without question, otoscopic examination, particularly with magnification, is the most important facet of accurate diagnosis in chronic otitis media. Complete examination should include critical scrutiny of the following areas:

1. The canal and drum must be cleaned carefully of wax and debris, which may prevent a complete view of the drum.
2. The pars tensa is observed in all quadrants, and the size and location of any perforation are noted.
3. The presence of retraction or perforation of the pars flaccida is investigated.
4. The presence of squamous epithelium in the middle ear should be noted. The presence of debris behind the eardrum is a clue to this pathologic condition.
5. The condition of the mucosa seen through the perforation is noted. Any secretion present in the middle ear is removed by suction to allow complete visualization.
6. The nature of any secretion is noted.
7. The bony canal walls should be observed for evidence of destruction. Widening of the notch of Rivinus is a significant early finding of cholesteatoma.
8. The presence and location of granulation or polyps (Fig. 48–6) should be noted.
9. Finally, the area of the mouth of the Eustachian tube should be inspected and evidence of patency noted. At this time, it is useful to have the patient auto-inflate the ear while the ear is being inspected.

Audiometric Evaluation

Audiometric evaluation is necessary to determine the status of conductive and cochlear function. By the use

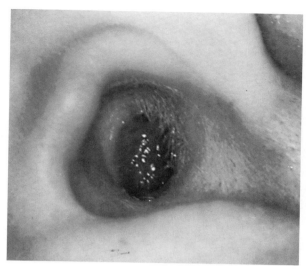

Fig. 48–6. Mucosal polyp filling the external ear canal in case of cholesteatoma. Surgical removal is necessary to secure drainage of middle ear and mastoid.

of air and bone pure tone audiometry and speech discrimination scores, the amount of ossicular damage present may be estimated, and the hearing benefit to be gained by reconstructive middle ear surgery can be judged.

To aid in this evaluation, the following observations will be of help.

1. A simple perforation usually causes no more than a 15- to 20-dB conductive hearing loss.
2. Damage to the ossicular chain causes a 30- to 50-dB conductive hearing loss if a perforation is present.
3. Discontinuity of the hearing chain behind an intact drum causes a flat 55- to 65-dB conductive hearing loss.
4. Marked impairment of speech discrimination, regardless of the bone conduction, indicates severe cochlear damage.

Radiology

A radiographic examination of the mastoid in chronic otitis media is of limited diagnostic value compared to the benefits of otoscopy and audiometry. Carefully controlled radiographic examination may be of great value in diagnosing congenital cholesteatoma, osteitis, or osteomyelitis. The status of the ossicular system may also be demonstrated through careful technique. In addition to CT (Fig. 48–7), the standard views are:

1. *The Schuller view*, which shows the extent of pneumatization of the mastoid from laterally and above. This becomes of value in surgery by defining the position of the lateral sinus and tegmen. This is particularly helpful in a sclerotic mastoid to forewarn the surgeon and thus prevent entry into the dura or lateral sinus.

2. *The Mayer's or Owen's view* is taken from above and anterior to the middle ear. This throws the ossicles and attic into view and allows one to determine whether bone destruction has involved these structures.
3. *The Stenver's view* shows the length of the petrous pyramid and is more useful in showing the internal auditory canal, vestibule, and semicircular canals. It also throws the antrum into cross section and may give evidence of enlargement from cholesteatoma.
4. *The third projection of Chausse* gives a longitudinal view of the attic and shows early evidence of destruction of the lateral attic wall. In summary, to be differentiated are the following conditions:

Chronic Suppurative Otitis Media. This diagnosis is made in a patient with a history of repeated attacks of aural discharge and the finding of a central perforation without evidence of squamous epithelial ingrowth or bone necrosis. Granulation tissue or mucosal edema may be present, and the discharge is usually mucoid or mucopurulent. Hearing loss is usually present in varying degrees of severity.

Atelectatic Otitis. This diagnosis is made when otoscopy reveals atrophy of the tympanic membrane accompanied by collapse into part or all of the middle ear space. The usual history is one of insidious onset of progressive hearing loss, although today many patients mention that one or more myringotomies and/or ventilating tube insertions have been performed in the past. Infection is not a prominent feature of the history and, when present, creates difficulty in differentiation from chronic suppurative otitis.

Secondary Acquired Cholesteatoma. This is added to the above picture when retraction of the atrophic membrane has resulted in pocketing with retention of keratin debris and further bone destruction. The presence of granulation at the posterior-superior margin immediately lateral to the anulus is a common finding. Infection with continuous discharge is more common when the disease has reached this stage.

Congenital Cholesteatoma. This diagnosis is usually made in young individuals who have had careful medical observation. They have a history of slowly progressive hearing loss without antecedent infection. Examination shows the presence of a whitish bulge of the eardrum, usually in the antero-superior quadrant. Until perforation of the drum takes place, hearing loss does not progress beyond 20 to 30 dB.

Primary Acquired Cholesteatoma. Infection in these cases often starts later in life, many times not until the second or third decade. Once aural discharge starts, it is persistent and usually constant. Examination reveals a perforation of the pars flaccida with destruction of the lateral attic wall. This area is often covered with a crust which must be removed to see the

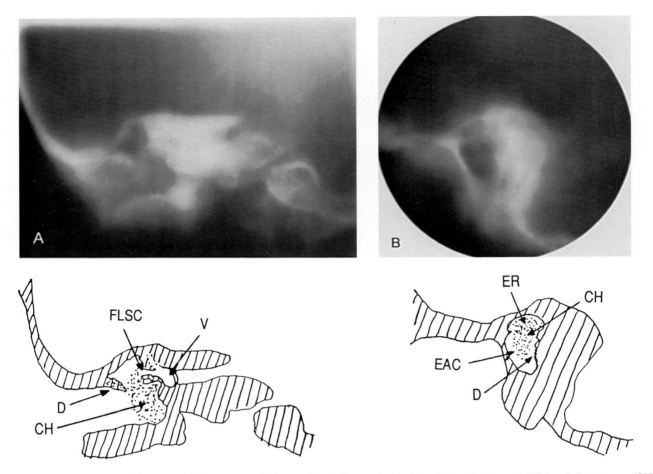

Fig. 48–7. Tomograms of middle ear in cholesteatoma. A. Front view indicates destruction of lateral attic wall (D) by cholesteatoma (CH). There is also erosion of the lateral semicircular canal causing a fistula (FLSC). B. Lateral view shows erosion of the attic (ER) with loss of ossicles. Destruction of the posterior anulus is indicated at D. EAC, External auditory canal; V, vestibule.

perforation. In advanced cases, there is a perforation of the postero-superior region of the pars tensa. Hearing loss is variable, depending on the amount of ossicular destruction and whether the cholesteatoma sac is in a position to transmit sound.

Treatment

Effective treatment in chronic otitis media must be based on definition of the causative factors involved and the stage in which the disease is found. Thus, the factors creating chronicity, the anatomic changes preventing good healing and proper function, and the infectious process involving the ear at the time of instituting treatment must be evaluated. When cholesteatoma is diagnosed, surgery is indicated, but the following regimen may be used to control infection if it is present preoperatively.

Eustachian Tube. The most important function to be considered is aeration and drainage of the middle ear by way of the Eustachian tube. The causes of interference with tubal physiology must be assessed and eliminated. Chronic infection or allergy affecting the

nose and pharynx should be diagnosed and treated. Residual adenoids creating mechanical obstruction should be removed. Sinus radiographs are indicated to find hidden areas of low-grade infection.

The adequacy of the Eustachian tube lumen is assessed by determining the ability of the tube to pass air. This may be done by having the patient auto-inflate the ear, by politzerization, or by special manometric study of the tube. Obstruction of the tympanic end of the Eustachian tube can often be determined by careful otoscopic inspection of this area while the patient is attempting to inflate the ear.

As a first step in treatment, the patient should be instructed how to clear the ear by auto-inflation and told to practice this many times each day. Anatomic changes preventing proper aeration must be treated surgically if the portion of the Eustachian tube involved is accessible.

Anatomic Factors. Permanent changes from normal anatomy commonly influence the response to medical treatment and cause chronic infection. Even as common a finding as a central perforation of the eardrum may be solely responsible for recurrent discharge from that ear and must be corrected surgically. Other types of purely surgical pathology are cholesteatoma, large polyps, masses of tympanosclerosis, and areas of bone necrosis from osteitis or osteomyelitis. Alteration of hearing function by damage to the sound conduction system must be corrected surgically to obtain satisfactory restoration of hearing.

General Factors of Host Resistance. In dealing with chronic infection of any part of the body, special efforts should be made to investigate local and systemic factors affecting host resistance. Included in this group are dietary insufficiency, diabetes, debility, agammaglobulinemia, allergic disorder, adrenal cortical insufficiency, chronic leukemia, liver or kidney disease, etc. The presence of these conditions can be suspected by the general appearance of the patient plus a failure of response to treatment.

Treatment of Infectious Process. In chronic ear infection, saprophytic as well as pathogenic organisms may be involved. Not only do the bacterial flora vary from time to time, but also the effects of prior or present antibiotic treatment are extremely potent in effecting a change of organism. Prolonged antibiotic administration causes the emergence of resistant strains and also causes overgrowth of organisms such as Pseudomonas or Pyocyaneous. For this reason, culture and sensitivity tests assume an important role in planning therapy.

The presence of discharge implies a perforation of the eardrum, and for this reason, topical application of antibiotic therapy becomes practical and efficacious. Agents that are unsuitable for systemic administration because of toxicity are often applicable topically.

To be effective, a solution for use in the ear should be suspended in a hygroscopic vehicle e.g. Propylene glycol. The antibiotics most frequently used are polymyxin B sulfate and/or neomycin sulfate. The preparation is more effective when acidified to a pH of 5 to 5.5. Occasionally, corticosteroids may be added to control local allergic manifestations.

Powders are chosen on the basis of bacterial sensitivity and solubility. An effective combination is 250 mg polymyxin B sulfate and 3 g of Chloromycetin and insufflated two or three times a day. The use of boric acid, either in solution or as a powder, is not indicated because it forms an insoluble cake that is difficult to clean out of the ear and prevents antimicrobial agents from reaching the mucosa. Alcohol in strengths greater than 70% should be avoided because it is both irritating and painful.

Before powder or drops are applied to the ear, discharge should be removed from the canal. Absorbent cotton wipes or suction are best for this. Cotton applicators are usually too bulky to be effective and sometimes cause external canal infection due to abrasion.

Systemic antibiotics, chose on the basis of sensitivity tests, are indicated in acute infections superimposed on the chronic infection. Infection of a cholesteatoma is difficult to treat because of the inability to obtain an antibiotic level within the sac where the infection exists. In these instances, removal of obstructing masses of debris or crusts from the mouth of the sac by gentle suction to obtain drainage is of great help. Water in the ear must be avoided; it causes the cholesteatoma to swell and may result in acute complication.

Granulations on the mucosa may be treated by applying a mild (5 to 10%) solution of silver nitrate and followed by 2% gentian violet, which is drying and bactericidal. These agents are also useful in treating the external otitis that exists in most cases of chronic otorrhea.

Polyps or large masses of granulations are best removed with a biting forceps or snare and the raw surface touched with 25 to 50% silver nitrate several times at intervals of 1 or 2 weeks to secure healing of the mucosa.

If the use of a thoughtfully applied regimen of therapy as outlined previously does not succeed in controlling the disease, surgical intervention is indicated to control areas of inaccessible or irreversible pathology.

UNUSUAL FORMS OF CHRONIC OTITIS MEDIA

Tuberculous Otitis Media

Otitis media caused by tuberculosis may arise from two sources: systemically through ingestion of nonpasteurized infected milk, and through direct contact with the bacillus from a patient with existent pulmonary tuberculosis. Both are becoming quite rare in this country.

Middle ear involvement begins with a painless and insidious onset. The tympanic membrane becomes thickened and infiltrated. This is followed by spontaneous perforation, which either slowly enlarges or becomes multiple, and is associated with a thin, odorless discharge and an indolent, afebrile course. Commonly there is a severe depression of hearing due to early labyrinthine involvement much out of proportion to the other symptoms and findings and is a good clue to the diagnosis.

Treatment involves the use of modern antituberculous agents. Once the disease has been arrested, tympanoplastic surgery may be utilized to repair permanent damage to the middle ear if useful cochlear function remains.

Pneumococcus Type III Otitis Media (Streptococcus Mucosus)

This is a subacute, indolent form of otitis media that assumes importance because of the frequency of associated intracranial complication. Fortunately, widespread use of early antibiotic therapy has made this a rare entity.

After a short, mild acute phase, a latent period ensues with only mild symptoms of hearing loss. The drum is dull and thickened. The disease then proceeds to intracranial complication by causing bone destruction and direct invasion of the meninges, brain, or lateral sinus.

Treatment with antibiotics in the early stages usually serves to prevent these complications.

SURGERY FOR CHRONIC OTITIS MEDIA

The present era of otologic surgery has seen marked technologic improvement. The basic concepts of eradication of irreversible disease and adequate drainage, as pioneered by Schwartze, Stacke, Zaufel, and many others and refined by the father of modern otologic surgery, Julius Lempert, remains the foundation of these advances (Austin & Smyth, 1964). The present methods of reconstruction and surgical conservatism have been made complete aural rehabilitation possible for the majority of individuals suffering from chronic ear diseases.

The indications for surgical intervention in chronic otitis media are basically twofold: control of infection and restoration of function. Because hearing improvement is not usually possible unless disease is eliminated from the involved ear, this remains a primary consideration in surgery. The severe handicap of hearing loss, however, demands every effort to improve hearing. With the potential of present-day techniques, this has become an equal consideration in the planning of surgical management.

Principles are either induced primarily or learned by trial and error. Both processes are related and both have occurred in otology. In general, the major innovations have been inductively initiated and improvements have evolved from trial and error. However initiated, the consequences of surgical decision can be appreciated only over time; and therefore each surgeon should analyze his results continuously and in relationship to the principles used in his surgical problem solving.

1. Ear surgery should proceed step by step. Each step should leave maximum freedom of choice in the decision to follow. The end state of such an operation, therefore, is unknown until its completion rather than preconceived. Such an approach requires more rigidly defined criteria for decision-making than does a set procedure. The flexibility of modern microsurgery should not be considered until these decision-making criteria are understood.
2. The simplest technique affording the greatest ease for the surgeon results in the fewest complications.
3. Underlay grafting results in a better functioning tympanic membrane and fewer serious complications.
4. Mastoidectomy should preserve the bony canal walls if possible. For proper exposure, this requires skill in the technique of posterior tympanotomy.
5. Ventilation of the middle ear space is impaired in chronic disease, and therapeutic effort is needed to improve this function.

Indications for Surgery

As mentioned, the basic reasons for surgery in this group of diseases are control of infection and restoration of function. Certain absolute indications for surgical intervention in the disease process may be defined, however. These indications are:

1. The presence of threatened or actual complication (see Complications of Chronic Otitis Media, Chap. 49).
2. The presence of irreversible pathologic condition in the mastoid or middle ear, such as cholesteatoma, osteomyelitis, or sequestration.
3. The lack of response to an adequate medical regimen, indicating the presence of a pathologic process requiring surgery.

Relative indications usually consist of milder and recurrent infection or the presence of a conductive hearing loss caused by past ear disease that may be surgically correctable. Absolute contraindications to surgery have not yet been defined, but it is agreed by most otologists that severe Eustachian tube dysfunction lessens the possibility of hearing restoration in most cases.

Medical Evaluation

Ear surgery is facilitated when it is possible to work on dry, noninflamed structures. To aid in obtaining this state, complete nose and throat evaluation must be carried out. Patients with coexistent disease of the nose, sinuses, and nasopharynx are more likely to suffer complications of healing that interfere with good postoperative function. The usual pattern is deficient ventilation, prolonged inflammatory response, scarring, and persistent conductive deficit. Chronic nasopharyngeal infection may indicate the need for adenoidectomy in both children and adults. Medical history may suggest the presence of otosclerosis, dietary deficiency, poor environmental conditions, or the presence of genetic or constitutional predisposition to upper respiratory disease. Hypothyroidism, hypoestrogenism, vitamin deficiency, and serum protein deficiency may all influence the operative result. Bleeding problems not only endanger success, but may create a severe problem of exposure. Culture of secretion from the middle ear is of little value because the administration of local or systemic antibiotics is not effective in chronic otitis media; rather, local cleansing, improved ventilation, and surgical repair are indicated. Radiological examination is of value in revealing hidden areas of mastoid disease or anatomic variations influencing the course of surgery.

On the other hand, freedom from infection is not and absolute necessity because most of these operations are performed to achieve a healthy ear. A necessary surgical procedure should never be delayed because of poor response to an adequate period of medical management.

Otoscopy

Otoscopic examination should provide not only the exact disease diagnosis, but also clues to possible surgical problems. Does squamous epithelium extend into or line the middle ear? Will this extension require mastoid exposure? Is the anterior margin of the perforation visible with a speculum? During otoscopy, the status of the Eustachian tube can be evaluated. The tubal region is visualized and the patient is asked to inflate the ear. The difficulty of inflation is gauged, and if none occurs, it is important to determine whether this is due to a functional problem or if a barrier to inflation has been created by an ingrowth of squamous epithelium. Most often the patient is unable to inflate his ear because of fear that it will do harm or because of the lack of practice. The Frenzel maneuver (contraction of the superior constrictor with a closed soft palate and nares) should be taught to all patients together with stressing the importance of ventilation in maintaining the health of the middle ear.

Approach to Surgical Management

Currently, there are two distinct philosophies in the surgical management of chronic otitis media. One group maintains the classic and time-honored idea that a fixed procedure is required to treat a certain ear disease and that deviation from this procedure jeopardizes the outcome. This is particularly applicable to the treatment of cholesteatoma, in which modified radical mastoidectomy is done in a standardized manner in each case. In some instances, this procedure, combined with forms of middle ear reconstruction, has been recommended as the operation of choice for all forms of chronic otitis media.

Another approach favored today adopts a less fixed attitude toward the exact operation needed to resolve the disease. This approach allows the nature and extent of the disease to determine the form the surgery will take. The surgical plan used to apply the foregoing principle is as follows:

1. The ear initially approached through the external canal, using a speculum and speculum holder. As an alternative, some surgeons prefer an initial approach through a post-auricular incision while still following the general plan outlined here.
2. The tympanic membrane remnant is prepared for grafting.
3. The middle ear is exposed through a tympanotomy incision, dissecting in continuity any pocketed squamous epithelium.
4. During step 3, the necessity for mastoidectomy is evaluated while controlling diseased portions of the middle ear. Criteria for this decision are the severity of mucosal disease, the accessibility of squamous epithelium, and the presence of cholestrin granuloma and attic cholesteatoma.
5. If preoperative mastoid radiographs have demonstrated a limited mastoid development (less than two mm^2 in area), a canal-down procedure is carried out through either an endaural or post-auricular approach. If there is more extensive mastoid development, a canal-up procedure is indicated, performed through a post-auricular incision. Complete posterior tympanotomy (facial recess dissection) is then used.
6. Removal of the disease process is attempted in toto through sharp dissection to preserve the continuity of the diseased capsule or squamous lining. The use of τ-chymotrypsin on small pieces of gelatin sponge facilitates this dissection as it melts the microadhesions holding the atrophic epithelium to the under layers.
7. Ossicular reconstruction is carried out, together with needed repair of the canal wall or meatoplasty.
8. Reconstruction of the tympanic membrane is the last step, using an underlay fibrous tissue graft supported on a blood-soaked Gelfoam packing.

These methods are more fully described in the sections that follow.

Terminology

The following definitions of operations have been accepted by the Committee on Conservation of hearing of the American Academy of Ophthalmology and Otolaryngology and include all the procedures to be discussed in this chapter.

1. *Myringoplasty.* An operation in which the reconstructive procedure is limited to repair of a tympanic membrane perforation.
2. *Tympanoplasty without Mastoidectomy.* An operation to eradicate disease in the middle ear and to reconstruct the hearing mechanism, without mastoid surgery, with or without tympanic grafting.

3. *Tympanoplasty with Mastoidectomy.* An operation to eradicate disease in both the mastoid process and middle ear cavity and to reconstruct the hearing mechanism with or without tympanic membrane grafting.

4. *Radical and Modified Radical Mastoidectomy.* An operation to eradicate disease of the middle ear and mastoid in which the mastoid and epitympanic spaces are converted into an easily accessible common cavity by removal of the posterior and superior external canal walls. Radical mastoidectomy also includes the mesotympanum in this cavity.

5. *Mastoid Obliteration Operation.* An operation to eradicate disease when present and to obliterate a mastoid or fenestration cavity.

Anesthesia

The level of anesthesia necessary in otologic surgery is related to the anxiety of the patient and the amount of stimulation inherent in the procedure. The most appropriate method of anesthesia varies with the individual situation of the surgeon and the degree of anesthetic skill available. All otologic procedures may be carried out with local anesthesia, but this may produce many difficulties caused by excessive bleeding and uncontrolled patient movement often arise.

In most instances, the combination of local anesthesia with basal narcosis is satisfactory. Difficult anesthetic problems in adults and children may best be handled with general anesthesia through an endotracheal tube, supplemented with local anesthesia so that a lighter plane of anesthesia may be used.

Local anesthesia for transcanal operations is placed in four quadrants in the outer portion of the cartilaginous ear canal. In mastoid procedures, the local anesthetic agent is infiltrated anterior to the helix and over the mastoid cortex posterior to the pinna to block the temporal region completely.

Preparation of the Ear

At surgery, the ear canal should be cleansed of loose debris and accumulated cerumen, but without trauma that will lower local tissue resistance to infection. A detergent soap is used to irrigate the canal without wiping, and after suction drying, a protein-iodine complex is used to paint the area. The external ear is prepared in the same manner. To prevent painful stimulus of the middle ear, gelatin sponges moistened with a physiologic solution may be placed through the perforation to protect the mucosa while the canal is being prepared. It is not usually necessary to remove hair, but hair should be kept out of the field with adhesive spray and drapes. Immediately before surgery, copi-

ous irrigation is used to eliminate all debris and foreign material.

Incisions

Three major approaches to the middle ear and mastoid are in use today: the transmeatal tympanoplasty incision, the endaural mastoid incision, and the post-auricular incision. The transmeatal incision is used to approach the middle ear directly and is used in tympanoplasty. The latter two incisions provide access to the mastoid cortex for mastoidectomy. The endaural incision has the advantage of fewer complications because of complete closure of the mastoid defect with periostium and a better cosmetic result. It is used primarily for canal-down surgery when restricted mastoid development is present. The post-auricular incision provides a much better view of the mastoid and middle ear together because of the angle of view may be changed over a greater range, particularly from the posterior direction. This incision is preferred over the endaural for most operations involving preservation of the ear canal.

The *transmeatal* incision is carried out through an endaural speculum secured with a speculum holder. It is triangular, starting 3 to 4 mm above the anterior spine of the malleus and extending posteriorly to an apex 8 to 10 mm lateral to the anulus at the posterosuperior region of the canal (Fig. 48–8). The incision is then carried to the inferior canal region, again 3 to 4 mm from the anulus. Elevation of the canal skin and anulus provides exposure of the posterior two thirds of the tympanum. Exposure anterior to this, if necessary, is carried out by dissecting the drumhead from its attachment to the malleus.

The *endaural* incision is started inferiorly at the junc-

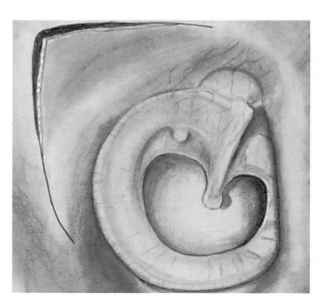

Fig. 48–8. The transmeatal incision.

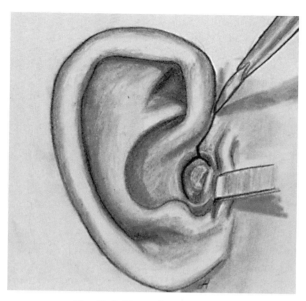

Fig. 48–9. The endaural incision.

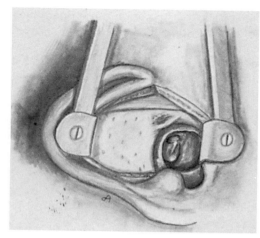

Fig. 48–11. The endaural retractor is placed to create a mobile window over the mastoid cortex.

tion of the cartilaginous and bony portions of the canal (Fig. 48–9). It is carried upward through the posterior canal wall and then brought out between the tragus and helix for at least 2 cm. This portion of the incision is carried down to the temporalis fascia. The periostium is elevated from the mastoid cortex and a self-retaining retractor inserted (Fig. 48–10). Before the retractor is spread, a relaxing incision is made through the anterosuperior canal to prevent the retractor from tearing the skin away from the posterior bony canal. Separation of the retractor blades then provides a movable window through which the entire mastoid cortex may be visualized (Fig. 48–11).

The *postauricular incision* is carried through the skin

a few millimeters posterior to the retroauricular fold in overlapping layers to mastoid cortex (Fig. 48–12). Its length should be sufficient to uncover the entire mastoid cortex. The periostium is then elevated anteriorly and posteriorly, after which a self-retaining retractor is placed. Care should be taken to avoid the region anterior to the mastoid tip to prevent injury to the facial nerve.

Myringoplasty

Because myringoplasty is a procedure that corrects a defect in the eardrum only when no other pathologic

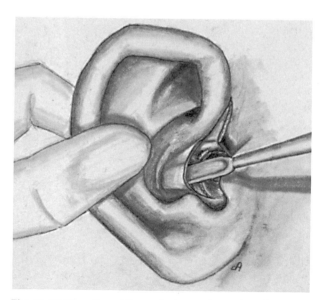

Fig. 48–10. Elevation of the periosteum after andaural incision.

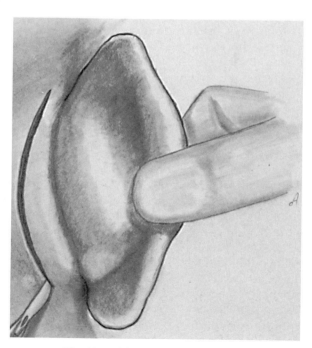

Fig. 48–12. The postauricular incision.

condition exists, this operation can properly be named only at its conclusion when it has been determined that these conditions were, in fact, present. Myringoplasty may be anticipated, however, in cases in which chronic or recurrent infection has not been present or in perforations of traumatic origin accompanied by a hearing loss of less than 15 dB. In every instance, the middle ear should be inspected because this adds little time to the procedure, does not increase the morbidity, and occasionally reveals the presence of hidden or unsuspected pathology.

Traumatic Perforation of the Tympanic Membrane

Traumatic perforation is a common reason for emergency care. The causes are varied, with water sports (diving or water skiing) being a frequent offender. Blows to the ear, usually with the cupped hand, and objects entering the ear with some force are also common causes. Occasionally, the patient has been injured by an explosion or by too forceful irrigation of the ear canal.

A high percentage of these cases are subject to litigation, so that complete and frequent examination of the ear and hearing is important. Because the energy of the traumatic force may be transmitted by the ossicular chain to the inner ear, an audiometric evaluation is important in each case. When severe force has caused the perforation, temporal bone and skull x-ray films should be made to determine if a fracture is also present.

Usually there is a severe but rapidly abating pain at the time of the injury. The tympanic membrane, on examination, is injected. The perforation is ragged or stellate in most instances and a clot of blood around or over the site of tearing, and hemotympanum is not common. Injuries caused by water may become rapidly infected, causing a seropurulent discharge. Without infection, there is usually a serous discharge for a few days after the injury. Welders are prone to perforation of hot chips of metal flying into the ear canal. These perforations are round with cauterized edges. This cauterization prevents healing in most of these cases, causing a persistent perforation.

During the first 2 weeks after a perforation, inspection only should be done, and instrumentation and cleaning avoided. The patient should wear a cotton plug in the ear to prevent water or dirt from entering the canal and be advised against washing his hair or the skin around his ear. Most of these perforations heal rapidly, and after 2 weeks any crust remaining on the tympanic membrane may be removed under magnification to see if healing is complete.

Infection of the middle ear, if present, should be treated with antibiotics as described in Chapter 53 for acute otitis media. A persistent perforation may follow infection, although in most cases closure of the perforation ensues as the infection subsides.

Persistent perforation calls for special measures. If the perforation has not healed within 1 month, an attempt may be made to close it in the office by the Derlacki method. The consists of stimulating the margin of the perforation and then covering it with a moist cotton disc for a few weeks. The margin is stimulated either with trichloroacetic acid or by incision with a tiny right-angled pick. A cotton patch moistened with Euthymol (a proprietary mixture of eucalyptol, methyl salicylate, menthol, thymol, boric acid, and benzoic acid in 20% alcohol) is placed over the perforation and remoistened two times a day at home with one or two drops of the same solution. Five percent urea in normal saline solution may be used in cases giving no response or reacting adversely to the Euthymol. This procedure is carried out at 10- to 14-day intervals until closure is accomplished. If there is no response after a 3-month period, or if there is intolerance of the treatment, as evidenced by repeated discharge after patching, surgical closure should be recommended. Variations on this technique using dry patching with cigarette paper, collagen film, or silastic film glued to the drumhead have been described. The moist technique seems to give the highest percentage of success—slightly more than 70%.

Graft Material

The first attempts to close drum perforations used split-thickness or full-thickness free skin grafts. Because of poor success rates, the predilection to infection, an the development of flap cholesteatoma (epithelial cysts originating from hair follicles and glands in the graft) with this material, its use has been largely abandoned. Today most grafts use connective tissue, either alone or in combination with canal wall skin. For this purpose, temporalis fascia or tragal perichondrium is frequently used. Other graft materials that have been used with satisfactory results are vein, periostium, and various preserved homograft materials, such as human tympanic membrane, dura, and heart valve. Preserved heterograft materials have also been used. The use of fresh autograft connective tissue such as vein or fascia avoids the complications of storage or transmission of disease and offers the greatest degree of success.

The connective tissue graft is used to replace the missing fibrous elements of the drum, and the squamous layer and mucosa are allowed to regenerate over it. The rapidly proliferative squamous layer carries blood to the graft, during which time it is able to survive by tissue perfusion. Using a fluorescein angiographic technique, Applebaum and Deutsch described the vascularization process during graft healing. The mallear artery is the major supply to the posterior half of the tympanic graft and the anterior annular vessel supplies the anterior segment. This study indicates that this process requires 2 to 4 weeks to complete, which suggests that cleaning or other manipulation should be avoided during this period. With the use of temporalis fascia, success rates as high as 98% have been reported.

Technique

Myringoplasty is usually performed by the transmeatal approach (see discussion of surgical incisions in previous section) or occasionally through a post-auricular incision. The procedure consists of four steps: obtaining the graft, preparing the drum to receive the graft, inspection of the middle ear, and finally placement of the graft. Perichondrial tissue is obtained from the meatal surface of the tragus through an incision just medial to its outer edge. In some instances, tragal cartilage is removed as well. Temporalis fascia is obtained through an incision above the hairline just superior to the auricle. Because these tissues contain little elastic tissue, they do not tend to shrink and may be taken immediately before being placed. Storage in physiologic solution or drying does not seem to alter the take rate.

The drum remnants are prepared by first splitting the edge of the perforation into two layers and then removing a 1- or 2-mm strip of mucosa from the undersurface of the drum (Figs. 48–13 and 48–14). This serves two purposes: to secure a raw edge of squamous epithelium around the entire periphery of the perforation from which regeneration will take place, and to ensure the removal of any ingrowth of squamous epithelium through the perforation into the middle ear.

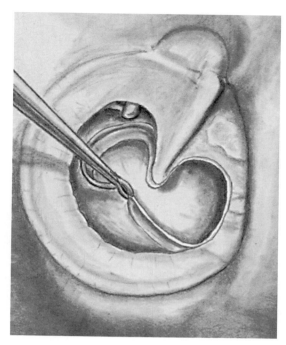

Fig. 48–14. Myringoplasty. The medial layer is stripped from the undersurface of the margin of the perforation.

Failure to secure either of these objectives may result in failure of the graft or in residual perforation.

An occasional difficulty encountered in this part of the operation is the inability to visualize the anterior margin of the perforation due to curvature of the ear canal. This problem is usually overcome by either elevating the anulus outward into view (Fig. 48–15) or removing this obstruction with a burr, after first re-

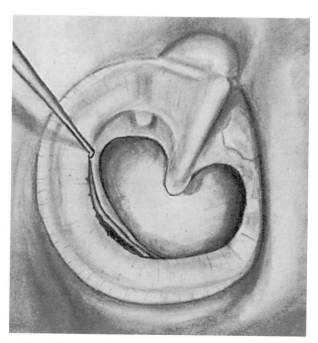

Fig. 48–13. Myringoplasty. The edge of the perforation is split into two layers.

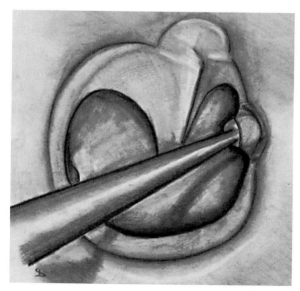

Fig. 48–15. The anterior margin of the perforation may be visualized by dissecting the anulus outward with a right-angled (reverse) elevator.

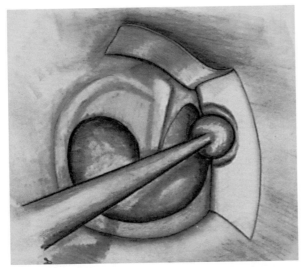

Fig. 48–16. When the anterior margin of the perforation is hidden behind a curved canal wall, it may be visualized by drilling or curetting away the bony canal after turning a skin flap.

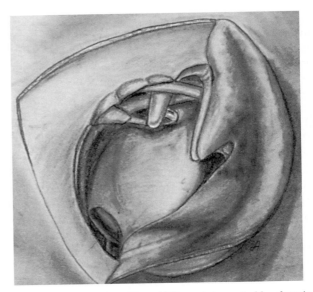

Fig. 48–17. Myringoplasty. The middle ear is inspected by elevation of a posterior tympanomeatal skin flap and, if necessary, by removal of a small amount of the posterosuperior lateral attic wall.

moving the skin from the area by turning a superiorly attached pedicle skin flap, which may be replaced at the end of the procedure (Fig. 48–16). A postauricular approach may be chosen in patients with a small or anteriorly angled canal. This provides a more direct view of the anterior region of the middle ear, but with some sacrifice of vision posteriorly.

Inspection of the Middle Ear

This is carried out by creating a tympano-meatal flap after making an endomeatal incision. A small amount of bone may be removed from the region of the posterosuperior anulus to visualize the lower portions of the posterior attic space, especially the long process of the incus and the incudostapedial joint (Fig. 48–17). Small mirrors or fiberoptic telescopes may also be used for inspection avoiding the loss of annular bone which may lead to attic collapse in some patients. Ossicular continuity and mobility should be checked at this time. Stapes fixation caused by otosclerosis may occasionally be noted but should not be surgically corrected until a healed, closed middle ear space has been obtained.

The creation of a skin flap is also great value in the presence of posterior perforations because a portion of the graft should be placed on the postero-superior canal wall under the skin flap.

Placing the Graft

To exclude squamous epithelium from the middle ear, the tissue graft is placed on the inner surface of the drum remnant. If vein is used, the intima is placed toward the promontory; with other tissues there is no distinction as to surface.

To support the graft, the middle ear is filled with a nutrient, gelatinous substance. A good choice for this mixture of tiny pieces of gelatin sponge combined with blood (Fig. 48–18). The graft is then trimmed to fit the perforation, leaving enough excess to tuck under its edge and to bring onto the postero-superior canal wall in the case of a large defect.

Another technique, evolved from the former method using skin grafts, is preferred by some surgeons. In this technique, the outer squamous layer of the drumhead is removed in continuity with canal skin flaps. The connective tissue graft is placed over the denuded tympanic membrane remnant and the canal skin replaced over this. This method has a higher complication rate. Anterior blunting of the canal-drum-

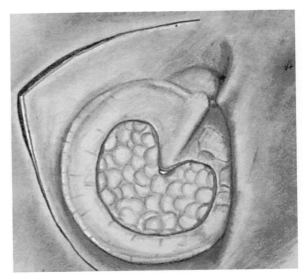

Fig. 48–18. Myringoplasty. To support the graft, the middle ear is filled with pledgets of gelatin sponge and blood clot.

head junction, lateralization of the graft, and iatrogenic cholesteatoma secondary to entrapment of squamous epithelium beneath the graft have all been reported as consequences of this procedure.

Tympanoplasty

Tympanoplasty may be performed with or without mastoid surgery as dictated by the disease process or preferred by the surgeon. The tympanoplastic portion of the procedure is intended to eliminate irreversible pathology and reconstruct the hearing mechanism by the method most appropriate to the pathology found. Because a perforation is usually present in these conditions, myringoplasty as just described becomes a part of the tympanoplasty.

Tympanoplasty Without Mastoidectomy

This is indicated in most cases of simple chronic otitis media, chronic adhesive otitis, and tympanosclerosis. The procedure may be divided into several basic steps, including obtaining the graft (see Myringoplasty), and preparation of the drum remnant. Often in these cases, an atrophic squamous epithelial layer has formed, and atrophic membrane may have retracted into the middle ear. This usually occurs in the posterosuperior portion of the middle ear (Fig. 48–19), but may involve the entire middle ear space and presents a special problem because the entire atrophic layer must be excised to prevent postoperative cholesteatoma formation and perforation of the drum. It has proved best to dissect this atrophic membrane from the middle ear spaces in continuity with the canal skin flap and then to excise it in its entirety to ensure the complete removal of the

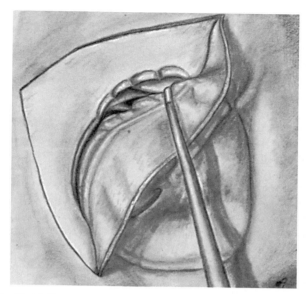

Fig. 48–20. Tympanoplasty. The atrophic epithelium is dissected free in continuity with the tympanomeatal flap, with care taken to maintain its integrity.

tissue (Fig. 48–20). The use of α-chymotrypsin is invaluable in this dissection. Pledgets of gelatin sponge moistened with α-chymotrypsin are used to peel the atrophic epithelium from its attachment to the underlying layers. This helps to insure the uninterrupted continuity of the epithelium so that it may be completely excised.

Exposure of the middle ear is accomplished by a tympano-meatal flap, as described previously. A small amount of the lateral attic wall may be removed to permit visualization of the attic and the contained ossicles. This exposure is necessary to determine the nature and extent of the pathologic condition so that the need for mastoid exposure can be carefully evaluated. If there is any question of irreversible disease extending into the mastoid cell system, mastoidectomy should always be performed as described in the next section entitled Tympanoplasty with Mastoidectomy.

Evaluation of the pathologic condition at surgery requires considerable experience to gauge its severity. It is always best to remove any questionable tissue rather than have it remain as a source of continuing infection. The main types of pathologic processes that may be encountered are squamous epithelium, mucosal infection, tympanosclerosis, osteitis, and osteomyelitis. Bone erosion may have caused dehiscence of normally protected areas such as the facial canal, oval window, lateral semicircular canal, promontory, or jugular bulb. These areas must be dissected carefully when mucosal disease or granulation obscures the state of bony integrity. The surgeon must be rigorous in appraising difficult-to-expose areas, such as the sinus tympani and the tubal region, because retained irreversible disease will result in surgical failure.

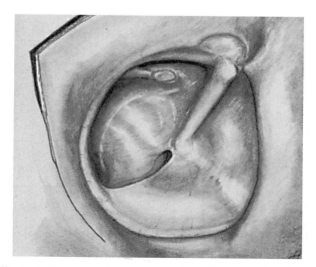

Fig. 48–19. Tympanoplasty. The presence of a retracted pocket of squamous epithelium in the posterior tympanum is a common surgical problem.

Squamous epithelial ingrowth has been discussed under preparation of the drum and its removal in continuity with the skin flap described. Another source of squamous epithelium in the mesotympanum is the downward extension of attic cholesteatoma under the drum, which may perforate the drum, usually postero-superiorly, before surgery. This type of squamous epithelium should not be removed in continuity but rather by carefully dissecting the drum or drum remnants from the lateral aspect of the cholesteatoma sac and then carefully removing the sac in toto from the mesotympanum. These techniques are necessary to ensure the complete removal of squamous epithelium. If the epithelium extends beyond visual control in the epitympanum, mastoid surgery with posterior tympanotomy should be carried out.

Mucosal disease may be encountered in every degree of severity from hyperemia and edema to thick fibrosis and tympanosclerosis. Polypoid degeneration is usually associated with the presence of squamous epithelium but may occur as an isolated finding. Granulation tissue is common and often covers osteitic bone. The milder forms of mucosal involvement are reversible and, unless associated with cholesteatoma or osteomyelitis, usually avoidable by proper preoperative care (see Chronic Otitis Media, Chap. 54). Irreversible pathologic processes such as polyps, fibrosed mucous membrane, or masses of tympanosclerosis, should be removed. Retained islands of mucosa in the hypotympanum and Eustachian tube allow rapid regeneration of mucosa even with extensive removal. Small plaques of tympanosclerosis may be left if they do not interfere with free transmission of sound energy. The antero-superior region of the mesotympanum should be carefully evaluated in this regard because extension into the attic with fixation of the malleus is common with tympanosclerosis in this area. Dissection should be carried out carefully in the region of the footplate, facial nerve, and lateral semicircular canal, since extension of infection in these regions carries severe consequences.

Bone disease is difficult to differentiate at surgery and in general should be removed until healthy tissue is reached. Osteomyelitis is irreversible, extending to sequestration, and unless eliminated completely will result in continued infection. It should be remembered in dealing with ossicular bone that its blood supply is derived from mucosal vessels so that damage to the mucosa may result in necrosis.

Ossicular Chain Reconstruction

Many techniques of ossicular reconstruction using both artificial materials, such as polyethylene, Teflon, hydroxyapitite, or stainless steel and transposition of ossicular remnants have been described. These methods depend, of course, on the particular ossicular

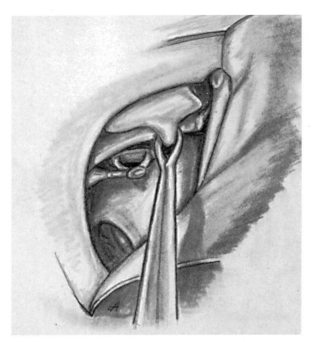

Fig. 48–21. Tympanoplasty: method of ossicular reconstruction. The incus is removed from the attic but is used for reconstruction only if healthy.

pathologic condition involved and will be so outlined in this section. The most commonly encountered ossicular defects, in order of their incidence, are: long process of the incus (36.4%); arch of the stapes (18.0%); entire incus (17.0%); entire malleus (8.6); head of the malleus (6.0%); handle of the malleus (4.3%). Congenital malformation, fixation, and combinations of these defects constitute another ten percent. In addition to these naturally occurring types of pathologic processes, the problem of disease control may require surgical excision of portions of the ossicles. In the case of cholesteatoma, it is often necessary to remove the head of the malleus and the body of the incus to ensure complete removal of matrix from the attic (Fig. 48–21). Severe tympanosclerosis with ossicular fixation often requires removal of the involved ossicles with subsequent replacement. It is especially true of the latter condition.

Use of Homograft Bone

Previous editions of this textbook have suggested the use of homograft ossicular bone as providing the tympanoplastic surgeon with the most useful material for ossicular reconstruction. The present era has seen this use to become negligible. The risk of transmission of AIDS, hepatitis and slow virus is responsible for this change. Although autograft bone is equally useful, in many instances it is not available because of the extensive disease present. Bone surrounded by cholesteatoma matrix, when examined histologically, is usually extensively involved with osteomyelitic degeneration.

Extension of squamous elements into the haversian system has also been found. Although some surgeons autoclave the diseased bone, it seems preferable to use bone not involved with disease. Other patients have extensive destruction caused by disease or past surgery and thus no ossicles are present for prosthetic use. Commercial bone banks have been established in several centers and can provide ossicles whose safety has been verified for prosthetic use.

For these reasons, the use of ossicular prostheses fashioned from hydroxyapitite has become widespread and are available in a variety of shapes as a substitute for ossicular bone. They may be further shaped using diamond burrs.

Systematic Reconstruction

Because reconstruction is based on the remaining elements of the ossicular system rather than the missing portions, and the critical portions are the malleus handle and stapes arch, a four square diagram may be used to illustrate the choices available for reconstruction (Fig. 48–22). The techniques to be described follow this scheme.

STAPES PRESENT, MALLEUS PRESENT: MALLEUS-STAPES ASSEMBLY. Falling within this category are two distinct types of ossicular problems. The first is *ossicular fixation,* either of the stapes or of the malleus head-incus body bloc located within the attic space. With this problem, the ossicular chain is intact but must be disrupted surgically to effect a hearing improvement.

Stapes fixation is often encountered in chronic ear surgery, caused by either otosclerosis or tympanosclerosis. In either case, stapedectomy is carried out as a staged procedure.

Fixation of the malleus head or body of the incus has a significant incidence as a cause of conductive hearing loss. When occurring together with other ossicular disease, it may be overlooked, and this causes postoperative hearing failure, necessitating revisional surgery. The cause of this fixation may be congenital because of lack of differentiation of the suspensory ligaments of the malleus and incus with consequent ossi-

fication. Acquired causes include hyperostotic healing of fracture of the tegmen, osteoma of the attic, and, particularly frequent in chronic otitis media, tympanosclerotic scarring of the attic. Tympanosclerosis has a predilection for the anterior attic space, often extending upward from the anterior-superior tympanic membrane and fixing the malleus because of involvement of the narrow premallear space. Effective treatment of all these conditions requires removal of the incus and malleus head, followed by reconstruction through malleus-stapes assembly described below.

The minimum defect of the incus is partial erosion of the tip of the long process or lenticular process. This erosion is often caused by osteomyelitis and progresses to complete loss of the end of the long process even after healing of the tympanic membrane. To avoid this complication, the incudo-stapedial region should be carefully examined to determine the health of the mucosa and underlying bone. Tiny erosions may be ignored, but greater amounts of necrosis necessitate sacrifice of normal ossicular continuity. A simple test of strength is to pull discreetly on the long process with a pick to see if it breaks easily. If the amount of disease falls between these two extremes, it is wise to proceed as though the long process were totally deficient. Erosion of the incus is uniformly associated with contact of retracted tympanic membrane and may be predicted when this is present. On the other hand, incus erosion is rare in simple central perforation without retraction and contact.

Reconstruction is carried out by fitting a prosthesis between the handle of the malleus and the stapes head: a malleus-stapes assembly. Bone, hydroxyapitite, and dense polyethylene sponge have all been used in this situation. The bony prosthesis may be constructed from either the malleus head or a portion of the incus body. Its length is sufficient to fit snugly between the malleus stapes without either slack, which will result in displacement or poor hearing, or excessive pressure, which might result in stapes subluxation. A groove is formed in one end of the prosthesis to fit against the malleus, and a socket is formed in the other end to fit over the stapes head (Fig. 48–23). A No. 4 diamond burr is the usual size used for this purpose. The socket of the prosthesis is placed over the stapes head. Then the malleus is gently pulled lateralward, using two instruments, while the prosthesis is "snapped" into position by a gentle push with the other instrument. Some practice necessary to obtain proficiency in the techniques of drilling and positioning the prosthesis. Figure 48–23 shows both a hydroxyapitite prosthesis designed by Kartush and one designed by Wehrs in a similar repair.

Compared to the former techniques of myringostapediopexy and incus repositioning, the results observed with this technique have been uniformly superior. Failures are usually technical, related to an

| | MALLEUS HANDLE | |
	Present	Absent
STAPES ARCH Present	A. Malleus-stapes assembly (59.2%)	C. Short columella (7.8%)
STAPES ARCH Absent	B. Malleus-footplate assembly (23.2%)	D. Long columella (8.2%)

Fig. 48–22. Classification of the types of ossicular defects encountered during surgery. Within each block is the method of reconstruction used for that defect. The number within the block indicates the percentage occurrence of the defect in relation to all ossicular defects.

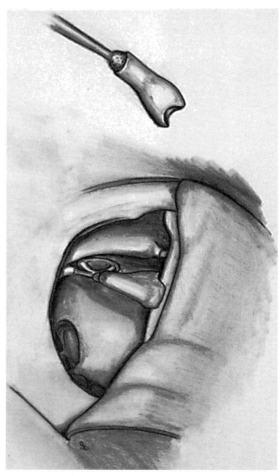

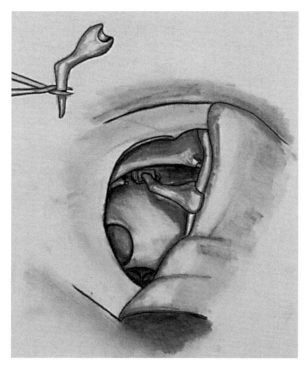

Fig. 48–24. Malleus-footplate assembly. A homograft malleus is carved as shown in the inset and fitted into place between the malleus handle and stapes footplate. It rests on a connective tissue pad over the footplate. This technique can also be used in revision of fenestration operations.

Fig. 48–23. Malleus-stapes assembly. A piece of ossicular bone, homograft or autograft, is drilled to fit between the malleus handle and stapes head (inset). It is then "snapped" into place as shown.

improper fit of the prosthesis. The good results reported are attributed to the excellent stability of the prosthesis because neither the malleus nor the stapes shifts during the healing period. This stability frees the ossicular graft from the shrinking process of the tympanic membrane graft during healing, which is responsible for many hearing failures occurring with former techniques.

MALLEUS PRESENT, STAPES ARCH DESTROYED: MALLEUS FOOTPLATE ASSEMBLY. The ossicular defect present in this category is found not only with destruction caused by the disease process but also postoperatively after the fenestration operation, and the reconstruction described applies to both situations. The disease process associated with destruction of incus and stapes arch, sparing the malleus handle, is caused by encroachment of squamous epithelium onto these ossicles, as seen in both primary acquired and secondary acquired cholesteatoma. Many surgeons use a total ossicular replacement prosthesis (TORP) in this situation, but I use malleus-footplate assembly (Fig. 48–24) as the recon-

struction for this type of defect. Again, the malleus handle serves as the lateral attachment for stability, the medial end resting on the footplate or oval window membrane. The first such reconstruction used a straight prosthesis, usually an incus body, angled between the malleus and footplate. Slippage and bony contact with fixation, however, were common complications with this method. Refinement of the technique involved the use of smaller angled prostheses to avoid poor results. The present method uses a hydroxyapatite prosthesis. The design of the hydroxyapatite prosthesis includes a vertical shaft extending from the oval window toward the TM and a angled portion extending to the undersurface of the malleus handle. Prostheses of this type have been designed by Wehrs, Goldenberg, and myself. The natural angle at the neck of the prosthesis allows the prosthesis to contact the undersurface of the malleus, always anterior to the midpoint of the oval window. Stability of the prosthesis may be further ensured by placing a piece of connective tissue as a "nonskid carpet" over the footplate. Again the prosthesis should fit snugly and be "snapped" into place and can be accomplished only by accurately gauging the individual dimensions encountered. If a fixed footplate is found at the time of reconstruction, staging is necessary, the prosthesis being placed and the tympanic membrane grafted at the first operation. A second procedure follows complete healing, and involves removal of the footplate and its replacement with a connective tissue graft on which is placed the already incorporated prosthesis.

MALLEUS ABSENT, STAPES PRESENT OR MALLEUS ABSENT, STAPES ABSENT. Loss of the malleus handle occurs as a sequel of necrotizing otitis media, cholesteatoma or prior surgery. As shown in Figure 48–21, presence or absence of the stapes arch is equally prevalent with the loss of the malleus. The results with this category of ossiculoplasty have been disappointing when compared to other results. Most reports indicate a 50 to 60% success rate. This author formerly used a homograft incus carved as either a long or short "slipper." Today most otologic surgeons use a columella to reconstruct these ossicular defects. These prostheses have been variously named TORP; TOP or PORP; POP for total ossicular (replacement) prosthesis or partial ossicular (replacement) prosthesis. To prevent extrusion, a graft of autogenous tragal cartilage is placed between the prosthesis and the drumhead. In spite of this precaution, extrusion occurs in 3 to 10% of patients, becoming more prevalent with increasing length of follow-up.

The prosthesis, when used, is carefully measured and cut to fit the ossicular defect. If it is placed on the footplate, a layer of connective tissue should be placed between the prosthesis and the footplate. This serves both to protect the vestibule and provide a "nonskid" pad to center and stabilize the medial end. A cartilage disk is formed from autograft tragal cartilage and placed between the prosthesis and tympanic membrane or graft. A perichondrial cover may remain on the cartilage disk and serve as the tympanic graft as well (Fig. 48–25). Dense porous polyethylene columellae contain a steel shaft, which allows the prosthesis to be angled to adapt to the curvature of the drumhead. Time has also taught that prostheses do not fare well in the presence of infection, and therefore staging may be indicated in patients with infection. Figure 48–25 illustrates both a short columella used when the stapes is present and a long columella used when the arch is destroyed. These are both fashioned from hydroxyapitite.

The present status of columellar repair is still in evolution. Methods using autograft cartilage as described by Goodhill and Sheehy offer reliable results that seem reasonably permanent when followed over time. Although the hearing results are not equivalent to those obtained when the malleus handle is present, they may be preferable to the continuing need for revision because of extrusion. Hydroxyapitite has given the best results for columellar reconstruction to date. This material, essentially similar to bone, has proven to be well tolerated and resistant to infection. The domed head columellae as first designed by Black are favored (Fig. 48–18A, B). Sade and Shering have both described a

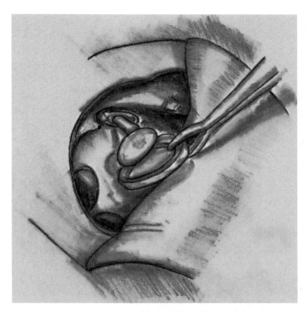

Fig. 48–25. A composite graft of thinned cartilage with attached perichondrium is placed over the TORP. This prevents extrusion while serving as the underlay graft. The components may also be placed separately.

prosthesis of ossicular bone (incus) with a fitted shaft for this purpose. This latter method allows the surgeon complete freedom of choice as to shaft material as plastics or ceramics may be used.

Finally, a word should be mentioned concerning the use of homograft tympanic membranes with en bloc ossicles. Conceptually, this is the ideal prosthesis for this type of reconstruction; however, when both the missing tympanic membrane and malleus are supplied, the hearing results have been disappointing. Although this is no worse than the results using the methods of reconstruction described above when coupled with grafting with autogenous connective tissue, the added expense of material preparation and banking seems to be much less cost-effective. A few centers are continuing research on these techniques, however, and may eventually show the superiority of this method after the problems have been resolved.

Tympanoplasty with Mastoidectomy

Extension of the pathologic process into the mastoid air cell system requires exposure and removal. It has been demonstrated in recent years that this may be done without removing the bony canal walls, thus maintaining normal tympanic anatomy and provides a great advantage in the reconstruction of a functional sound conductive system. The type of operation required (posterior tympanotomy) is difficult, dangerous, and time-consuming. Because the benefit of canal preservation is to avoid the morbidity and aftercare of a large mastoid cavity, canal preservation is most appropriate for patients with well developed air cell systems. The technical problems of this surgery are also minimal for patients with a well pneumatized mastoid. It is my practice to chose a canal-up operation when the air cell size is greater than 2 cm² on lateral radiographic examination. For patients with restricted mastoid development, modified radical mastoidectomy combined with tympanoplasty is the operation choice. This is performed through either an endaural or post-auricular incision (see Incisions, this Chap.) combined with meatoplasty. In some instances, the decision to proceed to mastoid exploration is made during the exploration of the tympanum. The presence of cholesteatoma or mucosal polyposus, or evidence of bone disease on radiographic examination, dictates mastoid exposure. The procedure to be described is carried out after removal of the tympanic pathologic condition and before ossicular reconstruction.

Posterior Tympanotomy

The incision for mastoid exposure is made postauricularly. Extensive simple transcortical mastoidectomy is performed, with the posterior and superior canal walls maintained (Fig. 48–26). The dissection is carried anteriorly to the anterior attic wall. A most important part of this dissection is that of the "facial triangle." The bone lying between the second turn of the facial nerve and the chorda tympani nerve is removed to expose the posterior aspect of the middle ear. This enables visualization of the stapes and the sinus tympani. The mastoid dissection should be sufficiently thorough to expose all diseased cell tracts but need not exenterate all cells because the mastoid is relined with normal mucosa.

The mastoid dissection is started in the region above the suprameatal triangle. The tegmen is found and fol-

lowed medially toward the antrum, the cavity being enlarged externally as the bone removal is carried deeper, so that the surgical defect is either straight-sided or funnel-shaped. The antrum is identified by the curve of the lateral semicircular canal on its floor. The dissection is then carried forward through the aditus ad antrum until the fossa incudis is reached and the short process of the incus is identified. The lateral attic wall is removed, and the superior canal wall is maintained until the space anterior to the malleus head can be completely visualized. The facial triangle is dissected by carefully removing the bone between the posterior anulus and facial nerve with diamond burrs to open the posterior sinus (Fig. 48–27). This allows a view of the posterior mesotympanum and sinus tympani from the mastoid aspect with much improved control of tympanic pathologic process. The mastoid dissection is completed by following the tegmen posteriorly to the lateral sinus, dissecting the sinodural angle in so doing, and then following the lateral sinus inferiorly toward the mastoid tip. When the pathologic condition has been encompassed, the dissection is completed. Since the second turn of the facial nerve has been well outlined by the initial dissection of the facial triangle, the position of the vertical segment of the nerve is defined, and injury should be no problem.

The mastoid cavity is allowed to fill with blood or may be filled with gelatin sponge unless there has been no extensive destruction of the lateral attic wall. In this case, either the canal should be repaired or the opera-

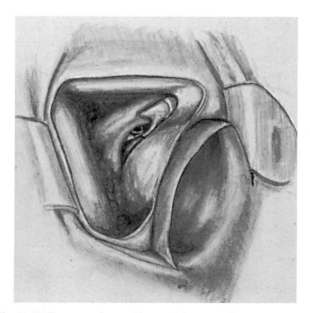

Fig. 48–27. Tympanoplasty with mastoidectomy. The entire attic and mastoid have been exposed and the diseased portion excised with the canal wall preserved. The facial recess (posterior sinus) has been opened to show a posterior view of the oval window niche and sinus tympani. In most cases with cholesteatoma, the incus and head of the malleus would have been removed.

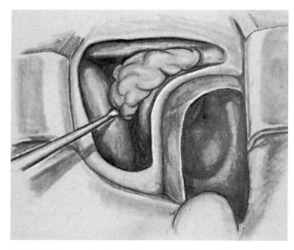

Fig. 48–26. Tympanoplasty with mastoidectomy. The mastoid cortex has been removed to expose a cholesteatoma, which is removed intact if possible. The bony canal wall has been preserved at this stage.

tion changed to "canal-down" (see subsequent section, Modified Radical Mastoidectomy). Often small bony defects are created in the canal wall during dissection. In other patients, cholesteatomatous erosion occurs, creating canal defects. In each case, repair must be carried out to prevent retraction through the defect and subsequent postoperative cholesteatoma formation. The most useful material for this purpose is autogenous tragal cartilage. A thin slice of cartilage is cut with a surgical knife and inserted between the meatal skin or tympanic membrane graft and the bony defect, usually at the conclusion of the procedure. Bone paste (bone dust combined with fibrin clot) is a useful adjunct in canal wall repair. Thin curved hydroxyapitite sheets are also available for this use. In most but not all instances, postoperative retraction will be prevented. Long-term observation is indicated to detect such occurrences because early intervention prevents the more severe complications of cholesteatoma. If retraction pockets become evident, mastoid obliteration seems to be the treatment of choice.

Prevention of Retraction Pockets

The major complication of operations that preserve the posterior bony canal wall is the formation of a retraction pocket. This may occur at any time after surgery, but is usually seen between 1 and 2 years postoperatively. This problem occurs because of a complex interrelationship between the disease process and technical details of the surgical method, and can never be completely eliminated. Careful attention to surgical techniques minimizes the occurrence of postoperative pocketing. The following steps have been found to be the most effective in lessening this incidence:

1. Defects of the canal wall at the posterior-superior scutum must be avoided. In a healthy ear (as in stapes surgery), a considerable amount of bone may be removed from this region without a problem. In chronic otitis media, however, this type of exposure must be avoided because it results in retraction of at least twice the normal incidence. Such defects are also commonly present because of bone destruction consequent to the disease. When such is the case, repair by cartilage and/or bone autograft should be performed.
2. Posterior-superior tympanic membrane retraction may be reduced by using a thicker graft material. Composite grafts of perichondrium is ideal for this purpose because a thin layer of cartilage may be left attached to the graft. This type of graft has a much greater resistance to atrophy and consequent retraction.
3. Efforts to secure ventilation of the middle ear and mastoid are important. Gelfilm had proven more useful than silicone or other types of film and is

used when apposition of raw surfaces may lead to adhesion.
4. Finally, frequent efforts to inflate the ear by the patient both pre- and postoperatively are important to restore and maintain the health of the ear. Both children and adults are instructed in the importance of this and are checked at each office visit for successful inflation to reinforce the patient's motivation in the chronic application of self-inflation.

Modified Radical Mastoidectomy

Because the classic radical mastoidectomy removed the entire middle ear, many attempts to modify the operation to preserve hearing have been described. One of the most successful of these was devised by Bondy. The pathologic indications for the operations were clearly delineated, but must be modified today owing to the refined surgical techniques now available. The object of radical mastoidectomy is to combine the middle ear, attic, and mastoid cavity into a single space draining through the external canal. The modified procedures preserved the middle ear space while draining the attic and mastoid. The element common to both these procedures is the removal of the posterior and superior canal walls.

Before and during the course of the surgery as described under Tympanoplasty with Mastoidectomy, the extent and severity of the disease process are evaluated. A decision to proceed with modified radical mastoidectomy may then be made based entirely on objective indications as to the extent of the disease. The most important indication for this procedure is difficulty in obtaining needed visualization in canal preservation surgery, particularly in a small, non-pneumatized mastoid. These conditions lead to unnecessary duration of surgery and increased risk of facial nerve injury or labyrinth exposure. Modified radical mastoidectomy should certainly be used by surgeons untrained in posterior tympanotomy.

Technically, the procedure entails removal of the superior canal wall, removal of the posterior canal wall to the level of the facial nerve, and creation of a canal skin flap, which will be turned down to line the mastoid cavity and attic space (Figs. 48–28 and 48–29). This is most simply accomplished through an endaural approach, following the disease so that its entire extent is visualized and exteriorized. Initially, the dissection is lateral to the anulus, exposing the attic and antrum in the process. The removal of the posterior and superior canal walls is carried gradually lateralward until the attic is completely exposed and the mastoid opened posteriorly.

After removal of the bony canal walls, incisions are made in the remaining canal skin from the region of the tympanic anulus outward to the endaural incision,

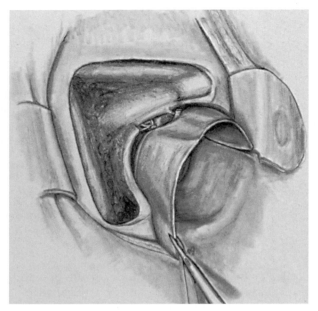

Fig. 48–28. Modified radical mastoidectomy. The superior and posterior canal walls have been removed, and the skin of the canal is being incised to fashion a pedicle flap attached near the anulus.

both anterosuperiorly and posteroinferiorly. This creates a tympanomeatal skin flap which, after the posterior anulus is dissected from the sulcus, is packed forward out of the way so that the remaining dissection of the facial ridge may be carried out. With diamond burrs, the remaining bone of the posterior canal wall is lowered to the inferior limit of the bony canal to create the facial ridge.

The severity of the pathologic conditions necessitating modified radical mastoidectomy has usually required the removal of the incus and the head of the

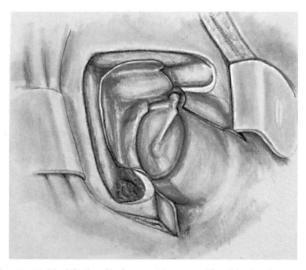

Fig. 48–29. Modified radical mastoidectomy. The skin flap is rotated over the facial ridge to line the mastoid cavity. If desired, a muscle flap may be placed behind the skin.

malleus. If not, the tympano-meatal flap may be draped over the attic ossicular mass. Usually, the flap is brought down to lie on the bare bone of the medial attic wall and backward to partially line the mastoid cavity. A trouble-free cavity is best obtained by the creation of a large meatus. Meatoplasty is carried out during the initial incision by removing a large semi-lunar segment of conchal cartilage. The conchal skin is maintained to facilitate rapid epithelialization of the cavity.

The modified radical procedure is concluded by repair of the tympanic membrane and ossicular chain, as described in the sections on myringoplasty and tympanoplasty. In some instances, staging is preferred, with the tympanic membrane grafted at the initial procedure and the ossicular repair performed at a second stage (see Staging in Chronic Ear Surgery).

The cavity is then packed with gelatin sponge and epithelialization allowed to proceed from the skin edges. Postoperative dressings and manipulation should be delayed for a minimum of 2 weeks in order not to interfere with this process. Mastoid pressure dressings are applied and remain for 24 to 48 hours to control postoperative hemorrhage.

Radical Mastoidectomy

Radical mastoidectomy is rarely indicated today because it involves severe loss of function. Its application is reserved for tumors of the middle ear or external meatus, and in these procedures it may extend far beyond the operation formerly used for control of ear infection. This operation removed all middle ear structures including the tympanic membrane, ossicles (with the exception of the stapes), tensor tympani muscle, and mucosa. The orifice of the Eustachian tube was occluded with bone chips or a cartilage plug. No grafting or skin flaps were used, the cavity being allowed to heal by secondary intention.

Mastoid Obliteration Operation

The usefulness of mastoid obliteration procedures has been recognized for many decades. The incidence of chronic infection of mastoid cavities has not been reported, but it appears with persistent regularity in all otologic practices. Many procedures have been reported for this purpose. Most have been used temporalis muscle for obliteration; others use fat or even space-occupying plastic materials, such as acrylic. Most early techniques have been abandoned because of failure to accomplish the primary purpose of obtaining a healthy ear.

The advantage of these procedures seems to be the enrichment of blood supply to the skin lining the cavity and the provision of a soft tissue layer between this skin and the underlying bone. Obliteration provides a small or nonexistent mastoid cavity, making the problem of aftercare much easier. These procedures are thus indicated in the treatment of any chronically infected mastoid cavity or the prevention of this complication by obliterating the mastoid primarily. The contraindications to these procedures are extension of the disease process beyond the confines of the mastoid, threatened complication, or a disease process that may not have been controlled during the mastoidectomy, such as widespread cholesteatoma. The decision to do an obliterative procedure must be made at surgery.

The technique to be described has been used by myself and others for several years with uniform success in obtaining a good, long-lasting result. This technique uses a soft-tissue, anteriorly based pedicle flap from the mastoid surface, supplemented when necessary by autogenous bone paste. The incision for mastoid obliteration is, of necessity, post-auricular. It is carried only through the skin, following which anterior and posterior undermining is done to expose a 4- to 5-cm area of subcutaneous fibrous tissue lying on the mastoid cortex. A pedicle flap is then outlined, leaving it attached anteriorly at the level of the posterior meatus (Fig. 48–30). This is elevated from the underlying cortex with a periosteal elevator and kept free of the bony field by insertion under the anterior blade of the self-retaining retractor. At the completion of the mastoid dissection, the flap is inserted into the cavity, terminating in the posterior attic and facial ridge to furnish a vascular connective tissue backing to the reformed canal wall. In small mastoid cavities, this flap is all that is necessary for obliteration.

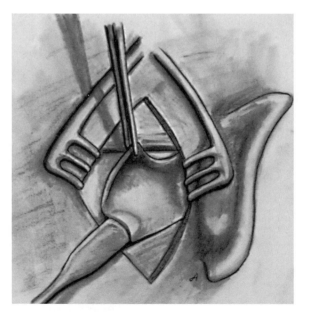

Fig. 48–30. Mastoid obliteration. After the postauricular incision, the soft tissue over the mastoid cortex is exposed and elevated as an anteriorly based pedicle flap. It must be long enough to extend into the most medial depth of the mastoid cavity.

The mastoid cortex is drilled away to expose widely the mastoid cavity. The bone dust is carried away through continuous suction irrigation, the aspirate being collected and saved in a sterile trap bottle. Care is taken during this drilling not to dissect any diseased bone or squamous elements. The presence of infected bone contraindicates the use of bone in an obliteration procedure. When sufficient bone has been collected, the bone dust is strained through a filter. The bony material then assumes the form of paste or mortar and is ideal for packing into the space behind the pedicle flap. Osteogenic activity is rapid, causing bony obliteration of the mastoid space.

The steps of mastoid obliteration are then as follows:

1. The incision and development of the pedicle flap.
2. The removal of mastoid cortical bone to expose the mastoid cavity or, in primary operations, the underlying mastoid cell system.
3. In primary procedures, the dissection is carried out as outlined under Modified Radical Mastoidectomy. In secondary procedures, the skin lining the mastoid bowl is dissected free as a sheet from posterior to anterior, leaving the membrane attached along the medial attic wall and facial ridge. This membrane serves as the new meatal wall skin and even if inflamed, rapidly heals. The excess mastoid skin is excised.
4. If tympanoplasty is required, it is performed as outlined earlier in this chapter.
5. The obliteration is performed as outlined in the paragraph above (Fig. 48–31).
6. The incision is closed without drainage to avoid the escape of the bone paste, and the canal is packed with moist Gelfoam pledgets as in other procedures. Prophylactic antibiotics are helpful to prevent postoperative infection in this procedure.

After care with this operation is minimal because healing is usually complete within 4 weeks postoperatively.

Staging in Chronic Ear Surgery

Hearing reconstruction may be carried out in either a one-stage or a two-stage procedure. The decision is based on the severity of the disease and the type of reconstruction necessary. It is essential to a functional sound conduction system to have an air-filled middle ear space. Failure in reconstructive surgery is more common in association with certain forms of pathology: total perforation, extensive and severe mucosal destruction, loss of the anulus through bone destruction, narrowing of the middle ear in modified radical mastoidectomy, and total atelectasis of the middle ear. In these and other forms of pathologic process, based

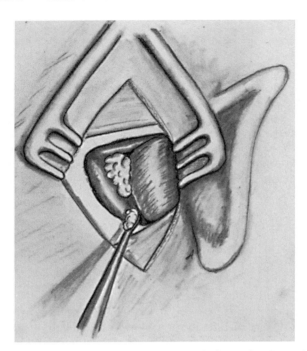

Fig. 48–31. Mastoid obliteration. The pedicle flap is fitted into the cavity, reforming the shape of the canal. Bone paste and bone chips (if needed) are packed in behind the soft tissue flap. The incision is closed without drainage.

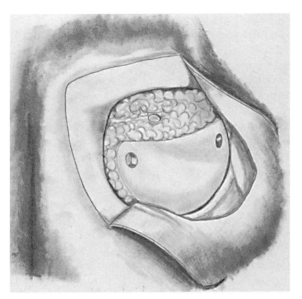

Fig. 48–32. Staged tympanoplasty. A plastic or paraffin mold is placed in the middle ear space and surrounded with gelatin sponge and blood clot.

on the surgeon's experience, an improved success rate may be expected through staged tympanoplasty.

In staged tympanoplasty, to achieve better hearing results, the initial procedure consists of grafting the tympanic membrane perforation, after first filling the middle ear space with an inert material such as silastic or supramid film. A thick material that resists folding or bending should be selected (Figs. 48–32 and 48–33). After the drumhead has healed and the mucosa has regenerated over the middle ear, a second procedure to repair the ossicular system is carried out, at which time the middle ear mold is removed. This method provides the obvious advantage of a healed, air-filled middle ear.

Suitable for the purpose of filling the middle ear are three materials available today. Teflon molds and crescents, as well as Silastic films, are commonly used. Gelfilm is an absorbable material that may be used for the same purpose, avoiding in many instances the need for a second operation. When placed in the middle ear, it persists unchanged for 6 to 12 weeks, allowing sufficient time for regeneration of the mucosal elements with re-aeration of the middle ear.

The second-look principle is another important indication for staging in chronic ear surgery. Used with canal preservation surgery performed when cholesteatoma is present, the second look is carried out 6 to 12 months after the initial procedure to detect the presence of residual disease. After this period, any residual disease is easily detected in a healed mastoid or middle

ear and may be removed without difficulty. These residua have the form of small pearls of cholesteatoma and thus can be completely eradicated without the need for radical surgery and has been reported to occur in 5 to 25% of cases. Cholesteatoma in a widely pneumatized mastoid is particularly prone to recurrence, and a second look is particularly essential in such patients. Another indication for re-exploration is cholesteatoma matrix left over a fistula, in the oval or round window niches, or in inaccessible areas of the sinus

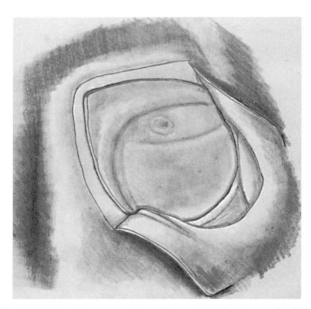

Fig. 48–33. Staged tympanoplasty. The graft is placed over the filled middle ear space. The mold is removed at a second operation after healing is complete.

tympani. At the conclusion of the primary surgery, the probability of residual disease is known to the surgeon, and reoperation should be indicated when this probability is present.

Postoperative Care

The use of prophylactic antibiotics has been the subject of much discussion in recent years. The most logical suggestion is to use antibiotics routinely, but only for the purpose of covering any possible contamination occurring at surgery (assuming that no active infection is present). For this purpose, 12 hour use of a broad-spectrum antibiotic is sufficient. The antibiotic should be given within two hours of the procedure to achieve a blood level at the time of the operation and discontinued 8 to 12 hours after the surgical procedure.

Dressings for tympanoplasty may be limited to cotton tampons loosely applied in the concha and changed daily. When mastoid incisions are made, a pressure dressing should be applied to prevent hematoma formation. This dressing may be removed after 24 hours and a cotton tampon substituted.

The duration of hospitalization must be individualized. In general, a patient undergoing a simple tympanoplasty may be able to leave the hospital 1 day following surgery, while those with more extensive procedures may require 3 to 5 days' recovery. The first dressing after surgery should be delayed for 2 to 3 weeks. This period allows adequate time for healing, so that cleaning the ear does not result in damage to the graft.

At the time of the first dressing, the state of healing of the ear canal and drum is assessed. Secondary infection of the canal is treated with topical antibiotics (see Chronic Otitis Media, Chap. 54). Excess granulation is painted with weak silver nitrate (5 or 10%), and 70% alcohol cleansing drops are prescribed to control the accumulation of serous discharge. Frequent inflation of the middle ear by the Frenzel technique (every 20 to 30 minutes) is reinstituted and continued for several weeks or months. Postoperative visits at bimonthly intervals should be made until healing is complete, after which examination should be done at 6-month intervals. These examinations should be carried out periodically for several years because a 10% regression rate is seen between the first and third years postoperatively, necessitating repeat surgery in some cases. A minimum of 5 years' observation should be advised in cases of cholesteatoma to guard against recurrence of the disease.

SUGGESTED READINGS

Applebaum EL, Deutsch EC: An endoscopic method of fluorescein angiography. Ann Otol Rhinol Laryngol 95:439–443, 1986.

Austin DF: Vein graft tympanoplasty. Trans Am Acad Ophthalmol Otolaryngol 67:198, 1963.

Austin DF: Cholesteatoma. J Laryngol Otol 78:384, 1964.

Austin DF: Present status of vein graft tympanoplasty. Arch Otolaryngol Head Neck Surg 81:20, 1965.

Austin DF (ED): Chronic ear disease. Surg Clin North Am 2:1972.

Austin DF: Transcanal tympanoplasty: A 15-year report. Trans Am Acad Opthalmol 82:30, 1976.

Austin DF: The off-centered Torp. Am J Otol 1:19, 1979.

Austin DF: Columellar tympanoplasty. Am J Otol 6:464, 1985.

Austin DF: Reconstructive techniques for tympanosclerosis. Ann Otol Rhinol Laryngol 97:670, 1988.

Austin DF: A decade of tympanoplasty; progress or regress? Laryngoscope 92:527, 1982.

Bellucci RJ: Dual classification of tympanoplasty. Laryngoscope 83:1754, 1973.

Bezold F, Siebenmann MD: Textbook of Otology, Trans. by J. Holinger. Chicago: E.H. Colgrove, 1908.

Black B: Ossiculoplasty prognosis; the SPITE method of assessment. Am J Otol 13:544, 1992.

Brockman SJ: Cartilage graft tympanoplasty. Laryngoscope 75:1452, 1965.

Derlacki EL, Clemis JD: Congenital cholesteatoma. Ann Otol Rhinol Laryngol 74:706, 1965.

Diamant M: Chronic middle ear discharge. Eye Ear Nose Throat Monthly 44:31–6, 77–83, 1965.

Diamant M: The "pathologic size" of the mastoid air cell system. Acta Otolaryngol (Stockh) 60:1, 1965.

Emmett JR, Shea JJ: Surgical treatment of tympanosclerosis. Laryngoscope 88:1642, 1978.

Committee on Conservation of Hearing: Standard classification for surgery of chronic ear infection. Arch Otolaryngol Head Neck Surg 81:204, 1965.

Corgill DA, Starrs LA: Intact canal wall tympanoplasty. Trans Am Acad Ophthalmol Otolaryngol 71:53, 1967.

Farrior JB: Stapedectomy and tympanoplasty. Arch Otolaryngol Head Neck Surg 76:140, 1965.

Farrior JB: Ossicular repositioning and prothesis. Arch Otolaryngol Head Neck Surg 71:443, 1960.

Glasscock ME, Jackson CG, Nissen AJ, et al: Postauricular undersurface tympanic membrane grafting: A follow-up report. Laryngoscope 92:718–727, 1982.

Goldenberg RA: Hydroxylapatite ossicular replacement prostheses: results in 157 consecutive cases. Laryngoscope 102(10):1091–1096, 1992.

Goodhill V, Harris I, Brickman SJ: Tympanoplasty with perichondrial graft. Arch Otolaryngol 79:131–137, 1964.

Grote JJ: Tympanoplasty with calcium phosphate. Arch Otolaryngol 110:197, 1984.

Grote JJ: Reconstruction of the ossicular chain with hydroxyapitite implants. Ann Otol Rhinol Laryngol Suppl 123:10, 1986.

Guilford FR: Preoperative evaluation in chronic ear disease. Arch Otolaryngol Head Neck Surg 78:271, 1963.

Guilford FR: Obliteration of the cavity in temporal bone surgery. Trans Am Acad Ophthalmol Otolaryngol 65:114, 1961.

Habermann J: Zur eitstehung des cholesteatoma des mittelohrs. Arch Ohrenh 27:42, 1888.

Jackson CG, Glasscock ME, Nisson AJ, et al: Ossicular chain reconstruction: The TORP and PORP in chronic ear disease. Laryngoscope 93:981, 1983.

Jako GJ: Posterior tympanotomy. Laryngoscope 77:306, 1967.

Jako GJ: Conservative middle ear surgery. Laryngoscope 76:1260, 1966.

Jansen C: Cartilage tympanoplasty. Laryngoscope 73:1288, 1963.

Jordan RE: Secretory otitis media in etiology of cholesteatoma. Arch Otolaryngol Head Neck Surg 78:261, 1963.

Juers AL: Cholesteatoma genesis. Arch Otolaryngol Head Neck Surg 81:5, 1965.

Juers AL: Modified radical mastoidectomy, indications and results. Arch Otol 57:245, 1953.

Kartush JM: personal communication.

Lang J, Kerr AG, Smyth GD: Long-term viability of transplanted ossicles. J Laryngol Otol 100:741–7, 1986.

Lempert J: Modern temporal bone surgery. Laryngoscope 60:740, 1950.

Lesinski SG (Ed): Symposium on homograft tympanoplasty. Otolaryngol Clin North Am 10:469, 1977.

Luetje CM, Denninghoff JS: Perichondrial attached double cartilage block: a better alternative to the PORP. Laryngoscope 97:1106, 1987.

Marquet J: Twelve year's experience with homograft tympanoplasty. Otolaryng Clin North Am 10:581, 1977.

McCabe B, Sade J, Abramson M (Eds): Cholesteatoma: First International Conference. Birmingham, Aescalapius, 1977.

McGuckin F: Chronic otitis media. Postgrad Med J 36:256, 1960.

McGuckin F: Concerning the pathogenesis of destructive ear disease. J Laryngol Otol 75:949, 1961.

McKenzie, D: Pathogeny of aural cholesteatoma. J Laryngol Otol 46:163, 1933.

Nager F: The cholesteatoma of the middle ear. Ann Otol Rhinol Larynol 34:1249, 1925.

Pennington CL: Incus interposition technics. In Proceedings of the Shambaugh Fifth International Workshop on Middle Ear Microsurgery and Fluctuant Hearing Loss. Huntsville, Strode, 1977, pp 323–334.

Perkins R: Human homograft otologic tissue transplantation buffered formaldehyde preparation. Trans Am Acad Opthalmol 74:278, 1970.

Portmann M: Etiology of chronic suppurative otitis media. Arch Otolaryngol Head Neck Surg 78:266, 1963.

Proctor B: Chronic middle ear disease. Arch Otolaryngol 78:276, 1963.

Rambo JHT: Musculoplasty. Ann Otol Rhinol Laryngol 74:535, 1965.

Rambo JHT: Use of paraffin. Laryngoscope 71:612, 1961.

Rambo JHT: Further experiences with musculoplasty. Arch Otolaryngol 71:428, 1960.

Ruedi L: Acquired cholesteatoma. Arch Otolaryngol Head Neck Surg 78:252, 1963.

Sade J (Ed): Cholesteatoma and Mastoid Surgery. Amsterdam: Kruger, 1982.

Shambaugh GE Jr: Surgery of the Ear. 2nd ed. Philadelphia: WB Saunders Co, 1967.

Shea JJ, Emmett, JR: Biocompatable ossicular implants. Arch Otolaryngol 104:191, 1978.

Sheehy JL: TORPs and PORPs in tympanoplasty. Clin Otolaryngol 3:451, 1977.

Sheehy JL: Surgery of Chronic Otitis Media in Otolaryngology. Hagerstown: WF Prior, 1972.

Sheehy JL: Ossicular problems in tympanoplasty. Arch Otolaryngol 81:115, 1965a.

Sheehy HL: Tympanic membrane grafting. Laryngoscope 74:985, 1964.

Shuring AG, Lippy WH: Semibiologic middle ear prosthesis: Ossicle cup and ossicle columella. Otolaryngol Head Neck Surg 90:629–634, 1982.

Smyth GDL, Kerr AG: Homologous grafts for ossicular reconstruction. Laryngoscope 77:330, 1967.

Smyth GD, Kerr AG, Goodey RJ: Tympanic membrane homograft: further evaluation. J Laryngol Otol 85:891–5, 1971.

Smyth GD: Tympanic reconstruction. Otolaryngol Clin North Am 5:111–25, 1972.

Smyth GD: Tympanic reconstruction. Fifteen year report on tympanoplasty. J Laryngol Otol 90:713–41, 1976.

Smyth GDL: Chronic Ear Disease. New York: Churchill Livingstone, 1980.

Teed RW: Cholesteatoma verum tympani. Arch Otol 25:455, 1936.

Thornburn IB: Experiences with pedicled temporal muscle flaps. J Laryngol 75:885, 1961.

Tumarkin A: Attic suppuration. J Laryngol Otol 64:611, 1950.

Tumarkin A: Pre-epidermosis. J Laryngol Otol 75:487, 1961.

Tabb HG: The surgical management of chronic ear disease. Laryngoscope 73:363, 1963.

Wehrs RE: Tympanoplasty with aeration. Arch Otolaryngol 82:18, 1965.

Wehrs RE: Homograft notched incus in tympanoplasty. Arch Otolaryngol 100:251, 1974.

Wehrs RE: Homograft ossicles in tympanoplasty. Laryngoscope 92:540, 1982.

Wehrs RE: Hearing results in tympanoplasty. Laryngoscope 95:1301, 1985.

Wullstein H: The restoration of function of the middle ear in chronic otitis media. Ann Otol Rhinol Laryngol 65:1020, 1956.

Wullstein H: Theory and practice of tympanoplasty. Laryngoscope 66:1076, 1956.

49 Complications of Acute and Chronic Otitis Media

David F. Austin

Modern chemotherapy has made otitic complications increasingly infrequent; however, they are encountered still and early recognition of the clinical patterns associated with these complications results in far more effective treatment. Formerly, a high percentage of complications were associated with virulent acute otitis media (56%). Today, most complications occur with chronic otitis media (76%) and are particularly frequent in conjunction with cholesteatoma. This has created a much more difficult therapeutic problem because the underlying otitic disease must be eliminated effectively to prevent recurrence of the complication.[1]

The complications to be considered involve extension of the disease process beyond the middle ear cleft to the meninges, lateral sinus, brain, or petrous portion of the temporal bone. The common extension of mastoid infection through the cortex to form a subperiosteal abscess has been discussed in this book.

The intracranial complications, in order of frequency, are meningitis (34%); brain abscess (25%—temporal lobe 15%, cerebellum 10%); labyrinthitis (12%); otitic hydrocephalus (12%); thrombosis of dural sinuses (10%); extradural abscess (3%); petrositis (3%); and subdural abscess (1%). Mortality and morbidity[1] have been completely altered with the advent of antibiotic therapy. The overall fatality rate with intracranial complications has fallen from 35% in the pre-antibiotic era to 5%, and the mortality rate for meningitis has been reduced from 80 to 22% and in brain abscess from 32 to 4%. These are remarkable advances indeed, but it must be remembered that the antibiotics have also made the diagnosis of these conditions more difficult because of the masking of the signs and symptoms of impending complication.

INTRACRANIAL COMPLICATION

Pathogenesis

In the progression of a middle ear infection to an intracranial complication, there are three phases through which it passes: 1) from the middle ear cleft to the meninges; 2) across the meninges; 3) into the brain tissue. Although hematogenous spread has been described on rare occasions, complication almost always occurs as a direct extension from the middle ear or mastoid. This results in involvement of either the middle or posterior cranial fossa with otogenic complication.[2,3]

Spread to the meninges may result from several factors (Fig. 49–1). Preformed pathways, such as a temporal bone fracture line, a bony dehiscence, or a surgical defect, may promote easy egress of infection. The labyrinth may also be considered a preformed pathway once it has become infected, resulting in the possibility of spread to the posterior cranial fossa. Another route of extension is by thrombophlebitis of emissary veins through the walls of the mastoid to the dura and dural sinuses.

Thrombophlebitis of the smaller haversian systems is a feature of osteomyelitis and osteitis and is the major factor in spread across the bony barrier of the mastoid and middle ear. This may result from a virulent otitis media and mastoiditis or a chronic otitis media. Complication in chronic ear disease usually follows an acute exacerbation of infection. The infection invades areas previously broken down or, in the case of cholesteatoma, spread through areas eroded by the cholesteatoma matrix which may be lying on bare dura.

The route of invasion[4] of the infection is thus determined by many factors: the extent and course of mastoid pneumatization, the location and areas of erosion

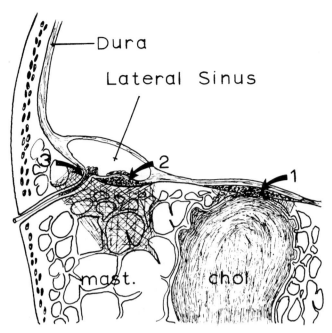

Fig. 49–1. Pathogenesis of complications; methods of spread to the meninges: 1) a cholesteatoma has caused erosion of the mastoid with the matrix lying against the dura; infection has resulted in an extradural abscess; 2) osteitis of the mastoid has caused thrombophlebitis of the haversian system with resultant perisinus abscess; a mural thrombus is forming in the lateral sinus adjacent to the abscess; 3) osteitis has involved a mastoid emissary vein; the infected thrombus is propagating into the lumen of the lateral sinus.

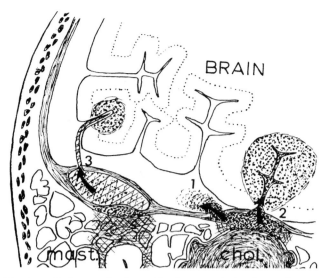

Fig. 49–2. Pathogenesis of complications; methods of spread across the meninges: 1) an extradural abscess has broken through the dura, resulting in a subdural abscess or spread into the subarachnoid space and diffuse meningitis; 2) the subarachnoid space has been obliterated through inflammatory reaction, resulting in direct invasion of the brain as the dura breaks down; this results in the "brain abscess with a stalk;" 3) the infected thrombus in the lateral sinus has extended along a communicating vessel, resulting in a cerebellar abscess.

of cholesteatoma, the areas of involvement in previous mastoid infection, and sites of predilection created by prior surgery. As suppurative infection extends to adjacent areas, local defense reactions are called into play, usually resulting in localized abscess formation. Extension through the mastoid cortex has been described previously. Extension across the tegmen results in extradural abscess of the middle fossa, whereas extension across the posterior wall of the temporal bone results in either extradural abscess or perisinus abscess. An osteitis without bone necrosis may cause a localized extradural abscess without an obvious communication with the middle ear cleft.

Spread across the meninges is initiated as the disease reaches the dura, with a resultant pachymeningitis (Fig. 49–2). The dura is extremely resistant to the spread of infection, becoming thickened, hyperemic, and more adherent to the adjacent bone. Granulation tissue forms on the exposed dura, and the adjacent subdural space may be obliterated. If an extradural abscess forms across the tegmen, it may become large because of the loose attachment of the dura to the temporal squama. In the posterior fossa, the dura is much more tightly attached, and an abscess in this location is much smaller. This is also true of the superior surface of the petrous bone medial to the arcuate eminence. If the primary area of involvement is adjacent to the

sigmoid sinus, abscess formation is termed "perisinus abscess." In this region, thrombophlebitis of the dural vessels may propagate, or local sinus wall irritation may lead to mural thrombus formation. Both of these processes may lead to sinus thrombosis, which may be either aseptic or suppurative.

If these first local measures to limit the spread of infection fail because of necrosis of the dura, invasion of the subdural space takes place. Although this space has usually been obliterated by the preceding inflammatory response, empyema may occasionally occur, with widespread diffusion through the entire plane, even to the opposite hemisphere. Subdural infection is most often localized but may increase in size to involve underlying cortical tissue by thrombophlebitis with the formation of multiple small brain abscesses. In direct extension of the infection to the brain, the subdural and subarachnoid spaces have been obliterated, usually resulting in a direct tract to the brain substance forming an "abscess with a stalk."

Infection of the dura and subdural space promotes reaction of the pia-arachnoid with serous meningitis. Attempts at localization often produce an arachnoid cyst, particularly in the posterior cranial fossa. Enlargement of this cyst may produce symptoms because of encroachment on the cerebellum. Rupture of localized dural, subdural, or arachnoid abscesses results in sudden diffuse meningitis. Meningitis often occurs by direct extension through the dura without prior abscess formation. This is particularly true with virulent microorganisms or markedly lowered resistance. Early in the development of meningitis, a serous effusion occurs which proceeds to suppuration if the infection is not quickly controlled. Serous meningitis may occur as a reaction to dural irritation, in which case the spinal fluid is sterile and the symptoms of meningitis are milder (meningismus). As infection develops, bacteria and acute inflammatory cells appear in the spinal fluid, and more marked symptoms and signs occur.

Spread into the brain tissue results in abscess formation, usually in the region midway between the ventricle and the surface of the cortex or in the center of the lobule of the cerebellum. This is a result of the method of progression of the infection into the brain tissue and occurs by either thrombophlebitis or extension of the infection into the Virchow-Robin spaces, terminating at the subcortical vascular area. Often sinus thrombosis results in thrombophlebitis of the communicating vessels with consequent cerebellar abscess explaining the frequent association of these complications.

Focal necrosis and liquefaction of the white matter are surrounded by an area of reaction. This edema and encephalitis may be extensive, causing more danger to life than the initiating abscess. Within several days, the process of encapsulation takes place by mobilization of microglia and fibrocytes. With capsule formation, the surrounding edema and encephalitis subside, resulting in a quiescent period.

Several courses may then follow. The capsule of the abscess may calcify with subsequent complete healing. The abscess may rupture, with the formation of one or more satellite abscesses. Rupture may take place into the ventricular system with subsequent meningitis. Enlargement of the abscess may result in external or internal hydrocephalus. Intermittent, inadequate drainage through the inflammatory tract into the subarachnoid space or mastoid cavity may cause intermittency in the symptoms.

The disease may be arrested at any phase or may involve the total process. This requires knowledge of the symptoms and signs of each specific complication and the ability to recognize an impending or beginning intracranial extension of the disease. Great watchfulness is required during the treatment of the complication to recognize the progression of one complication to another, so that suitable adjustment of therapy can be made.

Diagnosis of Impending Complication

Thorough acquaintance with the normal progress of both acute and chronic otitis media is a prerequisite to diagnosis of a threatened complication.[6] If a total program of treatment does not result in prompt remission of symptoms with cessation of discharge and otoscopic findings of resolution of the inflammation and fluid accumulation, the physician should become

watchful. Except in the initial stages of acute disease, the patient is not ill, so that continued elevation of temperature, pain, or signs of toxicity may be danger signals. The development of headache, usually parietal or occipital, is a grave warning and may indicate that intracranial involvement has already taken place. Malaise, drowsiness or somnolence, nausea and vomiting, and irritability all indicate extension of the disease. The signs of labyrinthine involvement will be discussed later. Children do not usually complain of headache and should be observed carefully. Their chief finding is signs of toxicity and a continued febrile state.

Findings in these cases may be the recurrence of aural discharge after initial response to treatment. Usually the drumhead remains inflamed, assuming at times a violaceous hue. In chronic otitis media, the signs of extension may occur after discharge has ceased, indicating the presence of purulent secretion under pressure. Persistence of temperature elevation while the patient is on therapy or following completion of therapy is a definite sign.

Computed tomography (CT) at this time may help by showing evidence of breakdown of the walls of the mastoid. For these findings to be reliable, however, they must be of excellent quality and taken in several planes. Evidence of bony breakdown is an absolute sign of complication and indicates immediate surgical intervention.

Lumbar puncture should be performed when it has been determined that the danger of complication exists. The patient will have been hospitalized, and these findings are extremely helpful in arriving at an exact determination of the type of complication occurring. Examination should include determination of the pressure level, smear, and culture for microorganisms, cell count, and chemical determination of protein, sugar and chloride content. Even if the findings are within normal limits, this information is of value as a base line if future spinal fluid examination becomes necessary.

Axial CT or magnetic resonance imaging (MR) is uniformly positive in obtaining both diagnosis and anatomic localization of the disease. Although expensive, the methods are cost-effective because of their ability to provide essential information.

Specific Symptoms and Signs

Because the formation of an extradural abscess is the initiating process in the extension of disease, this complication was formerly common. Now most acute infections or exacerbation of chronic infection are quickly treated with antibiotics, which often limits or prevents this initial type of spread. If the antibiotics have not been effective, the initial symptoms are headache, toxicity, and a persistent mild febrile state. The most significant clue is the persistence of infection in spite of adequate treatment. The abscess may spontaneously drain into the mastoid cavity, causing an increase in aural discharge.

Extradural abscess may be localized at the petrous apex, producing fifth and sixth nerve symptoms and signs of facial pain and lateral rectus paralysis (Gradenigo's syndrome). In the middle fossa, lateral to the arcuate eminence, the dura is rather loosely attached to the calvarium. Extradural abscess in this region may become extensive, involving the entire temporal squama. Breakdown of the squama may occur with involvement of the periosteum above the external ear. Subperiosteal abscess may then form at a distance above the pinna, causing a fluctuant swelling (Pott's puffy tumor).

The advent of chemotherapy has reduced the incidence of sinus thrombosis from 31% of complications in the pre-antibiotic era to 10%. This complication, though occurring less frequently, is dangerous because the former mortality rate of 38% seems to have been lowered only slightly. The reason for this is that sinus thrombosis is frequently (45%) associated with other complications, particularly meningitis, cerebellar abscess, and multiple sinus thrombosis occasionally extending to include the cavernous sinus.

Infection surrounding the lateral sinus causes the formation of a mural thrombus. This may progress to complete occlusion of the sinus lumen, with the possibility of growth in both directions and involvement of tributary vessels. Prompt treatment of the initiating infection may result in resolution, leaving a noninfected but thrombosed lateral sinus. This is usually asymptomatic, being discovered incidentally in later years at mastoid surgery. Invasion of the sinus by the infecting microorganism, usually hemolytic streptococci or type III pneumococci, results in purulent breakdown of the thrombus, septicemia, and bacteremia.

The onset of sinus thrombosis is marked by the appearance of a septic course typified by a high spiking temperature accompanied by marked toxicity, rapid pulse, chills, and sweating. During the frequent remissions, the patient looks and feels well, even euphoric. The fever quickly recurs, occasionally as often as every 4 hours. Nausea and vomiting may be present, and such severe symptoms as shock or convulsions occasionally occur. Headache, if present, is usually not severe and is not a prominent feature of this disease.

Involvement of the superior petrosal sinus may extend further into the cavernous sinus, causing the appearance of proptosis and chemosis, usually on the involved side. Pain in the lower jaw is frequently present. Involvement of the jugular bulb may lead to paralysis of the ninth, tenth, and eleventh cranial nerves.

The most typical and common finding in lateral sinus thrombosis is tenderness over the posterior mastoid at the exit of the mastoid emissary vein. Inflammatory response at this point may also cause redness and edema over the surface of the mastoid. Lumbar puncture shows normal spinal fluid, but the pressure may be increased, particularly with involvement of the larger sigmoid sinus or spread to the confluence of sinuses. With increase of the cerebrospinal fluid pressure, papilledema is often present. The Tobey-Ayer test (comparing the rise in CSF pressure with the alternate compression of each jugular vein) or the Queckenstedt test (bilateral simultaneous compression of the jugular veins) is helpful in determining the presence of lateral sinus thrombosis. The Lillie-Crow test gives the same indication by observing the retinal vein engorgement when the opposite jugular vein is compressed in the presence of lateral sinus thrombosis.

Blood cultures taken during the onset of a febrile period are positive in a high percentage of patients. This bacteremia may lead to the development of metastatic abscesses, particularly in the lung. The simultaneous occurrence of an ear infection with chest pain and productive cough should warn one of the possibility of pyogenic emboli from the lateral sinus.

Otitic hydrocephalus is most commonly a variant of sinus thrombosis. Typically, this complication follows an acute ear infection about 10 to 20 days after resolution. The increase in spinal fluid pressure may be accompanied by headache, nausea and vomiting, vertigo, and occasionally lateral rectus paralysis. These symptoms are usually quite mild. The marked increase in spinal fluid pressure (often above 300 mm H_2O) is accompanied by papilledema, while the spinal fluid chemistry remains normal.

The complication usually shows a slow resolution over a period of weeks to months without specific treatment. Persistence of papilledema may result in optic atrophy. To prevent this, frequent removal of cerebrospinal fluid by lumbar puncture may become necessary. In the case of bilateral sinus thrombosis with permanent increase of intracranial pressure, shunting procedures may be considered.

Subdural abscess, the purulent stage of pachymeningitis interna, is rare today. When it occurs, it must be regarded as a neurosurgical emergency, requiring immediate intervention to prevent a fatal termination. Purulent effusion collects rapidly in the subdural space over the ipsilateral cerebral hemisphere extending to or into the falx cerebri. Reaction may produce loculation or obliteration by adhesion of the dura to the pia-arachnoid.

The clinical picture is characterized by a rapid onset of severe headache, toxicity, and somnolence proceeding to coma. Irritation of the cerebral cortex produces Jacksonian seizures, whose pattern is a help in localizing the involved region. Paralysis of motor function consisting of contralateral hemiplegia or facial paralysis may occur. The cranial nerves may be affected by collections of purulent exudate causing, in many instances, oculomotor paralysis with ptosis and loss of conjugate deviation. Meningeal irritation is not predominant in this condition, and lumbar puncture helps to differentiate it from meningitis. The spinal fluid is usually clear without bacteria or change in chemistry. Spinal fluid pressure is usually moderately increased. Definite diagnosis is made by exploratory burr holes after a positive CT, which are therapeutic with evacuation of the purulent exudate.

Otogenic meningitis may occur at any time during the course of an ear infection. Meningitis may cause labyrinthitis by extension through the internal auditory canal or may follow labyrinthitis by the reverse route. The usual method of spread is by direct extension, seldom with thrombophlebitis. The mortality rate with meningitis has been reduced in the antibiotic era, but it is still a serious problem; death occurs in 25 to 35% of these patients. With multiple complications, the fatality rate is greater than 50%.

The development of meningitis is usually divided into three stages: serous, cellular, and bacterial. As the infecting microorganism, usually streptococci, pneumococci, or staphylococci, and less commonly H. influenzae, and coliform, bacillus, invades the subarachnoid space, the pia-arachnoid reacts with the exudation of serous fluid which raises mildly the level of CSF pressure. Clinically, this corresponds with mild symptoms of headache, slightly increased temperature, hyperirritability, and slightly positive signs of meningeal irritation. These signs are nuchal rigidity which occurs in all degrees from slight resistance to a fixed hyperextension; Kernig's sign, which is the inability to extend the leg on a flexed thigh due to pain in the back; and Brudzinski's sign, which is flexion of the legs at the knee when flexion of the head is attempted.

Progression may be arrested at this stage, or the disease may progress to the cellular stage in which there is an effusion of leukocytes into the spinal fluid. In addition to the increase in cells (often to a concentration of 1000/ml or more), there is an increase in the protein level and a mild decrease in chloride and sugar content. With the onset of the cellular stage, there is an increase in the severity of the clinical picture described as "bursting pain," the appearance of vomiting and cerebral hyperirritability with periods of delirium, confusion, and drowsiness. Photophobia and withdrawal from tactile stimulation will now occur. During periods of irritation, the patient lies on his side, in a fetal position facing the wall to avoid all stimulation. The temperature is continuously elevated, from 101 to 102 degrees Fahrenheit, usually with a lowered pulse rate.

The bacterial stage occurs with the appearance of frank pus in the spinal fluid. This is marked not only by the finding of bacteria on smear and culture of the fluid but also by the marked reduction (sometimes to zero) of spinal fluid sugar content because of the bacterial utilization. If the disease is not arrested at this stage, the previous hyperirritability progresses to somnolence and coma with cranial nerve paralysis appearing, most often involving the extraocular muscles. Incontinence and death may rapidly follow. Opisthotonos often occurs in these late stages, particularly in children.

The diagnosis of meningitis is usually not difficult with the classic picture presented. Lumbar puncture usually results in prompt accurate diagnosis. Sinus thrombosis or brain abscess coupled with meningitis may confuse the picture somewhat. In general, papilledema, epileptic seizures, or focal paralysis do not occur with uncomplicated meningitis and should point to no other disease. A leaking brain abscess may produce recurrent signs of meningeal irritation. The possibility of concurrent disease must not be forgotten when dealing with otogenic meningitis, and appropriate diagnostic measures should be taken in all such patients.

Brain abscess is the ultimate complication in both severity and difficulty of management. Combining, as it does, the aspects of both a space-occupying and a space-consuming lesion, its presence implies deficits that are often significant to the patient even after a cure is effected.

Because this complication occurs almost always as a direct extension from mastoid disease (usually chronic), the temporal lobe or cerebellum is involved on the side of the disease. Brain abscess often occurs as one of many complications, and carries a much greater risk to life than when occurring alone (50% versus 5 to 10% mortality). Cerebellar abscess usually occurs with preceding sinus thrombosis and temporal lobe abscess with subdural or extradural abscess. A leaking brain abscess may cause recurrent episodes of meningitis.

The initial stages of brain abscess are accompanied by a wide surrounding zone of encephalitis, causing marked edema and resulting in an increase in cerebrospinal fluid pressure. Marked variation in symptoms and signs may occur, principally owing to variation in the degree of edema present. If virulence of infection does not result in rapid demise, encapsulation of the abscess proceeds, with a definite walling off occurring within 10 to 14 days. A fibrous capsule is formed within a 5- to 6-week period. Encapsulation of the abscess is accompanied by a marked reduction of symptoms and signs because of regression of the surrounding encephalitis and edema. Exacerbation may take place, with rupture of the capsule and formation of satellite abscesses. Even after a firm fibrous capsule has formed, this may occur. Eventually calcification of the abscess wall takes place.

The general symptoms of brain abscess are those of a space-occupying lesion complicated by infection. There is an initial increase of intracranial pressure, with the accompanying symptoms of headache, nausea, and vomiting. Somnolence and confusion, sometimes combined with delusions or hallucinations, are often present. These symptoms characteristically vary in degree, depending on the state of edema, encapsulation, virulence, and response to treatment. Often these milder initial symptoms may be masked by the more striking features of other acute concomitant complications. With increasing severity, stupor and coma ensue, accompanied by a slow pulse and subnormal temperature. Papilledema does not appear until 10 to 14 days after onset, but with a rapidly progressive case, tentorial herniation or herniation of the cerebellar tonsils takes place, accompanied by fixation and dilation of the pupils and finally respiratory paralysis. In cases of milder severity, the varying general symptoms plus certain localizing symptoms and signs permit the diagnosis.

Localizing signs vary depending on the site and degree of involvement. The signs of temporal lobe abscess depend on whether the dominant side is involved. Dominant temporal lobe abscesses commonly cause aphasia, which may be complete or partial. Abscess in either temporal lobe may cause homonymous hemianopsia because of interference with the optic radiations. Spread upward from the temporal lobe initially causes a contralateral upper motor neuron facial paralysis with further progression resulting in upper limb and finally lower limb paralysis. Involvement of the minor temporal lobe, if small, is difficult to diagnose, causing vague symptoms of finger and body image agnosia. Often the general condition of these patients prevents the painstaking examination necessary to establish these aberrations.

The findings in cerebellar abscess may be few, even with one of massive size. The most typical findings are nystagmus, incoordination, and ipsilateral loss of muscle tone. Cerebellar nystagmus is spontaneous, slow, and coarse. It may be horizontal, usually with the quick component toward the involved side, rotatory, or vertical, which is an absolute sign of an intracranial involvement. Incoordination primarily involves the side of the lesion and is best tested by noting differences in fine motor coordination of the two sides. Such tests are grasping objects, finger-to-nose pointing, and one leg standing are most helpful in this regard. Dysdiadochokinesia is also present on the involved side. The patient falls to the side of the lesion, often telling of striking the door jamb when entering a room. Slurring of speech and difficulty in swallowing may also be present.

Diagnosis is based primarily on the clinical history, with confirmation helped by several forms of investigation. Lumbar puncture should be performed unless there is evidence of severely elevated intracranial pressure. This usually reveals some elevation of pressure, protein, and cell count, but may show no change from normal. Electroencephalography is of value and may show focal abnormality. A normal EEG does not rule out a brain abscess, however. Skull films may show shift of the pineal or even gas within the abscess. Arteriograms are of value in localizing the site of the lesion. Brain imaging performed with MR has improved diagnostic efficiency.

Treatment

The treatment of the intracranial complications of otitis media must be twofold; not only must effective care of the complication be instituted, but also resolution of the primary disease must be accomplished. Often the severity of the complication requires delaying necessary mastoid surgery until the patient is well enough to tolerate the procedure. On the other hand, the complication, especially if impending or early in its course, may be treated with the same procedure that controls the primary disease. In brief, the essence of treatment consists of rapid institution of large doses of antibiotics, surgical management of the primary mastoid infection at the optimum time, and neurosurgical control of the intracranial lesion when required. Because neurosurgical and otologic cooperation has been used in the investigative phase, this team should continue in the combined management.

The antibiotic management of these problems is complicated by the blood-brain barrier, which prevents achieving a high concentration of many antibiotics in the cerebrospinal fluid. As new antibiotics have appeared the efficacy of medical treatment has improved. Cephalosporins now are predominant in the treatment regime, ceftriaxone being the most used. This agent may be combined with others as needed. Chloramphenicol is still a useful adjunct. Every effort should be made to obtain a positive culture for sensitivity, either from the primary mastoid infection or the spinal fluid. If sensitivity tests or poor response to treatment indicate, another agent may be needed. Antibiotic therapy should be continued until the febrile course ends.

Surgical management, ideally, should be undertaken early in the course of the complication. The factors entering into this consideration are the diagnosis, the condition of the patient, and the response to antibiotic treatment. Continued spill or irritation from a cholesteatoma in the mastoid may cause a recurrent meningitis or progression in a brain abscess, so that control of the primary disease is essential for full recovery of the patient. In some instances, drainage of a subdural empyema or of an abscess must take precedence, but the mastoid surgery should be undertaken as soon thereafter as the patient's condition permits.

Surgical approach to the mastoidectomy in these cases should allow complete removal of the inciting pathologic condition. In most instances this requires modified radical mastoidectomy, although extensive simple mastoidectomy may be performed if control can be obtained. The essential part of the surgery is to expose and explore all possible routes of invasion of the infection. The bone overlying the sigmoid sinus should be thinned and removed. The posterior dural plate in Trautmann's triangle should be thinned, and the mastoid tegmen should be skeletonized in all cases.

Suspicion of underlying disease should be aroused by the presence of soft necrotic bone or violaceous granulation, sometimes covered by purulent exudate. The dura is normally firm and pale blue, with the sinus a deeper blue. A freely bleeding, inflammation of the dura indicates infection. Often the removal of necrotic bone releases the pus contained in a perisinus or extradural abscess.

Sinus thrombophlebitis is treated by opening the sinus after exposing it from the sinodural angle to the jugular bulb. All the necrotic or infected thrombus is aspirated and the sinus packed open. Surgicel is a good material for this purpose because it is slowly absorbed and obviates the necessity of delayed removal of gauze packing. Firm fibrous clot need not be removed because it helps prevent the extension of the infection.

The use of anticoagulants and jugular vein ligation has been advocated in the past to prevent the propagation of the thrombus but has been proved particularly effective in routine use. Anticoagulants may be used in situations in which growth of the thrombus becomes widespread with involvement of the petrosal and cavernous sinuses or the confluence of sinuses. Jugular ligation is rarely needed today with the control of septic emboli by antibiotics. Rather, a continued septic course calls for re-exploration of the sinus through the mastoid with further removal of the infected thrombus.

Jugular ligation, if indicated, is performed through a 2- to 3-inch incision at the anterior margin of the sternocleidomastoid muscle just below the mastoid tip. The vein is doubly ligated and divided between the ligatures.

The presence of otitic hydrocephalus may require repeated spinal taps, especially if optic atrophy is threatened. Usually, surgical treatment of the sinus thrombosis results in a gradual reduction of intracranial pressure.

Meningitis is treated primarily by antibiotic therapy. The possibility of an associated complication such as an abscess or thrombophlebitis should always be kept in mind and mastoid exploration undertaken if the expected response to treatment does not occur. Recurrence of otogenic meningitis is common, and it is felt that mastoid exploration should be performed in any case of recurrent meningitis regardless of the type of otitis media. In most cases, an area of bone necrosis is found, occasionally associated with an extradural collection of pus. This unresolved disease is undoubtedly responsible for the reinfection in these cases.

Subdural abscess is a severe and life-endangering complication whose treatment is a neurosurgical emergency. Bur holes are made above and below the involved area, and the purulent collection is aspirated. Irrigation, first with physiologic solution and then with an antibiotic-containing solution, is carried out, and the rubber drains are left in place so that frequent irrigation may be done. It is usually necessary to delay mastoid surgery until the empyema has resolved, but it should be done without more delay than is necessary for the neurosurgical treatment.

Brain abscess is again primarily a neurosurgical problem. Drainage of the abscess through the mastoid tegmen has been described in the past but is a risky procedure because of the possibility of herniation of the brain through the drainage site with the formation of a brain fungus. The best plan of management is to control the mastoid disease and associated extradural abscess through the mastoid and to treat the brain abscess from above through the cortex.

When the abscess has walled off and been localized, it is treated by either tapping or excision. Tapping is done through a bur hole. When the abscess has been reached, it is aspirated, and contrast material mixed with solution containing an appropriate antibiotic is instilled so that the progress of the abscess may be followed with radiographic examination. One aspiration may suffice, but usually several are required. A multilocular abscess presents a more difficult problem but is treated in essentially the same manner.

Excision of the abscess offers the opportunity to examine the dura and control the route of invasion, as well as the removal of the diseased area.

It is a great help in these situations to correlate closely the mastoid and neurologic surgery. A continuous spill of infection into the brain tissue from the involved mastoid delays the response to treatment. Ideally both areas should be treated concurrently. Severely ill patients, of course, cannot be treated in this way, but as soon as control of infection has resulted in reduction of cerebral edema, surgical care should be rendered.

INFLAMMATORY DISEASES OF THE LABYRINTH

Various circumscribed or diffuse forms of labyrinthitis are caused by most types of microorganisms capable of producing inflammatory reactions.[8] The most practical classification from a clinical and pathologic standpoint is:

1. Circumscribed
2. Diffuse serous
3. Diffuse suppurative
    a. Acute (manifest) stage
    b. Chronic (latent) stage

If toxins penetrate the labyrinth (usually through the round or oval windows), a serous type of labyrinthitis may result. A fistula is usually not present in this form. If the serous labyrinthitis is secondary to a cholesteatoma with erosion into the lateral canal, the fistula test is usually positive.

Circumscribed Labyrinthitis

Definition

A circumscribed labyrinthitis is, as its name implies, an infection or inflammation of a portion of the labyrinth, usually the external limb of the lateral canal. Theoretically, any portion of the vestibular or cochlear labyrinth may be involved.

Causes

The most common cause of circumscribed labyrinthitis is a cholesteatoma which has eroded into the lateral canal with the formation of a fistula. Occasionally, the oval window or the promontory is the pathway. At times, the superior or posterior canal is involved. The cochlea is less often affected, but when invasion does occur, the infection is more likely to cause a diffuse labyrinthitis. Either circumscribed or diffuse labyrinthitis may occur following mastoidectomy.

A circumscribed labyrinthitis with a positive fistula sign may be observed at times in congenital syphilis, the various granulomas, or temporal bone tumors if a softened area is formed in the bony capsule over a semicircular canal which exposes the membranous structure of the canal.

Extension to the labyrinth is more likely to occur during an acute exacerbation of a chronic otitis media than during a quiescent period of the otitis.

Pneumococcal type III infection of the middle ear and mastoid cells tends to break through one or more of the semicircular canals by way of the perilabyrinthine cells, especially the retrolabyrinthine group. In type III pneumococcal infection of the labyrinth, an epidural abscess of the posterior fossa is almost invariably present, and purulent meningitis frequently follows.

Pathology

A fistula, usually of the lateral semicircular canal, is present in probably more than half of the cases of circumscribed labyrinthitis. Fistulas may also form at the round and oval windows (Figs. 49–3 and 49–4), at the promontorium, or at the tympanic orifice of the Eustachian tube. No portion of the labyrinth, vestibular or acoustic, would be exempt, however, from possible fistula formation.

The fistula usually erodes only the bony labyrinth but may extend into the membranous portion. In the latter event, the pathologic process is much more likely to become diffuse. Fistulas located in the round or oval

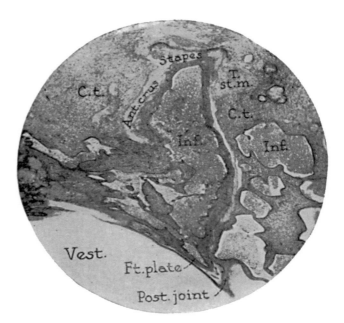

Fig. 49–3. Severe infection around the oval window. An acute suppurative process (Inf.) with some connective tissue (C.t.) in the region of the stapes and oval window. Mrs. T., aged 37, developed otitis media (right), mastoiditis, and intracranial complications (Streptococcus pyogenes). Autopsy, 16 days after the first symptoms, revealed a subdural abscess, thrombosis of the sigmoid and inferior petrosal sinuses, and meningitis. In spite of the severe infection about the stapes, the internal ear was not involved in that region, but a circumscribed labyrinthitis with a fistula of the round window (see Fig. 49–4) was found. The footplate and posterior joint of the stapes are shown. The anterior joint of the stapes and part of the crus do not show at this level of sectioning. The tendon of the stapedius muscle (T.st.m.) may be observed. ×36. (Courtesy of Dr. E. W. Hagens).

windows, the promontory, or the tympanic mouth of the Eustachian tube may involve the membranous cochlea and its nerves.

A fistula from any portion of the middle ear is formed by a primary breakdown of the middle ear mucosa, followed by resorption of a portion of the labyrinthine capsule to the endosteum. Bone resorption begins along the vascular canals. Erosion by a cholesteatoma may occur without a primary bacterial invasion of the labyrinth.

Symptoms

The acute stage of a circumscribed labyrinthitis lasts about a week. It begins with recurring attacks of dizziness and at times nausea, usually made worse by movements of the head and body. A spontaneous nystagmus toward the involved ear is present during the attacks. The temperature and hearing acuity are essentially normal. If there is any hearing loss, it is of the conductive type and of no greater degree than usually found in otitis media. The temporary hearing loss in the diffuse serous forms of labyrinthitis is usually greater than in the circumscribed type.

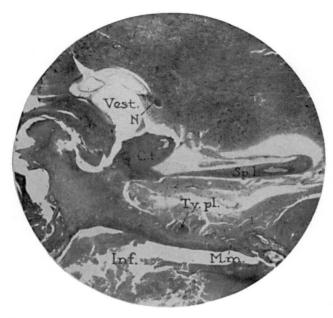

Fig. 49–4. Circumscribed labyrinthitis with a fistula of the round window. Horizontal section at the level of the start of the cochlea (same patient as in Fig. 49–3). Connective tissue (C.t.) formation has replaced the round window and grown into the vestibule (Vest.). The spiral ligament (Sp.l.) and the nerve (N) to the crista of the posterior semicircular canal are normal. Extensive infection (Inf.) in the tympanic cavity, with the thickened mucosa (M.m.) overlying the bony promontory, may be observed. The tympanic plexus (Ty.pl.) is normal. ×11. (Courtesy of Dr. E.W. Hagens).

In the chronic stage, intermittent attacks of vertigo, made worse or brought on by sudden movements of the head or at times by bending over, are usually noted. In some individuals, vertigo is absent. A low-grade spontaneous nystagmus may or may not be seen and, when present, may be in either direction.

The Fistula Sign

The presence of a fistula is determined by the fistula test, in which either compression or rarefaction of air in the external auditory canal is done. An airtight speculum of Siegle's otoscope or a rubber bag with an olive tip is inserted into the external auditory meatus. Compression of the bag or relaxation of the compressed bag produces increased or decreased air pressure within the canal, and if a patent fistula is present, a compression or expansion of the membranous labyrinth results. If a fistula is present, vertigo and nystagmus are caused by either compression or reduction of the air pressure, to one side by compression and to the opposite by decreased pressure. The fistula sign may be absent if the fistula is blocked by granulations or other obstructions.

Diagnosis

The clinical diagnosis of a circumscribed labyrinthitis is based on a history of recurrent attacks of vertigo and nystagmus in the presence of chronic otitis media and a positive fistula test. It is usually possible to demonstrate bony erosion of the labyrinth by CT.

Treatment

The treatment of a circumscribed labyrinthitis is directed primarily toward the chronic otitis media and/or the cholesteatoma. If the circumscribed labyrinthitis is in an acute stage, or before or after some surgical procedure, adequate treatment with antibiotics should be given.

Surgical treatment should be directed toward, and be adequate for, control of the primary disease process. Cholesteatoma matrix is usually removed from the eroded labyrinth with deft and sharp technique, and the area is immediately covered with connective tissue.

Diffuse Serous Labyrinthitis

The acute form of diffuse serous labyrinthitis (Figs. 49–5 and 49–6) is frequently secondary to a pre-existing circumscribed labyrinthitis, or may occur as a primary labyrinthitis following an acute middle ear infection in which toxins (and possibly bacteria) gain entrance to the labyrinthitis through the round and oval windows or through an erosion of the bony capsule. The erosion in this event reaches the endosteum by way of the vascular channels. The so-called diffuse serous induced labyrinthitis of Alexander and Ruttin frequently follows a mastoid operation, especially if the patient has had a previous circumscribed peri- or paralabyrinthitis. The symptoms in this event appear from the first to the fifth day after the operation. If serous labyrinthitis follows a direct injury to the labyrinth during the operation, the symptoms appear at once. This latter form may develop into a diffuse suppurative type within a few days. Edema of the middle ear may extend into the labyrinth, producing serous labyrinthitis. Probably the most common cause of serous labyrinthitis is the absorption into the labyrinth of toxic products from bacterial activity in the middle ear and mastoid.

A mild form of serous labyrinthitis follows surgery of the inner ear. This was almost universal after the fenestration or stapes operation or stapes surgery for otosclerosis. This form is short-lived and the high-tone hearing loss that occasionally follows this surgery is often ascribed to this cause.

Pathology

The essential pathology is that of a nonpurulent inflammation of the labyrinth. A section of the labyrinth examined histologically by Lindsay[9] showed an early cellular infiltration with a serous or a serofibrinous exudate.

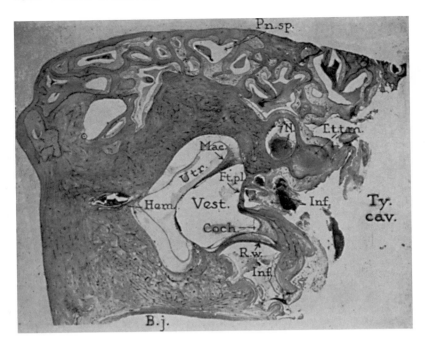

Fig. 49–5. Serous and suppurative labyrinthitis with extension of the infection to the labyrinth through the round window. M.I., a boy aged 3 years, gave a history of left otitis with fever and opisthotonus. Examination revealed left otitis media, mastoiditis (mastoid operated on), and meningitis (pneumococcal). At autopsy, a bilateral osteitis, otitis media, and labyrinthitis were found. The vertical coronal section shows the footplate of the stapes (Ft.pl.) resisting the extensive infection (Inf.), whereas the round window (R.w.) is infiltrated with cells. There is quite an accumulation of cells in the scala tympani at the start of the cochlea (Coch.). The utricle (Utr.) reveals a serous labyrinthitis. A hemorrhagic (Hem.) accumulation may be seen in the common crus of the semicircular canal. The facial nerve (7 N.), tendon of the tensor tympani muscle (T.t.t.m.), tympanic cavity (Ty.cav.), and jugular bulb (B.j.) may be seen. The extensive development of the infected pneumatic spaces (Pn.sp.) is unusual for a child 3 years of age. ×9. (Courtesy of Dr. E.W. Hagens).

Symptoms

The symptoms and signs of an acute labyrinthine upset are spontaneous, rotational vertigo, nystagmus, usually to the diseased side; and a beginning sensorineural hearing loss. These symptoms and signs come on suddenly if the labyrinthitis is of the induced type, that is, not associated with a fistula or due to a circumscribed labyrinthitis. In the former event, prodromal labyrinthine symptom are absent. The fistula sign would be absent. A history of a acute otitis media or a preceding mastoid operation is usually obtained.

A serous labyrinthitis secondary to a circumscribed labyrinthitis has similar but less severe symptoms because of some compensation that may have developed.

The fistula test is positive unless blocking of the fistula has occurred. A history of previous labyrinthitis from a circumscribed labyrinthitis may be obtained. The temperature in serous labyrinthitis is normal or near normal.

Differential Diagnosis

The degree and permanence of the hearing loss are important in differentiating serous from suppurative labyrinthitis. In the serous type, hearing loss is temporary, usually not great, whereas in diffuse suppurative labyrinthitis, it is total and permanent. If the hearing loss is great or complete in serous labyrinthitis, an early change into the diffuse suppurative type is possible.

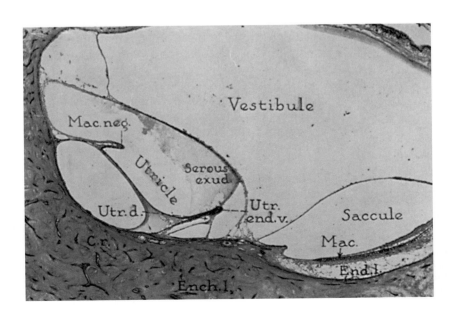

Fig. 49–6. Acute circumscribed serous labyrinthitis. C.S., a boy aged 10 years, gave a history of bilateral acute otitis media with headache and stiffness of the neck. The postmortem examination revealed a streptococcal meningitis with a bilateral osteitis of the temporal bone and a circumscribed serous labyrinthitis of the utricle on the left side. Various structures may be seen, such as the utricular duct (Utr.d.), utriculoendolymphatic valve (Utr.end.v.), macula neglecta (Mac.neg.), macula (Mac.) of saccule, endosteal layer (End.l.) of the bony labyrinth, and endochondral wider layer (Ench.l.) with the cartilaginous rests (C.r.). ×32.5. (Courtesy of Dr. E.W. Hagens).

If hearing loss is marked, masking of the good ear is necessary to prevent the transmission of sound to the better ear through the bone conduction. If some hearing, however small, is present in the affected ear, a diffuse suppurative labyrinthitis has not occurred, and the vestibular tests are not necessary to demonstrate a partially functioning labyrinth.

Diffuse serous labyrinthitis should be differentiated from noninflammatory diseases of the labyrinth and eighth nerve.

Prognosis

The prognosis in serous labyrinthitis is good in terms of survival and, usually, restoration of labyrinthine function unless the serous form changes into the suppurative type. A severe temporary type of deafness may cause some permanent hearing loss in serous labyrinthitis.

Treatment

Absolute bed rest is indicated during the acute stage. Mild sedation may be given. Antibiotics should be used in sufficient quantity and long enough to reach maximum efficacy.

Surgery is contraindicated. Adequate drainage of the middle ear should be maintained and in a later stage of an acute otitis media, simple mastoidectomy may be necessary. Tympanomastoidectomy may be advisable if a cholesteatoma with a fistula is present.

Acute Diffuse Suppurative Labyrinthitis

Acute diffuse suppurative labyrinthitis is characterized by complete deafness in the affected ear, associated with extreme vertigo (as a rule), nausea, vomiting, ataxia, and spontaneous nystagmus directed to the other ear (Figs. 49–5 and 49–7).

Causes

Suppurative labyrinthitis may follow a circumscribed type or develop from the induced serous form in which the infection enters through the round or oval windows. In many instances, the labyrinthitis is secondary to an acute or chronic otitis media or mastoiditis. In some cases, a subdural abscess or meningitis extends into the interior of the bony labyrinth with or without a middle ear involvement.

Pathology

The pathology consists of an infiltration of the labyrinth with polymorphonuclear leukocytes, combined with destruction of the soft tissue structures (Figs. 49–8 to 49–11). The osseous labyrinth may become carious in part. Granulation tissue forms and may at times wall off a portion of the necrotic bone, forming one or more sequestra. Paralysis of the facial nerve may occur, or the infection may extend to the intracranial structures if it is virulent.

Symptoms

Nausea, vomiting, vertigo, and ataxia are severe if the onset of the suppurative labyrinthitis is rapid. In the slower-developing form, these symptoms may be somewhat moderate because of the compensating action of the opposite labyrinth.

The quick component of the horizontal rotary nystagmus is directed to the other ear. If the patient is observed in the first few hours of the disease, before the function of the vestibular labyrinth has been destroyed, the nystagmus may be to the affected labyrinth.

Cochlear function is abolished. The temperature is normal or near normal, and if much elevation is present, it is probably due to other factors, such as the otitis

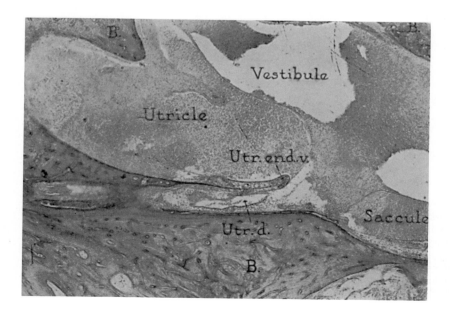

Fig. 49–7. Acute suppurative labyrinthitis. E.M., a girl aged 13 months, had a history of bilateral otitis media with fever and convulsions. A mastoid operation on the left ear was followed by death 2 weeks later. The postmortem examination revealed a pneumococcal meningitis and a bilateral osteitis and labyrinthitis. This section shows extensive purulent exudate throughout the vestibule, saccule, utricle,, and utricular duct (Utr.d.). The utriculoendolymphatic valve (Utr.end.v.) is shown clearly. The bony labyrinth (B) is normal. ×32.5. (Courtesy of Dr. E.W. Hagens).

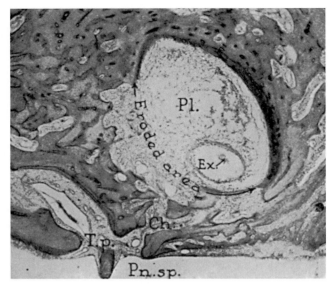

Fig. 49–8. Acute diffuse suppurative labyrinthitis. R.B., a boy aged 3 years, had a history of acute high fever and neck rigidity associated with a sudden onset of total bilateral deafness. The postmortem examination revealed a meningococcal suppurative meningitis and a bilateral suppurative labyrinthitis. The section through the superior semicircular canal shows the perilymph space (Pl.) practically filled with cellular material, which, as a result of the bone erosions, is in continuity through channels (Ch.) with the tunica propria (T.p.) of a large pneumatic space (Pn.sp.). A cellular exudate (Ex.) can be seen in the endolymphatic canal. ×18. (Courtesy of Dr. E.W. Hagens).

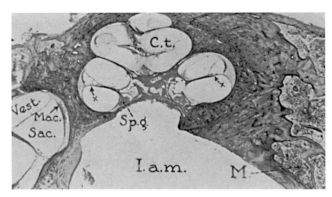

Fig. 49–10. Same patient as in Figure 49–8. Acute diffuse suppurative labyrinthitis. The section through the left ear shows the cochlea with only a rudimentary organ of Corti (x) in the basal coil. Considerable connective tissue (C.t.) is seen throughout, except in the scala tympani of the basal coil. The spiral ganglion (Sp.g.) is present in the basal coil but is mostly absent elsewhere. In the vestibule (Vest.), the saccule (Sac.) with its macula (Mac.) can be seen. At the level of sectioning, the eighth nerve does not appear in the internal auditory meatus (I.a.m.). Marrow spaces are seen (M.). ×8.9. (Courtesy of Dr. E.W. Hagens).

media or mastoiditis. As a rule, there is an absence of pain; if pain is present, it is probably caused by lesions other than the labyrinthitis.

During the acute stage, the position of the patient is characteristic. The patient lies on the other ear and directs his eyes toward the affected side, i.e., in the direction of the slow component of the nystagmus. This position reduces the vertigo.

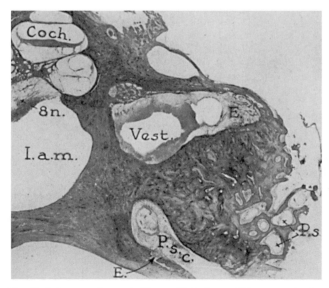

Fig. 49–9. Same patient as in Figure 49–8. Acute diffuse suppurative labyrinthitis with erosion through the posterior semicircular canal. Section through the right cochlea and vestibule shows extensive cellular exudate in the vestibule (Vest.). The utricle, saccule, and cristae are destroyed. Erosions (E.) are noted in the semicircular canal region. The cochlea in the left upper corner, the posterior semicircular canal, and the pneumatic space (P.s.) show cellular infiltration. I.a.m., Internal auditory meatus. ×7.05. (Courtesy of Dr. E.W. Hagens).

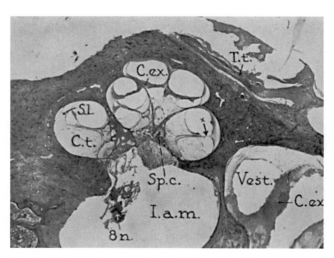

Fig. 49–11. Same patient as in Figure 49–8. Acute diffuse suppurative labyrinthitis. The section through the right ear shows connective tissue (C.t.) filling in the scala tympani of the cochlea and practically merging with the spiral ligamant (S.l.). The organ of Corti has been destroyed, leaving only the basilar membrane (x). Considerable cellular exudate (C.ex.) is noted in the middle and apical coils. The spiral ganglion cells are practically absent from the spiral canal (Sp.c.). A part of the eighth nerve (8n.) is in the internal auditory meatus (I.a.m.). An extensive cellular exudate in the vestibule (Vest.) and the tensor tympani muscle can be seen. ×8.9. (Courtesy of Dr. E.W. Hagens).

Reaction to caloric stimulus of the affected ear is absent. Neither caloric nor rotational tests should be done during the acute stage, because the vertigo would be greatly enhanced. If hearing in the involved ear is demonstrable, even though greatly reduced, it may be assumed that a diffuse suppurative labyrinthitis has not yet occurred. In other words, any hearing yet remaining indicates a partially functioning labyrinth, and the caloric and rotational tests are superfluous.

Diagnosis

The diagnosis is made from the history, symptoms and signs of a labyrinthine upset in which a complete and permanent loss of function (acoustic and vestibular) of the affected labyrinth occurs. CT of the middle ear, mastoid, and petrous pyramid may reveal some disease extraneous to the labyrinth. If meningeal irritation is suspected, spinal fluid examinations should be done.

Prognosis

An uncomplicated acute labyrinthitis treated with antibiotics has a favorable prognosis as far as life is concerned. If signs and symptoms of intracranial involvement persist despite adequate treatment, some form of labyrinthine drainage gives a better prognosis than if surgery is withheld.

Treatment

Absolute bed rest is essential during the acute phase, which may last for up to 6 weeks. Improvement usually occurs gradually, however. Mild sedation may be necessary in the early period. Phenobarbital, 32 mg, given three or four times a day, is satisfactory in most instances.

Adequate doses of antibiotics are given for an extended period, both to prevent an intracranial extension and to cure the labyrinthitis. Cultures should be obtained to identify the microorganism and demonstrate its antibiotic sensitivity. Prompt institution of treatment with either penicillin or an effective substitute if necessary. Large doses administered parenterally are required.

Drainage or removal of a sequestrum is indicated if intracranial complication is present and not responding to adequate antibiotic therapy. The presence of even a small amount of hearing in the affected side indicates a partially functioning labyrinth and contraindicates labyrinthine surgery.

Chronic (Latent) Diffuse Labyrinthitis

The chronic or latent stage of diffuse suppurative labyrinthitis begins at or shortly after the acute vestibular symptoms have subsided. This may be from 2 to 6 weeks after the onset of the acute period.

Pathology

About the end of the tenth week after the beginning of the acute stage, the internal ear is almost filled with granulation tissue. Some infected areas may still be present, however. The granulations gradually change into fibrous tissue with a beginning calcification. New bone formation may partly or completely fill the labyrinthine spaces in from 6 months to several years in about 50% of the cases. Figures 49–12 to 49–14 show different stages of latent labyrinthitis.

Symptoms

Complete deafness in the affected ear is present. A slight vertigo and spontaneous nystagmus, usually toward the other ear, may persist for several months or until compensation by the remaining labyrinth has occurred. Caloric tests elicit no response in the involved labyrinth, and the fistula test is negative even though a fistula may be present. The discharge from the ear may be absent, or may be present from a remaining focus in the labyrinth or other portions of the temporal bone.

Treatment

Local treatment should be directed toward any infection that may be present. Surgical drainage or exenteration of the labyrinth is not indicated unless a focus of infection in the labyrinth or perilabyrinthine region has extended to, or is suspected of extending to, the intracranial structures and is not responding to antibiotic therapy. A mastoidectomy may be done if indicated. If a focus of infection in the labyrinth or the petrosa is suspected, the labyrinth may be drained by one of the labyrinthine operations. Any loose sequestra found should be removed, with care to avoid injuring the facial nerve.

Sequestrum of the Labyrinth

Causes

Various degrees of sequestration of the osseous labyrinth may be associated with or follow:

1. An acute or chronic suppurative labyrinthitis.
2. An injury to the osseous labyrinth, especially after an operative procedure on the temporal bone.
3. Any of the granulomatous diseases affecting the ear, such as tuberculosis and syphilis.
4. A petrositis with necrosis extending to the bony labyrinth with sequestration of the labyrinth.
5. A dormant infection of the petrosal air cells becoming active and producing necrosis of the bony labyrinth.

Sequestration is more frequently observed in children but may be found at any age. Tuberculosis of the temporal bone in infants and children is especially

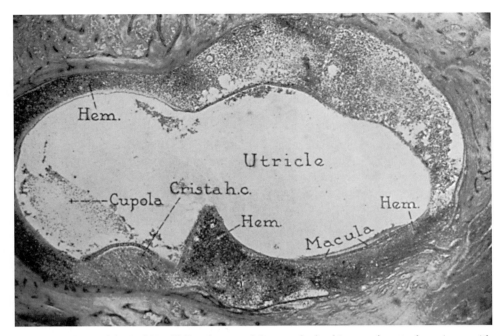

Fig. 49–12. Latent labyrinthitis. H.C., a boy aged 5 years, had a history of acute drowsiness with stiffness of the neck. The necropsy revealed an H. influenzae suppurative meningitis. The temporal bones showed a bilateral osteitis and labyrinthitis. The section through the vestibule demonstrates the characteristic findings of H. influenzae in a hemorrhagic (Hem.) condition of the perilymph space. The macula of the utricle is seen, as well as the crista of the horizontal semicircular canal (Crista h.c.), with cells infiltrating the cupola. ×35. (Courtesy of Dr. E.W. Hagens).

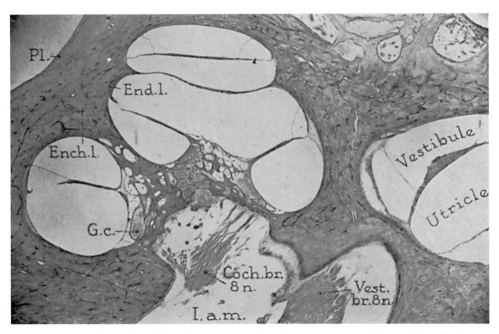

Fig. 49–13. Latent (atrophic) labyrinthitis. R.F., a girl aged 14 years, gave a history of measles 1 year before, followed by bilateral suppurative otitis media with bilateral deafness. There was an immediate history of headache, fever, and projectile vomiting accompanied by acute right mastoiditis. The necropsy revealed an early meningitis and a mixed-flora pneumonia. The temporal bones showed osteitis and atrophic labyrinthitis, with a total absence of the organ of Corti. In the basal coil are relatively few spiral ganglion cells (G.c.), and these are partly degenerated. In the internal auditory meatus (I.a.m.), the cochlear division of the eighth nerve, and also the vestibular branch, with Scarpa's ganglion cells, can be observed. The endosteal layer (End.l.) of the bony labyrinth, the wide endochondral layer (Ench.l.), and the periosteal layer (P.l.) are well demarcated. ×17. (Courtesy of Dr. E.W. Hagens).

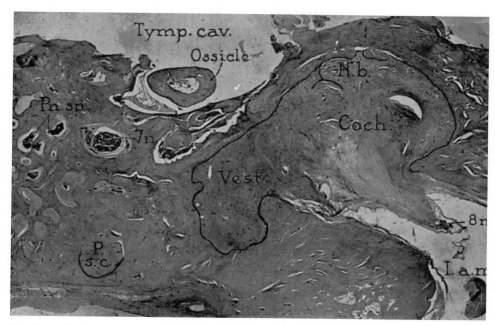

Fig. 49–14. Final stage of latent labyrinthitis. M.R., a woman aged 35 years, had a history of unilateral otitis media and mastoiditis with late intracranial complications. The postmortem examination revealed intracranial complications with a latent stage of unilateral labyrinthitis. The section through the labyrinth shows an extensive fibrosis and new bone (N.b.) filling in the cochlea (Coch.) and vestibule (Vest.). All traces of the membranous labyrinth are gone. The eighth nerve, in the internal auditory meatus (I.a.m.), is partially destroyed; only a few Scarpa's ganglion cells are present. Pus has infiltrated the fibers. The incus (ossicle) can be seen in the tympanic cavity (Tymp.cav.). Infected pneumatic spaces (Pn.sp.) may be seen, with the seventh nerve (7n.) close by. A cross section of the posterior semicircular canal (P.s.c.) is filled with fibrous tissue and bone. The border of the cochlea and vestibule and a portion of the posterior semicircular canal are outlined for better definition. ×8.5. (Courtesy of Dr. E.W. Hagens).

prone to necrosis with sequestration. A circumscribed labyrinthitis with a fistula secondary to a cholesteatoma or a granuloma may produce localized sequestra of the labyrinth of varying sizes.

Pathology

The scanty blood supply of the middle or endochondral layer of the otitic capsule results in a much reduced tendency to heal following an injury or an infection. This is not true of the thin, compact endosteal layer or of the outer or periosteal layer, which contains haversian lamellae with many blood vessels. If an infection reaches the middle or endochondral layer by way of an erosion or injury through either the periosteal or the endosteal layers, the development of a labyrinthine fistula or the formation of an endochondral sequestrum is possible. Healing of defects of endosteal or endochondral layers, the development of a labyrinthine fistula or the formation of an endochondral sequestrum is possible. Healing of defects of endosteal or enchondral layers is furnished from the periosteal layer by the formation of a compact lamellar bone.

The tendency toward a relatively greater pneumatization of the petrous pyramid superior and posterior to the labyrinth and medial to the arcuate eminence,

combined with a constricted exit from these air cells, predisposes to necrosis with sequestration of a portion or all of the labyrinth. A tendency toward intracranial invasion is also enhanced thereby.

Diagnosis

A sequestrum of the labyrinth, while difficult to diagnose preoperatively, may be suspected if a persistent otalgia, profuse otorrhea, exuberant granulations, and a marked or complete loss of labyrinthine function in the affected ear are present after a labyrinthitis or perilabyrinthitis. Probing of the necrotic ear, while not always advisable, may detect the sequestrum.

Imaging studies may indicate an erosion or even suggest a sequestrum of the bony labyrinth.

Prognosis

The sequestrum, in some instances, may be absorbed, or may be expelled spontaneously with or without alternations of the bony labyrinth. Drainage, surgical or otherwise, and removal of the sequestrum and all areas of infection in the temporal bone give a reasonably good prognosis. If drainage or removal of the infected and necrotic areas is not carried out, extension to the intracranial structures or the carotid artery may occur.

The facial nerve becomes involved in many instances, but complete recovery may take place after the subsidence of the infection, especially if the paralysis is only partial. If the nerve is partly destroyed, a nerve transplant may be necessary.

Treatment

If sequestration of the labyrinth is suspected, full and adequate doses of antibiotic should be given until there is evidence that further use of these agents is useless.

No hard and fast rule can be given as to the indications for surgical drainage and removal of the sequestrum. Each case should be judged by itself. In general, however, if a sequestrum can be diagnosed with reasonable certainty and total loss of labyrinthine function has occurred, some form of surgical drainage and removal of the necrotic areas should be done. If the sequestrum is firmly attached, removal may be deferred until the separation is more complete.

Surgery of Suppurative Labyrinthitis

The advent of effective antibiotic therapy, combined with early diagnosis and surgical correction of the causative otitis media, has made labyrinthine drainage a rare procedure. Suppurative labyrinthitis followed by signs of meningeal irritation, however, requires prompt surgical drainage of the labyrinth. Many authors have described specific procedures for opening various segments of the labyrinth, but the variations in these operations are not truly significant.

Technique

Before opening of the labyrinth, a complete radical mastoidectomy should be performed, particular care being taken to remove all diseased mastoid cells which may otherwise be a source of infection. The details of this procedure are given in, Surgery in Chronic Ear Disease.

The drainage of the labyrinth is carried out by first opening the ampullae of the horizontal and vertical semicircular canals and joining these openings at their junction with the vestibule. The membranous contents are then removed with a pick and suction. The stapes is then removed and the oval and round windows joined in one opening by removing the bone of the promontory between the windows (Fig. 49–15). The drainage thus accomplished achieves effective control of the labyrinthine infection and reduces the danger of spread to the meninges and brain.

Petrositis

Petrositis is not really a complication of ear infection but rather an extension of the infection into the mastoid cells surrounding the labyrinthine capsule. Not only may infection follow this course, but cholesteatoma may invade these cells, creating an extremely difficult therapeutic problem. Fortunately, the mastoid sclerosis accompanying chronic otitis media may block this avenue of spread, so that it is usually seen only in well-pneumatized temporal bones after acute otitis media.

Infection of the petrous cells occurs with most mastoid infections but does not constitute a separate prob-

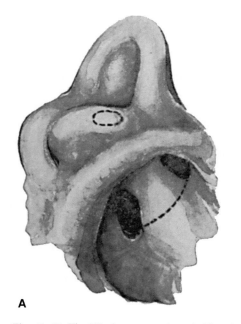 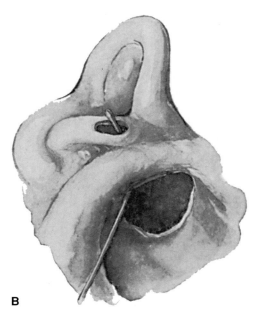

A **B**

Fig. 49–15. The Hinsberg operation. A. The plate of bone, separating the oval and round windows, to be removed. B. A probe has been inserted through the newly created opening into the vestibule and out through the opening into the lateral canal. The facial ridge separates the two openings.

lem because it resolves as the total infection is treated. In the pre-antibiotic era, resolution of infection in these cells was usually delayed because of poor drainage. This caused an important problem not always solved by the simple mastoidectomy performed in treating the mastoiditis. These same factors are present today in resistant infections not treated with thorough mastoidectomy to open all diseased cell tracts. The retained infection has a tendency to break through the posterior or superior walls of the petrous bone, and is a major source of otogenic meningitis.

Diagnosis

The diagnosis of petrositis is not made frequently today. The diagnosis should be first suspected in any case with persistent infection and discharge after adequate treatment of otitis media and mastoiditis, or following mastoidectomy. CT should be repeated to detect fluid density in and erosion of the petrous cells. Deep-seated ear pain accompanying the persistent discharge is an even more definite clue to the presence of petrositis.

Gradenigo's syndrome involves otorrhea, pain around the eye, and diplopia caused by abducens nerve paralysis and is an indication of disease in the petrous apex. Also accompanying petrositis may be mild vertigo, transient facial nerve paralysis, and low-grade intermittent fever.

Treatment

The treatment of persistent petrous cell infection is to provide adequate drainage by opening the diseased cell tracts to the petrous apex (Fig. 49–16). This is best done by initial adequate mastoidectomy to visualize the involved groups of cells. The posterior cells proceed medially from Trautmann's triangle, outlining the labyrinthine capsule superiorly and posteriorly. Cells opening in the attic region may run through the arch of the superior semicircular canal or anterior to the canal over the cochlea. There may be a cell tract opening below the posterior semicircular canal running to the region below the internal auditory canal. The most difficult cell tracts to follow are those running anterior to the cochlea from the Eustachian tube and carotid region. Opening these requires a preliminary radical mastoidectomy with sacrifice of the tympanic membrane and enlargement of the external auditory canal anteriorly. The cells are then followed by opening the medial wall of the Eustachian tube just above the carotid artery. Antibiotics selected by culture and sensitivity tests of the aural discharge are given for several days following the operation.

Facial Nerve Paralysis

Functional involvement of the facial nerve is not unusual in both acute and chronic infection of the middle ear and mastoid. This complication is discussed in Chapter 59 or 60.

REFERENCES

1. Yaniv E, Pocock R: Complications of ear disease. Clin Otolaryngol 13:357, 1988.
2. Proctor CA: Intracranial complications of otogenic origin. Laryngoscope 76:288, 1966.
3. Nissen AJ: Intracranial complications of otogenic disease. Am J Otol 2:164, 1980.
4. Lederer FL, Torok N: In Otolaryngology, Vol II. Edited by Schenk HP. Hagerstown: WF Prior Co, 1966.
5. Knauer WJ: Gradenigo's syndrome. Arch Otolaryngol 44:404, 1946.
6. Dawes JDK: In Diseases of the Ear, Nose and Throat. 2nd ed. Edited by Scott-Brown, Ballantyne, and Groves. London: Butterworths, 1965, p 479.
7. Ibekwe AO, Okoye BC: Subperiosteal mastoid abscesses in chronic suppurative otitis media. Ann Otol Rhinol Laryngol 97:373, 1988.
8. Lempert J: In Otolaryngology, Vol II. Edited by Schenk HP. Hagerstown: WF Prior Co, 1960.
9. Lindsay JR: Pathology of vertigo arising from the peripheral vestibular apparatus. Ann Otol Rhinol Laryngol 56:541, 1947.
10. Shambaugh G, Glasscock ME: Surgery of the Ear, 3rd ed. Philadelphia: WB Saunders Co, 1980.
11. Proctor B, et al: Sequestration of the osseous labyrinth. Arch Otolaryngol Head Neck Surg 37:819, 1943.

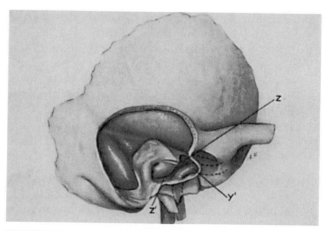

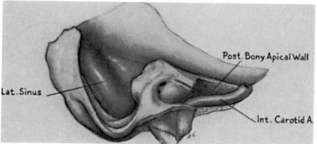

Fig. 49–16. A dissection showing the areas of cellular spaces in the petrous portion of the temporal bone. It may be necessary to open any or all of these in petrositis. y′, Transverse apical portion of internal carotid artery; z, bony wall of posterior fossa at petrous apex approached anterior to cochlea and above carotid artery; z′, jugular bulb.

50 Otosclerosis

David F. Austin

Otosclerosis is a primary disease of the labyrinthine capsule characterized by foci of new bone formation. Clinically, it is marked by conductive hearing loss (caused by stapedial fixation) and in many instances by progressive sensorineural hearing loss.

Although the basic factors initiating the formation of the otosclerotic focus are unknown, the disease is known to be inherited. There is a positive family history in 55% of patients with clinical otosclerosis.

Stacy Guild's investigations produced much of the primary knowledge of the epidemiology of otosclerosis. He studied temporal bones obtained at routine postmortem examination. He found histologic evidence of otosclerosis in 8.3% of 518 whites and 1% of 482 blacks. Other researchers have found the disease in as many as 12% of white patients' temporal bones. Clinical otosclerosis with stapedial fixation is seen in only 12% of those with histologic findings.

Even though there is no difference in the incidence of histologic otosclerosis between the sexes, clinical otosclerosis is seen more commonly in women—in 68%. This finding may be related to the fact that pregnancy stimulates the growth of the focus in some women, as well as to the fact the women seek help for their hearing problem more often than men.

PATHOLOGY

The otosclerotic focus is similar in most respects to normal fibrous bone. The major difference lies in the microstructure of the bony matrix, which in normal capsular bone is lamellar or mosaic in appearance but in otosclerotic bone has a warp and woof pattern similar to that seen in healing bone or a callus.

Otosclerotic foci have been described in all portions of the labyrinthine capsule. Most often (80 to 90% of cases), the focus occurs anterior to the stapes footplate in the region of the fissula ante fenestram—"the site of predilection." The border of the round window is the second most frequently involved site (30 to 50%). In about one half there is a single focus, and in the rest two or more foci. The endosteal layer of the capsule seems to limit the spread of the lesion, although an irritative hypertrophy of the endosteum has been described, and occasionally invasion of the vestibule or cochlea has been observed.

The otosclerotic focus consists of irregular areas of new bone formation with many vascular channels occurring on and within the dense bone of the labyrinthine capsule. The borders of the lesion are sharply defined but irregular, with projections along the vessels of the surrounding normal capsular bone. A border of blue-staining bone (with hematoxylineosin) is seen around a few of the vascular channels in the focus. These are called "blue mantles" and are typical of the otosclerotic lesion (Figs. 50–1 and 50–2).

The stages in the development and progression of the otosclerotic lesion have been described by Schuknecht as follows:

1. Destruction of enchondral bone with the formation of resorption spaces which contain a highly cellular fibrous tissue. This lytic phase may be caused by lysosomal hydrolases and osteoclastic activity.
2. Formation of mucopolysaccharide and osteoid deposits within the fibroblastic collagen of the resorption spaces leading to the production of immature basophilic bone.
3. Repetition of the remodeling process of resorption and new bone formation through several generations with the development of more mature acidophilic bone having a laminated matrix.
4. Formation of a highly mineralized acidophilic bone having a mosaic-like appearance because of the irregular patterns of resorption and new bone formation associated with the deposition of fatty deposits in the marrow spaces.

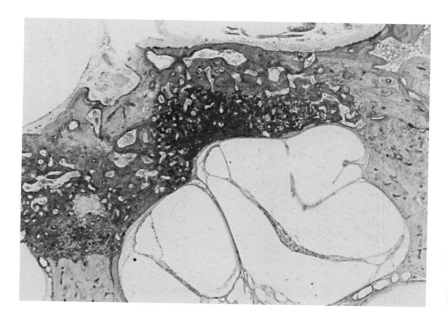

Fig. 50–1. Large otosclerotic focus lesion involving the lateral wall of the bony labyrinth and stapes footplate. The otosclerotic bone shows a varied histologic structure. Adjacent to the labyrinthine spaces, the bone has a feathery appearance and stains deeply with hematoxylin. More peripherally, there is a mosaic architecture with thick trabeculae staining with eosin. (Reprinted with permission from Schuknecht HF: Pathology of the Ear. Cambridge, MA, Harvard University Press, 1974.)

This process may become quiescent or active at random intervals. It is common also for an otosclerotic focus to contain both active and inactive regions (see Fig. 50–1).

PATHOGENESIS AND CAUSES

The cause of the development of the lesions is unknown, although investigations into this question have been undertaken since the lesion was first described (Politzer, 1893). The factors that influence the development of otosclerosis may be categorized as constitutional, local, and/or general activating factors.

The *constitutional* factors that have been best defined are heredity and race. A positive family history may be obtained in 50 to 60% of those suffering hearing loss from otosclerosis. This is indeed a high frequency because histologic otosclerosis is much more common than clinical otosclerosis. Because of the difficulty of recognizing otosclerosis in the absence of hearing loss, the mendelian pattern has yet to be defined because histologic study of temporal bones from complete families has not yet been done. The most thorough family studies indicate that otosclerosis is a monohybrid autosomal dominant inheritance with a penetrance of 40 to 50%.

Van der Hoeve syndrome of osteogenesis imperfecta, blue sclera, and otosclerosis is rare but definitely hereditary, and both Fowler and Shambaugh have

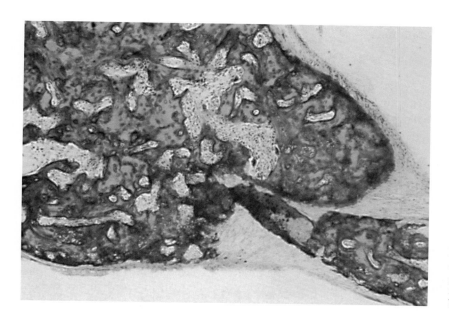

Fig. 50–2. Osteoclastic activity in an active otosclerotic lesion in the bony labyrinth at the anterior margin of the oval window. (Reprinted with permission from Schuknecht HF: Pathology of the Ear. Cambridge, MA, Harvard University Press, 1974.)

noted a correlation between blue sclera and otosclerosis in patients without frequent fractures.

Racial patterns have been noted in otosclerosis, with occurrence 10 times more frequent in whites than in blacks. The disease is also more prevalent in India than in China or Japan.

Local Factors

Many local conditions have been cited as influencing the development of the otosclerotic focus. The most prominently mentioned is the presence of the fissula ante fenestram at the site of predilection of the lesion. This is a small channel filled with connective tissue in the adult, but in early stages of development it is surrounded by cartilage, which may persist into adult life. It is felt that unstable cartilaginous elements may result in new bone formation or otosclerosis. Foci of otosclerosis posterior to the stapes may result from the presence of a similar structure—the fossula post fenestram—and foci at other areas result from cartilaginous rests that have been seen to persist in many regions of the labyrinthine capsule long after ossification is otherwise complete.

This explanation has not satisfied many workers, and the theory of bony stress caused by extrinsic forces or by intrinsic developmental torsion has been proposed by Mayer and by Sercer. These forces seem to develop the greatest strain at the site of predilection, and the tendency for new bone formation in this region is explained. Vascular and vasomotor influences on the bone of the labyrinthine capsule have also been mentioned as possible local causative factors.

Frost pointed out that the basic cause of otosclerosis must lie in the formation of cementum by the osteoblasts, as controlled by their enzyme systems. Abnormal chemical constituents have been identified in the matrix of otosclerotic bone. At present, a great deal of research is concentrated in this area that will hopefully be able to define the genetically determined abnormal enzyme systems responsible for this disease.

General Activating Factors

Sex and age seem to be interrelated factors. The incidence in women is double that in men (65 versus 35%), and the period of activity of the disease correlates closely with the period of fertility. Only in rare instances has the disease been found before puberty or with an onset after 50. On the average, onset occurs between the age of 20 and 25. In women, more rapid progression of the hearing loss during or shortly after pregnancy occurs in approximately 50%.

DIAGNOSIS

Typically, otosclerosis has its onset in early adult life, although the hearing loss may be ignored until middle age. After onset, the hearing deficit is slowly progressive. Women patients may tell of more rapid progression or onset during or shortly after pregnancy. Although a history of ear infection during childhood may be obtained occasionally, this is probably only a chance relationship. Only 1 to 2% of those with otitis media suffer a concomitant otosclerosis. Although the hearing loss may be severe, speech discrimination is preserved except in the rare case of cochlear involvement. The patient may tell of being able to hear better in a noisy environment than in quiet, and this is known as paracusia willisiana. Tinnitus is often present and is usually a low-frequency conductive type frequently accompanied by an audible pulse. Occasionally it is a high-pitched ringing, most often correlated with the presence of high-tone cochlear dysfunction. A positive family history of hearing loss occurring in early adult or middle age may be obtained in 50 to 60% of the cases.

Examination reveals a normal eardrum. Occasionally, a pinkish blush may be seen on the promontory, especially with a translucent drumhead. This is the Schwartze sign, indicative of a highly vascular otosclerotic focus. Pure tone hearing tests reveal a conductive loss of varying severity. Initially the major conductive component is in the lower frequencies caused by stiffness of the annular ligament. As the mass of the lesion accumulates and with increasing friction, the conductive loss involves all frequencies. In addition, stapes fixation influences the bone conduction thresholds due to increased impedance of the inner ear fluids, causing an apparent sensorineural hearing loss which is maximum at 2000 cp—the "Carhart notch." It averages 5 dB at 500 Hz, 10 dB at 1000 Hz, 15 dB at 2000 Hz, and 5 dB at 4000 Hz.

In recent times, with the advent of tomographic techniques, it has been possible to visualize the otosclerotic focus by radiographic examination. This technique is extremely useful in diagnosis of unusual symptoms, such as vertigo coupled with mild hearing loss, or in the severe cases in which bone conduction values cannot be obtained. Also of value in these latter cases is use of the speaking tube coupled with masking of the other ear with a Bárány noisemaker. In some of the patients with severe hearing loss, diagnosis is made by finding good discrimination with the speaking tube, a history of otosclerosis in the family, and a history of being able to use a hearing aid effectively in the past.

Otosclerosis must be differentiated from congenital conductive lesions and acquired ossicular defects caused by infection but with an intact drum. In unilateral congenital hearing loss which is stable, the date of onset may be equated with the date of discovery, and increasing severity may be mistaken for increasing notice of the defect. Acquired lesions may also be nonprogressive but occur later in life, and this may be a point of confusion. Aseptic necrosis of the long process of the incus is said to occur, but this is felt in most cases to be associated with mild ear infection not resulting in tympanic membrane perforation. Reliable differentiation of stapes fixation and discontinuity of the ossicular chain can be made with tympanometry.

LABYRINTHINE OTOSCLEROSIS

It has long been thought that there is a higher incidence of sensorineural hearing loss in patients with otosclerosis than in the general population. Statistical studies have not verified this, but temporal bone examination in otosclerosis has shown lesions that have definitely involved the cochlea. The major forms of pathology found in these instances are atrophy of the stria vascularis and degeneration of hair cells in the organ of Corti. In most cases, the otosclerosis has been diffuse throughout the capsule, or there has been a large focus with involvement of the endosteum. In only rare instances has the otosclerotic focus itself been found to be sufficient in extent to explain the severity of the hearing loss. The two major theories explaining the presence of cochlear hearing loss are that the otosclerosis releases toxic substances into the cochlea, or that the numerous arteriovenous shunts present in the otosclerotic focus impair the vascular supply of the stria vascularis. Because the degree of sensorineural hearing loss seems to correlate with the degree of involvement of the capsule adjacent to the stria, the latter idea seems to have much merit.

Many instances of labyrinthine hydrops have been reported in association with otosclerosis, with the typical symptoms and findings of Ménière's disease. In some cases this seems to be related to irritative involvement of the vestibule by the otosclerotic focus. In at least one temporal bone, a focus of otosclerosis was found obliterating the endolymphatic duct with associated cochlear hydrops. In most instances, stapedectomy will relieve the vertiginous symptoms.

Large-scale studies of patients treated with sodium fluoride over periods of up to 10 years suggest the ability of this agent to prevent sensorineural hearing loss. Although these studies did not incorporate an adequate control group, less than 20% of those given sodium fluoride demonstrated progressive sensorineural hearing loss, as compared to a much smaller group of untreated patients, 75% of whom had a progressive sensorineural hearing loss. These studies, conducted both in the United States and in France, have been taken as the basis for the recommendation for the administration of a 20 mg enteric-coated tablet of sodium fluoride twice daily. This dosage is combined with additional calcium intake, through use of either calcium gluconate or supplementary milk to prevent calcium depletion. This form of therapy should not be carried out without knowledge of the risk of the serious side effects of fluoride toxicity.

TREATMENT OF OTOSCLEROSIS

Treatment of otosclerosis has been largely restricted to surgical efforts to circumvent the conductive hearing loss characteristic of the disease. The lack of any basic therapy for otosclerosis is related only to the lack of exact knowledge concerning the etiology and pathogenesis of the disease. Undoubtedly, basic treatment will evolve as the nature of otosclerosis becomes clear, but until it does, our efforts must be directed toward the improvement of hearing in these cases.

Surgery in otosclerosis has an interesting history. Initial efforts at correcting the stapedial fixation were directed toward breaking through the bony lesion by palpation of the incus and stapes through an incision in the drumhead. This was pioneered by Miot, who reported a series of 200 such procedures in 1890. In 1892, both Blake and Jack reported their experiences with extraction of the stapes for otosclerotic deafness. Although many good results were reported, many prominent otologists expressed disapproval of these procedures in the early 1900s, and operative intervention was virtually abandoned. Holmgren, however, continued efforts to introduce sound into the cochlea by "decompressing the perilymph" through producing fistulas into the semicircular canals. Sourdille developed this work into a multistage fenestration of the lateral semicircular canal, which was later brought to perfection by Lempert with his one-stage fenestration operation. The reliability and predictability of this procedure (80% achievement of practical hearing in selected cases) made it the standard treatment for otosclerosis for 20 years.

In 1952, Rosen rediscovered stapes mobilization, and the obvious advantage of retaining the normal sound conduction mechanism made this a popular procedure. The process of bone healing with subsequent refixation of the stapes became apparent because less than 30% of these patients maintained hearing over a long term. The concept of bypassing the otosclerotic lesion at the oval window was introduced by E. P. Fowler, Jr., in 1956. He described the anterior crurotomy operation, in which the anterior crus was sectioned and an incision made through the footplate behind the focus of otosclerosis, thus freeing the posterior crus and attached segment of footplate. This procedure was much more successful in accomplishing permanent hearing improvement. A year later Shea reintroduced the concept of eliminating disease from the oval window by removing the stapes. Stapedectomy as defined by Shea with modern techniques and with application of auditory physiology has since become the universally applied operation for otosclerosis.

The time since stapedectomy was introduced is too short to be able to predict stabilization of surgical technique. With the passage of time and increasing permanency of results, it may be stated that stapedectomy is the standard procedure today for otosclerosis. The inconsistency of technique is caused by the nature of the surgical problem of restoring transmission of the maximum possible sound energy as complicated by the still active presence of the otosclerotic process.

SURGICAL LESION

The clinical lesion of otosclerosis at the oval window has several forms, each of which may present a distinct surgical problem. The Otosclerosis Study Group has defined these forms as localized and diffuse otosclerosis.

The *localized* form may be further differentiated as predominantly an anterior focus, a posterior focus, or with extension around the margins of the oval window.

The *diffuse* forms involve the footplate. They may be circumscribed, in which the footplate has a distinct margin, and may be thin or thick (also called "biscuit" type). Diffuse obliterative otosclerosis is that in which the annular ligament is invaded and therefore the footplate has lost a distinct margin. In extreme cases of this type, the entire oval window may be filled with otosclerosis mounding between the promontory and facial nerve. The character of the otosclerotic bone may also vary from a soft hypervascular lesion to a focus of dense bone with little vascularity. The round window may be involved, in some instances to complete obliteration.

INDICATIONS FOR STAPES SURGERY

The prediction of the hearing result in surgery for otosclerosis is of basic importance to both surgeon and patient. This prediction is based on an accurate estimate of the cochlear reserve and an accurate knowledge of the surgeon's own success rate in accomplishing the theoretic ideal result with the particular type of operation performed. Cochlear reserve must be calculated for the individual patient because pure tone bone conduction audiometry does not give an accurate measure of inner ear function. Fixation and increased mass of the stapes changes the mechanical impedance of the inner ear fluids and thus allows less energy transfer from the bone oscillator. Carhart has measured this loss in a large number of cases as based on bone conduction threshold change with surgery. As mentioned under Diagnosis, this loss has been estimated at 5 dB at 500 Hz, 10 dB at 1000 Hz, 15 dB at 2000 Hz, and 5 dB at 4000 Hz. Correcting the bone conduction

audiogram by these amounts gives a more accurate estimate of the functional capacity of the inner ear—the cochlear reserve. Comparing the speech discrimination ability with the pure-tone audiogram further defines the rehabilitative capacity of the surgical venture.

Ideally, because stapedectomy completely eliminates the conductive hearing loss, estimate of the cochlear reserve should serve as the predictive level of postoperative hearing. The ideal result would then be an average 10 dB better than the preoperative bone conduction average (overclosure of the bone-air gap). Approximately 50% of patients equal the predicted air conduction, and 90% will close the bone-air gap to within 10 dB. Loss of cochlear function occurs in less than 1% of stapedectomies. Because of this high probability of largely eliminating the conductive deficit in the otosclerotic patient, this procedure is not reserved for a particular category of patients but has been applied to patients with all degrees of hearing loss, including those with mild losses and those without measurable bone conduction. Stapedectomy may be used in patients with unilateral hearing loss, as well as in bilateral cases. It may be stated that stapedectomy may be applied to any patient with a conductive hearing loss whose correction will satisfy a definite need of the patient.

Surgery should be performed on the poorer-hearing ear in all but the most exceptional cases. In the instance of the only hearing ear being considered for surgery, the extreme disability of total deafness resulting from a bad result should indicate the recommendation of a hearing aid. Patients with severe hearing loss may be operated on with the understanding that a hearing aid will still be required after the operation. The great improvement in performance with a hearing aid is usually sufficient indication in these patients. Surgery may be performed on both ears, but only after a period of 6 to 12 months has passed since the initial surgery. This avoids the chance that a delayed complication might occur, resulting in a total hearing loss.

TECHNIQUE OF STAPEDECTOMY

Years have passed since the introduction of stapedectomy by Shea, but the technique has not yet stabilized to a point at which a "standard" operation exists. The basis of the procedure is to create a patent oval window, seal it with a membrane of either natural or artificial material, and provide a connection between the incus and the neomembrane cover of the oval window. When this is done, either all or a part of the stapes footplate is removed; the oval window is covered with vein, mucous membrane, connective tissue, fat, Gelfoam, or collagen membrane; and sound transmission is reestablished with a stapes crus, a Teflon, stainless steel, or titanium piston, stainless steel or tantalum wire, or platinum prosthesis. The preceding is *not* a comprehensive list of the variations of stapedectomy currently in use.

The technique of stapedectomy is further complicated by the variations in surgical pathology, as well as by variations in ossicular anatomy. Because of these factors, it has become apparent that a single technique is not suitable in all cases of otosclerosis, and the surgeon must be able to vary his method according to the conditions found at surgery. At present, most experts have selected the technique of "small fenestra stapedectomy" as offering the greatest permanency of good hearing with the least risk. When anatomic or surgical difficulties preclude this, total stapedectomy with tissue seal, using a piston, is performed. In the case of obliterative otosclerosis, the piston technique is used to reduce surgical trauma and prevent reclosure of the fistula.

The rationale for this series of procedures is based on the expected number of complications with each. Small fenestra stapedectomy has a reported rate of postoperative hearing loss of 1 in 200 patients. This increases to 3 to 4% in obliterative otosclerosis. Total stapedectomy has a complication rate of 1 to 2%. The vein graft with polyethylene tube method first used resulted in a 70% success rate and a 10% complication rate.

Preparation of the Ear

Stapedectomy is a transcanal operation, and because it is of great importance not to introduce pathogenic bacteria into the middle ear, care must be taken to evaluate the health of the external ear before surgery. All vestiges of external otitis must be eliminated because this is felt to be one of the factors responsible for complications. Because many patients will be wearing a hearing aid in the ear to be operated on, this should be removed at least 2 weeks before surgery. Patients with bilateral hearing loss should be advised to have an ear mold made for the other ear so that communication will be possible during the immediate postoperative period.

At surgery, the ear canal should be cleansed of loose debris and accumulated cerumen, but without trauma that will lower local tissue resistance to infection. A nonionic protein-iodine surgical scrub (Betadine, Purdue Frederick Co., Norwalk, CT) is used to irrigate the canal without wiping, and after suction drying, the same protein-iodine complex is used to paint the area. The external ear is prepared in the same manner. It is not usually necessary to remove any hair, but hair should be kept out of the field with adhesive spray and drapes.

Anesthesia

Local anesthesia injected in the outer third of the cartilaginous canal and into the incision site is used in these procedures. Adequate patient relaxation is important to avoid positional discomfort and bleeding from increased arterial and venous pressure. For this purpose, heavy premedication is necessary using a combination of a narcotic, a barbiturate, and a tranquilizer. Often it is necessary to supplement this during the operation. At these times the use of a short-acting narcotic agent and a short-acting barbiturate given intravenously is helpful. The thiobarbiturates should be avoided because of their depressant effect, hangover, and risk of laryngospasm. New forms of chemical narcosis are being developed, and time will bring even more ideal methods of patient preparation in stapes surgery.

Exposure

Exposure of the oval window region is essential for meticulous operative technique. In this, as in all temporal bone operations performed today, the operation microscope is essential. The use of a speculum holder is necessary to free both of the surgeon's hands.

The incision is made in the posterior and superior canal wall. This should be a sufficient distance from the annulus to provide an adequate skin flap to replace against bone regardless of the amount of bone removed from the canal wall for exposure. Bone is removed from the medial end of the posterosuperior canal wall until the entire oval window may be visualized. Curettes may be used for this purpose, but small diamond burs driven by a small electric-powered drill provide more speed and control of this dissection. Care should be taken to spare the chorda tympani nerve when possible. Needless sacrifice of the chorda results in a percentage of mild disability which may become more severe if surgery on the opposite ear results in loss of taste function. If the chorda tympani prevents good exposure of the oval window, however, it should be sectioned rather than stretched because the latter results in many postoperative complaints.

Evaluation of Pathologic Condition

The selection of surgical technique is based on evaluation of the extent and type of otosclerosis. The location and size of the otosclerotic foci, as well as the amount of footplate invasion, should be noted. Anatomic factors enter into technique selection. A narrow, deep oval window niche may require the use of a wire, which may be bent to avoid contact with the facial nerve.

Small Fenestra Stapedectomy

The initial step in stapedectomy is to remove the stapedial arch without mobilizing the footplate. The incu-

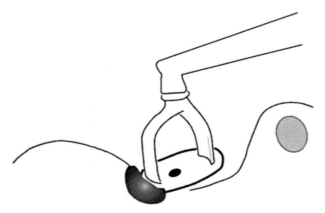

Fig. 50–3. The stapes is fixed by an anterior focus of otosclerosis (diagrammatic). A small opening has been made through the footplate to prevent hydraulic trauma to the cochlea.

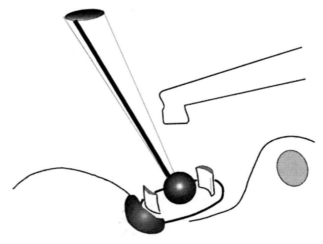

Fig. 50–5. The fenestra is created using a diamond bur rotating slowly or with hand-held hooks and rasps.

dostapedial joint is separated using a right angled knife. The stapedius tendon is sectioned with scissors. McGee, Perkins, and Silverstein, among others have described the advantages of the laser for this purpose. The crura can be vaporized and an accurate fenestra created with minimal trauma and consequent reduction in complications.

The more commonly used technique uses hand instruments or tiny motor-driven cutting tools. Initially, a small perforation is made through the footplate to prevent large pressure waves in case of inadvertent mobilization of the footplate. This opening is also helpful in recovering a displaced footplate. The crura are then transected with a small knife or a crurotomy saw. The fenestra is created in the posterior footplate which offers the safety of the largest clearance from the membranous labyrinth within the vestibule. Sharp hooks, rasps, or slowly turning burs are used to create a fenestra slightly larger in diameter than that of the piston. The distance between the incus and footplate is measured and a prosthesis selected whose length will extend 0.25 mm within the vestibule. A graft is placed over the opening by some surgeons, and others pack

areolar tissue around the piston after it is inserted. The piston is placed and secured tightly to the incus. These steps are illustrated in Figures 50–3 to 50–6.

Bleeding is controlled throughout the operation with pledgets of Gelfoam moistened with epinephrine 1:1000. If at all possible, there should be no hemorrhage during the time the oval window is open. This is not because blood injures the cochlea but because it increases the risk of surgical trauma because of poor visibility and increased technical difficulty. Often a pause of a minute or two immediately before opening the vestibule results in an entirely dry field and also relaxes the surgeon before this crucial phase of stapedectomy is undertaken.

The skin flap is carefully replaced and a small amount of packing placed over it to hold it in place. A piece or two of moistened Gelfoam is usually sufficient for this purpose. A small amount of antibiotic ointment is instilled in the canal. A cotton tampon placed in the outer meatus is an adequate external dressing.

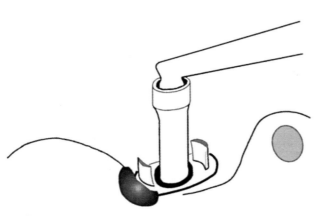

Fig. 50–4. The crura are divided with a crurotomy knife.

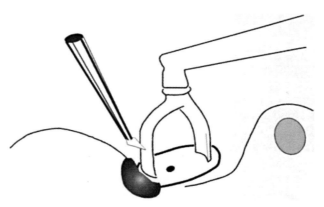

Fig. 50–6. The piston is placed between the fenestra and incus. It is secured to the incus and should extend no more than 0.25 mm into the vestibule.

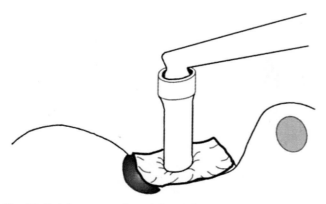

Fig. 50–7. A larger opening of the oval window is sealed with a connective tissue graft before placing the piston.

TOTAL STAPEDECTOMY

Total stapedectomy may prove necessary because of a narrow oval window or accidental loss of the stapes crura. This latter is especially apt to occur if the crura are atrophic. In these cases, the remainder of the stapes is removed by separating the incudostapedial joint. The entire footplate is removed, preferably in two pieces. The distance from the long process of the incus to the oval window is measured and the window immediately covered with a piece of connective tissue (Fig. 50–7). A prosthesis of the proper length is selected. This should extend to the level of the oval window and not enter the vestibule by more than 0.25 mm. The hook is crimped to fit firmly around the incus. If the prosthesis fits too loosely, it may cause necrosis of the long process. The prosthesis should be tight enough to prevent its dislodgment during the immediate postoperative period, after which mucosal scarring will hold it securely. The skin flap is then replaced as previously described. Figure 50–7 shows this technique.

Obliterative Otosclerosis

Partial stapedectomy with piston (Shea) has proved useful in cases of obliterative otosclerosis. Bony regrowth is not uncommon with this form of the disease, and the piston was designed to prevent this regrowth from immobilizing the prosthesis. Teflon is used because of its inertness and the smooth, self-lubricating nature of its surface. Stainless steel has also been used and has some advantage because the steel produces a slight adsorption of bone immediately surrounding it and in this way resists fixation. The main disadvantage of the steel piston is that its length cannot be adjusted, and a variety of slightly differing sizes must always be kept available.

A recently documented technique, popular in Europe, is the use of a small piston (0.4–0.6 cm in diame-

ter) placed through a precisely formed fenestra in the footplate. Some have used a surgical laser for this purpose. The technique is said to be safer, with fewer immediate side effects.

Some surgeons feel that any drilling on the otosclerotic focus stimulates bone growth and rapid recurrence of the lesion. These surgeons make a hole only large enough to admit the piston through the middle of the footplate with picks and chisel-knives. The experience of others has shown that removal of the mass of otosclerotic bone with burs until the niche of the oval window is completely delineated is not associated with an increased incidence of bony regrowth. Because of this latter view, the following technique is recommended (Sooy).

The incudostapedial joint is separated and the crura fractured after sectioning of the stapedius tendon. Small cutting burs used with constant irrigation are then used to remove the mass of otosclerotic bone filling the oval window niche. The footplate itself is *not* opened but merely thinned to a degree equaling a slightly thick otosclerotic footplate. The bone debris is completely removed, and all bleeding is controlled. The footplate is then removed in a routine manner by transection and piecemeal removal with small angled picks. The oval window need not be opened to its normal extent, a 1 to 2 mm fenestra being sufficient. The distance to the incus is then measured and the piston placed so that the end lies just below the level of the oval window. The opening is then sealed with small pledgets of Gelfoam placed around the piston.

Complications of Stapedectomy

The major complication of stapedectomy is further hearing loss caused by cochlear damage. As mentioned before, this occurs in about 1% of cases. Some of the other factors responsible for this secondary cochlear loss may be bone chips or bone dust in the vestibule, irrigation with an open oval window, rapid "uncorking" of the vestibule by removing the stapes in toto without a pressure-relief hole in the footplate, trauma with instruments to the vestibular contents, too rapid or violent aspiration of perilymph, and infection from bacteria entering or being implanted in the middle ear during surgical procedure.

Delayed cochlear losses seem to be associated with a fistula developing in the membrane covering the oval window, sometimes associated with infection. In some instances this has led to meningitis. An occasional delayed hearing loss has seemed to be caused by an immune response to foreign protein, although this is largely conjectural.

Tears of the tympanic membrane occasionally occur with creation of the tympanomeatal flap. These are repaired by approximation over Gelfoam or with a vein graft (see Chap. 55). Facial nerve paralysis sometimes occurs, but in most instances this is transient, being due to the local anesthesia. A persistent paresis may be caused by scarring or pressure of the prosthesis on a bare facial nerve. This is corrected by removal of the prosthesis and replacement with a wire, which may be bent to fit around an overhanging facial nerve.

FENESTRATION

This procedure is no longer used for restoration of hearing in patients with otosclerosis. The reader is referred to the thirteenth edition of this text for details of the operation. The incus was removed in the fenestration operation.

REVISION OF FENESTRATION

Today the best approach to the fenestration failure is with stapedectomy techniques. In these procedures, the stapes is removed, and the sound conduction mechanism is reconstructed with a prosthesis placed between the malleus handle and the oval window. Both preformed wire loops and Teflon pistons have been used for this purpose. With proper patient selection, at least 70% of this group may have their hearing restored to within 20 dB of measured bone conduction.

Patient Selection

The ideal patient for this procedure is one whose hearing improved temporarily after fenestration but regressed because of bony or fibrous closure of the fenestra. Patients who had a good surgical result but because of poor bone conduction did not achieve serviceable hearing are also good candidates. Those who had no result from fenestration despite a patent fenestra as evidenced by a fistula sign are poor candidates. Less than 1 of 4 of this group experiences a hearing improvement with revision.

Operative Technique

Although this is a transcanal procedure as in stapedectomy, the incision must be modified because of the previous mastoid surgery. The incision originates below the fenestra and is brought back onto the facial ridge. The second limb of the incision is carried from the first onto the remaining posteroinferior canal wall as in stapedectomy (Fig. 50–8). The skin flap is elevated, and after the middle ear is entered by dissecting out the annulus, the posterior spine is removed to improve visualization of the oval window region.

The entire stapes is then removed and the ossicular mechanism reconstructed with a prosthesis extending from the malleus handle to the oval window. Sheehy

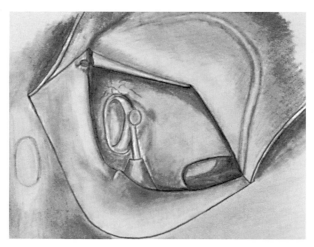

Fig. 50–8. Revision of fenestration. The middle ear is exposed by the indicated flap. Great care should be taken to avoid the fenestra.

has described the use of a preformed wire loop. A tunnel is formed by dissecting the tympanic membrane from the malleus handle, through which the upper end of the wire prosthesis is placed so that it may be crimped around the handle. The lower end is placed in the middle of a tissue seal covering the oval window (Fig. 50–9). Some surgeons prefer a plastic prosthesis inserted between the undersurface of the malleus and the oval window graft (Fig. 50–10).

A slightly easier method is to use the malleus-footplate assembly technique described in Chapter 55. The homograft bone prosthesis is carved to fit between the malleus handle and the oval window seal.

In the unusual instance in which the malleus handle is missing, a columella, may be used. In this situation, a tissue graft (vein or fascia) is used to cover the oval

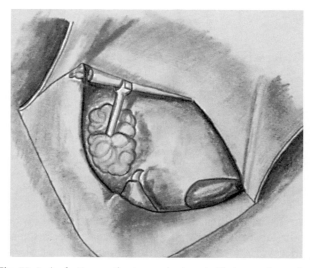

Fig. 50–9. A plastic prosthesis may be inserted between the undersurface of the malleus and the oval window graft. Several designs have been described for this purpose.

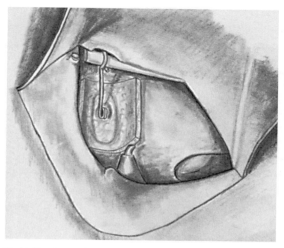

Fig. 50–10. Revision of fenestration. A preformed wire loop is placed between the malleus and the oval window after total stapedectomy (Sheehy).

window, and the columella is placed with its shaft resting on the oval window graft and its head under the tympanic membrane protected by an autograft cartilage disc under the drum membrane. This same technique may be used when the malleus is present.

The skin flap is returned to its former position and dressed, as in stapedectomy. A common problem is a small gap in the region in which the posterior spine has been removed owing to flap shrinkage. A tissue graft is used to fill this defect to prevent postoperative perforation.

A major contraindication to this procedure is the presence of infection of the mastoid cavity. This must be completely cleared before surgery, and in many instances a preliminary mastoid obliteration is advisable. Cochlear loss occurs in about 1% of these procedures.

SUGGESTED READINGS

Austin DF: Stapedectomy with tissue seal. In Controversy in Otolaryngology. Edited by Snow JB. Philadelphia: WB Saunders Co, 1980.

Bailey HAT, Pappas JJ, Graham SS: Small fenestra stapedectomy, a preliminary report. Laryngoscope 91:1308, 1981.

Goodhill V: Stapes Surgery for Otosclerosis. New York: Hoeber Medical Division, Harper & Row, 1961.

Guild SR: Histologic otosclerosis. Ann Otol Rhinol Laryngol 53:246, 1944.

Hough JVD: Partial stapedectomy. Trans Am Acad Ophthal Otolaryngol 66:412, 1962.

Hough JVD: Recent advances in otosclerosis. Arch Otolaryngol 83:379, 1966.

Hough JVD: A critique of stapedectomy. J Laryngol Otol 105:15, 1976.

House HP: Prefabricated wire loop—Gelfoam stapedectomy. Arch Otolaryngol 76:298, 1962.

Lempert J: Fenestra Nov-ovalis technique. Arch Otolaryngol 66:35, 1957.

Linthicum FH Jr: Correlation of sensorineural hearing impairment and otosclerosis. Ann Otol Rhinol Laryngol 75:512, 1966.

McGee TM: Comparison of small fenestra and total stapedectomy. Ann Otol Rhinol Laryngol 90:633, 1981.

Moon GN and Hahn MJ: Partial vs. total footplate removal in stapedectomy: A comparative study. Laryngoscope 94:912, 1984.

Nager GT: Sensorineural deafness and otosclerosis. Ann Otol Rhinol Laryngol 75:481, 1966.

Reudi L: Pathogenesis of Otosclerosis. Arch Otolaryngol 78:469, 1963.

Reudi L: Histopathological confirmation of labyrinthine otosclerosis. Laryngoscope 75:1582, 1965.

Reudi L and Spoendlin H: Pathogenesis of sensorineural deafness in otosclerosis. Ann Otol Rhinol Laryngol 75:525, 1966.

Schuknecht HF (Ed): Otosclerosis. Boston: Little, Brown and Co, 1962.

Schuknecht HF: Pathology of the Ear. Cambridge: Harvard University Press, 1974.

Shambaugh GE, Causse J: Ten years' experience with fluoride in otosclerotic (otospongiotic) patients. Ann Otol Rhinol Laryngol 83:635, 1974.

Shea JJ Jr: Fenestration of the oval window. Ann Otol Rhinol Laryngol 67:932, 1958.

Shea JJ Jr: Complications of the stapedectomy operation. Ann Otol Rhinol Laryngol 72:1109, 1963.

Shea JJ Jr, et al: Teflon piston operation for otosclerosis. Arch Otolaryngol 76:516, 1962.

Shea JJ Jr: A fifteen year report on fenestration of the oval window. Trans Am Acad Ophthalmol Otolaryngol 75:31, 1971.

Sheehy JL: Stapes surgery in advanced otosclerosis. Ann Otol Rhinol Laryngol 71:601, 1962.

Sheehy JL: Stapedectomy in the fenestrated ear. Arch Otolaryngol 78:574, 1963.

Silverstein H, Rosenberg S and Jones R: Small fenestra stapedectomies with and without KTP laser: A comparison. Laryngoscope 99:485–488, 1989.

Smyth GL, Hazzard TH: Eighteen years experience in stapedectomy. Ann Otol Rhinol Laryngol 87(Suppl 49):3, 1978.

Sooy FS, et al: Stapedectomy in obliterative otosclerosis. Ann Otol Rhinol Laryngol 73:679, 1964.

Wolff D, Bellucci RJ: Otosclerosis. Arch Otolaryngol 79:571, 1964.

51 Microtia, Canal Atresia, and Middle-Ear Anomalies

Simon C. Parisier and Charles P. Kimmelman

The child born with a malformed ear faces a lifelong hearing and communication impairment along with the social stigma of a facial deformity. Associated disturbances of the vestibular system may add the developmental hurdle of a motor delay. Frequently there are additional anomalies, such as mandibular hypoplasia as well as other facial and skeletal deformities. There may be dysfunction of associated neural pathways, including cranial nerves and intracranial structures. Additionally, there are psychological factors to be considered, including parental guilt, peer ridicule and the shame of "being different." Educationally and economically, these hearing-impaired children may have limited opportunities. The appropriate treatment of these patients involves recognizing the problems and limitations of therapy, which need to be thoroughly understood by the parents and, when appropriate, the patient.

EMBRYOLOGY OF ATRESIA AND MICROTIA

In the 3–4 mm embryo (3–4 weeks) the first indications of aural ontogenesis are the first and second branchiomeric structures and the otic placode, an ectodermal thickening on the lateral surface of the head opposite the fourth ventricle. The placode invaginates to first form a pit and then a vesicle detached from its surface origin. This otocyst forms the inner ear membranous structures, with the endolymphatic duct developing first at the 6 mm stage, followed by the appearance of the semicircular canals and the cochlear diverticulum at the 15 mm stage (6 weeks). By the end of the third month the cochlea is fully coiled.

The cranial nerves entering the otocyst exert an inductive influence to produce neuroepithelium, for which retinoic acid is a potent morphogen. Retinoic acid receptors are uniquely expressed in the developing organ of Corti; medications which affect retinoic acid metabolism, such as tritinoin (Acutane, Roche, Nutley, NJ), can lead to embryopathies, including inner ear malformation.[1]

The cochleovestibular ganglia develop from the otic placode epithelium. The nerve fibers themselves not only influence sensory cell development, but they are also directed to the developing inner ear by the sensory cells.[2]

As the membranous structures of the inner ear form, they become enveloped in a cartilagenous capsule, which eventually gives rise to the petrous portion of the temporal bone. Concurrently, the structures which originate from the first pharyngeal pouch develop separately, but adjacent to, the otic capsule structures. The pouch begins to form in the 3–4 mm embryo and expands into a tubotympanic recess, which will eventually give rise to the eustachian tube, middle-ear space, and mastoid air cell system. The third branchial arch migrates superiorly to the level of the recess, and its artery (the internal carotid) comes to lie dorsal to the eustachian tube. Variations in this relationship may result in a lateralized displacement of the internal carotid artery into the middle-ear space. In adults, an ectopic carotid artery can be mistaken for a middle-ear mass, such as a glomus tumor.

As the pharyngeal pouches form in the 3–4 mm embryo, corresponding grooves develop on the external surface of the nascent cervical region. The first of these branchial clefts deepens until it approaches the tubotympanic recess, being separated only by the thin layer of mesoderm destined to become the middle fibrous layer of the tympanic membrane. Subsequently, in the 30 mm embryo (8 weeks), the primordial external canal becomes occluded by an ectodermal plug. By the 21st week this begins to resorb to form the definitive external auditory canal replete with its hair and glandular appendages. Aberrations in the canalization process can lead to stenosis, canal tortuosity or fibrous/osseous obliteration. Since middle-ear structures develop independently, the tympanic cavity and ossicles may be normal.

Defects in the canalization process may also be associated with faulty formation of the pinna, which arises in the 8–11 mm embryo from six mesodermal thickenings. These hillocks surround the entrance of the first branchial cleft. The first branchial arch cartilage (Meckel's) forms the tragus and superior helical crus; the remainder of the pinna derives from the second arch cartilage (Reichert's), although some authorities posit a hyoid arch derivation for all but the tragus.[2] The developing auricular appendage migrates from its initial position in the lower face toward the temporal area. This movement occurs along the fusion plane of the first and second branchial arches. The auricle is initially located anteriorly in a horizontal axis; with development of the branchial structures it migrates from its original position in the lower face laterally, and, as its axis rotates, it assumes a more vertical angulation. Branchial cleft dysmorphogenesis can impede this migration and leave the pinna in a low, transverse orientation (Fig. 51–1).

As the middle ear forms, the separation between the first pharyngeal pouch and cleft is filled in by mesenchyme. In the 8 mm (6th week) embryo, part of the connective tissue condenses to form the malleus handle; the subsequent expansion of the tympanic cavity superiorly is delayed until the cartilaginous otic capsule fully forms. The expansion of the first pharyngeal pouch results in the envelopment of the ossicles in an endodermal epithelium. The ossicles predominantly originate from mesenchymal visceral bars of the first and second arches. The first arch forms the head of the malleus and body of the incus, with the second arch giving rise to the manubrium, long process of the incus, stapes superstructure and lateral portion of the footplate. The medial lamina of the footplate is derived from the otic capsule. The obturator foramen of the stapes forms around the stapedial artery, which usually remains diminutive while the stapes enlarges. If variations in vascular development cause enlargement of the artery, a conductive hearing loss may result from impairment of stapes motion. As the derivatives of the first pharyngeal pouch continue to extend into the developing temporal bone, the antrum, mastoid air cells, and petrous pyramid cells begin to form. Most mastoid development is postnatal; abnormalities which arrest middle-ear formation result in a poorly pneumatized bone.

The facial nerve is intimately related to the development of the middle- and inner-ear structures outlined above. The blastema of the stapes is adjacent to the seventh nerve, which divides the second (hyoid) visceral mesenchymal bar into a laterohyale, stapes blastema and interhyale. The interhyale forms the stapedius tendon, while the laterohyale forms part of the bony fallopian canal and pyramid. Thus, the development of the stapes is closely related to that of the facial nerve. Abnormalities in the development of the stapes frequently are associated with facial nerve anomalies. This relationship of facial nerve to developing middle-ear structures increases the likelihood of an anomalous course of the nerve in the malformed middle ear.[3,4]

ETIOLOGY OF AURAL ATRESIA

Atresia and microtia are associated with several known syndromes felt to be associated with inherited defects or acquired embryopathies due to intrauterine infection (rubella, syphilis) ischemic injury (hemifacial microsomia) or toxin exposure (thalidomide, tritinoin).

Although several inner ear abnormalities, such as Usher syndrome, Waardenburg syndrome and the neurofibromatoses are becoming understood on a molecular biologic basis, the genetic location of external and middle ear anomalies generally remains poorly characterized. Aural atresia occurs in approximately 1 in 20,000 live births. Although the inner and middle ears develop separately, inner ear abnormalities coexist in 12 to 50% of cases. Atresia is bilateral in 30% of cases, occurring more commonly in males and in the right ear.[5]

It is not surprising that an embryonic insult severe

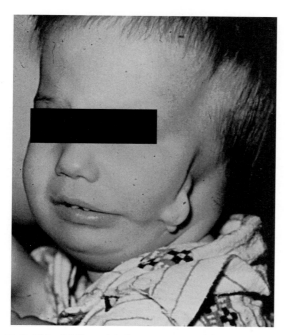

Fig. 51–1. This child's auricle has not migrated from its embryonic low, transverse positioning.

enough to cause aural atresia would also affect other organ systems. The following organs may be anomalous in patients with atresia: neurocranium defects (Crouzon's or craniofacial dysostosis), central nervous system (mental retardation), oral cavity (first and second branchial arch syndromes), the eye (Goldenhar's syndrome), the neck (branchial fistulas), the CHARGE association (**C**oloboma, **H**eart defect, choanal **A**tresia, **R**etarded growth, **G**enitourinary defects, and **E**ar anomalies), Treacher Collins syndrome (mandibulofacial dysostosis), Duane syndrome (abducens palsy with retracted bulb), VATER syndrome (probable disorganization of the primitive streak with impairment of early mesodermal migration causing **V**ertebral defects, **A**nal atresia, **T**racheoesophageal fistula, **R**enal defects and genital anomalies), and Pierre Robin syndrome. Chromosomal anomalies affecting the external and middle ears include Turner syndrome; Trisomies 13–15, 18, 21, and 22.

Anomalies of the ear in the absence of syndromes are usually not familial. From the above information it is obvious that other congenital anomalies should be assiduously sought; some, such as renal dysgenesis, may not be readily apparent. A chromosomal analysis may be indicated. As progress is made in molecular diagnosis, more definitive gene mapping may prove useful in identifying a genetic basis for many of these disorders.[6–8]

DIAGNOSIS AND EVALUATION

In the more severe cases of microtia, the diagnosis is apparent on inspection of the external ear. Depending on the degree of the abnormality, the microtic ear may be classified into three grades. In grade I, the auricle is developed and, though misshapen, has a readily recognizable, characteristic anatomy (Fig. 51–2). In grade II, the helix is rudimentary and the lobule developed (Fig. 51–3). In grade III, an amorphous skin tag is present (Fig. 51–4). In all stages, wide variations of morphology exist. The pinna may be fully formed with a transverse and low-set orientation. There may be accessory appendages of the pinna (pre-tragal tags with or without cartilage) and preauricular sinus tracts. The external canal may be stenotic or atretic to varying degrees (Fig. 51–5). In cases of stenosis, entrapped squamous epithelium may lead to a retention cholesteatoma with bone destruction. Schuknecht[9] observed that in 7 ears with congenital meatal stenosis, all had

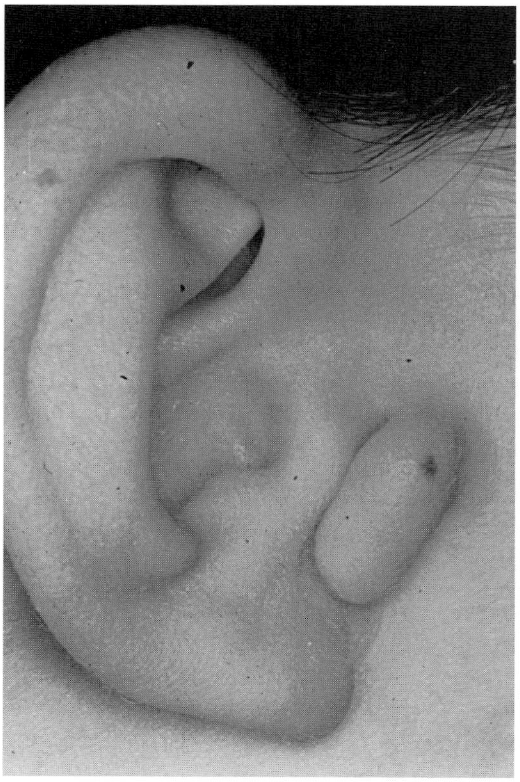

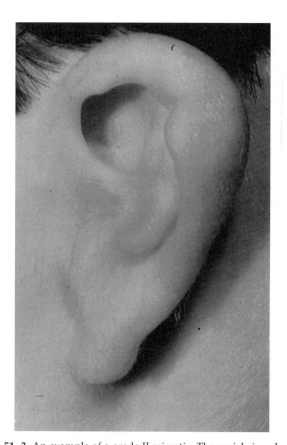

Fig. 51–2. This pinna exhibits a grade I microtia with canal atresia. The size of the auricle and the characteristic anatomical landmarks are fairly normal. A pretragal skin tag is present.

Fig. 51–3. An example of a grade II microtia. The auricle is reduced in size and has a characteristic recognizable shape. The inferior and superior crura have not developed, although the helix is well preserved.

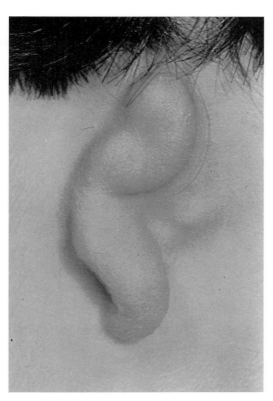

Fig. 51–4. Auricle showing a grade III microtia. An amorphous ridge of skin and nubbins of cartilage are present in place of a recognizable, well-developed auricle.

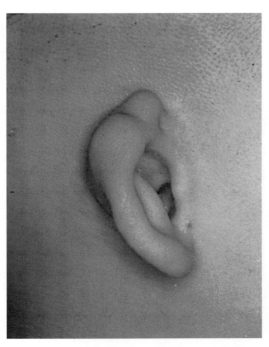

Fig. 51–5. A grade II-III microtia with poor formation of the superior third of the auricle and a preauricular pit, possibly because of a first branchial arch dysmorphism. The lower portion of the ear, which is derived from the second branchial arch, has a relatively normal appearance. The canal is stenotic, leading to the subsequent development of a retention cholesteatoma.

TABLE 51–1. Minor Congenital Middle Ear Abnormalities with Patent Ear Canal, Mobile Tympanic Membrane, and Conductive Loss

I. Ossicular Fixation
  A. Stapes Fixation
    1. Deficient annular ligament
    2. Elongated pyramidal process, ossified stapedial tendon
  B. Malleolar-Incudal Fixation
    1. Lateral epitympanic ankylosis
    2. Medial epitympanic ankylosis of body of incus, head of malleus
    3. Ossified anterior malleolar ligament
II. Ossicular Discontinuity
  A. Absent stapes arch
  B. Deficient lenticular process of incus
  C. Deficient long process of incus
III. Cochlear Capsule and Facial Nerve Anomalies
  A. Aplasia of oval or round window
  B. Facial nerve anomaly occluding oval window
  C. High jugular bulb occluding the round window niche

cholesteatomas, while 3 out of 11 ears with partial atresia and narrowed canals had cholesteatoma. In 50 ears with complete atresia, only two had cholesteatomas.

Abnormalities of the tympanic cavity alone may occur with a normal tympanic membrane and external ear. In ears with conductive hearing losses and normal otoscopic examinations, isolated ossicular anomalies should be suspected (Table 51–1). Ossicular fixation can be produced by a variety of abnormalities and may involve the stapes, incus or malleus (Table 51–1A,B). Alternatively, there may be a failure of bone development producing an ossicular discontinuity which generally involves the incus and/or stapes arch (Tables 51–1, 51–2). Ossicular malformations caused by abnormalities related to first or second branchial cartilaginous derivatives can frequently be surgically repaired (Table 51–1, Groups I and II). However, ossicular fixations due to cochlear capsule abnormalities, especially when associated with an aberrant facial nerve, may not be surgically correctable (Table 51–1, Group III). Otic capsule abnormalities producing stapedial fixation are frequently associated with abnormal communication between the inner ear and the subarachnoid space. In

TABLE 51–2. Congenital Atresia Classification

Class I. A. Aerated normal middle ear space
      B. Developed oval window with mobile stapes
      C. Oval window not obstructed by facial nerve

Class II. A. Narrowed, but aerated, middle-ear space
      B. Fixed stapes, oval window aplasia
      C. Oval window not obstructed by facial nerve

Class III. A. Nonaerated, hypoplastic middle ear space
      B. Oval window obstructed by facial nerve
      C. Tegmen low hanging, obstructs access to middle-ear space

these instances, manipulation of the stapes results in a persistent gusher of cerebrospinal fluid. Vascular malformations also occur in the middle ear, such as high jugular bulb, persistent stapedial artery and anomalous course of the carotid artery.

Further delineation of structural abnormalities requires computed tomography (CT).[10] Younger children may require sedation if they are unable to cooperate. The images are processed with a bone algorithm image enhancement using one and a half mm slices at either 1.5 or 1 mm intervals. Optimally, both axial and coronal scans are obtained, although reformatted coronal or sagittal images may be adequate. Three dimen-sional reconstruction[11,12] may be useful in visualizing the temporal bone topography in the more extensive malformations occurring in Treacher-Collins syndrome and hemifacial microsomia. CT studies allow determination of the degree of the canal atresia, the thickness of the atresia plate (Fig. 51–6A), the extent of pneumatization of the middle ear and mastoid, the distance between the glenoid fossa and mastoid, the intratemporal course of the facial nerve, the status of the malleus and incus and, in some instances, the presence or absence of the stapes and oval window (Fig. 51–6B). However, subtleties of oval and round window anatomy are often not revealed. An unsuspected

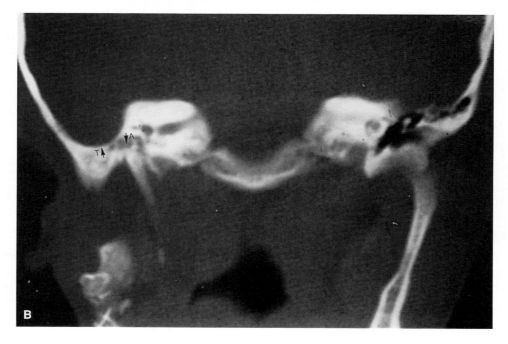

Fig. 51–6. A. Coronal CT scan showing a bony atresia plate (arrow). The middle ear space is normally pneumatized. B. Coronal CT scan showing a low-lying tegmen (T), which precludes construction of an external canal. The middle ear cleft has not developed. A rudimentary antrum is unaerated (A). Atresia surgery is contraindicated in this case.

cholesteatoma may also be apparent. The normalcy of the osseous inner ear structures is also revealed by CT.

Brainstem response audiometry should be performed neonatally in all children born with either microtia or atresia. In cases of microtia with fairly normal canals, an ossicular malformation producing a conductive hearing loss may be present. In patients with unilateral atresia, it is not unusual for the seemingly normal contralateral ear to have a hearing loss. Bilateral involvement may cause masking dilemmas; such is the case when one ear has a conductive loss and the other a sensorineural loss. These dilemmas may be minimized by using multichannel analysis of ipsilateral vs. contralateral responses to determine the laterality of wave I.[13] As the infant matures, behavioral audiometric evaluations must be obtained to confirm the neurophysiological tests of hearing. In children older than one year, conditioned free field play audiometry should help to quantify the overall hearing levels. Eventually, pure-tone and speech testing with masking should be obtained in children with fairly normal canals. Impedance and stapedial reflex measures in a seemingly normal ear can provide valuable information as well.

Evaluation of the function of other organ systems should be considered by the otologist. For example, some of the syndromal associations of atresia involve mandibular and laryngeal anomalies which can lead to airway obstruction; cardiac, renal, endocrine and immune function should be ascertained in selected instances.

MANAGEMENT OF AURAL ATRESIA AND MICROTIA

Nonsurgical

The prime concern in the young child is the assessment and improvement of hearing. When ear deformities are present, auditory brainstem response techniques outlined above are helpful in determining the type and severity of hearing loss and should be performed as early in life as possible. Early amplification, auditory training and speech therapy can improve speech and language skills. In children with bilateral atresia, amplification with bone conduction aids should be provided as soon as possible, preferably within the first few months of life. In infants with a unilateral atresia and conductive hearing loss in the seemingly normal ear, an air conduction aid should be fitted to the ear with a canal.

Surgical

In the unilateral case with normal contralateral hearing, repair of either the microtia or the atresia is consid-

ered elective and there is less urgency to intervene during childhood. When the atresia is bilateral with acceptable appearing auricles, reconstructive surgery can be performed at a fairly young age. However, in cases of microtia that require reconstruction, atresia repair should be deferred until the initial stages of the auricular repair are completed. Generally, microtia surgery requires a cartilage graft that is obtained from the lower costochondral region. An adequate graft requires sufficient growth and fusion at the donor site, which has usually occurred by 5–6 years of age. Additionally, in bilateral cases, many authorities recommend postponing surgery for the restoration of hearing until at least age 5 so that pneumatization can develop.[9] In children with frequent upper respiratory infections and suspected eustachian tube dysfunction, it may also be necessary to delay hearing reconstructive surgery.

Surgical Treatment of Congenital Conductive Hearing Loss

The success of the surgical correction of congenital conductive hearing losses is related to the abnormality, since a wide range of malformations is possible.[14,15] Surgery in an ear that has an isolated ossicular malformation with an otherwise patent canal, intact tympanic membrane, aerated middle ear cleft, normal facial nerve and mobile stapes has the potential for excellent hearing (Table 51–2, Class I). Conversely, an ear with canal atresia, a narrowed and poorly aerated middle-ear space, and an anomalously positioned facial nerve occluding the oval window is destined to have poor postoperative hearing (Table 51–2, Class III). Between these two extremes is an array of anomalies with variable surgical outcomes. Even with sophisticated imaging techniques, the preoperative prediction of what awaits the otologist is not always accurate.

Surgeons wishing to correct congenital conductive hearing losses are embarking on a procedure with significant potential complications. Generally, the initial attempt is the procedure most likely to improve the hearing. Unplanned revisions are often more complex and less successful. Additionally, if a significant sensorineural hearing loss occurs after surgery in a patient with bilateral malformations, the opposite ear is effectively excluded from surgical correction since it becomes the better hearing ear. Before assuming this responsibility, especially in children, the otologic surgeon must have sufficient experience to maximize the likelihood of a successful outcome.

The presence of a conductive hearing loss in an ear with a normal canal and mobile drumhead generally indicates that the ossicular chain is not transmitting sound energy to the cochlea. Isolated ossicular malformations involving the stapes arch and long process of the incus may not be appreciated on CT studies. In these cases, the middle ear can be explored by elevating a tympanomeatal flap and assessing the normalcy of the ossicular transduction mechanism. If the canal is small, a postauricular approach will improve operative exposure. Frequently, even the young child's ear canal has a sufficient diameter to admit an adequately sized ear speculum, even though the length of the canal is shorter.

Once the middle ear is entered, the surgeon needs to decide if the chain is fixed. If so, what is the cause of the fixation (Table 51–1). First, the motility of the incus and malleus is ascertained. Is the fixation in the epitympanum and if not, where (Fig. 51–7)? Drilling away the bone over the malleus head and body of the incus provides the required exposure to explore this area. Is the stapedial tendon ossified? If the stapes is fixed, mobilization may produce a sustained improvement. Alternatively, a stapedectomy using a replacement prosthesis with an oval window tissue graft to prevent a perilymphatic leak may be performed. In some cases, the surgeon may elect to defer stapes surgery until the child is grown.

A gap interrupting the ossicular chain's continuity occurs most commonly at the incudostapedial joint, either due to absence of the lenticular process and/or long process of the incus or the stapes arch. The presence of a mobile stapes facilitates the surgery and greatly improves the operative result. A variety of techniques have proven useful in the restoration of ossicular chain continuity by means of bridging an existing gap. If there is a small distance between the stapes capitulum and the long process of the incus, a tragal cartilage graft can successfully negotiate the gap. Deficiencies of the long process of the incus can be cor-

rected by either interposing the reshaped incus between the mobile stapes and the malleus handle or using an alloplastic prosthesis designed for this purpose (type III tympanoplasty). When the stapes arch is absent, similar procedures can be performed to bridge the gap from either the malleus handle or the undersurface of the drumhead to the mobile footplate (type IV tympanoplasty). A coexisting fixation of the stapes or obstruction of the oval window by the facial nerve increases the technical difficulty, yields poorer hearing results and increases the chance of complications, such as sensorineural hearing loss or facial nerve injury.

Surgery for Microtia and Canal Stenosis or Atresia

Congenital malformations of the auricle, external canal and middle ear may occur as isolated abnormalities or in various combinations. Reconstruction of the external ear is usually performed by a plastic surgeon while the external auditory canal and middle-ear defects are corrected by the otologist; both work as a team to achieve the optimal result.

Microtia surgery is technically difficult and not infrequently the results are somewhat disappointing. The surgery should be performed by individuals with special expertise. Auricular reconstruction is an elective procedure. The deformity can usually be masked by a longer hair style. Generally, the slight deformity of a grade I microtia may be cosmetically acceptable. Reconstruction of a moderately deformed grade II microtia must be individualized. Correction of a severe grade III microtia requires several staged procedures. During the first stage a segment of cartilage is obtained from the lower costochondral skeleton. It is then carved to the appropriate shape to form a scaffold for the new auricle. This process requires an artistic appreciation of the external-ear folds. The graft is implanted into a subcutaneous pocket at the appropriate position. A portion of the microtic skin tag is maintained to construct the lobule. The second stage is performed after several months. The auricle is freed from the scalp and a split thickness skin graft is applied to create a postauricular sulcus. At a third stage several months later the tragus is created. An alternative technique for the treatment of severe grade III microtia is to use a lifelike prosthetic ear which is attached to surgically implanted titanium posts that securely hold the auricle in a normal anatomical position.

The timing of the microtia and atresia repairs requires close communication between the surgeons. Because scarring interferes with the auricular repair, reconstruction of the atresia is deferred until the auricular cartilaginous scaffolding is completed. However, it is important to position the reconstructed auricle correctly so that it aligns with the meatal opening and the middle ear.

The meatal, canal and middle-ear reconstruction is

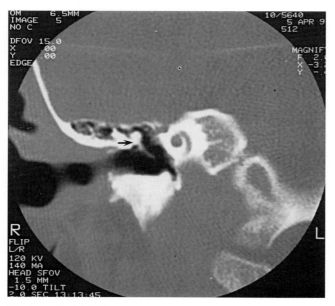

Fig. 51–7. Coronal CT scan in a patient with a congenital conductive hearing loss caused by osseous fixation of the malleus head to the lateral epitympanic wall (arrow).

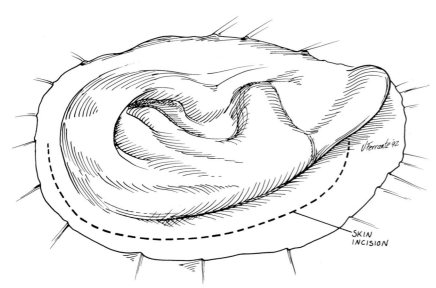

Fig. 51–8. Surgery for canal atresia. A postauricular incision is made. While exposing the mastoid cortex and dysmorphic tympanic bone, the previously implanted cartilaginous auricular scaffold should be protected during retraction.

frequently performed as part of the second or third stage of the auricular reconstruction. A postauricular approach is used, great care being taken to avoid exposing the scaffold (Fig. 51–8).[16,17] Temporalis fascia is harvested for reconstruction of the tympanic membrane. The periosteum of the lateral surface of the temporal bone is elevated. A bony circular canal is created by drilling between the glenoid fossa anteriorly and the tegmen plate superiorly while trying to avoid entering mastoid air cells posteriorly (Fig. 51–9). Continuous suction irrigation cools the bone and clears away blood and bone dust while the water enhances the translucency of the wet bone. This permits visualization of structures such as dura, facial nerve and glenoid fossa through the intact thinned bone. The surgeon should anticipate that the facial nerve will be located more anteriorly and more laterally than in the normal temporal bone. The nerve frequently follows a C-shaped path in its course between the geniculate ganglion and

its point of emergence from the temporal bone. The purposeful identification of the facial nerve will prevent inadvertent injury. A facial nerve monitor may facilitate identification of the nerve in atretic ears.

Visualization of the facial nerve as a landmark permits the opening of the atresia plate to approximate the size of a normal middle ear opening. While drilling on this plate, it must be remembered that the malleus handle may be fused to it. Precautions must be taken to avoid drilling on the mobilized atresia remnant, since this may transmit traumatic vibratory energy through the ossicular chain to the inner ear and result in a permanent sensorineural hearing loss.

The status of the ossicular chain is assessed (Fig. 51–10). If the stapes is mobile, an appropriate ossicular reconstruction is performed (Fig. 51–11). If it is fixed or the oval window is obscured by the facial nerve, the ossicular reconstruction should be deferred. Temporalis fascia is used to fabricate a new tympanic mem-

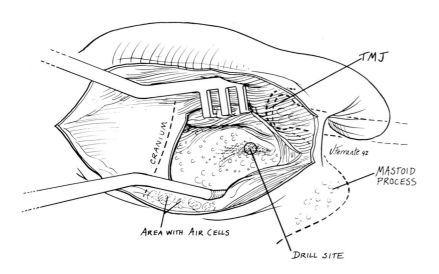

Fig. 51–9. Construction of a canal is begun by drilling between the glenoid fossa anteriorly and the superior temporal line. The latter roughly corresponds to the tegmen (floor of the middle cranial fossa). When possible, entry into the mastoid air cells is avoided.

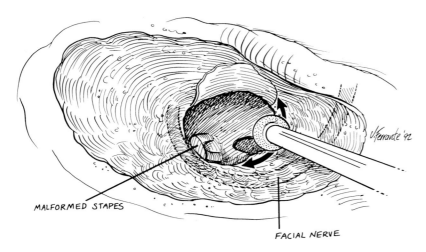

MALFORMED STAPES

FACIAL NERVE

Fig. 51–10. Drilling is continued until a normal sized middle ear opening has been created. Great care is taken not to drill on a mobile, deformed, but intact, ossicular chain. The anteriorly coursing facial nerve is identified.

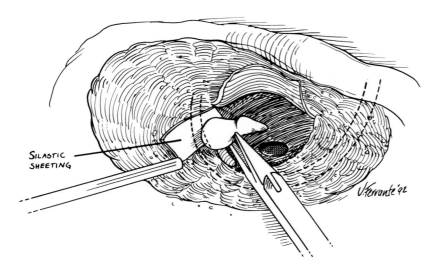

SILASTIC SHEETING

Fig. 51–11. The ossicular chain is reconstructed by interposing the malformed, sculpted ossicle onto the stapes. Silastic sheeting, 0.005 inches thick, is positioned to prevent bony ankylosis.

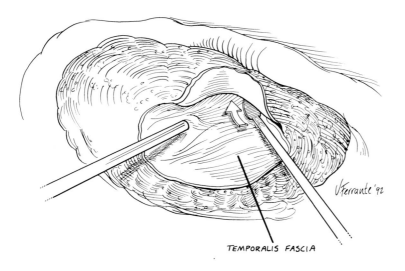

TEMPORALIS FASCIA

Fig. 51–12. Temporalis fascia is used to construct a tympanic membrane.

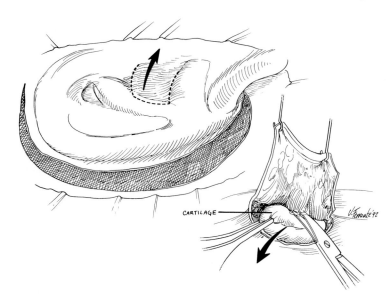

CARTILAGE

Fig. 51–13. A meatal opening is made through the imperforate conchal skin. A rectangular, anteriorly based skin flap is debulked and rotated to line the anterior lateral third of the new canal.

brane (Fig. 51–12). A meatal opening is made in the area of the imperforate concha, incising the skin to create a rectangularly shaped, anteriorly based conchal skin flap. The underlying cartilage and soft tissue are removed to debulk the flap and create an opening that communicates with the drilled out external canal (Fig. 51–13). The conchal flap is rotated to resurface the anterior third of the external canal and is stabilized by suturing to the adjacent soft tissues (Fig. 51–14). A thin split thickness skin graft is harvested from the lower abdomen and used to resurface the remaining ear canal. The canal is packed snugly with Gelfoam (Upjohn, Kalamazoo, MI) to compress the skin grafts against the underlying bone and soft tissue. The post-auricular incision is reapproximated using absorbable sutures.

Results of Atresia Surgery—Risks and Benefits

Atresia surgery is technically demanding. The results achieved are directly related to the experience and skill of the operating surgeon. Generally, hearing improvement to a serviceable level can be achieved in approximately 65% to 75% of selected cases. Complications of surgery include the small risk of facial paralysis, a severe to profound sensorineural hearing loss, stenosis requiring additional surgery, persistent otorrhea and tympanic membrane graft failure with perforation.

In children with a unilateral atresia and a normal contralateral ear, surgery may not be routinely indicated.[17] The potential benefit of this sophisticated surgery, i.e., achieving binaural hearing, may not justify the risk of complications. In binaural cases the successful creation of an external canal even when hearing cannot be improved will allow the use of an ear level air conduction hearing aid to restore hearing without using a cumbersome bone conduction aid. Thus, in bilateral cases in which the facial nerve obstructs the oval window or when a hearing improvement cannot be achieved, providing the patient with a stable, skin lined canal is a worthy goal in and of itself.

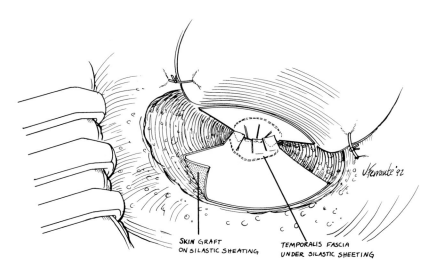

SKIN GRAFT
ON SILASTIC SHEATING

TEMPORALIS FASCIA
UNDER SILASTIC SHEETING

Fig. 51–14. A thin, split-thickness skin graft harvested from the lower abdomen is used to resurface the remainder of the canal. Handling and placement of the graft is facilitated by gluing the epidermal surface to thin (0.005 inch) Silastic sheeting. The raw surface of the graft is compressed against the bone by filling the canal lumen with Gelfoam.

REFERENCES

1. Lefebvre PP, Malgrange B, Staecker H, et al: Retinoic acid stimulates regeneration of mammalian auditory hair cells. Science *260*:692–695, 1993.

2. Anson BJ, Davies J, Duckert LG: Embryology of the ear. In Otolaryngology. Edited by Paparella MM, Shumrick DA, Gluckman JL, et al. Philadelphia: W.B. Saunders Co., 1991, pp. 3–21.

3. Williams GH: Developmental anatomy of the ear. In Otolaryngology. Edited by English GM. Philadelphia: J.B. Lippincott Co., 1990.

4. Nager GT, Proctor B: Anatomic variations and anomalies involving the facial canal. Otolaryngol Clin North Am *24*: 531–553, 1991.

5. Jafek BW, Nager GT, Strife J: Congenital aural atresia: an analysis of 311 cases. Trans Am Acad Ophthalmol Otolaryngol *80*: 588–595, 1975.

6. Snow JB: Preface. Otolaryngol Clin North Am *25*:xv–xvi, 1992.

7. Sando IS, Shibahara Y, Wood RP: Congenital anomalies of the external and middle ear. In Pediatric Otolaryngology. Edited by Bluestone CD, Stool SE. Philadelphia: W.B. Saunders Co., 1990, pp 271–302.

8. Bergstrom LB: Anomalies of the ear. In Otolaryngology. Edited by English GM. Philadelphia: J.B. Lippincott Co., 1990.

9. Schuknecht HF: Congenital aural atresia. Laryngoscope *99*: 908–917, 1989.

10. Curtin HD: Congenital malformations of the ear. Otolaryngol Clinics North Am *21*:317–336, 1988.

11. Jahrsdoerfer RA, Garcia ET, Yeakley JW, et al: Surface contour three-dimensional imaging in congenital aural atresia. Arch Otolaryngol Head Neck Surg *119*:95–99, 1993.

12. Andrews JC, Anzai Y, Mankovich NJ, et al: Three-dimensional CT scan reconstruction for the assessment of congenital aural atresia. Am J Otol *13*:236–240, 1992.

13. Jahrsdoerfer RA, Yeakley JW, Hall JW, et al: High-resolution CT scanning and auditory brain stem response in congenital aural atresia: Patient selection and surgical correlation. Otolaryngol Head Neck Surg *93*:292–298, 1985.

14. Jahrsdoerfer RA, Yeakley JW, Aguilar EA, et al: Grading system for the selection of patients with congenital aural atresia. Am J Otol *13*:6–12, 1992.

15. Teunissen EB, Cremers CWRJ: Classification of congenital middle ear anomalies. Report on 144 ears. Ann Otol Rhinol Laryngol *102*:606–612, 1993.

16. Shih L, Crabtree JA: Longterm surgical results for congenital aural atresia. Laryngoscope *103*:1097–1102, 1993.

17. Bellucci RJ: Congenital aural malformations: diagnosis and treatment. Otolaryngol Clin North Am *14*:95–124, 1981.

Crouzon Syndrome (Craniofacial Dysostosis)

Although Crouzon syndrome is an autosomal dominant form of hereditary hearing impairment, one-third of cases arise from new mutations.[13,14] Clinical features are limited to the cranium and face and include premature craniosynostosis, midface hypoplasia, ocular proptosis and hypertelorism producing a "frog face" appearance. Thirty percent of patients have a conductive hearing impairment secondary to either external auditory canal atresia or ossicular malformations. This syndrome has been mapped to the long arm of chromosome 10.[15]

Apert Syndrome (Acrocephalosyndactyly)

Like Crouzon syndrome, Apert syndrome is characterized by craniosynostosis. Most commonly, the coronal suture is involved, resulting in a high, steep forehead, flat occiput and broadening of the skull in the temporal area. However, in addition to cranial and facial malformations, Apert syndrome is associated with synostoses in the hands and feet. Mental retardation is present in most patients. Hearing loss is typically conductive and arises secondary to ossicular fixation. A case of perilymphatic gusher during stapedectomy in one patient has been reported.[16]

Stickler Syndrome (Hereditary Arthro-Ophthalmopathy)

This autosomal dominant syndrome is characterized by Marfanoid habitus, spondyloepiphyseal dysplasia, joint hypermobility, hypoplasia of the midface, severe myopia and varying degrees of Robin sequence. Because of the possibility of retinal detachment, ophthalmologic referral is mandatory. Approximately 15% of patients suffer a mixed form of hearing impairment. Gene linkage studies have shown that the syndrome is heterogeneous, with at least one locus mapping to chromosome 12; mutations of the precollagen type II gene (COL 2A1) have been described.[17–19]

Wildervanck Syndrome (Cervico-Oculo-Acoustic Dysplasia)

Inheritance of Wildervanck syndrome is believed to be multifactorial.[20,21] The phenotype is characterized by fusion of cervical vertebrae (Klippel-Feil anomaly), torticollis, abducens palsy with retracted bulbs (Duane syndrome), occasional cleft palate, and severe congenital sensorineural or conductive hearing loss. Middle ear and inner ear anomalies also have been reported.[22]

Melnick-Fraser Syndrome (Branchio-Oto-Renal Syndrome)

This autosomal dominant syndrome is estimated to affect 2% of children in schools for the hearing impaired. Although the phenotype can vary, full expression includes preauricular pits, external ear malformations, branchial cysts or fistulae, renal malformations and hearing loss. The hearing loss can be either conductive, sensorineural or mixed. Malformations of the ossicles and inner ears have been reported, including dilation of the vestibular aqueduct. The defective gene has been localized to chromosome 8.[23]

Pierre Robin Syndrome

This autosomal dominant syndrome occurs in approximately 1:30,000 live births. Clinical manifestations include cleft palate, micrognathia and glossoptosis, giving affected persons a bird-like appearance. Anomalies of the external ears, eyes, skeletal system and heart also can occur. Twenty percent of persons with Pierre Robin syndrome are mentally retarded.[24] Anomalies of the external, middle and inner ear have been described and cause conductive or mixed hearing loss.[25]

Syndromic Deafness with Ocular Abnormalities

Usher Syndrome

This disorder is the most common autosomal recessive syndromic form of hearing impairment. It affects approximately one-half of the 16,000 deaf-blind persons in the United States and 3–10% of the congenitally deafened population. The vision loss is progressive, usually heralded by complaints of night blindness or visual field defects, and occurs in both of the two clinically recognized forms of Usher syndrome.[26]

Usher syndrome type 1 (USH1) is characterized by retinitis pigmentosa, congenital profound hearing loss and absent vestibular function. It is genetically heterogeneous and has been mapped to both the short and long arms of chromosome 11[27,28] and the long arm of chromosome 14.[29] Usher syndrome type 2 (USH2) is characterized by retinitis pigmentosa and congenital mild-to-severe hearing loss. USH2 also is heterogeneous, with one locus on chromosome 1[30,31] and other loci as yet unmapped.[32]

USH1 and USH2 patients can be differentiated by tests of vestibular function. USH1 patients do not have any response to ice-water calorics, cannot perform tests of balance function, and show delayed psychomotor development. In contrast, USH2 patients have normal vestibular function and normal developmental milestones. Histopathological studies have shown widespread atrophic changes in the basal turn of the organ of Corti and in the spiral ganglia in a case of USH2. In addition to aural habilitation, since blindness ultimately develops, early intervention should include visual habilitation.

Alstrom Syndrome

This autosomal recessive syndrome is characterized by retinitis pigmentosa of infancy, obesity, diabetes mellitus and progressive sensorineural hearing loss that begins in late childhood. Variable degrees of nephropathy, acanthosis nigricans and premature baldness also can occur.[34]

Cockayne Syndrome

This autosomal recessive disorder is characterized by growth and mental retardation, joint contractures, photodermatitis, premature senility, retinal degeneration and progressive sensorineural deafness.[35] Affected persons appear normal at birth, although by the second year of life some anomalies begin to appear. Temporal bone histopathology shows loss of cells in the spiral ganglion and absence of hair cells particularly in the basal turn of the cochlea.[36] Patients with Cockayne syndrome have a defect in the mechanism of repair of DNA damage by ultraviolet light. This syndrome is genetically heterogenous. One gene that causes Cockayne syndrome has been mapped to chromosome 2q.[37,38]

Refsum Syndrome (Heredopathia Atactica Polyneuritiformis)

This autosomal recessive disorder is secondary to abnormal phytanic acid metabolism resulting in high levels of phytanate in the plasma, viscera and peripheral nerves. Affected persons appear normal until their second or third decades, when the first symptom, night blindness, develops. Widespread sensory disturbances, ataxia, weakness and wasting of muscles with cranial neuropathies develop. The insidious progression of the disease leads to complete incapacitation and a shortened life span. Approximately 50% of affected persons suffer a progressive, though usually asymmetric, form of hearing impairment.[39] The principal finding on temporal bone pathology is cochleosaccular atrophy.[40]

Syndromic Deafness Associated with Integument Abnormalities

Waardenburg Syndrome

Waardenburg syndrome is the most frequently diagnosed autosomal dominant form of hereditary deafness. It occurs with an estimated incidence of 2:100,000, although because expressivity is variable, this number may be an under-estimate. Three different phenotypes are recognized: Type 1 consists of dystopia canthorum, synophrys, heterochromia irides, broad nasal root, hair hypopigmentation (white forelock, premature graying), cutaneous patches of depigmentation and congenital deafness. Blue irides and vitiligo in dark-skinned persons are seen. In Waardenburg syndrome Type 2, dystopia canthorum is lacking. Waardenburg syndrome Type 3 includes limb deformities, such as syndactyly, and growth retardation (Klein-Waardenburg syndrome).

Hearing impairment is congenital and sensorineural, and is most commonly seen with Waardenburg syndrome Type 2. The degree of impairment may vary from mild to severe, and may be unilateral or bilateral. Histopathology of temporal bones has shown cochleosaccular degeneration secondary to absence of melanocytes in the intermediate layer of the stria vascularis.[41]

The gene responsible for Waardenburg syndrome Type 1 has been cloned and is known as PAX-3. It is located on chromosome 2 and is a transcription factor that plays an important role in tissue differentiation during development.[42–44] However, Waardenburg syndrome Type 1 is heterogeneous, and some families with the Type 1 phenotype fail to map to chromosome 2.[45] The chromosomal location for the gene responsible for Waardenburg syndrome Type 2 has not been established. Mutations of the PAX-3 gene also have been described for Waardenburg syndrome Type 3.[46]

LEOPARD Syndrome (Multiple Lentigines Syndrome)

LEOPARD is an acronym for the key features of this autosomal dominant syndrome characterized by hyperpigmented lentigines, electrocardiographic abnormalities, ocular hyperteliorism, pulmonary valvular stenosis, abnormalities of the genitalia, retardation of growth and sensorineural hearing impairment. Hearing loss occurs in about 25% of affected persons and can be mild to severe in degree.[47]

Neurofibromatosis

Two distinct autosomal dominant disorders encompass the neurofibromatoses. Neurofibromatosis Type 1, also known as Von Recklinghausen disease or peripheral neurofibromatosis, has an incidence of 33:100,000 population. Principal clinical manifestations are "cafe au lait" spots, intertriginous freckling, iris hamartomas (Lisch nodules), optic gliomas and multiple plexiform neurofibromas. Acoustic neurinomas occur in less than 1% of affected individuals. The gene for neurofibromatosis Type 1 has been localized to the pericentromeric region of the long arm of chromosome 17.[48]

Neurofibromatosis Type 2 or the central type of neurofibromatosis is characterized by bilateral cochleovestibular schwannomas. An increased incidence of other neoplasms of the central nervous system, such as meningiomas and astrocytomas, and ocular abnormalities, such as posterior subcapsular cataracts also occur. Approximately 4% of affected individuals develop acoustic neurinomas that lead to progressive sensorineural hearing loss in the second or third decades of life. Complete deafness often develops five to ten years later. The defective gene, which maps to chromosome 22,[49–52] has been cloned and named Merlin.[53] The product of this gene is homologous to several cytoskeletal proteins and represents a type of tumor suppressor gene. A marker for the presymptomatic diagnosis of neurofibromatosis type 2 has been proposed.[54]

Syndromic Deafness Associated with Cardiac Defects

Jervell and Lange-Nielsen Syndrome (Cardioauditory Syndrome)

The principal features of Jervell and Lange-Nielsen syndrome are autosomal recessive inheritance, congenital severe sensorineural deafness and recurrent syncopal attacks that begin in early childhood.[55] The syncopal attacks can vary in frequency and severity within the same individual, can be precipitated by physical or emotional exertion, and can lead to sudden death. Characteristic electrocardiographic findings include a prolonged QT interval and several T wave abnormalities. Prompt diagnosis and antiarrhythmic treatment has reduced significantly the high mortality rate associated with this disease.

Temporal bone findings have focused on the unusual PAS-positive spherical inclusions and eosinophilic hyaline substance in the stria vascularis. Atrophy of the organ of Corti, spiral ganglion and crista occur.[39] A gene that is associated with isolated long QT cardiac arrhythmias has been localized to the short arm of chromosome 11.[55]

Syndromic Deafness Associated with Renal Dysfunction

Alport Syndrome

This syndrome is characterized by progressive nephritis with uremia that is often heralded by hematuria in the first years of life. Renal insufficiency ultimately develops. Approximately 50% of patients have progressive sensorineural hearing impairment, although the degree of impairment varies widely. Histopathologic findings include degeneration of the stria vascularis, spiral ganglia and hair cells.[57] Hydrops often is present. The X-linked form of Alport syndrome is due to mutations in the alpha-5 (IV) collagen gene at Xq22-q23.[58] However, the disease is heterogeneous and autosomal mutations also can produce the disease phenotype.[20]

Syndromic Deafness Associated with Endocrine Dysfunction

Pendred Syndrome

Pendred syndrome is characterized by goiter and sensorineural hearing impairment. The thyroid enlargement results from an inborn error in thyroxine synthesis, although most patients maintain an euthyroid state. Thyroid enlargement occasionally can be appreciated at birth and appears before the age of five years

in at least 50% of affected persons. Intravenous perchlorate can be used to diagnose defective organic binding of iodine by the affected gland.[59]

Hearing impairment usually is congenital, bilateral and severe. Although there may be slight progression during early childhood, the loss generally remains fairly stable. Occasionally, vestibular function is depressed. Inner ear malformations such as Mondini dysplasia, may be diagnosed by computed tomography. Inheritance is autosomal recessive. The thyroglobulin gene has been mapped to the long arm of chromosome 8 and is a candidate gene for this syndrome.

Syndromic Deafness Associated with Metabolic Disorders

The mucopolysaccharidoses are the most common diseases in this category. Various genetically controlled pathways of lysosomal degradation are affected resulting in intracellular deposition of undegraded acid mucopolysaccharides like dermatan sulfate and heparin sulfate. High urinary concentration of these substances are found in affected individuals.

Hurler Syndrome (MPS-1H)

This autosomal recessive syndrome is caused by a deficiency in 2-L-iduronidase. It affects 1:100,000 persons who manifest disease symptoms in early childhood and usually die before their second decade. Physical findings include dysostosis multiplex, dwarfism, cloudy corneas, hepatosplenomegaly, mental retardation and conductive or mixed hearing loss. Otitis media, partial retention of mesenchyme precluding complete mastoid pneumatization, and basophilic deposits in the stria vascularis are seen on temporal bone histology. The defective gene has been cloned and localized to the short arm of chromosome 4.[60]

Hunter Syndrome (MPS-2)

This is the only mucopolysaccharidosis inherited in an X-linked fashion. The defect is due to idurono-2-sulfate sulfatase deficiency. A mild (Type A) and a severe (Type B) form have been described. Patients with Type A disease survive through childhood with minimal mental impairment, whereas Type B patients usually die before puberty after suffering progressive and severe psychomotor deterioration. Conductive or mixed hearing loss is present in about 50% of affected persons and usually is not severe. The defective gene has been cloned and localized to the long arm of the X chromosome.[61]

Syndromic Deafness Associated with Skeletal Dysplasia

Otosclerosis

Otosclerosis is a relatively common progressive disease of the otic capsule characterized by autosomal dominant transmission with incomplete penetrance. Biochemical abnormalities in the skin of affected persons suggest that the genetic defect may be related to collagen metabolism and that otosclerotic foci represent localized manifestations of a generalized connective tissue disorder.[62] However, other causes have been suggested, including persistent viral disease, a form of collagen autoimmunity, and defective control over bone remodeling.

Clinically, otosclerosis manifests with progressive conductive, pure sensorineural or mixed hearing loss. Cochlear otosclerosis is difficult to diagnose and should be suspected in the presence of a strong family history, a positive Schwartze's sign, stapedial disease in the contralateral ear, or periotic demineralization by computed tomography.

Osteogenesis Imperfecta

Osteogenesis imperfecta is a generalized connective tissue disorder resulting from mutations in genes that encode Type 1 collagen, the major structural protein in the body. Type 1 collagen contains two alpha-1 (I) chains (COL1 A1) and one alpha-2 (I) chain (COL1A2). The COL1A1 gene is located on the long arm of chromosome 17, and the COL1A2 gene is located on the long arm of chromosome 7.[63] Several different molecular defects have been found in persons with different types of osteogenesis imperfecta.[64] Type 1 disease (Van de Hove syndrome) is characterized by autosomal dominant inheritance, nondeforming fractures during childhood, normal stature, blue sclerae and hearing loss in 50% of affected persons. Studies of dermal fibroblasts from affected individuals demonstrate a decrease in the amount of Type 1 collagen due to a number of different gene mutations.

Osteogenesis imperfecta Type 2 is associated with severe fractures in utero and is lethal in the perinatal period. Affected infants can be recognized in early pregnancy by ultrasound examination or radiological studies. The latter demonstrate the characteristic bony changes of shortened long bones, beaded ribs, platyspondyly and marked calvarial demineralization.

The characteristic features of osteogenesis imperfecta Type 3 include progressive growth failure, frequent fractures, severe deformity, dentinogenesis imperfecta and hearing loss. Transmission is autosomal dominant in most instances. Osteogenesis imperfecta Type 4 is of intermediate severity between Types 1 and 3, with mild-to-moderate bone deformity and short stature.

Hearing impairment in osteogenesis imperfecta develops in early childhood and usually progresses. It is most commonly conductive but also can be sensorineural or mixed. Delayed enchondral and periosteal ossification, hypoplastic mastoid trabeculae and thin fragile stapedial crura have been noted on temporal bone histopathology.[33] The conductive deafness may be the re-sult of a deficient crural arch, stapes fixation by a focus of otosclerosis, or both. Otosclerosis occurring in association with osteogenesis imperfecta appears to have a more aggressive behavior, often leading to total obliteration of both windows and sensorineural deafness. This degree of pathology compromises the success of stapes surgery.[65]

Syndromic Deafness Associated with Chromosomal Abnormalities

Down Syndrome (Trisomy 21)

Deafness can be a component of some chromosomal abnormalities. Particularly noteworthy is the association of hearing impairment with trisomy 21 (Down syndrome). The incidence of Down syndrome is about 1:1,000 births in the United States. Hearing loss occurs in over 50% of patients and may be mixed or conductive. Temporal bone studies have shown shortened cochleae; residual mesenchyme in the middle ear, a wide angle of the facial genu, and small lateral semicircular canals. A case of typical Sheibe dysplasia has been described.[33] It is important to remember that because of mosaicism, affected patients may have normal intelligence, and only subtle signs of Down syndrome may be present.

Other Types of Syndromic Deafness

X-Linked Deafness with Stapes Fixation and Perilymphatic Gusher

This syndrome of mixed hearing loss may account for approximately one-half of all X-linked deafness. Its presence should be suspected if there is family history of perilymphatic gusher during stapedectomy. Deletions in the q21 region in chromosome X have been noted.[66–68]

Large Vestibular Aqueduct Syndrome, Congenital Perilymphatic Fistula

A mode of inheritance has not been described for these two syndromes associated with other congenital labyrinthine dysplasias that commonly present in early childhood as "idiopathic" progressive hearing loss with vertigo. It has been hypothesized that faulty embryogenesis of the temporal bone may be an etiological factor, thus predisposing affected patients to late-in-onset hearing loss. In children with unexplained recurrent meningitis or hearing loss, computed tomography of the temporal bones should be obtained to assess inner ear morphogenesis. The value of surgery has not been established.[69,70]

Refractory Otitis Media

Children may suffer from clinically significant conductive hearing loss as a result of refractory otitis media. It is important to consider an immunodeficiency in children with refractory infections involving several

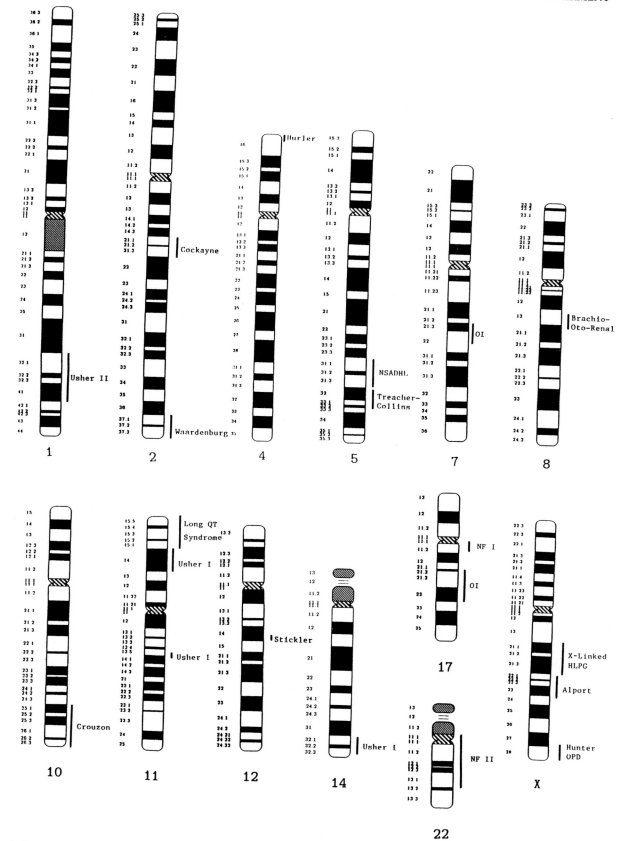

Fig. 52–1. Chromosomal assignments for many genes known to cause hearing impairment. Examples of heterogeneity include Usher syndrome type I and osteogenesis imperfecta. (NSADHL, Nonsyndromic autosomal dominant hearing loss; OI, osteogenesis imperfecta; NF, neurofibromatosis; X-linked HLPG, X-linked hearing loss with perilymphatic gusher; OPD, otopalatodigital syndrome)

areas of the respiratory tract (otitis, sinusitis, bronchitis, pneumonias). An example of an inheritable X-linked type of immunodeficiency is familial congenital agammaglobulinemia.

Mitochondrial Inheritance

Mitochondrial inheritance refers to the transmission of the mitochondrial genome via the female oocyte.[5] This pattern of inheritance has been described for familial aminoglycoside ototoxicity, some types of nonsyndromic deafness,[6,8] maternally inherited diabetes mellitus and deafness, and Kearns-Sayre syndrome (progressive external ophthalmoplegia, retinal pigmentary degeneration, cardiac conduction defects, and mixed hearing loss). Mutation of mitochondrial DNA may explain some complex pedigree patterns and may be important in late-in-onset degenerative diseases such as presbycuses.

Familial Aminoglycoside Ototoxicity

This entity refers to the development of sensorineural hearing loss after the administration of conventional doses of aminoglycosides for a short period. This abnormal response indicates an inherited susceptibility to the ototoxic effects of these drugs. In China, the prevalence of this disorder has been estimated at 1:10,000 persons.[7] Mutations of the mitochondrial genome have been described.[8]

Presbycusis

Hearing loss caused by the degenerative changes of ''aging'' is termed presbycusis. The clinical and audiological characteristics of presbycusis vary greatly. Current theories on the etiopathogenesis of presbycusis favor the interaction of both genetic and environmental factors.[71] Life-long accumulation of mitochondrial genomic mutations may be an important factor.[9]

Maternally Inherited Diabetes and Hearing Loss

Hereditary diabetes mellitus has many possible clinical presentations. One subtype, characterized by maternally transmitted diabetes and deafness, has been shown to be associated with a mitochondrial genome deletion. Both the diabetes and deafness result from impaired oxidative phosphorylation caused by this mutation.[72]

Nonsyndromic Deafness

Nonsyndromic hereditary hearing impairment implies the absence of additional phenotypic features to suggest genetic inheritance. Estimates suggest that more than 100 different genes may be responsible for the various types of nonsyndromic deafness, making linkage analysis an extremely difficult task. However, given the prevalence of this type of deafness, identifi-

cation of these genes is necessary for more precise disease classification, genetic counselling and intervention. To achieve this goal, attempts have been made to categorize some subtypes of nonsyndromic deafness based on mode of transmission, age-at-onset, type of audiogram, and severity.[20] Several loci for autosomal dominant nonsyndromic deafness and autosomal recessive nonsyndromic deafness have been identified.[73,74]

Genetic Counseling

Genetic counseling is essential to address personal concerns associated with the occurrence or chance of recurrence of a genetic disorder.[75] In most medical centers this information is provided by trained counselors, however clinicians usually are the first link to a patient and family. In providing appropriate health care, otolaryngologists must be cognizant of the ethical and cultural concerns of the deaf community and be aware of the implications and responsibilities associated with counseling persons with hearing impairment. Precise diagnostic information is necessary if associated conditions and habilitative options are to be presented. This information must be provided with the firm and clear emphasis that a hearing-impaired person can lead a happy and rewarding life. It is the counselor's responsibility to provide the counselee with information about organizations that deal with the psychological, cultural, genetic and legal aspects of hearing impairment.

Conclusion

Otolaryngologists must keep abreast of advances in this rapidly evolving field of medicine. The development of gene mapping technology has enabled scientists to localize many genes that cause hereditary hearing impairment (Fig. 52–1). In the future, markers will be available for the presymptomatic diagnosis of many of these disorders. Cloning these genes will improve our understanding of specific molecular defects and provide the basis for therapeutic intervention, perhaps making current nosologic classifications obsolete.

REFERENCES

1. Cremers CWRJ, Rijn PM, Hageman MJ: Prevention of serious hearing impairment or deafness in the young child. Proc Royal Soc Med 82:483, 1989.
2. Fraser GR: The causes of profound deafness in childhood. Baltimore: Johns Hopkins University Press, 1976.
3. Sank D, Kallman FJ: The role of heredity in early total deafness. Volta Rev 65:461, 1963.
4. Brown KS: The genetics of childhood deafness. In Deafness in Childhood. Edited by F. McConnell and P.H. Ward. Nashville: Vanderbilt University Press, 1967.

5. Anderson S, et al.: Sequence and organization of the human mitochondrial genome. Nature 290:457, 1981.

6. Jaber L, et al.: Sensorineural deafness inherited as a tissue specific mitochondrial disorder. J Med Genet 29:86, 1992.

7. Hu DN, et al: Genetic aspects of antibiotic induced deafness: mitochondrial inheritance. J Med Genet 28:79, 1991.

8. Prezant TR, et al: Mitochondrial ribosomal RNA mutation associated with both antibiotic-induced and non-syndromic deafness. Nature Genet 4:289, 1993.

9. Cortopassi GA, Arnheim N: Detection of a specific mitochondrial DNA deletion in tissues of older humans. Nucl Acids Res 18:6927, 1990.

10. Sando I, Hemenway WG, Morgan WR: Histopathology of the temporal bones in mandibulofacial dysostosis. Trans Am Acad Ophthalmol Otol 72:913, 1968.

11. Dixon MJ, et al: Genetic and physical mapping of the Treacher Collins syndrome locus:refinement of the localization to chromosome 5q32–33.2. Hum Molec Genet 1:249, 1992.

12. Gorlin RJ, Jue KL, Jacobsen U, et al: Oculoauriculovertebral dysplasia. J Pediatr 63:991, 1963.

13. Schiller JG: Craniofacial dysostosis of Crouzon: a case report and pedigree with emphasis on heredity. Pediatrics 23:107, 1959.

14. Vulliamy DG, Normandale PA: Craniofacial dysostosis in a Dorset family. Arch Dis Child 41:375, 1966.

15. Preston RA, et al: A gene for Crouzon craniofacial dysostosis maps to the long arm of chromosome 10. Nature Genet 7:149, 1994.

16. Bergstrom LV, Neblett LM, Hemenway WG: Otologic manifestations of acrocephalosyndactyly. Arch Otolaryngol 96:117, 1972.

17. Knowlton RG, et al: Genetic linkage analysis of hereditary arthro-ophthalmopathy (Stickler syndrome) and the type II collagen procollagen gene. Am J Hum Genet 45:681, 1989.

18. Ahmad NN, et al.: Stop codon in the procollagen II gene (COL2A1) in a family with the Stickler syndrome (arthro-ophthalmopathy). Proc Natl Acad Sci USA 88:6624, 1991.

19. Winterpacht A, et al: Kniest and Stickler dysplasia phenotypes caused by collagen type II gene (COL2A1) defect. Nature Genet 3:323, 1993.

20. Konigsmark BW, Gorlin RJ: Genetic and Metabolic Deafness. Philadelphia: W.B. Saunders Company, 1976.

21. Evenberg G, Rajten E, Sorensen H: Wildervanck's syndrome. Klippel-Feil's syndrome associated with deafness and retraction of the eyeball. Br J Radiol 36:562, 1963.

22. Eveberg G: Congenital absence of the oval window. Acta Otolaryngol (Stockh.) 66:320, 1968.

23. Smith RJH, et al. Localization of the gene for Brachiootorenal syndrome to chromosome 8q. Genomics 14:841, 1992.

24. Smith JL, Stowe FR: The Pierre Robin syndrome (glossoptosis, micrognathia, cleft palate). A review of 39 cases with emphasis on associated ocular lesions. Pediatrics 27:128, 1961.

25. Igarashi M, Filippone MV, Alford BR: Temporal bone findings in Pierre Robin syndrome. Laryngoscope 86:1679, 1976.

26. Smith RJH, et al: Clinical diagnosis of the Usher syndromes. Am J Med Genet 50:32, 1994.

27. Smith RJH, et al.: Localization of two genes for Usher syndrome type I to chromosome 11. Genomics 14:995, 1992.

28. Kimberling WJ, et al.: Linkage of Usher syndrome type I gene (USH1B) to the long arm of chromosome 11. Genomics 14:988, 1992.

29. Kaplan J, et al.: A gene for Usher syndrome type I (USH1A) maps to chromosome 14q. Genomics 14:979, 1992.

30. Kimberling WJ, et al: Localization of Usher syndrome type II to chromosome 1q. Genomics 7:245, 1990.

31. Lewis RA, et al.: Mapping recessive ophthalmic disease: linkage of the locus for Usher syndrome type II to a DNA marker on chromosome 1q. Genomics 7:250, 1990.

32. Dahl SP, et al.: Possible genetic heterogeneity of Usher syndrome type 2: a family unlinked to chromosome 1q markers. Am J Hum Genet 49(suppl):200, 1991.

33. Schucknecht HF: Pathology of the Ear, 2nd Ed. Philadelphia: Lea & Febiger, 1993.

34. Weinstein RL, Kliman B, Scully RE: Familial syndrome of primary testicular insufficiency with normal virilization, blindness, deafness, and metabolic abnormalities. N Engl J Med 281:969, 1969.

35. Cockayne EA: Dwarfism and retinal atrophy and deafness. Arch Dis Child 11:1, 1936.

36. Shemen LJ, Mitchell DP, Farkashidy J: Cockayne syndrome - an audiologic and temporal bone analysis. Am J Otol 5:300, 1984.

37. Weeda G, et al.: A presumed DNA helicase encoded by ERCC-3 is involved in the human repair disorders Xeroderma Pigmentosum and Cockayne's syndrome. Cell 62:777, 1990.

38. Weeda G, et al: Localization of the Xeroderma Pigmentosum group B-correcting gene ERCC3 to human chromosome 2q21. Genomics 10:1035, 1991.

39. Bergsmark J, Djupesland G: Heredopathia atactica polyneuritiformis (Refsum's disease). An audiological examination of two patients. Eur Neurol 1:122, 1968.

40. Smith RJH, et al: A histologic study of nonmorphogenetic forms of hereditary hearing impairment. Arch. Otolaryngol. Head Neck Surg 118:1085, 1992.

41. Nakashima S, Sando I, Takahashi H, et al: Temporal bone histopathologic findings of Waardenburg's syndrome: a case report. Laryngoscope 102:563, 1992.

42. Foy C, et al: Assignment of the locus for Waardenburg syndrome type I to human chromosome 2q37 and possible homology to the Splotch mouse. Am J Hum Genet 46:1017, 1990.

43. Baldwin CT, et al: An exonic mutation in the HuP2 paired domain gene causes Waardenburg's syndrome. Nature 355:637, 1992.

44. Tassabehji M, et al: Waardenburg's syndrome patients have mutations in the human homologue of the PAX-3 paired box gene. Nature 355:635, 1992.

45. Farrer LA, et al: Waardenburg syndrome (WS) type I is caused by defects at multiple loci, one of which is near ALPP on chromosome 2: first report of the WS Consortium. Am J Hum Genet 50:902, 1992.

46. Hoth CF, et al: Mutations in the paired domain of the human PAX3 gene cause Klein-Waardenburg syndrome (WS-III) as well as Waardenburg syndrome type I (WSI). Am J Hum Genet 52:445, 1993.

47. Gorlin RJ, Anderson RC, Blaw M: Multiple lentigines syndrome, complex comprising multiple lentigines, electrocardiographic conduction abnormalities, ocular hypertelorism, pulmonary stenosis, abnormalities of the genitalia, retardation of growth, sensorineural deafness, and autosomal dominant hereditary pattern. Am J Dis Child 117:652, 1969.

48. Barker D, et al.: Gene for von Recklinghausen neurofibromatosis is the pericentromeric region of chromosome 17. Science 236:1100, 1987.

49. Rouleau GA, et al: Genetic linkage of bilateral acoustic neurofibromatosis to a DNA marker on chromosome 22. Nature 329:246, 1987.

50. Rouleau GA, et al.: Flanking markers bracket the neurofibromatosis type 2 (NF-2) gene on chromosome 22. Am J Hum Genet 46:323, 1990.

51. Frazer KA, et al: A radiation hybrid map of the region on human chromosome 22 containing the neurofibromatosis type 2 locus. Genomics 14:574, 1992.

52. Wolff R, et al.: Analysis of chromosome 22 deletions in neurofi-

bromatosis type 2-related tumors. Am J Hum Genet *51*:478, 1992.

53. Trofatter JA, et al: A novel moesin-, ezrin-, radixin-like gene is a candidate for the neurofibromatosis 2 tumor suppressor. Cell *72*:791, 1993.

54. Narod SA, et al.: Neurofibromatosis type 2 appears to be a genetically homogeneous disease. Am J Hum Genet *51*:486, 1992.

55. Jervell A, Lange-Nielsen F: Congenital deaf-mutism, functional heart disease with prolongation of the QT interval, and sudden death. Am Heart J *54*:59, 1957.

56. Keating M, et al: Linkage of cardiac arrhythmia, the long QT syndrome, and the Harvey ras-1 gene. Science *252*:704, 1991.

57. Myers GJ, Tyler R: The etiology of deafness in Alport's syndrome. Arch Otolaryngol Head Neck Surg *96*:333, 1972.

58. Barker D, et al: Identification of mutations in the COL4A5 collagen gene in Alport syndrome. Science *248*:1224, 1990.

59. Illum P, Kiaer HW, Hvidberg-Hansen J, et al: Fifteen cases of Pendred's syndrome. Congenital deafness and sporadic goiter. Arch Otolaryngol *96*:297, 1972.

60. Scott HS, et al.: Chromosomal localization of the human alpha-L-iduronidase gene (IDUA) to 4p16.3. Am J Hum Genet *47*:802, 1990.

61. Le-Guern E, et al: More precise localization of the gene for Hunter syndrome. Genomics *7*:358, 1990.

62. Gordon MA, McPhee JR, Van De Water TR, et al: Aberration of the tissue collagenase system in association with otosclerosis. Am J Otol *13*:398, 1992.

63. Sykes B, et al: Consistent linkage of a dominantly inherited osteogenesis imperfecta to the type I collagen loci: COL1A1 and COL1A2. Am J Hum Genet *46*:293, 1990.

64. Byers PH, Steiner RD: Osteogenesis Imperfecta. Ann Rev Med *43*:269, 1992.

65. Garretson TJTM, Cremers CWRJ: Stapes surgery in osteogenesis imperfecta: analysis of postoperative hearing loss. Ann Otol Rhinol Laryngol *100*:120, 1991.

66. Cremers FPM, et al.: Physical fine mapping of the choroideremia locus using Xq21 deletions associated with complex syndromes. Genomics *4*:41, 1989.

67. Merry DE, et al.: Choroideremia and deafness with stapes fixation: a contiguous gene deletion syndrome in Xq21. Am J Hum Genet *45*:530, 1989.

68. Reardon W, et al.: A multipedigree linkage study of X-linked deafness: linkage to Xq13-q21 and evidence of genetic heterogeneity. Genomics *11*:885, 1991.

69. Levenson MJ, Parisier SC, Jacobs M, et al: The Large Vestibular Aqueduct syndrome in Children. A review of 12 cases and the description of a new clinical entity. Arch Otolaryngol Head Neck Surg *115*:54, 1989.

70. Reilly JS: Congenital Perilymphatic Fistula: A prospective study in infants and children. Laryngoscope *99*:393, 1989.

71. Salomon G (ed.): Hearing in the aged. In The European Concerted Action Project. Acta Otolaryngol (Stockh.) *476*(suppl), 1990.

72. Ballinger SW, et al.: Maternally transmitted diabetes and deafness associated with a 10.4 kb mitochondrial DNA deletion. Nature Genet *1*:11, 1992.

73. Leon PE, et al.: The gene for an inherited form of deafness maps to chromosome 5q31. Proc Natl Acad Sci USA *89*:5181, 1992.

74. Guilford P, et al.: A non-syndromic form of neurosensory, recessive deafness maps to the pericentromic region of chromosome 13q. Nature Genet *6*:24, 1994.

75. Ad Hoc Committee on Genetic Counseling. Genetic Counseling. Am J Hum Genet *27*:240, 1975.

53 Occupational Hearing Loss

Peter W. Alberti

Hearing loss produced by exposure to excessive sound is worldwide the most common cause of acquired adult sensorineural hearing loss. It is incurable, but should be entirely preventable. This chapter discusses the effect of noise on the ear, noise-induced hearing loss (NIHL) and its prevention, and other causes of occupational hearing loss.

Noise is any unwanted sound that by itself, may not be harmful unless its intensity is high. Noise has physical, physiologic, and psychologic connotations, all of which differ. Physically, sound can be measured and is defined in terms of duration, frequency (measured in Hz), and intensity (measured in sound pressure levels [SPL]), expressed in decibels (dB). Sound may be continuous, intermittent, impulsive, or explosive.

HISTORY

Although deafness produced by noise has been known for centuries, it first became a major problem with the discovery of gunpowder, and then with the industrial revolution, of which noise-induced hearing loss is a byproduct. It was recognized in the United States,[1] Germany and the United Kingdom[2] in the 1870s and 1880s. It was already well recognized in the last century when, in 1886, Thomas Barr[2] of Glasgow wrote, "It is familiarly known that boilermakers and others who work in very noisy surroundings are extremely liable to dullness of hearing. In Glasgow, we would have little difficulty finding hundreds whose sense of hearing has thus been damaged, by the noisy character of their work." Indeed, the riveting associated with shipbuilding gave the generic title "boilermakers' deafness" to NIHL. Barr's work stands the test of time as an excellent, well conceived and executed epidemiological survey.

As a result of the technical advances of the Second World War, machinery became larger, more efficient, and noisier. We are now seeing the additional harmful effects of this further increase in industrial sound levels.

The histology of noise-induced hearing loss in the organ of Corti was already described by Haberman[3] in 1890. Audiometrically, Fowler was the first to observe the 4 kz dip produced by noise, and Bunch[5] gave an excellent account of the audiometric features of noise-induced hearing loss in 1939. So, while NIHL has been well recognized for a century, its evaluation, accurate quantification, and prevention have only recently become important. An excellent historical review is given by Hawkins.[6]

THE EFFECT OF SOUND ON THE EAR

Sound, depending on its intensity, may produce 1) adaptation, 2) temporary threshold shift, and 3) permanent threshold shift.

Adaptation, which occurs whenever the ear is stimulated by sound, is a physiologic phenomenon, and for sounds of 70 db SPL or less, recovery occurs within half a second.

Temporary threshold shift (TTS) is a short-term effect usually measured in minutes and hours rather than seconds or days in which the hearing threshold elevates temporarily after exposure to noise. Temporary threshold shift occurs following intense sound stimulation, with a low frequency stimulus the maximum threshold shift may occur an octave above the centre frequency of the stimulating tone; as the stimulating frequency increases, the point of maximum shift moves close to the stimulating tone.[7] Tones of higher frequency cause more TTS than lower frequency tones of similar intensity. The amount of temporary threshold shift increases for the duration and intensity of the sound exposure. It lasts from minutes to hours and is also a physiologic phenomenon. For further details on adaptation and temporary threshold shift, the reader is referred to works by Mills[8] and Kryter.[9]

Permanent threshold shift is a permanent elevation of hearing threshold. It is usually confined to post-noise exposure.

The relationship between temporary threshold shift and permanent threshold shift has been the subject of much study. Mills[8] studied the development of the effect of sound stimulation and temporary threshold shift on certain psychophysic responses of the ear such as temporal integration, simultaneous masking, and so forth. He found that, as long as the sound continued, temporary threshold shift grew but the rate of growth varied according to the frequency of the sound. Periodic rest periods are protective. Thus, above a certain base level a 4 kHz sound produced an asymptotic threshold shift of 1.7 dB per each dB increase in sound level. The starting point at this frequency was 74 dB, and the lower the frequency, the higher the base level and the slower the growth of the TTS. Thus, at 1 kHz, there was no TTS below 82 dB. Figure 53–1 summarizes the findings of Mills and shows how difficult it is to define any one ''safe'' sound level in terms of a composite single intensity level. A safe sound varies according to its frequency components.

Most temporary threshold shift recovers in a few hours. If the noise exposure is sufficiently intense, however, TTS may last for several days or weeks. The cutoff point seems to be a TTS of approximately 40 dB. Below this, recovery is swift; above this, it is delayed.[10,11]

One of the practical problems of TTS is its effect on accurate quantification of hearing loss, in both audiometric screening and pension evaluation.

PERMANENT THRESHOLD SHIFT

The main purpose of this chapter is to discuss permanent threshold shift produced by exposure to intense sound. This is associated with pathologic changes in the cochlea, although the direct correlation between hearing loss and anatomic injury is not as clear-cut as was once thought.

HISTOPATHOLOGIC CHANGES RESULTING FROM EXCESSIVE SOUND EXPOSURE

The effect of sound stimulation on the ear has been studied by means of light microscopy and surface preparations, as well as scanning and transmission electronmicroscopy. Excellent reviews by Saunders et al[12,13] point out that acoustic injury to the ear has a dynamic and a static phase. The dynamic phase begins during acoustic stimulation which results in cellular elements in the ear undergoing structural and functional changes which may be permanent, or which may recover. Outer hair cells are more susceptible to damage. When the sound trauma ceases, the structure of the ear may recover completely or partially, scar, or disappear. This leads to a static phase in which hearing and the anatomic changes are stable. Bohne and Clarke[14] suggest that changes in the ear should be described as temporary/permanent/degenerative and reparative.

The difficulties of studying the cochlea should not be minimized. Human material is difficult to obtain and relatively unfresh; history regarding presbycusis and other ototoxic problems such as infection and drug exposure is usually unknown. Animal experimentation is essential. Unfortunately, there is no absolute correlation between animal experiments and man, or between electrophysiologic tests, behavioral audiograms, and histopathology in animals with noise-damaged hearing. Cytocochleograms performed for areas of hair cell loss frequently do not correlate with changes in behavioral hearing threshold. More recent

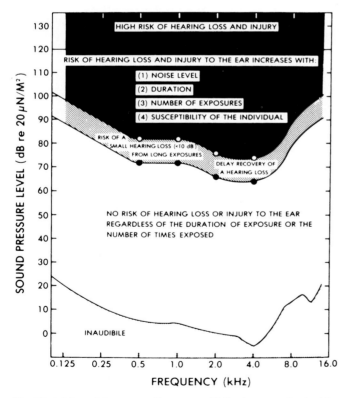

Fig. 53–1. Most of the range of human audibility is categorized with respect to the risk of injury and hearing loss. Reprinted with permission from Mills JH: Effects of noise on auditory sensitivity, psychophysical tuning curves and suppression. In New Perspectives on Noise Induced Hearing Loss. Edited by Hamernik RP, Henderson D, and Salvi R. New York, Raven Press, 1982, pp 249–263.

work, however, suggests that it is too crude merely to look at hair cell destruction and that when more subtle damage such as damage of the rootlet of the stereocilia is looked for there is much better correlation.[15,16] A critical level of noise exposure appears to exist. Below this level is biochemical and perhaps reversible change in the cochlea and above it major mechanical and irreparable damage. This is shown in both behavioral tests and histologic studies. The previously cited work by Mills[8] suggests that above a critical threshold for each decibel increase in intensity is a steady growth in hearing loss. Above a higher threshold, the increase in hearing loss suddenly grows much more rapidly, and histologic correlates[17] suggest that mechanical disruption occurs at this point.

A superb article by Lim[18] gives an overview of the structure of the cochlea as it is understood today. In turn, physiologic thinking about the structure of the cochlea has moved from a macro- to a microdynamic model. No longer is the main focus of attention the travelling wave. Current studies emphasize functional integrity of individual hair cells and their innervation; interaction between the outer and inner hair cells; and knowledge obtained from single auditory nerve fibers and their characteristic frequencies, both normal and noise-damaged. It is now apparent that the outer hair cells contract in response to a sound stimulus; this enhances and sharpens the mechanical displacement transmitted to the inner hair cells, which alone appear to transmit mechanical stimulation to initiate an VIIIth nerve afferent signal. The use of tracers such as horseradish peroxidase has allowed study of the concomitant central nervous system connection and damage. The reader is referred to work by Kiang et al.,[19] and for biochemical changes to work by Schacht and Conlon.[20]

HAIR CELL INJURY

Cochlear hair cells are damaged by exposure to excessive sound. The degree and type of damage are related to the amount of noise exposure. Until recently it was possible only to tell whether a hair cell was destroyed or not. Improved electron microscopy techniques have now allowed the demonstration of subtle changes that, when studied in conjunction with current views of cilia as containing actively contractile actin molecules, is beginning to lead to a better understanding of the damage that occurs. The first sign is shortening of the cilial rootlet.[16] This acute finding, produced by least damaging noise, is associated with floppy cilia and is partly reversible. The degree of resistance of cilia to deformation before and after noise stress has been measured by Saunders et al.[21] The first sign of an irreversible change is an actual fracture of the rootlet at the level of the cuticular plate, which leads to irreversible falling over of the cilia and ultimately cilial absorption. With these greater degrees of damage, intracellular changes also occur, including damage to lysosome granules, mitochondria, and the nucleus. As with other tissues in the body, there is a process of damage and repair. The repair with mild degrees of injury is within the cell itself, and with greater degrees of injury, healing and scar formation occur by migration from other cells.[22,23] An elegant series of experiments by Gao et al[24] demonstrates by means of electron photo micrographs, responses of hair cells to intense and very intense stimuli; in the former the cilia flop slightly but do not collapse: they appear to recover completely; in the former the cilia flop slightly but do not collapse acutely: they appear to recover totally; in the latter they flop significantly and never recover, indeed are scavenged and disappear.'

There has been much discussion in the literature about the role of other factors in noise damage, including the need for high levels of oxygenation and the effect of overstimulation on the stria vascularis and its ability to deliver nutrients. Certainly noise damage is metabolic as well as mechanical, but full correlations are yet to be made.[12]

AUDITORY NERVE AND CNS DAMAGE AFTER ACOUSTIC INJURY

There is also evidence of eighth nerve and central nervous system injury after chronic traumatic acoustic exposure. There certainly is good evidence of damage to the dendrites and nerve endings surrounding the hair cells following acoustic overstimulation, and in chronic preparations, spiral ganglion cell degeneration spreading into the cochlear nucleus.[24–27] Changes can be traced right up the central nervous system (CNS) after cochlear ablation, something that has important ramifications in terms of central processing of sound and the ability to rehabilitate following acoustic damage. In humans the psychophysical tuning of the cochlear nerve becomes broader with increasing hearing loss.[28]

PHYSIOLOGIC AND PSYCHOPHYSIC CHANGES TO NOISE EXPOSURE

This has been well reviewed by Schmiedt.[29] Views of cochlear function have been changed radically in the past decade by the appreciation that, of the afferent nerve fibers from the cochlea, which presumably carry information about sound stimulation to the central nervous system, 90% arise from the inner hair cells and yet damage to the outer hair cells is associated with hearing loss from noise exposure. The outer hair cells are overwhelmingly innervated by efferent fibers, and it is becoming clear that stimulation of the efferent fibers can alter the sensitivity of the cochlea by 20 or 30 dB. In other words, the outer hair cells have a tuning effect on the inner hair cells by a mechanism that is not yet clear. The outer hair cells themselves contract in response to sound stimulation, providing mechanical enhancement of the travelling wave motion transmitted to the inner hair cells. Micromechanical models of the cochlea are currently being intensively studied, and theoretic concepts change virtually month by month. Readers are referred to the book by Harrison[30] and article by Dallos[31] for a more detailed appreciation.

Much psychophysical work has been directed toward single nerve fiber tuning curves, which have demonstrated a broadening of tuning curves of individual nerve fibers following cochlear damage (Fig. 53–2). At their most sensitive, they are less frequency-selective than normal, and this is associated with outer hair cell damage. In humans, the tuning curve of the cochlear nerve becomes broader with increasing hearing loss, and certainly damage from noise is associated with reduced super-threshold hearing function.

NOISE-INDUCED HEARING LOSS

Intense acoustic overstimulation, whether acute or chronic, can produce noise-induced temporary threshold shift (TTS) and a noise-induced permanent threshold shift (PTS). The noise source may be continuous, intermittent, or mixed. Acoustic damage can also occur from a single intense sound such as an explosion or even a single gunshot. Typically, the first audiometric change in both TTS and PTS is a drop in hearing at 3, 4, or 6 kz, with normal hearing below and above these levels. This is known as an acoustic notch. In the early phases, the patient usually recovers. It has long been known that the previously unexposed ear is more easily damaged by noise than one accustomed to listening to loud sound,[32] (green ears) and there is recent evidence of the "toughening of ears" by noise exposure.[33] This is a topic of great current interest and has been well reviewed by Henderson et al,[33] Boetcher,[35] and Ryan et al.[36]

The recovery period following TTS is of interest. It has been studied in detail by Mill[37] in man and in many animal studies. Most recovery takes place within the first 12 hours after noise exposure and is overwhelmingly complete within 48 hours, although in detailed animal studies slight recovery continues for many weeks. This recovery is so slight that it is within the confidence limits of normal clinical audiometric tests. After a single massive insult such as an explosion, however, recovery may continue for many weeks until the hearing loss is stable.

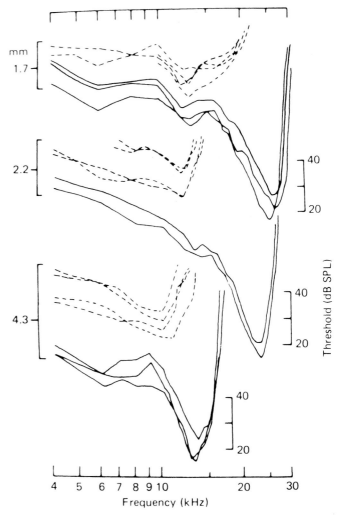

Fig. 53–2. Frequency-threshold curves (tuning curves) from single-spiral ganglion cells in guinea pigs with and without cochlear pathology. The solid curves were obtained from normal cochlear, whereas the dashed curves are associated with cell bodies innervating regions of the basal turn devoid of outer hair cells. The three sets of curves correspond to three cochlear locations; from top to bottom the locations are at 1.7, 2.2, and 4.3 mm from the basal end of the cochlear spiral. Note that the pathology not only desensitizes the tip of the curve, but also lowers the best (most sensitive) frequency. These results are indirect evidence that the mechanical tuning of the organ of Corti can be changed by damage. Reprinted with permission from Robertson D and Johnstone BM: Aberrant tonotopic organization in the inner ear damaged by kanamycin. J Acoust Soc Am 66:486, 1979.[117]

NOISE-INDUCED PERMANENT THRESHOLD SHIFT (NIPTS)

This has many synonyms, one of the earliest being boilermakers' deafness, and the current popular one being noise-induced hearing loss (NIHL). This is now probably the most common cause of acquired hearing loss in North American adults, and is overwhelmingly caused by chronic noise exposure in the workplace, whether civilian or military. It may be potentiated by additional social and recreational noise exposure. The speed of onset and the degree of loss are related to the total quantity of noise exposure, i.e., its intensity and duration, and to the individual's susceptibility to damage by the noise. In general terms, industrial noise exposure is less intense but more prolonged than military noise exposure.

It is difficult to quantify accurately the relationship between prolonged noise exposure and hearing loss because, over the years, workplace noise exposure changes, machinery is altered, jobs change, and hearing protection is provided. There are remarkably few long term longitudinal studies equating hearing loss with noise exposure, and the likelihood of such studies in the future is becoming increasingly remote because, as the hazards of noise have been recognized, companies that are interested enough to take regular noise measurements also provide hearing protection. The well-studied group of jute workers in Dundee in the 1960s is the benchmark against which most of this work is measured.[37] As a rule of thumb, in average workplace noise, say between 90 and 94 db, an almost stable hearing loss is achieved in the higher frequencies in about 10 years, and then gradually flattens into lower frequencies. The major part of the loss may occur quite early in the first 2 or 3 years,[39] and late losses are usually contaminated with presbycusis which becomes the dominant cause of worsening hearing.[40]

DAMAGE RISK CRITERIA

Many attempts have been made to define the relationship between noise exposure and hearing loss. It is currently accepted that, within a significant range with a lower boundary of safe sound and an upper boundary of sound so intense that it produces acute permanent damage, equal amounts of sound exposure produce equal amounts of damage. This is true whether sound exposure is spread over a short or long period. In other words, a given sound experienced for 8 hours does as much harm as twice that sound experienced for 4 hours or half that sound experienced for 16 hours. The reader must remember that decibels are a logarithmic scale. Doubling sound intensity is equivalent to increasing its intensity by 3 dB. Thus a 93 dB sound is twice as intense as a 90 dB sound, and a 103 dB sound is twice as intense as 100 dB sound. This equal energy concept, promulgated by Burns and Robinson,[41] has been widely adopted in Europe for many years and is gaining acceptance in North America. However, it is now suggested that if noise exposure is intermittent, as is usually the case in industry, the ear has time to recover and the 3 dB rule may be too strict. The best fit is probably a 4 dB halving and doubling. This issue is well reviewed by Ward.[42]

The appropriate technique of evaluating the harmful effects of impact sound is being debated. Rifle fire is a good example of military impact sound; a drop forge, a pile driver, and a hammer blow are all examples of industrial impact noise. The characteristics of impact sound vary widely; they are measured by rise and decay time and peak intensity and are difficult to measure because of the transient nature of the sound. Hammernik and Hsueh[43] give a good review of the nature and measurement of impulse sound. It is now suggested that impulse noise is more damaging than steady state noise.[44]

Attempts have been made to codify risks into national and international standards for noise exposure, which are used both to define the upper limit of safe exposure and to quantify the risk of hearing damage at various levels of intense sound. International standards have been based upon the equal energy (3 dB halving and doubling) concept and were initially embodied in ISO 1999 (1971) and revised as ISO 1999 (1984), which takes in account such factors as other ear disease and aging. In North America, tables based on 5 dB halving and doubling were introduced in the mid-1960s after a CHABA report in 1966 and codified in the Walsh-Healey Act of 1970. Here it is assumed that the trading relationship is 5 dB for halving and doubling of exposure, known as $L_{<OSHA>}$, as opposed to the European 3 dB loudness equivalent known as Leq. The historical basis for these differences is well reviewed by Shaw.[45] There is a significant, but in practical terms frequently unnecessary, debate about these trading relationships. It is important to know that with a 90 dBA* sound exposure for 8 hours a day, 5 days a week, 15% of the population is at risk for significant hearing loss after 10 years of exposure; and that for 85 dBA exposure 8 hours a day, 5 days a week, after 10 years only 7% of the population is at risk. It is prudent therefore to initiate hearing conservation measures from 85 dB upward, and from a hearing conservation standpoint little is to be gained from further dissection of these tables. Where they are significant is in attempting to equate total noise exposure in terms of medicolegal investigations. Few jobs have a steady noise exposure throughout the working day or working week, and attempts to equate actual noise measurements at work over a period of years in which several jobs have been held into a single risk figure for legal purposes are dramatically affected by which table of risk is used (Table 53–1, Loudness Equivalence). The tables of risk are based on human hearing threshold changes and are difficult to correlate with histologic damage and hair cell destruction in noise-exposed animals. The correlation between hair cell loss and permanent threshold shift is not good.[46] It is probable, however, that

---

* dBA is the sound level measured using an A-weighted filter, which approximates the 40 phon curve. It is the scale usually used because it approximates human hearing potential.

TABLE 53–1. Comparison of Hours of Equivalent Sound Exposure*

Hours of Permitted Exposure	L$_{OSHA}$	Leq
16	85	87
8	90	90
4	95	93
2	100	96
1	105	99
½	110	102
¼	115	105

* Using an 8-hour 90 dbA baseline as allowed by L$_{OSHA}$ and Leq.

better correlation will be found as more subtle changes in hair cells are sought. The human studies are based on large samples of workers including a big General Motors study by Baughn[47] and studies of Austrian industrial workers,[48] British steel workers,[49] and a number of Ontario, Canada industries.[50] They have been extensively evaluated in the literature by a series of studies performed by Passchier-Vermeer.[51]

NATURAL HISTORY OF NOISE-INDUCED PERMANENT THRESHOLD SHIFT (NIPTS)

There is interest in the progress of NIPTS over the years. What is the rate of growth of hearing loss; does it spread into other frequencies; does the rate of increase level off, accelerate or remain the same? These are difficult questions to answer because of the lack of good longitudinal studies. It is unlikely that PTS will occur without TTS, and it is also unlikely that PTS will be greater than TTS. Other than that, there is little relationship between the two, and attempts to predict PTS from TTS have not been successful. PTS usually starts in the higher frequencies, characteristically at 4 or perhaps at 3 or 6 kHz, and gradually spreads into neighboring frequencies. To begin with, it is asymptomatic, and only when it spreads into the lower frequencies such as 2 kHz is it a sufficient handicap to evince complaints. As time goes on, the notch disappears with hearing in the higher frequencies, also worsening so that the audiogram becomes indistinguishable from many other sensorineural hearing losses. It is stated, probably correctly, that after 10 years of exposure to a given noise, the loss in the higher frequencies stops worsening, but gradually the loss spreads into the lower frequencies (Fig. 53–3). The rate of spread and the degree of loss are related to both the intensity of sound and the individual's susceptibility to noise. This is as important with sound exposure as with other physical insults such as response to sunlight; individuals vary greatly and unfortunately there is no good way of predicting the unduly susceptible individual. If the ISO tables of risk are correct, it is probable that in later years too much hearing loss has been blamed on noise, and too little on presbycusis.

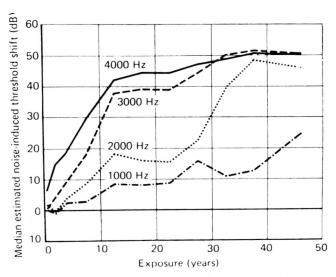

Fig. 53–3. Median hearing levels of small groups of subjects employed at the same textile mill. Controls had not been exposed to noise; spinners and weavers had both spent 10 years, on the average, in their respective occupations. Reproduced from Burns W, Hinchcliffe R, and Littler TS: An exploratory study: Hearing and noise exposure in textile workers. Ann Occup Hyg 7:323, 1964.[118]

TINNITUS

Tinnitus is distressing and a frequent concomitant of noise-induced hearing loss. Transient tinnitus is commonly experienced after exposure to intense sound and almost invariably after a blast injury but it usually clears. After years of exposure, however, it may become permanent and is present permanently in 50 to 60% of those with noise-induced hearing loss.[52–54] Alberti[54] found the incidence to be higher in those exposed to impact noise. The incidence and severity of tinnitus increases with increased hearing loss. This was not found by McShane et al,[55] highlighting the difficulty of distinguishing the organic from the nonorganic components of this distressing but unmeasurable complaint. Hinchcliffe and King[56] in a trenchant series of articles suggest that the symptoms of tinnitus associated with chronic noise exposure has only occurred since compensation was introduced. Their argument is well presented, but counter current opinion.

WORSENING OF HEARING AFTER NOISE EXPOSURE ENDS?

It is frequently asked if hearing loss from noise exposure can progress after removal from noise. Although hearing loss improves rather than worsens after removal of chronic noise exposure, there is considerable controversy in the literature about the interaction between noise, presbycusis, and progress of hearing loss. The overwhelming body of opinion, however, strongly suggests that hearing loss that progresses after removal of noise exposure is from some other cause. Tschopp and Probst[57] undertook a longitudinal study of hearing after exposure to a single sound; they found no worsening.

COMBINED EFFECTS OF OTOTRAUMATIC AGENTS

Many things are known to injure the ear, e.g., drugs, infections, trauma, age, and noise. The ear is also affected by premature degenerative disorders such as familial hearing losses. Most of these agents have a final common pathway: they damage the hair cells and other structures of the cochlea. There is great interest in and concern about how they interact: whether they are synergistic, additive, or protective. Is the noise-exposed ear more or less affected by aging or is the effect additive? "Is an old ear more likely to be damaged by noise than a young ear or is age irrelevant?" Matters are compounded by species differences among animals and between animals and man, and it is not always reasonable to extrapolate from one to the other. "Unfortunately, the ears that are most readily studied and about which there is a large body of knowledge, those of the guinea pig and chinchilla, do not necessarily behave in the same way as human ears." With this caveat, in guinea pigs it has been shown that kanamycin given after noise exposure is more damaging than kanamycin alone, although the reverse is not true. "The effect of loop diuretics on the ear appears not to be synergistic with noise, and the only human information available is that if salicylate is given at the same time as noise exposure, TTS is greater than without the drug."[58] The ototoxic cytotoxic drug cisplatin acts synergistically with other ototoxic drugs and noise.

Certain industrial solvents and chemicals are ototoxic. Jet fuel and styrene are predominant vestibulotoxic, but also appear to impair central auditory function.[59] Rybak[60] has published an exhaustive review in which he suggests that there may be a synergistic affect between inhaling styrene and noise exposure. He draws similar conclusions about inhaled carbon disulphide. Toluene is the most commonly used, most studied and probably the most ototoxic industrial chemical. It produces hearing loss and potentiates the effect of noise exposure.[61,62] Noise and vibration act synergistically in those who suffer from white hand and work in the cold such as foresters using chain saws or shipbuilders.[63–65] The interaction between noise exposure and aging is hotly debated. At most, it appears that presbycusis is additive to noise change, and even this is not demonstrated unequivocally. Studies by McCrae,[66] Novotny,[67,68] and Welleschik and Raber[69] give some evidence for additivity, although they also say that there is no interaction. This matter is of considerable concern in terms of pension assessments, which are frequently made only at a time when presbycusis might already be affecting the hearing. ISO 1999 implies an additive mechanism, which has been modeled by McCrae[66] and by Dobie[39] Robinson[70] reviews the subject at length. In later years, aging is a much more dominant cause of worsening hearing than further noise exposure, indeed at the higher frequencies by the age of 80, hearing is the same, whether the ear is noise exposed or not! The best model known to the author is that of Corso,[71] who gives a thoughtful discussion of the topic and concludes that, at best, there is limited additivity.

Is an already noise-damaged ear more or less susceptible to damage from further noise exposure than an undamaged ear? This question is frequently raised when a hearing-impaired worker attempts to move from one noisy industry to another, only to fail to find employment in the belief that, because of previous damage to their ears, their hearing is more likely to degenerate more rapidly than normal. The little existing evidence suggests that this is wrong and that the ear will continue to degenerate at a steady rate with a natural rate history appropriate for it.

The literature has also suggested that fair-haired, blue-eyed people are more susceptible to noise exposure than dark-haired, dark-eyed workers. Likewise, it has been suggested that black workers are less likely to experience noise damage than white workers. While the literature is large, it is not conclusive, and any effect that might be found is at best slight.[72,73]

ACOUSTIC TRAUMA

Explosions and other single loud sounds can cause hearing loss. Early examples of "telephone ear" produced by static were reported by Bunch.[5] Other examples include workers inside metal tanks, the outside of which is struck by sledge hammers, quarrymen too close to a blasting accident, and armed forces personnel near a single explosion. The most recent example is hearing loss produced by the inadvertent ringing of the cordless telephone into the ear of the listener.[74] Perhaps the most pervasive one at present is firecrackers.

SOCIO-ACOUSIS

The ear does not distinguish between occupational and social noise exposure. All noise is additive. Leisure pursuits may add significantly to total daily noise exposure and turn a marginally safe job, from a noise standpoint, to an acoustically hazardous one. The noise levels of everyday life are steadily increasing and to this should be added the voluntary sound levels of recreation. Transportation is the main cause—automobiles, particularly on throughways, motorcycles, trains, planes, and the substitution of diesel for gasoline engines have all helped to produce sound levels that, in some cities, for example Bangkok, exceed 100 dB in the city center. There is voluminous literature about this, and the reader is referred particularly to *The Effects of Noise on Man* by Krytes[9] and the publication *Noise as a Public Health Problem*.[75,76] The worker exposed to sound levels of 88 dBA for an 8-hour workday who then experiences 94 dBA for 2 hours traveling to and from work is at risk for hearing loss from noise because of the additive effects of the sounds. In the home, too, the blender, vacuum cleaner, and lawnmower all add to noise. In North American cities, ambient sound level ranges from 20 dBA on the north rim of the Grand Canyon to over 80 dBA in city centers near motorways. Noise levels within public transportation are high; some subway systems have sound levels above 90 dBA. Public opinion can be effective, and the quieting of airplanes is a major result of such pressure.

Recreational noise also is hazardous. Firecrackers can produce sudden deafness in children.[77,78] Recreational vehicles such as snowmobiles and motorcycles are frequently considered by their users to be more fun if loud. Chainsaws and radial-arm saws produce damaging sound levels for the hobbyist. There is much concern about the use of personal radios and cassette players, and the potential harmful effects of pop, rock, and disco music, although it would appear they are not a major cause of hearing loss.[79] Clark[80] has reviewed current North American sources of potentially harmful social noise: he highlighted the sound output of power tools and horticultural equipment. Children in rural areas appear particularly at risk from firearms, tractors and other farm equipment.[81]

MEDICAL NOISE

High-speed dental drills are almost certainly safe for dentists.[82] Other forms of medical noise include compression chambers, which may be an otologic hazard from both pressure equalization and noise near the air valves; there is at least one reported case of deafness inside such a chamber.[83] Drills and suction units at ear surgery have raised concern. While it appears that airborne sound levels from drills are safe,[84] bone-conducted sound levels are high, and Kylen et al.[85] conclude that, for the patient, the mixture of air- and bone-conducted sound may be damaging, particularly if large burrs are used. The smaller the burr, and the greater the number of teeth, the less the sound level. Man and Winerman,[86] however, studied bone conduction thresholds in operated and normal unoperated ears and found that the normal unoperated ear was unaffected by drilling. Because bone-conducted sound is transmitted across the skull without loss, this is strong evidence that sensorineural losses in chronic otitis media are caused by factors other than burr noise. Concern has also been raised about the noise of suction units which, at the ear, is extremely high.[87]

Hospitals contain many hazardous sound sources, of which the otologist should be aware. Apart from the normal industrial noises of steam plants, air conditioning units and commercial dishwashing equipment, certain medical equipment produces intense sounds, e.g., suction units, respirators, and incubators. The noise in ICUs can be intense,[88,89] and if not deafening is certainly disturbing. The background noise in an ICU may mask warning signals, from many life support devices, or at least make localising them more difficult. Magnetic resonance machines are very loud at the patient's head position and use of rubber or foam ear plugs is advocated.[90]

NONAUDITORY EFFECTS OF NOISE

There is great controversy about noise as a cause of hypertension. This is a difficult subject to untangle. Certainly sound may precipitate acute cardiovascular changes, but these are almost certainly normal physiologic responses to warning signals. Whether this leads in turn to chronic change remains debatable. Large population studies suggested that living in areas of high noise is more likely to produce hypertension, although a well-controlled study in the U.S. Air Force by Von Gierke et al.[91] failed to demonstrate such an effect. If there is a real effect, it is extremely small. The effect of noise on sleep deprivation is also a matter of concern. These and other factors are summarized by Kryter[9] and in recent volumes of the Quinquennial Symposium on Noise as a Public Health Hazard.[75,76]

There have been persistent reports of an association between excessive community noise exposure and mental disease. These have been extensively reviewed by Kryter.[9] There probably is no direct association. This has been confirmed by a careful study by Stanfeld et al.[92] There appears to be an effect on children's education of chronic noise exposure,[93] because of interference with speech perception and because of the development of strategies to block out sound. Behaviour of teachers may also be affected.[94,95]

CLINICAL FEATURES OF NIHL

There are no clear-cut clinical features that distinguish noise-induced hearing loss from several other causes of sensorineural hearing impairment. The diagnosis is based on history, physical examination, and appropriate laboratory tests including full hearing tests. Although there are audiometric configurations suggestive of the diagnosis, it may have many variations, and no one configuration fits all cases or excludes a case.

To compound matters, noise-induced hearing loss, like any other chronic disorder, may coexist with other lesions. The diagnosis, which is circumstantial, is largely based on a careful history and is frequently made by exclusion, i.e., if other causes of hearing loss have been excluded, noise exposure has been adequate, and there is an appropriate hearing loss, it is customary to attribute the loss to that cause. The diagnosis must be made individually, and one should avoid the statistical epidemiologic error of believing that noise exposure and hearing loss are necessarily causally related. To believe this is to believe that working in noise protects one from all other forms of ear disease. In a large consecutive series of claims for NIHL taken at random from a working population in Ontario, at least 5% had other ear disease as the major cause of their hearing loss.[96] NIHL may be superimposed upon other diseases such as chronic middle ear disease, Ménière's syndrome, familial hearing loss, otosclerosis, and the like. Unfortunately, people's memory about their own health is short, and little good information is available in the literature about the prevalence of ear disease in industrial populations at present.

The audiogram quantifies the hearing loss. Its pattern may give a clue toward the diagnosis because it may help to distinguish among various sites of lesion, conductive, cochlear or retrocochlear. The history includes questions about familial hearing loss, length of symptoms, childhood problems, school screening (whether school hearing screening has ever been failed), ear discharge, other diseases related to hearing loss such as renal problems, potential use of ototoxic drugs, and head injuries. Where indicated, further investigation should be initiated, including hematologic, serologic, and imaging, including, if necessary, CT or MRI. When noise exposure is believed to be the cause of the hearing loss, various causes of loss must be sought, e.g., recreational, military and occupational. Even within the realm of occupational hearing loss, it is often difficult to attribute the cause to a specific employer, and ultimately it may become a matter of clinical skill and exquisite judgement to establish both the cause of the hearing loss and the proportion of it which should be attributed to any given employer.

The responsibility of the assessing physician is to the patient: to quantify the hearing loss accurately, establish a diagnosis, and make a recommendation about treatment or rehabilitation. If physical signs or symptoms suggest other ear disease, this should be followed through and, in particular, causes of asymmetric hearing loss should be investigated. It is possible to have an asymmetric hearing loss from noise exposure such as, for example, individuals who fire guns off one shoulder, World War II DC3 pilots who wore a headphone over one ear and had the other ear exposed to engine noise and with the window open, workers who use certain industrial equipment such as rock drills, and people who drive farm tractors with one ear to the engine and the head constantly turned over the shoulder, protecting the other ear. Unequal hearing thresholds were present in about 10% of a large series of claimants for occupational hearing loss[97] which contained its fair share of serious ear disease such as acoustic neuroma, as well as asymmetric industrial exposure from machinery and unequal damage to ears from explosions at work. At least half of these had an explanation other than noise exposure; the relationship to work of the remainder was variable. The writer always asks if occupational exposure is asymmetric: it is surprising how often it is.

HEARING TESTS

Hearing tests used in occupational hearing loss are of two types, screening and diagnostic. Screening tests will be dealt with under the section entitled Hearing Conservation. This section deals with diagnostic tests. The degree of accuracy required here is greater than in routine clinical diagnostic audiology, and it cannot be overemphasized that the tester must be experienced in this type of work. The basis for most pension and compensation awards is the puretone audiogram, which must be accurate to be fair to both employer and employee. At the time of testing there should be no TIS. Authorities have legislated different time periods out of noise for this, ranging from 6 months to 48 hours. It is my view that if the claimant has been subjected to chronic noise exposure, a period of 48 hours free of noise is adequate for compensation assessment and, in fact, anything much longer is impractical, particularly if the employee is continuing to work. The situation is different after a major blasting accident or head injury, in which recovery may continue for a period of many weeks, and I believe that compensation assessment should not be undertaken for a minimum of 3 months after the episode.

The types of test to be undertaken vary by local usage rather than any intrinsic factors related to the tests. They must be undertaken with properly calibrated equipment and in appropriately calibrated sound proof enclosures. Although screening tests make much use of the automatic Békésy audiometry, a test to quantify accurately hearing loss overwhelmingly consists of routine behavioral audiometry: air conduction, bone conduction and speech reception thresholds. Further tests are undertaken as indicated. If there is an asymmetric loss, site-of-lesion tests are performed; if there is doubt about the accuracy of the behavioral test, the appropriate set of tests is performed.

Many audiometric tests are designed to identify exaggerated hearing loss but few which quantify it. Quantification for compensation purposes must be frequency-specific and parallel tonal audiometry. In unilateral hearing loss, the Stenger test is effective. In bilateral hearing loss, electric response testing is necessary, and in this group of patients, slow vertex response (SVR) audiometry is the most effective. This is more accurate and pleasant for the patient than psychogalvanic skin response audiometry. Auditory brainstem responses, currently much in vogue, usually provide only a click threshold, which gives a general idea of the level of hearing but not a simulacrum of an audiogram. To obtain this by means of brainstem audiometry requires expensive filtering techniques and a much lengthier test. The relative merits of various evoked response tests have been well described by Hyde et al.[98] and the slow vertex response audiometry in this type of patient by Alberti et al.[99] We use certain guidelines to identify the patient who should have SVR, and place considerable emphasis on the discrepancy between speech reception threshold and puretone average, and on the 500 Hz air conduction threshold. Klockhoff et al.[100] and Alberti et al.[101] both demonstrated that the probability of a hearing loss of 40 dB or greater at 500 Hz, being caused by something other than noise is high. These patients produce a high yield of other ear disease and of nonorganic hearing loss. A full review of the techniques of forensic audiology is given by Alberti.[102]

THERAPY AND REHABILITATION

The symptoms of an acute traumatic hearing loss can be helped by the use of hyperbaric oxygen[103,106] or carbogen. Some animal evidence supports this,[105] but this treatment does not have widespread acceptance in man.

The clinical onset of occupational hearing loss is usually insidious, but ultimately the complaints are those of any sensorineural hearing loss: difficulty in distinguishing one voice from many, difficulty in hearing in crowds, family complaints about the loudness of the television set, and inattentiveness. Much can be done to ameliorate the handicap with both specific and general devices. The psychological impact on the worker and their family has recently received considerable attention. Denial of problems, withdrawal and lack of family interaction may have a severe effect on interpersonal family relationships.[106,107]

We have found a telephone handset amplifier (obtainable from most telephone companies), a louder bell, and a specific television amplifier to be the most useful. Many patients use a hearing aid to amplify television, but this also amplifies all other sounds in the environment, such as paper rustling, children crying, dishes clattering, and other people talking. A specific amplifier for television such as a headphone or exten-

sion loudspeaker serves both to make the sound louder and to improve the signal-to-noise ratio.

A hearing aid is useful for and well accepted by those with noise-induced hearing loss.[108] They should not be withheld.

HEARING CONSERVATION PROGRAMS

Noise-induced hearing loss is incurable but preventable. The technique of prevention is known as hearing conservation. A hearing conservation program has four main features: sound measurement, engineering and administrative controls, personal hearing protection, and audiometric monitoring of the population at risk. A good hearing conservation program is multidisciplinary involving industrial hygienist, engineer, nurse, audiometric technician and frequently a supervisory audiologist and otologist. A good review of such programs is found in Feldman and Grimes[109] and in Berger et al.[110] Sound measurement is a skilled task devised to answer two questions: (1) what are the absolute sound levels in the plant, and (2) what is the sound exposure of the individual? Carefully performed sound surveys measuring sound levels throughout the plant and throughout the working day indicate the absolute levels in a plant and help identify those where there is potentially hazardous noise. The exposure of individual workers, if the job is static, may be extrapolated from these measurements, but it is far better to undertake individual noise dosimetry studies. These are small but expensive devices that store a measure of the total noise received. The measurement of impact and impulsive noise is particularly difficult and may require special laboratory equipment. A good hearing conservation program has the following elements.

1. Noise hazard identification
2. Engineering contacts
3. Personal hearing protection
4. Monitoring
5. Record keeping
6. Health education
7. Enforcement
8. Program evaluation

A great effort must be made to have total collaboration of the workforce; to be successful it requires bottom up planning and implementation and top down guidance.

SOUND ABATEMENT AND ADMINISTRATIVE CONTROL

The most effective way of reducing the risk of noise-induced hearing loss is to engineer out noise at the source by either silencing machinery or enclosing it. It is sometimes possible to retrofit machinery and provide sound-silencing barriers. Vicarious noise exposure should be eliminated; e.g., there is no need to have a workbench beside a drop forge and to expose the mechanic, as well as the forge operator, to the noise of the forge. This happens all too often. In many industrial plants, it is possible to put the equipment operator inside a sound-enclosed booth and separate him from noisy machinery, for example, in ships' engine rooms, hydroturbine halls, and paper-making plants.

For a further review of sound measurement, the reader should consult specialized texts.

PERSONAL HEARING PROTECTION

Protection methods are widely used where noise levels remain hazardous even after appropriate engineering and administrative controls have been put in place. It is, however, not enough to provide a protector; there must be a program to encourage their use and instruct in their proper fitting and maintenance. The plant physician has a major role to play in this area and should be familiar with the various types of protectors, their advantages and disadvantages, and their application. By far the most commonly used hearing protectors are earplugs, which constitute about 85% of personal protector devices in use in the U.S.[111] Earplugs should fit firmly and may require a few days of use before they are comfortable. The preformed plugs of the V51R or fir cone Comfit type must be sized appropriately for the individual user. Workers usually choose one size too small because it is more comfortable. Universal plugs, which are compressed before being placed in the ear canal and expand to close it, are widely used and range from waxed wool to the commonly used foam polyurethane EAR or Deci-Damp. They work well for most people but are difficult to fit into those with small ear canals, particularly some women.[112] Soft individually molded plugs, which were widely used, have not proven effective on a large scale. Theoretically, the most effective type of hearing protector is the ear muff, consisting of a solid cup containing a sound-absorbing material such as foam, sealed to the side of the head with a soft malleable gasket, and applied with sufficient pressure to produce an airtight seal. Muffs are, however, less comfortable to wear than plugs, and their performance is interfered with by hard hats and safety glasses. They tend to be reserved for heavy industry and industries in which intermittent use of a protector is appropriate. Figure 53–4 shows the average attenuation of a wide range of hearing protectors under average use conditions—a far cry from manufacturer's claims. Because the majority of industrial noise lies in the mid-90 dB range, however, 10 dB of attenuation is in fact effective. One must guard against

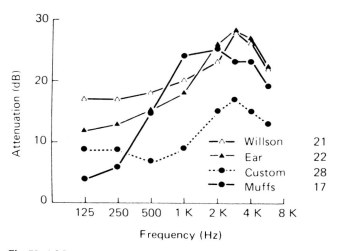

Fig. 53–4. Mean attenuation characteristics of three types of earplugs and a group of earmuffs, as issued to industrial workers and fitted by them. Reprinted with permission from Alberti PW, Riko K, Abel SM, and Kristensen R: The effectiveness of hearing protectors in practice. J Otolaryngol 8:354–359.[119]

inappropriate protection as well as underprotection. There is much literature about hearing protectors and their industrial use, which is summarized in the book Hearing Protectors in Industry.[113]

One of the problems with hearing protectors is that they distort external sounds by attenuating high frequency more than low frequency sound; another is that they exclude ambient signals as well as unwanted noise. Increasing use is therefore being made of active hearing protectors consisting of good quality muffs with built-in microphone and amplifier which, however, cut out above certain predetermined ambient noise levels. They act much like a good quality compression hearing aid with less and less amplification as the ambient noise rises, and, above a predetermined figure, usually 85 dB, the amplifier automatically cuts out when the device becomes a passive hearing protector. They are particularly useful in intermittent and impact noise and have been widely adopted by huntsmen who wish to hear the sounds of the countryside but to protect their ears from the sound of gunshots. These muffs have widening application.[114]

Modifications have also been made to passive muffs by the incorporation of filters which flatten the attenuation curve and provide a more natural environment for their user.[114]

HEARING SCREENING

A crucial feature of any conservation hearing program is the regular monitoring of workers' hearing.[115] New employees must be screened and the effectiveness of the program monitored by routine, usually annual, hearing tests. The annual hearing test has many functions; important among them is the opportunity it provides to re-enforce the hearing conservation program and to monitor proper use of hearing protectors. It detects those with hearing loss, identifies individuals' changes and whether a total programme is effective. This indicates whether a program is working, whether an individual worker needs counselling, or if the whole plant needs further instruction.

There are practical problems related to hearing screening. When should one do the test? Is temporary threshold shift a problem? It used to be taught that screening should not be performed unless the worker was out of noise for 16 and preferably 48 hours before the test. This is impractical, and now testing is done throughout the workday, for in an effective programme, there should be no TTS. Those who fail can be retested after a period in quiet.

What is a failure? Many suggestions have been made in the literature. The current belief is that a change of 15 dB or more in two or more frequencies should be an indication for a further referral. 10 dB changes are usually assumed to be within the realm of test/retest era of screening audiometry.

A further question is how, and for how long, to store records. This has been significantly helped by the introduction of computer programs designed to deal with the mass of figures generated, which are becoming widely used. The ideal system of hearing screening includes direct computer storage of the audiometric results from the audiometer and a printout of the current hearing test results, the most immediate prior one, and the first one on record.

MEDICAL, LEGAL, AND SOCIAL IMPLICATION

There is no clear-cut method of determining the handicap produced by hearing loss, and definitions vary. In turn, there is little congruity about levels at which compensation should be paid, for what, and for how long. One may compensate for loss of earnings or loss of enjoyment of life. Compensation may be paid only while retraining occurs or for life. Differences in philosophy have given rise to widely differing practices. The American Academy of Otolaryngology—Head and Neck Surgery suggests that hearing loss should be compensated if the average loss of the frequencies 500, 1000, 2000, and 3000 exceeds 25 dB. States vary widely in their interpretation of these recommendations.

OTHER CAUSES OF OCCUPATIONAL HEARING LOSS

Noise is not the only cause of occupational hearing loss. Head injury at work can produce hearing loss, sensorineural and conductive. Direct ear injuries also occur from slag or welding sparks,[116] which may be difficult to control. Perforations are common, and should be left to close spontaneously if they can, and if not, surgical repair should be done. Surgical repair gives disappointing results. If welders and braziers wore ear protection, perforations would not occur. Even stranger accidents happen; the author has seen two kitchen attendants who burned their ears when a tureen of hot soup tipped over and one man who burned his ear when he fell in a vat of chromic acid. Serious industrial burns may become infected and be treated by ototoxic antibiotics, and there is a suggestion that certain volatile chemicals experienced in the workplace may be ototoxic.

REFERENCES

1. Holt EE: Boilermaker's deafness and hearing in noise. Trans Am Otol Soc 3, 34–44, 1982.
2. Barr T: Transactions of the Philosophy Society of Glasgow 17: 223, 1886.
3. Habermann J: Uber die Schwerhortighkelt des Kesselschmiede. Archiv Ohrenhelikunde 30:1–25, 1990.
4. Fowler EP: Limited lesions of the basilar membrane. Arch Otolaryngol Head Neck Surg 8:151, 1928.
5. Bunch CC: Traumatic deafness. In Nelson Loose Leaf Medicine of the Ear. Edited by Fowler EP Jr. New York: Thomas Nelson, 1939, pp 349–367.
6. Hawkins JE Jr: Experimental noise deafness: Recollections and ruminations. *In* Hearing and Davis. Edited by Hirsch SK, Eldridge DH, Hirsch JJ, Silverman SR. Washington, DC: Washington University Press, 1976, pp 73–84.
7. McFadden D: The curious half-octave shift: evidence for a basalwood migration of the traveling-wave envelope with increasing intensity. In Basic and Applied Aspects of Noise-Induced Hearing Loss. Edited by RJ Salvi, D Henderson, RP Hamernik, V Colleti. New York: Plenum Press, 1986.
8. Mills JH: Effects of noise on auditory sensitivity, psychophysical tuning curves and suppression. *In* New Perspectives on Noise Induced Hearing Loss. Edited by Hamernik RP, Henderson D, Salvi R. New York: Raven Press, 1982, pp 249–263.
9. Kryter KD: The Effects of Noise on Man, 2nd edition. New York, Academic Press, 1985.
10. Melnick W: Human asymptotic threshold shift. In Effects of Noise on Hearing. Edited by D Henderson, RP Hamernik, DS Dosanj, JH Mills. New York: Raven Press, 1976, pp 277–289.
11. Melnick W: Human temporary threshold shift (TTS) and damage risk. J Acoust Soc Am 90:147–164, 1991.
12. Saunders JC, Dear SP, Schneider ME: The anatomical consequences of acoustic injury: A review and tutorial. J Acoust Soc Am 78:833–860, 1985.
13. Saunders JC, Cohen YE, Szymko YM: The structural and functional consequences of acoustic injury in the cochlea and peripheral auditory system: a five year update. J Acoust Soc Am 90:136–146, 1991.
14. Bohne BA, Clark WW: Growth of hearing loss and cochlear lesion increases of noise exposure. In New Perspectives on Noise Induced Hearing loss. Edited by Hamernik RP, Henderson, D, Salvi R. New York: Raven Press, 1962, pp 283–302.
15. Liberman MC: Chronic ultrastructural changes in acoustic trauma. Serial section reconstruction of stereocilia and cuticular plates. Hear Res 16:65–88, 1987.

16. Liberman MC, Dodds LW: Acute ultrastructural changes in acoustic trauma. Serial section reconstruction of stereocilia and cuticular plates. Hear Res 26:45–64, 1987.

17. Henderson D, Danielson RW, Farzi F: The critical level concept and impulse noise. In Noise as a Public Health Hazard. Swedish Council for Building Research, 1989.

18. Lim DJ: Functional structure of the organ of Corti: A review. Hear Res 22:117–146, 1986.

19. Kiang NYS, Liberman MC, Sewell WF, et al: Single unit clues to cochlear mechanisms. Hear Res 22:171–182, 1986.

20. Schacht J, Conlon B: Biochemistry of the inner ear. In: Otological Medicine and Surgery. Edited by Alberti PW, Ruben RJ. New York: Churchill Livingstone, 1988, pp 151–178.

21. Saunders JC, Canlon B, Flock A: Changes in stereocilia micromechanics following overstimulation in metabolically blocked hair cells. Hear Res 24:217–225, 1986.

22. Tilney LG, Saunders JC, Engleman H, et al: Changes in the organization of actin filaments in the stereocilia of noise damaged lizard cochlase. Hear Res 7:181–197, 1982.

23. Slepecky N: Overview of mechanical damage to the inner ear: Noise as a tool to probe cochlear function. Hear Res 22:307–321, 1986.

24. Gao W-Y, Ding D-L, Zheng X-Y, et al: A comparison of changes in the stereocilia between temporary and permanent hearing losses in acoustic trauma. Hear Res 62:27–41, 1992.

25. Spoendlin H: Primary structural changes in the organ of Corti after acoustic overstimulation. Acta Otolaryngol (Stockh) 71:166–176, 1971.

26. Liberman MC, Mulroy MJ: Acute and chronic effects of acoustic trauma: Cochlear pathology and auditory nerve pathophysiology. In New Perspectives on Noise Induced Hearing Loss. Edited by Hamernik RP, Henderson D, and Salvi R. New York: Raven Press, 1962, pp 105–135.

27. Morest DK, Bohne BA: Noise-induced degeneration in the brain and representation of inner and outer hair cells. Hear Res 9:145–151, 1983.

28. Patuzzi R: In: Noise Induced Hearing Loss. Edited by AL Dancer, D Henderson, RJ Salvi, RP Hamernik. St Louis: Mosby Year Book, 1992.

29. Schmiedt RA: Acoustic injury and the physiology of hearing. A review and tutorial. J Acoust Soc Am 76:1293–1317, 1984.

30. Harrison RV: The Biology of Hearing and Deafness. Springfield: Charles C Thomas, 1988.

31. Dallos P: Neurobiology of cochlear hair cells. In: Auditory Physiology and Perception. Edited by Y Cazals, K Horner, L Demany. Oxford: Pergamon Press, 3–17, 1992.

32. Glorig A: Noise and the Ear. New York: Grune & Stratton, 1958.

33. Flock A: The cochlear mechanisms. In Noise as a Public Health Problem, Swedish Council for Building Research, 5:337–338, 1990.

34. Henderson D, Campo P, Subramaniam M, et al: Development of resistance to noise. In: Noise Induced Hearing Loss. Edited by AL Dancer, D Henderson, RJ Salvi, RP Hamernik. St Louis: Mosby Year Book, 476–488, 1992.

35. Boettcher FA: Auditory brainstem response correlates of resistance to noise induced hearing loss in Mongolian gerbits. J Acoust Soc Am 94:3207–3214, 1993.

36. Ryan AF, Bennett TM, Woolf NK, et al: Protection from noise induced hearing loss by prior exposure to a nontraumatic stimulus: role of the middle ear muscles. Hear Res 72:23–28, 1994.

37. Mills JH: Threshold shifts as produced by a 90 day exposure to noise. In: Effects of Noise on Hearing. Edited by Henderson D, Hamernik R, Dosanjh D, Mills J. New York: Raven Press, 1976, pp 265–275.

38. Taylor W, Pearson JCC, Mair A, et al: Study of noise and hearing in jute weaving. J Acoust Soc Am 38:113–120, 1965.

39. Dobie RA: The relative contributions of occupational noise and aging in individual loss of hearing loss. Ear Hear 13:19–27, 1992.

40. Baughn WL: Relation between daily noise exposure and hearing loss based on the evaluation of 6835 industrial noise exposure cases. AMRL-TR-73-53, Wright-Patterson Air Force Base, Aerospace Medical Research Laboratory, 1973.

41. Burns W, Robinson DW: Hearing and Noise in Industry. London: HM Stationery Office, 1970.

42. Ward WD: The role of intermittence in PTS. J Acoust Soc Am 90:164–169, 1991.

43. Hamernick RP, Hsueh KD: Impulse noise: some definitions, physical acoustics and other considerations. J Acoust Soc Am 90:189–196, 1991.

44. Smoorenburg GF: Damage for low-frequency impulse noise: the spectral factor in noise-induced hearing loss. In: Noise-Induced Hearing Loss. Edited by AL Dancer, D Henderson, RJ Salvi, RP Hamernick. St. Louis: Mosby Year Book, 313–324, 1992.

45. Shaw EAG: Occupational noise exposure and noise-induced hearing loss: Scientific issues, technical arguments and practical recommendations. National Research Council Canada, Report 25051, Ottawa, 1965.

46. Ward WD, Turner CW, Fabry DA: The total energy and equal energy principles in the chinchilla. In Proceedings of 4th International Congress on Noise as a Public Health Problem. Edited by Rossi G. Turin, 1983, pp 399–405.

47. Baughn WL: Noise control—Percent of population protected. Int Audiol 51:331–338, 1966.

48. Rop I, Raber A, Fischer GH: Study of hearing losses of industrial workers with occupational noise exposure using statistical methods for the analysis of qualitative data. Audiology 18:181–196, 1979.

49. Burns W, Robinson DW, Shipton MS, et al: Hearing hazards from occupational noise: Observations on a population from heavy industry. Acoustic Report AC16, National Physics Laboratory, 1979.

50. Abel SM, Haythornthwaite CA: The progression of noise induced hearing loss—Survey of workers in selected Canadian industries. J Otolaryngol 13:2–36, 1984.

51. Pasachier-Vermeer W: Noise induced hearing loss from exposure to intermittent and varying noise. In Proceedings of International Congress on Noise as a Public Health Problem. Dubrovnick, US Environmental Protection Agency, Washington, DC, 1983, pp 169–200.

52. Man A, Naggan L: Characteristics of tinnitus in acoustic trauma. Audiology 20:72–78, 1981.

53. Axelsson A, Barreras ML: Tinnitus in noise induced hearing loss. In: Noise Induced Hearing Loss. Edited by AL Dancer, D Henderson, RJ Salvi, RP Hamernik. St Louis: Mosby Year Book 269–276, 1992.

54. Alberti PW: Tinnitus in occupational hearing loss: nosological aspects. J Otolaryngol 16:34–35, 1987.

55. McShane D, Hyde ML, Alberti PW: Tinnitus prevalence in occupational hearing loss claimants. Clin Otolaryngol 13:323–330, 1988.

56. Hinchliffe R, King PF: Medicolegal aspects of tinnitus. I, II, III. J Audiol Med 1, 38–58, 59–79, 127–147, 1992.

57. Tschopp K, Probst R: Acute acoustic trauma. A retrospective study of influencing factors in different therapies in 268 patients. Acta Otolaryngol 108:378–384, 1989.

58. McFadden D, Plattismier HS: Aspirin can potentiate the temporary hearing loss induced by intense sounds. Hear Res 9:295–316, 1983.

59. Odkvist LM, Moller C, Thuomas KA: Otoneurologic disturbances caused by solvent pollution. Otolaryngol Head Neck Surg 106:687–692, 1992.

60. Ryback LP: Hearing: The effects of chemicals. Otolaryngol Head Neck Surg 106:677–686, 1992.

61. Johnson AC, Canlon B: Toluene exposure affects the functional activity of the outer hair cells. Hear Res 72:189–196, 1994.

62. Morata TC, Dunn DE, Kretschmer LW, et al: Effects of occupa-

tional exposure to organic solvents and noise on hearing. Scand J Environ Health 19:245–254, 1993.

63. Iki M, Kurumatami N, Hirata K, et al: An association between vibration induced while finger and hearing loss in forestry workers. Scand J Work Environ Health 12:365–370, 1986.

64. Fyykko I, Koskimies K, Stark J, et al: Risk factors in the genesis of sensorineural hearing loss in Finnish factory workers. Br J Indust Med 40:439–440, 1989.

65. Stark J, Pekkaimen J, Pyykko I: Impulse noise and hand arm vibration in relation to sensorineural hearing loss. Scand J Work Environ Health 14:265–271, 1988.

66. Macrea JM: Presbycusis and noise induced permanent threshold shift. J Acoust Soc Am 90:2513–2516, 1991.

67. Novotny Z: Age factor in auditory fatigue in occupational hearing disorders due to noise. Ceskoslovenska Otolaryngol 24:5–9, 1975.

68. Novotny Z: Development of occupational deafness after entering into noisy job at an advanced age. Ceskoslovenska Otolaryngologie 24:151–154, 1975.

69. Welleschik B, Raber A: Einfluss von Expositionszeit und Alter auf den Irmbedingten Horverlust. Laryngol Rhinol Otol (Stuttg) 57:1037–1048, 1978.

70. Robinson DW: Relation between hearing threshold level and its component parts. Br J Audiol 25:93–103, 1991a.

71. Corso JF: Age correction factor in noise-induced hearing loss: A quantitative model. Audiology 19:221–232, 1980.

72. Humes LE: Noise-induced hearing loss as influenced by other agents and by some physical characteristics of the individual. J Acoust Soc Am 76:1318–1329, 1984.

73. Royster LH, Royster JD: Methods of evaluating hearing conservation program—Audiometric data bases. In Personal Hearing Protection in Industry. Edited by Alberti PW. New York: Raven Press, 1982, pp 511–540.

74. Singleton DT, Whitaker DL, Keim RJ, et al: Cordless telephones: A threat to hearing. Ann Otol Rhinol Laryngol 93:565–568, 1984.

75. Berglund B, Berglund V, Karlsson I, et al: Noise as a Public Health Problem. Swedish Council for Building Research, 1988.

76. Vallet M: Noise as a Public Health Problem. Bron: INRETS, 1993.

77. Gupta D, Vishwarama SK: Toy weapons and firecrackers: A source of hearing loss. Laryngoscope 99:330–334, 1989.

78. Axelsson A, Hellstrom PA, Altschuller R, et al: Inner ear damage from toy cap pistols and firecrackers. Int J Paediatr Otolaryngol 21:143–148, 1991.

79. Alberti PW: Noise and the ear. In Scott Brown's Otolaryngology, 5th ed. Vol. 2. Edited by Stephens D. Philadelphia: JB Lippincott, 1987, pp 594–641.

80. Clark WW: Noise exposure from leisure activities: A review. J Acoust Soc Am 91:175–181, 1991b.

81. Kramer MB, Wood D: Noise induced hearing loss in rural school children. Scand Audiol 11:279–280, 1982.

82. Coles RR, Hoare NW: Noise induced hearing loss and the dentist. Br Dent J 159:209–218, 1985.

83. Hughes KB: Sensorineural deafness due to compression chamber noise. J Laryngol 90:803–807, 1976.

84. Welles B: Noise risk due to dental turbine. Laryngol Rhinol Otol (Grenzgeb) 55:515–516, 1976.

85. Kylen P, Stjernvall JE, Arlinger S: Variables affecting the drill generated noise levels in ear surgery. Acta Otolaryngol (Stockh) 84:252–259, 1977.

86. Man A, Winerman I: Does drill noise during mastoid surgery affect the contralateral ear. Am J Otol 6:334–335, 1985.

87. Parkin JL, Wood GS, Wood RD, et al: Drill- and suction-generated noise in mastoid surgery. Arch Otolaryngol Head Neck Surg 106:92–96, 1980.

88. Ducel G, Suter T, Dupont B: The noise in an intensive care unit. Soz Preventive Med 21:135, 1976.

89. Bentley S, Murphy F, Dudley H: Perceived noise in surgical wards and an intensive care area: An objective analysis. Br Med J 2:1503–1506, 1977.

90. Brummett RE, Talbot JM, Charuhas P: Potential hearing loss resulting from MR imaging. Radiology 169:539–540, 1988.

91. Von Gierke HE, Harris CS: On the potential association between noise exposure and cardiovascular disease. In Noise as a Public Health Problem. 1989.

92. Stansfeld S, Gullacher J, Babish W, et al: Road traffic noise, noise sensitivity and psychiatric disorder: preliminary prospective findings from the Caerphilly study. In Noise as a Public Health Hazard, Vol. 3. Edited by M. Vallet, Bron: INRETS 268–273, 1993.

93. Evans GW: The nonauditory effects of noise on child development. In Noise as a Public Health Problem, 4. Edited by B Berglund, V Berglund, J Karlsson, T Lindvall. Stockholm: Swedish Council for Building Research 425–453, 1990.

94. Hetu R, Truchon-Gagnon C, Bilodau SA: Problems of noise in school settings. J Occup Speech Language Pathol Audiol 14: 31–39, 1990.

95. Bronzaft AL: The effects of noise on learning, cognitive development and social behaviour. In Noise and Health. Edited by TH Fay. New York: New York Academy of Medicine, 1991.

96. Alberti PW, Blair RL: Occupational hearing loss: An Ontario perspective. Laryngoscope 92:535–539, 1987.

97. Alberti PW, Symons F, Hyde ML: Occupational hearing loss: The significance of asymmetrical hearing thresholds. Acta Otolaryngol (Stockh) 87:255–263, 1979.

98. Hyde ML, Alberti PW, Matsumoto N, et al: Auditory evoked potentials in audiometric assessment of compensation and medical-legal patients. Ann Otol Rhinol Laryngol 95:514–519, 1986.

99. Alberti PW, Hydle ML, Riko K: Exaggerated hearing loss in compensation claimants. J Otolaryngol 16:6,362–366, 1987.

100. Klockhoff I, Drettner B, Svedberg A: Computerized classification of the results of screening audiometry in groups of persons exposed to noise. Audiology 13:326–334, 1974.

101. Alberti PW, Morgan PP, Czuba I: Speech and pure tone audiometry as a screen for exaggerated hearing loss in industrial claims. Acta Otolaryngol (Stockh) 85:328–331, 1978.

102. Alberti PW: Nonorganic hearing loss in adults. In Audiology and Audiological Medicine. Edited by Beagley H. London: Oxford University Press, 1981, pp 910–930.

103. Witter HL, Deko RC, Lipscomb DM, et al: Effects of pre-stimulatory carbogen inhalation on noise-induced temporary threshold shifts in humans and chinchilla. Am J Otol 1:227–232, 1980.

104. Demaertelaere L, Van Opstal M: Treatment of acoustic trauma with hyperbaric oxygen. Acta Otorhinolaryngol Belg 35: 303–314, 1981.

105. Dengerink HA, Axelsson A, Miller JM, et al: The effect of noise and carbogen on cochlear vasculature. Acta Otolaryngol (Stockh) 98:81–88, 1974.

106. Hetu R, Lalonde M, Getty L: Psychosocial disadvantages associated with occupational hearing loss as experienced in the family. Audiology 26:141–152, 1987.

107. Hallberg LR-M, Barreras ML: Living with a male with noise induced hearing loss: experiences from the perspective of spouses. Br J Audiol 27:255–261, 1993.

108. Riko K, McShane D, Hyde MI, et al: Hearing aid usage and requirements in occupational hearing loss claimants. J Otolaryngol 19:25–30, 1990.

109. Feldman AS, Grimes CT (Editors): Hearing Conservation in Industry. Baltimore: Williams and Wilkins, 1985.

110. Berger EH, Ward WD, Morrill JC, et al: Noise and Hearing Conservation Manual. Akron, Ohio, Am Indust Hyg Assoc, 1986.

111. Allen CH, Berger E: Development of a unique passive level-dependent hearing protector. J Acoust Soc (Suppl 1) 81:55, 1987.

112. Abel SM, Alberti PW, Rochas D: Gender differences in real-world hearing protector attenuation. J Otolaryngol *17*:86–92, 1988.

113. Alberti PW: Personal Hearing Protection in Industry. New York: Raven Press, 1982.

114. Alberti PW: Active hearing protectors. *In* Noise as a Public Health Problem. Edited by Berglund et al, 1989.

115. Royster LH, Royster JD: Effective hearing conservation programs (HCPs). What are the considerations? In Noise as a Public Health Problem. Edited by Berglund et al, 1988.

116. Frenkiel S, Alberti PW; Traumatic thermal injuries of the middle ear. J Otolaryngol *6*:17–22, 1977.

117. Roberston D, Johnstone BM: Aberrant tonotopic organization in the inner ear damaged by kanamycin. J Acoust Soc Am *66*: 466–469, 1979.

118. Burns W, Hinchcliffe R, Littler TS: An exploratory study: Hearing and noise exposure in textile workers. Ann Occup Hyg *7*: 323, 1954.

119. Alberti PW, Riko K, Abel SM, et al: The effectiveness of hearing protectors in practice. J Otolaryngol *8*:354–359, 1979.

54 Ototoxicity

Leonard P. Rybak and Hidetaka Kanno

Ototoxicity can be defined as the capacity of a drug or chemical to damage inner ear structure and/or function. The damage may occur in the auditory or vestibular portion or in both parts of the inner ear. There exists a large number of agents with the propensity for ototoxicity. This chapter deals with several of the more common drugs and chemicals likely to cause hearing loss and/or cochlear injury. These agents include the aminoglycoside antibiotics, the antineoplastic drugs cisplatin and carboplatin, the loop diuretics, salicylates, quinine, deferoxamine and toxic substances. For the therapeutic drugs, risk factors, pharmacokinetics, and monitoring of blood levels are discussed.

AMINOGLYCOSIDE ANTIBIOTICS

Pharmacokinetics

The pharmacokinetics of most aminoglycoside antibiotics are similar. Because only about 3% of an orally administered dose is absorbed from the gastrointestinal tract, these drugs usually are administered parenterally. Tissue concentrations of aminoglycosides are usually about one third of corresponding serum concentrations. Penetration of aminoglycosides across the blood-brain barrier is minimal, except in neonates. Previous literature has suggested that aminoglycosides are not metabolized. However, recent experiments have suggested that an ototoxic metabolite may be formed.

Aminoglycosides are excreted in the urine by glomerular infiltration, and therefore concentrations in the urine may exceed those in the serum. Impaired renal function reduces the rate of excretion and may lead to accumulation in the body. Doses are frequently adjusted downward in patients with decreased renal function.

Huang and Schacht[1] reported that a cytotoxic metabolite of aminoglycosides caused death of isolated guinea pig outer hair cells, whereas nonmetabolized aminoglycosides had no effect on cell viability. This may explain why ototoxicity associated with aminoglycoside antibiotics is delayed for days or weeks despite early peak drug levels in cochlear tissues.

The pharmacokinetics of aminoglycosides in the serum and perilymph have been investigated in human subjects under various conditions. The correlation has made it possible to extrapolate concentrations of aminoglycosides in the inner ear, which is relatively inaccessible, from concentrations of these drugs in serum, which is sampled easily.

Histopathology

In ototoxic doses, the cochleotoxic agents (neomycin, kanamycin, amikacin, sisomycin, livodomycin) appear to elicit patterns of injury to the cochlea in experimental animals that are similar to the patterns seen in human temporal bones. These compounds tend to cause selective destruction of the outer hair cells in the basal turn of the cochlea, with progression toward the apex as the dose and duration of treatment are increased.

In a well-documented clinical case of gentamicin ototoxicity, Keene et al[2] used graphic reconstruction of the Corti to obtain detailed information about the effect on cochlear and vestibular structures. The hair cells in the apex and middle coils were normal in the cochlea of this patient, who had bilateral high-frequency sensorineural hearing loss following gentamicin injections. Outer hair cells were extensively absent in the basal turn, and some loss of spiral ganglion cells was noted in the basal turn. Pathologic changes were also found in the vestibular sensory neuroepithelium.

Human studies also have shown netilmicin to be less likely to cause ototoxicity than some other aminoglycosides.

Several prospective studies of aminoglycoside ototoxicity have been carried out. Fee[3] and Smith et al[4] compared gentamicin ototoxicity with tobramycin ototoxicity and found cochlear damage in 10% to 16% of patients and vestibular toxicity in 5% to 15%.

Monitoring

Concentration of aminoglycosides are monitored for two reasons: 1) to ensure adequate levels for therapy and 2) to detect elevated or rising levels that may be associated with increased risk of ototoxicity and nephrotoxicity. The best indication of renal function is creatinine clearance, but the time required in its determination makes this test impractical for routine monitoring. In patients with constant metabolic production, serum creatinine level is a good indirect estimate of the glomerular filtration rate.

Suggested schedules for determination of serum levels are as follows:

1. For normal renal function: Peak level is determined the first one to two days of therapy, the trough level within one week, and peak-and-trough levels weekly thereafter. Peak levels are usually drawn one hour after administration, and trough levels are drawn 15 minutes before administration of the next dose.
2. For impaired but stable renal function: Peak-and-trough levels are determined within the first one to two days of therapy. Serum levels may have to be monitored daily when renal function remains unstable.

Since these relationships are somewhat different for each drug, reference books should be consulted for specific details.[5]

Moore et al[6] reported that bacteremia, elevated temperatures, liver dysfunction and serum urea nitrogen serum creatinine ratio were risk factors associated with ototoxicity in prospective double blind clinical trials of gentamicin, tobramycin and amikacin.

Ototoxicity is most likely to occur in patients with compromised renal function. The aminoglycoside antibiotics primarily affect the inner ear. Amikacin and kanamycin have more of an effect on the cochlea than on the vestibular system, whereas streptomycin and gentamicin appear to exert greater effects on the vestibular system, although auditory damage does occur with their use. However, with any of these drugs, both auditory and vestibular toxicity can occur simultaneously.

Acute damage to the cochlea is often preceded by tinnitus, although ototoxic effects can occur in the absence of tinnitus. The loss of hearing that results from the use of these drugs initially affects the high frequencies. Since patients do not complain about or have noticeable hearing losses until they have 30dB loss that includes frequencies as low as 3,000 to 4,000 Hz, the

detection of ototoxicity is difficult unless audiometric monitoring is performed.

The risk factors in ototoxicity are not fully established. Lerner and associates found an association of ototoxicity with elevated mean trough levels in a few of the studies, with nephrotoxicity. In another study, univariate and multivariate analysis of risk factors of ototoxicity show only age as a predisposing factor for toxicity.

One of the newly identified risk factors may be genetic susceptibility. Hypersensitivity to aminoglycoside antibiotics can be transmitted by mothers as a genetic trait. A mitochondrial DNA polymorphism, 1555^G, is associated with aminoglycoside-induced deafness.[8,9] The basis for this hypersensitivity to ototoxicity may be based on the three dimensional structure of the ribosome, favoring the binding of aminoglycoside, leading to disruption of protein synthesis and cell death in the cochlea.[9]

ANTINEOPLASTIC DRUGS/CISPLATIN AND CARBOPLATIN

After a 1 hour intravenous infusion of 70 mg/m2 of cisplatin, the plasma platinum concentrations were found to have a biphasic clearance with half-life values of 23 minutes and 67 hours. 17% of the administered dose was excreted in the first 24 hours. Renal excretion is primarily by glomerular filtration. Ninety percent of cisplatin is bound to serum proteins,[10] and this cisplatin-protein complex is inactive against tumor cells. The serum levels of non–protein-bound platinum display different kinetics than those found for total platinum levels in serum. It is not known whether toxic metabolites of cisplatin are formed either in the inner ear or in the other parts of the body. However, the liver has been shown to rapidly convert cisplatin into nontoxic metabolites within one hour.

Temporal bones removed from patients with cisplatin-induced hearing loss have demonstrated the following: large, fused stereocilia; damage to the cuticular plate of the outer hair cells; and extensive loss of sensory cells in the vestibular labyrinth in specimens studied by scanning electron microscopy.[11] In addition to noting outer hair cell degeneration in the basal turn of the cochlea, Strauss et al[12] reported degeneration of spiral ganglion cells and cochlear neurons in patients with documented cisplatin ototoxicity. However, the vestibular neurons appeared normal.

The exact incidence and severity of cisplatin-induced auditory effects is difficult to assess because of inconsistencies including variable dosing in previous studies and the lack of complete data from patients too ill to cooperate for pretreatment and post-treatment audiograms.[13]

Symptoms that strongly suggest cisplatin ototoxicity include otalgia, tinnitus, and subjective hearing loss. Tinnitus has been reported in 2% to 36% of patients receiving cisplatin. The tinnitus often is transient, lasting from a few hours up to a week after cisplatin therapy. The incidence of hearing loss among patients treated with cisplatin has been as low as 9% and as high as 91%.[13] In patients with head and neck cancer treated with cisplatin, about half develop hearing loss.[14] The hearing loss is usually bilateral and appears first at high frequencies (6000 and 8000 Hz). Progression to lower frequencies (2000 and 4000 Hz) may occur with continued therapy. The hearing loss may be asymmetric and may not appear until several days after treatment. Patients may experience some degree of reversibility, but when the hearing loss is profound, it appears to be permanent.[14] Because the hearing loss tends to occur at the higher frequencies, it may escape detection without audiometry. Cochlear toxicity may be detected earlier with high frequency audiometry (up to 20 kHz) than with conventional audiologic testing.[15] Speech discrimination scores may be markedly reduced when cisplatin ototoxicity occurs. The hearing loss may be gradual, progressive and cumulative, or may present suddenly. Several patterns of hearing loss have been recently described.[16]

The critical cumulative dose of cisplatin has been reported as 3–4 mg/kg body weight. Since ototoxicity may be more severe after bolus injection the ototoxic effects can be reduced by using slow infusion and dividing the doses over several months.[13]

Children receiving high cumulative doses of cisplatin (above 540 mg/m2) have a high incidence of hearing loss which is cumulative and dose dependent.[17] However, a plateau effect has been reported with no further deterioration of hearing at doses greater than 600 mg/m2. Still, a number of patients will develop more severe hearing losses in the 2 to 8 kHz range even after 1 or 2 courses of therapy, showing exceptions to the plateau effect.[18] Adults with a pre-existing history of otologic problems are said to experience a higher incidence of ototoxicity of cisplatin affecting both lower (1000–8000 Hz) and higher frequencies (10,000–18,000 Hz).[19] Ototoxicity of cisplatin appears to be enhanced by cranial irradiation.[20]

Early after its introduction, standard cisplatin doses were 50 mg/m2. Recently cisplatin treatment regimens have been developed using higher doses of cisplatin (100–120 mg/m2 = "high dose"; 150–225 mg/m2—"very high dose" regimen). These increased dosage regimens have resulted in a higher incidence of hearing loss than that observed with the lower dosage of 50 mg/m2 as well as some different perspectives on cisplatin induced hearing loss. In a study of 54 patients receiving "high dose" cisplatin, Laurell and Jungnelius[21] found that 81% of patients had significant threshold elevations (15 dB or more at one frequency or 10 dB or more in 3 frequencies). After therapy, which ranged from 1–7 courses, 41% of the patients had significant deterioration of hearing in the speech frequency range of 0.5–2 kHz. 25% of patients lost 25% of their remaining high frequency hearing after each course. Pre-existing hearing loss did not seem to predispose to ototoxicity, but advanced age was slightly associated with risk of hearing loss. The audiogram after the first course did not predict future deterioration of hearing later during treatment with "high-dose" protocols. In this study, the ototoxic risk was determined more by the amount of the single dose than by the cumulative dose levels. No ototoxic effects were seen at a peak plasma concentration of less than 1 mcG/L. Based on their findings, the authors recommended that patients undergoing "high-dose" cisplatin treatment undergo audiometric testing before the initiation of therapy and before each of the subsequent courses. Less frequent testing was deemed necessary for patients treated with low and moderate dose treatment.[21]

Kopelman et al[22] reported that all of their patients complained of decreased hearing after "very high-dose" cisplatin administration (150–225 mg/m2). Ototoxic reactions appear to be more likely in patients with low serum albumin, and in those with anemia.

New series of platinum anticancer drugs have been produced and tested clinically. Carboplatin is one such derivative. The principal toxicity of carboplatin is myelosuppression, especially thrombocytopenia. Renal toxicity is not usually a problem and neurotoxicity is minimal.[23]

Initial reports suggested a complete lack of ototoxicity. However, studies by Van Der Hulst et al[19] and Kennedy et al[23] have shown a significant incidence of hearing loss in carboplatin treated patients. 75% of patients treated with carboplatin had measurable hearing loss in the former study, whereas 20% of patients treated with carboplatin in the latter study had hearing loss. The authors in the latter study stated that no clinically significant hearing loss occurred.[23] On the other hand, cumulative sensorineural hearing loss has been shown in 11/22 children who received carboplatin chemotherapy.[24]

DIURETICS-LOOP DIURETICS

The loop diuretics are a group of potent synthetic drugs which act on the loop of Henly to inhibit the reabsorption of sodium, potassium and chloride ions by a Na-K-2Cl carrier. The ototoxicity of these agents has been reviewed.[25]

Most administered furosemide is excreted in the urine. Furosemide essentially follows a three compartment pharmacokinetic model, with an average half-life for renal elimination of 29½ minutes. Furosemide elimination decreases greatly in patients with advanced renal failure, in whom the half-life can be prolonged 10 to 20 hours. Long half-lives also have been observed in patients with congestive heart failure, especially those undergoing long-term furosemide treatment. The plasma half-life of furosemide is approximately 45–92 minutes in healthy subjects but is prolonged to approximately 3 hours in patients with renal failure. The gastrointestinal uptake of furosemide is high; most authors have concluded that approximately 65% of an oral dose of furosemide is absorbed. Plasma levels exceeding 50 mg/L frequently are associated with hearing disturbances.[25]

Although the usage of ethacrynic acid is very low currently, occasionally it is used in patients allergic to furosemide or refractory to its diuretic effect.

A study by Arnold et al[26] revealed some morphologic effects in the temporal bones from a patient who had received a total of 5000 mg of furosemide plus 250 mg of ethacrynic acid over 5 days before dying of renal failure. The inner and outer hair cells were normal at both the light and electron-microscopic levels, but the stria vascularis had marked cystic changes, as has been reported in animal studies. The dark cell areas of the vestibular system also were found to have marked cystic changes, with dilation of the intracellular fluid spaces, suggesting effects on fluid transport within the inner ear.

Tuzel[27] summarized the reported incidence of hearing loss, as documented by pure-tone audiometry in 179 patients treated with bumetanide and 62 patients receiving furosemide. Among patients receiving bumetanide, only 2 (1.1%) had audiometric changes of 15% dB or greater. Patients treated with furosemide had a 6.4% incidence of hearing loss. Tuzel did not report whether these hearing losses were temporary or permanent. Although most cases of loop-diuretic ototoxicity are temporary and fully reversible, some appear to be permanent. New loop diuretics are being developed and tested in animals, and some may prove to be even less ototoxic than bumetanide when clinical trials are performed.

A recent report of permanent, profound middle and high frequency sensorineural hearing loss in a transplant patient receiving ethacrynic acid illustrates that deafness from loop diuretics continues to be a problem which is clinically significant.[28] Permanent hearing loss has been reported in high risk premature neonates treated with furosemide.[29]

SALICYLATES

Pharmacokinetics and Biochemistry

Orally administered salicylates are absorbed very rapidly in the gastrointestinal tract, with an apparent half-life of 6 to 15 minutes. Absorption of salicylates is influenced significantly by gastric emptying time and by the presence of food in the stomach; food may more than double the absorption half-life of aspirin. Aspirin is broken down in the body to salicylic acid, with a biologic half-life of 15 to 20 minutes.[30] Salicylates are distributed mainly to the extracellular water compartments.[31] Concentrations of the salicylates are higher in the liver and kidney than in the serum, whereas brain concentrations are usually about 10% of those in the serum. Salicylates are excreted mainly in the urine.

Salicylate concentrations of 20–50 mg/dl in serum have been associated with hearing losses of up to 30 dB.[32] Human volunteers receiving aspirin at various doses experienced hearing loss and tinnitus at relatively low concentrations of total plasma salicylate. A linear relationship between hearing loss and unbound salicylate concentrations was reported.[33] Hearing loss can be observed at salicylate concentrations below 20 mg/dl, and there seems to be no threshold for salicylate-induced hearing loss. Severity of tinnitus increases as plasma salicylate concentrations exceed 40 mg/L.

No significant cellular alterations were found at the light-microscopic level beyond those attributed to the age of the patients in temporal bone studies.[34] Although the site-of-lesion testing of the auditory system in patients suffering from salicylate-induced hearing loss strongly suggests a cochlear pattern, histopathologic studies as yet have not pinpointed which cells are altered. These apparent inconsistencies, however, corroborate the typical clinical phenomenon of reversibility of the hearing loss, thus making it likely that salicylates have some temporary metabolic effect that is not severe enough to kill sensory receptor cells or neurons.

QUININE

Features of quinine ototoxicity have been recently reviewed by Jung et al.[35] Deafness, vertigo, tinnitus, headache, nausea and visual loss are symptoms of quinine intoxication. Prolonged daily doses of 200–300mg can result in sensorineural hearing loss in as many as 20% of patients. The hearing loss is frequently bilateral and symmetrical, but reversible. Usually, the high frequencies are affected first. High frequency audiometry has been advocated to monitor ototoxicity, because patients presenting with hearing loss in the speech frequencies may have permanent loss of hearing.

Human volunteers receiving quinine were found to have hearing impairment which correlated with the plasma concentration. Most frequently, when plasma drug concentration exceeded 15 micromol/L a subjective hearing loss or tinnitus occurred, but when drug levels were less than 5 micromol/L, there were no symptoms.[36] Chloroquine is used as an antimalarial drug and also to treat arthritis. Large doses may lead to permanent deafness.[37]

DEFEROXAMINE

The ototoxicity of deferoxamine has been recently reviewed by Kanno et al.[38] Deferoxamine mesylate (desferrioxamine:DFO) is a naturally occurring substance—a metabolite of Streptomyces pilosus—which forms a stable chelate with ferric iron. DFO was introduced as an iron-chelating agent in 1962. Since then, DFO has been used for the iron-overloaded patients, who need to receive multiple blood transfusions due to severe anemia such as thalassemia major, thalassemia intermedia or Diamond-Blackfan anemia. The cause is that iron-overload, especially iron deposition in the myocardium, has become the main cause of death in these patients although multiple transfusions have dramatically improved the prognosis, compared to no treatment. Over the years, DFO has remained the most efficient iron-chelating agent available, and recommendations for more intensive, high-dose administration have generally been accepted because it has been regarded as having minimal adverse effects.

In the 1980s, many authors have reported ototoxicity and ocular toxicity induced by DFO. In 1981, Marsh et al[39] reported reversible tinnitus in a woman with thalassemia intermedia. She developed tinnitus in clear association with chelation therapy with DFO. The cessation of the symptoms when DFO was stopped, and their return after further DFO therapy, strongly suggested a drug-related effect, although there was no evidence of hearing loss detected by audiometric testing. The number of reports associated with DFO ototoxicity has increased since a clinical comprehensive report by Olivieri et al in 1986.[40] They performed pure-tone audiometry or conditioned-play audiometry in 89 patients receiving DFO, of whom high-frequency sensorineural hearing loss (SNHL) was found in 22 patients. Of the patients with SNHL, 13 were symptomatic and 9 were asymptomatic. Clinical deafness developed acutely in four patients. Three patients regained normal hearing after drug administration was stopped, and one had partial improvement. The other patients had no recovery. In 1987, Gallant et al[41] reported a detailed series of the auditory thresholds of those patients which Olivieri et al[40] had reported. They showed that the changes of hearing threshold was highly related to receiving or not receiving varying doses of DFO. Guerin et al[42] described reversible acute SNHL in a patient receiving intravenous DFO treatment. In contrast, Orton et al[43] reported two younger sisters suffering permanent SNHL requiring hearing aids. Barratt and Toogood[44] reported audiograms in DFO-receiving patients with SNHL developing. Of nine patients with SNHL, six patients had high-frequency loss. The SNHL in three patients was predominantly unilateral. Albera et al[45] divided DFO-receiving patients into four groups based upon the degree of hearing loss and analyzed pure-tone

average results statistically. Papers by several authors showed that there was a uniform trend in the audiograms of patients treated with DFO characterized by a progressive sensorineural hearing loss at the higher frequencies. In the most affected group, the monthly DFO amount in relation to body weight, the actual DFO dose and the peak DFO dose were higher in the other groups. Positive recruitment results were found in all subjects of the most affected group. The SNHL of DFO ototoxicity can be divided into three different patterns: 1) asymptomatic hearing loss with audiogram showing high-tone hearing loss, which is similar to the loss found in occupational deafness, 2) low-tone loss, 3) severe hearing loss most pronounced at high frequencies. In order to give a therapeutic guideline for safe DFO administration, authors have described a therapeutic index (TI) which was indicated as the rate of mean daily dose DFO divided by serum ferritin level. They stated that if TI was less than 0.025, the incidence of DFO ototoxicity was reduced, and vice versa. SISI tests and auditory brainstem responses (ABR) results strongly suggest that the SNHL of DFO ototoxicity is of cochlear origin.

The incidence of DFO ototoxicity has varied from 3.8 to 57%. The majority of the SNHL was occurring at high frequencies similar to other ototoxic drugs such as aminoglycosides or cisplatin. The audiometric threshold in patients with severe SNHL exceeded 50 dB at all frequencies, indicating a 'flat' type of loss. The DFO-induced SNHL is, in most cases, accompanied by positive recruitment, not showing any abnormality by ABR tests. Consequently, the results suggest that the ototoxicity is of cochlear rather than of retrocochlear origin. Thus, it remains still controversial where DFO can act in the auditory pathway. The SNHL sometimes showed gradual development without any symptoms, and sometimes occurs acutely or suddenly. The SNHL in some patients recovered completely or improved within several weeks after cessation or withdrawal of the medication, but the other patients had no recovery of hearing and eventually needed hearing aids. It seems likely that the ototoxicity developed more and more severely if the earliest changes in cochlear function occurred at higher frequencies where patients would not clearly perceive hearing loss or symptoms. Therefore, periodic audiometric testing is important to detect early impairment of hearing due to DFO. Reversibility of the SNHL does not always appear to depend on the degree of initial SNHL.

Several investigators have postulated that risk factors for DFO ototoxicity were the following:

1. Younger patients
2. Higher dosage of the drug
3. Lower serum ferritin level
4. Peak DFO dose and monthly DFO amount
5. Better compliance with chelation therapy

The routes of drug administration or DFO concentration in serum may contribute to the sudden onset of SNHL if the ototoxicity is due to a direct effect of DFO on the cochlea. Moreover, although patients with hemodialysis sometimes receive DFO therapy, renal function in the patients is probably related to pathogenesis of DFO ototoxicity. In contrast, authors have described that total cumulative dose of DFO, chronic hypoxia originating from severe anemia and the presence of DFO ocular toxicity may not be considered as risk factors for DFO ototoxicity.

TOXIC SUBSTANCES

A recent paper reviewed the ototoxic effects of environmental chemicals.[46]

Various heavy metals have been associated with ototoxicity; arsenic, mercury, tin, lead, and manganese.

Persons living near a coal burning power plant were exposed to arsenic in the emitted smoke. They were found to have significant low-frequency sensorineural hearing losses.[47]

Mercury poisoning can result in hearing loss, ataxia, weakness and visual and sensory changes. Minimata disease is a syndrome of neurologic sequelae resulting from mercury poisoning. Up to 80% of patients with Minimata disease suffer from hearing loss. In the early and middle stages of the disease, cochlear lesions may be found. Hearing loss in the late stage may result from retrocochlear damage.

Organotin compounds have been ototoxic in animal studies. Leake-Jones and Rebscher[49] reported that a tin-containing catalyst (stannous octoate) used in curing the silicone rubber carrier for a cochlear implant, caused severe inflammation in the cochlea of cats implanted with this device, which would be likely to interfere with its function.

Occupational lead exposure has been reported to cause vertigo and sensorineural deafness. The hearing loss was greater at the higher frequencies, and the severity of hearing loss was proportional to the duration of exposure. Evaluation of children exposed to lead has resulted in interesting data. Blood lead levels were significantly related to delays in the age when children were able to sit up, to walk, and to develop speech, and the probability of hyperactivity. Children with higher blood lead levels had elevated hearing thresholds.[51]

Workers exposed to manganese have been reported to show low and high frequency sensorineural hearing loss, with preservation of middle-frequency thresholds.[52]

Various organic solvents have been associated with hearing loss. These include trichloroethylene, styrene, hexane, carbon disulfide and toluene.

Hearing loss and vestibular impairment have been attributed to trichloroethylene exposure. Exposed workers developing ototoxicity have bilaterally symmetrical sensorineural hearing loss in the higher frequencies, beginning at 2 or 3 kHz.[46]

Workers exposed to styrene may show abnormalities in central auditory tests. Hexane also appears to be neurotoxic. Workers chemically exposed to hexane have been found to have prolonged Wave V latency and Waves I-V interpeak latency on ABR testing.

Sensorineural hearing loss has been reported in workers exposed to carbon disulfide in the viscose rayon industry. The high frequencies appear to be affected most. The incidence and severity of hearing loss appears to increase over time.

Hearing loss has been reported in patients who sniff glue and in patients who are occupationally exposed to toluene. Noise exposure appears to increase the hearing loss associated with toluene exposure.

Toxic gases can also cause hearing loss. Carbon monoxide exposure has been associated with sensorineural hearing loss. The effects of carbon monoxide may be increased by simultaneous exposure to nitric oxide.

REFERENCES

1. Huang MY, Schacht J: Formation of a cytotoxic metabolite from gentmicin by liver. Biochem Pharmacol 40:R11, 1990.
2. Keene M, et al: Histopathological findings in clinical gentamicin ototoxicity. Arch Otolaryngol 108:65, 1982.
3. Fee WE, Jr.: Aminoglycoside ototoxicity in the human. Laryngoscope 90(Suppl. 24):1, 1980.
4. Smith CR, et al: Double blind comparison of the nephrotoxicity and auditory toxicity of gentamicin and tobramycin. N Engl J Med 302:1106, 1980.
5. Rybak LP, Matz GJ: Auditory and vestibular effects of toxins. In Otolaryngology, Head and Neck Surgery, 2nd Ed. Edited by C. Cummings, et al. St. Louis: Mosby, 1993.
6. Moore RD, Smith CR, Leitman PS: Risk factors for the development of auditory toxicity in patients receiving aminoglycosides. J Infect Dis 149:23, 1984.
7. Lerner SA, et al: Pharmacokinetics of gentamicin in the inner ear perilymph of man. In Aminoglycoside Ototoxicity. Edited by SA Lerner, GJ Matz, JE Hawkins, Jr. Boston: Little Brown & Co., 1981.
8. Prezant TR, Agapian JV, Bohlman C, et al.: Mitochondrial ribosomal RNA mutation associated with both antibiotic-induced and nonsyndromic deafness. Nature Genet 4:289, 1993.
9. Hutchin T, Haworth I, Higashi K, et al.: A molecular basis for human hypersensitivity to aminoglycoside antibiotics. Nucl Acids Res 21:4174, 1993.
10. Gormley PE, Bull JM, LeRoy AF, et al: Kinetics of cis-dichlorodiammineplatinum. Clin Pharmacol Ther 25:351, 1979.
11. Wright CG, Schaefer SD: Inner ear histopathology in patients treated with cisplatinum. Laryngoscope 92:1408, 1982.
12. Strauss M, et al.: Cisplatinum ototoxicity: clinical experience and temporal bone histopathology. Laryngoscope 93:1554, 1983.
13. Moroso MJ, Blair RL: A review of cisplatinum ototoxicity. J Otolaryngol 12:365, 1983.
14. Blakely BW, Gupta AK, Myers SF, et al: Risk factors for ototoxicity due to cisplatin. Arch Otolaryngol 120:541, 1994.

15. Fausti SA, et al: High-frequency monitoring for early detection of cisplatin ototoxicity. Arch Otolaryngol 119:661, 1993.

16. Blakely BW, Myers SF: Pattern of hearing loss resulting from cisplatinum therapy. Otolaryngol Head Neck Surg 109:385, 1993.

17. Kluba J, et al: Zur Uberwachung des Gehors wahrend der oto-toxischen. Cisplatin-Therapie Padiatr Grenzgeb 29:19, 1990.

18. Myers SF, et al: The "plateau effect" of cisplatinum induced hearing loss. Otolaryngol Head Neck Surg 104:122, 1991.

19. Van Der Hulst RFAM, Dreschler WA, Urbanus NAM: High frequency audiometry in prospective clinical research of ototoxicity due to platinum derivatives. Ann Otol Rhinol Laryngol 97:133, 1988.

20. Granowetter L, Rosenstock JG, Packer RJ: Enhanced cisplatinum neurotoxicity in pediatric patients with brain tumors. J Neuro-oncol 1:293, 1983.

21. Laurell G, Jungnelius V: High-dose cisplatin treatment: Hearing loss and plasma concentrations. Laryngoscope 100:724, 1990.

22. Kopelman J, et al.: Ototoxicity of high-dose cisplatin by bolus administration in patients with advanced cancer and normal hearing. Laryngoscope 98:858, 1988.

23. Kennedy ICS, et al: Carboplatin is ototoxic. Cancer Chemother Pharmacol 26:232, 1990.

24. Macdonald MR, et al: Ototoxicity of carboplatin: Comparing animal and clinical models at the The Hospital for Sick Children. J Otolaryngol 23:151, 1994.

25. Rybak LP: Ototoxicity of loop diuretics. Otolaryngol Clin North Am 26:829, 1993.

26. Arnold W, Nadol JB, Jr, Weidauer H: Ultrastructural histopathology in a case of human ototoxicity due to loop diuretics. Acta Otolaryngol (Stockh) 91:339, 1981.

27. Tuzel IJ: Comparison of adverse reactions to bumetanide and furosemide. J Clin Pharmacol 21:615, 1981.

28. Rybak LP: Ototoxicity of ethacrynic acid: (a persistent clinical problem). J Laryngol Otol 102:518, 1988.

29. Brown DR, Watchko JF, Sabo D: Neonatal sensorineural hearing loss associated with furosemide: A case control study. Dev Med Child Neurol 33:816, 1991.

30. Rowland M, Riegelman S: Pharmacokinetics of acetylsalicylic acid and salicylic acid after intravenous administration in man. J Pharm Sci 57:1313, 1968.

31. Hollister L, Levy G: Some aspects of salicylate distribution and metabolism in man. J Pharm Sci 54:1126, 1965.

32. Myers EN, Bernstein JM: Salicylate ototoxicity. Arch Otolaryngol 82:483, 1965.

33. Day RO, et al: Concentration-response relationships for salicylate-induced ototoxicity in normal volunteers. Br J Clin Pharmacol 28:695, 1989.

34. DeMoura LFP, Hayden RC, Jr: Salicylate ototoxicity: a human temporal bone report. Arch Otolaryngol 87:60, 1968.

35. Jung TTK, et al: Ototoxicity of salicylate, nonsteroidal anti-inflammatory drugs and quinine. Otolaryngol Clin North Am 26:791, 1993.

36. Alvan G, Karlsson KK, Hellgren U, et al: Hearing impairment related to plasma quinine concentrations in healthy volunteers. Br J Clin Pharmacol 31:409, 1991.

37. Toone EC, Jr, Hayden GD, Eliman HM: Ototoxicity of chloroquine. Arthritis Rheum 8:475, 1965.

38. Kanno H, Yamanobe S, Rybak LP: The ototoxicity of deferoxamine mesylate. Am J Otolaryngol 1994.

39. Marsh MN, Holbrook IB, Clark C, et al: Tinnitus in a patient with beta-thalassaemia intermedia on long-term treatment with deferrioxamine. Postgrad Med J 57:582–584, 1981.

40. Olivieri NF, Buncic JR, Chew E, et al: Desferal has significant audio-visual neurotoxicity. Annual meeting of American Society of Hematology, Abstr., 1984.

41. Gallant T, Boyden MH, Gallant LA, et al: Serial studies of auditory neurotoxicity in patients receiving deferoxamine therapy. Am J Med 83:1085–90, 1987.

42. Guerin A, London G, Marchais S, et al: Acute deafness and desferrioxamine. Lancet ii:39–40, 1985.

43. Orton RB, deVeber LL, Sulh HMB: Ocular and auditory toxicity of long-term, high-dose subcutaneous deferoxamine therapy. Can J Ophthalmol 20:153–6, 1985.

44. Barratt PS, Toogood IRG: Hearing loss attributed to desferrioxamine in patients with beta-thalassaemia major. Med J Aust 147:177–9, 1987.

45. Albera R, Pia F, Morra B, et al: Hearing loss and desferrioxamine in homozygous beta-thalassemia. Audiology 27:207–14, 1988.

46. Rybak LP: Hearing: The effects of chemicals. Otolaryngol Head Neck Surg 106:677, 1992.

47. Bencko V, Symon K, Chladek V, et al: Health aspects of burning coal with a high arsenic content. II. Hearing changes in exposed children. Environ Res 13:386–95, 1977.

48. Kurland LT, Faro SN, Siedler H: Minamata disease: The outbreak of a neurologic disorder in Minamata, Japan, and its relationship to the ingestion of seafood contaminated by mercuric compounds. World Neurol 1:370–95, 1960.

49. Leake-Jones P, Rebscher S: Cochlear pathology associated with chronically implanted scala tympani electrodes. Ann NY Acad Sci 405:203, 1983.

50. Ciurlo E, Ottoboni A: Variations of the internal ear in chronic lead poisoning. Minerva Otorhinolaryngol 5:130–2, 1955.

51. Schwartz J, Otto D: Blood lead, hearing thresholds, and neurobehavioral development in children and youth. Arch Environ Health 42:153–60, 1987.

52. Nikolov A: Hearing reduction caused by manganese and noise. J Oto-Rhino-Laryngol Audiophonol Chir Maxillofac 23:231–4, 1974.

53. Huang C-C, Chu NS: Evoked potentials in chronic n-hexane intoxication. Clin Electroencephalogr 20:162–8, 1989.

54. Morata TC: Study of the effects of simultaneous exposure to noise and carbon disulfide on workers' hearing. Scand Audiol 18:53–8, 1989.

55. Morata TC, Dunn DE, Kretschmer LW, et al: Effects of simultaneous exposure to noise and toluene on worker's hearing and balance. Proceedings of the Fourth International Conference on the Combined Effects of Environmental Factors. Baltimore: Johns Hopkins University, 81–6, 1991.

56. Groll-Knapp E, Haider M, Kienzl K, et al: Changes in discrimination learning and brain activity (ERPs) due to combined exposure to NO and CO in rats. Toxicology 49:441–7, 1988.

55 Sudden Sensorineural Hearing Loss, Perilymph Fistula, and Autoimmune Inner Ear Disease

Jeffrey P. Harris and Michael J. Ruckenstein

The treatment of sensorineural hearing loss often proves to be frustrating to the clinician as, in the majority of cases, the etiology is unknown and the underlying disease process is irreversible, with no effective therapy available. In these situations, therapy is focused primarily on rehabilitation. There are, however, several forms of sensorineural hearing loss in which the clinical course can be favorably influenced by medical intervention if it is provided in a timely fashion. This chapter focuses on three potentially treatable causes of sensorineural hearing loss—*sudden sensorineural hearing loss, perilymphatic fistula,* and *autoimmune inner ear disease*—and will emphasize practical approaches to their diagnosis and treatment.

SUDDEN SENSORINEURAL HEARING LOSS

Definition

A sensorineural hearing loss of greater than 30 dB in three contiguous frequencies that develops in less than three days is a practical and easily remembered definition of sudden sensorineural hearing loss.[1] The majority of patients with this entity will present a history of onset of hearing loss of considerably less than three days, and some flexibility should be maintained by the clinician with regard to the audiometric criteria.

Epidemiology

The incidence of sudden sensorineural loss has been estimated at one case per 5000–10,000 population per year[2,3] although the true incidence is likely to be higher as patients who experience a rapid spontaneous recovery likely never seek medical attention. This entity affects people of all ages although it more commonly occurs in patients between 30 and 60 years of age.[4] Males and females are evenly affected, and either ear is equally vulnerable.[5,6] The hearing loss is unilateral in approximately 90% of patients.[6]

Etiology

While circumstantial in nature, the bulk of the evidence supports a viral etiology as the cause of the majority of cases of sudden sensorineural hearing loss. Other proposed etiologies include vascular compromise and inner ear membranous rupture. It must be emphasized that these proposed etiologies pertain to idiopathic sensorineural hearing loss. It is imperative that the clinician rule-out known causes of auditory pathology prior to arriving at this diagnosis. The differential diagnosis of a patient with sudden sensorineural hearing loss will be considered below.

Viral Etiology

Sudden sensorineural loss has been documented to occur during cases of mumps, measles, rubella, and influenza, as well as during infection by the adenoviruses and cytomegalovirus (CMV).[2,7–10] Serologic studies of patients with idiopathic sensorineural loss have shown significantly increased titers of antibodies against a variety of viral agents not seen in a control population.[11] Between 25–30% of affected patients report an antecedent history of an upper respiratory infection within one month of onset of the hearing loss.[6] However, the significance of this association is questionable due to the ubiquity of viral upper respiratory infection. A recent study compared the clinical and audiometric characteristics of hearing loss in patients suffering from the viral infection known as Lassa fever to patients manifesting idiopathic sensorineural hearing loss.[12] The similarity of these two entities has been taken as support for a viral cause of idiopathic sudden sensorineural hearing loss.

Histopathologic analyses of temporal bones from patients who suffered from sudden deafness displayed atrophy of the organ of Corti, stria vascularis, and tectorial membrane.[13] These changes are similar to those seen in cases of viral labyrinthitis. Evidence that an inflammatory process results in sudden sensorineural loss has been provided by magnetic resonance imaging (MRI) studies with paramagnetic enhancement which have shown cochlear enhancement in cases on sudden deafness not seen in a control population.[14] Furthermore, the beneficial response of hearing loss to immunosuppressive therapy also provides support for the hypothesis that sudden sensorineural deafness is mediated by an inflammatory process.[15,16]

Vascular Etiology

The evidence to support the hypothesis that vascular compromise is a major cause of sudden deafness is less compelling. It stems from the analogy of sudden deafness and stroke and the known intolerance of the cochlea to ischemia. While vasospasm, thrombosis, embolism, hypercoaguability, and rheologic abnormalities have all been mentioned as potential causes of sudden deafness, the evidence to support this hypothesis is lacking. There have been reports of sudden deafness occurring in patients suffering from systemic diseases known to cause vascular compromise, including sickle cell anemia,[17] Waldenstrom's macroglobulinemia,[18] and systemic vasculitides.[19] In addition, sudden sensorineural loss is seen as a complication of cardiopulmonary bypass surgery, presumably as a result of an embolic phenomenon.[20,21]

While it is likely that, in certain instances, ischemia is the cause of sudden deafness, evidence suggests that it is not responsible for the majority of cases. Epidemiologically, the majority of patients with sudden deafness do not possess significant cardiovascular risk factors. To that extent, there is no conclusive evidence that patients with diabetes mellitus, a disease that is characterized by small vessel pathology, have an increased incidence of sudden sensorineural hearing loss. Experimental studies have shown that the ganglion cells are the most sensitive to ischemia, while the pathologic data presented above indicates that the organ of Corti, stria vascularis, and tectorial membrane are the predominant structures affected in cases of sudden sensorineural hearing loss.[22] Nadol and Wilson have commented that the most distal, and hence most susceptible portion of the cochlear blood supply feeds the apical turn.[23] Thus, if vascular compromise was a major etiologic factor in sudden hearing loss, one would expect the low frequencies to be the most severely and frequently affected. As will be described below, this is not the case. Lastly, no therapeutic regimen designed to enhance or augment vascular supply to the cochlea has been proven to have therapeutic value in the treatment of sudden deafness (see below). This is in contrast to the proven value of corticosteroid administration.

Rupture of the Labyrinthine Membranes

This potential cause of sudden sensorineural hearing loss will be addressed in separate section below on perilymphatic fistula.

Differential Diagnosis

As mentioned, it is imperative that the clinician expediently initiate the search for identifiable causes of sudden deafness. However, due to a narrow window of treatment opportunity, empirical therapy must be instituted prior to obtaining the results of various serological and radiological studies.

Congenital

Patients with Mondini deformity or enlarged vestibular aqueduct syndrome may present with sudden exacerbations of hearing loss.[24] These diagnoses should be considered in patients who present in their first to third decade of life with sudden deterioration in hearing. Evaluation is best performed with a high resolution CT scan of the temporal bone. If such a deformity is identified, most authorities would recommend the avoidance of potentially traumatic activities such as contact sports as sudden increases in CSF pressure could be directly transmitted into the inner ear with subsequent damage. There is no known benefit from any form of surgical intervention at the present time.

Infection

As discussed above, viral infection is thought to cause the majority of cases of "idiopathic" sudden deafness. There are, however, specific syndromes associated with particular infectious agents that should be identified. **Ramsey-Hunt syndrome,** caused by recrudescence of a Herpes Zoster infection, consists of painful herpetic eruption involving the auricle and canal, facial nerve paralysis, and hearing loss. The administration of oral acyclovir at the time of diagnosis is currently recommended as treatment for this disorder.

Lyme disease, caused by the tick-borne spirochete Borrelia burgdorferi, has been associated with a variety of cranial neuropathies including bilateral facial nerve paralysis and hearing loss. Similarly, **Syphilis** has long been known to affect the auditory system, either as part of a more diffuse syphilitic meningoneurolabyrinthitis or with symptoms of progressive auditory and vestibular dysfunction almost identical to that seen in Meniere's disease.[26] **Bacterial meningitis** is another well known cause of sudden deafness occurring either during the fulminant stages of infection or during the recuperative phase of the illness.

A considerable amount of information is accumulating concerning the affects of **HIV** infection on the auditory system.[27] In general Acquired Immunodeficiency Syndrome may result in hearing loss via direct neuropathic effects of the HIV virus, by opportunistic infection (e.g. bacterial or fungal meningitis, neurotropic viral infection such as cytomegalovirus) or via syphilitic infection, which has a much higher incidence in this patient population.

Neoplasm

In their extensive review, Shaia and Sheehy reported that approximately one percent of patients with sudden sensorineural deafness were found to have a vestibular schwannoma (acoustic neurinoma).[6] In addition, 15 percent of patients with vestibular schwannomas presented with sudden deafness.[28] These statistics may well change given MRI capacity to detect small tumors. Recovery in apparent response to corticosteroids does not rule out the presence of an VIIIth nerve tumor as a recent report has documented fluctuating, corticosteroid responsive hearing loss in the presence of an acoustic neurinoma.[29] Thus, it is imperative that all patients with asymmetric hearing loss undergo a work-up for retrocochlear pathology. Other benign lesions of the cerebellopontine angle (CPA) such as meningiomas, as well as primary or metastatic malignant lesions, may present with sudden deafness.

Trauma

Both acoustic and external temporal bone trauma are well recognized causes of sudden deafness. It is thus important to question the patient with regard to possible noise exposure, head trauma, and barotrauma (such as noseblowing, rapid painful descent in an airplane, or scuba diving).

Ototoxicity

A history of exposure to ototoxins (e.g. aminoglycosides, erthromycin, vancomycin, loop diuretics, cisplatin, nonsteroidal antinflammatories) should be sought.

Neurologic Disorders

While both multiple sclerosis and basilar migraines more commonly present with vertigo, they are also associated with hearing loss. Similarly strokes involving the anteroinferior cerebellar artery circulation (lateral pontomedullary syndrome) are associated with sudden hearing loss. These neurologic disorders present with a constellation of neurologic symptoms and their diagnosis should be considered in the appropriate clinical setting.[30]

Psychogenic

If the physician does not suspect a diagnosis of pseudohypocusis, he or she will likely miss it. This presentation is seen in the malingering population who are claiming to suffer from a hearing loss in order to derive some secondary gain and in patients undergoing a conversion reaction. This latter diagnosis is more common in the adolescent population.

Clinical Presentation

The majority of patients with sudden deafness either awake with the hearing loss or can pinpoint the exact time of onset.[31] Occasionally unilateral losses may go unrecognized by the patient until he or she is called upon to use the affected ear (e.g. using the telephone). Tinnitus is present in the majority of patients and may be the most distressing symptom. Vertigo is present in approximately 40% of cases and is usually transient and mild.[6] The presence of vertigo, however, carries with it a poorer prognosis for recovery.[1] A history of a viral prodrome may be present although the significance of this finding is questionable. It should also be remembered that the initial attack of Meniere's disease may present as sudden deafness. Clinical follow-up of these patients will document the emergence of the typical syndrome of Meniere's disease and allow for the correct diagnosis.

Investigations

Audiologic Investigations

A comprehensive audiologic assessment, including pure-tone thresholds, speech audiometry, and acoustic reflexes, is the cornerstone of the patient work-up. Sheehy has classified this patient population into four groups based on audiometric findings including a flat-type hearing loss (41%) high-tone loss (29%), low-tone loss (17%) and total loss (13%).[32] As mentioned above, a work-up to rule-out retrocochlear disease is required in any patient who manifests asymmetric persistent or progressive hearing loss. Thus, an ABR is required in any patient who does not completely recover their hearing loss or in whom hearing loss is recurrent, provided that the hearing loss is not so severe as to invalidate the results of this test. In such cases, an MRI should be obtained. Evoked potential audiometry is also indicated in cases of suspected pseudohypocusis.

Electronystagmography (ENG)

While the presence of abnormalities on ENG does have prognostic significance (see below), there seems to be little value in obtaining ENG evaluation during the acute phase of illness. Should residual vestibular dysfunction be present after stabilization of the patient's condition, ENG evaluation should be obtained.

Imaging Studies

As mentioned, a high resolution CT scan is indicated when a diagnosis of a congenital malformation of the temporal bone is being considered. Current standard of practice would dictate that an MRI with paramagnetic enhancement (Gadolinium) is required in patients with an abnormal ABR or in whom the hearing loss is so severe that an ABR would not be reliable. While MRI scans have provided some evidence that sudden deafness may arise from an inflammatory process (enhancement within the labyrinth), their routine use purely to document this event would not be cost effective.

Hematology, Biochemistry, and Serology

A CBC may provide evidence of an ongoing inflammatory process or occult hematologic malignancy. Similarly, an abnormal erythrocyte sedimentation rate may indicate the presence of ongoing inflammatory or autoimmune processes, and could lead to the performance of other diagnostic tests directed at uncovering these conditions. Serologic testing for syphilis should be employed almost routinely, as the incidence of syphilis in the population is increasing. An FTA-ABS is more sensitive than a VDRL in detecting late secondary or early tertiary syphilis. Lyme titers should be obtained in endemic areas. HIV serology should be obtained in those patients that are epidemiologically or clinically at risk. Serum cholesterol, lipid profiles, and blood sugar have been advocated in the past as part of a diagnostic work-up for sudden deafness. However, given that hypercholesterolemia has never been convincingly demonstrated to cause hearing loss, the routine use of this test can no longer be advocated. Similarly, given the virtual elimination of endemic goiter in North America, thyroid function tests are indicated only in a patient with signs of myxedema in whom a hearing loss has been demonstrated or in the pediatric population where Pendred's Disease would be diagnosed.

Treatment

The only therapy that has proven to be effective in the treatment of sudden sensorineural hearing loss is the administration of corticosteroids as soon after the onset of symptoms as possible.[15,16] Based on their studies, Laird and Wilson have demonstrated that corticosteroid responsiveness is more likely to be present in patients with a hearing loss of between 40–80 dB. Hearing losses beyond this range are significantly less likely to recover. Prednisone should be administered in the adult beginning at a dose of 60–80 mg and tapering over a several week course. Recurrence of symptoms after the taper is completed requires the resumption

of prednisone therapy at a dose of 40mg/day to continue for one month and the institution of a work-up for autoimmune inner ear disease (see below).

A variety of agents designed to improve cochlear circulation and oxygenation have been advocated as treatments for sudden deafness. These include carbogen gas inhalation, vasodilators, anticoagulants, antiplatelet agents, and plasma expanders. Despite their persistent popularity in certain centers, none of these agents have ever been shown to improve hearing beyond the known spontaneous recovery rate. A recent double-blind, placebo-controlled study evaluating the combination of Dextran and pentoxifylline failed to show any benefit from these drugs in patients with sudden deafness.[33] It is important to note that this study derived its population number by performing a power study, thus ensuring that an adequate number of patients were entered in the trial. These results are not surprising given the lack of evidence supporting the hypothesis that vascular compromise is a major etiologic factor in sudden deafness, as outlined above.

Prognosis

Several factors have been identified that influence patient prognosis.[34] Older patients are less likely to recover spontaneously. The presence of vertigo and/or ENG abnormalities also carry a worse prognosis. Severe to profound hearing losses were less likely to exhibit recovery, as were high-frequency losses. Flat and low- or mid-frequency losses displayed a better prognosis. The rapidity with which corticosteroid administration is initiated is also felt to be important in improving the chances of recovery.

PERILYMPH FISTULA

Definition

The maintenance of normal inner-ear function depends on the physical and electrochemical separation of the fluids in the endolymphatic and perilymphatic spaces from each other and the external environment. Abnormal communication of the perilymph with the middle-ear space results in inner-ear dysfunction and is known as a *perilymphatic fistula*. Considerable controversy surrounds this diagnosis, however, based on available data, a rational approach to management has evolved.

Epidemiology

Given the lack of definitive diagnostic criteria, it is impossible to estimate accurately the true incidence of perilymphatic fistulae. The consensus amongst otologists is that it represents a relatively rare entity.[35]

Etiology

Perilymphatic fistulae may arise via three basic mechanisms. Congenital dehiscences in the otic capsule or its associated membranes have been well documented in children. These more commonly occur in association with other abnormalities of the temporal bone (e.g. Mondini's dysplasia) or cranial skeleton (craniodysostoses), and the majority have been associated with middle-ear abnormalities which most commonly affect the stapes or round window.[36] A second group of patients report symptoms subsequent to experiencing external trauma to the ear or temporal bone. Trauma may be iatrogenic (e.g. stapes surgery) or as a result of blunt or sharp temporal bone trauma. Acoustic trauma and barotrauma have also been postulated to result in hearing dysfunction as a result of the transmission of rapid pressure changes to the round or oval windows via the middle ear (so called "implosive trauma"). However, in these latter conditions, hearing loss is more likely to result from intrinsic damage to inner-ear structures rather than perilymphatic fistulae.

More controversial are the fistulae referred to as "spontaneous." These have been postulated to be caused by increased intracranial pressure being transmitted to the labyrinth via the cochlear aqueduct or internal auditory canal (so called "explosive trauma"). Thus, it has been hypothesized that physical exertion such as straining, lifting, coughing, or sneezing can cause inner dysfunction.[37] Kohut has provided some evidence that ruptures may occur in the fissula ante fenestram, between the posterior semicircular canal and round window membrane, and through Hyrtl's fissure.[38] Alternatively, Simmons has postulated that rather than occurring between the perilymphatic spaces and the middle ear, intralabyrinthine ruptures may occur causing perilymphatic and endolymphatic mixture and inner ear dysfunction.[39] Data supporting the hypothesis of the spontaneous perilymphatic fistula have been challenged. Demonstration of increased intracranial pressure being transmitted to the labyrinth via the cochlear aqueduct were obtained in a cat model, an animal that possesses a wide and patent cochlear aqueduct.[40] In the human, the cochlear aqueduct is narrow and most often occluded by fibrous tissue. Furthermore, the round window of the human is much thicker and more resistant to rupture than that found in most animal models. In addition, the validity of the data described above indicating potential sites of fistula in the otic capsule has been challenged.[41] As will be described below, significant reservations also exist regarding the clinical data supporting the existence of the spontaneous perilymphatic fistula.

Clinical Presentation

Due to the lack of a definitive method of confirming the diagnosis of perilymphatic fistula, a wide gamut of symptomatology has been attributed to this pathology. Based on currently available data, a sudden sensorineural hearing loss, accompanied by tinnitus and vertigo that occurred immediately subsequent to an identifiable traumatic event would be suggestive of a diagnosis of perilymphatic fistula. Hearing loss may fluctuate; however, to support a diagnosis of perilymphatic fistula, such changes should occur in response to identifiable precipitating factors (e.g. pressure fluctuations, straining). Vertigo may be a prominent symptom. These represent conservative diagnostic criteria based on the lack of availability of a definitive diagnostic test. Some authors are more liberal in terms of the criteria they use to justify middle-ear exploration.[42,43] However, given our current inability to confirm the presence of a fistula, most otologists currently support a conservative approach to diagnosis.[35,41,44]

Diagnostic Evaluation

The Achilles' heel of perilymphatic fistula management is the lack of an objective, reproducible, and accurate method of diagnosis. For many years diagnosis was predicated on the direct observation of fluid accumulating in the region of oval or round windows on middle-ear exploration. However, this method of diagnosis has been recognized as being notoriously inaccurate, given the subjective nature of observational data and the propensity for a variety of fluids (e.g. injection, blood) to accumulate at the time of surgery.

The fistula test is the most well recognized clinical test utilized in the preoperative diagnostic evaluation. A pneumatic otoscope is used to obtain a firm seal on the external canal, and then positive pressure is applied to the tympanic membrane via the pneumatic attachment. A test is considered positive if vertigo and nystagmus are provoked by this maneuver. A positive fistula test may also be seen in cases of Meniere's disease and syphilis (Hennebert's sign). Some authorities consider the accuracy of the test to be improved if it is performed in conjunction with ENG evaluation or posturography, although others find this latter test to be unhelpful.[45] There are no specific findings on audiometric or vestibular testing associated with perilymphatic fistula. Electrocochleography (ECOG) may reveal an elevated SP/AP ratio. However, this test is nonspecific, and without a gold standard for diagnosis, it is difficult to interpret the meaning of these data particularly as the symptoms closely resemble atypical Meniere's disease in which ECOG findings are also common.[46]

Recent efforts have focused on the development of an intraoperative test that will confirm the presence of perilymphatic fluid. Intravenous fluorercein has been one method that has been proposed. However, animal experiments have failed to validate this technique.[47]

Intrathecal fluorescein has been shown to enter the perilymph, however, despite its popularity in the detection of CSF leaks, it has not become established as a method of detection of perilymph fistulae.[48] More promising are recent results pertaining to the detection of β2-Transferrin, a protein unique to cerebrospinal fluid and aqueous humor, in children with suspected perilymphatic fistulae.[49] The main disadvantage of this assay is that the results cannot be provided immediately at the time of exploration.

Radiologic studies, specifically a high resolution CT scan of the temporal bone, are indicated in cases of temporal bone trauma and in children in order to rule-out the presence of a congenital malformation.

Treatment

Most authorities agree that the initial management of a potential perilymphatic fistula should include bed rest, head elevation, and avoidance of straining or Valsalva for five to ten days. Should symptoms persist or progress, a middle-ear exploration under local anesthesia is advocated so that better hemostasis is achieved compared to general anesthesia. Meticulous attention should be paid to prevent blood or infiltration solution from entering the middle ear. The middle-ear contents should be observed for fluid accumulation in the region of the oval or round windows, with any fluid detected being absorbed in gelfoam pledgets and examined for fluorescein if intrathecal injection was employed or sent for β2-Transferrin assay (if available). Intraoperative Valsalva may aid in the promotion of fluid accumulation. Both the oval and round windows should be carefully examined, and if a fistula is detected, should be repaired with loose areolar tissue, fat, perichondrium, or muscle after the region is scarified. The use of fibrin glue to augment the repair is useful. Caution with regard to packing the oval window is required as inadvertent conductive hearing loss can develop. Therefore, the senior author only patches the oval window when definite pathology is seen.

Prognosis

Rizer and House, utilizing strict criteria for exploration, reported a 40% improvement in symptoms of vertigo and an approximately 20% improvement in audiometric data in patients undergoing perilymphatic fistula repair.[44] Importantly, patient history, findings on physical examination and audiometric and ENG results could not be correlated with successful surgical results as defined as intraoperative observation of a fistula and postoperative improvement of hearing loss and vertigo. The observation of a fistula at the time of exploration was a predictor of benefit from operation.

AUTOIMMUNE INNER EAR DISEASE

Definition

Defence against invading microorganisms is the prevalent concept explaining the evolution and need for the immune system. This system must possess the capacity to respond to potential environmental pathogens and must, therefore, maintain mechanisms that allow it to distinguish between foreign constituents and the host's own tissue. An autoimmune reaction ensues when the immune system's ability to distinguish between "self" and "nonself" is disturbed.

Autoimmune inner ear disease may occur as part of a symptom complex of multisystemic, organ-nonspecific autoimmune disease (e.g. Rheumatoid Arthritis, Wegener's granulomatosis) or as an organ-specific process, in which case it is referred to as primary autoimmune inner ear disease.

Epidemiology

With the exception of Cogan's syndrome, auditory and vestibular dysfunction is a well documented but rare complication of multisystemic, organ-nonspecific autoimmune disorders including rheumatoid arthritis, Wegener's granulomatosis, systemic lupus erythematosus (SLE), and vasculitides (see below). Due to the lack of a definitive diagnostic test for autoimmune inner ear disease, the precise incidence of this disorder cannot be estimated. Approximately 65% of the cases of this disorder afflict middle-aged women, a finding that is in keeping with the known predisposition of this autoimmune disorder.[50]

Etiology and Pathogenesis

In general, a variety of factors have been implicated in the origin of these diseases including a genetic predisposition, the presence of autoreactive CD4 (+)ve T helper (TH) cells and autoreactive B cells, and an initiating event such as a viral infection. It is hypothesized that an injurious event (trauma, viral or bacterial infection) may initiate the process by either exposing native antigens to the immune system, or by producing viral antigens that resemble host antigens and thus incite an immune response against both the virus and host tissue (molecular mimicry hypothesis).[51] The ensuing autoimmune reaction is then orchestrated by the autoreactive TH cell which is integral and essential promotor of any immune reaction. These cells may activate, or help to activate, a variety of immune effector mechanisms via the release of cytokines including autoantibody production (humoral arm) and/or a cellular response [autoreactive CD8 (+ve) cytotoxic T cells, Null Killer cells and macrophages].

Clinical Presentation

Organ-specific Autoimmune Inner Ear Disease

In 1979, McCabe reported on a group of patients with bilateral, asymmetric hearing loss that had been progressing from weeks to months.[52] Vestibular dysfunction was present in some of these patients, however, and manifestations were variable. McCabe hypothesized that these patients suffered from an autoimmune form of inner-ear dysfunction, and treated the patients with immunosuppressive therapy. Subsequent reports have confirmed this picture of rapidly progressive sensorineural hearing loss, which is asymmetric and bilateral in 80% of patients.[50,53] It is important to emphasize that hearing loss may fluctuate and that this, coupled with the presence of vestibular symptoms in 25–50% of the population, may initially suggest a diagnosis of Meniere's disease. The more aggressive course of autoimmune inner ear disease and the higher incidence of bilaterality early in the course of disease should alert the clinician to the possibility of autoimmunity. In fulminant cases, a serous otitis or mental confusion may be present initially which may serve to confound the diagnosis and lead to a delay in definitive treatment. Due to the slow progressive loss in bilateral vestibular function, the rare patient will present with ataxia typical of that seen in Dandy's syndrome. Multisystemic autoimmune abnormalities may be detected in up to 30% of patients.[50]

Multisystemic, Organ-nonspecific Autoimmune Disease

A variety of these disorders may result in audiovestibular dysfunction and will be discussed below.

Cogan's Syndrome

Cogan's syndrome represents the classic autoimmune disorder leading to inner-ear dysfunction[54,55] consisting of nonsyphilitic interstitial keratitis accompanied by vertigo, tinnitus, and hearing loss. Inner-ear dysfunction may be coincident with the ocular manifestations or occur up to six months before or after the onset of eye pathology. Other ocular abnormalities may occur, including episcleritis, uveitis, or conjunctivitis, in which case the disease is classified as atypical Cogan's syndrome. Progression of the disease occurs over several months.

Temporal bone histopathology in cases of Cogan's syndrome consists of plasma cell and lymphocytic infiltration of the spiral ligament, saccular rupture, degeneration of the stria vascularis, spiral ganglion cells and organ of Corti, osteoneogenesis of the round window, and endolymphatic hydrops.[56,57] The pathogenesis of the disease is unclear and may represent either a hypersensitivity response to infection with associated vasculitis or an organ-specific autoimmune reaction against an antigen with epitopes that are shared by the eye and inner ear, however, such antigens have yet to be identified.

Vogt-Koyanagi-Harada syndrome is similar to Cogan's syndrome and consists of hearing loss, vertigo, granulomatis uveitis, depigmentation of the hair and skin around the eyes, loss of eyelashes, and aseptic meningitis. It is felt to be an autoimmune reaction directed against melanin containing cells.

Other Autoimmune Diseases

Wegener's granulomatosis has been reported to cause serous otitis media in approximately 20% of cases and sensorineural hearing loss in less than 10% of patients.[58] Polyarteritis nodosa as well as other vasculitides may also affect the inner-ear circulation resulting in secondary damage to the vestibuloauditory apparatus.[59] Rheumatoid arthritis may occasionally affect the middle and inner ears and SLE may rarely cause chronic otitis media and inner-ear dysfunction secondary to vasculitis.[60] Ulcerative colitis, a presumed autoimmune disorder, may also cause a corticosteroid-responsive hearing loss.[61]

Diagnostic Evaluation

In patients with suspected autoimmune deafness, an appropriate review of systems would include questions concerning recurrent or chronic ocular disorders, chronic dermatitis, pneumonitis, pleuritis, cardiomyopathy, symptoms of inflammatory bowel disease, nephritis, and arthritis. In addition an immune profile consisting of a CBC with sedimentation rate, FTA-ABS, antinuclear antibody and rheumatoid factor, C1q-binding, Raji cell assay, cryoglobulins, and urinalysis has proven useful. If the review of systems or two or more of these blood tests are positive, then a diagnosis of autoimmune inner ear disease can be considered.

Considerable effort has been expended in developing a diagnostic test that is both sensitive and specific for autoimmune inner ear disease.[62] Research has focused on tests of cellular and humoral immunity directed against inner-ear constituents.

Tests of Cellular Immunity

McCabe originally advocated the lymphocyte migration inhibition assay in his diagnostic work-up.[52] However, it was never satisfactorily proven to be an accurate assay for this entity. Hughes has focused attention on the lymphocyte transformation test as a measure of organ-specific autoimmunity which measures the reaction of patient's own lymphocytes to crude inner ear antigen.[62] Unfortunately, controls for nonspecific reaction against human leukocyte antigens (HLA) have never been adequately documented. Furthermore, the stimulation elicited in patients with a known autoimmune inner ear disorder—Cogan's syndrome—is minimal.

Tests of Autoantibody Production

Immunofluorescence labeling of cadaveric temporal bones incubated with sera from patients suspected to have autoimmune inner ear disease has been advocated in several reports.[63–65] While a high degree of binding has been shown, the data must be interpreted with caution. Controls for binding against HLA were not adequately documented. Similarly degradation and alteration of cadaveric temporal bones subsequent to fixation can also significantly influence results. Lastly, the correlation of positive immunofluorescence microscopy with clinical response to immunosuppression has not been well correlated.

Western blot analysis is an immunologic technique utilized to detect antibodies directed against antigens of a particular molecular weight. In 1990, Harris and Sharp reported that 35% of patients with rapidly progressive sensorineural hearing loss possessed an antibody directed against a 68 kiloDalton (kD) antigen derived from bovine inner ear tissue that was also present in animals with experimental autoimmune inner ear disease.[66] Analysis has now been extended to 279 patients with rapidly progressive sensorineural hearing loss in whom 32% displayed this anti-68kD antibody on Western blot analysis. Only 5–8% of control patients manifested the same antibody, a difference that is both statistically and clinically significant.[67] Efforts are now being directed at defining this antigen and further refining this test.[68]

Treatment

Patients in whom a diagnostic work-up suggest an autoimmune etiology for their progressive inner ear dysfunction are treated initially with prednisone (60–80mg/day) for one month. If a clinical response is documented, treatment is continued for one to two more months with the corticosteroids then being gradually tapered. Recurrence necessitates the re-introduction of higher dose treatment. Given the complications of long-term corticosteroid use, cyclophosphamide (2–5mg/kg/day) may be substituted for prednisone at this stage. While on cyclophophamide, white blood cell counts should be maintained at approximately 3000 cells/mm.[3] Cyclophosphamide may also be considered in desperate, corticosteroid nonresponsive cases. However, in such cases it is preferable and more comforting to have some definite indicator of an autoimmune disorder directed against inner-ear antigens (e.g. a positive Western blot or lymphocyte transformation test) before initiating therapy with potent cytotoxic drugs. McCabe advocates an earlier introduction of cyclophosphamide, with patients who respond to a 3-week regimen of high-dose corticosteroids being

placed on a corticosteroid-cyclophosphamide combination for three months after which the cyclophosphamide is discontinued and the corticosteroids are slowly tapered.[53] Complications of cyclophosphamide use include bone marrow suppression, hemorrhagic cystitis, malignancies of the urinary tract, and possible future development of a hematologic malignancy. Other treatments, including methotrexate, azathioprine, cyclosporin, and plasmapheresis have been advocated, but their efficacy remains unproven. Cogan's syndrome is treated with high-dose prednisone (2mg/kg/day) for one week tapered to 1/mg/kg/day during the second week with the ultimate discontinuation of therapy being dictated by the clinical response.

Summary

One must maintain a high index of suspicion for treatable causes of sensorineural hearing loss. The use of specific diagnostic tests will certainly help the clinician rule-out several possible causes. However, those potential causes that cannot be immediately identified often require the institution of empirical treatment. It is hoped that over the next few years with advancements in such molecular biological techniques as rapid polymerase chain reaction (PCR) screening, our ability to define precisely the cause of sudden or rapid hearing loss will improve dramatically and allow for more precise and targeted therapeutic interventions.

SUGGESTED READINGS

1. Wilson W, Byl F, Laird N: The efficacy of steroids in the treatment of idiopathic sudden hearing loss. Arch Otolaryngol *106:* 772, 1980.
2. Van Dishoeck HAE, Berman TA: Sudden perceptive deafness and viral infection. Ann Otol Rhinol Laryngol *66:*963, 1957.
3. Byl F: 76 cases of presumed sudden hearing loss occurring in 1973: Prognosis and incidence. Laryngoscope *87:*817, 1977.
4. Megighian D, Bolzer M, Barien V, et al: Epidemiologic considerations in sudden hearing loss. Arch Otolaryngol *243:*250, 1986.
5. Mattox D, Simmons F: Natural history of sudden sensorineural hearing loss. Ann Otol Rhinol Laryngol *86:*463, 1977.
6. Shaia F, Sheehy J: Sudden sensorineural hearing impairment: A report of 1220 cases. Laryngoscope *86:*389, 1976.
7. Lindsay JR, Davey PR, Ward PH: Inner ear pathology in deafness due to mumps. Ann Otol Rhinol Laryngol *69:*918, 1960.
8. Lindsay JR, Hemenway WG: Inner ear pathology due to measles. Ann Otol Rhinol Laryngol *63:*754, 1954.
9. Jaffe BF, Maassab HF: Sudden deafness associated with adenovirus infection. NEJM *276:*406, 1967.
10. Veltri RW, Wilson WR, Sprinkle PM, et al: The implication of viruses in idiopathic sudden hearing loss: Primary infection or reactivation of latent viruses. Otolaryngol Head Neck Surg *89:* 137, 1979.
11. Wilson W, Veltri RW, Laird N, et al: Viral and epidemiologic studies of idiopathic sudden hearing loss. Otolaryngol Head Neck Surg *91:*650, 1983.
12. Liao BS, Byl FM, Adour KK: Audiometric comparison of lassa

fever hearing loss and idiopathic sudden hearing loss: Evidence for viral cause. Otolaryngol Head Neck Surg 106:226, 1992.

13. Schuknecht H, Donovan E: The pathology of sudden sensorineural hearing loss. Arch Otolaryngol 243:1, 1986.

14. Mark AS, Seltzer S, Nelson-Drake J, et al: Labyrinthine enhancement on gadolinium-enhanced magnetic resonance imaging in sudden deafness and vertigo: Correlation with audiologic and electronystagmographic studies. Ann Otol Rhinol Laryngol 101:459, 1992.

15. Wilson WR, Byl FM, Laird N: The efficacy of steroids in the treatment of idiopathic sudden hearing loss: A double-blind clinical study. Arch Otolaryngol 106:772, 1980.

16. Moskowitz D, Lee KJ, Smith H: Steroid use in idiopathic sudden sensorineural hearing loss. Laryngoscope 94:664, 1984.

17. Morganstein K, Manace E: Temporal bone histopathology in sickle cell disease. Laryngoscope 79:2172, 1969.

18. Platra E, Sara R: Deafness and Waldenstrom's macroglobulinemia. South Med J 72:1495, 1979.

19. Jenkins HA, Pollack AM, Fisch U: Polyarteritis nodosa as a cause of sudden deafness. Am J Otolaryngol 2:99, 1981.

20. Journeaux SF, Master B, Greenhalgh RM et al: Sudden sensorineural hearing loss as a complication of non-otologic surgery. J Laryngol Otol 104:711, 1990.

21. Millen SJ, Toohill RJ, Lehman RH: Sudden sensorineural hearing loss: Operative complication in nonotologic surgery. Laryngoscope 92:613, 1982.

22. Perlman HB, Kimura R, Fernandez C: Experiments on temporary obstruction of the internal auditory artery. Laryngoscope 69:591, 1959.

23. Nadol J, Wilson W: Treatment of sudden hearing loss is illogical. In Controversy in otolaryngology. Edited by JB Snow. Philadelphia, W.B. Saunders Co., 1980, pp 23–32.

24. Jackler RK, Luxford WM, House WF: Congenital malformations of the inner ear: A classification based on embryogenesis. Laryngoscope 97(suppl 40):2–14, 1987.

25. Mostacello AL, Worder DL, Nadelman RB, et al: Otolaryngologic aspects of Lyme Disease. Laryngoscope 101:592, 1991.

26. Darmstadt GL, Harris JP: Luetic hearing loss: Clinical presentation, diagnosis, and treatment. Am J Otolaryngol 10:410, 1989.

27. Chandrasekhar SS, Siverls V, Sekhar C: Histopathologic and ultrastructural changes in temporal bones of HIV-infected human adults. Am J Otol 13:207, 1992.

28. Berg HM, Cohen NL, Hammerschlag PE, Waltzman SB: Acoustic neuroma presenting as sudden hearing loss with recovery. Otolaryngol Head Neck Surg 94:15, 1986.

29. Berenholz LP, Eriksen C, Hirsch FA: Recovery from repeated sudden hearing loss with corticosteroid use in the presence of acoustic neuroma. Ann Otol Rhinol Laryngol 101:827, 1992.

30. Baloh RW, Harker LA: Central vestibular system disorders. In Otolaryngology, Head and Neck Surgery, ed. 2. Edited by CW Cummings. St. Louis, Mosby Co., 1993, pp 3177–3198.

31. Murai K, Tsuiki T, Kusano H, et al: Sudden deafness: An investigation of hearing loss. Acta Otolaryngol 456:12, 1988.

32. Sheehy JL: Vasodilator therapy in sensory-neural hearing loss. Laryngoscope 70:885, 1960.

33. Probst R, Tschopp K, Ludin E, et al: A randomized double-blind, placebo controlled study of Dextran/Pentoxifyllene medication in acute acoustic trauma and sudden hearing loss. Acta Otolaryngol (Stockh) 112:435, 1992.

34. Laird N, Wilson WR: Predicting recovery from idiopathic sensorineural hearing loss. Am J Otolaryngol 4:161, 1983.

35. Hughes GB, Sismanis A, House J: Is there consensus in perilymphatic fistula management? Otolaryngol Head Neck Surg 102:111, 1990.

36. Weber PC, Perez BP, Bluestone CC: Congenital perilymph fistula and associated middle ear abnormalities. Laryngoscope 103:160, 1993.

37. Goodhill V: Sudden deafness and round window rupture. Laryngoscope 81:1462, 1971.

38. Kohut RI, Hinojosa R, Budetti JA: Perilymphatic fistula: A histopathologic study. Ann Otol Rhinol Laryngol 95:466, 1986.

39. Simmons FB: Theory of membrane breaks in sudden hearing loss. Arch. Otolaryngol 88:41, 1968.

40. Harker LA, Norante JD, Ryu JH: Experimental rupture of the round window membrane. Trans Am Acad Ophthalmol Otolaryngol 78:448, 1974.

41. Shea JJ: The myth of spontaneous perilymph fistula. Otolaryngol Head Neck Surg 107:613, 1992.

42. Seltzer S, McCabe BF: Perilymph fistula: The Iowa experience. Laryngoscope 96:37, 1986.

43. Meyerhoff WL: Spontaneous perilymphatic fistula: Myth or fact. Am J Otol 14:478, 1993.

44. Rizer FM, House JW: Perilymph fistulas: The House Ear Clinic experience. Otolaryngol Head Neck Surg 104:239, 1991.

45. House JW, Morris MS, Kramer SJ, et al: Perilymphatic fistula: surgical experience in the United States. Otolaryngol Head Neck Surg 105:422, 1991.

46. Meyerhoff WL, Yellin MW: Summating potential/action potential ratio in perilymph fistula. Otolaryngol Head Neck Surg 102:678, 1990.

47. Bojrab DI, Bhansali SA: Fluorescein use in the detection of perilymphatic fistula: A study in cats. Otolaryngol Head Neck Surg 108:348, 1993.

48. Applebaum EL: Fluorescein kinetics in perilymph and blood: A Fluorophotometric study. Laryngoscope 92:660, 1982.

49. Weber PC, Kelly RH, Bluestone CD, Bassiouny M: ß2-Transferrin confirms perilymphatic fistula in children. Otolaryngol Head Neck Surg 110:381, 1994.

50. Hughes GB, Barna BP, Calabrese LH, et al: Clinical diagnosis of immune inner ear disease. Laryngoscope 98:251, 1988.

51. Ruckenstein MJ, Harrison RV: Autoimmune inner ear disease: A review of basic mechanisms and clinical correlates. J Otolaryngol 20:196, 1991.

52. McCabe BF: Autoimmune sensorineural hearing loss. Ann Otol 88:585, 1979.

53. McCabe BF: Autoimmune inner ear disease: therapy. Am J Otol 10:196, 1989.

54. Cogan DG: Syndrome of nonsyphilitic interstitial keratitis and vestibuloauditory symptoms. Arch Ophthalmol 33:144, 1945.

55. Haynes BF, Kaiser-Kupfer MI, Mason P, et al: Cogan's syndrome: Studies in thirteen patients, long-term follow-up, and a review of the literature. Medicine 56:426, 1980.

56. Wolff D, Bernhard WG, Tsutsumi S, et al: The pathology of Cogan's syndrome causing profound deafness. Ann Otol Rhinol Laryngol 74:507, 1965.

57. Zechner G: Zum Cogan-syndrome. Acta Otolaryngol 89:310, 1980.

58. McDonald TJ, DeRemee RA: Wegener's granulomatosis. Laryngoscope 93:220, 1983.

59. Bakaar LG: Polyarteritis nodosa presented with nerve deafness. JR Soc Med 71:144, 1978.

60. Campbell SM, Montanaro A, Bardana EJ: Head and neck manifestations of autoimmune disease. Am J Otolaryngol 4:187, 1983.

61. Jacob A, Ledingham JG, Kerr AI, Ford MJ: Ulcerative colitis and giant cell arteritis associated with sensorineural deafness. J Laryngol Otol 104:889, 1990.

62. Hughes GB, Moscicki R, Barna BP, San Martin JE: Laboratory diagnosis of immune inner ear disease. Am J Otol 15:198, 1994.

63. Arnold W, Pfaltz R, Altermatt HJ: Evidence of serum antibodies against inner ear tissues in the blood of patients with certain sensorineural hearing disorders. Acta Otolaryngol 99:437, 1985.

64. Soliman AM, Zaneti F: Improvements of a method for testing autoantibodies in sensorineural hearing loss. Adv Otorhinolaryngol 39:13, 1988.

65. Mayot D, Bene MC, Dron K, et al: Immunologic alterations in patients with sensorineural hearing disorders. Clin Immunol Immunpathol 68:41, 1993.

66. Harris JP, Sharp P: Inner ear autoantibodies in patients with rapidly progressive sensorineural hearing loss. Laryngoscope 97:63, 1990.

67. Gottschlich S, Billings PB, Keithley EM, et al: Assessment of serum antibodies in patients with idiopathic progressive sensorineural hearing loss and Meniere's disease. Laryngoscope 1995, in press.

68. Yamanobe S, Harris JP: Inner ear specific autoantibodies. Laryngoscope 103:319, 1993.

56 Meniere's Disease, Vestibular Neuronitis and Paroxysmal Positional Vertigo and Nystagmus

Douglas E. Mattox

Meniere's disease remains, in many ways, as much an enigma as it was when Prosper Meniere first reported patients with episodic vertigo attacks in 1861. Despite an abundance of published articles (according to a MedLine search 532 in 1985–90 and 522 in 1990–94) many aspects of the disease remain controversial.

CLASSIC MENIERE'S DISEASE AND ITS VARIANTS

According to the American Academy of Otolaryngology—Head and Neck Surgery's Committee on Hearing and Equilibrium "Guidelines for Reporting of Treatment Results in Meniere's Disease" published in 1985, Meniere's is characterized by (1) unilateral sensorineural hearing loss, typically fluctuating and predominantly in the low frequencies, (2) tinnitus, constant or intermittent with the hearing loss typically increasing in intensity before or during the vertiginous attacks, and a sense of fullness in the ear, and, (3) attacks of vertigo lasting minutes to hours with irregular intervals, and accompanied by nausea and vomiting. A sense of fullness in the ear is also experienced. The fluctuations in hearing often accompany the vertigo attacks. The patient is generally left exhausted and unstable for the subsequent one to three days after an acute vertigo attack. The tinnitus and fullness are generally constant, but frequently increase in severity just preceding or during the attack.

One difficulty in the diagnosis, and an issue of controversy, is that the auditory and vestibular symptoms may not develop simultaneously, and in many patients the full complement of symptoms never develops. "Vestibular Meniere's" disease is characterized by recurrent episodes of vertigo typical of classical Meniere's disease but without hearing loss. Twenty percent of patients with classical Meniere's disease will first present with vestibular symptoms alone.[1] Conversely, "cochlear Meniere's" disease consists of fluctuating low-frequency hearing loss without vertigo. Confusion developed when, in 1972, the Sub-committee on Equilibrium and Its Measurement of the American Academy Ophthalmology and Otolaryngology included both cochlear and vestibular variants in their definition of Meniere's disease.[2] This decision was reversed in 1985 when the Committee on Hearing and Equilibrium of the American Academy of Otolaryngology-Head and Neck Surgery limited the diagnostic term "Meniere's Disease" to those patients in whom the full complement of symptoms was present.[3] Evidence that cochlear Meniere's disease results from a similar physiologic process as classical Meniere's disease is based on positive glycerol tests and similar histologic findings as classical Meniere's.[4] Similarly, Dornhoffer and Arenberg[5] demonstrated increased summating potential to eighth nerve action potentials (SP:AP) ratios in 73% of 15 patients with vestibular Meniere's disease. It, therefore, would seem logical to consider these patients as falling within the continuum of Meniere's disease. It is important, however, to consider these patients separately for the purposes of treatment design and results reporting.

Other interesting variants of Meniere's disease include Lermoyez's syndrome, drop attacks, and otolithic crisis of Tumarkin. Lermoyez's syndrome has the same symptoms as classical Meniere's disease, however, they occur in reverse order—progressive hearing impairment is followed by a sudden vertiginous attack, and an immediate recovery of hearing after the attack. Lermoyez's syndrome is rare and only a few dozen cases have been recorded. Lermoyez's attacks can be interspersed with more typical Meniere's attacks.[6]

Tumarkin's otolithic crisis is characterized by a sudden drop attack without loss of consciousness, vertigo or autonomic signs. Patients describe the sensation of being pushed to the floor. These attacks are not accompanied by spinning vertigo or hearing fluctuations. Otolithic crises appear to occur either early or late in the course of Meniere's disease and occur in clusters lasting up to six months. These patients continue to have typical Meniere's episodes.[7,8] Baloh et al[8] hypothesized that the attack resulted from the sudden mechanical deformation of the otolithic membrane of the utricle or saccule due to pressure gradients within the inner ear. It is important to differentiate drop attacks associated with Meniere's syndrome from those caused by cardiac and neurological disorders.

Another important subgroup is "delayed" Meniere's disease. Delayed Meniere's is characterized by profound loss of hearing in one ear followed many years later by typical Meniere's attacks. The pre-existing hearing loss can be a result of disease causes including viral hearing loss (mumps or measles), head trauma, temporal bone fracture, sudden deafness, acoustic trauma or congenital or neonatal causes.[9] Schuknecht et al[10] distinguished between ipsilateral and contralateral delayed hydrops. The ipsilateral form occurs in the previously deafened ear whereas the contralateral form consists of typical Meniere's disease developing in the contralateral previously normal ear. In contralateral delayed Meniere's, Schuknecht et al[10] argue, on the basis of histologic findings, that the remaining ear had also suffered a mild viral attack when the opposite ear was rendered deaf. This would also suggest that subclinical viral disease may have an etiologic role in the development of all Meniere's disease. Labyrinthectomy is an excellent treatment for the vertiginous episodes in the ipsilateral form of delayed hydrops. Medical measures are most usually required in the case of an only hearing ear.[11]

PATHOGENESIS

Histologically, dilation of the endolymphatic spaces of the inner ear, or endolymphatic hydrops, is found in all temporal bones of patients suffering from Meniere's disease.[12] Guild proposed the concept of longitudinal flow of endolymph within the membranous labyrinth in 1927.[13] Hydrops is most severe in the pars inferior of the membranous labyrinth, that is the cochlear duct and the saccule. Distension of the saccule is commonly severe enough that it touches the stapes footplate. Hydrops of the utricle is rare. Individuals with severe hydrops can show evidence of previous rupture of the membranes.[14]

The fundamental assumption in the pathogenesis of endolymphatic hydrops is that there is either an overproduction or under-reabsorption of endolymph. The folded lining of the endolymphatic sac suggests that this is a reabsorptive organ. The pathogenesis of Meniere's disease could therefore be on the basis of abnormal reabsorptive function of the endolymphatic sac or

mechanical blockage somewhere in the endolymphatic system. Schuknecht and Ruther[15] performed histologic examinations on 46 human temporal bones to evaluate the status of the pathway of longitudinal flow to the endolymphatic sac. Blockages were found in the endolymphatic duct, endolymphatic sinuses, utricular ducts, saccular ducts and in the ductus reuniens. In total, these blockages arrested longitudinal flow from both the pars superior and inferior in 46%, pars superior alone in only 6.5%, and the pars inferior alone in 35%. Therefore, in total 87% of the temporal bones examined showed areas of blockage to longitudinal flow within the temporal bone. These cases would not be candidates for endolymphatic shunt surgery because the blockage was proximal to the region where the shunt was placed. It should be remembered that these were end-stage, severe cases of Meniere's disease and these blockages might not occur to this degree of severity in early cases.

Hebbar et al[16] and Masutani et al[17] examined temporal bones from patients with and without Meniere's disease and found the diameters of the endolymphatic duct and the proximal portion of the vestibular aqueduct were significantly smaller in those with Meniere's disease. Hebbar et al[16] found that the diameter of the endolymphatic duct was also smaller than normal in the contralateral ear and concluded that the smaller duct was not a result of the disease but might be an etiologic factor in the development of Meniere's disease. In Meniere's ears, the endolymphatic sacs were smaller and had fewer tubular epithelial structures in the interosseus portion than did control ears. The width of the external aperture of the vestibular aqueduct was also smaller in the Meniere's ears than in controls. These findings indicate that not only the size of the vestibular aqueduct, but also the endolymphatic sac is reduced in size in Meniere's disease. Similar findings were noted by Yamamoto and Mizukami[18] on 3-dimensional reconstruction of CT images of the external aperture of the vestibular aqueduct, which was found to be hypoplastic in Meniere's disease but not in controls or adults or children with chronic otitis media.

However, according to Oigaard et al,[19] a hypoplastic vestibular aqueduct may be a nonspecific sign of many inner ear disorders and can be observed in ears with chronic otitis media as well as in individuals without otologic diseases. Yuen and Schuknecht[20] did not find the diameter of the vestibular aqueduct to be different in Meniere's disease and control ears.

Ikeda and Sando[21] studied the vascularity of the endolymphatic sac in Meniere's and non-Meniere's temporal bones. They found fewer and smaller blood vessels in the endolymphatic sac of bones from individuals with Meniere's disease than in control bones.

Genetic and hereditary factors may also contribute to the development of Meniere's disease. A family history of a vertigo is commonly obtained in Meniere's patients, however, it is usually difficult to document the exact nature of the family member's problem. Morrison et al[22] evaluated human leukocyte antigen (HLA) in Meniere's patients and found the antigens A3, Cw7, B7 and DR2 were all in excess of that found in the general population. The Cw7 allele occurred in 70% of Meniere's patients compared to 26.5% of the general population. Analysis of these data led Morrison to conclude that a Meniere's associated gene resided on the short arm of chromosome 6 between HLA-C and HLA-A alleles. Other abnormalities of the immune status have been reported by other authors. Evans et al[23] found elevated IgM complexes and C1q component of complement in all age groups of Meniere's patients. Low levels of IgA complexes were a consistent finding and were significantly lower in the HLA Cw7 patients. Other authors have found similar trends in these genetic traits and in various tests of immune function. Although in individual studies many of these tests attain statistical significance, rarely are positive tests found in the majority of the patients nor are consistent findings seen across studies. Additional research will be required to determine the significance of these findings.[24–26]

Headaches have an increased incidence in the Meniere's population. The association between Meniere's disease and migraine appears to be much stronger for vestibular Meniere's than for classical Meniere's patients.[27]

ANIMAL STUDIES

Meniere's disease is a human condition; there is no spontaneously occurring or surgically induced animal model of Meniere's disease. Kimura and Schuknecht[28] obliterated the endolymphatic duct and reproducibly demonstrated the development of endolymphatic hydrops in guinea pigs. Similar results were found in the rat and rabbit, however, this finding could not be reproduced in the chinchilla or monkey.[29] Despite the development of hydrops, these animals do not show behavioral characteristics suggesting attacks of Meniere's disease.

In the endolymphatic space there are longitudinal gradients of endocochlear potential, potassium and chloride concentrations, and osmolality, all of which increase from the apex to the base of the normal cochlea. This osmotic gradient should drive water along the cochlear duct toward the base of the cochlea and eventually to the endolymphatic sac. The flow of endolymph from the cochlea to the endolymphatic sac was documented by the detection of macromolecules in the endolymphatic sac that had been injected into the cochlear duct.[30] The average linear speed of this flow was estimated using ion sensitive microelectrodes to be

about .01 Arguments for an absorptive role for the sac were drawn from morphological studies.[32]

Early changes after endolymphatic duct obliteration include a decrease in endocochlear potential and cochlear microphonics, but there is no apparent alteration in the major ion content of endolymph including potassium, sodium and chloride.[33,34] These changes initially occur in the apex and subsequently in the base of the cochlea.[35] Meyer zum Gottesberge proposed an imbalance of calcium hemostasis within the endolymph as a fundamental mechanism in the development of Meniere's disease. Calcium is normally 10–100 times lower in the endolymph than in perilymph or extracellular fluid. Calcium level increases in endolymphatic hydrops can lead to both an increase in osmotic pressure and a decrease in endocochlear potential.

Ruding et al[37] examined the cross linkages in the stereocilia of guinea pig cochlea after endolymphatic sac obliteration. Initial changes were restricted to the stereocilia of the outer hair cells and consisted of a derangement and bulging of the stereocilia with interruption of the cross-linkage systems. Subsequently the stereocilia fused and atrophied. Loss of both outer and inner hair cells started at the apex and progressed towards the base of the cochlea. This correlates with the low-frequency hearing loss seen in Meniere's patients. Sziklai et al[38] found that changes in auditory dysfunction preceded electrochemical changes in the composition of endolymph by more than two weeks. No change was observed in the regional or total cochlear blood flow after experimental hydrops.[39]

There is also an immunologic hypothesis for the pathogenesis of endolymphatic hydrops. Direct antigen challenge into the endolymphatic sac of systemically presensitized guinea pigs causes the development of endolymphatic hydrops.[40] Inoculations of the endolymphatic sac with keyhole limpet hemocyanin produced a paralytic nystagmus and suppression of the caloric reaction in guinea pigs.[41] In a study of endolymphatic sac tissue removed from patients, only a minority of specimens showed immunofluorescent reactions to IgG, IgA or IgM.[42] In summary, although an immunologic mechanism is interesting, there are still no human data supporting it.

NATURAL HISTORY

Before treatment possibilities are considered, it is important to gain a firm understanding of the natural history of the disease. Meniere's disease is characterized by remissions and exacerbations making it impossible to predict the future behavior of any individual patient based on the patient's own history, test results, or general population data. Meniere's disease has an average age of onset in the 40s, however symptoms can start in either extreme of life. The gender and the left/right ratios are nearly equal. Meniere's disease can be a self-limited, albeit protracted, problem. After a number of years, the vertigo attacks generally subside and the hearing loss stabilizes at a moderate to severe level. Green et al[43] reviewed 98 patients who had been followed for at least 14 years. At the end of this period, the vertigo attacks had disappeared completely in 50% of patients and somewhat resolved in another 28%. Hearing was absent in 48%, and worse in another 21%. After a 20-year follow up, Stahle et al[44] found that none of the patients had hearing better than 30 dB and in 82% the mean loss was more than 50 dB. Hearing appeared to stabilize around 50 dB, 5 to 10 years after the onset of the disease. Normal pure-tone audiograms were found in 21% of patients at the first examination. Caloric response decreased rapidly during the first decade of the disease and then stabilized at approximately 50% of the normal functioning level.[44]

A critical issue in the treatment of Meniere's disease with destructive procedures is the risk of developing symptoms in the contralateral ear. The incidence of bilateral Meniere's disease has been estimated between 7 and 78%.[45,46] The most commonly reported incidence of bilaterality ranges from 30 to 50%.[47] Several authors have claimed that the second ear usually becomes involved by Meniere's disease by the first 2 to 5 years after onset of symptoms.[48,49] This seems to be contradicted by longer term studies. Green et al. (1991)[43] noted bilateral disease was initially present in 13% of patients and subsequently developed in 45% of patients after a prolonged follow-up. Stahle et al[44] followed 34 patients for a minimum of 20 years. Forty-seven percent developed bilateral symptoms, and the development of disease in the second ear was almost linear with time.

The occurrence of Meniere's disease in children is infrequent and has been estimated to be less than 1% of all Meniere's patients. Hausler et al[50] reported 14 children under the age of 14 with Meniere's disease. Nine of these had no antecedent otologic disease, the other five had histories of initial hearing loss after mumps, haemophilus influenzae meningitis, temporal bone fracture or congenital hearing impairment. Otherwise the presentations and the course of the Meniere's disease itself were unremarkable compared to adults.

TESTING

Aside from standard audiometric and vestibular testing, the procedures most frequently used to corroborate the diagnosis of Meniere's disease are the glycerol dehydration test and electrocochleography. There is no test pathognomonic for Meniere's disease.

The glycerol dehydration test uses glycerol or mannitol as an osmotic diuretic and the patient's hearing thresholds and discrimination scores are serially tested during the diuresis.[51] Improvement in either is interpreted as consistent with Meniere's disease. Magliulo[52] found that animals subjected to blockage of the endolymphatic duct maintained better auditory thresholds when they were maintained on postoperative glycerol. This suggests that systemic glycerol is able to decompress the hydropic membranous labyrinth. Clinically, however, a positive glycerol test is found in roughly half the patients with clinically suspected Meniere's disease.[53,54] Some studies suggest that the glycerol test more likely to be positive in elderly patients, patients with more severe hearing loss, and those with fluctuating hearing loss.[53,55]

Sound evoked electrical potentials were first recorded from the inner ear by Wever and Bray in 1930.[56] The clinical application of recording these potentials has been named *electrocochleography* (ECOG). Potentials can be recorded from either the external auditory canal or tympanic membrane or with a trans-tympanic electrode on the promontory. Although the trans-tympanic technique is slightly more invasive, larger potentials and a better signal-to-noise ratio are obtained with this technique.

Three phenomena are measured by ECOG: the cochlear microphonic, the summating potential, and the nerve action potential. The use of ECOG for the diagnosis of endolymphatic hydrops has hinged on the relationship between the summating and action potential amplitudes. The potentials are obtained by alternating the presentation of condensation and rarefaction clicks, thus cancelling the cochlear microphonic. The summating potential is seen as a "knee" on the leading edge of the action potential response. Since the absolute amplitudes of the summating potential and action potential are highly variable from subject to subject, the SP/AP ratio is commonly used.[57] Schmidt et al[58] found that patients with Meniere's disease had larger summating potentials than patients with sensorineural hearing loss from other causes. Large summating potentials were also observed in animals with experimentally induced endolymphatic hydrops.[59] The mechanisms for the enlarged summating potential is thought to be displacement of the basal membrane toward the scala tympani from the abnormal endolymphatic pressure.[60]

Margolis et al[61] pointed out the difficulties in interpretation of ECOG data. If the basilar membrane was distorted, it would cause a large latency difference between condensation and rarefaction quick action potentials. This latency difference would cause distortion of the potentials averaged between condensation and rarefaction stimuli. As the disease progresses, the loss of sensory hair cells and nerve fibers would cause a decrease in the total response amplitude and could potentially result in an abnormal SP/AP ratio. In addition, uncancelled cochlear microphonics can falsely resemble abnormal summating potential in any stage of the disease.

These predictions are borne out by animal experiments. In experimental animals, an SP enlargement occurred in the early stage of experimental hydrops without an action potential threshold shift. In the later stages, there was a decrease in the action potential concomitant with loss of hair cells and cochlear neurons causing a decrease in the SP/AP ratio. No differences in SP amplitude between normals and controls were observed in chronic animals. Therefore it would appear that an enlarged summating potential should be expected only during the early stages of the disease when cochlear hydrops is present and hair cells and auditory neurons are intact.[62,63]

These studies are consistent with what has been found in humans. Enlarged summating potentials are found in Meniere's patients only when the hearing loss was relatively mild (less than 50 dB). Dauman et al[64] reported that SP amplitude was related to low-frequency hearing thresholds, which in turn fluctuate with displacement of the cochlear partition from the endolymphatic pressure. These changes in the endocochlear potentials during the course of the disease make interpretation of ECOG difficult and multiple testing paradigms should be used.[65]

ECOG findings can be difficult to correlate with clinical findings. Ohashi et al[66] followed 24 Meniere's patients with ECOG up to 8 years. Half the patients were treated surgically with endolymphatic sac decompression and the remainder were treated medically. Patients for the study were selected on the basis of abnormal SP/AP ratios. Interestingly, the ratios varied very little over time. Only one of the operated patients and two of the medically treated patients showed any significant variations, and these fluctuations did not coincide with changing medical or surgical interventions. Mori et al[67] failed to find a relationship between an abnormal summating potential and clinical symptoms including the duration of cochlear or vestibular symptoms, recent hearing fluctuation or recent vertigo attack. The abnormal summating potential did correlate with high-frequency hearing loss.

Attempts have been made to combine the glycerol test with electrocochleographic recording. Dauman et al[64] reported that when the summating potential was examined, 59% of Meniere's patients had a positive glycerol dehydration test, whereas only 29% had a positive test based on pure-tone threshold audiometry. This study also found that patients with large negative summating potentials at low frequencies also had larger action potentials and had short-term symptoms. Otherwise, there appeared to be no clear correlations between clinical observations and the electrocochleographic data either with or without glycerol.

MEDICAL MANAGEMENT

The wide variety of proposed treatments for Meniere's disease attests to the difficulty of finding a satisfactory therapeutic result in this difficult patient population. In 1977, Torok published a 25-year review of 834 papers concerned with the treatment of Meniere's disease.[68] Recovery occurred in 60 to 80% of patients. Another 20 to 30% of patients were considered improved, and 10 to 25% of patients were therapeutic failures. He concluded that while treating the patient was important, the specific nature of the treatment bore little relation to the therapeutic outcome.

The mainstay of current medical management is based on the regimen of Furstenberg et al. who proposed the avoidance of excess salt, caffeine, nicotine, alcohol and theophylline containing foods (chocolate).[69] This is similar to the dietary restrictions proposed in the management of migraine disorders. There are no controlled studies supporting the use of such a regimen. In some patients, however, the association between a salt, alcohol or chocolate load and a subsequent attack seems undeniable. The exact proportion of patients in whom such dietary triggers occur is unknown. Nonetheless, this seems an appropriate place to start medical therapy.

Almost all of the published studies of medical management of Meniere's disease suffer from common shortcomings including limited sample size, the highly variable nature of Meniere's disease from patient to patient, and the lack of appropriate staging of the disease to assure comparable populations in the experimental and control groups.

The most commonly used medical intervention in Meniere's disease is diuretics. Klockhoff and Lindblom[70] described a double-blind clinical trial of hydrochlorothiazide (HCTZ) in the treatment of Meniere's disease. This report studied 30 patients who were given four-month trials of HCTZ or a placebo. They concluded that the diuretic caused an improvement in hearing, tinnitus, vertigo and general condition over that obtained by placebo. A re-analysis of this data by Ruckenstein et al[71] questioned this conclusion based on the fact that in the original study, patients who had no change in their symptoms were excluded from analysis. Jackson, Glasscock et al[72] retrospectively compared a group of patients treated with vasodilators to a subsequent group treated with diuretics. The group treated with diuretics did marginally better with an improvement in 79% of patients compared to 61% in the former group. Ruckenstein et al. criticized this study based on the fact that the groups were sequential, not simultaneous, and the fact that the diagnosis and compliance with the therapy were not rigorously assured.[71] Van Deelen and Huizing[73] reported a small series of patients treated with diazide in a cross-over placebo controlled study. The diazide was found to have no effect on the hearing or tinnitus. However, vestibular complaints decreased on the diazide treatment. At the end of the two treatment periods, 17 of 33 patients had a distinct preference for the diazide, however three chose the placebo and 13 had no preference for either drug.

There is increasing enthusiasm among many investigators for the systemic or local application of aminoglycosides in the treatment of Meniere's disease because of the more profound effect of streptomycin and gentamicin on vestibular hair cells than on cochlear hair cells. Schuknecht was the first to establish a treatment regimen using systemic intramuscular streptomycin.[74] Intramuscular streptomycin was continued until ice water caloric responses were abolished; total doses ranged from 13.5 to 89 grams (mean: 39 g). Ninety-five percent of patients had no post-treatment vertigo, but 35% had persistent ataxia and 15% had persistent oscillopsia. Hearing loss after this treatment is uncommon. In a follow-up study on patients treated with intramuscular streptomycin, Wilson and Schuknecht[45] found that 90% of patients had stable hearing for an extended follow-up period. In an attempt to prevent the oscillopsia and ataxia that follow total vestibular ablation, Graham and Kemink[76] suggested "titrating" the dose by stopping treatment when symptoms ceased. Additional treatment would be given if the symptoms recurred. The disadvantage of this treatment is that both ears are similarly affected, thus it is applicable to unilateral Meniere's disease in an only hearing ear or bilateral Meniere's disease.

Unilateral disease has been treated with local application of aminoglycosides in the middle ear.[77,78] Beck and Schmidt[78] used gentamicin 30 mg/day for 6 days or until signs of ototoxicity and achieved control of vertigo in 90% of patients with preservation of hearing at the pretreatment level in 85%. Pyykko et al[79] treated 14 patients with bilateral Meniere's disease with intratympanic gentamicin. At a two-year follow up, 11 of the 14 had eliminated their vertigo attacks. Hearing was not adversely affected by the treatment.

Direct application of streptomycin into the inner ear has been proposed by Shea and Norris.[80] The rationale was to place the ototoxic drug as close as possible to the vestibular hair cells and at the same time spare hearing. The procedure involves a mastoidectomy, fenestration of the lateral semicircular canal with preservation of the membranous labyrinth, and infusion of streptomycin directly into the perilymphatic space. Shea and Ge[81] have reported excellent results using this technique. However, a multicenter study showed an unacceptably high incidence of worsening of the hearing loss (86%) and the hearing loss was at the severe to profound level in the majority of these.[82] The final results for the control of vertigo from this study have not been published. Within the first few postoperative months, 17% of patients underwent a secondary procedure for control of their vertigo. A significant problem with this procedure is the difficulty in determining the amount of drug infused into the labyrinth.[82]

SURGICAL THERAPY

A number of techniques have been attempted for the surgical treatment of Meniere's disease including the establishment of a permanent fistula between the endolymph and perilymph[83] and procedures to enhance the function of the endolymphatic sac. Decompression of the endolymphatic sac was first proposed by Portman in 1927;[84] this preceded the first description of the histopathology of Meniere's disease by 11 years. The hypothesis behind the procedure is that the endolymphatic sac is defective and unable to reabsorb endolymph, therefore an alternative drainage path should be provided. A number of modifications of sac surgery have developed over the years including simple decompression, decompression with insertion of muscle flaps, drainage and shunting of the endolymphatic sac into either the subarachnoid space or, more commonly, into the mastoid. Two recent reviews of this subject found more articles devoted to endolymphatic sac surgery in the recent literature than any other treatment of Meniere's disease.[71,85]

Most surgeons report a successful outcome from endolymphatic surgery ranging from 35 to 100% with an overall mean success rate of 72%.[85] Some recent literature suggests good results from endolymphatic sac surgery, however, a high rate of revision surgery was required. Monsell and Wiet[86] noted 19% of patients needed revision surgery, usually retrolabyrinthine vestibular neurectomy. Telischi and Luxford[87] reviewed 234 patients having at least 10 years follow-up after endolymphatic subarachnoid shunts. Twenty percent of these patients required a destructive procedure and another 17% required revisions of the original shunt procedure. Thus, approximately 60% of patients had control of vertigo by their original shunt surgery.

Among the numerous publications concerning endolymphatic sac surgery, only one has a true control group. This is the famous "sham" surgery study performed in Denmark.[88,89,90] This study included 30 patients who underwent a double-blind, placebo-controlled comparison of the endolymphatic mastoid shunt versus a simple cortical mastoidectomy. This study was controversial for many reasons, not the least of which was the fact that the patients involved in the study were not informed concerning their participation in the study, nor was there consent obtained for the possibility that they would be included in a control placebo group. The strength of this study is that the evaluating physicians also did not know to which group the patients belonged, thus eliminating their bias. Follow-up of the patients was published at 1, 3,

6, and 9 years. At 1 year, there was a significant improvement in the vertigo, nausea and vomiting, tinnitus, and aural fullness in both groups. There was a marginally significant improvement in vertigo in favor of the shunt procedure at 1 year. At the 3- and 6-year follow-ups, there were no statistically significant differences with regard to any of these parameters. A nine-year follow-up showed that successful control of vertigo had been maintained in 70% of patients in both groups and that there still were no statistically significant differences between the two groups in any measured parameter.[91]

Two other studies have compared the results obtained after endolymphatic sac surgery with patients who were recommended to have surgery but for various reasons did not have the procedure performed. Silverstein[92] found no long-term difference between the surgery and nonsurgery groups. More recently, Filipo and Barbara[93] found that vertigo and tinnitus were improved by sac surgery in a significant number of patients. Hearing function, which improved a few months after surgery in some patients, was found to deteriorate in the long run in both the surgical and nonsurgical groups.

Schuknecht and Ruther[15] questioned the logic of endolymphatic sac surgery in a study of temporal bones with Meniere's disease. They found 86% of 46 ears examined showed areas of blockage to longitudinal flow that are proximal to the region treated by the endolymphatic shunt. Cohen and Mattox[94] reported four endolymphatic shunts removed during surgery for other reasons. Findings included deterioration of the implant and fibrous tissue and cellular debris within the valve of the implant. None the less, endolymphatic sac surgery appears to be beneficial in at least half of the patients, and its risks and complications are minimal.

The "destructive" procedures for Meniere's disease include labyrinthectomy and vestibular neurectomy through either the middle or posterior fossa. The latter procedures are conceived to preserve hearing, the former sacrifices hearing at the same time that it destroys the vestibular peripheral end organ. Both procedures appear to be extremely effective in controlling the episodic vertigo attacks. A considerable number of patients, however, are left with complaint of persistent unsteadiness. Hammerschlag and Schuknecht[95] reported unsteadiness associated with quick head movements in 22% of their labyrinthectomy patients. This unsteadiness is likely a physiologic consequence of unilateral vestibular loss rather than residual disease. Willatt and Yung[96] found that the patients' chronic objective complaint of imbalance bore no relationship to the ability to perform a balance test. They concluded that the patients' psychology and personality also played an important part in recovery.

Five and ten years after labyrinthectomy, Levine et al[97] found 93% and 76% of patients respectively were free from episodic vertigo. The authors attributed the decline in results to aging with the development of vertebral-basilar insufficiency and poorer vision as well as the development of Meniere's disease in the second ear. Patient activity problems that were frequently cited in this series included difficulty in turning quickly, walking in poor lighting, and driving at night.

Both middle-fossa and posterior-fossa vestibular nerve sections are effective in eliminating the vertiginous episodes and also preserve preoperative hearing. Because it is technically less demanding, retrolabyrinthine or retrosigmoid vestibular neurectomy is more commonly performed than middle-fossa neurectomy. It had initially been hoped that dividing the efferent nerve fibers to the cochlea that ran along with the vestibular nerve would cause a long-term improvement or stabilization of hearing in patients after vestibular neurectomy. This has not been the case, and hearing appears to degenerate in postoperative patients similar to the natural history of the disease.[98] The results of vestibular neurectomy for management of vertigo appear to be similar to those for labyrinthectomy.[99]

BENIGN PAROXYSMAL POSITIONAL VERTIGO

In 1921, Barany described a characteristic paroxysmal vertigo and nystagmus that occurred in certain positions and suggested that this condition resulted from otolithic disease.[100] Dix and Hallpike agreed benign paroxysmal positional vertigo (BPPV) was a disorder of the otolith organs and described characteristics now used to clinically define this syndrome.[101] These characteristics include a critical provocative position with the affected ear-dependent, a mixed vertical-rotary (torsional) nystagmus, a brief latency of one to five seconds between the time of assuming the provocative position and the onset of symptoms, a crescendo-decrescendo in the severity of symptoms lasting up to 30 seconds, a reversal of the direction of nystagmus upon assuming sitting up, and a fatiguability of the response after multiple trials.[102]

Clinical complaints of patients with BPPV are easy to identify. Patients complain of symptoms occurring getting in and out of bed, and particularly when rolling from one side to the other. The initial complaint may be that the patient cannot recline in a dental chair or in a hairdressing salon. Frequently the patient is symptomatic when getting out of the bed as well as when bending down, straightening up or particularly when extending the head backwards to look up. In addition to the specific position related symptoms, patients may complain of a nonspecific disequilibrium or instability when they are up moving about. These symptoms may be the primary complaint, especially when the patient has unconsciously learned to avoid the eliciting position. A careful history is imperative to identify these patients.

Benign positional vertigo is a common disorder. One study estimated that 17% of new patients in a vestibular clinic carried this diagnosis.[102] A population based study in Minnesota suggested the instance was 64 per 100,000 population per year and that the incidence of benign positional vertigo increased by 38% with each decade of life.[103] The average age of onset of symptoms is in the early 50s.[104,105] BPPV usually has a spontaneous onset without antecedent otologic problems. However, it has been reported after head trauma, stapes surgery, viral labyrinthitis, and chronic otitis media.

Schuknecht and Ruby suggested the three common clinical courses for benign positional vertigo.[106] The most common is self-limited and subsides spontaneously over a few weeks to months. The second category of patients experience remissions and recurrences over weeks to years. The smallest group appears to have a permanent form of the disorder. Approximately 30% of patients had symptoms lasting 1 year or more.[105]

BPPV is a disorder of the posterior semicircular canal. Neural activity from the ampulla of the posterior semicircular canal is increased by deflection away from the utricle (ampulofugal) and decreased activity with motion toward the utricle (ampulopetal).[107] Experimental stimulation of the left posterior ampullary nerve results in a counter-clockwise deviation of the eye and a clockwise fast phase of the nystagmus. This suggests that BPPV could be produced by ampulofugal deflection of the posterior semicircular canal of the undermost ear. Schuknecht hypothesized that loose debris from the otoconia could settle on the ampulla of the posterior semicircular canal because it was the most dependent portion of the labyrinth.[108] Histologic sections showed basophilic deposits attached to the cupula of the posterior semicircular canal and coined the term "cupulolithiasis."[108] The increased mass of the cupula would make it sensitive to gravity, causing an ampulofugal deflection in the Hallpike position. Alternatively, Hall et al suggested the utricular debris could be free-floating within the long arm of the canal, a condition that has since been termed "canalithiasis."[109]

Regardless of whether the mechanism of BPPV is debris attached to the cupula or free-floating debris within the long limb of the posterior semi-circular canal, the physiologic response should be the same. The increased mass of particles attached to the cupula should deflect it away from the utricle in the Hallpike position. Similarly free-floating debris in the long arm near the cupula should fall away from the cupula during the Hallpike maneuver. As the particles move they should entrain endolymph to move in the same direction, and again displace the cupula away from the utri-

cle. An ampulofugal displacement of the cupula results in a rotary nystagmus with the upper pole of the eye moving away from utricle. The compensatory fast component (for which the nystagmus is named) is in the direction toward the stimulated ear, causing, for example, clockwise rotary nystagmus with stimulation of the left posterior canal.

Supporting the concept of canalithiasis, Parnes and McClure observed intraoperatively that there was free-floating debris in the posterior semicircular canal in 2 of 20 patients undergoing surgery for benign positional vertigo.[110] Interestingly, these two patients were the oldest in the series. However, debate exists concerning the significance of debris contained within the posterior semicircular canal. Kveton and Kashjarian found particulate matter in the endolymphatic space of the posterior semicircular canal in nine of ten patients undergoing translabyrinthine removal of acoustic neuroma.[111] None of these patients had a primary complaint of positional vertigo. Electron microscopic examination of this material was consistent with otoconia. The authors interpreted this finding as suggesting that debris within the posterior semicircular canal was not pathologic.

Although the vast majority of positional vertigo involves the posterior semicircular canal, a horizontal semicircular canal variant has been described.[112] Unlike the usual form of torsional-vertical nystagmus, there was an intense, direction-changing, horizontal, geotrophic nystagmus (beating toward the ground) that occurred in both left and right Hallpike positions. The individual episodes of vertigo typically last a minute and are usually associated with severe nausea. The direction-changing nystagmus begins abruptly and does not fatigue on repeated positioning. The nystagmus was stronger in one direction than the other. McClure speculated that this nystagmus resulted in accumulation of debris in the long arm of the horizontal semicircular canal.[112] Baloh et al described three key features of horizontal canal positional nystagmus: (1) a direction changing positional nystagmus induced in both lateral positions, (2) the peak of the slow phase velocity depends on the speed of the positional change, and (3) the same direction positional nystagmus is induced if the patient moves from the left lateral to supine position or from supine to the right lateral position.[113]

Drug therapy for benign positional vertigo has been uniformly disappointing, this is not surprising for a mechanical problem of the peripheral labyrinth.[114,115] However, the physical therapy approach has a long history and increasing success. Cawthorne proposed his "vestibular habilitation therapy."[116] This therapy consisted of having the patients assume head positions that provoked the symptoms of vertigo with a goal of increasing their tolerance rather than eliminating the cause. This modality has developed into habituation exercises commonly used today for patients suffering an acute unilateral loss from surgery (labyrinthectomy, acoustic neuroma), trauma, or neuronitis.

A specific treatment for BPPV was devised by Brandt and Daroff with the goal of dispersing debris within the posterior semicircular canal.[117] In this exercise the patient repeatedly went from the sitting to the supine position on the symptomatic side, to the supine position on the opposite side. The exercises were repeated three times a day. Although compliance was a problem, the authors reported successful treatment in many cases.

The first single treatment specifically designed to address the posterior semicircular canal was described by Toupet and Semont (Fig. 56–1).[118] In this "liberatory" maneuver, symptoms were initially provoked in the standard Hallpike position. After a brief period,

the patient was quickly brought to a sitting position and is immediately placed face down on the opposite side. In this way, debris in the posterior semicircular was "walked" out of the long arm of the posterior semicircular canal back into the utricle. Success with this technique ranges between 50 and 90%.[119,120]

Epley proposed another maneuver (Fig. 56–2) with a similar intent but somewhat less jarring to the patient.[121] In the Epley maneuver the patient initially assumes the provoking Hallpike position with the head in a dependent position. Next the patient is turned slowly toward the opposite ear until the patient is in a full face down position. After a few minutes, the patient is slowly returned to a sitting position. After either the Semont or Epley maneuvers, the patients are given a soft cervical collar to remind them to keep their head upright for 48 hours. They are instructed not to

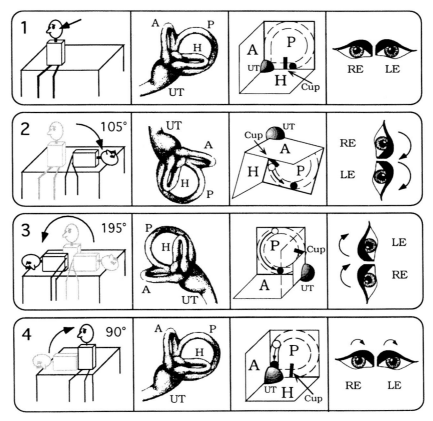

Fig. 56–1. Schematic drawing of the Semont liberatory maneuver in a patient with typical BPPV of the left ear. Boxes from left to right: position of body and head, position of labyrinth in space, position and movement of the clot in the posterior canal and resulting cupula deflection, and direction of the rotatory nystagmus. The clot is depicted as an open circle within the canal; a black circle represents the final resting position of the clot. (1) In the sitting position, the head is turned horizontally 45° to the unaffected ear. The clot, which is heavier than endolymph, settles at the base of the left posterior semicircular canal. (2) The patient is tilted approximately 105° toward the left (affected) ear. The head position change, relative to gravity, causes the clot to gravitate to the lowermost part of the canal and the cupula to deflect downward, inducing BPPV with rotatory nystagmus beating toward the undermost ear. The patient maintains this position for 3 minutes. (3) The patient is turned approximately 195° with the nose down, causing the clot to move toward the exit of the canal. The endolymphatic flow again deflects the cupula such that the nystagmus beats toward the left ear, now uppermost. The patient remains in this position for 3 minutes. (4) The patient is slowly moved to the sitting position; this causes the clot to enter the utricular cavity. Abbreviations: A, P, and H = anterior, posterior, and horizontal semicircular canals; Cup = cupula. UT = utricular cavity, RE = right eye, and LE = left eye.

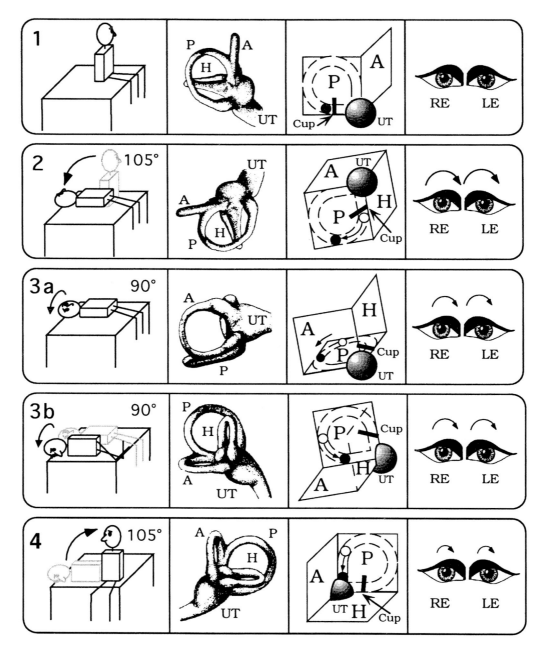

Fig. 56–2. Schematic drawing of modified Epley liberatory maneuver. Patient characteristics and abbreviations are as in figure 1. (1) In the sitting position, the head is turned horizontally 45° to the affected (left) ear. (2) The patient is tilted approximately 105° backward into a slight head-hanging position, causing the clot to move in the canal, deflecting the cupula downward, and inducing the BPPV attack. The patient remains in this position for 3 minutes. (3a) The head is turned 90° to the unaffected ear, now undermost, and (3b) the head and trunk continue turning another 90° to the right, causing the clot to move toward the exit of the canal. The patient remains in this position for 3 minutes. The positioning nystagmus beating toward the affected (uppermost) ear in positions 3a and 3b indicates effective therapy. (4) The patient is moved to the sitting position.

bend over, up or down with their head, or lie down. Of the subsequent 5 days patients are allowed to lie down but not on the affected side.[122] Epley reported complete resolution of symptoms in more than 85% of patients.[121] Although some authors have not been able to reproduce these results,[123] most authors have been able to obtain cure or substantial improvement in 70–90% of patients.[122,124,125]

A number of surgical procedures have also been proposed for the treatment of benign positional vertigo. These were more popular before the development of physical therapy techniques and are still useful in the small percent of patients who fail conservative therapy. Transection of the posterior ampullary nerve (singular neurectomy) was proposed by Gacek in 1974.[126] After an exploratory tympanotomy, bone is removed posterior and inferior to the round window membrane in order to identify and divide the singular nerve. This procedure is technically demanding and has a risk of sensorineural hearing loss. Recently, posterior occlusion of the semicircular canal has become the surgical procedure of choice.[127] The objective of the operation is to prevent flow of endolymph through the posterior canal thereby preventing cupular displacement. Posterior canal is fenestrated though the mastoid, avoiding opening the membranous labyrinth. The canal can then be obstructed with bone chips or bone wax. This procedure can usually be performed without causing sensorineural hearing loss.[128] Coagulating the membranous labyrinth with laser has also been suggested.[129] These procedures produce relief in 13 of 14 patients.[129] These surgical alternatives are viable in those few patients failing the positioning maneuvers.

Vestibular Neuronitis

The term vestibular neuronitis was coined by Dix and Hallpike.[101] Vestibular neuronitis is characterized by the acute onset of vertigo, nausea and often vomiting without concomitant hearing loss or other neurologic signs. Some patients may have a prodrome of instability. The acute phase of the attack lasts 24–72 hours during which any movement of the head precipitates severe vertigo. The most common clinical finding is a mixed horizontal and rotary nystagmus with the fast phase away from the affected part of the ear. The acute phase is followed by a period of slow resolution characterized by unsteadiness and disequilibrium, often lasting several weeks to months. Following the acute attack, transient episodes of dizziness may occur over the next 12–18 months. The clinical course of recovery is similar to that seen after a labyrinthectomy.

Vestibular neuronitis occurs most commonly in young and middle aged adults. Although a single attack and slow resolution is the most typical history, the syndrome can recur. The subsequent attacks are characteristically less severe than the initial event.

A viral etiology has been suggested. Vestibular neuronitis is well known to occur in small epidemics and has an increased incidence among disease contacts including family members and neighbors. There is limited histopathologic and serologic data supporting a viral etiology.[130]

The most common abnormal test is a decreased caloric response in the affected ear, although this is not mandatory for the diagnosis. Typically the caloric response recovers later in the course of the disease.[130,131]

Vestibular neuronitis is a self-limiting disease and will resolve without any specific intervention. A careful explanation of the process and reassurance of the patient is very helpful.

The use of vestibular suppressant drugs is controversial because of the theoretical possibility that early vestibular suppression may retard central compensation.[132] Most logical use of these drugs was suggested by Brandt who suggested that vestibular suppressants should be used to relieve the patient's vertigo but they should be used in a limited dosage for a short time so that they do not suppress the central vestibular compensation process. The compensation process is likely to be longer for older individuals.[133] In addition, recovery may be facilitated with a systematic plan of vestibular rehabilitation.[135-137]

There is slightly more concern about the possibility of a central lesion in patients with vestibular neuronitis than in BPPV or Meniere's disease. Magnusson and Norrving found one of four subjects above the age of 50 with symptoms typical of vestibular neuronitis had identifiable central nervous system lesions (cerebellar infarctions, vertebral artery occlusion) and therefore recommend imaging or Doppler blood flow studies on individuals in this age group.[138] Any patient with central or cranial nerve findings in clinical examination should have a more detailed evaluation.

SUMMARY

The etiology and pathogenesis of Meniere's disease have been reviewed with special attention to those factors that relate to current treatment regimens. A major limitation in the study and treatment of Meniere's disease is the high variability of the pattern of the disease among subjects and within a single subject over time. Future advances in the understanding of the pathogenesis of Meniere's disease should lead to more effective methods of treatment.

REFERENCES

1. Paparella MM, Mancini F: Vestibular Meniere's disease. Otolaryngology Head Neck Surg 93(2):148–51, 1985.
2. Alford BR: Report of the subcommittee on equilibrium and its measurement, Meniere's Disease: criteria for diagnosis and evaluation of therapy for reporting. Trans Am Acad Ophthalmol Otolaryngol 76:1462–1464, 1972.
3. Pearson BW, Brackmann D: Committee on Hearing and Equilibrium Guidelines for Reporting Treatment Results in Meniere's Disease. Otolaryngol Head Neck Surg 93:579–582, 1985.
4. Kohut RI, Lindsay JR: Pathologic changes in idiopathic labyrinthine hydrops. Acta Otolaryngol (Stockh) 73:402–412, 1972.
5. Dornhoffer JL, Arenberg IK: Diagnosis of vestibular Meniere's disease with electrocochleography. Am J Otol 14(2):161–4, 1993.
6. Schmidt PH, Schoonhoven R: Lermoyez's syndrome. A follow-up study in 12 patients. Acta Oto-Laryngol 107(5–6):467–73, 1989.
7. Janzen VD, Russell RD: Conservative management of Tumarkin's otolithic crisis. J Otolaryngol 17(7):359–61, 1988.
8. Baloh RW, Jacobson K, Winder T: Drop attacks with Meniere's syndrome. Ann Neurol 28(3):384–7, 1990.
9. Nadol JB, Jr, Weis AD, Parker SW: Vertigo of delayed onset after sudden deafness. Ann Otol Rhinol Laryngol 84:841–6, 1975.

10. Schuknecht HF, Suzuka Y, Zimmermann C: Delayed endolymphatic hydrops and its relationship to Meniere's disease. Ann Otol Rhinol Laryngol 99(11):843–53, 1990.

11. Hicks GW, Wright JW: Delayed endolymphatic hydrops: a review of 15 cases. Laryngoscope 98(8 Pt 1):840–5, 1988.

12. Hallpike C, Cairns H: Observations on the pathology of Meniere's syndrome. J Laryngol Otol 53:625–655, 1938.

13. Guild SR: The circulation of the endolymph. Am J Anat 39:57–81, 1927.

14. Paparella MM: Pathogenesis and pathophysiology of Meniere's disease. Acta Oto-Laryngologica—Suppl 485:26–35, 1991.

15. Schuknecht HF, Ruther A: Blockage of longitudinal flow in endolymphatic hydrops. Euro Arch Oto-Rhino-Laryngol 248(4):209–17, 1991.

16. Hebbar GK, Rask-Andersen H, Linthicum FH, Jr: Three-dimensional analysis of 61 human endolymphatic ducts and sacs in ears with and without Meniere's disease. Ann Otol Rhinol Laryngol 100(3):219–25, 1991.

17. Masutani H, Takahashi H, Sando I, Sato H: Vestibular aqueduct in Meniere's disease and non-Meniere's disease with endolymphatic hydrops: a computer aided volumetric study. Auris, Nasus, Larynx. 18(4):351–7, 1991.

18. Yamamoto E, Mizukami C: Development of the vestibular aqueduct in Meniere's disease. Acta Oto-Laryngol—Suppl 504:46–50, 1993.

19. Oigaard A, Thomsen J, Jensen J, Dorph S: The vestibular aqueduct in Meniere's disease. Acta Otolaryngol (Stockh) 82:279–81, 1976.

20. Yuen SF, Schuknecht HF: Vestibular aqueduct and endolymphatic duct in Meniere's disease. Arch Otolaryngol 96:552–5, 1972.

21. Ikeda M, Sando I: Vascularity of endolymphatic sac in Meniere's disease. A histopathological study. Ann Otol Rhinol Laryngol Suppl 118:6–10, 1985.

22. Morrison AW, Mowbray JF, Williamson R, Sheeka S, Sodha N, Koskinen N: On genetic and environmental factors in Meniere's disease. Am J Otol 15(1):35–9, 1994.

23. Evans KL, Baldwin DL, Bainbridge D, Morrison AW: Immune status in patients with Meniere's disease. Arch Oto-Rhino-Laryngol 245(5):287–92, 1988.

24. Koyama S, Mitsuishi Y, Bibee K, Watanabe I, Terasaki PI: HLA associations with Meniere's disease. Acta Oto-Laryngol 113(5):575–8, 1993.

25. Yazawa Y, Kitahara M: Immunofluorescent study of the endolymphatic sac in Meniere's disease. Acta Oto-Laryngol—Suppl 468:71–6, 1989.

26. Hughes GB, Barna BP, Kinney SE, Calabrese LH, Hamid MA: Nalepa NJ. Autoimmune endolymphatic hydrops: five-year review. Otolaryngol Head Neck Surg 98(3):221–5, 1988.

27. Rassekh CH, Harker LA: The prevalence of migraine in Meniere's disease. Laryngoscope 102(2):135–8, 1992.

28. Kimura R, Schuknecht HF: Membranous hydrops in the inner ear of the guinea pig after obliteration of the endolymphatic sac. Prac Otolaryngol 27:343–54, 1965.

29. Manni JJ, Kuijpers W. Experimental endolymphatic hydrops in the rat. Arch Otolaryngol Head Neck Surg. 112:423–6, 1986.

30. Manni JJ, Kuijpers W: Longitudinal flow of macromolecules in the endolymphatic space of the rat. An autoradiographical study. Hear Res 26:229–237, 1987.

31. Salt AN, Thalmann R, Marcus DC, et al: Direct measurement of longitudinal endolymph flow rate in the guinea pig cochlea. Hear Res 23:141–151, 1986.

32. Friberg U, Bagger-Sjoback D, Rask-Andersen H: The lateral intercellular spaces in the endolymphatic sac. A pathway for fluid transport? Acta Otolaryngol Suppl (Stockh) 426:1–17, 1985.

33. Cohen J, Morizono T: Changes in EP and inner ear ionic concentrations in experimental endolymphatic hydrops. Acta Otolaryngol (Stockh) 98:398–402, 1984.

34. Konishi T, Salt AM, Kimura R: Electrophysiological studies of experimentally induced endolymphatic hydrops in guinea pigs. In: Meniere's disease. Stuttgart: Thieme-Verlag, 1981;47–58.

35. Sziklai I: Ferrary E, Horner KC, Sterkers O, Amiel C. Time-related alteration of endolymph composition in an experimental model of endolymphatic hydrops. Laryngoscope 102(4):431–8, 1992.

36. Meyer zum Gottesberge AM: Imbalanced calcium homeostasis and endolymphatic hydrops. Acta Oto-Laryngol Suppl 460:18–27, 1988.

37. Ruding PR, Veldman JE, Berendsen W, Huizing EH: Scanning electron microscopy of hair cells, stereocilia and cross-linkage systems in experimentally induced endolymphatic hydrops. Euro Arch Oto-Rhino-Laryngol 248(6):313–8, 1991.

38. Sziklai I, Horner KC, Ferrary E, Sterkers O, Amiel C: Electrochemical composition of the cochlear fluids in the early experimental hydrops. Preliminary results. Acta Oto-Laryngol 107(5–6):371–4, 1989.

39. Larsen HC, Albers F, Jansson B, Angelborg C, Veldman J: Cochlear blood flow in endolymphatic hydrops. Acta Oto-Laryngol 106(5–6):404–8, 1988.

40. Tomiyama S, Yagi T, Sakagami M, Fukazawa K: Immunological pathogenesis of endolymphatic hydrops and its relation to Meniere's disease. Scan Microsc 7(3):907–19 discussion 919–920, 1993.

41. Tomiyama S, Nonaka M, Gotoh Y, Ikezono T, Yagi T: Immunological approach to Meniere's disease: vestibular immune injury following immune reaction of the endolymphatic sac. J Oto-Rhino-Laryngol Rel Special 56(1):11–8, 1994.

42. Yazawa Y, Kitahara M: Immunofluorescent study of the endolymphatic sac in Meniere's disease. Acta Oto-Laryngol Suppl 468:71–6, 1989.

43. Green JD Jr, Blum DJ, Harner SG: Longitudinal followup of patients with Meniere's disease. Otolaryngol Head Neck Surg 104(6):783–8, 1991.

44. Stahle J, Friberg U, Svedberg A: Long-term progression of Meniere's disease. Acta Oto-Laryngol Suppl 485:78–83, 1991.

45. Greven AJ, Oosterveld WJ: The contralateral ear in Meniere disease: A survey of 292 patients. Arch Otolaryngol 101:608–12, 1975.

46. Cawthorne T: Indications and results of labyrinthectomy via the oval window. In Pulec JL, ed. Meniere's disease. Philadelphia: WB Saunders Company, 557–61, 1968.

47. Paparella MM, Graiebie M: Bilaterality of Meniere's disease. Acta Otolaryngol (Stockh) 9:223–237, 1984.

48. Thomas K, Harrison MS: Long-term followup of 610 cases of Meniere's disease. Proc R Soc Med 64:853–6, 1971.

49. Rosenberg S, Silverstein H, Flanzer J, Wanamaker H: Bilateral Meniere's disease in surgical versus nonsurgical patients. Am J Otol 12(5):336–40, 1991.

50. Hausler R, Toupet M, Guidetti G, Basseres F, Montandon P: Meniere's disease in children. Am J Otolaryngol 8(4):187–93, 1987.

51. Klockhoff I, Lindblom U: Endolymphatic hydrops revealed by glycerol test. Acta Otolaryngol (Stockh) 61:459–462, 1966.

52. Magliulo G, Vingolo GM, Petti R, Cristofari P: Experimental endolymphatic hydrops and glycerol. Electrophysiologic study. Ann Otol, Rhinol Laryngol 102(8 Pt 1):596–9, 1993.

53. Mori N, Asai A, Suizu Y, Ohta K, Matsunaga T: Comparison between electrocochleography and glycerol test in the diagnosis of Meniere's disease. Scand Audiol 14(4):209–13, 1985.

54. Skalabrin TA, Mangham CA: Analysis of the glycerin test for Meniere's disease. Otolaryngol Head Neck Surg 96(3):282–8, 1987.

55. Yazawa Y, Kitahara M, Matsubara H: Clinical factors relating to the positive glycerol test for Meniere's disease. J Oto-Rhino-Laryngol Rel Special 52(3):149–55, 1990.

56. Wever EG, Bray CW: Auditory nerve impulses. Science 71:215, 1930.

57. Coats AC: The summating potential and Meniere's disease: I. Summating potential amplitude in Meniere's and non-Meniere's ears. Arch Otolaryngol 107:199–208, 1981.

58. Schmidt PH, Eggermont JJ, Odenthal DW: Study of Meniere's disease by electrocochleography. Acta Otolaryngol Suppl (Stockh) 316:75–84, 1974.

59. Aran JM, Rarey KE, Hawkins JR Fr: Functional and morphological changes in experimental endolymphatic hydrops. Acta Otolaryngol 97:547–57, 1984.

60. Durrant J, Dallos P: Modification of DIF: Summating potential comparison by stimulus biasing. J Acoust Soc Am 56:562–70, 1974.

61. Margolis RH, Levine SC, Fournier EM, Hunter LL, Smith SL, Lilly DJ: Tympanic electrocochleography: Normal and abnormal patterns of response. Audiology 31:8–24, 1992.

62. Van Deelen GW, Ruding PRJW, Veldman JE, et al: Electrocochleographic study of experimentally induced endolymphatic hydrops. Arch Otol Rhinol Laryngol 244:167–173, 1987.

63. Van Deelen GW, Ruding PRJW, Smoorenburg GW, et al: Electrocochleographic changes in relation to cochlear histopathology in experimental endolymphatic hydrops. Acta Otolaryngol 105:193–201, 1988.

64. Dauman R, Aran JM, Charlet de Sauvage R, Portmann M: Clinical significance of the summating potential in Meniere's disease. Am J Otol 9(1):31–8, 1988.

65. Levine SC, Margolis RH, Fournier EM, Winzenburg SM: Tympanic electrocochleography for evaluation of endolymphatic hydrops. Laryngoscope 102(6):614–22, 1992.

66. Ohashi T, Ochi K, Okada T, Takeyama I: Long-term follow-up of electrocochleogram in Meniere's disease. J Oto-Rhino-Laryngol Rel Special 53(3):131–6, 1991.

67. Mori N, Asai H, Sakagami M: The role of summating potential in the diagnosis and management of Meniere's disease. Acta Oto-Laryngol Suppl 501:51–3, 1993.

68. Torok N: Old and new in Meniere's disease. Laryngoscope 87:1870–1877, 1977.

69. Furstenberg AC, Lashmet FH, Lathrop F: Meniere's symptom complex: medical treatment. Ann Otol Rhinol Laryngol 43:1035–1047, 1934.

70. Klockhoff I, Lindblom U: Meniere's disease and hydrochlorothiazide: A critical analysis of symptoms and therapeutic effects. Acta Otolaryngol 63:347–365, 1967.

71. Ruckenstein MJ, Rutka JA, Hawke M: The treatment of Meniere's disease: Torok revisited. Laryngoscope 101(2):211–8, 1991.

72. Jackson CG, Glasscock ME, Davis We, et al. Medical management of Meniere's disease. Ann Otol Rhinol Laryngol 90:142–7, 1981.

73. van Deelen GW, Huizing EH: Use of a diuretic (Dyazide) in the treatment of Meniere's disease. A double-blind cross-over placebo-controlled study. J Oto-Rhino-Laryngol Rel Special 48(5):287–92, 1986.

74. Schuknecht HF: Ablation therapy in the management of Meniere's disease. Acta Otolaryngol (Suppl) Stockh 132:1–42, 1957.

75. Wilson W, Schuknecht S: Update on the use of streptomycin therapy for Meniere's disease. Am J Otol 2:108–111, 1980.

76. Graham MD, Kemink JL: Titration streptomycin therapy for bilateral Meniere's disease: A progress report. Am J Otol 5:534–35, 1984.

77. Odkvist LM: Middle ear ototoxic treatment for inner ear disease. Acta Otolaryngol Supp (Stockh) 457:83–6, 1989.

78. Beck C, Schmidt CL: Ten years of experience with intratympanically applied streptomycin (gentamicin) in the therapy of morbus Meniere. Arch Otorhinolaryngol 221:149–152, 1978.

79. Pyykko I, Ishizaki H, Kaasinen S, Aalto H: Intratympanic genta-

80. micin in bilateral Meniere's disease. Otolaryngol Head Neck Surg 110(2):162–7, 1994.

80. Shea JJ, Norris CH: Streptomycin perfusion of the labyrinth. In. Nadol JB (ed): Second International Symposium on Meniere's Disease, Cambridge, MA June 20–22, 1988. Amsterdam: Kugler & Ghedini, 1989.

81. Shea JJ Jr, Ge X: Streptomycin perfusion of the labyrinth through the round window plus intravenous streptomycin. Otolaryngol Clin North Am 27(2):317–24, 1994.

82. Monsell EM, Shelton C. Labyrinthotomy with streptomycin infusion: early results of a multicenter study. The LSI Multicenter Study Group. Am J Otol 13(5):416–22; discussion 422–5, 1992.

83. Schuknecht HF, Bartley M: Cochlear endolymphatic shunt for Meniere's disease. Am J Otol Suppl 20–22, 1985.

84. Portman G: Vertigo: Surgical treatment by opening the saccus endolymphaticus. Arch Otolaryngol 6:301–319, 1927.

85. McKee GJ, Kerr AG, Toner JG, Smyth GD: Surgical control of vertigo in Meniere's disease. Clin Otolaryngol 16(2):216–27, 1991.

86. Monsell EM, Wiet RJ: Endolymphatic sac surgery: methods of study and results. Am J Otol 9(5):396–402, 1988.

87. Telischi FF, Luxford WM: Long-term efficacy of endolymphatic sac surgery for vertigo in Meniere's disease. Otolaryngol Head Neck Surg 109(1):83–7, 1993.

88. Thomsen J, Bretlau P, Tos M, et al: Placebo effect in surgery for Meniere's disease. Arch Otolaryngol 107:271–77, 1981.

89. Thomsen J, Bretlau P, Tos M, et al: Placebo effect in surgery for Meniere's disease. Three year follow-up. Otolaryngol Head Neck Surg 91:183–6, 1983.

90. Thomsen J, Bretlau P, Tos M, et al: Endolymphatic sac-mastoid shunt surgery, a nonspecific treatment modality? Ann Otol Rhinol Laryngol 95:32–5, 1986.

91. Bretlau P, Thomsen J, Tos M, Johnsen NJ: Placebo effect in surgery for Meniere's disease: nine-year follow-up. Am J Otol 10(4):259–61, 1989.

92. Silverstein H, Smouha E, Jones R: Natural history vs. surgery for Meniere's disease. Otolaryngol Head Neck Surg 100:6–16, 1989.

93. Filipo R, Barbara M: Natural course of Meniere's disease in surgically selected patients. Ear Nose Throat J 73(4):254–7, 1994.

94. Cohen EJ, Mattox DE: Histologic and ultrastructural features of explanted Arenberg shunts. Arch Otolaryngol 120:326–332, 1994.

95. Hammerschlag PE, Schuknecht HF: Transcanal labyrinthectomy for intractable vertigo. Arch Otolaryngol 107:152–156, 1981.

96. Willatt DJ, Yung MW: Prognostic factors in labyrinthectomy. J Laryngol Otol 102(9):785–7, 1988

97. Levine SC, Glasscock M, McKennan KX: Long-term results of labyrinthectomy. Laryngoscope 100(2 Pt 1):125–7, 1990.

98. Glasscock ME III, Johnson GD, Poe DS: Long-term hearing results following middle fossa vestibular nerve section. Otolaryngol Head Neck Surg 100(1):35–40, 1989.

99. Magnan J, Bremond G, Chays A, Gignac D, Florence A: Vestibular neurotomy by retrosigmoid approach: Technique, indications, and results. Am J Otol 12(2):101–4, 1991.

100. Barany R: Diagnose von Krankheitserscheinungen im Bereiche des Otolithenapparatus. Acta Otolaryngol 2:434–437, 1921.

101. Dix M. Hallpike C: The pathology, symptomatology, and diagnosis of certain common disorders of the vestibular system. 61:987–1017, 1952.

102. Nedzelski JM, Barber HO, McIlmoyl L: Diagnosis in a dizziness unit. J Otolaryngol 15:101–4, 1986.

103. Froehling DA, Silverstein MD, Mohr DN, Beatty CW, Offord KP, Ballard DJ: Benign positional vertigo: Incidence and prognosis in a population-based study in Olmsted County, Minnesota. Mayo Clin Proc 66:596–601, 1991.

104. Katsarkas A, Kirkham TN: Paroxysmal positional vertigo: a study of 255 cases. J Otolaryngol 7:320–330, 1978

105. Baloh RW, Honrubia Y, Jacobsen K: Benign positional vertigo: clinical and oculographic features of 240 cases. Neurology 37: 371–378, 1987.

106. Schuknecht HF, Ruby RRF: Cupulolithiasis. Adv Otorhinolaryngol 20:434–43, 1973.

107. Cohen B, Suzuki JI, Bender MB: Eye movements from semicircular canal nerve stimulation in the cat. Ann Otolaryngol 73: 153–69, 1964.

108. Schuknecht HF: Positional vertigo: clinical and experimental observations. Trans Am Acad Ophthalmol Otolaryngol 66: 319–32, 1962.

109. Hall SF, Ruby RRF, McClure JA: The mechanics of benign paroxysmal vertigo. J Otolaryngol 8:151–158, 1979.

110. Parnes LS, McClure JA: Free-floating endolymph particles: A new operative finding during posterior semicircular canal occlusion. Laryngoscope 102:988–92, 1992.

111. Kveton JF, Kashgarian M: Particulate matter within the membranous labyrinth: Pathologic or normal? Am J Otol 15:173–6, 1994.

112. McClure JA: Horizontal canal BPV. J Otolaryngol 14:30–35, 1985.

113. Baloh RW, Jacobson K, Honrubia V: Horizontal semicircular canal variant of benign positional vertigo. Neurology 43: 2542–2549, 1993.

114. McClure JA, Willett JM: Lorazepam and diazepam in the treatment of benign paroxysmal vertigo. J Otolaryngol 9:472–477, 1980.

115. Fujino A, Tokumasu K, Yosio S, Naganuma H, Yoneda S, Nakamura K: Vestibular training for benign paroxysmal positional vertigo. Arch Otolaryngol Head Neck Surg 120:497–504, 1994.

116. Cawthorne T: The physiologic basis for head exercises. J Chart Soc Physiother 30:106–107, 1944.

117. Brandt T, Daroff RB: Physical therapy for benign paroxysmal positional vertigo. Arch Otolaryngol 106:484–485, 1980

118. Toupet M, Semont A: La physiotherapie du vertige paroxystique benin. In: Hausler R, ed. Les vertige d'origine peripherique et centrale. Paris: Ipsen, 21–27, 1985.

119. Norre ME, Beckers A: Exercise treatment for paroxysmal positional vertigo: comparison of two types of exercises. Arch Otolaryngol 244:291–4, 1987.

120. Semont A, Freyss G, Vitte E: Curing the BPPV with a liberatory maneuver. Adv Otorhinolaryngol 42:290–293, 1988.

121. Epley JM: The canalith repositioning procedure: For treatment of benign paroxysmal positional vertigo. Otolaryngol Head Neck Surg 107(3):399–404, 1992.

122. Blakley BW: A randomized, controlled assessment of the canalith repositioning maneuver. Otolaryngol Head Neck Surg 110:391–396, 1994.

123. Harvey SA, Hain TC, Adamiec LC: Modified liberatory maneuver: Effective treatment for benign paroxysmal positional vertigo. Laryngoscope 104:1206–1212, 1994.

124. Welling DB, Barnes DE: Particle repositioning maneuver for benign paroxysmal positional vertigo. Laryngoscope 104: 946–949, 1994.

125. Herdman SJ, Tusa R, Zee D, Proctor LR, Mattox DE: Single treatment approaches to benign paroxysmal positional vertigo. Arch Otolaryngol Head Neck Surg 119:450–54, 1993.

126. Gacek RR: Transection of the posterior ampullary nerve for relief of benign paroxysmal positional vertigo. Ann Otol Rhinol Laryngol 83:596–605, 1974.

127. Parnes LS, McClure JA: Posterior semicircular canal occlusion for intractable benign paroxysmal positional vertigo. Ann Otol Rhinol Laryngol 99:330–334, 1990.

128. Parnes LS, McClure JA: Posterior semicircular canal occlusion in the normal hearing ear. Otolaryngol Head Neck Surg 104: 52–57, 1991.

129. Anthony PF: Partitioning the labyrinth for benign paroxysmal positional vertigo: clinical and histologic findings. Am J Otol 14:334–342, 1993.

130. Ryu JH: Vestibular neuritis: An overview using a classical case. Acta Otolaryngol Suppl (Stockh) 503:125–130, 1993.

131. Okinaka Y, Sekitani T, Okazaki H, Miura M, Tahara T: Progress of caloric response of vestibular neuronitis. Acta Otolaryngol Suppl (Stockh) 503:18–22, 1993.

132. Zee DS: Perspectives on the pharmacotherapy of vertigo. Arch Otolaryngol 111:609–612, 1985.

133. Brandt T: Vestibular neuritis in vertigo: its multisensory syndromes. London: Springer-Verlag, 27–40, 1991.

134. Ishikawa K, Edo M, Togawa K: Clinical observation of 32 cases of vestibular neuronitis. Acta Otolaryngol Suppl (Stockh) 503: 13–15, 1993.

135. Cawthorne T, Cooksey FS: Vestibular injuries. Rehabilitation in vestibular injuries. Proc Soc Lond B Biol Sci 39:270–278, 1946.

136. Herdman SJ: Exercise strategies in vestibular disorders. Ear Nose Throat J 12:961–964, 1989.

137. Herdman SJ, Borello DF, Whitney SL: Treatment of vestibular hypofunction. In: Herdman SJ, ed. Vestibular rehabilitation. Philadelphia: FA Dans, 287–315, 1994.

138. Magnusson M, Norrving B: Cerebellar infarctions and 'vestibular neuritis'. Acta Otolaryngol Suppl (Stockh) 503:64–66, 1993.

57 Presbycusis

John H. Mills

Presbyacusis is defined generally as the hearing loss associated with increasing chronological age. It is a common problem today and will become even more significant in the future. Currently, according to the National Center for Health Statistics, some 20 million Americans have impaired hearing and approximately 75% of these people are over age 55. In the 25 year period between 1976 and 2000, the number of persons below age 75 will increase by 23%, the percentage between age 75 and 84 will increase by 57%, and the percentage over age 84 will increase by 91%. Indeed, by the year 2030 the elderly will comprise 32% of the population, an increase of 250%. As many as 60 to 75% of these older persons will be hearing impaired. Because of the increasing number of older Americans, high-prevalence problems such as age-related hearing loss and other chronic disabling conditions (balance, vision, arthritis) will place extensive and novel demands on the health care system.

BACKGROUND

The medical-scientific history of presbyacusis is relatively recent and rich. Although Toynbee[1] in 1849 is perhaps the first to write about age-related hearing loss and to prescribe a treatment (application of solutions of silver nitrate or mercurous chloride to the external auditory canal), Zwaardemaker[2] in 1891 is credited with the first accurate description of presbyacusis. With the clever use of Dalton whistles, Zwaardemaker demonstrated that older persons had far more difficulty detecting high-pitched sounds than younger persons. By the use of bone-conduction testing, he correctly considered age-related hearing loss to be of cochlear origin. Since the 1930's anatomic and histopathologic changes have been observed at nearly every location in the aging auditory system from the external ear with collapsing ear canals to neural degeneration of the auditory brainstem and temporal lobe.

Of the many investigations of presbyacusis, perhaps the most quoted and most extensive source of histopathologic data is the temporal bone studies of Schuknecht and colleagues.[3,4] In a number of studies, they have identified four types of categories of presbyacusis: 1) Sensory, characterized by atrophy and degeneration of the sensory and supporting cells; 2) Neural, typified by loss of neurons in the cochlea and central nervous system (CNS); 3) Metabolic, characterized by atrophy of the lateral wall of the cochlea, especially the stria vascularis; 4) Mechanical, where the inner ear changes its properties with a resulting inner-ear conductive hearing loss. Schuknecht has estimated the prevalence of each type as follows: Sensory, 11.9%; Neural, 30.7%; Metabolic, 34.6%; and Mechanical, 22.8%.[4] Each of these categories is hypothesized to have a characteristic audiometric configuration (i.e., sloping, flat) and, therefore, to be audiometrically identifiable. In subsequent studies, considerable difficulty was encountered in correlating the audiometric configuration with histopathologic observations and in differentiating one type of presbyacusis from another on the basis of the audiometric configuration.[5,6] The problem is that the audiometric configurations of older persons do not form clearly defined categories, and histopathologic changes at the level of light and electron microscopy are almost always observed at multiple sites in a given aging ear. Other studies suggest that the metabolic type of presbyacusis has a low prevalence, and that the mechanical type is purely theoretical and remains unobserved in temporal bone material.[7] Thus, although the research and clinical history of presbyacusis is rich, controversy and uncertainty remain. Much of the controversy and uncertainty can be explained, and in some instances resolved, whereas in other instances much additional research and careful clinical study are required.

TERMINOLOGY

One reason for uncertainty and controversy is that different authors use different definitions of the term presbycusis. Indeed, the correct spelling is an issue, i.e., presbyacusis versus presbycusis. Here we use "presbycusis" which is the technically, historically, and epistimologically correct spelling.

Another reason for confusion is that the term presbycusis is used loosely to describe a seemingly endless list of genetic, environmental, and disease states which can cause hearing loss in an older person. Oftentimes, presbycusis is used to refer to hearing loss due purely to the natural process of aging. More often, hearing loss is called presbycusis if the person is beyond the fifth decade, without consideration of disease, genetics, or other factors. In many studies older persons are considered homogeneous and are grouped regardless of hearing levels or are grouped if their hearing loss exceeds an arbitrary criterion.

Some of the uncertainty can be reduced by the use of the terms presbyacusis, socioacusis, and nosoacusis.[8] A generic definition of presbyacusic is age-related hearing loss (or threshold shift) which is the effect of aging in combination with lifelong exposures to nonoccupational noise, ototoxic agents, diet, drugs, and other miscellaneous factors. A more restrictive, precise definition of presbyacusis is hearing loss which increases as a function of chronological age and is attributable to "aging" *per se*. This "purely aging" hearing loss probably has a genetic basis. It may be correlated with age-related deterioration or declines in other senses especially balance, vision, and touch.

Socioacusis is defined as the hearing loss produced primarily by exposure to nonoccupational noise in combination with lifestyle factors such as diet and exercise. Nosoacusis is the hearing loss attributable to diseases with ototoxic effects. Thus, the hearing loss assessed in a person into the fifth decade and beyond is the combined result of aging, nosoacusis, socioacusis and possibly, for many persons, exposure to occupational noise as well. It is important for medical and legal reasons to differentiate presbyacusis from socioacusis, nosoacusis and occupational hearing loss.[9]

ADDITIVITY OF PRESBYACUSIS, SOCIOACUSIS, AND NOSOACUSIS

Most laboratory (with animals) and field studies indicate that hearing losses caused by exposure to noise are additive (in decibels) with the hearing loss attributed to presbyacusis (in the strict sense of the word).[9] A small sensorineural hearing loss of 25 dB at age 25, for example, seemingly has little social or medical relevance; however, by age 70 a hearing loss of 25 dB caused

almost totally by the aging process is added to the existing sensorineural hearing loss. The result is a moderate-severe sensorineural hearing loss of 50 dB. In other words, a seemingly minor hearing loss at a young age in combination with a number of seemingly minor noise exposures produces severe results when the effects of presbyacusis become evident. Clearly, the best protection from (prevention of) presbyacusis in the general sense of the word is to have highly organized hearing conservation programs and public education about the effects of noise and other ototoxic agents.

Rules for combining hearing losses attributable to presbyacusis, nosoacusis, and socioacusis are not always straightforward. In the medical-legal assessment of occupational hearing loss it is assumed that presbyacusic effects (aging plus socioacusis plus nosoacusis) add in decibels to the hearing loss produced by noise. This approach is supported by laboratory and field data for groups of subjects under a limited set of exposure conditions. For individual subjects and for complicated noise exposures, the procedures for allocation of hearing loss into different components are under development.[9]

EPIDEMIOLOGY

Over the past 25 years or so there has been a significant epidemiologic effort to describe hearing levels as a function of chronological age. Two sets of data have survived extensive scrutiny and are now part of an international standard, ISO 1999: "Acoustics: Determination of Occupational Noise Exposure and Estimation of Noise-Induced Hearing Impairment." Figure 57–1A age-related permanent threshold shifts at audiometric frequencies for males and females. These data are referred to as Data Base A in the ISO 1999 standard and are considered to represent highly-screened subjects. That is, the data in Figure 57–1A represent "pure aging" effects as well as socioacusis. Most of the hearing loss attributable to occupational hearing loss has been eliminated although a small nosoacusic effect may be present. Figure 57–1B gives epidemiologic data, referred to as Data Base B in the ISO 1999 standard, and are considered to reflect "pure aging" effects, socioacusis, some nosoacusis, and some effects attributable to occupational hearing loss. As shown in Figure 57–1, hearing loss in the higher frequencies is measurable by age 30, it increases systematically to age 60 (and beyond), it is largest at 4 and 6 kHz, and it is much larger in males than in females. There are also significant differences between Figure 57–1A (Data Base A) and Figure 57–1B (Data Base B), presumably due to differences in subject selection. Small effects due to occupational noise and nosoacusis were eliminated in Data Base A. Significant debate exists currently about the appropriateness and validity of Data Base A

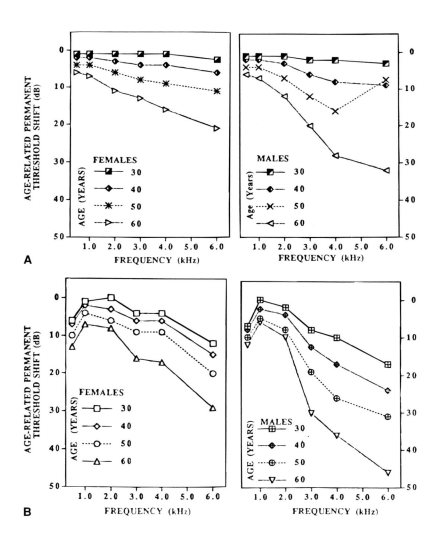

Fig. 57–1. Epidemiologic data showing hearing levels and chronological age. Data are from an international standard, ISO 1999. A is referred to as Data Base A and represents a sample that was highly screened in an effort to eliminate the potential influence of the effects of exposure to noise. B is also from ISO 1999 and is referred to as Data Base B. This sample is less well screened than Data Base A, and may contain data from persons with a history of exposure to noise.

and B, particularly in a medical-legal context involving the assessment of occupational noise-induced hearing loss.

Data from Figure Figure 57–1A and B have been replotted in Figure 57–2 to show the average hearing loss at 0.5, 1, 2, and 3 kHz as a function of chronological age. The mean hearing loss at these particular audiometric test frequencies is especially meaningful because this combination of test frequencies comprise those used in the computation of hearing handicap as recommended by the American Academy of Otolaryngology-Head and Neck Surgery (AAO). As Figure 57–2 shows, hearing loss increases systematically from age 20 through age 75. There are at least two remarkable features to Figure 57–2. One is that the largest difference between the worst case (males, Data Base B) and best case (females, Data Base A) is about 5 dB. One could suggest, perhaps strongly, that much of the debate about Data Base A and B is "much ado about nothing," i.e., 5 dB. This line of thinking is supported by the fact that, even at age 75, the hearing loss is only about 20 dB. According to the AAO, 1979 definitions

of hearing handicap, the average hearing loss at 0.5, 1, 2, and 3 kHz must exceed 25 dB to be considered a hearing handicap. In other words, according to the data of Figure 57–2 and the AAO 1979 definition of hearing handicap, substantially less than 50% of the population, male or female, have a hearing handicap even at age 75.

Other less selective epidemiologic data suggest that the prevalence of hearing handicap among older persons is substantially higher than that indicated by the epidemiologic data used in the ISO 1999 standard. Using 1662 subjects from the famous Framingham study of cardiovascular disease[10] Gates et al. reported that 55% met or exceeded the AAO, 1979 medical-legal definition of hearing handicap. The difference between results of Gates et al. and those of ISO 1999 reflect sampling differences, and the inclusion of subjects older than age 75 in the Gates et al. sample.

In addition to an audiologic assessment, hearing handicap can be assessed more subjectively using questionnaires such as the Hearing Handicap Inventory for the Elderly.[11] The correspondence between ob-

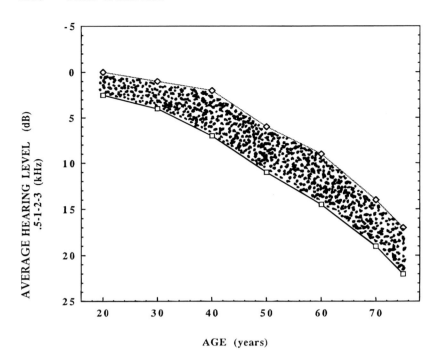

Fig. 57–2. Data from Figure 57–1 have been replotted to show the average hearing loss (0.5, 1, 2, and 3 kHz) as a function of age. The shaded area represents the difference between the "best case," i.e., women of Data Base A, and the "worst case," i.e., men of Data Base B.

jective, audiologic measures of hearing handicap and subjective measures from self-reports and questionnaires suggest that the AAO measure of handicap tends to overestimate handicap for older persons with mild-moderate hearing losses and to underestimate handicap for older persons with severe hearing losses.[11] Of course, there are many reasons for discrepancies between subjective and audiologic estimates of hearing handicap. One general rule emerges from questionnaires and epidemiologic studies of hearing handicap in older persons, namely, that the pure tone average of 0.5, 1, 2, and 3 kHz must exceed about 30 dB before most older persons consider themselves to have a hearing problem. Thus, there are indeed millions of older hearing handicapped persons in the United States.

Although much of the discussion has centered on the audiometric frequencies from 0.5 to 3 kHz, one of the more dramatic features of age-related hearing loss is the decline of auditory sensitivity at higher frequencies.[12,13] Figure 57–3A shows increasing hearing loss from age 20 to 29 to age 50 to 59 for test frequencies at and above 8 kHz. By age 50 to 59 the hearing loss at 16 kHz is greater than 60 dB. Figure 57–3B shows longitudinal threshold changes (the same group of observers) over the age range of 70 to 81 years, including thresholds for test frequencies up to 8 kHz. Hearing levels at 4 and 8 kHz exceed 50 dB by age 70 and exceed 70 dB at 8 kHz by age 79. Hearing loss at frequencies above 8 kHz is even more pronounced. Clearly, there is a dramatic age-related decline in auditory sensitivity at high frequencies. Indeed, it appears that hearing loss starts in the second decade (or earlier) in the frequency

range between 16 and 20 kHz, proceeds systematically in magnitude in the 16 kHz region, and spreads systematically downward in the frequency domain. By the eighth decade, the hearing loss is severe, even at 1 and 2 khz.

The interpretation of epidemiologic data which show a loss of high-frequency sensitivity at 16 to 20 kHz, when 10 and 19 year olds are compared with 20 to 29 year olds, is not straightforward. One point of view is that these age-related changes in hearing thresholds, as well as systematic declines in the number of outer-hair cells starting at birth and continuing throughout the lifetime of the individual,[14] are genetically determined, age-dependent events. That is, these age-related events are totally endogenous in origin. They are independent of exogenous events such as diet, exposure to environmental noise (socioacusis), and disease (nosoacusis). Another point of view is that these age-related changes in the ear and hearing reflect the combined effect of genetics, socioacusis, and nosoacusis. In this latter formulation socioacusis is given a major role, almost surely because of the famous Mabaan study.[15]

A hearing survey of Mabaans, a tribe located in a remote and undeveloped part of Africa, showed exceptionally good auditory sensitivity for males and females in their sixth-to-ninth decades. In addition to the lack of exposure to occupational nose, no exposure to firearms, and exposure only to very low-levels of environmental noise, the Mabaans were reported to lead a low-stress lifestyle, have a low-fat diet, and a very low prevalence of cardiovascular disease. This study was quoted widely in lay and professional publications, and became the scientific basis for the thesis that persons in Western industrialized societies were at risk of deafness because of socioacusis. Later analysis of the Mabaan data indicated very few differences between hearing levels of Mabaans and hearing levels of well-screened individuals from industrialized societies. One possible exception was that the hearing levels of Mabaan males over the age of 60 were slightly better in the high frequencies than their Western male counterparts. Additional criticism of the original Mabaan data involved the accuracy of the age of the Mabaan subjects. Apparently, the exact ages of the Mabaan subjects could not be confirmed. Lastly, important epidemiologic details of the Mabaan sample could not be determined, and thus the validity of the sampling was questionable, i.e., a highly biased sample. It is possible, for example, that only the healthiest subjects were

available and that these subjects also had the best hearing. Thus, the Mabaan data are equivocal in their support of the thesis of profound effects of socioacusis and nosoacusis on age-related hearing levels.

Whereas the Mabaan data are equivocal in their support of the role of nosoacusis and socioacusis in age-related hearing loss, experiments with laboratory animals clearly support the idea of an age-related hearing loss that is independent of socioacusis, nosoacusis, and exposure to occupational noise. In light of the complexities of the genetic, environmental, and disease-state factors which may affect the hearing of older persons, there are several ongoing efforts to develop animal models of presbyacusis. An appropriate animal model may allow identification and control of the most pertinent variables as well systematic studies of the biologic basis of presbyacusis.

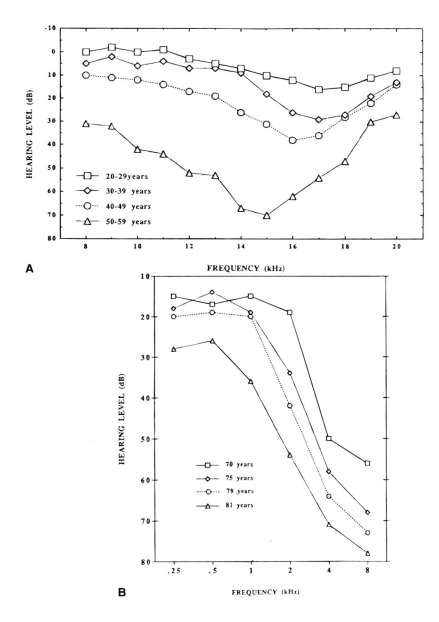

Fig. 57–3. Hearing loss at high frequencies. **A.** Hearing levels at test frequencies at and above 8 kHz over the age range from 20 to 59 (after ref. 12). **B.** Hearing levels at test frequencies of 0.25 to 8 kHz measured in a longitudinal study covering the age range from 70 to 81 (after ref. 13).

RESULTS FROM AGING LABORATORY ANIMALS

In many species of animals, auditory thresholds estimated from electrophysiologic potentials arising from the auditory nerve and brainstem increase as a function of chronological age.[16,17] The age-related decline in auditory function occurs in animals who are born and reared in acoustically controlled environments where sound levels rarely exceed 40 dBA. In addition to control of the acoustic environment, none of the animals received antibiotics or other drugs. Conductive hearing loss was eliminated as a potential source of the measured hearing loss. Clearly, environmental noise, drugs, disease, plus trauma did not have a causative role in the hearing losses observed in the aging animals. Thus, the notion that presbyacusis is not an aging effect *per se* but the combined effect of socioacusis and nosoacusis is not supported by laboratory experiments with several species of animals.

Perhaps the most dramatic feature of age-related hearing loss in laboratory animals is the variability between animals. For example, in a longitudinal study of aging gerbils, some animals, at the one extreme, had normal or nearly normal auditory sensitivity from 1 to 16 kHz, whereas at the other extreme, some animals did not respond to signals presented at levels of 80 dB SPL. Variability of this magnitude is remarkable given that chronological age, environment (temperature, humidity, air quality), acoustic history, and diet of the animals is virtually identical. These data and others involving different inbred strains of mice suggest a genetic basis for age-related hearing loss, at least in laboratory animals.[16,17]

In addition to a qualitative/quantitative correspondence between age-related hearing loss measured in aging rodents and audiograms of 60- to 70-year-old humans,[16] many of the histopathologic observations made on human temporal bones have been confirmed and extended on experimental animals.[17–19] In aging rodents, there is usually a small loss of sensory (outer) hair cells in the most basal and the most apical regions of the cochlea. Nerve loss, as indicated by loss of spiral ganglion cells, is most pronounced in the base of the cochlea. The lateral wall of the cochlea including the stria vascularis usually shows degeneration originating in both the base and apex and extending to mid-cochlear regions as the animal ages; however, in some animals there is a patchy loss of stria vascularis. Thus, in several species of animals, anatomic studies of cochlear material demonstrate at least three of the histopathologic conditions described in humans by Schuknecht and colleagues, namely, sensory, neural, and metabolic presbyacusis. In animals, all three types are usually present in each animal.

If there is a prominent (dominant) type of presbyacusis in laboratory animals, it is probably the metabolic category.[18] In addition to age-related, systematic degeneration of the stria vascularis starting in both the apex and base of the cochlea and proceeding medially, preceding and accompanying this degeneration is not loss of the protein, Na,K-ATPase. Sometimes the loss of this important protein, which is detectable using immunohistochemical techniques, occurs when the stria vascularis appears normal under light and electron microscopic examination. Thus, a normal appearing stria vascularis in an older ear is no assurance that the stria vascularis is normal. Accordingly, the prevalence of "metabolic presbyacusis" may prove to be substantially higher in humans when the appropriate immunohistochemical techniques are applied to the study of aging human temporal bones.

The most prominent changes in the physiologic properties of the aging ear are losses of auditory nerve function as indicated by increased thresholds of the compound action potential (CAP) of the auditory nerve.[17–19] This loss of CAP reflects a loss of sensory cells and spiral ganglion cells. Slopes of input-output functions of the CAP in aging animals are decreased even when the loss of auditory thresholds is only 5 to 10 dB. In other words, as the signal intensity is increased the amplitude of the CAP increases by a fraction of that observed in young animals with normal hearing or young animals with noise-induced or drug-induced hearing losses. These shallow input-output functions of the CAP are also reflected in shallow input-output functions of auditory brainstem responses. Thus, what appears to be abnormal function of the auditory brainstem in older animals reflects only the abnormal output of the auditory nerve. The reduced amplitudes of action potentials observed in aging ears is probably reflective of asynchronous or poorly synchronized neural activity in auditory nerve. The pathologic basis of asynchronized activity in the auditory nerve is unknown, but probably involves the nature of the synapse between individual auditory nerve fibers and the attachment to the inner-hair cell.

A second major difference between the presbyacusic ear and the ear with noise-induced hearing loss is the endolymphatic potential, i.e., the 80- to 90-millivolt, dc resetting potential in the scala media of the cochlea.[18] In aging animals, this dc potential is oftentimes reduced significantly and proportionally to losses/degeneration of the stria vascularis. Moreover, in experimental animals hearing losses can be eliminated by introducing a dc voltage into scala media and raising a low endolymphatic potential, i.e., 15 millivolts, to its normal value of about 80 millivolts.

A third difference between the physiology of the aging ear and the ear with noise-induced or drug-induced injury of the cochlea involves the nonlinear phenomenon of two-tone rate suppression, i.e., activity of the auditory nerve elicited by one tone is suppressed or eliminated by the addition of a second tone of different frequency.[19] In ears of quiet-reared aging animals, the mechanism of two-tone rate suppression appears to remain intact. In contrast, in noise-induced or drug-induced injury of the cochlea, a reduction or complete loss of two-tone rate suppression may be the first indicator of injury of the cochlea, usually outer-hair cells. These data are an excellent indicator that the pathologic bases of age-related hearing loss are fundamentally different from the pathologic bases of most forms of noise-induced or drug-induced hearing loss.

In summary, animal experiments conducted under strict conditions show age-related declines in auditory function that indicate a "pure aging" hearing loss. Most of the pathologic anatomy associated with this "pure aging" hearing loss is in the cochlea and includes loss of sensory cells and nerve fibers as well as a degeneration of the stria vascularis. In experimental animals most of the hearing loss can be accounted for by anatomic, physiologic, and biochemical changes in the auditory periphery. Indeed, there is no need to include the auditory CNS in an explanation of age-related hearing loss, even when the criterion measure of age-related hearing loss is derived from potentials arising from the auditory brainstem. Nearly all changes observed in auditory brainstem potentials can be explained by alterations in the auditory periphery.

Explanations of age-related changes in auditory brainstem potentials in terms of alterations in the auditory periphery run counter to the current dogma which is that there is a significant, perhaps dominant, component of presbyacusis which involves degeneration of the auditory CNS. To discuss the issue of CNS involvement in age-related hearing loss let us turn to data from human subjects, especially data on speech discrimination and auditory evoked potentials.

PERCEPTION OF SPEECH AND OTHER COMPLEX AUDITORY SIGNALS

The term "phonemic regression" was coined to describe a disproportionate difficulty in speech perception relative to the magnitude of hearing loss of older persons. Later, many studies of speech discrimination and other complex listening tasks showed results with older subjects that were difficult to interpret with respect to the audiogram alone.[20-21] With the ready availability of many published papers showing degenerative changes in the auditory brainstem and cortex of older persons, there evolved a viewpoint that a significant component of age-related hearing loss is attributable to the decline of the auditory CNS. Of course, the auditory CNS is involved in age-related hearing loss; however, the extent of the involvement of the CNS in presbyacusis is currently receiving much debate. Here, we should like to examine the CNS issue starting with data on speech discrimination by older persons.

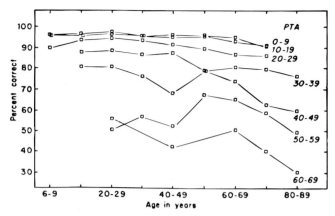

Fig. 57–4. Speech discrimination as a function of age with average hearing loss at 0.5, 1, and 2 kHz as the parameter. PTA represents the pure-tone average. Data are from 2162 persons (after ref. 20).

Perhaps the largest qualitative/quantitative description of speech discrimination as a function of age and hearing loss is provided by Jerger[20] from the clinical records of 2162 patients. Figure 57–4 shows percent correct on phonetically balanced (PB) words as a function of chronological age. The parameter on the figure is the pure-tone average of 0.5, 1, and 2 kHz. Figure 57–4 shows that speech discrimination declines systematically as a function of chronological age; however, the decline with age is dramatically dependent upon hearing loss. That is, for subjects with very little hearing loss (less than 30 dB) the decline with age is measurable but small through age 70. On the other hand, for subjects with moderate-to-severe hearing losses, the decline with age is noteworthy, particularly for persons between the ages of 45 and 85 with hearing losses of 40 to 49 dB, 50 to 59 dB, and 60 to 69 dB. In different words, when hearing loss as indicated by the pure-tone average is held constant, speech discrimination scores decreased between the ages of 40 and 80 for moderate (greater than 40 dB) to severe (60 dB) hearing losses. In contrast, age had very little effect as long as the pure tone average is less than about 30 to 39 dB. A remarkable and perhaps the most noteworthy feature of Figure 57–4 is that persons over the age range of 50 to 80 perform as well as 25 year olds as long as their average hearing loss at 0.5, 1, and 2 kHz is less than 35 dB or so. This fact runs counter to the stereotype of 70- to 80-year-old persons.

Performance on tests of speech discrimination by older persons is shown (Fig. 57–5) for PB words, two versions of the Speech Perception in Noise (SPIN) test, and synthetic sentence identification (SSI).[21] Figure 57–5A shows that the audiograms of groups of persons over the age range from 50 to 90 were nearly identical (±3 dB); however, statistical analysis of the speech discrimination data showed that performance on all tests (except the SSI) were not affected by age. That is, when

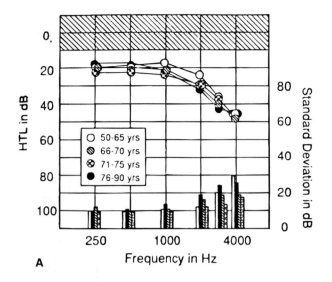

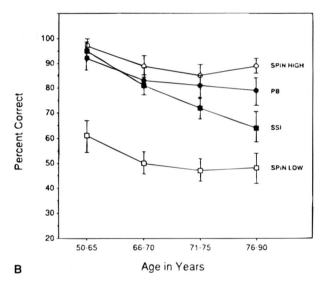

Fig. 57–5. Speech discrimination as function of age for four speech discrimination tests: SPIN (Speech Perception in Noise) high and SPIN low; PB (phonetically balanced); and SSI (synthetic sentence identification). **A.** Four age groups have nearly identical audiograms (after ref. 21.)

hearing levels were equated, there were no age-related declines in performance on tests of speech discrimination in persons over the age range of about 60 to 85. However, results on the SSI showed a significant decline with age.

There are many additional studies of speech discrimination using background noises, degraded speech signals, reverberation, and other variations which resulted in a more difficult listening task than the usual speech discrimination test which is done in quiet listening conditions.[22,23] Many of these studies show age-related effects; however, the interpretation of many of these data showing age-related declines in auditory behavior are not straightforward because the

subjects usually have significant hearing loss as indicated by the audiogram. Accordingly, some persons believe there is a large CNS component to presbyacusis whereas others believe and have shown that speech discrimination by older persons is predictable given the audiometric hearing loss, and the audibility of the speech material.[24] Indeed, as much as 95% of the variance in speech discrimination results can be accounted for on the basis of the audiogram.[24] In other cases where predictions of performance by older persons under noisy listening conditions are in error by 20 to 25%, it is still not necessary to invoke the involvement of the CNS although this is usually the interpretation.[23]

Although there are large individual differences in auditory behavior among individuals that are predictable by individual differences in auditory thresholds, there are many age-related declines in auditory behavior that are not strongly associated with auditory thresholds. This is most evident using the monaural SSI test and in binaural listening tasks conducted under acoustically stressful conditions.[21] In many binaural experiments using older subjects, age-related declines are observed that appear to be independent of peripheral hearing loss; however, it is oftentimes difficult to separate truly central processing disorders from disorders initiated by a pathologic input from the aging cochlea.

AUDITORY-EVOKED POTENTIALS

With the development of straightforward techniques to measure evoked potentials arising from the auditory nerve, brainstem and auditory cortex, one might expect there to have been significant progress in evaluating the aging auditory nervous system of human subjects. Whereas there indeed are many publications describing age-related declines in properties of evoked potentials,[16,17] namely, increased latencies and declines in amplitude as repetition rate is increased, most studies with aging humans show effects that are nearly, if not totally, explainable by peripheral hearing loss.[17] A noteworthy exception may be late cortical potentials (300 msec latency). Data from aging animals, however, show that evoked potentials from both the auditory nerve and brainstem are altered in amplitude and latency, and that these alterations are independent or nearly so of age-related changes in auditory thresholds. Moreover, the age-related changes observed in brainstem potentials nearly always reflect similar changes observed at the level of the auditory nerve. Thus, in humans (as in experimental animals) it is proving difficult to show age-related declines in the function of the auditory brainstem that are independent of age-related declines in the auditory periphery.

ALLEVIATION/TREATMENT

Assuming any problems with the external and middle ear are diagnosed and treated, assuming other medical issues are under control, assuming a diagnosis of presbycusis in the general sense, the best treatment currently available is a hearing aid. The successful use of hearing aids by older persons and the hearing-impaired in general is mixed. There is a literature of substantial magnitude which reports on the successful or unsuccessful use of hearing aids by the elderly. Many older persons who would clearly benefit from an aid do not use one. The reasons for not using an aid or being a dissatisfied user include cost, stigma of a hearing handicap and of being old, difficulty in manipulating controls, and too little benefit particularly in the presence of background noise.

In a large group of older persons (N = 210) who are participants in a longitudinal study of age-related hearing loss, 64% (N = 130) are candidates for a hearing aid. Candidacy by very conservative audiologic criteria is an SRT of 30 dB in the better ear, or hearing level greater than 40 dB at 3 and 4 kHz in the better ear. Using these criteria, more than half (N = 65 of 130) of those who are considered to be excellent candidates have never tried a hearing aid, and only one third (N = 40 of 130) of candidates were successful hearing aid users. The remaining persons (N = 25), for one or several reasons, were dissatisfied hearing aid users. Of those who did not meet the conservative criteria for a hearing aid (N = 80), our clinical judgment suggested that at least 40 to 50% of these persons (N = 40) would benefit from an aid. Clearly, the older persons in our longitudinal study were uninformed about hearing aids, poorly served, or underserved. Indeed, it is our opinion that as a result of excellent advances in hearing aid technology in the last five years, in combination with improved fitting techniques, nearly every older hearing-impaired person should be considered a potential candidate for a hearing aid.

Acknowledgments

Preparation of this chapter was supported by NIH (P01 DC00422). Judy R. Dubno provided helpful comments on the final document. Nancy Kinsley and Barbara Kranz-Dupree assisted in preparation of the figures and final document.

REFERENCES

1. Toynbee J: On the pathology and treatment of the deafness attendant upon old age. Mon J Med Sci 1849;1–12.

2. Zwaardemaker H: Der Verlust on hohen Tonen mit zunehmendem Alter. Ein neues Gesetz. Arch Ohren-nasen Kehlkopfheilkunde 32:53–56, 1891.

3. Schuknecht HF: Pathology of the Ear. Cambridge, MA: Harvard University Press, 1974;388–403.

4. Schuknecht HF, et al: Atrophy of the stria vascularis, a common cause for hearing loss. Laryngoscope 84:1777–1821, 1974.

5. Suga F, Lindsay JR: Histopathological observations of presbyacusis. Ann Otol 85:169, 1976.

6. Lowell SH, and Paparella MM: Presbyacusis: What is it? Laryngoscope 87:1710–1717, 1977.

7. Soucek S, and Michaels L (eds): Hearing Loss in the Elderly, New York: Springer-Verlag, 1990.

8. Ward WD: Effects of noise exposure on auditory sensitivity. In Handbook of Physiology, Section 9: Reactions to Environmental Agents, edited by Lee DHK. Bethesda, MD: American Physiological Society, 1977;1–15.

9. Dobie RA: Medical-Legal Evaluation of Hearing Loss. New York: Van Nostrand Reinhold, 1993.

10. Gates GA, et al: Hearing in the elderly: The Framingham cohort, 1983–1985. Ear Hear 11:247–256, 1990.

11. Matthews LJ, Lee FS, Mills JH, Schum DJ: Audiometric and subjective assessment of hearing handicap. Arch Otolaryngol Head Neck Surg 116:1325–1330, 1990.

12. Stelmachowicz PG, Beauchaine KA, Kalberer A, Jesteadt W: Normative thresholds in the 8- to 20-kHz range as a function of age. J Acoust Soc Am 86:1384–1391.

13. Moller MB: Hearing in 70 and 75 year old people: Results from a cross sectional and longitudinal population study. Am J Otolaryngol 2:22–29, 1981.

14. Bredberg G: Cellular pattern and nerve supply of the human organ of Corti. Acta Oto-Laryngologica Suppl 236:1–135, 1968.

15. Rosen S et al: Presbycusis study of a relatively noise-free population in the Sudan. Ann Otol 71:727, 1962.

16. Mills JH, Schmiedt RA, Kulish LF: Age-related changes in auditory potentials of mongolian gerbil. Hear Res 46:301–310, 1990.

17. Willcott JF: Aging and the Auditory System. In Anatomy, Physiology, and Psychophysics. San Diego, CA: Singular Publishing Group, 1991.

18. Schulte BA, Schmiedt RA: Lateral wall Na, K-ATPase and endocochlear potentials decline with age in quiet-reared gerbils. Hear Res 61:35–46, 1992.

19. Schmiedt R, Mills J, Adams J: Tuning and supresion in auditory nerve fibers of aged gerbils raised in quiet or noise. Haer Res 45:221–236, 1990.

20. Jerger J: Audiological findings in aging. Adv. Otorhinolaryngol 20:115, 1973.

21. Jerger J: Can age-related decline in speech recognition be explained by peripheral hearing loss? In Presbycusis and Other Age Related Aspects. 14th Danavox Symposium, Edited by J. H. Jensen. Hotel Faaborg Fjord, 1990.

22. Dubno J, Dirks D, and Morgan D: Effects of age and mild hearing loss on speech recognition in noise. J Acoust Soc Am 76: 87–96, 1984.

23. Schum DJ, Matthews LJ, and Lee FS: Actual and predicted word recognition performance of elderly hearing impaired listeners. J Sp Hear Res 34:636–642, 1991.

24. Humes LE, Christopherson L, and Cokely C: Central auditory processing disorders in the elderly: fact or fiction?'' In Central Auditory Processing. Katz J, Stecker N, and Henderson D, editors. St. Louis: Mosby Year Book 1992;141–149.

58 Cochlear Implants in Aural (Re)habilitation of Adults and Children

Richard T. Miyamoto, Mary Joe Osberger, and Kathy Kessler

Profound hearing loss poses a monumental obstacle to the acquisition of effective communication skills. The perception as well as the production of speech is highly dependent upon the ability to process auditory information. Early identification of hearing loss is an important first step in managing the effects of hearing impairment. Once identified, the level of residual hearing, if any, must be determined and an appropriate sensory aid recommended. In most cases, conventional amplification is the initial procedure of choice. If little or no benefit is realized with hearing aids, cochlear implants or vibrotactile aids become therapeutic options. This must be followed by the assessment of communication skills and needs, and the selection of a communication mode.

Cochlear implantation has been established as a therapeutic option for selected deaf adults and children. Device specific surgical techniques for placement of an intracochlear electrode array are required. However, successful application of this technology is highly dependent upon a sophisticated multidisciplinary team approach which addresses the varied needs of the deaf recipient. The aural/oral (re)habilitation program in which the patient is enrolled should include listening skill development, speech therapy, speechreading training, and language instruction.

PATIENT SELECTION

The selection of cochlear implant candidates is a complex process that requires careful consideration of many factors. Current selection criteria are as follows:

Two years of age and above
Profound bilateral sensorineural hearing loss (SNHL)
No appreciable benefit from hearing aids
No medical contraindications
High motivation and appropriate expectations
Enrolled in program that emphasizes development of auditory skills

Age Considerations

A lower age limit of 2 years was initially chosen for anatomic reasons. The cochlea is adult size at birth, and by age 2 years the mastoid antrum and facial recess, which provide access to the middle ear for active electrode placement, are adequately developed. However, because of the profound negative effect of early-onset deafness on the development of speech perception, speech production and language competence, an even younger age limit would be advantageous if profound deafness can be substantiated and the inability to benefit from conventional hearing aids demonstrated. No upper age limit is applied as long as the patient's health status will permit an elective surgical procedure.

Pediatric Cochlear Implantation
Pediatric cochlear implant recipients can be loosely divided into three main categories which significantly affect the anticipated outcomes when this technology is applied.

1. Postlingually deafened children. Children who become deaf at or after age 5 are generally classified as postlingually deafened. Even though

these children have developed many aspects of spoken language before the onset of their deafness, they demonstrate rapid deterioration in the intelligibility of their speech once they lose access to auditory input and feedback. Early implantation can potentially ameliorate this rapid deterioration in speech production and perception abilities. However, a postlingual onset of deafness is an infrequent occurrence in the pediatric population. If this were to be the only category for which cochlear implants positively impacted deaf children there would be limited applicability for this technology in children.

2. Congenitally or early-deafened young children. Congenital or early acquired deafness is the most frequently encountered type of profound sensorineural hearing loss. The acquistion of communication skills is a difficult process for these children. Whether sufficient acoustic input can be provided by cochlear implantation to perceive a speech signal linguistically is the focus of a comprehensive longitudinal study.

3. Congenitally or early-deafened adolescents and young adults. When cochlear implantation is considered in adolescence or young adulthood for a patient who has had little or no experience with sound because of congenital or early onset deafness, caution must be exercised because this group has not demonstrated high levels of success with electrical stimulation of the auditory system.

Adult Cochlear Implantation

Adult cochlear implantation has been focused primarily upon post-linguistically deafened patients. Only rarely is implantation recommended on prelingually deafened adults.

Audiological Assessment

The audiological evaluation is the primary means of determining suitability for cochlear implantation. Both unaided and aided thresholds using conventional amplification are determined. A period of experience with a properly fitted hearing aid and coupled with training in an appropriate aural (re)habilitation program is necessary. Hearing aid performance can then be compared to normative cochlear implant performance.

The children who have been the most obvious candidates for a cochlear implant are those who have demonstrated no response to warble tones in the sound field with appropriate hearing aids, or responses suggestive of vibrotactile rather than auditory sensation, i.e., aided responses at levels greater than 50 to 60 dB HL in the lower frequencies with no responses above 1000 Hz.

Not all children with profound sensorineural hearing losses are implant candidates. Hearing aid performance data collected in our laboratory have shown that most children with pure-tone thresholds between 90 to 105 dB HL with residual hearing through at least 2000 Hz demonstrate closed- and open-set speech recognition skills that are superior to multichannel implant users.

Sufficient receptive and expressive abilities to allow the child to learn to make a conditioned response will assist in accurately estimating the child's auditory potential and, if accepted as an implant candidate, will ultimately assist in device setting and permit the child to begin the extensive (re)habilitation program.

Medical Assessment

The medical assessment includes the otologic history, physical examination, and radiologic evaluation of the cochlea. The precise etiology for the deafness is determined whenever possible. However, experience with cochlear implants has demonstrated that stimulable auditory neural elements are nearly always present regardless of cause of deafness.[1] Two exceptions are the Michel deformity, in which there is a congenital agenesis of the cochlea, and the small internal auditory canal syndrome where the cochlear nerve may be congenitally absent.

Routine otoscopic evaluation of the tympanic membrane is performed. An otologically stable condition should be present prior to considering implantation in children. The ear proposed for cochlear implantation must be free of infection, and the tympanic membrane must be intact. If these conditions are not met, medical and/or surgical treatment prior to implantation is required. Because children are more prone to otitis media than adults, justifiable concern has been expressed that a middle-ear infection could cause an implanted device to become an infected foreign body requiring its removal. Of even greater concern is that infection might extend along the electrode into the inner ear, resulting in a serious otogenic complication such as meningitis or further degeneration of the central auditory system. To date, although the incidence of otitis media in children who have received cochlear implants parallels that seen in the general pediatric population, no serious complications have been documented.

The management of middle-ear effusions in children either under consideration for cochlear implantation or who already have cochlear implants deserves special consideration. A noninfected middle ear is a preoperative prerequisite. Conventional antibiotic treatment will usually accomplish this goal. When it does not, treatment by myringotomy and insertion of tympanostomy tubes may be required. Removal of the tube several weeks prior to cochlear implantation will usually result in a healed, intact tympanic membrane. When a middle-ear effusion occurs in an ear in which a cochlear implant device has been previously placed, no treatment is required as long as the effusion remains uninfected. Chronic otitis media, with or without cholesteatoma, must be resolved prior to considering implantation. Conventional otologic treatments are employed to accomplish this goal. Prior ear surgery which has resulted in a mastoid cavity requires special consideration but does not contraindicate cochlear implantation. This situation can be addressed by reconstructing the posterior bony ear canal or obliterating the mastoid cavity and closing the external auditory canal. These measures are taken to prevent delayed exposure of an implanted electrode.

Radiologic examination of the cochlea is performed to determine that the cochlea is present, patent, and of normal morphology.[2] High-resolution, thin-section CT scanning of the cochlea is the current imaging technique of choice. Congenital malformations of the cochlea, i.e. Mondini deformity, are readily identified and are not contraindications to cochlear implantation. Intracochlear bone formation as a result of labyrinthitis ossificans can usually be demonstrated by CT scanning. However, sclerosing labyrinthitis with soft tissue obliteration may not be accurately imaged. In these cases, magnetic resonance imaging (MRI) is an effective adjunctive procedure to determine cochlear patency. The T-2 weighted MRI will demonstrate loss of the endolymph/perilymph signal in sclerosing labyrinthitis. Intracochlear ossification (labyrinthitis ossificans) does not contraindicate cochlear implantation, but can limit the type and length of the electrode array which can be inserted into the scala tympani of the cochlea. When temporal bone fracture has resulted in profound sensorineural deafness, CT scanning may provide helpful information predicting the integrity of the cochlear nerve. Electrophysiological testing can confirm this finding.[3]

Although important information of special concern may be revealed, exclusionary factors are rarely encountered in the medical assessment.

Psychological Assessment

The psychological evaluation has proven invaluable in counseling the parents and providing information related to the management of the patient.[4] Information obtained regarding the patient's family dynamics and milieu is helpful in planning the rehabilitation program. Occasionally, exclusionary factors are identified such as undetected psychosis, organic brain dysfunction or mental retardation.

SURGICAL IMPLANTATION

Cochlear implantation in both children and adults requires meticulous attention to the delicate tissues and small dimensions. Skin incisions are designed to pro-vide access to the mastoid process and coverage of the external portion of the implant package while preserving the blood supply of the postauricular skin. The incision employed at the Indiana University Medical Center has eliminated the need to develop a large postauricular flap. The inferior extent of the incision is made well posterior to the mastoid tip to preserve branches of the postauricular artery. From here the incision is directed posterio-superiorly and then directed superior by a superior anterior limb. In children, the incision incorporates the temporalis muscle to give added thickness. A pocket is created for positioning the implant induction coil. Well anterior to the skin incision, the periosteum is incised from superior to inferior and a posterior periosteal flap is developed. At the completion of the procedure, the posterior periosteal flap is sutured to the skin flap compartmentalizing the induction coil from the skin incision.

Following the development of the skin incision, a complete mastoidectomy is performed (Fig. 58–1). The horizontal semicircular canal is identified in the depths of the mastoid antrum, and the short process of the incus is identified in the fossa incudis. The facial recess is opened using the fossa incudis as an initial landmark. The facial recess is a triangular area bounded by: 1) the fossa incudis (Fig. 58–2) superiorly; 2) the chorda tympani nerve laterally and anteriorly; and 3) the facial nerve medially and posteriorly. The facial nerve can usually be visualized through the bone without exposing it. The round window niche is visualized

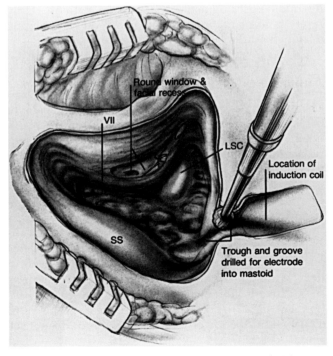

Fig. 58–1. Mastoidectomy performed to gain access to facial recess.

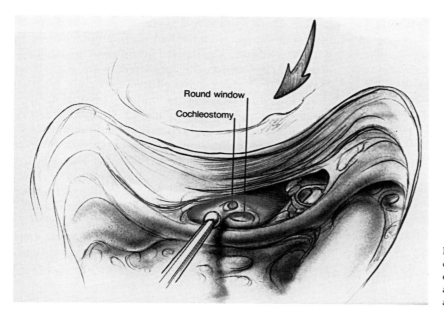

Fig. 58–2. Facial recess is bounded by the fossa incudis superiorly, the chorda tympani nerve laterally and anteriorly, and the facial nerve medially and posteriorly. A cochleostomy is created anterior and inferior to the round window.

through the facial recess approximately 2 mm inferior to the stapes. Occasionally, the round window niche is posteriorly positioned and is not well visualized through the facial recess or is obscured by ossification. Particularly in these situations, it is important not to be misdirected by hypotympanic air cells. Entry into the scala tympani is best accomplished through a cochleostomy created anterior and inferior to the annulus of the round window membrane (Fig. 58–3). A small

fenestra slightly larger than the electrode to be implanted (usually 0.5 mm) is developed. A small diamond burr is used to ''blue line'' the endosteum of the scala tympani, and the endosteal membrane is removed with small picks. This approach bypasses the hook area of the scala tympani allowing direct insertion of the active electrode array. After insertion of the active electrode array, the round window area is sealed with small pieces of fascia.

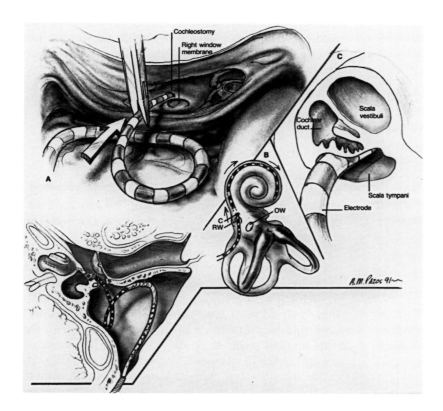

Fig. 58–3. Electrode is introduced through cochleostomy into scala tympani of the cochlea.

UNUSUAL SURGICAL CONSIDERATIONS

Intracochlear Ossification

Ossification at the round window is common in post-meningitic patients and has been encountered in approximately one-half of the children whose cause of deafness was meningitis who have received a cochlear implant at our center. In these patients, a cochleostomy is developed anterior to the round window and the new bone is drilled until an open scala is entered. A full electrode insertion can then be accomplished. Less frequently, labyrinthitis ossificans with extensive intracochlear bone formation may occur.[5] In these cases, the scala tympani of the cochlea may be entirely obliterated. Infrequently, the scala vestibuli may remain patent and in that case, the active electrode can be inserted into the scala vestibuli. When all scalae are obliterated or obstructed, a channel is drilled following the anatomic location of the scala tympani. The new bone is usually whiter and softer than the otic capsule bone. Care must be taken so as not to injure the internal carotid artery in its location anterior to the cochlea. The electrode array is then inserted as far as possible. This will allow insertion of approximately 8 to 10 electrodes of a multichannel electrode array. Satisfactory results were obtained in all patients implanted in this manner. The patients with multichannel implants demonstrate channel separation and are able to make pitch differentiations.

Cochlear Dysplasia

In cases of cochlear dysplasia, there is a significant risk of encountering a gusher upon fenestrating the cochlea while creating the cochleostomy.[6] A gusher is managed by allowing the CSF reservoir to drain off and inserting the electrode into the cochlea. A connective tissue plug is placed around the active electrode at the cochleostomy site sealing the leak. This has resulted in satisfactory performance with a single channel cochlear implant as well as with multichannel implants.[7] It is postulated that the source of the leak was through the lateral end of the internal auditory canal. Supplementally, a lumbar drain can be placed to reduce the spinal fluid reservoir until a satisfactory seal has occurred.

Complications

As with any surgical procedure, complications may arise with cochlear implant surgery.[8] Fortunately, complications have been infrequent and can be largely avoided by careful preoperative planning and meticulous surgical technique.

Among the most frequently encountered problems are those associated with the incision and postauricular flap. Using the above described incision in the pediatric population, we have had no flap breakdowns in over 100 children. The risks of performing the mastoidectomy and opening the facial recess are no greater than for other otologic procedures. Care must be exercised to avoid facial nerve injury. Potential mechanisms for facial nerve injury include direct burr injury while opening the facial recess and thermal injury secondary to friction generated heat from the burr or burr shaft. Adequate irrigation will usually dissipate the heat generated during drilling, but the surgeon must be cognizant of the fact that a diamond burr generates far more thermal energy than a cutting burr. Particularly when operating on congenitally deafened children, there is greater risk that the facial nerve may follow an abberant course within the temporal bone. This can usually be predicted by preoperative CT scan.

Delayed Considerations

Considerable concern was voiced at the outset of the pediatric cochlear implant program that the active electrode would be displaced by the lateral growth of the skull. Fortunately, this has not been a problem. By sealing the electrode into the cochlea with tissue seal and leaving a redundant loop of electrode in the air filled mastoid, the electrode has successfully accommodated skull growth. The author now has a number of pediatric patients who have had electrodes in place for a decade without evidence of growth related problems.

Also of concern was whether the connective tissue seal placed around the active electrode at the round window or cochleostomy would be adequate to prevent bacteria from entering the inner ear resulting in labyrinthitis or meningitis. To date, there have been no instances where this has occurred.

PERFORMANCE RESULTS IN ADULTS

Evaluation Procedures

Implant benefit in adults is measured using a battery of audiological tests that assess sound and speech detection and reception of speech with the implant compared to the patient's preoperative performance with hearing aids (Fig. 58–4). The least difficult tests are those that assess identification of environmental sounds and recognition of the prosodic characteristics of speech, such as temporal or intonation patterns. Speechreading enhancement is measured by comparing recognition of sentences or connected discourse with the implant turned off to performance with the implant turned on. Auditory word identification is assessed using a "closed-set" response format. In closed-set testing, the test (target) item is one of a limited number of choices, thus permitting guessing as in stan-

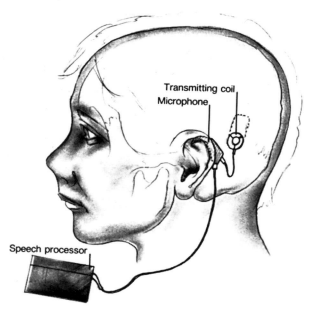

Fig. 58–4. External system consisting of induction coil, microphone, and speech processor.

dard multiple choice tests. The most difficult type of test is recognition of words or sentences in an "open set." In open-set testing, the test (target) stimulus is one of a large number of possible stimuli, and the listener has no alternatives from which to select the answer. Thus, guessing becomes a negligible factor. The ability of patients to perform auditory-only speech recognition tasks using an open-set response format is the ultimate goal of cochlear implantation.

Comparison of Single- and Multichannel Implants

Performance results in adults are reported in terms of benefits derived from particular implants as well as comparative benefits between different implant devices. An important study by Gantz and colleagues[9] compared the performance of five implant devices in postlingually deafened adults: two single-channel devices (3M/House and Vienna) and three multichannel (Ineraid, Nucleus and Storz) systems. The results revealed that patients with the multichannel devices achieved significantly higher scores on tests that assessed recognition of environmental sounds, speechreading enhancement, and word and sentence recognition than patients with the single-channel devices. An interesting finding was that the performance among the multichannel implant users was generally similar even though the devices employed different processing schemes.

The superiority of multichannel devices over single-channel systems was later substantiated in a prospective randomized study, funded by the Department of

Veteran Affairs. In this study with postlingually deafened adults, three devices were evaluated: the 3M/Vienna single channel implant and the Nucleus and the Ineraid multichannel devices.[10,11] The results showed that the two multichannel devices, the Nucleus (with the F0/F1/F2 scheme) and the Ineraid yielded clearly superior results over the single-channel device, with 60% of the multichannel users demonstrating some open-set speech recognition. Results were again similar between patients using the Ineraid and Nucleus devices. The study was extended to examine within-subject differences when the Nucleus processing scheme was upgraded to include fixed high frequency bands (MultiPeak coding strategy) as well as first and second formant information. Subjects demonstrated significantly higher scores on tests of word and sentence recognition when they were switched from the F0/F1/F2 strategy to the MultiPeak strategy. Moreover, significantly higher scores were observed for users of the Nucleus MultiPeak strategy than the Ineraid users on tests of auditory-only word and sentence recognition.

Variables Affecting Implant Performance in Adults

There are large between-subjects differences in implant benefit. For any given implant system, scores on speech recognition tasks can vary from 0% to 100%. The reasons for the large difference in patient performance are not clearly understood, and for this reason implant benefit cannot be reliably predicted from preoperative measures. One of the most important factors is auditory nerve survival, but preoperative tests for estimating the magnitude and location of surviving auditory nerve fibers are lacking. To date, neither radiographic nor electrophysiological measures are able to determine the condition of the auditory nerve.[12–14]

Postimplant speech recognition performance in adults has been moderately correlated with electrical thresholds, dynamic ranges, and the number of electrodes in use.[9,15] Moderate correlations between duration of profound deafness prior to implantation and speech recognition abilities also have been reported.[9] Standardized measures of intellectual ability have not been found to be predictive of implant outcome, but a measure of the patients' willingness to participate in their own health care was correlated significantly with speech understanding.[9,16]

Advances in Implant Technology

The first multichannel implant devices used either a feature extraction or a waveform speech coding strategy. The rationale underlying the feature-extraction approach was that patients with limited perceptual capabilities may not be able to use all of the information in the speech signal. Therefore, the most important features of speech were extracted, while other, presumably less important features, were eliminated. Feature extraction strategies have been employed in the Nucleus implant, beginning with the F0/F2 and F0/F1/F2 strategies and progressing to the MultiPeak strategy which actually encodes waveform information in the high frequencies in addition to extracting the first two formants. Processing schemes that employ a waveform strategy make no a priori assumption about the importance of individual speech features, but rather, provide a representation of the incoming acoustic waveform so that the listener can extract the relevant information needed for speech understanding. Devices that employed a waveform strategy are the Ineraid[17] and UCSF/Stroz implants.[18] These devices use a "compressed analog" (CA) strategy in which the incoming speech signal is analyzed using a vocoder (filter bank) strategy. In this scheme, the continuous acoustic waveform is preserved, and the site of electrode stimulation is determined by the frequency components in the input signal. Depending on that signal, any number of available channels are activated simultaneously, in simulation of the manner in which the normal ear processes sound. A problem encountered with CA strategies, however, is that the simultaneous stimulation of adjacent channels (i.e. electrodes) may produce interactions among channels, reducing channel independence and affecting speech recognition performance. A waveform strategy that addresses the problem of channel interaction is the continuous interleaved sampling (CIS) scheme developed by Wilson and colleagues.[19] Designed to reduce channel interactions through the use of interleaved nonsimultaneous stimuli, the CIS also attempts to retain the temporal information of the speech signal through the use of brief pulses and a high rate of stimulation on each channel that preserve the amplitude variations in the speech signal.

Both the CA and CIS strategies are implemented in the eight-channel CLARION Multi-strategy cochlear implant using either a monopolar or bipolar mode of stimulation.[20] Initial results from the clinical trial with the CLARION in adults revealed a median score of 65% on a test of open-set sentence recognition for the 61 patients tested after six months of device use. Roughly one-half of these patients obtained an open-set sentence recognition score higher than 70% with evidence of relatively rapid improvements in speech recognition performance after implantation.

PERFORMANCE RESULTS IN CHILDREN

Issues in Pediatric Implants

Unlike postlingually deafened adults who use the information transmitted by an implant to compare to previously stored representations of spoken language, pediatric implant users must rely upon the same information to first develop these representations. Because of this, perceptual skills develop over a relatively long time-course in prelingually deafened children.[21-23] Data suggest that substantial improvements in closed-set word recognition usually do not occur in prelingually deafened children until after they have used their multichannel implants for more than one year, and improvements in open-set speech recognition occur after an even longer period of device use.

Since pediatric implant work began, a number of new procedures have been developed to evaluate children's pre- and post-implant performance. Similar to work with adults, procedures were developed to assess perception of the prosodic information, speechreading benefit, and closed- and open-set speech recognition.

Comparison Between Single- and Multichannel Implants

Relatively few comparative single- and multichannel implant studies have been conducted with children. Most investigations with children have reported on the performance of either single-or multichannel implant users, whereas relatively few implant investigations have conducted comparative device studies. A study conducted by Miyamoto and colleagues[22] is one of the few that compared the performance of matched groups of children who used either the 3M/House device or the Nucleus multichannel cochlear implant over time. The results revealed that the performance of the Nucleus users was higher than that of the 3M/House users on every speech perception measure, even on those measures that assessed aspects of speech purportedly transmitted the best by the single-channel device (i.e., prosodic information). Thus, the multichannel implant not only permitted better word recognition without speechreading, but it also conveyed better information about the time-intensity cues in speech. Even though some reports have shown that a small percentage of children demonstrated open-set speech recognition with the 3M/House implant,[24] the highest level of performance achieved by the majority of single-channel users was the perception of stress pattern and syllable number in speech.

Performance with Multichannel Implants

The approach that has been used most often to evaluate implant benefit in children is a within-subject design wherein the subject serves as his or her own control in the pre-and post-implant conditions. The largest studies of this nature have been conducted as part of the clinical trials of the Nucleus multichannel implant in children.[25] After 12 months of multichannel implant use, Staller and colleagues[25] reported mean scores of 39% (n = 84) on a closed-set word identification test, 23% (n = 42) on a test of open-set sentence recognition, and 12% (n = 25) on a test of open set, monosyllabic word recognition. Examination of individual data revealed that 13% of the subjects demonstrated significantly above chance closed-set word identification before implantation, whereas, postoperatively, 62% of the subjects achieved this level of performance. Preoperatively, the subjects showed no open-set speech recognition, but 12 months after implantation, 45% of the subjects recognized one or more words in sentences administered in an open set.

Pediatric implant performance also is reported in terms of clinically descriptive categories of benefit. Geers and Moog[26] developed a classification system that describes performance along a hierarchy of speech perception abilities: (1) no pattern perception, (2) consistent pattern perception, (3) inconsistent word identification, (4) consistent word identification, and (5) open-set word recognition. Staller et al.[25] reported that the percentage of children reaching category 3 and above (i.e., closed- or open-set word recognition) increased from 12% to 80% postoperatively, and roughly half of the subjects demonstrated open-set speech recognition and were assigned a category rating of 5. Osberger et al.[27] developed a similar classification scheme, modified to describe performance on the tests in their assessment battery, and reported that roughly one-half of the subjects demonstrated open-set speech recognition after they had used their implants for an average of two years.

Variables Affecting Performance with Multichannel Cochlear Implants

Research has shown that there are large individual differences among implanted children on speech perception measures. Some children demonstrated relatively high levels of speech recognition, whereas others perceived primarily prosodic speech information from their devices.[25,27] The independent variables that have most often been examined to explain such performance differences are age at onset of deafness, duration of deafness before implantation, and educational setting. Studies by Staller and colleagues[25,28] reported that two factors, age at onset of deafness and duration of deafness, were significantly related to speech perception performance in children who used the Nucleus multichannel cochlear implant. Specifically, they found that subjects with later onset and shorter duration of deafness tended to perform better on measures of speech perception than did subjects with early onset and longer duration of deafness at the time of implantation.

The effect of age at onset of deafness on speech perception skills was examined by Osberger and colleagues[29] in children who received a single- or multi-channel cochlear implant. The results revealed that there were no significant differences in the mean postoperative speech perception scores as a function of age at onset of deafness unless the subjects were postlingually deafened (i.e., onset of deafness at or after age 5). Subjects with postlingual deafness achieved significantly higher speech perception scores on all measures than did the subjects with prelingually deafness (i.e., congenital or acquired deafness). In a more recent study which included only children with multichannel implants (i.e., the Nucleus device) with prelingual deafness who were implanted before age 10, the results showed no significant difference between the speech perception scores of a group of subjects with congenital deafness and the mean scores of a second group of subjects with deafness acquired before age three.[30] The general finding of similar performance between children with congenital and early acquired deafness is probably influenced by the secondary effects of meningitis (i.e., neurological problems and cochlear ossification) on the performance of the children with acquired deafness. These results indicate that children who are born deaf have the potential to derive the same benefit from multichannel implants as do children who had some exposure to spoken language before the onset of their deafness from meningitis.

The post-implant performance of children with postlingual deafness (i.e., onset of deafness at age 5 or later) differs from that of children with prelingual deafness in several important respects. Children with relatively late onset of deafness typically show rapid and marked improvement in speech perception abilities with an implant.[21,29] As noted earlier, speech perception performance improves very gradually in prelingually implanted children.

The results of several investigations have shown a significant relationship between the communication method used by the child and performance on speech perception measures. In these studies, more children who used oral communication achieved higher levels of implant performance than did children who used total communication (i.e., signs plus speaking and listening).[24,27] The relationship between communication mode and implant performance is less clear in other studies. For example, Miyamoto et al.[30] found that children who used oral communication obtained significantly higher scores on only two of the 13 speech perception measures. Clearly, additional research is needed to clarify this issue.

Comparison of Cochlear Implants, Hearing Aids, and Tactile Aids

A criticism of a within-subject research design is that it is difficult to interpret the results relative to the performance of other children with profound hearing impairments who have not received an implant. Even though there might be statistically significant differences between pre-and post-implant scores, it, nevertheless, can be difficult to determine the clinical significance of these changes. Comparison of implanted children's performance to that of a control group can address this issue. Osberger, Maso and Sam[31] developed a descriptive system to classify the range of hearing levels in children with profound hearing impairments. Previous research has shown that children with profound hearing impairments demonstrate a wide range of auditory capabilities.[32] Using the results of previous investigators as a guide, hearing-aid users were divided into three groups based on the unaided better-ear pure-tone thresholds at 500, 1000, 2000 Hz. Subjects classified as Gold hearing aid users demonstrated pure-tone thresholds of 90 to 100 dB HL at two of the three frequencies (with none of the thresholds greater than 105 dB HL). Silver hearing aid users demonstrated hearing levels of 101 to 110 dB HL at two of the three frequencies, whereas Bronze hearing aid users demonstrated two of three thresholds greater than 110 dB HL. Using this approach, the Gold hearing aid users were viewed as setting the "gold standard of performance" for children with profound hearing impairments because previous research has shown that children with this amount of residual hearing developed the most intelligible speech. At the other end of the continuum were Bronze hearing aid users who appeared to respond to auditory stimuli on the basis of vibrotactile sensation. To date, the majority of children who have received implants would be classified as Bronze hearing aid users.

Figure 58–5 shows cross-sectional data for 62 prelingually deafened children implanted with the Nucleus device. The mean age at onset of deafness of the subjects was .8 years and the mean age at implantation was 5.8 years. Whenever possible, subjects were tested in the pre-implant condition with hearing aids and at six-month intervals thereafter. Some subjects, however, entered the study after they had already been implanted or they were not available at every test session. Figure 58–5 also shows data for 21 Gold hearing aid users (mean pure-tone average of 94 dB HL) and 10 Silver hearing aid users (mean pure-tone average of 104 dB HL). Data for the Bronze hearing aid users actually reflects the preoperative performance of the implant users.

Figure 58–5 shows the performance of the implant and hearing aid users on the Minimal Pairs test, which assesses identification of words in a closed-set using only auditory cues. The words are contrasted on the basis of vowel or consonant distinctions, permitting examination of performance on the basis of these speech features. The results show relatively large and rapid improvement in the implanted children's recognition of words based on vowel distinctions. After two-and-a-half years of implant use, the mean score of the Nucleus subjects was the same as that of the Silver hearing aid users, and after three years of implant use, the performance of the implant users was better than that of the Silver hearing aid users. At the last interval, the mean score of the Nucleus group was slightly higher than that of the Gold group. Scores on the consonant items of the Minimal Pairs test were lower than those on the vowel items but the pattern of performance among the groups of subjects was similar for both consonants and vowels.

Figure 58–5 also shows performance on an open-set sentence recognition test, the Common Phrases test administered with auditory cues only. At the one-year post-implant interval, the mean score of the Nucleus users was higher than that of the Silver hearing aid users. In contrast, the mean score of the implant users

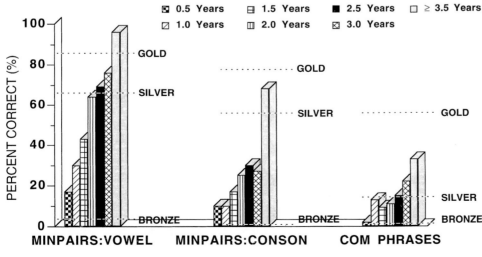

Fig. 58–5. Nucleus users.

remained lower than that of the Gold hearing aid users, even after more than three years of device use.

The data in Figure 58–5 suggest the following conclusions. First, children, who were classified as Bronze hearing aid users, preoperatively, achieved scores with their multichannel implants that were comparable to those of the Gold hearing aid users on most tests (except on a test of open-set speech recognition). Thus, it appears that deaf children, who did not even detect sound with hearing aids, derived substantial benefit from their multichannel cochlear implants. Secondly, the open-set speech recognition skills of the Gold hearing aid users might have remained better than those of the implant users because the former group had more experience with their devices than did the latter group. That is, the Gold hearing aid users received their sensory aids by the time that they were 2 years old, whereas the mean age at which the implant subjects received their devices was about six years. The mean score of the implant users on the open-set speech recognition test might have matched, or even exceeded, that of the Gold hearing aid users had the implant subjects received their devices at a younger age. Moreover, the performance of the implant users might exceed that of the Gold hearing aid users with further improvements in implant technology. Finally, the results suggest that children classified as Silver hearing aid users (i.e., pure-tone thresholds between 100–105 dB HL) might derive more benefit from multichannel implants than from continued use of only hearing aids.

An important issue in sensory aid research with profoundly deaf children has been determination of the benefits derived from non-invasive alternatives to cochlear implants, such as tactile aids. The results of a recent study by Miyamoto and colleagues[33] demonstrated that children who used multichannel implants derived substantially more speech perception benefit from their devices than did children who used multichannel tactile aids. Miyamoto et al compared the performance of two groups of subjects who either received a Nucleus implant or a multichannel vibrotactile aid, the Tactaid 7. There were 10 subjects in each group, matched on the basis of age at onset of deafness, age fit with a multichannel device, and nonverbal intelligence. Subjects were tested on a battery of speech perception measures in the pre-device interval and at one post-device interval (i.e., after an average of roughly one-and-a-half years of device use). The results revealed that the scores of the implant users improved significantly between the pre- and post-device intervals on all measures. Moreover, the scores of the Nucleus users were significantly higher than those of the Tactaid users on all measures. In contrast, the scores of the tactile aid users showed negligible change over time except on a test which evaluated open-set recognition of phrases with both auditory and visual cues. The results suggested that children learned to recognize words and understand speech without lipreading with a multichannel implant, whereas children who used a multichannel tactile aid demonstrated evidence of speech recognition only if tactile cues were combined with visual ones.

Speech Production

The primary role of a cochlear implant is to make speech sounds accessible auditorily. However, if cochlear implants are successfully to impact prelingually deafened children, they must also serve as aids to speech production. Previous research has demonstrated that profoundly hearing impaired children's phonetic repertoires increase after receiving a multichannel cochlear implant. For example, Osberger, et al.,[34] have demonstrated that children who have received a Nucleus 22-channel cochlear implant, are producing consonant and vowel features that are difficult for children with profound hearing losses to master (i.e., high vowels, diphthongs, alveolar consonants, and fricatives). Improvements in speech productions have also been documented by Tobey, et al.[35]

Children who are postlingually deafened or those who are implanted at an early age generally demonstrate large improvements in speech, whereas those with early onset of deafness who are not implanted until adolescence typically show more limited improvements in speech production performance.

The scores for the implanted subjects showed gradual improvement over time. After 2.5 years of cochlear implant use, the average speech intelligibility of the implanted subjects began to exceed that of the Silver hearing aid users. After 3.5 to 4 years of device use, the average intelligibility of the implant users was 40% which is approximately 20% higher than that of Silver hearing aid users. The majority of the children in this study were not implanted until they were 5 to 8 years old.[34] Further studies are underway to examine changes in speech intelligibility in children who were implanted at a younger age.

SUMMARY AND CONCLUSIONS

Cochlear implants are an appropriate alternative for selected deaf children and adults who do not benefit from conventional amplification. Improvements have been documented in both speech perception and speech production skills. However, the full impact of cochlear implantation will be determined only by detailed longitudinal studies. Multichannel systems which provide spectral information in addition to temporal and intensity cues have demonstrated performance advantages and it is anticipated that continued improvements in signal coding and processing will permit electrically transmitted information to even more effectively transcend the deafened peripheral auditory system. This requires refinements in assessing peripheral auditory neuronal survival and matching electrically transmitted signals to the future potential of the central auditory system in the deaf subjects.

REFERENCES

1. Hinojosa R, Marion M: Histopathology of profound sensorineural deafness. Ann NY Acad Sci 405:459–484, 1983.
2. Yune HY, Miyamoto RT, Yune ME: Medical imaging in cochlear implant candidates. Am J Otol 12(suppl)11–17, 1991.
3. Miyamoto RT: Electrically evoked potentials in cochlear implant subjects. Laryngoscope 96:178–185, 1986.
4. Quittner AL, Steck JT: Predictors of cochlear implant use in children. Am J Otol 12(suppl):89–94, 1991.
5. Jackler RK et al: Cochlear patency problems in cochlear implanation. Laryngoscope 97:801–805, 1987.
6. Miyamoto RT, et al.: Cochlear implantation in the Mondini inner ear malformation. Am J Otol 7:258–261, 1986.
7. Jackler RK, Luxford WM, House WF: Sound detection with the cochlear implant in five ears of four children with congenital malformations of the cochlea. Laryngoscope 97(suppl 40): 15–17, 1987.
8. Cohen NL, Rosenberg R, Goldstein S: Problems and complications of cochlear implant surgery. Ann Otol Rhinol Laryngol 96:14–15, 1987.
9. Gantz BJ, et al.: Evaluation of five different cochlear implant designs: Audiologic assessment and predictors of performance. Laryngoscope 98:1100, 1988.
10. Cohen NL, et al: A prospective, randomized study of cochlear implants. N Engl J Med 328:233, 1993.
11. Waltzman SB, et al: An experimental comparison of cochlear implant systems. Sem Hear 13:195, 1992.
12. Jackler RK: CT and MRI of the ear and temporal bone: Current state of the art and future prospects. Am J Otol 9:232, 1988.
13. Balkany TJ, et al: Workshop: Surgical anatomy and radiographic imaging of cochlear implant surgery. Am J Otol 8:195, 1987.
14. Stypulkowski P, Van den Honert C, Kvistad SD: Electrophysiologic evaluation of the cochlear implant patient. Otolaryngol. Clin North Am 19:249, 1986.
15. Kileny PR, Zimmerman-Phillips S, Kemink JL: Effects of active channel number and place of stimulation on performance with multichannel implant. Am J Otol 13:117, 1992.
16. Knutson J, et al: Psychological predictors of audiological outcomes of multichannel cochlear implants: Preliminary findings. Ann Otol Rhinol Laryngol 100:817, 1991.
17. Eddington DK: Speech discrimination in deaf subjects with cochlear implants. J Acoust Soc Am 98:1069, 1980.
18. Schindler RA, et al: The UCSF/Stroz multichannel cochlear implant: Patient results. Laryngoscope 96:597, 1986.
19. Wilson BS, et al.: Better speech recognition with cochlear implants. Nature 352:236, 1991.
20. Schindler RA, Kessler DK, Barker MJ: CLARION patient performance: An update on the clinical trials. Ann Otol Rhinol Laryngol, in press.
21. Fryauf-Bertschy H, Tyler RS, Kelsay DM, Gantz BJ: Performance over time of congenitally deaf and postlingually deafened children using multichannel cochlear implants. J Speech Hear Res 35:913, 1992.
22. Miyamoto RT, et al: Longitudinal evaluation of communication skills of children with single- or multichannel cochlear implants. Am J Otol 13:215, 1992.
23. Waltzman SB, et al: Long-term results of early cochlear implantation in congenitally and prelingually deafened children. Am J Otol 14(Suppl. 2):9, 1994.
24. Berliner KI, Tonokawa LL, Dye LL, House WF: Open-set speech recognition in children with a single-channel cochlear implant. Ear Hear 10:237, 1989.
25. Staller SJ, Dowell RC, Beiter AL, Brimacombe JA: Perceptual abilities of children with the Nucleus 22-channel cochlear implant. Ear Hear 12(Suppl.):34S, 1991.
26. Geers AE, Moog JS: Early Speech Perception Test. St. Louis: Central Institute for the Deaf, 1990.
27. Osberger MJ, et al: Independent evaluation of the speech perception abilities of children with the Nucleus 22-Channel cochlear implant system. Ear Hear 12(Suppl.):66S, 1991.
28. Staller SJ, et al: Pediatric performance with the Nucleus 22-Channel Cochlear Implant System. Am J Otol 12(Suppl.):126, 1991.
29. Osberger MJ, et al: Effect of age at onset of deafness on children's speech perception abilities with a cochlear implant. Ann Otol Rhinol Larynogl 100:883, 1991.
30. Miyamoto RT, et al: Prelingually deafened children's performance with the Nucleus multichannel cochlear implant. Am J Otol 14:437, 1993.
31. Osberger MJ, Maso M, Sam L: Speech intelligibility of children with cochlear implants, tactile aids, or hearing aids. J Speech Hear Res 36:186, 1993.
32. Boothroyd A: Auditory perception of speech contrasts by subjects with sensorineural hearing loss. J Speech Hear Res 27:134, 1984.
33. Miyamoto RT, et al: Comparison of tactile aids and cochlear implants in children with profound hearing impairments. Am J Otol, in press.
34. Osberger MJ, et al: Analysis of the spontaneous speech samples of children using a cochlear implant or tactile aid. Am J Otol 12(suppl):151–164, 1991.
35. Tobey EA, et al: Speech production performance in children with multi-channel cochlear implants. Am J Otol 12(suppl): 165–173, 1991.

59 Facial Paralysis

Kedar Karim Adour

When Sir Charles Bell first demonstrated in 1821 that the facial nerve is a motor nerve, unrelated to sensory enervation of the face, he erroneously named it the nerve of respiration. He had noted that, after he cut the facial nerve of his laboratory animal, the jackass, the nasal ala on the affected side collapsed and did not flare with respiration. The observation was correct, but the conclusion was erroneous. In 1895, Sir William Gowers noted that even after eliminating ear disease, skull fracture, damage during surgery, herpes zoster, and tumors, nearly two thirds of all cases of facial paralysis were labeled idiopathic. This type of facial paralysis, usually referred to as Bell's palsy, was clinically thought to be a neuritis due to exposure to cold and was often termed "rheumatic." The neuritic nature of Bell's palsy has been confirmed and the pathophysiology defined as an acute viral, inflammatory, autoimmune, demyelinating disease caused by the herpes simplex virus; the diagnosis is no longer one of exclusion. Even though it is estimated that 85% of all facial paralysis cases are true Bell's palsy, it is necessary to understand the fundamental dictum that facial paralysis is a sign and not a diagnosis. In the words of the late Sir Terrance Cawthorne, it cannot be overly emphasized that "All that palsies is not Bell's."

FACIAL NERVE ANATOMY

The motor nucleus of the facial nerve is situated in the pons, near the spinal tract and nucleus of the trigeminal nerve. The ventral cell group in this nucleus innervates the lower facial musculature, and the dorsal group the upper musculature. The sensory parasympathetic component (the intermediary nerve) emerges between the facial motor root and the vestibular division of the eighth cranial nerve. In the internal auditory canal, the motor root and intermediary nerve merge, entering the internal acoustic meatus accompanied by the cochlear and vestibular divisions of the eighth cranial nerve and the internal auditory artery and vein. This meatal portion occupies an anterior superior position as it traverses the short (8 to 10 mm) internal acoustic meatus, remaining anterior to the superior vestibular nerve and superior to the cochlear nerve. As it leaves the internal acoustic meatus, the facial nerve is superior to the transverse crest and anterior to a vertical landmark known to surgeons as "Bill's bar." On leaving the internal auditory canal, the labyrinthine segment (4 mm) of the facial nerve curves anteriorly around the basal turn of the cochlea, then greatly expands at the geniculate ganglion, proceeding 74 to 80 degrees posteriorly to form an angle known as "the knee." The greater superficial petrosal nerve leaves the facial nerve at the anterior edge of the geniculate ganglion and proceeds through the hiatus of the facial canal. The horizontal, tympanic segment (11 mm) begins just posterior to the geniculate ganglion and extends to the ampullary end of the horizontal semicircular canal. The pyramidal segment, known as "the elbow," forms an angle always greater than 90 degrees. In the newborn and the young child, this elbow appears to stretch backward, forming a loop. The vertical, mastoid segment (13 mm) begins below the posterior end of the horizontal semicircular canal and continues inferiorly through the facial canal, branching en route to become the nerve to the stapedius muscle and the chorda tympani. After leaving the skull through the stylomastoid foramen, the facial nerve passes through connective tissue septa in the parotid gland, where it divides into a number of branches to supply the muscles of the face (Fig. 59–1).

PHYSIOLOGY OF THE FACIAL NERVE

The facial nerve is known to carry three types of nerve fibers: branchial motor, visceral motor, and visceral

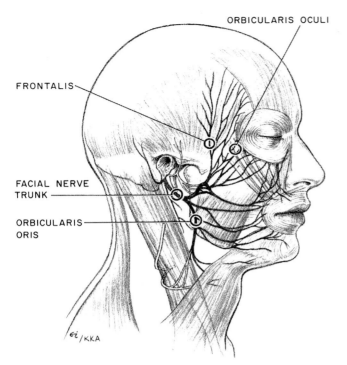

sensory (Fig. 59–2). The motor nucleus of the facial nerve provides branchial motor fibers to all the muscles of the face except the levator of the upper eyelid. The motor fibers also supply the stapedius muscle, the postauricular muscles, the posterior belly of the digastric muscle, and the platysma. Visceral motor preganglionic, parasympathetic fibers from the lacrimal nucleus pass by way of the intermediary nerve through the geniculate ganglion and greater superficial nerve, then through the vidian nerve, to the sphenopalatine ganglion. Postganglionic fibers from the sphenopalatine ganglion anastomose with the zygomaticotemporal branch of the fifth cranial nerve for tear production.

Visceral motor fibers from the superior salivatory nucleus provide preganglionic, parasympathetic fibers to the sphenopalatine ganglion, where postganglionic fibers traverse the palatine nerves to palatal glands, and the nasal nerve to nasal glands. Other visceral motor preganglionic, parasympathetic fibers from the superior salivatory nucleus leave the facial nerve through the chorda tympani nerve to the lingual nerve, then supply the submandibular and sublingual glands.

Visceral sensory fibers have their cell bodies in the geniculate ganglion and receive impulses from the taste buds (fungiform papillae) of the anterior two thirds of the tongue by way of the lingual and chorda tympani nerves. The proximal fibers terminate by way of the intermediary nerve in the nucleus of the solitary tract.

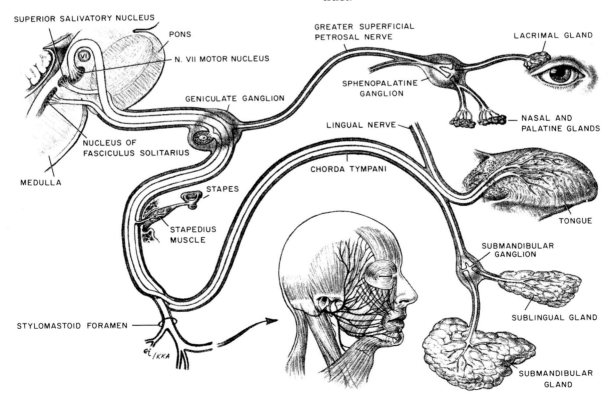

TABLE 59–1. Neurodiagnostic Tests Used to Evaluate Facial Paralysis*

Topographic tests (Site-of-lesion)
    Lacrimation
    Salivation
    Taste
    Electrogustometry
    Audiometric
        Brainstem-evoked auditory response
        Pure tone with speech discrimination
        Stapedial reflex
    Vestibular
        Electronystagmography
    Radiography
        Computerized tomography
        Magnetic resonance imaging
Physiologic tests (Prognostic)
    Electrical
        Nerve excitability
        Electromyography
        Evoked electromyography
        Facial nerve latency
        Strength duration curve
    Trigeminal facial reflex
    Submandibular salivary flow
    Lacrimation
    Stapedial reflex

* Based on House JW and O'Connor AF (eds): *Handbook of Neurological Diagnosis.* New York, Marcel Dekker, 1987, p 176.

NEURODIAGNOSTIC TESTS (TABLE 59–1)

Topographic Diagnosis

Topographic diagnosis is founded on the anatomic and physiologic anatomy of the facial nerve (Fig. 59–2). The particular motor, sensory, and secretory deficits that result from facial paralysis supposedly depend on the extent and site of the lesion. In addition to testing function of the facial nerve, topographic diagnosis includes audiometry, vestibular testing, radiography, and MRI (Table 59–1).

A lesion of the entire motor portion of the facial nerve as it leaves the stylomastoid foramen produces paralysis of all ipsilateral facial movements. On the side affected by the lesion, the patient is unable to wrinkle the forehead, close the eye, show the teeth, purse the lips, or whistle, but the palpebral fissure can be either widened or decreased. If there is minimal ptosis of the eyebrow, the fissure is usually widened. The nasolabial fold is flattened, and the corner of the mouth droops. Although corneal sensation is present, the corneal reflex is lost because motor fibers participating in this reflex are affected.

A lesion of the facial nerve lateral to the geniculate ganglion produces all the deficits found from the peripheral lesion and impaired sublingual and submandibular salivary gland secretion as well as impaired taste in the anterior two thirds of the tongue. The impaired salivary secretion results from interruption of preganglionic, parasympathetic fibers from the superior salivatory nucleus. Taste may not always be impaired by such lesions because some fibers may take an aberrant course through the major petrosal nerve. The stapedius muscle, which normally functions to dampen movement of the ossicles, may also be paralyzed. Such paralysis results in ablation of the stapedial reflex, which can be measured by impedance audiometry. Most important, noise intolerance (hyperacusis, loudness recruitment) on the affected side is *not* related exclusively to paralysis of the stapedius muscle, often occurs with a normal stapedial reflex, and probably represents loss of inhibition to the cochlea by way of the eighth cranial nerve.

Lesions of the facial nerve at or medial to the geniculate ganglion produce all the deficits described and impaired lacrimation on the side of the lesion as a consequence of destruction of the preganglionic, parasympathetic fibers leading to the sphenopalatine ganglion.

Central lesions affecting the corticobulbar and corticoreticular fibers that project on the cells of the facial nucleus produce marked muscle weakness in the contralateral lower half of the face, especially in the perioral regions. The facial paralysis is on the same side as the arm and leg weakness. Muscles of the upper facial region concerned with wrinkling the forehead, frowning, and some eye closure are not affected. Even in the presence of central facial paralysis, mimetic or emotional innervation of the facial muscles may be preserved. During the smiling or laughing response to genuine emotional stimulus, the muscles of the lower face contract symmetrically. Facial muscle contractions on the paralyzed side may even begin earlier and last longer than on the normal side. Mimetic or emotional innervation of the facial muscles is largely involuntary, and the neuroanatomic pathways mediating it are unknown.

The validity and reliability of topographic tests have not been confirmed, but there is consensus on how to perform the test.

Schirmer Tear Testing

The patient is informed that a branch of the facial nerve stimulates tear production; often, decreased tears are associated with the facial paralysis. The need to protect the eye is stressed, and the patient is informed that the test is harmless and painless although necessarily slightly irritating to the eyes. The patient is seated in an examining chair, preferably with head resting on a headrest. The test should be performed, preferably without topical anesthesia, before instilling topical medication or manipulating the eyelids. Care must be taken that the filter paper strips used in testing do not touch the cornea to avoid reflex lacrimation, which causes pain and invalidates the test. The patient is asked to look up while the physician draws the lower eyelid gently downward. The rounded end of the sterile strips is then hooked over each eyelid border at the junction of the middle and nasal third of the lower eyelid margin. The patient may continue normal blinking, although some prefer to keep their eyes closed during the test, which is permissible. The patient should be discouraged from squeezing the eyelids. After 5 minutes, the strips can be removed and the length of the moistened area measured. The measurement is recorded as the difference in millimeters between the two sides.

Modified Tear Test

Because the results of the standard Schirmer tear test vary greatly and are subject to divergent interpretations, a modified tear test was devised to give an indication of reflex tearing and baseline tearing and to shorten the time of the test. The steps are followed as outlined, and either the patient is allowed to inhale ammonia fumes or the patient's nose is stimulated with a cotton swab. The two filter paper strips are removed after 1 minute and compared. The results are recorded as equal, decreased, or increased on the affected side. This qualitative difference is sufficient to determine function.

Audiometry and Stapedial Reflex

A pure-tone audiogram must be recorded for all patients with facial paralysis. If the hearing is normal or if there is symmetric sensorineural hearing loss, speech discrimination and brainstem-evoked auditory response tests are not indicated to assess the paralysis. In a research setting, evoked auditory response can yield information confirming that the brainstem is involved in some cases of acute facial paralysis with normal hearing, but the finding has no therapeutic or prognostic significance.

Of all the topographic tests, the stapedial reflex test is the most objective and reproducible. In cases of severe sensorineural hearing loss, a nonacoustic reflex can be elicited by unilateral electrical stimulation of the external auditory canal. The stapedial reflex is valid only if the tympanic membrane is normal on the side tested. Latency, amplitude, and decay of the reflex can be determined. The accuracy of stapedial reflex testing in determining the site of the lesion is suspect, but the prognostic value is unquestioned.

Taste Tests

There are qualitative and semiquantitative methods of examining taste. The qualitative method records patient response in four categories of taste: sweet, sour, acid, and bitter. The semiquantitative method asks the patient to give a considered opinion about the taste of solutions of different concentration. To avoid subjective error, electrogustometry, which uses a galvanic electrode, was developed. All methods are comparative, using the unaffected side as a control for the abnormal side. Degrees of taste impairment are difficult to establish, however, because of wide variation in subject taste threshold.

For practical purposes, examination of taste is not necessary for diagnosis, but the clinical symptom of aberrant taste sensation (dysgeusia) is extremely important and confirms the diagnosis of cranial polyneuritis of viral origin.

Salivary Tests

There are multiple tests to measure functions of the chorda tympani nerve and the submandibular gland. All salivary flow tests require catheterization of both Wharton's ducts to compare salivary flow. Salivary flow is stimulated using 6% citric or acetic acid. The tubes are drained into collecting chambers and measured. Previous work suggests that measuring the salivary flow can be of value in predicting prognosis or in selecting cases for treatment but is not useful in determining the site of lesion. Pain and technical difficulties in duct cannulation have discouraged widespread measurement of salivary flow.

Radiography and Magnetic Resonance Imaging (MRI)

The facial nerve in Bell's palsy has a characteristic appearance on gadolinium-enhanced MRI (Gd-MRI) scans. Despite this important advance in imaging technology, the clinical presentation remains the mainstay of diagnosis, and radiography and MRI are not needed for the assessment of Bell's palsy and Ramsay-Hunt syndrome (herpes zoster cephalicus), which represent 85% of all cases of facial paralysis. But in 5% to 10% of the cases, radiography or MRI is critical to making a diagnosis. When a form of facial palsy has atypical features, the diagnosis of Bell's palsy should be questioned, and a Gd-MRI scan of the nerve should be obtained. The most common reason for obtaining a Gd-MRI scan is weakness which persists longer than would be expected in an uncomplicated case of Bell's palsy, that is, 3 months. Other atypical features include slowly progressive palsy, facial palsy accompanied by spasm, or other neurologic symptoms.

On Gd-MRI scans, the facial nerve in Bell's palsy appears bright because of gadolinium uptake in the inflamed segment. This appearance is usually pronounced in the region of the geniculate ganglion, but more diffuse enhancement of the entire infratemporal portion may be seen. This enhancement typically persists for several months and may not resolve entirely, even after paralysis has abated. The diameter of the nerve is the key difference between Bell's palsy and tumors which affect the nerve. In Bell's palsy, the nerve is bright but not swollen or otherwise distorted, but when a tumor is present, the nerve is typically bright and focally enlarged. A Gd-MRI scan of a patient with facial palsy should include the entire course of the facial nerve.

Polytomography has been phased out as resolution of the newer computerized tomography (CT) scans has improved. The capacity of CT to form coronal and sagittal reconstructions is invaluable for determining site of the lesion in temporal bone fractures. When a soft-tissue or inflammatory lesion is suspected, MRI is far superior. MRI produces unique high-resolution images using radio waves, magnetic fields, and computer processing. The technique both provides exquisite anatomic definition and distinguishes subtle biochemical changes. Both CT scanning and MRI have multiplanar and improved spatial resolution. CT scanning will probably be replaced by MRI, which is safe, noninvasive, uses nonionizing radiation, and has superior soft tissue contrast.

Vestibular Tests

Electronystagmography (ENG) and rotational tests of vestibular function are useful when facial paralysis is accompanied by unilateral hearing loss. Use of the rotational tests is based on auditory signs, not the facial paralysis, and these tests do not play a role in routine evaluation of a patient with facial paralysis.

Test Validity

Topographic tests are commonly considered simple and definitive. The results of such tests, however, show great discrepancy: marked decrease in lacrimation with normal stapedial reflex and normal taste, or absent lacrimation with absent stapedial reflex and normal submandibular salivation. These discrepancies occur in cranial polyneuritis, temporal bone fractures, and facial nerve tumors. In temporal bone fractures, the greater superficial petrosal and chorda tympani nerves are highly vulnerable to injury, independent of the facial nerve. In cranial polyneuritis of herpes simplex (Bell's palsy) and herpes zoster (Ramsay Hunt syndrome), there can be multiple sites of inflammation and demyelinization from the brainstem to the periphery. In addition, with tumors such as neurinomas, the tumor itself allows transmission of nerve impulses until late in the course of disease. Thus topographic diagnostic tests are useful only to supplement other diagnostic information; they are partial indicators of severity and therefore are relative indicators of prognosis.

NEURODIAGNOSTIC TESTS (PROGNOSTIC)

Electrical Tests

Neurodiagnostic tests are used not only to determine the site of the lesion producing the paralysis but also to evaluate the physiologic extent of nerve damage, predict prognosis, and determine treatment. Because reliability of the tests has been challenged, and newer forms of x-ray and magnetic resonance imaging have been developed, traditional testing has been modified and electrical tests are considered the best prognostic and physiologic tests.

Nerve Injury

To interpret electrical tests, it is necessary to understand the types of nerve damage. The most useful classification is Sunderland's five degrees of injury expressed in terms of damage to the endoneurium, perineurium, and epineurium. The five degrees of injury (Table 59–2) are of increasing severity according to the effect of the injury and not the cause of the injury. The older classification using neurapraxia, axonotmesis, and neurotmesis is not sufficiently precise but is in common usage. Again, it is emphasized that these are pathologic classifications and electrical tests are prognostic and not diagnostic tests.

Prognostic and Physiologic Tests

It is difficult to make a reliable prognosis in the early stages of facial paralysis. Electrodiagnostic testing attempts to predict prognosis by determining the physiologic extent of nerve damage. The results of available electrical tests (nerve excitability, facial nerve latency, evoked and volitional electromyography, and strength duration determination) show abnormality from days

TABLE 59–2. Sunderland's Classification of Nerve Injuries*

First degree	Conduction block	Neurapraxia
Second degree	Transection of axon with intact endoneurium	Axonotmesis
Third degree	Transection of nerve fiber (axon and sheath) inside intact perineurium	Neurotmesis
Fourth degree	Transection of funiculi, nerve trunk continuity being maintained by epineural tissue	Neurotmesis
Fifth degree	Transection of entire nerve trunk	Neurotmesis

* Sunderland S: Nerves and Nerve Injury. New York, Churchill Livingstone, 1978, p. 133.

up to weeks after degeneration, however. In the case of a severed nerve, nerve excitability, facial nerve latency, and evoked electromyography (ENog) results are normal for 72 hours. All stimulatory nerve tests reflect damage that has occurred three days earlier, and volitional electromyography (EMG) results do not become abnormal for 2 to 3 days. Moreover, once stimulatory electrical tests become abnormal, they remain so and cannot be used to monitor regeneration and reinnervation. In cases in which regeneration is expected, the electrical tests are good prognostic indicators but differ in interpretation based on the bias of various authors.

Methods of Electrical Testing

All electrical tests mentioned, except EMG, are performed percutaneously. Most electrical tests are comparative, using the normal side as a control for the abnormal side. Because neural degeneration is often neither acute nor complete, a single examination is not sufficient; re-examination days or weeks later is necessary.

Minimal Nerve Excitability Test (NET)

The minimal nerve excitability test (NET) requires simple percutaneous stimulation of the facial nerve at the stylomastoid foramen (Fig. 59–1) while raising the intensity of a short duration current to the threshold at which a just-visible muscle contraction is observed. Both the affected and the unaffected side are then stimulated and the two compared.

Maximal Nerve Excitability Test (MST)

Because the reliability of minimal nerve excitability testing was challenged, a modification called the maximal stimulation test was developed. The observer is placed to see both sides of the face simultaneously. The stimulating probe is applied to the nerve branch at the intensity that produces a just-visible muscle twitch. When the first contraction is observed, the area is explored to find the most sensitive point—that which displays the maximal amount of muscle motion. The current is then increased 1 to 2 milliamperes above this threshold to obtain maximal nerve excitability stimulation. Test results are expressed as the difference in facial muscle movement when comparing the affected side of the face with the normal side; these results are recorded as equal or decreased movement.

The amount of muscle movement on the affected side is compared with that on the normal side, and relative response is graded on a scale from 0 to 4. Zero is defined as no muscle response to stimulation of the peripheral nerve branch, and 4 is defined as equal response on the affected and normal sides. Intermediate numeric values were assigned to minimal, moderate,

TABLE 59–3. Maximal Stimulation Test (MST) Grading System Derived From Averaging Scores From Three Facial Sites Stimulated*

Difference	Grade
No response	0
Marked	1
Moderate	2
Minimal	3
Equal	4

* Resultant visible muscle contraction on affected side recorded relative to contraction on normal side.

and severe reduction in muscle response of the affected side compared with that of the normal side (Table 59–3). The degree of neural degeneration is not always equal in every branch of the facial nerve. This numeric method of recording MST results allows an average MST score for the entire face to be obtained by a simple computation. An example of such a computation is shown in Table 59–4. This method of reporting enables data to be entered into calculations for statistical analysis on the basis of the average score for stimulation of the three facial regions, thus more accurately reflecting the status of the entire peripheral nerve branch system. The hypothetical patient (Table 59–4) would suffer a "moderately" degenerated facial nerve, and recovery would be delayed and followed by sequelae.

A prospective research protocol was used to test reliability and prognostic accuracy of MST in patients with acute Bell's palsy who were followed for at least 4 months. The MST accurately predicted outcome in 94% of patients studied and was superior to facial nerve latency tests and evoked electromyography to a statistically significant degree. A score of ≤2.7 is 94% accurate in predicting incomplete final recovery marked by midface contracture with synkinesis. Final recovery can be predicted by using the average MST score obtained 2 weeks after onset of palsy (Table 59–5). Although facial nerve excitability testing is a simple procedure, determining the location of the peripheral branches requires experience (Fig. 59–1). The branch to the frontal muscle is usually found approximately 2.5 cm posterior to the outer canthus of the eye; the branch to the orbicular muscle of the eye is stimulated at the lateral border of the orbit. Location of the

TABLE 59–4. Method for Computing Average MST Results

Branch Tested	Visual Muscle Response	Numeric Score
Forehead	Minimal decrease	3
Eye	Moderate decrease	2
Mouth	Severe decrease	1
	Total score =	6
Average score (3 + 2 + 1 ÷ 3)		2

TABLE 5. Prediction of Recovery Based on Averaged MST Scores

MST Scores	% Recovery	Time (wks)	Sequelae (Severity)*
4	100	3–6	None
3–3.9	75–100	4–8	Minimal
2–2.9	75	6–12	Moderate
1–1.9	50–75	8–12	Moderate/severe
0–.9	<50	12 +	Severe

Contracture with synkinesis.

branch of the orbicular muscle of the mouth varies the most of all three branches but is usually just anterior to the notch where the facial artery traverses the mandible. The stimulating probe may have to be moved to determine the point of maximal response because the facial nerve can branch in many directions beyond the stylomastoid foramen (see Fig. 59–1).

Electromyography (EMG)

The term electromyography (EMG) refers in general medical usage to volitional electromyography, differentiated from evoked electromyography (ENog). The muscle action potentials produced by stimulating the nerve differ somewhat from those produced by voluntary effort. Muscle action potentials produced by voluntary effort are associated with a graded response that varies according to strength of the effort. A needle electrode is placed into the muscle to be tested, and the signal is monitored visually and audiographically on an oscilloscope. When muscle denervation has been present for 2 to 3 weeks, the muscle begins to fibrillate so that the needle electrode records fibrillation potentials, a sign of denervation. At a later stage, if recovery has begun, reinnervation potentials can be recorded.

Evoked Electromyography (ENog)

Evoked electromyography (ENog) not only permits study of muscle excitability and state of the muscle fibers but provides useful information regarding conduction properties of nerve fibers. It is the basis for determining conduction time, or latency (expressed in milliseconds) and motor nerve conduction, or velocity (expressed in meters/second). When testing the facial nerve, the distance between the stimulation and recording electrodes is only 10 to 12 cm, and tradition has established that facial nerve latency is preferable to conduction velocity as a measure of nerve function.

The stimulating electrode is placed over the nerve trunk at the stylomastoid foramen; the surface recording electrode, over the muscle group to be tested. The nerve is stimulated with a supramaximal stimulus. Functional status of the nerve is assessed by comparing amplitudes of the compound muscle action potentials on both sides of the face. The interval between the nerve stimulation and the start of the muscle potential—the facial nerve latency—can be accurately measured and is an acceptable indication of nerve function. This method is considered an improvement of the maximal stimulation test (MST). Instead of visual estimate, the muscle action potential is recorded. Although many advocate the use of ENog, the test has not been standardized. The test is labeled as electroneuronography, electroneurography (ENog), or neuromyography.

Strength Duration Curves

Determining the strength duration curve is tedious and somewhat painful and is not widely used. Briefly, this curve depicts the relationship between amplitude and duration of a stimulating impulse at the threshold for muscle response. If denervation has occurred, a stronger than normal stimulus is needed to activate the muscle, and the shape of the strength duration curve is thus changed.

Interpretation of Electrical Tests

In the surgical management of facial paralysis, stimulatory electrical tests are often used to select patients for treatment, and it is necessary to fully understand these tests to make the best decision. In the nonsurgical management of facial paralysis, these tests are used primarily to predict prognosis. Each test has limitations, and all tests show abnormality days to weeks after degeneration.

Minimal and maximal nerve excitability tests both have the disadvantage of relying on a visual end point. Evoked electromyography (ENog) has the advantage of possessing a recorded and often reproducible end point. Minimal nerve excitability testing (NET) and ENog, however, also have the disadvantage of reliance on stimulating the nerve trunk. Because the facial nerve trunk is deep in the stylomastoid foramen, an increased stimulus level is required that often triggers a reaction in the masseter muscle, the "trigeminal nerve artifact." Moreover, NET and ENog are interpreted on the basis of muscle reaction in only one part of the face. If the upper division of the facial nerve is cut, both procedures record muscle response equal to that of the other side. MSTs, which record the peripheral branches, accurately demonstrate the abnormal muscle response. The electrical impulse can stimulate only neurapraxic fibers; none of the tests distinguish between axonotmesis and neurotmesis. Therefore, the tests do not distinguish between injuries of second and third degree. The recorded compound action potential from a nerve with 25% of its fibers neurapraxic is the same regardless of whether the remaining fibers are in a stage of axonotmesis or neurotmesis.

Because stimulatory electrical tests remain abnormal even when volitional facial muscle action has returned, EMG may be of prognostic value in the regenerative period, but this is late in the entire course of the disease. During reinnervation, when there is visible facial muscle motion, obtaining an EMG is superfluous.

The findings from all electrical testing must be correlated with the clinical and pathologic process causing the paralysis. In general, the tests are useful only during the first weeks of the disease. If the nerve has been severed, regeneration cannot be expected unless repair is undertaken. Even then, stimulatory electrical tests are of no benefit because they cannot monitor regeneration. For the three most common causes of facial paralysis (cranial polyneuritis, temporal bone fracture, and acute otitis media), which account for 95% of all cases in which the facial nerve is intact, regeneration can be expected and is predictable. Because the degree of regeneration is related to the degree and rate of denervation, serial electrical tests are performed. If denervation has progressed from minimal to severe degeneration in 7 to 10 days, a greater and earlier return of volitional muscle motion can be expected than when progression from minimal to severe denervation occurs in 3 to 4 days.

If testing indicates equal muscle response on both sides of the face, the patient can be expected to have complete return of facial function in 3 to 6 weeks without complications of faulty nerve regeneration. The most common complications of faulty nerve regeneration are contracture, synkinesis (associated facial motion), and facial spasms (tics). An uncommon complication is gustatory tearing ("crocodile tears").

CLASSIFICATION OF FACIAL PARALYSIS

The most consistent attempts to classify facial paralysis rely on topographic diagnosis, which attempts to localize the "site of lesion" causing the paralysis. Some classify facial paralysis into types of disease processes, disregarding the possible site of involvement. Others have attempted to combine classifications, developing hybrid charts. For practical use, a utilitarian system (Table 59–6) offers a useful aid for diagnosis based on frequency of occurrence.

Onset of the paralysis must first be considered—was it acute or progressive? Acute cases include patients with paralysis that reaches maximum severity by 2 weeks after onset. These cases include patients with Guillain-Barré syndrome or the newly recognized entity of facial nerve involvement in Lyme disease and exclude neurologic disorders such as multiple sclerosis and amyotrophic lateral sclerosis. Progressive facial paralysis occurs during weeks, months, or years in pa-

TABLE 59–6. Proposed Pathologic Classification of Facial Paralysis in Order of Frequency

Acute Paralysis*	Progressive or Chronic Paralysis†
Polyneuritis	Malignancies
Bell's palsy (probably herpes simplex)	Primary parotid and adnexa
	Adenoid cystic
Herpes zoster	Acinic cell
Guillain-Barré syndrome	Squamous cell
Idiopathic autoimmune diseases	High-grade mucoepidermoid
	Undifferentiated
Lyme disease	Malignant mixed tumor
Trauma	Metastatic
Skull fracture or concussion	Breast, lungs, kidney, colon, skin
Surgery	
Facial and penetrating injury	Congenital Benign Tumors
Birth trauma	Schwannoma, neurofibroma, hemangioma, glomus tumor, cholesteatoma
Otitis Media	
Acute bacterial	
Chronic	
Bacterial	
Cholesteatoma	
Sarcoidosis	
Cerebrovascular Accident	
Neurologic Disorders	

Cases usually sudden in onset, reaching maximum severity within 2 weeks.

†*Cases increasing in severity after 2 weeks or persisting as flaccid paralysis beyond 4 months.*

tients who, if they do show recovery, never recover completely.

CRANIAL POLYNEURITIS (BELL'S PALSY AND HERPES ZOSTER)

Causes

In the past, Bell's palsy was defined as mononeuropathy of undetermined origin. The synonym for Bell's palsy was "idiopathic facial paralysis." Observations within the last few years have clarified this misconception. Bell's palsy is the clinically evident aspect of cranial polyneuritis probably caused by the herpes simplex virus (HSV-1). Neutralization antibody to HSV-1 reactivation in Bell's palsy indicates that HSV-1 is the cause. Also, the T-lymphocyte changes suggest an autoimmune reaction, and T2-weighted MRI has shown regions of increased signal intensity, indicating inflammation, in the brainstem as well as the intratemporal course of the facial nerve.

The clinical, neurologic, laboratory, and immunologic similarities between Bell's palsy and known manifestations of reactivated neurotropic HSV-1 in cranial ganglia supports the diagnosis. Although animal experimentation has been unable to support the compression hypothesis of Bell's palsy causation, an animal model using the mouse and the Kos strain of HSV-1 has succeeded in producing an acute, transient form of facial paralysis simulating Bell's palsy. Facial paralysis which developed between 6 and 9 days after virus inoculation continued 3 to 7 days, then resolved. The animals were killed between 6 and 20 days after inoculation. Histopathologically, severe nerve swelling, inflammatory cell infiltration, and vacuolar degeneration were manifest in the affected facial nerve and nucleus. HSV antigens were detected in the facial nerve, geniculate ganglion, and facial nerve nucleus. Latent HSV-1 infection in the geniculate ganglion was proven 3 weeks after the inoculation.

Cranial polyneuritis caused by herpes zoster is differentiated from that caused by HSV-1 by increased severity of symptoms, the presence of vesicles, and a rising antibody titer to herpes zoster virus. A "zoster-like form" of Bell's palsy exists without vesicles or rising titers to herpes zoster virus. Patients with this syndrome have a higher risk of nerve degeneration.

On Gd-MRI scans, enhancement of the geniculate ganglion was observed in 88% of Bell's palsy patients and in 100% with Ramsay Hunt syndrome. Paradoxically, no difference exists between the two diseases in terms of the pattern or intensity of enhancement of the facial nerve. In patients with internal auditory symptoms such as vertigo and tinnitus, enhancement was also seen in the cochleovestibular nerve.

Diagnosis of Bell's Palsy

Cases of Bell's palsy are similar in history, course, and outcome, and the diagnosis is not one of exclusion. Onset of the paralysis is often preceded by a viral prodrome. The symptoms and signs during the early phase of facial paralysis include facial numbness, epiphora, pain, dysgeusia, hyperacusis (dysacusis), and decreased tearing. The pain is usually retroauricular but sometimes radiates into the face, pharynx, or arm. These findings are usually unilateral but can be contralateral. The hyperacusis (dysacusis, phonophobia) occurs even with an intact stapedial muscle reflex. It probably represents dysfunction of the cochlear division of the acoustic nerve caused by interruption of the inhibitory fibers which traverse the cochlear ganglion. It is statistically significant that the presence of dysgeusia or hyperacusis in a patient with acute facial paralysis is sufficient for definitive diagnosis of Bell's palsy.

The physical findings include hypesthesia or dysesthesia of the fifth and ninth cranial nerves and of the second cervical nerve. Motor paralysis of branches of the tenth cranial nerve (the vagus nerve) are seen as a unilateral shift of the palate or shortening of one vocal cord with rotation of the posterior larynx to the affected side.

Thus, Bell's palsy can be diagnosed when facial paralysis is peripheral in origin, when systemic disease is not evident, when the history is of acute onset, and when concomitant sensory cranial polyneuritis is evident. No further diagnostic tests are needed. The dis-

ease is expressed as viral sensory polyganglionitis with secondary autoimmune demyelination, and the motor nerves are affected as they traverse the affected sensory ganglions.

Treatment

Discussing the diagnosis and prognosis should reassure most patients. Corticosteroids per se are considered excellent treatment for a viral, inflammatory autoimmune disease. Prednisone dramatically relieves the pain of Bell's palsy so that analgesics are usually not necessary. For adults, a total of 1 mg per kilogram of body weight daily (1 mg/kg/day) is suggested, to be taken in divided doses in the morning and evening. The patient should be seen on the fifth or sixth day after onset of the paralysis. If the paralysis remains incomplete (Type I), the dose of prednisone is tapered to zero during the next 5 days. If the paralysis is complete (Type II), the 1 mg/kg/day dose should be continued for 10 more days and tapered to zero over the next 5 days (total, 21 days). Prednisone is discontinued after day 21, even though return of facial function cannot be expected until 3 to 6 weeks after onset of the paralysis. Prednisone should never be stopped abruptly because rebound inflammation can lead to further denervation. Because Ramsay Hunt syndrome is more severe, with late neural degeneration, prednisone should be continued at the 1mg/kg/day level for 14 days and then tapered during the next week.

When the classic distribution of otic vesicles (Ramsay Hunt syndrome) is absent, the diagnosis of herpes zoster facial paralysis depends on the results of complement fixation tests weeks into the course of the disease. The presence of severe pain is a general indicator of poor prognosis, and such pain may represent a forme fruste of herpes zoster, or the zoster-like form of Bell's palsy. Therefore, the presence of severe pain is an indication for treating patients with the dose schedule advised for herpes zoster.

Acyclovir

Acyclovir and prednisone together is the preferred treatment of herpes zoster facial paralysis and Bell's palsy. In herpes zoster, prednisone alone causes reduction of pain and the resolution of vesicles. In Bell's palsy, the use of acyclovir in combination with prednisone leads to statistically significantly better final outcome than the use of prednisone alone (p ≤ .05). The acyclovir can be given intravenously or orally. If oral treatment is chosen, it is necessary to give 800 mg every 5 hours because absorption from the gut is limited. When treating HSV-1 Bell's palsy, acyclovir 200 mg every 5 hours for 10 days is suggested.

Facial Nerve Decompression

The history of facial nerve decompression reflects the lack of uniformity in selecting patients for surgery and the areas for decompression. In 1932, decompression of the distal 1 cm (3/8 of an inch) of the facial nerve at the stylomastoid foramen was proposed, but there was no consensus as to the timing of surgery. In 1939, decompression for the entire vertical segment was suggested. In the 1940s and 1950s, decompression of the vertical and pyramidal segments within 12 weeks of the onset of the paralysis was advocated when reaction of degeneration was present. In the 1960s, the iter chordae posterius was thought to be the most constricting area and chorda tympani neurectomy for "internal" facial nerve decompression began. And finally, in the late 1970s and early 1980s, decompression of the meatal and labyrinthine segments only through a middle cranial fossa approach is advocated. It is suggested that ENog and the clinical course of the paralysis are the best guidelines for selecting patients for facial nerve decompression. When ENog demonstrates 75 to 95% degeneration within 2 weeks after onset, urgent surgery may preserve the remaining axons. Surgery after day 14 is not advised because the active viral disease has abated and the early regeneration stage is beginning. Decompression should be limited to the meatal and labyrinthine segment through a middle cranial fossa approach. The transmastoid total facial nerve decompression as treatment for Bell's palsy has been invalidated.

Any discussion of the therapeutic options should include the mode of action, indications, contraindications, complications, and special considerations discussed.

Eye Care

Protection of the eye is paramount. It is necessary to protect the eye from foreign bodies and drying. Dark glasses must be worn during the day, artificial tears instilled at the slightest evidence of drying, and a bland eye ointment used during sleep. Taping the eye closed is not recommended, but early exposure keratitis may require patching or rarely a tarsorraphy.

Physiotherapy

Just as fewer clinicians are offering facial nerve decompression, fewer are offering electrical stimulation of the paralyzed muscles. Physiotherapy has been suggested as valuable for maintaining the morale of the patient. The cost to the community and to the patient of daily visits to the hospital for electrotherapy does not seem justified. An accurate diagnosis and a reliable estimate of prognosis, with careful explanation and reassurance, can give full confidence to the patient. Further, experimental research has shown that electrical stimulation of a denervated muscle retards ingrowth of neurofibrils to the motor endplates. Therefore, electrotherapy may be detrimental and should not be used.

TRAUMA

Trauma is the second most common cause of facial paralysis and is easily diagnosed. Traumatic facial paralysis, including that from iatrogenic causes, is classically divided into paralysis of "immediate" or paralysis of "delayed" onset. Although there is no consensus, an immediate-onset traumatic paralysis may be indication for urgent surgical exploration. In cases of basal skull fracture, topognostic tests are again highly inaccurate. Almost all of these cases of basal skull fracture with facial paralysis occur in highly pneumatized temporal bones. The greater superficial petrosal nerve and the chorda tympani are vulnerable to injury independently of the facial nerve. Further, such cases have associated hemotympanum, which obviates the use of tympanometry. Audiometric studies, however, are necessary for complete evaluation of the inner-ear and middle-ear damage.

High-resolution, thin-section CT scanning can accurately diagnose temporal bone fracture and is the best topognostic test. Coronal and sagittal reconstructions can often pinpoint disruption of the fallopian canal. If CT scanning reveals impingement of the bony canal on the facial nerve, exploration is essential. At time of exploration, bony spicules are removed and a severed nerve repaired.

Controversy still exists regarding incising an intact nerve sheath. The urge to look into the sheath is strong, but the sheath is a protective structure. It allows a direct path for neurofibril growth which aids regeneration and should therefore be preserved.

In cases of delayed facial paralysis after trauma, electrical tests are invaluable for determining prognosis and for selecting patients who do *not* need surgery. When delayed or partial paralysis progress to a complete clinical paralysis, the prognosis for full recovery is decreased. If CT scanning shows no impingement of bone, surgery is probably *not* indicated. Prognosis is determined by the rate and degree of denervation.

There is no study proving the beneficial effects of corticosteroid therapy in traumatic facial paralysis. In animal experiments using methylprednisolone, however, decreased time of recovery occurred when acute facial paralysis was produced by compression. On the basis of these animal experiments, it would seem justifiable to recommend corticosteroid therapy to treat facial paralysis caused by trauma.

ACUTE OTITIS MEDIA

In acute otitis media, the pathophysiologic mechanisms causing the facial paralysis are thought to be direct toxic effects and mechanical compression by the purulent exudate. The possibility exists, however, that the acute otitis media could activate the latent neurotropic HSV-1 virus and that the paralysis reflects "Bell's palsy" with concomitant otitis media. The two can be distinguished if there is an associated sensory deficit, such as facial hypesthesia. In any patient with facial paralysis and acute otitis media, CT scanning of the mastoid is indicated. In children, other diseases, such as eosinophilic granuloma, may manifest as acute otitis media.

For treatment, antibiotics, myringotomy, and corticosteroids are recommended. Corticosteroids with antibiotics improve the resolution of otitis media with effusion. The effect on return of facial nerve function is unknown, but it seems reasonable that reduction of the inflammation and resolution of the infection would be equally beneficial to the injured facial nerve.

As with most acute facial paralysis, clinically incomplete paralysis has an excellent prognosis for complete recovery. When the paralysis is clinically complete, the use of electrical tests aids in predicting recovery. Medical treatment for facial paralysis in acute otitis media in children is erroneously assumed to be 100% effective. Severe nerve degeneration and subsequent poor return of facial function with contracture and synkinesis does occur in children, and lack of tolerance to electrical tests makes it impossible to predict recovery.

PROGRESSIVE FACIAL PARALYSIS

Whereas acute facial paralysis such as cranial polyneuritis (HSV-1 Bell's palsy, herpes zoster), acute otitis media, and trauma are easily diagnosed, progressive facial paralysis requires extensive assessment. Such cases are usually caused by benign or malignant tumors (see Table 59–6) and require standard surgical treatment devoid of controversy. It has been stressed that occult neoplasms can present as an acute or recurrent ipsilateral facial paralysis, and therefore Bell's palsy should be considered a diagnosis of exclusion. This concept can be modified and reasonable diagnostic steps undertaken without subjecting a conservatively estimated 40,000 patients per year to unnecessary and prohibitively expensive evaluations and consultations.

Patients who have a slowly progressive paralysis or facial tics, or show no recovery by 4 months, require a full workup. Unfortunately, topognostic evaluation has been particularly disappointing with chronic or progressive facial paralysis. Operative findings during resection of discrete tumors have often been inconsistent with results of preoperative site-of-lesion testing. Electrodiagnostic tests may indicate tumor involvement. Incomplete paralysis with EMG fibrillation po-

tentials, decreased MST or ENog muscle amplitude potentials, complete loss of nerve excitability within 5 days, or prolonged facial nerve latency suggest tumor involvement. The definitive diagnosis for tumor involvement is made, however, by using high resolution CT scanning or MRI. When CT scanning and MRI results are negative, electrodiagnostic findings can aid in making decisions regarding surgery. Primary malignant or benign tumors can be resected and appropriate facial nerve grafting performed. Metastatic neoplasms require other modalities such as radiation or chemotherapy.

RECURRENT FACIAL PARALYSIS

Recurrent facial paralysis requires special attention because 10% of patients (approximately 4000) with one episode of Bell's palsy have a recurrence, which is ipsilateral in 50% of the cases. Because an ipsilateral recurrence of facial paralysis has been found with some tumors, the need for accurate diagnosis arises. The guidelines discussed under the section on Bell's palsy, the findings with electrodiagnosis, auditory abnormalities, and the clinical course aid in selecting patients requiring special assessment or treatment. CT scanning or MRI is not needed for every case of recurrent facial paralysis.

Melkersson-Rosenthal syndrome is a rare form of recurrent facial paralysis. Signs and symptoms include facial edema, furrowed tongue, and facial paralysis. It is thought to be an idiopathic autoimmune disease, and there is some evidence that this is the only form of acute facial paralysis that would benefit from a prophylactic total facial decompression.

OTHER CAUSES OF FACIAL PARALYSIS

There is a multitude of suggested causes (Table 59–7) of facial paralysis. With the exception of some neurologic disorders, most are rare and many questionable. The association of facial paralysis with benign parotid disease, various non-neurotropic viruses, and collagen-vascular disease needs re-evaluation. Any viral disease can and does activate HSV-1; it is impossible to assign the cause for the facial paralysis to the primary virus infection. A common example is mononucleosis, which invariably causes HSV-1 "fever blisters." Similarly, in patients with autoimmune collagen-vascular diseases, the HSV-1 virus reactivates more frequently than in the normal population. Because it is estimated that in the United States one case of Bell's palsy occurs every 13 minutes, concomitant presentation in a patient with a benign parotid tumor is likely.

TABLE 59–7. Described Causes for Paralysis of the Facial Nerve, in Alphabetical Order

Acoustic neurinoma
Amyloidosis
Amyotrophic lateral sclerosis
Anesthesia nerve block
Arachnoid cysts
Arterial embolization
Bannworth syndrome
Barotrauma
Branchial cleft cysts
Coxsackie virus
Cystic hygroma
Cytomegalovirus
Diabetes mellitus
Diphtheria
Eosinophilic granuloma
Glioma
Hemangiomas
Hydradenomas
Hypertension
Hyperthyroidism
Hypothyroidism
Influenza
Kawasaki's disease
Lead poisoning
Malaria
Melkersson-Rosenthal syndrome
Meningioma
Mobius syndrome
Mononucleosis
Mumps
Mycoplasma
Osteopetroses
Periarteritis nodosa
Polio
Polymyositis
Postvaccination
Relapsing polychondritis
Rhabdomyosarcoma
Rubella
Sarcoma
Stevens-Johnson syndrome
Teratoma
Tetanus toxin
Wegener's granulomatosis

SARCOIDOSIS

Sarcoidosis is one form of benign parotid disease that may cause facial paralysis. It is a systemic granulomatous disease of unknown cause, but many authorities suspect that tubercule bacilli are implicated in its causation. When sarcoidosis involves the nervous system, the clinical picture is either that of peripheral neuropathy or chronic meningitis with multiple cranial nerve palsies. In Heerfordt's syndrome, or uveo-parotid fever (uveitis, facial paralysis, and bilateral parotid swelling due to sarcoidosis), the facial paralysis may be attributed to the peripheral parotid involvement. The parotitis probably does not, but could, play a part in the facial paralysis. Treatment does not depend on the location of the lesion, and the response to corticosteroids is dramatic. The dosage is directly related to the clinical remission.

LYME DISEASE

Lyme disease, initially recognized in 1975, is caused by a newly identified spirochete that is transmitted by *Ixodes dammini* or related ixodid ticks carrying the spirochete, *Borrelia burgdorferi*. Facial paralysis is a reported complication of the infection. Like other spirochetal infections, Lyme disease has different clinical stages of remission and exacerbation. Stage 1 is associated with malaise, fatigue, headache, myalgias, and the classic erythema chronicum migrans. Stage 2 begins weeks or months later, when neurologic and cardiac abnormalities develop. The neurologic abnormality most commonly seen is seventh nerve palsy, which occurs in 5% of patients with untreated early disease and may be bilateral. Facial palsy may persist for many weeks, but gradual resolution generally follows, and residual weakness is typically mild. Stage 3 begins months or years later, and arthritis develops in many patients.

Acute Lyme disease must be diagnosed clinically because antibody titer results are usually negative early in the illness. Definitive diagnosis of Lyme disease requires a combination of compatible symptoms/ signs and reactive serology. Although serologic tests for Lyme spirochete IgG antibody appear quite specific for exposure to *B. burgdorferi*, they are not very sensitive. Treatment is most effective when given early and includes tetracycline or penicillin. Amoxicillin and erythromycin may also be effective. Treatment of secondary and tertiary Lyme disease may require prolonged therapy with intravenous antibiotics such as ceftriaxone sodium.

SUGGESTED READINGS

Adour KK, Hilsinger RL Jr, and Callan EJ: Facial paralysis and Bell's palsy: A protocol for differential diagnosis. Am J Otol (Suppl): 68–73, Nov 1985.

Adour KK, Hetzler DG: Current medical treatment for facial palsy. Am J Otol 5:499–502, 1984.

Adour KK: Current concepts in neurology, diagnosis and management of facial paralysis. N Engl J Med 307:348–351, 1982.

Adour KK, Sheldon MI, and Kahn ZM: Maximal nerve excitability testing versus neuromyography: Prognostic value in patients with facial paralysis. Laryngoscope 110:1540–1547, 1980.

Adour KK, Byl FM, Hilsinger RL Jr, Kahn ZM, and Sheldon MI: The true nature of Bell's palsy: Analysis of 1000 consecutive patients. Laryngoscope 88:787–801, 1978.

Adour KK, Boyajian JA, Kahn ZM, and Schneider GS: Surgical and nonsurgical management of facial paralysis following closed head injury. Laryngoscope 87:380–390, 1977.

Adour KK, Bell D, and Hilsinger RL Jr: Herpes simplex virus in idiopathic facial paralysis (Bell's palsy). JAMA 233:527–530, 1975.

Adour KK: Idiopathic facial paralysis (Bell's palsy): Factors affecting severity and outcome in 446 patients. Neurology 24:1112–1116, 1974.

Adour KK, Wingerd J, Bell D, Manning JJ, and Hurley JP: Prednisone treatment for idiopathic facial paralysis (Bell's palsy). N Engl J Med 287:1268–1272, 1972.

Alford BR, Jerger JF, Coats AC, Peterson CR, and Weber SC: Neurophysiology of facial nerve testing. Arch Otolaryngol 97:214–219, 1973.

Bell C: On the nerves, giving an account of some experiments of their structure and functions, which lead to a new arrangement of the system. Philos Trans R Soc Lond 111:398–424, 1821.

Citron D III, Adour KK: Acoustic reflex and loudness discomfort in acute facial paralysis. Arch Otolaryngol Head Neck Surg 104:303–306, 1978.

Coker NJ, Fordice JO, Moore S: Correlation of the nerve excitability test and electroneurography in acute facial paralysis. Am J Otol 13:127–133, 1992.

Esselen E: Electromyography and electroneurography. Facial nerve surgery. Proceedings of 3rd International Symposium on FN Surgery, J Fisch (ed), Zurich, Switzerland, 9–12 August 1976.

Fisch U: Surgery for Bell's palsy. Arch Otolaryngol Head Neck Surg 107:1–10, 1981.

Fujita H, Murakami S, and Matsumoto Y: Effect of steroid on experimental facial nerve injury. In Facial Nerve Research, Japan Society of Facial Nerve Research, Tokyo, 1983.

Gantz BJ, Gmuer AA, Holliday M, and Fisch U: Electroneurographic evaluation of the facial nerve. Method and technical problems. Ann Otol Rhinol Laryngol 93:394–398, 1984.

Glasscock ME: The facial nerve. Am J Otol 5:335–336, 1984.

Gowers WR: A Manual of Diseases: the Nervous System, Churchill, London, 1893.

House JW, and O'Connor AF (eds): Handbook of Neurotological Diagnosis. New York: Marcel Dekker, 1987.

Hughes GB, Nodar RH, and Williams GW: Analysis of test-retest variability in facial electroneurography. Otolaryngol Head Neck Surg 91:290–293, 1983.

Jansen JKS, et al: Hyperinnervation of skeletal muscle fibers: Dependence on muscle activity. Science 181:559–561, 1973.

Jonsson L: On the etiology of Bell's palsy, immunological and magnetic resonance imaging abnormalities. Comprehensive Summaries of Uppsala Dissertations from the Faculty of Medicine, 1987.

Kerbavaz RJ, Hilsinger RL Jr, and Adour KK: The facial paralysis prognostic index. Otolaryngol Head Neck Surg 91:284–289, 1983.

Kobayashi T, Kudo Y, Chow M-J: Nerve excitability test using fine needle electrodes, Acta Otolaryngol Suppl (Stockh) 446:64–69, 1988.

Lanser MJ, Jackler RK: Gadolinium magnetic resonance imaging in Bell's palsy, West J Med 154:718–719.

Liston SL, Kleid MS: Histopathology of Bell's palsy. Laryngoscope 99:23–26, 1989.

Matsumoto Y, Yanagihara N, Sadamoto M: Gd-DTPA-enhanced MR imaging in peripheral facial palsy. Facial Nerve Res Jpn 11:93–96, 1991.

May M, Klein SR: Facial nerve decompression complications. Laryngoscope 93:299–305, 1983.

May M, Blumenthal F, Klein SR: Acute Bell's palsy: Prognostic value of evoked electromyography, maximal stimulation and other electrical tests. Am J Otol 5:1–7, 1983.

May M: Nerve excitability test in facial palsy: Limitations in its use, based on a study of 130 cases. Laryngoscope 82:2122–2128, 1972.

Markby DP: Lyme disease facial paralysis: differentiation from Bell's palsy, BMJ 299:605–606, 1989

Mosforth J, Taverner D: Physiotherapy for Bell's palsy. Br Med J 2:675–677, 1958.

Murphy TP: MRI of the facial nerve during paralysis. Otolaryngol Head Neck Surg 104:47–51, 1991.

Neely JG, Alford BR: Facial nerve neuromas. Arch Otolaryngol Head Neck Surg 100:298–301, 1974.

Olson NR, Goin DW, Nichols RD, and Makim B: Adverse effects of facial nerve decompression for Bell's palsy. Trans Am Acad Ophthalmol Otolaryngol 77:67–71, 1973.

Pachner AR, Steere AC: The triad of neurologic manifestations of Lyme disease: Meningitis, cranial neuritis, and radiculoneuritis. Neurology 35:47–53, 1985.

Parisier SC, Som PM, Shugar J: Metastatic disease causing peripheral facial paralysis. In Disorders of the Facial Nerve. Graham M and House WF (eds). House Ear Institute Service. pp 197–205, 1982.

Pitts DB, Adour KK and Hilsinger RL Jr: Recurrent Bell's palsy: Analysis of 140 patients. Laryngoscope 98:535–540, 1988.

Rahn DW, Malawista SE: Clinical judgement in Lyme disease. Hosp Pract 25:39–56, 1990.

Robillard RB, Hilsinger RL Jr, and Adour KK: Ramsay-Hunt facial paralysis: Clinical analyses of 185 patients. Otolaryngol Head Neck Surg 95:292–297, 1986.

Ruboyianes JM, Adour KK, Santos DQ, Von Doersten PG: The maximal stimulation and facial nerve conduction latency tests: predicting the outcome of Bell's palsy. Laryngoscope 104(1 Pt 2) (Suppl 61):1–6, 1994.

Shiotani M, Yuda Y, Wakasugi B: Comparison of prognoses in Bell's palsy, Ramsay Hunt syndrome and zoster sine herpete. Facial Nerve Res Jpn 11:207–210, 1991.

Smith IM, Murray JAM, Prescott RJ, Barr-Hamilton R: Facial electroneurography: standardization of electrode position, Arch Otolaryngol Head Neck Surg 114:322–325, 1988.

Spector GJ: A targeted problem and its solution: Classification of facial nerve disorders. Laryngoscope 95:100–103, 1985.

Sunderland S: Nerves and Nerve Injury. New York, Churchill Livingstone, 1978, p 133.

Sugita T, Murakami S, Hirata Y, Fujiwara Y, Yanagihara N: Experimental facial nerve paralysis induced by herpes simplex virus. Facial Nerve Res Jpn 11:52, 1991.

Thomander L,d Stalberg E: Electroneurography in the prognostication of Bell's palsy. Acta Otolaryngol Head Neck Surg 92:221–237, 1981.

Tien R, Dillon WP, Jackler RK: Contrast-enhanced MR imaging of the facial nerve in 11 patients with Bell's palsy, AJNR Am J Neuroradiol 11:735–741, 1990.

Tschiassny K: Eight syndromes of facial paralysis and their significance in locating the lesion. Ann Otol Rhinol Laryngol 62:677–693, 1953.

Ushiro K, Yanagida M, Iwano T, Hosoda Y: Gd-DTPA enhanced MRI in patients with Ramsay Hunt syndrome. Facial Nerve Res Jpn 11:133–138, 1991.

Vahlne A, Edstrom S, Arstila P, et al: Bell's palsy and herpes simplex virus. Arch Otolaryngol Head Neck Surg 107:79–81, 1981.

Wayman DM, Pham HN, Byl FM, Adour KK: Audiological manifestations of Ramsay Hunt syndrome. J Laryngol Otol: 104–108, 1990.

Yanagihari N: Etiology and pathophysiology of Bell's Palsy. Ann Otol Rhinol Laryngol 97 (Suppl 137), 1988.

60 Surgery of the Skull Base

John J. Zappia, Alan G. Micco, and Richard J. Wiet

The skull base is a complex anatomic region that can be the site of a diverse group of pathologic processes. Surgical access to this area is necessary for a variety of neoplasms as well as non-tumorous conditions such as vertigo, facial paralysis and hemifacial spasm.

Treatment of skull base disorders can be quite complex, but recent advances allow more accurate assessment and more reliable outcomes. Improved imaging techniques (especially magnetic resonance imaging) allow more accurate planning of surgery and counseling of the patient. Diagnostic techniques such as auditory brainstem response (ABR) and electronystagmography (ENG) allow early identification of abnormalities. Intraoperative neural monitoring allows quicker, more reliable localization of important structures during surgery. As more experience is reported in this area, ideas and treatments are being refined and improved.

An important aspect of skull base surgery, and a large factor for optimal outcome, is cooperation among physicians. Consultation with a neuroradiologist maximizes the benefit of imaging techniques and allows interventional procedures such as embolization. Neurosurgical assistance is desirable when intracranial exposure is necessary. In selected cases, participation of other physicians such as vascular surgeons may also be beneficial.

ANATOMY

Superiorly the floor of the cranial cavity, or skull base, serves as a support for the brain and intracranial structures. Inferiorly, it attaches to the facial bones anteriorly and serves as the attachment for head and neck muscles laterally and posteriorly. The floor of the cranial cavity is composed of the frontal, ethmoid, sphenoid, temporal and occipital bones (Fig. 60–1) and is broadly classified into the anterior, middle and poste-

rior fossa. Numerous foramina allow passage of vascular and neural structures between the intracranial and extracranial space. The area below the midlateral portion of the skull base (essentially the temporal bone) is designated the infratemporal fossa.

Anterior Cranial Fossa

The anterior fossa is composed of the frontal bone anteriorly and laterally, the cribriform plate of the ethmoid bone centrally and the body and lesser wing of the sphenoid bone posteriorly and centrally. Immediately anterior to the cribriform plate is the foramen cecum through which an emissary vein passes to the nasal cavity. The perforated cribriform plate allows passage of the olfactory nerve fibers traveling from the olfactory epithelium of the superior nasal cavity to the olfactory bulb. The sella turcica contains the pituitary gland in the posterior central area of the anterior fossa at the junction with the middle and posterior fossae. The optic chiasm rests anterior and superior to the pituitary in the chiasmic groove. The cavernous sinus lies lateral to the pituitary gland and sella turcica.

Middle Cranial Fossa

The middle fossa is formed by the greater wing of the sphenoid bone anterocentrally and the temporal bone centrally, laterally, and posteriorly. It extends from the superior orbital fissure (greater wing of the sphenoid) anteriorly to the superior petrosal sinus along the petrous ridge posteriorly and from the cavernous sinus medially to the squamous portion of the temporal bone laterally. Anteromedially the foramen spinosum allows passage of the middle meningeal artery into the cranial space where it courses laterally along the outer surface of the dura. The trigeminal nerve originates in the posterior cranial fossa and enters the middle cranial fossa through a fold of dura over the medial petrous

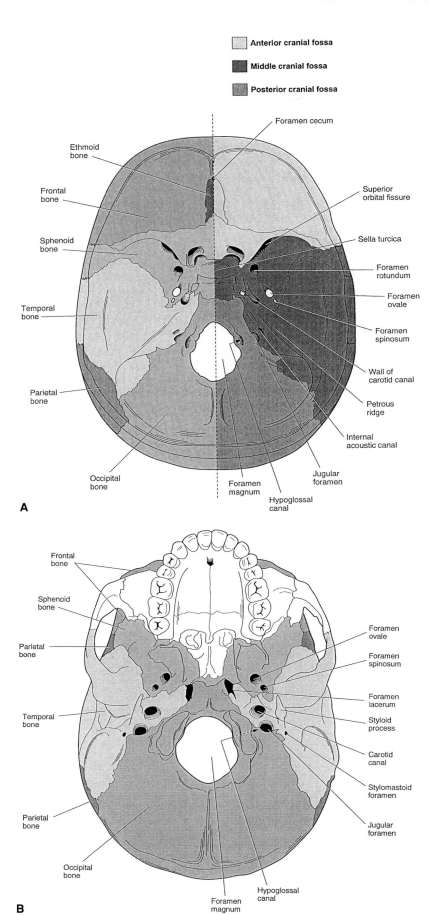

Anterior cranial fossa

Middle cranial fossa

Posterior cranial fossa

Foramen cecum

Ethmoid bone

Frontal bone

Superior orbital fissure

Sphenoid bone

Sella turcica

Foramen rotundum

Foramen ovale

Temporal bone

Foramen spinosum

Wall of carotid canal

Parietal bone

Petrous ridge

Internal acoustic canal

Occipital bone

Foramen magnum

Hypoglossal canal

Jugular foramen

A

Frontal bone

Sphenoid bone

Foramen ovale

Parietal bone

Foramen spinosum

Foramen lacerum

Styloid process

Temporal bone

Carotid canal

Stylomastoid foramen

Parietal bone

Jugular foramen

Occipital bone

Hypoglossal canal

Foramen magnum

B

Fig. 60–1. A. View of the skull base from above shows the foramina discussed in the text (right), the three basic divisions of the skull base (right), and the bones comprising this area (left). **B.** Inferior view of the skull base with the foramina labeled on the right side of the figure and the individual bones comprising the skull base on the left.

ridge, Meckel's cave. The Vth nerve (Gasserian) ganglion lies immediately anterior to this and rests over the horizontal portion of the carotid. From the Gasserian ganglion the three branches arise. The mandibular division of the trigeminal nerve exits the cranial cavity anteromedial to the foramen spinosum through the foramen ovale. Further anteromedially, the foramen rotundum allows for the exit of the maxillary branch of the trigeminal nerve in an anterior and horizontal direction to the pterygopalatine space. The ophthalmic branch of the trigeminal nerve, along with cranial nerves III, IV, VI and the ophthalmic vein, pass through the cavernous sinus and then enter the orbit through the superior orbital fissure. After entering the central portion of the temporal bone from the neck, the carotid artery curves medially 90° and runs a near horizontal course in a medial direction in the foramen lacerum before entering the intracranial space and passing through the cavernous sinus.

The middle cranial fossa is the one portion of the skull base with significant structures contained within the underlying bone, namely the VIIth nerve and the labyrinth. Their anatomy is reviewed elsewhere in this text. Access to and around these structures is a frequent issue in skull base surgery.

Posterior Cranial Fossa

The majority of the floor of the posterior fossa is composed of the occipital bone while the posterior face of the petrous portion of the temporal bone defines the anterior lateral extent. Centrally, the foramen magnum allows passage of the spinal cord and the vertebral arteries. Immediately lateral to the foramen magnum, each hypoglossal canal allows passage of a hypoglossal nerve from the intracranial cavity. Lateral to this, the jugular foramen lies at the junction of the occipital bone (medial posterior margin) and the temporal bone (anterolateral margin). The jugular vein (laterally) and the IXth, Xth and XIth cranial nerves (medially) traverse this foramen.

Superior to the jugular foramen, the internal auditory canal (IAC) serves as an entrance of the VIIth and VIIIth cranial nerves into the temporal bone. In the cerebellopontine angle (CPA) the VIIth nerve lies anteromedial to the VIIIth nerve. As the VIIIth nerve enters the IAC, it trifurcates into the auditory, the superior vestibular and the inferior vestibular nerves. In the lateral end of the IAC (fundus) these three nerves, along with the VIIth nerve fill each of the quadrants of the IAC (Fig. 60–2).

Infratemporal Fossa

The area below the temporal bones bilaterally is designated the infratemporal fossa. The internal carotid artery and the internal jugular vein pass through here in

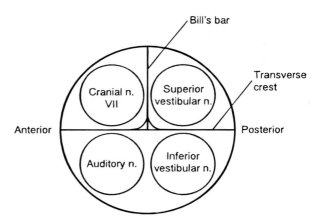

Fig. 60–2. Schematic drawing of the position of the four nerves at the lateral aspect of the internal auditory canal. The transverse crest and Bill's bar are important identifying landmarks.

a vertical direction. Medial to the internal jugular vein, cranial nerves IX, X and XI exit the jugular foramen and pass through the infratemporal fossa. The deep lobe of the parotid abuts the anterolateral margin of the infratemporal fossa.

EVALUATION

History and Physical Examination

Key aspects of history taking and physical examination as they relate to skull base disorders will be highlighted. A past medical history should always be taken to include use of medications, allergies, alcohol and tobacco use, and any past history of malignancy or neurological disorder such as multiple sclerosis. It is very important to rule out the possibility of metastasic neoplasms or systemic illness.

While some skull base lesions may be an incidental finding (on magnetic resonance imaging [MRI] scanning, for example), most patients will be symptomatic. Their complaints can range from nonspecific symptoms such as headache to very localized findings such as unilateral hearing loss. In directing questions to the patient, one should remember that most symptoms are related to encroachment on nervous and vascular structures along the skull base.

Evaluation of a patient with a skull base disorder requires a thorough head and neck examination, otologic/neurotologic exam and general neurological exam with emphasis on the cranial nerves. Specific signs, symptoms and findings will be discussed with each disorder.

Diagnostic Testing

Physiologic tests are also useful in diagnosis and treatment of skull base disorders. Patients with audioves-

**TABLE 60–1. Audiologic Evidence of
Retrocochlear Lesions**

Asymmetric SNHL
Reflex abnormalities
Tone decay
Rollover
Decreased discrimination out of proportion with hearing loss

tibular complaints or suspected cerebellopontine disorders undergo basic audiologic evaluation including pure-tone averages, speech reception thresholds, word recognition scores and tympanometry. These tests supply valuable information concerning the function of the external auditory canal, tympanic membrane, middle ear and ossicles, cochlea and auditory nerve. If a retrocochlear lesion is suspected, stapedial reflexes are obtained and rollover (decreasing discrimination with increasing intensity) is evaluated (Table 60–1). If there is suspicion of a retrocochlear lesion after initial evaluation, further testing (either ABR or MRI scan) is done (Fig. 60–3).

ABR testing is a very useful, noninvasive screening test used most commonly when an acoustic neurinoma is suspected. Although absolute latencies of the five obtained waves are helpful, the most commonly used measurement in evaluation of an acoustic neurinoma is the interaural comparison of wave V latencies. A difference of greater than 0.2 ms is considered significant. The sensitivity of ABR, using a click stimulus, is reported between 93 to 100%.[1] False positives range

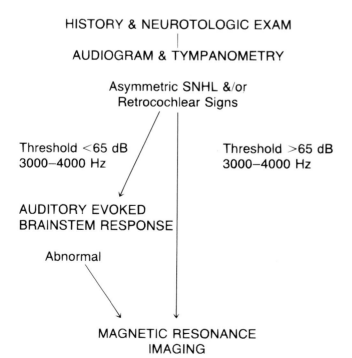

Fig. 60–3. Flow diagram demonstrates our procedure for evaluation of patients suspected of having retrocochlear disease.

from 8 to 25%.[2] Care must be used in evaluating a patient with pure-tone thresholds greater than 65 dB at 4K Hz, as an abnormal response may be due simply to the inability to activate the auditory system adequately.

The ABR is also useful in the identification of other disorders. In VIIIth nerve vascular compressive syndromes, the waves I–III latency tends to be prolonged. This is felt to be due to the irritation/compression from the pulsation of the blood vessel against the nerve. Abnormalities can also be seen in other disorders such as multiple sclerosis. Up to 93% of patients with multiple sclerosis have ABR abnormalities.[3] Various wave amplitude and latency abnormalities are possible, with wave V amplitude and waves III–V latencies being the most common.

The ENG is used to evaluate the vestibular labyrinth, the vestibular portion of the the VIIIth nerve and the central portions of the vestibular system. The caloric portion of the ENG allows each labyrinth to be evaluated individually. The information is very helpful when attempting to document objectively the side of vestibular abnormality when considering an ablative vestibular procedure such as labyrinthectomy or vestibular neurectomy.

Seventh cranial nerve status is frequently important in skull base disorder decision-making. Most commonly, the level of clinical function is the important feature. At times, in the completely paralyzed face, it is important to evaluate the integrity of the nerve. This provides useful prognostic information and is also helpful in Bell's palsy or herpes zoster oticus (Ramsay-Hunt syndrome) when surgical decompression of the VIIth nerve is being considered. Several tests are available including electroneuronography (evoked electromyography), maximal stimulation test, nerve excitability test and electromyography. The descriptions, indications and details of each of these tests are discussed in chapter 59.

Diagnostic Imaging

Imaging is frequently the key diagnostic method in skull base abnormalities. In mass lesions they are especially critical in treatment planning.

Magnetic resonance imaging (MRI) came into regular use in the late 1980s. Soft tissue detail is significantly improved from previous techniques. Gadolinium DTPA, a paramagnetic contrast agent, allows definition of many tissues and lesions. It is given intravenously and, unlike iodine compounds, adverse reactions to it are extremely rare. In the cerebellopontine angle, MRI has allowed identification of smaller acoustic neurinomas than in the past. Even very small acoustic neurinomas that do not show significant tissue distortion readily enhance with gadolinium (Fig. 60–4). One distinct advantage of MRI is that, in one "pass"

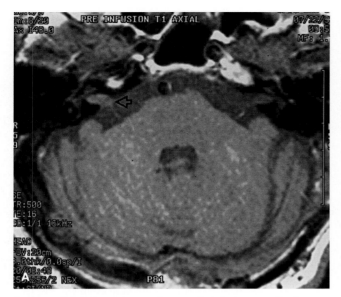

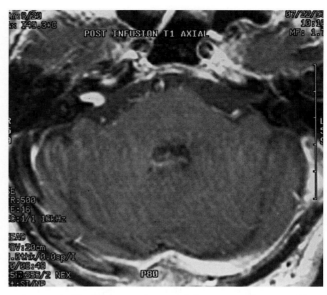

Fig. 60–4. MRI of a patient with a small right intracanalicular acoustic neurinoma. **A.** The T1 image shows subtle contrast changes without significant internal auditory canal enlargement (arrow). **B.** Gadolinium enhancement of the T1 image clearly delineates the tumor.

through the scanner, complete information is entered into the computer and an image can be created in any plane—most commonly the axial, coronal or sagittal planes. A drawback of MRI is the complete lack of visualization of bone, making it difficult to evaluate any bony abnormality or soft tissue bony interfaces. MRI scanning is contraindicated in patients with metal implants such as pacemakers and surgical clips. Claustrophobia and obesity can be relative contraindications although newer "open" scanners frequently allow enough room for obese patients and help alleviate claustrophobic symptoms.

Computerized axial tomography (CAT) became the prevalent imaging tool in the 1970s and although it allowed the best soft tissue detail at the time, it has subsequently been surpassed by MRI. High resolution CAT scanning of the temporal bone and skull base remains the best study of bony anatomy and of bone destruction by space-occupying lesions (Fig. 60–5). Intravenous iodine-based contrast can be used to enhance soft tissue visualization.

Angiography can be useful as both a diagnostic and treatment modality. Primary vascular abnormalities such as aneurysms, arteriovenous malformations and arteriovenous fistulas are readily seen on angiography. Vascular tumors such as glomus jugulare (Fig. 60–6) and glomus vagale can be clearly identified with their blood supplies delineated. Angiography is also useful to establish the patency, location and relationship of the adjacent blood vessels to the lesions.

In lesions that involve or are adjacent to the internal carotid artery, preoperative occlusion studies are of predictive value when considering resection of the artery. After catheterization of the internal carotid artery, the vessel is balloon occluded, and the patients are monitored. Patients tolerating occlusion are at lower risk for neurogenic sequelae postoperatively if the artery is resected or damaged during surgery.[4]

In vascular lesions such as glomus jugulare tumors, angiography with embolization has been used as an isolated treatment modality, but more commonly is used as a preoperative adjunct. Preoperative embolization has been shown to decrease intraoperative blood loss significantly in these patients.[5,6]

SKULL BASE DISORDERS

There is a large variety of skull base disorders. While many of these are mass lesions, other entities such as infectious diseases, inflammatory abnormalities and vascular compression syndromes must be considered. Although malignant lesions do occur, fortunately most of the skull base entities are benign. When evaluating a patient with a malignant skull base lesion, it is important to rule out the possibility of a metastasis from a regional or distant site.

Some mass lesions may be unique to specific areas of the skull base, while others can arise in more than one site. The following section will briefly review lesions by location. The more important entities will subsequently be discussed individually.

Lesions of the Anterior Skull Base

Mass lesions of the anterior skull base include benign fibro-osseous lesions and osseous lesions as well as

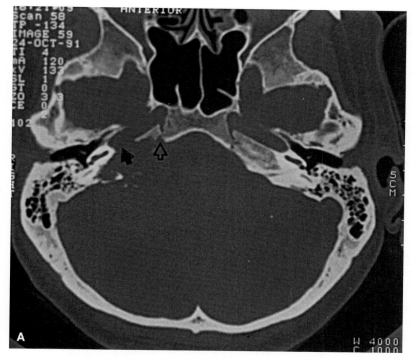

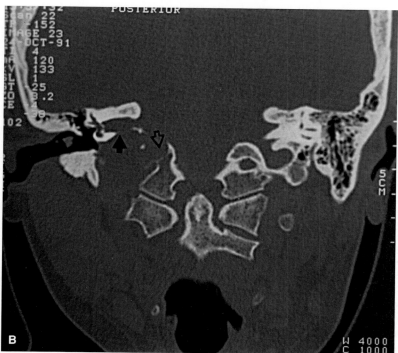

Fig. 60–5. CT of the temporal bone in which the chondrosarcoma arises from the right foramen lacerum. There is significant bone erosion of the petrous apex. **A.** Axial view demonstrates erosion of bone along the horizontal carotid canal (black arrow) and the clivus portion of the sphenoid bone (open arrow). **B.** Coronal view reveals bone erosion of the inferior aspect of the internal carotid artery (black arrow) and hypoglossal canal (open arrow).

malignant entities such as sinonasal tumors and esthesioneuroblastoma.

Fibro-osseous lesions, fibrous dysplasia and ossifying fibroma are common benign lesions of the anterior skull base. Fibrous dysplasia may occur in mono-ostotic (one site) or polyostotic (more than one site) forms. The mono-ostotic form is the most common. Ossifying fibromas have a higher growth rate than fibrous dysplasia. They are differentiated on CT from fibrous dysplasia by the appearance of a bony capsule. Another common lesion is the osseous lesion osteoma. They frequently arise in the frontal and ethmoid sinuses and involve the anterior skull base secondarily. Pathologic differentiation among these lesions is sometimes difficult. Treatment of these lesions is necessary only when functional problems arise or cosmetic deformity occurs.[7]

Two malignant lesions that can involve the anterior

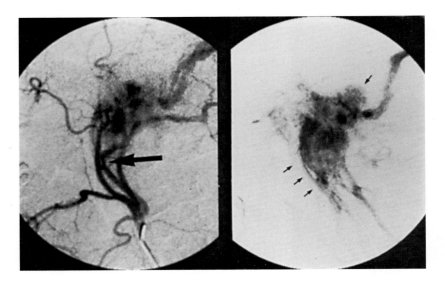

Fig. 60–6. Angiogram showing a large glomus jugulare tumor. The ascending pharyngeal artery (large arrow) is the dominant feeding vessel. Tumor fills the jugular vein (triple arrow) and extends into the posterior fossa (small single arrow). Reprinted with permission from Young N, Wiet R, Russell E, and Monsell EM: Superselective embolization of glomus jugulare tumors. Ann Otol Rhinol Laryngol 97:613–620, 1988.

skull base are paranasal sinus carcinoma and esthesioneuroblastoma. Ethmoid and, less commonly, frontal sinus tumors (most of which are squamous cell carcinomas) involve the anterior skull base through direct extension. Wide surgical removal, usually in combination with radiation or chemotherapy, is necessary when treatment for cure is planned. Esthesioneuroblastomas are of neural crest origin and represent about 2% of all malignant nasal neoplasms. The cribriform plate is involved early as this lesion arises from the olfactory epithelium.[8] Total gross removal may require craniofacial resection as well as orbital exenteration, in addition to sinus eradication.

Middle Fossa/Petrous Apex Lesions

Mass lesions of the middle cranial fossa and petrous apex include benign entities such as cholesterol granuloma, meningiomas, cholesteatomas and schwannomas. The latter three lesions will be discussed in more detail later in this chapter. Malignant lesions such as chordoma, chondrosarcoma and nasopharyngeal carcinoma can also affect this area.

Cholesterol granulomas are fluid filled cysts that may arise in any portion of the air cell system of the temporal bone, more commonly in the petrous apex. They occur in well pneumatized temporal bones in air cells that are poorly ventilated. The negative pressure causes a resultant hemorrhage in the air cell. Once the blood begins to break down, there is a foreign body reaction to one of the breakdown components, cholesterol.[9] Cholesterol granulomas have a propensity to affect cranial nerves. The patient usually presents with hearing loss although vertigo, facial paresis and diplopia may be present. Diagnosis is usually confirmed with a CT and MRI (Fig. 60–7). This lesion appears very bright on both T1 and T2 images. Treatment consists of surgical drainage with maintenance of ventilation.[10]

Of the malignant lesions, chordoma is relatively insidious. This neoplasm is thought to arise from the primitive notochord, and the majority involve the petroclival area. Symptoms are caused by progressive involvement of adjacent cranial nerves. The typical CT shows an irregular mass with bony destruction. MRI reveals a low intensity mass on T1 and T2 with variable enhancement. Extensive surgery in combination with high dose radiation therapy is the treatment of choice.[11]

Chondrosarcomas are rare, comprising less than 1% of skull base tumors.[12] They are thought to arise from trapped embryologic rests in and around the foramen lacerum. Hearing loss is the initial complaint of most patients although complaints may include tinnitus, vertigo, unsteadiness, diplopia and facial paresis. CT scanning shows irregular bony destruction with the contrast enhancement (Fig. 60–5). The lesion also brightly enhances on MRI. Total removal of the tumor is the optimum treatment. Radiation therapy is controversial.

Nasopharyngeal cancer has been discussed elsewhere in this text. Larger lesions can invade the skull base and present with symptoms of a skull base lesion.

Posterior Fossa/Internal Auditory Canal Lesions

Most mass lesions of the posterior fossa are benign. Acoustic neurinomas account for roughly 90% of the lesions while meningiomas account for about 5%. These will be discussed later. Other mass lesions include epidermoids, lipomas, and arachnoid cysts. The majority of the malignant lesions that do occur in this area are metastatic.

Epidermoids arise from trapped rests of stratified squamous epithelium and comprise 1% of CPA tumors.[13] Careful removal of all squamous cell elements

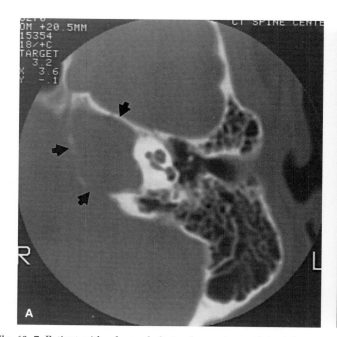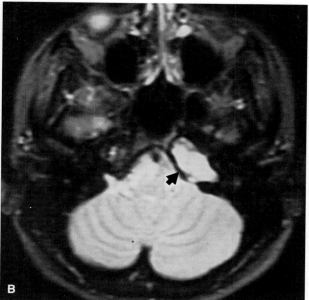

Fig. 60–7. Patient with a large cholesterol granuloma of the left petrous apex. **A.** Bone window axial CT shows soft tissue density replacing the entire left petrous apex (arrows). **B.** T1 MRI shows this bright lesion.

is necessary to prevent aseptic meningitis or recurrence. Lipomas can occur in the IAC and CPA. IAC lipomas tend to present earlier because of neural compression, while CPA lipomas may not cause symptoms until they are much larger. Diagnosis is made with MRI.[14] Arachnoid cysts, which are collections of cerebral spinal fluid (CSF) trapped by arachnoid granulations, comprise about 1% of CPA lesions. They are

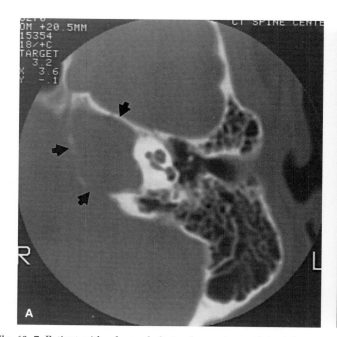

Fig. 60–8. T1 MRI image shows an apparent soft tissue mass (arrow) in the cerebellopontine angle in a patient who presented with headaches and vertigo. At the time of surgical resection an arachnoid cyst was identified.

very frequently asymptomatic and are incidental findings on MRI (Fig. 60–8). If symptomatic, surgical treatment involves opening of the cyst wall.[15]

Metastatic lesions from any other location to the CPA is possible. Fortunately, this occurrence is rare. Tumors most likely to metastasize are breast tumors, adenocarcinomas, prostate cancers and clear cell tumors of the genital organs.[16]

Infratemporal Fossa Lesions

Several primary neoplasms arise in the infratemporal fossa. The most common primary benign mass lesions are neurinomas of the V, IX, X, XI, and XII cranial nerves. This is also a common site of glomus jugulare and vagale tumors. Benign or malignant neoplasms of the deep lobe of the parotid gland can develop in this area. Of the remaining neoplasms that can arise in this location, lymphomas are the most common. Also regional metastases from head and neck primary sites may spread to the lymph nodes of this region.

SKULL BASE DISORDERS BY DIAGNOSIS

Neurinoma/Schwannoma

Acoustic Neurinoma

Acoustic neurinomas are the most common lesion of the CPA, representing 90% of all tumors in this area. Acoustic neurinomas constitute about 6% of all intracranial tumors. In the United States, there is an incidence of approximately 1:100,000 resulting in roughly 2,500 new cases diagnosed each year. The name is a misnomer because they actually arise from the Schwann cells surrounding the vestibular portion of the eighth cranial nerve. Since Schwann cells are peripheral nerve entities, then by definition these must arise in the IAC.

Acoustic neurinomas occur in two forms, sporadic and those associated with neurofibromatosis Type 2 (NF2). The sporadic form constitutes well over 90% of all acoustic neurinomas. NF2 is a rare autosomal dominant genetic disorder resulting in bilateral acoustic neuromas as well as other central nervous system neoplasms.

Unilateral hearing loss is the most common presenting symptom. Other symptoms that may occur are tinnitus, disequilibrium, vertigo, headache and aural fullness. Later symptoms can include facial numbness, facial weakness and diplopia. When the tumors are very large, neuropathies of III, IV, VI, IX, X, XI cranial nerves as well as cerebellar and brain stem compression can occur.

Acoustic neurinomas are relatively slow growing tumors. Grossly they appear yellow to gray and may have a cystic structure. Histopathologically, there are morphologic patterns: Antoni A and Antoni B. Antoni Type A is represented by small, densely packed spindle shaped cells with dark staining nuclei. In Antoni A the cells may have a whirled appearance referred to as Verocay bodies. They have no clinical significance. Antoni Type B refers to loosely packed vacuolated cells. Nuclei appear large and atypical and are densely staining. This is the predominant form in large tumors. There may also be a mixed pattern. The pattern does not correlate with the clinical presentation. Staining for S100 immunoperoxidase is confirmatory for a Schwann cell.

The introduction of MRI in the 1980s has revolutionized the diagnosis of acoustic neurinomas. Prior to MRI, CT was employed. CT was a valuable diagnostic tool if the tumor extended into the CPA or there was widening of the porous acousticus by the tumor. However, smaller intracanalicular tumors had to be diagnosed by air contrast CT requiring a lumbar puncture and injecting air in the subarachnoid space. MRI has made this procedure obsolete. Acoustic tumors readily enhance with the injection of gadolinium (Fig. 60–4). Tumors as small as 2 to 3 mm are easily seen. This allows for the diagnosis of acoustic neurinomas prior to the onset of severe clinical symptoms. Also, asymptomatic lesions which are contained in the IAC can be readily followed.

Surgical removal is the treatment of choice when the tumor is symptomatic or begins to extend beyond the IAC.[17] Total removal with the preservation of the facial nerve should be attempted. The choice of procedure—translabyrinthine, suboccipital or middle fossa—depends on the size of the tumor and the status of the hearing. These approaches will be discussed later in this chapter. In very large tumors and in high risk patients, there is a role for subtotal removal of the tumor to relieve symptoms.

Recently stereotactic radiation or gamma knife has been advocated for treatment of acoustic neurinomas. This involves a one-time dose of radiation focused on the center of the mass. The usual dose is 10 to 25 Gy. This causes shrinkage and necrosis of the mass. It has been employed in the elderly and other high-risk patients. The drawbacks are lack of elimination of the tumor and complications including hydrocephalus and cranial nerve neuropathies.

Facial Nerve Neuroma

Facial nerve neuromas are one of the few primary lesions of the nerve. Initial symptoms may include facial paresis or facial muscular fasiculations. They are found primarily in the intratemporal portion of the nerve, with the geniculate ganglion area being most common. MRI is helpful in the workup of patients with this lesion. These lesions are usually removed when facial weakness is present. Patients are usually reluctant to have them removed when they still have facial function, especially since the result will be a temporary total paralysis. These lesions are usually slow growing and can be watched for a period of time. Treatment is surgical removal with nerve grafting.

Other Neuromas

Schwannomas of the other cranial nerves are relatively unusual but Vth and IXth, Xth, XIth and XIIth nerve tumors must occasionally be treated. The petrous apex (especially with Vth nerve) and the infratemporal fossa can be involved. Symptoms are generally related to the involved nerve but can be caused by compression of adjacent structures. Trigeminal and vagal schwannomas are more common while IXth, XIth and XIIth cranial nerve schwannomas are rare. They are diagnosed with contrast MRI while CT can reveal expansion of the bone. Surgical removal is the treatment of choice for symptomatic lesions.

Meningiomas

Meningiomas are the most common benign intracranial tumors and can be found in all areas of the skull base. In the CPA they comprise 5% of all tumors. They are thought to arise from the arachnoid villi. Unlike acoustic neurinomas, they do not originate in the IAC but arise broadly from the petrous face. At presentation meningiomas are usually larger than acoustic neurinomas probably because they do not compress the contents of the IAC. Symptoms are related to the impingement on surrounding structures; however, compared to acoustic neurinomas, they more commonly spare hearing. The gross appearance of meningiomas shows a yellow to grey globular mass. Microscopically

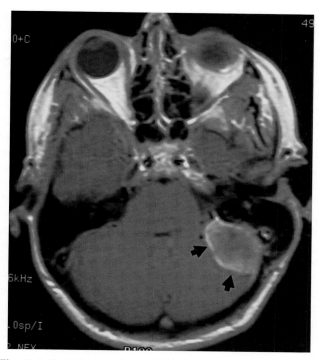

Fig. 60–9. Gadolinium-enhanced T1 MRI image of a large meningioma (arrows) originating from the posterior face of the left petrous bone.

it is characterized by sheets of polygonal cells. The boundaries of the cell are obscure. Nuclei contain chromatin and are pale staining. Histologically, calcifications known as psammoma bodies can be seen. On MRI, meningiomas appear as well circumscribed heterogenous masses that enhance with gadolinium (Fig. 60–9). On CAT the calcifications may be visible. Angiography may also be helpful as these lesions tend to be vascular. Surgical removal is necessary when symptoms appear.[18,19]

Cholesteatoma

Cholesteatomas of the petrous apex are thought to arise from epithelial rests trapped during development. The squamous cell debris begins to organize as a cyst which starts a destructive process that may erode bone. Another danger is secondary infection which can cause intratemporal as well as intracranial abscess formation. Presenting symptoms can include hearing loss, otorrhea, facial paresis or diplopia. This diagnosis is also confirmed with a combination of CT and MRI. CT shows a smooth expansile lesion with bony destruction. On MRI, the T1 intensity is low while the T2 intensity is usually increased. This lesion does not enhance with gadolinium. Surgical extirpation is the treatment of choice.[20]

Glomus Tumors

Glomus tumors are slow-growing vascular lesions with the majority (97%) being benign. They arise from

groups of chemoreceptor cells of neural crest origin which are predominantly found along the course of Jacobsen's nerve and within the adventitia of the jugular bulb. Tumors arising from Jacobsen's nerve and limited to the promontory are classified as glomus tympanicum tumors while those arising from the glomus bodies of the jugular bulb are classified as glomus jugulare tumors. The classification of these tumors can be seen in Table 60–2. Glomus tumors have been reported to be multicentric up to 10% of patients.[21] Glomus vagale tumors arise from the chemoreceptors along the vagus nerve. Glomus tumors may secrete vasoactive substances or be associated with other tumors, such as pheochromocytomas, which secrete these substances.

The diagnosis of glomus tumors is often difficult because the presenting signs and symptoms can be nonspecific, mimicking other otologic and neurologic conditions. By history, patients with glomus tumors typically present with pulsatile tinnitus followed by the development of hearing loss. The hearing loss is usually conductive because the middle ear is filled with tumor although a sensorineural hearing loss may develop if the cochlea is invaded.

Patients with glomus tympanicum tumors present with smaller tumors because the middle ear becomes involved earlier than with glomus vagale or jugulare tumors. On the other hand, patients with glomus jugulare tumors may present with dysfunction of jugular foramen contents (Vernet's syndrome).

Careful otoscopic evaluation, preferably with an operating microscope, is essential. Classically, a red tumor mass beneath an intact tympanic membrane is seen. If limited to the promontory with all tumor margins visible, it probably represents a small glomus tympanicum tumor. If the tumor extends beyond the level of the annulus (especially inferiorly), its classification cannot be made visually. A small mass seen in the floor

TABLE 60–2. Fisch Classification of Glomus Tumors

A	Limited to the middle ear
B	Involves the middle ear and mastoid, without infralabyrinthine involvement
C	Extends into the infralabyrinthine area and to the petrous apex. They originate in the jugular bulb and may erode overlying bone.
C1	May erode carotid foramen, but does not involve the artery.
C2	Involves vertical carotid canal.
C3	Invades vertical and horizontal carotid canal, but does not reach the foramen lacerum.
C4	Involves the whole intrapetrous carotid from the foramen lacerum to the cavernous sinus.
D	Intracranial extension.
De1	Extradural < 1 cm.
De2	Extradural > 1 cm.
Di	Intracranial, intradural
Di3	Intracranial, unresectable

of the middle ear may represent the "tip of the iceberg" of a large glomus jugulare tumor that may extensively involve the skull base. These tumors may blanch with positive pressure or pneumotoscopy (Brown's sign). The tumor also may extend through the tympanic membrane and present as an aural polyp. An audible bruit or evidence of vascular pulsations during tympanometry may also be present in these patients.

A glomus tumor filling the middle ear may also cause a diffusely discolored appearance of the tympanic membrane which may be mistaken for serous fluid. Other entities that can be confused with glomus tumors include a dehiscent jugular bulb or a rarely dehiscent carotid artery. Cholesterol granuloma can easily be confused with large glomus tumors because they can make the tympanic membrane appear reddish-blue. Judicious use of the appropriate diagnostic imaging techniques readily differentiates these possibilities.

Any attempt at biopsy should be deferred until a complete workup is done. A systematic protocol allows one to make the diagnosis and to define the extent of the tumor. These patients should undergo high-resolution CT with contrast injection. If the tumor is limited to the middle ear and there is no bony destruction, the tumor is classified as a glomus tympanicum tumor, and no further radiologic workup is needed. If the CT shows any bony destruction or connection with the jugular bulb, then an MRI is obtained which helps to define any intracranial extension, jugular or carotid involvement and also screens for the presence of a second glomus tumor in the head and neck. If workup reveals a glomus jugulare tumor and the patient is a surgical candidate, preoperative angiography is indicated. Superselective embolization of the tumor-feeding vessels is performed at the same time. During the angiography, the patency of the venous drainage system of the opposite side and the patency of the cerebral crossflow are evaluated. A combination of CT, MRI and angiography clearly defines the extent of the disease and, therefore, limits unexpected findings at the time of operation.

Surgical removal is the treatment of choice. Preoperative embolization can decrease operative morbidity. Radiation therapy can be used alone; however, it is usually reserved for patients with concurrent medical problems or the elderly who may be at higher risk for surgical complications.

Encephaloceles

Encephaloceles are defined as intracranial contents beyond the confines of the cranial vault. Various components may be extruding. In meningoceles, only the meninges and CSF have herniated. Encephalomeningoceles represent herniations of the brain along with meninges while hydroencephalomeningoceles represent the herniation of ventricles along with the brain.

Encephaloceles can be divided into acquired and spontaneous lesions. An acquired lesion is one that occurs secondary to an event such as trauma, chronic infection or surgery. Lesions are referred to as spontaneous if no preceding event is present. Spontaneous lesions can be further subdivided into congenital and idiopathic lesions. Congenital lesions occur in 1:3000 to 10,000 live births. They are more common in the anterior and posterior fossa. Congenital temporal lobe herniations are rare, but do occur. There are many theories to try to explain temporal lobe herniations. Most patients with a herniation are found to have multiple defects in the temporal bone. Arachnoid granulations greater than 3 mm are thought to cause bony erosion leading to herniation.[22]

Presentation is similar in all types of lesions. They can present with CSF rhinorrhea or otorrhea, recurrent meningitis, serous otitis media or a conductive hearing loss. Diagnosis is made with combination of CT for bony detail and MRI for soft tissue detail. Surgical repair is necessary if they become symptomatic. For lesions less than 2 cm in diameter, the repair can be done through a transmastoid approach. For lesions greater than 2 cm, the recommended treatment involves a transmastoid exposure of the lesion from below combined with a middle fossa craniotomy to expose the superior aspect of the defect.

Infectious Lesions

Petrous apicitis is a coalescence of the cells in the apex usually associated with a chronic infectious process, mastoiditis or cholesteatoma. Infectious agents include Staphylococcus, Hemophilus or Pseudomonas. Symptoms include aural discharge, retro-orbital pain and a VIth nerve palsy (Gradenigo's syndrome). Possible sequelae can include intracranial abscess formation, meningitis and further cranial nerve palsies. CT will reveal any bony destruction with irregular borders. On MRI the T1 image shows low signal intensity; however, the lesion is very bright on T2. Gadolinium infusion shows a ring enhancement around the lesion. Treatment includes intravenous antibiotics and surgical drainage to establish adequate and sustained drainage and ventilation of the petrous apex.

Vascular Compression Syndromes

Vascular compression syndromes are abnormal excitation of the nerve due to sustained contact with adjacent blood vessels. Prolonged contact of a blood vessel to a neural sheath causes chronic excitation and reorganization of the cranial nerve nucleus resulting in hyperfunction.[23] Depending on the involved cranial nerve, this condition may result in hemifacial spasm, trigeminal neuralgia or cochleovestibular compression syndrome.

Hemifacial spasm consists of involuntary facial muscle spasms. These usually begin with the orbicularis oculi and proceed to involve the lower parts of the face. Eventually the patient can develop facial weakness thought to be due to demyelination secondary to the compression. The unilaterality of this disorder helps to differentiate it from essential blepharospasm.

Trigeminal neuralgia is characterized by piercing facial pain. Tactile stimulation of the face, pain, cold, or dental work can cause hyperactivity in the nucleus resulting in the pain. Cochleovestibular compression syndrome has been reported to result in continuous vertigo, hearing loss, nausea, tinnitus and imbalance.

In these patients, all other potential causes must be ruled out. For those failing more conservative treatment (i.e. medical therapy to relieve symptoms), surgical exploration of the nerve and decompressing the offending vascular structure is an option. In the CPA, this is usually the anterior inferior cerebellar artery or posterior inferior cerebellar artery, but veins may also be the culprit.

MANAGEMENT

It is beyond the scope of this chapter to review the treatment issues for each of the skull base disorders, but a general overview of available modalities and techniques is designed to give the reader some basis for understanding their roles.

Some of the lesions discussed are malignant by definition. The majority are benign but clinically "malignant" either because of the debility of symptoms or their proximity to neural and vascular structures. The histologic classification, severity of symptoms and the proximity to important structures play a role in treatment decision making. Treatment options generally include surgery, radiation, chemotherapy or simple observation. Oncologic chemotherapy has a limited role in the management of skull base lesions aside from an occasional primary or metastatic cancer. This discussion will center around mass lesions that require intervention or pathophysiologic disorders that have failed medical therapy.

Radiation

External beam radiation has been used as an adjunct to surgery in certain lesions such as olfactory neuroblastoma. Primary radiation traditionally has been used in the more common benign lesions (such as acoustic neuroma) in the elderly or medically disabled, but treatment results vary. Primary risks include damage to the brain and nerves and the superficial structures such as skin as well as osteoradionecrosis of the bone.

More recently, stereotactically directed gamma radiation ("gamma knife") has been discussed as a treatment option.[24] Numerous cobalt sources (approx. 200) are positioned in a hemispherical pattern oriented towards a common point. In this technique, high doses of radiation are given to a more localized area in shorter periods of time than in traditional radiation therapy. Commonly patients receive their total radiation dose in a single treatment. Thus, the risks should be less than traditional radiation, and the time involved is greatly reduced (1 day vs. approx. 6 weeks). Its use is limited to somewhat smaller tumors (acoustic neurinomas <2 cm) and appears to be an option for surgically unsuitable patients with appropriate size tumors. The obvious benefit is avoidance of a large, usually intracranial surgical procedure. In the specific example of acoustic neurinoma, the initial risks are markedly less than surgical intervention, but over time the risks to adjacent structures such as the facial or cochlear nerves approach or exceed the surgical risks. Halting or limiting the growth of the tumor is the usual outcome with regression less commonly noted. An occasional problem arises when tumors do not respond to radiation and require surgical treatment. The surgical risks are increased since the radiation damaged tissue is generally more difficult to dissect.

Surgery

Considerations
The skull base is an area dense with important neural, vascular and structural entities. Preoperative discussions with the patients must include a thorough review of the pathologic entity as well as the potential and planned morbidity of the treatment. Each procedure and skull base area have their own individual structures at risk.

In the majority of accessible tumors, surgical removal is the treatment of choice. Surgery also allows access to particular structures such as the VIIth cranial nerve for microvascular decompression and the VIIIth cranial nerve for vestibular neurectomy. Success depends on many factors. Two important aspects are accurate assessment of the clinical entity preoperatively and, of course, the skill of the surgeon. The choice of surgical approach depends on the pathologic process as well as the expertise of the surgeon(s).

Expected morbidity, such as loss of any residual hearing in a translabyrinthine approach for acoustic neuroma removal, should be discussed and weighed against the benefits of surgery in general and specifically of a particular procedure/approach. In the case of the translabyrinthine approach, decreased risk to facial nerve and less cerebellar retraction are the primary advantages.

Complications

The more important complications result from alteration of function of the intracranial structures. Infarction of intracranial structures, such as the cerebellum or brainstem from excessive retraction or blood vessel damage, can result in significant morbidity or death. Intracranial hemorrhage may occur in the immediate or late postoperative period. Treatment usually includes immediate opening of the wound and return to the operating room for complete drainage of the blood with identification and control of the bleeding site. If identified and treated early, there may be no residual sequelae, but important functional defects are possible.

Complications may arise simply as a result of entrance into the cerebrospinal fluid containing space. Meningitis is a known risk and tends to occur between the third and seventh postoperative days. Because of the frequent postoperative malaise, head/neck discomfort and fevers from meningeal irritation, meningitis can be difficult to identify in this situation. A low threshold of suspicion and early lumbar puncture will allow early identification and rapid resolution with the institution of appropriate intravenous antibiotics.[25]

CSF leaks can occur at any time after the operation, but the risk is greatest in the first ten days. In high risk procedures, CSF lumbar drains may be placed at the time of operation to keep intracranial pressures low and decrease tension on wound closures. Drainage may occur through the nose (CSF rhinorrhea), through the ear (CSF otorrhea) or through the incision. In the anterior approaches (craniofacial), the fluid will generally drain through the nose anteriorly while in the posterior approaches the CSF reaches the nose through the eustachian tubes and may result in either anterior or posterior rhinorrhea. If a tympanic membrane perforation is present at the time of operation in the middle and posterior fossa approaches or occurs in the postoperative period, CSF otorrhea may occur. Initial treatment of CSF leak consists of head elevation and either lumbar puncture or placement of an in-dwelling lumbar spinal drain. If these conservative measures are unsuccessful, then surgical exploration and reclosure of the wound is necessary.

Injury to any of the vascular structures (i.e., carotid artery) or neural structures (i.e., cranial nerves) is possible and must be dealt with intraoperatively if the structure has been interrupted and postoperatively if there are significant sequelae. In the lateral and posterior approaches, altered function of the VIIth cranial nerve is a frequent postoperative problem. Transection of the nerve intraoperatively requires immediate primary repair or cable grafting, if possible. In this case delayed and incomplete recovery would be expected. If the continuity is maintained, but injury occurs secondary to stretching or contusion, recovery generally occurs, but time and completeness are variable. Risk to the cornea, which results from incomplete eye clo-sure, is the most important issue. For expected transient weaknesses, local eye care such as use of lubricants is all that is generally needed. For longer periods of altered function or permanent paralysis, procedures such as upper eyelid gold weight implantation, lower eyelid ectropian repair or tarsorrhaphy are frequently indicated for adequate corneal protection. In cases of permanent paralysis, nerve grafting, XIIth to VIIth end-to-side (jump graft) or end-to-end grafting, or muscle transposition (i.e. temporalis) may be useful for rehabilitation of the entire face.

Intraoperative Monitoring

Preservation of neural structures is a crucial part of skull base surgery. Although there is no substitute for surgical knowledge, neural monitoring is a useful adjunct. The motor nerve integrity can be followed by monitoring EMG activity in the appropriate muscles. Increased activity will be seen as the nerve is manipulated. The nerve of interest can also be electrically stimulated in the operative field to verify its identity. The VIIth nerve is probably the most commonly and easily monitored motor nerve.

In the hearing preservation approaches in acoustic neurinoma surgery, auditory function can be monitored in several ways. Most commonly, continuous ABR can be elicited. This has the advantage of being readily available and easy to set up but the disadvantage of requiring many averaged trials to detect an alteration. This can translate into a significant delay between the occurrence of a compromising action and the detection of the change in the ABR. The recording of electrocochleogram (ECoG) during a procedure is frequently used. As in ABR, stimulation is with repeated auditory clicks through an external auditory canal insert. Since recordings are generally obtained with a needle electrode on the promontory, the responses are more robust, require less trials and ideally require less time between the operative maneuver and the change in the observed waveform. Direct VIIIth nerve monitoring records nerve impulses traveling in the auditory nerve. The electrode is placed on the nerve proximal to the operative site so that any alteration in the physiologic status of the peripheral part of the auditory system will be immediately detected.[26]

Surgical Approaches

Because of the complexity of the skull base and the diversity of the possible abnormalities, many surgical approaches have been developed. They are continually being modified, and there are new ones being described.[27,28]

Craniofacial Approach

For lesions that involve the roof of the ethmoid sinuses or the superior nasal vault (cribriform area), visualization from above (cranially) and below (facially) can be

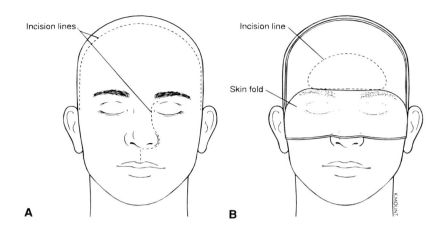

A   **B**

Fig. 60–10. A. The skin incisions for a craniofacial resection are shown here. **B.** After elevation of the forehead skin and retraction inferiorly, an approximate outline of the frontal craniotomy can be seen.

obtained through a craniofacial approach. The most common lesions include olfactory neuroblastoma and ethmoid sinus cancer.

PROCEDURE

The approach from above is initiated with a bicoronal incision originating anterior and superior to the auricles bilaterally followed by flap elevation over the forehead (Fig. 60–10). An anterior craniotomy exposes the frontal sinus, which is completely removed, and the frontal lobes which are gently elevated, necessitating transection of the olfactory nerves. This allows visualization of the floor of the anterior cranial fossa including the roofs of the orbits and cribriform plate area. Visualization can be obtained back to the area over the anterior portion of a fully pneumatized sphenoid sinus. The cribriform plate and various amounts of bone can be resected. Ideally, the tumors are extradural although dura (and even brain parenchyma) can be resected.

The approach from below is more variable but generally involves at least an ethmoidectomy. Most commonly, a lateral rhinotomy incision (Fig. 60–10) is used to allow a generous view of the nasal vault and associated paranasal sinuses. If necessary, the ethmoidectomy can be combined with maxillectomy or orbital exenteration. Reconstruction and closure vary, depending on the resection performed. At the completion of the procedure, dural repair can be accomplished with temporalis fascia, fascia lata or a local pericranial flap. In the most limited resections, the anterior cranial bone flap is replaced, and the upper and lower incisions are closed primarily. For more extensive resections, local or distant flaps may be required to reconstruct the defect and/or surgical prostheses may be necessary.

Infratemporal Fossa Approach
For access to the infratemporal fossa and the jugular foramen, the infratemporal fossa approach is available.

Glomus jugulare and vagale tumors, vagal neuromas and deep lobe parotid tumors may arise in this area.

PROCEDURE

A large curvilinear incision is made to allow access to the lateral skull and the upper cervical areas (Fig. 60–11). The skin flap is elevated anteriorly. The sternocleidomastoid muscle must be detached from its mastoid insertion to allow the generous exposure that is usually necessary. The VIIth nerve is identified exiting the stylomastoid foramen. The IXth, Xth, and XIth cranial nerves can be identified at the skull base exiting the jugular foramen into the neck. The hypoglossal nerve is seen crossing lateral to the carotid at approximately the level of the carotid bifurcation. The internal

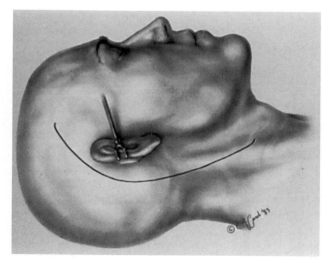

Fig. 60–11. A large C-shaped incision extending from the parietal area across the mastoid and inferiorly into the cervical area is necessary for complete exposure in the infratemporal fossa approach. Reprinted with permission from Wiet R, Causse J (eds): Complications in Otolaryngology: Head and Neck Surgery. Vol. 1. Philadelphia: BC Decker, 1986.

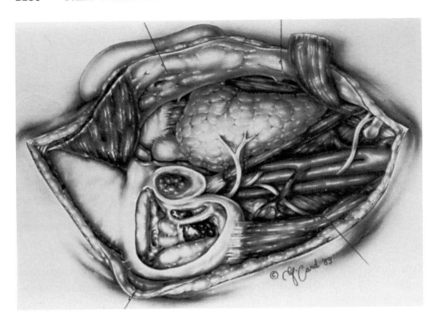

Fig. 60–12. After cervical exposure and mastoidectomy, most of the important structures are visible. In this drawing a glomus jugulare tumor can be seen medial to the facial nerve in the mastoid. Reprinted with permission from Wiet R, Causse J (eds): Complications in Otolaryngology: Head and Neck Surgery. Vol. 1. Philadelphia, BC Decker, 1986.

jugular vein and internal carotid artery are identified and isolated so they can be easily controlled.

Superiorly, the structures are located through a transmastoid approach. After the simple mastoidectomy, the sigmoid sinus, posterior and middle cranial fossa dura, and vertical facial nerve are identified (Fig. 60–12). In the majority of these procedures, the external auditory canal is removed, and the lateral canal skin is closed on itself. The facial nerve is skeletonized in the mastoid and middle ear, then completely mobilized. It is retracted anteriorly to allow direct visualization of the more medial structures. Having done this, the remaining infralabyrinthine bone is removed to

allow access to the tumor, the entire sigmoid sinus/jugular bulb/internal jugular vein and the internal carotid artery anterior medial to the jugular vein (Fig. 60–13). Removal of the tumor is then generally possible. In the case of glomus jugulare the sigmoid sinus, jugular bulb and the upper portion of the internal jugular vein are resected with the tumor. The operation may be continued intracranially in the same sitting or in a second stage for larger tumors. In glomus jugulare tumor operations, major blood loss is usually encountered although it is usually markedly decreased with preoperative embolization.

In most situations, the wound can be closed primar-

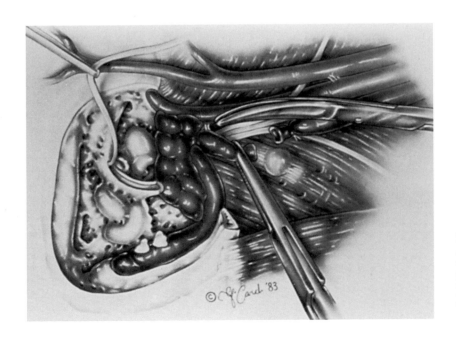

Fig. 60–13. After mobilization of the facial nerve and removal of additional bone medially, excellent visualization of the glomus jugulare tumor is possible. Reprinted with permission from Wiet R, Causse J (Eds): Complications in Otolaryngology: Head and Neck Surgery. Vol. 1. Philadelphia: BC Decker, 1986.

Translabyrinth   **Middle Fossa**   **Retrosigmoid**

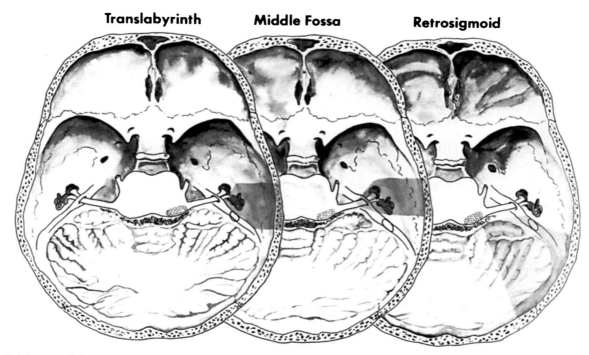

Fig. 60–14. Diagram of the the three main approaches to tumors of the cerebellopontine angle (CPA). The translabyrinthine approach gives the surgeon the best exposure but sacrifices hearing. The middle fossa offers the least exposure and thus is useful only for intracranial tumors in patients in whom hearing preservation will be attempted. The retrosigmoid approach gives good exposure of the CPA, but offers the least number of landmarks for identification of the facial nerve. We reserve it for small tumors of the CPA in patients in whom hearing preservation is worthwhile. Reprinted with permissions from Monsell EM, et al: Surgical approaches to the human cochlear nuclear complex. Am J Otol *8*:450–455, 1987.

ily. In more extensive resections, abdominal fat grafting, local tissue flaps such as temporalis muscle or free vascularized grafts may be necessary.

Internal Auditory Canal/Posterior Fossa Approaches

These surgical approaches overall are the most commonly used and designed to allow exposure of the IAC, the cerebellopontine angle and the petrous apex. The middle cranial fossa (MCF), the translabyrinthine (TL) and the retrosigmoid (RS) approaches can all be used for resection of acoustic neurinomas (Fig. 60–14). The MCF and RS approaches are classified as hearing preservation procedures since the labyrinth is preserved, and in many instances the cochlear division of the VIIIth nerve can be preserved, allowing at least the possibility of hearing postoperatively. In the TL approach the vestibular portion of the labyrinth is intentionally removed. Although this allows better visualization of the VIIth nerve and the IAC, any residual hearing is predictably and completely lost. Each has its advantages and indications.

Middle Cranial Fossa Approach

The middle cranial fossa procedure approaches the internal auditory canal from above, and here the labyrinth can be preserved in an attempt to conserve hearing. This procedure is commonly used in the resection

of acoustic neurinomas and for vestibular neurectomy. In the internal auditory canal, the vestibular portions of the VIIIth nerve are distinct from the cochlear division and at least theoretically, the vestibular nerve can be sectioned more precisely. In acoustic neurinoma surgery, the MCF approach is used when two main criteria are fulfilled: 1) the tumors should be completely within the internal auditory canal (intracanalicular), and 2) the patient should have preoperative hearing that is good enough to justify a procedure that is somewhat more complex than the other approaches.

This procedure can also be used to access the area medial to the IAC (petrous apex) for lesions such as cholesterol granulomas. For larger middle lobe encephaloceles, visualization through the MCF approach is necessary to bring the brain back into the intracranial cavity and to cover the bony defect adequately (generally with a bone flap). Additionally, this approach is used for exploration of the geniculate and labyrinthine portion of the VIIth nerve in cases of temporal bone trauma and for bony decompression for Bell's palsy.

PROCEDURE

With the surgeon at the head of the bed, the patient is placed in a supine position with the head turned so

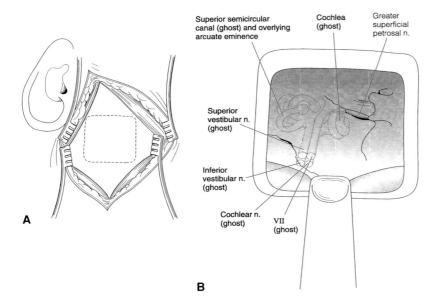

Superior semicircular
canal (ghost) and overlying
arcuate eminence

Cochlea
(ghost)

Greater
superficial
petrosal n.

Superior
vestibular n.
(ghost)

Inferior
vestibular n.
(ghost)

Cochlear n.
(ghost)

VII
(ghost)

A

B

Fig. 60–15. A. A view of the middle cranial fossa approach from the surgeon's position showing the area of planned craniotomy [dotted line] after a vertical incision has been opened. **B.** A view through the craniotomy allows exposure of the middle cranial fossa floor after retraction of the temporal lobe. The significant underlying structures are outlined.

the involved side is up. Although different incisions have been used, the simplest is a vertical incision extending from a point in the pre-auricular area one centimeter anterior to the auricle directly superiorly for 6 to 8 cm. The incision is carried down to the bone. A 3 cm square bone flap is created in the underlying bone and is removed to expose the dura overlying the temporal lobe. The temporal lobe is elevated off the floor of the MCF until the foramen spinosum and middle meningeal artery are seen anteriorly, the greater superficial petrosal nerve is seen anteromedially and the superior petrosal sinus is seen posteriorly (Fig. 60–15). The pertinent surface of the temporal bone can now be visualized. The arcuate eminence (the bony elevation over the superior semicircular canal) and the greater superficial petrosal nerve are the most common overt landmarks. From these the facial nerve and the internal auditory canal can be identified once drilling has begun. The superior semicircular canal (laterally) and the cochlea (medially) which lie on each side of the internal auditory canal must not be violated, or hearing will be lost.

In vestibular neurectomy, the superior and inferior vestibular nerves are identified in the IAC and transected. For VIIth nerve decompression exposure of the geniculate ganglion and labyrinthine portion of the VIIth nerve with opening of the nerve sheath is completed. In acoustic neurinoma resection, the tumor is carefully removed from the IAC with care being taken to preserve the VIIth nerve and the cochlear branch of the VIIIth cranial nerve.

Fascia and/or a muscle plug are used to close the dural defect, and the retracted temporal lobe is placed back in its anatomic position. The bone flap is replaced, and the incision is carefully closed.

Retrosigmoid Approach

In the retrosigmoid approach, the CPA is approached directly, and the IAC can be approached posteriorly. Because this approach allows a generous view of the CPA, it is useful in a variety of conditions and is used most frequently for CPA tumor resection, vestibular neurectomy and microvascular cranial nerve decompression. Because this is a hearing preservation approach, it is used in situations when serviceable hearing is present and the tumor is extracanalicular but is less than 2 cm. However, for intracanalicular tumors, the MCF approach is more appropriate. In tumors greater than 2 cm, hearing preservation is unlikely so the TL approach is used.

PROCEDURE

First, a curvilinear incision is made 4 cm posterior to the auricle to create an anteriorly based flap (Fig. 60–16). The bone of the mastoid and occipital area is exposed. A bone square is created with the sigmoid sinus defining the anterior limit and the transverse sinus defining the superior limit. Removal of the bone plug exposes the dura overlying the cerebellum. The dura is incised 5 to 10 mm. posterior to the sigmoid sinus and inferior to the transverse sinus. The cerebellum is retracted posteriorly to expose the CPA. In acoustic neurinoma resection, the posterior lip of the IAC must be drilled away to allow for visualization of the intracanalicular portion of the tumor.

Since the Vth to XIth nerves can be readily viewed, microvascular decompression of the Vth (for trigeminal neuralgia), VIIth (for hemifacial spasm) or VIIIth (for tinnitus or disabling positional vertigo) nerves can

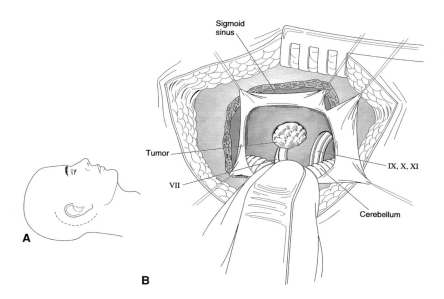

Fig. 60–16. **A.** With the patient in the supine position, approximate incision line for the retrosigmoid approach is identified [dotted line]. **B.** After craniotomy, dural incision and retraction of the cerebellum, cerebellopontine angle can be viewed. In this drawing, an acoustic neurinoma is seen extending out of the internal auditory canal.

be readily accomplished by gently placing a strip of Teflon® felt between the offending blood vessel and the nerve to prevent the irritating contact. Vestibular neurectomy is performed by identifying the longitudinal septum between the vestibular and the cochlear portion of the VIIIth nerve and transecting the upper (vestibular) half. With vestibular neurectomy, control of vertigo in Meniere's disease is generally reported to be greater than 90% regardless of the approach used.[29,30] CPA tumors such as acoustic neurinomas and meningiomas can be resected through this approach.

Upon completion of the procedure, the dura is closed in a water-tight fashion. If this is not possible, an abdominal fat graft is laid over the closure to seal the dural defect. Although some surgeons drill away the bone of the entire cranial defect, we prefer to preserve the bone square and replace it at the completion of the procedure. The skin is closed in the usual manner.

Translabyrinthine Approach

The translabyrinthine approach allows a generous view of the IAC, the CPA and the petrous apex if necessary. This approach is generally used in patients with poor hearing as any remaining hearing will be predictably and totally lost. Less brain retraction is required than in the MCF or the RS approach and unlike the RS approach, the facial nerve can be identified prior to tumor identification/removal. This approach is used in essentially all acoustic neurinomas that are larger

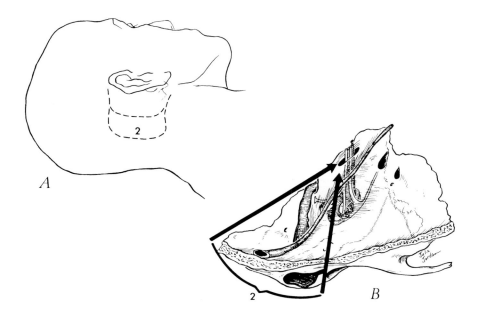

Fig. 60–17. **A.** Postauricular incision for translabyrinthine approach and its modification (2) for the combined approach. **B.** Combination of the translabyrinthine approach and retrosigmoid approach to the cerebellopontine angle may be used to excise larger tumors.

than 2 cm or in any patient with poor hearing regardless of the tumor size. Tumors greater than 4 to 5 cm. may require this approach combined with the RS approach for complete resection (Fig. 60–17).

PROCEDURE

With the patient in the supine position and the head rotated away from the side of interest, a postauricular incision is made 2 to 3 cm (Fig. 60–18) behind the postauricular sulcus. The mastoid bone is completely exposed, and a drill is used to remove completely the bone of the mastoid. The sigmoid sinus, posterior fossa dura, and middle cranial fossa are completely decompressed. The vertical portion of the facial nerve is identified and left with a thin bony covering. The facial recess (area between the vertical segment of the VIIth nerve and the chorda tympani nerve) is opened, and the incus is removed so the middle-ear space may be viewed and carefully packed at the end of the procedure. A labyrinthectomy is completed and as drilling continues medially, the internal auditory canal is exposed. The dura of the posterior fossa and internal auditory canal is opened, and the IAC and CPA are viewed (Fig. 60–18). In the fundus (lateral) portion of the IAC, a vertical crest of bone (Bill's bar) is present and is a useful landmark since the facial nerve is anterior and the superior vestibular nerve is posterior (see Fig. 60–2). After completion of the procedure, the middle ear space is carefully packed with pieces of temporalis muscle, and the remainder of the surgical defect is filled with fat obtained from the abdomen. The incision is meticulously closed, and a mastoid dressing is placed.

In selected situations the translabyrinthine approach can be "extended" to allow better access medially and anteriorly. In the *transcochlear* approach,[31] drilling is continued after a complete mastoidectomy and labyrinthectomy. The facial nerve is skeletonized and mobilized posteriorly from the stylomastoid foramen to the geniculate ganglion. The cochlea is then completely exenerated and the internal carotid artery skeletonized, allowing a generous view of the internal carotid artery, petrous apex, clivus, VIth and XIIth nerves and the basilar and vertebral arteries if necessary. A more extended view can be obtained through the *transotic* approach[32] with the tympanic membrane, malleus, incus and posterior external auditory canal wall removed in addition to skeletonization and mobilization of the VIIth nerve and exenteration of the cochlea. In the *modified transotic* approach,[33] the VIIth nerve is left in the fallopian canal decreasing the risk to it.

Approaches to the Temporal Bone

A large amount of skull base pathology occurs within the temporal bone. Frequently, there are specific approaches available that are generally simpler than the intracranial procedures.

Tympanotomy is performed through the external auditory canal and allows exposure of the mesotympanum. Frequently, glomus tympanicum and congenital cholesteatoma are limited enough to be removed through this approach. *Mastoidectomy* allows visualization of the mastoid air cell system and enables access to the antrum and epitympanum as well as the labyrinth and the deeper structures of the temporal bone. Exploration and/or decompression of the second genu and vertical segment of the VIIth nerve is possible.

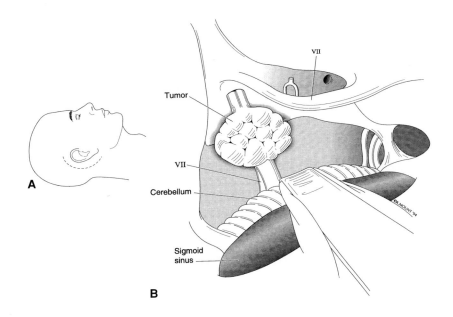

Fig. 60–18. A. The approximate postauricular incision for the translabyrinthine approach is shown (dotted line). **B.** After the drilling is complete, generous visualization of the cerebellopontine angle is possible. An acoustic neurinoma is seen arising from the eighth cranial nerve.

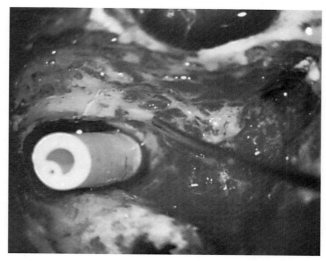

Fig. 60–19. Infralabyrinthine approach and stent placement into a cholesterol granuloma of the left petrous apex. This patient presented with vertigo, which resolved postoperatively.

Smaller tegmental encephaloceles can be repaired through this approach although ones larger than 2 cm will also require a middle fossa approach. Access to the tympanum is possible from the mastoid between the facial nerve and the chorda tympani via the *facial recess* approach. The *extended facial recess* approach requires sectioning of the chorda tympani nerve, extension of the facial recess opening inferiorly, and opening the bone around the posterior and inferior external auditory canal. A good view of the posterior and inferior tympanum can then be obtained, especially for larger glomus tympanicum tumors.

In specific situations, limited access of the petrous apex is all that is necessary. In petrous apicitis and petrous cholesterol granuloma drainage of the contents resolves the problem. If hearing is poor, the labyrinthectomy will allow a generous view medially. If useful hearing is present, the labyrinth must be avoided. The *retrofacial* approach is available after a complete mastoidectomy. Drilling is continued posterior to the facial nerve and inferior to the posterior semicircular canal. In the case of a cholesterol granuloma, the cyst is opened, and a stent is placed to maintain the drainage (Fig. 60–19). Multiple other paths are available and are chosen based on the location of the lesion and the aeration of the temporal bone.

REFERENCES

1. Hart RG, Davenport J: Diagnosis of acoustic neuroma. Neurosurgery *9*:450, 1982.
2. House WF, Luetje M (eds.): Acoustic Tumors I: Diagnosis. Baltimore: University Park Press, 1979.
3. Stockard JJ, Rossiter VS: Clinical and pathologic correlates of brainstem auditory response abnormalities. Neurology *27*: 608–613 (1977)
4. Sekhar LN, Janecka IP: Intracranial extension of cranial base tumors and combined resection: the neurosurgical perspective. In Surgery of Skull Base Tumors. Edited by C.G. Jackson. New York: Churchill-Livingston, 1991.
5. Young NM, Wiet RJ, Russel EJ, Monsell EM: Superselective embolization of glomus jugulare tumors. Ann Otol Rhinol Laryngol *97*:613–620 (1988)
6. LaRouere MJ, Zappia JJ, Wilner HI, Graham MG, Lundy LB: Selective embolization of glomus jugulare tumors. Skull Base Surgery *4*(1):21–25 (1994)
7. Harrison DFN: Osseous and fibroosseous condition affecting the craniofacial bones. Ann Otol Rhinol Laryngol *93*:199, 1984.
8. Harrison DFN: Surgical pathology of olfactory neuroblastomas. Head Neck Surg *7*:60;1984.
9. Nager GT, Vanderveen TS: Cholesterol granuloma involving the temporal bone. Ann Otol Rhinol Laryngol *85*:204, 1976.
10. Thedinger BA, et al: Radiographic diagnosis, surgical treatment and long term follow-up of cholesterol granuloma of petrous apex. Laryngoscope *99*:896, 1989.
11. Oot RF, et al: The role of MRI and CT in evaluating clival chordomas and chondrosarcomas. Am J Roentgerol *151*:567, 1988.
12. Kveton JF, et al: Chondrosarcoma of the skull base. Otolaryn Head Neck Surg *94*:23, 1986.
13. Nager GT: Epidermoids involving the temporal bone: clinical, radiological and pathologic aspects. Laryngosope *2*(suppl):1, 1970.
14. Christensen WN, Long DM, Epstein J: Cerebellopontine angle lipoma. Hum Pathol *17*:739, 1980.
15. Pappas DG, Brackmann DE: Arachnoid cysts of the posterior fossa. Otolaryngol Head Neck Surg *89*:328–332, 1981.
16. Hetselberger WE, Gardner G: Other tumors of the cerebellopontine angle. Arch Otolaryngol *88*:712, 1968.
17. National Institutes of Health Consensus Statement on Acoustic Neuroma. Washington, D.C. December, 1991.
18. MacCarty MR, Symen L: Meningiomas of the clivus and apical petrous bone, report of 35 cases. J Neurosurg *65*:160, 1986.
19. Nager GT, Masica DN: Meningiomas of the cerebello-pontine angle and their relation to the temporal bone. Laryngoscope *80*:863, 1970.
20. Pyle GM, Wiet RJ: Petrous apex cholesteatoma: exteriorization vs. subtotal petrosectomy with obliteration. Skull Base Surg *1*: 97, 1991.
21. Glasscock M, Jackson CG, Dickins Wiet R.: Panel discussion: glomus jugulare tumors of the temporal bone. The surgical management of glomus tumors. Laryngoscope *89*:1640, 1971.
22. Gacek R: Evaluation and management of the temporal bone arachnoid granulations. Arch Otolaryngol Head Neck Surg *118*: 327–332, 1992.
23. Moller AR, Jannetta PJ: On the origin of synkenesis in hemifacial spasms. Results of intracranial recordings. J Neurosurg *61*: 569, 1984.
24. Lunsford LD, Linskey ME: Stereotactic radiosurgery in the treatment of patients with acoustic tumors. *In* Acoustic Neuroma I. Edited by R.K. Jackler RK. Otolaryngol Clin North Am *25*(2):471, 1992.
25. Wiet RJ, Teixido MT, Liang JG: Complications in acoustic neuroma surgery. Otolaryngol Clin North Am *25*(2):389, 1992.
26. Wiet RJ, Liang JG, Teixido MT: Electrocochleography and direct nerve monitoring during vestibular neurectomy. *In* Intraoperative Auditory Monitoring. Edited by R. J. Wiet. Alexandria VA Am Acad Otolaryngol Head Neck Surg Foundation, 1992.
27. Sekhar S. Tumors of the cranial base. Diagnosis and treatment. Mount Kisco, NY: Future Publishing Co., Inc., 1987.

28. Jackler RK, Brackmann DE: Neurotology. St. Louis: Mosby, 1994.
29. Glasscock M, Kveton J, Christiansen S: Middle fossa vestibular neurectomy: an update. Otolaryngol Head Neck Surg 92:216, 1984.
30. Monsell E, Wiet RJ, Young N, Kazan R: Surgical treatment of vertigo with retrolabyrinthine vestibular neurectomy. Laryngoscope 98:835, 1988.
31. House WF, Hitselberger WE: The transcochlear approach to the skull base. Arch Otolaryngol 102:334, 1976
32. Jenkins HA, Fisch U: The transotic approach to resection of difficult acoustic tumors of the cerebellopontine angle. Am J Otol 2:70, 1980.
33. Gantz BJ, Fisch U: Modified transotic approach to the cerebellopontine angle. Arch Otolaryngol 109:252, 1983.

VI BRONCHOESOPHAGOLOGY

James B. Snow, Jr. and Joyce A. Schild

61 Introduction to Peroral Endoscopy

James B. Snow, Jr. and Joyce A. Schild

The advent of methods to visualize pathologic changes in the respiratory and alimentary tracts is undoubtedly a very important development in the care of patients with respiratory and alimentary diseases. Rational management of nearly all patients with pulmonary, upper respiratory, and digestive diseases requires endoscopic evaluation for diagnosis, and many commonly encountered disease processes are amenable to endoscopic management. Advances in lighting, flexibility, lens systems, video photography, ventilation, anesthesia, and magnification have made the benefits of peroral endoscopy available to more patients than ever before. Peroral endoscopy continues to increase in diagnostic and therapeutic importance and has the widest acceptance by both the medical profession and the public that it has enjoyed throughout its history.

HISTORY

The history of peroral endoscopy extends into the 19th century. Manuel Garcia, a Spanish singing teacher living in London, was the first to report the visualization of the larynx with mirrors and reflected sunlight. His discovery, reported in 1855, was followed by the independent development in 1856 of direct laryngoscopy by Türck and Czermak in Vienna. In Freiburg in 1868, Adolph Kussmaul, an internist, looked into the esophagus with reflected light after studying the technique of a sword swallower.[1] After this early inspiration, the relationship between esophagology and sword-swallowing came to resemble the one between astronomy and astrology. Nevertheless, careful observation of the sword swallower reinforces the lessons on neck position relative to the trunk and head position relative to the neck. Gustave Killian, also in Freiburg, demonstrated the endoscopic feasibility of removal of foreign bodies from the tracheobronchial tree in 1897 and has been recognized as the "father of bronchoscopy."[2]

Although Thomas Edison developed the electric lamp in 1878, the first distally lighted endoscope, the cystoscope, developed by Nitzi in 1879, used a platinum wire filament cooled by circulating water. At the turn of the century, Chevalier Jackson in Philadelphia introduced distally lighted laryngoscopes, bronchoscopes, and esophagoscopes, as well as telescopes with incandescent bulbs. His contributions to the whole understanding of bronchoesophagology were enormous, and he developed the art of the removal of foreign bodies from the air and food passages to the extent that there has not been any subsequent fundamental improvement.[3]

RECENT ADVANCES

Distal incandescent bulbs in hollow or open endoscopes have been replaced by fiber illumination carriers that provide steady, dependable, bright lighting.

The telescopic rod lens system of the British optical physicist H.H. Hopkins of Reading University, in which the air-containing spaces between the conventional series of lenses are replaced with glass rods with polished ends separated by small "air lenses," has been applied to endoscopy. This system transmits much more light and greater magnification. The depth and breadth of field is enhanced for detailed observation.[4] These telescopes have also been modified to view structures at various angles, i.e., 30°, 70°, 90°, 120°.

The recent application of the principles that Lamm developed in 1930 in the transmission of an image through a coherent bundle of small flexible glass threads has permitted the development of a truly flexible endoscope. Hirschowitz and his associates applied the fiberoptic principle to the gastroscope in 1958,[5] and Ikeda and his team,[6] as well as others, applied it to bronchoscopy and esophagoscopy. The fiberoptic bronchoscope has added greatly to the extent of the bronchial tree that can be visualized. Washings, brushings, curettage, and biopsy can be carried farther toward the periphery of the lung, especially in the upper lobes. Because the majority of early carcinomas of the bronchus arise in subsegmental bronchi of the third to sixth order of branching, this increased range is of critical importance. Visualization is often possible even if the bronchi are distorted, displaced, or stenotic. Longer, more detailed examinations can be carried out under local anesthesia. Fiberoptic bronchoscopy is reaching a level of perfection that brings it near the safety and effectiveness required for screening of selected populations. Miniaturization of the flexible bronchoscope to the 1.7 and 1.9 mm external diameter has made it possible to apply it to children also.[7,8]

Major contributions to documentation and teaching of bronchoesophagology were made by Holinger[9] with the Holinger-Brubaker camera. Marsh[10] has contributed to the concepts of early detection of bronchogenic carcinoma and photography through fiberoptic bronchoscopes, although the image resolution is not entirely satisfactory with coherent fiberoptics. Rayl's work with documentation through color television merits admiration.[11] Excellent endoscopic photography has been achieved by Ward[4], Benjamin[12] and others using the Hopkins rod lens telescope.

Yanagisawa and Yanagisawa[13] have developed videotape recording through laryngeal telescopes and nasopharyngolaryngoscopes, with and without stroboscopic lighting synchronized with the rate of vibration of the vocal cords, for studying laryngeal images. These video recordings, with audio recording of phonation, provide new insights in laryngeal pathophysiology. They provide unprecedented preoperative and postoperative documentation.

Microscopic evaluation and control of surgical procedures in the larynx have been developed under the leadership of Kleinsasser,[14] Ono and Saito,[15] Jako,[16] and Strong.[17] Kleinsasser clearly pointed out the contribution of magnification in detecting early pathologic changes suggestive of malignancy. Laryngoscopy under microscopic control provides excellent exposure, brilliant illumination, binocular vision, bimanual instrumentation, and magnification for precise surgical manipulation.[17]

Laser surgery of the larynx and bronchi has important application in the precise removal of lesions of the vocal cord for restoration of the voice; control of squamous cell papillomas of the larynx, trachea, and bronchi; management of subglottic hemangiomas and stenoses and detection and treatment of tracheobronchial lesions.[18–20]

Through the application of developments in the physics of optics, endoscopy has entered into a period of rapid expansion of new information and new therapeutic techniques that make it as exciting today as it

must have been when Kussmaul, Killian, and Jackson first began to look into the previously dark interior.

PREPARATION OF THE PATIENT

The patient should be carefully evaluated and prepared for peroral endoscopy. The present problem and all related and past medical problems should be assimilated. Of particular importance is the history of adverse reactions to drugs, especially to local or general anesthesia. As in other surgery, specific inquiry regarding a personal or family history of a bleeding tendency should be made, and a survey of the blood clotting mechanism, should be obtained in addition to the complete blood count, serologic test for syphilis, blood urea nitrogen, creatinine and glucose, and serum electrolytes. Blood gases should be obtained in individuals with airway obstruction or reduced pulmonary function from any cause. A complete physical examination should be performed. Unless the endoscopy is a true emergency, as in the case of certain foreign bodies of the trachea and bronchi, the preoperative evaluation should include the appropriate radiographic studies. Posterior-anterior and lateral chest x-rays are a necessity, and depending on the clinical problem, relevant computed tomography, magnetic resonance imaging or contrast studies may be obtained before endoscopy. Consultation with specialists in other fields should be obtained as indicated. If all of the information possible is available, the endoscopist will be in the best position to interpret the abnormal findings that may be encountered.

The psychologic preparation should begin at the first contact with the endoscopist, to instill confidence in the patient. The reasons for any special diagnostic studies and the endoscopic procedure should be presented in a thorough and rational way to gain the fullest understanding of the patient. The procedure should be described in positive terms. The possible benefits and risks must be discussed fully.

Food and fluids by mouth should be withheld for 8 hours before the procedure. The nature of the premedication depends on the type of anesthesia to be used.

As with other procedures on the respiratory and alimentary tracts, endoscopy may be accompanied by bacteremia. For this reason, patients with structural defects of the heart as evidenced by a heart murmur should have prophylactic antibiotic therapy before and after endoscopy to prevent bacterial endocarditis.

ANESTHESIA

The selection of local or general anesthesia for peroral endoscopy depends on a number of factors. Sometimes no anesthesia is appropriate. In most adults, either local or general anesthesia may be appropriate. Children are particularly sensitive to the toxicity of local anesthetics, and ordinarily should receive either general anesthesia or no anesthesia. Wrapping of the child for restraint is still occasionally appropriate, but as a rule, general anesthesia is preferred for direct laryngoscopy, tracheoscopy, bronchoscopy, and esophagoscopy in infants and children. In direct laryngoscopy and tracheoscopy in infants and children, the procedure is usually indicated by abnormalities that are slight variations from normal. Gross variations from normal are not compatible with life. General anesthesia is preferred for these examinations so that the patient is relaxed. Accurate observations of these slight variations from normal can then be made.[21]

In adults, local or general anesthesia may be used for any form of peroral endoscopy. Direct laryngoscopy for removal of lesions of the vocal cord to restore the voice and other procedures that require microscopic control are performed better under general anesthesia. Patients with large obstructive lesions, such as carcinoma of the larynx, may be managed with local anesthesia. The patient's personality and ability to cooperate are factors in the selection of the type of anesthesia. Patients with a tendency toward gagging with indirect laryngoscopy often do not make good subjects for direct laryngoscopy under local anesthesia.

Bronchoscopy in the adult, using a flexible bronchoscope, is usually well managed under local anesthesia. Coughing by the patient facilitates removal of obstructing secretions. A prolonged search with a flexible bronchoscope for locating an occult lesion in a patient with cytology characteristic of malignancy, removal of foreign bodies through an open tube, or laser resection of lesions are more readily done under general anesthesia.

Esophagoscopy and gastroscopy in the adult with the flexible upper gastrointestinal panendoscope can ordinarily be performed with local anesthesia. Generally, removal of foreign bodies of the esophagus and dilatation of esophageal strictures through open esophagoscopes are safer and more comfortable for the patient under general endotracheal anesthesia. Foreign body removal from the stomach with a flexible panendoscope is satisfactorily performed under local anesthesia.

Local Anesthesia

Local anesthetics are drugs that block nerve conduction anywhere in the nervous system. To be of practical value, their effect must be reversible but of sufficiently long duration to allow the procedure to be completed. The greatest hazard of local anesthetics is their toxicity. The ratio between the toxic and the effective dose is small. Most adverse reactions result from high blood levels caused by overdosage rather than allergic reactions. Not only the total dose administered but also the route, concentration, and rate of application contribute to the resultant blood levels. Adriani and Campbell[23] have shown that tetracaine and cocaine applied topically to the respiratory epithelium of the pharynx, trachea, and bronchi produce blood levels of the agent equal to 30% of the blood level obtained with intravenous administration. The absorption of topically applied local anesthetics is more rapid than from subcutaneous injection of these agents, and more toxic reactions occur when local anesthetics are applied topically than when they are infiltrated. The absorption is more rapid from pseudostratified ciliated columnar epithelium (respiratory epithelium), as in the trachea, than from stratified squamous epithelium, as in the esophagus. Unlike the situation with subcutaneously injected local anesthetics, the addition of epinephrine to the topically applied solution does not alter the rate of its absorption into the bloodstream.

Local anesthetic agents cause two types of toxic reactions. One is cardiovascular, caused by the direct depression of the myocardium and vasodilation. Depression of the myocardium and vasodilation lead to hypotension. The depression of the myocardium may result in asystole. The other is stimulation and subsequent depression of the central nervous system. The stimulation of the central nervous system produces restlessness, tremor, loquaciousness, and convulsions. The central nervous system stimulation is usually followed by profound depression and death caused by respiratory failure. The two forms of toxicity appear to occur simultaneously and are additive. Support of respiration is the essential feature in the management of toxic reactions.[24] Hypotension should be managed with intravenous sympathomimetic amines, and asystole should be managed by external cardiac massage. Convulsions should be controlled with neuromuscular blocking agents rather than central nervous system depressants, because the central nervous system stimulation is regularly and promptly followed by profound central nervous system depression.

Idiosyncratic and allergic reactions to local anesthetics are rare. Intolerance to local anesthetics is found in children, the aged, and debilitated and poor-risk individuals who cannot metabolize the agent at the usual rate. Contact dermatitis to tetracaine occurs not infrequently in medical personnel, and they should avoid skin contact with this agent.

Premedication for local anesthesia may include sedatives, narcotics, and cholinolytic agents, the type and dosage depending on the patient's age, debility and pulmonary function.

The psychologic preparation of the patient is as important as the premedication. Chevalier Jackson called it the "Sermon on Relaxation." The patient should be reassured that the procedure is designed for his benefit and that he will be able, with the aid of premedication and local anesthesia, to relax and cooperate in the procedure. One of the great advantages of local anesthesia is that it allows the surgeon and patient to cooperate in exploring the airway because motion, source of secretion, and changes in contour during respiration are important diagnostic clues.

Before application of any local anesthetic agent there must be in the operating room a laryngoscope, an endotracheal tube, the endoscopic instruments, and an anesthetic machine for delivery of oxygen under positive pressure. The patient's electrocardiogram, blood pressure and blood O2 saturation should be continuously measured. An intravenous catheter must be in place before local anesthesia is applied. Once topical anesthesia has been initiated the patient can not be left alone.

Cocaine, tetracaine, and lidocaine are the three topical local anesthetics in widest use for peroral endoscopy at this time. Various estimates of the maximum safe dose for a 70-kg adult exist, but the following are suggested and adequate:

cocaine	100 mg
tetracaine	40 mg
lidocaine	200 mg

The ratio between the toxic dose and the effective dose is more favorable for lidocaine, and it is the topical anesthetic of first choice.

The smallest volume and the lowest concentration possible to accomplish the desired effect should be used. Subsequent applications should be made deliberately, so that the blood level will not rise above safe levels and so that each application will achieve maximum surface anesthesia. Use stock solutions prepared by the manufacturer or the pharmacist.

The concentration of local anesthetics is customarily expressed in percentages. Tetracaine is effective in 0.5% and 1% solutions. Solutions of 1% are recommended for cocaine, and 1 or 2% solutions are recommended for lidocaine. It is absolutely essential to understand that a 1% solution means that there is 1 g of the agent in 100 ml or 10 mg per ml. In other words, 10 ml of a 1% solution of cocaine contains 100 mg. The safest way to handle a local anesthetic is to have only the maximum safe dose given to the operator. In other words, if the agent to be used is 1% cocaine and the maximum safe dose is considered to be 100 mg, the operator should ask for 10 ml of 1% cocaine and that exact amount should be poured into a graduated measuring glass. The operator should read the label of the stock solution including the expiration date and should verify that only the maximum safe dose has been delivered. It is possible to calculate the dose applied at any time by subtracting the amount remaining in the grad-

uated measuring glass from the maximum safe dose. Cocaine must not be injected. It should be tinted with methylene blue in the pharmacy as a further indication that it is not to be injected. Assuming 100 mg of cocaine is to be used as a topical agent in a 70-kg man for direct laryngoscopy or bronchoscopy, that amount should be enough for spraying the pharynx, for topical application into the piriform sinuses on cotton with Jackson cross-action forceps in the hope of establishing a conduction block of the superior laryngeal nerves, and for dropping the agent at first onto the vocal cords and then through them with a syringe and Abraham malleable cannula (Fig. 61–1). Not more than 1 ml or 10 mg should be applied at one time, and the applications should not occur more frequently than every 1 to 2 minutes. Less agent is needed if each application is given a chance to be effective before the next application. Once the larynx is anesthetized, the agent can be applied to the tracheobronchial tree more accurately. Positioning of the patient immediately after instillation of the agent into the tracheobronchial tree onto one elbow and then the other helps to distribute the agent to the bronchus on the same side. The maximum anesthetic effect of topically applied local anesthetics is not obtained until 5 to 10 minutes after the last application, and operative intervention should not begin until that latent period has elapsed.

Injection of a topical anesthetic agent with a fine ($1\frac{1}{2}$ inch #27) needle into the lumen of the trachea through the cricothyroid membrane is used when the anesthetic solution cannot be introduced through the lumen of the larynx.[25]

Anesthesia for direct laryngoscopy and bronchoscopy can be enhanced by infiltration of 1 to 2 ml of 1% lidocaine in the area of the thyrohyoid membrane where the superior laryngeal nerves enter the larynx. Whenever agents for infiltration are to be used in conjunction with topical agents, the use of the topical agent should be completed, and any residuum and the vessel that contained it should be removed from the operating table before the injectable agent is brought into the operative field. In this way, the chance of mistaking the topical agent for the injectable agent is minimized. As with topical agents, the operator should specify the volume and concentration of the injectable agent he wishes to use, whether or not it should contain epinephrine, and if so, in what concentration. Epinephrine in a concentration of 1/100,000 is preferred. The operator must read the label on the stock solution, supervise the pouring, and verify that the amount requested was delivered and did not exceed the maximum safe dose.

Local anesthetic agents have been shown to interfere with the growth of bacteria and modify the bacteriologic data obtained at bronchoscopy. Tetracaine and lidocaine have an inhibitory effect on the culture of fungi and bacteria, including *Mycobacterium tuberculosis*.[26]

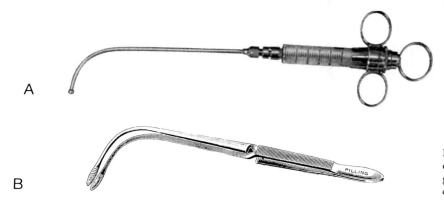

Fig. 61–1. A. Laryngeal syringe for introducing anesthetic solutions into the larynx by indirect laryngoscopy prior to peroral endoscopy. **B.** Jackson cross-action forceps.

Bronchoscopy under local anesthesia with an open bronchoscope produces arterial pCO_2 levels below the preoperative level, and arterial pO_2 levels on room air are sometimes above those encountered preoperatively. These effects probably result from hyperventilation and increased cardiac output.[27]

Bronchoscopy under local anesthesia with a flexible bronchoscope may be carried out through an open bronchoscope, tracheoscope, tracheotomy tube, or nasal or oral endotracheal tube, or the flexible bronchoscope can be introduced through the nose[28] or mouth. Hypoxia may occur under any of these circumstances if the flexible bronchoscope takes up too much of the airway.[29] Likewise, carbon dioxide retention occurs when a flexible bronchoscope is passed through a smaller endotracheal tube than 8.5 mm internal diameter. Oxygen can be delivered through a side arm to the endotracheal tube, and the flexible bronchoscope may be passed through a diaphragm over the lumen of the endotracheal tube. If the flexible bronchoscope is passed through an open bronchoscope or tracheoscope, oxygen can be delivered through the side arm of the open endoscope. If the flexible bronchoscope is introduced through the preferred nasal route or through the mouth, supplementary oxygen may be supplied through a face mask.

Topical anesthesia for esophagoscopy may be obtained by spraying the pharynx and periodically giving the patient small measured sips of the topically active local anesthetic to swallow. Systemic absorption from the esophagus and the stomach is negligible if the mucous membrane is intact. If there is ulcerative disease of the esophagus or stomach, special care must be taken.

General Anesthesia

Inhalation anesthesia can be safely used for direct laryngoscopy in infants and children if the airway is not compromised. For bronchoscopy in infants and children, positive pressure ventilation or adequate spontaneous respiration can be maintained through the ventilating side arm of a Holinger bronchoscope. For esophagoscopy in infants and children, general endotracheal anesthesia is preferred.

General endotracheal anesthesia is preferred for direct laryngoscopy in which microscopic control, surgery for restoration of the voice, or dilatation is to be employed. The cuffed endotracheal tube of small but adequate size comes to rest in the interarytenoid fold and presents no great problem for most endolaryngeal surgery. Esophagoscopy with an open esophagoscope is usually performed under general endotracheal anesthesia, especially if foreign body removal or dilatation is required.

General anesthetic techniques have been used in conjunction with the open bronchoscope. They include spontaneous respiration, ventilation through an endotracheal tube alongside the bronchoscope, ventilation through the side arm of the bronchoscope, entrainment of gas through the bronchoscope with Sanders' Venturi injector system,[30] and injection of gas through the ventilating side arm of the bronchoscope as described by Carden.[27]

General anesthesia with spontaneous ventilation through the bronchoscope has been widely used and is particularly suitable for bronchoscopy in children for therapeutic procedures, such as foreign body removal, as well as for diagnostic procedures. Nevertheless, significant increase in the arterial pCO_2 may occur, and the pH may decrease. It is less suitable for adults than for children.

A bronchoscope with a ventilating side arm can be used with a glass window or small telescope to occlude the bronchoscope, and the anesthetic gas and oxygen can be delivered through the ventilating side arm. Leakage of some gas does occur with this method and there is an increase in arterial pCO_2 when the window is removed to introduce instruments through the bronchoscope.

Sanders' Venturi injector system uses a small (16-gauge) high-pressure jet of oxygen in the long axis of the bronchoscope which causes entrainment of gas in the bronchoscope to ventilate the lungs.[30–32] The oxygen jet is introduced intermittently at a predetermined pressure, usually 50 pounds per square inch or less. The oxygen jet entrains anesthetic gases being fed through the ventilating side arm, as well as air from the open proximal end of the bronchoscope. Hence 100% oxygen is not delivered to the lungs. The jet of oxygen is controlled by an on-off toggle valve, which is connected to a single-stage variable pressure regulator. The pressure regulator is supplied with oxygen under pressure. The system is more efficient with proximally expanded bronchoscopes. It does not work as well in patients in whom pulmonary compliance is below normal. Carden modified this system by eliminating the 16-gauge jet and using a larger oxygen jet. This modification allowed the use of 100% oxygen and higher pressures at the proximal end of the bronchoscope. These systems may be used with adjunct intravenous agents.

General anesthesia may be needed for flexible bronchoscopy when the procedure is combined with other diagnostic procedures, when the search may be long, or when the patient cannot tolerate a procedure under local anesthesia for psychologic or other reasons. Application of positive pressure ventilation through the aspiration channel has proved dangerous because the tip of the flexible scope may make a tight seal with a segmental or subsegmental bronchus and produce a rupture of the parenchyma and pneumothorax.[34] If general anesthesia is to be used, a cuffed endotracheal tube is inserted. The flexible bronchoscope is inserted through an adapter with a diaphragm across the lumen of the endotracheal tube. In this way, an adequate seal is obtained for positive pressure ventilation during the general anesthetic. With a 5-mm flexible bronchoscope, endotracheal tubes larger than 8.5 mm internal diameter must be used to prevent hypoxia, hypercapnea, and high end expiratory pressures. Smaller endotracheal tubes may be appropriate with the 2.7-mm flexible bronchoscopes.

EQUIPMENT

The instruments of peroral endoscopy are vast, and a comprehensive listing is not intended here. Special instruments have been developed for special purposes. A beginning student should study the instruments presented in Jackson and Jackson's *Bronchoesophagology,*[3] as well as the recent catalogs of instrument manufacturers, to be aware of the special instruments available for particular endoscopic problems.

For direct laryngoscopy the standard Jackson laryngoscopes are useful in surveying the hypopharynx and larynx (Fig. 61–2A). The distal tip of the spatular portion is blunt and is intended for insertion posterior to the epiglottis to the level of the false vocal cords. The proximal end of the tube has a dorsal sliding portion

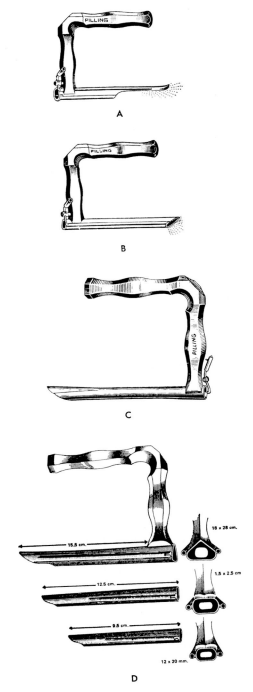

Fig. 61–2. Laryngoscopes. **A.** Standard Jackson laryngoscope. **B.** Jackson anterior commissure laryngoscope. **C.** Holinger anterior commissure laryngoscope. **D.** Jako laryngoscope.

that is detachable, so that a bronchoscope can be introduced through the laryngoscope and the laryngoscope can be removed without disturbing the bronchoscope. The standard Jackson laryngoscope is available in the infant (internal diameter 9 mm and overall length 9.5 cm), child (internal diameter 10.5 mm and length 10.3 cm), adolescent (internal diameter 10.6 and length 15.9 cm), and adult (internal diameter 13.0 mm and overall length 15.9 cm) sizes. Holinger has designed an infant or newborn laryngoscope (internal diameter 8.0 mm and overall length 8.1 cm) that is particularly useful in infants under 6 months of age. In the adult model of the standard Jackson laryngoscope, the handle is counter-balanced so that, when grasped properly, the spatular portion is maintained in the proper plane for inspection of the larynx. The standard Jackson laryngoscope does not permit adequate visualization of the anterior commissure in many patients. For visualization of the anterior commissure and laryngeal surface of the epi-glottis, the Jackson anterior commissure laryngoscope is preferred (Fig. 61–2B). It has a beveled distal end and is designed to be introduced below the false vocal cords, and this design permits excellent exposure of the ventricles, true cords, and anterior commissure. By rotating the handle 90 degrees so that the bevel will enter the glottis in the anterior-posterior plane, the sub-glottic area and trachea may be exposed. The Jackson anterior commissure laryngoscope is suitable for oper-ative work in the larynx. It is available in child (internal diameter 5.8 mm and overall length 13.3 cm) and adult (internal diameter 6.8 mm and length 15.5 cm) sizes. Holinger's hourglass modification of the anterior com-missure laryngoscope incorporates the principle of the Yankauer postnasal speculum (Fig. 61–2C). The distal end of the ventral surface of the tube rises obliquely and flares laterally. The proximal portion of the dorsal surface declines obliquely. It elevates the tuberculum of the epiglottis and provides additional working space for application of instruments.

Various laryngoscopes have been developed for lar-yngoscopy under microscopic control. The Jako laryn-goscopes, in adolescent and adult sizes, and the Dedo laryngoscope provide excellent working conditions with the Zeiss operation microscope (Fig. 61–2D). Gen-eral anesthesia is used through a cuffed endotracheal tube. The laryngoscope is supported by a holder over the patient. Binocular vision and bimanual manipula-tion are easily accommodated. Much endolaryngeal surgery that requires extensive manipulation, such as an arytenoidectomy, and which was formerly per-formed through the Lynch suspension laryngoscope is now performed under microscopic control. Jet ventila-tion attachments and bivalved laryngoscopes are also available for special situations.

The flexible nasopharyngolaryngoscope is useful for viewing the larynx and introducing endotracheal tubes in individuals in whom exposure of the larynx with an open laryngoscope is impossible or inadvisa-ble, as may be the case in patients with trismus, tempo-romandibular arthritis, mandibular fractures, pharyn-geal stenosis, and cervical spinal ankylosis and trauma.

The Jackson tracheoscope is an extra-long anterior commissure scope for examination of the cervical tra-chea. It has a working length of 18 cm.

Open bronchoscopes, such as the C.L. Jackson and Holinger models, have expanded proximal ends and ventilating side arms. The expanded proximal ends im-prove visibility and allow visual centering by the oper-ator with more ease. Instruments are introduced more easily into the funnel shape than into a cylindric proxi-mal end. A large ventilating side arm provides for the delivery of oxygen and anesthetic gases. Open bron-choscopes have fenestrations near the distal end to pro-vide ventilation to the other lung when the distal end of the bronchoscope is in a bronchus. Open broncho-scopes are designated by the number of millimeters of internal diameter and the number of centimeters of working length and range from 3–20 (3 mm × 20 cm) to 9–40 (9 mm × 40 cm). Modified bronchoscopes for use with lasers are also available. Telescopes with the Hopkins rod lens system are also used in open bron-choscopes and provide a brighter image and better res-olution. They are available as forward, forward-oblique, and lateral telescopes with a 5.5-mm external diameter and a viewing angle of what appears to be 90 degrees. The Hopkins telescopes are also available in a variety of pediatric sizes with the smallest outer diameter of 1.9 mm and the same angulations and viewing angle.

Flexible bronchoscopes have an insertion tube diam-eter of 2.2, 3.6, 4.9, 5.9, and 6.3 mm and are usually 55 cm working length. The distal ends have a bending angle of 180° up/130° down, with a visual field of 120°. The larger scopes have channels for forceps, cytology brush, lavage and suction.

Open esophagoscopes are oval or round in cross section and range in size from 3.5–25 (3.5 mm internal diameter × 25 cm in length) to 10–53 (10 mm × 53 cm). A light carrier channel and an aspirating channel are built into the wall. The oval open esophagoscopes, such as those designed by Mosher and Jesberg, are very suitable for foreign body removal, as well as for diag-nostic procedures. The distal end of the Jesberg esoph-agoscope is thickened to form a protective edge and molded to a smooth Haslinger sled runner shape for safety and ease of introduction. The round open esoph-agoscopes are more appropriate for negotiating ob-structions such as tumors and strictures and for their dilation.

The flexible upper gastrointestinal panendoscopes have an external diameter of 10 to 12.5 mm and are 100 to 105 cm long. The distal ends have a deflection capability of 270 degrees. The field of vision is 75 de-grees. There are channels for insufflation of air, brush-ing, biopsy, electrocautery snare and lavage and aspi-ration.

Tubes for application of suction are available in the size appropriate in length and diameter to the endo-scope being used. Aspiration tubes are of the open-end and velvet eye type. The open-end suction catheter applies stronger suction but is more traumatic. The vel-vet eye, because of its multiple openings, does not tend to pull mucous membrane into its lumen. Curved, flexible-tip aspiration tubes are helpful in certain situations, such as aspiration of the upper lobe bronchi.

Forceps are required for manipulation, biopsy, and foreign body removal. Alligator forceps of various lengths and sturdiness are available for direct laryngoscopy, bronchoscopy, and esophagoscopy and are very useful in various manipulations. Cupped, square, round, and oval basket and triangular forceps of various sizes and sturdiness are necessary for biopsy, depending on the clinical problem. Foreign body removal has been greatly improved by the development of the center-action foreign body forceps. This design allows the blades to close without retraction into the tubular sheath of the forceps. Foreign body forceps have been developed to deal with nearly every type of object that has become a foreign body. Forceps with integrated telescopes are especially helpful in removing foreign bodies from small airways.

For bronchoscopic diagnosis, lavage fluid collecting tubes, bronchial brushes, curettes, and aspirating needles, are also available. Sponges and sponge carriers are required for topical anesthesia and application of sympathomimetic amines to achieve vasoconstriction for visualization and control of bleeding.

For dilations, various bougies are needed. For the larynx, Jackson triangular brass dilators are very useful. For the esophagus, Jackson steel-stem woven filiform bougies from size 8 to 40 Fr are necessary for dilation through the esophagoscope. Plummer bougies from size 16 to 45 Fr may be passed over a thread but are now seldom used. Tucker retrograde bougies from size 12 to 40 Fr are passed from the gastrostomy to the mouth in long strictures of the esophagus, as occur with lye burns. Dilation done blindly with Hurst mercury-filled bougies from size 16 to 60 Fr is infrequently used. Maloney's tapered modification of the Hurst bougies from size 20 to 60 Fr is more frequently employed.

TECHNICAL FACTORS

Elective peroral endoscopy should be performed in an operating room. Endoscopic procedures should be carried out under the same circumstances as any other surgical procedure. All of the monitoring equipment and personnel of a general operating suite should be used and resuscitation equipment should be available.

Standard scrub facilities should be used. Good overhead lighting must be available. Two dependable sources of suction must be available. Instruments should be autoclaved, gas-sterilized, or soaked for sterilization with the same care as in any other operative procedure. The operative team should include as a minimum the surgeon, the assistant, the instrument technician, and the circulating registered nurse. They must mask, scrub, gown, and glove. All who look through the endoscope must wear protective eyeglasses to prevent tuberculous keratitis, conjunctivitis, hepatitis and AIDS as well as mechanical trauma to the eyes.[35] If local anesthesia is used, it should be administered in the same room as the operative procedure.

In peroral endoscopy in which upper airway obstruction is actually present or could potentially develop, there should be an awareness that the degree of obstruction may be increased by the procedure. For this reason, the operator must be prepared to relieve the obstruction promptly. A bronchoscope of suitable size for the patient should be lighted. A sterile tracheotomy set should always be at hand.[36]

The patient's head and body may be draped. For laser procedures protective face, eye, and body covers must be used. Operating room personnel must also wear appropriate eye protection.

It is convenient for a right-handed operator to sit with the stool slightly to the left of the long axis of the patient. The assistant should be at the operator's right. The illumination source should be to the left of the patient's chest. The instrument table should be placed behind the operator so that the operator may have access to it and see the instruments and the specimens. The microscope should be positioned to the right. If general anesthesia is used, the anesthesiologist can be at the patient's right.

The operator is seated, with the height of the stool and the height of the table adjusted so that the operator may lean forward to the endoscope from the hips with the back straight. The operator should not be required to take the right eye off of the operative field. Instruments including forceps, aspirating tube, spatula, scissors, dilators, applicators, knives, and syringes should be passed by the assistant, so that the tip of the instrument is placed into the endoscope and the handle is free for the operator to grasp. Most endoscopic instruments can be held like a pencil in the right hand of the assistant during the passing of the instrument to the operator, as illustrated in Figure 61–3. The tip can be accurately placed in the proximal end of the endoscope in this manner. As the instrument is brought out by the operator, it is taken from him by the right hand of the assistant, again as if the assistant were holding a pencil. Aspiration tubes, forceps, applicators, and so forth may all be passed in the same fashion. The instrument technician should keep the instrument table well organized.

The operating room should be lighted well enough to monitor the patients' color and general well-being without decreasing the operator's visual sensitivity.

The patient should lie flat on the operating table. The top of the patient's shoulders should be at the point where the main portion of the table and the headrest break to allow maximum mobility of the head and

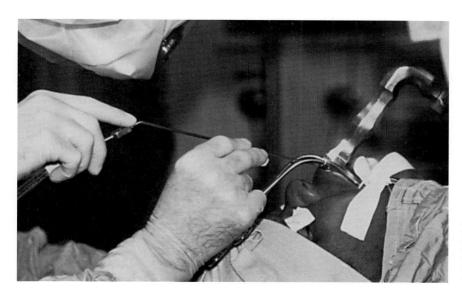

Fig. 61–3. Passage of endoscopic instruments to the operator. The assistant holds the instrument like a pencil and places the tip of the instrument in the endoscope so that the operator may take the instrument by the handle.

neck. For direct laryngoscopy, the neck should be flexed on the chest, and the head should be extended on the neck so that the chin points toward the ceiling.[31] This position brings the larynx, cervical esophagus, and trachea in a straight line with the thoracic esophagus and trachea. This Boyce position can be achieved with local or general anesthesia by positioning the head and the headrest of the operating table. It is the correct position for atraumatic introduction of the laryngoscope, bronchoscope, and esophagoscope. In bronchoscopy with an open bronchoscope, the head must be lowered when the bronchoscope is in the trachea. Lowering the head is accomplished by adjusting the headrest of the table. As the right bronchus is entered, the head should be shifted toward the left. As the left bronchus is entered, the head should be shifted toward the right.

In esophagoscopy with an open esophagoscope, the head must be lowered as soon as the esophagoscope has reached the thoracic portion of the esophagus. As the esophagoscope is advanced toward the lower portion of the esophagus, the head should be shifted to the right to allow for the leftward course of the distal portion of the esophagus, and the head must be lowered below the level of the thorax to allow for the anterior course of the distal portion of the esophagus. Failure to adjust to the anatomic course of the esophagus makes advancement of the open esophagoscope difficult and increases the possibility of perforation.

SUGGESTED READINGS

1. Huizinga E: On esophagoscopy and sword-swallowing. Ann Otol Rhinol Laryngol 78:32, 1969.
2. Major RH: A History of Medicine. Springfield, Charles C Thomas, 1954.
3. Jackson C and Jackson CL: Bronchoesophagology. 2nd ed. Philadelphia, WB Saunders, 1959.
4. Ward PH, et al: Advances in endoscopic examination of the respiratory system. Ann Otol Rhinol Laryngol 83:754, 1974.
5. Hirschowitz BI, et al: Demonstration of a new gastroscope, the fibergastroscope. Gastroenterology 35:50, 1958.
6. Ikeda S: Flexible bronchofiberscope. Ann Otol Rhinol Larnygol 79:916, 1970.
7. Silberman H, Tucker JA and Hampel A: Flexible neonatoloscope. Ann Otol Rhinol Laryngol 93:471, 1984.
8. Ward RF, Arnold JE and Healy GB: Flexible minibronchoscope in children. Ann Otol Rhinol Laryngol 96:645, 1987.
9. Holinger PH: Photography of the larynx, trachea, bronchi and esophagus. Trans Am Acad Ophthal Otolaryngol 46:153, 1942.
10. Marsh BR, et al: Flexible fiberoptic bronchoscopy: Its place in the search for lung cancer. Trans Am Broncho-Esophagol Assoc 1973, pp 101–110.
11. Rayl JF and Rourke D: Application of color television in bronchoesophagology. Trans Am Broncho-Esophagol Assoc 54:137, 1974.
12. Benjamin B: Eighteenth C. Baker, Jr. Memorial Lecture: Art and Science of Laryngeal Photography. Ann Otol Rhinol Laryngol 102:271, 1993.
13. Yanagisawa E and Yanagisawa K: Stroboscopic Videolaryngoscopy: A Comparison of Fiberscopic and Telescopic Documentation. Ann Otol Rhinol Laryngol 102:255, 1993.
14. Kleinsasser O: Microlaryngoscopy and Endolaryngeal Microsurgery. Philadelphia, WB Saunders Co, 1968.
15. Ono J and Saito S: Endoscopic Microsurgery of the Larynx. Ann Otol Rhinol Laryngol 80:479, 1971.
16. Jako GJ: Laryngoscope for microscopic observation, surgery and photography. Arch Otolaryngol Head Neck Surg 91:196, 1970.
17. Strong MS: Microscopic laryngoscopy, a review and appraisal. Laryngoscope 80:1540, 1970.
18. Simpson GT, Healy GB, McGill T and Strong, MS: Benign tumors and lesions of the larynx in children. Ann Otol Rhinol Laryngol 88:479, 1979.
19. Strong MS and Jako HJ: Laser surgery in the larynx. Ann Otol Rhinol Laryngol 81:791, 1972.
20. Strong MS, et al: Bronchoscopic carbon dioxide laser surgery. Ann Otol Rhinol Laryngol 83:769, 1974.

21. Snow JB: Clinical evaluation of noisy respiration in infancy. Lancet *85*:504, 1965.

22. Ferguson CF and Flake CG: Bronchography in the Diagnosis of Pediatric Problems. JAMA *164*:518, 1957.

23. Adriani J and Campbell D: The absorption of topically applied tetracaine and cocaine. Laryngoscope *68*:65, 1958.

24. Goodman LS and Gilman A: The Pharmacological Basis of Therapeutics. 3rd ed. New York, Macmillan Co, 1965.

25. Fry WA: Techniques of topical anaesthesia for bronchoscopy. Chest *73*:694, 1978.

26. Conte BA and Laforet EG: Role of topical anesthetic agents in modifying bacteriological data obtained by bronchoscopy. N Engl J Med *267*:957, 1962.

27. Carden E: Recent improvements in techniques for general anaesthesia for bronchoscopy. Chest *73*:697, 1978.

28. Harrell JH: Transnasal approach for fiberoptic bronchoscopy. Chest *73*:704, 1978.

29. Lindholm GF, Ollman B, Snyder JV, Millen BS and Grenvik A: Cardiorespiratory effects of flexible fiberoptic bronchoscopy in critically ill patients. Chest *74*:362, 1978.

30. Sanders RD: Two ventilating attachments for bronchoscopes. Del Med J *39*:170, 1967.

31. Morales GA, et al: Ventilation during general anesthesia for bronchoscopy: Evaluation of a new technique. J Thorac Cardiovasc Surg *57*:873, 1969.

32. Smith CO, Shroff PF and Steele JB: General anesthesia for bronchoscopy: The use of the Sanders' bronchoscopic attachment. Ann Thorac Surg *8*:348, 1969.

33. Gussack GS, Evans RF and Tacchi EJ: Intravenous anaesthesia and jet ventilation for laser microlaryngeal surgery. Ann Otol Rhinol Laryngol *96*:29, 1987.

34. Britton RM and Nelson KG: Improper oxygenation during bronchofiberscopy. Anaesthesiology *40*:87, 1974.

35. Lucente FE, Meiteles LZ and Pincus PL: Bronchoesophageal manifestations of acquired immunodeficiency syndrome. Ann Otol Rhinol Laryngol *97*:530, 1988.

36. McDowell DE and Maloney WH: Acute obstruction of the upper respiratory tract. Arch Otolaryngol *61*:29, 1955.

37. Vaughan C: Vocal Fold Exposure in Phonosurgery. J. Voice *7*: 189, 1993.

62 Laryngology

Joyce A. Schild

Evaluation of the larynx is mandatory in any individual with symptoms referable to the voice or upper airway: dysphonia, pain in the larynx or stridor. The examination begins with attention to voice characteristics of pitch, volume, and clarity. Hoarseness, breathiness, whisper, faintness, variable pitch, sudden stops or starts are all symptoms of vocal and, thus possibly, laryngeal abnormality. Once alerted to the symptoms the larynx can be visualized in most adults by the technique of indirect laryngoscopy. A round mirror attached at approximately 45° to a handle long enough to reach the posterior pharynx is warmed to body temperature and inserted perorally and directed caudally to expose the larynx. Light is reflected from the mirror to the larynx and back to the observer. The entire larynx and surrounding hypopharyngeal structures must be observed during respiration and phonation of simple sounds. To see the true vocal cords in phonation, a high pitched "E" is preferable because it results in adduction and maximal tension of the vocal cords, with simultaneous elevation of the epiglottis to allow visualization of the entire length of the phonating edges of the true vocal cords. The false vocal cords, the laryngeal surface of the epiglottis, and the pyriform sinuses are also seen during this action. Abduction of the vocal cords is observed during respiration. In addition to these observations of motility, any contour asymmetries are easily seen by this simple technique. Topical anesthetic sprayed onto the palate, pharynx and tongue base may be necessary in some people to abolish the gag reflex and allow for longer examination. A variation of this mirror technique is the use of a rod telescope, of either 70° or 90° viewing angle. These instruments provide brighter light and an enlarged image, inverted 180° from mirror view due to the optical properties of the system (Fig. 62–1). Simple diagrams of the larynx drawn at the time of each examination can be very helpful in following the course of the patient's lesion. It is advisable to label the right and left vocal cords in these diagrams to prevent confusion between images derived from differing optical systems.

For those who cannot tolerate indirect instruments or whose anatomy precludes it, flexible fiberoptic examination is invaluable. The 3.2 mm diameter fiberscope is small enough to be used in nasal passages constricted by septal deviations or enlarged turbinates, or even for neonates and young children who would otherwise need the more physically taxing direct procedures to view the larynx. Tolerance of the fiberscope is enhanced by using a combination of topical anesthesia and decongestant in the nose, supplemented by pharyngeal topical anesthesia if necessary. The image orientation through the fiberscope is the same as that of the rod telescope. In addition to visualizing contour changes and simple voicing, sustained speech, singing, and swallowing can be observed over several minutes if necessary. Either rod telescopes or flexible fiberoptic scopes can easily be adapted to lightweight photo or TV cameras to obtain recorded images for later review and comparison of several observations done at separate times. Stroboscopic light may also be utilized for 'slow motion' images.

Radiographic examination of the larynx is helpful in supplementing information gathered by physical examination. Postero-anterior and lateral views of the soft tissues of the neck provide overall information regarding size, shape and location of the larynx. For greater detail computerized tomography (CT) is excellent for visualizing calcified cartilage while magnetic resonance imaging (MRI) in three planes shows soft tissue structures exceptionally well.

Direct laryngoscopy is necessary for those individuals who cannot be evaluated by the above methods, but it is more commonly utilized for operative procedures such as polyp removal or biopsy. Direct laryngoscopy is indicated, not only for obvious benign or malignant lesions, but also for subtle lesions found on x-ray and

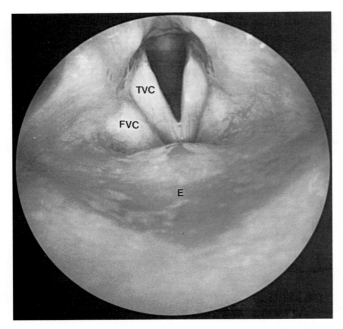

Fig. 62–1. Normal adult larynx in inspiration, viewed with a 90 degree telescope. E, Epiglottis; TVC, true vocal cord; FVC, false vocal cord. All endoscopic photographs in this chapter obtained at direct laryngoscopy unless otherwise noted.

for persistent symptoms not explained by any other examination. Additionally, direct palpation through the laryngoscope can reveal induration discernable only by this method. Use of tissue stains such as Toluidine blue may divulge areas of epithelial abnormality not previously identified. Small subglottic lesions hidden by normal proximal structures, and upper tracheal disease unseen on standard x-rays can be exposed by inspection with angled telescopes at direct laryngoscopy.

DIRECT LARYNGOSCOPY

For direct examination, the larynx and pharynx are rendered thoroughly numb by topical or regional bloc anesthesia, or the patient undergoes general anesthesia which allows a more lengthy manipulation without discomfort for the patient. A laryngoscope is chosen to suit both the patient's anatomy and the needs of the surgeon. A blunt-bladed Jackson laryngoscope with removable slide is helpful in retracting the epiglottis and false cords but may not reveal the anterior commissure, subglottis, or even the piriform sinuses as well and as safely as an anterior commissure laryngoscope can. The narrow waist of an 'hour-glass' laryngoscope overcomes the difficulties associated with large teeth or macroglossia and also exposes the anterior commissure very well. However, if needed, a ventilating bronchoscope can be passed through the Jackson laryngoscope and the laryngoscope can then be removed by separat-

ing the slide from the superior blade allowing the bronchoscope to be utilized for distal airway examination. Large-lumen laryngoscopes are needed for binocular vision when the operating microscope is used; both straight and flared-tip scopes are available. Panoramic views can be obtained with curved blade or expanding laryngoscopes, especially when combined with a support mechanism. This support allows the operator to use both hands while the laryngoscope is maintained in a stable, motion-free position.

With any laryngoscope, the technique for exposure of the larynx is similar. The supine patient is best positioned with the head elevated on a pillow or head rest with the nose and chin parallel to the floor, the Boyce or 'sniffing position.'[1] For the right handed operator, the laryngoscope is grasped in the left hand leaving the right hand free to use delicate instruments or to help in positioning the scope. The scope is inserted along the right lingual sulcus and advanced (while keeping pressure off of the teeth) into the pharynx to examine it and the base of the tongue, valleculae and lingual surface of the epiglottis (Fig. 62–2A). After a slight forward shift of the hand along the horizontal handle, the laryngoscope is advanced just under the tip of the epiglottis, then lifted and advanced further to view the pyriform sinuses. Further advancement of the laryngoscope into the vestibule of the larynx gently separates the aryepiglottic folds and false cords to expose the entire entire length of the true vocal cords, as well as the shape and size of the glottic opening (Fig. 62–2B). Inspection is done by the unaided eye or with a straight 0° telescope. The underside of the vocal cords may be seen better with a 30° or 90° telescope. All contours and mucosal surfaces exposed are inspected during these maneuvers and, if necessary, documented with video or photography. The binocular operating microscope with a 400 mm lens enlarges the view for even more detailed inspection or manipulation. Biopsies of lesions, removal of polyps, or delicate microsurgical repair procedures can then be accomplished. Passive mobility of the arytenoids on the cricoid cartilage can be assessed by palpating them with the tip of a fine suction or forceps. Patients examined under topical anesthesia can phonate or breathe on request to demonstrate intact neuromuscular activity. Those who are under general anesthesia may need the level of anesthesia lightened in order to evaluate this activity.

At the conclusion of the procedure, as the laryngoscope is removed, all blood and excess secretions must be aspirated from the larynx, upper trachea and pharynx to prevent soiling of the lower airways. If the patient has been intubated for the procedure, spontaneous respirations, swallow, cough and response to simple commands must have returned before the patient is extubated and transferred to the recovery area for further observation. When the patient is able to drink and eat, discharge home is often possible the same day as the laryngoscopy.

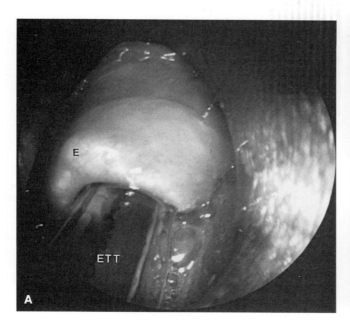
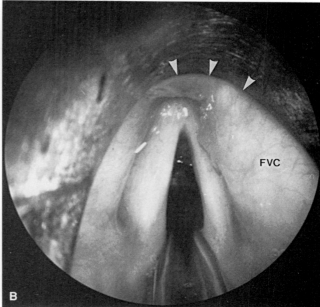

Fig. 62–2. A. Direct laryngoscopy of a normal adult larynx showing epiglottis (E) and endotracheal tube (ETT). B. Same patient with epiglottis lifted anteriorly with the tip of the laryngoscope (arrows). There is a slight bulge at the anterior end of the right false vocal cord (FVC) caused by pressure of the laryngoscope.

LARYNGEAL DISEASE

Abnormalities of the larynx necessitating evaluation include masses, inflammations, trauma, congenital abnormalities, neurologic disturbances, and malignancies.

Mass lesions are probably the most common reason for laryngeal examination including direct laryngoscopy. Of these, benign **polyps** (Fig. 62–3) occur most often on the phonating edge of one or both of the vocal cords and rapidly result in hoarseness. This may be the only symptom the patient reports unless the polyp size increases to obstruct the glottic airway. Polyps may be either broad based or pedunculated (Fig. 62–4). The latter may be freely mobile, resulting in sudden change in voice or airway symptoms if the position of the polyp changes. Polypoid swelling involves the subepithelial loose layer of connective tissue of the vocal cord described by Reinke in 1897,[2] and is therefore referred to as "Reinke's edema" or as polypoid degeneration of the vocal cord. Histologic examination typically shows smooth non-ulcerated epithelium covering an underlying stroma of connective tissue, amorphous ground substance and scattered chronic inflammatory cells.[3] Variations of the polypoid change contain old hemorrhage or organizing thrombosed vessels ("hemorrhagic" polyps) or dense connective tissue ("fibrous" polyp) (Fig. 62–5). The etiology of polyps is not definitely known but may involve residual edema from prior URI, acute vocal trauma such as shouting which causes a ruptured blood vessel, or long term vocal abuse. Occasionally, severe vocal abuse results in ulcerations or pedunculated granulomas at the vocal process of one or both arytenoid cartilages. Chronic gastroesophageal reflux or the trauma of prolonged use of endotracheal tubes have also been found to play a role in similar lesions at the arytenoids[4] (Fig. 62–6). Altered phonatory habits may also be the end

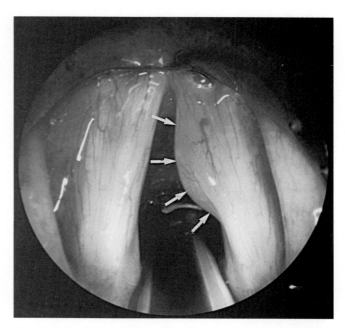

Fig. 62–3. Sessile polyp (arrows), right true vocal cord with an enlarged vessel at its base.

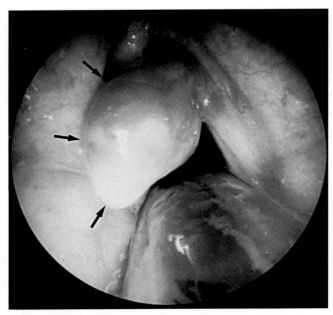

Fig. 62–4. Large pedunculated polyp (arrows), right true vocal cord displaced proximally and obscuring visualization of the left cord. Histologically, the polyp contained hyaline material amid a highly vascular stroma.

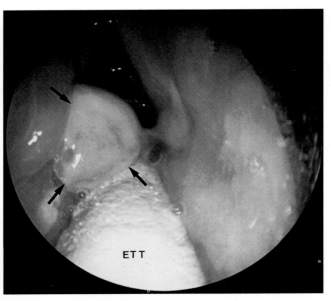

Fig. 62–6. Granuloma (arrows) on the vocal process and medial surface, left arytenoid. Lesion occurred after prolonged endotracheal intubation. A similar smaller lesion is obscured by the operative endotracheal tube (ETT), which is lying in the usual position in the posterior glottis.

result of vocal polyps and, therefore, these patients must have the benefit of speech therapy, before and after surgical removal of the lesion.

Direct laryngoscopy is necessary to remove polyps. Simple cup forceps can be used for small pedunculated masses. In case of large or sessile polyps, a knife, laser or scissors used with grasping forceps may give improved control of the direction of incision and the amount of tissue removed. If both cords are involved with polypoid degeneration, it is best to remove tissue only from one cord. When the contralateral change is still large enough to occlude the airway, tissue may be

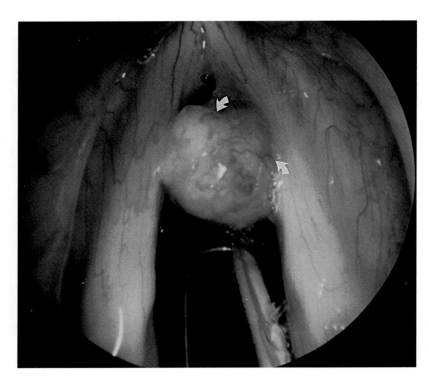

Fig. 62–5. Polyp, right true vocal cord with prominent vascularity (curved arrows). Right false cord is retracted exposing the lateral extent of the superior surface of the true vocal cord. Muscle mass appears slightly atrophic.

removed from the posterior half of the remaining polyp leaving intact mucosa to cover the anterior commissure, effectively preventing synechia formation at this critical area.

Vocal abuse is also responsible for vocal **nodules.** Abusive voice production occurs as the result of speaking consistently at the wrong pitch, repeatedly speaking for long duration, and using too much sound volume. Many vocal abusers combine all three. Typically persons using such vocal abuse are teachers, lawyers, coaches, and workers in noisy industry. Children who shout frequently or who use habitual vocal overemphasis can also develop nodules. Vocal nodules occur as bilaterally symmetric elevations on the vocal cords (Fig. 62–7). The typical location is at the junction of the anterior and middle thirds of the phonating margin of the vocal folds. This is the mid point of the membranous cords, the area of maximal excursion of the vocal cord edges, and of maximal impact on phonation. Therefore, vocal abuse from extra stress, loudness, or duration has maximal effect at this point. The result is edema, followed by organizing reaction of acute and chronic inflammation and eventual cornification localized to the impact point. Primary intervention for vocal nodules is voice correction therapy.[5] However, for those nodules which are cornified, direct laryngoscopy and removal of the nodules may be necessary. *Only the local tissue elevations should be removed,* not the entire mucosal cover, leaving the remaining mucosa intact with only minimal raw surface areas to heal. The patient must return to the speech therapist to empha-size the importance of correct voice usage to prevent recurrence of nodules.

Other benign masses occur less frequently, but they also present with the primary symptom of hoarseness. Cellular activity resulting in benign neoplasm may involve any of the types of tissue which form the laryngeal structure. Muscle-derived tissue typical of **rhabdomyoma** can form large masses anywhere in the larynx, distorting the shape and flexibility of the true vocal cords with resultant voice change even though the overlying mucosa is usually normal. Histologically, the tissue appears very cellular with uniform elongated or round to oval cells with eosinophilic cytoplasm and often eccentric nuclei. Cross striations can be difficult to identify without electron microscopy.[6] Treatment is by local excision.

Chondroma, a very slow growing cartilaginous tumor of the larynx, forms most often in the cricoid cartilage,[3] and may interfere with arytenoid mobility in some patients. If the chondroma is large and in the subglottic area, it can cause airway obstruction. Because of the slow growth and hypocellularity, it can be difficult to differentiate benign chondromas from low grade chondrosarcomas. Radiographs can be helpful because they characteristically show a pattern of scattered calcified areas within the mass if it is sarcomatous. Imaging with CT or MRI can also delineate the size, shape, location and integrity of the walls of the tumor.[7] The endoscopic appearance is that of intact mucosa with an underlying smooth, hard mass sometimes associated with mucosal hyperemia. Biopsy forceps often slip off of the hard mass and obtain only mucosa. For this reason punch biopsy forceps may be needed to obtain true tumor tissue. Complete removal is recommended to prevent recurrence.

Another unusual benign tumor of the larynx is the **granular cell tumor.** In the head and neck this tumor is more frequent in tongue, but when in the larynx it occurs mainly on the true vocal cord causing hoarseness. If it arises elsewhere in the larynx, it can remain asymptomatic for extended time periods. Formerly called granular cell myoblastoma because of its superficial resemblance to muscle tissue, it is now considered to be of neurogenic origin. A generous biopsy is important because superficial epithelial hyperplasia can cause confusion with squamous cell carcinoma if the biopsy specimen is too small.[8] Special histologic stains or electron microscopic examination may be necessary to differentiate it from rhabdomyoma. Local excision is curative.

Other rare neurogenic tumors include neuromas, neurilemmomas, neurofibromas, and paragangliomas. **Neuromas,** usually of traumatic origin, arise from regenerating nerve cells and scar tissue at transected peripheral nerves; they can occur after surgery in or near the larynx, often following laryngectomy or neck dissection. They cause severe pain or cough especially

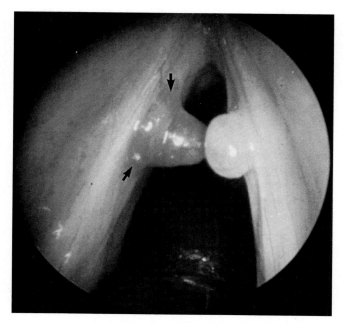

Fig. 62–7. Bilateral vocal nodules in a 42-year-old factory worker. The left nodule is discolored by resolving hemorrhage (arrows) caused by shouting.

with stimulation of the mass. If symptoms are debilitating they may be excised.

Neurofibromas contain nerve sheath cells, along with trapped nerve fibers and collagen; they generally are not encapsulated. Laryngeal neurofibroma can occur as an isolated tumor or as part of the classical Neurofibromatosis Type 1 of von Recklinghausen.[9] The clinical symptoms and endoscopic appearance vary, depending on the location of the tumor. Those on or near the vocal folds will cause voice change, large ones in the pyriform sinus will cause dysphagia. Complete surgical removal is preferred, when possible, since regrowth may be aggressive.

Neurilemmoma (also known as Schwannoma, neurinoma, and peripheral fibroblastoma) arise from nerve sheath (Schwann) cells and usually are encapsulated. They are rare in the larynx. Surgical resection, usually by an external approach, is necessary.

Paragangliomas of the larynx are extremely rare. They have arisen from both the superior and recurrent laryngeal nerves.[10] The tumor is related in neural crest origin to carotid body tumors and glomus tympanicum. These paragangliomas, unlike pheochromocytomas, rarely produce clinically measurable catecholamines. Closely related tumors with similar appearance and symptoms include carcinoid tumor and hemangiopericytoma. They are distinguishable from paragangliomas by subtle histochemical reactions.[11] Grossly the laryngeal paraganglioma mass is usually smooth, dull, and red or blue in color. The patient may complain of excruciating local pain even before the tumor is apparent. Histologically the tumor characteristically shows organoid groups of cells ("Zellballen") with interspersed extensive vascular channels that have few contractile cells in the vascular walls. Biopsy can produce very severe hemorrhage due to the extensive vascularity. Therefore direct examination of the patient with severe pain must be preceded by vascular imaging such as MRI with gadolinium infusion. The patient should have preparation for hemorrhage control and blood volume replacement even for direct laryngoscopy. Treatment is by surgical excision; total laryngectomy may be necessary in some instances.

Teratomas and **hamartomas** also are very rare in the larynx. Tissue arising from any germ cell layer can be found in these lesions, either common to the site and of more than one germ cell layer (hamartoma), or unusual to the location (teratoma) (Fig. 62–8). These masses are usually located on the true vocal cord, epiglottis or the ventricle.

Laryngeal manifestations of systemic disease processes may also affect the larynx and require direct laryngoscopy and biopsy. In some patients, the diagnosis may be the result of a single appearance in the larynx, though most have widespread locations. One such group of systemic abnormalities includes granulomatous diseases which appear typically in the subglottis

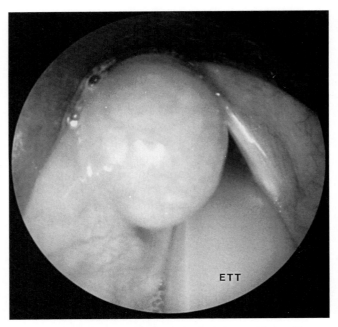

Fig. 62–8. Hamartoma protruding from the left ventricle in a 13-year old patient. The mass was removed totally with a large cup forceps. The remainder of the larynx was completely normal. ETT, Endotracheal tube.

and proximal trachea as reddened, roughened, friable infiltrates that interfere with voice production or air flow. **Sarcoidosis,** a non-caseating granuloma, can involve the larynx as well as skin, salivary glands, tracheobronchial tree, nose and lymph nodes. Angiotensin-converting enzyme (ACE) level is increased in 60% or more of patients with sarcoidosis; the ACE level can also be used to follow the course of the disease in these patients.[12] After progression from the initial friable infiltrate, long-standing laryngeal sarcoidosis can cause severe swelling and deformity of the soft tissues, leading to voice alteration and airway obstruction. Treatment with corticosteroids improves the patient's condition.

Scleroma is a granulomatous reaction to infection by Klebsiella rhinoscleroma which affects the mucosa of the upper and lower air passages.[13] As its earlier name (rhinoscleroma) implies, the infection frequently results in nasal disease as well as larynx and tracheal mucosal changes. The early appearance is that of nonspecific inflammation, followed by granulations and slowly progressive scarring. Histologically, the tissues contain large macrophages with vacuolated cytoplasm (Mikulicz cells) which enclose the causative organism. Eventually, scarring can cause laryngeal or tracheal stenosis as well as nasal collapse. At this late stage the organisms are often difficult to identify. Scleroma is rare in the U.S. except in former residents or travelers from Egypt, central Europe and Central America. Antibiotic therapy must be continued for months and is most effective in the early stages of the disease.

Wegener's disease is a granulomatous vasculitis involving the lungs, kidneys, nose, and larynx. It may appear in the larynx alone in its early stages when diagnosis can be difficult even with a generous biopsy. The antineutrophil cytoplasmic autoantibody, (C-ANCA), predominantly that with fine granular cytoplasmic flourescence test may be the key to diagnosis in such patients (Ref 4 Batsakis). In the more common widespread form, lung and kidney biopsies provide the relevant information. Long term chemotherapy is necessary for control of this systemic disease.

Amyloidosis can also affect the larynx. Originally thought to be a starch-like deposit due to the tissue reaction to iodine stain, amyloid is now known to be a fibrous protein with varying subunits.[15] It may be localized, occur systemically, or be associated with chronic illness. Amyloidosis presenting in the larynx is usually localized, though systemic involvement must be ruled out by thorough workup including serum and urine electrophoresis and immunoelectrophoresis. Biopsy of other organs may also be necessary in some cases.[16] In either form, laryngeal amyloid deposits appear as yellowish submucosal plaques or nodules. The false cord is the site involved most often, however true cords, ventricle or subglottis have also been affected. In the true cord, deposits result in altered motility and cause hoarseness. When circumscribed, the lesion may be removed totally to improve the voice. Larger or more widespread airway plaques can cause persistent problems due to respiratory obstruction. In such cases, the offending mass may be reduced by cup forceps excision or laser ablation of the obstructing projection.

The systemic autoimmune disease **rheumatoid arthritis,** as well as other arthritides, can be found in the larynx where it affects the cricoarytenoid joint with swelling, pain, stiffness and ultimate fixation of one or both joints.[17] Early in the course of the joint destruction pain often radiates to the ear, but may not be bothersome later if fixation occurs. Medical management of early rheumatoid arthritis can maintain joint mobility when started promptly. In later stages, symptoms vary. If unilateral fixation occurs, the severity of the eventual voice change depends on the final position of the immobilized cord which can be remedied by surgical medialization when necessary. If both arytenoids become fixed in the midline, the airway will be compromised and surgical lateralization or arytenoidectomy may be required to enlarge the glottis but at risk of voice deterioration.

Acute **inflammation** of the larynx is most often the result of acute virus infection, which causes edema and vascular engorgement. Because it usually resolves spontaneously, it rarely requires attention unless the resultant hoarseness and discomfort are sustained beyond the expected 2–3 week duration. Simple 'home remedies' of humidification, analgesia, and decreased

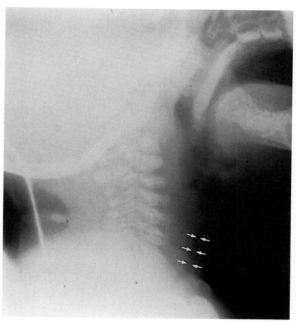

Fig. 62–9. Lateral radiograph of the neck in an 8-month-old infant with croup. There is a narrowing of the subglottic air column (arrows) but a normal epiglottis.

vocal activity suffice in the adult. However in children, especially those less than 1 year old, the inflamed subglottis may be so severely edematous that it can be life threatening (Fig. 62–9). Rapidly worsening 'barking' cough, hoarseness, and airway obstruction with biphasic/stridor and air hunger are the hallmarks of croup and *must* be addressed promptly. High humidity delivered by ultrasonic nebulizer, provides soothing mucus-thinning effects in most children. A mucosal decongestant such as racemic epinephrine added to the nebulized inhaled moisture decreases the swelling and opens the airway. A few babies may require direct laryngoscopy for diagnosis (to differentiate an unsuspected foreign body, congenital stenosis or hemangioma) and short term intubation.[18]

Bacterial infection of the larynx can also occur. Infection with Hemophilus influenza type B (HiB) notoriously causes involvement of either the epiglottis alone ('**epiglottitis**'), or of the false vocal cords, arytenoids and surrounding pharynx too ('**supraglottitis**') (Fig. 62–10). Children as well as adults can be affected. The severely swollen tissues cause airway compromise with resultant muffled voice, inspiratory stridor, retractions and decreased oxygenation. The patient prefers to sit upright and would rather drool than swallow. In less severe cases, when the patient's physical condition permits, a portable 'cross-bed lateral' neck x-ray may be obtained to aid in diagnosis. The more severely affected patient will need *immediate* management by a direct laryngoscopy and intubation or, more rarely, tracheotomy. Adults with this infection can

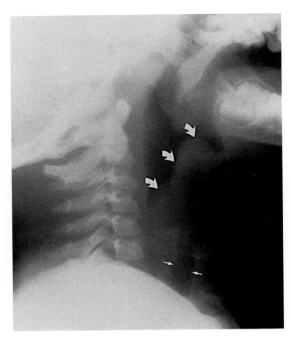

Fig. 62–10. Lateral radiograph of a 22-month-old child with epiglottitis. There is marked swelling of the epiglottis, aryepiglottic folds, and arytenoid areas (curved arrows). The subglottic air shadow is widely patent (small arrows). There is "ballooning" of the pharyngeal air shadow as a result of this child's effort to inhale.

often be managed by close observation because the airway is larger, and because the adult patient can communicate any increase in symptoms. Once the airway is secure, appropriate antibiotics and fluid replacement can be administered. The recently available HiB vaccines have decreased the incidence of this disease in children, though not yet in adults.[19]

Other bacterial infections of the larynx have become less common with the advent of preventive immunizations or antibiotic treatment: diphtheria and tuberculosis are two good examples.

Laryngeal papillomatosis, a chronic viral infection of the mucous membranes of the airway has increased in recent years, and is most often found in the larynx, especially in children. Because of its tendency to return after removal, this disease is also called recurrent respiratory papillomatosis (RRP). The causative agent, human papilloma virus (HPV), induces tissue response in the form of warty exophytic masses which can be located anywhere in the larynx from the tip of the epiglottis to the subglottic region (Fig. 62–11). Each projection has a central capillary with surrounding connective tissue covered by normal squamous cell epithelium. Scattered virus particles have been identified in both affected and normal mucosa (Ref 20 Abramson). Papillomas on the phonating edges of the true vocal cords cause hoarseness. Larger papillomas can occlude the airway at any level. Papillomas may also occur in the tracheobronchial tree, pharynx, and nose.

RRP affecting the larynx is commonest in the pediatric age group but can also appear for the first time in adults. The natural history of RRP is that of repeated regrowth, of variable rapidity for each individual. In many prepubertal children, the recurrence rate slows and then stops, but in some patients the papillomas do not regress or they reappear in later years. Direct laryngoscopy, therefore, is undertaken only as often as symptoms become prominent. The papillomas must be removed carefully to preserve underlying structures. Cup forceps can be used to remove tissue for biopsy and rapid debulking of large masses. The operating microscope coupled to the CO_2 laser combines good visualization with delicate removal of tissue and hemostasis, for maintenance of normal structures. Periodic examination of other areas of the upper and lower airways should be done to monitor possible spread to other sites. Removed tissue from any area must be examined histologically to insure continued accurate diagnosis. Human papilloma virus typing further identifies the involved virus, which in the larynx is most often HPV types 6 and 11. Other pediatric laryngeal problems involving voice problems or airway obstruction may also require detailed evaluation and are discussed in chapter 21.

External trauma to the larynx occurs as the result of suicide, homicide or accidents.[21] Penetrating injury from knife or gunshot wounds and compression injury from blunt objects, vehicular impact, or falls can crush the supporting cartilages and tear the soft tissues. The

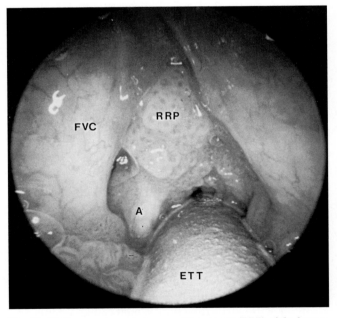

Fig. 62–11. Recurrent respiratory papillomatosis (RRP) of the larynx of a 6-year-old child entirely covering the membranous true vocal cords, extending to the subglottis and left false vocal cord (FVC) adjacent to the endotracheal tube. An area of smooth mucosa at the arytenoid (A) is the only indication of true vocal cord level. ETT, Endotracheal tube.

resultant symptoms vary in severity from slight hoarseness to severe airway disruption. Assessment of the injuries must be done as soon as possible in order to plan appropriate treatment, always keeping in mind the possibility of severe injuries to other areas. Examination of the larynx by flexible fiberoptic endoscope or mirror is preferred initially but direct laryngoscopy is necessary eventually in many victims. Radiologic evaluation must also be done to determine the extent of fractures, possible displacement of fragments, amount of soft tissue injury and integrity of adjacent skull and cervical spine. MRI in 3 planes will demonstrate the extent of soft tissue damage, CT identifies bone and cartilage deformity, angiography may be needed for vascular injuries.[22] Minor trauma resulting in simple contusion can be managed by close observation only. Severe fractures, displaced fragments, and extensive soft tissue damage require open surgical correction to reposition structures, reline mucosal surfaces and provide support with appropriate stents when necessary. When open reduction is required, tracheotomy is also necessary until healing occurs.[23] Trauma to the larynx is considered further in chapter 30.

Neurologic dysfunction can also affect the larynx. Patients with nerve palsies are seen by the otolaryngologist because of the vocal or respiratory effects.[24] *Unilateral vocal cord paralysis* will result in a breathy, weak voice, aspiration of swallowed liquids, and an ineffectual cough due to lateral position of the affected vocal cord and incomplete closure of the glottis. In some patients, the mobile cord will gradually ''compensate'' for its partner's lost activity, and symptoms will abate unless the patient is fatigued. In *bilateral vocal cord paralysis* both true vocal cords are positioned at or near the glottic midline, which obstructs the flow of air with inspiration. Voice, cough and swallow are usually less symptomatic due to the close apposition of the cords. Because the vocal cords are pushed apart by the airflow of exhalation, it can be difficult for the neophyte examiner to differentiate *passive* lateral displacement of the cords due to exhaled air, from *active* muscular abduction on inhalation in the intact patient. To overcome this confusion, a second observer may be needed to indicate the inhale-exhale cycle as the examiner is viewing the larynx. A second source of confusion arises if the arytenoids are fixed in position by scar, rather than by paralysis. Such immobility is often caused by prior extended endotracheal tube placement, or by severe inflammation. Laryngeal EMG may be helpful to evaluate the integrity of the intact neuromuscular connection (Ref 25 Miller and Rosenfeld). Direct laryngoscopy may also be required whereby palpation of the arytenoids will differentiate mobility from rigidity of the joints. Any evaluation of unilateral or bilateral vocal cord palsy requires a thorough investigation of the course of the recurrent and superior laryngeal nerves from their central origins to their pe-

ripheral neuromuscular junctions. In obvious localized trauma to the nerves from iatrogenic or other source, such evaluation may be limited. However in obscure diagnoses, investigation may extend from intracranial (Complete neurologic examination with brain imaging), to chest (x-ray and endoscopy), and to periphery (evaluation for systemic disease, or examination of the neck for primary or metastatic tumors). Chapter 32 covers Functional and Neurologic Disorders of the Larynx.

Management of vocal cord palsies depends on the position of the affected vocal cord. Unilateral cord paralysis may be corrected by surgical medialization. Under local anesthesia, through an external incision, a window is made in the ipsilateral thyroid cartilage ala and a wedge is placed lateral to the internal perichondrium which therefore moves the cord medially.[26] The size and position of the wedge can be adjusted as the cord position is monitored by observing it via a flexible endoscope passed through the nose into the pharynx, and by listening to the patient's voice. For the high-risk patient, an alternative rapid endoscopic method is available using inert material injected lateral to the vocal process of the arytenoid on the affected side.[27] Bilateral palsy which results in compromise of the glottic opening often must be treated acutely by tracheotomy to by-pass severe airway obstruction, but definitive management can be difficult. At the time of acute recurrent nerve injury it may be possible to re-anastomose the severed nerve ends if they are identifiable. If the etiology is unknown but generalized neuro-muscular disease is not present, or when late scarring prevents identification of the affected nerves, nerve transfer or nerve-muscle pedicle grafting may be successful. If these methods are not available, the glottis may be widened by lateralizing one cord by excising an arytenoid and adjacent cord via endoscopy,[28] or by means of open surgery. The resultant open glottis causes some voice deterioration and mild cough and swallow disability, but allows the patient of be rid of the tracheotomy.

Other neurologic dysfunctions are also familiar to otolaryngologists. The weak voice of the Parkinsonian patient; the strained, strangled quality of the spasmodic dysphonia patient; the dysarthria of spinocerebellar degeneration and the altered speech and voice of the stroke victim may require evaluation by direct or indirect means though successful treatment will not always be possible.

Malignancy of the larynx occurs in all tissue types present in this organ. All of the benign tumors discussed earlier have malignant variants with local invasion, and local or distant metastases. Laryngeal malignancy strikes approximately 1.5% of total cancer victims in the United States.

Very early lesions may appear innocuous to the untrained observer, therefore, any persistent abnormality seen on preliminary examination should be investigated further. CT and MRI studies are invaluable in disclosing cartilage invasion and soft tissue involvement. Direct laryngoscopy must be done to obtain more information. Endoscopic examination of the tracheobronchial tree and esophagus are performed also, to identify any synchronous lesions. All areas of the larynx and adjacent structures must be examined thoroughly in order to accurately stage the lesion and plan therapy. Motility evaluation is an essential part of the staging process but can be done more accurately by preoperative indirect examination or videostroboscopy. It is especially important to view obscure sites such as the underside of a curled epiglottis and the interior of the ventricles. Angled telescopes are particularly helpful for subglottic areas which cannot be seen otherwise. Histologic examination of the tissue samples will show deep invasion of atypical epithelial cells of varying differentiation. In the in situ carcinoma, the changes will be present only above the epithelial basement membrane. Treatment options for SSCA depend on the location and extent of the lesion. Very small tumors on the membranous vocal cord may be removed endoscopically, while larger tumors and metastatic disease require various combinations of surgery, radiation, and chemotherapy.

SUGGESTED READINGS

1. Vaughan CW: Vocal fold exposure in phonosurgery. J Voice 7: 189, 1993.
2. Reinke F: Über die funktionelle Struktur der menschlichen Stimmlippe mit besonderer Berücksichtigung des elastischen Gewebes. Anat Hefte 9:105, 1897.
3. Shanmugaratnam K: Histological Typing of Tumours of the Upper Respiratory Tract and Ear, 2nd Ed. Berlin: Springer-Verlag, 1991.
4. Feder RJ, Michell MJ: Hyperfunctional, hyperacidic, and intubation granulomas. Arch Otolaryngol 110:582, 1984.
5. Murry T, Woodson GE: A comparison of three methods for the management of vocal fold nodules. J Voice 6:271, 1992.
6. Battifora HA, Eisenstein R, Schild JA: Rhabdomyoma of larynx: Ultrastructural study and comaparison with granular cell tumors (myoblastomas). Cancer 23:183, 1969.
7. Mishell JH, Schild JA, Mafee MF: Chondrosarcoma of the larynx: Diagnosis with magnetic resonance imaging and computed tomography. Arch. Otolaryngol. Head Neck Surg 116: 1338, 1990.
8. Cree IA, Bingham BJG, Ramesar KCRB: View from beneath: Pathology in focus: Granular cell tumour of the larynx. J Laryngol Otol 104:159, 1990.
9. Riccardi VM: Von Recklinghausen neurofibromatosis. N Engl J Med 305:1617, 1981.
10. Barnes L: Paraganglioma of the larynx: A critical review of the literature. J Otorhinolaryngol Rel Spec 53:220, 1991.
11. Ferlito A, Friedmann I: Contribution of immunohistochemistry in the diagnosis of neuroendocrine neoplasms of the larynx. J Othorhinolarynogol Rel Spec 53:235, 1991.
12. DeRemee RA, Rohrbach MS: Serum angiotensin-converting enzyme activity in evaluating the clinical course of sarcoidosis. Ann Intern Med 92:361, 1980.
13. Shum TK, Whitaker CW, Meyer PR: Clinical update on rhinoscleroma. Laryngoscope 92:1149, 1982.
14. Batsakis JG, El-Naggar AK: Wegener's granulomatosis and antineutrophil cytoplasmic autoantibodies. Ann Otol Rhinol Laryngol 102:906, 1993.
15. Glenner GG: Amyloid deposits and amyloidosis: The B-fibrilloses. N Engl J Med 302:1333, 1980.
16. Lewis JE, Olsen KD, Kurtin PJ, Kyle RA: Laryngeal amyloidosis: A clinicopathologic and immunohistochemical review. Otolaryngol Head Neck Surg 106:372, 1992.
17. Montgomery WW: Cricoarytenoid arthritis. Laryngoscope 73: 801, 1963.
18. McEniery J, Gillis J, Kilham H, Benjamin B: Review of intubation in severe laryngotracheobronchitis. Pediatrics 87:847, 1991.
19. Takala AK, Peltola H, Eskola J: Disappearance of epiglottitis during large-scale vaccination with Haemophilus influenzae type B conjugate vaccine among children of Finland. Laryngoscope 104:731–735, 1994.
20. Abramson AL, Steinberg BM, Winkler B: Laryngeal papillomatosis: Clinical, histopathologic and molecular studies. Laryngoscope 97:678, 1987.
21. Line WS Jr, Stanley RB Jr, Choi JH: Strangulation: A full spectrum of blunt neck trauma. Ann Otol Rhinol Laryngol 94:542, 1985.
22. Schild JA, Denneny EC: Evaluation and treatment of acute laryngeal fractures. Head Neck 11:491, 1989.
23. Olson NR: Laryngeal Trauma. Washington, D.C., American Academy of Otolaryngology—Head and Neck Surgery Foundation, 1982.
24. Dedo HH: The paralyzed larynx: An electromyographic study in dogs and humans. Laryngoscope 80:1455, 1970.
25. Miller RH, Rosenfield DB: The role of electromyography in clinical laryngology. Otolaryngol Head Neck Surg 92:287, 1984.
26. Isshiki N, Taira T, Kojima H, Shoji K: Recent modifications in thyroplasty type I. Ann Otol Rhinol Laryngol 98:777, 1989.
27. Arnold GE: Vocal rehabilitation of paralytic dysphonia. IX. Technique of intracordol injection. Arch Otolaryngol 76:358, 1962.
28. Ossoff RH, et al.: Endoscopic laser arytenoidectomy revisited. Ann Otol Rhinol Laryngol 99:764, 1990.

63 Bronchology

Joyce A. Schild and James B. Snow, Jr.

INDICATIONS FOR BRONCHOSCOPY

Individuals suffering respiratory problems such as chronic cough, difficulty breathing, stridor, hemoptysis, excessive sputum production, and chest pain are candidates for thorough diagnostic evaluation of their tracheobronchial tree including bronchoscopy. Such evaluation may also be necessary in patients with vocal cord paralysis, metastatic neck masses, and for determination of possible synchronous tumors in patients with squamous cell carcinoma of other parts of the aerodigestive tract (Ref Levine and Nielson 8). Additional history will often reveal clues to the cause of the symptoms. Sudden choking followed by dyspnea or persistent cough would arouse suspicion of the presence of a foreign body, long standing allergies in the patient or the family would suggest asthma in someone with new onset of dyspnea or cough, while information relating to toxins or work-related materials might direct attention to these substances. Physical examination of the chest must include careful auscultation of all lung fields in order to note unusual or absent breath sounds, rhonchi, rales and local or generalized wheezes. Percussion is important to help discern localizing signs such as dullness or tympany (Fig. 63–1).

Radiographs of the chest are essential to provide further information about the patient's condition. They can demonstrate pulmonary masses; segmental, lobar, and pulmonary atelectasis or emphysema; cavitary lesions; coin lesions; parenchymal densities; pleural effusions; and radiopaque foreign bodies. Both posteroanterior and lateral exposures are needed to localize any lesions (Fig. 63–2). Atelectasis and obstructive or compensatory emphysema suggest bronchial obstruction and are of special concern to the endoscopist. Atelectasis may occur distal to bronchial obstruction of any cause. If the atelectasis is massive, as with the collapse of a lobe or lung, compensatory emphysema occurs in the other lung areas. Obstructive emphysema may occur with any form of partial bronchial obstruction, as seen with some foreign bodies or exophytic tumors. Computerized tomography (CT) of the chest, including the techniques of ultrafast scanning[9] and spiral volumetric CT[10] can provide even more details, not only regarding the lumen of the tracheobronchial tree and pulmonary parenchyma such as in lung nodules and bronchiectasis, but also the adjacent structures such as enlarged mediastinal lymph nodes or vascular abnormalities impinging on the airways.

Pulmonary function testing is extremely helpful in diagnosing the effect of lung lesions. The most useful observations of abnormalities in distal airways are the measurements of forced expiratory volume in 1 second (FEV1) and forced vital capacity (FVC), expressed as a ratio FEV1/FVC. The normal limits for these indices are usually set at 80% of the predicted values of the local reference standards. Additionally, the display of flow/volume loops can graphically indicate disruption of normal aerodynamics in the larger airways of the tracheobronchial system, often suggesting whether the abnormality is intra- or extrathoracic. As an example, fixed obstruction of the extrathoracic trachea would result in flattening of both the inspiratory and expiratory portions of the flow-volume loop. Gas exchange abnormalities are reflected in alterations of the pH, pO_2 and pCO_2 in arterial blood samples.[11] Other tests such as sputum cytology or bacteriology can be obtained before bronchoscopy but often are more revealing when specimens are gathered during the procedure.

Bronchoscopy is necessary for therapeutic reasons when the patient is unable to cough effectively to maintain clear passages, as can occur in postoperative periods or with severely debilitating but short-term illness; for removal of foreign bodies; for drainage of some abscesses or bronchiectatic debris; for dilatation of stenosis and placement of stents; and for removal of benign endobronchial masses such as papilloma or

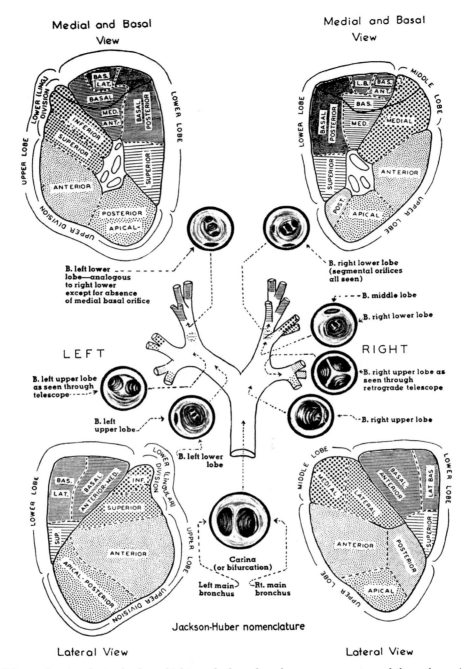

Fig. 63–1. Schema showing the tracheobronchial tree, the bronchopulmonary segments, and the endoscopic landmarks.

chondroma. Palliative removal of obstructive malignancies can also be done. In such cases cup forceps can be used to remove exophytic tumor but this is often followed by bleeding. Such bleeding can be controlled with vasoconstrictors or by tamponade with the bronchoscope against the bleeding area or, in the smaller bronchi, with an inflatable balloon catheter or gauze packing.[12] Tumor removal is especially effective with the use of lasers because of better control of bleeding. CO_2 lasers are now available in many operating suites but require specially adapted endoscopes and micro-

manipulators. YAG laser, though less widely available, has the advantage of energy delivery through a flexible fiber so that it can be used with either open tube or flexible bronchoscopes. The method selected will depend on the patient's condition, the location of the lesion, the availability of specialized ancillary instruments, and the training and skills of the endoscopist.

Bronchoscopy can be totally or relatively contraindicated. In patients with severe heart disease or recent myocardial infarction, physical stress can precipitate cardiac decompensation. Manipulation in patients

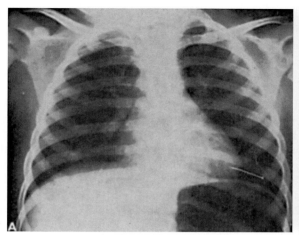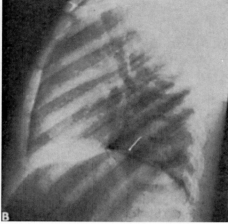

Fig. 63–2. Posteroanterior (A) and lateral (B) chest roentgenograms of a patient with a straight pin in the lateral basal segment of the left lower bronchus.

with uncontrolled blood clotting abnormalities risks hematoma or hemorrhage, and therefore must be avoided until the condition can be corrected. Recent massive hemoptysis must be approached with caution, and careful preparations made for control of any new hemmorhage.[13] Open tube bronchoscopes are the better choice in these cases because of the ability to rapidly clear the airways of blood and clots rapidly with large-bore aspirators and to tamponade the bleeding source until surgery can be carried out. Thoracic aortic aneurysm precludes aggressive instrumentation of the bronchial tree with a rigid bronchoscope because of the risk of rupture of the thin-walled vessel and exsanguination. However a flexible fiberoptic instrument might be substituted to lessen the chance of such trauma in a patient needing minimal intervention, for example simple aspiration of secretions to clear the tract. Patients with severe body deformity or rigidity often are impossible to bronchoscope with rigid instruments and therefore require flexible instruments to circumvent the anatomic barrier.[14] In acute bacterial infection, manipulation of the bronchi can induce excessive edema and respiratory obstruction and it is advisable to delay endoscopic examination if possible. However when a foreign body is suspected in a patient with a respiratory infection, especially a child, delayed removal is not possible and any endoscopy must be followed with rigorous postoperative management to prevent edema and obstruction.

TECHNIQUE OF BRONCHOSCOPY

Bronchoscopy can be accomplished with either general or topical anesthesia, though the former is now preferred when using the open tube bronchoscope. The position of the patient varies depending on the instrument selected. For open-tube bronchoscopy, the patient is supine with the head on a movable headrest and the shoulders at the 'break' of the table. With flexible fiberoptic instruments (FFO) the patient can be either upright or recumbent. Patients must be comfortable, cooperative (or sedated), and monitored carefully in all instances, since hypoxia may be associated with this procedure even in an otherwise healthy patient.[15]

When using an open-tube bronchoscope, general anesthesia is the current method of choice though thorough application of topical anesthetic agents to the mouth, pharynx, larynx and tracheobronchial tree can also be utilized alone or to supplement general anesthesia. (See Chapter 61 for local anesthesia technique.) The bronchoscope can be passed either through a Jackson laryngoscope which is then removed, or it can be introduced directly into the patient's mouth. In the latter method, the bronchoscope is held in the operator's left hand in such a way as to protect the patient's teeth. The patient's head should be elevated above the level of the table and hyperextended at C1-C2 to straighten the lumen of the mouth and pharynx and facilitate the advancement of the tube. With direct visualization through the bronchoscope, and using the right hand to guide it, the bronchoscope is inserted into the right side of the patient's mouth, between the tongue and the mandible, and advanced until the base of the tongue and the tip of the epiglottis are seen. The tip of the bronchoscope is lifted to raise the epiglottis and expose the laryngeal inlet. The bronchoscope is rotated so that its beveled edge acts gently to displace the left vocal cord as the tip is inserted into the glottis and advanced into the airway. When using general anesthesia, it can thereafter be administered through the ventilating side channel of the bronchoscope. Supplemental topical anesthetic can be instilled directly through the bronchoscope as needed.

The patient's head is then repositioned and lowered slightly to allow inspection of the entire circumference of the trachea as the bronchoscope is advanced to the carina. The head must now be tilted laterally to allow further visualization of either main bronchus. The endoscopist must decide whether to evaluate the diseased side first, or to inspect the uninvolved side while it is still clear of secretions or blood. However, it is technically easiest to pass the bronchoscope into the right side initially as the lumen is almost a direct extension of the trachea. The lobar bronchial orifices can be inspected directly. Segmental and subsegmental bronchi are viewed best with telescopes of varying viewing angles passed into the bronchoscope through an adapter to maintain a seal for anesthesia. The middle and lower lobe segments are best viewed with a 120° telescope, while the right upper segments can be seen with a 90° telescope. After completing the inspection on the right, the scope is retracted to the carina. The patient's head is then rotated to the right while the scope is advanced into the left main bronchus and then into the lobar orifices. Segmental bronchi on the left are seen well through the 90° or 120° telescope.

Video or photographic cameras can be attached to the eyepiece of any of the telescopes used for viewing the bronchial tree. Videocameras are particularly helpful in teaching endoscopic technique because they allow students to view the airways directly before doing the procedure themselves. The actual introduction and advancement of the endoscope can then be accomplished with more confidence for the student and less trauma for the patient. A second benefit of video is the instantaneous information available to the anesthesiologists and other operating personnel, which maximizes their ability to respond to any event that may occur. Video recordings can be retained for comparison to subsequent examinations or to other patients with similar pathology. Images taken from the video can also be made for the patient's record, but photographs record clearer images of pathology and are better for presentations and other permanent records.

When using a flexible bronchoscope in the awake patient, it can be inserted via the mouth, but is tolerated better when passed via the nose if there is no major nasal abnormality. The instrument can also be inserted through an open bronchoscope or through an endotracheal tube when the need for frequent removal and reinsertion is anticipated, or when the patient requires ventilatory support and general anesthesia during the procedure. In patients with distorted anatomy that makes laryngeal exposure difficult, small flexible endoscopes can also be used inside an endotracheal tube to provide visualization of the larynx and trachea for insertion of the tube.

When inserting the FFO, topical anesthetic spray allows comfortable passage of the instrument. More anesthetic can be applied as needed by instilling it through the instrument channel of the FFO before it is advanced. Whether inserted via the nose or mouth, any

upper airway abnormality should be noted during the insertion. By flexing and rotating the FFO it can be maneuvered around obstructions until the larynx is recognized and entered. The scope is then advanced into the trachea and distal bronchial tree. Minimal movement of the patient's head is needed during the procedure. Indeed, the flexibility of this instrument is a major advantage in patients who are immobile. However, if the bronchial tree itself is distorted severely, it may be necessary to rotate or tilt the patient's head so that the FFO can be maneuvered around a "tight" corner. In this manner the FFO can be advanced into the segmental and even subsegmental bronchi to view directly the affected region. Secretions can be retrieved from the specific area involved; for extremely adherent material the FFO tip can be wedged in place and large amounts of fluid instilled and aspirated to clean the site. Tiny biopsy forceps or brushes are passed through the instrument channel to obtain material for histologic examination. If the lesion is beyond the viewable range, radiologic guidance can assist in positioning the forceps or brush to obtain the needed specimen.

The size, shape, motility, and mucosal lining of the tracheobronchial tree must be continuously and closely examined as the bronchoscope is advanced and withdrawn. The trachea is inspected for intrinsic lesions or external compression. The carina is evaluated for sharpness, deviation, and mobility with respiration and cardiac contraction. The presence of subcarinal lymphadenopathy is indicated by carinal displacement, immobility, induration, or broadened base and blunted edge. Similar distortions in more distal areas must be identified as well. Mucosal changes can be very subtle due to obscure location, small size or minimal surface changes. Slight surface irregularity or friability may be the only visual clue to a neoplasm. Often the best site for biopsy can be determined with telescopic magnification, but in vivo tissue staining has yielded diagnostic information in special circumstances.

A generous biopsy of a visible exophytic lesion is readily accomplished through an open bronchoscope using straight or angled cup forceps. Any mild bleeding can be readily controlled with gentle pressure of the bronchoscope tip or a bronchoscopic sponge carrying a drop or two of epinephrine. Flat endobronchial lesions may also be sampled in the same manner, provided one keeps in mind the anatomic position of major blood vessels near segmental branchings, and avoids deep biopsies in these areas. Small sized cup or brush biopsies can be obtained through a flexible bronchoscope. This instrument is particularly useful in obtaining samples from peripheral sites or from areas impossible to reach with an open scope, such as the apical segmental bronchi. Transbronchial biopsy of lung parenchyma may be performed through a flexible bronchoscope under topical anesthesia with acceptable complication rates.[16] In addition to malignancy, it is common to diagnose diffuse or bilateral lung disease in this manner. The specimen is obtained by inserting the flexible biopsy forceps into the instrument channel and advancing it until it can be felt to engage tissue without pain, which would indicate the pleura has been touched. The forceps position changes with respiration and it is best to open the cups on inspiration and close them on expiration when the tissue has contracted against the blades. The right middle lobe is avoided because of the direction of many bronchi leading to the oblique fissure with its pleura and the possibility of pneumothorax. It is also best to perform a biopsy of only one lung, if possible, to preclude the occurrence of bilateral pneumothorax. Bronchial brushing is an alternative sampling method in some cases. The tiny brush is passed via the instrument channel and advanced to the area of involvement, when small movements of the brush within the tissue obtain scrapings of the lesion and retain them within the bristles. The material is then processed for histologic or cytologic examination. Care must be taken to avoid pneumothorax during brushing also.

Secretions retrieved from simple aspiration of loose material in the larger airways must be sent for microbiologic as well as cytologic examination. Bronchoalveolar lavage (BAL) is fruitful in diagnosis and management of inspissated mucus and other extensive disease of the smaller respiratory airways.[17] In this technique the FFO is firmly placed into the indicated subsegmental bronchial lumen and 50 ml aliquots of saline are instilled and immediately collected into a trap. Commonly 100 ml to 200 ml of lavage fluid is instilled to obtain a sample, but amounts up to 400 ml may be used, until the area is deemed clear of the offending substance. The return volume varies, but can be as much as 60% of the amount instilled in normal individuals. BAL has become a major tool of clinical investigators since it can provide information about cellular and molecular components in normal individuals as well as in disease processes. BAL is used in diagnosing mycobacterium tuberculosis and pneumocystis carinii; in managing bacterial, viral, and fungal infections; and in diagnosing and managing diffuse problems such as alveolar proteinosis, pneumoconiosis, sarcoidosis and other idiopathic lung diseases.

Any endoscopy must be described thoroughly for the patient's medical record. Both positive pathologic findings and areas of normality are important to note. A statement should be made about each segment to indicate whether it was normal, abnormal or not seen. The size and type of instruments used should be recorded as well as any difficulties encountered.

COMMON CONDITIONS REQUIRING ENDOSCOPY

As in the larynx described in Chapter 62, lesions of the tracheobronchial tree (TBT) and lung can derive from any of their tissues. These lesions can be inflammatory, neoplastic, acquired, or congenital.

Inflammatory lesions of the TBT are frequently encountered in clinical situations, though they rarely need bronchoscopy unless the condition persists, exacerbates, or the diagnosis is not clear. The "garden variety" acute viral tracheobronchitis is of short duration and resolves spontaneously in most cases. However in young children, viral inflammation may cause edema severe enough to require intubation or it may be complicated by bacterial infection, which can require bronchoscopy to remove dry crusts and purulent secretions that have not responded to antibiotics. Bronchiolitis, which is most often caused by the respiratory syncytial virus, is an illness which involves the lower airways. It results in edema leading to the accumulation of mucus, and to decreased airflow which causes prolonged expiration and air trapping. Complete obstruction of localized areas can also cause atelectasis. Bronchoscopy or intubation is not indicated in bronchiolitis because the obstruction is peripheral, but other supportive measures are utilized such as cool humidified oxygen, semi-upright position, and IV fluids. The antiviral agent, Ribavirin, is also required in the severely ill young child.[18]

In contrast, bacterial inflammations in either children or adults can necessitate endoscopy to provide secretion for bacteriologic examination and to identify any associated condition. Community acquired bacterial pneumonia is most often caused by *S. pneumoniae*, *H. influenzae*, or *S. aureus* which are rapidly responsive to antibiotics.[19] Those infections that do not respond will require further evaluation which should include bronchoscopy if radiography and morning sputum collection do not prove helpful. The inflammatory process set off by infection results in edema with increased amounts and viscosity of bronchial secretions, to the point that ciliary activity is no longer able to clear the excess. When ciliary mechanisms fail, cough occurs but it too may fail to remove viscous material, especially in debilitated or neurologically impaired patients. The resulting mucus plug can completely obstruct the bronchus leading to atelectasis of a segment, a lobe, or the whole lung depending on the location of the obstruction. These retained secretions must be removed by aspiration because the longer atelectasis persists, the greater the chance of irreversible damage to the lung parenchyma. The aspirate is processed to identify the causative microorganisms. The larger bronchi can be rapidly cleared of retained secretions by means of the open bronchoscope and large bore aspirating tubes. Smaller bronchi are effectively cleared with flexible scopes because only small amounts of local anesthetic can be used, enabling voluntary cough effort which brings material from distal areas. At the same procedure, any other cause of secretion retention such as benign stenosis, foreign body, or tumor can be identified and managed.

Bronchiectasis, the irreversible dilation of medium to small bronchi, is thought to be the end result of severe or recurrent infection. Fibrosis and destruction of the supporting muscle and cartilage leads to tubular or saccular enlargement of the bronchi. Important predisposing factors include cystic fibrosis; ciliary dyskinesia; genetic immune defects such as hypogammaglobulinemia; and mechanical obstruction from foreign bodies, tumor or stenosis.[20] Less common causes include severe pneumonia, allergic bronchopulmonary aspergillosis and, rarely, intralobar sequestration. The accumulation of pools of pus leads to chronic cough and copious sputum, with dyspnea and orthopnea in advanced cases. The complications of hemoptysis, brain abscess and cor pulmonale have become rare since antibiotics are used extensively to treat any bacterial infection. In addition to the history and physical findings, radiologic examinations are basic to making the diagnosis of bronchiectasis. Chest CT has become the most effective imaging technique, since it is noninvasive, rapid, and clearly indicative of all areas of involvement. Bronchography is reserved for evaluation of localized disease in patients who may be surgical candidates (Fig. 63–3). Bronchoscopy is rarely used

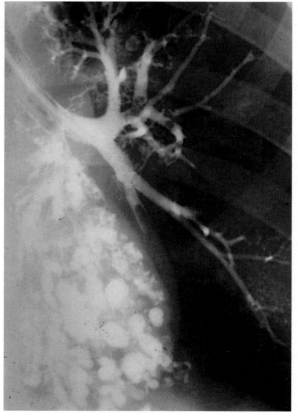

Fig. 63–3. Left posteroanterior bronchogram of a 10-year-old child with bronchiectasis and atelectasis of the left lower lobe subsequent to severe pneumonia.

now in the diagnosis of this disease, but can effectively remove large collections of material in the proximal airways in the patient with overwhelming accumulations of sputum. Bronchoscopy is also useful to identify and treat stenotic areas and to obtain mucosal biopsies in the patient with abnormal cilia.

Cystic fibrosis is particularly apt to result in secretion retention because of the viscid nature of the mucus in these patients. It is estimated to be the cause of half of the bronchiectasis in children in the United States. This hereditary condition causes large amounts of very tenacious material to gather in all the bronchi, obstructing the smaller ones completely. Atelectasis occurs, along with fibrosis, bronchiectasis, and patchy emphysematous areas. Extremely vigorous cough is necessary to expel the sputum but this must be supplemented by mucus thinning agents, chest physical therapy and postural drainage maneuvers to be effective. Bronchoscopy with lung lavage has also been helpful in older children and adults. Though the newer techniques of gene therapy may be the answer to this vicious problem in the future,[21] selected patients are now undergoing lung transplant to survive.[22]

Lung abscess may also be the end result of severe infection, however here the process is localized to a limited area. In general the treatment is prolonged antibiotic therapy in addition to postural drainage and chest physiotherapy. Bronchoscopy is indicated for diagnostic purposes to rule out an underlying carcinoma or foreign body and to obtain secretions for culture from the most specific source possible. It is also used to provide drainage of the abscess in some cases where the appropriate segmental bronchus can be determined radiologically.

In lung infections of obscure origin, flexible fiberoptic bronchoscopy is especially effective in determining the cause when the microorganism is sparse or difficult to identify. In such cases the technique of lung lavage can be utilized to gain enough material to attain the diagnosis. This is particularly true for Mycobacterium tuberculosis and Pneumocystis carinii infections as well as Toxoplasma gondii, Legionella, Histoplasma, Influenza, and Respiratory Syncytial Virus where isolation from BAL fluid is considered to be diagnostic.[17]

Noninfectious inflammatory disorders of the lower respiratory tract also occur and require bronchoscopy for diagnostic purposes. Also known as interstitial lung disease (ILD), they are a group of varied conditions that result in thickening of the alveolar walls, with fibrosis and epithelial changes that include the vascular walls as well as the alveoli.[23] Some occur as isolated entities, others are associated with systemic disease. There is slowly progressive loss of functioning alveoli-capillary relationships until respiratory compromise ensues with dyspnea and cough. As fibrosis progresses, the lung gradually develops intervening cystic spaces and becomes less and less functional, until final failure occurs. Unfortunately, as a result of the insidious progress of ILD, these patients may go undiagnosed for prolonged periods. Known causes of ILD include inhalation of organic and inorganic dusts, use of medications of various classes, radiation, inhalation of certain toxins, and some infectious agents. ILD of unknown etiology is most often idiopathic pulmonary fibrosis, sarcoidosis or associated with collagen vascular disorders. Once the diagnosis is suspected from the history, physical examination or chest x-ray, further studies must include screening for liver, renal, muscle and collagen vascular disorders. Pulmonary function tests and ventilation/perfusion scans will help to define the extent of the respiratory impairment. Bronchoscopy is usually accomplished with flexible fiberoptic endoscopy to rule out neoplasm or infection. Transbronchial biopsy may be utilized in some patients with sarcoidosis, but open lung biopsy may be necessary in obscure diagnoses. However in many patients BAL will be helpful in determining the cell type involved in the alveolitis, as well as the offending inhalant in some cases.

Probably the most frequent reason for diagnostic endoscopy in adults is to identify the presence and histologic diagnosis of a neoplasm.[24]

Benign neoplasms of the trachea or bronchi may be removed through an open bronchocope. Neoplasms with narrow pedicles are the most suitable for endoscopic resection. Papillomas, fibromas, granulomas and lipomas can be treated in this way. Broad-based or vascular lesions will require laser control, or resection via thoracotomy. Some endobronchial masses of amyloidosis can be palliatively resected at bronchoscopy. In tracheopathia osteochondroplastica, multiple submucosal nodules form which consist of calcified cartilage and lamellar bone. The masses occur throughout the TBT and can cause obstruction by their size and by alteration in airflow and mucus retention. The obstructive masses can be bronchoscopically reduced in size to improve the airway, though the widespread distribution of these masses precludes their total removal.

Suspected malignant neoplasm of the tracheobronchial tree is the most serious indication for bronchoscopy (Fig. 63–4). Since the mid-1950s, lung cancer rates and mortality have risen drastically in the United States and other industrialized countries.[25] In 1987 lung cancer became the leading cause of death for women in the U.S., overtaking that of breast cancer. Cigarette smoking is the major risk factor. Histologic types of bronchogenic cancer are grouped as small cell cancer (SCC) and non-small cell cancer (NSCC). The NSCCs include adenocarcinoma, squamous cell carcinoma, and large cell carcinoma. Early detection is vital since the growth and spread of these tumors can be rapid, especially that of SCC.[26,27] Clinical symptoms of lung cancer are absent in occult tumors, but include

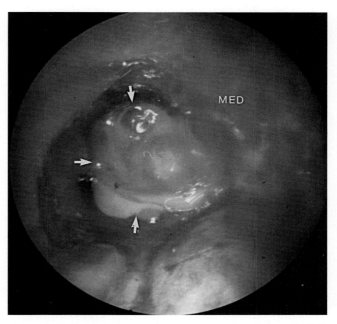

Fig. 63–4. Endoscopic view of cancer (arrows) occluding the left main bronchus of a 41-year-old man. Following partial resection using the carbon dioxide laser, the lung reexpanded rapidly. MED, Medial wall.

cough, pain, weight loss, obstruction, hemoptysis and paraneoplastic manifestations in more advanced lesions. Prognosis is dependent on the histologic type, the stage at presentation of the tumor and by the treatment which can be given. SCC is responsive to chemotherapy and radiation though its growth rate and dissemination often place it in the advanced stages at diagnosis, with the poorest prognosis. In NSCC, surgery is the treatment of choice if the tumor is resectable, with radiation and chemotherapy included for more advanced lesions.[28]

Endoscopy in these patients can be done with the open bronchoscope for lesions that are in the trachea, main bronchi, segmental and some sub-segmental bronchi where large forceps can be used effectively to obtain generous biopsies. Large bore telescopes of appropriate angle improve the visualization of the tumor's surface elevation, ulceration, vascularity, and bronchial wall invasion. Telescopes also help to identify any associated changes such as induration, nodal compression, carinal distortion, secondary infection, and pulsation of any adjacent large vessel. In more peripheral lesions FFO is the better choice because it is possible to obtain samples by brush technique or transbronchial biopsy even in very small lesions. Endoscopic therapy of obstructing lesions can also be accomplished using either the CO2 laser coupled to the open-tube bronchoscope for central tumors, or the YAG laser fiber delivery system with the flexible instrument for peripheral or more angulated locations. The obstructing mass must be exophytic not extrinsic compression, must contain only small vessels, and must be within the viewing range of the bronchoscope.

Pediatric airway disease, whether congenital or acquired, is another major reason to use diagnostic and therapeutic bronchoscopy. The most common findings mandating endoscopy include stridor, atelectasis, and suspicion of foreign body.[29] Open-tube bronchoscopy remains the best method for many procedures, however FFO is used more frequently since the development of small diameter instruments. Although the techniques are similar to those used in adult bronchoscopy, the procedures require even greater delicacy of touch because of the small size of the airways and because the child is often severely ill. Magnification available through telescopes and television has greatly improved the ability to see lesions and to speed the entire procedure, making it safer for these small patients. Secretions from acute or chronic infections can be removed and cultured, the degree of expiratory collapse of any bronchomalacia can be evaluated, vascular compressions can be recognized, the rare tumor mass or cyst can be identified, and possible intubation trauma (especially in tiny babies) can be verified. In addition to diagnostic gains, therapeutic goals can also be accomplished in children. Mucus plugs can be removed, some stenoses can be dilated either with the bronchoscope itself or with bougie and balloon dilators,[30] and small exophytic growths such as papilloma can be removed or laser vaporized.

Additionally and importantly, foreign bodies can be retrieved expeditiously. Foreign bodies of the tracheobronchial tree occur mainly in children, particularly those under two years old. Children this age are actively exploring their world and all the interesting objects in it. Carelessness accounts for most foreign body accidents.[31] Caregivers must watch that children not play while eating, must prepare the food to avoid slippery vegetable and seed fragments, must remove small hardware items and tiny toy parts from the child's reach, must close all safety pins immediately, and must not allow teeth to be used to remove small objects from other sites. Physicians should advise that children under six not be allowed to eat nuts, and no one should be allowed to run, roughhouse or laugh while eating. Though sharp objects like pins or fishbones are more likely to lodge at or above the larynx, smooth objects such as nuts, corn kernels, watermelon seeds and small toys can pass through the glottis to lodge in the TBT.

Foreign bodies entering the airways induce immediate severe coughing, often with cyanosis. The coughing lasts for a short time and then subsides as the object finally comes to rest in one area. Although the foreign body often lodges in the right bronchus because of its more direct extension from the trachea and its larger size, the left bronchus or any segmental bronchus can also become the site of lodgement. A relatively quiet period ensues during which the foreign body may be forgotten. Eventually a more persistent cough may resume, and other signs and symptoms occur which vary depending on the kind of obstruction produced (Fig. 63–5). Inspiratory or expiratory wheeze, altered or absent breath sounds, and tympany or dullness to percussion can occur. The child may be fussy or less active. PA radiographs in inspiration and expiration, as well as lateral projections should be taken to define the location and degree of obstructive emphysema or atelectasis (Fig. 63–6). Alternatively, chest fluoroscopy with permanent cine or video recording can be done. It must always be remembered that a long-indwelling foreign body of the bronchus can produce emphysema, recurrent pneumonitis, bronchiectasis and lung abscess.

Large foreign bodies of the trachea may cause rapid suffocation. A young child who collapses at play is likely to have a tracheal foreign body. Smaller foreign

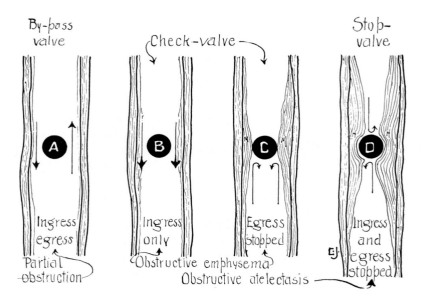

Fig. 63–5. Valve mechanisms in bronchial obstruction. Bypass valve (A) permits the passage of air on inspiration and expiration. No distal collapse or emphysema develops. Expiratory check or one-way valve permits the ingress of air during inspiration (B) but prevents the egress of air during expiration (C) owing to contraction of the bronchus. This form of obstruction traps air in the lung distal to the foreign body, and the repetition of this process with each respiratory cycle produces obstructive emphysema. Inspiratory check or stop valve (D) prevents the movement of air on inspiration or expiration. Absorption of the air distal to the obstruction results in atelectasis. Reprinted with permission from Jackson C: Bronchoscopy and Esophagoscopy. Philadelphia, WB Saunders, 1950.

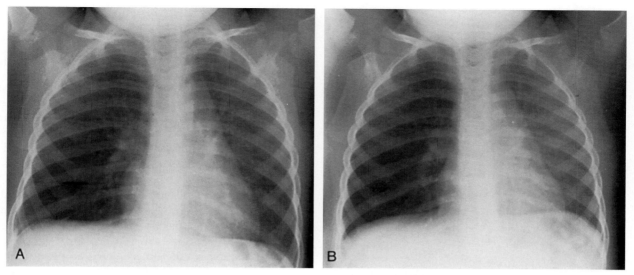

Fig. 63–6. Inspiratory (A) and expiratory (B) posteroanterior chest roentgenograms demonstrating obstructive emphysema of the right lung caused by a peanut in the right bronchus. The difference between the two lung fields becomes more marked on expiration.

bodies may move in the trachea on each inspiration and produce an audible slap at the carina, and a palpatory thud as the object strikes the subglottic area on expiration. Radiography is not usually helpful with tracheal foreign bodies. By listening at the open mouth and palpating the trachea, one can confirm the diagnosis by these telltale signs.

Vegetable foreign bodies produce severe inflammatory reactions in the respiratory tract. These reactions occur rapidly and are particularly severe with peanuts and other nuts. On the other hand, metallic and plastic objects that cause only partial obstruction of a bronchus may be tolerated for long periods (Fig. 63–7). Grassheads present a special problem because of their tendency to migrate toward the periphery of the lung owing to the ratchet action of their barbs during the respiratory cycle.[32] Some grassheads can even penetrate lung, pleura, and chest wall to form a sinus. These foreign bodies often require thoracotomy for removal.

Dried vegetables such as beans are especially dangerous since their small size on entrance allows easy inhalation, but they immediately begin to absorb water and can expand to completely fill the airway. The resulting stop valve action completely occludes the bronchus and causes the rapid development of atelectasis with resulting shift of the mediastinum, and decreased respiratory efficiency (Fig. 63–8). Severe respiratory distress with cyanosis can take place within 30 minutes following the aspiration. Cardiorespiratory failure occurs unless the foreign body is removed. The bean may have swelled larger than the glottic aperture and usually it must be broken into smaller pieces for removal through the glottis, thus turning one object into several potentially obstructive foreign bodies!

In a patient in whom the history and symptoms are thought to be caused by aspiration of a foreign body, the situation usually demands bronchoscopic investigation. If no foreign body is found at bronchoscopy, repeat bronchoscopy is indicated if the symptoms and physical signs do not disappear or radiography does not return to normal. It is very helpful to have a duplicate object in order to study its mechanical properties and avoid problems involved in the removal of the foreign body. Unlike dried vegetables where speed is

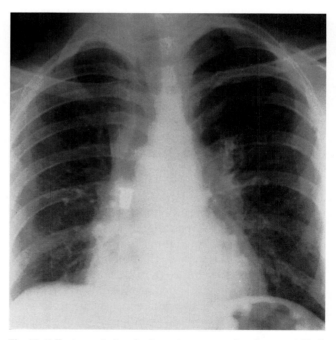

Fig. 63–7. Posteroanterior chest roentgenogram showing a metal bolt in the right bronchus intermedius. The object was hollow, allowing almost normal airflow with respiration.

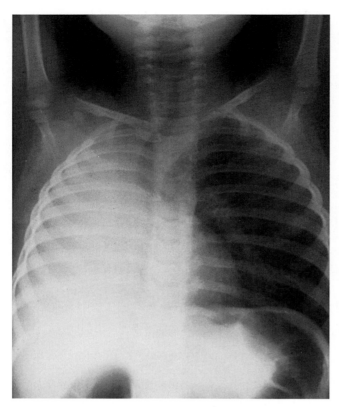

Fig. 63–8. Posteroanterior chest roentgenograms of an 18-month-old child who had aspirated a dry pinto bean only a short time earlier. The bean swelled to occlude the right main bronchus and resulted in respiratory distress. Note total atelectasis of the right lung, markedly deviated trachea, mediastinal shift toward the occluded right side, and hyperaeration of the left lung.

essential, most airway foreign bodies do not present a need for urgent intervention, and one may take time to prepare the patient optimally and gather the equipment that might be particularly useful in the problem at hand. In a patient with a foreign body indwelling more than 24 hours, attention to adequate hydration and control of secondary infection and other coincident medical problems makes the removal safer and more likely to be successful. General anesthesia is used in most patients for foreign body removal, but local anesthesia is appropriate in some adult cases.

The size of the ventilating bronchoscope should be appropriate to the size of the patient. It should be small enough in diameter to reach the level of the object and yet provide as large a working lumen as possible. Forceps specifically designed for each type of foreign body should be used. Forceps with integrated magnifying telescopes markedly improve visualization though, as yet, only a few blade styles are available to remove foreign bodies. Videocameras can also be used with these telescopes to provide even larger images for the endoscopist.

Once the foreign body has been visualized, it is important to avoid any maneuver that might displace the object distally and thereby make its removal more difficult. Surrounding secretions should be carefully suctioned away, and the object studied to achieve the best exposure and to determine the best position of the bronchoscope for forceps application. In general, the distal tip of the bronchoscope should be as close as possible to the object without touching it in order to avoid interfering with the space needed for application of the forceps. Careful consideration should be given to the plane in which the forceps are opened and the manner in which they are advanced to encompass the foreign body.

As a general rule, foreign bodies are removed by placing the distal ends of the forceps' blades beyond the equator of the object so that it cannot be propelled distally as the forceps close. Care must be taken to avoid crushing fragile objects such as peanuts. Fragmentation complicates the problem because it creates several smaller foreign bodies. When possible, bronchial foreign bodies are withdrawn through the bronchoscope, but in some instances the object is too big and must be removed as a trailing foreign body. In this method the object is withdrawn to the bevel of the bronchoscope, fixed in place with the thumb and forefinger of the left hand holding the forceps against the bronchoscope, and all are removed as one unit. Chances of success in withdrawing the unit are best during inspiration. The longer axis of the cross section of the object should be rotated into the anterior-posterior plane at the glottis so that the foreign body is not sheared from the forceps by the vocal cords.

Some foreign bodies either produce subglottic swelling or expand sufficiently to make their exit through the cricoid cartilage impossible. Under these circumstances, a tracheotomy should be performed so that the foreign body may be removed through the opening. In such a situation, the tracheotomy should be maintained until the subglottic edema subsides. Most bronchial foreign bodies may be removed safely on the first effort. This must be accomplished quickly to avoid edema and trauma. The risk of leaving a foreign body for a while longer must be weighed against the risk of the effects of undue endoscopy trauma. After a period of unsuccessful manipulation, it may be better to wait for a day or two and try again, when the reaction to the initial manipulation has subsided, thus avoiding intubation or tracheotomy.

Fluoroscopic guidance can be used for the removal of some opaque foreign bodies located so far in the periphery of the lung that they cannot be removed under direct vision through the bronchoscope (Fig. 63–9). A biplane fluoroscope is needed to enable forceps application in the correct direction. It requires close cooperation between endoscopist, anesthesiologist and radiologist to minimize the difficulties of fluoroscopic bronchoscopy.

Tracheal foreign bodies may produce little or no re-

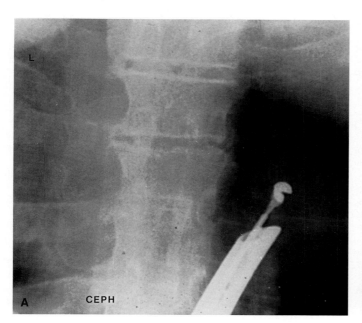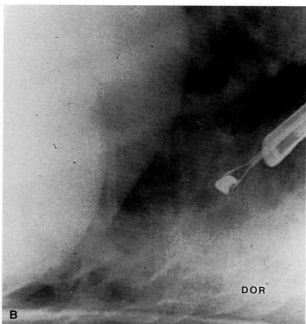

Fig. 63–9. Simultaneous fluoroscopic views of the right chest obtained during the retrieval of a gold tooth onlay. Posteroanterior (A) and lateral (B) images are deliberately rotated to the same position as the patient so that the endoscopist can direct the bronchoscope and apply the forceps correctly without delay. R, Right; L, left; CEPH, cephalad; DOR, dorsal.

spiratory distress and then suddenly become impacted in the subglottic area. With the introduction of the bronchoscope, they can be inadvertently bypassed or displaced into the distal portion of the trachea. However in some cases it may be life-saving to deliberately bypass the object with the bronchoscope in order to ventilate the patient. After a foreign body has been removed, it is necessary to reintroduce the broncho-scope and inspect the whole tracheobronchial tree for a possible second foreign body.

In looking for a foreign body, it is important to know what part of the foreign body is likely to be seen. Pointed foreign bodies, such as nails, tacks, and pins, are almost always situated with the point directed superiorly, and it is the point one must look for, not the whole foreign body. The point must be ensheathed within the bronchoscope or enclosed in the blades of the forceps before traction is made to prevent perforation of the bronchus. If embedded, the foreign body must be pushed distally with the forceps to disengage the point, and then aligned with the long axis of the bronchoscope for removal (Fig. 63–2).

Wood screws usually lodge with the head proximally located and are difficult to remove because there are no forceps spaces around the head for application of the forceps blades. The tips of head-holding forceps may be passed over the head of the screw to obtain a secure grasp. Hollow foreign bodies may also have no external forceps spaces but may be handled by placing one blade of an alligator forceps inside and one out-side. Alternatively, expanding hollow objects forceps

can be used. Some foreign bodies can be removed with a flexible bronchoscope with forceps passed through the instrument channel, but only a few small forceps are currently available and no ventilation is possible through these bronchoscopes.

Complications are rare after the prompt removal of foreign bodies, and recovery is swift. The resolution of obstructive emphysema, if present initially, occurs rapidly. All other physical and radiographic signs of the foreign body should disappear. If that is not the case, repeat bronchoscopy should be carried out. The recovery after removal of a long indwelling object is more variable but is often surprisingly complete and rapid. Recovery depends on the amount of permanent bronchial damage.

SUGGESTED READINGS

1. Jackson CL, Huber JF: Correlated applied anatomy of the bron-chial tree and lungs with a system of nomenclature. Dis Chest 9:319, 1943.
2. Boyden EA: Segmental Anatomy of the Lungs: A Study of the Segmental Bronchi and Related Pulmonary Vessels. New York: McGraw-Hill, 1955.
3. Weir N: Anatomy of the larynx and tracheobronchial tree. *In* Scott-Brown's Otolaryngology, 5th Ed. Edited by A.G. Kerr. Butterworth Somerset, Great Britain, 1987.
4. Harris JH Jr: The clinical significance of the tracheal bronchus. Am J Roentgen 79:228, 1958.
5. Myer CM III, Cotton RT, Holmes DK, Jackson RK: Laryngeal and laryngotracheoesophageal clefts: Role of early surgical re-pair. Ann Otol Rhinol Laryngol 99:98, 1990.

6. Weibel ER: Morphometry of the Human Lung. New York, Academic Press, 1963.

7. Ikeda S: Flexible bronchofiberscope. Ann Otol Rhinol Laryngol *79*:916, 1970.

8. Levine B, Nielsen EW: The justifications and controversies of panendoscopy--a review. Ear Nose Throat J *7*:335, 1992.

9. Mori M, et al: Accurate contiguous sections without breath-holding on chest CT: Value of respiratory gating and ultrafast CT. Am J Roentgenol *162*:1057, 1994.

10. Paranjpe DV, Bergin CJ: Spiral CT of the lungs: Optimal technique and resolution compared with conventional CT. Am J Roentgenol *162*:561, 1994.

11. Grant BJB, Saltzman AR: Respiratory functions of the lung. *In* Textbook of Pulmonary Diseases. 5th Ed. Volume 1. Edited by G.L. Baum and E. Wolinsky, Boston: Little Brown, 1994.

12. Cordasco EM Jr, Mehta AC, Ahmad M: Bronchoscopically induced bleeding: A summary of nine years' Cleveland clinic experience and review of the literature. Chest *100*:1141, 1991.

13. Selecky PA: Evaluation of hemoptysis through the bronchoscope. Chest *73*:741, 1978.

14. Marsh BR, et al: Flexible fiberoptic bronchoscopy: Its place in the search for lung cancer. Ann Otol Rhinol Laryngol *82*:757, 1973.

15. Council on Scientific Affairs, American Medical Association: The use of pulse oximetry during conscious sedation. JAMA *270*:1463, 1993.

16. Andersen HA: Transbronchoscopic lung biopsy for diffuse pulmonary diseases: Results in 939 patients. Chest *73*:734. 1978.

17. American Thoracic Society Official Statement of ATS: Clinical role of bronchoalveolar lavage in adults with pulmonary disease. Am Rev Respir Dis *142*:481. 1990.

18. Stern RC: Acute bronchiolitis. *In* Nelson Textbook of Pediatrics. 14th Ed. Edited by R.E. Behrman, et al. W.B. Saunders, 1992.

19. Donowitz GR, Mandell GL: Acute pneumonia. *In* Principles and Practice of Infectious Diseases. 3rd Ed. Edited by GL Mandell, RG Douglas, Jr, and JE Bennett. New York: Churchill Livingstone, 1990.

20. Bone R: Bronchiectasis. *In* Cecil Textbook of Medicine. 19th Ed. Edited by J.B. Wyngaarden, LH Smith, Jr., and JC Bennett. Philadelphia, W.B. Saunders. 1992.

21. Weinberger SE: Recent advances in pulmonary medicine. Part 1. N Engl J Med *328*:1389, 1993.

22. Weinberger SE: Recent advances in pulmonary medicine. Part 2. N Engl J Med *328*:1462. 1993.

23. Crystal RG: Interstitial lung disease. *In* Cecil Textbook of Medicine, 19th Ed. Edited by JB Wyngaarden, LH Smith, Jr., and JC Bennett. Philadelphia, W.B. Saunders. 1992.

24. Prakash UBS, Offord KP, Stubbs SE: Bronchoscopy in North America: The ACCP survey. Chest *100*:1668. 1991.

25. Samet JM: The epidemiology of lung cancer. Chest *103*:20S, 1993.

26. Martini N: Operable lung cancer. CA Cancer J Clin *43*:201, 1993.

27. Hinson JA, Jr, Perry MC: Small cell lung cancer. CA Cancer J Clin *43*:216. 1993.

28. Ihde DC: Chemotherapy of lung cancer. N Engl J Med *327*:1434–1439, 1992.

29. Hoeve LJ, Rombout J: Pediatric laryngobronchoscopy: 1332 procedures stored in a database. Int J Pediatr Otorhinolaryngol *24*:73–82, 1992.

30. Skedros DG, Chan KH, Siewers RD, Atlas AB: Rigid bronchoscopy balloon catheter dilation for bronchial stenosis in infants. Ann Otol Rhinol Laryngol *102*:266. 1993.

31. Jackson C, Jackson CL: Bronchoesophagology. Philadelphia, W.B. Saunders, 1950.

32. Clery AP, Ellis FH, Jr, Schmidt HW: Problems associated with aspiration of grass heads (inflorescences). JAMA *171*:1478, 1959.

64 Esophagology

Joyce A. Schild and James B. Snow, Jr.

Esophagoscopy is a primary method of investigating diseases of the esophagus. In addition to open tube esophagoscopes which are used to examine and treat esophageal disease, the flexible fiberoptic upper gastrointestinal panendoscopes allow examination of the upper gastrointestinal tract to the duodenum.

ANATOMY OF THE ESOPHAGUS

The esophagus is a vertical muscular tube that extends from the hypopharynx to the stomach. It measures 23 to 25 cm in length in the adult, beginning at the lower border of the cricoid cartilage at approximately the level of the sixth cervical vertebra. It passes through the neck, superior mediastinum, and posterior mediastinum anterior to the cervical and thoracic vertebrae, terminating at the cardiac orifice of the stomach at the level of the eleventh thoracic vertebra.

The esophagus starts in the midline but then curves slightly to the left. In the mediastinum, it returns to the midline at the level of the fifth thoracic vertebra. In the inferior portion of the mediastinum, it deviates to the left as it passes anteriorly into the esophageal hiatus of the diaphragm. Importantly, the curvatures in the anterior-posterior plane follow the convexity of the bodies of the cervical vertebrae and the concavity of the bodies of the thoracic vertebrae. The abdominal portion of the esophagus, which is only 1.25 cm long, is in the esophageal groove on the posterior surface of the left lobe of the liver. The left and anterior surfaces of the abdominal esophagus are covered with peritoneum.

The esophagus is posterior to the trachea and in contact with the common carotid arteries. The recurrent laryngeal nerves lie in the angle between the esophagus and the trachea. The thoracic duct lies on its left side. Both lobes of the thyroid gland come in contact with the esophagus, more so on the left. In the superior mediastinum, the esophagus passes posterior to and to the right of the arch of the aorta and then descends on the right side of the descending aorta until the inferior portion of the mediastinum is reached, where it passes anterior to and slightly to the left of the aorta. Inferior to the arch of the aorta, the left bronchus crosses and indents the esophagus anteriorly. The thoracic duct is posterior to the lower portion of the esophagus. It passes to the right of the esophagus and is posterior to it at the level of the fourth thoracic vertebra as it passes to the left of the esophagus to enter the neck. The azygos vein is to the right side of the esophagus in the thorax. The right vagus nerve descends posterior to the esophagus, and the left vagus descends anterior to the esophagus.

The esophagus is lined by nonkeratinizing stratified squamous epithelium covering a thin lamina propria. The muscularis mucosae is composed of smooth muscle fibers arranged longitudinally. It becomes thicker in the lower third of the esophagus. The submucosa consists primarily of thick collagenous and coarse elastic fibers and contains mucus glands and Meissner's plexus.

The muscle of the esophagus is composed of an inner circular layer which is continuous with the inferior constrictor of the pharynx and an outer longitudinal layer. The longitudinal fibers are arranged proximally into fascicles which attach to the cricoid cartilage. Distally the fascicles blend to form a uniform layer surrounding the esophagus. Auerbach's myenteric plexus lies between the two muscle layers. The muscle is striated in the upper third, mixed in the middle third, and nearly all smooth in the lower third. The outer coat, or fibrosa, consists of loose fibroelastic tissue rather than a true strong serosa like that found in the gastrointestinal tract distal to the esophagus. The circular layer of muscle is slightly thicker at the level of the cricoid cartilage and blends with the cricopharyngeus muscle, which is attached to the cricoid cartilage. This upper esophageal sphincter is a high-pressure zone in esophageal manometry and corresponds with the cricopharyngeal muscle.[1] The lower esophageal sphincter is approximately 3 cm long and may descend 1 to 3 cm with normal respiration. A single distinct muscle responsible for the lower sphincter action has not been identified.

ENDOSCOPIC ANATOMY

Normally the lumen of the esophagus is collapsed in a flattened or stellate pattern. The wall of the esopha-

gus is thin, and lined by shiny, pale pink mucosa. The diameter of the esophagus is reduced at four points: the cricopharyngeus, the crossing of the aorta, the crossing of the left bronchus, and the diaphragm. The average distances to these points from the upper teeth, according to age, are shown in Figure 64–1.

The cricopharyngeus muscle periodically relaxes and contracts in the nonparalysed patient. This action can be viewed through an open tube esophagoscope placed posterior to the cricoid cartilage. As the esophagoscope is advanced, the impression of the arch of the aorta and the left bronchus are usually seen only

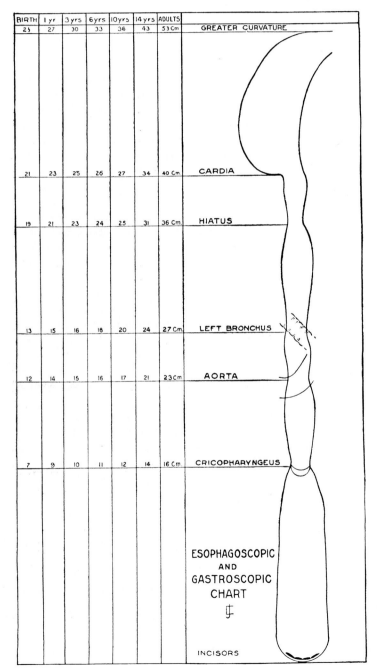

BIRTH	1 yr	3 yrs	6 yrs	10 yrs	14 yrs	ADULTS	
23	27	30	33	36	43	53 Cm	GREATER CURVATURE
21	23	25	26	27	34	40 Cm	CARDIA
19	21	23	24	25	31	36 Cm.	HIATUS
13	15	16	18	20	24	27 Cm.	LEFT BRONCHUS
12	14	15	16	17	21	23 Cm	AORTA
7	9	10	11	12	14	16 Cm.	CRICOPHARYNGEUS

ESOPHAGOSCOPIC
AND
GASTROSCOPIC
CHART

INCISORS

Fig. 64–1. Distances from the upper incisor teeth to esophageal landmarks. Reprinted with permission from Jackson C and Jackson CL: Bronchoesophagology. Philadelphia, WB Saunders, 1950.

faintly, but pulsations can be felt readily through the endoscope. Further down, the hiatus is usually apparent as an anteriorly placed narrowing. As the hiatus is passed, the stellate pattern of the esophagus is replaced by the deeper red, velvety gastric mucosa with prominent rugal folds.

INDICATIONS FOR ESOPHAGOSCOPY

Esophagoscopy for diagnosis is indicated in nearly all patients with unexplained symptoms and signs of esophageal and mediastinal diseases. It is specifically indicated in the diagnosis of dysphagia, odynophagia, aphagia, a sensation of a lump or 'sticking' in the throat, vocal cord palsies, retrosternal pain, heartburn, hematemesis, persistent regurgitation or vomiting, and caustic ingestion. It is also indicated to look for a second primary carcinoma in patients with squamous cell carcinoma of other aerodigestive areas, and in patients with neck masses thought to be metastatic disease.[2] Endoscopy may also be helpful in patients with radiologic evidence of extrinsic or intrinsic esophageal abnormality, abnormal motility, or altered esophageal pH. In a pregnant patient, endoscopy under local anesthesia can replace radiologic evaluation of GI symptoms.

Esophagoscopy for therapeutic purposes is indicated in patients with foreign bodies, achalasia, diverticula, and stenoses of various causes. Strictures can be dilated under visual control, and indwelling tubes of various types can be inserted for nutrition maintenance in carcinoma of the esophagus.

Contraindications to esophagoscopy include uncorrected coagulopathy, and recent perforation of the esophagus from trauma or spontaneously as in the Mallory-Weiss syndrome. Cervical spine rigidity may allow only flexible endoscopy, while trismus may prevent any examination unless a small diameter endoscope can be passed nasally. The diagnostic accuracy of upper gastrointestinal panendoscopy in upper GI bleeding is high for the first 12 to 24 hours after the bleeding episode, but must be delayed until vital signs are stable and blood volume is replaced. If bleeding is persistent, endoscopy can be performed under general anesthesia just before operation.

RADIOLOGIC DIAGNOSIS

Radiologic studies are usually done prior to endoscopy because the procedure can be carried out more safely if the structure and function of the esophagus is known. Radiologic evaluation should include PA and lateral chest films to screen for other abnormalities such as mediastinal widening, pulmonary masses, pneumo-

nia, atelectasis, pulmonary or soft tissue emphysema, pleural effusion and radiopaque foreign bodies.

Neck images are particularly helpful in evaluating the patient with cervical esophageal lesions. A good lateral view is one in which the neck is slightly flexed on the thorax, the head is extended on the neck, and the shoulders are positioned caudally and dorsally. The tissues between the cervical vertebra and the larynx and trachea are well seen and can be evaluated for swelling or other abnormality. Foreign bodies can be seen directly if radiopaque, or inferred by intraluminal air in the cervical esophagus surrounding a nonradiopaque object. Paraesophageal swelling and air from a perforation, and displacement of the larynx and trachea by neoplasm can be readily appreciated. Cervical spine osteophytes, that may cause dysphagia, can also be detected.

Contrast materials are utilized to outline the contours of the esophagus. Barium sulfate suspensions of various consistencies are usually used, but water-miscible solutions are appropriate if a perforation is suspected, and water or oil-based contrast is preferred where aspiration is likely. Contrast studies are useful in demonstrating congenital or acquired atresia, stenosis, and aerodigestive fistulas; external compression caused by vascular abnormalities, and cervical or mediastinal masses; and intraluminal abnormality such as foreign body, varices, esophagitis, tumor, ulceration, and stenosis. Cineflouroscopy is particularly valuable in demonstrating deglutition problems in the pharynx,[3] and motility and mucosal disturbances in the esophagus.[4] A permanent record of the details, progress and response to treatment can be obtained in achalasia, gastroesophageal reflux, intraesophageal dysmotility, esophageal spasm, Schatzki rings, hernias, diverticuli, and scleroderma.

TECHNIQUE OF ESOPHAGOSCOPY

The examination can be performed with either an open esophagoscope or with a flexible panendoscope. It should be done in a well equipped endoscopy suite, and the patient should not have taken anything to eat or drink for at least 8 hours prior to the examination. Premedication as described in Chapter 62 should be administered. General anesthesia with an endotracheal tube is preferred for the majority of patients requiring open tube esophagoscopy, but topical anesthesia is satisfactory for flexible endoscopy. With general anesthesia, the introduction of the esophagoscope is eased by the use of a muscle relaxant and is safer than any other technique in preventing perforation of the cervical esophagus. Under local anesthesia, the patient is encouraged to swallow the lubricated esophagoscope as it is gently advanced. Once the esophagus is entered, gentle insufflation of air through the endoscope facilitates the advancement of the scope and the inspection of the mucosal walls of the esophagus. The position of the patient is not important for flexible endoscopy.

Position of the patient for open esophagoscopy is critical, and initially is the same as for open bronchoscopy in the Boyce position (Chapter 64). The patient's shoulders should be at the edge of the main portion of the operating table so that the head and neck may be moved freely on the headrest. The cervical esophagus is almost vertical in the Boyce position; therefore, the open esophagoscope should be held nearly vertically at first. The tip of the esophagoscope is lightly coated with lubricant before introduction. As the esophagoscope is introduced to the level of the junction of the hypopharynx and esophagus, with the thumb of the left hand a gentle lift and forward pressure may be applied through the tip of the esophagoscope at the posterior plate of the cricoid cartilage. As the cricopharyngeus relaxes, one can see several centimeters into the lumen of the esophagus and observe some motion with respiration. The esophagoscope is carefully advanced only during a period of relaxation, NEVER forced while the muscle is in contraction, and is never advanced unless there is a distinct lumen ahead. If the lumen remains closed, a small Jackson bougie can be introduced to serve as a 'lumen finder'. Considerable patience is required here because this site is the one most frequently perforated. Under local anesthesia, the cricopharyngeus can be seen to open and close periodically. Under general anesthesia with muscle relaxant, the esophagus is patent any time the cricoid cartilage is displaced anteriorly, and the instrument may be advanced gently.

As the esophagoscope is advanced through the cervical esophagus, care must be taken to keep pressure off the posterior wall. It is easy to tear the posterior wall of the esophagus by impinging the tip of the esophagoscope onto the cervical vertebrae, especially in patients with calcified spurs on the vertebrae. Lifting the esophagoscope, with the operator's thumb as a fulcrum, will keep the tip of the instrument from lacerating the posterior wall. As the esophagoscope is advanced, it begins to impinge on the posterior wall of the esophagus, and therefore the head is lowered gradually to allow passage of the esophagoscope through the mid portion of the esophagus. At this stage of the examination, the head, neck, and chest are resting in the same plane. In the lower third of the esophagus, the course of the esophagus is slightly anterior and to the left, and the esophagoscope begins to impinge on the posterior wall again. The head must be further lowered to allow the tip of the open esophagoscope to be angled anteriorly and advanced. At this point, the head is depressed relative to the thorax, and rotated slightly to the right. The esophagogastric junction must be negotiated gently and only if a lumen is visible ahead of the endoscope. The lumen appears as a slit or rosette where the esophagus goes through the diaphragm. In some patients, particularly if there is dilatation of the thoracic esophagus, it may be difficult to find the hiatus without a bougie used as a lumen finder. Once the hiatus is found, the abdominal esophagus and cardia are easily passed if they are normal. If coughing occurs here, the instrument should be withdrawn to avoid the risk of perforation. Many abnormalities occur in this area and predispose to perforation of the esophagus unless gentleness and judgement are exercised. As the stomach is entered, gastric juice usually flows down the esophagoscope and obscures the light. Once this fluid is removed, the color and texture change of the mucosa can be noted. The stomach can be safely entered with the open endoscope in most patients, but occasionally this is not possible, and the procedure must be terminated at this level. In flexible endoscopy, the stomach is usually well seen before advancing into the duodenum. Perforation of the esophagus is a serious complication and can be avoided by the use of the most conservative judgement, particularly in the manipulation of the open esophagoscope.

On withdrawing the instrument everything should be examined again. The esophagoscope can be gently rotated to give a panoramic view as the instrument is removed.

ENDOSCOPIC DIAGNOSIS AND MANAGEMENT

Motility disturbances can occur as a primary disorder or as part of systemic illness. Achalasia, a primary neurogenic abnormality, results in failure of normal peristalsis with absent lower esophageal sphincter relaxation. The cause of this disease is as yet unclear in the primary form, however a similar disease in South America, known as Chagas' disease, occurs as the result of infection by Trypanosoma cruzi. In both forms, the end result is progressive dilation of the esophagus above the inferior sphincter. Dysphagia, regurgitation and substernal pain of variable severity occur and progress. The initial onset is usually in middle years, although even children have been diagnosed with achalasia. The esophagus retains amazing amounts of food which is emptied into the stomach only when the intraluminal pressure is greatly elevated. Retained contents may be regurgitated in the recumbent position, especially during sleep, resulting in aspiration, pneumonia and progressive pulmonary disability. Fluids are often taken in large quantities with meals, probably in order to raise the intraesophageal pressure and trigger relaxation of the sphincter which empties the esophageal contents and relieves substernal pressure. Cold liquids are usually less well tolerated than warm ones. Because of the dysphagia and regurgitation, many patients will suffer severe weight loss in addition to their other symptoms. Diagnosis is made on radiographic findings, esophageal motility studies, and esophagoscopy. Chest roentgenograms may show mediastinal widening with a visible air-fluid level in some individuals. An absent gastric air bubble is common. On barium swallow, the dilatation of the esophagus is obvious, along with a beaklike taper in the nonrelaxed lower sphincter area. In later stages, the esophagus may attain a sigmoid contour with poste-

rior folding (Fig. 64–2). Absent peristalsis and delayed emptying of the esophagus are noted on cineflouroscopy. Differentiation from carcinoma can be difficult in the early stages. Esophageal motility studies are necessary to differentiate the early stages of achalasia from diffuse esophageal spasm. In achalasia, motility studies characteristically show slight elevation of esophageal pressure, absence of peristaltic activity, failure of esophageal sphincter relaxation with swallow, and in-

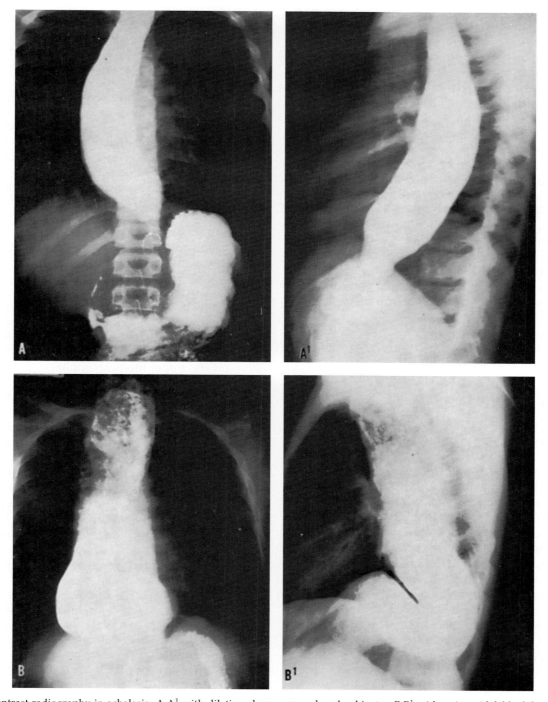

Fig. 64–2. Contrast radiography in achalasia. A,A¹ with dilation above a nonrelaxed sphincter. B,B¹ with a sigmoid fold of the esophagus.

creased sensitivity to cholinergic agonists such as methacholine. Esophagoscopy is helpful in evaluating the degree of dilatation, as well as in identifying the presence of carcinoma which may occur in long-standing disease.[5] In the patient under general anesthesia, relaxation may lead to flooding of the pharynx and overflow into the trachea. Esophagoscopy should be done after the esophagus is emptied of retained contents to avoid aspiration pneumonia. In the patient examined after topical anesthesia, the elevated cricopharyngeal pressure may require slightly more 'push' with the esophagoscope at this level before the esophagus is entered. Caution must be exercised here to avoid complications.

Medical management of achalasia has not been effective, but esophagoscopy can be of use in treatment to allow placement of Jackson style dilators under direct vision at the initial diagnostic esophagoscopy if no important mucosal lesion is found. Subsequently the use of mercury weighted bougies of the Hurst or Maloney type may be effective. Often, forceful dilation with pneumatic dilators may be needed to attain more lasting relief.[6] This must be done with the esophagus empty and under flouroscopic observation for correct placement and inflation of the dilator bag. The patient may have some temporary pain following dilation and must be observed for several hours after the procedure to be certain that perforation has not occurred. Relief of symptoms after dilation may last for months or years. If relief is not obtained, the patient must undergo esophagomyotomy via transthoracic, transabdominal or laparoscopic approach.[7]

Diffuse esophageal spasm is characterized by pain rather than dysphagia. The pain is substernal and may be severe, with radiation in a pattern that mimics cardiac pain. It may occur with tension, while eating, or during sleep and is more common in men. The diagnosis may be elusive because the spasms are not present continuously. When seen radiographically, it has been described as corkscrew, curling, pseudomuscular hypertrophy and pseudodiverticulosis. Nutcracker esophagus is similar to diffuse spasm, but is confined to the lower esophagus and has otherwise normal peristalsis.[8] Treatment should emphasize explanation and reassurance, with sedation, long-acting nitrates and nifedipine as adjuncts. Esophagoscopy is necessary to rule out other conditions which may mimic these conditions. Dilation may be helpful in some patients.

Cricopharyngeal muscle dysfunction is the result of an incoordination of the cricopharyngeus muscle with inability to relax during deglutition. First recognized in patients with bulbar poliomyelitis, this entity subsequently has been recognized in patients with bulbar paralysis of other causes including cerebrovascular accidents, intracranial trauma and neoplasms, amyotrophic lateral sclerosis, and multiple sclerosis. Similar clinical symptoms occur in myopathies such as muscu-

lar dystrophy, myasthenia gravis, dermatomyositis, thyrotoxicosis, and oculopharyngeal muscular dystrophy. Increased resting tone or spasm of the cricopharyngeus, giving rise to the globus sensation, can occur as an isolated symptom, however reflux esophagitis has been found in many of these patients. Extensive resections of the pharynx and larynx can also result in similar symptoms though as a result of fibrosis as well as muscular incoordination. Cricopharyngeal muscle dysfunction may be accurately diagnosed by esophageal motility studies,[9] or by contrast radiography done with specific attention to deglutition phases.[3] In these patients, if esophagoscopy is normal, cricopharyngeal myotomy is often worthwhile. Those patients with chronic, severe aspiration may require laryngeal closure, laryngotracheal separation, or laryngectomy to protect the lower airways.

Diverticula of the esophagus occur at several different levels and are categorized by location and mode of development. Pharyngoesophageal or Zenker's diverticula and lower esophageal diverticula are thought to be related to disordered motility of the cricopharyngeus and esophagus and to congenital or acquired weakness of the muscular walls. They do not contain a muscle layer and are classified as pulsion diverticula.[10] Traction diverticula, containing muscle, are thought to result from inflammatory processes adjacent to the esophagus causing contracture and deformity of the entire wall, usually in the mid third of the esophagus. Tuberculous mediastinal nodes are often cited as an etiologic factor. Traction diverticula are frequently asymptomatic and often found incidently on radiographic studies of the upper gastrointestinal tract.

Zenker's diverticula tend to occur in older male patients. They produce symptoms by compressing the cervical and upper thoracic esophagus because of their position posteriorly and to the left. They enlarge over time to produce progressive dysphagia, noisy swallowing, and regurgitation of undigested food. Because these diverticula always remain distended by food or liquids and are without a sphincteric closure, they are likely to empty into the hypopharynx when patients are recumbent. Aspiration pneumonitis is a frequent complication and may be the major presenting complaint. Diagnosis is made with contrast radiograpy to outline the extent of the diverticular sac (Fig. 64–3). The study should include the lower esophagus to define the extent of gastroesophageal reflux and hiatus hernia which frequently are associated with Zenker's diverticula.

Treatment of a Zenker's diverticulum is by operation which should include preliminary esophagoscopy to aspirate the contents of the sac, and to exclude any possible associated neoplasm.[11] Because it is easier to enter the loose sac than the tightly closed esophagus, it is best to examine with an open endoscope for better control, thus avoiding perforation. Under direct visualization, a mercury-filled bougie may be inserted into

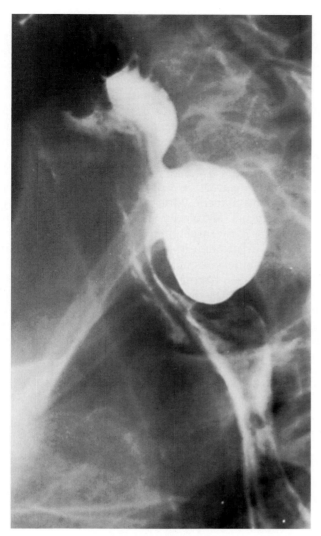

Fig. 64–3. Lateral view of contrast radiography of a pharyngoesophageal diverticulum. Note aspiration of contrast material.

the esophagus to define its course, to determine the amount of tissue to be removed, and to have a firm surface against which the cricopharyngeus may be divided. The diverticulum may be temporarily distended with gauze packing, or lighted with a fiberoptic instrument to make identification and dissection easier.[12] The approach is generally through the left side of the neck with the head turned to the right. The sternocleidomastoid and thyroid lobe are retracted after identifying the recurrent laryngeal nerve to avoid injury to it.

The diverticulum is identified and dissected to its origin. The cricopharyngeal myotomy is performed. When the gauze packing or transilluminator has been removed, the sac is excised. After the bougie is withdrawn to relax the edges of the excision, the pharyngeal wound can be closed without tension. The wound is drained with a suction catheter.

Alternative approaches are also available. Very

small diverticula may be treated by cricopharyngeal myotomy alone, or with myotomy and diverticulopexy. In some debilitated patients endoscopic diverticulotomy, described by Dohlman and others,[13] has been modified for use with lasers.[14] The technique has an acceptable complication rate and is useful for those patients requiring rapid management without open operation.

Inflammation of the esophagus has many causes. Gastroesophageal reflux (GER), with or without demonstrable hiatus hernia, is probably the commonest cause of inflammation of the esophagus. The normal pressure relationships of the lower esophagus and stomach favor GER, because the pressure in the stomach is higher than that of the esophagus. Though the anatomic basis for the lower esophageal sphincter (LES) has been elusive, its physiologic existence is well established. Pressure studies have shown a high intraluminal pressure zone over approximately 3.5 cm at the level of the diaphragm, with the highest pressure at the level of the diaphragm corresponding to the LES. Here the pressure is higher than either the esophagus or the stomach. However, within seconds after swallowing, as the peristaltic wave passes downward, the pressure at the LES falls quickly for 4 to 6 seconds and then returns to normal. When the gastric pressure exceeds that of the LES for long periods of time or if the normal coordination of the LES is deranged, gastric content can reflux into the esophagus. If this refluxate, containing digestive enzymes and other low pH material, is not promptly cleared by peristalsis, inflammation can occur. This inflammation may proceed to ulceration and stricture formation in severe cases. If the material refluxes high enough, it can reach the larynx and pharynx causing inflammation in these areas as well. In some patients whose GER is otherwise asymptomatic, aspiration of refluxate has also been found to be the cause of chronic cough and wheezing, wrongly suggesting asthma.[15] The relationship of sliding hiatal hernia to the reflux of gastric content remains unclear, since the frequency of hiatal hernia in the general population exceeds the frequency of documented GER, and GER does not always produce symptoms or esophagitis in normal individuals or those with esophagogastric incompetence. However, there is a relationship between duodenal ulcer and peptic esophagitis, as shown by the occurrence of peptic esophagitis in roughly 30% of patients with peptic ulcers.[16]

The early changes in peptic esophagitis are limited to the epithelium and lamina propria, but erosion, pseudomembrane formation, and ulceration penetrating into the muscularis occur in the later stages. Finally, fibrosis and epithelial acanthosis occur, causing the formation of a web if superficial or a stricture of the ulcer penetrates deeply (Fig. 64–4). A Schatzki ring may be the result of such formation at the gastroesophageal junction. The deep ulceration of Barrett's ulcer

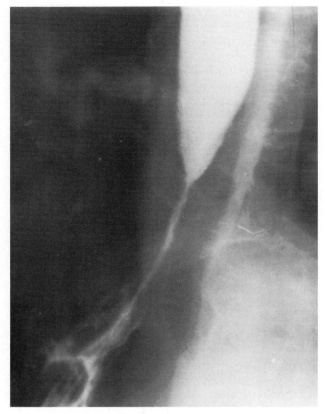

Fig. 64–4. Contrast radiography shows a stricture of the lower one third of the esophagus caused by peptic esophagitis.

tends to occur in areas of columnar epithelium, which may be either a congenital anomaly or an acquired condition. The symptoms of peptic esophagitis are substernal pain or heartburn, dysphagia, and regurgitation. Symptoms are aggravated by stress, spicy food, alcoholic beverages, vomiting, leaning forward, and nasogastric intubation. Some individuals may also be worsened by aspirin or other nonsteroidal anti-inflammatory medication, tetracyclines, and slow-release potassium chloride. This is especially a problem in dehydrated patients and in the elderly who may be taking multiple medications.

The diagnosis of esophagitis is confirmed by radiography of the lower esophagus. The changes are those of ulceration, spasm, and narrowing, as well as the sometime associated hiatal hernia and possible obvious reflux of gastric contents (Fig. 64–5). Esophagoscopy will establish the diagnosis and exclude other causes. The mucosa is red and friable, often with patchy fibrinous exudate. Inflammatory pseudopolyps may occur at the GE junction and appear as inflamed gastric mucosa.

Treatment should consist of a bland diet with frequent small feedings; antacids; H2 blockers; gastric acid suppressant in severe cases; and posture instruction, including avoidance of postprandial recumbency,

and elevation of the head of the bed.[17] Weight reduction, alcohol avoidance, and cessation of smoking are also helpful. Gastric motility-enhancing medications may be of use in those patients with persistent fullness, nausea and belching.

Stricture formation is usually satisfactorily managed with bougienage, but surgical repair may be necessary in patients with persistent symptoms, or complex problems. Antireflux procedures combined with hiatus hernia repair or esophageal lengthening maneuvers can be done.[18]

Infectious causes of esophagitis also occur, especially in the diabetic patient. Candida albicans may produce ulcers, nodularity, and intramural pseudodiverticulosis. Oral thrush may be present causing odynophagia in addition to the dysphagia of esophageal disease. Diagnosis is confirmed by biopsy and cultures obtained at esophagoscopy. Other infections causing esophagitis are less frequent, but include herpes simplex, cytomegalovirus and other virus infections. They are recognized increasingly in immune compromised patients, including those with AIDS. Treatment is by medical management, with dilatation if strictures develop.

Corrosive esophagitis is caused by the ingestion of

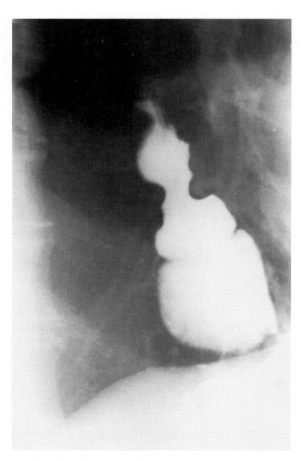

Fig. 64–5. Contrast radiography of a hiatal hernia.

concentrated alkali or acid. In children the ingestion is usually accidental, but in adult the corrosive may be swallowed purposely.[19] Alkaline caustics include sodium hydroxide, found in household lye as in drain cleaners; sodium carbonate in washing soda; sodium metasilicate; sodium triphosphate in cleaners used in home, farm and industry; and ammonia. Acids include compounds such as nitric acid, hydrochloric acid, found in toilet bowl cleaners; sulfuric acid; silver nitrate; and phenol. Sodium hypochlorite, found in household chlorine bleach, has the potential to cause a severe burn in high concentrations but usually is not clinically a problem.[20] Alkaline caustics penetrate deeply into tissue and produce liquifaction necrosis that may extend through all layers of the esophagus depending on the amount and concentration ingested. Acid caustics produce a coagulation necrosis, but may still produce severe burns that result in severe strictures. The purposeful ingestion of any caustic is particularly dreadful because of the extensive damage and resulting scar formation. Initially, the burn may show hyperemia, ulceration, or perforation. Luminal surface changes are prominent by 24 hours. When ulceration occurs, repair by granulation occurs and the granulation may persist for 2 to 3 weeks or longer. Circumferential scarring and subsequent contracture into stricture become apparent from 2 to 6 weeks after the ingestion.

Caustic material is ingested in both liquid and granular form. Even tiny amounts of granular caustic may cause stricture in a small child. Liquid caustic placed in familar containers such as soft drink bottles are particularly tempting to children and have also fooled unsuspecting adults. Prevention depends on proper storing and handling of these ubiquitous and powerful substances. Parents must childproof their own homes and be continuously alert to their child's activities in other locations. Careful disposal of all caustics and use of child-proof packaging could save a lot of grief.

Patients who have ingested caustics present with burns of the lips and oral cavity, drool, and refuse food and fluids because of pain. There may be burns of the hands which must be washed thoroughly to avoid burns of the eyes. Antidotes are not effective; emetics may cause further burns if the regurgitated material has residual caustic activity. Both should be avoided. Fever and pain in the substernal and abdominal areas are signs of possible perforation. Laryngeal burns may result in upper airway obstruction requiring tracheostomy. The correlation between the degree of a burn of the lips, oral cavity, and pharynx and the esophageal burn is poor. There may be no burns of the lips, mouth, and pharynx and yet a massive burn of the esophagus. Conversely, severe upper area burns may occur without esophageal damage.

Initially following ingestion of a caustic, the patient should be supported with parenteral fluids and ob-

served for signs of involvement of areas outside of the esophagus. Within 24 hours of the ingestion, esophagoscopy under general endotracheal anesthesia should be performed to determine the presence of an esophageal burn.[21] If no burn is found, the patient may be discharged when oral intake is adequate. If a burn is found at, or distal to, the cricopharyngeus, the examination is terminated without advancing the endoscope further for fear of perforating the esophagus. A course of corticosteroid therapy should be started, and a broad-spectrum antibiotic such as ampicillin should be given. An esophagram should be performed at 2 to 3 weeks to evaluate mucosal healing and possible stricture formation. Once the patient is able to swallow liquids, usually 3 to 4 days after the burn, liquid medication and nourishment can be taken by mouth. Food containing particulate matter that might be retained in the granulation tissue is withheld until the mucosa is healed. The next esophagram is performed for any clinical indication and routinely at 6 weeks. If evidence of stricture formation is present after the corticosteroid therapy has been terminated, bouginage is started carefully. A feeding tube or string may be kept in the esophagus with a developing stricture to prevent the loss of the lumen. Early bouginage, as introduced by Salzer,[22] is now rarely used except in patients who have delayed seeking treatment.

Other stenoses of the esophagus occur as the result of nonmalignant systemic disease. Systemic sclerosis or scleroderma, is an autoimmune disorder that involves connective tissue throughout the body.[23] The skin thickens, causing external manifestations in the face, trunk and extremities. It may be associated with polyarthritis, Reynaud's phenomenon, pulmonary changes of fibrosis and cyst formation, and renal and cardiac failure. In the esophagus, dense fibrous tissue accompanies muscle atrophy to cause stiffness. As peristalsis decreases, there may be GER and distal esophageal narrowing. The symptoms of esophageal involvement are the same as in other causes of esophageal stenosis. Diagnosis is based on the general manifestations of the disease, contrast radiography (Fig. 64–6), esophageal motility studies and laboratory findings of elevated erythrocyte sedimentation rate, anemia, hypergammoglobulinemia, and increased antinuclear antibodies. Glucocorticoids and cytotoxic therapy are used to control the general disease. Esophageal dilation may be of value in patients with localized strictures but must be done carefully because of the general rigidity of the esophageal wall. Antireflux precautions and H2 blockers may be helpful in patients with GER. Antireflux surgery may be necessary if GER is severe. Resection and esophageal replacement may be needed in some patients.

Dermatomyositis is a rare disease with similarities to systemic sclerosis. It produces polymyositis and cutaneous changes which may mimic scleroderma. The

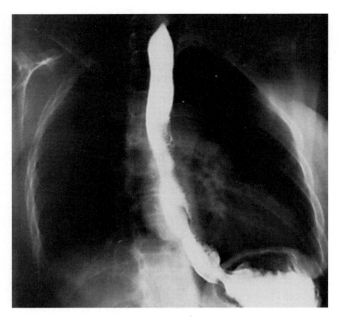

Fig. 64–6. Contrast radiography of the esophagus in scleroderma showing dilatation.

similarity of radiographic and motility studies makes the differential diagnosis difficult[24]; however, the LES may be more protective against GER. Dysphagia, with sensation referred to the pharynx, is a frequent symptom and is improved with corticosteroid therapy.

Other epithelial diseases may also involve the esophagus leading to ulceration and stenosis such as pemphigus and pemphigoid, Behcet's disease, epidermolysis bullosa, and Steven's-Johnson syndrome. Radiation and chemotherapy likewise can result in esophagitis leading to stricture formation.

Corrosive and other strictures of the esophagus may be managed with dilation or reconstruction of the esophagus. Short single strictures may be managed with Jackson bougies passed through an esophagoscope, followed subsequently by dilations using Maloney's mercury-filled bougies of increasing diameter, at increasing time intervals until the patient is able to eat in a near normal manner. Some patients may require repeated dilations at long intervals for many years and must always be alert while eating to avoid food foreign bodies.

In patients with more severe and extensive strictures of the esophagus, dilation with Tucker bougies is safer.[25,26] The Tucker bougie is made of soft rubber that is tapered at both ends surrounding a cord that runs through the length of the dilator with a loop each end. A gastrostomy is required to enable the passage of a strong silk suture through the entire esophagus, out through the nose and tied in a loop that the patient wears between dilations. At the time of dilation, a bougie and a new silk are attached to the old silk and the bougie drawn through the esophagus in retrograde or prograde direction. Two to three bougies are drawn through the stricture in tandem. Each one may be left in the area of the stricture for a brief period to exert maximum dilating effect. The new silk suture is drawn through the nose and tied under the clothing to the end coming out of the gastrostomy so that the loop of silk is available for the next dilation. The dilation may be repeated as frequently as necessary, increasing the interval when possible. Patients with extensive, nonresponsive strictures are candidates for esophageal reconstruction. Carcinoma of the esophagus occurs more frequently in patients with strictures than in the general population. The diagnosis may be difficult because of the distortion and inaccessibility of the lesion for biopsy.

Neoplasms of the esophagus may occur at any level. Less than 1% of neoplasms are benign, and include leiomyoma, lipoma, hemangioma and papilloma. All can produce dysphagia, regurgitation and aspiration. Of the benign tumors, leiomyoma is the most common, usually arising in the lower third of the esophagus in young individuals.[27] A smooth filling defect, or later the appearance of extrinsic compression, is found on contrast studies. Endoscopically the mass appears mobile and covered with normal mucosa. Surgical excision is necessary.

In contrast, lipomas appear as polypoid intraluminal lesions which may attain great size before becoming symptomatic.[28] If pedicled on a long stalk, they may be regurgitated and cause dyspnea as well as dysphagia.[29] Small lipomas may be removed endoscopically, larger ones must be resected by open operation. Hemangiomas and papillomas of the esophagus are rare. Symptoms can include bleeding. Treatment has included corticosteroids, localized resection or laser therapy.

Squamous cell carcinoma is the primary malignant neoplasm of the esophagus. Adenocarcinomas may also occur, usually in the lower third of the esophagus where they may be confused with superior invasion from a primary neoplasm of the stomach. Sarcomas occur infrequently, most often in the young.

Squamous cell carcinoma occurs predominantly in the sixth and seventh decade and more frequently in males, except for cervical esophageal lesions which are more common in women in those areas where the Plummer-Vinson syndrome is found. Other predisposing conditions include achalasia, hiatus hernia, Barrett's esophagus, and caustic or other long-standing strictures. Various foods, ethanol abuse and tobacco have also been implicated. As in other obstructive conditions, symptoms include dysphagia, especially for solids; regurgitation; and retrosternal discomfort. The symptoms are progressive, and in later stages of the disease are accompanied by weight loss, pain, and distant metastases. Metastasis occurs to jugular, supraclavicular and mediastinal lymph nodes. Hoarseness sig-

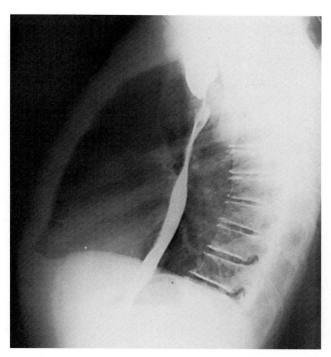

Fig. 64–7. Contrast radiography demonstrates an annular constriction with sharp irregular edges caused by carcinoma of the upper third of the esophagus.

nals involvement of the recurrent laryngeal nerves. Cough can be due to aspiration of retained esophageal content or to tumor penetration of the trachebronchial tree with fistula formation.

Radiographic contrast studies of the esophagus will demonstrate a filling defect, ulceration, impaired peristalsis, and abrupt or irregular narrowing of the lumen with proximal dilatation (Fig. 64–7). Chest films are mandatory to rule out the presence of metastatic disease. Computerized tomography can be utilized to show tumor thickness locally, as well as possible mediastinal and liver involvement. Esophagoscopy is required to establish the histologic diagnosis and exclude other possibilities and may be helpful in palliation with the introduction of an indwelling tube to allow peroral liquid nourishment. Biopsy of the lesion may be difficult if the lumen is severely narrowed by infiltration or if the lesion is spreading submucosally. Inflammation may also interfere with obtaining a diagnostic specimen. Brushing and lavage specimens can improve diagnostic accuracy. Specimens must be secured carefully because of the possibility of perforation through friable tumor tissue. Bronchoscopy should be performed at the same time to rule out tracheobronchial involvement.

Treatment of carcinoma of the esophagus is surgical in localized tumors but may be combined with radiation and chemotherapy for more extensive lesions to prolong palliation. The type of surgical procedure de-

pends on the location and extent of the lesion and reconstructive techniques when possible.

Foreign bodies of the esophagus are common in young children and in the older age group, particularly in denture wearers who have less oral sensation. Because the muscular activity of the upper portion of the esophagus is weak in comparison to the pharyngeal musculature, foreign bodies propelled into the hypopharynx are most likely to lodge just below the cricopharyngeus. The next most common site is just above the gastroesophageal junction. Other locations are the indentations of the esophagus caused by the aortic arch and the left bronchus. Pre-existing esophageal disease, particularly strictures, predispose to the retention of foreign bodies. Coins, poorly chewed food, safety pins, bones, and toy parts are common foreign bodies. As with bronchial foreign bodies, prevention is the key to avoidance of esophageal foreign bodies. Careful food preparation with scrutiny of food for bones or uncooked areas, keeping safety pins and other inedible objects out of the mouth and keeping inappropriate food and toys away from small children are important for prevention.

The history surrounding the foreign body ingestion is extremely important. When and how it occurred, as well as a description of the object, and subsequent symptoms can give the endoscopist valuable information. If available, a duplicate of the object can be helpful in choosing the most appropriate instruments for esophagoscopy and removal of the foreign body.

Symptoms of a foreign body vary with its position and make-up. Upper esophageal objects produce dysphagia and suprasternal pain on swallowing. With more distal objects, the symptoms are vague and the position level may not be describable. Rough objects may produce a superficial abrasion or laceration of the mucosa in their jouney to the stomach, causing pain which subsides within 24 hours. Persistent pain suggests that the foreign body has remained lodged. Large objects will obstruct the esophagus causing salivation, regurgitation of any swallowed liquid including saliva, cough due to aspiration, and dyspnea if the trachea is compressed by their bulk. Sharp foreign bodies can cause perforation of the esophagus, either initially or as the object's sojourn increases. Occasionally the symptoms are minimal, and a long-indwelling foreign body is discovered in the evaluation of a patient with progressive dysphagia or weight loss. Disc batteries may lodge in the esophagus and react with the mucosa. The resulting esophageal burn may be severe enough to cause perforation and mediastinitis.[30] They must be removed as soon as possible, with careful technique to reduce the possibility of increasing the caustic leak.

Once suspicion of a foreign body has been aroused, its presence must be proved or disproved. Radiologic studies are necessary (Fig. 64–8). Radiopaque objects

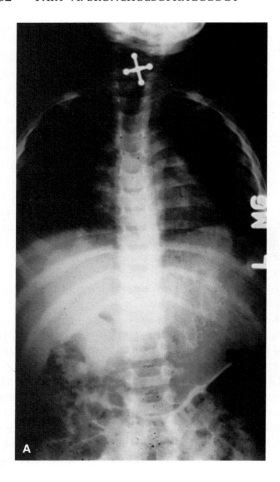

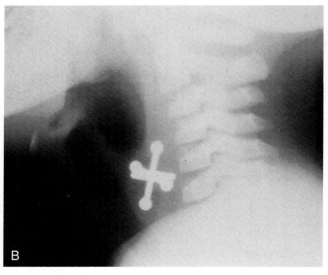

Fig. 64–8. Roentgenograms of a 4-year-old child with a jack in the cervical esophagus. The postero-anterior view (A) demonstrates the location of the jack as well as the absence of any other radiopaque object. The lateral view of the neck (B) shows the position of the pointed projections and the resulting tracheal compression.

can be identified in most instances with posterior-anterior and lateral neck films from the skull base to the thoracic inlet. These films will delineate the general shape of the object, as well as its location. For radiopaque objects that may have passed beyond the cervical esophagus, a single anterior-posterior roentgenogram from clavicles to pubis can be helpful. Evidence of nonradiopaque objects may also be found, such as increase in the distance between the cervical vertebrae and the larynx and trachea or air in the cervical esophagus. If the foreign body cannot be located in this manner, a contrast study of the esophagus with barium sulfate solution or a water-miscible solution may demonstrate it. However, it is preferable to avoid contrast material because it can obscure the foreign body during endoscopy. Very small radiodense objects can sometimes be demonstrated with CT. If the patient's symptoms persist, even in the instance of negative radiologic studies, it is safest to perform esophagoscopy in order to exclude the possibility of a foreign body.

Foreign bodies that have passed beyond the esophagus, generally pass through the GI tract without problem. If the object is seen in the stomach radiographically, the patient's stools can be examined for 5 days until it is recovered. If this does not occur, another film should be obtained to locate the object. Foreign bodies

that remain in the stomach (most likely with objects that are held in a mucosal fold, or that are too long to negotiate the duodenum) should be removed endoscopically. A sharp object, such as a pin, which passes beyond the stomach but then does not progress for several days may require laparotomy for removal to preclude perforation of the bowel.

Foreign bodies of the esophagus are removed most safely with an open esophagoscope under general endotracheal anesthesia. An esophagoscope of appropriate size for the patient should be used. The oval Jesberg esophagoscopes are preferred by some endoscopists for foreign body removal. However the rounder Jackson esophagoscopes can be rotated around their long axis, if necessary, for better maneuverability. Forceps specifically designed for the type of foreign body should be readied before the procedure begins. Care must be taken not to override the foreign body to avoid driving the object through the esophageal wall. Secretions should be suctioned carefully to avoid displacing the object distally and the object studied to determine the best forceps application for removal. The distal tip of the esophagoscope should be close to the object, without touching it, and any space around the object should be maintained in order to leave room for application of the forceps. More room exists for forceps application during inspiration if the patient is breathing spontaneously.

A sharp foreign body, such as a pin, with proximal point impaled in mucosa must be disengaged before withdrawal by grasping and moving it distally until it is freed. It is helpful to grasp the shaft near the point, rather than at the point, with side-grasping jaws that allow visual monitoring as the object is grasped, disengaged, and brought into the lumen of the endoscope to guard the point from being impaled again. Rotation forceps can be used with an open safety pin to carry it distally into the stomach and rotate it, so it can be removed with the point trailing.

Mucosa must not be grasped when removing any foreign body, to avoid perforation of the esophagus. Often, esophageal foreign bodies are too large to be retrieved into the esophagoscope, and must be brought out as trailing objects. This is accomplished by bringing the foreign body to the end of the esophagoscope and then fixing the forceps to the endoscope with the thumb and index finger of the left hand; the forceps, esophagoscope, and foreign body are then removed as one unit. The esophagoscope serves as a deflector to prevent the proximal mucosa and cricopharyngeus from stripping the foreign body from the forceps. Some irregular objects such as toy jacks are removed by grasping the knobbed end with forceps having cupped blades and tumbling the object from the esophageal walls. After any foreign body has been removed, the esophagus should be reexamined for trauma, a possible second foreign body, or previous condition such as stenosis. Patients may need follow-up contrast studies to evaluate the condition further.

Forcing a foreign body into the stomach by eating bread, use of a probang, and blind removal of cervical esophageal foreign bodies with Foley catheters are condemned for the following reasons: foreign bodies are often multiple; a smooth, opaque foreign body may be accompanied by a nonopaque sharp foreign body; esophageal foreign bodies are often associated with previously unrecognized esophageal abnormalities; loosened foreign bodies may be aspirated into the tracheobronchial tree; and safe methods of removing foreign bodies with open esophagoscopes exist.[31] The use of proteolytic enzymes to digest meat foreign bodies has been abondoned because of the mortality associated with their use.

Several other esophageal conditions occur that must be recognized in order to be treated effectively. In 1929, Mallory and Weiss described massive upper gastrointestinal bleeding caused by a longitudinal tear through or below the esophagogastric junction.[32] Severe retching usually precedes the hematemesis. The differential diagnosis includes hemorrhagic gastritis, peptic ulcer, esophageal varices, and spontaneous rupture of the esophagus, or Boerhaave syndrome. The bleeding in Mallory-Weiss tears is usually not life threatening but can require blood transfusions in preparation for diagnostic endoscopy.

In contrast, esophageal varices may result in massive bleeding leading to shock if not treated. Hematemesis and melena may also be produced. The varices result from hypertension in the portal venous system as a result of intrahepatic obstructive disease, such as posthepatic or alcohol-related cirrhosis and neoplasms, or from extrahepatic causes including portal vein thrombosis, congenital atresia or stenosis, and extrinsic pressure. Increased portal vein pressure causes enlargement of the collateral circulation leading to huge dilatation of the esophageal veins which may then rupture. Radiologic contrast studies demonstrate longitudinal, irregular indentations of the contrast medium. The varices may be further distended by Valsalva maneuver. Endoscopy is necessary for a definitive diagnosis, and for treatment by injection of sclerosis agents in selected cases. Balloon tamponade can be useful in the acute management of bleeding varices but should be avoided in patients who have had recent sclerosing injections due to the possibility of breakdown and perforation.

Congenital vascular anomalies may produce dysphagia by compression of the esophagus. Double aortic arch or right arch with a left ligamentum arteriosum cause circumferential compression and cause symptoms in infancy, characteristically as the child's diet is advanced to solid food. In contrast, an aberrant right subclavian vein passing posterior to the esophagus may cause only intermittent symptoms (dysphagia lusoria) later in life, or may be completely asymptomatic. Other extrinsic compression may arise as a result of an aneurysm of the descending aorta, mediastinal masses and primary or metastatic lymphadenopathy.

The Plummer-Vinson syndrome, or sideropenic dysphagia, is an ill-defined association of dysphagia, iron deficiency anemia, upper esophageal webs, glossitis, cheilitis, spoonshaped fingernails, splenomegaly, and a 10% incidence of postcricoid and oral cavity carcinoma. It tends to occur in older edentulous women of Scandinavian or Irish descent. Not all patients have all of the findings. Treatment consists of administration of iron and vitamins and esophageal dilation of webs when they occur.

COMPLICATIONS OF ESOPHAGOSCOPY

The main complications of esophagoscopy are bleeding and perforation. Preoperative evaluation of the blood coagulability should be done and any abnormalities corrected before endoscopy. Bleeding otherwise is usually the result of biopsy or dilation, and in rare instances can be severe enough to require transfusion.

Esophageal perforation may occur with ANY manipulation of the esophagus. The esophagus is a deli-

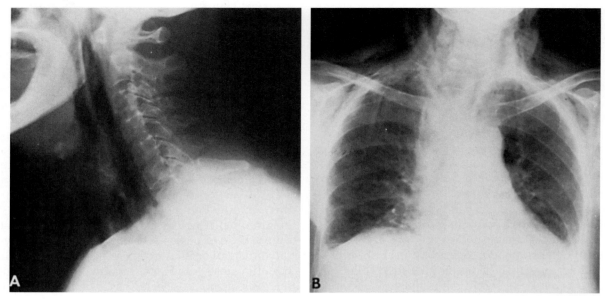

Fig. 64–9. Roentgenograms of a patient with perforation of the esophagus which demonstrate mediastinal and subcutaneous emphysema. A. Lateral view of neck. B. Posteroanterior view of chest.

cate structure, made more vulnerable to injury by disease, and must be treated gently. Areas at greatest risk are the hypopharynx just above the cricopharyngeus, the cervical esophagus, and the GE junction. Proximal perforations are the result of instrument impinging on the cervical vertebrae, particularly when spinal rigidity or calcified spurs have developed. Distal perforations can result when the lumen of the esophagus is difficult to identify, especially when it is deviated from its usual course or markedly dilated as in achalasia. Perforations may occur with biopsy of the esophagus because of its thin wall. All types of dilation carry the risk of perforation whether done under direct visualization with a Jackson dilator through an esophagoscope, with an indwelling string guided Tucker dilator, with an unguided mercury weighted bougie, or with vigorous pneumatic dilator.

Perforation of the esophagus is usually apparent within several hours. It is prudent to keep the patient from taking anything by mouth, while maintaining intravenous fluids, until certain that perforation has not occurred.

Perforation of the cervical esophagus or hypopharynx is characterized by steady pain and tenderness in the neck. Swelling and subcutaneous crepitus can be palpated and subcutaneous emphysema seen radiographically (Fig. 64–9). Water-miscible contrast can be used to demonstrate the location of the perforation. The infection can spread to the mediastinum, should be treated promptly with intravenous antibiotics, withholding of all oral intake, and exploration and drainage of any pus through a low cervical incision. Since it is rarely possible to repair a perforation at this level, a drain is often left in the wound until it heals.

Perforations of the thoracic esophagus are more serious but early recognition and management has improved the morbidity and mortality in this complication.[33] Thoracic perforations are characterized by high fever, tachycardia, hypotension, pain in the chest radiating to the back, tenderness on sternal pressure, and subcutaneous emphysema in the neck. Chest roentgenograms demonstrate mediastinal widening emphysema and unilateral or bilateral pleural effusion. Water-miscible contrast may be given to define the exact point of perforation. Treatment includes intravenous alimentation and broad-spectrum antibiotics, nothing by mouth, surgical drainage of the mediastinum, and repair of the perforation when possible.

SUGGESTED READINGS

1. Meyer GW, Castell DO: Current concepts of esophageal function. Am J Otolaryngol 1:440, 1980.
2. Maisel RH, Vermeersch H: Panendoscopy for second primaries in head and neck cancer. Ann Otol Rhinol Laryngol 90:460, 1981.
3. Logemann JA: Evaluation and Treatment of Swallowing Disorders. San Diego, CA, College-Hill Press, Inc., 1983.
4. Meyer GW, Castell DO: Evaluation and management of diseases of the esophagus. Am J Otolaryngol 2:336, 1981.
5. Wychulis AR, et al: Achalasia and carcinoma of the esophagus. JAMA 215:1638, 1971.
6. Heimlich HJ, O'Connor TW, Flores DC: Case for pneumatic dilatation in achalasia. Ann Otol Rhinol Laryngol 87:519, 1978.
7. Soper NJ, Brunt LM, Kerbl K: Laparoscopic general surgery. N Eng J Med 330:409, 1994.
8. Cuschieri A, Clark J: Hiatal hernia and reflux oesophagitis. *In* Surgery of the oesophagus. 2nd ed. Edited by Hennessy TPJ and Cuschieri A. Oxford Butterworth-Heinemann Ltd., 1992, pp. 170–214.

9. Blakely WR, et al: Section of the cricopharyngeus muscle for dysphagia. Arch Surg *96:*745, 1968.

10. van Overbeek JJM: Meditation on the pathogenesis of hypopharyngeal (Zenker's) diverticulum and a report of endoscopic treatment in 545 patients. Ann Otol Rhinol Laryngol *103:*178, 1994.

11. Garlock JH, Richter R: Carcinoma in a pharyngo-esophageal diverticulum: A case report. Ann Surg *154:*259, 1961.

12. Hulshof JH, van der Meij AGL: A helpful device in cricopharyngeal surgery. Arch Otolaryngol Head Neck Surg *114:*907, 1988.

13. Dohlman G, Mattsson O: The endoscopic operation for hypopharyngeal diverticula. Arch Otolaryngol *71:*744, 1960.

14. Benjamin B, Gallagher R: Microendoscopic laser diverticulotomy for hypopharyngeal diverticulum. Ann Otol Rhinol Laryngol *102:*675, 1993.

15. Ing AJ, Ngu MC, Breslin ABX: Chronic persistent cough and clearance of esophageal acid. Chest *102:*1668, 1992.

16. McHardy G: Reflux esophagitis. Ann Otol Rhinol Laryngol *81:*761, 1972.

17. Pope CE II: Acid-reflux disorders. N Engl J Med *331:*656, 1994.

18. Nissen R, Rossetti M: Surgery of the cardia ventricle. CIBA Symposium *11:*195, 1963.

19. Schild JA: Caustic ingestion in adult patients. Laryngoscope *95:*1199, 1985.

20. Hook CT, Lowry LD: Effect of chlorine bleach on the esophagus: A review and study. Ann Otol Rhinol Laryngol *83:*709, 1974.

21. Cardona JC, Daly JF: Current management of corrosive esophagitis. Ann Otol Rhinol Laryngol *80:*521, 1971.

22. Salzer H: Frühbehandlung der Speiseröohren-verätzung. Wein Klin Wochenschr *33:*307, 1920.

23. Gilliland BC: Systemic sclerosis (scleroderma). *In* Harrison's Principles of Internal Medicine, 13th ed. Edited by Isselbacher KJ, et al., New York, McGraw-Hill, Inc., 1994, pp 1655–1661.

24. Donaghue FE, et al: Esophageal defects in dermatomyositis. Ann Otol Rhinol Laryngol *69:*1139, 1960.

25. Tucker GF: Cicatricial stenosis of the esophagus with particular reference to treatment for continuous string retrograde bouginage with the author's bougie. Ann Otol Rhinol Laryngol *33:*1180, 1924.

26. Hawkins DB: Dilation of esophageal strictures: Comparative morbidity of antegrade and retrograde methods. Ann Otol Rhinol Laryngol *97:*460, 1988.

27. Lo NN, Nambiar R: Leiomyoma of the oesophagus. Aust. NZ J Surg *61:*757, 1991.

28. Zschiedrich M, Neuhaus P: Pedunculated giant lipoma of the esophagus. Am J Gastroenterol *85:*1614, 1990.

29. Cochet B, et al: Asphyxia caused by laryngeal impaction of an esophageal polyp. Arch Otolaryngol *106:*176, 1980.

30. Maves MD, Carithers JS, Birck HG: Esophageal burns secondary to disc battery ingestion. Ann Otol Rhinol Laryngol *93:*364, 1984.

31. Ritter FN: Questionable methods of foreign body treatment. Anne Otol Rhinol Laryngol *83:*729, 1974.

32. Weiss S, Mallory GK: Lesions of cardiac orifice of the stomach produced by vomiting. JAMA *98:*1353, 1932.

33. Bladergroen MR, Lowe JE, Postlethwait RW: Diagnosis and recommended management of esophageal perforation and rupture. Ann Thorac Surg *42:*235, 1986.

INDEX

Note: Page numbers followed by f indicate figures; page numbers followed by t indicate tables.